Current Veterinary Therapy

Food Animal Practice 2

Edited by

Jimmy L. Howard, M.S., D.V.M.

Diplomate, American Board of Veterinary Practitioners
(Food Animal Practice)
Professor of Veterinary Medicine
Botswana Agricultural College
Gabarone, Botswana, Africa
Formerly, Head of Diagnostic Services
Texas A & M Veterinary Medical Diagnostic Laboratory
Amarillo, Texas
and Former Assistant Professor of Food Animal Medicine at
Kansas State University and the University of Illinois

1986

W.B. Saunders Company

Philadelphia   London   Toronto   Mexico City
Rio de Janeiro   Sydney   Tokyo   Hong Kong

W. B. Saunders Company: West Washington Square
Philadelphia, PA 19105

Library of Congress Cataloging in Publication Data

Main entry under title:

Current veterinary therapy.

Includes index.

1. Veterinary medicine.   I. Howard, Jimmy L.
   II. Title: Food animal practice 2.

SF745.C784 1986   636.089′55   85–2006

ISBN 0–7216–1526–0

Editor: Darlene Pedersen
Designer: Terri Siegel
Production Manager: Laura Tarves
Manuscript Editor: Mary Anne Folcher

CURRENT VETERINARY THERAPY: Food Animal Practice 2   ISBN 0–7216–1526–0

Last digit is the print number: 9   8   7   6   5   4   3   2   1

The editor would like to dedicate this second volume of *Current Veterinary Therapy: Food Animal Practice* to the authors and consulting editors who had confidence enough in the work to add their names to such an endeavor. Most of these men and women are personal friends and colleagues, and my heartfelt thanks go out to them. The success of this volume will be the result of their efforts.

CONTRIBUTORS

BRUCE ABBITT, D.V.M., M.S.
Theriogenologist, Texas Veterinary Medical Diagnostic Laboratory, College Station, Texas.

D. SCOTT ADAMS, D.V.M., Ph.D.
Adjunct Assistant Professor and Veterinary Medical Officer, USDA-ARS, Department of Veterinary Microbiology and Pathology, Washington State University, Pullman, Washington.

R. S. ADAMS, B.S., Ph.D.
Professor of Dairy Science, The Pennsylvania State University, University Park, Pennsylvania.

WILLIAM MAURICE ALLEN, DVSc., Ph.D., M.Sc., M.R.C.V.S.
Private Consultant.

N. KENT AMES, D.V.M., M.S.
Associate Professor, Large Animal Clinical Sciences, Michigan State University, East Lansing, Michigan.

JOHN J. ANDREWS, D.V.M., M.S.
Professor of Veterinary Pathology, College of Veterinary Medicine, Iowa State University, Ames, Iowa, Iowa State University Veterinary Diagnostic Laboratory, Ames, Iowa.

C. H. ARMSTRONG, D.V.M., Ph.D.
Professor of Veterinary Microbiology, School of Veterinary Medicine, Purdue University, West Lafayette, Indiana.

ROBERT ASSAF, Agr., M.Sc.V.
Professor, Universite du Quebec, Institut Armand-Frappier, Ville de Laval, Quebec, Canada.

JESS L. AYERS, D.V.M., Ph.D.
Practitioner, Los Olivos, California.

ERVIN J. BAAS, D.V.M., Ph.D.
Staff Veterinarian, National Institute of Arthritis, Diabetes, and Digestive and Kidney Diseases, Bethesda, Maryland.

PETER A. BACHMANN, D.V.M.
Professor of Microbiology and Infectious Diseases, Institute of Medical Microbiology, Infectious and Epidemic Diseases, University of Munich Veterinary Facility, Munich, FRG.

GEORGE M. BAER, D.V.M., M.P.H.
Chief, Rabies Laboratory, Viral and Rickettsial Zoonoses, Division of Viral Diseases, Centers for Disease Control, Atlanta, Georgia.

C. V. BAGLEY, D.V.M.
Associate Professor, Utah State University, Logan, Utah.

DON E. BAILEY, D.V.M.
General Practitioner, Rosenburg, Oregon.

E. MURL BAILEY, JR., D.V.M., Ph.D.
Professor of Toxicology, College of Veterinary Medicine, Texas A&M University, College Station, Texas.

B. J. H. BARNARD, B.V.Sc., M.Med.Vet.
Veterinary Research Institute, Onderstepoort, Republic of South Africa.

KAREN H. BAUM, D.V.M.
Assistant Professor, Large Animal Medicine, V-M R CVM-Virginia Tech, Blacksburg, Virginia.

JAMES T. BAXTER, M.S., Ph.D., F.I.Biol., M.R.C.V.S.
Professor of Veterinary Medicine, Royal (Dick) School of Veterinary Studies, University of Edinburgh, Scotland, United Kingdom.

DARRELL E. BAY, Ph.D., R.P.E.
Professor of Entomology, Department of Entomology, Texas A&M University, College Station, Texas.

VAL R. BEASLEY, D.V.M., Ph.D.
Assistant Professor of Toxicology, University of Illinois, College of Veterinary Medicine, Urbana, Illinois.

DAVID BECHTOL, B.S., D.V.M.
Practitioner, Canyon, Texas.

DWIGHT G. BENNETT, D.V.M., Ph.D.
Professor of Clinical Sciences, College of Veterinary Medicine and Biomedical Sciences, Colorado State University, Veterinary Teaching Hospital, Colorado State University, Fort Collins, Colorado.

G. J. BENSON, D.V.M., M.S., D.A.C.V.A.
Diplomate, American College of Veterinary Anesthesiologists, Associate Professor of Veterinary Clinical Medicine, Department of Veterinary Clinical Medicine, College of Veterinary Medicine, University of Illinois, Urbana, Illinois.

JOHN N. BERG, D.V.M., Ph.D.
Professor, Department of Veterinary Microbiology, Diplomate, American College of Veterinary Microbiology, College of Veterinary Medicine, University of Missouri-Columbia, Columbia, Missouri.

MARTIN E. BERGELAND, D.V.M., Ph.D.
Professor of Veterinary Diagnostic Investigation, University of Minnesota, College of Veterinary Medicine, St. Paul, Minnesota.

ERNST L. BIBERSTEIN, D.V.M., Ph.D.
Professor of Microbiology, School of Veterinary Medicine, University of California, Microbiology Service, Veterinary Medical Teaching Hospital, University of California, Davis, California.

LEROY G. BIEHL, D.V.M., M.S.
Swine Extension Veterinarian, University of Illinois, Urbana, Illinois.

STEPHEN BISTNER, D.V.M.
Professor, Comparative Ophthalmology, University of Minnesota, School of Veterinary Medicine, St. Paul, Minnesota.

LEONARD BLACK, B.V.Sc., Ph.D., F.R.C.V.S.
Head, Vaccine Evaluation Section, The Wellcome Foot and
Mouth Disease Vaccine Laboratory, Pirbright, Surrey, England.

EDWARD H. BOHL, D.V.M., Ph.D.
Professor Emeritus, Food Animal Health Research Program,
Ohio Agricultural Research and Development Center, The Ohio
State University, Wooster, Ohio.

ROBERT BOHLENDER, D.V.M.
Practitioner, North Platte, Nebraska.

R. KENNETH BRAUN, D.V.M., M.S.
Diplomate, A.C.T., Professor and Chairman Department of
Preventive Medicine, College of Veterinary Medicine, University
of Florida, Gainesville, Florida.

ROGER BREEZE, B.V.M.S., Ph.D., M.R.C.V.S.
Professor and Chairman, Department of Microbiology and Pathology, College of Veterinary Medicine, Washington State University, Associate Director, Washington Technology Center,
Seattle, Washington.

JANICE C. BRIDGER, B.Sc., Ph.D.
Research, Principal Scientific Officer, Department of Microbiology, A.F.Rc. Institute for Research on Animal Diseases, Compton, Nr. NewBury, Berks., United Kingdom.

TALMAGE T. BROWN, JR., D.V.M., Ph.D.
Professor of Veterinary Pathology, School of Veterinary Medi-
cine, North Carolina State University, Pathologist, Veterinary
Medicine Teaching Hospital, School of Veterinary Medicine,
North Carolina State University, Raleigh, North Carolina.

CINDY J. BRUNNER, Ph.D., D.V.M.
Assistant Professor, Auburn University School of Veterinary
Medicine, Auburn, Alabama. Director, Veterinary Clinical Im-
munology Laboratory, Auburn, Alabama.

WILLIAM B. BUCK, D.V.M., M.S.
Diplomate, American Board of Veterinary Toxicology, Professor
of Toxicology and Director, National Animal Poison Control
Center, College of Veterinary Medicine, University of Illinois,
Urbana, Illinois.

CHRISTOPHER BUTTON, M.Med.Vet.(Med.), Ph.D.
Associate Professor, Faculty of Veterinary Science, University
of Pretoria, Republic of South Africa.

JERRY CALLIS, D.V.M., M.S., D.Sc.
Adjunct Professor, Cornell University, Ithaca, New York, Adjunct Professor, Pennsylvania State University, University Park,
Pennsylvania, USDA-ARS, Director, Plum Island Animal Disease Center, Greenport, New York.

IVAN W. CAPLE, B.V.Sc., Ph.D.
Professor of Veterinary Medicine, University of Melbourne
School of Veterinary Science, Department of Veterinary Clinical
Sciences, Werribee, Victoria, Australia.

EDWARD A. CARBREY, V.M.D., M.S.
Chief, Diagnostic Virology Laboratory, National Veterinary
Services Laboratories, Veterinary Services, APHIS, USDA,
Ames, Iowa.

JAMES R. CARLSON, Ph.D.
Professor and Chairman, Department of Animal Sciences, Col-
lege of Agriculture and Home Economics, Washington State
University, Pullman, Washington.

WILLIAM W. CARLTON, D.V.M., Ph.D.
Professor, Veterinary Pathology and Toxicology, School of Vet-
erinary Medicine, Purdue University, Department of Veterinary
Microbiology and Pathology, School of Veterinary Medicine,
Purdue University, West Lafayette, Indiana.

ROBERT L. CARSON, D.V.M., M.S.
Assistant Professor of Veterinary Medicine, Auburn University
School of Veterinary Medicine, Theriogenologists Department,
Large Animal Surgery and Medicine, Auburn University, Au-
burn, Alabama.

T. L. CARSON, D.V.M., M.S., Ph.D.
Professor of Veterinary Pathology, College of Veterinary Medi-
cine, Iowa State University, Veterinary Toxicologist, Iowa State
University Veterinary Diagnostic Laboratory, Ames, Iowa.

ARTHUR A. CASE, M.S., D.V.M.
Professor Emeritus of Veterinary Medicine and Surgery, College
of Veterinary Medicine, University of Missouri-Columbia, Columbia, Missouri. (Retired from regular veterinary faculty.)

ANTHONY E. CASTRO, D.V.M., Ph.D.
Associate Professor, College of Veterinary Medicine, Oklahoma
State University, Stillwater, Oklahoma.

DONALD R. CLARK, D.V.M., Ph.D.
Professor of Veterinary Physiology, Texas A&M University,
College Station, Texas.

N. ANDY COLE, Ph.D.
Research Animal Scientist, U.S.D.A., A.R.S., Bushland, Texas.

ROBERT W. COPPOCK, D.V.M., M.S., Ph.D.
Head, Clinical Investigation Group, Animal Sciences, Alberta
Environmental Centre, Vegreville, Alberta, Canada.

CREIGHTON N. CORNELL, D.V.M., M.S.
Assistant Professor, Biochemistry, University of Missouri, Columbia, Missouri.

THOMAS M. CRAIG, D.V.M., Ph.D.
Professor, Department of Veterinary Microbiology and Parasi-
tology, Texas A&M University, Veterinary Teaching Hospital,
Texas A&M University, College Station, Texas.

ROBERT A. CRANDELL, B.S., D.V.M., M.P.H.
Head, Diagnostic Microbiology, Texas Veterinary Medical Diagnostic Laboratory, Visiting Professor, Department of Veterinary Public Health, College of Veterinary Medicine, Texas A&M
University, College Station, Texas.

STANLEY E. CURTIS, M.S., Ph.D.
Professor of Animal Science, University of Illinois, College of
Agriculture, Urbana, Illinois.

RANDALL C. CUTLIP, D.V.M., Ph.D.
Veterinary Pathologist, Research, National Animal Disease Center, Ames, Iowa.

S. J. CYSEWSKI, D.V.M., M.S.
(deceased).

A. H. DARDIRI, D.V.M., M.V.Sc., M.Sc., Ph.D.

LLOYD E. DAVIS, D.V.M., Ph.D.
Professor of Veterinary Clinical Medicine and Pharmacology,
University of Illinois College of Veterinary Medicine, Veterinary
Medical Teaching Hospital, Urbana, Illinois.

P. MIKELL DAVIS, D.V.M.
Associate Clinical Professor, College of Veterinary Medicine, Mississippi State University, Mississippi State, Mississippi.

A. J. DELLA-PORTA, B.Sc., Ph.D.
Principal Research Scientist, Commonwealth Scientific and Industrial Research Organization, Australian National Animal Health Laboratory, Geelong, Victoria, Australia.

STANLEY M. DENNIS, B.V.Sc., Ph.D., F.R.C.V.S., F.R.C.Path.
Professor of Pathology, Kansas State University, College of Veterinary Medicine, Manhattan, Kansas.

GARY D. DIAL, D.V.M., Ph.D.
Assistant Professor, Department of Food Animal and Equine Medicine, North Carolina State University, Raleigh, North Carolina.

STEPHEN G. DILL, D.V.M.
Assistant Professor, Large Animal Medicine, New York State College of Veterinary Medicine, Large Animal Clinic, Cornell University, Ithaca, New York.

JOSEPH A. DIPIETRO, D.V.M., M.S.
Associate Professor of Veterinary Clinical Medicine, Departments of Veterinary Clinical Medicine and Veterinary Pathobiology, College of Veterinary Medicine, University of Illinois, Urbana, Illinois.

THOMAS J. DIVERS, D.V.M.
Assistant Professor of Medicine, New Bolton Center, University of Pennsylvania, Kennett Square, Pennsylvania.

KEVIN J. DOBSON, B.V.Sc., M.A.C.V.Sc.
Principal Veterinary Officer, Epidemiology and Preventative Medicine, Department of Agriculture, Adelaide, South Australia.

JOSEPH L. DORNER, D.V.M., Ph.D.
Professor, Veterinary Pathobiology, Veterinary Clinical Medicine, University of Illinois College of Medicine, Urbana, Illinois.

MAARTEN DROST, D.V.M.
Professor of Reproduction, College of Veterinary Medicine, University of Florida, Clinician, Veterinary Medical Teaching Hospital, Gainesville, Florida.

R. A. EASTER, Ph.D.
Associate Professor of Animal Nutrition, Department of Animal Science, College of Agriculture, University of Illinois, Urbana, Illinois.

B. C. EASTERDAY, D.V.M., Ph.D.
Professor and Dean, School of Veterinary Medicine, University of Wisconsin, Madison, Wisconsin.

WILLIAM C. EDWARDS, D.V.M., M.S.
Diplomate, American Board of Veterinary Toxicology, Associate Professor, Oklahoma Animal Disease Diagnostic Laboratory, Department of Surgery and Medicine, College of Veterinary Medicine, Oklahoma State University, Stillwater, Oklahoma.

R. G. ELMORE, D.V.M., M.S.
Professor, Large Animal Medicine and Surgery, College of Veterinary Medicine, Texas A&M University, College Station, Texas.

PAUL G. ENESS, D.V.M.
Professor, Department of Veterinary Clinical Sciences, College of Veterinary Medicine, Iowa State University, Ames, Iowa.

BENNIE G. ERWIN, D.V.M., M.S.
Associate Director of Veterinary Medicine, Coopers Animal Health Inc., Kansas City, Kansas.

A. KONRAD EUGSTER, D.V.M., Ph.D.
Head, Texas Veterinary Medical Diagnostic Laboratory, Texas A&M University, College Station, Texas.

W. H. FALES, M.S., Ph.D.
Associate Professor of Veterinary Microbiology, College of Veterinary Medicine, Clinical Microbiologist, Veterinary Medical Diagnostic Laboratory, College of Veterinary Medicine, University of Missouri, Columbia, Missouri.

HAROLD E. FARRIS, JR., D.V.M., M.S.
Associate Professor, Division of Laboratory Animal Medicine, University of Arkansas Medical School, Little Rock, Arkansas.

THOMAS M. FOLKERTS, D.V.M.
Head, International Animal Science Field Research, Lilly Research Laboratories, Eli Lilly and Company, Greenfield, Indiana.

MURRAY E. FOWLER, D.V.M.
Professor, Veterinary Medicine, School of Veterinary Medicine, University of California, Chief of Zoological Medicine Service, Veterinary Medical Teaching Hospital, University of California, Davis, California.

F. H. FOX, D.V.M.
Professor of Veterinary Medicine and Obstetrics, New York State College of Veterinary Medicine, Ambulatory Clinic, Cornell University, Ithaca, New York.

GLYNN H. FRANK, D.V.M., M.S., Ph.D.
Immunology Research Laboratory, National Animal Disease Center, Central Plains Area, United States Department of Agriculture, Ames, Iowa.

MERWIN L. FREY, D.V.M., Ph.D.
Professor of Veterinary Science, Department of Veterinary Science, University of Nebraska, Lincoln, Nebraska.

JIM FULLER, B.S., M.S.
Fuller Farms, Huntley, Wyoming.

ALLAN FURR, D.V.M., M.S.
Chief Staff Veterinarian, Animal Imports, USDA-APHIS-VS, Hyattsville, Maryland.

JOSEPH H. GAINER, D.V.M.
Veterinary Medical Officer, Food and Drug Administration, Beltsville, Maryland.

GEORGE B. GARNER, Ph.D.
Professor, College of Agriculture, University of Missouri, Columbia, Missouri.

E. PAUL J. GIBBS, B.V.Sc., Ph.D., F.R.C.V.S.
Professor of Virology, Department of Infectious Diseases, College of Veterinary Medicine, University of Florida, Gainesville, Florida.

DONALD R. GILL, Ph.D.
Extension Animal Nutritionist, Professor of Animal Science, Oklahoma State University, Stillwater, Oklahoma.

DANIEL A. GINGERICH, D.V.M., M.S.
Director of Research, Bristol Animal Health Care Division, Bristol Laboratories, Syracuse, New York.

ROBERT D. GLOCK, D.V.M., Ph.D.
Central Arizona Veterinary Laboratory, Casa Grande, Arizona.

DAN E. GOODWIN, D.V.M., Ph.D.
Director, Oklahoma Animal Disease Diagnostic Laboratory, College of Veterinary Medicine, Oklahoma State University, Stillwater, Oklahoma.

ROBERT A. GREEN, D.V.M., Ph.D.
Professor of Veterinary Pathology, College of Veterinary Medicine, Texas A&M University, Director of Clinical Pathology Laboratory, Veterinary Teaching Hospital, Texas A&M University, College Station, Texas.

WALTER M. GUTERBOCK, D.V.M., M.S.
Chino Valley Veterinary Associates, Ontario, California.

RALPH F. HALL, D.V.M.
Professor, Department of Rural Practice, College of Veterinary Medicine, University of Tennessee, Knoxville, Tennessee.

MICHAEL S. HAND, D.V.M., Ph.D.
Associate Professor of Clinical Nutrition, School of Veterinary Medicine, North Carolina State University, Raleigh, North Carolina.

LYLE E. HANSON, D.V.M., Ph.D.
Professor, Department of Veterinary Pathobiology, College of Veterinary Medicine, University of Illinois. Urbana, Illinois.

EDWARD T. HENRY, D.V.M.
Assistant Professor, Department of Food Animal and Equine Medicine, School of Veterinary Medicine, North Carolina State University, Raleigh, North Carolina.

R. P. HERD, M.V.Sc., Ph.D.
Professor of Parasitology, College of Veterinary Medicine, Ohio State University, Columbus, Ohio.

WERNER R. HEUSCHELE, D.V.M., Ph.D.
Adjunct Professor, College of Veterinary Medicine, The Ohio State University, Columbus, Ohio, Adjunct Clinical Professor, School of Veterinary Medicine, University of California, Davis, California, Adjunct Professor, College of Veterinary Medicine, The Oklahoma State University, Stillwater, Oklahoma, Head, Microbiology and Virology, Research Department, Zoological Society of San Diego, San Diego, California.

CLAIR M. HIBBS, D.V.M., Ph.D.
Director, New Mexico Veterinary Diagnostic Services, Research Professor, University of New Mexico Medical School, Albuquerque, New Mexico.

HARVEY D. HILLEY, D.V.M., Ph.D.
Associate Professor, Swine Section Leader, Department of Food Animal and Equine Medicine, North Carolina State University, Raleigh, North Carolina.

ROBERT B. HILLMAN, D.V.M., M.S.
Senior Clinician, Department of Reproductive Studies, New York State College of Veterinary Medicine, Cornell University, Ithaca, New York.

F. C. HINDS, Ph.D.
Head, Division of Animal Science, University of Washington, Laramie, Wyoming.

C. A. HJERPE, D.V.M.
Professor, Veterinary Medicine, School of Veterinary Medicine, University of California, Davis, Director, Veterinary Medical Teaching Hospital, University of California, Davis, California.

ALVIN B. HOERLEIN, D.V.M., Ph.D.
Professor Emeritus, Microbiology, Colorado State University, College of Veterinary Medicine and Biological Sciences, Fort Collins, Colorado.

WALTER E. HOFFMAN, D.V.M., Ph.D.
Associate Professor, Veterinary Clinical Pathology, University of Illinois, College of Veterinary Medicine, Veterinary Medical Teaching Hospital, Urbana, Illinois.

GLEN F. HOFFSIS, D.V.M., M.S.
Professor, Ohio State University, Columbus, Ohio.

G. R. HOLLIS, Ph.D.
Professor, Animal Science and Extension Specialist, Swine, University of Illinois, Department of Animal Sciences, Urbana, Illinois.

BARBARA S. HOOK, B.A., D.V.M.
Postdoctoral Fellow, Department of Pathology, Cornell University, Ithaca, New York.

J. R. HOWARD, D.V.M., Ph.D.
Practitioner, Brawley, California.

JIMMY L. HOWARD, D.V.M., M.S.
Diplomate, American College of Veterinary Practitioners, Food Animal Practice, Professor, Animal Health, Botswana Agricultural College, Gaborone, Botswana, Africa.

J. T. HUBER, Ph.D.
Professor of Animal Nutrition, University of Arizona, Tucson, Arizona.

ROBERT S. HUDSON, D.V.M., M.S.
Diplomate, American College of Theriogenologists, Alumni Professor, Large Animal Surgery and Medicine, Auburn University, Head, Beef Section, Auburn, Alabama.

BRUCE L. HULL, D.V.M., M.S.
Diplomate, American College of Veterinary Surgeons, Professor, Food Animal Surgeon, Ohio State University College of Veterinary Medicine, Columbus, Ohio.

ELAINE HUNT, D.V.M.
Diplomate, A.C.V.I.M., Assistant Professor, North Carolina State University, School of Veterinary Medicine, Department of Food Animal and Equine Medicine, Raleigh, North Carolina.

RAYMOND J. HUSMANN, D.V.M.

ALBERT A. ILEMOBADE, D.V.M., M.S., Ph.D.
Dean, School of Agriculture and Agricultural Technology, Professor of Animal Production and Health, Federal University of Technology, Akure, Nigeria.

CYNTHIA HOMAN JACOBS, D.V.M.
Assistant Professor, Division of Laboratory Animal Medicine, University of Arkansas Medical School, Little Rock, Arkansas.

LYNN F. JAMES, Ph.D.
Research Leader, USDA-ARS Poisonous Plant Research Laboratory, Logan, Utah.

WILLIAM L. JENKINS, B.V.Sc., M.MED.VET., Ph.D.
Professor, Department of Veterinary Physiology and Pharmacology, College of Veterinary Medicine, Texas A&M University, College Station, Texas.

MICHAEL M. JOCHIM, D.V.M., Ph.D.
Veterinary Medical Officer, USDA-ARS, Denver, Colorado.

A. EARL JOHNSON, M.S.

TIMOTHY JORDAN, B.S., D.V.M.
Herd Health Consultant, Palo Duro Veterinary Services, P.C., Canyon, Texas.

ROBERT A. KAINER, D.V.M., M.S.
Professor of Anatomy, College of Veterinary Medicine and Biochemical Sciences, Colorado State University, Fort Collins, Colorado.

ARNOLD F. KAUFMANN, D.V.M., M.S.
Chief, Bacterial Zoonoses Activity Division of Bacterial Diseases, Center for Infectious Diseases, Centers for Disease Control, Atlanta, Georgia.

RICHARD F. KEELER, Ph.D.
Research Chemist, USDA, Logan, Adjunct Professor of Veterinary Sciences, ADVS Department, Utah State University, Logan, Utah.

GEORGE A. KENNEDY, D.V.M., Ph.D.
Diplomate, American College of Veterinary Pathologists, Associate Professor, Diagnostic Laboratory, Kansas State University, Manhattan, Kansas.

CLEON KIMBERLING, D.V.M., M.P.H.
Extension Veterinarian, Colorado State University, Fort Collins, Colorado.

CARL A. KIRKER-HEAD, M.A., VET.M.B., M.R.C.V.S.
Resident in Surgery, Tufts University, New England Veterinary Medical Center, Resident in Surgery, Large Animal Clinic, Boston, Massachusetts.

S. K. KNELLER, D.V.M., M.S.
Associate Professor, Radiology, Department of Veterinary Clinical Medicine, College of Veterinary Medicine, Chief of Radiology, University of Illinois, Urbana, Illinois.

L. D. KONYHA, D.V.M., M.S.
Assistant Director, Northern Region USDA-APHIS, Veterinary Services, Scotia, New York.

GARY D. KORITZ, D.V.M., Ph.D.
Associate Professor of Veterinary Pharmacology, College of Veterinary Medicine, University of Illinois, Urbana, Illinois.

BARBARA KOTT, D.V.M., M.S.

PALLE KROGH, D.V.M., Ph.D.
Professor, Veterinary Pathology and Toxicology, School of Veterinary Medicine, Purdue University, Department of Veterinary Microbiology and Pathology, School of Veterinary Medicine, Purdue University, West Lafayette, Indiana.

JERRY P. KUNESH, D.V.M., Ph.D.
Professor, Department of Veterinary Clinical Sciences, College of Veterinary Medicine, Iowa State University, Ames, Iowa.

HAROLD J. KURTZ, M.S., D.V.M., Ph.D.
Professor, Veterinary Pathology, College of Veterinary Medicine, University of Minnesota, Diagnostic Pathologist, Veterinary Diagnostic Laboratory of Minnesota, St. Paul, Minnesota.

GARRY LACEFIELD, M.S., Ph.D.
Professor, Agronomy Department, Extension Forage Specialist, University of Kentucky, Research and Education Center, Princeton, Kentucky.

AUBREY B. LARSEN, D.V.M., M.S.
Project Leader of Mycobacteriosis, U.S.D.A., Animal Disease Center, Ames, Iowa. (Retired.)

VAUGHN L. LARSON, D.V.M., Ph.D.
Professor, Large Animal Medicine, University of Minnesota, St. Paul, Minnesota.

H. W. LEIPOLD, D.V.M., Ph.D.
Professor, Kansas State University, Manhattan, Kansas.

NORMAN D. LEVINE, Ph.D.
Professor Emeritus, College of Veterinary Medicine, University of Illinois, Urbana, Illinois.

PETER B. LITTLE, D.V.M., M.S., Ph.D.
Diplomate, American College of Veterinary Pathologists, Professor of Pathology, University of Guelph, Ontario Veterinary College, Guelph, Ontario, Canada.

CHARLES W. LIVINGSTON, JR., D.V.M., Ph.D.
Professor, Texas Agricultural Experiment Station, Texas A&M University, Research and Extension Center at San Angelo, San Angelo, Texas.

W. EUGENE LLOYD, D.V.M., Ph.D.
President, Vet-A-Mix, Inc., Shenandoah, Professor (Collaborator), College of Veterinary Medicine, Iowa State University, Ames, Iowa.

THOMAS O. MANNING, D.V.M., M.S., A.C.V.D.
Assistant Professor of Dermatology, School of Veterinary Medicine, North Carolina State University, Raleigh, North Carolina.

W. B. MARTIN, Ph.D., M.R.C.V.S., D.V.S.M., F.R.S.E.
Scientific Director of Moredun Research Institute, Edinburgh, England.

DONALD MATTSON, D.V.M., Ph.D.
Associate Professor of Veterinary Medicine, College of Veterinary Medicine, Veterinary Diagnostic Laboratory, Oregon State University, Corvallis, Oregon.

DAVID McCLARY, D.V.M., M.S.
Diplomate, American College of Theriogenologists, Assistant Professor of Veterinary Medicine, Auburn University, School of Veterinary Medicine, Head, Dairy Section, Auburn, Alabama.

ALYN McCLURE, D.V.M.
Practitioner, Gilbert, Arizona.

STEWART McCONNELL, D.V.M., M.Sc.
Professor of Veterinary Urology, College of Veterinary Medicine, Texas A&M University, College Station, Texas.

JOHN McCORMACK, D.V.M.
Professor of Large Animal Medicine, University of Georgia, College of Veterinary Medicine, Field Services Section, Athens, Georgia.

H. A. McDANIEL, D.V.M., Ph.D.
Chief of Technical Support Staff, Animal Health Programs, Veterinary Services USDA, APHIS, Hyattsville, Maryland.

SHEILA M. McGUIRK, D.V.M., Ph.D.
Assistant Professor, Department of Medical Sciences, Large Animal Internal Medicine, University of Wisconsin School of Veterinary Medicine, Madison, Wisconsin.

JAMES D. McKEAN, D.V.M., M.S.
Extension Veterinarian (Swine), Professor, Veterinary Pathology, Iowa State University, Ames, Iowa.

D. G. McKERCHER, D.V.M., Ph.D.
Professor of Virology, School of Veterinary Medicine, University of California, Davis, California. (Retired.)

J. G. McLEAN, B.V.Sc., Ph.D.
Senior Lecturer in Veterinary Biochemistry, University of Mel-

bourne School of Veterinary Science, Department of Preclinical Sciences, Parkville, Victoria, Australia.

T. A. McPHERRON, D.V.M., M.S.
Consultant Veterinarian, St. Joseph, Illinois.

CHARLES A. MEBUS, D.V.M., Ph.D.
Research Leader, Pathobiology, USDA-ARS, Plum Island Animal Disease Center, Greensport, New York.

WILLIAM L. MENGELING, D.V.M., Ph.D.
Chief, Virological Research Laboratory, National Animal Disease Center, Ames, Iowa.

H. DWIGHT MERCER, D.V.M., Ph.D.
Professor of Pharmacology and Toxicology, Clinical Pharmacology Consultant, Clinical Toxicology Consultant, Mississippi State University Veterinary Clinic, Mississippi.

M. MERRALL, B.V.Sc., Ph.D., M.A.C.V.Sc.
Ambulatory Clinician, Farm Service Clinic. Senior Lecturer of Veterinary Medicine, Faculty of Veterinary Science, Massey University, Palmerston North, New Zealand.

DUANE MIKSCH, D.V.M., M.S.
Associate Professor, Department of Veterinary Science, Extension Veterinarian, University of Kentucky, Research and Education Center, Princeton, Kentucky.

JANICE M. MILLER, B.S., D.V.M., M.S., Ph.D.
Veterinary Medical Officer, National Animal Disease Center, USDA-ARS, Ames, Iowa.

R. B. MILLER, D.V.M., M.S., Ph.D.
Associate Professor of Veterinary Medicine and Surgery and Veterinary Pathology, College of Veterinary Medicine, Food Animal Clinician, Veterinary Teaching Hospital, University of Missouri, Columbia, Missouri.

SASHI B. MOHANTY, B.V.Sc.&A.H., Ph.D.
Professor of Veterinary Virology, Virginia-Maryland Regional College of Veterinary Medicine, University of Maryland, College Park, Maryland.

CECIL P. MOORE, D.V.M.
Assistant Professor, Department of Surgical Sciences, School of Veterinary Medicine, University of Wisconsin, Madison, Comparative Ophthalmology Service, Veterinary Medical Teaching Hospital, Madison, Wisconsin.

EDWIN W. MOSS, D.V.M., M.S.
Practitioner, Bassano Veterinary Clinic, Bassano, Alberta, Canada.

JOHN O. MOZIER, D.V.M.
Division Vice President, Research and Development, Bayvet Division of Miles Laboratories, Inc., Shawnee Mission, Kansas.

PETER C. MULLOWNEY, M.V.B., M.R.C.V.S.
Diplomate, American Board of Veterinary Practitioners, formerly, Assistant Professor, Department of Rural Practice, University of Tennessee, Knoxville, Tennessee. Melcomb House, Newport, County Mayo, Ireland.

JONATHAN M. NAYLOR, M.R.C.V.S., D.A.C.V.I.M., Ph.D.
Associate Professor, Veterinary Internal Medicine, University of Saskatchewan, Chief, Large Animal Services, W.C.V.M., University of Saskatchewan, Saskatoon, Saskatchewan, Canada.

DALE R. NELSON, D.V.M., M.S.
Associate Professor, Food Animal Medicine and Surgery, Department of Veterinary Clinical Medicine, College of Veterinary Medicine, University of Illinois, Urbana, Illinois.

DALLAS L. NELSON, D.V.M., Ph.D.
Consultant for Agriculture and Toxicology, Wakefield, Kansas.

PAUL NICOLETTI, D.V.M., M.S.
Professor, Department of Infectious Diseases, College of Veterinary Medicine, University of Florida, Gainesville, Florida.

CELESTINE O. NJOKU, D.V.M., Ph.D., F.R.V.C.S.
Professor of Veterinary Pathology, Ahmadu Bello University, Faculty of Veterinary Medicine and Fellow of the Royal Veterinary College of Sweden, Consulting Pathologist, Veterinary Teaching Hospital, Ahmadu Bello University, Zaria, Nigeria.

MELITON N. NOVILLA, D.V.M., M.S., Ph.D.
Senior Pathologist, Toxicology Division, Lilly Research Laboratories, Eli Lilly and Company, Greenfield, Indiana.

FREDERICK W. OEHME, D.V.M., Ph.D.
Professor of Toxicology, Medicine, and Physiology, College of Veterinary Medicine, Kansas State University, Director, Comparative Toxicology Laboratories, College of Veterinary Medicine, Kansas State University, Manhattan, Kansas.

A. E. OLSON, M.S.
Research Associate, Veterinary Science, Utah State University, Logan, Utah.

CARL OLSON, D.V.M., Ph.D.
Department of Veterinary Science, College of Agricultural and Life Sciences, and Department of Pathobiology, School of Veterinary Medicine, University of Wisconsin, Madison, Wisconsin.

DAVID P. OLSON, D.V.M., M.S., Ph.D.
Professor, Department of Veterinary Science, University of Idaho, Moscow, Idaho.

BENNIE I. OSBURN, D.V.M., Ph.D.
Professor of Pathology and Associate Dean Research, School of Veterinary Medicine, University of California, Davis, California.

GARY D. OSWEILER, D.V.M., M.S., Ph.D.
Professor, Veterinary Diagnostic Laboratory, Iowa State University, Ames, Iowa.

RANDALL S. OTT, D.V.M., M.S.
Diplomate, American College of Theriogenologists, Associate Professor, Department of Veterinary Clinical Medicine, College of Veterinary Medicine, University of Illinois, Urbana, Illinois.

J. S. PALMER, D.V.M., M.P.H.
(Deceased, formerly Veterinary Medical Officer, USDA-ARS Veterinary Toxicology and Entomology Research Laboratory, College Station, Texas).

ROGER J. PANCIERA, D.V.M., M.S., Ph.D.
Professor, Veterinary Pathology, College of Veterinary Medicine, Oklahoma State University, Stillwater, Oklahoma.

JOHN W. PAUL, D.V.M., M.S.
Manager, Professional Services, American Hoechst Corporation, Animal Health Division, Somerville, New Jersey.

H. B. PETERSON, Ph.D.
Professor Emeritus, Department of Agriculture and Irrigation Engineering, Utah State University, Logan, Utah.

ALLAN C. PIER, D.V.M., Ph.D.
Professor and Head of Department of Microbiology and Veterinary Medicine, University of Wyoming, Director, Wyoming State Veterinary Laboratory, Laramie, Wyoming.

ROBERT E. PIERSON, D.V.M. (retired)
Colorado State University, Fort Collins, Colorado.

THOMAS A. POWE, D.V.M., M.S.
Diplomate, American Board of Veterinary Practitioners, Associate Professor of Veterinary Medicine, Auburn University School of Veterinary Medicine, Food Animal Medicine, Large Animal Clinic, Auburn, Alabama.

MARSHALL R. PUTNAM, D.V.M., M.S.
Diplomate, American College of Theriogenologists, Assistant Professor, Department of Large Animal Surgery and Medicine, School of Veterinary Medicine, Auburn University, Auburn, Alabama.

OTTO MARTIN RADOSTITS, D.V.M., M.S.
Professor, Veterinary Medicine, Western College of Veterinary Medicine, University of Saskatchewan, Saskatoon, Saskatchewan, Canada.

F. K. RAMSEY, D.V.M., Ph.D.
College of Veterinary Medicine, University of Iowa, Ames, Iowa.

W. C. REBHUN, D.V.M.
Associate Professor of Veterinary Medicine and Ophthalmology, New York State College of Veterinary Medicine, Veterinary Medical Teaching Hospital, Cornell University, Ithaca, New York.

HUGH W. REID, B.V.M.&S., D.T.V.M., Ph.D., M.R.C.V.S.
Principal Veterinary Research Officer, Animal Diseases Research Association, Moredun Institute, Edinburgh, Great Britain.

IAN M. REID, B.Sc., Ph.D., M.N.S.
Agricultural and Food Research Council, Institute for Research on Animal Diseases, Compton, Newbury, Berkshire, United Kingdom.

E. J. RICHEY, D.V.M.
Veterinary Practitioner, Pawhuska, Oklahoma.

JACK G. RILEY, Ph.D.
Professor of Animal Science, Kansas State University, Manhattan, Kansas.

C. JEREMY ROBERTS, B.V.Sc., Ph.D., M.R.C.V.S.
Agricultural and Food Research Council, Institute for Research on Animal Diseases, Compton, Newbury, Berkshire, United Kingdom.

DAVID ROBERTSHAW, M.R.C.V.S., Ph.D.
Professor of Physiology and Head of Department, Colorado State University, Fort Collins, Colorado.

BRUCE D. ROSENQUIST, D.V.M., Ph.D.
Professor, Department of Veterinary Microbiology, College of Veterinary Medicine, University of Missouri, Columbia, Missouri.

LOYD D. ROWE, D.V.M.
Veterinary Medical Officer, USDA-ARS Veterinary Toxicology and Entomology Research Laboratory, College Station, Texas.

LAWRENCE P. RUHR, D.V.M., Ph.D.
Associate Professor of Veterinary Toxicology, School of Veterinary Medicine, Louisiana State University, Baton Rouge, Louisiana.

IVAN G. RUSH, Ph.D.
University of Nebraska, Panhandle Station, Scottsbluff, Nebraska.

JULIE M. SANDERSON, M.S.
Research Assistant in Plant Pathology, Department of Plant Pathology, University of Wisconsin, Madison, Wisconsin.

BERNARD FREDERICK SANSOM, M.A., D. Phil.
Free-lance Scientific Editor.

VICKI JO SCHEIDT, D.V.M., A.C.V.D.
Assistant Professor, Dermatology, School of Veterinary Medicine, North Carolina State University, Raleigh, North Carolina.

LAVERNE M. SCHUGEL, D.V.M.
Vice President, Technical Services and Research, Zinpro Corporation, Chaska, Minnesota.

ROY A. SCHULTZ, D.V.M., M.S.
Swine Consultant, Avoca Veterinary Clinic, Avoca, Iowa.

R. D. SCOGGINS, D.V.M.
Associate Professor, Extension Veterinarian, University of Illinois, Urbana, Illinois.

RICHARD C. SEARL, D.V.M.
Veterinary Consultant, Mesa, Arizona.

J. W. SEXTON, D.V.M., M.S.
Associate Professor of Veterinary Medicine (Retired), Department of Veterinary Medicine, Iowa State University, Ames, Iowa.

JAMES A. SHMIDL, D.V.M., M.S.
Director, Toxicology and Regulatory Affairs, Bayvet Division of Miles Laboratories Inc., Shawnee Mission, Kansas.

J. L. SHUPE, D.V.M.
Professor, Veterinary Medicine, Utah State University, Logan, Utah. Adjunct Professor, University of Illinois, Urbana, Illinois.

ROBERT L. SIEBER, D.V.M., M.S.
All Creatures Animal Hospital and Dairyland Management Services, Appleton, Wisconsin.

JOHN C. SIMONS, D.V.M.
Director, Animal Health Technician Program, Eastern Wyoming College, Torrington, Clinician, Goshen Veterinary Clinic, Torrington, Wyoming.

EUGENE B. SMALLEY, Ph.D.
Professor of Plant Pathology, Department of Plant Pathology, University of Wisconsin, Madison, Wisconsin.

A. R. SMITH, D.V.M., Ph.D.
Associate Professor, University of Illinois, College of Veterinary Medicine, Urbana, Illinois.

ALVIN W. SMITH, D.V.M., Ph.D.
Professor of Veterinary Medicine and Director of Research, Oregon State University, College of Veterinary Medicine, Research and Administration, College of Veterinary Medicine, Oregon State University, Corvallis, Oregon.

DEAN H. SMITH, D.V.M., M.S.
Professor, Oregon State University (1956–1976), Corvallis, Oregon, Washington State Department of Agriculture, Olympia, Washington.

J. P. SMITH, D.V.M., M.S.
Associate Professor, Veterinary Parasitology, Department of Veterinary Microbiology and Parasitology, Texas A&M University, College of Veterinary Medicine, College Station, Texas.

JOHN A. SMITH, D.V.M., M.S.
Diplomate, American College of Internal Medicine, Assistant Professor, Food Animal Medicine, College of Veterinary Medicine and Biomedical Sciences, Colorado State University, Fort Collins, Colorado.

M. H. SMITH, D.V.M., Ph.D.
Professor and Chairman, Department of Veterinary Science, North Dakota State University, Fargo, North Dakota.

MARY C. SMITH, D.V.M.
Associate Professor of Large Animal Medicine, Ambulatory Clinic Teaching Hospital, New York State College of Veterinary Medicine, Cornell University, Ithaca, New York.

PAUL C. SMITH, D.V.M., M.S., Ph.D.
Professor and Head, Department of Microbiology, School of Veterinary Medicine, Auburn University, Auburn, Alabama.

ROBERT A. SMITH, D.V.M., M.S.
Diplomate, American Board of Veterinary Practitioners, Food Animal Practice, Associate Professor of Medicine and Surgery, Large Animal Clinic, College of Veterinary Medicine, Oklahoma State University, Stillwater, Oklahoma.

J. GLENN SONGER, Ph.D.
Associate Professor of Veterinary Science, University of Arizona, Tucson, Arizona.

MARK F. SPIRE, D.V.M., M.S.
Diplomate, American College of Theriogenologists, Associate Professor, Kansas State University, Director, Embryo Transfer Unit, Department of Surgery and Medicine, Manhattan, Kansas.

P. B. SPRADBROW, B.V.Sc., Ph.D., D.V.Sc.
Professor of Veterinary Virology, University of Queensland, Brisbane, Australia.

J. STORZ, D.V.M., Ph.D.
Louisiana State University, School of Veterinary Medicine, Baton Rouge, Louisiana.

BARBARA STRAW, D.V.M., Ph.D.
Associate Professor, New York State Diagnostic Laboratory, Cornell University, Ithaca, New York.

S. P. SWANSON, M.S.
Senior Chemist, Department of Veterinary Biosciences, College of Veterinary Medicine, University of Illinois, Urbana, Illinois.

RAYMOND W. SWEENEY, V.M.D.
Lecturer in Large Animal Medicine, University of Pennsylvania, School of Veterinary Medicine, New Bolton Center, Kennett Square, Pennsylvania.

BRINTON L. SWIFT, D.V.M.
Professor of Veterinary Medicine, University of Wyoming, Laramie, Wyoming.

PETE D. TEEL, Ph.D., R.P.E.
Assistant Professor, Department of Entomology, Texas A&M University, College Station, Texas.

RICHARD H. TESKE, D.V.M., M.S.
Associate Director for Science, Center for Veterinary Medicine, Food and Drug Administration, Rockville, Maryland.

JAMES R. THOMPSON, D.V.M., M.S.
Associate Professor, Department of Veterinary Clinical Sciences, Iowa State University, College of Veterinary Medicine, Ames, Iowa.

LINDA S. THOMPSON, D.V.M.
Equine Practitioner, Ames, Iowa.

JOHN C. THURMON, D.V.M., M.S.
Professor, Veterinary Clinical Medicine, Department of Veterinary Clinical Medicine, College of Veterinary Medicine, University of Illinois, Urbana, Illinois.

KENNETH S. TODD, JR., Ph.D.
Professor and Chairperson, Veterinary Parasitology, Assistant Head, Department of Veterinary Pathobiology, College of Veterinary Medicine, University of Illinois, Urbana, Illinois.

DAVID G. TOPEL, Ph.D.
Professor and Department Head, Animal and Dairy Science, Auburn University, Auburn, Alabama.

DEOKI N. TRIPATHY, B.V.Sc.&A.H., Ph.D.
Professor, Department of Veterinary Pathobiology, College of Veterinary Medicine, University of Illinois, Urbana, Illinois.

H. H. VAN HORN, Ph.D.
Professor, Dairy Science Department, University of Florida, Gainesville, Florida.

KENT R. VAN KAMPEN, D.V.M., Ph.D.
Professor and Head, Department of Animal, Dairy, and Veterinary Sciences, Utah State University, Logan, Utah.

W. A. VESTRE, D.V.M., M.S.
Associate Professor, Ophthalmology, Department of Small Animal Clinics, School of Veterinary Medicine, Purdue University, West Lafayette, Indiana.

JEROME G. VESTWEBER, D.V.M., Ph.D.
Professor of Surgery and Medicine, Kansas State University, Manhattan, Kansas.

J. S. WALKER, D.V.M., M.S.
Program Leader, International Research Division, Office of International Cooperation and Development, USDA, Washington, D.C.

JACK WARD, D.V.M.
Practitioner, Hamilton, Montana.

WALLACE M. WASS, D.V.M., Ph.D.
Professor, Department of Veterinary Clinical Sciences, College of Veterinary Medicine, Iowa State University, Ames, Iowa.

BIMBO WELKER, D.V.M.
Assistant Professor, Division of Agricultural and Urban Practice, Large Animal Surgery, Virginia—Maryland Regional College of Veterinary Medicine, Virginia Tech, Blacksburg, Virginia.

D. M. WEST, B.V.Sc., Ph.D., F.A.C.V.Sc.
Clinician Farm Service Clinic, Senior Lecturer in Veterinary Medicine, Faculty of Veterinary Science, Massey University, Palmerston North, New Zealand.

MAURICE E. WHITE, D.V.M.
Associate Professor of Medicine, New York State College of Veterinary Medicine, Ambulatory Clinic, New York State College of Veterinary Medicine, Cornell University, Ithaca, New York.

HOWARD W. WHITFORD, D.V.M., Ph.D.
Veterinary Bacteriologist, Texas Veterinary Medical Diagnostic Laboratory, College Station, Texas.

R. DAVID WHITLEY, D.V.M., M.S.
Diplomate, American College of Veterinary Ophthalmologists,

Assistant Professor of Comparative Ophthalmology, Department of Comparative Ophthalmology, College of Veterinary Medicine, Chief of Ophthalmology Services and Veterinary Ophthalmologist, Veterinary Medical Teaching Hospital, College of Veterinary Medicine, University of Florida, Gainesville, Florida.

ROBERT H. WHITLOCK, D.V.M., Ph.D.
Chief of Medicine, Professor of Medicine, Chief of Section of Large Animal Medicine, School of Veterinary Medicine, University of Pennsylvania, Philadelphia, Pennsylvania.

CHRISTINE S. F. WILLIAMS, B.V.Sc., M.R.C.V.S.
Director, Laboratory Animal Care Service, Michigan State University, East Lansing, Michigan.

DON E. WILLIAMS, D.V.M., M.S.
Private consultant in beef herd management, Guymon, Oklahoma.

MICHAEL R. WILSON, B.V.Sc., Ph.D., M.R.C.V.S.
Professor, University of Guelph, Guelph, Ontario, Canada.

JOHN K. WINKLER, D.V.M.
Associate Professor Emeritus, Auburn University School of Veterinary Medicine, Clinician, Large Animal Clinic, Auburn, Alabama.

DWIGHT F. WOLFE, D.V.M., M.S.
Assistant Professor, School of Veterinary Medicine, Auburn University, Large Animal Surgery and Medicine, Auburn, Alabama.

RICHARD L. WOOD, D.V.M., Ph.D.
Veterinary Medical Officer, USDA-ARS, National Animal Disease Center, Ames, Iowa.

R. J. YEDLOUTSCHNIG, D.V.M.
Section Head, Diagnostic Services Section, United States Department of Agriculture, Animal and Plant Health Inspection Service, Foreign Animal Disease Diagnostic Laboratory, Orient Point, New York.

PREFACE TO THE SECOND EDITION

The second edition of *Current Veterinary Therapy: Food Animal Practice* is for the purpose of update and improvement of the information contained in the first edition. Over 250 authors and 15 consulting editors have contributed to this edition. Numerous new authors and consulting editors add a new dimension. The response to the first edition has been excellent; therefore, the format has not been drastically changed. [However, in order to include in one volume all that is current in food animal practice, the decision has been made to add references to articles in the previous edition when little or no changes have taken place in therapy or management.]

The responsibility for scientific material contained in each article is solely that of the author. Attempts were made by the editor and consulting editors to standardize the manuscript without affecting the content.

Note should be taken of the purpose of the text. It is designed to be used as a quick, concise resource book concerning the prevention, therapy, and management of food animal disease. It is not intended, because of lack of space, to be an encyclopedia of medicine, surgery, toxicology, nutrition, and so forth. However, it is an excellent source of concise material in these areas.

It is impossible to individually thank everyone who had a part in producing this new edition. However, I must thank God for giving me both the time and the energy to complete this work and to thank my wife, Sammie, who again was my stenographer and my source of encouragement. Very special thanks go to the excellent consulting editors, who helped outline, critique, and proofread the manuscripts, and to the authors themselves who made the whole thing possible. The excellent staff of W. B. Saunders, who have been outstanding to work with and who do such superb work in editing and putting the final touch to the book, are to be commended. Finally, the editor must also thank the several thousand readers who bought the first edition and who sent the hundreds of favorable comments.

The editor hopes you, the reader, will find this a worthwhile addition to your library and welcomes your constructive comments and criticism of this edition.

JIMMY L. HOWARD, EDITOR

CONTENTS

SECTION 10

SECTION 11

SECTION 13

DISEASES OF THE REPRODUCTIVE AND URINARY SYSTEMS 765
Robert S. Hudson, D.V.M., M.S., Consulting Editor

SPECIAL THERAPY AND PROCEDURES

WILLIAM L. JENKINS
Consulting Editor

Fluid, Shock, and Blood Therapy

DANIEL A. GINGERICH, D.V.M., M.S.

The health of the body is dependent on the maintenance of normal volume and composition of fluids in the vascular, intercellular, and intracellular compartments. These are physiologically interrelated in such a manner that an abnormality in one compartment is reflected as abnormalities in the others. Normal volume and composition of body fluids are maintained by balancing oral intake of water, dietary nutrients, and electrolytes with output of fluids and electrolytes, primarily in urine and feces. The intake of water, regulated by the phenomenon of thirst, and the output of fluids and electrolytes, regulated chiefly by the kidney, are under the control of an exquisite neuroendocrine system that responds to increases or decreases in volume, sodium concentration, and osmotic pressure of circulating fluid. The respiratory system also plays an indispensable role in the maintenance of normal acid-base composition of the fluid.

The physiologic consortium consisting of thirst, renal mechanisms, and respiratory mechanisms is so effective that the normal animal can maintain life-supporting body fluid balance despite seemingly overwhelming challenges to the system. This is well illustrated by the adaptive mechanisms that enable animals such as camels, cattle, and sheep to survive for long periods in hot climates without water. An examination of the physiologic nature of disturbances that *do* cause life-threatening fluid imbalances provides insight into normal physiology as well as a basis for understanding fluid therapy.

Volume Deficits

The most common reason for instituting fluid therapy in food animals is to restore the volume of fluids to normal. *Dehydration,* in the strictest sense, refers to a deficit of body water but is usually used to describe a deficit of both water and electrolytes in the body.

Water Deficits

Dehydration can arise from either a deficit of water intake, an increase in water loss, or a combination of both. This form of dehydration is sometimes encountered in range herds under drought conditions, in confined animals denied access to water, or in diseased animals that are unable to drink. The deficit of water is shared by all body compartments, but efforts are made to maintain circulating volume at the expense first of extracellular fluid and then of intracellular fluid. As the condition becomes more advanced, the circulating fluid volume is also reduced, leading to hemoconcentration, increased blood viscosity, and, finally, peripheral circulatory failure.

Loss of Water and Electrolytes

The more usual form of dehydration arises from excessive loss of water and electrolytes in certain diseases. In food-producing animals, diarrhea is probably the most frequently encountered disease condition in which serious loss of fluids and electrolytes occurs. Vomiting in monogastric animals and functional intestinal obstructive conditions in ruminants also lead to fluid and electrolyte loss.

Acid-Base and Electrolyte Imbalances

Virtually all conditions in which body fluid volume is reduced are associated with characteristic acid-base and electrolyte imbalances. Acid-base and electrolyte balances are intricately interrelated in the body, in that the various anions and cations participate in physicochemical buffering of body fluids against sudden changes in pH. In addition to physicochemical buffering, acid-base status is maintained physiologically by balancing the acid and alkali gains with losses. The kidney regulates the excretion of nonvolatile acids as well as electrolytes, and the respiratory system regulates the excretion of volatile acids in the form of CO_2.

Metabolic Acidosis

Abnormally high acidity (or low alkalinity) in the body is referred to as *acidosis.* Acidosis has been conventionally classified as "respiratory," referring to acidity due to an accumulation of CO_2 in the body, and "metabolic," referring to acidity due to a relative excess of nonvolatile acids in the body. From a fluid therapy point of view, only metabolic acidosis need be considered. Respiratory acidosis occurs only in rare cases of respiratory center depression, in conditions of extreme loss of pulmonary function, or under prolonged general anesthesia. Physiologically, there are two ways in which metabolic acidosis can occur: (1) gain of acid and (2) loss of base (Table 1).

Table 1. Causes of Metabolic Acidosis

General Causes	Physiologic Mechanisms	Examples
Gain of acid	Gain of exogenous acid (lactic acid)	Engorgement toxemia
	Incomplete oxidation of fat (ketoacids)	Acetonemia, diabetes
	Incomplete oxidation of carbohydrates (lactic acid)	Dehydration (ischemia)
	Tissue catabolism (phosphoric, sulfuric acids)	Dehydration, starvation
	Decreased renal function (all of the above)	Dehydration, kidney disease
Loss of base	From the G.I. tract	Diarrhea
	From drooling saliva	Pharyngitis

Gain of Acid. In the normal animal, the dietary and metabolic acids that enter the system are buffered or excreted and therefore do not appreciably change the acid-base status of the body. If abnormally large amounts of acid enter the system or if the normal regulatory mechanisms are compromised, acidosis may occur. This situation arises in a number of disease conditions that are frequently encountered in food animal practice (Table 1). Engorgement toxemia is an example of a disease characterized by acidosis due to the absorption of abnormally high amounts of lactic acid (which arise as a result of fermentation of soluble carbohydrates) from the gastrointestinal tract. The incomplete oxidation of fats, as in acetonemia, results in the accumulation of ketoacids in the body. The incomplete oxidation of carbohydrates, due to anaerobic metabolism when tissues are inadequately perfused during dehydration, results in higher production of organic acids such as lactic acid. Increased tissue catabolism and cellular breakdown result in the release of inorganic acids, chiefly phosphoric and sulfuric acids. Finally, any or all of the preceding acids may accumulate and contribute to severe acidosis if renal function is in any way impaired. It should be noted that dehydration is the common feature of this type of acidosis, which compromises the body's ability to regulate acid-base balance.

Loss of Base. Acidosis due to the loss of base is frequently encountered during diarrhea and is caused by the loss of bicarbonate or its equivalent in diarrheic feces. Less frequently, extensive salivary losses of bicarbonate may occur in ruminants that cannot swallow. Although actual losses of base contribute to the acidosis, the dehydration that usually develops concurrently also leads to a gain of acid, as explained previously.

Electrolyte Shifts During Acidosis. Regardless of the specific cause, metabolic acidosis has profound effects on the electrolyte balance in the body. As the hydrogen ion concentration in extracellular fluids increases, hydrogen tends to move into cells in exchange for the intracellular cations sodium and potassium (Fig. 1). This tendency has the effect of lowering intracellular pH and decreasing the concentration of intracellular cations, principally potassium. If the acidosis develops acutely, as in neonatal diarrhea in calves, plasma potassium concentrations often increase to dangerous levels. In older animals, however, decreased plasma potassium concentrations are a common finding during acidosis.

Metabolic Alkalosis

Abnormally high alkalinity (or low acidity) in the body is referred to as *alkalosis*. Alkalosis has been conventionally classified as "respiratory," referring to alkalinity due to an abnormally low CO_2 content in the blood, and "metabolic," referring to alkalinity due to an abnormally high bicarbonate concentration in the blood. In practice, only metabolic alkalosis need be considered, since respiratory alkalosis is rarely recognized in conjunction with the need for fluid therapy. Although metabolic alkalosis could theoretically be caused either by a gain of base or by a loss of acid (Table 2), alkalosis due to a gain of base is likely to occur only iatrogenically with overzealous administration of bicarbonate or bicarbonate precursors.

Loss of Acid. Metabolic alkalosis almost invariably arises as a result of a loss of acid from the body. The loss of gastric secretions containing hydrochloric acid during vomiting can lead to metabolic alkalosis. Less obvious, but more frequently encountered in food animal practice, is the loss of abomasal hydrochloric acid in ruminants with intestinal obstructive disease. For every molecule of hydrochloric acid that is secreted, one chloride ion is removed from the plasma and one new bicarbonate ion is synthesized and returned to the circulation, as depicted in Figure 2. The hydrochloric acid normally moves on into the intestinal tract to be buffered and reabsorbed. If these secretions cannot, because of some disease condition, move into the intestinal tract, the fluid becomes trapped and accumulates in the abomasum and is refluxed into the forestomach. Even though ruminants do not ordinarily vomit, the chloride-rich acid fluid that becomes sequestered in the abomasum and forestomach is lost to the systemic circulation as effectively as from vomiting in monogastric animals. This pattern is common in cattle suffering from a wide variety of digestive disorders, including (1) abomasal displacement, torsion, and impaction, (2) high intestinal obstruction such as intussusception

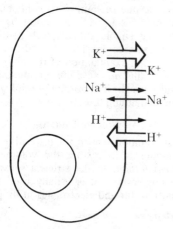

Figure 1. Intracellular-extracellular cation shifts that occur during acidosis, depicting the movement of hydrogen into the cell in exchange for potassium.

Table 2. *Causes of Metabolic Alkalosis*

General Causes	Physiologic Mechanisms	Examples
Gain of base	Gain of exogenous base Oxidation of endogenous organic acids	Iatrogenic Convalescent lactic acidosis
Loss of acid	Loss of hydrochloric acid from the stomach or abomasum	Vomiting Abomasal disorders (e.g., torsion) Vagal indigestion (G.I. stasis) Intussusception (intestinal obstruction)

of the jejunum, and (3) generalized gastrointestinal stasis such as in vagal indigestion (Table 2).

Electrolyte Shifts During Alkalosis. As the hydrogen ion concentration in extracellular fluids decreases, intracellular-extracellular shifts of cations in exchange for hydrogen (in a direction opposite to that described for acidosis) have been postulated. Plasma potassium concentrations are usually markedly reduced during metabolic alkalosis, but this phenomenon is thought to be due principally to continued urinary losses in the face of sudden reductions in dietary intake of potassium rather than to intracellular movement of potassium.

FLUID AND ELECTROLYTE THERAPY IN PRACTICE

The objective of fluid therapy is to aid in restoring the volume and composition of body fluids to normal. It should be emphasized that the clinician does not reestablish fluid and electrolyte balance; the body does. The clinician merely administers fluids and electrolytes in proportions likely to assist the body's own physiologic mechanisms in restoring normal balance in less accessible fluid spaces. The practice of rational fluid therapy depends on a working knowledge of:

1. The pathogenesis of both acidosis and alkalosis in diseased animals.

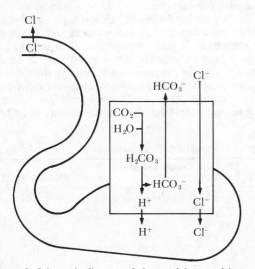

Figure 2. Schematic diagram of abomasal (or gastric) mucosal cell, depicting secretion of hydrochloric acid. The net process removes chloride from and returns bicarbonate to the circulation. Hypochloremic metabolic alkalosis results if these secretions are lost or trapped.

2. The electrolyte disturbance patterns associated with both acidosis and alkalosis.

3. The composition of electrolyte solutions suitable for treatment of acidotic patients as well as solutions suitable for alkalotic patients.

Route of Administration

Fluid therapy has been skillfully practiced in human patients, with undeniable success, for decades. However, adult humans weigh an average of only 70 kg, rarely need more than two or three liters over 24 hours, and willingly lie quietly while fluids are infused intravenously. In contrast, adult cattle often weigh 500 kg, may need as much as 20 liters of fluids over 24 hours, and not only refuse to lie quietly but frequently seem intent on destroying whatever IV apparatus an ingenious clinician may have devised.

Because of such difficulties, fluid replacement has too often been dismissed as impractical in food animal practice. Likewise, in human medicine, particularly in epidemics of diarrhea in underdeveloped countries, sophisticated fluid therapy technologies are too cumbersome to be applied to large populations of impoverished patients. Fortunately, in the 1960's, application of knowledge from laboratory studies on carrier-mediated sodium and water absorption led to the discovery that oral therapy during human cholera with glucose-electrolyte solutions could improve fluid balance. It has now been established beyond reasonable doubt that water and electrolytes are readily absorbed by the small intestine of animals with diarrheal diseases.

Oral Absorption

Three absorptive mechanisms are currently recognized, each of which is dependent on and coupled to the absorption of sodium (for review see Schultz, 1981). The mechanism that has aroused the most interest in food animal practice is the so-called carrier-mediated absorptive process, whereby sodium absorption is coupled directly to the absorption of organic solutes such as glucose and neutral amino acids. Water accompanies the sodium-solute absorption passively, rendering the absorbate isotonic with plasma. In order for fluid absorption to occur by this mechanism, isotonic fluids containing approximately 100 mEq of sodium per liter along with readily absorbable solute such as glucose and neutral amino acids in amounts reasonably consistent with isotonicity (300 to 350 mOsm/L) are optimal. Electrolyte solutions lacking glucose or amino acids are not as readily absorbed. More recently, it has been found in both pigs and calves that providing volatile fatty acid radicals such as acetate and propionate as anions replacing chloride further enhances absorption, particularly from the colon.

The volume of fluids absorbed by the above mechanisms

Table 3. *Electrolyte Solutions for Oral Therapy in Neonatal Diarrhea*

			Electrolyte Content					Amino	
			Na^+ (mEq/L)	*K^+ (mEq/L)*	*Cl^- (mEq/L)*	*HCO_3^- (mEq/L)*	**Glucose (mM/L)**	**Acids* (mM/L)**	**Total (mOsm/L)**
Optimal for absorption			100	10	70	40	80	60	Isotonic
Electro-Plus A*		q. s. 2L	100	15	75	40†	60	60‡	350
Homemade formula:		q. s. 4L	99	13	73	39	60	60‡	344
NaCl	14 gm								
KCl	4 gm								
$NaHCO_3$	13 gm								
Glucose	43 gm								
Glycine	18 gm								

*Available from Pitman-Moore, Inc., Washington Crossing, NJ 08560.
†As citrate.
‡Glycine.

is directly related to the total amount of sodium and solute transported across the intestine. It is therefore difficult to envision a physiologic rationale for the use of hypertonic oral fluids, since such a use implies a shortage of water relative to sodium and solute. Because the absorbate is always isotonic when delivered to the serosal side, if *all* the available sodium and solute were absorbed, extra water would have to be obtained from another source. The standing osmotic gradient theory of local hypertonicity in the lateral intercellular spaces now has been refined by the finding that the apical tight junctions are manyfold more permeable to water and small ions than originally supposed. Thus, only modest increases in osmolality (perhaps 3 to 5 mOsm/L) of fluid within paracellular spaces are required to drive water absorption. At least in severely dehydrated neonates, hypertonic solutions would appear to be dangerous. Healthy 300-kg heifers do not tolerate five-fold hypertonic (1500 mOsm/L) fluids orally even though they have free access to water.

In neonatal diarrheic pigs and calves, which have very little reserve within the intestinal tract, it is important that oral fluids be balanced so as to provide optimal amounts of sodium and other solute. Examples of a commercially available solution and of a suggested homemade formula that fulfills most of these requirements are presented in Table 3. The usual dose for neonatal calves is 2 liters of solution orally 2 to 3 times per day. Baby pigs with diarrhea will often drink oral electrolyte solutions from a shallow pan, the major drawback being that the glucose in the solution makes the piglets and their pen a sticky mess.

In the adult ruminant, in contrast to the neonate, the intestinal tract contains a tremendous reserve of water and electrolytes equivalent to 12 to 20 per cent of the body weight. For this reason, the precise balance of the oral fluids administered is much less critical in larger animals. Specifically, it is difficult to imagine a circumstance in which shortage of suitable organic solute in intestinal contents would be a limiting factor in the absorption of sodium and water. Therefore, electrolyte solutions for adult animals are designed to be balanced and isotonic and yet to contain an excess of those electrolytes likely to be deficient according to the condition of the animal. The compositions of several commercially available solutions, in comparison with normal plasma, are listed in Table 4. They are roughly divided into those most suitable for acidotic patients, those most suitable for hypochloremic alkalotic patients, and a neutral solution.

Parenteral Fluids

In cases of advanced dehydration, shock, persistent vomiting, or upper G.I. obstruction or in cases in which the rate of fluid and electrolyte loss exceeds the oral absorptive capacity, fluids should be administered parenterally. If peripheral vasoconstriction (as evidenced clinically by cold extremities) has not occurred, fluids given subcutaneously or intraperitoneally will be absorbed over a 5 to 6 hour period. The intravenous route of administration represents the most direct access to the circulating fluid space and should be utilized whenever other routes are inadequate. Considerable ingenuity is required to prepare and administer fluids intravenously in sufficient

Table 4. *Electrolyte Composition of Fluids in Comparison with Plasma*

		Electrolyte Content (mEq/L)						
Condition	**Fluid**	*Na^+*	*K^+*	*Ca^{++}*	*Mg^{++}*	*Cl^-*	*HCO_3^-*	**Total**
	Normal plasma	142	5	5	3	104	28	310
Acidosis	Electro-Plus B*	145	10			104	55	310
Hypochloremic alkalosis	Ringer's injection†	147	4	5		156		312
	Electro-Plus C*	145	10	5	3	155		329
	Physiologic saline	154				154		308
Neutral	Lactated Ringer's solution†	130	4	3		109	28‡	274

*Available from Pitman-Moore, Inc., Washington Crossing, NJ 08560.
†Available from Abbott Laboratories, North Chicago, IL 60064.
‡As lactate.

quantities over a sufficiently long period, but the procedure is often life-saving. Balanced, isotonic electrolyte solutions are recommended as a starting point for parenteral therapy, although extra electrolytes, glucose, amino acids, and other ingredients can be added to intravenous solutions to meet the specific needs of the patient.

The solutions listed in Table 4 are entirely satisfactory for intravenous infusion, provided that reasonable sanitary precautions are observed. Solutions that do not contain bicarbonate may be sterilized by autoclaving.

Fluid Therapy in Acidotic Patients

Metabolic acidosis, as discussed in the preceding section, may be caused by a gain of acid, a loss of base, or a combination of both (Table 1).

Diagnosis

Careful clinical examination along with shrewd physiologic reasoning will usually provide the necessary diagnostic clues suggestive of acidosis. If the animal has severe diarrhea a loss of base should be presumed. If the animal is severely dehydrated, a gain of acid should be presumed. The plasma electrolyte pattern characteristic of metabolic acidosis in adult animals includes normal sodium, usually decreased potassium, normal chloride, and markedly decreased bicarbonate concentrations, as depicted in Figure 3. Because of the intracellular-extracellular shifts of potassium and other cations, a loss of potassium from the cells should be presumed regardless of the plasma potassium concentration.

Therapy

Fluid therapy for acidotic patients should include balanced electrolyte solutions containing excess bicarbonate or other alkalinizing agents. Efforts to drive potassium into cells can be made by including glucose in the solution along with a small excess of potassium. Of the solutions listed in Table 4, it is clear that the electrolyte composition of Electro-Plus B would be most suitable as a starting point for fluid therapy, although lactated Ringer's solution could also be used. The use of bicarbonate precursors such as acetate or lactate should be avoided in the patient with severe metabolic acidosis, because under these conditions they may not function as alkalinizing agents. The use of freshly prepared Electro-Plus B either orally or intravenously, or the use of a solution of similar composition, would be an optimal approach to fluid therapy in cases of metabolic acidosis. The inclusion of 1 per cent glucose in the electrolyte solution should be a routine practice.

Dosage

Attempts to calculate doses of fluids on the basis of estimated needs of large animal patients have not been rewarding. However, it should be noted that a severely dehydrated animal may have lost fluids equivalent to 10 per cent of the body weight, which would represent 50 liters in a 500-kg cow. The extent to which this hypothetical 50 liters needs to be supplied by the clinician depends entirely on the response of the patient and its willingness to drink. As a very general guideline, fluids should be given in increments of 1 liter per 25 kg of body weight and repeated as necessary until the animal responds and begins to drink on its own. This would represent 20 liters or more for an adult cow, given either intravenously (over several hours) or orally. Some acidotic animals may drink the electrolyte-glucose solution on their own.

Fluid Therapy in Neonatal Diarrhea

Neonatal animals with acute diarrheal diseases are more likely to succumb to the effects of extensive loss of water and electrolytes with its consequential dehydration and metabolic acidosis than to the infectious agent itself. For this reason, fluid therapy is of fundamental importance to the management of these patients.

Electrolyte Abnormalities

The plasma electrolyte pattern typical of acute neonatal enteritis includes normal sodium, increased potassium, normal chloride, and markedly reduced bicarbonate concentrations, as depicted in Figure 4. Plasma electrolyte changes do not, however, reflect the drastic reduction in plasma volume nor the development of intracellular acidosis and reduction in intracellular potassium concentration.

Oral Therapy

At the earliest sign of diarrhea in the newborn, a sodium-glucose/amino acid solution, such as those shown

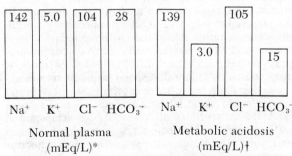

Figure 3. Plasma electrolyte profile typical of metabolic acidosis in adult animals, depicting bicarbonate deficit and hypokalemia (*Normal values for cattle, B. J. McSherry and I. Grinyer, Am. J. Vet. Res. *15*:509, 1954; †Average values from two acidotic cattle. D. A. Gingerich, Proc. Am. Assoc. Bov. Pract., Columbus, Ohio, 72, 1974.)

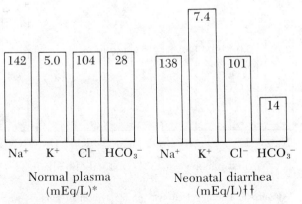

Figure 4. Plasma electrolyte profile typical of neonatal animals with metabolic acidosis due to acute diarrhea, depicting bicarbonate deficit and hyperkalemia. (*Normal values for cattle, B. J. McSherry and I. Grinyer, Am. J. Vet. Res. *15*:509, 1954; ††Mean values from calves with acute enteric infections. B. Tennant, *et al.* J. Am. Vet. Med. Assoc. *161*:993, 1972.)

in Table 3, should be given orally. The usual dose for calves is 2 liters repeated 2 or 3 times per day. Milk should be withheld if signs of diarrhea persist but must be reintroduced within 2 days to avoid the effects of inadequate nutrition.

Parenteral Therapy

If the animal becomes moribund, intravenous therapy should be instituted using a bicarbonate-containing solution, such as one of those listed in Table 4, supplemented with glucose to a final concentration of 1 to 1½ per cent. The use of acetate or lactate as a substitute for bicarbonate should be avoided in these patients. Intravenous fluids should be given at the rate of 1 liter per hour in calves and usually must be continued for several hours for maximum benefit. Intravenous therapy can be supplemented by subcutaneous administration of fluids and by oral fluids as discussed above.

Fluid Therapy in Alkalotic Patients

Hypochloremic metabolic alkalosis is commonly encountered in cattle as a result of entrapment of hydrochloric acid in the abomasum and forestomach (Fig. 2).

Diagnosis

If clinical examination reveals an abomasal displacement, torsion, or impaction, a state of hypochloremia should be presumed. If an intestinal obstruction such as an intussusception or cecal volvulus is diagnosed, or if generalized gastrointestinal stasis is present, hypochloremia should be suspected. The plasma electrolyte pattern characteristic of hypochloremia includes normal sodium, decreased potassium, markedly decreased chloride concentrations, and a reciprocal increase in bicarbonate concentrations, as depicted in Figure 5.

Therapy

Fluid therapy for alkalotic patients should include balanced electrolyte solutions containing excess chloride. Excess potassium would also appear to be indicated. Of the solutions listed in Table 4, it is clear that the electrolyte

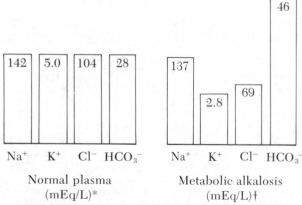

Figure 5. Plasma electrolyte profile typical of animals with hypochloremic metabolic alkalosis, depicting chloride deficit and reciprocal increase in bicarbonate concentration. (*Normal values for cattle, B. J. McSherry and I. Grinyer, Am. J. Vet. Res. *15*:509, 1954; †Average values from three alkalotic cattle, D. A. Gingerich, Proc. Am. Assoc. Bov. Pract., Columbus, Ohio, 72, 1974.)

composition of Ringer's solution (not lactated Ringer's) or Electro-Plus C would be most suitable as a starting point for fluid therapy, although physiologic saline could also be used. These solutions are equally appropriate for oral or intravenous administration and may be sterilized by autoclaving. The solution used should also contain 1 per cent glucose. Cattle with obstructive diseases such as abomasal disorders, for which surgical intervention is the treatment of choice, often develop serious hypochloremia and attendant imbalances, making them poor surgical risks. In these patients, intravenous administration of chloride-rich fluids prior to and during surgery is beneficial. The usual rate of administration is 4 liters or more per hour. After surgical correction of the obstructive condition and after gastrointestinal motility is at least partially restored, most of the electrolyte imbalances associated with hypochloremia usually are corrected spontaneously within 24 to 48 hours. Oral electrolyte therapy appears clinically to be beneficial in speeding recovery during this time. The usual dose is 20 liters or more for an adult cow. Some alkalotic animals may drink the chloride-rich electrolyte-glucose solution on their own.

SHOCK THERAPY

Pathophysiology of Shock

Shock is an extreme form of the body fluid imbalances characterized by a diminishing circulating blood volume relative to the capacity of the vascular system. In food animal species, shock is frequently encountered as a result of (1) severe and acute loss of blood or other body fluids (hypovolemic shock), (2) overwhelming infections with gram-negative organisms (endotoxic shock), or (3) a combination of both. Hypovolemic shock may occur owing to acute blood loss, severe diarrhea, or other conditions such as fluid loss from the uterus in hydrops cases. Acute coliform mastitis, septicemic colibacillosis, toxic metritis, salmonellosis, and pasteurellosis are examples of diseases in which endotoxic shock may occur. Although the precise pathogenesis of shock varies according to the initiating mechanism, the physiologic consequences are similar. These include a drastic deficit of blood volume, catecholamine-mediated vasoconstriction, severe metabolic acidosis, and terminal respiratory failure.

In the initial or compensatory stages of shock the decreases in circulating volume are balanced by vasoconstriction, and blood pressure tends to be maintained. In the progressive stages of shock, compensatory mechanisms are no longer able to cope with the reduced blood volume, and blood pressure and cardiac output are progressively reduced. The irreversible stage of shock is characterized by failure to respond favorably to infusion of blood or fluids and is due to myocardial depression and the pooling of blood in capillary beds. Clinical signs of shock are not specific, but decreased body temperature, cold extremities, blanched mucous membranes, rapid weak pulse, and profound depression are clinical findings consistent with a state of shock.

Shock in Neonatal Colibacillosis

The confusion in terminology that has arisen with regard to colibacillosis in calves and pigs may be due to failure to take note of the two principal forms in which the disease occurs, *septicemic* colibacillosis and *enteropathogenic* colibacillosis.

Septicemic colibacillosis occurs in neonatal animals that are hypogammaglobulinemic because of the failure either to ingest or to absorb colostrum. In these animals shock occurs as a result of *endotoxins* released from dying bacteria directly into the blood stream. Endotoxins cause primary vascular changes resulting in shock due to redistribution (pooling) of blood within capillary beds rather than to an absolute reduction in blood volume. Diarrhea may also occur in septicemic colibacillosis but is not necessarily a characteristic feature.

Enteropathogenic colibacillosis is the diarrheal form of the disease. Enteropathogenic strains of *E. coli* colonize the small intestine and release *enterotoxins* that cause the intestinal mucosa to secrete excessive quantities of isotonic fluid. Intestinal hypersecretion leads to severe diarrhea, rapid depletion of body water and electrolytes, and ultimately, shock due to the reduction of blood volume.

The physiologic consequences as well as the therapeutic approach in the two forms of colibacillosis are similar, but it is useful conceptually to recognize the differences in pathogenesis.

Treatment of Shock

The therapeutic goal in shock is to restore normal perfusion to as much of the tissue mass as possible. The most universally accepted treatment is the restoration of blood volume by infusion of whole blood, plasma, or electrolyte solutions. Prior to initiation of therapy, however, the clinician should recognize and the owner should be advised that shock is sometimes irreversible.

Expansion of Circulating Volume

Intravenous infusions of fluids should be started immediately in animals in shock. Catheterization of the jugular or other peripheral vein is recommended. Catheter placement may require a surgical cutdown in severe cases.

Intravenous infusion of whole blood or plasma in cases of shock is of proven benefit in humans and has been used successfully in neonatal calves. Transfused blood or plasma is retained well in the vascular system, and volumes of up to one third of the normal blood volume are often required in shock patients. This would represent just over 1 liter in a typical newborn calf but 12 liters or more in an adult cow. Since collection and storage of whole blood are limiting factors and separation of large enough quantities of plasma is technically difficult, whole blood or plasma is usually used in conjunction with infusion of electrolyte solutions. The simultaneous administration of whole blood through one catheter and an electrolyte solution through a separate catheter is an ideal approach to fluid volume expansion in shock patients.

Balanced electrolyte solutions containing excess bicarbonate are indicated for intravenous infusion in shock patients. Bicarbonate is important in combating the severe metabolic acidosis that is a consistent finding in animals in shock (Table 1). The use of bicarbonate precursors such as lactate, which must be oxidized in the liver before it can serve as a physiologic buffer, should be avoided in shock therapy. Furthermore, bicarbonate should not be added to electrolyte solutions such as lactated Ringer's solution that contain calcium, because insoluble precipitates form. Balanced electrolyte solutions containing excess bicarbonate (Table 4) are ideal for intravenous infu-

sion during shock. The total volume of intravenous electrolyte solutions required is massive, often approaching 10 or even 20 per cent of body weight. The rate of infusion should be rapid at first. As a guideline, an infusion rate of 1 liter per 25 kg of body weight during the first hour would represent 2 liters per hour in a newborn calf and up to 20 liters per hour in an adult dairy cow. After the first hour, the infusion rate should be reduced to avoid the likelihood of pulmonary edema and other iatrogenic fluid and electrolyte imbalances. Considerable ingenuity is required to prepare and administer sufficient quantities of appropriate intravenous fluids, but the results are often rewarding in shock patients.

Corticosteroids

The use of corticosteroids in shock therapy is controversial but has been shown to be beneficial in certain experimentally induced endotoxic and other shock systems. The beneficial effects of steroid therapy in shock are thought to include protection against the effects of endotoxins, decreased peripheral resistance, decreased capillary permeability, stabilization of lysosomal membranes, and increased cardiac output. Current consensus is that if steroids are used in shock therapy they should be given early, in a readily available form, and in massive doses. Prednisolone sodium succinate (Solu-Delta-Cortef)* injected intravenously at dosages of 11 mg/kg is clinically effective in small animal patients in shock but is not available in large enough dosage forms for routine use in large animals. Dexamethazone (Azium)† injected intravenously at a dosage rate of 4 to 10 mg/kg has a slower onset of activity but is also clinically effective.

Corticosteroids should receive due consideration as a part of the therapeutic approach to shock in valuable animals. There is no evidence that one or two so-called shock doses of steroids are harmful, although steroids are contraindicated in pregnant animals.

BLOOD THERAPY

Indications for Blood Transfusion

In food animal practice, blood transfusions are usually given only as a life-saving therapeutic measure. The value of blood transfusions in the treatment of shock has been discussed in the preceding section. In addition to its value as a fluid (blood plasma is the most physiologic fluid available for expansion of the circulating fluid volume), whole blood or plasma from healthy donors can be used as a source of other constituents that are often overlooked. These include (1) plasma proteins, (2) immunoglobulins, (3) coagulation factors, and (4) hemoglobin.

Acute Blood Loss

Whole blood transfusions are indicated as an emergency life-saving measure in cases of acute blood loss associated with trauma, hemolytic syndromes, certain parasitic diseases (e.g., coccidiosis), or hemorrhagic disorders. Besides the life-saving effect of expanding circulating volume, blood transfusion augments the restoration of normal plasma proteins and provides platelets, prothrom-

*Available from The Upjohn Company, Kalamazoo, MI 49001.
†Available from Schering Corporation, Kenilworth, NJ 07033.

bin, and other factors that may reduce bleeding in hemorrhagic diseases.

Whole blood transfusion can also be life saving in that transfused red blood cells *temporarily* increase the oxygen-carrying capacity of the blood. The word "temporary" should be emphasized, since the mean survival half-time of transfused homologous erythrocytes is only around 2 days in cattle and 2 weeks in swine. Despite the short survival time of transfused erythrocytes themselves, however, the iron and other hemoglobin breakdown products should be available to the animal as a nutritional boost in regenerating new erythrocytes and hemoglobulin during longer term recovery from acute anemia. Blood transfusions are of little if any value in chronic, progressive anemias.

Colostrum-Deprived Neonates

The infusion of blood or plasma in neonatal animals that have failed to ingest colostrum early in life and therefore are deprived of their normal source of immunoglobulins has been suggested. Although it is estimated that 2 to 3 liters of plasma would be required to make up the gamma globulin deficit in a colostrum-deprived calf, some practitioners report that a liter or two of whole blood given intravenously is beneficial. Because adequate gamma globulin concentrates are not available commercially for food-producing animals, the potential benefits of blood or plasma transfusions for valuable animals should not be overlooked. In very small animals such as piglets, intraperitoneal injections of blood or plasma can be substituted for intravenous infusion, although this route of administration is second best.

Transfusion Incompatibilities

It is indeed fortunate that cattle and swine rarely have demonstrable natural isoagglutinins that cause transfusion reactions on an initial transfusion of blood. Blood groups do exist, however, that present the threat of transfusion reactions on subsequent transfusions. Exceedingly complex blood group systems have been described, most active of which, from a transfusion compatibility point of view, are the J system in cattle and the A system in swine. Transfusion reactions that do occur following repeated transfusions of incompatible blood are immediate anaphylactic reactions characterized by arched back, straining, muscular trembling, dyspnea, coughing, salivation, lacrimation, tachycardia, hemoglobinuria, and hyperthermia. These reactions are usually epinephrine responsive. Since serious transfusion reactions can be avoided by (1) avoiding repeated transfusions and (2) discontinuing the transfusion and administering epinephrine should signs of a reaction appear, the practitioner should not be hesitant about giving blood transfusions in food animal species.

Collection of Blood

Because collection, typing, and banking of animal blood are not feasible with present technology, blood must be collected from another animal at the time of transfusion. Selection of a suitable donor depends partly on the purposes of the tranfusion. For transfusions in neonatal animals, the dam of the recipient is usually the most suitable donor. In cases of hemorrhagic disease affecting the entire herd, a donor from outside the herd should be sought. For transfusions in large animals with infectious diseases, such as coliform mastitis, for example, a herd-

mate that has fully recovered from the disease may be the most suitable donor. Larger quantities of blood can be collected from slaughtered animals at the time of stunning. Great care must be taken that donors are healthy and completely free of diseases that may be transmissible in the blood.

Various blood collection techniques have been described for large animals, including direct transfusion from donor to recipient by the use of a Shikle's syringe, vacuum pump–assisted collection into closed containers, collection into commercially available vacuum bottle systems, and collection by gravity flow. Sodium citrate is the anticoagulant of choice and should be placed in the collection container in an amount sufficient to give a final concentration of 0.3 per cent (3 gm per liter of blood). The blood should be swirled during collection to assure proper mixing with an anticoagulant. Plastic bag blood collection sets containing anticoagulant are commercially available and are entirely satisfactory for both collection and transfusion of small quantities (500 ml) of blood. For larger transfusions, sterilized glass or plastic containers with the proper amount of sodium citrate should be routinely carried as a part of the practitioner's equipment. Blood should be filtered through sterile gauze before it is used for transfusion.

Relatively large quantities of blood can be collected from healthy donors without endangering the animal's life. A safe upper limit for blood withdrawal is 1 liter per 200 kg of body weight. A mature cow could safely donate 4 liters of blood.

Supplemental Reading

Brasmer, T. H. (ed.): Shock. Vet. Clin. North Am. 6:171–309, 1976.
Bywater, R. J.: Evaluation of an oral glucose-glycine-electrolyte formulation and amoxicillin for treatment of diarrhea in calves. Am. J. Vet. Res. 38:1983–1987, 1977.
Dell, R. B.: Normal acid-base regulation. In Winters, R. W. (ed.): The Body Fluids in Pediatrics. Boston, Little, Brown & Co., 1973.
Gingerich, D. A.: Practical fluid and electrolyte therapy and its pathophysiological basis. In Proceedings of the 7th Annual Convention of the American Association of Bovine Practitioners, 1974, pp. 72–80.
Schultz, S. G.: Salt and water absorption by mammalian small intestine. In Johnson, L. R. (ed.): Physiology of the Gastrointestinal Tract. New York, Raven Press, 1981, pp. 983–989.
Swan, R. C., and Pitts, R. F.: Neutralization of infused acid by nephrectomized dogs. J. Clin. Invest. 34:205–212, 1954.
Tennant, B., et al.: Physiological and metabolic factors in the pathogenesis of neonatal infections in calves. J. Am. Vet. Med. Assoc. 161:993–1007, 1972.
Winters, R. W.: Physiology of acid-base disorders. In Winters, R. W. (ed.): The Body Fluids in Pediatrics. Boston, Little, Brown & Co., 1973.

Antimicrobial Therapy

WILLIAM L. JENKINS, B.V.Sc., M.Med.Vet., Ph.D.

Large animal practitioners constantly face the problem of bridging the gap between theoretical information available and the actual treatment of the animals under their care. This dilemma is perhaps most evident in the selection of an antibacterial agent or combination of agents to treat infections located in an organ or tissue. Ideally, one should ensure an appropriate and safe concentration of the antibacterial drug at the site of infection for a sufficient period to prevent damage or to eliminate the pathogenic organism and thus allow recovery to commence. However, to achieve this seemingly simple goal, a substantial number of factors and considerations often come into play. They concern the animals involved, the causative microorganism(s), the antibacterial agent(s), and the experience of the attending veterinarian. This article covers some of the major features associated with the clinical use of antimicrobial drugs, with special emphasis on the rational selection of such agents and the pitfalls that may be encountered when using drugs of this class.

Fate of Antibacterial Agents in the Body

Most antibacterial agents not only exert a detrimental effect on the pathogen but also are subject to the same processes as other drugs within the body. They often also exert a pharmacodynamic or even toxic effect on the animal.

Antimicrobial drugs are administered or applied in a variety of pharmaceutical forms, from which they become available for absorption and subsequent delivery to their sites of action. Following absorption, these compounds are distributed, to a greater or lesser degree, to various body fluid spaces and tissues. During this distribution phase, a drug must attain the concentration required at the site of infection in order to destroy or inhibit invading pathogenic microorganisms. Various metabolic reactions and excretory mechanisms are utilized to eliminate the drug and its metabolites from the body. These processes lead to a progressive decline of the antibacterial agent's concentration in the body fluids, and repetitive administration at fixed intervals is necessary to maintain the level of the drug within its therapeutic range. Under-dosing leads to subtherapeutic levels at the sites of infection, whereas over-dosing or too-frequent administration is likely to produce toxic manifestations.

A number of special pharmacokinetic features must be appreciated in order to make optimal use of antimicrobial agents. As far as oral administration is concerned, it is important to be cognizant of the degree of absorption that takes place (bioavailability), the multitude of factors that may alter the rate of absorption, the role that the disease process may play in modifying the absorption process, and the effects of the agent selected on the resident intestinal or ruminal microflora. Parenteral administration should be carried out with an awareness of the pharmaceutical factors that may influence the rate of absorption, the blood flow at the site of delivery, the local and systemic reactions that might occur, and any *in vitro* incompatibilites of drugs that are inadvisedly mixed in the same syringe.

The intracorporeal distribution features of note include the relative dispersion of the antibacterial agents into the various fluid and tissue compartments of the body, the percentage of binding to plasma proteins, the degree of specific tissue binding, and the distribution of the drugs into the CNS, mammary gland, and fetus. The alteration of distribution patterns by the disease process, age, and nutritional status as well as potential interactions between concurrently administered drugs must also be borne in mind.

As far as biotransformation is concerned, the site of metabolic transformation, the degree of biotransformation, the activity and fate of metabolites, and potential interactions with other drugs are the major features of concern. The influence of the disease state, inter-species differences, and age are additional factors that should receive attention in each case.

The primary and secondary routes of excretion and mechanisms involved also should be known, so that the influence of disease processes on elimination kinetics can be appreciated. The role of age and potential interactions involving excretion rates are also important.

Although many pharmacokinetic parameters have been determined in food animals for a number of the commonly used antibacterial agents, only a limited number of these terms are needed for the purpose of understanding the basis of rational chemotherapy and the problem of residues. These terms are:

1. *Volume of distribution* (Vd), which relates the amount of drug (A_B) in the body to the concentration of drug (C_p) in the plasma, or $Vd = A_B/C_p$. The units are usually liters.

2. *Clearance* (Cl), which at the simplest level represents the rate of elimination by all routes relative to the concentration (C) of a drug in any body fluid, or Cl = rate of elimination/C. The units are usually in milliliters per minute. Total body clearance (Cl_B) may be derived from 0.693 Vd/t½.

3. *Half-life* (t½) indicates the time necessary for the plasma concentration to decline by 50 per cent during the elimination (or β) phase. t½ = 0.693/β. The units are usually in minutes or hours.

It is important to realize that disease processes may modify all three of these important pharmacokinetic parameters.

PRINCIPLES OF ANTIMICROBIAL THERAPY

General Aspects

Rational chemotherapy is based on four essential factors: (1) an effective concentration of the selected antimicrobial agent for the particular organism at the site of infection; (2) a dosage rate and frequency that will ensure an adequate drug concentration for a sufficient period between doses; (3) a duration of therapy sufficient to achieve cure and to prevent relapse in an immunologically competent animal; and (4) supportive therapy and adequate nutritional intake, which are often critical for success.

The minimal inhibitory concentration (MIC) given for a particular bacterial species may not be consistent. Methodology, different strains, media used, time (regrowth), bacteriostatic *versus* bactericidal concentrations, rate of diffusion of antibiotic, and degree of bacterial inhibition required for effective therapy are all noteworthy considerations.

A crucial question is whether it is in fact necessary to maintain effective concentrations of antimicrobial drugs throughout the dosage period. Persistent antibacterial effects at subinhibitory concentrations have been demonstrated for penicillins, cephalosporins, macrolides, and tetracyclines, but *not* for aminoglycosides. Antibiotic-damaged organisms are usually more susceptible to leukocidal activity.

The clinical relevance of additive, synergistic, or antagonistic effects of antimicrobial combinations remains speculative to some degree, but general guidelines should be followed.

Additional drugs that may compromise host defense (immunosuppressants and antineoplastics) often complicate effective antimicrobial therapy and should be introduced judiciously.

Requirements for Successful Antimicrobial Therapy

1. Clinical diagnosis. Successful chemotherapy requires specific diagnosis if it is to be rational. However, a reasonable preliminary diagnosis is often all that is possible.

2. Bacteriologic diagnosis. Treatment should be aimed at the specific pathogen. The problems associated with polymicrobial infections, compared with the problems associated with monomicrobial infections, are always greater. The ideal is a conclusive bacteriologic diagnosis. Often, however, such a diagnosis must be presumptive (at least initially), and therapy based on past experience. Rational deduction is frequently necessary under field conditions. However, the examination of a direct smear stained with Wright's or even Gram's stain may prove to be very helpful.

3. Culture and sensitivity testing with the determination of MIC, if possible.

4. Appropriate selection of antimicrobial agent. Many factors should be considered—causative microorganism(s), results of sensitivity tests, pathogenicity of organism(s), acuteness of infection, kinetics, expense, potential toxicity of the drug(s) indicated, organic dysfunctions (especially renal function), and possible interactions with concomitantly administered drugs.

5. Correct dosage and route of administration of the chosen agent. The dose must result in adequate therapeutic concentrations at the sites of infection for a sufficient period. The advocated dosage schedules should always be carefully followed for at least 3 to 5 days, longer if needed.

6. Supportive and accompanying treatments, which are often critical for success.

7. Laboratory control of the effects of treatment, a goal that is, unfortunately, often difficult to attain under field conditions.

Reasons Why Failure May Follow Antimicrobial Therapy

1. The diagnosis is wrong, e.g., viral rather than bacterial infection.

2. Bacteria are not susceptible to the action of the antibiotic selected or are in static phase and therefore unresponsive. Phenotypic resistance is also seen with L-forms of bacteria (loss of cell wall).

3. Although originally susceptible, the organism has developed resistance.

4. Polymicrobial infection is present with insufficient antibiotic cover.

5. A combination of incompatible antibiotics has been administered.

6. Superinfection has taken place.

7. Reinfection by original or other pathogenic bacteria has occurred.

8. Drainage is inadequate in a surgical infection or a foreign body is present.

9. Defense mechanisms of the patient have been jeopardized by disease or concurrent therapy.

10. Detrimental changes in infected tissue, such as hypoxia, acidosis, and tissue debris, have reduced the effectiveness of the antibiotic or sulfonamide.

11. Inappropriate route of administration or incorrect dosage rate or interval has been chosen.

12. Expired or substandard products have been used.

13. Early withdrawal of selected agent has been necessitated by toxicity or adverse side effects.

14. Selected agent(s) has interacted with other concurrently administered drugs, diminishing the antimicrobial effect or altering the pharmacokinetics.

Combination Therapy

Treatment with antibacterial combinations may be necessary for success in certain instances. The administration of two or more agents may be beneficial in the following situations: (1) to treat mixed bacterial infections in which the organisms are not susceptible to a common agent; (2) to achieve synergistic antimicrobial activity; (3) to overcome bacterial tolerance; (4) to prevent the emergence of drug resistance; (5) to minimize toxicity; and (6) to prevent enzymatic inactivation of an antibiotic.

Additive and/or synergistic effects do occur when antibacterial agents are used in combination, but antagonism may also occur, sometimes with serious consequences.

Generally speaking, bacteriostatic agents act in an additive fashion, whereas bactericidal agents are often synergistic. However, antibacterial effects of several bactericidal antibiotics are substantially impaired by the simultaneous use of a bacteriostatic agent. These interactions should serve as general guidelines, because many exceptions are known, and a large number of confounding factors may play a role. A general classification of some common antimicrobials as bactericidal or bacteriostatic is shown in Table 1.

Examples of combination therapy for mixed infections include the use of clindamycin, metronidazole, or the semisynthetic penicillins for their anaerobic coverage in combination with aminoglycosides for their gram-negative efficacy.

Synergism against certain bacterial pathogens frequently can be achieved with combinations of penicillins or cephalosporins and aminoglycosides. The combined use of trimethoprim and selected sulfonamides also leads to a synergistic effect.

Preventing the development of resistance with combination antimicrobial therapy is best exemplified by the use of carbenicillin or ticarcillin together with gentamicin or tobramyin for the treatment of *Pseudomonas* infections.

Bacterial enzymatic inactivation of beta-lactam antibiotics such as the penicillins and cephalosporins can be prevented by the concurrent administration of a beta-lactamase inhibitor such as clavulanic acid. This fairly recent innovation promises to be a major advance in combination therapy.

Table 1. *Some Common Bactericidal and Bacteriostatic Antibacterial Agents*

Classification	Agents
Bactericidal*	Penicillins
	Cephalosporins
	Aminoglycosides
	Peptides
	Nitrofurans
	Trimethoprim/sulfonamides
Bacteriostatic*	Tetracyclines
	Chloramphenicol
	Macrolides
	Lincosamides
	Sulfonamides

*At usual concentrations.

Resistance of Microorganisms to Antibacterial Agents

Bacteria have two types of genetic structures that may confer resistance—a chromosome and plasmids. Both consist of double-stranded DNA, and both are associated with the inner cell membrane of the bacteria at some time. Plasmids are not essential for survival but carry genetic determinants that confer antibiotic resistance on bacteria.

Chromosomal Resistance to Antibacterial Agents (Mutation)

Mutation can occur in bacterial chromosomal genes, leading to resistance to particular antimicrobial agents. Several mechanisms have been identified:

1. Alteration of target site in the bacterial cell so that attachment by the antibiotic is blocked. Examples: resistance to streptomycin and to erythromycin.

2. Development of alternate metabolic pathways which then bypass the site of inhibition. Examples: resistance to trimethoprim and sulfonamides.

3. Changes in the permeability characteristics, which then exclude the antibacterial from the cell. Examples: resistance to chloramphenicol, tetracycline, and aminoglycosides.

4. Increased production of antibiotic inactivating enzymes otherwise present in low concentration. Examples: resistance to ampicillin and cefamandole.

Note that in these cases the antibacterial drugs act only as selective agents, allowing the resistant mutants to emerge either by a single step or by sequential mutations. Their genesis is independent of the presence of the agent. Mutated bacteria are often metabolically deranged and are at a selective growth disadvantage, so they usually disappear with time.

Plasmid-Mediated R Factor, or Acquired, Resistance

The occurrence and persistence of antibiotic resistance is far more complex when the resistance determinant is carried by a plasmid, or R factor. Plasmids may contain from 20 to 500 genes and can carry resistance to a number of different antibacterial agents (3 to 6 is quite a common number, but up to 9 have been recorded).

There are three possible mechanisms by which plasmids may migrate from one bacterium to another, namely, transformation, transduction and conjugation. In transformation, naked DNA seems to pass from the donor to the recipient through the growth medium. This process appears to be confined to a limited range of bacteria. In transduction, the transfer is mediated by a bacteriophage

that makes use of its specialized molecular equipment adapted for inserting DNA into recipient bacteria. Normally it is phage DNA that is transferred in this way. In certain cases, however, some DNA from the episome in the bacterial cell replaces the proper phage nucleic acid sequence. Phage-mediated transduction may occur between gram-positive as well as gram-negative species. In conjugation, the DNA passes from the donor cell to the recipient, assisted by a bridge formed during direct cell-to-cell contact. This is the most sophisticated form of transmission, because for transfer to occur at all, the donor has to have the necessary surface appendages to form the bridge (coded for by the resistance transfer factor, or RTF).

General facets of conjugation make it a very important process as far as gene transfer under natural conditions is concerned. Many types of bacteria can act as recipients, and resistance can pass freely from organisms normally saprophytic in the gut of animals to pathogenic bacteria. Pasteurella and Pseudomonas transfer seems to occur at a lower efficiency. In general, transfer occurs more frequently between gram-negative bacteria, although gram-positive organisms may also be involved. Conjugation allows the passage of a number of distinct genes at one time. Thus, resistance to several antibiotics, all mediated by different biochemical means, may be acquired in a single step. The great efficiency of the conjugation process ensures that the probability of gene transfer to a super-infecting pathogen is very high.

As with mutational resistance, the loss in susceptibility associated with acquired resistance is based on similar mechanisms, some of which are listed in Table 2.

The clinical relevance of plasmid-mediated resistance in veterinary medicine principally concerns (1) enteric infections, in which the reservoir of R-factors may be carried by saprophytic flora in the gut; (2) the use of low levels of antibiotics (as in animal feeds), which may lead to a high incidence of R-factors in a given population; and (3) the indiscriminate use of antibiotics, which may well eliminate the future usefulness of many antimicrobial agents.

The therapeutic guidelines to minimize the emergence of bacterial resistance are as follows:

1. A broad-spectrum antibacterial agent should not be used if a narrow-spectrum agent is also active against the causative organism.

2. Information regarding endemic infections and sensitivity patterns should be regularly sought and used for the rational choice of an antibiotic.

3. Appropriate dosage rates should always be followed.

4. When a combination regimen is used to prevent the

Table 2. Mechanisms by Which Organisms Acquire Resistance to Common Antibacterial Agents

		Organisms	
Antibacterial Agent	Mechanism	Gram-Positive	Gram-Negative
Penicillin, ampicillin, carbenicillin	Beta-lactamase hydrolysis	Yes	Yes
Oxacillin, methicillin	Beta-lactamase hydrolysis	No	Yes
Cephalosporins	Beta-lactamase hydrolysis	Yes	Yes
Chloramphenicol	Acetylation by acetyltransferase	Yes	Yes
Tetracycline	Permeability block	Yes	Yes
Aminoglycosides	Acetylation, phosphorylation, or adenylation	Yes	Yes
Macrolides, lincosamides	Structural protein change	Yes	No
Sulfonamides	Drug-insensitive dihydropterate synthetase	Yes	Yes
Trimethoprim	Drug-insensitive dihydrofolate reductase	Yes	Yes

development of resistant strains, the individual agents should be used in full dosage.

5. Antibacterials for topical application should be selected from those to which development of resistance is uncommon.

6. For prophylaxis, an antibacterial agent should be used that will prevent colonization of a specific organism or will eradicate it shortly after it has become established.

7. To the extent that it is consistent with the reasonable practice of medicine, every effort should be made to reduce the use of antibiotics to clear medical indications and to avoid the overuse of newer agents when previously available agents are effective in a given clinical situation.

CLINICAL PHARMACOLOGY OF THE ANTIBACTERIAL AGENTS

A relatively limited number of antibacterial agents are commonly used in food animals. Thus, it behooves the practitioner to be familiar with the substantive clinical characteristics of these drugs in order to derive the optimal therapeutic benefits for the cases under his or her care. Some of the key pharmacologic features of frequently employed antibiotics, sulfonamides, and nitrofurans are reviewed here.

Penicillins

Penicillins continue to be among the most important antibiotics available because of their remarkable antibacterial activity, relative safety, and low cost. The penicillins share many characteristics with the cephalosporin group, and these two classes, together with the new monobactams, are often referred to as beta-lactam drugs or cell wall inhibitors.

GENERAL PROPERTIES

The penicillins are sensitive to heat, light, extremes in pH, heavy metals, and oxidizing as well as reducing agents. They often lose activity in aqueous solution and should not be stored at temperatures exceeding 30°C. Care should thus be taken with the handling of penicillin preparations.

Penicillins are weak acids derived from 6-aminopenicillanic acid (6-APA), and because of their poor aqueous solubility and instability, they are most often available as salts or esters for parenteral administration. Sodium and potassium salts are absorbed rapidly from injection sites, whereas aqueous or oily suspensions of organic salts, such as procaine and benzathine, are absorbed much more gradually (repository or long-acting preparations). The trihydrate forms of the semisynthetic penicillins possess greater aqueous solubility than the parent compounds and are often preferred for both parenteral and oral use.

Penicillins contain a beta-lactam nucleus that when cleaved by a beta-lactamase (penicillinase) produces penicilloic acid derivatives with a resultant loss of biological activity. Derivatives of penicilloic acid formed in the body are the major antigenic determinants for penicillin hypersensitivity.

Alterations of the penicillin side chain can produce differences in resistance to enzymatic breakdown, modifications of antibacterial spectra, and, finally, changes in pharmacokinetic fate.

ANTIMICROBIAL FEATURES

Penicillins interfere with the development of bacterial cell walls by impairing the formation of cross-links between peptidoglycan strands. Deprived of its rigid cell wall, the bacterial cell loses the protection it requires because it has a high intracellular osmotic pressure. The effect of penicillins is generally bactericidal although bacteriolysis may also take place. However, at subminimal inhibitory concentrations, beta-lactam antibiotics also exert residual effects on bacteria (minimal antibiotic concentrations, or MAC) that may, in turn, alter the cell structure and enhance phagocytosis by host cells.

Beta-lactam antibiotics have no effect on existing bacterial cell walls, and susceptible organisms must be actively multiplying to be affected. Understandably, penicillins are most effective during the logarithmic phase of bacterial growth.

Various penicillins possess different quantitative activity against certain organisms. Gram-positive bacteria are usually more susceptible than gram-negative bacteria, in part owing to the latter's more complex cell wall. However, the susceptibility patterns can vary a great deal among bacterial strains, and many factors play a role, not the least of which is the concentration of a penicillin at the site of infection. Substitutions on the 6-APA nucleus have produced various novel classes of penicillin with activity against a wide variety of bacteria.

Bacterial resistance to penicillins may take a number of forms:

1. Intrinsic resistance—inability of the penicillin to penetrate or bind to specific bacterial protein.

2. Beta-lactamase resistance—either plasmid or chromosomally mediated.

3. "Tolerance"—autolytic enzymes in bacterial cell wall are not activated.

4. L-forms of bacteria—absence or incompleteness of cell wall.

Penicillins as a group tend to be more active in an acidic environment (pH 5.5 to 6.5).

ANTIBACTERIAL SPECTRA

Benzylpenicillin, or penicillin G, and its oral congeners, such as penicillin V, are generally active against both aerobic and anaerobic gram-positive organisms and, with few exceptions, are inactive against gram-negative organisms at usual therapeutic concentrations. Organisms sensitive to benzylpenicillin in vitro include Streptococci, penicillin-sensitive Staphylcococci, *Corynebacterium, Clostridium, Bacteroides* (non-fragilis strains), *Erysipelothrix rhusiopathiae, Actinomyces bovis,* and *Leptospira canicola.*

The semisynthetic beta-lactamase–resistant penicillins such as cloxacillin, flucloxacillin, oxacillin, and nafcillin have spectra similar to penicillin G but are also effective against penicillinase-producing strains of *Staphylococcus aureus.* However, the MICs for members of this group may be higher for both Streptococci and sensitive Staphylococci strains than for penicillin G.

Ampicillin and amoxicillin are the most frequently used semisynthetic broad-spectrum penicillins in food animal practice. These penicillins are active against a large number of gram-positive and gram-negative organisms, including species of Staphylococci, Streptococci, *(Streptococcus fecalis), Corynebacterium, Clostridium, Escherichia coli, Klebsiella, Shigella, Salmonella, Proteus,* and *Pasteurella.*

However, they are susceptible to beta-lactamase attack (Staphylococci and some gram-negative strains), and a recent development has been to combine a beta-lactamase inhibitor, such as clavulanic acid or sulbactam, with a semisynthetic penicillin in order to enhance its spectrum. An example of this approach is the combination of potassium clavulanate and amoxicillin.

The anti-*Pseudomonas* penicillins such as carbenicillin and ticarcillin have spectra similar to that of ampicillin but also are effective against strains of *Pseudomonas* and *Proteus vulgaris*. They are not as effective against some Streptococci and Staphylococci but do possess a modicum of beta-lactamase resistance.

KINETIC FATE

Absorption. Most penicillins in aqueous solution are rapidly absorbed from parenteral sites. Absorption is delayed when the inorganic penicillin salts are suspended in oil vehicles or when the sparingly soluble repository organic salts such as procaine penicillin G and benzathine penicillin G are administered. These latter preparations should never be injected intravenously. Only some penicillins are acid stable and may be administered orally. Absorption occurs from the upper gastrointestinal tract, but the degree and rate of absorption differ greatly among the various penicillins. Peak serum concentrations are generally achieved within 2 hours of oral administration. Absorption of penicillins also takes place following intrauterine infusion.

Distribution. Following absorption, penicillins are widely distributed in body fluids and tissues. The volume of distribution tends to reflect extracellular compartmentalization, although some penicillins, such as amoxicillin, penetrate into tissues quite well. Significant levels of the various penicillins are generally encountered in the liver, kidney, muscle, and lungs, but only very low concentrations occur in poorly perfused areas such as the cornea and synovial fluid. In plasma, penicillins are reversibly and loosely bound to plasma proteins. The extent of this binding varies with particular penicillins and their concentration. For example, ampicillin is usually about 20 per cent bound, whereas cloxacillin may be 80 per cent bound. The penicillins do not usually readily traverse the normal blood-brain, placental, mammary, and prostatic barriers. However, massive doses or the presence of inflammation will often allow diffusion to occur into the respective fluids. Inflammation also permits effective levels of some penicillins to be reached in abscesses as well as in pleural, peritoneal, and synovial fluids.

Biotransformation. Penicillins are generally excreted unchanged, but small fractions of a given dose undergo metabolic transformations by unknown mechanisms. Penicilloic acid derivatives that are formed tend to be allergenic.

Excretion. Between 60 and 90 per cent of a parenterally administered penicillin will be eliminated in the urine within a short time; e.g., up to 90 per cent of penicillin G can be removed in the urine within 6 hours. However, the biliary route may also be a major excretory pathway for the broad-spectrum semisynthetic penicillins. About 20 per cent of renal excretion occurs by glomerular filtration and about 80 per cent by tubular secretion—a process inhibited by probenecid and other weak organic acids. Clearance values for penicillins are considerably lower in neonates than in adults, and anuria may increase the half-life of penicillin G from about 30 minutes to 10 hours. Penicillins are also eliminated in milk, though often only in trace amounts in the normal udder, and may persist for up to 90 hours after injection. Penicillin residues in milk also have been found following intrauterine infusion of the antibiotic.

SIDE EFFECTS AND TOXICITY

Direct toxic reactions are very rare. The penicillins are among the safest of the antibiotics.

The salt form that is used may occasionally be responsible for adverse effects. For example, potassium penicillin G administered intravenously to a severely acidotic calf could precipitate fatal hyperkalemia.

Hypersensitivity reactions are the most frequent cause for concern. They may manifest as urticaria, angioedema, anaphylaxis, drug fever, serum sickness, or the Arthus reaction. Anaphylactic reactions are not uncommon in cattle, and if the preparation contains a carboxymethylcellulose adjuvant, the likelihood of an allergic response seems to be increased. Cross-reactivity between penicillins, and even some cephalosporins, is quite frequent.

Superinfections may occur when broad-spectrum penicillins are used orally. Staphylococci, *Pseudomonas, Proteus* or yeasts are most often involved.

POTENTIAL DRUG INTERACTIONS

Ampicillin sodium should not be mixed with any other preparation, and penicillin G is incompatible *in vitro* with many other drugs. Carbenicillin and ticarcillin inactivate the aminoglycosides by a chemical interaction.

Neomycin decreases the absorption of certain penicillins by an unknown mechanism.

Displacement of penicillins from plasma protein-binding sites and delayed tubular secretion occur when drugs such as salicylates, phenylbutazone, sulfonamides, and other weak acids are administered concurrently.

The presence of food decreases the absorption of ampicillin.

SPECIFIC PREPARATIONS (CURRENTLY USED)

Procaine Penicillin G
SPECTRUM: Gram-positive organisms.
ROUTE. Intramuscular injection or intramammary infusion.
DOSAGE. IM 10,000–20,000 IU/kg every 12 or 24 hours.
WITHDRAWAL TIMES. Cattle, 10 days; sheep, 9 days; swine, 7 days.*
MILK DISCARD TIME. 72 hours.*

Benzathine Penicillin G
SPECTRUM. Gram-positive organisms.
ROUTE. Intramuscular or subcutaneous injection.
DOSAGE. 10,000–20,000 IU/kg every 48 hours.
WITHDRAWAL TIME. Cattle, 30 days.*

Ampicillin
SPECTRUM. Broad.
ROUTE. Intramuscular injection or oral administration.
DOSAGE. IM 4–10 mg/kg every 24 hours; PO 4–10 mg/kg every 12 or 24 hours.
WITHDRAWAL TIMES. Cattle, IM 6 days, nonruminant calves, PO 15 days.*

---

*Withdrawal and milk discard times will depend upon the regulations in the practitioner's country. The times listed here are general guidelines only.

Amoxicillin
SPECTRUM. Broad.
ROUTE. Intramuscular or subcutaneous injection.
DOSAGE. 6–10 mg/kg every 24 hours.
WITHDRAWAL TIME. Cattle, 30 days.*
Cloxacillin
SPECTRUM. Gram-positive organisms, including penicillinase-producing Staphylococci.
ROUTE. Intramammary infusion (dry cow).
DOSAGE. 500 mg/quarter.
CAUTION. Use no later than 30 days prior to calving.

NEWER SEMISYNTHETIC PENICILLINS AND RELATED BETA-LACTAMS

Mecillinam. Specifically gram-negative spectrum.
Bacampicillin, Pivampicillin, and Talampicillin. Ampicillin precursors with improved absorption characteristics.
Sulbenicillin and Ticarcillin. Carbenicillin derivatives active against *Pseudomonas* and *Proteus*.
Meclocillin and Piperacillin. Ureido-type penicillins, potent broad-spectrum antibiotics that are effective against *Pseudomonas* and many gram-negative Enterobacteria.
Thienamycin, Clavulanic Acid, and Sulbactam. Beta-lactamase (penicillinase and cephalosporinase) inhibitors.
Aztreonam and Sulfazecin. Monobactam antibiotics that are very active against aerobic gram-negative bacteria and are highly resistant to beta-lactamase hydrolysis.

Cephalosporins and Cephamycins

Few classes of antibiotics have proliferated as rapidly as the cephalosporins, but as a group they have enjoyed little attention in food animal medicine. Until recently, these beta-lactam antibiotics differed from one another with respect to their pharmacology rather than their antibacterial spectra. The newer generations of cephalosporins have a broader range of activity, although their cost is prohibitive for routine use in veterinary medicine.

GENERAL PROPERTIES

The physical and chemical properties of the cephalosporins are similar to those of the penicillins. Cephalosporins as weak acids (derived from 7-aminocephalosporinic acid) are used either as the free bases or as sodium salts. The beta-lactam nucleus of the cephalosporins is also susceptible to beta-lactamase hydrolysis (cephalosporinases). Modifications of the cephalosporin side chain have produced differences in beta-lactamase susceptibility, antibacterial spectrum, and pharmacokinetic fate.

ANTIMICROBIAL FEATURES

Cephalosporins and cephamycins inhibit bacterial cell wall synthesis much as the penicillins do and are thus usually bactericidal. A residual antibacterial effect is also evident with the cephalosporins.
Bacterial resistance may occur for one of three reasons:
1. Intrinsic resistance, for example, *Pseudomonas aeruginosa* is resistant to all first- and second-generation cephalosporins.
2. Beta-lactamase resistance, either plasmid or chromosomally mediated.

3. Cleavage of 3-acetyl group found in some cephalosporins.
Cephalosporins as a group tend to be most stable at a pH between 6 and 7.

ANTIMICROBIAL SPECTRUM

Cephalosporins are generally effective against most gram-positive aerobic cocci and several gram-negative organisms, including *Escherichia coli, Proteus mirabilis, Klebsiella, Salmonella, Shigella, Enterobacter,* and other *Proteus* organisms. All strains of *Pseudomonas* are resistant.
The newer cephalosporins possess a broader spectrum, being effective against many gram-negative pathogens as well as *Pseudomonas aeruginosa* and *Bacteriodes fragilis* isolates. They are often beta-lactamase–resistant.
Although cephalosporins and cephamycins are generally resistant to penicillinase produced by *Staphylococcus aureus,* some beta-lactamase enzymes (cephalosporinases) inactivate either cephalosporins alone or both cephalosporins and penicillins (cross-resistance).

KINETIC FATE

Absorption. Only a few cephalosporins are acid stable and thus may be administered orally (cephalexin, cephradine, cefadroxil, and cefachlor). The others are administered either intravenously or intramuscularly, with peak plasma concentrations occurring about 30 minutes following injection.
Distribution. Cephalosporins are widely distributed throughout most body fluids and tissues, including kidneys, lungs, joints, bone, soft tissues, and the biliary tract. However, poor penetration into the CSF, even in the presence of inflammation, is a notable feature of the standard cephalosporins. The degree of plasma protein-binding is variable.
Biotransformation. Several cephalosporins (cephalothin, cephapirin, cephacetrile, and cefotaxime) are desacetylated, primarily in the liver. Few of the other cephalosporins are metabolized to any appreciable extent.
Excretion. Most cephalosporins are excreted by renal tubular secretion although glomerular filtration is important for some agents (cephaloridine, cephalexin, and cefazolin). Biliary elimination may be significant in the excretion of the newer cephalosporins. These beta-lactam antibiotics are generally short-acting drugs that may maintain effective blood levels for 6 to 8 hours. Their plasma half-lives are often in the range of 30 to 90 minutes, but there are exceptions.

SIDE EFFECTS AND TOXICITY

The cephalosporins are relatively nontoxic, although cephaloridine may be nephrotoxic in some species.
Hypersensitivity reactions of several forms may occur, particularly in animals with a history of penicillin allergy.
Superinfection may arise with the use of cephalosporins, and *Pseudomonas* is a likely opportunistic pathogen.

POTENTIAL DRUG IINTERACTIONS

In vitro incompatibilities are quite common for cephalosporin and cephamycin preparations.
Potential pharmacokinetic interactions are similar to those of the penicillin group.
Aminoglycosides may enhance cephaloridine nephrotoxicity, but there is some doubt about this particular

---

*Withdrawal times will depend upon the regulations in the practitioner's country. The times listed here are general guidelines only.

interaction. Furosemide, however, does appear to potentiate the nephrotoxicity of cephaloridine.

SPECIFIC PREPARATIONS (CURRENTLY USED)

Although the cephalosporins are being used with increasing frequency in veterinary medicine, only one intramammary preparation has been approved for use in food animals in the United States.

Cephapirin

SPECTRUM. Broad, including penicillinase-producing *Staphylococcus aureus*.

ROUTE. Intramammary infusion.

DOSAGE. 200 mg/quarter. Repeat once in 12 hours.

MILK DISCARD TIME. 96 hours after last treatment.*

NEWER CEPHALOSPORINS AND CEPHAMYCINS

Cefamandole, Cefoxitin, Cefuroxime, Ceforanide. Second-generation cephalosporins and a cephamycin. Broad-spectrum antibiotics moderately resistant to beta-lactamase.

Ceftriaxone, Cefoperazone, Cefmenoxime, Cefsulodin, Cefotaxime, and Moxalactam. Third-generation group. Moderately active against gram-positive organisms, very active against gram-negative bacteria, and highly resistant to beta-lactamase.

Aminocyclitols (Aminoglycosides)

The aminoglycoside-aminocyclitol antibiotics are compounds with a broad spectrum of activity against many bacterial species, although their clinical use should be restricted to gram-negative bacterial infections when possible. The naturally occurring as well as semisynthetic aminoglycosides are all chemically very similar. Spectinomycin is not an aminoglycoside and is discussed separately.

GENERAL PROPERTIES

The aminoglycosides are bases, containing aminosugars, that have high aqueous solubilities and low lipid solubilities. The group characteristically is chemically and heat stable within reasonable limits. Modification of substituents on each basic ring structure accounts for the differences in antimicrobial spectrum, patterns of resistance, and toxicity seen with different aminoglycosides.

ANTIMICROBIAL FEATURES

Aminoglycosides are actively transported across the cytoplasmic membrane and then bind to ribosomes in susceptible bacteria. Because the impairment of protein synthesis that results is usually lethal, this class of antibiotics is considered to be bactericidal, although at lower concentrations bacteriostatic effects may be evident. Rapidly multiplying bacteria are more sensitive than static organisms, and no residual effect is evident with the aminoglycosides.

Bacterial resistance to aminoglycosides may take a number of forms:

1. Ribosomal binding mutants—alteration of binding site for aminoglycosides. Occurs in a single step for streptomycin.

2. Aminoglycoside-modifying enzymes—three classes of enzymes involved, mostly plasmid-mediated. Chemical

*Milk discard time will depend upon the regulations in the practitioner's country. The times listed are general guidelines only.

alteration in drug structure may render a compound relatively stable to enzymatic attack; e.g., kanamycin modified to amikacin is relatively resistant to inactivating enzymes.

3. Mutants defective in drug accumulation because of metabolic or structural defects. The failure of uptake in anaerobic and facultative organisms grown anaerobically may be explained on this basis.

4. Cross-resistance is common among this group of antibiotics.

The aminoglycosides are much more active in an alkaline environment (MIC's often 20- to 80-fold greater at a pH of 6 than at a pH of 8). The beta-lactam antibiotics and aminoglycosides often act synergistically when used in combination.

ANTIBACTERIAL SPECTRUM

Streptomycin and dihydrostreptomycin possess a relative narrow spectrum, and bacterial resistance to streptomycin is becoming very prevalent. Many gram-negative bacilli and some Staphylococci are still susceptible.

Neomycin, framycetin (neomycin B), and kanamycin possess a much broader spectrum, but their clinical use is mainly directed against gram-negative organisms such as *Escherichia coli, Klebsiella, Salmonella, Enterobacter,* and *Proteus.*

Gentamicin, tobramycin, amikacin, sisomicin, and netilmicin as a group have somewhat extended spectra compared with those above. They are often effective against *Pseudomonas.*

Resistance and cross-resistance emerge with continuous use of aminoglycosides, and susceptibility patterns change with the passage of time.

Anaerobic bacteria are not appreciably affected by aminoglycoside antibiotics.

KINETIC FATE

Absorption. The aminoglycosides are poorly absorbed from the gastrointestinal tract; usually less than 10 per cent of an orally administered dose is absorbed. However, severe enteritis may permit greater absorption. Absorption from intramuscular or subcutaneous sites is rapid, achieving significant blood levels within 60 minutes. Intravenous administration is potentially hazardous and should be carried out with caution by slow infusion.

Distribution. The distribution of aminoglycosides is primarily extracellular, with little penetration of any tissue except the renal cortex, where they accumulate in the proximal renal tubular epithelial cells. They are not appreciably bound to plasma proteins in most cases. Generally speaking, the aminoglycosides do attain therapeutic concentrations in synovial, pleural, and even peritoneal fluid, particularly if inflammation is present. Therapeutic levels are not attained in cerebrospinal fluid, tracheobronchial secretions, ocular fluids or fetal tissue in most species.

Biotransformation. The aminoglycoside antibiotics are not metabolized in the body and are excreted unchanged.

Excretion. Renal elimination by glomerular filtration, with close to 100 per cent of administered drug ultimately recovered in the urine, is the excretory pathway for all aminoglycosides. The accumulation in the renal tubular epithelial cells results in prolonged low tissue levels—for up to 90 days in the case of neomycin. All the aminoglycosides have relatively short plasma half-lives of 1 to 2½ hours, and administration 2 or 3 times a day is often required to maintain effective inhibitory concentrations at sites of infection. Doses should be reduced in patients with renal impairment and in neonates.

SIDE EFFECTS AND TOXICITY

Nephrotoxicity is of major concern when use is made of the aminoglycosides and is most frequently manifested as a nonoliguric renal failure with proteinuria and urinary sediment changes consistent with tubular injury. The occurrence is related to both dose and duration of treatment, being infrequently observed in less than 7 days. Several factors predispose to aminoglycoside nephrotoxicosis. These include prior renal insufficiency, dehydration and hypovolemia, metabolic acidosis, exposure to other nephrotoxins, concurrent furosemide administration, and severe sepsis or endotoxemia.

Ototoxicity due to vestibular and cochlear impairment can occur with all aminoglycosides but is rarely encountered in food animals.

Aminoglycosides in doses producing high plasma levels have been associated with respiratory arrest attributable to neuromuscular blockade. Calcium will antagonize this effect, as will an anticholinesterase agent such as neostigmine.

Superinfection may occur following oral or topical use.

Neomycin appears to be capable of producing a malabsorption syndrome in susceptible animals.

Hypersensitivity reactions are uncommon but may be seen with constant topical contact.

POTENTIAL DRUG INTERACTIONS

Enhanced nephrotoxicity may become evident with concurrent administration of aminoglycosides and other potentially nephrotoxic agents.

An increased tendency to neuromuscular blockade is evident when neuromuscular blocking agents are administered at the same time as an aminoglycoside.

Aminoglycoside ototoxicity is enhanced by the simultaneous administration of furosemide.

High concentrations of carbenicillin have been shown to inactivate aminoglycosides *in vitro* and even *in vivo* in the presence of renal failure.

SPECIFIC PREPARATIONS (CURRENTLY USED)

Neomycin
SPECTRUM. Broad.
ROUTE. Oral administration, intramammary infusion, and intrauterine use.
DOSAGE. PO 10–20 mg/kg every 12 hours (general guideline only).
WITHDRAWAL TIMES. Cattle, orally, 30 days; swine and sheep, 20 days.*

Streptomycin and Dihydrostreptomycin
SPECTRUM. Limited; resistance common.
ROUTE. Intramuscular injection, oral administration, intramammary infusion.
DOSAGE. IM 10 mg/kg every 12 hours; PO 20 mg/kg every 8 to 12 hours.

---

*Withdrawal times will depend upon the regulations in the practitioner's country. The times listed here are general guidelines only.

NEW AMINOGLYCOSIDES

Amikacin. Broad spectrum; less cross resistance.
Netilmicin. Broad spectrum; effective against many aminoglycoside-resistant organisms; less toxic.
Sisomicin. Very similar to gentamicin.

Spectinomycin

Spectinomycin is an aminocyclitol antibiotic, but its structure differs from that of the aminoglycosides.

ANTIMICROBIAL FEATURES

Spectinomycin binds to bacterial ribosomes and thus interferes with protein synthesis, but the effect is bacteriostatic rather than bactericidal. Spectinomycin can be inactivated by an enzyme coded for by an R factor, but mutant resistance due to diminished ribosomal binding is perhaps more common.

ANTIBACTERIAL SPECTRUM

Spectinomycin is active against several strains of Streptococci and a wide range of gram-negative bacteria. It is also active against *Mycoplasma* spp., but most *Chlamydia* are resistant.

KINETIC FATE

Absorption. Spectinomycin is poorly absorbed from the gastrointestinal tract but is rapidly absorbed after intramuscular administration, with peak blood levels occurring within 1 hour.
Distribution. Spectinomycin penetrates tissues rather poorly, and its distribution is principally extracellular.
Biotransformation. Metabolic transformation of spectinomycin is very limited, and 80 per cent of an administered dose can be recovered unchanged in the urine over 24 to 48 hours.
Excretion. About 75 per cent of spectinomycin is eliminated by glomerular filtration in about 4 hours.

SIDE EFFECTS AND TOXICITY

At usual doses, no major toxic reactions to spectinomycin have been reported.

SPECIFIC PREPARATION (CURRENTLY USED)

Spectinomycin
SPECTRUM. Broad, including *Mycoplasma* spp.
ROUTE. Intramuscular and oral administration.
DOSAGE. IM 5–10 mg/kg every 12 hours; PO 20 mg/kg every 12 hours.
WITHDRAWAL TIME. Swine, 21 days.*

Tetracyclines

The tetracyclines are a group of broad-spectrum antibiotics, some of which occur naturally (oxytetracycline, chlortetracycline, and demethylchlortetracycline) and several of which are derived semisynthetically (tetracycline, methacycline, minocycline, and doxycycline).

GENERAL PROPERTIES

All tetracycline derivatives are crystalline, yellowish, amphoteric substances that in aqueous solution form salts with both acids and bases. Most are available in acidic solutions as hydrochlorides. Tetracyclines are stable as dry powders, but at higher temperatures they rapidly lose activity. Aqueous solutions are unstable, especially at an alkaline pH. Propylene glycol is commonly used as a vehicle for parenteral preparations, and pyrrolidone polymers, such as povidone, are also employed as dispersing and suspending agents for aqueous solutions intended for injection.

The tetracyclines typically chelate divalent and trivalent cations, such as calcium, magnesium, iron, and aluminum, to form insoluble complexes. Substitutions on the tetracycline nucleus produce some differences in kinetic characteristics among the members of this group and somewhat better penetration of bacteria such as *Staphylococcus aureus* by the more lipid-soluble tetracyclines. Overall, though, the tetracyclines are about equally active.

ANTIMICROBIAL FEATURES

Tetracyclines reversibly bind to subunits of bacterial ribosomes and so interfere with protein synthesis. They also affect the cytoplasmic membrane, which may leak cell contents. In high doses, tetracyclines tend to be bactericidal, but usually they exert only a bacteriostatic action.

This group of antibiotics enters bacterial cells by passive diffusion as well as by a specialized transport process. Mammalian cells are also sensitive to the action of tetracyclines, but very much lower intracellular concentrations are achieved than in susceptible bacteria. The tetracyclines are most effective against actively multiplying microorganisms, and adequate host defense is often essential for their successful clinical use.

Resistance develops predominantly because the bacterial cell becomes less permeable to the antibiotic. Two forms are recognized:

1. Intrinsic resistance—mutant strains do not possess the transport mechanism.

2. Plasmid-mediated resistance—can be transmitted either by transduction (e.g., *Staphylococcus aureus*) or by conjugation (many gram-negative bacteria). Resistance develops slowly in a multistep fashion but is widespread today because of the extensive use of the tetracyclines, particularly in animal feeds. R factors generally carry multiple resistances, e.g., to aminoglycosides, chloramphenicol, sulfonamides, and penicillins.

There is usually cross-resistance between tetracyclines. As a group, these agents tend to be more effective at a pH of about 6.5.

ANTIBACTERIAL SPECTRA

The tetracyclines are typically very-broad-spectrum drugs. The spectra comprise gram-positive and gram-negative bacteria, including some anaerobes, *Rickettsia, Chlamydia, Mycoplasma, Actinomyces,* spirochetes, *Anaplasma,* and even some protozoa. *Pseudomonas aeruginosa, Serratia,* and many *Proteus* strains are frequently naturally resistant. Doxycycline and minocycline tend to be more effective against *Staphylococcus aureus.*

KINETIC FATE

Absorption. Orally administered tetracyclines are absorbed somewhat irregularly from the upper small intestine. Chlortetracycline is not well absorbed (about 35 per cent), compared with oxytetracycline and tetracycline (60 to 80 per cent) and minocycline and doxycycline (90 to 100 per cent). Effective blood levels are reached in 2 to 4 hours. Several factors influence absorption, including milk, food, calcium, magnesium, aluminum, iron and sodium bicarbonate. The tetracyclines may be administered orally to swine and young preruminant herbivores. Once ruminal fermentation is established, tetracyclines at therapeutic levels will suppress cellulolytic and other microfloral functions, although in time some adaptation may take place. Specially buffered tetracycline solutions can be administered intramuscularly and intravenously. Through pharmaceutical manipulation, the absorption of oxytetracycline from intramuscular sites may be substantially delayed and thus produce a long-acting effect. The tetracyclines are irritant substances, and necrosis at the site of injection occurs and takes some time to heal. Residues at the injection site may persist for up to 3 weeks. Absorption of tetracyclines also takes place from the uterus and udder.

Distribution. The tetracyclines distribute quite extensively throughout the body, with the highest concentrations found in the kidneys, liver, bile, spleen, and lungs. Lower levels occur in serosal fluids, synovial fluids, CSF, and vitreous humor. Because of their propensity to bind calcium ions, these antibiotics tend to be deposited irreversibly in growing bones and teeth of young animals (and even in the fetus). Doxycycline and minocycline penetrate cells very readily owing to their lipid solubility. Tetracyclines are bound to plasma proteins to a greater or lesser degree (25 to 80 per cent).

Biotransformation. Metabolic degradation is limited for most tetracyclines but may be extensive for some members of the group (up to 40 per cent for doxycycline).

Excretion. The majority of the tetracyclines are excreted by glomerular filtration, although biliary elimination and enterohepatic cycling are also involved. The feces is always a significant excretory route (often about 10 per cent of a dose), even when these antibiotics are injected parenterally. Intestinal elimination is the major process in the case of doxycycline. The tetracyclines are also eliminated in milk, attaining about 50 per cent of the plasma concentration in most instances but the levels are higher in mastitic milk. Peak concentrations occur in milk 6 hours after a parenteral dose, but traces may be found even 48 hours following drug administration. The plasma half-lives of the tetracyclines in adult cattle vary from about 6 to 12 hours, and once-daily injections are usually sufficient to maintain effective inhibitory concentrations at the sites of infection when standard dosage rates are employed. A long-acting formulation of oxytetracycline, if injected intramuscularly, provides plasma concentrations above 0.5 µg/ml for approximately 72 hours. The elimination of tetracyclines is prolonged in the very young (less than a month old) calf and in the presence of acute disease processes, especially when renal function is impaired (doxycycline being an exception in this case).

SIDE EFFECTS AND TOXICITY

High doses of tetracyclines administered orally will depress ruminal microfloral activity and produce ruminoreticular stasis.

In monogastric animals (swine and young ruminants), gastrointestinal disturbances may result from superinfection due to non-susceptible microbial species (fungi, yeasts, and bacteria such as resistant Staphylococci).

Intravenous administration of undiluted propylene glycol–based preparations leads to intravascular hemolysis and subsequent hemoglobinuria.

The rapid intravenous injection of a tetracycline may produce sudden collapse due to acute hypotension. This depression of cardiovascular function appears to be related to the ability of the tetracyclines to chelate ionized calcium, though reaction to the carrier may also be involved. This reaction can be avoided by giving the injection slowly (longer than 5 minutes) or by pretreatment with calcium gluconate intravenously.

Tetracyclines chelate calcium in teeth and bones and thereby become incorporated into these structures, inhibiting calcification and staining them yellow. In extreme cases the healing of bone is impaired.

This group of antibiotics is anti-anabolic by virtue of their ability to interfere with protein synthesis. Azotemia may be aggravated by the tetracyclines. The combined use of a tetracycline with a glucocorticosteroid can lead to pronounced weight loss.

Hepatosis due to fatty infiltration of the liver, particularly during pregnancy, has been described in some species.

Reactions, necrosis, and yellow staining at injection sites are frequently seen.

The administration of outdated tetracycline products may lead to acute renal tubular nephrosis. Excessive doses of oxytetracycline also produce nephrotoxicity.

Hypersensitivity reactions have been observed but are not common.

POTENTIAL DRUG INTERACTIONS

The absorption of tetracyclines from the gastrointestinal tract is impaired by milk and milk products, antacids, kaolin, and iron preparations.

Tetracyclines gradually lose activity when diluted in infusion fluids.

The possibility of chelation with divalent or trivalent cations should always be borne in mind when tetracyclines are mixed with any other medications.

SPECIFIC PREPARATIONS (CURRENTLY USED)

Oxytetracycline
SPECTRUM. Broad.
ROUTE. Oral and parenteral administration, intrauterine infusion.
DOSAGE. IM 5–10 mg/kg every 24 hours (or 20 mg/kg every 48–72 hours if depot form); IV 2.5–5 mg/kg every 24 hours; PO 10–20 mg/kg every 12 hours.
WITHDRAWAL TIMES. Cattle, 18 days; swine, 18 days. (Long-acting oxytetracycline, 28 days.)*
Chloretetracycline
SPECTRUM. Broad.
ROUTE. Oral.
DOSAGE. PO 5–10 mg/kg every 12 hours.
WITHDRAWAL TIMES. Cattle, 10 days; swine, 1–7 days (depends on form).*

NEW TETRACYCLINES

Doxycycline. Longer plasma half-life; excellent tissue penetration; greater activity against most bacteria.
Minocycline. As for doxycycline but more active, even against tetracycline-resistant Staphylococci.

*Withdrawal times will depend upon the regulations in the practitioner's country. The times listed here are general guidelines only.

Macrolides

The macrolides are a large group of structurally related antibiotics, but only a few have been found to be clinically useful, namely erythromycin, spiramycin, oleandomycin, leucomycin, and tylosin. Their antibacterial spectra and pharmacokinetic fates are generally similar.

GENERAL PROPERTIES

The macrolides are weak bases that have low aqueous solubility but are soluble in organic solvents. The group is unstable in both alkaline and acidic environments. Erythromycin is even inactivated at pH 4. Macrolides can undergo a large number of chemical reactions, and more stable ester forms are commonly used in pharmaceutical preparations—acetylates, estolates, succinates, and stearates being examples.

ANTIMICROBIAL FEATURES

Macrolides interfere with protein synthesis in bacteria at the ribosomal level, where they bind and block transpeptidation and translocation reactions. The effect is essentially confined to rapidly dividing cells. Though commonly regarded as being bacteriostatic, macrolides at higher concentrations may be bactericidal, especially against gram-positive organisms.

Bacterial resistance to macrolides can occur by the following mechanisms:
1. Inability to penetrate microbe (gram-negative organisms).
2. Alteration of the receptor site on the ribosome (gram-positive organisms). This form of resistance may develop quite rapidly, particularly for erythromycin.
3. Cross-resistance between macrolides is well recognized.

These weak bases are significantly more active at an alkaline (pH 8.0) than at neutral or acidic pH levels. Macrolides (erythromycin), lincosamides (clindamycin), and chloramphenicol may compete for the same site on the ribosome and thus may impair one another's antibacterial actions.

ANTIBACTERIAL SPECTRUM

The macrolides' spectrum of activity is essentially against gram-positive organisms (Streptococci, Staphylococci, *Corynebacterium*, *Clostridium*, *Listeria monocytogenes*, etc.).

Some strains of gram-negative bacteria may be sensitive (*Haemophilus*, *Neisseria*, and *Pasteurella*).

Mycoplasma, *Chlamydia*, *Rickettsia*, and *Actinomycetes* may be susceptible.

KINETIC FATE

Absorption. Members of this group of antibiotics are often well absorbed following oral administration, but gastric acid and the particular ester or salt used may modify intestinal availability of the drug. Peak plasma levels occur within an hour in most instances. Absorption from the ruminoreticulum can be delayed and is unreliable. Erythromycin and tylosin are also administered intramuscularly to food animals. However, pain and swelling may occur at the injection site.

Distribution. The macrolides diffuse well into tissues and body fluids but do not readily cross the intact blood-brain barrier. Relatively low serum concentrations at usual dosage rates reflect a substantial distribution to the peripheral compartments. High concentrations of these antibiotics generally occur in lung, liver, kidney, spleen, and reproductive tract, with quite low levels in skeletal muscle. The degree of plasma protein binding of macrolides is usually between 20 and 40 per cent.

Biotransformation. Metabolic inactivation of the macrolides is often extensive, but the relative proportion depends on the route of administration and the particular macrolide. With oral administration, about 80 per cent of an erythromycin dose undergoes metabolic inactivation, whereas tylosin appears to be eliminated in an active form.

Excretion. Macrolide antibiotics and their metabolites are excreted mainly in bile, with enterohepatic cycling being a common component of the biliary elimination process. Urinary clearance is often slow and variable. Milk, though a minor route of excretion (up to 4 per cent), often has macrolide concentrations several-fold greater than plasma, especially in the presence of mastitis. In cattle, the plasma half-life of erythromycin has been shown to be about 3 hours and that of tylosin about 1.8 hours. Effective inhibitory concentrations are maintained for about 8 hours following oral administration and for about 12 to 24 hours following intramuscular injection.

SIDE EFFECTS AND TOXICITY

Side effects and toxicity due to macrolide antibiotics are uncommon in food animals.

Gastrointestinal disturbances may occur, and rectal edema with partial anal prolapse has been observed in swine.

Allergic reactions may occasionally occur, and severe shock reactions may result from overdosage in baby pigs.

Pain and tissue irritation are associated with intramuscular injections.

POTENTIAL DRUG INTERACTIONS

Macrolides should not be used concurrently with chloramphenicol or lincosamides.

Acidic solutions will depress the activity of macrolides, whereas alkalinization will enhance their effects.

Erythromycin and tylosin are incompatible with many pharmaceutical preparations, including hydrocortisone, streptomycin, tetracyclines, and sulfonamides.

SPECIFIC PREPARATIONS (CURRENTLY USED)

Erythromycin
SPECTRUM. Gram-positive organisms and *Mycoplasma*.
ROUTE. Parenteral administration, intramammary infusion.
DOSAGE. IM 4–8 mg/kg every 12–24 hours.
WITHDRAWAL TIME. Cattle, 14 days.*
MILK DISCARD TIME. 72 hours.*

Tylosin
SPECTRUM. Gram-positive organisms, a few gram-negative strains, and *Mycoplasma*.
ROUTE. Oral and parenteral administration.
DOSAGE. IM 4–10 mg/kg every 24 hours; PO 10 mg/kg every 8 hours.
WITHDRAWAL TIMES. Cattle, 21 days; swine, 14 days.*

---

*Withdrawal and milk discard times will depend upon the regulations in the practitioner's country. The times listed here are general guidelines only.

NEW MACROLIDES

Spiramycin. Has been used in Europe for many years against *Mycoplasma* infections and *Treponema hyodysenteriae* in swine.

Rosamicin. Spectrum similar to that of erythromycin but more effective against some gram-positive organisms.

Miscellaneous Antibiotics

A number of additional antibiotics are employed in food-producing animals in various parts of the world. A selection of these agents are reviewed in a synoptic manner.

Lincosamides (Lincomycin and Clindamycin)

Lincomycin has been employed in swine and cattle for systemic infections. This antibiotic is primarily bacteriostatic (inhibits protein synthesis) and possesses an antimicrobial spectrum that includes only gram-positive organisms, several anaerobes, and some *Mycoplasma* species. Resistance to lincomycin develops gradually, but a characteristic cross-resistance with the macrolides has been identified. Lincomycin is rapidly but not completely absorbed following oral administration but is well absorbed from intramuscular injection sites. Plasma protein–binding is very low, and diffusion into tissues takes place readily. Effective concentrations occur in most tissues and fluids, including bone. The CSF is an exception to this pattern in the absence of meningitis. Biotransformation of lincomycin seems to be very limited, and the unchanged antibiotic is excreted in bile, urine, and milk. Lincomycin is generally administered orally every 12 hours and intramuscularly every 24 hours. Side effects are rare, though a transient diarrhea may be observed. A 2-day withdrawal time has been set for swine.

Polymyxins (Polymyxin B, Polymyxin E or Colistin, and Colistimethate)

Polymyxins have been used for the treatment of enteritis in young calves and pigs and of bovine mastitis as well as for preputial irrigation in bulls. This class of polypeptide antibiotic is somewhat toxic and is rarely employed systemically. Polymyxins are bactericidal owing to their ability to disrupt bacterial cell membranes, but their antibacterial spectrum consists of only gram-negative bacilli, including most isolates of *Pseudomonas*. They may also inactivate endotoxins *in vivo*. Polymyxins are synergistic against gram-negative bacteria when combined with potentiated sulfonamides or oxytetracycline. The development of resistance to the polymyxins is uncommon. These polypeptides are not absorbed following oral administration. Parenteral administration produces peak plasma levels in about 2 hours. Blood and interstitial levels are usually low, because polymyxins bind to cell membranes as well as cell debris and purulent exudates. Very low concentrations are attained in transcellular fluids. Excretion is primarily renal. Plasma half-lives for polymyxins range from 3 to 6 hours but will be longer in the presence of renal insufficiency. Dosage rates for the polymyxins vary, and the following are only guidelines: IM 5,000 units/kg every 12 hours; PO 20,000 units/kg every 12 hours; intramammary 50,000–100,000 units per quarter; intrauterine 100,000 units. The polymyxins are notably nephrotoxic and neurotoxic. Neuromuscular blockade has been reported. Intense local pain on injection is common.

Chloramphenicol

The use of chloramphenicol in food-producing animals is no longer permitted in the United States. Chloramphenicol is a broad-spectrum antibiotic that inhibits ribosomal protein synthesis and is usually bacteriostatic but may be bactericidal against some organisms. Its antimicrobial spectrum includes the majority of gram-positive and gram-negative organisms, several anaerobes, *Rickettsia,* and *Chlamydia* species. Of particular note is this agent's efficacy against *Salmonella.* Bacterial resistance to chloramphenicol may be due to an occasional resistant mutant that emerges relatively slowly in a population but more commonly is due to R factor–mediated resistance. These plasmids often carry multiple drug resistance (chloramphenicol, tetracycline, streptomycin, erythromycin, ampicillin, and others). Chloramphenicol may be given parenterally or orally. The water-soluble sodium salt of the succinate ester can be administered intramuscularly but may not be as effective when administered by this route. Chloramphenicol is rapidly absorbed after oral dosage in nonruminants, with peak plasma concentrations being recorded in 1 to 2 hours. It is rapidly distributed into all tissues and body fluids, and inhibitory concentrations are present in most instances. The majority of chloramphenicol (80 to 90 per cent) is eliminated in the urine as an inactive form following hepatic biotransformation. However, an enterohepatic cycle may also be present. The plasma half-life of chloramphenicol in cattle is about 2 hours and is even less in swine (1.3 hours), so administration is required 2 or 3 times a day. Withdrawal times in those countries where the use of chloramphenicol is allowed vary considerably and are as long as 14 days. Chloramphenicol is a potentially toxic antibiotic that produces a dose-dependent, reversible depression of bone marrow function as well as a dose-independent, irreversible form of blood dyscrasia, which is seen in humans. It is principally this toxic effect that has led to the elimination of chloramphenicol's use in food animals. This antibiotic inhibits microsomal enzyme function and is potentially immunosuppressive with respect to the anamnestic response. Chloramphenicol is inactivated by ruminal microflora.

Novobiocin

Novobiocin is a narrow-spectrum antibiotic with a bacteriostatic action against gram-positive organisms. Its principal use in food animal medicine is for the intramammary treatment of bovine mastitis.

Tiamulin

Tiamulin is a medium-spectrum antibiotic with activity against gram-positive bacteria and mycoplasmas. It has been used with success against mycoplasmal infections in cattle and swine as well as for the treatment of *Treponema hyodysenteriae* infection in swine.

Bacitracin

Bacitracin is a narrow-spectrum peptide antibiotic active against a range of bacteria similar to those affected by penicillin G. Its main use in food animals has been as a feed additive.

Rifamycins

Rifamycins are extended-spectrum antibiotics, two members of which (rifampin and rifanide) have enjoyed some clinical use in veterinary medicine. Susceptible organisms include gram-positive bacteria, a limited number of gram-negative bacteria, some anaerobes, *Chlamydia* species, and *Mycobacterium.* The rifamycins are bactericidal, but resistance develops readily. Because rifamycins penetrate tissues and cells to a substantial degree, they are particularly effective against susceptible intracellular pathogens.

Synthetic Antibacterial Agents

Several classes of antibacterial agent are not naturally occurring antibiotics but are produced synthetically. Of these, the sulfonamides, potentiated sulfonamides, and nitrofurans are discussed here.

Sulfonamides

A large number of sulfonamides have been synthesized since their discovery, but only a handful are of therapeutic importance in food animal medicine. Although there are some differences among various sulfonamides with respect to kinetic fate and toxicity, the group will be reviewed from a generic perspective.

GENERAL PROPERTIES

Sulfonamides are more soluble in an alkaline than in acidic pH and are usually prepared as sodium salts for intravenous administration. Such solutions are highly alkaline, are not very stable, and precipitate out with the addition of polyionic electrolytes. In a mixture of sulfonamides, each component drug exhibits its own solubility; therefore, a combination of sulfonamides is more soluble than one drug used alone. This is the basis of "triple" sulfonamide mixtures. Certain sulfonamides are designed for low solubility so that they will remain in the lumen of the intestine for an extended period. These are the "gut-active" sulfonamides such as pthalylsulfathiazole and succinylsulfathiazole.

ANTIMICROBIAL FEATURES

The sulfonamides are structural analogs of para-aminobenzoic acid (PABA) and competitively inhibit the enzymatic step in the synthesis of folic acid during which PABA is utilized. This inhibition impairs metabolic processes in susceptible bacteria, stopping growth and multiplication in those organisms that cannot utilize preformed folate. The effect is bacteriostatic, though a bactericidal action may be evident at the high concentrations that occur in urine.

Owing to their basic mode of action, sulfonamides are effective against growing and proliferating but not against dormant microorganisms. Growth can also resume when the sulfonamide is displaced by an excess of PABA or when drug concentrations become too low to affect the enzyme. Thus, adequate cellular and humoral defense mechanisms are critical for successful sulfonamide therapy.

Only after a latency period of a few hours do sulfonamides affect bacteria, and their chemotherapeutic action directly depends on their concentration at the site of infection.

Although all of the sulfonamides possess the same mechanism of action, differences are evident with respect to activity, pharmacokinetic fate, and even spectrum of activity at usual dosage rates. These differences are due to the variety of physiochemical characteristics seen among sulfonamides.

Bacterial resistance to sulfonamides generally emerges gradually but does become limiting with the promiscuous use or misuse of sulfonamides. Several forms of resistance are recognized:

1. Intrinsic resistance—inability of bacteria to synthesize their own folate.

2. Mutant resistance—bacterial strains produce an excess of PABA or have a reduced enzyme affinity of sulfonamides because of a structural difference.

3. Plasmid-mediated resistance—R factor resistance that may become widely disseminated.

4. Cross-resistance—very prevalent between the sulfonamides.

Blood concentrations between 5 and 15 mg/dl are regarded as being safe and efficacious.

ANTIBACTERIAL SPECTRA

Sulfonamides can inhibit both gram-positive and gram-negative bacteria, a few *Rickettsia, Nocardia, Actinomyces,* and some protozoa, such as Coccidia and *Toxoplasma.* The more active sulfonamides may include Streptococci, Staphylococci, *Escherichia coli, Salmonella,* and *Pasteurella* in their spectra.

Exceptional sulfonamides possess some activity against *Pseudomonas, Proteus,* and *Clostridium* species.

KINETIC FATE

Absorption. Sulfonamides are as a rule administered orally or intravenously to food animals. Other parenteral routes have been employed, but most sulfonamide solutions are strongly alkaline and therefore tissue-irritant. Sulfamethazine sodium and specifically buffered sulfonamide solutions are exceptions to this generalization. Oral absorption rates depend on age, the species involved, the relative solubility of the sulfonamide used, gastrointestinal content, the disease process, the degree of dehydration, and several other compounding factors. Sulfonamides may be either rapidly absorbed, with peak plasma levels occurring within 1 to 2 hours, or barely absorbed, as in the case of the "gut-active" group. Absorption occurs quite readily in pigs, young calves, and lambs but is delayed in adult cattle and sheep. Ruminal stasis prolongs absorption even further. Slow-release bolus forms of several sulfonamides are used orally in cattle to prolong blood levels. Absorption also takes place from the uterus and from treated wounds.

Distribution. Following absorption, most sulfonamides become widely distributed to tissues and body fluids (even the CSF in some instances). A distribution quotient (DQ), i.e., the relationship between tissue and serum concentration, is typical for each sulfonamide, and plasma concentrations usually reflect tissue levels. The DQ is generally below 1 in tissues and fluids, but high sulfonamide levels are usually encountered in kidney, liver, and lung, and somewhat lower levels in bone and muscle. Sulfonamides become bound to plasma proteins to an extent varying from 20 to over 90 per cent. The degree of plasma protein–binding influences tissue concentrations (only the unbound fraction is free to diffuse into tissues) and the elimination rate (a high level of binding delays excretion). Several sulfonamides (e.g., sulfamethazine and sulfathiazole) diffuse into the intestinal lumen following parenteral administration.

Biotransformation. Sulfonamides generally undergo extensive metabolic transformation in the liver. The extent of biotransformation depends on water solubility. A few sulfonamides are excreted rapidly in an active form, whereas most are eliminated either unchanged or as inactive metabolic products, many of which are conjugates. Paradoxically, the acetylates of most sulfonamides are far less water-soluble than the parent compounds; this is not true for sulfadiazine, sulfamerazine, and sulfamethazine.

Excretion. The sulfonamides undergo biliary and urinary excretion and may also diffuse directly into intestinal content (feces) and milk. The kidneys are the major organ of elimination, with glomerular filtration, active tubular secretion, and tubular reabsorption the main processes involved. Urine pH, renal clearance, and the concentration as well as solubilities of the respective sulfonamides and their conjugates will determine whether solubilities are exceeded and crystal precipitation occurs. This event can be prevented by alkalinization of the urine, high fluid intake, reduction of dosage rates in the presence of renal insufficiency, and use of triple-sulfonamide combinations. The elimination half-lives of sulfonamides differ and should not be extrapolated between species; e.g., the half-life for sulfadiazine is 10.1 hours in cattle and 2.9 hours in swine. The recommended dosage rates and frequencies reflect this disparity in elimination kinetic patterns.

SIDE EFFECTS AND TOXICITY

Hypersensitivity reactions—skin rashes, urticaria, angioedema, anaphylaxis, and drug fever—have been reported.

Crystalluria, with hematuria and even tubular obstruction, can occur but is rare in food animals. Sulfonamides with long plasma half-lives and high intrinsic solubilities tend not to produce crystalluria, particularly if water intake is high and the urine is alkaline.

Acute toxic manifestations may be observed following too-rapid intravenous administration or an excessive dose of several sulfonamides. Clinical signs include muscle weakness, ataxia, blindness, and collapse.

Gastrointestinal disturbances may occur when sulfonamides attain sufficiently high levels in the gastrointestinal tract to disturb the normal microfloral balance.

Sulfonamides will depress normal cellulolytic function in the ruminoreticulum, but the effect (unless very high levels are present) is usually transient and adaptation occurs.

Several toxic effects have been recorded following prolonged courses of sulfonamides. Included among these are bone marrow depression, icterus, peripheral neuritis, and myelin degeneration in the spinal cord and peripheral nerves.

POTENTIAL DRUG INTERACTIONS

Sulfonamide solutions are incompatible with calcium-containing fluids and many other preparations.

Sulfonamides may displace concurrently administered drugs, such as the nonsteroidal anti-inflammatory drugs, from plasma protein-binding sites.

Alkalinizing agents and antacids tend to inhibit the gastrointestinal absorption of sulfonamides.

PRINCIPLES OF SULFONAMIDE THERAPY

Sulfonamides are much more effective when administered early in the course of a disease. Chronic infections, especially with large amounts of exudate or tissue debris, are often not responsive.

In severe infections, the initial dose should be administered intravenously to reduce the lag time between dose and effect to a minimum.

The initial dose should be greater than (often double) the subsequent regular maintenance doses.

It is important to monitor urine output and to ensure a ready source of drinking water. Concurrent administration of urinary alkalinizers will prevent crystalluria.

A course of treatment should not exceed 7 days under usual circumstances, but a beneficial response within 72 hours is a requirement for therapy to continue. The problem of sulfonamide resistance should always be borne in mind. Treatment should be continued for 48 hours after remission of clinical signs to prevent relapses.

It is imperative to appreciate that sulfonamides are bacteriostatic and that the adequacy of immunological and other defense mechanisms must be assisted (nutrition, supportive therapy) and never impeded (corticosteroids, starvation).

SOME SPECIFIC PREPARATIONS (CURRENTLY USED)

Sulfamethazine
ROUTE. Parenteral and oral administration.
DOSAGE. IV, IM, or IP 110–200 mg/kg (initial) and 100–110 mg/kg every 24 hours (maintenance).
WITHDRAWAL TIME. Cattle, 10 days or up to 28 days (slow-release boluses); swine, 14 days.*
MILK DISCARD TIME. 96 hours.*

Sulfabromethazine
ROUTE. Oral administration.
DOSAGE. PO 130–200 mg/kg every 48 hours (2 doses).
WITHDRAWAL TIME. Cattle, 10 days.*
MILK DISCARD TIME. 96 hours.*

Triple Sulfonamide Solution (8% sodium sulfamethazine, 8% sodium sulfapyridine, 8% sodium sulfathiazole)
ROUTE. Parenteral administration.
DOSAGE. IV 45 ml/50 kg (initial) and 15 ml/50 kg every 24 hours (maintenance).
WITHDRAWAL TIME. Cattle, 10 days.*
MILK DISCARD TIME. 96 hours.*

Sulfadimethoxine
ROUTE. Parenteral and oral administration.
DOSAGE. IV or PO 55 mg/kg (initial) and 27.5 mg/kg every 24 hours (maintenance).
WITHDRAWAL TIME. Cattle, 7 days.*
MILK DISCARD TIME. 60 hours.*

Pthalylsulfathiazole and Succinylsulfathiazole
ROUTE. Oral administration.
DOSAGE. PO 100–200 mg/kg every 8–12 hours.

Potentiated Sulfonamides

A fairly recent advance in chemotherapeutics has been the development of a group of benzylpyrimidines (trimethoprim, methoprim, pyrimethamine) that inhibit dihydrofolate reductase in bacteria and protozoa far more efficiently than in mammalian cells. As a single substance, trimethoprim has little effect against bacteria (rapid development of resistance), but combining it with sulfonamides such as sulfadiazine (cotrimazine), sulfadoxine (cotrimoxine), and sulfamethoxazole (cotrimoxazole) potentiates both components.

---

*Withdrawal and milk discard times will depend upon the regulations in the practitioner's country. The times listed here are general guidelines only.

GENERAL PROPERTIES

Trimethoprim is a basic drug (pKa 7.6) that tends to accumulate in more acidic environments—acidic urine, milk, ruminal fluid.

ANTIMICROBIAL FEATURES

In susceptible bacteria, the sulfonamide component blocks the synthesis of dihydrofolic acid (as discussed previously) and trimethoprim inhibits the next enzyme in the sequence (dihydrofolate reductase) to prevent the formation of tetrahydrofolic acid (folinic acid). Folinic acid is required for the synthesis of DNA. This sequential blockade produces a bactericidal rather than a bacteriostatic effect under usual conditions, but in the presence of thymidine, only bacteriostasis is evident because the block is circumvented.

Mammalian enzyme systems have a very much reduced affinity for trimethoprim.

The optimal ratio for the combination of sulfonamide and trimethoprim depends on the type of microorganism in question. However, the commercially available preparations employ a trimethoprim:sulfonamide ratio of 1:5.

Bacterial resistance to trimethoprim has been recognized, but resistance to the combinations has yet to be shown to be a problem. The presence of a sulfonamide appears to delay the emergence of bacterial resistance. Resistance may take two forms:

1. Mutant resistance—bacteria become dependent on exogenous folinic acid or thymine.
2. Plasmid-mediated resistance based on enzyme modification—has been described for trimethoprim but has not become widespread.

ANTIBACTERIAL SPECTRUM

The sulfonamide-trimethoprim combinations that are available are active against gram-negative and gram-positive organisms, including *Actinomyces, Bordetella, Clostridium, Corynebacterium, Escherichia coli, Fusobacterium* spp., *Haemophilus, Klebsiella, Pasteurella, Proteus, Salmonella, Shigella, Campylobacter,* and Streptococci and Staphylococci. Some streptococcal strains are only moderately sensitive, as are *Brucella, Erysipelothrix, Nocardia,* and *Moraxella*. The antibacterial spectrum does not include *Pseudomonas* or *Mycobacterium*.

KINETIC FATE (OF TRIMETHOPRIM)

Absorption. Trimethoprim is rapidly absorbed following oral administration (peak plasma levels in about 2–4 hours) except in ruminants, in which case trimethoprim tends to be trapped in the ruminoreticulum and even appears to undergo a degree of microbial degradation. Following parenteral administration, absorption occurs readily, effective antibacterial concentrations being reached within about an hour and peak levels in about 4 hours.

Distribution. Trimethoprim diffuses extensively into tissues and body fluids. Tissue concentrations are often higher than the corresponding plasma levels—especially in the lungs, liver, and kidney. About 30 to 60 per cent of trimethoprim is bound to plasma proteins.

Biotransformation. The extent of metabolic transformation of trimethoprim in food animals has not yet been established, although there is a suggestion that hepatic biotransformation may be very extensive in adult ruminants. This is not the case in most species, in which more than 50 per cent of a dose is often excreted unchanged.

Excretion. Trimethoprim is largely excreted in the urine by glomerular filtration and tubular secretion. A substantial amount may also be found in the feces. The concentration in milk is often 1 to 3.5 times higher than in plasma. The plasma half-life of trimethoprim is quite prolonged in most species; effective levels are maintained for over 12 hours, with the result that the frequency of administration is usually 12 to 24 hours. The elimination kinetic parameters are not yet available for cattle and sheep but seem to be much shorter than for monogastric species.

SIDE EFFECTS AND TOXICITY

Side effects of this combination are rare in large animals—up to 10 times the recommended dose has been given with impunity. However, the sulfonamide components do retain their intrinsic toxicity as discussed earlier.

Prolonged administration of trimethoprim at reasonably high levels leads to maturation defects in hematopoiesis. This occurrence has been described in foals.

SPECIFIC PREPARATIONS (NOT APPROVED FOR FOOD ANIMALS IN THE U.S.)

Trimethoprim-Sulfadiazine Formulations
ROUTE. Parenteral and oral administration.

DOSAGE. PO 15 mg/kg of combination every 12 hours or 30 mg/kg of combination every 24 hours; IV or IM 15–60 mg/kg every 24 hours (depending on severity of infection).

Nitrofurans

The nitrofuran derivatives (such as nitrofurazone, furazolidone, and nifuraldezone) are a group of relatively small antimicrobial drugs with activity principally against gram-negative bacteria, including *Salmonella,* though they are also often effective against some gram-positive organisms, fungi, and protozoa (coccidia). Many strains of *Proteus* and all strains of *Pseudomonas aeruginosa* are resistant. The mechanism of action is not entirely clear, but nitrofurans appear to inhibit bacterial carbohydrate metabolism and thereby to exert a bactericidal effect. The activity of nitrofurans is greatly enhanced in a more acidic environment. Resistant mutants are rare, and clinical resistance emerges slowly. There is no cross-resistance between nitrofurans and other antibacterial agents.

Nitrofurans are used only orally or topically. Nitrofurazone's main indications include the treatment of bovine mastitis, bovine metritis, and wounds (pus, blood, and milk reduce the antibacterial activity) and use as a feed additive to control enteric bacterial and coccidial infections. The withdrawal time of nitrofurazone in swine is 5 days. Furazolidone has been used to control enteric bacterial infections, principally by *Salmonella* but also other gram-negative pathogens, as well as coccidiosis. It is poorly absorbed from the intestinal tract, as are most of the nitrofurans except nitrofurantoin, which is not used in food animals. Nifuraldezone also has been employed to control bacterial enteritis in calves.

Toxic signs encountered with excessive doses of nitrofuran derivatives include CNS involvement (excitement, tremors, convulsions, peripheral neuritis), gastrointestinal irritation, poor weight gain, and depression of spermatogenesis. Hypersensitivity reactions have also been known to occur.

The oral dose of furazolidone in calves is generally 10–12 mg/kg every 12 hours.

Supplemental Reading

Booth, N. H., and McDonald, L. E. (eds.): Veterinary Pharmacology and Therapeutics, 5th ed. Ames, Iowa, Iowa State University Press, 1982.

Brander, G. C., Pugh, D. M., and Bywater, R. J.: Veterinary Applied Pharmacology and Therapeutics, 4th ed. London, Bailliere Tindall, 1982.

Colloquium on Clinical Pharmacology: J. Am. Vet. Med. Assoc. *170*:1049–1115, 1980.

Colloquium on Recent Advances in the Therapy of Infectious Diseases: J. Am. Vet. Med. Assoc. *185*:1058–1225, 1984.

Edberg, S. C., and Berger, S. A.: Antibiotics and Infection. New York, Churchill Livingstone, 1983.

Hjerpe, C. A.: Systemic antimicrobial therapy in beef cattle; pharmacologic and therapeutic considerations. Proc. Ann. Conv. Am. Assoc. Bov. Pract. *15*:92–108, 1983.

Kuemmerle, H. P.: Clinical Chemotherapy. Vol. II: Antimicrobial Chemotherapy. New York, Thieme-Stratton Inc., 1983.

Therapeutic Management of Inflammation

GARY D. KORITZ, D.V.M., Ph.D.

Inflammation is a dynamic process by which living tissues respond defensively to irritants, whether physical, chemical, infectious, or immunologic. The protective nature of inflammation is apparent when it results in the removal of an irritant and repair of damaged tissues. If the inflammatory process becomes excessive or unduly prolonged, however, it may cause greater harm than the original insult.

The signs of inflammation are redness, swelling, heat, pain, and loss of function of the affected tissue. The release of histamine from mast cells and basophils is an immediate response to tissue irritation that results in local vasodilation, increased blood flow, and, thus, hyperemia. Histamine produces this early vascular response for only 30 to 60 minutes before it becomes less important than various delayed mediators of inflammation such as the prostaglandins, thromboxanes, leukotrienes, 12-HETE (a chemotactic factor), superoxide, kinins, complement, and lysosomal enzymes. The first five of these substances are synthesized in the damaged tissue as a result of increased availability of arachidonic acid from phospholipids in the membranes of injured cells (Fig. 1). The kinins and prostaglandins sustain the hyperemia and, in addition, produce pain and increased capillary permeability. Plasma proteins then escape through the capillary walls, leading to local edema formation by osmotic retention of exudated fluids. These fluids dilute toxic substances and carry immunoglobulins into the region. As serum loss continues, blood flow slows and leads to passive congestion of the tissue. White blood cells adhere to and emigrate through the vascular endothelium in response to locally produced chemotactic factors. Platelets will also adhere to the endothelium in response to intimal damage as well as thromboxane production, resulting in local thrombosis. Decreased blood flow, cell necrosis, pain, and swelling all contribute to the loss of tissue function. Fever may be

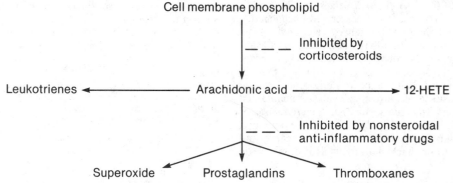

Figure 1. Inflammatory mediators arising from cell membranes and the sites of action of various anti-inflammatory drugs.

associated with the inflammatory process if sufficient pyrogenic substances are released into the general circulation to stimulate prostaglandin production in the hypothalamic thermoregulatory center.

Subsequent events lead to either healing or chronic inflammation. If the causative irritant has been eliminated, the inflammatory debris is removed by phagocytosis, liquefaction, and absorption. Damaged tissues either regenerate or are replaced by scar tissue. If the irritant remains, however, chronic inflammation and the associated disruption of tissue function will persist.

THERAPEUTIC INTERVENTION

The clinician may elect not to intervene pharmacologically in an inflammatory process that (1) is not causing serious discomfort and (2) appears to be eliminating the irritant with the restoration of normal function. Moderate pain and fever are beneficial when the former serves to limit the movement of an injured tissue and the latter inhibits bacterial growth. Excessive pain, fever, swelling, and loss of function call for therapeutic intervention, as does chronic inflammation. Of course, all efforts should be made first to diagnose the cause of inflammation and then to remove or control the irritant, if possible.

Antihistaminic Drugs

The commonly used antihistaminic agents (Table 1) competitively block the action of histamine at H_1 receptors. They are well absorbed orally by monogastric but not by ruminant animals. Intramuscular rather than intravenous administration is recommended in order to avoid CNS stimulation.

The administration of antihistaminics to counter some of the signs associated with allergic and anaphylactic reactions is a widely accepted clinical practice. (Epinephrine injection will be required if the condition is life-threatening.) Empirically, the antihistaminic agents seem to be of value in the treatment of various forms of dermatitis, laminitis, asthma, bloat, mastitis, and metritis. However, there are no well-controlled clinical studies to support these proposed indications. Because the antihistaminics only partially block the very early stages, administration of nonsteroidal anti-inflammatory drugs or corticosteroids may be required for adequate control of acute inflammatory reactions.

Nonsteroidal Anti-Inflammatory Drugs

These drugs, which include aspirin, phenylbutazone, dipyrone, meclofenamic acid, naproxen, and flunixin, inhibit the conversion of arachidonic acid to prostaglandins and thromboxanes. As is evident from Figure 1, this inhibition results in decreased formation of some, but by no means all, of the mediators of inflammation. Nonsteroidal anti-inflammatory drugs are effective analgesics only for pain of low to moderate intensity. Their antipyretic action is due to the inhibition of prostaglandin production in the hypothalamic thermoregulatory center.

Only aspirin and phenylbutazone have been studied sufficiently in food-producing animals for informed use (see Table 1). Phenylbutazone is not approved for food-producing animals in the United States; aspirin may be used, because it is a "grandfather" drug.

Aspirin is absorbed slowly by ruminants and rapidly by swine following oral administration. The half-life of salicylic acid, the major metabolite of aspirin, is about 1 hour in ruminants and 6 hours in swine. Following cessation of aspirin therapy, most of the drug will be cleared from the body in ruminants in 1 day and in swine in 2 days. Aspirin is an effective and inexpensive anti-inflammatory, analgesic, and antipyretic agent that has been used in the treatment of lameness and mastitis in cattle.

Phenylbutazone is highly bound to both plasma and tissue proteins. Drug interactions may occur through the displacement by phenylbutazone of other drugs from plasma proteins. The binding of phenylbutazone to tissue proteins might result in detectable drug residues for as long as 2 weeks after the cessation of therapy. Phenylbutazone has been used to treat lameness in cattle.

Corticosteroids

More of the reactions associated with inflammation are suppressed by the corticosteroids than by any of the other classes of anti-inflammatory drugs. Cell membranes are stabilized, and the formation of many inflammatory mediators is prevented (see Fig. 1). Cellular responses are also inhibited, resulting in decreased leukocyte infiltration, impairment of phagocytosis, and decreased fibroplasia. Thus, both inflammation and healing are retarded.

The synthetic corticosteroids may be thought of as derivatives of the natural hormone hydrocortisone (cortisol). Relative glucocorticoid and anti-inflammatory potencies increase and mineralocorticoid effects decrease as specific sites on the drug molecule are altered by the

Table 1. Some Common Anti-inflammatory Drugs and Their Dosages

Generic Name	Trade Name	Source	Species	Dosage
Antihistaminic Drugs				
Pyrilamine maleate	Histavet-P	Burns-Biotic, Omaha, NB	Large animals	1–2 mg/kg q 6–12 hr
Tripelennamine hydrochloride	Re-covr Injection	E. R. Squibb, Princeton, NJ	Cattle*	1 mg/kg IV or IM q 6–12 hr
			Swine	1 mg/kg IV or IM q 6–12 hr
Diphenhydramine hydrochloride	Benadryl	Parke-Davis, Morris Plains, NJ	Large animals	0.5–1 mg/kg IV or IM
Nonsteroidal Anti-Inflammatory Drugs				
Aspirin	Veterinary Aspirin	Craig Laboratories, Norwich, CT	Cattle*	100 mg/kg orally q 12 hr
			Swine	10 mg/kg orally q 6 hr
Phenylbutazone	Butazolidin	Burroughs Wellcome, Kansas City, MO	Cattle	4 mg/kg IV or orally q 24 hr
			Swine	4 mg/kg IV or orally q 24 hr
Corticosteroids				
Dexamethasone	Azium	Schering Corporation, Kenilworth, NJ	Cattle*	5–20 mg IM or orally q 24 hr
Flumethasone	Flucort Solution	Diamond Laboratories, Des Moines, IA	Cattle	1.25–5 mg IV or IM q 24 hr
Isoflupredone acetate	Predef 2X	Upjohn Company, Kalamazoo, MI	Cattle*	10–20 mg IM q 12–24 hr
			Swine*	5 mg/136 kg IM
Triamcinolone acetonide	Vetalog Parenteral Injection	E. R. Squibb, Princeton, NJ	Cattle	12–30 mg IM or SC

* Approved for use in the United States.

addition of double bonds, fluorine, or other functional groups. As the potency of the synthetic corticosteroids is increased, however, their biological half-lives and potential to produce detrimental suppression of the pituitary-adrenal axis are increased.

The free alcohols of the corticosteroids are poorly water soluble. Esterification of these drugs provides a means to control solubility and, thereby, the rate of absorption. Thus, esters such as dexamethasone phosphate and prednisolone succinate are highly water soluble and are often administered intravenously for the rapid attainment of high concentrations in body fluids. When given intramuscularly or subcutaneously, these esters are absorbed in minutes to hours. Because esters such as isoflupredone acetate are poorly water soluble, they are administered intramuscularly or intrasynovially, with absorption occurring in days to weeks. Trimacinolone acetonide is insoluble in water, generally is injected intramuscularly, and is absorbed very slowly.

The poorly soluble corticosteroids are often formulated as suspensions, which should not be administered intravenously.

Considerations to be made prior to the administration of a corticosteroid should include (1) whether or not the drug is indicated for the treatment of the disorder diagnosed, (2) the seriousness of the disorder, (3) the predisposition of the patient to side effects, and (4) the specific contraindications.

The large variety of corticosteroids available makes selection a difficult process (see Table 1). The decision should be based on the route of drug administration, drug formulation as it influences the onset and duration of effects, the relative importance of sodium retention, and cost *versus* effectiveness as an anti-inflammatory agent (Table 2).

The major principles of corticosteroid therapy are as follows:

1. A single large dose is usually harmless.
2. Multiple doses for a few days, if not specifically contraindicated, are unlikely to be injurious.
3. Therapy for weeks or months at doses much greater than replacement needs significantly increases the risk of side effects.
4. The dosage for chronic conditions is frequently determined by trial and error and must be re-evaluated periodically.
5. Abrupt termination of prolonged corticosteroid administration may precipitate signs of adrenal insufficiency.

In summary, one should administer the smallest effective multiple dose in chronic conditions and large doses for short periods in acute conditions to ensure maximum efficacy and benefit.

Some of the inflammatory diseases that have been treated with corticosteroids are allergy, hepatitis, nephri-tis, cerebral or spinal edema, mastitis, metritis, and lameness. There is still considerable controversy as to the safety and efficacy of corticosteroids in the treatment of these diseases.

Dimethylsulfoxide

When applied topically, dimethylsulfoxide (DMSO) is a potent anti-inflammatory agent that also increases the dermal penetration of a number of other drugs. Whether or not intramammary administration of DMSO diminishes inflammation is equivocal; however, the distribution of antibiotics infused into the gland does appear to be enhanced. DMSO is not approved in the United States for use in food-producing animals.

In the bovine, DMSO is metabolized to its sulfone and sulfide, both of which are normally present in meat and milk. Following the application of DMSO to cattle, these metabolites return to their usual concentrations within 3 to 7 days.

CONTRAINDICATIONS TO AND COMPLICATIONS OF ANTI-INFLAMMATORY THERAPY

In general, because anti-inflammatory drugs mask the signs of inflammation, they should not be administered prior to a diagnosis of its cause. Furthermore, they are contraindicated if reduction of fever is to be used to monitor the response of antibacterial therapy.

Antihistaminic Drugs

At therapeutic doses, antihistaminics may produce depression and ataxia. Higher doses or rapid intravenous injection may result in convulsions and even death. Gastrointestinal side effects, although uncommon, include anorexia, nausea, and constipation or diarrhea.

Nonsteroidal Anti-Inflammatory Drugs

Signs of aspirin toxicity include gastrointestinal ulceration, severe acid-base disturbances, and prolonged bleeding time. Aspirin therapy should be stopped at least 7 days prior to elective surgery. Use of the drug in pregnant animals is not advisable because of potential teratogenesis and prolongation of gestation by interference with prostaglandin synthesis.

Phenylbutazone is less toxic in animals than in humans, in whom fatal blood dyscrasias can occur. Gastrointestinal ulceration may be produced in animals with repeated high doses.

Both aspirin and phenylbutazone may cause renal papillary necrosis. This lesion is usually associated with prolonged therapy or dehydration with decreased urine output and concentration of the drugs in the renal papillae.

Corticosteroids

Some of the corticosteroids retain significant mineralocorticoid activity which might result in water and electrolyte disorders. Edema may occur in some instances, and polydipsia and polyuria are often observed. Increased renal tubular secretion of potassium may produce hypokalemia, and renal loss of calcium and phosphorus impairs bone homeostasis. The latter condition may lead to reduced bone growth, prolonged fracture repair, or osteoporosis.

Stimulation of gluconeogenesis may produce a number

Table 2. *Characteristics of Some Common Corticosteroids*

Corticosteroid	Sodium Retention	Anti-Inflammatory Activity
Hydrocortisone	+ +	1.0
Prednisolone	+	4.0
Triamcinolone	Slight	5.0
Isoflupredone	Slight	10.0
Dexamethasone	Slight	30.0
Flumethasone	Slight	40.0

of undesirable effects. Skeletal muscle may decrease in size as a result of protein catabolism. Further weakening occurs in the presence of hypokalemia. Muscle wasting, poor wound healing, and osteoporosis will occur with prolonged therapy. Body fat depots also decrease and redistribute. Fatty infiltration of the liver is favored.

The CNS is affected in several ways. Behavioral changes may be expressed as euphoria and improved appetite or, less frequently, as mania or depression. Increased cerebral excitability lowers the convulsive threshold. Decreased fever may mask the presence of an infectious disease.

The corticosteroids have widespread effects on the endocrine system. Parturition has been induced in sheep, cattle, and horses by the more potent drugs, such as dexamethasone and flumethasone. All of the synthetic corticosteroids have the ability to suppress ACTH production, which with prolonged administration may result in adrenocortical hypoplasia. Abrupt cessation of glucocorticoid therapy in the presence of a pituitary-adrenal axis unable to respond to external stresses may precipitate a shock-like state and collapse of the animal.

The hemoglobin content of red cells is increased, as is the number of circulating polymorphonuclear leukocytes. However, the leukocytes exhibit decreased phagocytic ability. Eosinopenia, lymphopenia, and a decrease in lymphoid tissue mass also occur. These changes increase susceptibility to infection by a variety of pathogens. Furthermore, immune responses are impaired. Vaccines may or may not produce immunity. Latent infections may be activated.

There are a number of specific contraindications to corticosteroid therapy. They include pregnancy, renal insufficiency, decreased cardiac reserve, rapid body growth (in young animals), bone healing, corneal ulceration, and chronic infection.

Dimethylsulfoxide

A potential teratogen, DMSO should not be used in pregnant animals. Rubber gloves should be worn to prevent dermal absorption when applying DMSO in order to avoid the possible development of cataracts with repeated exposure. Industrial-grade DMSO should not be used, because it could contain chemical contaminants that might be injurious if absorbed through the skin.

Supplemental Reading

Booth, N. H., and McDonald, L. E. (eds.): Veterinary Pharmacology and Therapeutics, 5th ed. Ames, Iowa, Iowa State University Press, 1982.
Gilman, A. G., Goodman, L. S., and Gilman, A. (eds.): Goodman and Gilman's The Pharmacological Basis of Therapeutics, 6th ed. New York, Macmillan Publishing Co., Inc., 1980.
Upson, D. W.: Upson's Handbook of Clinical Veterinary Pharmacology, Bonner Springs, Kansas, VM Publishing, 1980.

Immunologic Disorders and Immunotherapy

CINDY J. BRUNNER, Ph.D., D.V.M.

The concept of the immune system as an organ susceptible to disease and responsive to therapy is rapidly gaining acceptance in veterinary medicine. Clinical evaluation of immunologic function is now possible, as is identification of specific immunologic disorders. One of the newest and most exciting applications of immunologic research comes from the development of techniques to modify the immune response through immunotherapy.

COMPONENTS AND FUNCTION OF THE IMMUNE SYSTEM

The immune system can be divided into nonspecific and specific sectors. The nonspecific sector includes phagocytic leukocytes and the complement cascade. The specific sector consists of lymphocytes, which can be divided into at least two categories. T lymphocytes are those dependent upon the thymus and thymic hormones for maturation; with essential help from macrophages, T lymphocytes react with antigens and participate in cell-mediated immune reactions. B lymphocytes develop under the influence of the "mammalian bursa equivalent," which has not been clearly identified. With T lymphocyte help, most B lymphocytes mature into plasma cells, each producing antibodies of unique antigenic specificity.

The most vigorous interactions between invading agents and cells of the immune system occur along mucosal surfaces and in regional lymphoid tissue. Successful invasion beyond this barrier usually incites a systemic immune response.

An immune response is the product of a well-integrated system. Many internal factors are involved, the most critical being (1) possession of appropriate genetic information for recognizing and responding to an antigen, (2) balanced participation of all components of the system, and (3) effective regulatory mechanisms to control the response. External factors such as drugs, nutritional status, age, hormone levels, and unique characteristics of an invading agent will also strongly influence the outcome of the response.

DETECTION AND TREATMENT OF IMMUNOLOGIC DISORDERS

As with any other organ system, the immune system may become diseased; abnormalities may occur in either its development or its function. In some cases these aberrations can be detected by using standard diagnostic procedures, but most require specialized techniques available only at major veterinary hospitals or diagnostic facilities. Three major types of abnormalities can occur: immunodeficiencies, hypersensitivity reactions, and autoimmune disorders.

Immunodeficiencies

The most common form of immunodeficiency is failure of a newborn animal to absorb colostral antibodies. This lack of passive protection results in higher susceptibility to infections. A simple assay of serum gamma globulins by zinc sulfate turbidity analysis may indicate whether passively transferred immunoglobulin (Ig) is present; a concentration less than 1 gm/dl is considered low. Other more sensitive and specific tests include quantitation of serum IgG by radial immunodiffusion and field tests such as BOVA-S and EQUI-Z.* If the animal is more than 24 to 48 hours old, Ig will no longer be absorbed across the intestinal mucosa, and replacement therapy must be pro-

*Available from V.M.R.D., Inc., Pullman, WA 99163

vided parenterally. In that case, serum (approximately 14 ml/kg body weight) or whole blood (20 ml/kg) should be injected subcutaneously or intravenously.

Congenital absence or dysfunction of components of the immune system (primary immunodeficiency) results in chronic, debilitating disease. After disappearance of passive protection, the young animal will be susceptible to severe and recurrent infections. One often sees disease caused by opportunistic or mildly pathogenic agents, such as cryptosporidia, *Pneumocystis carinii*, streptococci, *Aspergillus* spp, and yeasts, or generalized infections with herpes or papilloma viruses. Bacterial and fungal infections may be controlled temporarily with chemotherapy but usually recur. Some animals also become infected with microorganisms from attenuated live vaccines (BVD, IBR, *Brucella abortus*). Congenital immunodeficiency may be hereditary or may be induced by infection or toxicity *in utero*; in many cases, however, the cause is not evident.

Tests commonly used to detect immunodeficiencies are listed in Table 1. As is noted, some routine procedures may be used to diagnose immunodeficiency presumptively, but if precise diagnosis is desired, a clinical immunology laboratory should be contacted.

Congenital immunodeficiencies are not common in large animals, although a few have been identified: Chédiak-Higashi syndrome, an inherited neutrophil defect in partial-albino Hereford cattle; severe combined immunodeficiency in Arabian foals; thymic aplasia from a zinc malabsorption syndrome in Black Pied Danish cattle; and IgG_2 deficiency in Red Danish cattle. Single cases of other congenital disorders have also been reported.

Successful treatment of congenital immunodeficiencies

Table 1. *Diagnostic Tests for Immunodeficiencies*

Nonspecific compartment (neutrophils and monocytes)	Differential leukocyte count*
	Phagocytosis of latex beads or bacteria†
	Chemotaxis†
	Bactericidal activity†
	Iodination†
	Nitroblue tetrazolium reduction†
Specific compartment (lymphocytes) T lymphocytes	Differential leukocyte count*
	Intradermal injection of mitogen or antigen*
	DNCB sensitization*
	Lymph node biopsy*
	Skin allo(iso)graft rejection*
	Post-mortem examination: lymphoid hypoplasia*
	T lymphocyte count†
	Lymphocyte blastogenesis test (PHA, Con A)†
	Lymphokine production (MIF, LMIF)†
B lymphocytes	Lymph node biopsy*
	Electrophoresis of serum proteins*
	Radial immunodiffusion for specific Ig class*
	Specific antibody response following vaccination*
	Immunoelectrophoresis†
	B lymphocyte count†

*Can be performed with standard equipment and technical skills in a clinical laboratory.

†Special test requiring submission of samples to a clinical immunology laboratory at a veterinary college, major veterinary hospital, or appropriately equipped diagnostic facility.

Table 2. *Causes of Secondary Immunodeficiencies*

Infectious agents	Viruses (BVD, IBR, influenza)
	Pasteurellosis
	Trypanosomiasis
Drugs	Corticosteroids
	Antimetabolites (azathioprine, mercaptopurine)
	Alkylating agents (cyclophosphamide)
	Folic acid antagonists (methotrexate)
	Cyclosporines
Nutritional imbalance	Vitamin deficiency (A, B, C, E)
	Mineral deficiency (zinc, iron, selenium)
	Protein/calorie malnutrition
Toxicoses	Aflatoxicosis
	Iodine toxicity
Neoplasia	Lymphosarcoma
	Multiple myeloma
	Any metastasis to bone marrow
Other	Failure to absorb colostral antibodies
	Heavy parasite infestation
	High plasma cortisol levels at parturition
	Protein-losing enteropathy
	Renal failure

in animals is extremely difficult. Bone marrow transplantation has been attempted, but the usual outcome is a fatal graft-versus-host reaction. Immunodeficiency disorders in young animals occasionally disappear spontaneously after several weeks if adequate supportive care is provided.

Secondary, or acquired, immunodeficiencies are much more common than primary disorders in food-producing animals. In a secondary disorder, the immune system has developed normally but its function is depressed. Factors such as vitamin deficiency, infection, pregnancy, and physiologic changes due to "stress" may suppress function of the immune system. As a result, the animal is susceptible to infection with many of the same agents encountered in primary immunodeficiency disorders. The course of an infection may be prolonged or more severe than in normal animals. Agents or factors that can produce secondary immunodeficiencies are listed in Table 2.

Secondary immunodeficiencies should be differentiated from primary disorders. The diagnosis of secondary deficiencies is based on the same tests of immunocompetence as those of primary disorders (see Table 1), although emphasis may be on function rather than on numbers of cells. The best therapeutic measure is removal of the underlying cause of the defect. One should also consider restorative immunotherapy, such as administration of hyperimmune serum.

Hypersensitivity Reactions

Excessive or inappropriate response to an antigen creates a condition in which immune-mediated tissue damage can occur. Four immunopathologic mechanisms have been described. Some of the clinical manifestations of these mechanisms are given in Table 3.

Type 1 reactions, also called immediate, anaphylactic, or atopic reactions, occur when antigen combines with IgE located on mast cells. This binding triggers the release of vasoactive amines, including histamine, from the mast cell granules. The vascular changes that occur as a result are typical of acute inflammation and may be localized or

Table 3. *Clinical Manifestations of Hypersensitivity Reactions*

Type of Reaction	Manifestations
Type 1	Eczema Allergic inhalant dermatitis (atopy) Milk allergy (Jersey cattle) Hypersensitivity pneumonitis Drug allergy (also vaccine reactions) Insect bites and stings Urticaria
Type 2	Bullous skin disorders (pemphigus complex) Hemolytic anemia, thrombocytopenia Drug allergy Neonatal isoerythrolysis Blood transfusion incompatibility Myasthenia gravis Anemia due to hemoparasitism
Type 3	Glomerulonephritis Serum sickness Rheumatoid arthritis Vasculitis Hypersensitivity pneumonitis Drug allergy
Type 4	Allergic contact dermatitis (dyes, metals, plant resins) Encephalomyelitis Tuberculin skin reaction Hypersensitivity pneumonitis Orchitis, epididymitis Granulomatous inflammation (Mycobacteria, Actinobacilli)

systemic. Intradermal injection of a panel of suspected antigens (allergens) is the most common diagnostic test for type 1 reactivity. Development of focal edema and erythema after 10 to 15 minutes indicates sensitivity to the injected allergen. Measurement of antigen-specific IgE with the radioallergosorbent test (RAST) is currently being evaluated in veterinary medicine, but its clinical usefulness is limited by the scarcity and cost of reagents.

Type 2 reactions result from the binding of antibodies to cell membranes or cell surface receptors. Cellular damage may result if complement is activated, as is the case in immune-mediated hemolytic anemia. Binding of antibodies to a receptor for a hormone or other small molecule may result in either blockage or continual triggering of the receptor. Myasthenia gravis and certain endocrinopathies, including some forms of thyroiditis and diabetes mellitus in humans, are thought to be the result of receptor binding. Antibodies on erythrocytes are detected with the Coombs' direct antiglobulin test, and antibodies on other cell surfaces or on receptors are detected by immunofluorescence microscopy or radioimmunoassay.

Type 3 reactions involve activation of complement by antigen-antibody complexes in the circulation or in tissues. Biologically active complement components induce vasodilation, increase vascular permeability, and cause local influx of leukocytes (particularly neutrophils). Tissue damage results from release of enzymes from the neutrophils. Vasculitis and glomerulonephritis are characteristic of systemic type 3 reactions and are often seen during certain viral infections, including hog cholera, African swine fever, and bluetongue. Diagnosis of type 3 reactions is based on observation of typical histologic features and on detection of immune complexes in affected tissues by immunofluorescence microscopy.

Type 4 reaction, or delayed hypersensitivity, is generated by the response of T lymphocytes to antigens. Granulomatous inflammation is typical of type 4 reactivity and is seen, for example, in histoplasmosis, actinobacillosis, and mycobacterial infections. Delayed hypersensitivity is most often identified with an intradermal antigen test that is read at 48 to 72 hours, such as the tuberculin test. Occasionally a blastogenic response by lymphocytes cultured with an antigen may be used to identify type 4 reactivity *in vitro*.

The most obvious therapy for immune-mediated tissue damage is elimination of the antigen, if it can be identified. Glucocorticoids are commonly used to suppress mild reactions, such as atopic dermatitis and allergic contact dermatitis. Stronger immunosuppressive drugs, including azathioprine, methotrexate, cyclophosphamide, and cyclosporine, are in experimental use. Hyposensitization by repeated subcutaneous injection of antigen is effective in some type 1 reactions but might be harmful in diseases involving the other types of reactions.

Autoimmune Disorders

Specific immunologic reactivity against the body's own antigens is seldom seen in food-producing animals. Autoimmunity may develop as a result of loss or bypass of the normal regulatory mechanisms of the immune system. The tissue damage that occurs in autoimmunity is due to one or more of the immunopathologic mechanisms discussed in the previous section (i.e., types 1 to 4 reactions.)

Examples of autoimmune disorders in animals include cytolytic disorders (hemolytic anemia, thrombocytopenia); reactions against solid tissues (polyneuritis, encephalitis, sympathetic ophthalmia, pemphigus-type bullous skin diseases); and generalized autoimmune reactions of unknown origin (lupus erythematosus, rheumatoid arthritis).

Potent immunosuppressive therapy is usually required to suppress autoimmune reactions.

IMMUNOTHERAPY

Advances in understanding the regulation of the immune system have made possible the development of methods to control immune responses. The two general objectives of these techniques are to augment deficient reactivity and to suppress hyperactive responses.

Potentiation of an immune response may be as simple as using an adjuvant to enhance the immunogenicity of a vaccine. Many commercial vaccines are administered with aluminum-containing adjuvants such as aluminum hydroxide. Newer synthetic adjuvants may be useful with inactivated viral vaccines or vaccines produced with recombinant DNA technology.

Immunologic activity can be stimulated nonspecifically with cells or cell wall products from mycobacteria (Regressin,* and bacillus Calmette-Guérin or BCG) and *Propionibacterium acnes* (Immunoregulin†). It must be emphasized that the clinical use of these agents is usually restricted to certain animal species and defined medical

*Available from Ragland Research, Inc., Athens, GA 30601.
†Available from Immuno Vet Inc., Tampa, FL 33630.

conditions for which regulatory agency approval has been granted. In many cases, use of such treatments is still experimental, and reliable information about their safety and effectiveness is not yet available.

General suppression of immune function is much easier to achieve than immunopotentiation. Corticosteroids are commonly used to suppress immunologic reactivity, although their effectiveness may vary with the animal species. Cytotoxic drugs (methotrexate, cyclophosphamide, azathioprine, cyclosporine) destroy lymphocytes or inhibit their function. It should be noted that use of these agents may increase the susceptibility of the patient to infectious diseases.

Administration of antibodies is also a form of immunotherapy. Plasma and hyperimmune serum provide protection against infection in animals that did not absorb colostral antibodies or that fail to produce their own immunoglobulins. Monoclonal antibodies against specific structural components or virulence factors of microorganisms may temporarily prevent colonization or invasion by those microorganisms. Specific antibodies may also inhibit active immunization and may limit the intensity and duration of an immune response. Much still needs to be learned about these opposing roles of antibody molecules.

Technologic advances in molecular biology have made available moderate numbers of immunologically active molecules for clinical evaluation. Various interferons and lymphokines that normally serve a regulatory role in the immune system are being tested in patients with immunologic disorders. The clinical usefulness of substances produced with the "new" technologies will depend on parallel advances in the knowledge of regulation within the immune system.

Supplemental Reading

AVMA Council on Biologic and Therapeutic Agents: Colloquium on clinical immunology. J. Am. Vet. Med. Assoc. *181*:971–1182, 1982.

Butler, J. E. (ed.): The Ruminant Immune System. New York, Plenum Press, 1981.

Salvaggio, J. E. (ed.): Primer on allergic and immunologic diseases. J. Am. Med. Assoc. *248*:2579–2772, 1982.

Tizard, I. R.: An Introduction to Veterinary Immunology, 2nd ed. Philadelphia, W. B. Saunders Company, 1982.

Hypersensitivity

LEONARD BLACK, B.V.Sc., Ph.D., F.R.C.V.S.

Hypersensitivity reactions are those provoked in animals that have been previously sensitized. By convention, these reactions are detrimental to the hosts, producing, for example, hypotension, respiratory distress, and urticaria but excluding those responses that are benign (humoral antibody anamnestic responses). This definition, however, requires qualification. The tuberculin reaction is regarded as an example of delayed hypersensitivity even though it is not in itself detrimental and is a usual manifestation of cell-mediated immunity. Only hypersensitivity produced by immune mechanism is discussed here. For a discussion of photosensitization see Environmental Skin Conditions.

CLINICAL SIGNS

Cattle

Incidence is difficult to determine because many hypersensitivity reactions probably pass unnoticed. When animals are kept under surveillance during the critical period, for instance after vaccination, reactions have been estimated at less than 0.1 cases per 1000. However, the incidence is unpredictable, and in certain areas the frequency is far greater.

Immediate reactions usually develop 10 to 20 minutes after exposure to an allergen, and the early signs include licking of the lips, salivation, and lacrimation. Cattle show manifestations of pruritus, including swishing the tail, stamping the feet, licking the coat, shaking the head, scratching with the horns, scratching the ears with a hind foot, and, in severe cases, frenzied rubbing against stationary objects. There is urination, defecation, frothing at the mouth, and edema around the eyes, muzzle, anus, and vulva. Bloat occasionally occurs.

Respiratory signs also develop which may be mild or so severe as to terminate fatally. Initially, there is only hyperpnea and an occasional cough, but later severe respiratory distress may develop. Large volumes of froth pour from the mouth (Fig. 1), the head and neck are extended, and the tongue protrudes. Rarely does cyanosis occur, but collapse and death may follow. The relative prominence of respiratory and dermal signs varies from case to case.

The clinical signs usually subside without treatment, although urticaria may persist for 12 to 24 hours. Abortions sometimes occur 1 or 2 days after the acute reactions have subsided.

Late reactions set in 1 to 3 weeks after exposure. Papules 3 to 20 mm in diameter develop between the hindlegs and on the dewlap, neck, and flanks, and sometimes they cover most of the body (Fig. 2). Hair becomes sparse, and the papules exude serum and scab over. Rubbing the lesions leaves open bleeding sores, which attract flies and become infected. Milk yield drops, there may be abortion, and over the next 3 months, wasting can be so severe as to warrant destruction. As a general rule, however, slow recovery takes place.

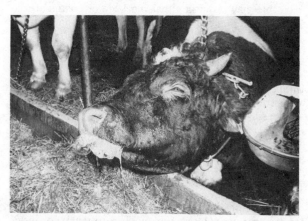

Figure 1. Severe anaphylaxis in a Friesian cow. Note periorbital edema, frothing at the muzzle, and collapse.

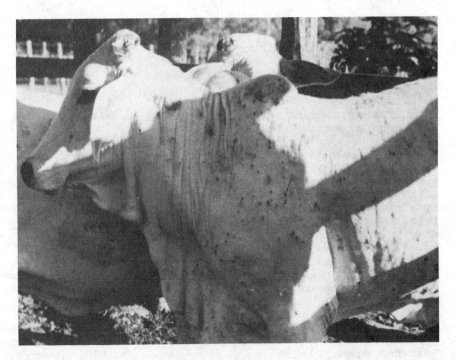

Figure 2. Late allergic skin reactions that occur 1 to 3 weeks after exposure to allergen. In this case the animals had been vaccinated about 10 days previously. (The photograph was taken by Dr. D. Baumgarten of Cooper Paraguay S. A. Laboratories, whose kind permission to publish it is acknowledged with thanks.)

Pigs

The occurrence of hypersensitivity reactions in pigs is rare. Moist, noisy breathing sounds may be audible several meters away. Muscle tremors are often followed by staggering, collapse, loss of consciousness, apnea, and cyanosis. The animal appears to be dying, but recovery usually follows.

PATHOGENESIS

Four types of hypersensitivity reactions, analogous to those recognized in humans, are identifiable in cattle. In practice, however, reactions are often not clear-cut, and the four types occur in various combinations.

Type I (anaphylaxis). Immediate reactions, as described previously, fall into this category. They are associated with reaginic (IgE) antibodies. These antibodies develop after first exposure to the sensitizing substance (allergen) and fix onto the surface of mast cells and basophils. On subsequent exposure, the allergen triggers release of the anaphylactic mediators (histamine, bradykinin, serotonin, leukotrienes, and/or prostaglandins) from the cells, which in turn are responsible for the clinical signs (Fig. 3).

Type II. Initial exposure provokes the production of cytotoxic (IgG) antibodies, which react with antigens on cell membranes and produce cytolysis or hemolysis. Hemolytic icterus of the newborn is an example of this type of reaction.

Type III. Arthus reactions, serum sickness, late reactions as described, and bovine farmer's lung are thought to be of this type. On first exposure, the antigen provokes precipitating antibodies, which form soluble complexes with available antigen. These circulate in the serum and, in circumstances that are not fully understood, form deposits in the skin, lungs, small blood vessels, and/or glomerular membrane. The clinical signs depend on their site of deposition; for instance, proteinuria and wasting follows accumulation in the glomerular membranes, whereas thrombosis and local necrosis follow deposition in the blood vessels of the skin.

Type IV. First exposure provokes a population of immune cells and re-exposure, for instance by intradermal antigen injection (tuberculin reaction) or by application of an antigen impregnated swab (patch test), produces local cellular infiltration and swelling that reaches maximum size 48 to 72 hours later.

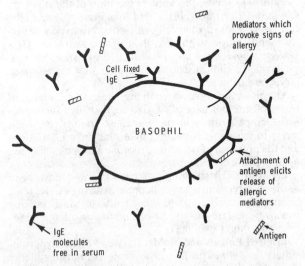

Figure 3. Mechanism of immediate, Type 1, or anaphylactic reactions: First exposure to allergen provokes reaginic (IgE) antibodies that fix onto tissue mast cells and basophils. At re-exposure, the antigen reacts with these cell-fixed reagins and elicits the release of mediators that produce the allergic manifestations.

PROVOCATION OF REACTIONS

Macromolecules (proteins and polysaccharides) with molecular weights of about 35,000 daltons are often responsible for provocation, although smaller molecules may also act in this way after fixing to large molecules in the animal's body.

The following factors have been implicated as causes of hypersensitivity reactions in food animals.

Drugs. Penicillin, streptomycin, dihydrostreptomycin, neomycin, oxytetracycline, chloramphenicol, and sulfonamides.

Hormones. Diethylstilbestrol and corticosteroids.

Vaccine Components. Horse serum, hamster serum, cattle serum denatured by formalin, gelatin, egg albumen, bovine serum albumin, chick embryo and baby hamster kidney cell (BHK 21) derivatives have been incriminated. Reactions against vaccines for salmonellosis, pasteurellosis, rabies, brucellosis, leptospirosis, contagious bovine pleuropneumonia, and foot and mouth disease vaccines also have been documented.

Additives. Carboxy- and hydroxypropyl-methylcellulose. (These widely used additives may be responsible for reactions sometimes attributed to other components of injectable pharmaceutical preparations.)

Infectious Agents. Type IV reactions have been reported after intradermal injection of inactivated viruses/bacteria or their derivatives into sensitized cattle. Such reactions could be demonstrated in animals sensitized by human, bovine, and avian tuberculosis, Johne's disease, glanders, streptococci, parainfluenza 3, *Brucella melitensis*, leptospira, and Q fever.

Anaphylactic-type reactions have also occurred after an intravenous injection of inactivated IBR/IPV virus and *E. coli* endotoxin. Hypersensitivity may actually play a role in the pathogenesis of husk, focal necrotizing encephalitis, louping ill, malignant catarrhal fever, brucellosis, arthritis, mastitis, and colibacillosis.

Parasites. Severe reactions to the bites of the stable fly (*Stomoxys calcitrans*), black fly (*Simulium* spp.) and blue tick (*Boophilus* spp.) have been ascribed to hypersensitivity. Sensitization to the gut fluid of the warble fly (*Hypoderma bovis*) has also been held responsible for anaphylaxis-like clinical signs that develop after the encysted larvae are damaged.

The tissue reactions surrounding the cysts or migration tracts of internal parasites (*Ascaris, Fasciola, Dictyocaulus, Oesophagostomum* spp.) are also thought to be allergic in nature, as indicated by eosinophilic infiltrations and the presence of circulating reaginic antibodies directed against extracts of the parasites.

Feedstuffs. Urticaria and dyspnea in calves have been ascribed to feedstuffs and milk proteins acting as allergens. Similar signs, observed in dairy cattle in which milking was overdue, are thought to be due to autoallergic sensitization to their own milk.

Inspired Pollens and Molds. Ragweed pollen hypersensitivity was one of the first forms of bovine allergy documented. Inspired hay mold (*Micropolyspora faeni*) is responsible for bovine farmer's lung, which produces dyspnea in cattle housed in dusty conditions.

Other Considerations

Occasionally, substances seem to provoke reactions after first exposure. These may be anaphylactoid reactions, that is, anaphylaxis-like reactions unassociated with immune mechanisms. On the other hand, the presence of possible allergens (antibiotics, for instance) in a wide variety of injectable preparations and feed substances may make the source of first sensitization difficult to trace.

PATHOLOGY

Postmortem findings include edema of the lungs, froth in the trachea, cyanosis, and petechiae on the mucosal surfaces.

Late-type skin lesions are infiltrated with eosinophils and polymorphonuclear cells in the early stages, which later give way to mononuclear cells. However, mixed cell infiltrations are common, and histopathologic examinations are generally not helpful.

DIAGNOSIS

In acute cases, conditions producing acute lung edema, such as East Coast fever and malignant catarrh, must be eliminated. Late skin reactions must be differentiated from dermatomycoses, mange, and pediculosis.

Tests to identify the allergen responsible include intradermal injections of suspect substances, passive cutaneous anaphylaxis, passive cutaneous anaphylaxis inhibition, and provocation tests. All may give rise to inconclusive results but can be regarded as useful adjuncts to a diagnosis made on subjective or circumstantial evidence.

TREATMENT

In acute cases, the first priorities are to clear respiratory edema and restore blood pressure. Epinephrine injection (1 in 1000), 8–16 μg/kg IM or 4–8 μg/kg IV, should be given to cattle and repeated 30 to 40 minutes later if needed. (Subcutaneous injections are inadvisable.) Atropine sulfate, 30–60 μg/kg body weight for cattle and 80–160 μg/kg for sheep IM, has also been recommended.

Late skin lesions can be treated with corticotropin (ACTH), 200–600 units in gel or oil injected IM every 2 to 3 days, and/or flumethazone, 0.01 per cent, penicillin, 1 million units, and streptomycin, 1 gm in 90 per cent aqueous dimethylsulfoxide, applied topically. Provided it is certain that they are not causally involved, parenteral antibiotics (procaine penicillin G, 12–20 million units IM daily for 3 to 4 days) can be used against secondary bacterial invaders.

Supplemental Reading

Black L, Pay TWF. The evaluation of hypersensitivity tests in cattle after foot and mouth disease vaccination. J. Hyg. (Cambr.) 74:169–181, 1975.
Black L. Hypersensitivity in cattle. Part II. Clinical reactions. Vet. Bull. 49:77–88, 1979.

Vaccination and Veterinary Biologic Products

RICHARD C. SEARL, D.V.M.

Biologics are needed for diagnostic, prophylactic, and therapeutic use in the prevention, control, treatment, and eradication of diseases affecting food animals. There are 48 licensees in the United States and one permittee, under

USDA-APHIS-VS supervision, licensed to produce 502 biologic products. In calendar year 1982, 21,762,135,367 doses of such biologics were produced and 782,493,254 doses destroyed.[1]

The virus, serum, toxin, and analogous products provisions of the Act of Congress of March 4, 1913, prohibit the production for sale or interstate movement of worthless, contaminated, dangerous, or harmful biologics intended for use in the diagnosis or treatment of animal diseases. The act is now administered by the United States Department of Agriculture (USDA), Animal and Plant Health Inspection Service (APHIS-USDA), Veterinary Services, through Biologics Staff (licensing), Biologics Laboratories, and Biologics Operations.

The consumer or livestock owner who uses USDA-licensed veterinary biologic products is assured that there exists a need for the product, it is not worthless, and it meets requirements for purity, safety, potency, and efficacy as shown by scientifically proven, valid evaluation procedures.

Biologics are intended for use in healthy animals as an aid in the prevention of disease. Properly used, they increase resistance to disease but do not provide absolute immunity to or freedom from infectivity. All descriptive information, dosages, recommendations for use, claims, warnings, and contraindications contained on labels and in package inserts are supported by data submitted to and accepted by APHIS-USDA.

When these products are properly used as directed, unchanged, and according to label directions, the licensed producer is responsible for their safety, efficacy, and purity. If they are repackaged or misused, or label directions are not followed, the user assumes responsibility.

BIOLOGICAL CLASSIFICATIONS

Biologics for many years have been generally classified according to the antigens and microbial agents included in their formulas. With scientific advances and newer techniques, such simple classifications are no longer precisely correct. In general, biologic classifications are as follows.

Vaccines: Products including or derived from viruses; they may be live or inactivated.

Bacterins: Products containing bacterial organisms and antigens derived from bacterial organisms; they may be live or inactivated.

Toxoids: Products containing antigens as toxoids produced by inactivating toxins produced by bacteria.

Sera: The clear sera derived from animals; may be normal serum derived from healthy animals or hyperimmune serum from animals that have been hyperimmunized; they may be standard or concentrated.

Diagnostics: Antigens or antibodies purified and variously processed for use in diagnostic test procedures.

Antigens: Substances foreign to the recipients so that when introduced into the body result in the production of antibodies.

Antibodies: Immunoglobulins (Ig) produced by the animal in response to the stimulus of an antigen.

BIOLOGICS—KILLED VERSUS LIVE

Although the early biologics were killed products, with the advent of tissue culture systems there followed the development of many live products that were derived from virulent organisms and were attenuated or modified by various procedures until they had lost their virulence but still stimulated a protective immune response.

In the 1970's, with increased knowledge and technology, came the development of many new inactivated biologics. There are desirable and undesirable features of each class, and it cannot be said that one group is better than the other. In general, the following statements can be made:

Live products (1) produce a quicker immune response; (2) usually require only one dose; (3) produce fewer local reactions; (4) produce more systemic reactions; (5) infect the recipient; and (6) have a potential for transmitting vaccinal antigen to other animals and reverting to virulence.

Killed (inactivated products) (1) require a longer time to produce a protective response; (2) usually require two doses; (3) have a potential to induce more local reactions; (4) produce fewer systemic reactions; (5) are safer and cannot produce disease; and (6) do not transmit vaccinal antigen to other animals and cannot revert to virulence.

It has been stated, with good reason, that the use of killed products is compatible with efforts to minimize and eradicate disease. It seems obvious that if a killed product is available, that is as efficacious as its live counterpart there is good reason for using the killed product.

In comparing vaccines within a class, such as modified live vaccines or killed vaccines, or comparing killed with modified live vaccines, only general comments may be made. Numerous differences between products within a general class exist as well as between the same or similar products produced by different manufacturers.

With inactivated products, such differences arise as a result of
1. Bacterial or viral strains used.
2. Method of inactivation used.
3. Whether whole culture or washed and resuspended bacteria are used.
4. The antigenic mass per dose.
5. Type and amount of adjuvant used.
6. Presence or absence of immunomodulators.
7. Preservatives, stabilizers, antifoaming agents, and other chemicals.

With live products, such differences arise as a result of
1. Strain selection.
2. Method of attenuation.
   a. By number and type of tissue culture passages and absence or use of passages in alternate hosts.
   b. By chemical attentuation.
3. Selection and cloning.
   a. Selection of avirulent strains.
   b. Selection of temperature sensitive strains.
4. Antigenic mass per dose.
5. Addition of stabilizers and preservatives.

With all of the factors just listed, and perhaps other factors, it is not surprising that there can be marked differences among the antigens contained in biologics for use against certain infective organisms. Some of these important differences are (1) transmission to non-vaccinates; (2) safety of use in pregnant animals; (3) type of immune response, i.e., whether local secretory, systemic, or both, or cell-mediated immune (CMI) response; (4) degree of modification and attenuation of modified live virus (MLV) products; (5) action of MLV antigens on the immune system, such as immunosuppression; (6) antigen blockage or interference in multiple-antigen products; and (7) latency, shedding, transmission, and reversion potential.

SUBUNIT VETERINARY BIOLOGICS*

A subunit biologic is one that contains only those immunogenic components necessary to elicit an immune response. A primary requirement for subunit products is knowing which particular immunogen is responsible for the production of immunity by the host.

Methods of Production

Basically, three methods are available for large-scale production:

1. Large-scale production of the biologic agent followed by extraction and purification of the subunit immunogen. This method has been used successfully with influenza types A and B. Its major disadvantage is high cost.

2. Synthesis of the specific immunogen by chemical means. This method requires high technology that does not yet have a practical application. In this technique, the determinant sites, which involve only a few amino acids, can be coupled to a carrier protein such as bovine serum albumin. This coupled hapten is then used as the subunit vaccine.

3. Recombinant DNA technology. This procedure involves insertion of DNA specific for the immunogen into bacterial plasmids. Organisms so engineered then produce the subunit immunogen.

Advantages of Subunit Technique

1. Safety. No living infectious agent present, plus no oncogenic, pyrogenic, or allergenic activity.

2. Efficacy. Large amounts of immunogen may be given without danger of antigen interference, immunosuppression, or overloading the immune system.

3. Identification of vaccinates. Serologic test procedures can be developed that will differentiate vaccinates from infected animals.

Disadvantages of Subunit Technique

1. Adjuvants are required to bind the antigen and produce depot slow release of antigen to obtain the immune response. Subunits may be of low molecular weight and require aggregation or linkage to carrier molecules.

2. The subunit approach is expensive owing to the multidisciplinary high-technology, equipment, and research and development work involved. However, actual production expense will be reduced.

3. It may not be possible to stimulate precisely the production of specific classes of immunoglobulins or the cell-mediated immune response necessary to provide protection to certain diseases.

In the future, the subunit technology together with monoclonal antibody technology should make available a new class of antigens and eliminate some of the objections to currently available biologics.

BIOLOGIC CONSTITUENTS

Any biologic contains substances other than the organism or antigen in the formula. Live, modified live, and avirulent live products usually contain substances such as stabilizers to protect the antigen and preservatives to prevent inadvertent contamination. They may also contain

*Abstracted from Reed, D. E.: A Subunit Approach. 84th USAHA Meeting, 1980.

an additive such as a color indicator, which serves as a pH determinant for detection of contamination.

Inactivated products may contain trace amounts of the chemicals used to inactivate the antigen and preservatives to prevent contamination, and most contain adjuvants necessary to enhance the immune response. They may or may not contain additive pH color indicators. If desiccated, they may also contain additives used as stabilizers.

VACCINE USE

Vaccines, bacterins, and toxoids are meant to be used in programs of immunoprophylaxis and are not recognized as being therapeutic agents.

They act by stimulating the animal's immune system to minimize or negate the effects of invading microorganisms whose antigens are included in the formula.

All vaccines contain biologic substances that can be rendered useless, harmful, or nonimmunogenic by improper handling and storage, mixing, or administration. One should always read the labels and package insert direction slips prior to use for dosage, method of administration, warnings, and contraindications.

The capabilities and limitations of all vaccines depend upon the quality, content, and type of antigen and the type, degree, and duration of the immune response they produce.

VACCINATION PROGRAMS

Owing to the extreme diversity of management and environmental conditions under which livestock are raised and held, including the purpose, types, class, and species, no precise vaccination program suits all purposes.

The objectives of preventive programs are to reduce and, if possible, eliminate the economic loss, disease incidence, and risks associated with livestock production. Vaccines and vaccination programs are to be used in conjunction with good management, sanitation, nutrition, and environmental control programs. The objectives are to protect the adult breeding stock, the reproductive capabilities and the fetus, neonates during the early growth periods, and the growth of marketable animals and breeding replacements.

The disease prevalence and severity in a given area or the diseases to which the animals will be exposed when sold or moved will largely govern which vaccines will be included in any control program. Because economics are involved, it will usually be necessary to make risk-benefit evaluations on what vaccines and vaccine types are to be used. All biologics are used as preventives, so programs must be planned and proper vaccinations accomplished prior to disease exposure. If the agents are used after disease exposure, or in the face of an outbreak, additional judgment decisions must be made. When vaccine use, safety, efficacy, or compatibility with other products is in doubt, the manufacturer should be contacted for definitive information.

VACCINES AND LACTOGENIC PROTECTION

Certain diseases may occur at such an early age that the use of biologics to stimulate an active immune response to them is not practical. In many such diseases, early passive protection may be given to neonates by ensuring active immunization of the pregnant dam. Antibodies against diseases to which the female is immune may be expected to be concentrated and contained in the colostrum, providing passive protection to the neonate for variable periods of time.

Variables are inherent in the results obtained by such passive protection. Some of these variables are as follows:

1. Some females may concentrate serum antibodies in colostrum more efficiently than others.

2. Some newborns absorb and utilize antibody in the colostrum better than others.

3. It is important that the newborn nurse colostrum as soon after birth as possible and in adequate amounts.

4. It has been shown that the colostral antibody level of the cow 24 hours after calving, if milked out or nursed during that period, is only 5 per cent of the level immediately after freshening.

5. Inability of the neonate to absorb colostral antibody into the system ("gut closure") occurs 18 to 36 hours after birth. Antibody consumed after this time is active only within the gut lumen.

6. In the bovine it has been shown that different quarters may actually produce different quantities of antibody. Similar observations have been made in swine.

PASSIVE PROTECTION—DISEASES AND VACCINES

Transmissible Gastroenteritis (TGE)

No evidence exists to show that the available MLV or killed TGE vaccines will induce the production of IgA in the colostrum and milk when used in susceptible recipients. It has also been suggested that when susceptible vaccinated gilts or sows are exposed, they suffer intestinal infection, which tends to reduce milk flow. IgA is the important antibody in milk, whereas IgG levels are present mainly in colostrum and decrease rapidly in milk. Although TGE vaccines are an aid in reducing the severity of disease, they are lacking in that they do not produce IgA and thus protect the gut of the neonate nursing milk. The vaccinate that has been previously exposed and infected may be expected to develop an anamnestic response resulting in the production of IgA, IgG, and IgM, and hence her litter will be better protected.

Enterotoxigenic Colibacillosis (ETEC)

Vaccines against ETEC that produce IgG antibody passed to the calf via the colostrum and milk are now available for use in pregnant cattle. IgG is the important immunoglobulin in the bovine, providing intestinal protection; IgA function is not well known in cattle. Because ETEC infections occur in the first few days of the calf's life, the vaccines available have proven to be effective. It is important that the vaccines be given at the times specified, namely, just prior to the calving, for best results.

Vaccines are also available to prevent porcine ETEC strains from adhering to gut enterocytes, thus preventing attachment, colonization, and disease. Challenge and field reports indicate that these vaccines are also effective.

Clostridial Diseases

Clostridial toxoids for preventing *C. tetani* and *C. perfringens* (types C and D) are effective and widely used. Available data in lambs indicate that passive protection against these diseases is afforded up to the usual time of castration and docking procedures if the pregnant ewe is vaccinated.

General Passive Protection

It is recognized that most other vaccines, when given to pregnant females, provide for passive protection of the neonate that may then persist for variable times. The titers of such passive antibodies and their persistences vary between individuals and between diseases and depend on the half-life of homologous antibodies. Because passive antibodies may negate and interfere with vaccinal antigens, neonates vaccinated at an early age should be revaccinated later. Passive antibodies to infectious bovine rhinotracheitis and parainfluenza are usually absent at 5 to 6 months of age, although it has been reported that bovine viral diarrhea passive antibody may persist for up to 8 months.

ADVERSE REACTIONS

Any biologic product, to be effective, must produce a beneficial reaction in the recipient. However, in certain instances the reaction produced is undesirable.

Local Reactions

Local reactions are visible at the site of injection and may occur hours, days, or weeks after the injection. Arthus reactions are type III hypersensitivity reactions manifested as a soft, boggy swelling at the injection site. They are the result of an immune-mediated reaction that occurs when the injected antigen combines in an immune complex with complement-fixing antibody present in the recipient. This immune complex releases substances irritating to the tissues. If treated early, these reactions are usually responsive to antihistaminic agents and corticosteroid therapy. Untreated, they slowly subside and are usually not apparent after 3 or 4 days. Such reactions occur with both live and inactivated antigens.

Local Inflammatory Reactions

Local inflammatory reactions may occur with either live or inactivated products but in nearly all cases are a result of adjuvants or irritants present in inactivated products. Adjuvants, which are included to enhance the immune response, accomplish their goal by providing for a slow release of the antigen and the creation of a mild local inflammatory reaction. There are many types of adjuvants in use, and in some instances an individual may be sensitive to a particular compound. Many local reactions are unavoidable and due to no fault of the administrator. The occurrence of local reactions may be minimized or negated by: (1) selecting a site where sufficient muscle mass is present; (2) avoiding injections in intermuscular septas; (3) avoiding subcutaneous injections, and (4) avoiding leakage to subcutaneous tissue by not vaccinating severely dehydrated animals, using too large or too short a needle, and by ensuring absence of air bubbles in the syringe.

On occasion, an abscess will develop at the site of injection. It may become apparent 7 to 10 days after vaccination or may develop even more slowly, becoming apparent 3 weeks after injection. Early-developing abscesses may be caused by septic techniques. Sterile abscesses, unrelated to technique or contamination but due to the irritating action of adjuvants and the animal response to an irritant, may also occur. Most abscesses that develop slowly and occur 3 weeks after injection are due to a combination of factors. Often, the animal or animals involved have recently recovered from or are undergoing a bacterial infection. If the tissues become devitalized by the injection, organisms present as a low grade bacteremia, then settle out, colonize, and reproduce in the devitalized tissues.

Systemic Reactions

Systemic reactions occur with either killed or, more commonly, live products. Systemic reactions are variously manifested as overt illness, abortions, diarrhea, fever, myositis, temporary reduced milk yield, ataxia, and death. Such reactions may be caused by inappropriate vaccination of subjects with debilitating conditions or incubating or overt disease. They may also be associated with a lack of attenuation or modification of live antigens when used in stressed animals or with immunosuppressive effects of the antigen used, or they may be immune mediated.

Immune-Mediated Reactions

Acute Anaphylaxis

Acute anaphylaxis is a well-known and potential hazard with the use of any antigen in an animal sensitized to that antigen.

Arthus Reactions

Arthus reactions are less well recognized but may be manifested as stiffness or myositis as well as edema and swelling in areas unrelated to the injection sites, such as the face, an extremity, the underline, or the scrotum. Such a reaction may cause deranged consciousness or marked ataxia. The immune complex involved in Arthus reactions releases irritants that cause tissue swelling, edema, and extravasation of fluids at the site of the lesion, resulting in edema and pressure. The signs observed are determined by the site or sites involved and the severity of the lesions.

Endotoxic Shock

It is this author's observation that animals receiving injections of biologics containing gram-negative organisms may undergo endotoxic shock. Animals of any age may be involved, but signs are usually apparent in young animals on farms where pasteurellosis or colibacillosis has been diagnosed. Some animals in the group seem to be sensitized to endotoxin as a result of prior contact; upon vaccination, the biologic provides the challenge or exciting antigenic dose. These reactions are usually associated with pasteurella, coliform or hemophilus antigens and may be sudden or require hours to develop. The responses resemble acute anaphylaxis but persist for longer periods.

Affected animals manifest various clinical signs, with the severity of the reaction usually inversely related to body weight. The following features have been observed:

1. Clinical signs apparent in minutes or hours or delayed until 12–18 hours after injection.
2. Rapid respiration, froth in trachea and mouth, and temperature up to 40°C.
3. Sawhorse stance, ataxia, or recumbency.
4. Marked myositis, generalized stiffness, and reluctance to move.
5. Transient diarrhea.
6. Marked reduction of milk yield in dairy cows, lasting from 4 to 7 days.

7. Animals found dead the day following vaccination with no apparent cause of death.

This condition is usually unresponsive to anaphylaxis therapy, but favorable responses to antihistaminic agents and steroids have been reported. Recovery may be slow, requiring 3 or 4 days for a return to normal.

Overt Disease Following Vaccination

It is not always possible to restrict vaccinations to healthy, unexposed animals as specified in product direction pamphlets. The veterinarian must therefore make immunization decisions on the basis of risk-benefit ratios. Overt or post-vaccinal disease may occur as a direct or an indirect result of the vaccine being used. Such reactions are usually related to the use of live vaccines.

Licensed producers of vaccines conduct in-house safety tests on healthy, susceptible animals with multiple doses of vaccine. The vaccines are injected and the animals are observed according to guidelines established and accepted by APHIS-USDA. The products then undergo field testing using recommended dosages. With various products, post-vaccinal disease may be observed related to one or more of the following circumstances:

1. Animals that are sick, incubating disease, or stressed by environmental and management conditions are injected.
2. Lack of attenuation of the product occurs when it is used under field conditions.
3. The antigen has an immunosuppressive action.
4. The product is used in pregnant animals or in animals permitted to commingle with pregnant animals, which is contraindicated in product direction pamphlets.
5. A risk and potential for inadvertent contamination with virulent adventitious agents exists. These are usually the result of low-level, non-cytopathic viruses which cannot be detected or are difficult to detect by available *in vitro* testing procedures.
6. Although it has not been known to occur with all live antigens, the possibility remains that some live antigens may shed or sequester and later shed to susceptible animals and, with several animal passages, revert to virulence. The fate and action of all antigens following injection is not fully known.
7. Evidence indicates that the use of some antigens may result in an increased incidence and severity of the disease when animals are challenged by the virulent organism. Two mechanisms may be involved, sensitization and immunosuppression.
8. Biologicals that contain antigens derived from animal tissues used in their production may provoke an immune reaction in the newborn inheriting the specific antigen. These reactions usually arise as a result of improper use or of repeated use of the product in breeding females.

IMMUNIZATION AND THE IDEAL VACCINE

Users of vaccines should be aware of possible failure to immunize or protect even though they use vaccines recognized as being effective. Some 2 to 5 per cent of a given animal population may be incapable of mounting a protective immune response. A proportion of vaccinations may be negated by interference from maternally derived passive antibodies. Some animals will show abnormal responses when vaccinated in the incubative stage of disease or if under treatment with immunosuppressive drugs.

The ideal vaccinal strain should be inactivated or, if live, genetically stable. If living, the vaccinal strain should undergo only limited replication and then should be completely eliminated by the recipient's defense mechanisms with no opportunity for spread to other animals. Its use should not interfere with the host's ability to respond to other antigens in the vaccine or to other infectious agents regardless of the dosage used. It should be free from local and systemic adverse reactions. A single dose should produce both cell-mediated immunity and humoral responses. The resulting protection should be long-lasting and should prevent infection, latency, and carrier states. The potency should be sufficient to override passive antibody interference. The product should be stable, should have a long shelf life, and should be resistant to heat and poor storage conditions.

Reference

1. Biological Products. Notice No. 36, USDA Veterinary Services, 1983.

Therapeutic Management of Gastrointestinal Diseases

JOHN W. PAUL, D.V.M., M.S.,
and WILLIAM L. JENKINS, B.V.Sc.,
M.Med.Vet., Ph.D.

The purpose of this discussion is to provide an overview of gastrointestinal (GI) medication. In some instances, the reader is referred to other articles in the section for a more detailed discussion on particular subjects.

Oral administration of drugs is the oldest method of medication and for many GI conditions remains the preferred route. Various dosage forms are available for the oral administration of drugs. These include powders and pellets for mixing with or top dressing feed as well as soluble powders and liquids for addition to drinking water. An obvious limitation to this method of medicating feed and water occurs in an animal that is unable to consume adequate amounts of the drug to achieve the desired effect, particularly diseased animals that tend to be anorectic or oligodipsic. Other oral dosage forms include powders, tablets, boluses, capsules, solutions or suspensions for administration via stomach tube or drench gun and, of newer vintage, oral pastes. Parenteral administration of certain drugs may also be useful for the treatment of GI disorders.

APPETITE STIMULANTS

The stimulation of appetite in sick or debilitated animals is often highly beneficial, particularly in ruminants in which feed promotes fermentation in the forestomach and the act of feeding markedly enhances ruminoreticular motility. Agents that have been used as appetite stimulants, often on an arbitrary basis, include B complex vitamins, bitters such as gentian, quassia, and nux vomica, corticosteroids, anabolic steroids, and benzodiazepines, such as elfazepam (not approved). The therapeutic benefit of some of these agents remains obscure. Others, such as the corticosteroids, may also possess distinctly deleterious side effects, and the risk:benefit ratio needs to be carefully considered in each case for which they are used.

STOMACHICS AND RUMINATORICS

Stomachics and ruminatorics promote the functional activity of the stomach, or abomasum, and the ruminoreticulum, respectively.

The therapeutic use of stomachics is limited in food animal medicine. Cholinergic agents such as neostigmine and carbachol have been used to stimulate gastric motility and secretions. More recently, metoclopramide, a dopamine antagonist, has been shown to enhance motility of the upper gastrointestinal tract without increasing secretions.

Few drugs, if any, have proved to be useful ruminatorics. Parasympathomimetic agents have been employed in an attempt to promote forestomach motility, but their effects are often unpredictable and unreliable. Frequently, uncoordinated and irregular ruminoreticular contractions occur, and the benefit to overall forestomach function is questionable. Metoclopramide has been suggested as an alternative agent to correct ruminoreticular atony, but its usefulness has yet to be proven. The optimal manner in which to enhance forestomach motility and function is to encourage affected animals to eat, since reflex responses associated with feeding increase both the strength and frequency of primary ruminoreticular movements. In addition, moderate ruminoreticular distention promotes forestomach motility.

In dealing with ruminoreticular stasis, the therapeutic goals should include the following:

1. Provide readily fermentable substrate for microbial digestion.

2. Ensure a highly fluid medium within the ruminoreticulum.

3. Provide an abundant supply of viable ruminal microflora from an animal on similar ration.

4. Adjust the intraruminal pH with either alkalinizing or acidifying agents, depending upon the etiology and clinical findings.

5. Promote active ruminoreticular motility as noted previously.

This physiologic approach is frequently of greater benefit than reliance on so-called ruminatoric drugs.

CARMINATIVES AND ANTIZYMOTICS (ANTI-BLOAT REMEDIES)

Carminatives facilitate the eructation of free gas, whereas antizymotics decrease microbial fermentation and gas production. The major uses of these classes of agent in food animal practice is in the prevention and treatment of acute and subacute (feedlot) frothy bloat in ruminants.

Anti-frothing agents used for prophylactic purposes include oil of turpentine in linseed oil, formalin, creolin, antibiotics, and, most commonly today, pluronics such as poloxalene. However, the only sure way to prevent frothy bloat is to avoid grazing stock on pastures known to produce bloat. Appropriate management will also reduce the incidence.

For treatment of acute cases of frothy bloat, surfactant

agents should be administered. These include poloxalene or other pluronics, polymerized methyl silicones such as simethicone, household detergents, and even common vegetable oils such as peanut and sunflower oils. Oil of turpentine also has been employed for many years but tends to taint meat and milk.

ANTACIDS AND AGENTS TO TREAT GASTRIC ULCERS

The principal use of oral antacids in food animal medicine is as a part of the treatment regimen for ruminal lactic acidosis. Alkalinizing agents promote an elevation of intraruminal pH and thereby retard the absorption of lactic acid directly from the ruminoreticulum into the portal circulation. Many compounds have been employed to neutralize excess acidity in cases of ruminal acidosis following excessive soluble carbohydrate engorgement. They include sodium bicarbonate, magnesium oxide, magnesium hydroxide, magnesium trisilicate, magnesium carbonate, calcium hydroxide, calcium carbonate, and aluminum hydroxide. Of these, magnesium oxide is the most potent, with a potential danger of causing severe ruminal alkalosis. Magnesium hydroxide is commonly employed, but the carbonate salt may be more effective. Sodium bicarbonate is not particularly effective; it produces a rapid genesis of carbon dioxide, leading to free gas bloat in an atonic ruminoreticulum.

Gastric and abomasal ulceration occurs quite frequently in food animals. In fact, abomasal ulcers are also not uncommon in exotic ruminants. Besides oral alkalinizing agents, H_2-receptor blockers such as cimetidine and, more recently, ranitidine also have been used with apparent success to treat abomasal ulcers in young animals.

MODULATION OF INTESTINAL MOTILITY AND INGESTA FLOW

The two major therapeutic goals of modifying gastrointestinal motility and ingesta flow are: (1) to stimulate motility or passage of ingesta associated with constipation or stasis (laxatives and purgatives), and (2) to inhibit motility and ingesta flow associated with diarrhea (antidiarrheal agents).

Laxatives and Purgatives

Stimulation of GI motility or increased passage of ingesta may be accomplished by a variety of means. The parasympathomimetics, such as carbachol, arecoline, and neostigmine, stimulate GI secretions as well as motility, thus increasing GI fluid content as well as ingesta movement.

Other cathartics useful in stimulating motility of the GI tract include irritants such as castor oil, cascara sagrada, and danthron. The irritant cathartics may produce a rather drastic effect on the intestinal tract; hence, other laxatives and cathartics that are equally effective are more commonly used. For instance, saline cathartics are poorly absorbed salts of magnesium or sodium. They exert their effect by remaining in the lumen of the intestine while absorbing and retaining water, thus increasing the bulk of the intestinal contents and softening the feces. Saline cathartics are not highly effective in ruminants and do not stimulate rumen motility. Magnesium sulfate, magnesium hydroxide, and sodium sulfate are the more commonly used saline cathartics.

The bulk-forming laxatives are hydrophilic and thus increase bulk by virtue of their water uptake. This action helps to maintain soft feces. The full laxative effect of this group of compounds is usually not observed until the second to third day of administration. Bulk-forming laxatives include methylcellulose, sodium carboxymethylcellulose, and wheat bran, but these are of limited use in mature ruminants because of the cellulolytic activity of ruminal microflora.

The lubricant laxatives, including mineral oil and dioctyl sodium sulfosuccinate, are either inert oils or surface-active agents. Their action is to soften feces without stimulating peristalsis. Continued use of mineral oil can result in deficiencies of the fat-soluble vitamins. Mineral oil is administered orally, whereas dioctyl sodium sulfosuccinate may be given *per os* as well as *per rectum* in enema form. Dioctyl sodium sulfosuccinate may be useful for the emulsification and removal of oil and petroleum products from the ruminoreticulum. It has also been used for the treatment of abomasal impaction.

Laxatives and cathartics should not be used in cases of intestinal obstruction or when the viability of intestinal tissue is in question. Drinking water must always be readily available to animals that have been given a purgative, especially when saline purgatives are administered.

Antidiarrheal Agents

Diarrhea is a common and often life-threatening medical problem, particularly in young animals. The therapeutic management of diarrhea is complex and demanding for a number of reasons, not the least of which is the high incidence of multifactorial causes of diarrheic syndromes. Rational therapy requires a specific diagnosis, but this is often not possible under field conditions so, initially at least, therapeutic measures are based on general principles and clinical experience. The major approaches to treatment include the use of modulators of intestinal motility, gastrointestinal protectants and adsorbents, gastrointestinal astringents, secretion-inhibiting drugs, anti-infective agents, fluid therapy (see "Fluid, Shock, and Blood Therapy") and microbial modifiers.

Modulators of gastrointestinal motility include parasympatholytic agents such as atropine, methscopolamine, glycopyrrolate, aminopentamide, and benzetimide. These anticholinergic drugs, which diminish motor and secretory activity of the gastrointestinal tract, have been used with success in some cases, especially in combination with antibiotics. However, recent evidence suggests that inhibition of colonic motility may paradoxically precipitate diarrhea. Opiates and opiate derivatives diminish propulsive motility but enhance tone of the GI tract and are also employed for the nonspecific treatment of diarrhea. Opiate drugs used for this purpose include codeine and the tincture and camphorated tincture of opium. Diphenoxylate and difenoxin are meperidine derivatives used specifically to control diarrhea, often in combination with anticholinergic agents. Loperamide, with a wider margin of safety than diphenoxylate, not only increases smooth muscle tone and decreases propulsion but possesses antisecretory activity as well.

Several compounds are used as protectants and adsorbents in the GI tract. Their function is to adsorb ingested or bacterial toxins produced in the gut, thus preventing or reducing systemic absorption of the toxins. They also provide a coating of the intestinal mucosa that protects the mucosal surface from irritating substances. There is some indication that adsorbents, when administered in conjunction with other drugs such as the antimicrobial agents, may adsorb a portion of the dose, thereby reducing the effectiveness of the antimicrobial therapy. Compounds commonly used as GI adsorbents and protectants are activated attapulgite, kaolin, magnesium trisilicate, activated charcoal, pectins, and salts of bismuth or magnesium. The subsalicylate salt may be especially beneficial because of an antiprostaglandin and thus antisecretory action.

Gastrointestinal astringents precipitate proteins, alter surface characteristics, and form a protective layer on the GI epithelium. The metallic astringents are rarely used today, but astringents of plant origin, such as tannic acid and catechu, remain useful adjuncts in antidiarrheal therapeutic regimens. Catechu is preferable to tannic acid because the slow release of catechutannic acid in the gut reduces its toxicity.

Secretion-inhibiting drugs are used in combination with adsorbents and antibiotics in order to reduce secretion, particularly in the neonatal diarrheic syndromes caused by enterotoxin-producing bacteria. Anticholinergic agents do not inhibit enterotoxin-induced secretion, but several types of drugs do possess this capability. Examples include nonsteroidal anti-inflammatory drugs (such as flunixin meglumine, salicylates, and indomethacin), chlorpromazine, methylprednisilone and loperamide.

A wide variety of antimicrobial agents are used for the treatment of bacterial enteritis (see Antimicrobial Therapy). Medication may be administered in the drinking water, added to feed, or given as individual treatments in the form of boluses and capsules. Several chemotherapeutic agents will also achieve therapeutic levels in the GI tract following parenteral administration. Gram-negative bacteria are common bacterial pathogens of the GI tract; therefore, agents that possess gram-negative activity should be given primary consideration for therapeutic use. The most rational selection, however, should be based on culture and sensitivity test results. Ampicillin, aminoglycosides, tetracyclines, sulfonamides, nitrofurans, and the quinolines have been widely used for the treatment of GI bacterial infections. Carbadox and virginamycin are also available as feed additives for the control of swine dysentery.

Although the benefits of microbial enteric modifiers remain obtuse, it seems that in certain refractory enteritis cases, oral use of lactic acid–producing organisms does promote recovery. Cultures of *Lactobacillus acidophilus* and *L. bulgaris* are most commonly employed. These organisms may produce an unfavorable pH in the GI tract for offending pathogens or may successfully compete with them for available nutrients. *L. bulgaricus* also has been shown to exercise specific anti-enterotoxin activity.

INTERNAL PARASITICIDES

Probably the most common requirement for GI therapy is the prevention or treatment of internal parasites. Anthelmintic therapy is reviewed in length in the next article.

Supplemental Reading

Booth, N. H., and McDonald, L. E. (eds.): Veterinary Pharmacology and Therapeutics, 5th ed. Ames, Iowa, Iowa State University Press, 1982.
Brander, G. C., Pugh, D. M., and Bywater, R. J.: Veterinary Applied Pharmacology and Therapeutics, 4th ed. London, Bailliere Tindall, 1982.

Anthelmintic Therapy*

JOHN W. PAUL, D.V.M., M.S.

Efficacy of an anthelmintic drug is determined by two types of experimental procedures. First, effectiveness is determined by critical or controlled-critical tests in which experimental animals are necropsied at a specified period of time after drug treatment; the parasites remaining in the carcasses are compared either with those parasites passed prior to necropsy or with the parasitic burdens found in untreated (control) animals. Second, and less precise, anthelmintic efficacy is estimated by a qualitative and quantitative fecal examination for parasite eggs before and after drug treatment of the animal. In either case, it is incumbent upon the investigator to employ well-designed protocols for proper anthelmintic drug evaluation.

In spite of well-designed studies, a review of the literature reveals variability of activity for any given anthelmintic agent. Some of the factors that contribute to variation in anthelmintic drug action are as follows:

Stage of Parasite Development at Treatment Time. Not all anthelmintic drugs possess activity against immature stages of parasites, perhaps because (1) immature forms have different biochemical requirements or (2) they may be spared the effects of drug action because of their location in the host during tissue migration phases. In general, the newer benzimidazoles demonstrate high activity against immature as well as adult stages of most of the common nematode parasites.

Treatment during different phases of a parasitic infection may not yield true efficacy. For instance, administration of a placebo may appear effective during the declining phase of a self-limiting infection such as *Strongyloides westeri* of young foals. In a controlled study, treatment of this type of infection must be evaluated during the ascending phase of the parasitic infection.

Climatic Conditions. Climatic conditions favorable to parasites may lead to rapid reinfection, thereby causing difficulty with anthelmintic evaluation when performed on pasture. In addition, certain climatic conditions can induce hypobiotic or inhibited stages of some parasites. An example is that of inhibited early fourth stage larvae of *Ostertagia ostertagi,* which are refractory to most anthelmintics with the exception of some of the second-generation benzimidazoles.

Drug Metabolism and Kinetics. Differences in pharmacokinetics and metabolism of a given drug are known to vary between animal species; however, sufficient work has not been done to detect possible variation between individuals, which may in turn affect anthelmintic varia-

*Author's note: All statements made in this chapter are those of the author and do not reflect any position of the American Hoechst Corporation.

bility. Some anthelmintics are most effective when administered in low doses over a long period, owing, perhaps, to the kinetic pattern of certain drugs with short half-lives. Repeated treatment with low doses enhances exposure of the parasites to these drugs.

Physical Aspects of the Host. In ruminants, the reticular groove reflex may affect anthelmintic performance. Some anthelmintics appear to be more active when administered directly into the abomasum, a function of reticular groove closure. Anthelmintic activity of the newer benzimidazoles may be enhanced when they are delivered into the rumen, which serves as a drug reservoir, thus providing sustained release of the drug; however, this is only a hypothesis and more work needs to be performed in order to clarify this subject. Age and its influence on immune factors is another example of a physical characteristic of the host related to anthelmintic variability. Controlled experiments have clearly shown that newborn calves are more susceptible than older calves to induced parasitic infection.

Nutrition. The nutritional status of the host plays an important role in the establishment of parasitism and removal of those parasites. Studies conducted in animals with protein and iron deficiencies have demonstrated decreased anthelmintic effectiveness, which is probably due, at least in part, to impaired host-defense mechanisms.

Genetics. Modern knowledge of genetics has led to selective breeding of animals in an attempt to develop natural host resistance to parasitism. Some progress has been made in this respect, but much more work is needed. An excellent example of the interaction of genetic factors and anthelmintic drugs is seen in what appears to be individual sensitivity of sheep to haloxon, which may then affect toxicity. A genetically related esterase that is involved in detoxification of haloxon may be present or absent in sheep. The LD_{50} value for haloxon in sheep with the esterase was determined to be 11,392 mg/kg, whereas the corresponding value in sheep lacking the esterase was 765 mg/kg.

Parasite Resistance to Drugs. Drug resistance is a topic of current concern. Obviously, some parasites are innately resistant to certain drugs, because they may possess metabolic or biochemical characteristics not affected by the mode of action of a particular drug. However, emergence of drug-resistant strains of parasites previously susceptible to a given drug has been reported frequently. Drug-resistant strains of *Haemonchus* spp, *Trichostrongylus* spp, and *Ostertagia* spp in sheep have been reported in recent years with the benzimidazoles and even more recently with levamisole and morantel. To date, drug-resistant parasites of cattle have not been identified or documented. The difference of resistance patterns in parasites of sheep and cattle is not fully understood; however, the difference is possibly due to management systems and parasite control programs. Sheep are likely to be subjected to more intensive deworming procedures than cattle, resulting in greater drug pressure on the sheep parasites. A similar situation can be cited with drug-resistant small strongyles of horses, which are often subjected to repeated drug exposure. There is a need to better understand the mechanism of acquired drug resistance and to develop anthelmintic, management, and selective breeding programs to minimize the emergence of drug-resistant parasitic strains.

An appreciation of the preceding concepts is important to fully understand anthelmintic therapy as well as interpretation of reports in the literature on anthelmintic safety and efficacy. The remainder of this discussion is devoted to anthelmintics currently approved for use in food animals in the United States.

BENZIMIDAZOLES

Thiabendazole (Omnizole, TBZ, Thibenzole)*

Since its discovery in the early 1960's, thiabendazole has found widespread acceptance as a highly effective and safe broad-spectrum anthelmintic for the treatment of most of the major gastrointestinal nematodes of livestock. Thiabendazole is available in a variety of product forms, including suspension, paste, bolus, crumble, pellet, premix, and medicated concentrate.

Thiabendazole is approved for use in cattle, sheep, goats, and swine. In cattle, the recommended dosage of 66 mg/kg is indicated for the treatment of *Haemonchus* spp, *Trichostrongylus* spp, *Ostertagia* spp, and *Oesophagostomum radiatum*. A dose of 110 mg/kg is recommended for severe infections of the above parasites and for the control of *Cooperia* spp. Treatment may be repeated within 2 to 3 weeks if indicated. Milk from treated cows must be withheld from market for 96 hours after treatment. Cattle should not be treated within 3 days of slaughter.

A thiabendazole dosage of 44 mg/kg is recommended in sheep and goats for control of *Haemonchus* spp, *Trichostrongylus* spp, *Ostertagia* spp, *Cooperia* spp, *Nematodirus* spp, *Bunostomum* spp, *Strongyloides* spp, *Chabertia* spp, and *Oesophagostomum* spp. In goats with severe infections of these parasites, 66 mg/kg is recommended. Milk from dairy goats must be withheld from market for 96 hours; sheep and goats must be withheld from slaughter for 30 days after treatment.

Thiabendazole is approved for limited indications in swine. For baby pigs infected with *Strongyloides ransomi*, thiabendazole paste is recommended at a dosage of 62 to 83 mg/kg, with retreatment in 5 to 7 days if necessary. To aid in the prevention of *Ascaris suum*, thiabendazole is added to the feed at a level of 0.05 to 0.1 per cent per ton of feed for 2 weeks, and then at a level of 0.005 to 0.02 per cent per ton for 8 to 14 weeks. Pigs cannot be slaughtered for 30 days following treatment.

Thiabendazole is generally considered to be a very safe drug. A dose of nearly 20 times the therapeutic level has been shown to be safe even for debilitated and very young animals. Thiabendazole is safe to use in pregnant animals.

Fenbendazole (Panacur)†

Fenbendazole was approved for use in cattle in the United States in 1983. At a dosage of 5 mg/kg, fenbendazole is indicated for removal and control of adult *Haemonchus contortus*, *Ostertagia ostertagi*, *Trichostrongylus axei*, *Bunostomum phlebotomum*, *Nematodirus helvetianus*, *Cooperia* spp, *Trichostrongylus colubriformis*,

*Available from MSD AGVET, Division of Merck & Co., Inc., Rahway, NJ 07065.

†Available from American Hoechst Corporation, Animal Health Division, Somerville, NJ 08876.

Oesophagostomum radiatum, and the lungworm, *Dictyocaulus viviparus.* The same dosage is also highly effective against immature stages of most of the common nematodes of cattle, although this particular use is not approved at this time in the United States. At a dosage of 10 mg/kg, fenbendazole generally has excellent activity against inhibited fourth stage larvae of *Ostertagia ostertagi* (type II ostertagiasis) and the tapeworm *Moniezia* spp; these two uses are also not approved at this time.

Fenbendazole is available as a 10 per cent suspension and in a multidose 10 per cent paste cartridge for cattle. Cattle must not be slaughtered within 8 days following the last treatment. Because a withdrawal time in milk has not been established, fenbendazole should not be used in dairy cattle of breeding age.

For use in swine, fenbendazole was introduced to the United States in 1984 and is indicated for removal and control of *Ascaris suum* (large roundworm), *Oesophagostomum dentatum,* and *O. quadrispinulatum* (nodular worms), *Hyostrongylus rubidus* (small stomach worm), *Trichuris suis* (whipworm), immature and adult *Stephanurus dentatus* (kidney worm), and *Metastrongylus apri* (lungworm). The recommended dosage is 3 mg/kg daily for 3 consecutive days. Fenbendazole for swine is available as 4 per cent and 20 per cent premixes for use in complete feeds. There is no slaughter withdrawal time in pigs when this agent is used as directed.

Fenbendazole enjoys an exceptionally broad margin of safety; 100 times the recommended dose in cattle is not toxic. Because the drug is not teratogenic or embryotoxic, and because it has no deleterious effects upon sperm, fenbendazole can safely be used in all breeding animals. Fenbendazole has been administered concurrently with vaccinations, growth implants, and organophosphate treatments in cattle, without adverse effects. It has also been tested and found compatible when given concurrently with the commonly used feed additive antibiotics in swine.

Albendazole (Valbazen)*

Albendazole is available as an oral suspension for use in the United States and only under special conditions as an emergency investigational new animal drug for treatment of liver flukes in cattle and sheep. The drug is available only in certain states where liver fluke infection has been documented as a problem. The recommended dosage under the special emergency provision is 10 mg/kg for cattle and 7.5 mg/kg for sheep.

In one efficacy study with cattle naturally infected with *Fasciola hepatica,* albendazole was administered in different formulations, but all were given at the rate of 10 mg/kg. On the basis of necropsy findings, removal of adult flukes ranged from 87.1 to 98.6 per cent, whereas the range of immature fluke removal was 74.5 to 91.0 per cent. In sheep, a dosage of 7.6 mg/kg was 91 per cent effective against adult liver flukes.

Other conditions specified under the emergency use provisions require that animals not be treated within 180 days of slaughter; the drug is not to be used in animals intended for veal or in lactating animals producing milk for human consumption. Further restrictions include the warning that cows and ewes should not be treated during the first 45 days of pregnancy and that albendazole should not be used in combination with other anthelmintics, because albendazole has efficacy against parasites other than liver flukes. Indeed, when albendazole is administered to cattle and sheep at the doses stated previously, high efficacy against the common GI nematodes, lungworms, and tapeworms would be expected.

IMIDAZOTHIAZOLES

Levamisole (Ripercol-L,* Tramisol,* Levasole†)

Levamisole is the l-isomer of dl-tetramisole. Following its discovery in the late 1960's, levamisole has come to prominence as a broad-spectrum anthelmintic for use in food-producing animals and is approved for use in cattle, sheep, and swine. The drug is available as the phosphate salt for subcutaneous injection in cattle, as the hydrochloride salt in an oral gel for cattle, as oral boluses for cattle and sheep, and as a soluble powder for drenching cattle and sheep as well as for use in the drinking water of pigs. Levamisole resinate is available as a feed premix.

In cattle, levamisole is indicated for the removal of *Haemonchus* spp, *Trichostrongylus* spp, *Ostertagia* spp, *Cooperia* spp, *Nematodirus* spp, *Bunostomum* spp, *Oesophagostomum* spp, and the lungworm *Dictyocaulus viviparus.* At the recommended dosage of 8 mg/kg, levamisole is highly effective against the adult forms of these parasites but less effective in removal of the immature stages. Cattle treated with levamisole orally must not be slaughtered within 48 hours of treatment or within 7 days following subcutaneous injection. The drug is not to be used in dairy cattle of breeding age.

The bolus and soluble drench formulations of levamisole are approved for use in sheep and, at 8 mg/kg, are indicated for efficacious treatment of *Haemonchus* spp, *Trichostrongylus* spp, *Ostertagia* spp, *Nematodirus* spp, *Bunostomum* spp, *Oesophagostomum* spp, *Chabertia* spp, and *Dictyocaulus viviparus.* Sheep must be withheld from slaughter for 3 days after treatment.

When administered to swine in the drinking water or feed at the rate of 8 mg/kg, levamisole is indicated for removal of *Ascaris suum, Oesophagostomum* spp, *Strongyloides, Stephanurus,* and the lungworm *Metastrongylus.* A withdrawal period of 3 days must be observed after treatment with levamisole.

Levamisole has a much narrower margin of safety than thiabendazole and the other benzimidazoles. When the agent was administered orally to cattle and sheep at 3 times the recommended dosage, no adverse effects were observed. At 2 times the recommended dosage injected subcutaneously in cattle, slight muzzle foaming may occur, but it disappears within 1 hour. Five times the recommended dosage has been administered to swine without apparent adverse reactions. Occasional swelling may occur at the site of injection but will usually subside in 7 to 28 days. Salivation or muzzle foam may occasionally occur following oral administration to cattle and swine. The reaction will disappear within a short time. Levamisole is not contraindicated in pregnant animals.

*This drug is no longer available in the United States.

*Available from American Cyanamid, Princeton, NJ 08540.
†Available from Pitman-Moore, Inc., Washington Crossing, NJ 08560.

AVERMECTINS

Avermectins are a group of related agents that possess anthelmintic activity. They are produced by the soil microorganism *Streptomyces avermitilis* and, as such, are antibiotics. However, their antimicrobial potency is not significant.

Ivermectin (Ivomec)*

Ivermectin is a specific avermectin chosen for development for use in animals as a parasiticide. Its mechanism of action is to stimulate gamma-aminobutyric acid (GABA), which causes paralysis and slow death of the parasite. Depending on the particular parasite, complete kill may require several days or even a few weeks. GABA is a neuromuscular transmitter in many internal and some external parasites. Because tapeworms and liver flukes do not possess GABA, ivermectin has no effect on them. In the mammalian host, GABA is present only in the central nervous system. In the normal, healthy animal, foreign substances such as ivermectin do not cross the blood-brain barrier. The recommended dosage for cattle, 200 mcg/kg, is effective for the treatment and control of adults and fourth-stage larvae of *Ostertagia ostertagi* (also the inhibited fourth stage larvae), *O. lyrata*, *Haemonchus placei*, *Trichostrongylus axei*, *T. colubriformis*, *Cooperia oncophora*, *C. punctata*, *C. pectinata*, *Oesophagostomum radiatum*, *Nematodirus helvetianus* (adults only), and *N. spathiger* (adults only). The drug is also effective against the lungworm, *Dictyocaulus viviparus;* the parasitic stages of cattle grubs, *Hypoderma bovis* and *H. lineatum;* as well as the lice, *Linognathus vituli* and *Haematopinus eurysternus;* and scabies mites, *Psoroptes ovis* and *Sarcoptes scabiei var. bovis.*

Ivomec is available as a 1 per cent solution for subcutaneous injection in cattle only. The product is not for intramuscular or intravenous injection. Doses greater than 10 ml should be divided between two injection sites to reduce the potential for injection site reaction. Each ml of Ivomec per 110 lbs (50 kg) body weight will provide the recommended dose of 200 mcg/kg. To reduce the potential of injection site infections, use of sterile equipment and disinfection of the injection site is recommended. Clients should be instructed to observe treated cattle for injection site reactions, which may consist of swelling and discomfort or may progress to clostridial infection requiring aggressive antibiotic therapy. As with any grubicide, proper timing of treatment is necessary to avoid killing the grubs when they are located in tissues surrounding the esophagus or in the vertebral canal. In safety studies, toxic signs appeared with doses exceeding 30 times the recommended dose. The recommended dose did not affect breeding performance in bulls or cows.

Cattle must not be treated with Ivomec within 35 days of slaughter. Because a withdrawal time has not been established in milk, this agent should not be used in female dairy cattle of breeding age. Ivermectin binds to soil and is inactivated over time. Free ivermectin may adversely affect fish and certain water-borne organisms; contamination of lakes, streams, and ponds should be avoided.

TETRAHYDROPYRIMIDINES

Pyrantel (Banminth)*

Pyrantel, a tetrahydropyrimidine, was discovered in the mid-1960's. In the United States, pyrantel tartrate is approved for use only as a swine premix.

Pyrantel tartrate is recommended for addition to the ration of swine at the rate of 800 mg/ton (22 mg/kg) as a single treatment for the removal and control of *Ascaris suum* and *Oesophagostomum* spp. It is also recommended for addition to the ration at the rate of 96 gm/ton (2.6 mg/kg) for a 3-day treatment to remove and control *A. suum;* this dosage is most commonly employed in a continuous feeding program to aid in the prevention of migration and establishment of *A. suum* as well as the prevention of *Oesophagostomum* spp. Pigs may not be slaughtered within 24 hours after treatment. When pyrantel is fed in combination with carbadox to swine up to 34 kg, the withdrawal period is 10 weeks.

Pyrantel is a moderately safe drug, with a safety margin of approximately 7 times the therapeutic dose. The drug should be used with caution in severely debilitated animals. Pyrantel does have some cholinergic activity; however, there is no clinical evidence to show that it should not be used with other cholinergic drugs. The drug is safe to use during the growth phase and during pregnancy.

Morantel (Rumatel, Nematel)*

The tartrate salt of morantel, an analog of pyrantel, is commercially available for use in cattle as an oral bolus or medicated premix. The premix is added to complete feeds to provide 0.968 mg/100 kg of morantel tartrate. It should not be mixed in feeds containing bentonite. At the approved dosage of 4.4 mg/lb. (9.68 mg/kg), mature forms of *Haemonchus* spp, *Ostertagia* spp, *Trichostrongylus* spp, *Cooperia* spp, *Nematodirus* spp, and *Oesophagostomum radiatum* are effectively removed.

Morantel tartrate is considered a very safe drug. The LD_{50} in mice is 5 gm/kg, compared with 170 mg/kg for the related compound, pyrantel tartrate. The user of morantel is cautioned to consult a veterinarian before treating severely debilitated animals and not to use the drug in dairy cows of breeding age. Cattle treated with morantel are not to be slaughtered within 14 days after treatment.

HYGROMYCIN

Hygromycin B (Hygromix)†

Hygromycin B, an antibiotic produced by a fermentation process, possesses limited anthelmintic activity. It exerts its action by elimination of egg production by female worms and has a cumulative lethal effect against adult worms. This drug is aproved for use in swine in the United States but is not approved for use in ruminants. Hygromycin B is available for use as a premix.

For the control of *Ascaris suum, Oesophagostomum*

---

*Available from MSD AGVET, Division of Merck & Co., Inc., Rahway, NJ 07065.

*Available from Pfizer, Inc., New York, NY 10017.
†Available from Elanco Products Co., Indianapolis, IN 46206.

spp, and *Trichuris suis* in swine, hygromycin B is added to the complete feed at the rate of 12 gm/ton. The medicated feed is given to sows continuously for 8 weeks, beginning 3 weeks prior to farrowing, and fed continuously to the pigs for the first 6 months of life or up to 100 to 120 lbs. Swine may not be slaughtered for 48 hours after withdrawal of hygromycin B. When hygromycin B is fed to swine in combination with chlortetracycline or tylosin, the withdrawal period is 15 days.

The only known toxic manifestation of hygromycin B is impaired hearing, which appears to be reversible upon withdrawal of the drug.

ORGANOPHOSPHOROUS COMPOUNDS

Coumaphos (Baymix)*

Coumaphos is approved for use in dairy and beef cattle. This organophosphate is commercially available as crumbles for feed top-dressing at the rate of 2 mg/kg daily for 6 consecutive days. A premix is also available for addition to complete feeds at the same dosage, which can be achieved by supplying coumaphos at 0.200 gm/100 kg/day for 6 consecutive days.

At the recommended dosage, coumaphos is indicated for the control of adult *Haemonchus* spp, *Trichostrongylus* spp, *Ostertagia* spp, *Cooperia* spp, and *Nematodirus* spp. Treatment may be repeated at 30-day intervals if required. There are no withdrawal requirements for coumaphos for either slaughter or milk.

Doses of coumaphos at 4 to 5 times the recommended level have been fed to cows without harmful effects, and it is safe to use in pregnant animals. The drug is contraindicated in cattle that are stressed or under 3 months of age. Coumaphos should not be administered with other cholinesterase-inhibiting chemicals nor within a few days before or after treatment with those compounds. Coumaphos should not be added to feed containing phenothiazine. Feeds containing coumaphos should not be pelleted.

Dichlorvos (Atgard, XLP-30)†

The organophosphorous drug dichlorvos (DDVP) is formulated in a polyvinyl chloride resin that adds stability to and delays release of the drug, hence reducing its toxicity. Within the food-producing animal group, dichlorvos is approved for use only in swine. The resin pellets of dichlorvos are available as two formulations: Atgard is a litter-pack intended to be added to the ration at time of use; Atgard-C provides added stability that is suitable for bulk manufacture of feeds containing dichlorvos.

Dichlorvos is indicated for the removal and control of the following adult and immature swine parasites: *Ascaris suum, Oesophagostomum* spp, *Trichuris suis,* and *Ascarops strongylina.* Dichlorvos (Atgard-C) may be mixed in the feed at the rate of 348 gm/ton and given for 2 consecutive days. For a single treatment, 479 grams of dichlorvos (Atgard-C) is mixed with 1 ton of feed. For pregnant sows, dichlorvos (XLP-30) is mixed with the

feed at the rate of 334 to 500 gm/ton and given for the last 30 days of gestation to provide 1 gram of dichlorvos per head daily. Dichlorvos (Atgard), when added to the feed and administered shortly after mixing, achieves a dosage of approximately 17 mg/kg as a single treatment that may be repeated in 4 to 5 weeks if required. There are no withholding requirements for slaughter of pigs treated with dichlorvos.

Dichlorvos is generally quite safe in swine. Transient softening of the stools may be expected in approximately 4 per cent of treated animals. At high doses, typical signs of organophosphorus toxicosis can be expected. The LD_{50} for the polyvinyl chloride resin formulation of dichlorvos in pigs is approximately 2500 mg/kg, compared with 300 to 500 mg/kg for unformulated dichlorvos. Scouring pigs should not be treated with dichlorvos. This agent should not be used in conjunction with other cholinesterase inhibitors. When dichlorvos is mixed with complete feeds, the feeds must not be pelleted and must remain dry. Poultry should not be allowed access to feed containing dichlorvos or to feces of treated swine.

Haloxon (Halox, Loxon)*

In the early 1960's, the organophosphate compound haloxon was discovered. Haloxon is approved in the United States for use in cattle only. It is available as a bolus or as a powder to be added to water for drenching.

Haloxon may be administered as the bolus or drench at the rate of 35 to 50 mg/kg and is indicated for control of *Haemonchus, Ostertagia, Trichostrongylus,* and *Cooperia.* Treatment should be repeated in 3 to 4 weeks for most effective results. Dairy animals of breeding age must not be treated with haloxon, and cattle must be withheld from slaughter for 1 week after treatment.

Haloxon is relatively safe in cattle, with a therapeutic index of approximately 5; however, in sheep, toxicity can be quite variable owing to a genetic trait of that species. Those sheep possessing esterase A are capable of metabolizing haloxon and are able to tolerate high doses of the drug. Conversely, sheep deficient in esterase A are susceptible to neurotoxic effects of haloxon and may develop posterior paralysis, anorexia, or diarrhea or may die. The drug is no longer approved for use in sheep and goats because of this toxic potential. Haloxon is safe to use in pregnant animals. As with all organophosphates, haloxon should not be used with other cholinesterase inhibitors.

PHENOTHIAZINE†

Phenothiazine was first used as an anthelmintic in the late 1930's and has been used extensively since that time; however, with the introduction of thiabendazole and, later, levamisole, the use of phenothiazine has abated. Phenothiazine powder is available for mixing in the feed or adding to water as a drench. Micronized phenothiazine is more efficacious but also tends to be more toxic, owing to more complete absorption of the drug from the gastrointestinal tract. Parasite resistance to phenothiazine has been recognized for several years.

*Available from Bayvet-Cutter, Shawnee Mission, KS 66201.

†Available from SDS Biotech Corp., Animal Health Business, Painesville, OH 44077.

*Available from Wellcome—Animal Health Division, Kansas City, MO 64141.

†Generic brands are available.

In cattle, phenothiazine is highly effective against susceptible strains of adult *Haemonchus* and *Oesophagostomum* but is less effective against *Ostertagia, Trichostrongylus axei,* and *Chabertia* with a single dose of 10 gm/45 kg. A dose of 20 gm/45 kg (10 gm/kg if micronized) is required to effect removal of *Bunostomum*. A continuous daily dose of 2 gm/cow helps control gastrointestinal nematodes partly by the larvicidal and ovicidal action of phenothiazine in the feces. The drug must not be administered to lactating dairy cows or within 4 days of slaughter.

Phenothiazine is used as a drench in sheep and goats, at the rate of 12.5 gm per animal weighing 11 to 27 kg or 25 gm per animal over 27 kg for removal of susceptible strains of adult *Haemonchus, Oesophagostomum, Ostertagia, Trichostrongylus axei, Bunostomum,* and *Chabertia*. Phenothiazine is also added to the feed of sheep at 1 gm/head/day on a continuous basis for the control of these parasites. The drug must not be given to lactating dairy goats or to sheep or goats within 4 days of slaughter.

Phenothiazine is seldom used in swine because of its very narrow spectrum (only *Oesophagostomum*) and the high susceptibility of swine to toxic effects of the drug.

The toxicity of phenothiazine varies among species. Sheep and goats tolerate phenothiazine quite well, cattle are more susceptible, and swine are highly susceptible. There appears to be an individual sensitivity to phenothiazine. The risk of intoxication increases in debilitated and, especially, anemic animals. Hemolytic anemia is the usual toxic manifestation of phenothiazine. Phenothiazine also plays a role in the induction of photosensitivity, which is manifest when the animal is subsequently exposed to bright sunlight; it is a problem in calves but may also affect goats and sheep. In sheep (and, to some extent, cattle) deprived of water, phenothiazine can cause a fatal renal papillary necrosis. Phenothiazine should not be administered to pregnant animals during the last 4 weeks of pregnancy nor used in conjunction with organophosphates. The maximum recommended total dose for cattle is 80 gm, or 60 gm of micronized phenothiazine.

PIPERAZINE*

Piperazine has been recognized for its anthelmintic properties for over 30 years. There are several salts of piperazine, including adipate, citrate, hydrochloride, phosphate, sulfate, and tartrate. The salt derivatives have stability and solubility advantages over the base. Efficacy of the piperazine salts is similar, provided that the dose is calculated according to the activity of the base content. Piperazine is available as powders and premixes for mixing with the feed as well as solutions for treatment of the drinking water.

Because of its very limited spectrum against the common parasites of ruminants, piperazine is not used to any great extent in cattle or sheep.

As a swine anthelmintic, piperazine is moderately effective in the control of *Ascaris suum* and *Oesophagostomum* with a single dose of 110 mg/kg. Herd treatment is accomplished with 0.2 to 0.4 per cent piperazine in the feed or 0.1 to 0.2 per cent in the drinking water. All medicated feed or water should be consumed in 8 to 12

hours; therefore, fasting and/or withholding water overnight may be useful prior to treatment. Retreatment is recommended after 2 months. Drug withdrawal times have not been established for swine.

Piperazine enjoys a wide margin of safety even in very young animals; it is also safe to use during pregnancy.

Supplemental Reading

Georgi, J. R.: Parasitology for Veterinarians, 3rd ed. Philadelphia, W. B. Saunders Company, 1980.
Jones, L. M., et al. (eds.): Veterinary Pharmacology and Therapeutics, 4th ed. Ames, Iowa, Iowa State University Press, 1977.

External Parasiticides

JAMES A. SHMIDL, D.V.M., M.S.,
JOHN O. MOZIER, D.V.M.,
and DALLAS L. NELSON, D.V.M., Ph.D.

External parasiticides are compounds used in the control of insects or arachnids (mites, ticks, etc.). They are more commonly referred to as animal insecticides. External parasiticides are normally used on food-producing animals (1) to treat severe infestations that result in clinical disease; (2) to increase production of meat and other products of animal origin; and (3) to stop or prevent the spread of insect- or arachnid-borne disease.

BOTANICAL AND CHLORINATED HYDROCARBON COMPOUNDS

The first products that were used for the control of external parasites of food-producing animals were of plant origin. Examples of such botanical compounds are rotenone, nicotine, and natural pyrethrin. These compounds had limited application and usefulness. The first highly effective compounds were the chlorinated hydrocarbon compounds such as DDT and toxaphene. The development of the chlorinated hydrocarbon insecticides coincided with the beginning of what is considered to be the modern era of agriculture. At that time there was a great increase in agricultural productivity. Humanity was no longer at the mercy of parasitic pests affecting domestic plants or animals. The chlorinated hydrocarbon insecticides were highly effective insecticides, but they had some serious shortcomings. They were highly persistent because they were usually chemically stable and degraded very slowly in the environment. In addition, a stable body residue developed in exposed organisms. With some compounds there was an interesting phenomenon termed biologic magnification. Biologic magnification, which led to harmful consequences in the environment, was the result of a residue in the lowest or the first organism in the food chain. For example, an aquatic insect that has a residue is eaten by a fish, which is consumed by a larger fish, which is eaten by a bird. Each succeeding species accumulates a greater body residue than the organism that it consumed. In some cases this process has resulted in a toxicologic manifestation in the species at the top of the food chain. An additional problem with chlorinated hydrocarbons was that even after years of extensive study, their toxic mode of action was poorly understood, and there were no effective antidotes.

*Generic brands are available.

ORGANOPHOSPHOROUS AND CARBAMATE COMPOUNDS

The subsequent discovery and development of organophosphorus and carbamate compounds gave the agriculturist and veterinarian very effective tools for the control of pests on plants or animals. These compounds are said to be systemic in action, i.e., the compound will be translocated in the body of the plant or animal. This characteristic allows the dermal application of an organophosphorus compound to control a parasite in a remote anatomic location. The most important toxic mode of action of both carbamate and organophosphorus compounds is cholinesterase depression. Both classes of compounds are in general more acutely toxic than the chlorinated hydrocarbon compounds. Atropine is an effective antidote for both organophosphorus and carbamate parasiticides. The oxime compound 2-PAM, in combination with atropine, is effective for treating intoxication by the organophosphorus compounds. The carbamates and organophosphorus compounds are rather unstable after application and do not magnify in the environment. They are rapidly metabolized and eliminated from the body. Some of the more recently developed external parasiticide compounds are synthetically derived pyrethroid compounds. They are more highly effective and economic than the pyrethrins of plant origin.

AVERMECTINS

The newest animal parasiticides that have been developed are the avermectin family of compounds. They have a broad spectrum of activity against both internal and external parasites. These compounds were isolated from the fermentation of the soil organism *Streptomyces avermitilis* and have a neurotoxic action on the parasite. At the time of this writing, registration in the United States has been granted for the use of avermectins in cattle and horses. The compound ivermectin is registered for use in several countries and has been shown to be very effective in the control of both internal and external parasites. Among the external parasites it controls are grubs, lice, and mites.

PARASITICIDE USE

Modern chemistry has given the veterinarian highly effective external parasiticides, but it is very important that they be used according to the label recommendations. The product should be used solely on the animal species for which it is labeled, and only the prescribed dose should be applied for the specific parasite infestation for which the product is labeled. The use of animal medications has had some unfavorable publicity because of illegal residues in human food. When examining a label, one must pay strict attention to the time after treatment during which milk cannot be saved for human consumption or animals may not be slaughtered for food. To adhere to all label recommendations is the professional responsibility of every veterinarian who uses or recommends the use of an animal medication. Often a veterinarian finds a product labeled for the control of a parasite on one species of animal when the same parasite may infest other host species. The product should not be used on a host species for which there is no label recommendation. There could be several reasons for the lack of label recommendations, including a lack of residue data, too high a residue of the compound or its metabolites in the host, and an insufficient safety margin between safe and harmful doses. Different products have different safety factors. In any occurrence of toxicity associated with an external parasiticide, there is usually a history of accidental exposure or use contrary to label directions. Veterinarians are often required to make difficult clinical decisions when they encounter a severe infestation that is causing a pathologic condition in host animals and often is complicated by adverse climatic conditions. A product and method of application must be selected that will control the parasite without causing undue stress to the host animal. The products that are available as external parasiticides for use on food animals have all been reviewed and approved by a governmental agency to ensure that the product is effective as labeled, is safe to the host species, and will not result in an unacceptable residue.

Treatment

Active ingredients (carbamate or organophosphorus compounds) have been formulated into a number of products for application by several treatment methods. These include the following approaches.

"Pour-on" products are formulated in a dilute solution so that they may be poured down the back of the animal. They are easy to use and have become a popular method for treating cattle for grubs (*Hypoderma* spp). Some of these products are also approved for control of cattle and swine lice.

The low-volume products such as SPOTTON* (brand of fenthion) and Dursban† (brand of chloropyrifos) are formulated with a higher concentration of active compound than the "pour-on" products. They are also applied to the skin of the backs of cattle. They are easy to apply, and their spectrum of activity is similar to that of "pour-on" products.

Solutions for a dip vat and the whole-body spray applied with a high-pressure sprayer have similar uses, advantages, and disadvantages. These treatment methods are effectively used for ticks, flies, grubs, lice, and mange control. The dip vat is a very effective application method and is widely used in cattle feedlot operations. Whole-body sprays, although still used, are not as popular as they were in earlier times. The main disadvantage of both treatment methods is the question of their use during severe cold weather.

The backrubber is one of the oldest "self-treatment" methods used for applying parasiticides to cattle or hogs. There are several types on the market. This application method has several advantages, among which is ease of application, because infested animals tend to seek out and use a rubber. The disadvantage of the backrubber is that it must be serviced regularly to ensure proper dispensing of the parasiticide.

Dust bags have generally the same advantages as the backrubber but are usually more effective because they require less servicing and dispense the parasiticide more consistently when used by cattle. The dust bags are especially effective for horn fly and lice control, and their

Text continued on page 51

---

*Available from Haver Laboratories, Shawnee, KS 66201.
†Available from Fort Dodge Laboratories, Fort Dodge, IA 50501.

Table 1. Some Common Products Used For External Parasite Control on Cattle

Product	Company and Address	Marketed Formulation	Pest	Method of Application	Withdrawal Period Prior to Slaughter (Days)	Comments
Chlorpyrifos Dursban	Fort Dodge Laboratories, Fort Dodge, IA 50501	Low-volume pour-on	Lice and horn flies	Backline treatment	14 (after initial treatment)	Read precautions statement.
Coumaphos All formulations	Bayvet Division of Miles Laboratories, P.O. Box 390, Shawnee Mission, KS 66201	Wettable powder	Horn flies, lice, ticks, grubs, screw-worms, and mites	Spray or dip	0	Treat lactating dairy cattle only at lower dilution.
		Flowable	Horn flies, lice, ticks, screw-worms, and mites	Spray or dip	0	Treat lactating dairy cattle only at lower dilution.
		Liquid	Horn flies, face flies, lice, ticks, and grubs	Spray or backrubber	0	Treat lactating dairy cattle only at lower dilution.
		Pour-on	Grubs	Backline treatment	0	Do not treat lactating dairy cattle.
		Dust (1%)	Horn flies and lice	Dust bag or shaker can	0	Apply no more than 2 oz. per animal per day.
		Dust (5%)	Screw-worms and ear ticks	Spot treatment	0	Treat wounds with light, but thorough coverage.
		Spray foam	Screw-worms, fly maggots, and ear ticks	Aerosol spray	0	Spray wound until complete coverage is obtained.
Crotoxyphos/dichlorvos Ciovap	SDS Biotech Corporation, 1100 Superior Avenue, Cleveland, OH 44114	Liquid	Horn flies, face flies, stable flies, lice, ticks, and mites	Spray or backrubber	0	Repeat as necessary, but not more than once weekly.
Simax	Zoecon Corporation, 12200 Denton Drive, Dallas, TX 75234	Liquid	Horn flies, face flies, stable flies, lice, ticks, and mites	Spray, backrubber, or pour-on	0	Repeat as necessary, but not more than once weekly.
Dioxathion Delnav	Anchor Laboratories, St. Joseph, MO 64502	Liquid	Horn flies, lice, and ticks	Spray or backrubber	0	Do not use more than every 2 weeks.
Del-Tox	Burroughs Wellcome Co., Kansas City, MO 64108	Liquid	Horn flies, lice and ticks	Spray, dip, pour-on, or backrubber	0	Do not use on dairy animals.
Dioxathion/dichlorvos Lintox-D	Zoecon Corporation, 12200 Denton Drive, Dallas TX 75234	Liquid	Horn flies, lice, and ticks	Spray, dip, or backrubber	0	Do not use on dairy animals.
Dichlorvos Vapona	SDS Biotech Corporation, 1100 Superior Avenue, Cleveland, OH 44114	Liquid	Horn flies, face flies, stable flies, and house flies	Spray	0	Do not exceed 2 oz. per animal daily as a fine-mist spray.
Famphur Warbex	American Cyanamid Co., P.O. Box 400, Princeton, NJ 08540	Pour-on	Grubs and lice	Backline treatment	35	Do not treat lactating dairy cattle or within 21 days of freshening. Do not treat Brahman bulls.
Fenthion Spotton	Bayvet Division of Miles Laboratories, P.O. Box 390, Shawnee Mission, KS 66201	Low-volume pour-on	Grubs and lice	Backline treatment	45	Do not treat dairy cattle of breeding age.

Product	Manufacturer	Formulation	Controls	Application	Days to slaughter	Comments
Tiguvon	Same	Pour-on	Grubs and lice	Backline treatment	35 (single treatment)	Do not treat lactating dairy cattle.
Lysoff	Same	Pour-on concentrate	Lice and horn flies	Backline treatment	21 (single treatment)	Dilute with water prior to use. Do not treat lactating dairy cattle within 28 days of freshening.
Fenvalerate	SDS Biotech Corporation, 1100 Superior Avenue, Cleveland, OH 44114 (and others)	Ear Tags	Horn flies, face flies, and ticks	Attach to ear	0	Remove tags before slaughter.
Lindane — Linspray	Norden Laboratories, Lincoln, NB 68501	Liquid	Horn flies, lice, and ticks	Spray or dip	30 (spray), 60 (dip)	Do not apply to dairy cattle.
Lindex	Tech America, P.O. Box 338, Elwood, KS 66024	Pressurized spray	Screw-worms, blow flies, and ear ticks	Direct application	0	Do not use on dairy cattle.
		Powder	Horn flies and lice	Direct application	0	Read directions for treating dairy cattle.
Malathion	Salsbury Laboratories, Charles City, IA 50616	Liquid	Horn flies, lice, and ticks	Spray or backrubber	0	Do not treat dairy cattle.
Methoprene	Moorman's Manufacturing Co., Quincy, IL 62310	Mineral mix	Horn flies	Mixed with feed	0	Daily in feed.
Methoxychlor/malathion	Anchor Laboratories, St. Joseph, MO 64502	Dust	Horn flies, lice, and ticks	Direct application	0	Read directions for use in dairy animals.
Permethrin — Ectiban	ICI Americas Inc., Wilmington, DE 19897 (and others)	Ear tags, tape, or strips	Horn flies, face flies, and ticks; aids in control of stable flies	Attach to ear	0	Remove before slaughter.
Permectrin	Anchor Laboratories, St. Joseph, MO 64502	Liquid	Horn flies, face flies, stable flies, horse flies, lice, ticks, and mites	Spray	14	Retreat not more than once every 2 weeks.
Phosmet — Prolate	Zoecon Corporation, 12200 Denton Drive, Dallas TX 75234	Liquid	Grubs, lice, horn flies, ticks, and mites	Spray, dip, or pour-on	21	For use on beef cattle only.
Lintox	Same	Dust	Horn flies and lice	Dust bags or hand-dusting	0	1 oz. per adult animal.
Stirofos — Rabon	SDS Biotech Corporation, 1100 Superior Avenue, Cleveland, OH 44114	Wettable powder	Horn flies, lice, and ticks	Spray	0	Do not treat dairy cattle.
		Oral larvacide premix	Horn flies, face flies, horse flies, and stable flies	Mixed into feed	0	Mix uniformly into cattle feed ration.
		Dust	Horn flies and lice; aids in control of face flies	Dust bag or shaker can	0	Apply 2 oz. per animal per treatment.
Trichlorfon — Neguvon	Bayvet Division of Miles Laboratories, P.O. Box 390, Shawnee Mission, KS 66201	Pour-on	Grubs and lice	Backline treatment	21	Do not treat lactating dairy cattle or within 7 days of freshening.
Pour-On Cattle Insecticide	Tech America, P.O. Box 338, Elwood, KS 66024	Pour-on	Grubs and lice	Backline treatment	21	Do not treat lactating dairy cattle or within 7 days of freshening.

Table 2. Some Common Products Used For External Parasite Control on Sheep and Goats

Product	Company and Address	Marketed Formulation	Pest	Method of Application	Withdrawal Period Prior to Slaughter (Days)	Comments
Coumaphos						
All formulations	Bayvet Division of Miles Laboratories, P.O. Box 390, Shawnee Mission, KS 66201	Wettable powder	Lice, ticks, horn flies, screw-worms, fleeceworms, and keds; mites in sheep only	Spray or dip	15	Do not treat lactating dairy goats.
		Dust	Screw-worms and ear ticks	Spot treatment	0	Dust into the infested wound or ear.
		Spray Foam	Screw-worms and fly maggots	Aerosol spray	0	Spray wounds until complete coverage is obtained.
Crotoxyphos/dichlorvos						
Ciovap	SDS Biotech Corporation, 1100 Superior Avenue, Cleveland, OH 44114	Liquid	Lice, ticks, and mites	Spray	0	Repeat as necessary, but not more often than every 7 days.
Simax	Zoecon Corporation, 12200 Denton Drive, Dallas, TX 75234	Liquid	Lice and ticks	Spray	0	Repeat as necessary, but not more often than once weekly.
Dioxathion						
Delnav	Anchor Laboratories, St. Joseph, MO 64502	Liquid	Lice, ticks, horn flies, keds, and wool maggots	Spray or dip	0	Treat as required, but not more often than every 2 weeks.
Dioxathion/dichlorvos						
Lintox-D	Zoecon Corporation, 12200 Denton Drive, Dallas, TX 75234	Liquid	Lice, keds, and wool maggots	Spray or dip	0	Wet thoroughly.
Lindane						
Linspray	Norden Laboratories, Lincoln, NB 68501	Liquid	Ticks and mites	Spray	30	No label directions for goats.
Lindex	Tech America, P.O. Box 338, Elwood, KS 66024	Pressurized spray	Screw-worms, fleeceworms, and ear ticks	Direct application	0	Treat wound thoroughly.
Malathion	Salsbury Laboratories, Charles City, IA 50616	Dust	Lice and keds	Dust application	0	Not for use in dairy goats.
Methoxychlor/malathion	Anchor Laboratories, St. Joseph, MO 64502	Dust	Lice and keds	Dust or powder duster	0	Do not apply to lactating goats.
Permethrin						
Permectrin	Anchor Laboratories, St. Joseph, MO 64502	Liquid	Lice, ticks, and blowflies	Spray	14	No label directions for goats.

Table 3. Some Common Products Used For External Parasite Control on Swine

Product	Company and Address	Marketed Formulation	Pest	Method of Application	Withdrawal Period Prior to Slaughter (Days)	Comments
Coumaphos All formulations	Bayvet Division of Miles Laboratories, P.O. Box 390, Shawnee Mission, KS 66201	Wettable powder	Lice, ticks, horn flies, and screw-worms	Spray	0	Repeat as necessary.
		Liquid	Lice	Spray	0	Apply to complete wetting.
		Dust	Lice	Shaker can	0	Repeat as necessary, but not more than once every 10 days. Bedding may be treated.
		Spray foam	Screw-worms and fly maggots	Aerosol spray	0	Spray wounds until complete coverage is obtained.
Crotoxyphos/dichlorvos Simax	Zoecon Corporation, 12200 Denton Drive, Dallas, TX 75234	Liquid	Lice and ticks	Spray	0	Make second application in 14 days if needed.
Ciovap	SDS Biotech Corporation, 1100 Superior Avenue, Cleveland, OH 44114	Liquid	Lice and ticks	Spray	0	Repeat as necessary, but not more than once every 7 days.
Dioxathion Delnav	Anchor Laboratories, St. Joseph, MO 64502	Liquid	Lice, ticks, and horn flies	Spray or dip	0	Thoroughly wet animals.
Dioxathion/dichlorvos Lintox-D	Zoecon Corporation, 12200 Denton Drive, Dallas TX 75234	Liquid	Lice	Spray or backrubber	0	Do not treat sows less than 2 weeks before farrowing or while nursing.
Fenthion Tiguvon	Bayvet Division of Miles Laboratories, P.O. Box 390, Shawnee Mission, KS 66201	Ready-to-use pour-on	Lice	Pour-on	14	Pour uniformly along the animal's back.

Table continued on following page

Table 3. *Some Common Products Used For External Parasite Control on Swine* (Continued)

Product	Company and Address	Marketed Formulation	Pest	Method of Application	Withdrawal Period Prior to Slaughter (Days)	Comments
Lindane Linspray	Norden Laboratories, Lincoln, NB 68501	Liquid	Lice and mange	Spray	30	Do not treat sows less than 2 weeks before farrowing nor for at least 3 weeks after farrowing.
Malathion	Salsbury Laboratories, Charles City, IA 50616	Powder	Lice	Direct application	0	Use as individual treatment.
		Liquid	Lice and mites	Spray	0	Animal should be kept out of sun and wind for a few hours after spraying.
Methoxychlor/malathion	Anchor Laboratories, St. Joseph, MO 64502	Dust	Lice	Direct application	0	Repeat in 10 days or thereafter as needed.
Permethrin Permectrin	Anchor Laboratories, St. Joseph, MO 64502	Liquid	Lice, ticks, horn flies, and mites	Spray, paint, or dip	14	Retreat after 4–6 weeks.
Ectiban	ICI Americas Inc., Wilmington, DE 19897	Dust	Lice	Direct application	0	A second treatment in 14 days is recommended.
		Liquid	Lice and mites	Spray	5	Apply a second spray in 14 days.
Phosmet Lintox	Zoecon Corporation, 12200 Denton Drive, Dallas, TX 75234	Dust	Lice	Direct application	1	Repeat in 10 days as needed.
Stirofos Rabon	SDS Biotech Corporation, 1100 Superior Avenue, Cleveland, OH 44114	Wettable powder	Lice	Spray	0	Repeat in 2 weeks if necessary.

use has grown in recent years. They may be hung where cattle are forced to dust themselves, such as in gateways to pastures, or they may be located where cattle congregate and use them at will.

The medicated ear tag is the most recent development. It has proved to be a very useful method for horn fly control, especially when continuous control is important, as in a herd of cattle. Approved insecticidal ear tags are purported to give season-long control.

Other methods of application, such as mist sprayers, foggers, and treadle sprayers, do not have wide application. They may be of use in special situations.

In determining what product or treatment method to use, several considerations need to be made. It is obvious that the treatment of choice should be effective in the control of the parasite, cause no untoward reaction in the host, and be easy to apply and economical to use. These several considerations are the reasons that so many products and methods of application have been developed.

Tables 1 to 3 list common products used for external parasite control on cattle, sheep, goats, and swine. The products are listed by common (generic) name and trade name when possible. These tables are not intended to be an all-inclusive listing of products for the noted indications, but only to be representative. The current label must be studied thoroughly, prior to the use of any external parasiticide, for specific use directions, safety considerations, and proper meat or milk withdrawal periods.

Anesthesia in Ruminants and Swine

JOHN C. THURMON, D.V.M., M.S., D.A.C.V.A., and G. J. BENSON, D.V.M., M.S., D.A.C.V.A.

Progress in the development of anesthetic agents, equipment, and techniques for ruminants and swine has been notoriously slow in the United States. Most advances in development of injectable agents have come from European countries or researchers using food-producing animals as models for development of surgical techniques that could eventually be employed in humans. With the advent of cardiac bypass and the subsequent use of ruminants for development of surgical techniques and equipment, safe general anesthetic techniques for calves have evolved.[1-6] Studies of the influence of selected anesthetic agents on maternal-fetal circulation[7-10] and of anesthetic requirements during pregnancy[11] have contributed a great deal to our understanding of maternal-fetal responses to anesthetic-related agents.

Although these methods offer relatively safe and reliable anesthesia for major surgical intervention, it must be emphasized that they are expensive and time consuming and require a large investment in equipment and are therefore not readily adaptable to field use. Nonetheless, it would be naive to imply that procedures requiring major surgical intervention (e.g., thoracic surgery, orthopedic surgery), can be safely performed when appropriate anesthetic agents and equipment are unavailable.

Owing to economic influences, most minor surgical procedures in food-producing animals are performed under field conditions, where local or regional analgesia or a brief period of general anesthesia is satisfactory. Because ruminants are docile by nature, they are rather easy to handle and restrain with proper equipment. Cattle will accept mechanical restraint (e.g., cattle chute, head catch, nose tongs) without inflicting severe injury upon themselves or their handlers. It is partly for this reason that local analgesic and mechanical restraint techniques have been highly developed and are widely employed in ruminants. Most field operations are completed using regional analgesia in cattle,[12] because local analgesics are economical and many surgical manipulations can be performed best with the animal in a standing position. Another factor contributing to the refinement of local analgesic techniques is the untoward physiologic alterations of respiratory and cardiovascular function in large ruminants placed in an unnatural postural position. These potential problems can be avoided when surgery is performed with the animal standing. Valuable animals requiring major procedures are generally transported to large animal hospitals, where appropriate facilities, equipment, and drugs are available.

The objective of this article is to review anesthetic techniques reported as satisfactory for use in ruminants and swine. Because of limited space, heavy emphasis is not placed on physiologic and pharmacologic responses to drugs. A number of well-written textbooks are available for those wishing greater detail.[13-16]

Relatively few anesthetic and anesthetic-related agents are currently approved for use in ruminants and swine, so we will review techniques employing nonapproved as well as approved drugs. Perhaps in the future some of the nonapproved agents will become legal for use in food-producing animals.

PHYSICAL CHARACTERISTICS OF RUMINANTS

When ruminants are restrained in either dorsal or lateral recumbency, their massive abdominal contents are shifted, placing pressure upon the major abdominal vessels and the diaphragm. This pressure may impede venous blood flow returning to the heart, resulting in decreases in cardiac output, blood pressure, and, ultimately, blood perfusion of tissue. In spite of these changes, blood pressure is reasonably well maintained in cows anesthetized with halothane in oxygen. Musewe and colleagues[17] have investigated the influence of sternal recumbency on ventilatory function in nonanesthetized adult cows. From their studies, they learned that in cows placed in sternal recumbency intraruminal and intrapleural pressures increased. The higher intraruminal pressure forced the diaphragm forward into the pleural cavity, increasing its length and decreasing pulmonary functional residual capacity. The cows responded to this functional insult by increasing tidal volume and by slowing and prolonging inspiration. These responses appeared in part to offset the functional embarrassment caused by increased intraruminal pressure and permitted the animals to maintain adequate pulmonary function. Rumen insufflation to a pressure of 40 torr caused a significant decrease in arterial oxygen and a significant increase in arterial carbon dioxide, thus illustrating the influence of increased intraruminal pressure on pulmonary function.[17] Hypoxemia and hypercapnia (causing respiratory acidemia) can become life-threatening in ruminants that are not properly prepared prior to long-term general anesthesia.

Clinical observations suggest that lateral or dorsal recumbency is more detrimental to pulmonary function than sternal recumbency. Abnormal positioning (lateral or dorsal recumbency) leads to mismatching of pulmonary ventilation and perfusion. Alterations in ventilation-perfusion are progressive, leading ultimately to right-to-left shunting of blood and hypoxemia. In addition, hypoventilation and hypercapnia can result because diaphragmatic excursion is limited by the weight of the abdominal contents. Deep sedation or general anesthesia enhance the insults to pulmonary function induced by abnormal body position through depression of the central nervous systems and of the muscles of respiration. Anesthetic-induced depression of the cardiovascular system decreases tissue perfusion.[1] Large quantities of ruminal gas are produced by the unfasted animal. Normally, these gases cannot be eructated when the animal is in lateral or dorsal recumbency. Thus, intraruminal pressure can become extremely high, further limiting diaphragmatic excursion and the animal's ability to breathe.

To a degree, these untoward cardiopulmonary alterations can be avoided by preanesthetic patient preparation, supplemental administration of oxygen, and mechanical ventilation. Availability and cost of equipment often precludes use of these measures. In cows breathing room air, given xylazine (0.22 mg/kg IM), and restrained in dorsal recumbency, we found arterial oxygen levels to be dangerously low (45–60 torr). Supplemental oxygen given by nasal tube (flow rate, 20–30 L/min) helped decrease hypoxemia. However, placing the animals in sternal position or returning them to a standing position was ultimately found to be the most effective means of correcting hypercapnia and hypoxemia.

ANESTHETIC HAZARDS

Regurgitation

In the anesthetized ruminant, regurgitation is common and of major concern.[18] It may be classified as either active or passive, with passive regurgitation also being referred to as "silent regurgitation." In light planes of anesthesia, active regurgitation is more likely to occur, whereas passive regurgitation is associated with deep surgical anesthesia. Active regurgitation, as the term implies, is characterized by explosive discharge of large quantities of ruminal ingesta. At the time of regurgitation, ruminal contents are frequently aspirated deep into the respiratory passages. Massive amounts reaching the smaller airways often initiate acute bronchial constriction, hypoxia, and finally asphyxiation. If the animal does not succumb to asphyxia, the subsequent development of progressive foreign body pneumonia (in spite of all therapeutic measures) is a real possibility. The successful outcome of aspiration pneumonia probably depends more on the amount and pH of foreign material aspirated than on methods or drugs employed in treating it. Bronchospasm occurring at the time of aspiration may be treated with bronchodilators. Aminophylline (2–4 mg/kg) injected slowly intravenously (over a 5-minute period) may be helpful. A more rapid rate of administration causes myocardial stimulation, accompanied by increased oxygen requirements.[19] Suction may be employed for aspirate

removal, but because of particulate size and aspiration into the deep recesses of the respiratory passages, suction has not proved to be of much value. Oxygen should be administered by mask or nasal tube. If the animal survives the acute stages of aspiration, corticosteroid and broad-spectrum antibiotic therapy may be helpful. To decrease the likelihood of regurgitation, the following measures have been advocated:

1. Withhold food and water for 24 hours prior to induction of anesthesia in adult animals. Young calves (i.e., prior to full rumen development) should be starved of food and water for no more than 12 hours.

2. Position animal in left lateral or sternal recumbency during the intubation procedures.

3. Avoid rough manipulation of the rumen and other internal abdominal organs during surgery.

4. Place a sand bag or some other device beneath the animal's neck to elevate the occiput above overall body level.[13] This measure will tend to prevent passive regurgitation and allow saliva to flow out of the animal's mouth, thus avoiding aspiration.

Because regurgitation cannot be totally prevented, either a cuffed endotracheal tube or a correctly fitting Cole's tube should be placed into the trachea of any ruminant subjected to general anesthesia. Regurgitation occurring in animals in which the trachea has been properly intubated does not pose a major hazard, if upon recovery the tube is removed with the cuff inflated. This extubation technique allows removal of massive amounts of regurgitant that may have accumulated in the trachea cephalad to the tube cuff. Before the tube is removed, the mouth, nares, and pharynx may be flushed safely with water to remove regurgitation and decrease the likelihood of aspiration.

Regurgitation may occur during intubation, often being precipitated by poor induction and intubation techniques. Some have sought to avoid this problem by intubating prior to induction. This requires good patient restraint (i.e., cattle chute or strapping animal to surgical table) and the use of a mouth wedge held securely in place to prevent the animal from chewing the tube and one's hand and fingers during intubation. Generally, the hazards of regurgitation prior to intubation are avoided by not attempting intubation until surgical anesthesia has been attained. At this point, the tube is quickly and accurately placed in the trachea and the cuff quickly inflated. In the lightly anesthetized animal, accidental insertion of the endotracheal tube into the esophagus with to-and-fro movement to ascertain its location is sure to initiate active regurgitation. In the event that the onset of regurgitation is recognized before intubation can be completed, the endotracheal tube can be quickly passed into the esophagus and the cuff inflated, allowing ruminal contents to flow out of the mouth while another tube is being placed in the trachea.

Ruminal Tympany (Bloat)

Bloat commonly occurs in anesthetized ruminants,[13, 20] but it is not always serious. In a series of 99 cattle in which general anesthesia was maintained with halothane in oxygen, Weaver[21] considered bloat not to be a serious problem. The use of a stomach tube to relieve bloat was required in one animal only. However, in this study, anesthesia lasted an average of only 80 minutes, and 11 of the animals were starved of food for 1 to 5 days and denied water for 24 hours.

Although bloat cannot be totally prevented, its incidence and severity can be decreased by starving ruminants of food and water for 24 hours prior to anesthesia. Fasting does not cause a major decrease in ruminal contents, but it appears to decrease the rate of fermentation and thus the rate of ruminal gas production.

Should acute bloat occur, provided that it is not of a "frothy" type, pressure can be relieved by passing a stomach tube or by trocarization of the rumen. This latter method is discouraged except under the severest of circumstances, for fear of gross contamination of the peritoneal cavity and subsequent peritonitis. Some veterinarians routinely pass a stomach tube into the rumen prior to or shortly after induction of anesthesia. This precaution may lead ultimately to a more acute problem, because the tube, acting as a foreign body in the esophagus, may initiate regurgitation. For this reason we employ a stomach tube for bloat relief only when it is absolutely necessary and when the animal has an endotracheal tube in place. An alternative method is to position the animal in sternal recumbency. In this position, ruminal decompression occurs naturally. Positional relief of bloat is usually unacceptable during an operation, but it is the most acceptable means once the procedure has been completed. Moderate external pressure applied to the abdominal wall over the rumen will aid initiation of eructation.

Salivation

Ruminants normally produce copious quantities of saliva, which continue to flow during anesthesia. The amount produced is increased by some anesthetic agents (e.g., ether), whereas it is decreased by others (e.g., halothane).[22]

Hall[13] suggests that using atropine as an antisialagogue is of little value because it does not decrease the amount of saliva secreted and because atropine causes an increase in saliva viscosity, rendering it more difficult to remove from the respiratory passages if inhaled. Clinical observations suggest, however, that the oropharynx is drier in cattle given atropine, although the period of decreased saliva production is indeed brief. Weaver[21] found that atropine, when given at a dose of 30 mg to adult cattle, decreased saliva production from between 5 and 10 ml/100 kg/min to between 1 and 5 ml/100 kg/min.

When inhalation anesthesia is to be employed, atropine should be given 10 to 20 minutes prior to induction. Once the trachea has been intubated, the amount and consistency of saliva produced is of minor importance. However, in animals with decreased respiratory passage secretions (e.g., bronchitis, tracheitis), the drying effect of atropine will inhibit the effectiveness of ciliated cell activity.

PREANESTHETIC MEDICATION

Table 1 contains a list of tranquilizers and sedatives used as preanesthetic medications in large animals.

Parasympatholytic Agents

Atropine sulfate is given to decrease saliva production and alleviate bradycardia. Atropine should be given at a higher dose than is recommended in some texts. The following doses of atropine have been found to be helpful for short periods of decreased saliva secretion in ruminants and swine.

Cattle. 0.06–0.12 mg/kg IM.
Sheep and Goats. 0.15–0.3 mg/kg IM.
Swine. 0.04 mg/kg IM.

Ataractics-Tranquilizers

In general, phenothiazine tranquilizers induce a number of undesirable side effects while decreasing apprehension in nervous animals, rendering them easier to handle.

In some instances, the desirable characteristics may be overshadowed by undesirable effects, including hypotension and hypothermia. Such effects are more likely to occur in ill animals or when an actual or relative overdose of the tranquilizer has been given. Tranquilizers given to cattle prior to induction of general anesthesia will decrease the amount of anesthetic agent required, but recovery time will generally be increased. Because a rapid return of protective mechanisms (i.e., cough and swallowing reflex) and righting reflexes in ruminants recovering from anesthesia is highly desirable, tranquilizers should be given only to animals that are unruly and cannot otherwise be handled safely. Further, these agents may induce relaxation of the esophagus and cardia, thus promoting regurgitation.[27]

Tranquilizers are commonly given to cattle undergoing surgery in a standing position and rendered analgesic with a regional or field block. Under these circumstances, the tranquilizer dosage must be greatly decreased; otherwise, the animal is likely to lie down during the operation.

Phenothiazine tranquilizers should be avoided in the ill or debilitated animal because of their tendency to complicate such existing conditions as hypovolemia, anemia, hypothermia, shock, and hepatic dysfunction. Finally, all tranquilizers cross the placenta, causing fetal depression.

Administration of Tranquilizers

These agents may be given intramuscularly or intravenously. For intramuscular administration, a small-bore needle of sufficient length (i.e., 3.8 to 5.1 cm) to allow drug deposition in muscle tissue should be used. Depositing the agent in fat, which has low blood flow, will result in slow absorption and in delayed and often decreased animal response. The amount should be decreased to the lowest recommended dose when given intravenously, and the injection should be given slowly. Rapid administration can cause severe reactions. Jones[27] suggests the intravenous route for phenothiazine tranquilizers should be avoided because a number of deaths following intravenous injection have been reported in cattle.

Tranquilizers should be given under circumstances that cause the least possible distress to the patient. The animal should be in a quiet place and left undisturbed until maximal drug response occurs. Repeated stimulation of the animal for assessment of degree of tranquilization prior to full onset of action will be accompanied by excitement, often resulting in less than a desirable response. Although phenothiazine tranquilizers are useful agents, they should be used judiciously in ruminants in order to assure a desirable response.

Specific Sedatives

Xylazine Hydrochloride (Rompun)*

Xylazine is probably one of the most useful sedatives for use in ruminants.[32] However, it has not been approved

---

*Available from Haver Laboratories, Shawnee, KS 66201.

Table 1. Preanesthetic Medication: Tranquilizers and Sedatives (mg/kg)*

Generic Name	Trade Name (Manufacturer)	Cattle†		Sheep and Goats†		Swine†		Comments
		IV	IM	IV	IM	IV	IM	
Chlorpromazine hydrochloride	Thorazine (Pitman-Moore, Inc., Washington Crossing, NJ 08560)	0.22–1.0[14]	1.0–4.4[14]	0.55[14]	2.2	0.55–3.3[23,24]	2.0–4.0[25]	Use IV route with caution; give lowest effective dose.
Promazine hydrochloride	Sparine (Wyeth Laboratories, Division of American Home Products Corp., Philadelphia, PA 19101)	0.44–1.0	0.4–1.0	0.44–1.0	0.44–1.0	0.44–1.0	0.44–1.0	Intravenous route in cattle may nullify sedative effect.
Triflupromazine hydrochloride	Vetame (E. R. Squibb & Sons, Inc., Princeton, NJ 08540)	0.1 (maximum: .40 mg)	0.2 (maximum: 150 mg)	0.1 (maximum: 40 mg)	1.0 (maximum: 40 mg)	0.88	1.3	Not as effective as chlorpromazine in cattle.
Acepromazine maleate	Acepromazine maleate injectable (Ayerst Laboratories, Division of American Home Products Corp., New York, NY 10017)	—	0.03–0.1[13]	—	0.03–0.1[13]	—	0.03–0.1	Use of IV route questionable in cattle; injections require approximately 35 minutes for full onset of tranquilization.
Propiopromazine hydrochloride	Tranvet (Diamond Laboratories, Inc., Des Moines, IA 50304)	0.22–1.0[14]	0.22–1.0[14]	0.5[14]	—	0.55–1.0[14]	0.55–1.0[14]	Do not give to young calves.
Ethyl isobutrazine	Diquel (Jensen-Salsbery Laboratories, Division of Richardson-Merell, Inc., Kansas City, MO 64141)	0.55[14]	0.55–1.10[14]	—	—	1.25	2.2–4.4[14]	

Xylazine hydrochloride	Rompun (Haver-Lockhart Laboratories, Shawnee, KS 66201)	0.05–0.15	0.1–0.33	0.05–0.11	0.1–0.22[29]	—	—	IV route can be hazardous; dosage should be decreased to ½ of that given IM; xylazine is not an effective sedative when used alone in swine. Usually combined with ketamine.
Azaperone	Stresnil (Pitman-Moore, Inc., Washington Crossing, NJ 08560)	—	—	—	—	—	4.0–8.0 small swine[30] 2.0 large swine[31]	When given at 2.5 mg/kg, azaperone will prevent fighting in newly mixed animals.[31]
Diazepam	Valium (Hoffman-LaRoche, Inc., Nutley, NJ 07110)	—	—	0.4–1.0	0.8–2.0	—	5.5–8.5	In miniature swine, maximal sedation occurs in approximately 30 mins;[25] the use of diazepam at this dose will decrease the anesthetic dose of pentobarbital about 50%.
Chlorprothixene	Taractan (Hoffman-LaRoche, Inc., Nutley, NJ 07110)	—	—	—	—	0.3–1.0[27]	—	Optimal effect 5–10 minutes after injection.
Fetanyl citrate and droperidol	Innovar-Vet (Pitman-Moore, Inc., Washington Crossing, NJ 08560)	—	—	—	—	—	1 ml/12–25 kg body wt.	Atropine pre-medication is required to prevent severe bradycardia. Droperidol alone may be just as effective as the combination.

*Read package insert for approval of use in food-producing animals, and for milk discard and slaughter withdrawal times.
†Superscript numbers in dosage columns indicate references.

for use in food-producing animals in the United States. Xylazine is generally classified as a sedative[13, 33] with strong analgesic, hypnotic, and autonomic properties.[34]

Because xylazine is in broad use in European and other countries, a great deal of clinical information on its use has been published. As with most anesthetic and anesthetic-related agents, some undesirable side effects accompany the use of xylazine. It abolishes ruminal motility at high dose,[36] and bloat often occurs in unfasted animals. The respiratory and pulse rates are decreased, as is cardiac function. These responses are more severe following intravenous administration. The profuse salivation and bradycardia that accompany its administration can be counteracted to a large degree by atropine. Postadministration diarrhea is common, but it is generally self-limiting, clearing in approximately 36 hours.[37] Xylazine has been used as preanesthetic medication and as a sedative combined with local analgesia for a wide variety of surgical procedures. It has also been used to immobilize bulls for electroejaculation and semen collection.[35]

Precautions. Xylazine given to cows in the last trimester of pregnancy may cause premature parturition[27] and retention of fetal membranes.[37]

The use of xylazine should be avoided in ruminants with pronounced debilitating disease. More specifically, it should not be given to animals that are hypovolemic or have urinary tract blockade. Xylazine has been shown to increase urine output by 6.7 times over a 2-hour period when given at a rate of 0.22 mg/kg intramuscularly in cattle.[38]

If given intravenously, particularly in young ruminants and when used at 10 per cent (100 mg/ml) concentration, xylazine should be diluted in 5 to 10 ml saline and given over 2 to 3 minutes. The dosage should not exceed 0.11 mg/kg.

After being given xylazine, ruminants should be observed closely for 30 minutes to 2 hours. Some animals may remain recumbent for more than 2 hours if undisturbed.[34] Bloat appears to be of greater concern in animals that have not been properly fasted of food and water and when a high dosage of xylazine has been given. Because animals recovering from xylazine sedation may appear to be in a general state of wakefulness but later may lie down in lateral recumbency and die from acute bloat, it is advisable to observe them closely for a time and to encourage them to move about until they have fully recovered.

Administration. Xylazine may be given intravenously[39] or intramuscularly. With the intravenous route, onset of action is immediate. The intravenous route stresses cardiovascular function and is, therefore, recommended to be given only to healthy animals and in low dosage.

When xylazine is given intramuscularly, a small-bore needle (i.e., 18- to 20-gauge) sufficient in length to penetrate muscle tissue (3.8 to 5.1 cm) must be used, or drug deposition will occur in fatty tissue. When a large-bore needle is used, drug may leak from the needle puncture site. Moveover, when the high concentration (100 mg/ml) is used, the needle employed to withdraw the calculated dosage from the xylazine vial should not be removed from the syringe prior to intramuscular needle placement, because the xylazine filling the needle dead space will be lost, decreasing total dose injected. Even though it is known that the degree of sedation induced by xylazine will vary from animal to animal, drug loss at the needle puncture site, drug deposition in fat, or loss of drug from needle dead space may be responsible for failure of the level of sedation normally induced with a given dose to occur. Additionally, it is suspected that xylazine potency may decrease as storage time increases.[33]

Because xylazine is available in 2 per cent (20 mg/ml) and 10 per cent (100 mg/ml) concentrations, dosage should be calculated on the basis not of ml/kg but rather of mg/kg of body weight. When dosage calculation is based on ml/kg of body weight, inadvertent substitution of the 10 per cent concentration for the 2 per cent concentration will result in gross overdosage.

Xylazine has not proved to be an acceptable sedative when employed alone in swine. It does, however, appear to be a useful agent when given in combination with ketamine. Combining xylazine with ketamine enhances muscle relaxation and appears to increase visceral analgesia, which is considered to be poor with ketamine. Appropriate dosages for xylazine are as follows:

Cattle. 0.05–0.15 mg/kg IV; 0.10–0.33 mg/kg IM.
Standing Surgery. 0.05 mg/kg IM.
Sheep and Goats. 0.05–0.10 mg/kg IV; 0.10–0.33 mg/kg IM.

Because the sedative response to xylazine is due primarily to its agonistic effect upon alpha-2 receptors located in the central nervous system, drugs that block these receptor sites may be used to antagonize xylazine sedation effectively. Yohimbine* and 4-aminopyridine,* given intravenously at dosages of 0.125 mg/kg and 0.3 mg/kg, respectively have been proved to be effective for this purpose.[64] Another compound used to reverse the sedative effect of xylazine is tolazoline,* 0.2–2.0 mg/kg IV. These antagonists have proved to be very useful agents when animals have been accidentally overdosed or when rapid recovery from xylazine sedation is desirable.

AGENTS FOR CAPTURE OF FREE-RANGING CATTLE

A number of agents used singularly and in various combinations have been used to capture wild cattle.[28] Xylazine, though not an ideal agent, has been used extensively for this purpose.[40] Free-ranging wild cattle do not respond to xylazine with the same degree of sedation and immobilization as do docile animals. Therefore, after the free-ranging animal has become recumbent, it should be approached quietly from its blind side and a mechanical restraint should be applied at once, or the animal may regain its feet and flee.

For capture purposes, xylazine may be administered with a Cap-Chur-type rifle.† However, in large animals, the rifle may be incapable of delivering an immobilizing volume of 2 per cent xylazine. Use of the 10 per cent concentration helps to overcome this problem. When high doses are administered, the sedated animal should be observed closely for several hours so that side effects such as bloat and prolonged recumbency can be effectively treated. Wild cattle captured by Stewart[40] were given an estimated dose of xylazine ranging from 0.66 to 0.88 mg/kg. Recumbency occurred in 3 to 7 minutes, but the animals were not always sufficiently sedated to prevent fleeing when they were approached. Subsequently, a

---

*Available from Sigma Chemical Company, St. Louis, MO 63178.
†Available from Palmer Chemical and Equipment Co., Inc., Douglasville, GA 30134.

second dose was given, estimated to be from 0.52 to 0.53 mg/kg. The interval between first and second dose ranged from 2 to 70 minutes. Total dosages of the magnitude given by Stewart[40] should be used with extreme caution and employed only when absolutely necessary. Further, a specific antagonist (e.g., yohimbine), should be readily available and administered when required to reverse excessive sedation and other responses (e.g., bloat) that could prove to be life-threatening.

Kidd and associates[28] reported on the use of various combinations and dosages of muscle relaxants, parasympatholytics, tranquilizers, narcotics, and dissociative agents. In trials involving a large number of cattle (approximately 125), none of the combinations was found to be entirely satisfactory. After a great number of trial-and-error studies, the following combination of agents was considered to be acceptable: acepromazine, 25 μg/kg; phencyclidine hydrochloride, 200 μg/kg; atropine sulfate, 90 μg/kg; and etorphine,* 2.5 μg/kg.

Phencyclidine has been withdrawn from the United States market. Ketamine, 2 mg/kg, may be used as a replacement for it in this combination. Total volume then becomes a concern. This problem can be overcome to a limited extent by freeze-drying ketamine and reconstituting it at a higher concentration (i.e., 200–300 mg/ml).

In England, a neuroleptanalgesic combination of acepromazine and etorphine (Immobilon)† is used to immobilize cattle. The concentration ratio is 10 mg/ml of acepromazine to 2.45 mg/ml of etorphine, along with an antagonist, diprenorphine (Revivon).† The dosage in cattle is as follows: acepromazine, 100 μg/kg; etorphine, 22.5 μg/kg; and the antagonist, diprenorphine, 30 μg/kg. This drug combination may cause a moderate degree of excitement when given in a dosage insufficient to induce rapid immobilization. In addition, excitement may appear some hours after the antagonist has been given. Post-recovery excitement is thought to be due to enterohepatic cycling of etorphine. Because of this possibility, animals should be kept under surveillance in a well-secured enclosure for 12 hours following reversal.[41] In our experimental studies with etorphine in ponies, we observed post-remobilization excitement in one animal. The excitement was adequately controlled by intravenous administration of acepromazine. A more rational approach to the problem would be to administer a dose of diprenorphine.

Etorphine is available in the United States; however, it is approved for use in zoo animals only. Because etorphine is a very potent narcotic, it must be handled with extreme caution. The antagonist should be drawn into a syringe and should be immediately available in case a person is accidentally injected while working with etorphine.

Cyprenorphine and diprenorphine[41] are specific antagonists of etorphine. To reverse etorphine's effects, these agents are given intravenously at a dosage approximating 1.5 to 2 times the dosage of etorphine.

CHLORAL HYDRATE

Because the stages and planes of anesthesia are not well-defined and its analgesic qualities are poor, chloral hydrate is seldom used to induce and maintain surgical

anesthesia in cattle. This compound can be used safely to induce light narcosis and can be supplemented with local analgesia for minor surgeries.

Chloral hydrate is highly irritating to tissues and will cause necrosis if injected perivascularly. For this reason, the vessel into which it is administered should be well cannulated and of large size with free-flowing blood. The time required for maximal narcosis is longer than for barbiturates. Therefore, chloral hydrate should be given slowly in order to assess patient response as narcosis progresses, thus avoiding overdose. Full effects of an intravenous dose of chloral hydrate occur approximately 5 minutes after its injection.

Chloral hydrate has been used effectively to sedate confined animals that could not otherwise be approached or handled. Denying animals water for 24 to 36 hours makes them thirsty enough to consume water containing chloral hydrate. General dosages are as follows:

Oral Administration for Sedation. Adult cattle, 100–150 gm in 8–10 liters of water.

Light to Medium Narcosis. IV administration, 5–7 gm/100 kg body weight.

Note: Chloral hydrate has been given intraperitoneally in pigs for general anesthesia at a dose of 4 to 6 ml of a 5 per cent solution per kg body weight. The incidence of peritonitis appears to be rather high. For this reason, intraperitoneal administration cannot be recommended.

PENTOBARBITAL SODIUM

Satisfactory sedation can be achieved with pentobarbital in cattle. The concentration that can be given intramuscularly without causing severe tissue necrosis (approximately 3 per cent) requires too large a volume for practical use; therefore, it is generally given intravenously. By this route, pentobarbital is given slowly until noticeable unsteadiness and rear limb weakness occur. This response generally occurs after 1 to 2 gm have been given to an adult cow. Usually 3 gm will induce recumbency.

With the advent of xylazine, sedation with pentobarbital has been less commonly employed. In some instances the combined use of these two agents may be advantageous.

INJECTABLE ANESTHETIC AGENTS FOR RUMINANTS AND SWINE

Barbiturates

The barbiturates have been popular agents for induction of general anesthesia since the 1930's. The period of surgical anesthesia induced by the short-acting and ultra-short-acting agents is brief, but complete recovery may be exceedingly long in young calves, lasting up to 24 hours.[26] When used for induction of anesthesia and followed by maintenance with an inhalation agent, the barbiturates are nearly ideal and are widely employed for this purpose, both alone and in combination with other agents (e.g., glyceryl guaiacolate). It is not advisable to use barbiturates alone for anything more than the briefest of surgical procedures.[22] Although anesthesia can be prolonged by repeated injections, regurgitation with aspiration, apnea, and death are likely to occur unless proper preventive measures are employed.

Once a barbiturate has been injected, control of anesthetic depth and rate of recovery is clearly out of the hands of the veterinarian and depends on tissue redistri-

---

*Available from Lemmon Co., Sellersville, PA 18960.
†Available from Reckitt and Colman, Pharmaceutical Division, Hull, England.

bution and metabolism of the drug. In cattle, rate of metabolism of the agent has been reported to have a stronger influence on recovery time than tissue redistribution. The reverse appears to be true for sheep, goats, and swine.[42] In either case, the precise control of anesthetic depth achievable with inhalation agents of relatively low solubility is not possible with barbiturates.

Barbiturates rapidly cross the placenta. Severity of fetal depression is directly related to total dose administered to the dam. Barbiturates are not recommended for cesarean section when given in high dosage. An ultra-short-acting agent (e.g., thiopental) may be used safely as an induction agent in animals destined for cesarean section when an inhalation agent (e.g., halothane) is to be employed as the maintenance anesthetic.

Specific antagonists are not available for barbiturates. Analeptics, such as doxapram hydrochloride (Dopram-V)* will stimulate the respiratory centers, increasing respiration rate and tidal volume in barbiturate depressed animals. Subsequently, the animal may revert to a deep state of depression because of decreased arterial carbon dioxide content. Apnea is more appropriately treated with mechanically assisted or controlled ventilation until adequate spontaneous breathing resumes. Barbiturate overdose may be treated by administering sodium bicarbonate (to increase blood pH) and balanced electrolyte solutions in conjunction with a diuretic. Peritoneal dialysis should be considered as well as administration of fresh whole blood. Although hemodialysis is used in human medicine, its practicality in large animals is doubtful. Aside from therapeutic measures, the patient should be kept warm and should not be allowed to remain in one position for a prolonged period. Adequate ventilation and oxygen supplementation are important. Prophylactic antibiotics will help avoid secondary bacterial infection.

Endotracheal intubation is essential in ruminants subjected to barbiturate anesthesia. A properly placed endotracheal tube with inflated cuff will provide protection from aspiration of saliva and regurgitated ruminal contents. In addition, apnea, which is common with barbiturate anesthesia, can be dealt with effectively.

PENTOBARBITAL SODIUM

Pentobarbital is not a suitable agent for general anesthesia in adult cattle but may be used in calves more than 1 month of age.[13] A prolonged recovery time is to be expected in animals younger than 1 month.[14] In adult sheep and goats (that have been properly fasted) and in swine, pentobarbital will provide 20 to 30 minutes of relatively safe anesthesia. Supplemental injections to prolong anesthesia are not recommended unless given under ideal hospital conditions with appropriate respiratory support equipment available. Analgesia and muscle relaxation are poor, except in deep planes of anesthesia, and recovery is prolonged and requires close patient surveillance if satisfactory results are to be achieved. Recommended doses are:

Calves. 15–30 mg/kg IV (over 1 month of age).
Sheep and Goats. 20–30 mg/kg IV.
Swine. 15–30 mg/kg IV.

Thiobarbiturates

With the increasing popularity of inhalation anesthesia, thiobarbiturates are used more extensively as induction agents in cattle, sheep, goats, and swine than is pento-

barbital. When surgical anesthesia is to be maintained with an inhalation agent, such as halothane in oxygen, thiopental sodium (Penthothal)* or thiamylal sodium (Surital)† is given by rapid intravenous injection. This method of administration is often referred to as a "crash induction" and is generally preferred in large, thrifty animals because uncontrollable excitement is seldom encountered. If thiobarbiturates are given slowly, a much larger dose will be required and recovery will be prolonged. A 10 per cent concentration of either of these agents is desirable to allow the required volume to be contained in a single large syringe. Such a high concentration is caustic and will likely cause varying degrees of phlebitis. This development is seldom recognized unless one has occasion to examine the vessel into which the barbiturates was injected a few days later. Accidental perivascular injection (occurring in inappropriately restrained animals and with faulty vessel cannulation) can cause tissue necrosis and slough. For these reasons it is probably safer to use a 5 per cent concentration.

For induction of anesthesia, a precalculated dose of either thiopental sodium or thiamylal sodium is drawn into a syringe and injected rapidly into the jugular vein. In cows, the milk vein has been used, although it should be realized that phlebitis would be potentially more harmful in this vessel. The vein employed should be well cannulated. A 7.5- to 10-cm needle of 16 to 18 gauge should be used in order to assure ease of injection and decrease the possibility of perivascular injection.

When a lower concentration (e.g., 5 per cent) is to be used, one end of a short (25 to 30 cm) length of plastic tubing is attached to the intravenous needle or catheter, and a three-way stop-cock is connected at the other end. Two syringes containing the calculated dose of barbiturate are attached, one at each of the open stop-cock ports (Fig. 1). The contents of one syringe are injected rapidly, the stop-cock valve is rotated, and contents of the second syringe are injected rapidly. The entire injection procedure should be completed in 5 to 10 seconds. Fifteen to 20 seconds after completion of the injection, the animal will develop posterior limb weakness followed by rapid collapse to its sternum. Apnea lasting 15 to 30 seconds is not uncommon but should give rise to little concern in the physically fit animal. Intubation should be completed at once. Inappropriate jaw relaxation, chewing, and the likelihood of regurgitation can occur if intubation is delayed or prolonged.

Because the potency of thiamylal sodium is somewhat greater than that of thiopental sodium, a slightly smaller dose of the former should be given. Recommended dosages vary among reports, but in our experience, the following dosage schedule has proved safe for induction in thrifty animals unpremedicated with tranquilizers:

Cattle. Thiopental sodium, 6–12 mg/kg IV, thiamylal sodium, 4–8 mg/kg IV.
Sheep and Goats. Thiopental sodium, 10–16 mg/kg IV; thiamylal sodium, 8–14 mg/kg IV.

The higher dose is used in vigorous lightweight animals and the lower dose in older heavy animals. When cattle have been premedicated with a tranquilizer or sedative such as xylazine, the doses of thiobarbiturates should be decreased by approximately 1/4 to 1/3. Animals with circulatory shock or uncompensated cardiovascular dis-

*Available from A. H. Robins Company, Richmond, VA 23220.

*Available from Abbott Laboratories, North Chicago, IL 60064.
†Available from Parke-Davis and Company, Detroit, MI 48232.

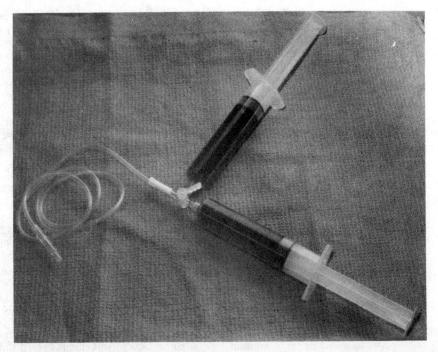

Figure 1. Syringes, stop-cock, and plastic tube extension used for rapid intravenous administration of a large volume of anesthetic.

ease should not be subjected to barbiturate "crash induction." A safer method is to use glyceryl guaiacolate combined with a low level of barbiturate.

In swine, anesthesia is induced by injecting a barbiturate into an ear vein. The anterior vena cava has been used but cannot be recommended because of the likelihood of perivascular injection or possibly direct intracardiac injection. "Crash induction" is not generally employed in this species because of the lack of a vein large enough for rapid injection. A lesser concentration of barbiturate (5 per cent or less) should be used in order to avoid phlebitis and ear slough. Swine are difficult to restrain for venipuncture unless they have been properly premedicated with a tranquilizer or sedative. They frequently shake their heads and ears, causing needle dislodgement and perivascular injection.

For injection into a pig's ear vein, a small-bore needle or catheter (18 to 22 gauge, 2.5 to 3.8 cm in length) is suitable. It is helpful to use a short length of plastic tubing (Butterfly)* between the needle and syringe, to avoid dislodging the needle if the pig struggles during the injection procedure.

For intravenous injection, the vein is raised by placing a tight-fitting rubber band at the base of an ear. When the vessel has been suitably cannulated, the rubber band is cut free. Aspiration of a small quantity of blood into the syringe will assure that the needle has not been dislodged and injection can begin. One-third to 1/2 of the calculated dose is given rapidly. Swine restrained with a nose snare will sink down on their rear quarters 15 to 20 seconds after the initial injection. Close observation at this time is important to ensure that the animal is breathing. The injection is continued, with anesthesia slowly increased to the desired depth. Surgical anesthesia from the initial injection will last for 10 to 15 minutes, with

recovery requiring approximately 1 hour. If inhalation anesthesia is to be used, there will be adequate time for tracheal intubation. Extending anesthesia time with supplemental injections of barbiturates will greatly prolong the recovery period and increase the likelihood of apnea.

Induction doses for swine are: thiopental sodium, 10–20 mg/kg IV; thiamylal sodium, 6–18 mg/kg IV.

Thiobarbiturate and Glyceryl Guaiacolate Combination

Glyceryl guaiacolate (GG) is a muscle relaxant acting at the level of the internuncial neurons located within the spinal cord and on polysynaptic fibers. Respiratory function is little affected by this agent beyond the changes associated with abnormal postural position. Cardiovascular function remains stable in the healthy animal.

It should be clearly understood that glyceryl guaiacolate induces little if any analgesia. When combined with a low level of barbiturate to maintain surgical anesthesia, it should be supplemented with local analgesia. Thiopental sodium and thiamylal sodium may be combined with glyceryl guaiacolate and used as an induction agent for cattle.[43, 44] For sheep and goats, this combination probably does not offer any great advantages over thiobarbiturates alone when employed specifically for induction. In cattle, it has the advantage of being effective when administered more slowly than thiobarbiturates alone, thus allowing titering of anesthesia to the desired depth. This combination has proved safe for immobilization of mature cattle for procedures that require only a minimal degree of analgesia. For example, the application of a plaster-of-Paris cast can safely be performed with a barbiturate and GG drip. Light anesthesia with adequate muscle relaxation is easily and safely achieved if painful manipulations are not required.
Administration:

GG solution is prepared by adding 50 gm to 1 L of 5 per cent dextrose in water to make a 5 per cent solution.

*Available from Abbott Laboratories, North Chicago, IL 60064.

The mixture is heated in a water bath to put the GG into solution. Thiopental sodium or thiamylal sodium is generally added at the rate of 2 gm per liter. Greater amounts of barbiturate (3–4 gm/L) may be added if immobilization is to be continued for longer than 45 minutes to an hour. Another alternative is to continue with a second liter of the standard solution. In either event, the greater the total dose of barbiturate, the longer the recovery. Recovery to the point that an animal will regain its righting and protective reflexes usually does not extend beyond 45 minutes to 1 hour once administration is discontinued.

For induction, the GG-barbiturate combination must be administered rapidly by gravitational flow or by pressurizing the administration vial. A 12-gauge needle or catheter is required for rapid administration in adult ruminants. Once immobilization, muscle relaxation, and light general anesthesia have been achieved, the flow rate is decreased to a slow drip just sufficient to sustain immobilization. At this point, the animal's trachea should be intubated, a prerequisite to general anesthesia in ruminants. The GG-barbiturate combination drip can be continued for short minor procedures, or the animal can be connected to an inhalation machine for induction and maintenance of deep surgical anesthesia.

For safety's sake, the dose of GG-barbiturate combination should not exceed 2 ml/kg of a 5 per cent solution for induction purposes. The total dose should not exceed 4 ml/kg when used as a drip to extend immobilization time. For 5 per cent solution of GG with 2 gm of thiobarbiturate per liter, the total dosages for specific purposes are as follows:

Induction. 1.5–2 ml/kg given rapidly IV.

Maintenance. Should not exceed 4 ml/kg over the entire course of administration, usually 45 minutes to 1 hour and 45 minutes.

Cyclohexylamines

Members of this group of nonbarbiturate anesthetics induce a peculiar state of unconsciousness often referred to as "cataleptoid" or dissociative anesthesia. This anesthetic state differs markedly from that induced by barbiturates. Generally, the animal's eyelids remain open, front limbs are extended, rear limbs are flexed, and pupils are dilated. Nystagmus is not uncommon, and muscle tone is increased, particularly in light planes of anesthesia. Protective reflexes (i.e., cough, swallowing), to a degree, remain intact. The myotactic reflexes are hyperexcitable, thus decreasing the usefulness of these agents for operations on or about tendinous structures. Somatic analgesia is profound, but visceral analgesia is poor. Patient movement during anesthesia is rather common and does not necessarily indicate pain perception unless the reaction corresponds to surgical manipulation.

With ketamine, we have observed postanesthetic excitement in mature cattle and in swine.[45] It is most likely to occur when the drug is given intramuscularly and when the animal is not permitted to recover in a quiet, darkened environment. A sedative dose of barbiturate (e.g., 2–4 mg/kg pentobarbital) will adequately control this side effect.[45]

KETAMINE HYDROCHLORIDE

Cattle. Ketamine, although not approved by the United States Food and Drug Administration (FDA), has been investigated more than any of the cyclohexylamines for use in food-producing animals. Fuentes and Tellez[46] reported on the use of ketamine in 10 cows undergoing minor and major surgeries ranging from toe amputation to laparotomy. Subsequently, the use of ketamine and xylazine for cesarean section was reported by the same authors.[47] The neonate had tachycardia and tachypnea that disappeared shortly after delivery. In their study, cows for elective surgery were starved of food and water for 24 hours. Atropine was not given. They reported that regurgitation, bloat, and salivation were "absent." Anesthesia was induced by rapid intravenous injection of ketamine, 2 mg/kg, followed by constant intravenous infusion. The infusion was prepared by adding ketamine (2 mg/ml) to normal saline. The ketamine-saline solution was infused intravenously at a rate of 10 ml/min in adult cattle.

Our clinical experience suggests that in cattle premedicated with atropine and xylazine, anesthesia can be induced safely with ketamine, 2 mg/kg administered as a bolus IV. Although jaw muscle relaxation is not as profound as that induced by barbiturates and GG, tracheal intubation can be accomplished by the use of a mouth wedge when surgical anesthesia is to be maintained with an inhalation agent. Recently, we have conducted clinical trials with GG solution (5 per cent in 5 per cent dextrose) containing 1 mg/ml of ketamine and 0.1 mg/ml of xylazine. This combination of drugs, when given IV, induced safe and reliable general anesthesia in cattle, sheep, and goats. Initially, 0.55 ml/kg of this solution was given rapidly IV. Thereafter, the solution was given at a rate of 2.2 ml/kg/hr. We have maintained satisfactory general anesthesia for up to 2 1/2 hours in calves and mature cattle with this drug combination. Surgical procedures, including femoral fracture plating and pinning, umbilical hernia repair, and cesarean section, were performed. For these procedures, the trachea was intubated and supplemental oxygen (5–15L/min) was given during the surgical procedure. Increased inspired oxygen concentration is necessary only for prolonged procedures (i.e., longer than 1 hour) or in debilitated patients.

Sheep and Goats. Numerous reports have appeared on the use of ketamine in sheep.[48–54] Although the results are generally good, two major limiting factors remain: lack of FDA approval for use in food-producing animals and high cost.

Taylor and colleagues[52] reported on the successful use of ketamine in pregnant ewes. Initially, 2 mg/kg of ketamine was given intravenously for induction; anesthesia was maintained by drip infusion with 2 mg/ml of ketamine in 5 per cent glucose given at a rate of 4 ml/min. Surgical procedures ranged from 1 to 2 hours in length. In their study, animals were not starved or given premedication. Regurgitation, salivation, and bloat were not reported to be problems. Thurmon and co-workers[53] found that ketamine, 22 mg/kg given IM, will induce satisfactory anesthesia in sheep premedicated with atropine 0.22 mg/kg and acetylpromazine 0.55 mg/kg. The duration of analgesia is brief, but muscle relaxation is good. In this study, duration of surgical anesthesia was extended to 1 to 1 1/2 hours by intermittent intravenous administration of ketamine at a rate of 2 to 4 mg/kg. Total dosage required was from 33 to 44 mg/kg.

In goats, a combination of atropine, xylazine, and ketamine has been used to induce and maintain surgical anesthesia for a wide variety of surgical procedures (laparotomy, eyeball enucleation, amputation of claws, abomasotomy, and enterotomy).[29] Atropine 0.4 mg/kg was given initially, followed in 20 to 25 minutes by xylazine 0.22 mg/kg given IM. After 8 to 10 minutes had elapsed, 11 mg/kg of ketamine was given IM. Surgical anesthesia was maintained for 2 1/4 to 2 3/4 hours by supplemental increments of ketamine or a mixture of xylazine and ketamine. When ketamine alone was used to extend surgical anesthesia, it was given IM at a rate of 6 mg/kg. When the xylazine-ketamine mixture was used, it was given IM at the rates of 0.045 mg/kg of xylazine and 2.45 mg/kg of ketamine. For extending surgical anesthesia, ketamine supplementation was preferred over the xylazine-ketamine mixture. Clinical experience suggests that ketamine 2 to 4 mg/kg should be given intravenously to extend surgical anesthesia for brief periods, whereas the intramuscular route should be employed if longer duration is required.

Even though regurgitation has not been reported to be a serious problem with ketamine anesthesia, tracheal intubation complements sound judgment in the wise use of all general anesthetic agents in ruminants.

A combination of steroids—alphaxalone and alphadolone (Saffan*)—has been used in sheep and goats to induce and maintain surgical anesthesia. Saffan is generally given at 2–4 mg/kg IV. It will provide 10 to 20 minutes of anesthesia. Anesthesia time may be extended by continuous IV infusion, 0.23–0.24 mg/kg/min.[13] Recovery will occur in approximately 30 minutes once the infusion is discontinued.

Swine. Ketamine has been used rather extensively in swine for minor operations.[45] Atropine will control the excessive salivation caused by ketamine, which may be given intramuscularly or intravenously. Immobilization following intramuscular injection (11 mg/kg) occurs in 3 to 5 minutes. Muscle relaxation is only fair, and analgesia is brief. To increase the degree of analgesia and prolong the duration of surgical anesthesia, small increments (2–4 mg/kg) may be given intravenously. Injection of 2 per cent lidocaine at the surgical site can be safely used to enhance analgesia.

Clinical trials suggest that the intravenous route is safe, and recovery is less likely to be accompanied by excitement than when ketamine is given intramuscularly, particularly in older sows and boars. We have successfully used ketamine injected intratesticularly, 3–5 mg/kg, to immobilize large boars for castration. Surgical removal of the testicle also removes a significant portion of the ketamine dose and hastens recovery. The testicles should not be discarded where they may be consumed by other animals, lest the latter become anesthetized.

Physical restraint sufficient for intravenous injection is often difficult to achieve in swine. Premedication with a tranquilizer may be helpful. Forty to 60 minutes after 1 to 2 mg/kg of chlorpromazine is injected intramuscularly, pigs will object less to venipuncture and injection.[13, 23] European reports indicate that the butyrophenone tranquilizers are most effective when employed for this purpose.[30, 55] Of this group, azaperone (Stresnil)† appears to be the most useful. The degree of sedation with azaperone is dose related. A 2-mg/kg dose given intramuscularly will induce mild tranquilization. At a dose of 4 to 8 mg/kg,

deep sedation and immobilization will occur, provided that the animal is left undisturbed for 15 to 30 minutes. Because analgesia with azaperone alone is only fair, painful manipulations can cause animals to awaken in an agitated state.[56] When sows are disturbed during the recovery period, they may become excited. However, ketamine and azaperone seem to be a workable combination of agents in swine when used judiciously. Ketamine should not be given until full sedation from azaperone is present. The combination of azaperone and metomidate (Hypnodil)* has been used extensively for anesthesia of swine in European countries. Azaperone is given intramuscularly at a rate of 1 to 2 mg/kg. In 10 to 15 minutes, metomidate, 10 mg/kg, is injected intraperitoneally or 4 mg/kg is given IV. Some reports indicate that analgesia and relaxation are adequate for cesarean section,[57] but other reports indicate that a local anesthetic is required for adequate analgesia.[55]

Recently, we have investigated the use of glyceryl guaiacolate (a 5 per cent solution in 5 per cent dextrose and water) containing 1 mg/ml of ketamine and 1 mg/ml of xylazine given IV (via central ear vein by 16- to 18-gauge catheter) to induce and maintain surgical anesthesia in mature swine. This combination of drugs is initially given rapidly at a dose of 0.5–1 ml/kg to induce anesthesia. Thereafter, the infusion is continued at a rate of 2ml/kg/hr. This combination of drugs has been used to maintain surgical anesthesia for 2.5 hours. Muscle relaxation and analgesia are quite profound. Recovery is rapid (30–40 minutes) once infusion is discontinued. A combination of ketamine 2 mg/kg, xylazine 2 mg/kg, and oxymorphone 0.075 mg/kg mixed in the same syringe and given IV has been used to induce and maintain surgical anesthesia. When the IM route was chosen each of the drug doses was doubled.[65] In our limited experience with this combination, we have found it to induce relatively good analgesia and muscle relaxation. Recovery was smooth and could be hastened by administration of naloxone.† Major drawbacks to use of this combination center on hypoventilation, cost, and lack of FDA approval.

Saffan (alphaxalone and alphadolone) given intravenously or intramuscularly has been used to induce general anesthesia in swine. Unlike barbiturates, this agent does not cause profound respiratory depression. Intravenous injection induces only a brief period of anesthesia; thus, frequent supplemental increments are required if anesthesia is to be extended. Even with repeated injections, recovery is smooth and brisk. Premedicating pigs with a tranquilizer (azaperone, 4 mg/kg IM) will decrease the initial dose of Saffan required to induce anesthesia by approximately half.[13] The initial intravenous dosage is 4 to 6 mg/kg. The IV route is generally used because intramuscular administration requires a higher dose, necessitating a large volume of the agent.

A neuroleptoanalgesic combination fentanyl citrate and droperidol (Innovar-Vet)† has been used as preanesthetic medication in swine. Atropine is given to depress salivation and prevent bradycardia. Fifteen to 30 minutes after intramuscular injection, pigs are easily restrained for intravenous injection. Ear vein puncture will elicit little if any head shaking. Squealing, usually associated with

*Available from Glaxo Laboratories, Greenford, Middlesex, England.
†Available from Pitman-Moore, Inc., Washington Crossing, NJ 08560.

*Available from Janssen Pharmaceutical, Beerse, Belgium.
†Available from Pitman-Moore, Inc., Washington Crossing, NJ 08560.

physical restraint, is generally absent. The sedative response to this combination of drugs is attributed primarily to the actions of droperidol, because fentanyl citrate has a fleeting action.

A favorable response has been observed in pigs given ketamine after premedication with Innovar-Vet. The recommended preanesthetic dosage of this agent is 1 ml/12–25 kg IM after 0.04 mg/kg of atropine IM.

INHALATION ANESTHESIA

Without question, the use of inhalation agents is the safest and most satisfactory means of maintaining general anesthesia in ruminants and swine. Until recently, inhalation anesthesia was widely employed only in research laboratories and in hospitals dealing with valuable animals requiring major surgical intervention. The reasonable cost of halothane has stimulated a renewed interest in inhalation anesthesia for food-producing animals as well as in the progressive development of advanced surgical techniques being employed in valuable animals. At this time, equipment cost, the economic value of the average animal, and the inconvenience of transporting equipment to the field are major disadvantages of the use of inhalation anesthesia in general food animal practice. However, it should be emphasized that there is no satisfactory substitute for inhalation anesthesia in valuable animals requiring general anesthesia for major surgical procedures.

Surgical Table Padding

Cattle do not appear to be as susceptible as horses to generalized myositis. This does not mean that padding is unnecessary, because partial radial nerve paralysis may occur in heavy cattle kept deeply anesthetized for prolonged periods. The usual 5 to 7.5 cm of foam rubber padding or air mattress is not adequate in all cases. Clinical experience has shown in both horses and cattle that an automobile tire inner tube strategically placed beneath the animal's shoulder, combined with a moderate amount of table-top padding, will prevent radial nerve paralysis. For proper placement of the inner tube, the animal is rolled to its back and the tube is fitted over the dependent leg. The animal is turned back to its side, and the tube is inflated. Inflation of the tube tends to raise the animal's front quarters, taking body weight off the radial nerve where body contact is made with the table-top padding. With this position, the scapula is allowed to fall away from the thoracic wall, thus relieving pressure on and around the brachial plexus.

Inhalation Agents

Ether, chloroform, and cyclopropane were the first inhalation agents used in ruminants and swine. They have, for the most part, been replaced by two major halogenated compounds, halothane and methoxyflurane. Two agents of newer vintage, enflurane and isoflurane, possess physical characteristics that promote rapid induction and recovery, but they are currently too expensive to assume an important role in anesthesia of ruminants and swine.

HALOTHANE

This compound is a potent, volatile agent with a rather broad safety margin. The physical and pharmacologic characteristics of halothane make it a highly desirable agent for use in large animals. Owing to halothane's high volatility, high potency, and relatively low solubility, the depth of anesthesia can be regulated quickly and within a rather precise range. Rapid adjustment of anesthetic depth, a highly desirable characteristic, is possible with halothane but cannot be achieved with methoxyflurane nor with most injectable agents.

Recovery from halothane anesthesia is relatively rapid. Ruminants in light surgical anesthesia are generally able to assume sternal recumbency 10 to 15 minutes after administration is discontinued. Excitement during the recovery period is rarely observed.

Halothane crosses the placental barrier and induces fetal depression. However, once respiration is initiated after birth, halothane blood levels decrease rapidly, and central nervous depression disappears. Because of high vapor pressure, it is unsafe to use halothane as an open drip. Safety can be ensured only when halothane is used in a precision vaporizer; this arrangement usually employs a circle rebreathing system.

METHOXYFLURANE

Surgical anesthesia has been induced and maintained with methoxyflurane in all species of food-producing animals. Many of the desirable characteristics of halothane are absent with methoxyflurane. This agent, although more potent than halothane, has a lower vapor pressure and a higher solubility. The latter two physical characteristics are responsible for the slow induction and recovery common with methoxyflurane.[58] Because safety of general anesthesia in ruminants depends largely upon rapid induction and recovery, methoxyflurane cannot be considered to be a highly desirable anesthetic agent for this species. When the matter is examined from a different point of view, however, the low vapor pressure of methoxyflurane may be considered desirable. This characteristic allows the agent to be used with a relatively high degree of safety in a nonprecision vaporizer located in the breathing circuit. Also, although terribly wasteful and not totally safe, the open drip method can be used. This method is expensive and is commonly associated with patient hypoxia as well as environmental pollution. Analgesia and muscle relaxation are considered to be better in light planes of anesthesia with methoxyflurane than with halothane. Methoxyflurane crosses the placental barrier and causes prolonged fetal depression. For this reason, it should not be employed as the major anesthetic agent for cesarean section.

Inhalation Anesthetic Equipment

Today, several companies manufacture anesthesia machines designed for use in large animals. These machines are well constructed and durable but extremely expensive. Although originally designed for use in the horse, they are ideal for adult cattle. Machines designed for use in human medicine or veterinary small animal practice are large enough for calves, sheep, goats, and swine. Details of these machines have been described in numerous texts.[13–16]

Rebreathing Systems

The machine shown in Figure 2 is equipped with calibrated vaporizers for halothane located out of the breathing circuit. With this arrangement, a precise volume percentage of anesthetic vapor can be delivered to the

The original rebreathing system employed with inhalation agents was the to-fro canister (Fig. 3). The term "to-fro" means that inhaled and exhaled gases travel back and forth through the carbon dioxide absorbent, instead of in a circular pattern as in the circle system. Although not as satisfactory as a circle system, it is an economical substitute that can easily be "home made." Details for construction of a large to-fro canister have been published.[63]

When a small animal machine equipped with a precision vaporizer is available, a to-fro canister can be used to administer inhalation anesthesia economically in large animals. To use a to-fro system with a small animal machine, the fresh gas delivery line is disconnected from the circle rebreathing system and attached to the fresh gas inflow port of the to-fro canister. Oxygen flow rate and concentration of anesthetic vapor delivered to the to-fro canister are determined by flow meter and vaporizer setting respectively, on the small animal machine.

Nonbreathing systems (e.g., Ayres T piece, Norman elbow) can be used in small food-producing animals. But owing to the high fresh gas flow rates required, they are uneconomical in all but the smallest patients (e.g., piglet, newborn lamb) and cause excessive environment contamination unless properly scavenged.

Oxygen Flow Rates and Anesthetic Vapor Concentration

Because the concentration of nitrogen in the lungs is approximately 80 per cent in animals breathing ambient air, high oxygen flow rates are necessary for rapid denitrogenation during the induction period. An alternate method is to flush the rebreathing system and the animal's lungs several times with oxygen as soon as the endotracheal tube is connected to the rebreathing system of the

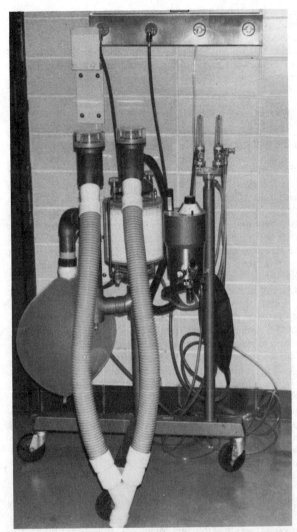

Figure 2. Inhalation anesthetic machine designed for use in large animals (i.e., adult cattle and horses). North American Drager, Telford, PA 18969.

rebreathing circuit. The out-of-circuit vaporizer is preferred, particularly with highly volatile and highly potent agents such as halothane. This machine uses a circle rebreathing system, which routes expired gases through a soda lime canister for removal of exhaled carbon dioxide. The rebreathing systems are used as either semiclosed or closed. Generally, the semiclosed method is preferred. The term semiclosed means that the volume of fresh gas delivered to the rebreathing system (i.e., oxygen and halothane vapor) is greater than that required for patient metabolic needs. To prevent overfilling of the system and production of excessive airway pressure, the exhaust valve is left open as an escape route for the excess inflow of fresh gas.

With the closed system, the exhaust valve is closed, and fresh gas inflow to the rebreathing system just meets the patient's metabolic needs. This method is more economical than the semiclosed method but requires closer scrutiny and precise gas flow adjustment. Hypercapnia and hypoxemia are more likely to be a problem with the closed method.

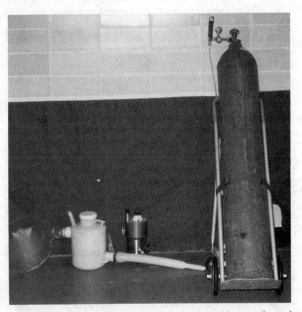

Figure 3. Home-constructed to-fro rebreathing canister is shown here with reservoir bag and Cole's endotracheal tube attached. A precision vaporizer is employed to supply anesthetic vapor to the breathing system. An oxygen tank with pressure regulator–flow meter combination makes this a simple but complete anesthetic delivery system for large animals.

anesthetic machines. Denitrogenation will ensure against early hypoxia and promote rapid induction of anesthesia. Following induction with an injectable agent (e.g., barbiturate, GG-barbiturate), the oxygen flow meter should be adjusted to deliver oxygen at 5 to 8 L/min in mature cattle and 2 to 4 L/min in small ruminants and swine. The out-of-circuit vaporizer is adjusted to deliver 3 to 5 per cent halothane, depending on the rate of induction desired. When a 5 per cent setting is used, particularly in small animals (i.e., sheep, goats, pigs, and calves), the patient should be observed closely in order to prevent overdose. The oxygen flows and vaporizer settings are gradually decreased as the animal approaches surgical anesthesia, which will usually require 15 to 20 minutes. When surgical anesthesia has been attained, the oxygen flow rate should be decreased to 3 to 5 L/min in adult cattle and 1 to 2 L/min in small animals. Vaporizer settings of 1.5 to 3 per cent will be required to maintain surgical anesthesia in most animals. In a mature cow, the higher vaporizer setting will be required with low oxygen flow rates. It is more appropriate to rely on patient response than on specific oxygen flow and vaporizer setting to determine induction rate and anesthetic depth.

Termination of Anesthesia

Shortly before completion of the surgical procedure, the anesthetic vapor concentration is decreased to approximately half of that required for maintenance. Just prior to completion of surgery, the anesthetic vaporizer is turned off and the rebreathing system is flushed with oxygen. The animal should be left connected to the anesthetic machine and breathing oxygen until signs of recovery—active palpebral reflex, limb movement, chewing, and swallowing—are readily apparent, at which time it should be moved to a quiet, darkened recovery area. The animal should be observed closely for character and rate of respiration and color of mucous membranes until it is able to support itself in sternal recumbency. The endotracheal tube should not be removed until strong protective reflexes—chewing and swallowing—are present. If a cuffed endotracheal tube is used, it should be removed with the cuff inflated in order to remove foreign material (e.g., saliva, regurgitant) that may have accumulated in the trachea proximal to the cuff.

Animals are usually able to stand within 30 to 40 minutes after being moved to the recovery area.

Endotracheal Intubation

Whenever general anesthesia is employed, the importance of tracheal intubation cannot be overemphasized. Tracheal intubation has the advantages of assuring a patent airway, preventing aspiration of saliva or regurgitant, providing a rapid and safe means for controlling ventilation if apnea occurs, and establishing a route for delivery of oxygen or inhalation agents. Assisted or controlled ventilation is effective only when the trachea is intubated. Even with the best-fitting face mask, there will be leaks, and positive-pressure ventilation with a mask will force gas into the rumen or stomach, particularly in swine, increasing intra-abdominal pressure and decreasing the effectiveness of positive pressure ventilation or normal breathing.

Death during general anesthesia occurs most often from respiratory arrest. When the trachea is intubated, simple measures can be employed to support ventilation. In small

ruminants and swine, one has only to blow into the endotracheal tube until the respiratory pattern is reestablished. A hand-operated resuscitator is economical and effective and can be used to support respiration with room air (Fig. 4). Oxygen supplementation by connecting an oxygen line to the resuscitator may be used when necessary.

Types of Endotracheal Tubes

Two types of tubes are used in adult cattle: the cuffed tube and the Cole's tube (Fig. 5). The cuffed tube provides a complete seal between the tube and tracheal wall when the cuff is properly inflated. The cuff should be inflated to a pressure that will just prevent escape of gas between cuff and tracheal wall when 25 to 30 cm H_2O positive pressure is applied. Most foreign material (i.e., saliva, regurgitant) accumulating in the trachea anterior to the cuff will be extracted to the oropharynx when the tube is removed with the cuff inflated; it is for this reason that cuffed tubes are generaly used. However, the Cole's tube has been used satisfactorily in large numbers of cattle. Instead of a cuff, it has an air seal, which is adequate for positive pressure ventilation and is achieved between tube and airway wall in a rather unique way. In adult cattle, the large diameter of the tube extends through the larynx, where the shoulder presses upon the first tracheal ring. The smaller diameter of the tube extends into the trachea. A snug fit inside the larynx and impingement on the first tracheal ring create an effective air seal. If foreign material should proceed distal to the tube's impingement on the tracheal rings, it would not be extracted with tube removal. On the other hand, tracheal contamination has not been identified as a problem when the Cole's tube is properly placed and anchored to the lower or upper jaw with adhesive tape or gauze.

Sizes of Endotracheal Tubes

The largest tube that can be placed into the trachea without injury to the delicate airway tissues should be used. It is the internal diameter that determines the amount of breathing resistance created by a given size tube. Thin-walled tubes are desirable, but if the wall is too thin, the tube can become kinked easily if the animal's neck is flexed. Over-inflation of the cuff can cause thin tube walls to collapse, creating airway obstruction.

Endotracheal tube sizes for cattle are listed in Table 2.[22] Although the diameters listed in the table have been found to be appropriate, the lengths are a bit excessive in some animals. The portion of endotracheal tube extending out of the animal's mouth is mechanical dead space and should be removed in order to promote effective ventilation. Connecting the Y-piece of the rebreathing

Table 2. *Endotracheal Tube Sizes for Use in Cattle**

	Internal Diameter (mm)	Approximate External Diameter (mm)	Length (cm)
Large bulls	30	38	100
Average cows	25	31	80
Yearling cows	20	26	80
Calves 6 mos	18	22.5	60
3 mos	16	19.5	60

*Adapted from L. R. Soma (ed.). Textbook of Veterinary Anesthesia. Baltimore, Williams & Wilkins, 1971.

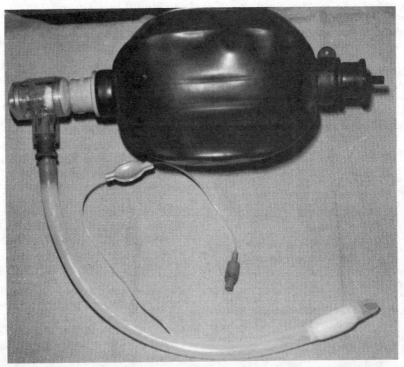

Figure 4. Hand-operated resuscitator with cuffed endotracheal tube attached. When desirable, oxygen can be metered into the resuscitator at a port located on the end opposite the endotracheal tube connection.

system as closely to the animal's mouth as possible eliminates most of the unnecessary dead space.

Large sheep and goats will require a tube having an internal diameter of 10 to 16 mm. Tubes with internal diameters of 6 to 10 mm will be adequate for smaller ruminants. For the latter group, the disposable tubes used in humans and dogs are quite satisfactory. In general, tubes required for goats will be one to two sizes smaller than those required for sheep of the same weight.

Proportionately, swine will require considerably smaller tubes than goats or sheep. For example a 50-kg pig will require a 9-mm tube.[22] A 10- to 14-mm internal diameter is satisfactory for adult sows, whereas smaller swine will require tubes of 6 to 10 mm.

Before induction of anesthesia, tube size for ruminants can be approximated by external palpation of the treachea. It is wise to have three tubes at hand: one the size judged to be appropriate by tracheal palpation, one a size larger, and one a size smaller.

Technique
INTUBATION OF CATTLE

Two basic techniques are employed for tracheal intubation in cattle. With either method a dental wedge* is essential to prevent injury to the anesthetist's hand and

---

*Available from Jorgensen Laboratories, Loveland, CO 80538.

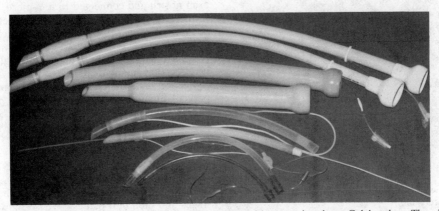

Figure 5. An assortment of endotracheal tubes. The two large tubes with tapered end are Cole's tubes. The plastic stylet (in the tube third from the bottom) is used as an aid to tracheal intubation.

damage to the endotracheal tube by the animal's teeth (Fig. 6). The mouth wedge should be left in place during anesthesia and until the tube is removed. Adhesive tape or gauze placed around the animal's muzzle in front of the mouth wedge will prevent its dislodgment if the animal becomes lightly anesthetized and begins chewing.

The first method for tracheal intubation has been well described.[13] A mouth wedge is inserted and held in place by an assistant who also extends the animal's head, decreasing the orotracheal angle and creating a straight pathway from mouth to the trachea. The animal's tongue is drawn out of the mouth, and the anesthetist's hand is passed between the dental arcades until contact is made with the epiglottis and arytenoid cartilages. The tube is then passed alongside or beneath the anesthetist's arm and is gently guided with the fingertips through the laryngeal opening and into the trachea. The cuff is quickly inflated.

The procedure for the second method is the same as that for the first, up to the point of passing the endotracheal tube. At this point, a small stiff tube (horse stomach tube three times longer than the endotracheal tube) is passed into the trachea. The operator's hand is removed from the animal's mouth, and the endotracheal tube is passed over the small tube into the trachea (Fig. 7).[20] The small tube is removed. This method is preferred in medium-sized cattle and in all animals in which the Cole's tube is used.

INTUBATION OF CALVES, SHEEP, AND GOATS

In animals with a small oral cavity, a laryngoscope with a long illuminated blade (Rawson or extension on human blade) (Fig. 8) can be used for direct visualization of the laryngeal opening and tracheal intubation. Because the mouth of herbivores cannot be opened widely, the combination of laryngoscope blade and large endotracheal tube may occlude one's view of the laryngeal opening. In such cases, a rather fine plastic catheter can be passed into the trachea to act as a stylet over which the endotracheal tube is passed (see Fig. 5). When the endotracheal tube is in place, the stylet is removed and the cuff is inflated.

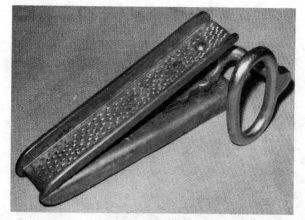

Figure 6. Dental wedge used to hold the mouth of adult cattle open for tracheal intubation.

FETAL TRACHEAL INTUBATION

Apnea may be encountered when a fetus is delivered by cesarean section. Tracheal intubation prior to delivery provides a means of dealing with this problem.

When the fetal head is delivered through the uterine wall incision, the laryngoscope is used to visualize the laryngeal opening for tracheal intubation. With the tube in place, fluids can be aspirated from the upper airways. Mechanical ventilation using a hand-operated resuscitator (see Fig. 4) is commenced and may be continued until a normal respiratory pattern is established. Oxygen may be delivered to the fetus via the resuscitator when available and required. These maneuvers can all be completed prior to disruption of the placental-umbilical circulation, if so desired.

When apnea persists in the presence of a strong fetal heartbeat, a small dose of doxapram (0.2–0.4 mg/kg IV) or some other analeptic may aid in the establishment of spontaneous breathing.

INTUBATION OF SWINE

Pigs are more difficult to intubate than small ruminants because of the several physical features, including a relatively small larynx, inability to open the mouth widely, blending of cricoid cartilage into the laryngeal orifice, and a ventral slope from larynx to trachea. With light basal anesthesia, laryngeal spasms often occur when endotracheal intubation is attempted. Spraying the laryngeal membranes with 4 per cent lidocaine shortly before proceeding with intubation will usually prevent laryngeal spasms, making the procedure less hazardous. A muscle relaxant (e.g., succinylcholine, 1–2 mg/kg) will induce muscle paralysis and prevent laryngeal spasms.

The technique for tracheal intubation in swine is essentially the same as that for small ruminants. A mouth wedge can be used to keep the mouth open. An alternative is to place loops of small-diameter rope around the upper and lower jaws immediately behind the canine teeth. An assistant applies traction on each loop, opening the mouth widely. A laryngoscope is nearly essential for intubation unless one has had a great deal of experience. With the laryngoscope, the laryngeal opening can be directly visualized and the tube passed into the trachea. As in sheep and goats, a small-gauge plastic catheter can be passed into the trachea first serving as a stylet over which the endotracheal tube may be passed (see Fig. 5).

A technique whereby a small cuffed tube is placed into each nostril and connected to a Y-piece, which in turn is connected to the Y-piece of the anesthetic machine, has been used as a substitute for endotracheal intubation. Tape or gauze is placed around the animal's snout to prevent open-mouth breathing. Although anesthesia can be effectively maintained, this technique does not provide protection against aspiration of foreign materials nor prevent inflation of the stomach when positive-pressure ventilation is employed. It is, therefore, no less hazardous than a well-fitted nose cone.

STAGES AND PLANES OF ANESTHESIA

Traditionally, general anesthesia has been divided into stages and then into planes.[62] These signs associated with

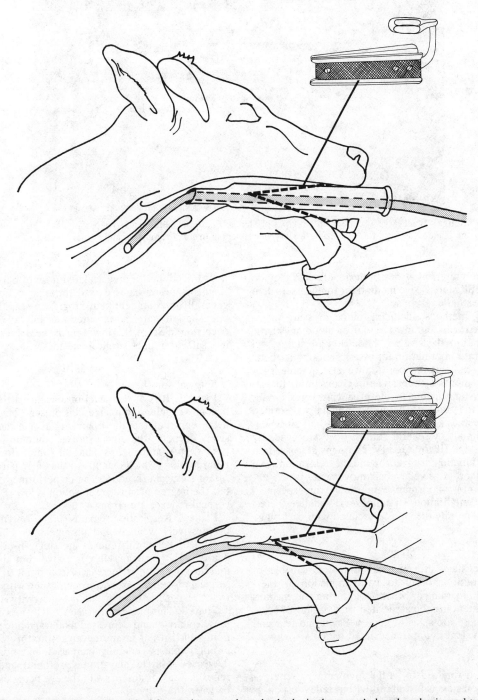

Figure 7. These drawings illustrate a method for passing an endotracheal tube in the cow. A dental wedge is used to prevent injury of hand and arm, and a small tube three times the length of the endotracheal tube is inserted into the trachea. This tube serves as a guide for directing the endotracheal tube into the trachea.

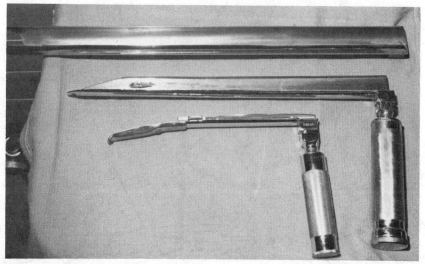

Figure 8. *Top,* Large animal laryngoscope with two types of blades. *Bottom,* The human laryngoscope has been modified by adding an extension to the blade. It is ideal for visualizing the laryngeal opening in small ruminants and swine.

each stage are empirical at best, but nonetheless they do serve as a useful noninvasive method for rough assessment of patient anesthetic response.

Monitoring methods, including blood pressure measurement, electrocardiogram, alveolar or blood anesthetic concentration, blood gas values, and acid-base status, will provide accurate information for assessment of anesthetic depth and physiologic response; however, equipment for these measurements is expensive, time-consuming to use, and generally unavailable to the practicing veterinarian. As a result, the traditional signs as originally described for ether anesthesia in humans (Guedel) and since described in animals by several authors[13, 14, 43] are generally used. From Stage III to Stage IV, the signs are based on vital system function, degree of muscle relaxation, eye reflexes, and progressive eyeball movement, which appears to be most informative in the bovine species.[44] Preanesthetic medication (tranquilizers, sedatives, etc.) unpredictably modify the signs associated with each stage of anesthesia.

Stage I

This is the stage in which an animal is capable of resisting restraint in order to avoid induction of anesthesia. Rapid breathing or breath-holding may be encountered. Excitement may be associated with voiding of urine and feces. These are signs of apprehension and fear and are more prevalent in unpremedicated patients.

Stage II

This is often referred to as the involuntary excitatory stage. Consciousness is lost abruptly, but reflex responses to stimuli are exaggerated. The respiratory pattern is irregular, and struggling is associated with breath-holding. The jaw muscles are unrelaxed, and attempts to intubate will initiate chewing and coughing. Reflex responses, other than poor muscle relaxation, chewing movements, coughing, and likelihood of active regurgitation, are not as bothersome in ruminants as in other domestic animals at this time.

When surgical anesthesia is attained by rapid intrave-

nous injection of a precalculated dose of barbiturate, this stage of anesthesia is passed through so quickly that it generally goes unidentified. Progressing rapidly from consciousness to surgical anesthesia usually avoids problems occurring in Stage II. However, in the debilitated animal, it is safer to induce surgical anesthesia slowly.

Stage III

Surgical anesthesia.

Plane 1. It is at this level of anesthesia that breathing becomes regular and analgesia is present. Nystagmus may be evident but rapidly disappears as anesthesia progressively deepens; this sign is not as common in cows as in horses. In ruminants, esophageal stimulation may evoke regurgitation, which extends to the early part of Plane 2. Minor surgical procedures can be performed at this plane, but the degree of muscle relaxation is low. Palpebral and corneal reflexes are strong.

Plane 2. Respiration remains stable. Laryngeal reflexes progressively weaken and disappear as Plane 3 is approached. Palpebral reflexes are sluggish or have disappeared. The corneal reflex is active, but the degree of muscle relaxation is increased to a point at which most surgical procedures can be accomplished without initiating reflex responses. Intercostal muscle activity is diminished.

Plane 3. This plane is characterized by loss of intercostal muscle activity and depressed diaphragmatic muscle function, which result in an uneven respiratory pattern. Respiration rate is generally increased, but tidal volume is decreased. Muscle relaxation is profound, and the corneal reflex is weak or absent, with the eye being fixed centrally between the palpebra.

Stage IV

The pupil is widely dilated, and all other eye reflexes have disappeared. Respiration is purely diaphragmatic in character, with excessive abdominal movement occurring with each agonal breath. Cardiac function is rapidly failing. The anus is dilated, and feces and urine may be passively voided. At this point, if respiration is not supported, anesthetic concentration is not decreased, and fluids are not administered rapidly to support the failing cardiovascular system, death is inevitable.

ANESTHESIA AND EYEBALL ROTATION IN CATTLE

Rotation of the eyeball in cattle has been described in detail[22, 44] and has been shown to be a reliable means of monitoring anesthetic depth as well as progression of recovery from halothane anesthesia.

The eyeball is normally centered between the palpebra in the unanesthetized cow in lateral recumbency (Fig. 9A). As anesthesia is induced, the eyeball rotates ventrally, with the cornea being partially obscured by the lower eyelid (Fig. 9B and C). As depth of anesthesia is increased, the cornea becomes completely hidden by the lower eyelid (Fig. 9D); this sign indicates Stage III, Plane 2 to 3 anesthesia. A further increase in the depth of anesthesia is accompanied by dorsal rotation of the eyeball. Dorsal movement is complete when the cornea is centered between the palpebra (Fig. 9E); this sign indicates deep surgical anesthesia with profound muscle relaxation. With this depth of anesthesia, the patient's vital signs must be monitored closely and the anesthetic per-

centage must be decreased to a maintenance level. Otherwise, anesthesia may progress rather quickly to Stage IV.

During recovery, eyeball rotation occurs in reverse order to that observed during induction.

MALIGNANT HYPERTHERMIA (MH) IN SWINE

Malignant hyperthermia is a condition occurring in some strains of swine subjected to stress. The predisposition to MH appears to be inherited as an autosomal dominant gene with incomplete penetrance.[59] It is encountered most often in animals with a high proportion of muscle to body mass. The incidence of MH is higher in confined animals of Pietrain, Landrace, Spotted Swine, Large White, and Hampshire breeding. Other breeds are not immune, but the incidence does appear to be less in Durocs.[60]

MH is characterized by rapid onset of tachycardia, muscle rigidity, hyperthermia, tachypnea that progresses to dyspnea, and, finally, apnea, cardiac dysrhythmias, bradycardia, and death. In susceptible animals, MH usually occurs shortly after exposure to halothane. Although we have observed MH with methoxyflurane anesthesia,

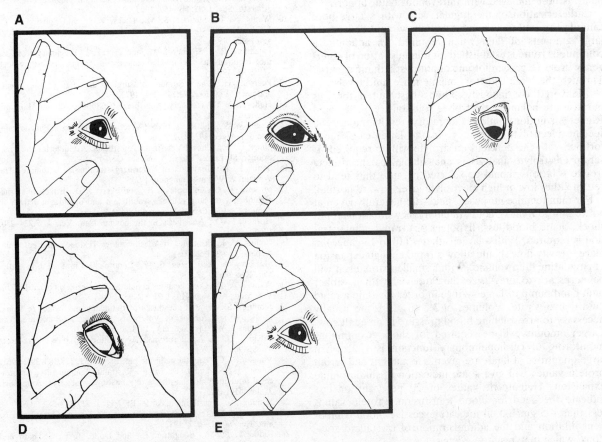

Figure 9. Eyeball position during induction and maintenance of general anesthesia of cattle. A, Position of eye when cow is unanesthetized and positioned in lateral recumbency. B, and C, With induction of anesthesia, the eye rotates ventrally, the cornea being partially obscured by the lower eyelid. D, As depth of anesthesia is increased (Stage III, Plane 2–3), the cornea is completely hidden by the lower eyelid. E, Further increases in the depth of anesthesia cause the eye to rotate dorsally to a central position between the palpebra. At this point, deep surgical anesthesia has been attained, and muscle relaxation is profound. Decreasing the depth of anesthesia is accompanied by eye movements occurring in a reverse order.

the onset was slower than with halothane anesthesia. MH can be precipitated by subjecting susceptible swine to any stressful condition. This syndrome is not peculiar only to stress induced by halothane or methoxyflurane anesthesia.

The muscle relaxant succinylcholine has been shown to induce MH in susceptible swine, but dantrolene (Dantrium)* 1–2 mg/kg, a muscle relaxant, has been shown to prevent the syndrome.[61]

The body temperature of swine subjected to general anesthesia should be monitored closely. A sudden increase indicates the likelihood of MH onset. Treatment after the condition is clinically evident is generally unsuccessful. If MH is detected in the earliest stage, elimination of halothane, ventilation with oxygen, administration of sodium bicarbonate, and rapid body cooling with ice packs may be helpful.

SUPPORTIVE FLUID THERAPY DURING ANESTHESIA

In the healthy patient subjected to short-term, light surgical anesthesia, administration of supportive fluids is not considered to be absolutely necessary unless the animal has been starved of food and water for over 24 hours. Prolonged deep surgical anesthesia, on the other hand, is best managed with intravenous fluid support.

Catheterization of the jugular vein with a large-bore cannula (i.e., 10 to 13 gauge) will allow rapid delivery of large amounts of fluid when required. In addition, a continuous route is established for administration of emergency drugs (e.g., cardiotonic or antidysrhythmic agents). Through the large catheter, maintenance fluid levels can be delivered continuously. Fluids best suited for this purpose are balanced electrolyte solutions (e.g., lactated Ringer's solution) unless laboratory results indicate a specific electrolyte deficiency. In the latter case, fluids fortified with the deficient electrolyte will be required. If serum electrolyte analysis is unavailable, balanced electrolyte solutions should be selected because they tend to return either low or high electrolyte levels toward normal.

For maintenance purposes, fluids are generally given at a rate of 4 to 8 ml/kg/hour. In emergency situations (e.g., shock, acute blood loss, hypotension), rapid administration is required. With a large catheter (10 to 13 gauge) in place, gravity flow should allow a rapid enough expansion of circulating fluid volume. With a smaller catheter, it will be necessary to pressurize the fluid vial with a rubber bulb hand pump or large syringe in order to attain a rapid fluid delivery rate. Volumes of 3.5 to 7.5 L are usually necessary to arrest falling blood pressure in an adult cow. Larger amounts will be required for shock. Continuous monitoring of cardiopulmonary function is vital when large quantities of fluids are given. Hematocrit and serum protein values will give some indication of fluid volume expansion. Hematocrit values of 20 per cent or less indicate the need for blood transfusion. Protein values less than 4.5 gm/100 ml indicate excessive blood component dilution and the administration of crystalloid solutions, which may result in edema.

Fluid loading is essential in sows that are hypotensive or demonstrate other signs of shock. With a 16-gauge, over-the-needle catheter placed in a large central ear vein,

2 to 3 L of fluid can be given rather rapidly by pressurizing the fluid vial. This procedure is often the single most important measure that can be taken to promote safe anesthesia in a sow presented for cesarean section; this is particularly true if the sow is toxic from dead piglets *in utero* and epidural anesthesia is to be employed.

References

1. Donawick, W. J., Hirmath, I., and Baue, A. E.: Anesthesia, ventilation, and experimental thoracotomy in the calf. Am. J. Vet. Res. 30:533–541, 1969.
2. Gerring, E. L., and Scarth, S. C.: Anesthesia for open heart surgery in the calf. Br. J. Anaesth. 46:455–460, 1974.
3. McFarlane, J. K., Robillard, F. A., and Blundell, P. E.: Anesthesia for cardiopulmonry bypass in calves. Can. Anaesth. Soc. J. 14:240–245, 1967.
4. Nishzawa, T., Morris, D. T., and Couves, C. M.: Surgical techniques for total artificial heart replacement in calves. Can. J. Surg. 17:261–265, 1974.
5. Short, C. E., Keats, A. S., Liotta, D., and Hall, W.: Anesthesia for cardiac surgery in calves. Am. J. Vet. Res. 29:2287–2294, 1968.
6. Steffey, E. P., and Holland, D.: Halothane anesthesia in calves. Am. J. Vet. Res. 40:372–376, 1979.
7. Kumar, A.: Physiologic, Biochemical and Clinical Effects of Ketamine Hydrochloride in Goats (Capra hircus) With and Without Premedication. Ph.D. Thesis, University of Illinois, 1973.
8. Palahniuk, R. J., and Shnider, S. M.: Maternal and fetal cardiovascular and acid-base changes during halothane and isoflurane anesthesia in the pregnant ewe. Anesthesiology 41:462–472, 1974.
9. Smith, J. B., Manning, F. A., and Palahniuk, R. J.: Maternal and foetal effects of methoxyflurane anaesthesia in the pregnant ewe. Can. Anaesth. Soc. J. 22:449–459, 1975.
10. Wallis, K. L., Shnider, S. M., Hicks, J. S., and Spivey, H. T.: Epidural anesthesia in the normotensive pregnant ewe. Anesthesiology 4:481–487, 1976.
11. Palahniuk, R. J., Shnider, S. M., and Eger, E. I.: Pregnancy decreases the requirement for inhaled anesthetic agents. Anesthesiology 41:82–83, 1974.
12. Pearson, H.: The treatment of surgical disorders of the bovine abdomen. Vet. Rec. 92:245–254, 1973.
13. Hall, L. W.: Veterinary Anesthesia Textbook, 8th ed. London, Bailliere Tindall, 1983.
14. Lumb, W. V., and Jones, E. W.: Veterinary Anesthesia. Philadelphia, Lea & Febiger, 1973.
15. Short, C. E.: Clinical Veterinary Anesthesia: A Guide for the Practitioner. St. Louis, The C. V. Mosby Co., 1974.
16. Soma, L. R.: Textbook of Veterinary Anesthesia. Baltimore, The Williams & Wilkins Company, 1971.
17. Musewe, V. O., Gillespie, J. R., and Berry, J. D.: Effects of sternal recumbency on lung volumes, ventilation and diaphragm activity in domestic cattle. Personal communication.
18. Horney, F. D.: Anesthesia in the bovine. Can. Vet. J. 7:224–230, 1966.
19. Collins, V. J.: Principles of Anesthesiology Textbook, 2nd ed. Philadelphia, Lea & Febiger, 1976.
20. Masservy, A., and Jones, E. W.: Endotracheal intubation in cattle. Vet. Rec. 68:32–33, 1956.
21. Weaver, A. D.: Complications in halothane anaesthesia of cattle. Zbl. Vet. Med. A. 8:409–416, 1971.
22. Jennings, S.: General anesthesia of ruminants and swine. In Soma, L. R. (ed.): Textbook of Veterinary Anesthesia. Baltimore, The Williams & Wilkins Company, 1971.
23. Ritchie, H. E.: Chlorpromazine sedation in pigs. Vet. Rec. 69:895–900, 1957.
24. Vaughn, L. C.: Anesthesia in the pig. Br. Vet. J. 117:383–391, 1961.
25. Regan, H. A., and Gillis, M. F.: Restraint, venipuncture, endotracheal intubation and anesthesia of miniature swine. Lab. Anim. Sci. 23:409–419, 1975.
26. Jennings, S.: Anesthesia in cattle. Br. Vet. J. 117:377–382, 1961.
27. Jones, R. S.: A review of tranquilizers and sedation of large animals. Vet. Rec. 90:613–617, 1972.
28. Kidd, A. R. M., Boughton, E., and Done, J. T.: Sedation and immobilization of cattle in the field. Vet. Rec. 88:679–687, 1971.
29. Kumar, A., Thurmon, J. C., and Hardenbrook, H. J.: Clinical studies of ketamine HCl and xylazine HCl in domestic goats. Vet. Med. Small Anim. Clin. 71:1707–1713, 1976.
30. Ferguson, A. R.: The use of azaperone in pig practice. Ir. Vet. J. 25:61–64, 1971.
31. Callear, J. F. F., and Van Gestel, J. F. E.: An analysis of the results

*Available from Norwich-Eaton Pharmaceuticals, Norwich, NY 13815.

of field experiments in pigs in the United Kingdom and Ireland with the sedative neuroleptic azaperone. Vet. Rec. 89:453–458, 1971.

32. Reynolds, W. T.: Anesthesia in cattle. Aust. Vet. J. 51:270–272, 1975.
33. Clarke, K. W., and Hall, L. W.: "Xylazine"—a new sedative for horses and cattle. Vet. Rec. 85:512–517, 1969.
34. Hopkins, T. J.: The clinical pharmacology of xylazine in cattle. Aust. Vet. J. 48:109–112, 1972.
35. Rickard, L. J., Thurmon, J. C., and Lingard, D. R.: Preliminary report on xylazine hydrochloride as a sedative agent in bulls for electroejaculation and semen collection, Vet. Med. Small Anim. Clin. 69:1029–1031, 1974.
36. Seifelnasr, E., Salch, M., and Soliman, F. A.: In vivo investigations on the effect of Rompun on the rumen motility in sheep. Vet. Med. Rev. 2:158–165, 1974.
37. Rosenberger, G., Hempel, E., and Baumeister, M.: Contributions to the effect and applicability of Rompun in cattle. Vet. Med. Rev. 2:137–142, 1969.
38. Thurmon, J. C., Nelson, D. R., Harsfield, S. M., and Rumore, C. A.: Effects of xylazine hydrochloride on urine in cattle. Aust. Vet. J. 54:178–180, 1978.
39. Lane, D. R.: The sedation of cattle. Vet. Rec. 86:358, 1970.
40. Stewart, J. M.: Observations on the restraint and immobilization of uncontrollable cattle with Rompun. Vet. Med. Rev. 3:197–204, 1972.
41. Dobbs, H. E., and Ling, C. M.: Reversible immobilization and analgesia in the bullock. Vet. Med. Rev. 91:11–15, 1973.
42. Sharma, R. P., Stowe, C. M., and Good, A. L.: Studies on the distribution and metabolism of thiopental in cattle, sheep, goats, and swine. J. Pharmacol. Exp. Ther. 172:128–137, 1970.
43. Garner, H. E., Mather, E. C., Hoover, T. R., Brown, R. E., and Halliwell, W. C.: Anesthesia of bulls undergoing surgical manipulation of the vas deferentia. Can. J. Comp. Med. Vet. Sci. 39:250–255, 1975.
44. Thurmon, J. C., Romack, F. E., and Garner, H. E.: Excursions of the bovine eyeball during gaseous anesthesia. Vet. Med. 63:967–970, 1968.
45. Thurmon, J. C., Nelson, D. R., and Christie, G. J.: Ketamine anesthesia in swine. J. Am. Vet. Med. Assoc. 160:1325–1330, 1972.
46. Fuentes, V. O., and Tellez, E.: Ketamine dissociative analgesia in cattle. Vet. Rec. 94:482, 1974.
47. Fuentes, V. O., and Tellez, E.: Mid-line caesarean section in a cow using ketamine anesthesia. Vet. Rec. 99:338, 1976.
48. Ivankovich, A. D., Miletich, D. J., Reimann, C., Albrecht, R. F., and Zahed, B.: Cardiovascular effects of centrally administered ketamine in goats. Anesth. Analg. 53:924–931, 1974.
49. Kumar, A., Thurmon, J. C., and Dorner, J. L.: Hematologic and biochemical findings in sheep given ketamine hydrochloride. J. Am. J. Vet. Med. Assoc. 165:284–287, 1974.
50. Kumar, A., Thurmon, J. C., Nelson, D. R., and Link, R. P.: Effects of ketamine hydrochloride on maternal and fetal arterial blood pressure and acid-base status in goats. Vet. Anesth. 5:28–33, 1978.
51. Levinson, G., Shnider, S. M., Gildea, J. E., and DeLorimier, A. A.: Maternal and foetal cardiovascular and acid-base changes during ketamine anesthesia in pregnant ewes. Br. J. Anaesth. 45:1111–1115, 1973.
52. Taylor, P., Hopkins, L., Young, M., and McFadyen, I. R.: Ketamine anesthesia in the pregnant sheep. Vet. Rec. 90:35–36, 1972.
53. Thurmon, J. C., Kumar, A., and Link, R. P.: Evaluation of ketamine hydrochloride as an anesthetic in sheep. J. Am. J. Vet. Med. Assoc. 162:293–297, 1973.
54. Thurmon, J. C., Kumar, A., and Cawley, A. J.: Changes in the acid base status of sheep anesthetized with a combination of atropine sulphate acepromazine and ketamine hydrochloride. Aust. Vet. J. 51:484–487, 1975.
55. Anderson, I. L.: Anesthesia of swine. N. Z. Vet. J. 25:319–321, 1977.
56. Cox, J. E.: Immobilization and anesthesia of the pig. Vet. Rec. 92:143–147, 1973.
57. Ravaud, M.: Une nouvelle méthode d'anésthesie de la truie lors de césariennes realisées pour obtenir des animaux. S. P. F. Recl. Med. Vet. Ec. Alfort 148:1245–1249, 1972.
58. Douglas, T. A., Longstreeth, S. J. J., and Weaver, A. D.: Methoxyflurane anesthesia in horses and cattle. Vet. Rec. 76:615–623, 1964.
59. Nelson, T. E., Jones, E. W., Hendrickson, R. L., Falk, S. N., and Kerr, D. D.: Porcine malignant hyperthermia. Observation on the occurrence of pale, soft, exudative musculature among susceptible pigs. Am. J. Vet. Res. 35:349–350, 1972.
60. Wagner, A. J.: The porcine stress syndrome. Vet. Med. Rev. 1:68–77, 1972.
61. Gronert, G. A., Milde, J. H., and Theye, R. A.: Dantrolene in porcine malignant hyperthermia. Anesthesiology 44:488–495, 1976.
62. Jones, L. M.: Veterinary Pharmacology and Therapeutics, 3rd ed. Ames, Iowa, Iowa State University Press, 1965.
63. Thurmon, J. C., and Benson, G. J.: Inhalation anesthetic delivery equipment and its maintenance. Vet. Clin. North Am.: Large Anim. Pract. 3:73–96, 1981.
64. Kitzman, J. V., Booth, N. H., Hatch, R. C., and Wallner, B.: Antagonism of xylazine sedation by 4-aminopyridine and yohimbine in cattle. Am. J. Vet. Res. 43:2165–2169, 1982.
65. Breese, C. E., and Dodman, N. H.: Xylazine-ketamine-oxymorphone: An injectable anesthesic combination in swine. J. Am. Vet. Med. Assoc. 184:182–183, 1984.

Regional Analgesia of Food Animals

G. J. BENSON, D.V.M., M.S., D.A.C.V.A.,
and J. C. THURMON, D.V.M., M.S., D.A.C.V.A.

Regional analgesia is a deliberately induced, temporary loss of sensation in a defined body area without loss of consciousness. It is induced by agents that act upon the nerve endings or nerve trunks, causing paralysis of function and relaxation of muscles. Economically, regional analgesia is well suited for use in food-producing animals. Regional techniques may be used for a variety of surgical procedures, for a number of reasons. Postoperative sequelae are few, as physiologic alterations due to the analgesic agent are minimal. Major procedures can be done with the animal standing, thereby avoiding casting and prolonged recumbency in the large patient. The techniques, although requiring skill, are easily learned. Finally, regional analgesia may be induced with a minimal amount of help, an important consideration for surgery in the field, for which assistants are unavailable.

The major disadvantage of regional analgesia is that the patient is not immobilized. The judicious use of sedatives and physical restraint may be used to control the patient. Regional techniques are contraindicated in patients with pathologic processes involving the site of injection such as infection, fibrosis, scarring, and deficient blood supply.

The major objective of this article is to review the pertinent anatomy, physiology, and pharmacology associated with regional analgesia and to describe common regional analgesic techniques.

CLASSIFICATION OF REGIONAL ANALGESIA

Regional analgesia may be classified by the site of anesthetic-nerve contact.

Terminal analgesia occurs when analgesic agents are applied directly upon the nerve ending as a result of:

1. Absorption of the agent from surface application with subsequent diffusion to the nerve endings. Examples of such surfaces are mucous membranes, the cornea, and the synovial membranes of joints and tendon sheaths.

2. Infiltration of the operative field to place the agent in contact with the nerve endings. An example is a line block for abdominal incision, in which the analgesic is injected beneath the skin and onto the peritoneum.

3. Intravenous injection of the agent into a limb around which a tourniquet has been applied. This technique is most commonly used in people for operations involving the extremities and may be utilized in animals as well.

Field analgesia results from injection of the agent around the periphery of the operative field, which causes nerve impulse blockade within. It avoids the presence of the agent in incised tissue and its subsequent effect upon healing. An example is the "backwards 7" block for left paralumbar laparotomy.

Conduction analgesia results from infiltration of the agent around major nerve tracks innervating large regions of tissue. Examples are:

1. Spinal analgesia: deposition of the agent within the spinal canal.

2. Paravertebral analgesia: infiltration of spinal nerves where they emerge from intervertebral foramen.

3. Infiltration of peripheral nerves, e.g., pudendal, digital.

ANATOMY

Successful induction of regional analgesia is in large part dependent upon an understanding of the spinal cord, the meninges, and the spinal and peripheral nerves. The central nervous system comprises the brain and spinal cord. The spinal cord is encased within the vertebral canal and extends from the foramen magnum to approximately the last lumbar vertebrae, depending upon the species. Spinal nerves leave the cord at each spinal segment and exit the canal at the intervertebral foramen. The spinal nerves are composed of an efferent ventral motor branch and an afferent dorsal branch. The caudal portion of the vertebral canal contains the cauda equina, which contains descending spinal nerves. In the fetus, all spinal nerves exit at right angles to the spinal cord. In the adult, however, owing to differential growth rates between the spinal cord and bony vertebral canal, the nerves must run posteriorly to reach their respective intervertebral foramina. This feature is significant and affects the level of analgesia induced by the deposition of analgesic agent within the spinal canal. Variations of innervation occur among and within species. Table 1 gives a summary of the areas of motor and sensory innervation supplied by the spinal nerves.

The meninges (dura mater, arachnoid, and pia mater), which surround the spinal cord, are important in uptake and distribution of analgesic agents injected into perivertebral areas. Various spaces are associated with the meninges and are important to understanding spinal anesthetic techniques and nomenclature (Fig. 1). The dura mater has two layers within the cranial vault, an inner or visceral layer and an outer layer adherent to the cranial periosteum. The inner or visceral layer invests the spinal cord and dorsal and ventral nerve roots; the outer layer is absent in the vertebral canal of some species. The epidural space is the space within the spinal canal outside the visceral layer of dura mater. It has also been referred to as the extradural space, and in those species having both layers of dura, it is called the intradural space. The dura adheres to the periosteum of the foramen magnum, thereby preventing the passage of fluid from the spinal epidural space to the cranial epidural space. The epidural

Table 1. Sensory and Motor Innervation Related to Spinal Cord Segments

Spinal Segment	Nerves	Sensory Innervation	Motor Innervation
Coccygeal	All	Tail	Coccygeal muscles
Sacral	5,4	Tail base and croup Anal region and sphincter Vulva Perineum	Anus Terminal rectum Vagina Penis, bladder, and urethra
Lumbar	3,2,1 6,5,4	Croup	Parts of lumbosacral plexus
Lumbosacral plexus	Posterior gluteal	Lateral/posterior aspect of hip/thigh	Extensors of hip
	Greater sciatic	Mid-tibia to digits	Flexors of stifle Flexors/extensors of hock and digit
	Anterior gluteal	Lateral thigh	Flexor/abductors of hip
	Obturator	Medial aspect of thigh	Abductors of hip
	Femoral	Anterior aspects of limbs as low as hock	Flexors of hip Extensors of stifle
Lumbar	3	Loins Croup Anterior stifle Scrotum, prepuce Inguinal region of mammary gland	Sublumbar muscle group Posterior parts of abdominal muscles
	2	Loins, flank Anterior/lateral thigh Prepuce Mammary gland	Sublumbar muscle group Posterior parts of abdominal muscles
	1	Loins Posterior abdomen Lateral thigh	Posterior parts of abdominal muscles
Thoracic	Last two	Abdominal wall and flank posterior to umbilicus	Abdominal muscles
	Mid to last	Anterior/ventral abdominal wall	Intercostal muscles Anterior abdominal muscles

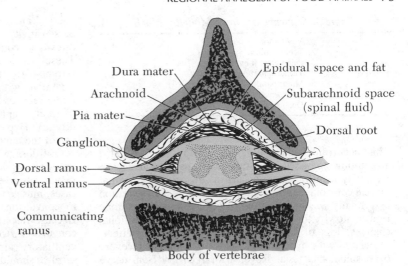

Figure 1. Anatomic detail of cross-section of spinal canal at level of intervertebral foramen.

space contains blood vessels, lymphatics, and fat, and it communicates with the paravertebral tissues via the intervertebral foramina. This communication may be interrupted in older animals by fibrous connective tissue, bony malformation, or arthritis and in obese patients by fat.

The subarachnoid space is located between the arachnoid and pia mater. The subarachnoid space contains cerebrospinal fluid and is continuous with the cerebral subarachnoid space. Because no direct communication occurs between the subarachnoid and epidural spaces, analgesic agents cannot pass directly from the epidural space to the cerebrospinal fluid. However, epidural analgesic agents can diffuse through the dura and arachnoidea to reach the cerebrospinal fluid. Arachnoid granulations protrude through the dura into the epidural space at the dural root sleeve and may afford a preferential pathway for passage of agents between the epidural space and the cerebrospinal fluid.

The pia mater is one cell layer thick and lies directly on the spinal cord. Diffusion of agents from the cerebrospinal fluid to the spinal cord itself is relatively unimpaired.

At each segment, dorsal and ventral nerve roots emerge from the cord to form the bilateral spinal nerves. The spinal nerves contain autonomic nerve fibers that supply vasoconstrictor activity to the skin, viscera, and muscle tissue. As the nerve roots leave the spinal cord, they pierce the meninges and carry a layer of each with them. These nerve roots with their meningeal covers join to form the spinal nerves. The meningeal covers fuse at their junction and extend no further peripherally.

The number of vertebrae and the terminations of spinal cord and spinal meninges vary among species and influence the application of spinal analgesic techniques (Table 2). Either spinal or epidural injection may be given at the lumbosacral junction in ruminants and in swine.

In nonmyelinated nerve fibers, conduction of impulses is relatively slow but increases as the fiber's diameter increases. In fibers in which frequent, rapid transmission occurs, a myelin sheath that insulates the fiber has evolved. This myelin sheath is broken at intervals (i.e., the nodes of Ranvier) to allow direct contact between the cell membrane and the extracellular fluid. Depolarization can occur only at the nodes of Ranvier, so the impulse "jumps" from node to node along the course of the fiber, increasing rate of conduction.

Onset and duration of blockade of peripheral nerves is a function of fiber type and number within the nerve. Myelin limits the area of immediate contact between cell membrane and local analgesic agent to the nodes of Ranvier. Therefore, a higher concentration of agent is needed to block myelinated fibers than to block nonmyelinated fibers. Large-diameter fibers present less surface area per unit of volume for absorption of analgesic agent than small-diameter fibers, which have a large surface area per unit volume. Therefore, small-diameter fibers are blocked more readily than large-diameter fibers. Onset of blockade depends upon diffusion of the local analgesic agent into the nerve trunk and fixation or stabilization of the cell membrane in individual fibers. Conduction of impulses is prevented by stabilization of the membrane potential precluding depolarization. Thus, in a large mixed nerve, the fibers will be blocked in order to their susceptibility to the agent (Table 3). Autonomic paralysis and vasomotor tone are lost first followed by analgesia and last by motor paralysis. Not uncommonly, pain sensation will be lost while motor function and touch perception are retained, a phenomenon known as differential block.

Table 2. *Anatomical Features of the Spinal Cord and Vertebrae of Ruminants and Swine*

Species	Spinal Cord Termination	Meningeal Termination	Number of Lumbar Vertebrae	Number of Sacral Vertebrae
Cow	*S2	S4	6	5
Sheep	S2	S2–4	6–7	4
Goat	S2	S2–4	6–7	4
Pig	S1	S2–3	6–7	4

*S = sacral vertebra.

Table 3. *Sequence of Nerve Modality Block*

1. Vasomotor blockade
2. Temperature
3. Pain (slow, then fast)
4. Tactile sensation
5. Motor paralysis
6. Joint sensation, proprioception
7. Deep pressure

This occurrence may be confusing to the anesthetist attempting to assess the degree of patient analgesia. Recovery from blockade occurs in reverse order, so that muscle control is regained first, followed by pain sensation and finally vasomotor tone. Because vasomotor tone returns slowly, the patient may be intolerant of positional changes, loss of body fluid, and systemic drug effects associated with hypotension following apparent recovery from spinal analgesia. Reversal or recovery from nerve blockade depends upon diffusion of the drug from a high concentration in the nerve fiber into the blood vascular system, where it will subsequently be redistributed, metabolized, and excreted.

ANALGESIC DRUGS

Local analgesics are drugs that, when applied to a nerve, temporarily block conduction without producing permanent damage. The rates of diffusion and absorption may be altered by the addition of epinephrine or hyaluronidase. By delaying absorption, epinephrine prolongs the duration of action and decreases systemic toxicity of local analgesic agents. Conversely, hyaluronidase, by promoting diffusion and absorption, increases the area of infiltration affected by the agent. Because hyaluronidase is of little benefit in conduction-type techniques and because of its cost, it is seldom used in veterinary practice. Table 4 compares some commonly used agents.

The commonly used local analgesics are weak bases. They are generally marketed as acid solutions of the water-soluble salts. Their acidity increases the stability of the solution and of the vasoconstrictor when present. In tissue, the acid salt is neutralized, liberating the base. Because it is the basic form that can penetrate cell membranes, causing blockade, it is readily apparent that a local analgesic will be less effective in inflamed tissue, where pH is decreased, because less of the basic form is liberated.

Local analgesics may cause untoward side effects. Hypersensitivity reactions may be seen as a result of using ester-type compounds, particularly upon repeated use. These reactions may appear as allergic-type dermatitis, asthma-like attacks (in humans), and anaphylaxis. Pretreatment with antihistaminic agents will decrease systemic reaction. Epinephrine and aminophylline are used to treat anaphylaxis and bronchospasm (asthmatic syndrome). Hypersensitivity reactions are rarely seen with use of the amide group.

Overdosage causes central nervous system stimulation followed by depression. Varying degrees of stimulation may be observed preceding depression. In the most severe cases, muscle twitching and opisthotonus rapidly progress to convulsions and subsequent death due to asphyxia. Because respiratory muscle function is ineffective during convulsions, treatment is directed at seizure control and ventilatory support. Patients suffering from convulsive seizures should receive anticonvulsants. Diazepam or barbiturates have been used for this purpose, followed by tracheal intubation and ventilation with an oxygen-enriched gas mixture. An alternative approach would be the use of a muscle relaxant and positive-pressure ventilation until the local analgesic and muscle relaxant are metabolized and excreted.

If the dosage of a local analgesic agent is sufficiently high, depression will follow stimulation. Cortical centers are affected first, followed by medullary depression. Clinical signs include deep sedation, generalized analgesia, loss of consciousness, muscle flaccidity, hypotension, tachycardia, and a weak, thready pulse. Death ensues owing to cardiovascular collapse and hypoventilation. Treatment is aimed at supporting the cardiovascular and respiratory systems and rapidly restoring the homeostatic mechanisms. This entails the establishment of a patent airway, administration of oxygen, and the rapid intravenous administration of balanced electrolyte solutions combined with vasopressors that have central effects, such as ephedrine and mephentermine. In general, the therapy is commensurate with that for any form of central cardiovascular collapse.

Regardless of the route of administration, the toxicity of local analgesic agents is the direct result of drug blood levels. Plasma concentrations are a function of site of administration, total dose of the drug (volume × concentration), concurrent use of vasoconstrictor, rate of injection, rate of tissue redistribution, degree of protein binding, and rate of metabolism. Depending upon local blood flow, infiltration of tissues with lidocaine HCl results in

Table 4. *Some Commonly Used Analgesic Agents*

	Esters		Amides		
	Procaine (Novocain)	Tetracaine (Pontocaine)	Lidocaine (Xylocaine)	Bupivacaine (Marcaine)	Mepivacaine (Carbocaine)
Potency*	1:1	10:1	1.5–2:1	3–4:1	3:1
Toxicity*	1:1	10:1	1.0–1.5:1	3:1	0.75:1
Recommended Concentration (%)					
Spinal	2	0.2–0.5	2–5	0.5–0.75	2
Epidural	1–2	0.2	2–4	0.5–0.75	1.5–2
Large Nerve	2	0.2	2	0.5	2
Infiltration	0.5	0.1	0.5	0.25	0.5–1
Onset (minutes)†	1–3	5–10	1–3	5–25	3–10
Duration (hours)†	1–1.5	2–3	0.75–1	3.5–6	2.5–4

*Procaine = 1.
†Of spinal analgesia.

maximum blood levels within 30 minutes. The toxic dose of lidocaine so administered is approximately 6 gm in the adult horse or cow.

Biotransformation and detoxification of local analgesics vary with the drug and the species. Amides are primarily metabolized by the liver, with the rate of metabolism being increased by enzyme induction. Lidocaine is slowly metabolized, but because of its high lipid solubility it is 90 per cent redistributed within 1 hour of administration. Ester metabolism is species-dependent, being metabolized by pseudocholinesterase in some species and by the liver in others.

SPINAL ANALGESIA

The nomenclature of various types of spinal analgesia in human and veterinary literature is confusing. For purposes of this discussion, *spinal analgesia* refers to all types of analgesia resulting from deposition of a local analgesic agent within the spinal canal. There are two types of spinal analgesia: (1) subarachnoid or "true" spinal analgesia, in which the agent is deposited in the subarachnoid space and, therefore, into the cerebrospinal fluid, and (2) epidural analgesia, the technique more commonly utilized in veterinary medicine, in which the agent is deposited within the epidural space. This latter technique is further described by the site of injection; thus, *caudal epidural* describes the epidural injection of an agent at the sacrococcygeal or intercoccygeal spaces. Caudal epidural analgesia is said to be either high or low, being differentiated by the total dose of local analgesia administered. *High caudal epidural analgesia* results when the agent is injected at the tail head in a dose sufficient to cause paralysis of the rear limbs. In *low caudal epidural analgesia*, the dose is small and results in analgesia of the perineal region only, without affecting motor function to the rear limbs. *Lumbosacral subarachnoid* and *lumbosacral epidural* analgesia result from injection at the lumbosacral junction. Either technique causes paralysis of the rear limbs. *Segmental epidural analgesia* results from the epidural injection of an agent in the lumbar or thoracic region, resulting in a belt or band of analgesia encircling the body. Motor function anterior and posterior to the area contacted by the agent within the epidural space is generally not affected, so the patient remains standing. Although this technique was first reported in cattle, it is not commonly used because alternative methods of producing analgesia of the same regions (e.g., paralumbar block) are easier to perform.

Because the epidural space usually communicates with the paralumbar space, and arachnoid villi in the spinal meninges allow diffusion of agents from the epidural space into the cerebrospinal fluid, local analgesics injected into any one of the three spaces may be found in the other two. Probably, there are multiple sites of action for local analgesics around the spinal cord, including the cord itself, the dorsal and ventral nerve roots, and the spinal nerves. Analgesia induced by epidural injection of procaine coincides with the rise and fall of procaine levels in cerebrospinal fluid. Diffusion of the agent through the dural root sleeve may allow the subperineural (submeningeal) blockade of the nerve roots. After repeated injections in the cow, procaine may be recovered from the cerebrospinal fluid; this finding would indicate that the meninges are not an effective barrier to diffusion. Analgesia induced by epidural injection depends upon complex diffusion processes but is principally due to the agent's effects on nerves and nerve roots within the epidural and paravertebral spaces.

The effect of analgesics in the epidural space is influenced by: (1) the size of the epidural space, i.e., condition, age, pregnancy, and length, (2) the volume of solution, (3) the concentration of solution, (4) the speed of injection, (5) gravity, and (6) technique.

The epidural space contains blood vessels, lymphatics, and fat. Engorgement of vessels, which occurs in pregnancy, or increased quantities of fat, as in obesity, will decrease the volume of epidural space available for the analgesic agent. Therefore, a given volume of agent migrates farther from the site of injection in pregnant or fat animals. For this reason, the dose of analgesic agent should be decreased by $\frac{1}{3}$ during late pregnancy and in obesity. Anterior migration of epidural drugs is also enhanced by transfer of negative pleural pressure to the epidural space.

The larger the epidural space, the larger the dose of drug required for a given level of blockade. Thus, patients with longer "crown to rump" measurements will require larger doses of epidural agents than those having short "crown to rump" measurements. The epidural space attains maximum size in the young adult. It is smallest in young (immature) and old patients.

Extent of blockade is a function of total mass (volume × concentration) of drug injected. Increasing either volume or concentration without changing the other parameter will increase the extent of blockade, but concentration has a more profound effect than volume on extent of blockade. Increasing the speed or force with which injection is made increases migration of the agent but may result in uneven distribution of agent within the epidural space and "patchy" block. In subarachnoid injections, intermittent injection and withdrawal ("barbotage") of the agent with cerebrospinal fluid increases the spread of blockade. Migration of drugs in the epidural space is influenced by gravity, whereas that of drugs placed in the cerebrospinal fluid occurs according to their specific gravity relative to that of cerebrospinal fluid. Drugs with a lower specific gravity than cerebrospinal fluid (hypobaric) will "float" like oil on water and migrate anteriorly if the head or forequarters are elevated. Mixing of local analgesic agents with 50 per cent dextrose renders them hyperbaric. Thus, they sink in cerebrospinal fluid, migrating to the dependent portions of the subarachnoid space.

In general, arterial blood pressure is decreased in proportion to the areas of the blockade during subarachnoid or epidural analgesia. The exact mechanism has not been conclusively identified, but it appears to be related to blockade of autonomic nerve fibers. If blockade does not extend anterior to the fifth thoracic segment, compensation occurs to maintain normal arterial blood pressures. Skarda and Muir[1] reported no effects upon arterial blood pressure, blood gases, or pH in healthy unsedated cows following segmental subarachnoid analgesia extending from T9 to L4 on both sides of the spine. Concurrent use of sympatholytic drugs such as the phenothiazine derivative tranquilizers will prevent compensation. Decreased venous return due to alpha$_1$-receptor blockade will promote venous pooling of blood in relaxed skeletal muscle and will result in reduced cardiac output. Opening the peritoneal cavity, hypoxia, hemorrhage, and surgical packing pressure may also decrease venous return. In all likelihood, the fall in arterial blood pressure is caused primarily by preganglionic sympathetic blockade and secondarily by decreased cardiac output. Patient positioning influences the alterations in blood pressure, with horizontal or head-down positions causing the least hypotension. In unsedated patients, centrally mediated and adrenal-mediated effects play a role in pressure regulation. Circulatory effects are more pronounced in patients experiencing stress of late pregnancy, parturition, and hypotension, for example.

Subarachnoid or epidural analgesia compromises respiratory function as the level of blockade progresses anteriorly. There is progressive depression of the intercostal muscles and depression of the diaphragm as phrenic roots are blocked. Medullary depression and respiratory arrest can occur with excessive subarachnoid injections. When correct analgesic dosages and techniques are employed, such complications are unlikely. Other effects of subarachnoid or epidural techniques are bowel contraction, splenic engorgement, and gastrointestinal sphincter relaxation.

Circulatory and respiratory changes should be treated if they endanger the patient. Respiratory failure necessitates establishment of a patent airway by endotracheal intubation and controlled ventilation with an oxygen-enriched atmosphere. Analeptic agents are of no use in respiratory failure induced by subarachnoid or epidural analgesia. Increased intra-abdominal pressure caused by abdominal packs, large abdominal tumors, a gravid uterus, or severe retraction may further increase respiratory embarrassment. Decreased arterial blood pressure and cardiac output are best treated by enhancing venous return. Rapid administration of balanced electrolyte solutions via a large venous catheter may be used to treat hypotension or to prevent its occurrence in the "at risk" patient. Should hypotension occur, vasopressors and a head-down tilt are helpful.

The inadvertent subarachnoid injection of large doses of local analgesic, which occurs when epidural technique and dosage are intended, results in "total spine." Controlled ventilation and cardiovascular support with fluids and vasopressors are indicated until the agent is eliminated. The patient should be positioned to restrict or prevent anterior migration of the agent. If a hypobaric agent is injected subarachnoidally, the patient is placed in a head-down position so that the agent is concentrated caudally. If a hyperbaric agent is administered in excess into the cerebrospinal fluid, the head is elevated above the rest of the body to prevent the agent from reaching the brain and upper spinal cord.

Other untoward sequelae of subarachnoid or spinal techniques include emesis due to unobtunded vagal reflexes arising from visceral manipulation; damage to spinal veins, arteries, or nerves; meningitis; and transient neurologic sequelae. In people, headaches, urine retention, fecal incontinence, loss of peripheral sensation, and loss of sexual functions have been reported. Spinal cord and meningeal injury or infection may result from improper technique or the analgesic agent itself. Paraplegia has been reported in people and animals, possibly as a result of exacerbations of pre-existing spinal disease. Inadvertent intravascular injection of an agent may result in cardio-vascular collapse. Although the reported incidence of severe complications is relatively low, care should be taken to avoid intravascular injection.

In patients that are toxemic or are experiencing cardiovascular collapse or shock, subarachnoid and epidural techniques should be viewed in light of their cardiovascular effects. Indiscriminate use of these techniques may result in cardiac decompensation and death. In such patients, subarachnoid or epidural techniques must be used judiciously, with particular attention given to cardiopulmonary function. Circulatory support should begin prior to induction of spinal analgesia.

Extreme obesity with excessive epidural fat or venous engorgement favors greater anterior migration of the agent in the epidural or subarachnoid spaces. Orthopedic spinal disease may result in partial closure of the paravertebral foramina, causing increased retention and anterior movement of the agent within the epidural space.

Specific Technique for Subarachnoid and Epidural Analgesia

Local and regional analgesia techniques should be preceded by aseptic preparation of the site for needle introduction. Because drugs used for subarachnoid or epidural analgesia come in direct contact with the spinal cord, spinal nerves, and meninges, meticulous care must be taken to ensure that chemical or bacterial contamination does not occur. Although the degree of asepsis practiced will be dictated by the surroundings, the cleanest possible technique should be used in order to avoid contamination and sequelae such as meningitis. The injection site should be clipped free of hair and scrubbed as for a surgical incision. The anesthetist should perform a surgical scrub on his or her hands and should wear sterile gloves. Syringes, needles, and drugs should be sterile. The smallest amount of detergent left on a needle entering the cerebrospinal fluid can cause permanent neurologic damage. Therefore, needles and syringes should be steam-autoclaved with stylets and plungers removed. The area may be draped with an "eye" drape.

A spinal needle should be used. It has a stylet to prevent clogging with tissue plugs, a short bevel to enhance tactile sensation as various tissues are penetrated, and a notch on the hub to indicate the bevel direction. The bevel should be directed toward the area to be rendered analgesic, usually anterior. Needle size and length vary with the species and size of the patient. The technique for continuous epidural analgesia requires a special type of needle. The Tuohy needle opens at an angle to the shaft for introduction of a catheter into the epidural space. The analgesic agent can be repeatedly injected through this fine-gauge catheter.

Epidural and Subarachnoid Analgesia Techniques in the Cow

In principle, any surgical procedure caudal to the diaphragm may be performed under epidural or subarachnoid analgesia. These techniques are commonly used for laparotomy and operations on the hindquarters of cattle, swine, and small ruminants. Epidural and subarachnoid analgesia may be indicated when general anesthesia is contraindicated. Geriatric patients may tolerate these techniques better than general anesthesia. Contraindications for epidural and subarachnoid techniques include:

1. Damage to lumbar or sacral vertebrae.

2. Damage to spinal cord or meninges.

3. Stenotic orthopedic processes of the vertebral canal.

4. Infection at the site of injection or within the spinal canal.

5. Congenital or acquired deformities of the spinal canal.

6. Paresis or lameness of nervous origin of the hindquarters.

7. Hypotension or circulatory collapse.

8. Cardiovascular disease.

Epidural analgesia in cattle is most commonly induced at the caudal region, either at the sacrococcygeal junction or between the first and second coccygeal vertebrae (Fig. 2). Raising and lowering the tail enables the anesthetist to locate the space between the vertebrae. The needle is inserted on the midline in the center of the space. If insertion is between the first two coccygeal vertebrae, the needle is directed anteriorly at a 45° angle. At the sacrococcygeal junction, the angle should be steeper, about 60° to the skin. Penetration of the interarcual ligament can be felt at a depth of 2 to 4 cm in the adult. If the needle strikes bone, insertion is too deep, and the needle should be withdrawn about 0.5 cm. With the tip of the needle in the epidural space, there should be no blood in the needle or resistance to air injection. Glass syringes are especially helpful because of their low resistance to plunger movement. Low caudal epidural analgesia, suitable for operations of the tail, anus, rectum, vulva, and perianal skin in the standing patient, may be induced by injecting 8 to 15 ml of 2 per cent procaine or 5 to 7 ml of 2 per cent lidocaine in adult cows. High caudal epidural analgesia resulting in hindlimb paralysis and recumbency is suitable for most procedures caudal to the diaphragm. Dosage depends on the surgical site and patient size. Sixty to 100 ml of 2 per cent lidocaine is sufficient for laparotomy incisions reaching the umbilicus in adult cows.

Lumbosacral epidural analgesia can be readily induced in the cow. The site for injection is the lumbosacral space, which is located between the dorsal iliac spines and between the lumbar spinous process arteriorly and the sacral spines caudally (see Fig. 2). The patient is restrained in the standing position. The skin and underlying tissues over the lumbosacral space are infiltrated with a small amount of analgesic. The needle is inserted on the midline perpendicular to the skin. Resistance will be noted as the needle pierces the ligamentum flavum at a depth of 11 to 13 cm. At that point, the needle will be in the epidural space. Neither blood nor cerebrospinal fluid will be observed upon withdrawal of the stylet nor by aspiration. There will be no resistance to the injection of air or analgesic agent. If the needle is advanced farther, the meninges may be penetrated. Removal of the stylet allows the escape of cerebrospinal fluid from the needle. If the position of the needle is in doubt, the anesthetist should attempt to aspirate cerebrospinal fluid. Aspiration of cerebrospinal fluid confirms penetration of the dura and arachnoid, and "true" spinal analgesia may be induced. Thirty-five to 50 ml of 2 per cent lidocaine is sufficient to induce lumbosacral epidural analgesia extending anteriorly to the umbilicus in mature cows. For subarachnoid analgesia, the dose is decreased by 50 per cent. Injection is made with the bevel of the needle facing forward.

Epidural and Subarachnoid Analgesia in the Goat, Sheep, and Pig

Lumbosacral, subarachnoid and epidural analgesia may be readily induced in the goat, sheep, and pig. The landmarks for injection are the same as for the cow. In the goat and sheep, the dose is 1 ml per 5 kg body weight of 2 per cent lidocaine for epidural analgesia caudal to the umbilicus. Total dosage should not exceed 15 ml of 2 per cent lidocaine in any size sheep or goat.

In the pig, the landmarks for location of the lumbosacral space are more difficult to identify. However, with practice the technique is readily mastered. Depth of spinal needle insertion depends on the size and condition of the patient, ranging from 2 to 3.5 cm in 10- to 20-kg pigs to 9 cm in 100-kg pigs. In heavy boars and sows, depth of penetration may be 10 to 13 cm. The dose for lumbosacral epidural analgesia with 2 per cent lidocaine is 1 ml per 10 kg body weight to a maximum of 20 ml in the adult. This will provide analgesia caudal to the umbilicus suitable for laparotomy and cesarean section.

Paravertebral Analgesia

Paravertebral analgesia is regional analgesia of the spinal nerves induced either proximally, at their exit from the intervertebral foramina, or distally, as they cross the tips of the transverse processes of the lumbar vertebrae. The primary indication for paravertebral analgesia is laparotomy in the standing patient. The advantages of paravertebral over infiltration techniques include: a lower total dosage of agent producing a wide area of analgesia; better muscle relaxation, allowing easier manipulation of

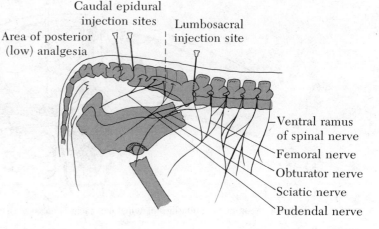

Caudal epidural injection sites

Lumbosacral injection site

Area of posterior (low) analgesia

Ventral ramus of spinal nerve

Femoral nerve

Obturator nerve

Sciatic nerve

Pudendal nerve

Figure 2. Anatomic relationships and injection sites for epidural analgesia in cattle.

viscera and decreasing intra-abdominal pressure; no interference by the agent with healing; and the procedure is simple, safe, and yet elegant enough to discourage the use of feed store drugs by the owner.

The paralumbar fossa is innervated principally by the 13th thoracic and first and second lumbar spinal nerves. Occasionally, fibers of the 12th thoracic nerve supply cutaneous innervation to the cranial portion of the fossa. Infrequently, the 3rd lumbar nerve supplies fibers to the caudal portion of the fossa, but blockade of the 3rd lumbar nerve should be avoided, because it supplies motor fibers to the rear limb. The nerves routinely blocked to provide paralumbar analgesia are T13, L1, and L2.

As the spinal nerves emerge from the intervertebral foramen, they divide into dorsal and ventral branches. The dorsal branch further divides into medial and lateral branches. The medial-dorsal branch innervates the dorsal lumbar muscles (loins). The lateral-dorsal branch provides cutaneous innervation to the dorsal half of the paralumbar fossa. The ventral branch of the spinal nerves innervates the skin of the ventral half of the paralumbar fossa to the ventral midline and innervates the muscles and peritoneum of the abdominal wall. As the spinal nerves run laterally, they sweep posteriorly to pass above and below the tip of the lumbar transverse processes. Thus, the lateral-dorsal branch passes above and the ventral branch of T13 passes below the tip of the transverse process of the first lumbar vertebra. The branches of the first lumbar nerve are located in a like manner at the tip of the transverse process of the second lumbar vertebra, and the branches of the second lumbar nerve are located at the tip of the transverse process of the fourth lumbar vertebra (Figs. 3 and 4).

The proximal technique has been described by several authors. The tips of the transverse processes of L1 and L2 are palpated. The skin is infiltrated above the anterior and posterior border of the transverse process of L1 and the posterior border of L2, 2 to 5 cm off the midline, depending on patient size. After an analgesic skin bleb, a 14-gauge, 1.0-cm needle is inserted through the skin to act as a guide. An 18-gauge, 15-cm needle is used for injection. This needle is inserted through the guide needle perpendicular to the skin. The authors have found it best to "walk" the needle off the transverse process by repeated insertion in order to ascertain the depth and

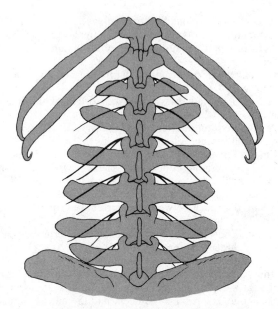

Figure 3. Anatomic relationships of spinal nerves and lumbar vertebrae for paravertebral analgesia in cattle.

location of the nerves. The 13th thoracic nerve is located just anterior to the edge of the transverse process of L1. As the needle is advanced, the intertransverse ligament can be felt as it is penetrated at the depth of the transverse process. The injection is made above and below the ligament over an area of 2.5 to 5 cm from top to bottom (see Fig. 4). This process is repeated over the posterior border of the transverse process of L1 and L2 to block the corresponding nerves. If necessary, T12 may be blocked by injecting just anterior to the edge of the 13th rib at the level of the tips of the transverse processes of L1. Ten to 30 ml of 2 per cent lidocaine is injected at each site. As the anesthetist becomes more adept at locating the spinal nerves, less agent will be required. Analgesia is evident within 5 to 10 minutes of injection. Induction time is a function of dose and accuracy in placement of the drug upon the spinal nerves. Because the dorsal branch of the spinal nerve is blocked, scoliosis

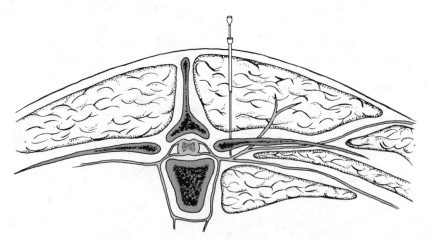

Figure 4. Anatomic relationships of spinal nerves and lumbar vertebra for paravertebral analgesia in cattle.

is induced as the muscles of the back relax on the side to be operated.

The distal block (Cakala block) is performed at the tips of the transverse processes of L1, L2, and L4. In this technique, an 18-gauge, 6-cm needle is inserted horizontally, and 15 ml of 2 per cent lidocaine is infiltrated directly above and below the tips of the transverse process. Because only the ventral and lateral-dorsal branches are affected, scoliosis does not occur; this is an advantage in the very sick or debilitated individual, who might not be able to stand following relaxation of the dorsal-lumbar muscles.

Either the proximal or distal paralumbar technique can be utilized in goats or sheep.

ANESTHESIA OF THE PENIS

Pudendal Nerve Block

The pudendal nerve may be blocked in ruminants for exposure and analgesia of the penis, relaxation of the retractor penis muscle, and analgesia to at least a portion of the prepuce. This block has also been recommended for relief of straining induced by vaginitis or prolapse of the uterus; however, in these situations low caudal epidural analgesia works equally well. Caudal epidural techniques have been used for exposure and analgesia of the penis but have the disadvantage of causing hindlimb paresis or paralysis at effective dosage levels. Therefore, the pudendal block is preferred for examination and treatment of the penis in the standing patient.

The pudendal nerve is located by rectal palpation at the lesser sciatic notch and foramen medial to the sacrosciatic ligament. The nerve lies caudal and dorsal to the internal pudendal artery at the cranial angle of the notch and is the size of a wheat straw. The site for injection is the ischiorectal fossa, which is bounded laterally by the sacrosciatic ligament (sacrotuberous ligament), ventrally by the ischial tuberosity (pin bone), and medially by the rectum and tail head. The area should be clipped and prepared as for surgery. A skin bleb or wheal is made at the deepest part of the fossa. In the bull, a 14-gauge, 1.0-cm guide needle is inserted through the skin. With one of the anesthetist's hands in the rectum, an 18-gauge, 15- to 30-cm needle is passed through the guide needle and directed cranially and somewhat ventrally to the pudendal nerve. Correct placement of the tip of the needle is determined by palpation. Twenty-five ml of 2 per cent lidocaine are deposited on the pudendal nerve, and 5 to 10 ml is deposited 2 to 3 cm caudal and dorsal on the middle hemorrhoidal nerve. The process is repeated on the opposite side. Care must be taken to avoid intravascular injections. Maximum analgesia and relaxation occur in 30 to 40 minutes and last several hours.

Pudendal nerve block can also be performed in the sheep and goat. The nerve is located by digital palpation per rectum. The injection site is the same as for the bull, and 7 ml of 2 percent lidocaine is sufficient at each side. Analgesia and relaxation occur within 5 to 10 minutes of injection.

Dorsal Penile Nerve Block

Alternative blockade of the dorsal nerve of the penis may be used to induce analgesia and relaxation of the penis. This technique is somewhat easier to perform than

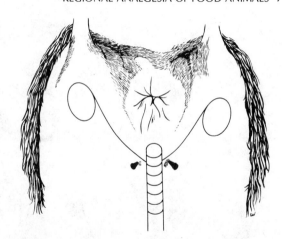

Figure 5. Injection site for blockade of the dorsal nerve of the penis in the bull.

the pudendal nerve block and is equally effective. The nerve is blocked as it crosses the ischial arch and gives rise to branches innervating the retractor penis muscle. The injection site is approximately 10 cm below the anus at the level of the ischial tuberosities (pin bones) and about 2.5 cm off the midline, just lateral to the penis on each side (Fig. 5). The skin is infiltrated. The needle is inserted and is directed cranially and somewhat medially to contact the pelvic floor at the ischial arch near the midline. The needle is withdrawn 1 cm, and 20 to 30 ml of 2 per cent lidocaine is injected. The procedure is repeated from the opposite side. Care must be taken to avoid intravascular injection of the agent, since the nerve is accompanied by the dorsal artery of the penis. Onset of analgesia and relaxation occurs in 20 to 30 minutes and lasts 1 to 2 hours. This procedure is applicable to the sheep and goat.

ANESTHESIA OF THE HORN

The cornual nerve supplying sensory innervation to the bovine's horn is blocked for dehorning. The nerve is located just off the edge of the frontal crest, beneath the skin and fascia. It is best blocked in the upper third to half of the frontal crest. The needle is inserted off the lateral edge of the crest and directed medially, being kept ventral and as close to the crest as possible. Five ml of 2 per cent lidocaine is injected at a depth of 0.5 to 1 cm. The cornual artery and vein run just lateral to the nerve; intravascular injection will prevent nerve blockade. In exotic breeds, especially the Simmental, it is also necessary to block the infratrochlear nerve, which innervates the medial aspect of the horn. This nerve is best blocked by infiltrating a line of analgesic agent subcutaneously from the midline to the facial crest dorsal to the eye across the forehead. The infratrochlear nerve in cattle divides into several branches that pass around the supraorbital process and then across the forehead; a line block, as illustrated in Figure 6, provides effective blockade of this nerve.

The horn of the goat is made analgesic by blocking the cornual and infratrochlear nerves (Fig. 7). The cornual nerve is located just posterior to the root of the supraorbital process beneath the skin, fascia, and frontalis muscle.

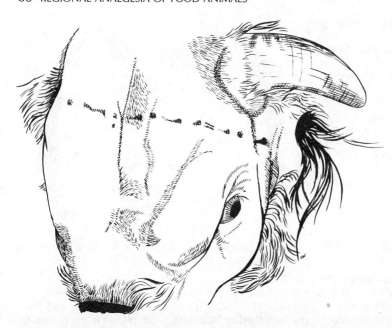

Figure 6. Injection sites for induction of analgesia of the horn in cattle. Cornual and infratrochlear nerves.

The infratrochlear nerve may be palpated beneath the skin above the dorsomedial margin of the orbit. In the adult, 1 to 2 ml of 2 per cent lidocaine is used at each site. Care must be taken to avoid overdosing young kids, particularly during infiltration of nerves about the head. One to 2 ml of 2 per cent lidocaine is sufficient to block all four sites in a young kid. Volume could be increased by diluting with saline in order to keep the dose to a minimum. In addition to blockade of the nerve supply to the horn, it is helpful to sedate goats to be dehorned or disbudded. Sedation renders them more tractable and also prevents vocalization, which may be distressing to the owner.

ANESTHESIA OF THE EXTREMITIES AND DIGITS

The digital nerve supply in the ruminant is complex and variable, making regional conduction analgesia of the

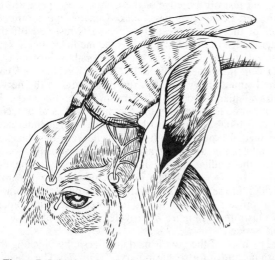

Figure 7. Injection sites for induction of analgesia of the horn in the goat. Cornual and infratrochlear nerves.

digits difficult. Precise location of the nerves by palpation is not easy, because the skin is tense distal to the carpus, and the subcutaneous tissues are fibrous. Therefore, many believe that simple ring block, in which local analgesic agent is infiltrated through a transverse plane around the limb, is the most reliable method of inducing analgesia of the digits. Nevertheless, precise blockade of the digital nerves may be accomplished below the fetlock joint. There are 4 sites for injection to induce analgesia of 1 digit, or 6 sites to induce analgesia of the entire foot (Fig. 8). Injection sites are located on the midline of the anterior and posterior aspects of the pastern at the middle of the first phalanx. Injection at these two points will induce analgesia of the interdigital tissues and the medial aspect of the digits, which is suitable for removal of corns or other interdigital procedures. To induce analgesia of the entire digit, a line is drawn between the anterior and posterior injection sites around the digit. The line is divided into thirds, and injection is made at ⅓ and ⅔ of the distance between the initial injection sites. This will induce analgesia to the entire digit for amputation of the digit or extensive procedures involving the sole and third phalanx. Injection is made with the needle perpendicular to the skin at a depth of 2 to 3 cm. Five ml of 2 per cent lidocaine at each site is sufficient.

Intravenous regional analgesia has been recommended for analgesia of the extremites and digits. This technique provides good cutaneous analgesia of the limbs and digits but in our experience does not consistently induce adequate interdigital analgesia for such procedures as amputation of the digit. Increasing the dosage to 50–60 ml will often overcome this problem. A tourniquet is placed around the limb proximal to the tarsus or carpus. For analgesia of the rear limbs, a roll of gauze should be placed in the depression between the tibia and the tendocalcaneus to improve the efficacy of the tourniquet (Fig. 9). The hair is clipped and the skin scrubbed over the radial or metatarsal vein. Thirty ml of 2 per cent lidocaine is administered intravenously as close to the surgical site as possible. Analgesia occurs within 10 minutes. The tourniquet is left in place until the operation is

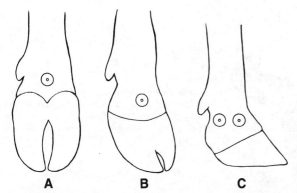

Figure 8. Injection site for induction of analgesia of the bovine foot by blockade of the digital nerves. *A,* Volar (plantar); *B,* dorsal; *C,* lateral and medial.

completed. The tourniquet may be left in place up to 75 minutes with no ill effects; lameness and edema have been reported after 2 hours. Upon completion of the operation, the tourniquet should be slowly released and left off for 15 seconds, then reapplied for 2 minutes. This sequence should be repeated several times to prevent the analgesic agent from being released too rapidly into the systemic circulation.

Analgesia and paralysis of the forelimb distal to the elbow may be induced by blockade of the brachial plexus. This procedure is ideal for closed reduction and external fixation of fractures in the distal limb. The site for injection is 12 to 14 cm in front and at the level of the acromion. The needle is advanced horizontally and posteriorly to the lateral aspect of the first rib. Care should be taken to avoid intravascular injection. The needle is serially withrawn and redirected ventrally so that an area 6 to 8 cm long is infiltrated along the lateral aspect of the first rib with 10 to 15 ml of 2 per cent lidocaine in calves, sheep, and goats. A total of 40 to 60 ml is required in a mature cow.

ANALGESIA OF THE UDDER

In ruminants, operations involving the udder may be carried out under high caudal or lumbosacral epidural or subarachnoid analgesia. However, if the procedure is to be done in the standing patient, regional analgesia must be used. Principal innervation of the udder is derived from the second and third lumbar nerves and the perineal nerve. Occasionally, the skin of the anterior aspect of the udder receives fibers from the first lumbar nerve. Therefore, the first three lumbar nerves and the perineal nerves are blocked to render the udder analgesic. Blockade of the lumbar nerves has been discussed previously. The perineal nerve is blocked at the ischial arch just beneath the skin and fascia, about 2 cm lateral to the midline, with 5 ml of 2 per cent lidocaine. If analgesia of the entire udder is desired, the nerves should be blocked bilaterally. In this situation, it is best to use a distal paravertebral technique to preserve tone in the dorsal lumbar musculature.

Surgery of the teats may be done with subcutaneous infiltration around the base of the teat. Procedures involving the teat orifice and canal will also require analgesia of the mucous membrane. The quarter is drained, and 10 ml of 2 per cent lidocaine is infused via the teat canal. In goats, the dose is 2.5 ml of 2 per cent lidocaine. Analgesia extends to the milk cistern.

ANALGESIA AND AKINESIS OF THE EYE AND EYELIDS OF THE RUMINANT

The eyelids receive motor innervation from the auriculopalpebral branch of the facial nerve. Blockade of the auriculopalpebral nerve results in akinesis (paralysis) of the upper and lower eyelids, but no analgesia is induced. This nerve block is useful for allowing easy examination of the eyeball and topical application of medications. The nerve runs from the base of the ear rostrally along the dorsal border of the facial crest. It may be blocked in the cow with 10 ml of 2 per cent lidocaine injected at the base of the ear, just dorsal to the zygomatic arch beneath the fascia. An alternative method is to infiltrate around the orbital rim. With either method, the third eyelid is unaffected.

Analgesia of the eyelids is induced by infiltrating along the dorsal and ventral rims of the orbit to block the fibers of the ophthalmic and maxillary nerves. The needle is inserted dorsal to the medial canthus and directed laterally to deposit 5 ml of 2 per cent lidocaine. The procedure is repeated ventral to the medial canthus.

Innervation of the eye is complex. The lids and conjunctiva receive sensory innervation from the ophthalmic nerve and the maxillary branch of the trigeminal nerve.

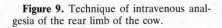

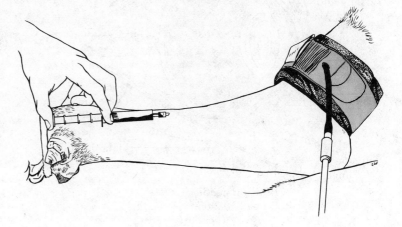

Figure 9. Technique of intravenous analgesia of the rear limb of the cow.

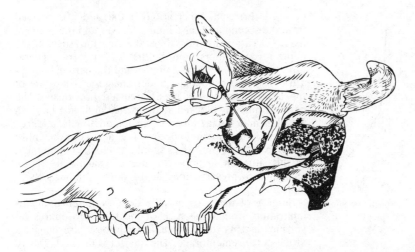

Figure 10. Insertion of needle at the trochlear notch for injection of agent at the foramen rotundum orbital.

The straight and oblique muscles of the eyeball receive motor fibers from the oculomotor, abducens, and trochlear nerves. The eyeball itself receives sensory innervation from the ciliary branch of the ophthalmic nerve. The oculomotor, trochlear, ophthalmic, and maxillary branches of the trigeminal and abducent nerves may be blocked as they emerge from the foramen rotundum orbitale. Injection at this point results in analgesia of the eyeball, conjunctiva, eyelids, and skin of the forehead, and paralysis of the ocular muscles. The auriculopalpebral nerve must be blocked as previously described to induce motor paralysis of the eyelids and because it occasionally gives rise to some sensory fibers as well. Clinical experience suggests that subcutaneous infiltration completely around the orbital rim will eliminate patient response when the eyelids are incised for complete eye enucleation.

There are several techniques for approaching the nerves as they emerge from the foramen rotundum orbitale. An approach made 1.5 cm lateral to the medial canthus has been described.[2] Topical analgesia of the conjunctiva is induced with either lidocaine or proparacaine. The needle is inserted through the conjunctiva below the eyeball and directed toward the base of the horn of the opposite side. After crossing the floor of the bony orbit, the needle is directed 10 to 15° more ventrally to a depth of 10 to 11 cm. Deeper penetration may result in the needle's entering the foramen rotundum orbitale and reaching the brain. In the adult cow, 20 ml of 2 per cent lidocaine will induce analgesia.

An alternative method is the Peterson technique. A curved needle 12 cm long with a 25-cm radius of curvature is used. The needle is inserted at the angle between the supraorbital process and the zygomatic arch, with the concave surface posterior and the hub slightly above the point of insertion. The needle is pushed ventrally to strike the coronoid process and then past it until the needle contacts the bony floor of the pterygopalatine fossa.

A third method is insertion through the trochlear notch on the mediodorsal aspect of the orbit (Fig. 10). The needle is inserted at the notch and directed medially and

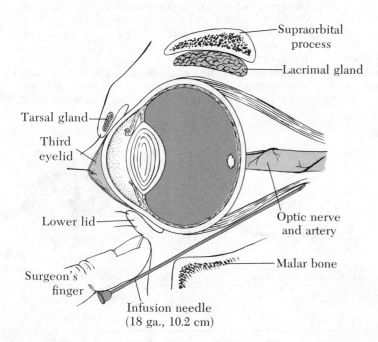

Supraorbital process

Lacrimal gland

Tarsal gland

Third eyelid

Lower lid

Surgeon's finger

Infusion needle (18 ga., 10.2 cm)

Optic nerve and artery

Malar bone

Figure 11. Retrobulbar injection of the bovine eye.

ventrally to a depth of 10 to 12 cm, where it contacts the floor of the pterygopalatine fossa. Deeper insertion may result in the needle's entering the foramen. Twenty ml of 2 per cent lidocaine will induce analgesia suitable for enucleation or for surgical procedures of the eyeball and conjunctiva.

Retrobulbar injections may be used to induce proptosis of the eyeball for exposure and immobilization as well as to induce global analgesia. Topical analgesia of the conjunctiva is also required. An 18-gauge, 38-mm needle is inserted through the conjunctiva at either the medial or lateral canthus to its full depth. The needle is inserted tangential to the eyeball so that the tip penetrates the periorbital tissue, giving the sensation of penetrating a drum head (Fig. 11). Ten ml of 2 per cent lidocaine and 5 to 15 ml of sterile saline are deposited behind the eyeball. Analgesia of the eyeball and cycloplegia are induced. Exophthalmus is induced, and retraction of the eyelids results in proptosis. The procedure is satisfactory for removal of small tumors of the cornea or sclera but should be avoided if there are corneal ulcers or lacerations that would predispose to rupture of the globe. Following completion of the surgical procedure, the eyeball can be returned to its normal position. An antibiotic ophthalmic ointment should be applied to prevent drying. Suturing the eyelids closed for 24 hours will insure eyeball protection while the anesthetic-saline mixture is being absorbed.

References

1. Skarda, R. T., and Muir, W. W.: Effects of segmental subarachnoid analgesia on arterial blood pressure, gas tensions, and pH in adult conscious cows. Am. J. Vet. Res. *42*:1747–1750, 1982.
2. Schreiber, J.: Die anatomische Grundlagen der Leitungsänasthesie beim Hund, I. Die Leitungsänasthesie der Kopfnerven. Wien. Tierärztl. Fortschrift. *42*:129, 1955.

Supplemental Reading

Evans, L. H.: Regional analgesia in large animals. *In* Soma, L. R. (ed.): Textbook of Veterinary Anesthesia. Baltimore, Williams & Wilkins, 468–488, 1971.
Hall, L. W.: Wright's Veterinary Anesthesia and Analgesia, 7th ed. Baltimore, Williams & Wilkins, 32–146, 1971.
Lumb, W. V., and Jones, E. W.: Veterinary Anesthesia. Philadelphia, Lea & Febiger, 371–425, 1973.
Rueben, L. F., and Gelatt, K. N.: Analgesia of the eye. *In* Soma, L. R. (ed.): Textbook of Veterinary Anesthesia. Baltimore, Williams & Wilkins, 489–499, 1971.
Westhues, W., and Fritsch, R.: Spinal anesthesia. *In* Westhues, W., and Fritsch, R. (eds.): Animal Anesthesia. Edinburgh and London, Oliver and Boyd, 1960.
Skarda, R. T., and Muir, W. W.: Segmental thoracolumbar subarachnoid analgesia in cows. Am. J. Vet. Res. *42*:632–638, 1981.
Skarda, R. T., and Muir, W. W.: Hemodynamic and respiratory effects of segmental subarachnoid analgesia in adult Holstein cows. Am. J. Vet. Res. *42*:1343–1348, 1982.
Skarda, R. T., and Muir, W. W.: Hemodynamic effects of unilateral segmental lumbar epidural analgesia in cattle. Am. J. Vet. Res. *40*:645–650, 1979.
Skarda, R. T., Yeary, R. A., Muir, W. W., and Burt, J. K.: Appearance of procaine in spinal fluid during segmental epidural analgesia in cows. Am. J. Vet. Res. *42*:639–646, 1981.

Drug Interactions

JOHN W. PAUL, D.V.M., M.S.

The subject of drug interactions is a complex issue with many facets. The objective of this discussion is to present a concept of drug interactions that includes four basic categories: reactions caused by a single drug, which may be more appropriately described as adverse drug reactions; interactions caused by multiple drug usage, which may be referred to as drug incompatibilities; drug interactions with laboratory tests, which could result in an incorrect diagnosis or clinical evaluation; and incompatibilities of drugs *in vitro*. The concept is founded on the veterinarian's basic understanding and awareness of the practical significance of drug interactions.

Recent reports from veterinary teaching hospitals in the United States indicate that from 0.3 to 2.5 per cent of the animals treated by those institutions undergo some form of adverse drug reaction. These figures are somewhat lower than the percentage of drug reactions reported in human hospitals, which may be as high as 18 per cent. Because many animal patients are in large herds, minor drug reactions may not be recognized. Therefore, it is difficult to make an accurate assessment of animals that experience drug reactions. Nevertheless, the potential for drug interactions in animals is sufficient to warrant serious consideration of the subject.

REACTIONS CAUSED BY A SINGLE DRUG

An adverse drug reaction is generally considered to be an unfavorable response to the interaction of a drug with a biochemical or physiologic process in the patient. Anaphylactoid reactions are not uncommon in animals. Penicillin and its semisynthetic derivatives are known to elicit anaphylactoid reactions in sensitive individuals. On occasion, a single treatment of penicillin is believed to serve as the sensitizing as well as the challenging shock dose. Owing to the longer duration of effect from the benzathine salt of penicillin, the duration of shock potential is proportionately longer and should be considered following administration of this form of the drug. Parenteral administration of oxytetracycline has also been reported to cause anaphylactoid reactions. The interaction of antimicrobial agents with microorganisms can contribute to undesirable responses in the animal patient. Suppression of normal flora by chemotherapy may permit establishment of a pathogen or may disturb digestive processes. Development of bacteria resistant to various antimicrobial agents presents a problem in selection of appropriate drugs to effect a cure of an infectious process.

Another example of an adverse reaction is produced by the interaction of a drug with an enzyme system. The organophosphorous compounds inhibit the action of cholinesterase in the host as well as the parasite. Overdosage or treatment of debilitated animals provides a greater potential for adversity. Haloxon generally is considered one of the safer organophosphates; however, an interaction in sheep has been reported. In lambs possessing esterase A, the LD_{50} of haloxon was 11,392 mg/kg, whereas in lambs lacking esterase A, the LD_{50} was only 763 mg/kg. This phenomenon, associated with genetically controlled enzymes, helps explain unexpected and sporadic neurotoxicity in lambs following treatment with haloxon.

Some drugs interact with specific organ functions. For example, xylazine administered at recommended clinical doses has been reported to produce increased blood glucose levels associated with increased hepatic glucose production and diminished hepatic blood flow. Arsanilic acid has been reported to cause blindness in swine. The aminoglycoside antibiotics possess a potential for ototoxicity and cause some degree of neuromuscular blockade that can result in cardiovascular depression and respiratory distress. The mechanism of this drug interaction apparently involves competitive inhibition of calcium by the aminoglycosides. A recent report demonstrated that total blood calcium was reduced by one third following parenteral administration of aminoglycosides to dairy cows; therefore, caution is advised in the use of these drugs in postpartum cows, especially those with a history of milk fever.

The subject of cell-mediated immunity is of vast interest. The corticosteroids interfere with this important process by inhibiting the actions of macrophages and lymphocytes. This is the likely mechanism by which corticosteroids are associated with recrudescence of viruses, especially the herpesviruses and the fulmination of quiescent fungal infections.

The corticosteroids and prostaglandins interact with pregnancy in animals. For this reason, these drugs can be used to induce abortion or early parturition when administered during the last trimester of pregnancy; however, this procedure may be complicated by placental retention, metritis, and weakness in calves if the parturition is induced too early.

INTERACTIONS CAUSED BY MULTIPLE DRUG USAGE

Some examples can be cited whereby drug combinations will result in a synergistic or more favorable response. For instance, the combination of trimethoprim and certain sulfonamides produces a synergistic antimicrobial effect through a sequential inhibition of bacterial metabolism of PABA and folic acid. Penicillin and streptomycin may be synergistic in their actions against some bacteria. Probenecid competes with penicillin for renal elimination pathways, thus prolonging penicillin blood levels. Tranquilizers used with barbiturates provide for a smoother induction of and recovery from anesthesia.

There are many examples of antagonistic or undesirable effects associated with multiple drug therapy. Adverse effects of the aminoglycoside antibiotics were cited previously. These reactions are additive when two or more of these agents are used concomitantly. When they are administered in conjunction with neuromuscular blocking agents, such as succinylcholine, this action of the aminoglycosides is intensified.

Chloramphenicol offers another example of a drug interaction associated with the metabolism of drugs. Chloramphenicol inhibits specific hepatic microsomal enzymes that are responsible for the biotransformation of barbiturates. This interaction results in prolonged barbiturate anesthesia. The opposite type of interaction exists between steroids and barbiturates. The steroids induce hepatic microsomes, thereby shortening the duration of barbiturate anesthesia.

Another type of interaction involves protein-binding of drugs. A particular drug, a sulfonamide for example, may be bound, to a large extent, to plasma proteins. In a sense, this serves as a depot of the drug since only the unbound portion is biologically active. If another drug that has a strong affinity for protein binding were to be administered concurrently, the sulfonamide could be displaced from its binding site. This would result in a transient potentiation of the sulfonamide effect, but a more rapid elimination from the body. The overall effect would be manifested as a decreased duration of sulfonamide availability.

The absorption or availability of some drugs can be impaired by interactions with other compounds. Tetracyclines chelate various bivalent and trivalent cations, such as calcium, magnesium, aluminum, and iron. Thus, calcium gluconate, milk products, and antacids can bind with tetracycline, thereby rendering it ineffective.

Although clinical evidence is not clear, there is a strong suggestion that bactericidal drugs, such as penicillin, and bacteriostatic drugs, such as tetracycline, have an antagonistic effect. Until more data is available in veterinary medicine, caution should be exercised with this type of combined chemotherapy.

The anthelmintic levamisole exerts its mode of action by interfering with ATP metabolism, whereas the organophosphorous compounds act by inhibition of cholinesterase. Despite the different modes of action, it has been observed clinically that when these two types of compounds are used concomitantly, an adverse reaction may occur. The exact mechanism of this interaction is not clear. It is well understood, however, that when more than one organophosphate is administered concurrently or shortly after administration of other cholinesterase inhibitors, a potentiated depletion of cholinesterase occurs.

DRUG INTERACTIONS WITH LABORATORY TESTS

An often overlooked but extremely important aspect of drug interactions involves the alteration of hematologic, blood chemical, or urologic tests results by drugs. Deviation from normal test values may be caused by pathologic changes in organs or alteration of enzyme systems by certain drugs. Drugs that are hepatotoxic or nephrotoxic are examples of agents capable of causing this type of drug interaction. In addition, some drugs may interact with the chemistry of the test procedure. For instance, different anticoagulants added to blood collection tubes can interfere with laboratory tests. In a recent report, it was found that heparin had little or no effect on laboratory tests, but EDTA produced a marked reduction of several

Table 1. *Potential Effects of Drugs on Laboratory Test Values*

Drug(s)	Test Values Increased	Test Values Decreased
Acetylpromazine	Glucose, bilirubin, alkaline phosphatase	Cholinesterase, RBC count, WBC count, platelet count, hemoglobin, PCV
Ampicillin	Alkaline phosphatase, eosinophil count, SGOT, SGPT	None
Anabolic steroids	Ca, P, BUN, total protein, total bilirubin, SGOT, SGPT	Glucose, T_4
Corticosteroids	Bilirubin, glucose, Na, Cl	Coagulation time, prothrombin time, WBC count, K
Erythromycin	Alkaline, phosphatase, SGOT, SGPT	Cholesterol
Furosemide	BUN, glucose	Na, K, Ca
Gentamicin	BUN, SGOT, SGPT	None
Nitrofurantoin*	Bilirubin, eosinophils count, SGOT, SGPT	None
Penicillin	Alkaline phosphatase, protein, Coombs test	RBC count, WBC count
Phenothiazine†	Bilirubin, glucose, SGOT, SGPT	None
Phenylbutazone	BUN, creatinine, glucose, bilirubin, SGOT, SGPT, Na, Cl	RBC count, hemoglobin, PCV
Sulfonamides‡	Amino acids, bilirubin, BUN, SGOT, WBC count, prothrombin time, urine glucose	Protein-bound iodine, RBC count
Tetracycline	BUN, coagulation time, WBC count, urine glucose, urine protein	Ca, K
Thiabendazole	Cl, glucose, SGOT	WBC count
Xylazine	Blood glucose, urine glucose, BUN	RBC count, hemoglobin, PVC, blood insulin

*Also causes brownish urine.
†Also causes red-brown urine.
‡Also causes brownish urine and urine crystals.

test values. The use of corticosteroids represents an important cause of erroneous laboratory results, especially in regard to leukocyte counts and immunologic tests.

Sound clinical judgment must be exercised in the interpretation of laboratory test results when the patient is on medication or when the blood sample has been treated with anticoagulants. When considering laboratory test values, one might pose the following questions: Am I aware of the patient's complete medication history? Am I sufficiently familiar with the laboratory procedure to be able to rule out the possibility of drug interference? Am I making a diagnostic or therapeutic decision on the basis of the most specific laboratory determination?

Table 1 provides examples of some commonly used drugs and their effects on laboratory test results.

Table 2. In Vitro *Drug Incompatibilities*

Drug	Incompatibility
Ampicillin	*Do not mix with other drugs.*
Acepromazine	Chloramphenicol, phenylbutazone, sulfonamides
Ca gluconate	Na bicarbonate, tetracyclines, phenylbutazone, sulfonamides
Chloral hydrate	Alkaline solutions
Chloramphenicol	Erythromycin, hydrocortisone, tetracycline, procaine, vitamin B complex
Erythromycin	Hydrocortisone, penicillin G, streptomycin, chloramphenicol
Furosemide	Ringer's solution
Gentamicin	*Do not mix with other drugs.*
Hydrocortisone	Chloramphenicol, erythromycin, kanamycin, promazine, tylosin, tetracycline
Kanamycin	*Do not mix with other drugs.*
Levamisole	Neomycin, phenylbutazone, sulfonamides, tetracyclines
Lincomycin	*Do not mix with other drugs.*
Penicillin G	Sulfonamides, erythromycin, tetracycline
Sulfonamides	Acepromazine, Ca gluconate, dextrose, kanamycin, penicillin G, procaine, tylosin
Tetracyclines	Many solutions, including Ca
Tylosin	Hydrocortisone, tetracycline, streptomycin, sulfonamides
Vitamin B complex	Many solutions, especially antibiotics
Xylazine	Thiamylal

IN VITRO DRUG INCOMPATIBILITIES

In vitro drug incompatibilities may properly be classified as iatrogenic drug interactions. Many drugs are physically or chemically incompatible. Drug incompatibilities in admixtures often become readily apparent, as evidenced by precipitation, color change, or gas formation. However, in some cases, even though no visible signs of interaction are apparent an ingredient(s) may be rendered inactive. For instance, sulfonamides inactivate penicillin without visible signs when mixed *in vitro*, owing to the high pH of the sulfa. Extreme temperatures during storage, specifically freezing, can adversely affect the integrity of a drug. The need to examine drugs that have been frozen for physical or chemical changes must be emphasized.

There may be some justification for admixing drugs on certain occasions to save time or to avoid multiple injections. Clinicians should check a reliable reference or consult a pharmacist before combining drugs *in vitro* to avoid possible interactions.

Table 2 lists *in vitro* incompatibilities of some commonly used drugs.

CONCLUSIONS

The clinical significance of drug interactions in animals is often minor, although in some cases they may be fatal. In the critically ill patient, the temptation to employ relatively large doses, particularly of antimicrobials or corticosteroids, or to use multiple-drug therapy is enhanced. These two factors, combined with a debilitated state of the patient, increase the probability of severe drug interactions that could mean the difference between recovery and death. It would be prudent to consider the possibility of drug interactions during selection of drugs for concomitant use, evaluation of adverse reactions or laboratory test results, or mixing of drugs *in vitro*.

Supplemental Reading

1. Adams, H. R.: Acute adverse effects of antibiotics. J. Am. Vet. Med. Assoc. *166*:983, 1975.

2. Aronson, A. L.: The use, misuse, and abuse of antimicrobial agents. Mod. Vet. Pract. *56*;383, 1975.
3. Davis, L. E., et al.: Pharmacologic basis of adverse drug reactions. Bov. Pract., No. 12, 1977.
4. Evaluation of Drug Interactions, 2nd ed. Washington, D.C., American Pharmaceutical Association, 1976.
5. Hansten, P. D.: Drug Interactions, 4th ed. Philadelphia, Lea & Febiger, 1979.
6. Jawetz, E.: Synergism and antagonism among antimicrobial drugs. West. J. Med. *123*:87, 1975.
7. Martin, E. W., et al.: Hazards of Medication—A Manual on Drug Interactions, Incompatibilities, Contraindications, and Adverse Effects. Philadelphia, J. B. Lippincott Co., 1971.
8. Veterinary Values '81. New York, Ag Resources, 1981.

Cryosurgery and Hyperthermia

HAROLD E. FARRIS, JR., D.V.M., M.S.,
and CYNTHIA HOMAN JACOBS, D.V.M.

CRYOSURGERY

Cryosurgery is the medical application of cold to destroy tissue. Since the first veterinary reports in 1970, cryosurgery has become a widely accepted modality for the treatment of skin cancer in animals.[1] In food animal practice, this modality is widely used to treat bovine ocular squamous cell carcinoma. A preliminary report on the cryosurgical treatment of interdigital fibromas, papillomatosis, and fibromas of glans penis is presented in this discussion. A treatment protocol that has resulted in a cure rate of more than 90 per cent of bovine ocular squamous cell carcinomas and the cryosurgical instrumentation required in veterinary practice are also discussed in detail.

Instrumentation

Both liquid nitrogen and nitrous oxide units have been designed for veterinary use. Since nitrous oxide provides a working temperature of -70 to $-90°C$, the depth of freeze with nitrous oxide units is limited. Lesions greater than 1 cm in depth have to be excised or removed by electrosurgery prior to freezing with nitrous oxide units. Therefore these authors do not recommend nitrous oxide units for clinical use. Liquid nitrogen has a working temperature of $-196°C$, and spray application of liquid nitrogen can rapidly lower tissue temperature to $-25°C$ at depths of 2 to 4 cm.

The ideal veterinary unit should have the following features: (1) portability and sturdy construction for field use; (2) precise control of the spray (on-off application); (3) both closed probe and spray tips; (4) tissue temperature monitor; and (5) large reservoir to eliminate frequent filling with liquid nitrogen.

Two units used in our investigations and practice are the C76* and Cryogun.† The cost of a reliable cryosurgical unit complete with a tissue temperature monitor and storage Dewar will range from approximately $800 to $1500.

---

*Available from Frigitronics, Inc., Shelton, CT 06484.
†Available from Brymill Corporation, Vernon, CT 06066.

Cryosurgical Protocol for Bovine Ocular Squamous Cell Carcinoma (BOSCC)

Small premalignant lesions, including focal ulcerations and papillomas on eyelids, are treated without anesthesia. Eyelid lesions larger than 0.5 cm are treated following sedation with xylazine. Multiple applications of topical anesthesia either alone or in conjunction with retrobulbar anesthesia are used for treatment of lesions on the bulbar conjunctiva or cornea. If metastasis has occurred, the lesion is greater than 5 cm in diameter with poorly defined margins, or the adjacent bones have been invaded, treatment should not be attempted. The skin around the lesions is clipped to remove debris and provide better exposure of lid lesions. The boundary of the lesion is then marked with a felt marking pen. A thermocouple needle is placed at the base of the lesion, and when possible, a second thermocouple needle is placed 0.5 to 0.7 cm beyond the margin of the lesion. To prevent destruction of adjacent normal tissue, a polystyrene plastic shield is placed over the cornea, and the skin below the lesion is covered with a 0.2 to 0.5 cm layer of petroleum jelly.

Liquid nitrogen spray is used on all eyelid lesions and on most ocular lesions. A spray tip is selected that provides the most rapid rate of freezing without excessive runoff of liquid nitrogen droplets. A 20-gauge or smaller spray tip is used for lesions less than 1 cm in diameter, whereas an 18-gauge tip is used for lesions larger than 1 cm. The spray tip is held at a distance of 0.5 to 1.0 cm and directed toward the center of the lesion. This distance not only assures the greatest depth of freeze at the thickest portion of the lesion but also prevents underfreezing (less than $-25°C$) of areas if a rotating motion around the tumor is used. In experimental studies in which porcine, bovine, and equine skin was frozen with various units and various-sized spray tips held 0.5 to 1.0 cm from a central point, the iceball formed had a depth slightly more than one-third the diameter of the surface iceball.

Tissue temperature monitoring is not used for corneoscleral lesions. Otherwise the method of treatment of corneoscleral lesions is the same as that of eyelid lesions. Freezing is terminated when the iceball extends 0.2 to 0.3 cm beyond the margins of the ocular lesions. Following a thaw to $+5°C$, all lesions are rapidly refrozen. Within 1 hour after the double freeze-thaw cycle, the frozen area appears erythematous and edematous. Within 24 hours, the area becomes dark because of the accumulation of blood cells from damaged microvessels; this condition persists until the third or fourth day after freezing, at which time necrosis occurs. Frequently, papillary lesions undergo necrosis and slough completely within 1 week of freezing. Often the frozen area remains covered with an eschar that separates 4 to 6 weeks after freezing, leaving a smooth, slightly erythematous scar. The rate of healing is directly related to the size of the original area frozen. Postoperative care is not required after freezing.

Ocular Squamous Cell Carcinoma

In 1975, Farris and Fraunfelder[2] reported the treatment of 718 cases of ocular squamous cell carcinoma in cattle with various cryosurgical units and techniques. Tumors ranged in size from less than 0.5 cm to 7 cm in diameter and depth. A single freeze at $-25°C$ at the base of the lesion or until the iceball enveloped the tumor and a surrounding 0.2 to 0.4 cm of normal tissue resulted in a

66 per cent cure at a 6-month follow-up evaluation of 609 lesions. In 109 lesions treated with a double freeze-thaw cycle to −25°C, a cure rate of 97 per cent was achieved.

Because a large number of cows were sold following a "cure," long-term follow-up has not been possible on a significant number of animals. However, a 4-year follow-up of 25 cattle with from 1 to 3 squamous cell carcinomas on the lids or the corneoscleral junction has shown development of primary tumors at other sites on the lids or the corneoscleral junction in approximately 25 per cent of cases. All recurrences were treated before tumor size had exceeded 1 cm in diameter.

Interdigital Fibroma

Cattle are sedated with xylazine and treated in the standing position in a restraint chute. The claws are separated by placing a block of wood between the toes. A thermocouple needle is placed at the central base of the fibroma, and strips of styrofoam are placed between the fibroma and the wall of the digits. Using a large (18-gauge) spray aperture, the fibroma is rapidly frozen to −25°C. Following an unaided thaw to +5°C, the fibroma is refrozen.

The treated animal is then returned to pasture without postoperative care. However, lameness from postoperative edema and the subsequent tissue slough has been observed in approximately 50 per cent of the animals treated. Of 30 interdigital fibromas treated, 80 per cent were ablated after a double freeze-thaw and 13 per cent were ablated following a second freezing 30 to 45 days after the primary double freeze-thaw. Because of the sale of the animals, follow-up was not obtained on 7 per cent of the animals treated.

Fibroma of the Glans Penis and Bovine Papillomatosis

Cryosurgery shows particular promise in the treatment of fibroma of the glans penis and bovine cutaneous papillomatosis. Animals are restrained while standing and either tranquilized or treated without anesthesia. A double freeze-thaw cycle, as described previously, is used. However, tissue temperature monitoring is not required. The rapid freezing is terminated when all of the neoplastic mass and 0.2 to 0.3 cm of surrounding normal tissue are included in the iceball. Only the base of any large wart attached by a narrow stalk is frozen. To protect normal tissue, either 7.5-cm discs of 0.3-cm Teflon with punched-out centers of various diameters can be placed over the mass to be frozen, or petroleum jelly can be applied around the lesion. A significant advantage of cryosurgical treatment of fibroma of the glans penis is the minimal scarring that occurs after cryosurgery.

Summary

Cryosurgery has become the treatment of choice of bovine ocular squamous cell carcinoma. In addition, cryosurgery is a modality that should be considered for treatment of other neoplastic and non-neoplastic lesions in cattle.

Cryosurgical units that deliver liquid nitrogen provide a more rapid freezing rate of large lesions and thus a higher cure rate than units designed for delivery of nitrous oxide.

Cryosurgery is a simple, rapid procedure; it is economical, provides analgesia itself owing to sensory nerve injury, requires minimal preoperative and no postoperative medication, has few side effects, and may be repeated if necessary.

HYPERTHERMIA

Hyperthermia therapy for the treatment of neoplasia has received considerable attention in the past decade both in human and in veterinary medicine. The application of heat for the purpose of tissue destruction is not new to medicine. However, advances in our understanding of the biology and technology of hyperthermia therapy have elucidated some of its potential as an adjunct if not the sole mode of therapy for a variety of cancer forms.

There are two forms of hyperthermia therapy: local hyperthermia and systemic, or whole-body, hyperthermia. Local application is used for superficial, discrete, and well-defined tumors. Whole-body hyperthermia is directed against internal or widespread cancer forms. Although whole-body hyperthermia may find applications in companion animal medicine, for a number of reasons it is unlikely to become prominent in food animal medicine in the near future. Thus, only local hyperthermia therapy for treatment of bovine ocular squamous cell carcinoma is considered here.

Local Hyperthermia Therapy and Instrumentation

It has been demonstrated that certain cancer cells *in vivo* can be selectively destroyed at temperatures of 42 to 43°C, these temperatures being tolerated by most normal tissues. *In vitro*, malignant cells may be more sensitive to heat than normal cells owing to certain biochemical differences. Discrete solid tumors are believed to be especially susceptible to local heating because of their abnormal vasculature.

There are a number of ways to accomplish local tissue heating: (1) radiofrequency energy (100 KHZ to 100 MHZ), (2) microwave (1 KHZ), (3) ultrasound, and (4) local tumor perfusion baths. Radiofrequency is used most often for small, well-defined tumors that are easily accessible. At present, it seems to offer the greatest advantage, particularly with respect to application in food animal medicine. Radiofrequency (rf) sources, amplifiers, and electrodes are cheap and simple to operate. Recent studies *in vitro* have attempted to define precisely the limits of tissue destruction surrounding radiofrequency electrodes, thus making this mode of hyperthermia therapy better controlled. A commercial rf unit is available.*

It has been shown that nonuniform heating of tumors may enhance tumor growth or even stimulate metastasis. For this reason, thermometry is an important facet of hyperthermia therapy. The radiofrequency units described in the literature for use in food animal therapy have a thermister within one electrode that limits electrode temperature (and therefore presumably tissue temperature) to 50°C. Although this thermister may not measure tissue temperature very accurately, the rf device cited is used in treatment of bovine ocular squamous cell carcinoma, in which penetration thermocouples may be contraindicated.

---

*ID 4A Thermoprobe, available from Ideal Instrument Co., Chicago, IL 60612.

Ocular Squamous Cell Carcinoma (OSCC)

In a study by Grier and colleagues,[3] 45 ocular squamous cell carcinomas (17 cattle and 8 horses) were treated with a local current field (LCF) radiofrequency device that heated the tumor tissue to 50°C for 30 seconds. The device has both surface and piercing probes, allowing treatment of tumors of varying depths. All tumors treated in the study were diagnosed histologically as squamous cell carcinoma. They were approximately 5 cm in diameter and without deep conjunctival or scleral penetration. The animals with corneal OSCC were anesthetized with 0.5 per cent proparacaine hydrochloride. Those with eyelid OSCC received 2 per cent lidocaine infiltration, and those with extensive corneal and lid involvement required retrobulbar blocks. The eyeballs were immobilized by use of an ocular spoon designed for the purpose. Corneal lesions were treated at 50°C for 30 seconds with a surface probe that was applied with firm pressure to ensure uniform heating. Conjunctival and third eyelid lesions were also treated with piercing probes. When tumor size was greater than could be covered by one application of the probe, treatment was simply repeated in the adjacent tissue. Overlapping treated areas on or near the cornea may, however, lead to perforation. Atropine and antibiotic ointment were used for 1 to 3 days after treatment.

Following therapy, most animals were blepharospastic and had ocular discharge for up to 10 days. Slough of tumor occurred at 3 to 10 days, leaving a red, granular bed. If the tumor area was large, this granular bed became encrusted. The encrustations fell off in 14 to 21 days, leaving pink, healthy tissue. Complications included hypopyon and uveitis that was responsive to topical mydriatics, antibiotics, and corticosteroids. One animal developed depression and anorexia.

Treatment resulted in 80 per cent complete and 16 per cent partial regressions at 2 to 10 months after treatment. Twelve of 37 tumors were treated a second time. Fifty per cent of the tumors had not responded previously to surgery, cryosurgery, radiation, or immunotherapy. The tumors treated in the experiment were diagnosed histologically as squamous cell carcinoma to emphasize the fact that 25 per cent of ocular squamous cell tumors will regress spontaneously.

In a similar study by Kainer and associates[4] 56 benign squamous cell tumors and 20 OSCC (confirmed by exfoliative cytology) were treated with a radiofrequency device. The tumors were heated to 50°C for 30 seconds. A report from the Los Alamos Scientific Laboratory was cited as reference that this short term high temperature had a cytotoxicity equal to that of 42°C for 64 minutes. Restraint, anesthesia, and globe immobilization were as described previously. Lesions greater than 1 cm were treated with multiple overlapping probe applications. Tumors 4 mm thick were pared away with a scalpel, then flushed with 50 per cent povidone-iodine solution before hyperthermia treatment. Adjacent normal tissue exhibited an inflammatory response for up to 2 weeks after treatment. Tumors treated on the cornea or corneoscleral junction developed a leukematous zone owing to heat-induced edema. Occasionally, small scars resulted. Conjunctival and palpebral sites healed by granulation and epithelialization. This study reported that when second-treatment tumors were included, 90.8 per cent of 76 tumors regressed completely following hyperthermia therapy.

As evidenced by these two studies, local hyperthermia therapy is an effective and technically simple means of treating OSCC in the bovine. A disadvantage, however, is that irregularly shaped tumors are difficult to heat uniformly. Grier and colleagues[3] recommended that eyelid tumors be treated 3 to 4 mm beyond the tumor.

In a number of studies, it has been shown that hyperthermia used in combination with other modes of cancer treatment (chemotherapy, radiation, surgery, and immunotherapy) can produce a synergistic therapeutic response. Either alone or in combination with other forms of cancer treatment, hyperthermia is likely to continue to increase in use as treatment of neoplasia.

References

1. Krahwinkel, D. J., Jr., Merkley, D. F., and Howard, D. R.: Cryosurgical treatment of cancerous and noncancerous diseases of dogs, horses, and cats. J. Am. Vet. Med. Assoc. *169*:201–207, 1976.
2. Farris, H. E., Jr., and Fraunfelder, F. T.: Cryosurgical treatment of ocular squamous cell carcinoma of cattle. J. Am. Vet. Med. Assoc. *168*:213–216, 1976.
3. Grier, R. L., Brewer, W. G., Paul, S. R., and Theilen, G. H.: Treatment of bovine and equine ocular squamous cell carcinoma by radiofrequency hyperthermia. J. Am. Vet. Med. Assoc. *177*:55–61, 1980.
4. Kainer, R. A., Stringer, J. M., and Lueker, D. C.: Hyperthermia for treatment of ocular squamous cell tumors in cattle. J. Am. Vet. Med. Assoc. *176*:227–233, 1980.

NEONATAL DISEASE AND DISEASE MANAGEMENT

OTTO MARTIN RADOSTITS, D.V.M., M.S.
Consulting Editor

Congenital Defects in Cattle

H. W. LEIPOLD, D.V.M., Ph.D.

Various structural and functional defects have been described in calves, ranging from variant and blemish, to imperfection and deviant, to malformation and monstrosity. Losses from such defects are usually of limited concern and are unlikely to be reported. Only under unusual circumstances, as when the defect occurs repeatedly in the same herd, is an affected neonate likely to come to the attention of investigators concerned with congenital anomalies. Thus, most defective neonates are unrecorded and unnoticed by veterinarians, animal scientists, and geneticists. The thalidomide-induced congenital defects in humans during the 1960's proved that defects need not be hereditary. This information attracted the interest of a wider group of medical, veterinary, and animal science researchers to the field of teratology. Only recently, however, has there been a perceptible change in attitude by veterinarians, geneticists, animal scientists, and livestock industrialists toward the importance of congenital defects in cattle.

Much of the attitude change stemmed from the experiences of artificial insemination (AI) and breed registry organizations, which recognized that they and their consulting experts required more scientific information about congenital defects than was available. The threat of litigation altered the processes by which these organizations reached and disseminated policy decisions relative to congenital defects in cattle. Organizations involved in litigation shared their experiences with other organizations and, consequently, most United States AI breed registry organizations now have programs to monitor undesirable genetic traits and to control specific genetic traits. These programs include sharing the names of cattle known to transmit the defect with herd owners. As a result, many more herd owners seek advice from veterinary practitioners relative to appropriate genetic control measures. This change has also been assisted by a genetic disease consulting program at Kansas State University that utilizes a combination of diagnosis, pathology, research, and data contained in a central congenital defects file.

The concept of genetic defects as basically structured defects is changing as the number of metabolic anomalies identified in cattle increases. Prenatal viral infections, plants, and other environmental factors are now recognized as causes of specific congenital defects in calves. This review focuses on the environmental factors causing congenital defects and localized defects due to single mutant genes, since much work in the past has been directed toward the nature and effects of these malformations in cattle. Metabolic defects and localized malformations due to multifactorial inheritance also are included, as they are beginning to emerge as problems in bovine medicine.

DEFINITION

Congenital defects or diseases are abnormalities of structure or function present at birth. They may affect a single anatomic structure or function, an entire system, parts of several systems, all of several body systems, or possess both functional and structural defects (syndrome). All body structures and functions may be affected. Defects may be obvious grossly, but some are not recognized without careful radiologic, clinico-pathologic, or necropsy examination. A description of syndromes found in veterinary medical genetics is important because it allows for more accurate diagnosis of some of these troublesome diseases. The frequency with which various parts of the body are affected varies according to breed, geographic location, season, sex, age of parent, and nutrition. Normal structural and functional variants, commonly identified as "defects" by breeders, are excluded.

NATURE

Congenital defects pose a diagnostic challenge to the practicing veterinarian. They also may act as sentinels of the human environment and are of comparative significance for other species. A defective neonate is an adapted survivor from a disruptive event of genetic or environmental cause or from a genetic-environmental interaction at one or more stages in the complex integrated sequences of embryogenesis or fetal development. If the disruptive event is not immediately lethal, it is followed by the normal developmental sequences, which must then accommodate the event and its sequelae. Often this is not possible, and the affected embryo or fetus dies before completing development and is resorbed or is aborted. These events are ofen undetected in cattle.

Susceptibility to injurious environmental or genetic agents varies with the stage of development and decreases with increasing fetal age. In the period of pre-attachment, the zygote or embryo is resistant to teratogens but susceptible to genetic mutations and chromosomal aberrations. During the embryonic period, the embryo is highly susceptible to teratogens. Susceptibility to teratogens declines with increasing embryonic age, as the critical periods for development of various organs or organ systems are passed. The fetus becomes more resistant to the action of teratogenic agents with greater fetal age with the exception of later differentiating structures, such as the cerebellum, palate, and urogenital system.

Although losses caused by congenital defects are less than those losses caused by nutritional deficiency, infectious agents, or neoplasia, defects may result in considerable economic losses to individual breeders. Congenital defects produce economic losses by increasing perinatal mortality. In addition, loss of value of relatives of genetically defective cattle can be serious. Developmental defects may be lethal, semi-lethal, compatible with life, or impair viability. They may have little effect or an esthetic effect that lowers economic value. Additional losses occur when congenital defects are only one manifestation of a syndrome that also includes embryonic and fetal mortality. Congenital defects also may be an added source of confusion in diagnosing other diseases or abortions. Finally, control measures may require extensive and expensive adjustments in breeding programs if the defect is caused genetically, since such a defect may recur generation after generation.

Until recently, the study of such congenital defects has been an accepted, though little emphasized, opportunistic research activity of veterinarians. A current assessment reveals some major problems in this area: inadequate information, i.e., too few case reports, inadequate anatomic and pathologic investigations or descriptions, inadequate and inappropriate genetic analysis, and failure to integrate underlying processes of embryologic, pathologic, and genetic nature.

FREQUENCY

The frequency of congenital defects in animals is not a fixed proportion of all births but varies owing to genetic and environmental factors or to their interactions. Frequency also is influenced by breed, geographic location, and season. In addition, the interest of the observer may bias data collection. Frequencies of all congenital defects, as well as those of individual structures or functions, are difficult to obtain because many defects can be identified only by necropsy. Many defects go unnoticed, others are not reported for economic reasons, and others occur so rarely as to defy accurate accounting. It has been estimated that 0.5 to 1 per cent of calves born have congenital defects. The incidence reported ranges from 1 in 500 to 1 in 100, with 40 to 50 per cent born dead, and only a small fraction of the defects are not visible externally. For comparison, congenital defects in humans are estimated from 1 to 3 per cent. The most frequently encountered congenital defects involve the skeletal, central nervous, and muscular systems. The relative frequency of the

various defects involved in 2293 congenitally defective calves collected over a 9-year period was central nervous system (21.6 per cent), musculature (13.7 per cent), facial bones (8.8 per cent), anomalous twins (10.0 per cent), hydrops (9.7 per cent), large body cavities, such as schistosomus reflexus (6.9 per cent), bones of the leg (6.9 per cent), digestive (4.3 per cent), urinary and reproductive (4.3 per cent), bone and cartilage (2.8 per cent), heart and vessels (2.7 per cent), skin (2.0 per cent), and others (1.7 per cent).

CAUSES

Many congenital defects have no clearly established cause, others have environmental causes, and others have genetic causes. In addition, the interaction of environmental and genetic factors may account for a considerable proportion of defects.

Environmental Factors. Teratogenic factors reported for domestic animals include toxic plants, viruses, drugs, trace elements, and physical agents, such as irradiation, hyperthermia, and pressure during rectal examination. They are difficult to identify but often follow seasonal patterns, stressful conditions, and maternal disease. They do not have a familial pattern as do genetic causes. They occur in any genotype during the appropriate critical period. Maternal disease patterns vary, but abortion incidence may be increased and morbidity may be observed. Field studies usually have led to observations on the frequency and pattern of a defect in a population that suggest what kind of teratogen appeared to be the most likely cause.

Crooked calf disease in Utah and on Kodiak Island, Alaska, characterized by joint contractures and additional defects, such as torticollis, scoliosis, or kyphosis, and various degrees of cleft palate, is caused by ingestion of *Lupinus caudatus*, *L. sericeus*, or *L. nootkatensis*. The alkaloid anagyrine is identified as the teratogen, and the greatest risk of disease development is between 40 and 70 days of gestation.

Not all cases of crooked calf disease can be explained by ingestion of lupines during the critical phases of development, since feeding *Conium maculatum* to pregnant cows between days 50 and 75 of pregnancy causes similar defects. *Coniine* was identified as the possible teratogen. Other plants suspected of causing defective calves are *Senecio*, *Indigofera spicata*, Cycadales, *Blighia*, loco plants, Papaveraceae, *Colchicum*, *Vinca*, and tobacco. Sudan grass pasture *(Sorghum sudanese)* in Australia may have caused arthrogryposis in calves.

Locoweed poisoning *(Oxytropis* and *Astragalus)* in range livestock (most commonly cattle, sheep, and horses) may cause emaciation, visual impairment, neurologic deficit signs, habituation, abortion, and congenital defects. Locoweed has produced musculoskeletal defects in calves. Locoweed poisoning in growing cattle may have similarities to the genetic mannosidosis of Angus cattle, as the alkaloid indolizidine-1,2,8-triol is a potent and specific inhibitor of the hydrolytic enzyme α-D-mannosidase.

Rectal palpation between days 35 and 40 of gestation may cause atresia coli. In one study, of 125 calves born in the "pre-42 day group," 6 had intestinal atresia whereas not one of the 103 calves born in the "post-43 day group" had atresia. It was concluded that palpation and pressure on the amnion during organogenesis (days 33 to 40) can cause atresia coli and, occasionally, atresia jejuni. Male calves were affected more frequently.

Prenatal viral infections, such as intrauterine Akabane virus infections, may be teratogenic in cattle, causing abortions, premature births, and congenital defects, and arthrogryposis and hydranencephaly (A-H syndrome) in Japan, Israel, Australia, and Kenya. The bovine viral diarrhea (BVD) virus induced congenital defects in calves, such as cerebellar dysplasia, ocular defects, brachygnathia inferior, alopecia, dysmyelinogenesis, internal hydrocephalus, dysmaturity (intrauterine growth retardation), and impaired immunologic competence. Blue tongue virus caused congenital defects in calves. Experimental transmission to pregnant heifers via insects resulted in abortions, stillbirths, and congenital defects, such as arthrogryposis, campylognathia, and prognathism with domed cranium. Hydranencephaly and a "dummy-calf" syndrome (inactivity, dullness, behavioral disturbances) also have been seen. In Oklahoma, abortions and congenital defects, such as arthrogryposis, kyphosis, and scoliosis, occurred.

In South Africa, Wesselsbron virus caused congenital porencephaly and cerebellar hypoplasia in calves.

Genetic Factors. Genetic defects are the pathophysiologic results of mutant genes or chromosomal aberrations occurring in any environment. Except for chromosomal aberrations, genetic defects are recognized only when they occur in characteristic intragenerational familial frequencies and intergenerational patterns.

One chromosomal defect in cattle encountered in high frequency is centric fusion of acrocentric chromosomes to form Robertsonian translocations. Chromosomal defects and aberrations in chromosomal number are becoming increasingly important for determining the cause of congenital defects in cattle.

Causes of many congenital defects are unknown, but many follow simple Mendelian inheritance, mostly simple autosomal recessive inheritance. Other monofactorial inheritance patterns may be encountered and characterized as overdominant, dominant, incomplete dominant, and polygenic.

Diagnosis of the genetic causes of congenital defects is based on the rule that genetic diseases run in families. Thus, congenital defects occur in typical intergenerational patterns and intragenerational frequencies. Recognizing these patterns and frequencies requires enumerating normal and abnormal offspring and identifying their familial relationships. Various statistical methods are used to analyze such data. Breeding trials are necessary to confirm inheritance patterns. Cattle have 30 pairs of chromosomes and all pairs but 1 (sex chromosomes) are exactly the same size and shape. Genes, in turn, occur in pairs and are found in the same location (locus) on the matching chromosome pairs. Genes at the same locus are referred to as alleles. When genes of the given locus are the same, they are referred to as homozygous. A gene has the property to mutate, while the other allele remains unchanged. If this mutation has no visible effect on its carrier (heterozygote), it is referred to as a recessive mutation. However, this recessive mutation may be carried along for several generations until by chance two carriers are mated, and a defect will be exposed in about one fourth of the offspring. If the mutation modified the heterozygote, it is referred to as a dominant mutation.

Statistical methods are used to analyze genetic data. Analysis is complicated when there are several diagnostic entities, as when a syndrome of defects is found. The family can be identified through one or more defective offspring called the index cases (propositi or probands). This step is important because, under certain modes of inheritance, some normal parents can produce both normal and abnormal young, while others can produce only normal calves. In genetic analysis, only families of parents that produce a defective offspring are included, and families of parents that can, but do not, produce defects are excluded. This truncated selection increases the frequency of defectives over that expected theoretically from the complete selection possible in experimental matings.

The recessive inheritance pattern involves only two kinds of calves—normal and defective. Only a few normal carriers or heterozygotes can transmit the disease. Although two defective parents produce only defectives, most defectives do not reproduce; hence, most defectives are born to normal parents. Each normal parent heterozygous for a defect transmits one of the two abnormal genes necessary to produce the defective offspring (homozygous abnormal). But most normal cattle do not transmit the defect (homozygous normal). When the carriers are mated with noncarriers, they produce only normal offspring.

When normal carriers (heterozygotes) that produced a defective offspring are mated repeatedly, 25 per cent of their progeny should be defective and 75 per cent should be normal. Two of every three normal offspring from such parents carry a hidden recessive gene that they again may transmit to their progeny, just as their parents transmitted the abnormal gene to them. Thus, recessive defects are carried generation after generation by normal phenotypic carriers (heterozygotes), and this results in the insidious spread of the undesirable gene through the population. Carriers (or heterozygotes) for a defect, transmitted as an autosomal recessive, are identified only after they have had defective offspring.

Eliminating defective progeny usually keeps recessive genes at low frequencies. But breeds in which only a few animals produced most breeding animals or in which many animals are closely related to a single outstanding animal are vulnerable to an outbreak of genetic defects. This may happen when the foundation animal carries an unknown recessive gene.

Dominance, the reverse of a recessive inheritance pattern, is a less common pattern, and dominant genes are passed from one generation to the next. They do not "skip" generations as recessive genes may do and usually are seen in parent and offspring. With dominant inheritance, normal unaffected animals breed true, but those with the defect may produce both normal and abnormal offspring. Dominant defects are controlled easily by eliminating all defective animals.

Incomplete dominance creates three kinds of animals: normal, slightly defective, and severely deformed. The normal and the severely deformed animals breed true. Slightly abnormal animals, when mated together, produce one-fourth normal progeny, one-half slightly defective progeny, and one-fourth severely deformed progeny. The disease can be controlled easily by eliminating all defective progeny.

Overdominance is similar to incomplete dominance in that three classes are produced: normal, superior, and deformed. Normal and deformed animals breed true. The superior animals, when mated with other superior animals, produce one-fourth normal, one-half superior, and one-fourth defective offspring. The superior animals usually are selected as replacements in preference to normal animals, but this is at the cost of losing 25 per cent of their offspring from like mates, because these offspring are defective. Overdominant traits are difficult to control because all superior animals also carry the undesirable gene, and owners are reluctant to choose inferior breeding animals.

A few reports describe characteristics linked with sex, i.e., the genes are carried on the sex chromosomes. Another class of genetic diseases is caused by chromosomal aberrations. However, structural and numerical aberrations of chromosomal material in cattle have not reached the diagnostic significance encountered in humans.

Congenital defects also may be inherited in a polygenic manner, with or without a threshold. Multiple gene defects may be inherited as dominant characteristics but most of these are recessive. The control measures are the same, to breed families with little or no defects of the kind needing control.

DIAGNOSIS

Determining the cause of congenital defects may be difficult, as the cause usually exerts its effects some time before the defect is recognized. All defects should be thoroughly examined and documented.

Histories should be obtained and carefully evaluated: breed, time of year, exposure to or suspected exposure to teratogens, feeding and management practices, type of breeding, previous breeding records, maternal medical and vaccination records, disease status of herd, periods of stress, drugs administered, congenital defects observed previously, and any history of similar congenital defects. Breeding records should be examined for characteristic intragenerational and intergenerational hereditary patterns of genetic disease, as discussed earlier.

Defective calves should be subjected to standard necropsy, and the defects should be classified by the body system that is primarily involved. Sections of brain, spinal cord, lungs, liver, kidneys, and other appropriate tissues should be collected and fixed in 10-per cent buffered neutral formalin for histopathologic examination.

If a viral teratogen is suspected, serum samples should be taken and checked for viral antibodies, and sections of spleen, liver, and brain should be taken for possible virus isolation. Serologic and fluorescent antibody techiques are more reliable than isolation when a viral teratogen is suspected.

Live defective calves' leukocytes and various tissues should be collected for culture and for examination of possible chromosomal aberrations. Blood samples also should be drawn from live calves produced by artificial insemination to verify parentage. Please consult with AI center or breed organization for proper handling of blood samples and where to send them.

SPECIFIC DEFECTS

Organs or structures may show arrested development, may be absent (agenesis or aplasia), or may be small (hypoplasia). An embryonal or fetal structure may fail to disappear when it normally should, e.g., the ductus arteriosus or the thyroglossal duct and the overlying skin of the anal opening—atresia ani. Certain openings, grooves, and fissures may fail to close properly, especially those in the midline. Examples of resulting conditions are cranioschisis and rachischisis from lack of closure of the neural groove, palatoschisis or cleft palate, patent foramen ovale in the heart, ventricular septal defect in the heart, persistent cloaca due to the rectal and external genital openings not separating, and ventral abdominal wall defects. Closure defects such as hernias are common. Aberrant (ectopic or heterotopic) structures occur, involving displacement of tissues, e.g., adrenal and thyroid, to a location where they are not normally found. Islands or foci of pancreatic tissue are found in the wall of the stomach, and adrenal tissue is found in the kidney or pelvic tissue. Displacement of cutaneous and mucosal tissue is considered to be the cause of dermoid cysts. Embryonic remnants of developmental vestiges are useless structures in adult animals but are of phylogenetic importance, and embryogenetically, the organs are formed but regress later. Duplication may involve many parts of the body. Diprosopus, dicephalus, cranial or caudal duplication, incomplete twinning, penis and prepuce duplication, or polydactyly of the feet may be seen. Hypertrophy and hyperplasia are other mechanisms, causing double muscling in cattle. Disturbances of cartilage and bone formation may lead to chondrodystrophy fetalis or dwarfism.

It is difficult to arrive at a single system suitable for classifying congenital defects in animals. Three principal systems have been used: etiology, affected embryonic tissue, and most involved defective body system. The last system is used in this chapter.

The next section defines defects of various body systems in domestic and feral animals. It places emphasis on defects of current interest and concern.

Skeletal System

The skeletal system is involved in many congenital defects of animals. Parts of the system may be affected with single, isolated osseous defects, or the whole skeleton may be affected.

Single, Isolated Skeletal Defects

Among 331 animals with cleft palate in a veterinary hospital population, Charolais cattle had cleft palate as part of a syndrome of multiple malformations, such as arthrogryposis. Cheilognathoschisis (cleft lip) and brachygnathia inferior (short lower jaw) may be of concern in some breeds of cattle.

Axial skeletal defects have been rarely described. One example, however, is atlanto-occipital fusion.

Localized defects of the appendicular skeleton usually are inherited and are of considerable economic importance. Tibial hemimelia in Galloway cattle is due to homozygosity of a simple autosomal recessive gene. Tibial hemimelia has associated defects: bilateral agenesis or reduction in length of the tibia, bilateral agenesis of the patella, nonclosure of the pelvic symphysis, cranioschisis, meningocele, internal hydrocephalus, ventral abdominal hernia, nonunion of the müllerian ducts in females, and cryptorchidism in males.

Polydactyly, increase in number of digits, may affect all four feet, but there is a tendency for the front feet only to be involved. The mode of inheritance is polygenic, requiring a dominant gene at one locus and recessive genes at another locus. Rare congenital defects, like common ones, may be genetic or environmental in origin, or may reflect a combination of both. Although of modest economic importance, ectrodactyly, partial absence of phalanges, is important because externally it is similar to hereditary bovine syndactyly.

Syndactyly, fusion or nondivision of functional digits, is due to homozygosity of a simple autosomal recessive gene with incomplete penetrance and varying degrees of expressivity and pleiotropism. It is the commonest inherited skeletal defect of Holstein cattle in the United States. It is also encountered in Angus, Chianina, Simmental, and crossbred cattle.

Syndactyly in Holstein cattle usually follows a particular pattern of fusion or nondivision. If one leg is affected, it is first the right front, followed by the left front. If three legs are affected, the pattern is right and left front, followed by right hind leg. Rarely, four feet are affected. The degree of fusion or nondivision is always more advanced in the right front foot when more than one foot is affected. Hereditary bovine syndactyly is associated with a functional defect (malignant hyperthermia) that requires special environmental conditions for expression. The defect is allelic in Holstein, Angus, and Chianina breeds in the United States, however, beef breeds seem to be more severely affected.

The development of syndactylous carriers and normal Holstein-Friesian embryos, 31 to 45 days of age, has been studied. The anlagen of the metacarpal bones were close together in the 37-day-old syndactylous embryo, and the distal ends had started to fuse. The normal 39-day-old embryo had widely separated blastemata of the future phalanges, while the syndactylous embryo had a single mass of blastema.

A program to test syndactyly in Holstein, Angus, and Chianina cattle uses superovulation of homozygous, affected, syndactylous cows; insemination with the semen of bulls to be tested; embryo transplant; and preterminal cesarean section at 60 days of gestation. Females can be tested by using semen from affected bulls, by embryo transfers, and by early fetal recovery.

Systemic Skeletal Defects

Various classification schemes have been proposed for the chondrodysplasia-dwarfism complex. Chondrodysplasia is basically a defect of interstitial growth of epiphyseal, articular, and basocranial cartilages, resulting in variable shortness of legs, cranial base, and vertebral column. Various types of dwarfism are distinguished, such as short-headed, long-headed, and Telemark, all considered to result from recessive genes. In addition, the Dexter, comprest, and compact mutants (considered dominants) are part of a complex of conditions from more than one locus and seem to be related to the recessive types.

Several gross features have been described for diagnosis of dwarfism in cattle.

1. Normal closure of the spheno-occipital synchondrosis occurs between 24 and 36 months, whereas in dwarfism it may occur from birth to 5 months of age.

2. Projection of the orbitosphenoid (ala minor) into the cranial cavity in a medial and dorsal direction is typical for dwarf cattle.

3. In calves younger than 10 days of age, compression of the ventral borderline of lumbar and thoracic vertebrae can be of diagnostic help.

4. Three groups of calves may be distinguished: those with normal vertebral columns, those with abnormal vertebral columns, and intermediates with normal and abnormal overlaps.

Osteopetrosis, a recessive hereditary defect encountered in black and red Angus calves, is characterized grossly by small body size and weight, brachygnathia inferior with impacted molar teeth, misshapen coronoid and condyloid processes, open fontanelle, thickened cranial bones, agenesis or hypoplasia of major foramina of the skull, and absence of bone marrow cavities. There is a lack of remodeling of primary spongiosa that persists throughout the metaphyseal and diaphyseal areas. Calves affected with osteopetrosis are born prematurely at 251 to 272 days (mean 262) gestation and may be mistaken for an abortion problem rather than osteopetrosis. Affected calves are stillborn, and the only external characteristics may be small body size and short lower jaw. Osteopetrosis in Hereford, in Dutch Holstein-Friesian, and in European Simmental calves had similar morphologic features.

Acroteriasis congenita, described as a recessive trait in Europe, involved low birth weight, defects of all four legs, defects of the facial skeleton, cleft palate, brachygnathia inferior, microtia, and hydrocephalus. Other findings were deficient ossification of the skeleton of the head and kyphosis or scoliosis of the vertebral column.

Crooked calf disease, reproduced by feeding lupines (*Lupinus sericeus* and *L. caudatus*) to pregnant cows between days 40 and 70 of gestation, is similar to a skeletal defect syndrome of arthrogryposis, kyphoosis, torticollis, scoliosis, and cleft palate. This cattle defect may be due to homozygosity of recessive genes. The only difference between crooked calf disease and the skeletal defect syndrome was cleft palate, which was always manifested in the genetic forms but only seen occasionally in the lupine-induced disease. Calves born to cows fed a manganese-deficient diet had similar skeletal deformities.

Congenital disorders of joints may be generalized or restricted to a single joint. Ankylosis, abnormal union of the ends of bones forming the joint, may involve one or more joints. Arthrogryposis and congenital contracture of muscles have been reported many times as ankylosis. Fifteen cows were irradiated with 200 roentgens between 27 and 34 days of gestation; two calves that were irradiated at day 31 and three calves that were irradiated at day 32 were born with osseous fusion of humeroradial joints. Bilateral spontaneous osteoarthritis of the stifle joint in Holstein-Friesian and Jersey cattle has been described as an autosomal recessive trait. Occurrence of hip dysplasia in Hereford cattle seemed to be compatible with an hereditary etiology.

Central Nervous System

Congenital defects of the CNS are common, and most can be recognized by a structural change involving both the skeletal and central nervous systems or only the latter.

CNS defects are classified into five groups by combining anatomic and functional approaches: (1) cerebral defects and malformations, involving only or mainly the cerebrum, (2) defects of cerebellum and brain stem, involving only or mainly the cerebellum and brain stem, (3) spinal cord defects, (4) spastic and paralytic diseases, and (5) storage diseases.

Nature, cause, and frequency of congenital malformations of the CNS reported in two separate studies indicated that internal hydrocephalus is common in certain beef breeds. Agenesis of corpus callosum, anencephaly, hydranencephaly, and Arnold-Chiari deformity, although rare, may be confused clinically with hydrocephalus.

Meningoencephalocele is protrusion of meninges and brain tissue through the cranial cleft, usually forming a large liquid-filled sac located in the frontal region, but some are midfrontal, parietal, or occipital.

Hydrocephalus results from excessive fluid accumulating in the cranial cavity within the ventricular system (internal hydrocephalus) and appears to be inherited in many breeds as a simple autosomal recessive trait. Affected calves had reduced body size and weight, narrow, refined facial features, cranial doming, caudodorsal-rostroventral angulation of palpebral fissures, microphthalmia, and protruding edematous tongues. Micropolygyria of the cerebral convexities resulted from dorsal elevation of gyri located within the longitudinal fissure to the cerebral surface, and shallow sulci formed secondarily. Attentuation of the convolutions on the dorsal cerebral surface and cystic dilation of the optic chiasma were presumably due to pressure. Mesencephalic kinking at the anterior portion of the aqueduct, lateral splaying of the dorsal thalamus, and absence of the interthalamic adhesion were features. The sigmoid configuration of the brain and the splaying configuration of the thalamus resembled the cephalic flexure and diencephalon of 40-day-old bovine embryos, respectively. Cerebellar hypoplasia and dysplastic lesions were present.

Cerebellar hypoplasia has been described as a genetic defect in many breeds of cattle. Whereas all earlier investigators invariably incriminated hereditary causes in cerebellar disease, recent evidence points to intrauterine fetal infection with BVD virus causing cerebellar hypoplasia combined with ocular defects.

The pathological changes in the allegedly genetic form of cerebellar hypoplasia differ from those of the BVD virus-induced cerebellar defect. The ocular lesions and large irregular cavities in the folial white matter and the inflammatory processes observed in cases of BVD viral origin have not been described in the genetic form, while cerebellar aplasia has not been seen in virus-induced cerebellar hypoplasia and degeneration.

BVD virus may cause cerebellar hypoplasia and degeneration along with other anomalies in calves. The critical period during gestation for viral infection to precipitate cerebellar hypoplasia was between 146 and 150 days. Calves carried to term were either stillborn, mummified, or born alive with "cerebellar ataxia" (generalized ataxia, malpositioning of the limbs, and difficulty in rising or apparent weakness). In addition, blindness, nystagmus, and head tremors may occur. Gross lesions of varying degrees consisted of decreased cerebellar size, ocular lesions, and occasional skeletal defects. Microscopically, there was mild to severe depletion of the cortical layers to complete destruction of the cortex and folial white matter. In severe forms, only neuropil and meninges were intact. Large irregular cavities occurred in the severely affected white matter. Depending upon time of inoculation, there was more disruption of normal architecture of the cerebellar cortex and formation of spheroids or swelling of Purkinje cell axons (torpedos) in the granular layer. Other changes observed were glial nodules in the deep cortical tissue and white matter of the telencephalon.

Progressive ataxia in Charolais cattle is characterized by weakness of hind legs, which is first noticed at 8 to 24 months of age and progresses from slight ataxia involving all four limbs to recumbency. Histologic examination reveals lesions throughout the white substance of brain and spinal cord, and reduced density or stainability of all circular or ovoid areas, often with one or more axons centrally or eccentrically placed.

Congenital cerebellar atrophy has been reported in Holstein calves and in a Charolais calf.

Hereditary neuraxial edema, described in polled Hereford calves, was characterized by extensor spasms and inability to stand. Histologically, it was characterized by edema of the terminal portions of myelinated bundles and by gray substances containing heavily myelinated fibers. Genetic analysis in two herds indicated autosomal recessive transmission.

Various developmental spinal cord defects of calves have been described under the terms spina bifida and spinal dysraphism (status dysraphicus). Spina bifida implies a defect of vertebrae with or without spinal cord defects. Spinal dysraphism is a myelodysplasia or malformation of the spinal cord especially of the central canal, with or without involvement of vertebrae.

Clinically, cattle are affected from birth with complete hind leg paralysis, severe ataxia, or sometimes hopping gait. In cattle able to stand, stance is extremely wide, and there is overextending (goose stepping) and crossing of hindlegs while walking or standing. Some calves may appear to be weak in the hind legs with a deficit in placing reflexes, without considerable crossing or overextending.

Gross morphologic changes may not be obvious in intact spinal cords. When concurrent spina bifida is present, defective vertebrae in the affected spinal column segment are observed. The spinal cord may require sectioning to demonstrate the lesion, which is generally manifested as a cavitation, with or without fluid, in the affected portion of the spinal cord. Histologically, syringomyelia, and anomalies of the dorsal septum and ventral median fissure, central canal, and gray matter, or any combination are observed. The causes of spinal dysraphia and spina bifida are unknown.

Congenital or familial disorders of cattle may clinically mimic degenerative spinocerebellar disorders, especially spinocerebellar degenerations, but as of yet, most are without demonstrable histopathologic CNS lesions of a progressive, systemic degenerative nature.

Not all of these conditions are both familial and congenital, but all are suspected to be either one or the other. Clinical onset is not always at birth or even early in life, and the outcome is not invariably fatal, as are most progressive, degenerative CNS disorders in cattle. Each condition is of some if not major economic importance to the cattle industry.

Epilepsy is defined as a sudden, brief, or prolonged loss of consciousness usually preceded by a convulsion. Epilepsy can be further classified into symptomatic and idiopathic, whereas in symptomatic epilepsy there is some associated disease process or lesion, and in idiopathic (true) epilepsy there is no demonstrable cause or lesion. Epilepsy was described in Brown Swiss cattle, however, no histologic examination was reported.

Spastic Disorders

Both spastic paresis and spastic syndrome imply CNS involvement and a hereditary basis. However, CNS lesions have not been described, and the dysfunction has been suggested recently to be merely a functional CNS disorder, thus implying a lack of specific lesions.

Spastic paresis has been recognized in many breeds of cattle ("contraction of the Achilles tendon," "Elso heel," straight hock") and appears to be worldwide in distribution.

Clinically, signs were usually not present at birth. Most cases were first observed in calves from 2 to 18 months of age, the usual sign being related to difficulty in ambulation. Generally, only one hind leg was affected, and it was stated that there was a predilection for the right hind leg, with bilateral involvement being less common. The cause of impaired locomotion and difficulty in rising was related to chronic spastic contraction of the quadriceps femoris, gastrocnemius, and adductor muscles. Additionally, the superficial flexor, semitendinosus, and semimembranosus muscles may be involved, resulting in tautness of the flexor (Achilles) tendons that causes the tuber calcis to draw inward, towards the tibia, and produce an overly straight limb and a weak hock. The limb may appear shorter than normal; only the toes seem to contact the walking surface, and the limb swings freely when the affected cattle walk. Arching of the back and a raised tail may be observed.

Spastic syndrome has been observed in most breeds of cattle and dairy breeds, but Holsteins are affected more frequently than beef breeds. It is also known as crampy (Krämpfigkeit), neuromuscular spasticity, posterior paralysis, progressive posterior paralysis, stretches, and other names.

Signs occurred later in life, most cattle were at least 3 to 6 or more years of age before clinical dysfunction was noted. Following the initial onset of spasms, which were usually only slight muscle spasms, progression to more severe, advanced dysfunction was usually prolonged over a period of several months to years. Clinical signs were reported to be elicited by "irritating or painful" stimuli to the feet, joints, spinal column, udder, penis, and abdomen, including infectious and inflammatory disorders of these structures.

Both sexes may be affected, but the majority of cases have been described in bulls, especially those in AI units. Spastic syndrome has been considered a disorder of "postural reflex mechanism." Characteristic clinical signs were spastic contractions of muscles of the hind legs and back when affected cattle were walking or standing. The spasms lasted for only seconds or minutes or were prolonged for days or months. Spasms often were severe enough to cause the hind legs to remain in complete extension, stretched caudally. Recovery was not known to occur, and affected cattle were eventually unable to ambulate normally. Gross microscopic examinations of CNS tissue revealed no lesions. Treatment with CNS depressant drugs has proven moderately successful in relieving spasms in some cattle. It was suggested that the disorder is a functional derangement of the CNS. Genetic analyses of selected cases have indicated spastic syndrome was familial, but the exact mode of inheritance was unknown.

The "weaver syndrome" (bovine progressive degenerative myeloencephalopathy, BPDM) is a hereditary disease of both male and female purebred Brown Swiss cattle. Clinical signs are ataxia, hind leg weakness, abnormal positioning of the hind feet, and eventual recumbency. Because of the peculiar, weaving gait of affected cattle, the disease is referred to colloquially as the weaver syndrome. Gross pathologic changes are limited to atrophy of large muscle groups of the loin and hind legs.

Epidemiologic studies failed to indicate any specific geographic or environmental factors common to the occurrence of BPDM in purebred Brown Swiss cattle in the United States. The incidence of recorded cases of BPDM increased greatly during the past 6 to 7 years.

Clinical and laboratory findings were reported for a large group of purebred Brown Swiss cattle affected with BPDM. Three sires were incriminated in 48.6 per cent of the cases; one was incriminated in 31.4 per cent of the cases, indicating a definite familial predilection and possible hereditary nature for the disease. Hallmarks of the disease were hind leg weakness, ataxia, and dysmetria, with an onset of 5 to 8 months of age, progressing to eventual recumbency and frequently death from rumen tympany. Hind leg weakness, ataxia, and dysmetria were present. A deficit of unconscious proprioception was postulated as the cause of hind leg signs. Laboratory analyses revealed no hematologic abnormalities. Elevation of certain serum enzymes was found, however, no enzyme alteration was considered specific for this disease. Limited cerebrospinal fluid (CSF) analyses demonstrated detectable creatine phosphokinase (CPK) activity.

Microscopic lesions were confined to the white matter of the spinal cord, the axons of some brain stem nuclei, and the Purkinje cells of the cerebellar cortex. Spinal cord lesions consisted of axon degeneration, loss of axons and myelin, vacuolation of white matter due to large, empty intercellular spaces, and axonal spheroid formation. Both ascending and descending fibers were involved, and lesions were most severe in thoracic spinal cord segments. Cerebellar lesions showed selective degeneration and loss of Purkinje cells and occasional torpedos in the granular layer of the cerebellar cortex. Brain stem lesions were inconsistent and limited to occasional axonal swelling in the brain stem nuclei.

Axonal changes were primarily degenerative but also included reactive and dystrophic forms, as evaluated with transmission electron microscopy. In addition, recent transmission electron microscopy studies of the cerebral cortex also demonstrated abnormalities of synapses in affected animals. It was postulated that BPDM of purebred Brown Swiss cattle may be a congenital metabolic defect of axon transport that is familial and possibly inherited but not manifested until a certain stage of development in affected cattle.

Another neurodegenerative inherited disease has been described recently in horned Hereford calves. It was characterized in newborns by tremulous shaking of the head, body, and tail, difficulty in arising, a wobbly spastic gait, and lack of bellow. Transient improvement was followed by deterioration with a progressive spastic paraplegia. Generalized tremors were induced easily by a variety of stimuli, and spinal reflexes may be exaggerated or depressed. The major pathologic finding was excessive accumulation of neurofilaments within neurons of the central, peripheral, and autonomic systems.

Storage Diseases

A lysosomal storage disease is associated with accumulation and storage of some substance within lysosomes owing to a specific enzyme deficiency preventing specific catabolism. Criteria for a disease to be classified as an inborn error of lysosomal catabolism are (1) it should be a storage disease, (2) it should be inherited, (3) the storage substance, not necessarily homogeneous, should be stored at least initially within lysosomes, and (4) there should be partial or absolute deficiency of one lysosomal enzyme that is normally responsible for hydrolyzing the storage material.

Among the recorded storage diseases involving the CNS of cattle are GM_1 gangliosidosis, glyconeogenesis, and mannosidosis.

Generalized glyconeogenesis Type II in cattle has been reported in Beef Shorthorn and Brahman.

GM_1 gangliosidosis results from reduction (70 to 80 per cent) in β-galactosidase activity and occurs as a hereditary defect in Friesian calves of both sexes. It probably is analogous to Type II GM_1 gangliosidosis (Derry's disease) in humans, because GM_1 ganglioside accumulates in the brain but not in the liver and spleen of affected calves. Clinical signs of slight swaying of hindquarters, reluctance to move, and stiffness of gait appear during the first few weeks of life.

Mannosidosis, originally reported as pseudolipidosis, is associated with a deficiency of α-mannosidase and occurs in Angus cattle as a simple recessive. A deficiency of mannosidase results in storage of an oligosaccharide containing glucosamine and mannose.

Mannosidosis in Angus and Murray Gray cattle, originally described in Australia and New Zealand, has recently been recognized in the United States. Mannosidase activity is used to test cattle for normal activity (homozygous) and reduced activity (heterozygous).

Mannosidosis is characterized by ataxia, incoordination, head tremor, aggression, and failure to thrive. Calves may be affected at birth, but clinical signs usually do not appear until they are several weeks or months old. Most affected cattle die within the first 12 months of life, or mannosidosis may be a cause of neonatal mortality. Neuronal vacuolation takes place with vacuoles formed from saccular dilations of the Golgi apparatus. Secondary lesions include spheroidal swellings of axons caused by local accumulations of electron-dense bodies, mitochondria, and local proliferation of neurofilaments. Periodic acid-Schiff (PAS)-positive, lipofuscin-like globules may be observed within astrocytes, microglia, and pericytes of blood vessels.

Ocular Defects

Relatively few ocular defects have been described in cattle. Single or multiple defects restricted to the eye, defects observed in conjunction with defects in other organs, and defects associated with pigment deficiencies, however, have been described.

Frequency of ocular defects, such as anophthalmia and microphthalmia, was estimated in six United States breeds to be, maximally, 1 in 7500 births and, minimally, 1 in 50,000 births. The cause of these bovine ocular defects is unknown. BVD virus has been demonstrated to cause cerebellar hypoplasia combined with ocular defects, such as retinal atrophy, acute and chronic neuritis, cataract, and microphthalmia with retinal dysplasia.

Ocular dermoids in Hereford cattle are a genetically transmitted defect characterized by autosomal recessive and polygenic inheritance. Calves typically are affected bilaterally with multiple, interconnected ocular growths that clinically, histologically, and ultrastructurally mimic normal skin with hair. Sites most commonly involved include ventro-lateral limbus, third eyelid, medial canthus, eyelid, and conjunctiva. Central corneal and anterior segmental dermoids also are observed.

Muscular System

Congenital defects of muscle are common in cattle, and all are economically important. Muscular hypertrophy ("Doppellender," double muscling, muscular hyperplasia) is encountered in most major beef herds. Double-muscled calves vary widely, and few calves have all the characteristics. A few characteristics in a herd, however, indicate the presence of the trait, the most noticeable being the rounded outline of the hindquarters. The tail is attached more cranially than normal. The muscles of the shoulder, back, rump, and hindquarter are separated by deep creases, especially those between the semitendinosus and biceps femoris and between the longissimus dorsi muscles of either side. Necks are shorter and thicker, and heads are smaller and lighter. Double-muscled cattle stand in a stretched position. Diaphyses of the long bones tend to be shorter. Macroglossia may be present. Additional problems are abnormal genital tracts, impaired reproduction, slow sexual maturity, long gestation, and greater birth weight combined with dystocia. Double-muscled calves are less viable and susceptible to rickets and joint disease.

Differentiation of skeletal muscle tissue, neuromuscular junction, and peripheral nerves was studied in fetal and neonatal arthrogrypotic Charolais calves. Muscular rigidity was caused by impaired neurogenic function, involving mechanisms exerting influence on the motor activity of neurons in the spinal cord. Another study described abnormal nerve-muscle interaction. Focal accumulation of 16 S acetylcholinesterase in endplate regions of the muscle was not observed, as in the normal control calves. Silver nitrate impregnation of motor innervation revealed abnormal features, such as preterminal branching and ultraterminal sprouting in affected calves.

Records of 944 calves affected with arthrogryposis were compiled according to localization of the deformity, sex, Belgian province, months of birth, degree of retraction, therapy, and complications. In 50 per cent of cases, the defects affected both carpi. The condition was more common in male calves and in those calves born during December to April. The most common complications were decubitus sores and omphalitis.

Arthrogryposis includes more than one etiologic and pathologic entity. It is a worldwide problem and has been described in all major breeds of cattle. Usually, all four legs are symmetrically arthrogrypotic in Charolais calves. Cleft palate is associated with the defect. Some calves also have kyphoscoliotic deformities of the vertebral column. The muscular system is characterized by moderate to marked wasting and widespread replacement of fat cells. Tetramelic arthrogryposis associated with cleft palate is inherited as a simple autosomal recessive in Charolais calves.

Skin

Developmental defects involving skin, adnexa, and pigment are not uncommon in cattle and may be either generalized or localized.

Albinism may be classified as partial, incomplete, and complete. In partial albinism, the iris is blue and white centrally and brown peripherally, and the coat color is usually characteristic of the breed or more dilute. Incomplete albinos have colobomas of the nontapetal fundus and tapetal fibrosum hypoplasia.

A new albinotic color deficiency, recently identified in Angus cattle, appears to be inherited as a simple autosomal recessive trait. It is characterized by brown hair over the entire body surface instead of the typical black hair. The muzzle, hooves, and scrotum in males also are brown. The skin surface is brownish to gray. This is particularly obvious at the glabrous skin, such as around eyelids, ear openings, muzzle, and anal and reproductive openings. The dark black iris of Angus cattle is replaced by a light, usually two-colored iris. This gives a double-ringed appearance to the iris when viewed closely, i.e., an outer, faintly brown ring and an inner, light blue ring circling the pupil. The pupils always appear constricted in daylight. From a distance, the eyes appear white. The ocular fundus is albinotic.

Fragility of skin and epitheliogenesis imperfecta are genetic defects of bovine skin. Protoporphyria is found in Limousin cattle.

Hypotrichosis was studied in horned and polled Hereford cattle, ranging from slightly to severely affected. The skin was thin and pliable with only a few hairs observed per unit area on the lateral and ventral neck, face, ears, thorax, flank, rump, and forehead. The hair coat over the eyelids and around the prepuce, umbilicus, and switch of tail was thin, wavy, and silky. Microscopic examination revealed an epidermis 2 to 3 cell layers thick and poorly differentiated dermal papillae. Frequently, the hair shafts were fragmented and did not conform to the internal contours of the hair follicles.

Six different kinds of hypotrichosis are distinguished in cattle.

1. Hairless lethal is encountered in exotic breeds. Affected calves die shortly after birth owing to this simple autosomal recessive.

2. Semi-hairlessness has been reported only in polled Herefords and is characterized by thin coat at birth. Later, the hair coat is sparse and patchy, and the skin is wrinkled and scaly. It is inherited as a recessive trait.

3. Hypotrichosis associated with anodontia has been described in Maine-Anjou calves as a recessive trait.

4. Viable hypotrichosis, encountered in Guernseys and exotic breeds, characterized by partial to complete absence of hair at birth, is due to homozygosity of simple autosomal recessive genes.

5. Hypotrichosis with missing incisor teeth has been reported in Holstein-Friesian calves. The trait is possibly dominant.

6. Streaked hairlessness in Holstein-Friesians, characterized by vertical hairless streaks over hip joints and sometimes over the body and legs, is due to a dominant sex-linked gene.

Congenital hypertrichosis has been described in European cattle. Polypnea occurs during hot weather. Abnormal curliness of hair transmitted as an autosomal dominant has been reported in Ayrshire calves.

Cardiovascular System

Like humans and other domestic animals, cattle are affected with several different cardiovascular defects. With few exceptions, most congenital cardiac defects are reported as single cases. Descriptions of series of cases are few. During routine meat inspection of 50,742 bovine hearts, congenital anomalies were found in 88 (0.17 per cent). The cause of cardiovascular defects has received little study in calves.

Digestive System

Recent work indicated that atresia coli may be caused by rectal palpation. Results obtained thus far incriminated palpation of the amniotic sac between day 36 and 40 of gestation as a cause of atresia coli in calves.

Large Body Cavities

Although scrotal, inguinal, and, in particular, umbilical hernias are considered common in cattle, little is known about their cause.

From 323,961 case abstracts submitted by 12 United States and Canadian Veterinary College hospital clinics, 1315 cases were diagnosed as being affected with congenital umbilical hernia, 705 with congenital inguinal hernia, and 57 with congenital scrotal hernia. Several breeds of cattle were at risk for one or both types of hernia. The introduction of American Holsteins into northern Germany has led to increasing reports of umbilical hernias.

Reproductive System

An intersex individual is one with congenital anatomic variations, including some reproductive organs of both sexes, or it is genetically one sex but phenotypically the other sex. Hermaphrodites, by definition, have the gonads of both sexes, either as an ovary and testis or combined into an ovotestis. A pseudohermaphrodite has the gonads and reproductive organs of one sex with some characteristics of the opposite sex.

Freemartins are heifer calves born as a co-twin with a bull calf. About 93 per cent are affected with variable hypoplasia or agenesis of organs, developing from müllerian ducts and stimulating development of the wolffian duct system. They are usually sterile. Bovine freemartins may not be caused by humoral factors but may be a function of sex chromosome mosaics. Recent investigations of freemartin embryos and fetuses revealed two successive phases in development. The initial phase of inhibition from day 50 to 75 of gestation was characterized by the arrest of gonadal development in the female and regression of müllerian duct development. The fetuses were considered to be under the influence of an inhibiting factor. A phase of masculinization followed at day 75.

Various deviations of the penis and prepuce have been described, and all are rare with unknown causes. Penile agenesis is uncommon. Duplication of the penis has been described. Persistent penile frenulum, considered common in Shorthorn and Angus, is thought to be inherited.

Numerous investigators have reported testicular hypoplasia, which is bilateral or unilateral and partial or complete.

Cryptorchidism, or incomplete descensus of the testicle, may be unilateral or bilateral. The available evidence indicates possible genetic transmission.

Segmental aplasia of the wolffian duct, usually unilateral, is characterized by aplasia of segments located mostly in the head of the epididymis.

Ovarian aplasia has been reported with and without associated anomalies of the tubular reproductive structures. Ovarian hypoplasia in the Swedish Highland breed may be total or partial and unilateral or bilateral. Defects of oviducts, uterus, cervix, and vagina have been described in several breeds. In many, fusion of the müllerian ducts is either lacking or exaggerated. A high incidence of duplication of the cervix in Hereford cattle was reported to be caused by a sex-limited, simple autosomal recessive gene with low penetrance and varying expressivity. Segmental aplasia of the müllerian duct system has been described by many workers. White heifer disease, inherited as a polygenic trait, falls into two distinct classes of morphologic aberrations, both with partial or total persistence of the hymen and one with additional defects cranial to the hymen. Common to both types are functional ovaries and accumulation of secretion products.

Prolonged gestation has been recorded for most dairy breeds as hereditary, and two distinct pathologic conditions have been distinguished. In the first type, caused by a single autosomal recessive gene, the calf continues to grow in utero and is carried up to 100 days past normal term. Calves born or taken by cesarean section are weak and die in hypoglycemic crisis. In the second type, also caused by homozygosity of a recessive gene, the fetus ceases to grow beyond 7 months and may be affected with craniofacial defects.

Rectovaginal constriction (RVC) due to a simple autosomal recessive, which affects the anus and the vulvovestibular area of Jersey females, is characterized by inelastic constrictions at the junction of the anus, rectum, vestibule, and vulva. The affected male has anal stenosis. The calves of cows with dystocia are delivered following episiotomy or cesarean section. Rectal examinations are difficult to perform on affected cattle. In addition, Jersey cows with RVC are prone to develop udder edema at calving, frequently followed by severe mastitis.

The constricting tissues associated with RVC in Jersey cattle were studied clinically, grossly, and microscopically in affected and 2 control cows. Common to RVC cows were nonelastic fibrous tissue bands located at the anorectal junction and within the vestibular muscularis. Light microscopic and scanning electron microscopic examinations revealed variable amounts of fibrosis affecting the external anal sphincter muscle. Both fibrous tissue bands were composed of well vascularized, irregular connective tissue containing randomly distributed myofibers and adipose tissue. No abnormalities in ultrastructure examination of the tissue bands were observed. The collagen had normal periodicity, and striated muscle had normal cross banding.

Metabolic Diseases

Protoporphyria is a photosensitizing disease in Limousin cattle caused by homozygosity of a simple autosomal recessive gene. Heterozygote cattle may be detected by breeding trials, by determination of ferrochelatase activity in a variety of tissues or fibroblast cultures, and by quantification of free protoporphyrin circulating red blood cells. Protoporphyric Limousin cattle kept at Kansas State University had convulsions, ataxia, and protoporphyric liver cirrhosis.

The recent description of the consequences of UMP (uridine monophosphate) synthase deficiency in cattle is interesting. Cows deficient in UMP synthase secreted milk with abnormally high levels of orotate, i.e., 300 to 1000 μg/ml orotate compared with 80 μg/ml orotate for normal cows. There was a lactation-induced orotic aciduria. Plasma orotate also was elevated. Genetic transmission

was suggested by a common bull in the pedigrees of all deficient animals. Cows with half the normal level of UMP synthase are probably heterozygotes. For these putative heterozygotes, the condition is apparently benign. However, the existence of a gene for UMP synthase deficiency in the dairy cow population poses a hazard analogous to the human population, in which homozygosity is associated with high perinatal morbidity and mortality.

EFFECTS OF CONGENITAL DEFECTS

There are a number of effects of congenital defects to consider: (1) reduced value of affected animals, (2) neonatal mortality, (3) possible component of embryonic and fetal mortality syndrome, (4) lower productivity as a result of longer calving intervals, (5) common maternal sequelae of dystocia and infertility, (6) decreased herd improvement as a result of loss of replacements and consequent reduction in culling potential, (7) alterations in breeding programs as a result of control measures, and (8) inaccurate differential diagnosis.

CONTROL OF CONGENITAL DEFECTS

Control of congenital diseases is difficult. Environmentally induced defects may be eliminated by adjusting management practices. Control of genetically caused defects requires accurate diagnosis of the defect and identification of the genetic transmission patterns. Once a sire has been identified as a carrier of a recessive defect, it is the breeder's responsibility to notify customers of the presence of the defective gene in this bull.

Animal breeders and veterinarians are involved every day in improving animal health and production. Accurate diagnosis of defects, partly or wholly caused by genetic factors, is necessary before control measures can be established. Such diagnosis involves understanding hereditary patterns of disease. Many different congenital defects, caused by genetic, environmental, environmental-genetic, and unknown factors, have been identified in cattle. It is also important to recognize that congenital defects are economically significant to the cattle breeding industry.

Supplemental Reading

Greene, H. J., Leipold, H. W., Huston, K., et al.: Congenital defects in cattle. Ir. Vet. J. 27:37–45, 1973.

Johnson, J. L., Leipold, H. W., Snider, G. W., and Baker, R. D.: Progeny testing for bovine syndactyly. J. Am. Vet. Med. Assoc. 176:549–550, 1980.

Johnson, J. L., Leipold, H. W., Schalles, R. R., et al.: Hereditary polydactyly in Simmental cattle. J. Hered. 72:205–208, 1981.

Jolly, R. D.: Two models lysosomal storage diseases. In R. J. Desnick, D. F. Patterson, and D. G. Scarpelli (eds.), Animal models of inherited metabolic diseases. New York, Alan R. Liss Inc., 145–164, 1982.

Jones, J. M., and Jolly, R. D.: Dwarfism in Hereford cattle: a genetic, morphological and biochemical study. N.Z. Vet. J. 30:185–189, 1982.

Leipold, H. W., Watt, B., Vestweber, J. G. E., and Dennis, S. M.: Clinical observations in rectovaginal constriction in Jersey cattle. Bovine Pract. 16:76–79, 1981.

Leipold, H. W., Huston, K., and Dennis, S. M.: Bovine congenital defects. Adv. Vet. Sci. Comp. Med. 27:197–271, 1983.

Pearson, H.: Changing attitudes to congenital and inherited diseases. Vet. Rec. 105:318–323, 1979.

Robinson, J. L., Drabik, M. R., Dombrowski, D. B., and Clark, J. H.: Consequences of UMP synthase deficiency in cattle. Proc. Natl. Acad. Sci. 80:321–323, 1983.

Rousseaux, C. G., Klavano, G. G., Johnson, E. S., et al.: "Shaker" calf syndrome: a newly recognized inherited neurodegenerative disorder of horned Hereford calves. Vet. Path. (in press), 1983.

Ruth, J. R., Schwartz, S., and Stephenson, B.: Diagnostic tests for the carrier of bovine protoporphyria. Proc. Am. Assoc. Vet. Lab. Diag. 23:79–82, 1980.

Shanks, R. D., Dombrowski, D. B., Harpestad, G. W., and Robinson, J. L.: The inheritance of UMP synthase among dairy cattle. J. Dairy Sci. 66(Suppl. 1):122, 1983.

Stuart, L. D., and Leipold H. W.: Bovine progressive degenerative myeloencephalopathy "weaver" of Brown Swiss cattle. I: Epidemiology. Bovine Pract. 18:129–132, 1983.

Stuart L. D., and Leipold, H. W.: Bovine progressive degenerative myeloencephalopathy "weaver" of Brown Swiss cattle. II. Clinical and laboratory findings. Bovine Pract. 18:133–146, 1983.

Swartz, H. A., and Vogt, D. W.: Chromosome abnormalities as a cause of reproductive inefficiency in heifers. J. Hered. 74:320–324, 1983.

White, J. M., Vinson, W. E., and Pearson, R. E.: Dairy cattle improvement and genetics. J. Dairy Sci. 64:1305–1317, 1981.

Wilson, T. M., deLahunta, A., and Confer, L.: Cerebellar degeneration in dairy calves: clinical, pathologic, and serologic features of an epizootic caused by bovine viral diarrhea virus. J. Am. Vet. Med. Assoc. 183:544–547, 1983.

Colostrum and Passive Immunity in Food-Producing Animals

JONATHAN M. NAYLOR, M.R.C.V.S.,
D.A.C.V.I.M., Ph.D.

Lack of colostral immunity continues to be a major predisposing factor to neonatal disease and ecomonic loss in food-producing animals. In recent years, our knowledge of colostrum feeding has advanced, but a completely reliable method for preventing hypogammaglobulinemia has yet to be described.

DEFENSE MECHANISMS IN CALVES, LAMBS, AND PIGLETS

Neonates are born with incompletely developed host defense mechanisms, and colostral protection plays an important role in early neonatal life. In general, the lymphoid, neutrophil, and macrophage populations are well developed at birth. However, antigenic stimulation following birth is necessary to complete the development of lymphoid tissue in organs, such as the gut and spleen. The protected uterine environment produces a calf that is immunologically naive at birth. The lymphoreticular system has not encountered foreign antigens, and there is very little circulating preformed immunoglobulin (antibody) at birth. Furthermore, when lymphocytes meet a foreign antigen for the first time, their immunoglobulin production is somewhat slow. Future challenges, however, are met with rapid responses. This occurs because the initial antigenic challenge stimulated responsive lymphocytes to multiply and the population of responsive lymphocytes expanded. In other words, the initial challenge "tooled up" the antibody synthesis machinery, and subsequent demand stimulated mass production. There is also evidence that the ability of lymphocytes to respond to challenge—as measured by the response to exposure to mitogens—is diminished in the immediate perinatal period, particularly in calves born to dams fed an energy deficient diet. Feeding colostrum provides the neonate with a source of preformed immunoglobulin, some of which is actively absorbed across the small intestine and provides passive (because the immunoglobulin was acquired, not synthesized by the neonate's own immune system) protection against systemic disease. Part of the immunoglobulin remains in the gut where it can neutralize pathogenic bacteria and help prevent the development of diarrhea.

The phagocytic defenses of the neonatal calf and lamb are depressed at birth. This improves rapidly in the first days of life, particularly if colostrum is fed. It is possible that these improved phagocytic defenses may be due to improved serum complement concentrations; complement binds to bacteria and opsonizes their engulfment by neutrophils. Colostrum feeding enhances the neutrophilia that occurs in the first day of life in calves and also enhances the neutrophilic response to endotoxin challenge. These results suggest that colostrum may contain a factor that stimulates neutrophil production by the bone marrow.

In addition, colostrum contains transferrin and lactoferrin, which bind iron and thus restrict bacterial growth. These factors, together with colostral complement and immunoglobulin, help limit growth of bacteria in the gut.

FORMATION AND COMPOSITION OF COLOSTRUM

Cow colostrum contains about 22 per cent solids compared with the 12 per cent solids of milk. Much of this extra solid is immunoglobulin, but colostrum is also a rich source of casein, fat, and vitamins, especially A and E. There is also a trypsin inhibitor, which helps protect immunoglobulin from digestion in the calf's gut as well as protein fractions that facilitate absorption of immunoglobulins in both calves and piglets.

In cows and ewes, IgG_1 is the principal colostral immunoglobulin. IgG also dominates in sow and mare colostrum. In cows, immunoglobulin is concentrated in colostrum from about 5 weeks prepartum, probably in response to rising estrogen concentration in the dam. Special receptors on the mammary epithelium selectively bind serum IgG_1, and this is taken into the cell by micropinocytosis and transported to the lumen of the mammary gland where it is released into colostrum. Serum IgG_1 concentrations fall to 50 per cent, as colostral concentrations rise to 3 to 12 times that of serum. Colostral IgM and IgA also reach higher concentrations than are found in serum, and they are derived partly from the serum pool and partly from local synthesis by lymphocytes within the mammary gland.

A number of factors influence the total amount of immunoglobulin found in colostrum. The volume of colostrum produced is affected by breed, i.e., dairy cows produce much more than beef cows. Cows produce more than heifers. Feeding dams protein deficient diets does not appear to affect colostrum, but energy deficient diets markedly reduce colostral volume (Table 1).

Colostral immunoglobulin concentration is not related to the volume of colostrum produced, and feeding energy deficient diets does not affect immunoglobulin concentration. There are marked breed differences in colostral immunoglobulin concentration. Low colostral IgM and

Table 1. *Volume of Colostrum Produced by Cows at First Milking or First Suckling by Calf*

Breed	Management	Average Colostrum Yield (L)
Beef—Hereford Cross*	Outwintered: poor nutrition	0.6
	Inwintered: silage ad lib	1.7
Dairy—Aryshire†		2.2
Jersey		2.2
Holstein-Friesian		2.4

*Logan, E. F.: The influence of husbandry on colostrum, yield and immunoglobulin concentration in beef cows. Brit. Vet. J. *133*:120–125, 1977.

†Petrie, L.: Maximizing the absorption of colostral immunoglobulins in the newborn dairy calf. Vet. Rec. *114*:157–163, 1984.

IgA concentrations in Guernseys have led to the speculation that this may result in high calf mortality in this breed. Cows also affect the colostral immunoglobulin concentrations and serum immunoglobulin concentrations of their 1-day-old calves. An important factor that influences colostrum quality (immunoglobulin concentration) is the age of the cow. Heifers have poor quality colostrum while older cows have the best quality colostrum. Another very important factor is milking stage. In general, colostral immunoglobulin content is halved with each successive milking, therefore the first milking colostrum has twice the immunoglobulin content of the second milking colostrum. Colostrum leakage and premilking will both adversely influence colostrum quality. Administration of long-acting corticosteroids, which takes 9 to 19 days to induce parturition, will depress colostral immunoglobulin concentration. Limited evidence suggests that the commonly used North American corticosteroid preparations, which take about 2 days to induce calving, do not adversely affect the immunoglobulin concentrations attained by calves if the cow was over 260 days into gestation at induction. However, in one study, both induced and control calves had a very high incidence of hypoimmunoglobulinemia.

There are similarities between colostrum production in cattle and sheep. Ewe colostral immunoglobulin concentration decreases by about half with every feeding in systems where lambs are allowed to suckle only every 6 hr. Interestingly, the total volume of colostrum and the total amount of immunoglobulin produced by ewes tend to increase with demand, i.e., the number of lambs. This greater production of immunoglobulin only partially compensates for the fact that it has to be shared among more lambs, and so the immunoglobulin content of the lamb's serum at 30 hr of age falls with litter size.

Swine colostral samples have the highest immunoglobulin content if the sow has had 4 to 10 parturitions.

ABSORPTION OF COLOSTRAL IMMUNOGLOBULIN

Immunoglobulins are fairly resistant to digestion by intestinal enzymes and are further protected by the presence of a trypsin inhibitor in bovine colostrum. In the lamb, at least, parietal cell development is not complete until 3 days after birth, and this helps protect colostral protein from acid denaturation and peptic digestion.

Colostral proteins are absorbed in the small intestine, particularly in the distal portion. Specialized epithelial cells, which are present at birth, take up immunoglobulin by micropinocytosis and transport it into the body. This uptake is nonspecific—a variety of macromolecules can be absorbed. Colostrum is rich in the enzyme γ-glutamyl transpeptidase. This is absorbed along with immunoglobulin and gives rise to high serum concentrations of the enzyme, which persist for 5 weeks of life in calves. Alkaline phosphatase is also found in the serum of lambs and calves that have suckled, and elevated serum levels can persist for weeks in calves but are normal at 2 days of age in lambs. Some of this alkaline phosphatase is probably derived from the intestinal brush border enzyme, which is transported into the neonate along with colostral proteins. High serum levels of γ-glutamyl transpeptidase and alkaline phosphatase in young neonates may result because of colostral absorption not liver disease.

Closure occurs when macromolecules are no longer released into the circulation, and this occurs before the specialized absorptive cells are sloughed from the gut epithelium. In piglets, uptake of macromolecules from the gut into epithelial cells persists long after the ability to release the macromolecules intact into the serum is lost. In calves and lambs, closure is about 24 hr after birth, although efficiency of absorption declines from birth, particularly after 12 hr, and some calves fail to absorb immunoglobulin if fed after 12 hr of age. Feeding may induce earlier closure, but there is little colostral absorption after 24 hr of age even if the calf is starved. Piglets are different, since they can absorb colostral immunoglobulins just as well at 24 hr of age as they can at birth provided they have been starved. Feeding lactose solutions after birth, however, induces closure, and the piglets fail to absorb immunoglobulin if subsequently fed colostrum. If parturition is induced in cows using very slow-acting corticosteroids (9 to 19 days), the efficiency of absorption of colostral immunoglobulin is reduced in the calf. However, there is no evidence that more rapid-acting corticosteroid preparations (2 days) induce closure or that treating calves with ACTH or cortisone at birth affects immunoglobulin absorption.

Behavioral factors are very important in determining the final immunoglobulin concentration attained by calves. Following birth the cow licks the calf dry and may eat the placenta: the calf then nuzzles upwards, along the dark underside of the cow, and in this way ends up in the region of the udder. In cows with good conformation, the teats are set at a high point between the thighs and so are in the calf's path. Cows with poor udder conformation have dropped teats, and the calf has trouble finding them as it nuzzles up into the darker region of the thighs. The initial licking of the calf dry appears to be very important to the cow-calf bond, and the dam will not allow the calf to suck if this phase of behavior has not been successfully completed. Calves born in stalls can mistake walls for the dam and orient to the dark corners. This is particularly likely to happen if the cow remains lying down. In general, beef cows mother their calves better than dairy cows, and cows have better maternal instincts than heifers. If the calf does not suck its dam in the first 8 hr of life it will be hypoimmunoglobulinemic. Despite behavioral differences, calves born to dairy heifers attain serum immunoglobulin concentrations similar to calves born to cows—better mothering behavior in cows is compensated by better udder conformation in heifers. Calves born to beef and dairy animals also attain similar immunoglobulin concentrations, possibly because while beef cows are better mothers, they do not produce as much colostrum.

Mothering has a tremendous beneficial effect on the efficiency of absorption of immunoglobulin. Mothered calves absorb 70 per cent more immunoglobulin from a standard feed than nonmothered calves. This benefit is still seen if the calf obtains the colostrum by sucking its dam but is separated from its dam between feeds. Field surveys implicate separating the calf from its dam as one cause of hypoimmunoglobulinemia in calves. Dairy calves kept with their dams attain higher serum immunoglobulin concentrations than hand fed calves even though the mothered calves may suckle less colostrum than hand fed calves.

Temperature stress adversely affects colostral immunoglobulin absorption. Cold environments decrease calf vigor, although absorption is normal if the calf ingests colostrum. Heat stress lessens immunoglobulin absorption efficiency.

Dystocia does not appear to adversely affect immunoglobulin uptake by calves, but cesarean section does.

Timing of colostrum feeding is important because the efficacy of absorption of immunoglobulin from colostrum decreases linearly from birth.

Amount of immunoglobulin ingested is also a major determinant of final serum immunoglobulin concentration. The calf's final immunoglobulin status improves linearly with the amount of immunoglobulin fed. The upper limit for the volume of colostrum that has to be fed to saturate the absorption mechanisms has not been accurately determined. One study suggests that the best serum immunoglobulin levels are attained by feeding calves 4.0 L of colostrum at their first meal. High colostral immunoglobulin concentration also improves the calf's serum immunoglobulin status. Interestingly, better results are obtained by feeding highly concentrated colostrum than by feeding the same total amount of immunoglobulin in a larger volume of more dilute colostrum.

Miscellaneous effects include better absorption in certain breeds and inhibition of absorption if enterotoxigenic *Escherichia coli* invade the gut before colostrum is fed.

Although there was once hope that feeding potassium isobutyrate might improve colostral immunoglobulin absorption, it does not improve the immunoglobulin status of conventionally fed calves.

Immunoglobulin is well preserved in fermented colostrum, but absorption is less effective than in fresh colostrum. Correcting the pH to 6.15 will partially correct this problem.

DISEASE IN HYPOIMMUNOGLOBULINEMIC NEONATES

Colostrum-fed calves attain peak immunoglobulin levels 24 hr after birth. Serum immunoglobulin concentrations decline with a half-life of 20 days for IgG, 4 days for IgM, and 2 days for IgA. Colostrum-deprived calves synthesize immunoglobulin from birth, but it takes 3 months before they reach similar immunoglobulin levels to those found in colostrum-fed calves. The immunoglobulin profile becomes comparable to the adult between 3 and 6 months of age.

In general, receiving colostrum on the first day of life helps protect the calf for the first 3 to 5 weeks of life. Severely deprived calves tend to die of colisepticemia in less than 4 days or suffer from chronic polyarthritis. Moderately hypoimmunoglobulinemic calves are susceptible to diarrhea and other diseases. In addition, saving colostrum and continuing to feed it after the gut has closed gives additional local protection. For example, feeding immunity-producing colostrum can protect against rotaviral diarrhea. Presumably, protection against enterotoxigenic *E. coli* diarrhea, obtained by vaccinating the dams in late pregnancy to boost colostral antibody levels, is mainly due to local effects.

There is evidence that colostral immunoglobulin can give partial protection up to 5 months of age. In one survey, death from pneumonia was reduced in calves that had high serum levels of colostral immunoglobulin. Experimental challenge studies with parainfluenza type 3 virus produced less severe clinical signs in colostrum-fed calves. Antibody to infectious bovine rhinotracheitis (IBR) virus appears in nasal secretions within 1 day of colostrum ingestion and persists for 15 to 20 days. Serum antibody persists longer. Colostrum-fed calves with intranasal IBR antibodies were resistant to experimental IBR infections. Colostrum-derived immunoglobulin also helps protect against infectious bovine keratoconjunctivitis. Cows vaccinated at 5 to 6 months of gestation with a *Moraxella bovis* vaccine produced colostrum that partially protected calves against signs of pinkeye when experimentally challenged at 2 months of age.

In piglets and lambs, colostrum feeding helps protect against septicemia, diarrhea, and death. These benefits are not entirely due to the immunologic properties of colostrum. Neonatal piglets and lambs that fail to suck from birth are very prone to death in the first few days of life due to hypothermia and hypoglycemia caused by cold stress and starvation. In addition, small size predisposes piglets and lambs to death and is associated with poor serum immunoglobulin concentrations in piglets. The immunologic benefits of colostrum feeding in piglets are probably due to both local and systemic effects. Piglets can attain maximal serum immunoglobulin concentrations after 1 hr of suckling but are still susceptible to enteric disease if removed from colostrum feeding at 12 hr of age. Although the immunoglobulin content of sow's colostrum is similar to milk by 24 hr post partum, continued feeding of immunoglobulin fortified milk can give local protection against enteric disease for the first 5 to 10 days of life.

Methods of Detecting Colostral Immunoglobulin Status

Single radial immunodiffusion is the most specific method for detecting immunoglobulin. It requires 18 to 48 hr before the results are available. The costs of this assay can be reduced if samples are run in batches of 6 to 12 samples and if only IgG is quantified. Serum IgG_1 concentrations below 4 and 8 gm/L indicate poor and marginal immunoglobulin status, respectively. Care is suggested if IgG plates are used because these may give 2 rings and unreliable results, as shown in Figure 1. One advantage of single radial immunodiffusion is that it can

When cow serum is applied to Ig G radial imunodiffusion plates, one ring is usually seen. This represents two superimposed patterns, one due to IgG₁ and the other to IgG₂.

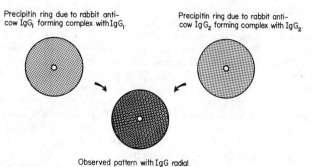

When calf serum is applied to IgG radial immunodiffusion plates two rings are seen because IgG₁ is present in much greater quantities than IgG₂ in calf serum.

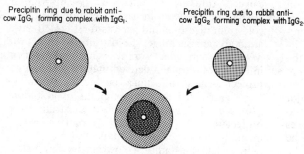

Figure 1. Results of application of cow and calf sera to IgG radial immunodiffusion plates. Immunodiffusion plates that give 2 rings with calf sera overestimate the amount of IgG present. Naylor, J. M.: Large Animal Practice, 1. Vet. Clin. North Am.: 331–361, 1979. (With permission.)

be used to estimate immunoglobulin concentration in whole colostrum.

Refractometric measurement of total protein is the simplest and quickest field test for immunoglobulin status. The principle of the test is that the neonate has a fairly constant amount of albumin and other proteins (about 40 to 45 gm/L) at birth, and this level rises following absorption of colostral proteins. The test is not specific for immunoglobulin but has the advantage that it is also influenced by such nonimmunoglobulin defense proteins as complement. Serum protein measurement is easier than plasma protein measurement because a centrifuge is not required, and it also correlates slightly better with immunoglobulin content. Serum protein concentrations below 55 gm/L or plasma concentrations below 60 gm/L are associated with disease and death, as shown in Figure 2. Calves with low protein concentrations also grow slower.

Electrophoresis allows serum proteins to be fractionated and the gamma globulins to be quantified. Gamma globulin concentrations below 5 and 10 gm/L indicate severe and partial immunoglobulin deficiency, respectively.

The zinc sulfate turbidity (ZST) test precipitates immunoglobulins. The density of the precipitate can be measured spectrophotometrically and compared to standard solutions of bovine gamma globulin in precolostral calf serum. Another method is to compare the density of the precipitate to standard solutions of barium sulfate and to record the result as ZST units. For field use the density can be gauged visually. The test can only be performed

on serum, since hemolysis and carbon dioxide both interfere with the test. ZST scores below 10 and 20 indicate severe and partial hypoimmunoglobulinemia, respectively.

The sodium sulfite precipitation test uses solutions of 14 per cent, 16 per cent, and 18 per cent sodium sulfite; 0.1 ml of serum is added to 1.9 ml quantities of each of these solutions, and the mixtures are allowed to stand for 1 hr at 22° C. Samples containing less than 5 gm/L of immunoglobulin precipitate with the 18 per cent solution, samples with 5 to 15 gm/L of immunoglobulin precipitate with 16 and 18 per cent solutions, and samples with more than 15 gm/L precipitate with all 3 solutions.

In general, testing for serum immunoglobulin status is done between 1 and 8 days of age. The calves have finished absorbing colostral immunoglobulin and have not synthesized appreciable endogenous immunoglobulin at this age range. Results from all the tests will be spuriously elevated by dehydration or spuriously lowered by protein-losing enteropathies (a rare occurrence in sick calves). Problems in interpretation due to dehydration can be avoided by rehydrating the calf prior to sampling. Alternatively, serum albumin and immunoglobulins can be measured concurrently, and immunoglobulin values can be corrected to a normal serum albumin concentration of 30 gm/L. Serum immunoglobulin estimation in chronically sick calves is unreliable because of the effects of antigenic stimulation on immunoglobulin synthesis.

Care is needed when making predictions about a calf's

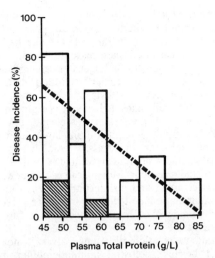

Figure 2. Disease susceptibility can be predicted from plasma total protein. The test can be rapidly performed in the field. Naylor, J. M., Kronfeld, D. S., Bech-Nielsen, S., et al.: J. Am. Vet. Med. Assoc.: *171*:635–638, 1977. (With permission.)

individual performance on the basis of its immunoglobulin status. Such factors as management and novel pathogens influence disease incidence. Group rearing and a dirty environment predispose colostrum-deprived calves to disease and death. Some severely colostrum-deprived calves are reared without problems—particularly if the calf is kept in an isolated single pen. Calves with high serum immunoglobulin concentrations can still become sick, especially when there is a lack of specific immunoglobulins to pathogens newly introduced onto the farm or to pathogens found in the calf's environment but not in the dam's environment.

RECOMMENDATIONS

Cows calve under a variety of management systems, but hypoimmunoglobulinemia can be a problem under any system. A number of recommendations can be made when a farm is experiencing disease problems associated with hypoimmunoglobulinemia, and these fall into 5 categories.

1. Optimizing cow-calf management to diminish the incidence of hypoimmunoglobulinemia.
2. Detecting cows with poor quality colostrum and offering the calf substitute colostrum.
3. Boosting immunoglobulin status of calves by transfusion.
4. Reducing exposure to pathogens during calving and calf rearing.
5. Boosting specific immunity by vaccination.

In addition, there may be a case for providing additional local immunity during the first weeks of life by feeding preserved or fermented colostrum until weaning.

Cow-calf management can be handled in a number of ways. Beef cattle have strong maternal instincts and are generally left to mother their calf. It is important to provide a windbreak during cold weather and shade during very hot weather to reduce temperature stress on the calf. Cows should be fed well in late pregnancy and given additional grain if the weather is very cold, because poorly fed cows do not produce enough colostrum for their

calves. Indiscriminate handling of calves and separation of calf from dam can lead to mismothering and reduce serum immunoglobulin concentration. Farmers should observe their cattle, preferably every 2 to 3 hr, and assist the calves that have not nursed to suck.

Dairy cows should be allowed to mother their calves for the first 24 hr of life. Calves separated at birth attain only about 65 per cent of the serum immunoglobulin concentration of nursed calves. Management systems that restrain cows by the head prevent the cow from licking her calf clean and establishing a good cow to calf bond. Calves can also have difficulty getting up if they are born in the gutter behind the cow. Free stall systems offer poor footing and a dirty environment for the calf. Cows can calve satisfactorily in a good loose box. The straw bedding should be packed well so that it doesn't interfere with the calf's movements. Concrete floors can present problems if they are smooth and the straw gets scraped away from them at parturition; calves have difficulty rising if born onto wet smooth concrete. Calves that are born in loose boxes may explore the walls and end up in dark corners rather than at the cow's dark underside where the udder is located. A field offers the best environment. Footing is good and dark corners are absent. Another problem that can inhibit successful sucking is overly large teats.

Surveys record the highest serum immunoglobulin concentration and lowest mortality in suckled calves and in field-born calves.

In any management system some calves fail to nurse. Signs that indicate colostrum intake include a slack quarter where the calf has suckled, the calf will have a muzzle wet with saliva and milk, and the belly will be full. Calves that do not appear to have nursed and orphaned calves should be assisted to nurse. If this assistance fails, one can try hand feeding, but this can be a frustrating process until the calf learns to suck well. Calves with swollen heads secondary to difficult parturition can be a special problem. Leaving the calf alone for an extra hour or two sometimes helps. If time is at a premium, tube feeding can be used, and an enema bag is useful for this purpose. Tube-fed calves can satisfactorily absorb immunoglobulin. The volume of colostrum that should be fed has not been adequately established. A minimum of 2 L should be given, but 3 L may be more appropriate. Serum immunoglobulin concentrations rise with the volume of colostrum given. It is very important that only first milking colostrum is offered, as second milking colostrum is lower in immunoglobulin. Also, cows are better donors than heifers. High immunoglobulin colostrum is best because more immunoglobulin is presented in a given feed, and there is also better immunoglobulin absorption from a volume of full-strength colostrum than from double the volume of half-strength colostrum. Veterinarians and managers of large dairy herds can gauge colostral immunoglobulin content from its specific gravity, as shown in Figure 3. Colostrum samples with specific gravities of less than 1.036 have a poor immunoglobulin content, and samples with specific gravities of more than 1.047 have an excellent immunoglobulin content. Milk has a relatively high specific gravity—1.032 on average—but little immunoglobulin. The specific gravity test is only valid when applied to colostral samples obtained within 24 hr postpartum. Special colostrometers can be purchased, but a regular hydrometer can also be used. Checking colostrum would identify one important source of low calf immu-

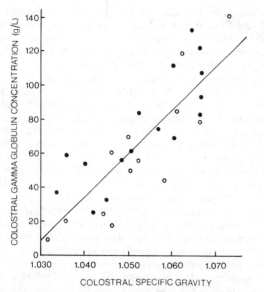

Figure 3. Colostral gammaglobulin concentration can be predicted from its specific gravity. A hydrometer can be used in the field to detect poor quality colostral samples. Immediate postpartum colostrum indicated with solid circles. Twenty-four hours old postpartum colostrum indicated with open circles. (Modified from Fleenor, W. A., Stott, G. H.: Hydrometer test for estimation of immunoglobulin concentration in bovine colostrum. J. Dairy Sci.: 973–977, 1980.)

noglobulin concentration. If it is not possible to test colostrum, it is important to supplement the first feeding of calves born to cows that have been premilked or have leaked colostrum prepartum, because these cows have low colostral immunoglobulin concentrations. Cows with infections also have poor colstral immunoglobulin concentrations and an increased incidence of mortality in their calves. Their calves would benefit from colostrum supplementation. Calves born by cesarean section attain poor serum immunoglobulin concentrations when fed dam's milk and might also benefit from supplementation. Colostrum for supplementing calves should always be first milking and is best obtained from multiparous cows. It can be frozen in 3 L containers and is stable for about a year. Involving calf-rearing personnel in the early management of the calf might be one way of ensuring that calves are given the best possible attention.

Recently, a product containing a monoclonal antibody against the K99+ antigen has been introduced as an aid in the prevention of E. coli scours. This product is given orally to the neonatal calf. A recent experimental study showed it would reduce the severity of E. coli diarrhea and would reduce mortality when given 2 to 4 hr prior to K99+ E. coli challenge. The product is expensive, however, and it does not stop scouring. A field trial would be helpful in evaluating its usefulness.

Transfusion has been practiced to boost serum immunoglobulin levels in hypoimmunogobulinemic calves that are too old to further absorb immunoglobulin across the gut. Three L of blood or 2 L of plasma are given by slow intravenous infusion. Giving blood increases the packed cell volume to very high levels, and in consequence the serum immunoglobulin concentrations are higher because the immunoglobulins are contained in a smaller volume of serum. The total *amount* of immunoglobulin gained by the calf is similar whether blood or plasma is given. Transfusion is logical therapy, but controlled studies showing a decrease in disease susceptibility do not exist.

Reducing exposure to pathogens at calving is achieved by cleaning loose boxes regularly. Outdoor calving probably offers the cleanest environment. Calves that are removed from their dams at 1 day of age are best reared in *single* pens. Calf hutches offer a cleaner environment than barns, but they require more labor, and there is more opportunity for cold stress. Feeding has to compensate for this, and a high fat, veal quality, milk replacer is best during cold seasons. Moving calves to a new environment and cleaning and disinfecting the environment reduce contamination and disease incidence. Hypoimmunoglobulinemic calves can do well in a low disease environment.

Systemic vaccination of young calves is not usually practiced because colostral immunoglobulin interferes with immunity. The best use for vaccination is on the dam in the last trimester of gestation to boost colostral immunoglobulin levels. Administration of E. coli vaccines containing the K99 antigen to cows successfully boosts colostral anti-K99 antibody concentrations and protects calves against experimental challenge with enterotoxigenic E. coli in early life. A controlled field trial showed that a six-strain enterotoxigenic E. coli vaccine reduces mortality from severe diarrheal disease in early life.

Vaccinating cows and ewes can boost colostral titers against rotavirus antigens experimentally. A European trial found that administration of an experimental rota-corona virus vaccine to pregnant cows reduced the incidence of diarrhea in calves. However, tests of 2 commercially available vaccines in North America have been very disappointing. In one test a commercial vaccine did not significantly increase colostral antirotaviral antibody. A field trial with a commercial rota-corona virus and E. coli vaccine found that there was no difference in incidence of diarrhea, mortality, or growth rate between calves of cows receiving vaccine and calves of cows receiving adjuvant alone. In a second trial, in which vaccine was randomly administered on a farm to farm basis, the incidence of diarrhea in calves was higher on "vaccinated" farms than "nonvaccinated" farms. Beware of claims for vaccine efficacy on the basis of trials using historical controls. If a farm has a bad problem with scours one year, there is usually less of a problem the next year irrespective of whether or not the farm institutes vaccination.

Colostrum feeding after closure can provide additional local protection and may be useful in controlling diarrhea in calves on problem farms. This is most practicable on dairy farms where male calves are sold in the first few days of life. Enough surplus colostrum will be available to feed the heifer calves through the first 5 weeks of life. However, feeding half the ration as colostrum would give some protection to calves on farms where all calves are kept. The system works best on large farms where colostrum supply is fairly continuous. Colostrum can be preserved by refrigeration, by acid or formaldehyde preservation, or by fermentation. Fermentation works well. Most systems use 3 buckets: one for filling, one for fermenting, and one for feeding. They should be thoroughly cleaned between batches. It is important to stir colostrum well before feeding. It is usually diluted 2:1 or

1:1 with water and fed at the rate of 10 per cent of body weight in 2 divided feeds daily. Hay and calf starter should be introduced at 1 week of age. Water should always be available. Feeding immune colostrum until weaning has been recommended for the control of rotaviral diarrhea.

Lambs are usually left to obtain colostrum from their dam. In cold weather they may fail to suck and succumb to hypothermia in the first hours of life. These lambs can be resuscitated by giving them 10 ml/kg of a 20-per cent dextrose solution intraperitoneally (IP) (maximum volume of 50 ml) and then placing them in a 40° C environment. When the lambs have regained strength and rectal temperature has reached 38° C, they should be removed and fed 100 to 200 ml of colostrum. Initially, orphaned lambs can be maintained on colostrum fed at 50 ml/twice daily. Administration by stomach tube avoids problems with aspiration. Experimental studies show that if the catheter tip is in the thoracic esophagus, the esophageal groove will close. If this technique is used, however, there is greater potential for aspiration in weak lambs. Cow's colostrum can be used instead of ewe's colostrum, but there can be problems with a fatal anemic syndrome at 1 to 3 weeks of age. This is believed to be secondary to extravascular hemolysis, as the result of bovine immunoglobulin reacting with serum proteins and the immune complexes adhering to the red blood cells.

Sows are usually left to farrow and nurse their young with minimal assistance. Extensive handling of the piglets should be avoided, as this interferes with colostral antibody uptake. The farrowing area should be clean, warm, and provide sure footing for the piglets. Colostrum banks are rarely feasible, but there might be a place for saving 50 ml aliquots of first milking colostrum. This could be fed by stomach tube to weak piglets, late born piglets, or piglets born to sows with agalactia. A portion of colostrum should also be added to subsequent hand feedings until the piglets are at least 36 hr old. Bovine colostrum might be an alternative to sow colostrum, but there have been problems when bovine colostrum was used in lambs.

References available from the author upon request.

Neonatal Diarrhea in Ruminants (Calves, Lambs and Kids)

O. M. RADOSTITS, D.V.M., M.S.

Acute diarrhea is a common disease of newborn calves, lambs, and kids. It is characterized clinically by abnormal fecal discharge, progressive dehydration, and death in a few days. The emphasis in this article will be on the disease in calves. The condition is similar in lambs and kids.

ETIOLOGY

The etiology of neonatal diarrhea is complex and involves interactions between enteropathogenic strains of *Escherichia coli*, *Salmonella* spp., *Clostridium* spp., rota-

viruses, corona-like viruses, *Cryptosporidia* spp., and the level of colostral immunity, the nature of the diet, and the system of management.

Specific serotypes of *E. coli* are the causative agents of enteric colibacillosis in calves. These serotypes have the ability to dilate ligated loops of intestine because they produce enterotoxin. They differ from the serotypes that are responsible for coliform septicemia. Certain *Salmonella* spp. may cause enteritis and diarrhea in newborn farm animals. *Clostridium perfringens* Types A, B, C, and E have been associated with acute hemorrhagic enteritis and rapid death in calves and lambs. The rotavirus and coronavirus are now known to be major causes of diarrhea in calves. *Chlamydia* spp. have also been associated with diarrhea in newborn calves, but only rarely. *Cryptosporidia* spp. are intracellular protozoan parasites that have been considered as causative agents of diarrhea in calves. Occasionally, fungi are recovered from diarrheic calves, but their presence is considered to be secondary to prolonged diarrhea in calves that have been on a course of oral antibacterial therapy for several days.

EPIDEMIOLOGY

Acute neonatal diarrhea occurs commonly wherever farm animals are maintained and is a significant cause of economic loss in raising livestock. There are many epidemiologic factors that influence the disease, each one of which must be considered and evaluated when investigating the cause of an outbreak, so that effective clinical management and control of the disease may be achieved. The disease is most common in animals from 2 to 10 days of age; it may occur as early as 12 to 18 hr after birth and occasionally occurs in animals up to 3 weeks of age.

Enterotoxigenic colibacillosis occurs primarily in calves under 3 days of age. Rotavirus and coronavirus causes diarrhea in calves from 5 to 15 days of age. *Cryptosporidia* spp. usually affects older calves from 15 to 35 days of age.

Immunity

Farm animals are born agammaglobulinemic and must ingest colostrum and absorb colostral immunoglobulins within hours after birth to obtain protection against septicemic and enteric colibacillosis. The mortality rate from enteric colibacillosis is much higher in calves with low levels of serum immunoglobulins than in calves with adequate levels. Based on surveys, up to 25 per cent of newborn dairy and beef calves have low levels of serum immunoglobulins because they do not receive sufficient colostrum early enough after birth, which makes them very susceptible to neonatal disease, especially colibacillosis. Colostral immunoglobulins are absorbed for up to 24 hr after birth in calves, but maximum efficiency of absorption occurs during the first 6 to 12 hr after birth and decreases rapidly from 12 to 24 hr after birth. Newborn calves, lambs, and kids should ingest approximately 50 ml/kg body weight within the first 8 to 12 hr.

The maximum level of serum immunoglobulins is reached in the calf at 24 hr after birth, and the factors that reduce those levels below an adequate value include the effects of maternal behavior and conformation, the vigor of the calf, and the influence of the environment. Calves that receive their first colostrum by bucket do not acquire the same high levels of serum immunoglobulins as calves that receive their first colostrum by natural sucking of the teat. In both cases, the presence of the dam improves absorption. Calves that are weak or have an edematous tongue from a prolonged, difficult parturition may not be able to suck for several hours, resulting in a markedly decreased ability to absorb colostral immunoglobulins. Beef calves born outdoors may be subjected to several influences that affect colostral intake: (1) they may be born during a snowstorm and suffer severe cold exposure, (2) when born they may be dropped in a snow bank and be unable to get up even with the assistance of the dam, or (3) in crowded calving grounds, mismothering due to mistaken identity may occur, resulting in the calf's receiving no or very little colostrum.

Rotavirus and coronavirus antibodies are present in the colostrum of about 90 per cent of cows for the first few days after parturition and provide the calf with protection against these viruses for the first several days of life. However, the antibody levels decline rapidly to low levels when the mammary secretions change from colostrum to milk, which accounts for the occurrence of viral diarrhea in calves after several days of age when the antibody titers in the milk are too low to provide protection.

Effect of Meteorologic Influences

While little epidemiologic data is available to support the claim, many veterinarians have observed a relationship between adverse climatic conditions and acute neonatal diarrhea in calves and lambs. During inclement weather, such as a snowstorm, a common practice in beef herding is to confine the calving cows in a small area where they can be fed and watered more easily. The overcrowding is commonly followed by an outbreak of enteric colibacillosis in the calves. There is evidence that cold, wet, windy weather during the winter and hot, dry weather during the summer has a significant effect on the incidence of dairy calf mortality.

Nutrition and Feeding Methods

Dairy calves fed milk substitutes appear to be more prone to diarrhea than those fed cows' whole milk. Extreme heat treatment of the liquid skim milk in the processing of dried skim milk for use in milk substitutes for calves results in denaturation of the whey protein. This interferes with digestibility of the nutrients and destruction of any lactoglobulins that are present and may have a protective effect in the young calf.

Standard of Housing and Hygiene

Housing and hygienic practices are probably the most important epidemiologic factors influencing the incidence of colibacillosis in dairy calves and lambs born in sheds. As the size of herds has increased and as livestock production has become more intensified, the quality of hygiene and sanitation, particularly in housed animals, assumes major importance. In beef herds, overcrowded calving grounds are a major contributing factor.

Source of the Pathogen and Its Ecology and Transmission

In most species, the primary source of infection is the feces of infected animals. Calves obtain the pathogens from contaminated bedding and calf pails, dirty calf pens, diarrheic calves, overcrowded calving grounds, and the perineal skin and udder of the cow. The pathogen is spread within a herd through the feces of infected animals and through all of the inanimate objects that can be contaminated by feces, including bedding, pails, boots, tools, clothing, and feed and water supplies. The organism is one of the first encountered by newborn farm animals within minutes after birth. The high population density of animals that occurs in overcrowded calving grounds in beef herds and heavily used calving pens in dairy herds contributes to a large dynamic population of E. coli. The population of bacteria in an animal barn will continue to increase unless there is animal depopulation, cleanout, disinfection, and a period of vacancy. In some countries where lambing must be done in buildings to avoid cold weather exposure, the lambing sheds may become contaminated within a few weeks, resulting in outbreaks of septicemic and enteric colibacillosis.

PATHOGENESIS

Enterotoxigenic strains of $K99^+$ E. coli have the ability to colonize in the small intestine and produce enterotoxin, which causes an increase in net secretion of fluid and electrolytes from the systemic circulation into the lumen of the intestine. Large volumes of fluid containing sodium, chloride, potassium, and bicarbonate become sequestered in the lumen of the intestine, and there is minimal if any structural change in the intestinal epithelial cells. Infection with Salmonella spp. may result in an acute hemorrhagic fibrino-necrotic enteritis. Bacteremia may occur with localization of the organisms and development of lesions elsewhere in the body, such as the meninges, eyes, feet, tail, and bones. The rotaviruses infect only the mature columnar epithelial cells covering the distal one third of the small intestinal villi. Infected cells are eventually sloughed into the lumen, exposing the lamina propria and resulting in villous atrophy. The cells are replaced within 72 to 96 hr, but their temporary absence results in a loss of intestinal lactase, a digestive enzyme located in the brush border of the villous cells. The deficiency in lactase causes a malabsorptive diarrhea. With normal villous cell renewal, most cases of rotavirus diarrhea should resolve spontaneously in 2 or 3 days unless there is a concurrent infection with enteropathogenic strains of E. coli. The pathogenesis of coronavirus infection is similar to rotavirus but is commonly affected by crypt destruction, which makes regeneration of villous epithelial cells much longer, resulting in persistent diarrhea for several days.

The pathogenesis of cryptosporidiosis in calves is not well understood. The cryptosporidia appear free in the lumen of the intestine and attached to the microvilli of the villous epithelial cells of both the small and large intestines.

The loss of fluids and electrolytes into the lumen of the intestine results in electrolyte imbalance, dehydration, acidosis, hyperkalemia if the acidosis is severe, circulatory failure, shock, and death. An adequate level of serum immunoglobulins will protect calves from death due to diarrhea but not necessarily from the diarrhea. The fatality rate will be high in calves that are deficient in serum immunoglobulins in spite of intensive antimicrobial and fluid therapy.

CLINICAL FINDINGS

The major clinical findings are diarrhea, abnormal feces, dehydration, weakness, and death within one to several days after the onset. It is usually difficult, based on clinical findings alone, to make a definitive etiologic diagnosis. However, by consideration of the case history, the age of the animals affected, and the character of the feces, it may be possible to make a presumptive diagnosis.

In diarrhea caused by the calves' diet, the feces are voluminous, pasty to gelatinous in consistency, and the animal is bright, alert, and usually able to suck or drink from a pail. Calves that are fed milk replacers containing heat-denatured skim-milk protein will be affected with a chronic persistent diarrhea that does not respond to treatment except the feeding of cows' whole milk. Continued feeding of the inferior milk replacer usually results in emaciation and death from starvation in 2 to 4 weeks.

Acute enterotoxigenic colibacillosis occurs in calves under 5 days of age and rarely later. The onset is acute, and previously healthy, vigorous calves may be in a state of collapse in 12 to 24 hr. The feces are profuse and watery, pale yellow or green in color, and only rarely contain blood. The temperature is usually normal but may become subnormal as the disease progresses. In the early stages, there may be mild abdominal distention due to fluid-filled intestines, which are detectable on succussion and auscultation. Mild to moderately affected calves may be diarrheic for a few days and recover spontaneously without treatment. However, many calves that are inadequately treated become progressively dehydrated, anorexic, and toxemic. Severely affected calves may lose up to 16 per cent of body weight in a few days and, terminally, they are unable to stand or maintain sternal recumbency, their extremities are cold, and they may have bradycardia or cardiac arrhythmia associated with hyperkalemia.

Enteric salmonellosis usually occurs in calves from 2 to 6 weeks of age. The feces are often foul smelling and commonly contain frank blood, fibrinous casts, and excessive amounts of mucus. A fever is common, and affected calves are depressed, anorexic, and lose considerable weight in a few days.

Hemorrhagic enterotoxemia in calves is characterized by an acute onset of depression, weakness, dysentery, abdominal pain, and death in a few hours. Nervous signs occur occasionally.

Diarrhea due to rotavirus infection usually occurs in calves from 1 to 2 weeks of age. In cases uncomplicated by E. coli, there is a profuse, watery diarrhea that lasts up to several hours with recovery in 18 to 24 hr. In calves with mixed infections, the diarrhea may persist for a few days, and dehydration, acidosis, and weakness will occur as in enterotoxigenic colibacillosis. Coronavirus infection occurs in calves from a few days to several weeks of age and is indistinguishable clinically from diarrhea due to rotavirus. Cryptosporidiosis may cause a diarrhea in calves from 5 to 35 days of age, but it cannot be distinguished clinically from the other common causes of diarrhea in calves. However, diarrhea caused by rotavirus, coronavirus, and cryptosporidia is usually persistent, lasting several days, and recovery may not occur.

CLINICAL PATHOLOGY

The effects of the loss of electrolytes and fluids can be evaluated in the laboratory. The packed cell volume and the total solids concentration of the blood will indicate the degree of dehydration, and the blood urea nitrogen level may be increased in severe cases owing to inadequate renal perfusion. The blood bicarbonate values are markedly reduced, blood pH values represent acidosis, and the levels of other serum electrolytes are variable. There is usually a decrease in levels of serum sodium, chloride, and potassium, but potassium values may be elevated in severe cases of acidosis.

The determination of the level of serum immunoglobulins of diarrheic calves is considered valuable in assessing prognosis and in determining the intensity of the therapy required for survival. The level of serum immunoglobulins as a measure of susceptibility is most accurate at 24 hr after birth and can be used as an aid in surveillance of the colostral intake of calves.

NECROPSY FINDINGS

Because of rapid postmortem autolysis and bacterial invasion, necropsies should be done on freshly killed animals affected with the disease, particularly in herd outbreaks where an etiologic diagnosis is desirable.

There are no gross lesions characteristic of any of the common causes of diarrhea in calves. Dehydration, fluid-filled intestines, distention of the abomasum with fluid, and varying degrees of emaciation are common. There are no gross lesions that will differentiate diarrhea caused by enterotoxigenic E. coli, rotavirus, coronavirus, or cryptosporidia. In animals with salmonellosis, there may be a hemorrhagic fibrinonecrotic enteritis. Clostridium perfringens Type C causes a characteristic hemorrhagic enteritis. In enterotoxigenic colibacillosis, there are large numbers of E. coli covering the villi, and there may be minimal or no visible change in the villous epithelial cells. Rotavirus and coronavirus infections result in villous atrophy. In cryptosporidiosis, the parasites are visible on the brush border of the cells in the distal half of the small intestine. In chlamydial enteritis of calves, there are lesions in the abomasum and in the small and large intestines. There is desquamation of villous cells at the levels of the small intestine, and intracytoplasmic inclusion bodies are visible. In mycotic abomasitis and rumenitis in calves, there are congestion, hemorrhage, and necrosis of the mucosae of the abomasum and rumen, and fungal elements are readily visible.

Calves that have been fed on inferior quality milk replacers are emaciated. A notable lack of body fat, serious prominent atrophy, and an absence of milk clot in the abomasum are also possible.

DIAGNOSIS

It is often difficult to make a definitive etiologic diagnosis because (1) the diarrheas caused by different enteropathogens are not characteristic but similar, (2) mixed intestinal infections are common, (3) previous treatment with antimicrobials may alter the intestinal and fecal flora, (4) fast, reliable diagnostic techniques are not yet available for all of the possible enteropathogens, and (5) enteropathogens can often be isolated from normal animals, which makes interpretation of their isolation from diarrheic animals difficult.

When only a few animals are involved and when no

deaths are occurring, the submission of fresh fecal samples for isolation and characterization of the enteropathogens may be sufficient. When outbreaks of the disease occur, it may be necessary to submit affected animals for necropsy without treatment. This will allow accurate counts of bacteria at different levels of the intestine, examination of fresh intestinal mucosa for viruses, and preparation of a reliable histologic section of intestinal mucosa.

In the case of animals fed on milk-replacer diets, the composition of the diet's ingredients should be examined for evidence of factors that result in inadequate digestibility and subsequent diarrhea. The clotting of a milk-replacer solution (as fed) may be tested with rennet and compared with the clotting of cows' whole milk as a control. Whole milk (10 ml) will clot in a few seconds following the addition of a few drops of dairy rennet, while no clotting will occur even after a few hours in the case of milk replacers made with heat-denatured skim-milk powder.

TREATMENT

The treatment of acute neonatal diarrhea may include one or more of the following: (1) isolation of affected animals from the herd, (2) alteration of the diet, (3) fluid and electrolyte replacement, (4) antimicrobial and immunoglobulin therapy, and (5) the use of antiparasympathomimetics and intestinal protectants. During herd outbreaks, affected animals should be identified with a tag so that hourly and daily progress can be monitored.

Isolation

Diarrheic animals should be isolated from the herd as soon as they are detected. When calves are raised indoors, diarrheic cases should be removed to a separate pen as far away from healthy animals as possible. This applies even to herds where calves are housed individually in separate pens if inadequate ventilation and drainage appear to be promoting dissemination of the disease. With calves raised on pasture, diarrheic calves should be removed to a separate pen or paddock for treatment. Healthy animals should be fed and examined before attending to sick calves, and separate feeding facilities should be used to feed diarrheic calves. Most enteropathogens may be carried by inanimate objects, and it may be necessary for animal attendants to change or disinfect boots and protective clothing after coming into contact with diarrheic calves.

Alteration of the Diet

In viral and probably other types of diarrhea, the digestive and absorptive capacities of the intestinal tract are reduced. Hence, it would seem logical not to feed milk during the acute diarrheic period, but rather to provide readily absorbable substances such as oral glucose-electrolyte mixtures. Under experimental conditions, restricting milk intake to calves with rotavirus diarrhea reduced deaths. In contrast, one study, done on diarrheic calves received in a clinic, showed that offering milk to diarrheic calves when they were willing to drink following rehydration with intravenous fluids resulted in a slight but insignificant increase in survival rate over calves that were starved for 24 hr following rehydration.

Balance studies in diarrheic calves have shown that continued milk intake helps to maintain plasma volume, which suggests that calves should receive a source of oral fluid during the periods of diarrhea. Oral glucose-electrolyte mixtures are commonly used as a source of energy, fluid, and electrolytes during such times. These mixtures are inexpensive, easy to use, readily available, and if given by the farmer when diarrhea is first noticed will usually successfully treat existing dehydration and prevent further dehydration and acidosis.

In individual cases, it is common practice to withhold milk from diarrheic dairy calves for up to 24 hr and to maintain hydration by feeding oral glucose-electrolyte solutions. Beef calves are commonly left with the cow in an enclosure, and the cow is milked every few hours to reduce the amount of milk available to the calf during the acute stage of the diarrhea. However, there are no data to support this recommendation, and some workers feel that milking the beef cow with a diarrheic calf will aggravate the disease.

Following recovery, hand-fed calves may be offered small quantities of whole milk 3 times daily (no more than total daily intake equivalent to 8 per cent of body weight) on the first day and increase this amount to the normal daily allowance in the next few days. Milk should not be diluted with water, as this may interfere with the clotting mechanism in the abomasum.

Fluid and Electrolyte Replacement

Regardless of cause, the physiologic changes that occur in most diarrheic calves can be summarized as follows: varying degrees of dehydration that may reach 16 per cent of body weight in severe cases; loss of sodium, chloride, bicarbonate, and potassium; moderate to severe metabolic acidosis. These changes are corrected by the parenteral and oral use of simple or balanced electrolyte solutions. When dehydration and acidosis are severe, solutions containing bicarbonate ion are indicated. Acute cases in which there is kidney failure are often accompanied by hyperkalemia, which may cause cardiac arrest; therefore, solutions containing potassium should not be administered until kidney function is restored. Conversely, when diarrhea has been chronic, total body potassium may be depleted and solutions containing potassium are indicated. Solutions containing lactate are undesirable because they must be converted to the bicarbonate ion by the tissues, which may or may not be functioning normally, and because plasma lactate levels may already be increased.

Many oral and intravenous fluids are available for treating diarrheic calves. No single electrolyte mixture is ideal for treating all calves and, while guidelines are available, the particular fluid, dose, and method of administration that are most likely to be successful for each calf are best learned by experience.

Oral Fluid Therapy

Many diarrheic calves can be treated successfully on the farm by the stockman using oral fluid therapy. Calves that have been taken off milk for a period of 24 hr but that are still willing to suck should be fed a volume of oral fluids equal to 3 to 4 per cent of body weight every 6 to 8 hr using a nursing bottle. Moderately dehydrated calves that will not suck but are strong enough to maintain sternal recumbency require 1 to 2 L by stomach tube every 6 to 8 hr until they are able to stand or until the diarrhea stops. When body temperature is below normal, fluids should be warmed before administration and heat from heat lamps provided. When the consistency of the feces begins to improve, calves should be returned to a full milk diet slowly. Many oral electrolyte solutions are available commercially. Those that contain glucose and glycine in addition to other electrolytes have been found useful in controlled trials.

Intravenous Fluid Therapy

Severely dehydrated calves, calves that cannot maintain sternal recumbency, and calves with chronic persistent diarrhea should be given fluids intravenously. These calves often experience a marked drop in body temperature and should be covered and kept warm if transported. Three types of solutions that are useful in such cases are outlined next.

Isotonic Sodium Bicarbonate. A solution that contains 156 mEq/L HCO_3 and 156 mEq/L Na^+ can be made by dissolving 13 gm of $NaHCO_3$ in 1 L of sterile water. This solution is very effective for the treatment of acidosis in calves when the blood pH is reduced to 7.2 or lower.

These calves are usually comatose, 10 to 16 per cent dehydrated, and have cardiac arrhythmias. In these cases, 2 L (equal to 312 mEq/HCO_3) can be given to an average sized calf in the first 1 to 2 hr before changing to isotonic saline and sodium bicarbonate or a balanced electrolyte solution.

Isotonic Saline and Sodium Bicarbonate. This solution can be made by dissolving 26 gm of sodium bicarbonate in 4 L of half-normal (0.425 per cent) saline or by mixing 1 L of isotonic sodium bicarbonate (13 gm $NaHCO_3^-$/L) and 1 L of isotonic (0.85 per cent) saline. This provides a solution containing 78 mEq/L HCO_3, 79 mEq/L Cl^-, and 156 mEq/L Na^+ and hence supplies an excellent ratio of fluid and bicarbonate to correct the 2 life-threatening defects of acidosis and dehydration. Most diarrheic calves that are 6 per cent or more dehydrated can be given 4 L of this solution without making them alkalotic. Depending on the severity of the case, a further 1 to 2 L may be given before changing to one of the balanced electrolyte solutions. Once calves have had 3 to 4 L of this fluid, they brighten considerably, maintain sternal recumbency, and may stand.

Balanced Electrolyte Solutions. The so-called balanced electrolyte solutions provide electrolytes in amounts that approximate those normally present in body fluids. They are used to maintain calves once a severe acid-base imbalance has been corrected or to correct minor imbalances. Examples are Ringer's solution and several commercial preparations.

Most acutely scouring calves do not require glucose at the time of initial therapy. In contrast, calves that have been diarrheic for several days and calves that have been fed a poor quality milk replacer do require energy, and glucose, amino acids, and vitamins should be given once the animal is rehydrated and the acid-base imbalance is corrected.

Fluids should be administered to effect; however, guidelines for estimating the dose and rate of administration should be followed during the initial stages of therapy.

For *severe dehydration* (8 to 12 per cent of body weight) fluids should be replaced as follows:
Hydration therapy: 100 ml/kg body weight administered intravenously in the first 4 to 6 hr.

Maintenance therapy: 140 ml/kg body weight administered over the next 20 hr.
For *moderate dehydration* (6 to 8 per cent of body weight) fluids should be replaced as follows:
Hydration therapy: 50 ml/kg body weight administered intravenously in the first 4 to 6 hr.
Maintenance therapy: 140 ml/kg body weight administered over the next 20 hr.
The techniques for long-term intravenous administration of fluids to the calf have been described. Maintenance therapy may be given orally if the calf is well enough to suck from a nursing bottle or drink from a pail. Oral fluids may also be given by stomach tube, with the daily dosage being divided into small doses given every 6 to 8 hr.

Calves that respond and recover usually show marked improvement from intravenous or oral fluid therapy or both within 24 to 36 hr. Signs of a beneficial response are muscular movement, head lifting, urination within 1 to 2 hr, and evidence of correction of the dehydration. Calves that do not respond will not hydrate normally. They may not begin to urinate because of irreversible renal failure, they remain depressed, they are not strong enough to suck or drink, and their feces remain watery. Continued fluid therapy beyond 3 days is usually futile in these calves.

Antimicrobial and Immunoglobulin Therapy. Antibiotics, sulfonamides, and other chemotherapeutics have been used routinely for the treatment of diarrhea in calves, because it has been assumed that a bacterial infection of the intestine was present that could develop into bacteremia or septicemia. However, there is a noticeable lack of well-conducted clinical trials demonstrating the efficacy of antibacterials in treating diarrhea in newborn farm animals. Conversely, there is no information that indicates that they are not useful. In one study that evaluated the efficacy of antimicrobial agents given to newborn calves with acute undifferentiated neonatal diarrhea, there was a slight improvement in survival rate when chloramphenicol was given parenterally combined with nitrofurazone given orally compared with the survival rate in calves that received no antimicrobial therapy.

One of the major difficulties confronting the veterinarian in the field is deciding if diarrheic calves are bacteremic. Many diarrheic calves that die not uncommonly have primary or secondary infections of internal organs, such as kidney, liver, brain, joints, and lungs. Since calves that are likely to develop bacteremia cannot be clinically differentiated from those that are not, more animals than necessary are treated systemically. Time does not usually permit pretreatment culture of the organism and determination of drug sensitivity, so that broad-spectrum antibiotics and selected chemotherapeutics are used based on the veterinarian's previous experience. Some of the commonly used antibiotics are chloramphenicol, ampicillin, and trimethoprim-sulfonamide combinations. Neonates may be unable to metabolize drugs as effectively as adults, and care must be taken to avoid toxicity. The maximum effective doses for these drugs in calves have not been determined, but using the adult doses based on body weight appears to be successful without causing toxicity in calves.

Many oral preparations are available for the treatment of diarrhea in calves. Some consist of a single drug, while others are mixtures with or without absorbents, astringents, and electrolytes. They have been used on an empiric basis, since controlled trials have not been conducted. Chloramphenicol, neomycin sulfate, tetracyclines, sulfonamides, trimethoprim-sulfonamide mixtures, nifuraldezone, and ampicillin are in common use in different mixtures. Any of these drugs may be used but should be discontinued after 4 to 5 successive treatments to avoid eliminating too many species of drug-sensitive intestinal bacteria. If response to an oral antibacterial preparation does not occur within 24 to 48 hr, it is unlikely that further treatment will be beneficial. In such cases, diarrhea is not caused by bacteria, such as enteropathogenic E. coli (EEC) or Salmonella spp., or it is caused by bacteria that are resistant to the antibiotic. Excessive antibacterial treatment may result in fungal gastritis caused by Candida, Aspergillus, Mucor, and Rhizopus spp., and in intestinal overgrowth caused by Proteus and Pseudomonas spp.

In outbreaks of enterotoxigenic colibacillosis, the causative organism may be isolated from feces or intestinal fluid, identified as an enteropathogen, and a drug sensitivity obtained. Since EEC do not usually invade the systemic circulation, a separate culture and drug sensitivity must be done on the internal organs if bacteremia is present. When the EEC and the invasive E. coli are not sensitive to the same drug, different antibacterials may have to be administered orally and parenterally.

Trimethoprim-sulfonamide is the drug of choice for salmonellosis in calves.

In acute cases of hemorrhagic enterotoxemia caused by Clostridium perfringens Type C, calves are found dead or are found in the terminal stages, and treatment is therefore often unsuccessful. Large doses of penicillin combined with type specific C. perfringens type C antiserum or antitoxin may be administered to calves with less acute cases or to calves prophylactically in the event of an outbreak.

Fungal gastritis is difficult to diagnose and treat. Limited success has been reported using sodium iodide or feed-grade griseofulvin. Cryptosporidiosis may be treated with oral sulfonamides, but to date there is insufficient information available to make this recommendation.

In some countries it may be illegal to use some of the antimicrobials mentioned here because of the regulations regarding their use in food-producing animals. Some are available to farmers on a prescription basis only, which makes examination of the animals and a diagnosis necessary before recommendations are made. The indiscriminate use of antibiotics in milk replacers or for treatment of newborn calves is widespread and must be viewed with concern when the problems of drug resistance transfer from animal to animal and from animal to human are considered.

One of the most important factors determining whether or not calves survive diarrhea is the serum immunoglobulin status of the animal before it develops the disease. Most of the veterinary literature on therapy omits this information, and it is therefore difficult to assess. There is considerable evidence that the mortality rate is significantly higher in diarrheic calves that are deficient in serum immunoglobulins, particularly IgG, in spite of exhaustive antimicrobial and fluid therapy than in calves with adequate levels of serum immunoglobulins. This finding stimulated interest in the possible use of purified solutions of bovine gamma globulin in diarrheic calves that are hypogammaglobulinemic. However, since bovine gamma globulins must be given intravenously and in large amounts, the cost is often prohibitive. In addition, they are much more protective than they are curative and therefore unlikely to be of value once the calf is affected with diarrhea. Whole-blood transfusions given to severely affected calves may be used as a source of gamma globulins, but unless given in large quantities (2 L for a 50-kg calf) would not significantly elevate the serum immunoglobulin levels in deficient calves. This emphasizes the importance of the calf's ingesting liberal quantities of colostrum within the first few hours after birth.

Antiparasympathomimetics and Intestinal Protectants. Benzetimide has been used for the treatment of diarrhea in newborn calves. The use of this drug and similar drugs may seem rational, but the apparent clinical effect is difficult to evaluate and generally not impressive. Intestinal protectants, such as kaolin and pectin, are in general use for diarrheic animals, but likewise their beneficial value is difficult to evaluate. Kaolin and pectin will decrease the volume of feces passed, but the total amount of water excreted in the feces will not be significantly reduced.

MANAGEMENT OF OUTBREAKS

When outbreaks of diarrhea occur, each affected calf should be identified so that the time it become ill, how often it has been treated, and to which cow it belongs can be recorded. Ear tagging each calf at birth is the most useful system. An alternative method is to mark calves on different parts of the body or with different colors at each treatment. Every effort should be made to isolate affected animals from susceptible calves, and recently born calves should be housed or pastured away from diarrheic calves. All new cases should be treated immediately. Beef calves with the disease should be removed from the calving grounds to an isolation pasture. Outbreaks of diarrhea in beef calves can often be stopped or controlled by removing animals from crowded calving grounds and dispersing them onto well-drained pasture or rangeland.

PREVENTION AND CONTROL

Because of the complex nature of neonatal diarrhea, it is unrealistic to expect total prevention, and control at an economic level should be the major objective. *The incidence of clinical disease and the case fatality rate will be dependent on the balance between the level of infection in the environment and the level of colostral immunity present in the calf before it becomes ill.* Differences in herd size, availability of facilities, land, and labor, and general management objectives make it impossible to recommend specific management procedures that are applicable to all situations. However, there are three broad management principles that should be applied in all herds.

1. *Reduce the degree of exposure of newborn animals to the infectious agents.*

2. *Provide maximum nonspecific resistance with adequate colostrum and optimum animal husbandry.*

3. *Increase the specific resistance of the newborn by vaccination of the dam or the newborn.*

Reducing Exposure to Infectious Agents

Dairy Calves. These comments apply particularly to calves born indoors, where contamination is usually higher than outdoors.

Calves should be born in well-bedded box stalls that were previously cleaned and disinfected. The perineum and udder of the dairy cow should be washed shortly before calving. Do not allow cows to calve in stanchions and deliver their calves into the gutter. This results in gross contamination of the calf before it ingests colostrum.

Immediately after birth the umbilical vessels of the calf may be swabbed in 7 per cent solution of tincture of iodine. Tying off the vessels with cotton thread or applying a plastic clip at the level of the abdominal wall is also practiced. Strict hygiene must be employed when handling the umbilical vessels. Gross contamination, septicemia, or navel ill, or all three, may occur if the animal attendant handles the vessels with dirty hands.

If weather permits, tether or house affected calves outside in individual stalls for 1 to 2 weeks before mixing them with other calves. If calves must be raised indoors, they should be housed in individual pens constructed to reduce spread of infectious agents. Diarrheic calves should be removed from the main calf barn if possible and treated in isolation.

Beef Calves. These calves are usually born outside on pasture or on confined calving grounds.

Calving grounds should have been free of animals previous to the calving period. The grounds should be well drained, dry, and scraped free of snow if necessary. A top dressing of the calving grounds with straw or wood shavings will provide a comfortable calving environment.

Avoid prolonged or excessive confinement of the calving cows and calves in the calving area. Population density may be kept to a minimum by dividing the main herd into smaller groups, each into a separate calving area. In a few days following birth, when the calf is nursing successfully, the cow-calf pair should be moved to a nursery pasture to avoid overcrowding in the calving grounds.

Veal Calves. These calves are usually obtained from several different sources and 25 to 30 per cent or higher may be deficient in serum immunoglobulin. The level of management must be excellent. Emphasis must be on minimizing the amount of infection in the calf barn. There is no practical, economical method of correcting hypogammaglobulinemia.

On arrival, calves should be placed in their individual calf pens that were previously cleaned, disinfected, and left vacant to dry. Feeding utensils are a fequent source of pathogens and should be cleaned and air-dried daily. Calves affected with diarrhea should be removed and isolated immediately. High quality milk replacers should be used, and calves should be slightly underfed for the first 2 to 4 days after arrival.

Provision of Maximum Nonspecific Resistance and Liberal Quantities of Colostrum

This measure begins with the provision of optimal nutrition to the pregnant dam that will result in a vigorous newborn animal and adequate quantities of colostrum. The next most important control measure is to ensure that colostrum is ingested in liberal quantities within minutes after birth. At least 50 ml/kg body weight should be ingested within 2 to 5 hr after birth. However, a major difficulty under practical conditions is determining how much colostrum a particular newborn animal has consumed at a certain time after birth.

Under natural conditions, when the calf sucks within 1 hr after birth, at least 5 hr are required for the calf to acquire protective levels of immunoglobulins, during which time the calf is essentially agammaglobulinemic and highly susceptible to systemic infection.

The behavior of the newborn is a major topic in applied ethology, and every economical effort must be made to foster a strong neonatal bond immediately after birth. In large herds where economics permit, a laboratory surveillance system may be used on batches of calves to determine the serum levels of immunoglobulin acquired. An accurate analysis may be done with single radial immunodiffusion or standard electrophoresis, or an estimation may be done with refractometry or the ZST test. For the most accurate assessment, blood should be collected from all calves at 24 hr of age. Samples taken a few days later may not be a true reflection of the original serum immunoglobulin levels. The information obtained from determination of serum immunoglobulin levels in calves at 24 hr of age can be used to improve management practices, particularly the early ingestion of colostrum.

Dairy Calves. Immediately after birth, unless the calf is a vigorous sucker, colostrum should be milked from the cow and fed by nursing bottle or by stomach tube at the rate of at least 50 to 80 ml/kg body weight in the first 2 hr. Alternatively, the calf can be assisted to suck, which can result in ingestion of adequate quantities of colostrum.

The calf should be left with the cow for at least 2 days. This contact will improve the absorption of immunoglobulin.

Following the colostrum feeding period, dairy calves are usually placed in individual stalls until weaning. A recent development is the feeding of fermented colostrum to newborn calves for up to 3 weeks after birth. This provides a constant source of lactoglobulins in the intestinal tract and reduces the incidence of neonatal diarrhea of calves due to a wide variety of pathogens.

Calves should be fed regularly and preferably by the same person. One of the most important factors affecting dairy calf mortality is the concern and care provided by the calf rearer.

Beef Calves. Beef calves should be assisted at birth, if necessary, to avoid exhaustion and weakness due to a prolonged parturition.

Normally, beef calves will make attempts to get up and suck within 20 min after birth, but this may be delayed for up to 8 hr or longer. Beef calves that do not suck within 2 hr should be fed colostrum by nursing bottle or, if necessary, by stomach tube. Beef calves deserted by indifferent dams also need special attention.

Constant surveillance of the calving grounds is necessary to avoid overcrowding, to detect diarrheic calves that should be removed, to avoid mismothering, and to ensure that every dam nurses its calf. Although up to 35 per cent of beef calves may not have sufficient serum levels of immunoglobulins, the provision of excellent management will minimize the case fatality rate from acute diarrhea.

Increasing Specific Resistance of the Newborn by Vaccination of the Pregnant Dam or the Newborn

The immunization of calves against colibacillosis by vaccination of the pregnant dam or by vaccination of the fetus has received considerable research attention in recent years, and the results appear promising. The pregnant dam is vaccinated 6 and 2 weeks before parturition to stimulate antibodies to strains of enteropathogenic *E. coli,* which are then passed on to the newborn through the colostrum.

The use of an *E. coli* vaccine containing an enterotoxigenic strain of the organism provides protection against experimentally induced enterotoxigenic colibacillosis using the same homologous strain. The mechanism of protection is now considered to be the production of antibodies against the pilus antigens that are responsible for colonization of *E. coli* in the intestine. These favorable results suggest that vaccination may become a valuable method of aiding in the control of enteric colibacillosis of calves, especially in problem herds. A major limitation of vaccines is that calves must still ingest colostrum in sufficient quantities early enough to acquire the protection afforded by the vaccine.

The antibody response of newborn calves to a vaccine depends on their colostral antibody status. There is a marked failure of the colostrum-fed calf to respond to injected antigens, not because of the relatively immature lymphoid system, but rather because the presence of maternal antibody to the antigens used interferes with specific antibody stimulation.

Viral vaccines containing the modified-live rotavirus and coronavirus are available for administration to the cow in late pregnancy with the aim of increasing the level of colostral and milk antibodies available to the calf. However, experimental trials have indicated that the level of antibodies is increased to protective levels only during the period of colostrum production. The levels of antibodies to rotavirus and coronavirus decline very rapidly when the mammary secretions change from colostrum to milk within 2 to 3 days after parturition. This accounts for the failure of the vaccines and of the naturally occurring antibodies to provide protection in calves that commonly develop the disease after several days of age. Some recent work has shown that the combined intramuscular and intramammary vaccination of pregnant cows with a rotavirus and coronavirus vaccine containing an adjuvant will result in the stimulation of protective levels of antibodies in the milk for several days.

Supplemental Reading

Cryptosporidiosis

Anderson, B. C.: Cryptosporidiosis—a review. J. Am. Vet. Med. Assoc. *180*:1455–1457, 1982.

Anderson, B. C. and Hall, R. F.: Cryptosporidial infection in Idaho dairy calves. J. Am. Vet. Med. Assoc. *181*:484–485, 1982.

Anderson, B. C., Donndelinger, T., Wilkins, R. M. and Smith, J.: Cryptosporidiosis in a veterinary student. J. Am. Vet. Med. Assoc. *180*:408–409, 1982.

Angus, K. W., Appleyard, W. T., Menzies, J. D., et al.: An outbreak of diarrhea associated with cryptosporidiosis in naturally reared lambs. Vet. Rec. *110*:129–130, 1982.

Campbell, I., Tzipori, S., Hutchinson, G., and Angus, K. W.: Effect of disinfectants on survival of cryptosporidium oocysts. Vet. Rec. *111*:414–415, 1983.

Moon, H. W., Woode, G. N., and Ahrens, F. A.: Attempted chemoprophylaxis of cryptosporidiosis in calves. Vet. Rec. *110*:181, 1982.

Pearson, G. F. and Logan, E. F.: Scanning and transmission electron microscopic observations on the host-parasite relationship in intestinal cryptosporidiosis of neonatal calves. Res. Vet. Sci. *34*:149–154, 1983.

Sanford, S. E. and Josephson, G. K. A.: Bovine cryptosporidiosis: clinical and pathological findings in forty-two scouring neonatal calves. Can. Vet. J. *23*:343–347, 1982.

Tzipori, S.: Cryptosporidiosis in animals and humans. Microbiol. Rev. *47*:84–96, 1983.

Tzipori, S., Campbell, R., and Angus, K. W.: The therapeutic effect of 16 antimicrobial agents on Cryptosporidium infection in mice. Aust. J. Exp. Biol. and Med. Sci. *60*:187–190, 1982.

Tzipori, S., Smith, M., Halpin, E., et al.: Experimental cryptosporidiosis in calves: clinical manifestations and pathological findings. Vet. Rec. *112*:116–120, 1983.

Willson, P. J. and Acres, S. D.: A comparison of dichromate solution flotation and fecal smears for diagnosis of cryptosporidiosis in calves. Can. Vet. J. *23*:240–246, 1982.

Escherichia coli

Acres, S. D., Isaacson, R. E., Babiuk, L. A., and Kapitany, R. A.: Immunization of calves against enterotoxigenic colibacillosis by vaccinating dams with purified K99 antigen and whole cell bacterins. Infect. Immun. *25*:121–126, 1979.

Acres, S. D., Isaacson, R. E., Khachatourians, G., et al.: Vaccination of cows with purified K99 antigen, K99+ anucleated live *E. coli* and whole cell bacterins containing enterotoxigenic *E. coli* for prevention of enterotoxigenic colibacillosis of calves. Proc. Second Int. Symp. Neonatal Diarrhea. Vet. Inf. Dis. Org., Saskatoon, 443–455, 1979.

Bellamy, J. E. C. and Acres, S. D.: Enterotoxigenic colibacillosis in colostrum fed calves: pathologic changes. Am. J. Vet. Res. *40*:1390–1397, 1979.

Bywater, R. J.: Evaluation of an oral glucose-glycine-electrolyte formulation and amocillin for treatment of diarrhea in calves. Am. J. Vet. Res. *38*:1983–1987, 1978.

Cleek, J. L. and Phillips, R. W.: Evaluation of a commercial preparation for oral therapy of diarrhea in neonatal calves: administration by suckling versus intubation. J. Am. Vet. Med. Assoc. *178*:977–981, 1981.

Isaacson, R. E., Moon, H. W., and Schneider, R. A.: Distribution and virulence of *E. coli* in the small intestines of calves with and without diarrhea. Am. J. Vet. Res. *39*:1750–1755, 1978.

Moon, H. W., and McDonald, J. S.: Antibody response of cows to *E. coli* pilus antigen K99 after oral vaccination with live or dead bacteria. Am. J. Vet. Res. *44*:493–496, 1983.

Myers, L. L.: Vaccination of cows with *E. coli* bacterin for the prevention of naturally occurring diarrhea disease in their calves. Am. J. Vet. Res. *37*:831–834, 1976.

Myers, L. L.: Passive protection of calves against experimentally induced and naturally occurring enteric colibacillosis. Am. J. Vet. Res. *41*:1952–1956, 1980.

Nagy, B.: Vaccination of cows with a K99 extract to protect newborn calves against experimental enterotoxin colibacillosis. Infect. Immun. *27*:21–24, 1980.

Radostits, O. M. and Acres, S. D.: The prevention and control of epidemics of acute undifferentiated diarrhea of beef calves in Western Canada. Can. Vet. J. *22*:243–249, 1980.

Rotavirus and Coronavirus

Myers, L. L. and Snodgrass, D. R.: Colostral and milk antibody titers in cows vaccinated with a modified live-rotavirus-coronavirus vaccine. J. Am. Vet. Med. Assoc. *181*:486–488, 1982.

Raif, L. J. and Smith, K. L.: A review of rotavirus immunization of cows and passive protection in calves. Proc. Fourth Int. Symp. Neonatal Diarrhea. Vet. Inf. Dis. Org., Saskatoon, 1983.

Raif, L. F., Redman, D. R., Smith, L. K., and Thiel, K. W.: Passive immunity to bovine rotavirus in newborn calves fed colostrum supplements from immunized or nonimmunized cows. Infect. Immun. *41*:1118–1131, 1983.

Snodgrass, D. R., Nagy, L. K., Sherwood, D., and Campbell, I.: Passive immunity in calf diarrhea: vaccination with K99 antigen of enterotoxigenic *E. coli* and rotavirus. Infect. Immun. *37*:586–591, 1982.
Tzipori, S., Smith, M., Halpin, C., et al.: Intestinal changes associated with rotavirus and enteropathogenic *E. coli* infection in calves. Vet. Microbiol. *8*:35–43, 1983.

Neonatal Diarrhea in Pigs: Pathogenesis and General Therapeutic Approaches

JOHN J. ANDREWS, D.V.M., M.S.

Diarrhea in baby pigs is a common and important economic problem in swine rearing. Today, in spite of improvements in management and veterinary care, gastroenteritis is still the most common swine disease in many herds.

The practicing veterinarian should therefore understand how the important agents cause enteritis in baby pigs, should know how to recognize the presence of these agents, and should be able to identify the host's defense mechanisms that may be employed to control and minimize losses.

MECHANISMS OF GUT PROTECTION

The pig has a number of protective mechanisms by which diarrhea is either prevented or controlled. Soon after birth, the sterile intestine is rapidly populated with usually nonpathogenic organisms. These organisms directly compete with pathogenic organisms for nutrients and attachment sites and thus are extremely helpful in blocking the successful colonization of pathogenic organisms. *Lactobacillus* spp. generally colonize the stomach; some lactobacilli and fecal streptococcal organisms colonize the small intestine; and *Clostridium* spp., *Escherichia coli*, streptococci, and lactobacilli heavily colonize the colon. The presence of these agents, in addition to blocking colonization of pathogenic organisms, also stimulates local immune responses. The acidic environment of the stomach and upper duodenum limits the types of organisms that can survive in these areas.

Ingested immunoglobulins in the colostrum and lactational milk have a major role in preventing the pathogenic effects of many infectious agents. Plasmacytes located in the lamina propria of the duodenum and jejunum, once stimulated antigenically, secrete locally active immunoglobulins (mainly IgA and IgM) and thus provide additional immunologic protection of the gut as early as 5 to 10 days following parturition.

Nonimmunologic protective mechanisms include (1) gut motility that keeps most organisms located in the lower ileum and colon; (2) the gut wall itself that, when irritated, secretes large amounts of fluid that dilute harmful bacteria and toxins; (3) local interferon production and so-called cell block mechanisms that act to reduce virus penetration and infection of intestinal epithelium; (4) rapid replacement of damaged epithelium by proliferating crypt cells, resulting in rapid healing for injured gut; (5) contraction of the lamina propria when intestinal epithelium has been lost and has not, as yet, been replaced, thereby minimizing the amount of eroded surface exposed; (6) an inflammatory response including infiltration of inflammatory cells, exudation of fibrin and, in many cases, hemorrhage in response to severe irritation; and (7) the capacity of the colon to absorb excessive fluid (diarrhea results only when the amount of fluid presented to the colon exceeds its resorptive capacity).

MECHANISMS OF THE PRODUCTION OF DIARRHEA

There are a limited number of ways in which agents or substances can cause diarrhea. In the neonatal pig the most important and common of these include the following:

1. Destruction and loss of intestinal epithelial cells.
2. A high osmolarity (osmotic pressure) of gut contents thereby drawing fluid into the gut lumen.
3. Toxic effects on the gut epithelial cells, causing fluid loss into the gut lumen.
4. Local necrotizing effects on the epithelium, lamina propria, and underlying tissues.
5. Invasion of organisms into the lamina propria and underlying tissues (usually inciting a host-inflammatory response).

Recognition of These Mechanisms and Their Etiologic Significance

Loss of Intestinal Epithelium. The loss of intestinal epithelium results in the contraction of the underlying lamina propria. This can be recognized grossly by the thin-walled appearance of the intestine and by the loss of the intestinal villi (so-called villous atrophy as observed by a number of different techniques). This loss of effective absorptive surface and mature absorptive cells results in decreased absorption of ingested food. Lactose (milk sugar) is converted to lactate in this situation by gut bacteria, and an acid pH in the lower ileum and colon results. (This can be recognized in the acute watery stages of the diarrhea by using litmus paper.) The increased concentration of lactate is osmotically active, and fluid is "drawn" into the gut lumen, resulting in diarrhea. Because of the loss of absorptive epithelial cells, other substances such as fat are not absorbed well and, therefore, the mesenteric lacteals either contain less than the normal amount of chyle or may be completely lacking in chyle when observed grossly.

Acute transmissible gastroenteritis (TGE) is the classic example of this type of damage. In TGE, the damage is so extensive in the jejunum and ileum that the thin-walled fluid-filled gut can usually be recognized grossly, and the diagnosis can be further substantiated by observing the marked villous atrophy in the small intestines, the acid pH of the watery colon contents, and the lack of chyle in the lacteals. Since autolysis rapidly destroys intestinal villous epithelium, it is essential to examine a freshly killed, acutely affected piglet at necropsy when attempting to view these changes.

Endemic TGE virus infections and rotavirus infections produce less damage to the intestinal epithelium, and this damage is generally limited to the lower jejunum and ileum. Therefore, the resulting intestinal wall is not as thin, the villous atrophy is not quite as marked and may be found only in the ileum, and the change in the pH of the colon contents may be only slight or undetectable when compared with "typical" TGE infections.

Coccidia replicate in the jejunum and ileum of young swine and produce a loss of intestinal epithelium. Apparently, they produce diarrhea in a manner similar to TGE and rotavirus but with a greater inflammatory reaction in the lamina propria. Usually, the damage caused by coccidia when observed grossly is quite minimal (although a fibrinonecrotic exudate is occasionally seen on the mucosal surface), and the diarrhea that results resembles the mild "dribbling" type of diarrhea seen in swine infected with endemic TGE and rotavirus. Coccidial infections in pigs less than 2 weeks of age do not produce, as yet, oocysts in the feces, and therefore infections have been confirmed only by observing immature coccidial forms in histologic sections of infected jejunum or ileum or in stained mucosal impression smears taken from jejunum or ileum.

Osmotic Overloading. Osmotic diarrhea may result from a loss of the intestinal epithelium as explained earlier but also may result from an overloading of the absorptive capacity of the intestine with osmotically active substances. This may occur iatrogenically when a diet containing high levels of undigestible osmotic agents, such as sucrose (table sugar), is fed to young animals as a replacement therapy or, more commonly, when a young animal has simply ingested too much lactose by overloading its digestive system with mother's milk.

Although these animals seldom die, the expected changes include an intestine filled with fluid and an acidic pH of the colon contents. The lacteals will be full, and the intestinal villi will be of normal length. Bacteria may be present, but unless there are secondary infections, the pure populations of pathogenic organisms normally isolated from animals with infectious bacterial diarrhea cannot be isolated. The feces produced is generally whitish to whitish-yellow in color.

Bacteria. Bacteria such as enteropathogenic *E. coli* cause diarrhea because of their ability to secrete locally active enterotoxins. These toxins do not usually kill the intestinal epithelial cells but rather alter the electrolyte and fluid balance of these cells. The lesion observed in piglets with *E. coli* enteritis is a gut dilated by fluid (but with thicker walls than in TGE infections) with intestinal villi still intact (these can be easily observed). In chronic colibacillosis, some shortening of villi, especially in the ileum, may occur. Because the ability of the intestinal epithelial cells to absorb fat is not altered, the intestinal lacteals will contain white chyle. This is easily observed in piglets less than 1 week old but is less apparent in older pigs. The yellowish to greenish fluid in the intestinal lumen will frequently have a basic or neutral pH. In order to confirm the diagnosis, a pure population of piliated *E. coli* should be isolated from the upper jejunum or lower duodenum of a freshly killed, acutely affected, untreated piglet. Most enteropathogenic *E. coli* isolated from neonatal swine can be typed according to pilus antigens, such as K88, K99, or 987P.

Other Organisms. Other organisms also affect the intestinal epithelium and may produce locally effective toxins or toxins that are absorbed and produce systemic effects or both.

Organisms such as *Clostridium perfringens* type C produce a locally active necrotizing toxin (beta toxin) that causes nonselective necrosis of the epithelium and the underlying lamina propria. The diarrhea produced by this type of agent causes watery feces in its early stages but rapidly progresses to a diarrheic feces containing fibrin, necrotic debris, and blood. The lesions produced by *C. perfringens* Type C are fairly easy to recognize at necropsy and consist of severe necrosis of the epithelium and lamina propria that is normally limited to the small intestines and often accompanied by surface and lumenal hemorrhage and by gas bubble formation in the wall of the intestine.

Subacute lesions of *C. perfringens* Type C may resemble those produced by severe coccidiosis. A useful differential feature is the location of the lesion. Coccidiosis generally affects the lower jejunum and the ileum, while lesions of clostridial enteritis affect the upper one half of the small intestines.

THERAPY

Antibiotic Therapy

Antibiotic therapy has been and continues to be a widely used approach for diarrhea in baby pigs. The basic theory is simply to kill or inhibit the offending organisms. However, there are many situations in which this approach simply doesn't work. It works poorly or not at all (1) when the offending organisms are viral, (2) when rapid reinfection with the original bacterial pathogens occurs because of environmental contamination, (3) when the intestinal mucosa, and possibly submucosa, has been severely damaged prior to antibiotic therapy (e.g., *C. perfringens* Type C infections), (4) when the killed organisms release powerful toxins (probably endotoxins) as they die that may subsequently harm or even kill the pig (as in 10-day hemolytic *E. coli* enterotoxemia), and (5) when the offending organism is resistant to the antibiotic used.

Competitive Colonization

A second therapeutic approach is to populate the intestines with high numbers of nonpathogenic organisms that compete with the colonization of pathogenic bacteria. This therapy has met with variable degrees of success using oral dosing of baby pigs with high numbers of organisms, such as *Lactobacillus* sp., enterococci, and nonpathogenic *E. coli*. The use of antibiotics in combination with this type of a program is counterproductive because of the loss of nonpathogens killed by the antibiotics.

Physiologic Therapy

Physiologic approaches to correcting diarrhea problems include rehydrating the animals with electrolytes and decreasing the ingestion of osmotically active agents. Practically speaking, the subcutaneous and intraperitoneal

limit expulsion of *E. coli* from the lumen of the intestine, and prevent antibodies in milk from reaching the distal half of the intestines where they might protect against the effects of the organism.

Factors affecting the challenge include nutrition, chemotherapy, crate design, ventilation, quarantine and, notably, hygiene. It is possible but difficult to control the disease through hygiene alone. This single approach to control leaves the animal very susceptible to infection. Therefore, it is wise to use hygiene in conjunction with enhanced immunity. Under natural circumstances, sows will become infected with *E. coli*. The infection will act as a vaccine to enhance immunity. The probability of infection is to some extent related to the hygiene standards of the environment that the sows are kept in. The more emphasis on hygiene, the less likelihood that sows will acquire immunity. This contradiction of the requirements is overcome by maintaining hygiene standards, especially in the farrowing house, and enhancing immunity through vaccination of pregnant sows.

Recently, a number of effective *E. coli* vaccines have been introduced. The important antigens are those associated with the pili K88ac, K99, and 987P, and of less significance are the Types 1 and K88ab pili. There does not appear to be a major advantage in using purified pili vaccines over whole-cell bacterins containing the pili. Many United States veterinarians successfully use oral live cultures to stimulate immunity in the sow, hoping that the resulting immunity overcomes the possibly increased challenge. In both the oral-live and parenteral-killed vaccinations, immunity is acquired from the sow through colostrum and the continuous ingestion of milk. Anything that interferes with milk production, such as mastitis, will therefore reduce immunity to enteric colibacillosis.

Where effective bacterins or vaccines are available, intelligent management of the hygiene-challenge-immunity relationship can all but eliminate enteric colibacillosis as a significant swine disease.

TREATMENT

Treatment should be instituted as soon as swabs have been taken for confirmation of the diagnosis. Specific treatments cannot be detailed in this article because of the variation in sensitivity among different *E. coli* strains. A broad-spectrum antibiotic could be used until an antibiogram is completed. A piglet may lose 30 per cent of its body weight in fluid loss in colibacillosis; therefore, oral electrolytes should be made available immediately. Piglets of any age will drink from open bowls if they are dehydrated. The fluid should be changed and bowls cleaned frequently. Piglets continue to have diarrhea for several hours after the offending organisms have been eliminated.

Neonatal Polyarthritis in Swine

JAMES McKEAN, D.V.M., M.S.

Polyarthritis is the concurrent inflammation of the intra-articular components of several joints in an individual animal. The joints most commonly affected in swine are the knees, elbows, and hock joints. The stifle, shoulder, hip, and occipital joints are less frequently affected. A variety of organisms have been shown to cause polyarthritis, including *Streptococcus*, *Corynebacterium pyogenes*, *Staphylococcus*, and *Escherichia coli* in suckling pigs and *Erysipelothrix insidiosa*, *Mycoplasma hyorhinis*, *M. hyosynoviae*, *Haemophilus parasuis*, and occasionally *E. coli* in older animals. The septicemic distribution of these organisms may cause coexistent meningitis, polyserositis, or endocarditis.

CLINICAL SIGNS

Swelling of periarticular tissues with accompanying pain and lameness is generally the first sign of polyarthritis, with knees and hock joints the most commonly observed sites. In young pigs, signs may appear from 1 to 8 weeks of age but most commonly occur by 2 to 3 weeks. Individual pigs or entire litters may be affected. Purulent intra-articular exudate is seen with streptococcal, staphylococcal, and corynebacterial infections, while *E. coli* produces a fibrinous to fibrinopurulent exudate. With chronic infection, organization and induration of the exudate occurs, often causing permanently reduced joint function.

EPIDEMIOLOGY AND PATHOGENESIS

The incidence of polyarthritis is sporadic. Variability among herds is influenced by the presence of pathogenic organisms, environmental conditions, and trauma to infected pigs. No seasonal incidence has been reported, although adverse environmental or sanitary conditions predispose animals to clinical disease. Gilt litters may have a slightly higher frequency of infection than sow litters. Apparently, large numbers of pigs are exposed to pathogenic agents, but disease is evident only in those pigs lacking adequate antibody protection or under stressful conditions, or both. Skin abrasions of knees and of faces caused by struggling for nursing position may open a path for infection.

Hemolytic streptococcal invasion is most commonly observed in suckling pigs. *Streptococcus equisimilis* is observed most frequently, but other Group C and Groups D and L streptococcal species have been reported. Exposure occurs early, primarily from dam to litter. Aerosol transmission and vaginal contamination during birth are the primary sources of infection, with the nasopharynx, umbilicus, and skin abrasions as the primary entry sites from which infection spreads. Occasionally, infection results in sudden death with no premonitory signs. Lesions are those associated with acute septicemia. Initially, synovial fluid volume increases and appears creamy or white. Subacute to chronic infection results in a fibrinopurulent synovitis, pericarditis, or meningitis, or all three. In an outbreak of streptococccal meningitis, the meninges may become opaque and hyperemic. In some cases, gross changes are not notable. Internal hydrocephalus may occur. Pericarditis results in a fibrinopurulent exudate on the pericardial surfaces.

Streptococcus suis II infection may cause meningitis and polyarthritis. Pigs between 4 and 8 weeks of age that have recently undergone the stress of mixing and moving are most susceptible. Morbidity is low, but mortality is high in clinically affected pigs. Infection is by aerosol transmission from carrier swine. The incubation period may be as short as 24 hr. Sudden death and lesions of generalized septicemia may be observed. Affected pigs may have acute manifestations, resulting from localization of the organism in the meninges. Death occurs shortly after onset of signs including incoordination, paralysis, and tetanic spasms. In younger animals, a less acute course encourages polyarthritis.

Corynebacterium pyogenes infection causes a chronic lesion with periarticular fibrosis and a pasty greenish purulent exudate. Periarticular muscle necrosis and articular structure destruction may also be seen. *C. pyogenes* exudate tends to become crumbly in texture over time.

Coliform invasion from the intestinal tract may cause polyserositis, meningitis, and arthritis. Clinical signs are depression, rough hair coat, labored breathing, and death within several days of initial signs. Suckling pigs are most likely affected. Diarrhea is not a consistent sign. The *E. coli* strains isolated have been predominantly O strains and have not been enteropathogenic. Postmortem examination reveals large volumes of fibrinous exudate in the pleural, pericardial, and peritoneal cavities. Fibrinonecrotic pneumonia may be present with this septicemic form. Meningitis and polyarthritis are less often observed. Mortality is generally low, although sporadic outbreaks resulting in high morbidity and mortality can occur.

Staphylococcus species produce polyarthritis similar in appearance to that caused by *Streptococcus* species, but incidence is quite low in comparison to streptococcal involvement.

Septicemia caused by any of the aforementioned bacteria may result from invasion of the umbilical cord, of the castration site, of other skin wounds, or of the small intestine by the pathogenic serotypes.

DIAGNOSIS

Differential diagnosis can be made from clinical signs and by isolation of the causative organism from affected joints, meninges, and pleural peritoneal or pericardial cavities. Blood culture results are generally unrewarding because the number of circulating bacteria declines following initial septicemia. Smears of exudates stained with Gram's stain may also be helpful. Small abscesses at the umbilicus, castration or tail docking sites, or the presence of necrotizing gingivitis may be helpful in determining the portal of entry. However, in affected swine, the portal of entry is often not easily identified.

TREATMENT AND PREVENTION

Because of the sporadic nature of neonatal polyarthritis syndrome, prevention can be quite difficult. Introduction of new nonimmune breeding females may result in increased incidence of the syndrome in their offspring. As immunity develops in these adults, incidence should fall to the previous levels. Each herd should be evaluated as to the costs of the disease and the costs of proposed preventive programs. Sensitivity patterns of isolates will indicate which drugs may be effective for parenteral treatment and for prevention. With streptococcal infections, prophylactic treatment of each piglet with 22,000 IU/kg penicillin, 11 mg/kg lincomycin, or 8.8 mg/kg tylosin

has proven effective. Treatment of existing infections utilizing the same drugs can be successful occasionally if started early and continued for 2 to 3 days. For severe streptococcal infections in herds, use of high doses of tetracycline (200–400 gm/ton) in feed for 2 to 4 weeks prior to farrowing may be justified to reduce the carrier state in the sow population. Control of streptococcal and coliform septicemias may require use of autogenous bacterins in prefarrowing sows or in suckling pigs. Corynebacterial and staphylococcal infections rarely are of sufficient economic significance to warrant a vaccination program.

Good nursing care and adherence to sanitary practices are important measures to minimize the spread of disease. Sanitizing farrowing and nursing facilities between groups, dipping umbilical cords at birth in strong tincture of iodine solutions, farrowing in dry, comfortable facilities, and placing rugs or mats for 1 to 3 days after birth to reduce knee abrasions in suckling pigs are management practices used to minimize disease spread. Owners should be cautioned to avoid opening new routes of infection by improper or unsanitary tail docking and castration, or by clipping needle teeth.

Internal Parasitism in Neonates

DWIGHT G. BENNETT, D.V.M., Ph.D.

Because of the parasite's short prepatent period (period before sexual maturity), the parasitic problems of neonatal food animals are in most cases quite similar to those of older animals, as discussed in other articles of this book. For more detailed discussions, refer to the articles by Drs. Todd and Herd. In this article, only those problems applying particularly to neonates are presented.

PARASITISM IN NEONATAL RUMINANTS

Among the major gastrointestinal strongyles and trichostrongyles of ruminants, those of the genera *Ostertagia, Haemonchus, Trichostrongylus, Cooperia,* and *Nematodirus* have prepatent periods of 2 to 4 weeks, and those of the genera *Bunostomum, Chabertia,* and *Oesophagostomum* have prepatent periods of 5 to 8 weeks. All of these parasites produce harmful effects before reaching sexual maturity (patency), so all are a potential danger to neonates. *Bunostomum* presumably is capable of prenatal infection. The phenomena of larval inhibition and spring rise, which are closely related to each other, serve to provide large number of infective larvae on pastures when neonates are born.

However, parasitism is perhaps not generally as early as would be supposed from the prepatent periods. The largely milk diet in the suckling may reduce the exposure to larvae on pastures. In addition, milk in the gastrointestinal tract seems to inhibit development of the parasites. It has been demonstrated that twin lambs are parasitized earlier and more severely than single lambs, presumably because of less milk consumption and earlier commencement of grazing by twins. Early weaning (30 days) and complete removal of lambs from their dams to clean areas have resulted in very minimal parasite loads. Also, when lambs are weaned early, the weather in the temperate zone prior to weaning is not optimal for transmission of parasites.

Pathogenesis and clinical signs in the neonate are similar to those in the adult, but the effects are more severe because there is no resistance developed in the young. The finding of parasitism in the neonatal ruminant, when heavily exposed, may depend upon necropsy because the animal often dies before eggs are passed in the feces. Treatment of strongyles and trichostrongyles in neonates may be accomplished using thiabendazole and cambendazole in the same way as in adults. Levamisole may also be used in the neonatal ruminant. Ivermectin at 200 µg/kg has been effective against fourth stage larvae of strongyli, trichostrongyli, and lungworms in young calves.

The cattle ascarid, *Neoascaris vitulorum,* is most common in the tropics and subtropics. Prenatal infection is apparently the only route of infection. It is impossible to establish patent infection by ingestion of the eggs, so calves are already infected at birth. Patency occurs 3 weeks after birth. Verminous pneumonia, depression, and poor growth are signs in the prenatally infected calf. Piperazine adipate at 200 to 400 mg/kg is effective against the intestinal stages.

Coccidia may affect very young calves, especially *Eimeria zurnii,* in which the schizonts may develop as early as 2 days after ingestion of oocysts. Sanitation is the only very effective method of prevention of coccidiosis. Treatment is often of little value once signs develop, though amprolium at doses of 10 mg/kg has been reported as curative.

PARASITISM IN NEONATAL SWINE

Ascaris suum is apparently not capable of prenatal infection of pigs, but the larvae may enter the liver as early as 18 hr and the lungs as early as 5 days after ingestion of infective eggs. So there is the potential of damage in very young pigs. At least partial immunity against migrating larvae is transferred in the colostrum. Colostral antibody may persist up to 3 weeks.

The pulmonary phase of the infection is generally the most severe in the very young pig. In fact, when ascarid infections are fatal, deaths generally occur during the pulmonary migration. Necropsy is required for diagnosis because the worms have not developed to the stage of egg production. Confinement facilities for farrowing and nursing greatly reduce problems with *A. suum* in neonatal pigs. Pyrantel tartrate at 96 gm/ton of feed may help prevent ascarid migration.

Both transplacental and transcolostral infection of pigs with *Strongyloides ransomi* apparently occur. Following transplacental infection, the larvae rest in the liver, lungs, and possibly other tissues of the fetus and rapidly complete their migration to the intestine within 2 to 4 days after birth. The parasites then develop in the intestine with no further migration. Enteritis and diarrhea with death losses as high as 75 per cent have been reported in pigs less than 2 weeks old. Eggs may be found in the feces, but frequently necropsy is required for diagnosis because no eggs are passed.

Oral thiabendazole, in a paste formulation at 60 to 80 mg/kg, is effective against *Strongyloides* in pigs. Thiaben-

dazole, when given in the feed to sows at 50 mg/kg of body weight at 2 days before and at 3 days after parturition, has markedly reduced infections in neonatal pigs.

Supplemental Reading

Benz, G. W. and Ernst, J. V.: Anthelminthic efficacy of Ivermectin against immature gastrointestinal and pulmonary nematodes of calves. Am. J. Vet. Res. *42:*2097–2098, 1981.

Cold Stress of Calves and Lambs

DAVID P. OLSON, D.V.M., M.S., Ph.D.

Conventional livestock management schemes often result in birth of calves and lambs during late winter and early spring. As a result, these newborn animals may be exposed to adverse weather conditions, such as cold, fluctuating air temperature, excessive wind, and moisture. Beef calves and lambs born under range conditions in less temperate regions of North America often have little opportunity for natural or man-made protection and are especially susceptible to weather-related stress. In some cases, dairy calves from poorly managed herds may also suffer the consequences of exposure to severe climatic conditions. Field and laboratory studies have shown a direct relationship between increased incidence of respiratory and enteric diseases and reduced survival of calves and lambs subsequent to their exposure to adverse weather conditions.[1-4] In addition, field data suggest that the weak calf syndrome is caused in part by inclement weather.[5]

Homeothermic animals are those that maintain their core body temperature (CBT) within narrow limits despite variation in environmental temperature.[6] Animals readily maintain a balance between heat production and heat loss within the thermoneutral temperature zone. Temperatures within the thermoneutral zone vary among species; however, the overall limits range between 10 and 35°C. The thermoneutral zone is that zone in which heat production in the body is independent of air temperature. Ambient temperatures toward the lower end of this zone evoke responses such as crowding, active searching for warmer environments, and piloerection and peripheral vasoconstriction to conserve body heat. Critical temperature is defined as the lower limit of the thermoneutral zone. Temperatures below this point induce increased heat production by shivering and nonshivering thermogenesis, since animals exposed to these temperature extremes are no longer able to maintain their CBT by heat conservation measures alone. Hypothermia results when heat loss exceeds normal or depressed heat production and heat conservation and may be directly responsible for death. Newborn calves and lambs have normal stores of brown adipose tissue that is thermogenic when directly stimulated by catecholamines. However, experiments have shown that these animals are more susceptible to the effects of cold exposure than are their adult counterparts, in spite of this fat-derived source of heat. Factors that may contribute to excessive heat loss by cold-exposed young calves and lambs include a high ratio of body surface to body mass, thin skin, small quantity of hair or fleece, reduced amount of subcutaneous fat, poor neural control of cutaneous vasculature, and accelerated heat loss owing to evaporation of water from wet skin.

COLD STRESS IN CALVES

Clinical Condition, Behavioral Reaction, and Temperature Response

There is a direct relationship between severity of the cold exposure and the extent of changes seen in calves. The most severe weather-related conditions often include a combination of excessive wind and moisture and near-freezing air temperature. Exposure of 1- to 3-day-old calves to severe cold and moisture will cause rapid and progressive hypothermia despite intense shivering and attempts to minimize heat loss.[7, 8] Shivering will cease or become greatly diminished after the CBT is lowered by 6 to 8°C. Calves will also show signs of depression, somnolence, muscular weakness, and reluctance to stand and to nurse as CBT decreases. Calves usually die if their CBT has been lowered more than 10°C. These animals are either recumbent or comatose and have a poor response to pain stimuli before death. Cause of death is usually due to respiratory arrest. The time required to cause profound hypothermia and eventual death under field conditions may vary between 6 and 24 hr and will depend on the ambient temperature, wind velocity, and moisture content of the environment. Calves from 1 to 4 days of age are most susceptible to the effects of profound cold exposure, although animals as old as 7 days of age may also be affected in a similar manner provided the cold stress conditions are sufficiently severe. Data so far suggest no significant differences between breeds in susceptibilities to cold.

The CBT is the most reliable indicator of the ability of cold stressed animals to regulate their body temperature and maintain homeothermy. However, various tissues of severely cold stressed calves may cool at different rates, depending on the region of the body. For example, rectal and oral temperatures decrease linearly with time and closely approximate (within 0.5°C) the concurrent temperatures obtained for CBT. In contrast, temperatures within muscles in the shoulder and thigh regions decline in a curvilinear fashion. Thus, muscle temperatures in these locations are lowered despite heat produced from shivering thermogenesis. The most profound and rapid decrease in temperature occurs in subcutaneous tissues owing to conductive, convective, radiative, and evaporative heat losses. Here, tissue temperatures may nearly approximate those of the environment.

Calves exposed to moderate cold but not to excessive moisture are likely to show signs of intermittent shivering and dehydration and only slight depression and muscular weakness.[9] Their CBT and postural, sensory, and motivational responses are usually unchanged, although temperatures of subcutaneous tissues of the extremities are likely to decrease to an extent similar to that seen in severely cold stressed animals. It is also possible for calves exposed to moderate cold to die, particularly if they have been stressed for prolonged periods.

Clinical Pathologic Response

Various clinical pathologic changes have been noted in cold stressed calves. Although these changes are nonspecific, they nonetheless serve as useful indicators of the health status of cold stressed animals. Severely cold stressed calves tend to become dehydrated.[10] Thus, there is a corresponding slight increase in hematocrit value, hemoglobin concentration, and total number of erythrocytes. In contrast, there is a tendency for these calves to become leukopenic, owing primarily to neutropenia, although numbers of other leukocytes decrease as well. The most consistent cold-induced serum chemical changes include significant increases in plasma concentrations of glucose, cortisol, and catecholamines.[11, 12] These plasma constituents rise early and rapidly with onset of cold stress and, with the possible exception of glucose level, are likely to remain elevated throughout the stress period. Large increases may also be seen in concentrations of phosphorus, iron, alkaline phosphatase, aspartate aminotransferase, and lactate dehydrogenase, whereas minor increases occur in concentrations of calcium, total protein, albumin, and blood urea nitrogen (BUN). Of interest is the tendency for serum insulin level to lessen during severe cold stress. Thus, a paradox seems to develop in cold stressed calves whereby there is an increase in plasma concentration of readily metabolizable glucose for heat production, yet this substrate cannot be utilized because of depressed, levels of insulin. Similar changes in hematologic and serum chemical values may be seen in calves subjected to moderate cold stress, although the magnitude of most of the respective changes is not likely to be as great as those in severely cold stressed animals. Nonetheless, even moderate cold is likely to induce significant elevations in concentration of glucose, cortisol, and catecholamines.

Cardiovascular Response

Exposure of young calves to severe cold causes profound changes in cardiovascular function.[13] Initially, as the CBT decreases 2 to 3°C, there is a slight increase in aortic blood pressure and a significant increase in heart rate. Then, as hypothermia becomes more pronounced, there is a rapid and significant lowering in aortic blood pressure and heart rate. During the decline in aortic blood pressure, the systolic pressure in particular changes from the normal sharp peak to one that is curved and blunt. In addition, the normal electrocardiographic waveforms are obscured by extraneous and erratic peaks. Exposure of young calves to moderate cold temperature tends to elevate and sustain heart rate, whereas little change would be expected in arterial blood pressure or electrocardiographic activity of these animals.

Host Defense

Specific and nonspecific host defense mechanisms are affected in cold exposed calves. For example, there is a delay in onset and a significant decrease in rate of absorption of colostral immunoglobulins for the first 15 hr of life in hypothermic calves.[14] Beyond this early age, however, their efficiency of absorption is similar to that of nonstressd calves. Nevertheless, this early and temporary cold-induced failure of passive transfer type of immunodeficiency disease may result in a serious compromise of host defense. In contrast, normothermic cold stressed calves are able to absorb colostral immunoglobulins in a manner similar to nonstressed calves.[15] Exposure of calves to moderate cold during the first 3 days of life has no major effect on complement activity[16] or on the *in vitro* bactericidal activity of their neutrophils,[17] whereas lymphocytes from these animals tend to have a higher stimulation response to mitogens.[18] The clinical relevance of these findings is not totally clear except to suggest that cellular host defense mechanisms of young calves are probably not adversely affected by exposure to moderate cold. In contrast, exposure of 3- to 5-week-old calves to moderate cold does cause suppression of contact sensitivity skin test reactions and variable delayed-type hypersensitivity responses.[19] Data are not available concerning the effects of severe cold stress and hypothermia on cellular defense mechanisms of young calves.

Lesions

Exposure of young calves to either moderate or severe cold will consistently induce lesions. These lesions are subcutaneous hemorrhage and edema. They are common in the limbs, ventral to the sternum, and occasionally in the head region.[7, 9] Similar lesions have not been reported in either the thoracic or abdominal organs of cold stressed calves. Localization of these cold-induced lesions to the extremities may be explained in part by direct damage to endothelium of the peripheral vasculature and also by almost constant contact of these tissues to cold surfaces, since the cold stressed calves tend to remain recumbent for long periods. Moderate to severe hemorrhage has also been reported in the synovial cavity and membranes of the hock joints of cold stressed calves.

COLD STRESS IN LAMBS

Clinical Condition and Temperature Response

Numerous field and laboratory studies have shown that newborn lambs are highly susceptible to severe climatic stress. High mortality rates of young lambs have clearly been correlated with exposure to cold temperature, wind, and excessive moisture. Continuous as well as short periods of severe weather can cause high mortality among newborn lambs.[20] Lambs of certain breeds, such as the Cheviot and Scottish Blackface, are more resistant to experimental and natural cold exposure than are those of other breeds, such as Merino and Finnish Landrace.[21] In addition, lambs with long birth coats have lower weather-related mortality than do those with short birth coats.[22] Cold-exposed newborn lambs readily become hypothermic within the first few hours of life owing to severe hypoxia during birth[23] and to excessive heat loss.[24] Later, hypothermia in lambs up to 3 days of age can result from depressed heat production due to starvation and excessive mobilization and depletion of energy stores. Those that are at a high risk for development of hypothermia include lambs born to ewes in poor condition or to very young or very old ewes, twin or triplet lambs, and lambs that are small, premature, or weak at birth. Weak and hypothermic lambs also have poor teat seeking and sucking abilities, which further limit their heat production capabilities. The metabolic rate of cold-exposed lambs increases by approximately 3 to 4 times[25] and is due to shivering (60 per cent) and nonshivering thermogenesis (40 per cent).[26] Nonshivering thermogenesis is due to the presence of brown adipose tissue that disappears in lambs at an early age.[27]

Clinical Pathologic Response

Plasma concentrations of glucose, lactic acid, free fatty acids, and glycerol are initially elevated in lambs exposed to severe cold.[28] Later, however, plasma concentrations of glucose and free fatty acids lower, suggesting a depletion of important energy reserves.[29] Muscle glycogen is also rapidly depleted in cold stressed lambs.

Cardiovascular Response

Cold exposure of lambs causes important changes in cardiovascular function and oxygen consumption.[30] For example, cardiac output declines, whereas oxygen consumption of the animal remains high as body temperature decreases. In addition, there is an elevation in blood flow to brown adipose tissue, myocardium, diaphragm, and the major muscles involved in shivering, whereas blood flow is lowered to peripheral tissues and major internal organs, such as spleen, kidneys, liver, and intestine.[31]

Lesions

Lesions found in cold and starvation stressed lambs include peripheral subcutaneous edema, especially in the distal forelimbs and hindlimbs.[32] Reduced body weight, elevated catabolism of fat, and changes in the adrenal glands, such as smaller size, darkened cortex, and subcapsular hemorrhage, may also be found in cold and starved lambs.

TREATMENT FOR COLD STRESSED CALVES AND LAMBS

The discussion so far has clearly indicated that cold temperature, wind, and excessive moisture may be highly detrimental to the health of young calves and lambs and that these weather-related stresses may be directly responsible for the deaths of affected animals. Cold stressed and starved young calves and lambs are often affected later with secondary respiratory or enteric diseases or both, which is consistent with the known detrimental effects that these stresses have on specific and nonspecific host defense mechanisms. As a result, the veterinary practitioner must diagnose and treat not only the more obvious secondary complicating diseases but also the primary weather-related disorders. Practical rewarming methods have been described for treatment of cold stressed calves[8] and lambs.[24] These rewarming methods supplement shivering thermogenesis and are designed to raise the body temperature of cold stressed animals by application of various forms of external heat to the exterior of the body. Rewarming methods that have been tested are immersion in warm water, heat lamps, and electrical heat pads. Data indicate that these methods are effective in reversing the detrimental effects of cold exposure.[8, 10, 12, 13, 24] Another method of rewarming is to allow the cold stressed animal to breathe warmed and water-saturated air. In this way, the body core is rewarmed first. Hypoglycemia in cold stressed calves and lambs must also be treated by oral feeding or injection of glucose. Finally, other methods of nursing care, including protective housing, handfeeding, and antibiotic and replacement fluid therapy, may also be indicated during recovery.

References

1. Martin, S. W., Schwabe, C. W., and Franti, C. E.: Dairy cattle mortality rate: influence of meteorologic factors of calf mortality rate in Tulare County, California. Am. J. Vet. Res. 36:1105–1109, 1975.
2. Withers, E. W.: Mortality rates and disease incidence in calves in relation to feeding management and other environmental factors. Br. Vet. J. 108:382–405, 1952.
3. Slee, J.: Cold stress and perinatal mortality in lambs. Vet. Ann. 16:66–69, 1976.

4. Webster, A. J. F.: Weather and infectious disease in cattle. Vet. Rec. *108*:183–187, 1981.
5. Stauber, E. H.: Weak calf syndrome: a continuing enigma. J. Am. Vet. Med. Assoc. *168*:223–225, 1976.
6. Webster, A. J. F.: Physiological effects of cold exposure. *In* D. Robertshaw (ed.): Environmental Physiology. Baltimore, University Park Press, 33–69, 1974.
7. Olson, D. P., Papasian, C. J., and Ritter, R. C.: The effects of cold stress on neonatal calves. I. Clinical condition and pathological lesions. Can. J. Comp. Med. *44*:11–18, 1980.
8. Olson, D. P., South, P. J., and Hendrix, K.: Regional differences in body temperature in hypothermic and rewarmed young calves. Am. J. Vet. Res. *44*:564–571, 1983.
9. Olson, D. P., Bull, R. C., Kelley, K. W., et al.: Effects of maternal nutritional restriction and cold stress on young calves: clinical condition, behavioral reactions, and lesions. Am. J. Vet. Res. *42*:758–763, 1981.
10. Olson, D. P., South, P. J., and Hendrix, K.: Hematologic values of hypothermic and rewarmed young calves. Am. J. Vet. Res. *44*:572–576, 1983.
11. Olson, D. P., Ritter, R. C., Papasian, C. J., and Gutenberger, S.: Sympathoadrenal and adrenal hormonal responses of newborn calves to hypothermia. Can. J. Comp. Med. *45*:321–326, 1981.
12. Olson, D. P., South, P. J., and Hendrix, K.: Serum chemical values in hypothermic and rewarmed young calves. Am. J. Vet. Res. *44*:577–582, 1983.
13. Olson, D. P., South, P. J., and Hendrix, K.: Cardiovascular and shivering responses in hypothermic and rewarmed young calves. Am. J. Vet. Res. *44*:969–974, 1983.
14. Olson, D. P., Papasian, C. J., and Ritter, R. C.: The effects of cold stress on neonatal calves. II. Absorption of colostral immunoglobulins. Can. J. Comp. Med. *44*:19–23, 1980.
15. Olson, D. P., Bull, R. C., Woodard, L. F., and Kelley, K. W.: Effects of maternal nutritional restriction and cold stress on young calves: absorption of colostral immunoglobulins. Am. J. Vet. Res. *42*:876–880, 1981.
16. Woodard, L. F., Eckblad, W. P., Olson, D. P., et al.: Hemolytic complement levels of neonatal calves delivered from protein-energy malnourished dams and subjected to cold stress. Cornell Vet. *70*:266–271, 1980.
17. Woodard, L. F., Eckblad, W. P., Olson, D. P., et al.: Effects of maternal protein-energy malnutrition and cold stress on neutrophil function of bovine neonates. Am. J. Vet. Res. *41*:1208–1211, 1980.
18. Woodard, L. F., Eckblad, W. P., Olson, D. P., et al.: Effects of maternal protein-energy malnutrition on lymphoblastogenic responses of bovine neonates subjected to cold stress. Am. J. Vet. Res. *41*:561–563, 1980.
19. Kelley, K. W., Greenfield, R. E., Evermann, J. F., et al.: Delayed-type hypersensitivity, contact sensitivity, and phytohemagglutinin skin-test responses of heat- and cold-stressed calves. Am. J. Vet. Res. *43*:775–779, 1982.
20. Slee, J.: Cold stress and perinatal mortality in lambs. Vet. Ann. *16*:66–69, 1976.
21. Slee, J., Griffiths, R. G., and Samson, D. E.: Hypothermia in newborn lambs induced by experimental immersion in a water bath and by natural exposure outdoors. Res. Vet. Sci. *28*:275–280, 1980.
22. Slee, J.: The effects of breed, birth coat and body weight on the cold resistance of newborn lambs. An. Prod. *27*:43–49, 1978.
23. Eales, F. A., Gilmour, J. S., Barlow, R. M., and Small, J.: Causes of hypothermia in 89 lambs. Vet. Rec. *110*:118–120, 1982.
24. Anonymous: Detection and treatment of hypothermia in newborn lambs. Practice. *4*:20–22, 1982.
25. Alexander, G. and Bell, A. W.: Maximum thermogenic response to cold in relation to the proportion of brown adipose tissue and skeletal muscle in the body and to other parameters in young lambs. Biol. Neo. *26*:182–194, 1975.
26. Alexander, G., Bell, A. W., and Williams, D.: Metabolic response of lambs to cold. Effects of prolonged treatment with thyroxine, and of acclimation to low temperatures. Biol. Neo. *15*:198–210, 1970.
27. Thompson, G. E. and McEwan-Jenkinson, D.: Nonshivering thermogenesis in the newborn lamb. Can. J. Physiol. Pharm. *47*:249–253, 1969.
28. Alexander, G., Bell, A. W., and Hales, J. R. S.: The effect of cold exposure on the plasma levels of glucose, lactate, free fatty acids and glycerol and on the blood gas and acid-base status in young lambs. Biol. Neo. *20*:9–21, 1972.
29. Eales, F. A., Small, J., and Armstrong, R. H.: Plasma composition in hypothermic lambs. Vet. Rec. *106*:310, 1980.
30. Koivikko, A.: Experimental hypothermia in neonatal lambs. Poor cardiac response to increased oxygen consumption during shivering. Acta Physiol. Scand. *78*:571–573, 1970.
31. Alexander, G., Bell, A. W., and Hales, J. R. S.: Effects of cold exposure on tissue blood flow in the newborn lamb. J. Physiol. *234*:65–77, 1973.
32. Haughey, K. G.: Cold injury in newborn lambs. Aust. Vet. J. *49*:554–563, 1973.

HERD HEALTH MANAGEMENT

T. A. Mc PHERRON, D.V.M., M.S.
Consulting Editor

Dairy Cow Herd Health Management

RAYMOND J. HUSMANN, D.V.M.

Successful dairy herd health management requires a veterinary medicine-agribusinesss relationship that is unparalleled in any other aspect of veterinary medicine. The veterinarian must first realize that he or she is but a part of a management and delivery service team that must have a commonly agreed upon and dedicated goal of economic success of the dairy herd enterprise.

In many instances, dairy herd owners, especially in family owned enterprises, must be made to realize that their future financial success depends on a reasonable profit margin. Many family-owned dairies are operated solely to satisfy a "way of life." Regardless of the owners' personal goals, they must be readily interpreted and defined in ways that all management contributors and the owners readily understand. Further, the definition must be in terms that are accessible and easily evaluated. The monetary profit margin satisfies these criteria most readily and completely. If the herd owner does not have an appreciation, understanding, acceptance, and dedication to this principle, attempts at total dairy herd health management result in futility.

Once realistic goals, interpreted in terms of profit margin, have been set, definite accomplishment time limit guides must be established. With well-understood, time-limited goals, members of the management group can more readily function at the level of performance expected of them. Without well-understood, time-limited goals, management team success is determined by the lowest performing member. As an example, mastitis control may be aimed at 70 pounds daily milk production per lactating cow, but if nutrition management is directed at 50 pounds daily milk production per lactating cow, general management will soon be led to conclude that high levels of mastitis control do not yield satisfactory profit returns.

Since total dairy herd health management is such a broad, complex task, it must be defined and broken into component areas before it can be appreciated and dealt with. There must be a definitive understanding of the difference between the business of management and the management delivery system. A common problem may illustrate the point. Many dairy farmers equate measures to lower somatic cell counts to total dairy herd health management. An increased somatic cell count is but a

tree, while total dairy herd health management is indeed a forest!

Consequently, composition of the management team must vary according to the demands of the dairy herd and the desires and expectations of the owner. Generally speaking, there must be management expertise available, which is essential for the successful operation of any business. Accounting, banking, legal, nutritional, and veterinary medical services are the key areas that must be available. Individuals with skills satisfying these broad categories must have additional resource experts readily accessible. The most successful management teams appear to be those that collect large amounts of pertinent information and interpret them in terms the owner readily understands and can readily base decisions on.

In order for the management team to set goals, it must appreciate the expectations and desires of the owner. For example, is peak individual animal performance a main consideration or is the owner interested primarily in "doubling the size" of the operation? Philosophies, desires, and expectations must be rephrased in monetary terms and placed in a reasonable time frame.

There must be an agreement on how and when goal evaluations are to be completed and interpreted. In addition, it must be decided how much effort and money are to be directed and dedicated to the "business aspect" of dairy herd management, and what is to be set aside for funding and staffing a management delivery system.

Veterinarians are normally considered a vital part of both the general management and management delivery teams. In the role as a member of the management delivery group, they are routinely asked to interpret general management directives in terms of "day-to-day" routines that the management and delivery system members can understand and handle. The scope of such technical assistance may range from milking procedure evaluation through artificial insemination and ventilation. The veterinarian is also required to perform in the more traditional role of the dairy herd veterinarian, i.e., provision of technical services.

Maintenance of a viable veterinarian-client relationship is of utmost importance in dairy herd health management. This relationship must be nurtured by communication. Client veterinarian contact and exchange must be conducted at different levels and intensities such as the following:

1. General management meetings, possibly semiannually.
2. Regularly scheduled client-veterinarian management

123

meetings at which general management goals and directives are compared with current achievements.

3. Client-veterinarian exchange in which management delivery systems are evaluated and changed to meet requirements of general management.

4. Client-veterinarian contact in which specific areas of management delivery such as milking procedures are evaluated, discussed, and altered to meet production levels.

5. Client-veterinarian contact in dealing with specific technical problem areas, such as calf pneumonia. The level of counsel must be adjusted to the desires and capacities of the owner.

The veterinarian must also be prepared and capable of communicating with the other management delivery system personnel in dealing with daily operational problems in the following areas:

I. Individual animal.
   A. Calf management. See the next article, Dairy Calf Health Management.
   B. Open heifer. All aspects of management should lead to the goal of breeding a healthy heifer with 750 pounds body weight (large breeds) at 15 months of age or less. This goal may be attained by closely following the management recommendations dealing with grouping by age and size, adequate housing, parasite control, and balanced nutrition.
   C. Bred heifer. Of prime importance in this area is attention directed to practical growth without abnormal weight gain. Inseminating heifers with "calving-ease" bulls will help to reduce the percentage of first calving dystocia.
   D. Dry cow. Areas of particular importance in management delivery to the dry cow are mastitis control using practices such as dry cow udder infusion, trimming feet, balanced nutrition, adequate housing, and optimal exercise.
   E. Breeding bull. Whether a bull is used as the primary genetic source or in a clean up capacity, he must be physically and sexually mature enough to handle the assigned cow numbers and must meet the requirements of semen evaluation and breeding soundness tests.

II. Herd production. Dairy herd improvement association testing or monthly owner milk weighing is necessary to make certain that individual cow profitability is maintained. Culling standards have to be set for the individual farm. The veterinarian usually requires general management support in enforcing the culling schedule pressure.

III. Herd reproduction. The management delivery system must provide adequate reproductive care commencing with delivery of the newborn. The veterinarian should set the standards of management delivery for the parturient cow. Clean calving pens and utensils are basic. Management and delivery service should handle the requirements of dystocia, retained placenta, and so forth, with the thought of making it possible for the new mother to begin a profitable lactation and a normal reproductive cycle. Management delivery must be able to provide instruction of and supervision of all drug administration procedures, such as uterine boluses, uterine flushes, hormone treatments, and parenteral antibiotics.

The recently freshened cow should be observed frequently each day. Cows exhibiting abnormal vaginal discharges should be infused. Indiscriminate, routine uterine infusion of all fresh cows is not recommended. Those cows with calving injuries such as vaginal tears must have corrective care provided. All heat dates must be detected and recorded.

Routine reproductive examinations are concerned primarily with the following:
A. The cow that has freshened since the last scheduled reproductive examination visit.
B. The cow that has been fresh 28 to 56 days and has not been pronounced "O.K. to breed" or has not shown heat.
C. The noncycling cow that has not been bred 35 days or more.
D. Problem cows may include animals with stubborn metritis, pyometra, urine pooling in the anterior vagina, wind-sucking, nonfunctional ovaries, reproductive tract adhesions, and hormonal imbalance. Hormonal imbalances may involve luteal cysts, follicular cysts, or progesterone deficiencies.
E. Pregnancy diagnosis.

Artificial insemination in the small dairy herd often requires technical assistance from the management and delivery system veterinarian. Heat detection is usually one of the problems that must be effectively and profitably handled. Various tail-head detecting devices, bright-colored paint sticks used on the tail head, "gomer" bulls, implanted steers, vasectomized bulls, and implanted follicular cystic cows are sometimes helpful aids. All efforts should be directed to detecting, identifying, and recording cows in heat. Heats detected prior to 60 days post-calving help to establish the cycle dates so that a cow may be detected, identified, and inseminated according to an optimal reproductive schedule.

IV. Disease prevention. All management and management-delivery personnel must focus primarily on disease prevention rather than on disease treatment. Disease prevention areas are listed next to provide examples of the varying degrees of importance that management must direct the delivery team to place upon problems at hand.
A. Mastitis control is essential and involves general management directives, management delivery, and technical services. The veterinarian is usually involved at all levels. Possibly one of the most important veterinary functions is to help establish the existing level of mastitis control and the desired level of mastitis control. Some portions of the following survey format may be helpful.

Mastitis Control Survey

1. Premises
   a. Pasture
      (1) Area
      (2) Type vegetation
      (3) Drainage
      (4) Debris
   b. Lots
      (1) Number and size
      (2) Surface
      (3) Windbreak
      (4) Shade
      (5) Drinking water
      (6) Grouping by production levels

(7) Protected feedbunk spaces
    (a) Hay
    (b) Silage
c. Housing
  (1) Loose
    (a) Total area
    (b) Bedding type
    (c) Bedding condition
    (d) Ventilation
      1. Ridgecap
      2. Forced air
  (2) Free stalls
    (a) Number
    (b) Size
    (c) Surface
    (d) State of repair
    (e) Ratio of cows to free stalls
  (3) Alleyways
    (a) Surface
    (b) Width
    (c) Drainage
  (4) Maternity pens
    (a) Size
    (b) Surface
    (c) Cleanliness
  (5) Heat pen
  (6) Dry cow lot
    (a) Surface type
    (b) Bedding type
    (c) Drainage
  (7) Holding pen
    (a) Size
    (b) Surface
    (c) Slope
    (d) Length of time cows are in holding pen per day
  (8) Bred heifer lot
d. Manure disposal interval
  (1) Lots
  (2) Pens
  (3) Alleyways
  (4) Holding pens
  (5) Free stalls
2. Milking equipment
a. Vacuum pump
  (1) Measured CFM (cubic ft/min)
  (2) Vacuum reserve tank capacity
  (3) Belt wear and tension
  (4) Manufacturer's specifications
b. Vacuum pump motor size (recommendation of 1 hp/20 CFM required)
c. Vacuum system installation
efficiency = *CFM wash manifold* / *CFM vacuum pump*
d. Pulsator
  (1) Brand
  (2) Model
  (3) Number of units
  (4) Pulsation
    (a) Single action
    (b) Alternating action
  (5) Pulsations per minute
  (6) Graph
    (a) Not milking
      1. Milk phase to rest phase ratio
      2. Pulsator vacuum level

    (b) Milking
      1. Pulsator vacuum level configuration
      2. Stability of teat end vacuum
  (7) Length of milking period
  (8) Milking duration per cow
e. Vacuum line
  (1) Origin (reserve tank)
  (2) Diameter
  (3) Looped to source
  (4) Moisture drain
f. Milk line
  (1) Location (high or low)
  (2) Looped to receiver jar
  (3) Weigh jars installed—height with reference to teat end
  (4) Unit number
  (5) Slope
  (6) Diameter uniformity
g. Automatic detachers
  (1) Brand name
  (2) Model
h. Inflations
  (1) Brand name
  (2) Model
  (3) Manufacturer's recommended frequency of change
  (4) Current frequency of change
  (5) Visual inspection
    (a) Cracks
    (b) Rough surfaces
    (c) Breaks
    (d) Vents
3. Milking herd
a. Number of cows being milked
b. Current daily milk production per cow
c. 305-day production average
  (1) Butterfat
  (2) Milk
d. Average age
e. Current somatic cell count
f. Average somatic cell count
  (1) Lactation 1
  (2) Lactation 2
  (3) Lactation 3
  (4) Lactation 4
  (5) Lactation 5
  (6) Lactation 6
  (7) Lactation 7 and over
g. Average stage of lactation _____days
h. Stage of lactation somatic cell count
  (1) Less than 50 days
  (2) 50 to 200 days
  (3) Over 200 days
i. Milking procedure
  (1) Total time required to milk entire herd
  (2) Sanitation
    (a) Udder
      1. Type germicide used in udder wash
      2. Concentration of germicide used in udder wash
      3. Method of determining germicide concentration
      4. Individual paper towels for drying used

        5. Teats and udder drying prior to milking
- (b) Teat visual inspection
  - *1.* Ends clean prior to milking
  - *2.* Protrusions evident
  - *3.* Type teat dip used
  - (c) Claw sanitized between cows
  - (d) Claw sanitizing agent
- j. Tank sampling history
  - (1) Somatic cell counts and dates collected
  - (2) Total bacteria counts and dates collected
  - (3) Bacterial isolates and dates collected
  - (4) Sediment rating and dates taken
- k. Dairy bacterial counts and collection dates
  - (1) Pre-incubation
  - (2) Total
- l. California mastitis teat (CMT) quarter scores (positive quarters divided by total quarters sampled)
- m. Bacteriologic survey of positive CMT quarters
  - (1) Organism identity
  - (2) Percentage of quarters infected
  - (3) Percentage of cows infected
  - (4) Sensitivity
- n. Drug history—quarter treatment
  - (1) Lactating
  - (2) Dry

B. Areas such as parasite control may need direction by the general management group. If flies are a major problem, definite goals need to be established and determined amounts of management delivery time and money need to be directed toward fly control. Most of the effort and funds should be spent in elimination of breeding areas, e.g., timely manure removal and disposal or storage. If internal parasites are a potential problem, management delivery measures must be directed toward prevention by draining adequately, grouping of animals, assaying parasite levels, and instituting mechanisms for satisfactory control.

C. Other infectious disease problems must be identified and equated to a dollar value. Only then can management at all levels decide how to cope with the particular situation.

V. Nutrition. Management must realize that an economical, balanced ration is one of the prerequisites of profit in the dairy business. Afterward, all levels of management and management delivery must be dedicated to satisfying the varying requirements of each individual animal. The following format may help establish some of the data input essential for the nutritionist servicing the dairy herd.

A. Roughage
  1. Hay
     a. Type
     b. Analysis
     c. Quantity consumed per cow per day
  2. Silage
     a. Type
     b. Analysis
     c. Quantity consumed per cow per day
B. Concentrate
  1. Balanced to roughage

    2. Distribution
  a. Parlor
  b. Magnet feeder—cow pressure
  c. Computer feeder—cow pressure
  d. Hand fed over ensilage
  e. Frequency
  f. Time with reference to milking time
C. Water
  1. Availability
  2. Source
  3. Accessibility
  4. Bacterial assay

VI. Stress. Stress may be defined as any influence that attempts to cause an individual animal or system within that animal to deviate from a range of function that is normal. Recognition that stress may be the deciding factor for the health and well-being of the animal and also may determine profit or loss for the entire operation is needed. Stress control may well be the keystone for herd health management. Some examples of factors that may cause stress are as follows:

A. High humidity
B. Abnormal temperature
C. Chilling wind
D. Abnormal sounds in the milking parlor
E. Stray voltage in the milking parlor
F. Electrical shock at the water fountain
G. Finely ground roughage
H. Slippery walking surfaces
I. Uncomfortable free stalls
J. Inadequate feed bunk space

In summation, although the problems presented by the dairy herd are diverse and complex, they can be met, identified, and satisfied by proper owner, general management, and management-delivery team actions.

Dairy Calf Health Management

R. KENNETH BRAUN, D.V.M.

Replacement heifers are the economic basis for the future of the dairy cattle industry. Therefore, it is important that dairy farmers, and all other individuals responsible for replacement rearing programs, perform their duties in an optimal manner. Herd health is not the sole responsibility of veterinarians any more than production control is the sole responsibility of dairy farmers and other agricultural consultants. Veterinarians, like dairy owners and other agricultural specialists, must work as team members, and each member must be concerned with replacement rearing in its broadest sense, making decisions based upon the animal's well-being and agricultural economics.

A replacement rearing program is not appropriate for every dairy farmer, and some should be strongly encouraged to discontinue their programs. An exception to this statement would be if dairy replacements are unavailable or are more expensive than raising them. A rule of thumb to be used as a criterion for deciding on whether a dairy farmer should or should not be rearing replacements is the level of herd milk production. When herd milk production level is below the state or region average, dairy owners should be encouraged to use their management efforts to increase milk production rather than to dilute these efforts with a replacement rearing program. Additional factors to be taken into consideration when deciding the merits of replacement rearing are

1. Land availability and its cost or its value for alternate use.

2. Genetic potential of heifers reared vs. heifers purchased.

3. Heifers grown on the farm have the advantage of being climatized and purchased heifers do not.

4. Heifers with advantages 2 and 3 are produced at a lower cost than purchased replacements.

Replacement rearing programs are not rigid sets of guidelines that if strictly adhered to will ensure success. Each farm differs in its level of management ability, physical plant facilities, geographic location, and the owner's desire to reach attainable goals. The success of a replacement rearing program is determined by the interplay of management and environmental and biologic factors.

If veterinarians want to meet the challenge as consultants for herd health and production control of today's ever enlarging, highly mechanized dairy enterprises, then they must broaden their interest and knowledge from traditional veterinary medicine to include the improvement of healthy animals, whereby these individuals can attain their genetic potential within the agricultural-economic framework. In addition, veterinarians must be capable of and willing to provide assistance in training managers and members of the farm labor force. Unless these people understand the capabilities of veterinarians, have confidence in them, and feel comfortable communicating with them, they will not play a major role in the program.

A rapidly emerging dimension related to veterinarians monitoring and strengthening their role as a herd health consultant is that they must have a good knowledge of finance and must be competent in analyzing and evaluating herd performance records so that deficiencies can be recognized and appropriate changes can be recommended for implementation by management. By performing much of the physical work (physical examinations, treatment, necropsy) of gathering information on which veterinarians base their advice, then and only then, can they advise clients to make appropriate adjustments when attainable goals are not being achieved. Accurate and complete record keeping is a prerequisite to the optimal function of a replacement rearing program.

I set individual performance goals for each dairy owner. These goals are designed to include the following: first, they must be economically justified and provide comfort for cattle; second, they must be attainable; and third, they must be measurable. Veterinarians and dairy farmers should realize that production goals will vary among regions of the country, herd size, and the level of management intensity that the owner wishes to or can attain.

Dairy farmers, with assistance from veterinarians and other agricultural consultants, have to maintain an accurate and up-to-date record system on individual replacements as well as the adult herd. These data must be handled and processed to make them relevant. Dairy owners, along with their consultants, must be able and willing to monitor replacement heifer performance in relation to attainable goals.

The objective of this article is to identify the parameters that are of assistance to the management team in increasing heifer replacement rearing efficiency and to provide information on how to analyze data in relation to realistic goals attainable by dairy farmers. The essentials for a dairy replacement rearing program include

1. Setting goals—what are we aiming for on a particular farm?

2. Implementation—what are the tools and techniques that are needed to meet these goals?

3. Evaluation and analysis—how can we translate accurate records, obtained during a short period of time, into relevant information for the benefit of dairy owners?

4. Control—how can we control and improve profitable animal production by optimal decision making? Consultative decisions regarding profitable animal production must be made in writing to the dairy farmer as soon as an unwanted situation is detected or anticipated.

With the implementation of these guidelines, a momentary profile of the performance of a replacement rearing program on a farm can be shown.

I. Replacement Rearing Guidelines and Methods: Goals. Dairy owners, veterinarians, and other agricultural specialists should collectively establish goals for a particular farm that are attainable, economically justified, and measurable. These goals should include 4 to 6 parameters that are the framework for an optimal replacement rearing program. An example of these goals includes the following:

A. Rearing replacement heifers should be based on improving herd genetic level. We expect the projected ME 305 day milk for first lactation heifers to be 75 to 125 lb, higher during the current 12 months as compared with first lactation heifers calving during the previous 12 months. This increase is due to genetic improvement of their parents (AI sires). We expect an additional yearly increase of 50 to 100 lb because of improved management factors (nutrition, culling, mastitis control, reproductive efficiency, and so forth).

B. Rearing costs for home-reared heifers should be justified economically, otherwise replacement heifers should be purchased. In this latter case, attention must be paid to genetic potential, age at calving, body weight, conformation, acclimation, and health status.

C. Of all the female calves born, more than 92 per cent should survive the first 24 hr of life. Of those heifers selected for herd replacements prior to birth, more than 80 per cent should survive and calve at 24 to 25 months of age.

D. Replacement heifers (Holstein-Friesian breed) should be inseminated at first heat beginning at 14 months of age at a body weight of 750 lb (340 kg) and a pelvic height of 51 in (125 cm).

E. Replacement heifers (Holstein-Friesian breed) should calve at 24 to 25 months of age, weigh 1150 lb (525 kg) after calving, and have a pelvic height of 56 in (136 cm).

F. Replacement heifers should be reared if milk production level of the herd is above the state or regional average. Dairy farmers with below average milk production should use their management efforts and resources to increase production rather than dilute efficiency with a replacement rearing program.

II. Tools and techniques. Implementation procedures

utilizing various tools and techniques that discuss or outline are a reflection of my successful experience and biases. In no way should it be construed that different procedures would not be equally successful.

A. Calf rearing chart with the following headings:
1. Identification, date of birth, flap tag, tattoo, sire and dam.
2. Dates of weaning, moving to group pen, vaccinations, deworming, and moving to pasture.
3. Date of weighing and deviation from growth chart.
4. Health disorders—type and date.
5. Advised month of insemination, insemination dates, results of pregnancy checks, expected calving date, service sire identity.
6. Remarks, e.g., culling date and reasons.

B. Farm checklist
1. A calendar with time-related veterinary and agricultural items to examine or to discuss with the dairy farmer.
2. Target growth curve or table.
   a. Scale or heart girth tape.
3. Colostrometer to measure immunoglobulin (Ig) level of colostrum.
4. Refractometer to measure calf total serum protein level for evidence of colostrum absorption.
5. Feeding standards.
   a. NRC requirements, pasture management.
6. Clinical examination.
   a. Supplementary examination (blood, feces, and so forth).
7. External information.
   a. Laboratory reports (necropsy results and so forth).
   b. Slaughter house checks.
   c. Sire summaries.

C. Replacement rate—optimum use of herd genetics. The number of replacements to be reared on a particular farm will depend on various factors, some of which are listed as follows:
1. Herd genetic improvement level can be greatly influenced by the pressure applied to culling for low production (voluntary). Herd genetic improvement level will be slow, however, when a high rate of culling (involuntary) occurs for the following reasons: reproduction, disease, injury, mastitis, feet and legs, and mortality. When involuntary cull rates are high, dairy owners tend to rear all available herd replacements.
2. Herd size—owners that are increasing herd size tend to raise all their herd replacements. Owners maintaining or decreasing in herd size tend to rear fewer replacements.
3. Calf mortality rate—when calf mortality rates are high, numbers of calves available to be reared will be low.
4. Calving interval—for every 30 days, a herd calving interval is increased, and 8 per cent fewer calves will be born.

D. Breeding period—selective mating for superior progeny.
1. Bull choice—selection should be made on the following criteria:
   a. Use of AI program.
   b. Production, i.e., fat, protein, milk.
   c. Prevention of calving difficulties.
   d. Pregnancy rate (in herd comparison of AI bulls).
2. Cow choice.
   a. Identification.
   b. Listing cows' and heifers' genetic merit and conformation qualities.
   c. Prebreeding examination (cows and heifers).
      (1) Reproductive tract (rectal examination).
      (2) Hoof trimming.
      (3) Condition scoring (extremes).
      (4) Heifers—age and weight according to standards.
3. Vaccinations—prebreeding.
   a. IBR, PI_3, BVD.
   b. Leptospirosis (5-way).
   c. Vibrio (natural service).

E. Gestation period. Goal. Prevent extremes in body condition,[8] i.e., overcondition and undercondition.
1. Condition scoring (end of lactation, end of dry period) on a scale of 1 to 5.
   a. At drying off, 3.5 to 4.0.
   b. At calving (cows), 3.5 to 4.0.
   c. At calving (heifers), 3.0 to 3.5.
2. Udder edema.
   a. K and Na may be present in excessive amounts when feeding high levels of high energy feedstuffs.
   b. Genetic relationships.
3. Drying-off period.
   a. Mastitis prevention.
      (1) Colostrum quality.
      (2) Abortion (stress).
   b. Vaccinations.
      (1) *Escherichia coli* (K99 pili), K85, K35, K30 (capsular).
      (2) Rota-corona virus.
   c. Nutrition.
      (1) 12 per cent crude protein.
      (2) Feed complete ration at a rate of 1.5 per cent of body weight during last 3 weeks of gestation.
      (3) Condition score.
4. Milk fever prevention.
   a. Calcium phosphorus levels and ratios.
   b. Colostrum production (5 mg Ca/L).
   c. Maintenance of appetite during parturition period (feed for maintenance plus 5 kg of milk).

F. Parturition period (12 hr before parturition to end of parturition): Goal. Calf born healthy and cow ready to meet demands of optimal lactation.
1. Maternity pen should be cleaned and disinfected prior to each calving.
2. Maternity pen should be bedded with straw.
3. Perineum and udder should be washed prior to cow's placement in maternity pen (10 to 12 hr prior to calving).
4. Avoid stress, i.e., sudden changes in feeding and climate.

5. To assist at calving clean perineum, equipment, hands, and forearms well. Use lubrication other than soap in vagina during delivery.
6. Disinfect calf's navel with iodine at birth and repeat 12 hr later.
7. Monitor per cent of umbilical stumps larger than 10 mm in diameter.
8. Mammary gland evaluation.
    a. Mastitis—use strip plate.
    b. Colostrum quality (colostrometer).[4]

G. Colostrum period (first 72 hr of life): Goal. Newborn calf to receive adequate amounts of high quality colostrum within the first hr of life.
1. Colostrum feeding.
    a. Colostrum collecting and feeding should be conducted under good sanitary conditions (clean teats, hands, and equipment).
    b. Calf should receive 2 quarts of high quality colostrum (first milking) as soon after birth as possible. A second feeding (2 quarts) should be 8 to 10 hr later.
    c. The remainder of first milking after calving is colostrum that should be fed to calf for first 2 to 3 days of life.
    d. The second to sixth milkings are fresh cow milk and should be fed to the calf following the colostrum period.
    e. When 2 or more cows calve the same day, colostrum should be pooled prior to feeding newborn calf.
    f. Colostrum can be held under refrigeration (sanitary conditions) for 3 days. However, colostrum should be placed in a refrigerator within 1 hr of collection. Excess, high quality colostrum should be stored in 2 quart containers, dated, and frozen for future use. Colostrum from mature cows has a wider spectrum of antibodies than first-calf heifers.
    g. Levels of immunoglobulins (Igs) absorbed from colostrum are dependent upon
        (1) Interval between birth and suckling.
        (2) Concentration of Igs in colostrum.
        (3) Birth weight—a 78-lb calf needs to absorb 50 gm of Igs for protection against septicemia.
    h. Level of Igs absorbed by a calf can be monitored by collection of a serum sample obtained between 2 and 7 days of life.[5, 7] When using a refractometer to determine total serum protein levels, a calf with less than 5.0 gm per cent should be considered colostrum deprived.
2. Calf identification.
    a. Ear tag and tattoo at birth to assure proper identification.
    b. Start record keeping!
3. Housing (birth to weaning).
    a. Remove newborn calf from maternity pen as soon as possible and place in an individual stall that is clean and well-ventilated.
    b. Calves should remain in an individual stall untill 2 weeks following weaning.
    c. Sanitation, bedding, and ventilation are extremely important during this period for disease control.
    d. On large farms, milk-fed calves can be individually grouped according to age, and youngest calves attended to first each day.
    e. Separation of weaned calves from milk-fed calves is essential for disease control.
4. Vaccination (2 to 3 days of age).
    a. Calves should be given 500,000 IU of vitamin A and 75,000 IU of vitamin D (IM).
    b. In areas with soils marginally deficient in selenium, calves should be given 100 mg vitamin E and 10 mg of selenium IM to prevent nutritional muscular dystrophy.
    c. Administer IBR and PI₃ intranasally (optional).

H. Milk feeding period (3 days of age to weaning or 6 to 8 weeks of age): Goal. Maintenance of good health with daily weight gain of 1.45 lb (0.7 kg).
1. Milk replacer.
    a. When a high quality milk replacer is available, it can be fed in place of fermented or whole milk.
    b. It is important to mix and feed as directed.
    c. It is advised to feed 2 times daily. To save labor, it is possible to feed once daily after 21 days of age.
2. Whole milk.
    a. Feed daily at the rate of 8 per cent of body weight.
    b. Feed 2 times daily for first 21 days. If calves are growing well at 21 days, labor can be saved by feeding once daily until weaned.
    c. Milk replacer can be fed once daily following whole milk feeding for 21 days.
    Feeding milk (or milk replacer) free-choice to a calf or group of calves may limit concentrate intake and be a cause of indigestion and delay in growth after weaning.
3. Mastitic milk.
    a. Secretions looking like milk can be fed the same as whole milk with similar results.
4. Nipple pails can be used to feed milk to calves until weaning, but maintenance of nipple orifice size and sanitation of pail between calves is essential.
5. For disease control, calves should be fed milk beginning at 3 to 6 days of age from individual pails, washed daily.
6. Concentrates.
    a. A commercial calf starter ration with good digestibility, palatability, and composition should be fed free-choice beginning at 3 days of age.
    b. Avoid contamination of concentrates with milk or water by separation of the 2 buckets.
    c. When daily consumption exceeds 2.5 lb, calves can be weaned from milk.
7. Roughage.
    a. Fine stem, high quality hay can be fed free-choice beginning at 1 week of age. If good quality hay is not available, wait until calf is 4 to 6 months of age before feeding.
8. Vaccinations.
    a. 7-way *Clostridium* toxoid (4 to 6 weeks of age).
    b. Lungworm vaccination (if available).

9. Dehorning.
   a. At 4 to 6 weeks of age use electric dehorner and do not dehorn at or near weaning.
10. Remove extra teats.
    a. At 4 to 6 weeks of age (at dehorning) or later if more convenient.
11. Enteric disease control (see III).
12. Respiratory disease control (see IV).
13. Parasitic disease control (see V).
I. Group rearing (time of weaning until 6 to 8 months of age): Goal. Maintenance of good health with average daily weight gains of 1.6 lb (0.73 kg).[6]
   1. Housing.
      a. Two weeks following weaning, calves should be moved to group pens, preferably separated from milk-fed calves to avoid horizontal infection.
      b. The stocking rate of calves between weaning and 6 to 8 months of age is important for control of respiratory and parasitic diseases.
      c. Optimum stocking rate is 10 to 15 calves of similar size and age.
      d. Space allocation (minimum requirements).
         (1) Rearing outdoors group pen: 500 to 1000 ft²/animal.
         (2) Rearing in a barn or paved pen: 75 to 100 ft²/animal.
      e. Calves reared outdoors need protection from the sun in warm climates. In temperate climates, they need protection from sun, cold draft, rain, and snow.
   2. Nutrition program.
      a. Free-choice calf starter ration (concentrate) should be continued for first 2 to 3 weeks in group pen.
      b. A growing ration can then be fed free-choice until 6 months of age.
      c. Good quality hay, if available, should be fed free-choice. If good quality hay is not available increase fiber content of calf starter to control bloat and body condition. Hay, when fed, should be placed in rack for prevention of waste and control of internal parasites.
      d. Provide fresh, clean water ad lib.
      e. Monitor growth rate by comparing age and body weight to standard table (Table 1)[2, 3] If a scale is not available, a chest circumference measurement can be made with a special tape. It is preferred to compare body weight with the standard table at 1 to 3, 3 to 6, 12 to 15, and 15 to 24 months (Table 2).
   3. Parasitic disease control (see V).
   4. Respiratory disease control (see IV).
   5. Vaccinations.
      a. *Brucella abortus* strain 19 vaccine.
      b. 7-way *Clostridium* toxoid (4 to 6 months of age).
      c. Intramuscular IBR, PI₃, BVD at 4 to 6 months of age.
      d. Lungworm vaccination (if available).
   6. Remove extra teats at the time of *Brucella abortus* vaccination (if not done earlier).

Table 1. *Growth Rate—Calves (Holstein-Friesian)*

Age		Weight (lbs (gm)/day)
Week	1	0.14 (64)
	2	0.45 (204)
	3	0.71 (322)
	4	0.86 (390)
	5	1.40 (636)
	6	1.60 (726)
	7 (weaned)	1.30 (590)
	8	1.90 (863)
Month	2–5	1.57 (714)
	6–10	1.66 (756)
	11–15	1.45 (657)
	16–20	1.30 (591)
	21–24	1.45 (657)

7. Pinkeye control (*Moraxella bovis*).
   a. Fly control—dust bags, ear tags.
   b. Remove eye irritation—weeds, dust, direct sun.
   c. Vaccination.
J. Six to fourteen months of age: Goal. Maintenance of good health, average daily weight gain of 1.5 lb (0.68 kg), normal estrus cycle, and optimum body size 750 lb (341 kg) for breeding by 14 months of age.
   1. Housing.
      a. No special measures need to be taken for housing during this period. In hot climates, shade should be provided for protection from sun. In temperate climates a barn (open on 1 side) is adequate for protection from inclement weather during winter months.
      b. Stocking rate of not more than 60 to 80 head per pen is recommended. Group according to size.

Table 2. *Optimum Growth Rate and Chest Circumference Measurements (Birth to 24 Months)*

Age (months)	Weight (pounds)	Weight (kilograms)	Chest Circumference (inches)	Chest Circumference (centimeters)
Birth	79–84	36–38	28	70
1	99	45	32	82
2	143	65	35	90
3	209	95	41	103
4	264	120	44	103
5	320	145	48	121
6	374	170	50	126
7	429	195	52	132
8	484	220	54	138
9	528	240	56	143
10	572	260	59	150
11	616	280	60	153
12	660	300	61	155
13	704	320	63	159
14	748	340	64	163
15	792	360	65	166
16	836	380	67	170
17	880	400	68	172
18	924	420	69	175
19	957	345	70	177
20	990	450	70.5	179
21	1034	470	71	181
22	1100	500	73	185
23	1155	525	74	188
24	1210	550	75	190
After calving	1155	525	77	195

2. Feeding program.
   a. When available, good quality pasture and roughage is adequate to provide nutritional needs for this group. Overconditioning can be a problem on occasion.
   b. Supplemental feeding must be provided when pasture or roughage is inadequate.
   c. Many different compositions of feedstuffs can be fed to this group. Of importance is the amount of energy, protein, fiber, vitamins, and minerals (refer to standards) available in feedstuffs to provide optimal weight gains at lowest cost.
   d. Provide fresh, clean water ad lib.
   e. Monitor growth rate (see Tables 1 and 2). Be aware that overconditioning can cause reduced levels of milk production.[6]
3. Vaccinations (administer 2 to 3 weeks prior to start of breeding period).
   a. Leptospirosis (5-way).
   b. IBR, PI_3 and BVD intramuscularly.
   c. *Staphylococcus aureus* (in problem herds).
4. Parasitic disease control (see V).
   a. Cattle grubs *(Hypoderma bovis)*, pour-on at time of vaccination.
5. Respiratory disease control (see IV).
6. Pinkeye control (see I 7).
7. Identification such as ear tags and tattoos must be legible for individual identification.

K. Fourteen to twenty-four months of age: Goal. Conception between 14 and 15 months of age. Prevent extremes in body condition. Average daily weight gains of more than 1.3 lb. Calve at 24 months of age, weighing 1150 lb with a condition score of 3.5.
1. Bull choice (see D 1).
2. Housing (see I 1).
3. Nutrition program (see I 2).
4. Late gestation.
   a. Ten to 14 days prior to expected parturition date move heifer to a springer pen for close observation and assistance at calving, if needed.
   b. Clip hair on flanks and udder for sanitation control.
   c. Feeding program at this time should be similar to lactation ration. Feed complete ration at the rate of 1.5 per cent of body weight by calving.
   d. Udder edema (see E 2).
5. Age at calving (see Tables 1 and 2).

L. Parturition period (see F).

III. Enteric disease control.
A. Occurrence—1 day to 3 weeks of age.
B. Causes.
  1. Bacterial.
    a. *E. coli.*
    b. *Salmonella.*
    c. *Clostridium.*
  2. Viral.
    a. Rotavirus.
    b. Coronavirus.
    c. BVD.
    d. Enterovirus.
    e. Adenovirus.
    f. Parvovirus.

  3. Sporozoa.
    a. *Cryptosporidium*
  4. Nutritional.
    a. Milk replacer.
      (1) Poor quality.
      (2) Improper preparation.
C. Prevention.
  1. Colostrum management. Feed adequate amounts of high quality colostrum as soon after birth as possible, and continue for at least the first 72 hr of life.
  2. Proper sanitation, housing, and climate.
  3. Monitor preparation of milk replacer, quantity, and interval fed (whole milk to milk replacer).
  4. Vaccinations (dry cow period).
    a. *E. coli* (K99 pili), K85, K35, K30 (capsular).
    b. *Salmonella.*
    c. Rota-corona virus.
D. Monitor.
  1. Immunoglobulin absorption.[1, 5, 7]
  2. Clinical signs.
    a. Early recognition of illness (calf feeder).
    b. Lack of appetite.
    c. Fecal consistency and character.
    d. Dehydration.
  3. Bacterial and virologic examination of fecal or intestinal contents or both.
E. Treatment. The successful treatment of neonatal diarrhea is dependent upon the calf being born in a sanitary environment and absorbing adequate levels of colostral immunoglobulins early in life. In addition, observation of calves twice daily for early detection of diarrhea is essential. The 2 most reliable therapeutic measures that I recommend are oral electrolytes (commercial products) and bismuth subsalicylate.* The recommended dosage of bismuth subsalicylate is 2 to 3 oz administered orally 2 to 4 times daily. Frequency and duration of treatment are dependent upon severity of signs. Oral electrolytes should be administered as instructed on label. Calves having diarrhea caused by salmonellosis may respond favorably when treated early with oral chloramphenicol or trimethoprim-sulfamethoxazole. However, these antimicrobial agents are not approved for food animals in the United States.
  1. Electrolyte therapy.
  2. Antidiarrheal therapy.
  3. Maintain body temperature.
  4. TLC (Tender Loving Care).

IV. Respiratory disease control.
A. Occurrence—1 to 60 days of age (milk feeding period).
B. Causes.
  1. Viral, bacterial, mycoplasmic.
    a. Colostrum deprived calves.
    b. Lack of specific antibody in colostrum.
  2. Close contact with older animals.
  3. Climatic and environmental conditions.

---

*Corrective mixture—Beecham Laboratories, Bristol, Tennessee; Antidiarrheal mixture—Affiliated Labs; Pepto-Bismol—Norwich Eaton Pharmaceuticals, Inc., Norwich, New York; Bactrim DS—Roche Laboratories, Nutley, New Jersey.

a. Stocking rate.
b. Nutrition.
c. Sanitation.
d. Humidity, draft, and temperature.
e. Bedding.
4. Other.
a. Premature birth.
b. Breech presentation, inhalation pneumonia.
C. Prevention.
1. Ensure contact between pregnant heifers and cows for at least 2 months. Through this contact it is anticipated that colostrum quality in heifers will be improved owing to active specific or nonspecific agents present in herd.
2. Vaccination of problem herds for specific agents (cows or calves or both).
3. Colostrum management. Feed adequate levels of high quality colostrum as soon after birth as possible.
4. Rear unweaned calves separately from weaned calves and older cattle.
5. Provide optimum housing, sanitation, climatic conditions, and stocking rate.
6. Provide optimum nutrition.
7. Aureomycin S700.* Add to feed at 700 mg/head/day for 21 to 28 days. Use when moving animals from individual stalls to group pens during stressful weather conditions.
D. Monitor.
1. Clinical signs.
a. Off feed.
b. Coughing.
(1) At rest.
(2) At exercise.
c. Physical examination.
2. Nasal swabs (culture).
3. Necropsy results.
4. Colostrum absorption at birth (serum proteins).
E. Treatment. Successful treatment of respiratory disease is primarily dependent upon the factors discussed in Prevention (see C). Early detection of respiratory disease, appropriate treatment, and segregation from healthy animals is extremely important in controlling clinical outbreaks.
1. Antimicrobial therapy.
a. Systemic.
b. Oral.
(1) Bolus.
(2) Medicated water or feed or both.
2. Isolation and good climate.
3. Good nutrition and small amounts of feed frequently.
F. Occurrence.
1. Two to twelve months of age.
2. Causes.
a. Viral, bacterial, mycoplasmic.
b. Lungworms.
c. Fungi.
d. Toxins.
e. Climatic and environmental conditions.
(1) Stocking rate.
(2) Mixed-age groups.

(3) Nutrition.
(4) Sanitation.
(5) Humidity, drafts, and temperature.
f. Other.
(1) Breed predisposition.
G. Prevention. Pneumonia is infrequently observed among calves being reared individually in hutches. Pneumonia can be a serious problem in heifers when they are placed in group pens after moving from hutches. The 5 most important factors to be considered in preventing pneumonia are
1. Group calves according to age.
2. Stock 10 to 15 calves per pen, 2 to 6 months of age; 30 to 50 calves per pen, 6 to 10 months of age; and 50 to 100 heifers per pen thereafter.
3. Ensure optimum ventilation and housing in colder climates, shade in sun belt climates along with sanitation.
4. Provide at 2 to 6 months of age: 500 to 1000 ft^2 per head when reared outdoors and 75 to 100 ft^2 (minimum) per head when reared indoors (northern climate).
5. Allow adequate feed bunk space 1.5 linear feet per head. Feed bunks must be cleaned daily, and calves 2–6 months old should be fed calf-growing ration free-choice. Water should be clean and accessible at all times.
6. Vaccinate. BVD, IBR, PI$_3$, and BRSV (Bovine Respiratory Syncytial Virus).
7. Deworm.
H. Monitor.
1. Clinical signs.
a. Off feed.
b. Coughing.
(1) At rest.
(2) At exercise.
c. Physical examination.
2. Nasal swabs (culture).
3. Blood samples (serology).
4. Fecal samples (lungworms, gastrointestinal parasites).
5. Necropsy results.
I. Treatment.
1. Antimicrobial therapy.
a. Systemic.
b. Oral.
(1) Medicated water or feed or both.
2. Deworming.
3. Isolation and good climatic conditions.
4. Good nutrition and feed small amounts frequently.
5. Move to clean pasture or house in case of lungworm infection (see V A 2).
J. Occurrence.
1. Twelve months and older.
2. Causes.
a. Viral.
(1) IBR.
b. Bacterial.
(1) *Pasteurella.*
(2) *Haemophilus.*
c. Climatic conditions.
3. Prevention.
a. Closed herd.
b. Vaccination.
c. Optimum housing.

*Available from American Cyanamid Co., Princeton, NJ 08540

4. Monitor.
  a. Clinical signs.
  b. Off feed.
  c. Loss of production.
  d. Nasal swabs (culture).
  e. Blood samples (serology).
  f. Necropsy results.
5. Treatment.
  a. Antimicrobial therapy.
  b. Isolation and good climatic conditions.
  c. Good nutrition and feed small amounts frequently.

V. Parasitic disease control.
  A. Endoparasites.
    1. Gastrointestinal parasites.
      a. Coccidiosis.
        (1) Occurrence—1 week to 4 months.
        (2) Prevention.
          (a) Sanitation.
            1. Place calves in clean, disinfected pen.
            2. Prevent fecal contamination of feedstuffs and water supply.
          (b) Preventive therapy (medicated feedstuffs).
            1. Amprolium*.
            2. Decoquinate.
            3. Chlortetracycline-sulfamethazine.
        (3) Monitor.
          (a) Clinical signs (loose feces and poor condition).
          (b) Fecal examination.
        (4) Treatment.
          (a) Coccidiostats.
          (b) Move to clean pen.
          (c) Improve overall sanitation.
      b. Nematodes—*Ostertagia, Cooperia, Trichostrongylus.*
        (1) Occurrence—young cattle during first pasture period.
        (2) Prevention of parasitism due to overwintered larvae.
          (a) Use of pastures that had no young stock on them in the previous year (consult grassland calendar of past year).
          (b) Start grazing at the end of May in temperate climates.
          (c) Mow pastures for hay or silage prior to grazing (consult grassland calender for current year).
        (3) Prevention of reinfection.
          (a) Move animals every 2 weeks to different parcels of pasture that have been mowed for hay or silage prior to grazing.
          (b) If (a) is not possible, graze calves behind adult cattle but not yearling cattle.
          (c) House calves at end of pasture season or earlier if pasture growth is slow.
          (d) Stocking rate depends upon pasture growth rate (number of animals per acre).
        (4) Monitor parasite level by
          (a) Fecal examination 4 to 5 weeks following placement on pasture for first time.
          (b) Clinical signs are rough hair coat, lack of weight gain, and possible diarrhea.
          (c) Review of pasture management (grassland calendar).
        (5) Treatment.
          (a) Deworm at 5 weeks of age if eggs per gram of feces (epg) are 100 to 200.
          (b) Repeat treatment every 4 weeks when pasture management is poor.
          (c) Deworm at the time of housing in temperate zones (treat for inhibited *Ostertagia* larvae).
    2. Other internal parasites.
      a. Lungworm infection *(Dictyocaulus).*
        (1) Occurrence of disease in young cattle and in older nonimmune cattle.
        (2) Prevention.
          (a) On infected farms (herd history) prevention is only possible by properly conducted vaccination.
          Use of pasture management as recommended for gastrointestinal parasite control does not provide adequate protection against lungworm infection.
          (b) Lungworm larvae overwinter on pastures and are a source of infection to susceptible cattle. Mowing pastures does not prevent infection.
          (c) Yearling cattle that are immune carriers are a source of infection to the pasture.
        (3) Prevention of reinfection.
          (a) Moving to newly seeded pasture.
          (b) Housing under good climatic conditions and feeding of silage or hay.
        (4) Monitor parasite level.
          (a) Clinical signs include coughing, abdominal breathing, and poor growth rate.
          (b) Fecal examination (refrigerate and examine within 24 hr).
          (c) Saliva examination.
          (d) ELISA or IHA test (serum sample).
        (5) Treatment.
          (a) Deworm as soon as possible after first clinical signs are observed.
          (b) House for remainder of season when growth rate is retarded.
          Pay special attention to climatic conditions in barn, as prior damage due to lungworm infection predisposes respiratory system to other infectious respiratory pathogens.
      b. Liver fluke.
        (1) Occurrence—during first pasture season and continues to adulthood.

*Available from Merck, Sharp & Dohme, Rahway, NJ 07065

(2) Prevention.
    (a) Good drainage of pasture.
    (b) Fence off poorly drained portions of pasture.
    (c) Snail control.
(3) Monitor parasite infection.
    (a) Fecal examination (1 egg = positive).
    (b) Slaughterhouse examination of liver.
    (c) Blood test (serum IHA).
(4) Treatment
    (a) Anthelmintics (January and April) such as Albendazole, Norden Laboratories, Inc., Lincoln, Nebraska.
        1. For most of these infections it is desirable for a low level of infection to exist during the susceptible period so that immunity can develop without overt signs of disease or lack of efficient and optimum weight gains.
        2. Control of gastrointestinal parasites will vary with type of housing, climatic conditions, and stocking rate.
        3. Use of anthelmintics has been a part of gastrointestinal parasite control. Kinds of products used will vary according to cost and ease of application. Deworming interval will vary according to rate and level of infection.

B. Ectoparasites.
  1. Lice—*Damalinea, Haematopinus, Linognathus,* and *Solenoptes.*
    a. Occurrence—1 month of age and older.
    b. Prevention.
      (1) Young stock: clip hair over midline.
      (2) Adults: clip hair completely.
      (3) Use clean grooming equipment.
      (4) Disinfect grooming equipment between use on adult and young cattle.
      (5) Provide good nutrition.
    c. Monitor.
      (1) Clinical signs: licking, itching, bald spots, and loss of body condition or production or both.
      (2) Inspection for lice and nits by pulling out and examining some hair.
    d. Treatment.
      (1) Ectoparasiticides (all animals in herd).
      (2) Repeat treatment in 3 weeks to kill newly hatched lice.
  2. Mange mites—*Chorioptes, Psoroptes,* and *Sarcoptes.*
    a. Occurrence.
      (1) 1 month of age and older.
      (2) Localized.
        (a) *Chorioptes*—tailhead and escutcheon.
        (b) *Psoroptes*—midline, tailhead to shoulder.
        (c) *Sarcoptes*—neck and shoulder.
    b. Prevention.

(1) Sanitation.
(2) Good nutrition.
(3) Segregation of young from adults.
(4) Disinfection of grooming equipment.
c. Monitor.
  (1) Clinical signs: skin changes, itching, bald areas, and production and condition losses.
  (2) Microscopic examination of skin scraping. Keep in mind *Ajueszky's disease.*
d. Treatment.
  (1) Ectoparasiticides (repeat in 8 to 10 days).
  (2) Disinfect grooming equipment.
3. Fungal infections (ringworm and *Trichophyton*).
  a. Occurrence—cattle of all ages.
  b. Prevention.
    (1) Sanitation.
  c. Monitor.
    (1) Clinical signs.
    (2) Microscopic examination of skin scrapings.
  d. Treatment.
    (1) Fungicides.
      Natural immunity is probably most important for recovery.

C. Flies (stable flies, horn flies). Goal: prevent irritation of skin, eyes, and teat end.
  1. Occurrence—cattle of all ages on pasture.
  2. Prevention.
    a. Repellants (synthetic pyrethrins).
    b. Sanitation (remove breeding sites).
    c. Biologic (wasps).
  3. Monitor.
    a. Observation.
  4. Treatment.
    a. Insecticide.
    b. Dust bag.
    c. Spray.
    d. Back rubber.
    e. Ear tags.
D. Cattle grubs *(Hypoderma lineatum, H. bovis).* Goal: prevent losses owing to excitement, decreased milk production, and value of hides.
  1. Occurrence—cattle of all ages on pasture.
  2. Prevention.
    a. Control of adults by treating cattle to kill larvae.
  3. Monitor.
    a. Observation and herd history.
  4. Treatment.
    a. Insecticides (organophosphates).

EVALUATION AND ANALYSIS IN RELATION TO OBJECTIVES SET

This can be performed by using the following items:
1. Number of calves born per month and per year .... ____
2. Number of calves at 2 to 10 days of age with total serum protein levels > 5 gm ..... > 95 %
3. Number of calves with enlarged umbilical stumps (> 10 mm) .... < 10 %

4. Number of calves born dead and number that have died by 24 hr following birth:
   a. Cows .... < 8 %
   b. First lactation heifers .... < 10 %
5. Number of calves that died
   a. between 24 hr and 2 months of age ...... < 6 %
   b. between 2 and 5 months of age .... < 2 %
   c. > 5 months of age .... < 2 %
6. Number of calves and heifers culled up to calving .... < 2 %
7. Number of calves and heifers sold for veal or breeding purposes .... ____
8. Frequency distribution of mortality in relation to age and diagnosis .... ____
9. Number of calves and heifers treated for diarrheal disease, birth to 4 weeks old...... < 20 %
10. Number of calves and heifers treated for pneumonia, birth to 10 months old........ < 10 %
11. Frequency distribution of calves and heifers above and below optimum weight according to age (target growth curve) .. ____
12. Average age of heifers at calving (months)...................................... < 25
13. Frequency distribution of heifers above and below optimum age at calving .... ____
14. Average condition score of heifers at calving (scale 1 to 5) 3.0–3.5
15. Estimation of economic losses due to mortality, rearing costs, and missed production days (heifers calving after 25 months of age............................... ____
16. DHIA (Dairy Herd Improvement Association) records (projected ME 305 days, milk).
    a. Projected ME 305 day milk records favor second and later lactations by approximately 500 lb milk as compared with first lactation heifers. With average genetic improvement, we would anticipate a difference in projected ME 305 days milk production records of first lactation heifers compared with second and later lactations of milk .... < 400 lb (183 kg)

CONTROL

The information, evaluation, and analysis obtained from farm visits must serve to optimize calf rearing methods. In addition, this information will show a momentary profile of the replacement rearing program that will enable farm management to become more understandable. Therefore, advice given on farm management practices regarding health status, treatment and prevention of health disorders, nutrition, and growth can be justified. A written report including recommendations should be sent to the dairy owner within 3 days of each scheduled farm visit. If necessary, goals should be reset.

CONCLUSIONS

Replacement rearing programs can only be applied if simple and practical guidelines are available. Objectives,

conditions, or data may differ between farms, states, and countries.

Guidelines for the implementation of a replacement rearing program must be adjustable to specific farm conditions or management goals. Apart from these guidelines, accurate and complete record keeping is a prerequisite to the optimal function of replacement rearing programs. Within this framework, data collected by the dairy farmer, veterinarian, and other agricultural consultants must be handled and processed so that they are relevant. This information has to be transferred to the dairy owner with a minimum loss of time in order to be functional for daily decision making.

Without the assistance of computers on large dairy farms, such information will be retrospective in nature. Computerization of data handling and analysis is an important management tool. With its use, unwanted situations regarding replacement rearing, herd health, and production control can be prevented or identified early so that optimum farm income is realized.

Supplemental Reading

1. Braun, R. K., and Tennant, B. C.: The relationship of serum gamma gobulin levels of assembled neonatal calves to mortality caused by enteric diseases. Agri-Practice 4:14–24, 1983.
2. Clapp, H. J.: What height and weight should your heifer be? Hoards Dairyman, September 25, 1981.
3. Clapp, H. J.: Charting heifer growth. Ontario Ministry of Argiculture and Food. Fact Sheet, June, 1982.
4. Fleenor, W. A., and Stott, G. H.: Hydrometer test for estimation of immunoglobulin concentration in bovine colostrum. J. Dairy Sci. 63:973–977, 1980.
5. Pfeiffer, N. E., and McGuire, T. C.: A sodium sulfide precipitation test for assessment of colostral immunoglobulin transfer to calves. J. Am. Vet. Med. Assoc. 170:809–811, 1977.
6. Sejrsen, K., et al.: Influence of nutrition on mammary development in pre- and post-puberal heifers. J. Dairy Sci. 65:793–800, 1982.
7. Tennant, B. C., et al.: Use of the glutaraldehyde coagulation test for detection of hypogamma-globulinemia in neonatal calves. J. Am. Vet. Med. Assoc. 174:848–853, 1979.
8. Wildman, E. E., et al.: A dairy cow body condition scoring system and its relationship to selected production characteristics. J. Dairy Sci. 65:495–501, 1982.

Beef and Herd Health Management

JIMMY L. HOWARD, D.V.M., M.S.,
JACK WARD, D.V.M.,
and JOHN C. SIMONS, D.V.M.

The need to develop ongoing herd health programs in beef cow and calf production units is less apparent than in dairy or feedlot operations. Ranch life is relatively pleasant and traditionally glamorous. The tendency has been for ownership and management to pass from one generation to the next. A built-in apprenticeship is readily available to interested persons who live on ranches. The procedures that make for success have evolved through trial and error. A considerable amount of empirical knowledge has been accumulated, and much of it continues to be valid. The vicissitudes of droughts, blizzards, and unstable markets have placed cow herds in strong hands and helped develop a unique and independent philosophy in the survivors. People who raise beef cattle have been traditionally reluctant to become involved with detailed records and formal contracts.

In recent times, economic pressures and tax reporting procedures are making necessary a better coordination of the many facets of the beef industry.

Those who study the problem soon become aware of the need for individual consideration for each specific situation. If a herd health program is to be meaningful, a correlated effort is needed that includes ownership, management, labor, and appropriate specialists. Specialists include the veterinarian, the nutritionist, the laboratory diagnostician, the data analyst, the tax consultant, and the banker. The area of beef nutrition is not a vastly complicated one, and veterinarians may be capable of training themselves and managers in the essentials.

The goal of the herd health program is to maintain and to improve profit margin. Good records and accurate analysis of these records are essential.

This article largely concerns itself with the role of the veterinarian. If veterinarians are to justify their existence in the herd health program, they must have general knowledge of management finance. Training of the managers and of the labor force is a prime responsibility. Unless these people understand the capabilities of veterinarians and have confidence in them, they will not be part of the program.

The essentials of the total herd health program for cow and calf production in beef cattle include the following:

1. Production goals.
2. Selection and maintenance of breeding stock.
3. Identification of problems.
4. The record-keeping system.
5. Outlining and implementing the program.

PRODUCTION GOALS

Someone has said that if you aim at nothing you will hit it every time. The first consideration of animal production is to determine and establish attainable goals. Such goals must reflect the productivity of the land, and the land should finally determine the type of livestock and the production objective. Many ranchers have gone broke attempting to irrigate with insufficient water supply or to produce livestock with insufficient energy supply. Every improvement and every new procedure costs something. It is necessary to ask and to validly answer the question "Will it pay?" before damming the creek, buying the supplement, or changing the breed.

Reasonable goals for a cow herd on a well-watered ranch of the western plains might include the following:

1. A 12-month calving interval.
2. A 95 per cent weaned calf crop.
3. A 60-day calving season.
4. Weaning weights equal to 40 per cent of the mother's normal weight.
5. Preweaning death loss < 2 per cent.
6. Postweaning death loss < 1 per cent.
7. Annual death loss in cows < 0.5 per cent.
8. Ongoing reduction of losses from disease.

Goals for a cow herd on a 12-month grazing program on mountain and desert may need to be more modest.

SELECTION AND MAINTENANCE OF THE BREEDING STOCK

The selection of the individual breeding females is generally after the fact. The question is "What are we going to do with this herd of animals?" Individuals or the entire herd can be sold and replaced, but this is not the ordinary situation. Mostly we are asking about the following:

1. Type and number of bulls.
2. A female replacement program.
3. An immunization program.
4. A program to update the status quo.
5. An emergency program.
6. Special programs for specific situations, including estrous synchronization, artificial insemination, and crossbreeding.

If advice is asked concerning breed selection, the veterinarian should probably be conservative. Reproductive efficiency, availability of replacement stock, and market preference are prime considerations. Intermediate weights and solid colors have some advantages. Conformation that lends itself to a high percentage of red meat is a sound concept that can be sought with any breed. Hereford cattle have lost ground in the market place but are still quite popular in crossbreeding programs using Angus, Simmental, Charlais, or Saler breeds as the other breed of the cross. Shorthorn cattle are said to be gaining in popularity, and Angus cattle have a solid place at the market. *Bos indicus* cattle have a place in many climates and also lend themselves to successful crossbreeding programs. The so-called exotic breeds have both advantages and disadvantages. Chianina crosses have done very well in the fat, show calf area. Temperament is an important consideration. Veterinarians should be cautious about recommending embryo transplant or exotic show calf programs in which champion prices are essential to success.

The Selection of Bulls

The average bull:cow ratio is probably about 1:25. This ratio can undoubtedly be lowered by careful selection and culling. Managers need to be specifically trained in this area. A few simple rules should be followed:

1. Introduce only virgin bulls.
2. Do not buy problems. Bulls must be able to see, eat, and walk. They also must be able to mount and intromit. Generally, if he needs surgery, he needs to be culled.
3. The testicles are the most important anatomic structures. A good buyer should be able to measure testicular size and to recognize an obvious inflammatory process. Do not buy bulls whose testicles are of less than average size for age and breed. Also do not buy bulls with detectable testicular lesions.
4. It is preferable to buy bulls that have been subjected to a meaningful breeding soundness evaluation. Such an evaluation should include the following:
   a. A general physical examination.
   b. An internal examination by rectal palpation.
   c. Semen collection and evaluation. Semen collection may be induced by rectal massage, electroejaculation, or artificial vagina. If rectal massage is used, make sure that the penis is extended and visible. The criteria for semen quality include productivity (estimated indirectly from scrotal circumference), per cent of normal spermatozoa, and degree of spermatozoa vigor. Using the Society for Theriogenology and the American College of Theriogenology scoring system, do not buy the bull if either his scrotal circumference score or his

spermatozoa morphology score is less than 24. Also do not buy him if his total score is less than 60.

5. After reproductive capability has been assured to the best extent possible, the buyer should look for conformation, pedigree, and price.

Morbidity rates on bulls are relatively high. Foot problems, eye problems, and traumatic problems from fighting or breeding all take their toll. Constant surveillance is necessary, especially in the breeding season. Only sound bulls should be over-wintered in the bull battery. Sound bulls may be used indefinitely, but the average turnover is probably less than 3 years.

The Female Replacement Program

Female replacements should be chosen for reproductive efficiency, disease resistance, and feed conversion efficiency. These are interrelated criteria that are at least somewhat measurable and lend themselves to programming. A suggested program may include the following:

1. Identification of the cow and calf: Keep it simple. Numbers under 1000 or combinations of a letter and a number under 100 work well. Plastic ear tags for the calves and plastic ear tags or carefully applied freeze brands for the cows are practical. It is a good idea to keep 2 books, including 1 of pocket size to be carried in the vehicle and 1 of a handy size to be kept in the office. Each person involved in the calving process must have a means of recording information that can be placed in the permanent record. Training a cowhand to write such information down is difficult but necessary.

2. Keeping the record: All births, deaths, abortions, retained membranes, genital prolapses, infectious diseases, and surgical processes (paste dehorning) should be recorded on both cow and calf records.

3. Branding and initial immunization procedures: Calves are ordinarily branded 2 to 6 weeks after birth. Recommended immunization procedures are controversial, and 2 schools of thought are prevalent:

   a. Vaccinate for blackleg, malignant edema, IBR, PI_3, and pasteurellosis.*

   b. Vaccinate only for blackleg and malignant edema. Proponents of this procedure hope it will aid in selection for disease resistance.

4. Grub control and continuing immunization procedures:

   a. In September, use a pour-on grub and lice control procedure or an organophosphate suspension dip for grub, lice, and mite control. Injectable parasiticides are now available and satisfactory.

   b. Vaccinate for brucellosis and revaccinate for blackleg and malignant edema.

   c. Further immunizations are optional and may include revaccination for IBR, PI_3, and pasteurellosis. Leptospirosis, *Clostridium haemolyticum*, and *C. novyi* immunizations may also be considered in special situations.

5. Weaning and selection of female replacement prospects:

   a. Keep more prospects than the ultimately required

number of replacements (generally about 150 per cent).

   b. Select for size, conformation, maternal production, and disease resistance. Generally, the largest heifers will have the other criteria.

   c. In the 4 to 6 weeks postweaning period feed a 50 per cent concentrate ration. Use a natural protein source in a complete supplement that will produce about 14 per cent crude protein in the dry matter ration. Energy values for the complete ration include

   NE_m = about 1.7 Mcal/kg DM and
   NE_g = about 1.12 Mcal/kg DM*

   Gain should equal 1 to 1.5 lb/day (0.45 to 0.7 kg).

   d. Treat any sick animals (shipping fever) with chemotherapeutic agents. Record all treatments and response.

6. Postweaning nutrition (6 weeks postweaning to breeding season): Feed to gain 0.5 to 0.7 kg/day. In northern climates, net energy for maintenance requirements will average from 0.080 to 0.095 Mcal/kg $BW^{0.75}$ (body weight) during winter. In moderate climates, the NE_m requirement will be about 0.077 Mcal/kg $BW^{0.75}$. Thus, more energy is required in cold weather. As the calves grow, the protein requirement as a per cent of the ration will decrease. A 300-kg animal requires about 35 per cent more feed than does a 200-kg animal, but the protein requirement will increase only 12 per cent, assuming a 0.6 kg/day gain. Additives such as rumensin, antibiotics, and Zeranol (Ralgro) may give positive effects. Use of additives with prospective replacement heifers is questionable. Calcium requirement will be 15 to 20 gm/day, and phosphorus requirement will be 15 to 17 gm/day. There is no need to exceed these amounts. Vitamin A requirement will be 13,000 to 16,000 IU/day. When the calves weigh over 250 kg, urea can be used as a protein supplement if the limitations for use of urea are not exceeded.

7. Prebreeding immunization:

   a. 30 to 60 days before the breeding season, vaccinate for vibriosis.

   b. Initial or booster immunizations for IBR and leptospirosis should be given concurrently with vibriosis vaccine.

   c. Booster immunizations for *Clostridium haemolyticum* or *C. novyi* or both may be given in special situations.

8. The breeding season:

   a. Breeding season for virgin heifers begins 2 to 3 weeks ahead of the cow herd to provide a longer recovery period before rebreeding after initial parturition.

   b. Breed for 2 estrus cycles (about 45 days).

   c. If artificial insemination is used, estrous synchronization with prostaglandins or a combination of progestins and estrogens should be considered. Synchro-mate† is reputed to produce good results. Care must be taken to follow the manufacturer's directions. If the calving season is subject to violent

---

*Two problems cloud the issue: a really dependable immunization procedure against the shipping fever complex has not been demonstrated, and neither has it been demonstrated that failure to contract shipping fever is a reliable method of measuring heritable disease resistance.

---

*NE_m = net energy for maintenance
DM = dry matter
NE_g = net energy for gain
†Available from Searle Animal Health Division.

weather, estrous synchronization should be considered with a degree of caution.

9. Examination of pregnancy: Best results will be achieved if the heifers are palpated 40 to 70 days after the breeding season. At this time, the final selection of the desired number of replacement heifers is made. The recommended criteria, in order of importance, are as follows:
   a. Heifers bred in the first half of the breeding season.
   b. Heifers that have a negative disease history.
   c. Heifers that come from highly productive mothers.
   d. Heifers that have desirable conformation and color.

10. Wintering the pregnant heifer: After the summer grazing season, the pregnant heifer must maintain condition and grow at a normal rate. The growth rate equals about 0.25 to 0.3 kg/day. An additional 0.4 kg/day can be expected in the last trimester, resulting from the products of conception. Through fall and winter, the pregnant heifer will require a daily intake of about 0.85 Mcal NE_m/kg $BW^{0.75}$, 1.5 to 2.5 Mcal NE_g, and the crude protein content of the DM ration should equal about 8.5 per cent. Daily mineral and vitamin requirements include calcium 20 gm, phosphorus 16 gm, potassium equal to 0.7 per cent of the dry ration, and 20,000 IU of vitamin A. Such can be provided by 20 lb of high quality prairie hay plus 0.5 to 1 lb of soybean meal or equivalent daily. Crop residues, alfalfa hay, or haylage and corn ensilage are all acceptable forage sources. Additional needs in late gestation include $0.024 \times BW/kg^{0.75}$ in Mcal NE_m, $\dfrac{1.136 \times kg\ BW/kg^{0.7}}{0.45}$ in grams crude protein, 5 gm Ca, 5 gm P, and 3000 to 5000 IU of vitamin A. It should be remembered that when the ration is in negative energy balance, additional protein will be utilized as energy. In these cases, the ration should be balanced for energy and then re-evaluated for protein. In many cases, the additional energy source will bring the protein into balance.

11. Preparturient immunization procedures:
    a. About 60 days before the calving season, the replacement heifers should receive booster immunizations for vibriosis.
    b. *Clostridium perfringens* type C bacterin may be used concurrently and 3 weeks later.

12. The calving season: The heifers will begin calving 2 to 3 weeks ahead of the cow herd and will continue for 6 to 7 weeks. Constant surveillance (every 2 hr) is necessary for optimum results. If the bulls have been carefully selected, heifers needing assistance should not exceed 10 per cent, and those requiring a cesarean section or fetotomy should not exceed 1 per cent. All cases of dystocia, genital prolapse, and retained membranes (beyond 72 hr) should be recorded. Heifers that require assistance at calving should receive systemic and intrauterine chemotherapy. Heifers that have retained membranes for more than 72 hr should also receive systemic and intrauterine chemotherapy. There is little need to manually remove fetal membranes from an intact bovine uterus.

The heifer calving pasture should have a barn that has a hot and cold water source, a place to tie up the animal and assist, some recovery stalls, and a convenient place to load on a low trailer. Standard equipment includes obstetrical chains and handles, a head snare, and a calf puller. Cleaning materials should include mild disinfectants and lubricant soaps. Hypodermic equipment should be available, such as plastic syringes (10 to 60 ml) and needles (16, 18, and 20 gauge) 1 to 1.5 in long. Drugs needed are antibiotics (penicillin and terramycin), a local anesthetic (lidocaine), a corticosteroid, oxytocin, and epinephrine. Those who are to assist in the calving process must be carefully trained in epidural anesthesia, the importance of posture and positioning, and the judicious use of a calf puller. The importance of cleanliness is a difficult concept to teach, but people who have been trained in animal health technology grasp the concept with relative ease. It is also very important that lay people recognize their limitations and that they get help when progress using normal procedures ceases.

The scourge of the calving season is calf diarrhea. The infectious causative agents are many and variable. Simple chemotherapy is often disappointing, and symptomatic treatment for dehydration and acidosis early and often is necessary for acceptable results. Oral administration of fluids is relatively convenient and is generally effective if used early. Salt, sodium bicarbonate, and nutrients can be incorporated in the treatment. Systemic and enteric use of chemotherapeutic agents and vitamins give variable results. Gut relaxants (paregoric) and protectants (mineral oil or Kaopectate*) may be used to some advantage.

Subcutaneous fluids containing dextrose and electrolytes are effective if dehydration is slight to moderate. Large amounts of isotonic fluids will absorb water from subcutaneous sites if water balance mechanisms are functional. Calves that are in a state of dehydration, where water loss approaches or exceeds 8 per cent of body weight, will need intravenous (IV) rehydration. IV rehydration requires special facilities and technical skills. Unless there is someone on the ranch skilled in animal health technology, it is probably wise to haul these calves to drive-in clinics for 24- to 48-hr treatments. However, re-uniting such calves with their mothers can be a problem. Best results will be achieved if the calf is returned precisely to the spot where it was picked up, and flagging the spot is a worthwhile procedure.

The practical essentials of fluid therapy for diarrheic calves are relatively simple. Time and economics will limit monitoring, so a number of assumptions must be made.
   a. Calves requiring IV therapy will be in states of dehydration, acidosis, hypoglycemia, generally hyperkalemia, and often shock.
   b. The specific molecules and ions that will be in deficit are water, dextrose, Na^+, Cl^-, HCO_3^-, and K^+.
   c. Do-it-yourself formulation of fluid preparations is a highly economical procedure. If recipes are provided, animal health technicians can be trained to mix and use them. The sources of the deficient molecules and ions include the following:
      (1) Distilled water.
      (2) Sterile 50-per cent dextrose solution.

---

*Available from The Upjohn Co., Kalamazoo, Michigan 49001.

(3) Sterile sodium bicarbonate solution (8.4 per cent).*

(4) Pure KCl.

(5) Concentrated (10×) electrolyte solutions that contain NaCl, NaHCO$_3$, and KCl. A dilution of 1:9 with distilled water yields an isotonic solution of Na$^+$ 142 Meq, Cl$^-$ 117 Meq, and HCO$_3^-$ 30 Meq/L.

The rehydrating solutions should be hypertonic (600 to 700 Meq/l). Maximum rates of infusion can equal normal total blood volume per hour until rehydration is complete.

Example: If dehydration is equal to 10 per cent of normal body weight (the calf is weak, the corneas are dry, and the skin is not pliable), the water loss from an 80-lb calf will be about 4 L (4000 ml). The normal blood volume is estimated as 7 per cent of normal body weight (0.07 × 80 = 5.6 lb, 2.55 kg, 2550 gm, or 2550 ml).†

Thus, the rehydration fluid can be administered at a rate of 2500 ml/hr. Rehydration can be achieved in $\frac{4000}{2500} \times 60 = 96$ minutes. This rate of infusion should not be exceeded, but slower rates are acceptable and may be desirable.

After rehydration is complete, a maintenance preparation (400 to 450 Meq/L) is used at a rate of about 300 ml/hr until the calf is discharged.

Table 1 presents a usable recipe for a hypertonic rehydration fluid formulation, showing amounts of ingredients, ion concentrations, and total milliequivalents for each molecule or ion.

Table 2 has a usable recipe for a hypertonic maintenance fluid formulation, showing amounts of ingredients, ion concentrations, and total milliequivalents.

Recent research at Colorado State University indicates that hypertonic IV solutions may contain higher concentrations of glucose or potassium or both. Up to 800 ml of 50-per cent glucose and 3 gm of KCl per 4000 ml of solution may produce a positive effect. Also, the maintenance solution can contain up to 120 ml of 8.4-per cent NaHCO$_3$ solution and 1.5 gm of KCl per 4000 ml for as long as the diarrhea persists without producing problems.

13. Immunizations in the calving season: The use of coronavirus and rotavirus oral vaccines in newborn calves have generally been effective when the viruses are present and cause problems. The products are expensive, however, and a positive diagnostic laboratory test result should be established before their routine use is implemented. More recently, a combination of lyopholized rota-corona virus has been prepared for injection into pregnant cows in late gestation. The vaccine is reconstituted in a liquid bacterin containing antibodies against a specific strain of E. coli selected for its high K99 pili content. Two injections of the vaccine (2 ml each) is required for maximum efficacy. The second dose may be given 2 to 3 weeks after the first dose. The entire procedure should be completed not later than 3 weeks prior to calving. This vaccine is reputed to cut morbidity rates by 50 per cent and mortality rates by 75 per cent.

*Commercial NaHCO$_3$ solutions must be used to avoid the toxicity of Na$_2$CO$_3$ that forms with simple mixing procedures.

†The specific gravity of extracellular fluid is assumed to be 1 (1 gm/ml).

Table 1. *Hypertonic Rehydration Fluid Formulation*

Ingredient	Amount	Meq/gm or L*	Total Meq
50 % dextrose	400 ml	2750/L	1100
10X electrolyte solution	400 ml	2940/L	1176
8.4 % NaHCO$_3$	120 ml	2000/L	240
Pure KCl	1.5 gm	27/gm	40
Distilled water	3080 ml	—	—
Total	4000 ml		2556

*Meq/L = $\frac{2556}{4}$ = 639

The principle involves the production of more effective colostrum by the cows.

THE IMMUNIZATION PROGRAM

A wide variety of biologics are available for use in cattle. Some are used routinely in practically all cattle, some are used only in special situations in which the causative organisms are expected to be present in significant numbers, and some are of doubtful value. Immunization procedures can generally be applied while the cattle are being handled for other purposes, including branding, grub control, or pregnancy examination. A common year-round program may include the following:

1. At branding time for the calves.
   a. *Clostridium chauvoei* and *C. septicum* bacterins.
   b. IBR and PI$_3$ vaccines (optional).
   c. *Pasteurella* bacterin (optional).
2. In conjunction with grub control procedures.
   a. Booster shots for IBR, PI$_3$, and *C. chauvoei*, *C. septicum*, and *Pasteurella* bacterins.
   b. Give brucellosis vaccine to heifer calves.
   c. Yearly boosters for vibriosis and *C. perfringens* type C if the cows are examined for pregnancy.
3. At weaning time.
   a. Intranasal applications of IBR and PI$_3$ agents if previous immunization has not been possible.
   b. Yearly boosters for vibriosis and *C. perfringens* type C if pregnancy examination is done at this time.
4. In the last trimester of gestation.
   a. Initial vaccination for vibriosis and *C. perfringens* type C in purchased replacements that are pregnant.
   b. Initial vaccination for *C. perfringens* type C and boosters for vibriosis in pregnant first calf heifers.
   c. Rota-corona virus and *E. coli* bacterin in all pregnant cows and heifers (includes 2 injections, 2 to 3 weeks apart).
5. In the calving season.
   a. Oral coronavirus and rotavirus vaccines for baby calves.
   b. Booster immunizations for IBR in adult cows in some situations.

Table 2. *Hypertonic Maintenance Fluid Formulation*

Ingredient	Amount	Meq/gm or L*	Total Meq
50 % dextrose	300 ml	2750/L	825
10X electrolyte solution	300 ml	2940/L	882
8.4 % NaHCO$_3$	60 ml	2000/L	120
Pure KCl	1 gm	27/gm	27
Distilled water	3340 ml	—	—
Total	4000 ml		1854

*Meq/L = $\frac{1854}{4}$ = 463.5

SURVEILLANCE OF THE COW HERD

Daily surveillance by management or labor or both is necessary. The veterinarian will likely see the adult cow herd once a year if no significant emergency situation arises. The cows should be examined for pregnancy and age in conjunction with grub control or weaning procedures. The cow herd will be culled at this time. Cows to be removed from the breeding herd are open cows, cows that have weaned a substandard calf, and cows that have a history of prolapsed genitalia, eye problems, lumps, mastitis, or chronic foot problems.

Nutritional considerations for adult cows are very similar to those of heifers, but they are not complicated by an NE_g requirement for growth.

Ordinarily, the quality of the forage ration will be at its best when the requirements are highest (peak lactation and the breeding season). Droughts or late springs may complicate the situation. The areas of most concern are energy and phosphorus deficiency in late gestation and early lactation, energy and magnesium deficiency when the grass is lush, and energy deficiency in the breeding season. Generally, if energy is not in negative balance, the protein need is being met.

THE EMERGENCY PROGRAM

Emergency situations are most likely to be avoided if they are anticipated. Management and technical help need to be properly informed about a number of possibilities.

1. Pulmonary emphysema: Do not move cows from dry upland pastures to wet meadows without expecting problems and planning alternatives.

2. If outside replacements must be introduced, check anaplasmosis, brucellosis, and leptospirosis titers, and vaccination history (especially vibriosis and brucellosis). Do not introduce used bulls.

3. See bulls every day, especially in single sire mating situations.

4. Do not introduce the cow herd to cornstalks without checking on how much corn is still in the field.

5. Approach the use of legume pastures with extreme caution. Use detergent supplements and fill the cows before turning them on the pasture.

6. If winter calving is part of the program, a positive energy balance and adequate phosphorus and magnesium levels in the ration are important.

Prepare for emergencies. Some dependable person on the ranch should be knowledgeable in venipuncture, the use of stomach tubes, the principles of restraint, the importance of reading labels and other instructions, and the dangers of hurrying.

Perhaps the best contribution to be made by the veterinarian is to gain the confidence of the cowhands and to educate them.

A well cared for and updated drug supply is needed on the ranch, including a sympathetic stimulant, 2 or more chemotherapeutic agents, a corticosteroid preparation, a local anesthetic, a tranquilizer, and a laxative.

A refrigerator makes a good, clean storage place for all drugs except high volume entities (mineral oil and magnesium oxide preparations).

A portable branding chute and portable corrals can be lifesavers. A great deal can also be accomplished with a snow fence and steel posts.

SPECIAL PROGRAMS

AI presents a number of advantages, including the use of outstanding sires and better control of venereal diseases. However, there are some significant limitations. Acceptable results will be obtained only if the AI technician is adequately trained. Basic courses are available at a number of colleges and universities. The various business groups of the AI industry also provide training courses. A special type of individual is necessary: the inseminator must be methodical, meticulous, and understand 3 principles:

1. The cow is made of living tissue that is subject to injury and infection.

2. Semen contains living cells that can easily be killed.

3. A technique must be developed that minimizes risk both to the semen and the cow.

AI will not enhance the fertility of the cow herd. The handling of the cows is time consuming and expensive. The cows must be confined in pastures of a handy size that are designed to accommodate movement. Nutrition must be complete and balanced, and a weight gaining situation is necessary for optimum results.

The advent of prostaglandins and progestin-estrogen combinations has made estrous synchronization a practical possibility, and the AI process can be accomplished with a minimum amount of time. The cows need handling 2 to 3 times, so care must be exercised in planning and building the facility. If the calving season is subject to violent weather, the use of estrous synchronization should be approached with caution. In most cases, the insemination program will include only 1 estrous cycle. A cleanup bull program must be planned to include 40 to 50 per cent of the cow herd.

There are distinct advantages to crossbreeding. Greater disease resistance and feed conversion efficiency are expected consequences. F-1 breeding cows are reputed to be superior to straight bred counterparts in milk production, disease resistance, and feed conversion efficiency.

The disadvantages of crossbreeding lie in the complications of the replacement program. Ordinarily, 3 generations of cows exist in a cow herd. Using the same bulls, 3 dilutions are produced that will provide a lot of variety in the calf crop. This may not be serious in large herds that can be conveniently divided or in calves that can be sorted into saleable groups for uniformity. Hereford-Angus and Hereford-Simmental crosses continue to be popular. In recent years, infusions of Chianina genes is common, particularly in Angus cattle. Charolais and Limousine crosses are especially sought after by cattle who are interested in early finishing programs. The production of F-1 replacement heifers may be a lucrative program, and the purchase of F-1 replacements may be a viable alternative.

IDENTIFICATION OF PROBLEMS

Problems are more easily solved if they are recognized early. The opportunity to see early signs of trouble is greatest first for the cowhand, second for the manager, and last for the veterinarian. For optimum results, the cowhand must be taught to observe and report. Significant observations are dead, sick, and lame animals, animals off by themselves, lonely cows without calves, lonely calves without mothers, abortions, signs of estrus at times other than the breeding season, and problems with the water supply. Astute observation and reporting must be commended if it is to be a fact of the program.

The veterinarian will be on the ranch for emergency situations and for some routine procedures (breeding soundness evaluations for bulls and pregnancy examinations for females). Ongoing records and yearly comparisons will identify trends and progress.

The diagnostic process is a veterinary responsibility. The complete physical examination, necropsy, sampling for laboratory analysis, and interpretation of findings cannot easily be delegated to lay people. Each death and abortion should be investigated as a possible herd problem. The complete diagnostic process is not infallible, but it is vastly superior to random guessing. Paired serology samples are inconvenient, and fluorescent antibody identification is beset with gray areas of interpretation. In many cases, it is probably advantageous to use both of these techniques. Bacterial culture is still a valid procedure. Basic techniques can be used at the clinic level if laboratory service is inconvenient. Recently, diagnostic kits have been developed that enable performance of 16 differential tests for common pathogenic bacteria. In addition, a number of kits are being devised to help diagnose specific viral agents in the field.

The most prevalent and expensive disease in the cow and calf operation is the shipping fever complex. Morbidity rates in excess of 20 per cent are common, and mortality rates of 2 per cent are probably average. The primary causes are multiple and are triggered by stress. Death is largely from secondary bacterial infection. The most common isolates are *Pasteurella multocida* and *P. haemolytica*. A *Haemophilus*-like organism tentatively classified as *H. somnus* is often involved, especially late in the season. The ordinary syndrome is characterized by elevated temperature, nasal discharge, and respiratory distress. *H. Somnus* infections often produce central nervous system disturbances from thromboembolic meningoencephalitis (TEME).

Necropsy results of *Pasteurella* infected calves generally reveal fibrinous pleuritis and lobar pneumonia. Microscopically, the lesions are typical of an acute exudative fibrinous bronchopneumonia.

Antibiotics and sulfa drugs provide the basics of therapy. Susceptibility to specific chemotherapeutic agents is not always predictable. A recommended procedure includes the following steps:

1. Treat the calves with maximum doses of a bactericidal agents, such as penicillin, penicillin derivatives, or tetracycline compounds, and collect laboratory samples, including nasal swabs from live animals or lung samples from dead ones or both. Epinephrine should be available to treat anaphylactic reactions.
2. Send the samples to a laboratory for culturing and sensitivity testing. The local veterinary clinic may have this capability.
3. Continue treatment for 3 to 4 days.
   a. If the response is positive, continue to use penicillin or the specific derivative as a primary therapeutic agent if other animals become affected.
   b. If the response is negative, change chemotherapeutic agents according to the results of the sensitivity tests.

Supportive treatment involves whatever can be done to provide comfort and nutrition. A shed or windbreak, potable water, adequate bedding, and high quality dry forage are essential. The use of corticosteroids, vitamins, and diuretics is common. Experimental studies have generally failed to show definite positive results from the use of these agents. In fact, the use of corticosteroids is contraindicated.

No really satisfactory immunization program has been demonstrated. IBR and PI$_3$ vaccines and *Pasteurella* and *Haemophilus* bacterins are commonly used. Experimental results are generally positive in terms of long-time gain and profit, but there seems to be little effect on morbidity or mortality in the weaning season. The use of biologics as treatment is not generally recommended.

Weaning procedures designed to minimize stress offer apparent advantages, but morbidity and mortality have occurred using every known program. Recommended procedures include the following:

1. Creep feed the calves using 0.5 to 1.5 kg of concentrate /calf/day for the last 30 to 40 days of the preweaning period.
2. Provide a good forage source for the cows and calves at weaning time.
3. Wean the cows from the calves in 2 or more groups over a period of about 1 week.
4. If forage is abundant, wean the calves late (at 8 or 9.5 months of age).
5. Calves receiving a significant amount of milk and some grain are conditioned to concentrates. Postweaning rations containing 50 to 70 per cent concentrates may be used and are generally economically advantageous.
6. Early weaning (3 to 5 months of age) may be desirable. These calves do well on oats and high quality forage if a natural protein source is used to support the desired gain.

THE RECORD KEEPING SYSTEM

Uniform record systems are being marketed by several sources. Data analysis by computers has arrived in the realm of ordinary business. Microcomputers or access to network minicomputers or both have come into common use, and software covering every facet of agricultural practice is readily available. There is little excuse for not keeping good records, but getting them written down when they happen continues to be a problem. Neither the veterinarian nor the rancher is famous for keeping meticulous records. It is probably necessary that someone be specifically accountable. This person will generally have to nag cowhands, managers, technicians, and veterinarians for information on a daily basis. Keeping track of vital information for registration purposes has long been a problem but a necessary practice for purebred operations. Systems have evolved that provide models for commercial units.

The essence of record keeping for the beef cow and calf operation is simplicity. The vital information is less complex than in the case of dairy or purebred operations.

Vital information for individual cows is birth date, complete immunization records, complete medical records, the dates and status of pregnancy examinations, and weaning weights for the calves.

For calves, it is necessary to record birth dates, sex, complete immunization and medical procedures, and weaning weights.

For prospective replacement heifers, continuing immunization and medical records and the results of the initial pregnancy examination are needed. If a heifer is chosen as a replacement, she acquires a permanent individual cow record.

For a bull the date of acquisition, the original breeding soundness evaluation record, ongoing immunization and medical records, subsequent breeding soundness evaluation records, and the identification of the cows that he is exposed to, especially in single mating programs, are necessary.

Most record systems stress feed conversion efficiency. The concern is with weight and weight gain. Immunization, medical, and pregnancy examination records are often overlooked or kept separately. It is a simple matter to design a 5×8 card that will show all vital information if both sides of the card are used. It is convenient to use code systems for immunization procedures and problems. If a usable computer program is not available, a filed record system that can be analyzed both on an individual and on a herd basis is necessary. We recommend an alphabetic or numeric card file or both for individual cows. The first 2 cards should contain a herd summary and a coding system. The physiologic states, such as pregnancy, parturition, and problems, can be designated by colored metal clip tags on the cards. Examples are blue for pregnancy, green for postparturition, and red for problems. Examples of usable codes are listed next.

Immunization Code

Antigen	Code
Blackleg and malignant edema	B
Brucellosis	Br
Clostridium perfringens type C	Cp
IBR	I
Leptospirosis	L
Pasteurella	Pa
PI$_3$	P
Rota-corona virus	Rc
Vibriosis	V

Problem Code

Antigen	Code
Actinomycosis or bacillosis	Ac
Anaplasmosis	An
BVD	Bvd
Brucellosis	Br
Calf diarrhea	Cd
Cancer eye	Ce
Foot rot	Fr
IBR	I
Pulmonary emphysema	Pe
Shipping fever	Sf
TEME	Te
Trichomoniasis	Tr

IMPLEMENTING THE HERD HEALTH PROGRAM

The involvement of veterinarians in beef cow and calf herd health programs can largely be classified into 3 categories.

1. Veterinarians are employed full time. They may be the owner, part owner, manager, or full time specialist.

2. Veterinarians are regularly employed part time on a fee basis for each specific need.

3. Veterinarians are employed on a contract basis for a monthly salary based on projected time spent or numbers of cases involved.

Full Time Employment

The most successful involvement by veterinarians is full time employment. Close relationships with lay help, in-service training, and correlation with specialists are relatively easy to achieve. Generally, management will have more trust in veterinarians if they are not involved elsewhere, especially with competing institutions or endeavors that distract their attention. In these cases, instruction can be given with authority, and pressure can be brought to bear to implement the principle. Equipment and drugs can be purchased on a wholesale basis, and the veterinarian is likely to be on the property when he or she is needed. Unfortunately, the number of opportunities for such employment is limited. Generally, basic veterinary education is deficient in this area. Students training to be veterinarians have a definite advantage if they are from a ranch, and have additional education in animal science, genetics, and nutrition.

Part Time Employment

The most prevalent situation is for veterinarians to be involved in a limited way. They operate general or limited practices and are used on the ranch in specific situations. If there is sufficient interest and dedication, the involvement can be quite sophisticated. Voluntary in-service training for ranch help and printed recommendations can be of considerable help. The areas of responsibility may include the following:

1. Veterinarians outline the immunization programs in writing and sell the biologics to the ranch at a competitive markup. They instruct the ranch employees in the use and storage of these products and inspect the storage facilities when they are there.

2. They recommend and furnish the drug and equipment inventory at competitive prices and give specific instructions in care and usage.

3. They provide special technology as needed.
   a. The pregnancy examination of heifers and cows.
   b. Breeding soundness evaluations for bulls.
   c. Complicated surgery. He or she may provide instruction for ranch employees in a number of techniques, including branding, castration, dehorning, abscess drainage, hemostasis, and animal restraint.

4. Veterinarians can be knowledgeable in the area of nutrition, including mathematical computation of rations. They may be the nutrition specialist or they may need to understand what the nutrition specialist does.

5. They need access to the ranch records and to understand them. Veterinarians also need access to the ranch calendar for scheduling.

6. His or her advice may be sought in the disposition of cull animals.

7. The veterinarian will be called in the case of an epizootic situation, will perform necropsies on all dead animals, and will act as a liaison between the ranch and the diagnostic laboratory.

8. They may conduct seminars for ranch employees from specific ranches or communities on a free service or fee basis. They will also use routine visits and emergency calls as in-service training opportunities for ranch employees.

Text continued on page 147

Cow Card

Cow no. A32			Year Born: 1972						

Year	Day calf born	Sex	Age at weaning	Wean-ing weight	Index	Acc. index	Other data and remarks	Sire	Grade
72									
73									
74	3/10	M	220	380				A6	
75	3/23	M	207	410				B9	
76	3/15	F	215	415				?	
77	4/1	F	200	390				?	
78	3/28	M	203	410				?	
79	3/22	F	208	400				?	
80	4/2	M	198	405				?	
81	4/6	M	194	390				?	

Figure 1. Cow card (front of 5 × 8 card).

Other data and remarks

		Heifer replacements		Year	Ck. pg	Immunizations			
		Year born	Herd no.	1972		3 Rc	6 B I P Pa	9 B I P Pa	Br
Cow no. A32	Year born: 1972								
Cow record				1973	Aug. 20	$V^1, ^2V$			
Day born	3/22			1974	Oct. 25	V^1 Cp	C^2_p	V^{10}Cp	
Age at weaning	208 days			1975	Oct. 20		V^{10}Cp		
Weaning weight	410			1976	Oct. 21		V Cp		
Index				1977	Oct. 22		V Cp		
Grade	A			1978	Oct. 23		V Cp		
12-month weight				1979	Oct. 20		V Cp		
18-month weight				1980	Oct. 22		V Cp		
Sire	74 or 80			1981	Oct. 20				
Dam	A 140								
Final record									
Age	9								
No. calves weaned	8								
Avg. index									

Figure 2. Cow card (back of 5 × 8 card).

Individual Cow Record

Cow no. | Birth date

Grand sire

Grand sire

Sire

Dam

Grand dam

Grand dam

Cow's Performance Record | Other data and remarks

Weaning age
Actual weaning weight
Daily gain
Adjusted weaning weight
Weaning grade
12-month weight
Daily gain
18-month weight
Daily gain

Figure 3. Individual cow record (front).

Cow-Calf Performance Record

Cow no. | Birth date

Calf Performance Record

	Herd		Birth				Weaning						Disposal, Remarks, Other Data
Year	number	Sex	Day	Wt.	Sire's number	Age in days	Actual weight	Daily gain	Adjusted weight	Grade	12-month weight	18-month weight	

Figure 4. Cow-calf performance record (back).

University of Wyoming — College of Agriculture — Agricultural Extension Service

WEANING RECORD
FORM PT-3 (1-73-1M-2)

Ranch... Dates: From.............................. to..............................

Cow Number	Year Cow Born	S E X	WEAN WT.		Grade	Index	Remarks	Cow Number	Year Cow Born	S E X	WEAN WT.		Grade	Index	Remarks
			Steer	Heifer							Steer	Heifer			

Figure 5. Weaning record.

University of Wyoming — College of Agriculture — Agricultural Extension Service

BREEDING HERD INVENTORY
FORM PT-1 (4-72-1M-2) (1-73-1M-2)

Ranch_____ Dates: From_____ to_____

Cow Number	Year Cow Born			Remarks	Cow Number	Year Cow Born			Remarks

Figure 6. Breeding herd inventory.

CALF CROP WEANING WORK SHEET
Use separate sheets for heifers, bulls and steers

Name_____

Address_____   Sex_____

1	2	3	4	5	6	7	8	9	10	11	12	13	14	15	16	17
Dam No.	Sire No.	Calf No.	Day of Wean.	Day of Birth.	Wean. age Days	Actual Wean. Wt.	Birth Wt.	Gain in Wt.	Daily Gain	Age Adj.	Adj. Gain	Adj. Wean. Wt.	Age of Dam	Dam Adj.	Adj. Dam Wt.	Grade

Figure 7. Calf crop weaning work sheet.

The disadvantages of the part time, fee basis involvement is insecurity and unavailability. Veterinarians so involved will be subjected to both competition and distractions. Distractions come from the "fire engine" part of the practice and the competition comes from the itinerant, self-styled specialist who can outpromise them. Group practice and quality service tend to dilute these problems.

Contract Employment

In this case, the service rendered is identical to the fee service program. The advantages are said to be in greater security derived from a signed contract and a better awareness of veterinary responsibility by everyone concerned. Educational institutions seem to favor this arrangement. The situations in which this arrangement exist are far outnumbered by more loosely structured fee basis programs. Possible reasons include the following:

1. The rancher traditionally fears the formal contract and sees it as a trap.

2. Contracts may be overcomplicated and imply loss of flexibility.

3. Progress is generally slow and contains some ups and downs.

4. The calf market is also full of rather sensational ups and downs, and the enthusiasm of the rancher follows the market.

5. Inexperienced veterinarians have been inclined to outpromise their capability and produce some disenchantment.

Undoubtedly, the future trend will be toward more formal and sophisticated arrangements. The advantage will be to those who have sincere concepts of complete veterinary service and to those who can make adjustments between abstract theory and complex situations and between personal aims and ideas and a world full of interests, opinions, and ideas that are different from their own.

Supplemental Reading

Agricultural Extension Service: University of Wyoming, Laramie: Measure Up, a performance testing program for Wyoming commercial beef producers. Bulletin 556: September, 1971.
Annual Conference for Veterinarians: Proceedings of Seminar. Management, Nutrition and Diarrhea of the Newborn Calf, CSU, Fort Collins, Colorado. January 11, 1976.
Bierschwal, C. J., and deBois, C. H. W.: Fetotomy in Large Animals. Bonner Springs, Kansas, VM Publishing, Inc.
Lofgreen, G.: Feeding the Sick Feeder Calf. Bovine Nutrition, Preconvention Seminar II, Eleventh Annual Conference AABP, Seminar Proceedings. Baltimore, 102–112, 1978.
National Academy of Sciences, National Research Council, no. 4. Nutrient Requirements of Beef Cattle. 1976.
Roberts, S. J.: Veterinary Obstetrics and Genital Diseases (Theriogenology). Ann Arbor: Edwards Brothers, Inc., 1971.
The Society for Theriogenology. A Compilation of Current Information on Breeding Soundness Evaluation and Related Subjects. vol. VII, 2nd ed., 1976.
USDA. Guidelines for Uniform Beef Improvement Programs. Beef Improvement Federation Recommendation Program Aid 1020, 1970.
Zemjanis, R.: Diagnostic and Therapeutic Techniques in Animal Reproduction. Baltimore: Williams & Wilkins, 1962.

Beef Cow and Calf Herd Health Management (Large Range Herds)

ROBERT BOHLENDER, D.V.M.

A herd health program is a series of disease prevention procedures and of efficiency control measures that are each economically justifiable. We could well refer to the program as economical performance medicine.

Economic pressures have encouraged both the cattle and the industrialist veterinary practitioner to move toward programmed veterinary care. The end result must be a positive impact on the profit margin for the cattle producer and the veterinarian. An important factor in the evolution and success of programmed medicine is the development of constructive attitudes in all parties involved.

The various production systems and their individual complexities require the practitioner to become familiar with each ranch operation. Veterinarians must be realistic, however, in developing workable herd programs. Herd size, facilities, available labor force, disease problems, and degree of sophistication are all factors to consider when working with the client.

Local practitioners are more aware of area attitudes, climate, nutrition, disease problems, parasite levels, and management trends than any other professionals in their area. Through contact with a ranch, the practitioner can encourage preventive procedures with each diagnosis. The program must be reactive with a constant consideration of cost-benefit factors.

An adequate, tailor-made program for a large cow herd must be well structured. Because of the large number and high investment per cow unit extensive diagnostic efforts are justified. Any added procedure or program alteration must be based on a cost-benefit factor. This often requires diagnostic backup to project potential loss.

The veterinarian's role becomes extensive and multifaceted. It will include diagnosis, training personnel, outlining and supervising the preventive program, and detection and treatment of individual animals. The veterinarian will be responsible for the control and eventually the prevention of emergency situations. He or she will also be responsible for routine procedures, such as breeding soundness evaluation of the bulls and pregnancy palpation of the cows.

In recent years, the veterinarian has played an increasingly important role in the marketing of calves, yearlings, and culled cows. As retained ownership becomes more popular and as the computerized feedlots identify producers with poor health performance, sound preventive health programs will receive more credibility.

A cow and calf program by necessity is complex because it involves a wide range of ages and breeds, both sexes, and the seasonal nature of calving, breeding, weaning, wintering, and marketing.

An effective herd health management program is a form of management by objectives. The producer and the veterinarian should establish goals, create an action plan within a time frame, establish areas of responsibility, and evaluate the results of the program. Additions, deletions, or modifications of the health program should be made based on the evaluation.

Client education is a key part of evolving and maintaining the program. It is important to expose clients to modern veterinary medicine. They must be aware of all the various services, their costs, and their advantages.

As a herd health program evolves, some transfer of responsibility for various phases of the veterinary care must occur. The practitioner becomes more involved with the herd and the producer becomes more involved with the individual animal. Properly structured, individual animal care will be improved, and the properly trained producers will become more adept at recognizing sick calves. Producers will also develop an ability to detect early symptoms of disease and recognize a case that is not routine and call upon the veterinarian for a diagnosis.

GOALS

As the herd health management program evolves, the veterinarian and the producer should establish goals. Set down long-term production goals along with more specific goals, within a time frame, of percentages, weights, and marketing. These must be closely monitored with good, usable record keeping.

The long range goals of the herds health program should include the following:

1. Improve and maintain reproductive performance.
2. Improve calving performance and calf survival.
3. Improve control of disease and parasites.
4. Maximize production of marketable calf weight per cow unit.
5. Improve marketing and efficient cow herd culling.
6. Prevent drug residues and adverse reactions.

It would be difficult to establish realistic percentages for all regions of the United States. However, attempts should be made to maximize production using all the available resources.

REPRODUCTIVE PERFORMANCE

The most important single demand in the cow and calf operation is a high conception rate in the shortest possible breeding season.

A workable record keeping system is imperative if progress is to be attained in reproductive performance. These records should reflect pregnancy rate, length of calving season, calf mortality, and culling rates. This data should indicate diagnosis of problems, and age groups in which performance is low. Individual animal identification is important to maintain adequate records to assist in making culling and selection decisions.

Nutrition is a key management factor for achieving a high pregnancy rate and a short calving season. In many cow and calf operations, including many large ranches, the nutritionist is not utilized properly. Veterinarians should prepare themselves to recognize problems or inefficiencies in nutrition and encourage consultations or corrections.

The limiting factor related to reproduction is usually energy. The level of energy prior to calving influences the calving to estrous interval, while the level of energy after calving primarily influences the conception rate. The cow age, weight, and condition along with the level of milk production influence the nutritional demands to maintain performance.

Feed requirements vary during the reproductive cycle and should be broken down by stages:

Period 1 of 82 days (interval from calving to breeding). This is the period of greatest nutritional demand. The cow is at her maximum milk production, in many areas is under adverse weather conditions, and is recovering from parturition and should be pregnant by the end of the period. The cow will utilize by priority available nutrients for (1) maintenance, (2) lactation, and (3) reproduction.

Period 2 of 123 days (interval from rebreeding to weaning). The cows should gain weight while still producing milk enough to have the calf gain to its genetic potential.

Period 3 of 110 days (from weaning to 50 days before calving). This is the period that is significant in economizing the year's feed costs. The requirements are less than at any other stage of the cycle, but in many regions weather conditions are variable. The cow should be able to maintain condition, and the fetus should develop.

Period 4 of 50 days (a critical stage preceding calving). The requirements are greater in this period because 75 per cent of fetal growth occurs during the last 50 days. The return to estrum will be delayed in a cow that is losing weight or not gaining weight during this period.

There are significant variations in nutrient values of roughages and feed gains from year to year, so feed analysis and balancing rations are important. Changeable trace mineral concentrations within or among different geographic regions also support the use of feed analysis information.

Replacement Heifer Selection and Preparation

The producer has considerable expense in developing a replacement heifer until her first calf is marketed. This expense along with the genetic impact the replacement has in an aggressive breeding program makes the selection and preparation of heifers another key part of ranch management.

By breeding the yearling heifer 3 weeks before the main cow herd, they receive the extra attention they need at calving time and have the extra time to rebreed. Puberty is a function of age, breed, and weight, so heifers should be sufficiently developed. Adequate growth must be achieved without too much fat to avoid jeopardizing potential milk production.

The worming and vaccinating programs are designed to control diseases in heifers through weaning and winter as well as through the breeding season, pregnancy, and colostral production to protect her calf.

Pelvic evaluation can be done before breeding to aid in control of dystocia. By using a square centimeter (cm²) to birth weight ratio, the approximate weight of the calf that the 2-year-old heifer can deliver can be estimated. Determine the total cm² by multiplying the distance between the right and left shaft of the ilium by the distance from the pubic symphysis to the sacrum. Divide the answer by 2.2 to obtain the weight the heifer can deliver. By using a 2:1 ratio, and by selecting bulls to sire calves of a predictable weight, cases of dystocia can be reduced. Pelvic evaluation can also be done at the same time as the pregnancy palpation. The timing of pelvic evaluation should fit the individual herd's needs.

Bull Management

In most large cow and calf operations bulls are the only herd additions. Care must be taken to prevent the introduction of disease into the cow herd at this time. Adequate selection, testing, worming, vaccination, and isolation of the new bulls is mandatory. Only virgin bulls should be introduced into the herd.

The new bulls should be purchased early enough (60 days before the breeding season) to allow them to adapt to the environment and to establish their position in the herd's "pecking order."

Management of bull selection and evaluation of the bull's performance are important aspects of beef improvement. The use of performance tested bulls is recommended, especially in large range herds where individual performance testing might be difficult.

A breeding soundness evaluation of all new bulls should be a prerequisite of purchase. Be sure to counsel the client to buy sound bulls with good scrotal circumferences. A positive relationship between scrotal circumference and sperm production exists. Bulls with small testes tend to produce a higher percentage of abnormal spermatozoa, and young bulls with small testes usually also have small testes at maturity. Young bulls with above average scrotal circumference and good sperm morphology tend to sire heifers that reach puberty at an early age. The average scrotal circumference may vary appreciably for different breeds.

The breeding soundness evaluation must include a complete physical examination, rectal examination, scrotal circumference measurement, and semen collection and evaluation. Using the Society for Theriogenology scoring system, a bull must score higher than 60 to be considered satisfactory.

The bull should be observed closely during the breeding season for proper mating behavior and libido. When available, a libido evaluation is a valuable way to more accurately assign the bull:cow ratio. In many range areas, this ratio is 25 cows per mature bull and 20 cows or less for yearlings and 2-year-old bulls. This ratio will also vary in relation to terrain, watering facilities, and desired length of calving season.

The use of yearling bulls has become common practice and requires close management. If possible, these bulls should be used on a rotation basis, with a rest period every 2 to 3 weeks. If not possible, the yearling bull should be removed from the breeding pasture after 6 to 8 weeks, segregated, and fed back to condition before returning to the bull battery.

PROGRAM PROCEDURES

This program is an action plan to accomplish the various procedures needed by the cow and calf herd with minimal handling.

For ranches that have very minimal herd health programs, some procedures can be applied during traditional handling times. However, as specific needs arise, certain procedures must be timed, so as not to compromise immunity or disease exposure. This may require additional processing time. An attempt should be made to consolidate all the procedures as much as possible to minimize handling cost and stress.

I. Cow Herd
  A. Pre-weaning procedures (performed in the alleyway).
    1. Insecticide pours, sprays, or dips for grub, lice, and fly control.
    2. Observe eyes for squamous-cell carcinoma to preserve culled cow salvage value or retain reproductive performance. Perform cryosurgery or thermal treatment for severe eyelid lesions.
    3. Evaluate crippled cows.
    4. Check for abscesses and treat those needing it.
    5. Identify poor producing cows, as evidenced by their calves.
  B. Fall and winter procedures (animals caught in a chute).
    1. Pregnancy palpation.
      a. Identify open cows for culling.
      b. Evaluate any pelvic pathologic condition.

This examination will help control cow deaths or calving problems. Cows that have had vaginal prolapse should be culled. Pelvic evaluation of first calf heifers will help control severe cases of dystocia and help judge maternal performance of new herd sires.

   c. Determine the cause of open and late cows and record age, condition, and breed groups.

2. Physical examination. This is facilitated by having the cows confined (usually the only time during the year that they will be confined).

Examine the following closely:

   a. Crippled cows. Check feet and legs. Long toes should be trimmed or marked for culling.

   b. Udder pathologic conditions. Examine for teat hair rings, "warty teats," large teats, and bad quarters.

   c. Examine horns. Watch for stub horns growing into the head.

   d. Examine teeth. Cows with marginal teeth should be marked for special feeding or early culling after calves are born. Broken mouth cows should be culled.

   e. Examine eyes for cancer. Perform surgery or provide treatment as needed. Cull if not responding to treatment.

3. Perform blood tests for cows if they are to be marketed soon. This will avoid extra handling, and the brucellosis status will be determined and identified for a particular cow unit, enhancing marketing.

4. Ear tags.

   a. Replace lost and illegible tags.

   b. Clip hair away from tag for easy visibility at calving time.

5. Vaccinations. This varies with region and production systems. A typical example of vaccinations in some areas is as follows:

   a. Leptospirosis bacterin (5-way).

   b. *Clostridium perfringens* type CD toxoid. First dose—initial year.

   c. Rota-corona scour virus vaccine. First dose—initial year.

   d. Vibriosis bacterin (if needed).

6. Insecticide pours. Give if not performed previously and if the time is correct for grubicide.

7. Deworm as needed. Timing and products vary with region.

C. Precalving procedures (performed in the alleyway). Some producers resist handling heavy gravid cows; however, very few problems are encountered.

1. Insecticide pours. These will be needed in some herds to obtain good lice control in cold climates. Previous grubicide application should avoid problems with extraneous grub kill. You can use lice and grub pour-on or specific lice pour-on.

2. Vitamin ADE injection if needed to enhance colostral quality and calving performance.

3. Vaccinations.

   a. Rota-corona scour virus vaccine. Second dose—initial year or annual booster.

   b. *E. coli* bacterin. Second dose—initial year or annual booster.

   c. *Clostridium perfringens* type CD toxoid. Second dose—initial year or annual booster.

   d. Vibriosis bacterin is given if not given previously.

   e. Leptospirosis bacterin (5-way) is given if not given previously.

4. Deworm if needed.

5. Check for cancer of the eyes, lumps, and crippling. Sort cows according to age and poor condition. Review calving facilities, supplies, and inventory.

D. Postcalving procedures.

1. Vaccinations.

   a. IBR-BVD. Initial vaccination or booster. IBR is used almost universally. BVD is used only in certain areas. Modified Live Virus (MLV) vaccine must be given only to open cows.

2. Palpation for estrous synchronization.

3. Injection or implantation for synchronization.

4. Artificial insemination.

5. Apply fly tags.

II. Calf Program Procedures

A. Procedures at birth.

1. Apply identification tags to assist mating, pairing, performance testing and so forth.

2. Give *Clostridium perfringens* CD toxoid in selected cases in which enterotoxemia or abomasal ulcerations are a problem.

3. Give rota-corona scour virus vaccine orally in selected cases in which cow vaccination was not used. This vaccine is only used in areas where the related diseases are problems.

4. Implant with growth stimulants.

5. Dehorn if desired. Paste is preferred in young calves.

6. Castrate at this time if preferred.

B. Procedures at branding time. In western range areas this is done at 2 to 9 weeks of age or occasionally at weaning.

1. Vaccinations.

   a. *Clostridium chauvoei-septicum* or *C. chauvoei-septicum-novyi-sordelli* bacterin.

   b. *Clostridium perfringens* type CD toxoid if needed.

   c. IBR (or IBR-PI$_3$) is used selectively.

   d. Leptospirosis bacterin is given in special cases.

   e. *Haemophilus* bacterin is administered discriminatingly.

2. Castrate.

3. Dehorn.

4. Brand.

5. Implant.

6. Deworm.

7. Apply fly tag.

C. Preweaning procedures.

1. Insecticide pours for grub, lice, and fly control.

2. Implant or re-implant.

3. Vaccinations.

   a. IBR-PI$_3$.

   b. BVD.

   c. Leptospirosis bacterin (5-way) given at this time or at postweaning, as needed.

   d. *Haemophilus* bacterin given selectively.

   e. Brucellosis vaccination. It is very important

to give at an early age to avoid stress and residual titers. This will facilitate marketing.
  f. Bovine respiratory syncytial virus vaccine given selectively.
  g. *Pasteurella* bacterins given in some cases.
  h. Clostridial vaccine boosters if needed.
D. Procedures at weaning (minimize handling as much as possible).
  1. Vaccinations.
    a. *Haemophilus* bacterin—first or second dose if required.
    b. *Pasteurella* bacterin—first or second dose if needed.
    c. Bovine respiratory syncytial virus vaccine—first or second dose if needed when necessary.
E. Postweaning procedures (after weaning stress).
  1. Insecticide pour for winter lice control.
  2. Implant growth stimulant.
  3. Deworm.
  4. Vaccinations.
    a. IBR booster.
    b. BVD if needed.
    c. Clostridial boosters if not given earlier.
    d. Leptospirosis bacterin if not administered previously.
  5. Vitamin ADE injection.
  6. Calf tag identifying preconditioning if applicable.
F. Replacement heifers.
  1. Place ear tags.
  2. Give year brand.
  3. Clean up scur horns or missed horns.
  4. Pelvic evaluation to predict weight of calf the heifer will be able to deliver. This allows more accurate bull selection or culling.
  5. Vaccinations.
    a. Vibrio bacterin.
    b. Leptospirosis bacterin (5-way).
    c. IBR booster.
    d. Clostridial bacterin booster.
    e. BVD selectively.

As the herd health management level becomes more sophisticated on a ranch, the assignment of definite responsibility can be accomplished. The daily surveillance of the various cattle groups becomes more worthwhile. Problems will be detected early and resolved or brought to the attention of the veterinarian for prompt action. A good example is respiratory disease at weaning. In these cases, early treatment is needed. If the outbreak is significant, diagnostic laboratory work will help determine treatment and possibly justify preventive additions or changes. A similar situation exists with calf scours and abortions.

The veterinarian who is responsible for large herds must develop a plan for each ranch to recognize and to react to emergency situations. As individual treament responsibility is transferred to ranch personnel, they better recognize unique problems. They also need to be instructed regarding whom to call and when to call for advise or assistance.

Client Education

The seasonal nature of ranching provides a logical client education opportunity for the practitioner. A meeting to review calving or weaning problems and procedures is popular with cattle workers. Over a period of years these meetings become motivational as well as educational, and they remain popular and important. Most large ranches have some turnover in cowhands, so these sessions are important to their indoctrination.

New drugs, treatment, procedures, or vaccines can be introduced to a number of people through these meetings. A discussion of diagnostic techniques also helps cowhands understand their role in diagnosis.

Records

An effective herd health program record system developed by the veterinarian should be compatible with the record system kept by the producer. These records should reflect the significant disease problems and diagnoses in the herd. They also should show the percentages that will provide a basis of evaluation of the health program. A variety of systems are available, including computerized programs. Many of these record individual performance, however, and may overlook the total herd impact of the health program.

In order to maintain a herd health program the producer must gain an economic advantage. In many instances, the percentage increases in productivity are rather subtle and could go unnoticed by management. The veterinarian should provide a progress report to the ranch managers pointing out areas of improvement. The report can be verbal or written and can incude recommendation for additions or alterations in the program.

Several methods of veterinary involvement are used, with fee basis work being the most common. Most health programs evolve from individual animal service work up to a full program. Another arrangement is a contractual agreement. This type is more complex and requires a definite outline as to what procedures and responsibilities are to be covered and what the charges are to be made.

The other alternative is full time employment. Few operations are large enough to justify this arrangement.

Farm Herds*

DUANE MIKSCH, D.V.M., M.S.

A large proportion of United States beef originates in small (farm) cow herds. Two-thirds of beef breeding herds in the United States have fewer than 50 cows, and 41 states have an average herd size of fewer than 50 cows. Of the North Atlantic states, 9 have an average herd size of only 4 cows. Only 2 per cent of all United States beef herds have more than 500 cows. However, a minimum of 200 cows is generally considered necessary for an "economic unit" or a "primary enterprise." These figures contrast with over 40 per cent of United States cattle "finished" being fed in fewer than 200 feedlots.

CHALLENGES

When beef cattle are part of an agronomic farming operation, they seldom command the majority of the farmer's attention. Cows are usually kept to utilize existing

*Presented under title "An Idealistic Cow-Calf Herd Health Program" at the 16th annual conference of the American Association of Bovine Practitioners, Oklahoma City, Oklahoma, Nov. 30–Dec. 1, 1983.

forage rather than forage being produced to feed the cows. As important as records are, farmers will keep records on cattle only to the extent that they enjoy record keeping.

This does not suggest that cow and calf operations are not important. It shows, really, that a lot of people like to own cattle. People who own cattle usually care about the cattle's health and appearance, and cattle are produced even when a profit is very unlikely. This situation creates a challenge for veterinarians to provide acceptable and affordable preventive health programs in sometimes difficult or improbable circumstances. Health programs will necessarily vary somewhat, depending on locale, inherent disease or health problems, and management preferences.

The smaller the herd, the greater will be the cost per animal for health maintenance. Adequate handling facilities can be especially expensive in small herds. Yet having "adequate" facilities is often the key to implementing and continuing a variable health maintenance program. The first challenge to the veterinarian may be to design adequate and affordable handling facilities for clients with small beef enterprises of varied descriptions. Handling facilities, like health maintenance programs, must be tailored to individual needs.

The smaller the herd, the less opportunity there is for the cattle owners to gain needed experience in distinguishing between normal and abnormal animal behavior, castrating and dehorning calves, giving injections, and handling calving. Frequency of repetition may be insufficient to adequately reinforce learning. Likewise, many veterinarians serving farmers have a practice involving less than 50 per cent food-animal medicine. Care of beef cattle is often a rather small part of the practice of the veterinarian supplying their health services. As a result, the veterinarian may be given little opportunity to become proficient in rectal palpation. Purchase of special equipment such as an electroejaculator may also be hard to justify.

OPPORTUNITIES

Despite the difficulties of delivering adequate veterinary service at an affordable cost, preventive health programs are very important to the productivity of small beef herds. The death of 1 or a few animals before the cause is identified is relatively more costly in a small herd. Herd replacements are more apt to be bought than raised in a small herd, thereby increasing the risk of introducing disease. A 1-bull herd is in the greatest jeopardy of delayed calving if the bull is not sound at breeding time.

Owners of small herds can benefit greatly from the use of artificial insemination. They cannot afford to keep a variety of bulls to breed cows and to breed heifers and to produce the best breed combinations. They can afford to use better bulls through artificial insemination (AI) than they can afford to own.

The operator of a small herd will probably not become a proficient inseminator. Once-a-year breeding of a few cows is not sufficient for most people to develop and retain adequate proficiency. Professional inseminators are usually only available in areas with considerable dairy farming. More often, dairy owners who inseminate their own cows will inseminate a neighbor's beef cows. Superior health management is essential for AI to be successful.

The veterinarian may be the appropriate supplier of AI service. It brings the practitioner and producer together on the positive note of improved production rather than on the more negative note of disease prevention. As provider of both herd health and AI service, the veterinarian will become better acquainted with the herd and its management. The availability of products to synchronize breeding, some of which are prescribed drugs, have made veterinarian provided AI service more practical and appropriate.

In some regards, a group practice may be better able to provide programmed preventive health service than a veterinarian practicing alone. One veterinarian in the group may be able to specialize in cattle or, at least, in food animals. In group practice, there is less interference with appointments by emergencies. This can be very important in keeping a client on a preventive health program. A producer should, however, be the client of 1 veterinarian. Rotating veterinarians on herd work, or sending whoever is available, negates much of the advantage of a herd health program.

Veterinarians providing health care to beef herds should be active members of local and state cattle producing organizations and participate in planning sessions of the County Extension Council beef commodity group. Veterinarians within a geographic area should strive to give uniform recommendations to producers, and they should also actively work toward uniform recommendations with other professionals giving advice in disciplines that overlap. Credibility and effectiveness are diminished when producers receive conflicting advice. Conversely, repetition and replication reinforce good advice.

Products used in herd health maintenance are available to the cattle producers from a variety of suppliers. Veterinarians providing health care must directly address discrepancies in prices between sources. They must (1) convince clients that their advice provided with the product warrants a higher charge, (2) write prescriptions and direct clients to a least cost source, or (3) find a way to be cost competitive with other sources. Disguising products or suggesting that 1 trade name is superior to another trade name of the same product is generally counterproductive. All nonprescription products widely used by veterinarians in herd health work are available as over-the-counter products.

CLIENT EDUCATION

One of the greatest challenges to veterinarians serving farm beef herds is to be adequately compensated for producer education and consultation in a way acceptable to the producers. Client education is a necessary and desirable part of an effective herd health program. As important as client education is, many veterinarians, especially those in mixed practice, don't find time to provide it. Some veterinarians are not convinced that client education is mutually beneficial. The fact is, the better producers understand their problems and the proper solutions to those problems, the more they realize the benefits of good veterinary service. Client education will be rewarded by better results from the veterinarian's efforts and, in most cases, it will lead to more demand for services.

It is important for veterinarians to understand and to

emphasize to their clients the relative merit of each health management practice. For example, proper feeding is relatively more important than vaccination. Stress load should be considered when scheduling herd work. Age and condition of animals, weather, and harshness of each intended procedure are all important considerations. Weaning results in considerable stress to calves and should not be combined with other stressful procedures. Weaning should follow or precede major processing of calves by a minimum of 3 weeks.

The veterinarian providing health recommendations and services must remain acutely aware of the need to constantly caution against animals with potential drug residues being slaughtered. For example, cows are quite often treated with a pour-on for grub control at the same time they are examined for pregnancy and physical soundness. Treated cull cows may be immediately sent to slaughter if the owner is not reminded of withdrawal requirements for drugs.

Raising herd replacements should be encouraged for disease prevention and genetic improvement. Buying replacements increases the risk of introducing disease into the herd and makes genetic progress difficult. The necessity for adequate quarantine and retesting of animals being introduced to a herd must be emphasized.

Cattle handlers should be trained in calving management as follows: (1) they need to know the importance of frequent observation, (2) they must be able to distinguish between normal parturition and dystocia, (3) they should develop competence and confidence within their capabilities, and (4) they should be taught to seek professional help at the proper time.

Calf scours during calving season should be anticipated and prevented. Cattle workers should be taught the principles of calf scours prevention. They should learn the importance of prompt and adequate treatment. Timely treatment should seldom require parenteral administration or a visit by the veterinarian. The relatively greater importance of combatting dehydration and acidosis compared with controlling the causative organism must be emphasized.

Castrating and implanting with a growth stimulant may be best done by the educated herd handler on an as-born

Table 1. *Beef Cow Year by Nutrient Requirement Periods*

Period 1 (82 days)	Period 2 (123 days)	Period 3 (110 days)	Period 4 (50 days)
Calving to breeding	Breeding to weaning of calf	Weaning of calf to 50 days	Last 50 days of pregnancy

basis. Dehorning and castration should not be put off until weaning or fall roundup. The earlier they can be done, the easier it is on the calf. Dehorning can be done without attracting flies, and using implants favors early castration. Calves need blackleg protection early. The importance of revaccination for long-term protection must be stressed.

NUTRITION

A short calving season is prerequisite to a workable preventive health program. Nutritional management is the most important factor in maintaining a short calving season. Heifers must be fed adequately from weaning to breeding if they are to calve at 2 years of age. Puberty is a function of both age and weight. Failing to feed heifers adequately before breeding results in delayed skeletal development and calving difficulty in addition to a low pregnancy rate. If feed levels are excessive, heifers will become overly fat, dystocia will increase, milk production may be lowered, productive life span may be shortened, and feed costs will be prohibitive.

The limiting factor related to reproduction is usually energy. Feed requirements of cows vary during the reproductive cycle. The greatest demand occurs from calving to breeding. Protein is also an important consideration in feeding. Young growing animals are often underfed protein, whereas mature dry cows are often overfed protein. Lactating cows require twice as much protein as dry cows. Other nutrients that are frequently deficient and require supplementation are phosphorus and selenium. The beef cow's reproductive cycle and her varying nutrient requirements are illustrated in Tables 1 and 2.

Table 2. *NRC Requirements for Beef Cows of Various Weights by Period*

			Daily Requirements				
Body wt.	TDN	NE$_m$	Crude Protein (lb)	Digestible Protein (lb)	Ca (gm)	P (gm)	Vitamin A (Ux1000)
Period 1—Calving to Breeding*							
900	11–14	10.7–13.6	1.8–2.6	1.1–1.6	25–45	25–41	21–34
1100	12–15	11.6–14.6	2.0–2.8	1.2–1.7	27–46	27–43	24–38
1300	13–16	12.6–15.5	2.2–3.0	1.3–1.8	28–46	28–44	27–43
Period 2—Breeding to Weaning Calf*							
900	9–11	8.7–10.7	1.5–2.1	0.9–1.3	22–41	22–37	21
1100	10–12	9.7–11.6	1.6–2.3	1.0–1.4	24–42	24–39	24
1300	11–13	10.7–12.6	1.7–2.4	1.1–1.5	25–42	25–39	27
Period 3—Weaning Calf to 50 Days before Calving							
900	8.0	7.8	.82	.43	13	13	21
100	8.5	8.2	.90	.45	13	13	24
1300	9.0	8.7	.99	.49	14	14	27
Period 4—Last 50 days of pregnancy							
900	8.8	8.5	1.0	.48	14	14	21
1100	10.0	9.7	1.1	.53	15	15	24
1300	11.1	10.8	1.2	.58	17	17	27

*Requirements depend on milking ability, age, and condition.

HERD HEALTH CALENDAR

A preventive health program is most easily understood and communicated using a calendar. Adjustments in practices can be recorded on the calendar for geographic area, for calving season, and so forth. The calendar concept emphasizes the need for a concise calving season. It provides a framework for integrating the recommendations from persons in the various disciplines serving beef herd enterprises. It is a starting place for veterinarians within a geographic area to work toward uniformity in their recommendations. An example of a health calendar for March to April calving is presented next.

January

Vaccinate fall weaned calves against BVD, IBR, and PI$_3$. This revaccination should be scheduled sometime between 30 days postweaning and 30 days prebreeding for replacement heifers that were vaccinated prior to weaning since (1) they will be over the stress of weaning, (2) they will be old enough to develop a solid, lasting immunity, (3) they should be away from the cows so there will be no danger of exposing pregnant cows to vaccine virus, and (4) there will be no danger of interference with conception or pregnancy in the vaccinates.

Halter and tie replacement heifers. Having halter-broken cows is worth the effort.

Feed supplemental magnesium to cows from 60 days before calving until the start of breeding in areas where grass tetany is a problem.

Treat for lice twice within 21 days to break the louse life cycle if lice were not adequately controlled in the fall.

Inject vitamin A if feed is deficient and dietary supplementation is impractical.

February

Begin calving heifers about 3 weeks ahead of calving cows because (1) they can be given the extra attention they need, and (2) they will have the extra time they need to be in an estrous cycle at start of breeding.

First colostrum from older cows should be available for heifers' calves that require it. This may necessitate keeping frozen colostrum from the previous year.

March to April

Calve cows and remainder of heifers.

See that calves get colostrum immediately for maximum absorption of immunoglobulins.

Have an effective calf-scour prevention program in place.

Identify calves and record calving events for use in selection and culling.

Evaluate bulls for breeding soundness. This should include fertility determinations, physical examinations, and mating behavior observations.

Dehorn and castrate calves early, i.e., before they reach 4 months of age.

Implant steer calves with a growth stimulant at the time they are castrated.

Vaccinate breeding herd against leptospirosis and vibriosis.

Table 3. *Livestock Weather Safety Index*

Temperature °F	\	Relative Humidity (%)																			
	5	10	15	20	25	30	35	40	45	50	55	60	65	70	75	80	85	90	95	100
75									70	70	71	71	72	72	73	73	74	74	75	75
76							70	70	70	71	72	72	72	73	74	74	74	75	76	76
77						70	70	71	71	72	72	73	73	74	74	75	75	76	76	77
78				70	70	71	71	72	72	73	74	74	75	75	76	76	77	78	78	78
79				70	70	71	72	72	73	73	74	74		76	77	77	78	78	79	79
80			70	70	71	72	72	73	73	74	74	75	**Alert** 76	77	78	78	79	79	80	
81		70	70	71	71	72	73	73	74	75	75	76	77	77	78	78	79	80	80	81
82		70	71	71	72	73	73	74	75	75	76	77	77	78	79	79	80	81	81	82
83	70	71	71	72	73	73	74	75	75	76	77	78	78	79	**Danger**	81	82	82		83
84	70	71	72	72	73	74	75	75	76	77	78	78	79	80	80	81	82	83	83	84
85	71	72	72	73	74	75	75	76	77	78	78	79	80	81	81	82	83	84	84	85
86	71	72	73	74	74	75	76	77	78	78	79	80	81	81	82	83	84	84	85	86
87	72	73	73	74	75	76	77	77	78	79	80	81	81	82	83	84	85	**Emergency**		87
88	72	73	74	75	76	76	77	78	79	80	81	81	82	83	84				87	88
89	73	74	74	75	76	77	78	79	80	80	81	82	83	84	85	86	86	87	88	89
90	73	74	75	76	77	78	79	79	80	81	82	83	84	85	86	87	87	88	89	90
91	74	75	76	76	77	78	79	80	81	82	83	84	85	86	86	87	88	89	90	91
92	74	75	76	77	78	79	80	81	82	83	84	84	85	86	87	88	89	90		
93	75	76	77	78	79	80	80	81	82	83	84	85	87	87	88	89	90			
94	75	76	77	78	79	80	81	82	83	84	85	86	87	88	89	90				
95	76	77	78	79	80	81	82	83	84	85	86	87	88	89	90					
96	76	77	78	79	80	81	82	84	84	86	87	88	89	90	91					
97	77	78	79	80	81	82	83	84	85	86	87	88	90	91						
98	77	78	79	80	82	83	84	85	86	87	88	89	90							
99	78	79	80	81	82	83	84	86	87	88	88	90								
100	78	79	80	82	83	84	85	86	87	88	90	91								
105	80	82	83	84	86	87	88	90	91											

April to May

Deworm yearlings 3 weeks and 6 weeks after they are turned on pasture.

Deworm cows in areas where a "periparturient rise" is a problem. Worms do survive winter—both on pasture and in cattle.

Initiate hornfly and facefly control. Apply insecticide-containing ear tags at full recommended dosage. Rotate products and take every precaution available to delay insecticide resistance in the fly population.

May, June, and July

Breed replacement heifers 45 days only. Begin breeding heifers 3 to 4 weeks before starting to breed cows. Expose 50 per cent more heifers than needed as replacements.

Breed cows for 65 days only.

Vaccinate calves for blackleg and malignant edema soon after all calves are born.

Complete castrating, implanting, and dehorning calves.

August

Examine heifers for pregnancy. Select replacements from heifers that become pregnant after 45 days of breeding. Cull open heifers from the breeding herd.

Halter and tie all replacement animals. This should include pregnant yearlings and heifer calves that are prospective replacements.

Observe Livestock Weather Safety Index (Table 3) when working with cattle in hot weather.

Deworm suckling calves if location and environment indicate a need.

Re-implant steer calves according to schedule recommended for the product use.

September to October

Examine cows for pregnancy and physical soundness. Mark for culling those that are open, old, or impaired.

Collect blood samples from the breeding herd. Achieve and maintain a "Brucellosis Certified Free Herd." Request blood samples be screened for anaplasmosis, leptospirosis, and other diseases of concern for which tests are reliable.

Vaccinate calves for leptospirosis, IBR-PI$_3$, BVD, blackleg and malignant edema, *Haemophilus somnus*, and pasteurellosis.

Certify calves as "preconditioned" where a program is available. This will enhance the value of feeder calves. It will also encourage extended ownership of stockers and development of replacements for the breeding herd.

Halter and tie all bred heifers and heifer calves that are prospective replacements.

Treat all cattle for grubs and lice. Retreat within 21 days to preclude necessity of treating during the winter.

Vaccinate heifer calves against brucellosis. Age at vaccination will depend on other management practices and current regulations. Don't combine brucellosis vaccination with weaning or other severe stresses.

November to December

Wean and deworm calves.

Plan winter feeding program completely and carefully.

References

1. AABP–NCA: Recommendations to improve reproductive performance in beef cattle.
2. AABP–NCA: Recommended practices for the control of bovine respiratory disease in the cow-calf herd.

Cattle Feedlot Health Management

DAVID T. BECHTOL, B.S., D.V.M.
and TIMOTHY JORDAN, B.S., D.V.M.

The cattle industry has rapidly expanded in the past 2 decades to meet the consumer's demand for a year-round supply of choice beef. As a result, the management of feedyards is challenged to operate their cattle feeding facilities efficiently in order to produce a wholesome, nutritious product at an acceptable price to the consumer and to return a profit to both the commercial feedyard and its clients.

The industry, therefore, has become highly specialized to meet these challenges. The manager must be well versed in many facets of cattle feeding. Rarely does any one manager have all the required knowledge, and therefore he or she contracts with private, independent specialized consultants. The purpose of feedlot consultants is to provide objective advice and recommendations that are confidential and tailored to meet the requirements of individual feedlots.

With respect to the increasing number of large commercial feedyards, the role of veterinarians has changed over the past few years. Rather than have them do the actual processing and treating of individual animals, veterinarians are now contracted to advise, supervise, and teach these procedures. They are more involved in management decisions, and they are more concerned in feedlot economics—herd health cost and performance for maximum results and profits.

A veterinary consultant's primary objective and responsibility is to maximize cattle performance through prevention and control of disease.

Health problems in feedlots are never static; they require constant monitoring with evaluation and re-evaluation. For a veterinary consultant to evaluate complex problems, he or she must be totally involved with management of the feedyard, from feedlot receiving programs, which process the animal and put it into its home pen, to feedyard treatment programs. The feedyard veterinarian must also employ a record system to assist in the maintaining and monitoring of the factors causing diseases.

When initially formulating or evaluating a feedlot health program, one should divide the crucial health areas into 5 broad phases—receiving, processing, starting, finishing, and medication. By viewing the feeding period with these 5 areas in mind, one can better identify and understand the problems of the animal in the feedlot environment. Let us examine these areas and include them in a comprehensive health program.

RECEIVING PHASE

The primary purpose of the receiving period is to allow recovery time from shipment and to prepare the cattle for processing and subsequently starting on feed. This period begins as the cattle are unloaded from the truck into the feedyard. At this point, one must evaluate the cattle visually and correlate this examination with past experience and present practices. Also, one must ask questions about the history of the load of cattle pertaining to procurement, past treatment, and handling and use this in the subjective evaluation of the cattle.

Per cent shrink (defined as the differene between purchase weight and receipt weight) is an important factor in the receiving period. Cattle with greater than 7 per cent shrink should be considered predisposed to infectious disorders and handled accordingly. Lightweight younger calves have different problems than older yearlings or aged cattle. Country or local cattle have different problems than sale-barn cattle. These areas must be addressed and resolved when receiving cattle in the feedyard.

Upon receipt, cattle are routinely weighed and put in a holding pen supplied with fresh hay and water. Native grass hays that are of good quality and not moldy function well in these pens where feeding is for management and maintenance rather than performance. The hay and water should be supplied along the fence line, as most newly received cattle will wander and pace the outermost edge of any confined areas. Once the cattle have adequately consumed hay and water, they will be more ready for initial working.

PROCESSING PHASE

Processing of cattle in the feedyard entails all necessary vaccinations, anthelmintics, acaricides, growth implants, and any compound deemed necessary in a particular feedyard for maximizing performance. Antibiotics may also be incorporated at processing, and this will be discussed later. Processing recommendations and procedures are one of the prime areas that are directly under the auspices of the feedyard veterinarian. There must be communication with the manager and the consulting nutritionist in this area because of the overlap in the action of both of these agents.

In order to specify a processing program, the veterinarian must first identify all problems present in a particular area and feedyard and then formulate a workable plan of action for prevention and correction of these problems. The solution and eventual prevention of a problem will lie in a combination of prophylactic procedures (such as vaccination) as well as good cattle management and medication or treatment.

One must remember that respiratory disease accounts for 80 to 85 per cent of overall mortality and 75 to 80 per cent of morbidity in the feedlot industry. The veterinarian must also recognize that bovine respiratory disease is usually a secondary bacterial problem initiated by a combination of stress and primary virus infection. Although a workable research model is lacking for respiratory disease, one must be well acquainted with the pathogenesis and pathophysiology of this disease complex in order to formulate a comprehensive preventive program.

The processing program should include products that are efficacious, relatively nonstressful, and easy to administer, and that provide an excellent cost to benefit ratio. This program should not be completely static but should allow for alteration, refinement, and customizing where and when deemed necessary.

Viral vaccinations may include single or combination inoculation for IBR, PI$_3$, BVD, or BRSV. Bacterial vaccination may include clostridial inoculation as well as vaccination for *Pasteurella haemolytica* and *P. multocida*, and *Hemophilus somnus*. In highly stressed calves, response to vaccination is questionable at this time. The use

of multiple antigens at processing may potentiate a poor immune response, and this must be kept in mind when using multiple antigen exposure at processing. This area of multiple antigen exposure is extremely controversial but can be sorted out in any feedyard after a complete evaluation of problems. Table 1 lists what should be considered a basic feedyard processing program.

All procedures used in processing are usually done within 24 hr of receipt into the feedyard. Acaricide treatment should be done as quickly upon arrival as possible to prevent spread of external parasites. Only in highly stressed calves are surgical procedures such as castration and tip dehorning delayed until the cattle have acclimated to the feedyard environment.

Recently, revaccination with important viral antigens at 5 to 7 days postprocessing has received renewed attention and evaluation. The initial results with this practice have looked very encouraging.

STARTING PHASE

After cattle are processed they are placed in a feeding pen that may be used for starting, or they are placed in the ultimate finishing pen. This is of paramount importance in the feeding period. How the cattle are handled at receiving and processing is realized during this phase. In order to devise an adequate starting program let us divide this period into 2 sections—nutrition and health.

Nutrition

Nutrition of feedlot cattle is discussed elsewhere in this book, but the important interaction of starting cattle on feed and overall health is so intertwined that it deserves further discussion. The important aspect of starting cattle on feed is to get as much energy and usable nutrients into the cattle as quickly as possible without precipitating secondary digestive and metabolic disorders. Usually the cattle are acclimated to full feed by 21 to 25 days after receipt.

Table 1. *Basic Feedyard Processing Program*

Yearling Program
Vaccinations: IBR, MLV inoculation, four-way clostridial
   (*Clostridium chauvoei, C. septicum, C. sordelli, C. novyi*)
   inoculation
Growth implant
Anthelmintic
Vitamin ADE (at least 1.5 million units)
Surgery
   Tip dehorning
   Castration
Acaricide

Calf and Sale-Barn Program
Vaccinations: IBR, PI$_3$ killed or MLV inoculation, four-way
   clostridial inoculation
Growth implant
Anthelmintic
Vitamin ADE (at least 1.5 million units)
Surgery
   Tip dehorning
   Castration
Acaricide
Other: revaccinate with IBR, PI$_3$, MLV booster inoculation at 5 to
   7 days postprocessing

Optional vaccinations may include: BVD, BRSV, intranasal IBR
   and PI$_3$, *P. haemolytica, P. multocida,* and *H. somnus*

Hay is used primarily in the starting period as a management tool to attract cattle to the feedbunk and secondarily to supply a readily available energy source. Native grass hay and, less commonly, alfalfa hay are used for this purpose. The hay is put in the bunk, and the ration lightly topdressed, thus forcing the cattle to nose through the feed in order to get the hay. The ration is increased as the hay is decreased. Hay is usually supplied in this fashion for 2 to 3 days but may be used longer with a poor starting pen, with the addition of new cattle to an existing pen, or with highly stressed sick cattle.

Round hay bales are also used in the pen, which are fed in steel feeders to minimize waste. Hay may also be fed inside the feedbunk on the apron. Care should be used in this respect, as feeding on the ground may allow for the transmission of infectious enteritis.

A good working relationship between the veterinarian and the nutritionist will help ensure the success of a starting program as much as anything else. Health problems commonly occur secondary to lack of adequate consumption in the feedlot environment. The health program in the starting period is a combination of nutrition, management, and medication. Nutrition has been briefly discussed, medication will be discussed later, so let us now look at the management considerations of the starting period.

Health

Pen checkers and doctoring crews will be the persons handling this portion of the program, so consulting veterinarians must educate them to be their eyes and ears. Education, communication, and motivation are keys to a successful working relationship. Supply these workers with all the necessary information needed to adequately diagnose and treat the common problems encountered in the feedyard. Also, impress upon them the need to realize the limit of their knowledge and to call on the veterinarian when additional expertise is needed. Starting pens should be examined on a daily basis, and problem pens checked twice daily. Sick cattle should be removed from the pen, identified by tagging, and given appropriate treatment. Questionably sick animals should be examined further in the treatment facility and not left in the pen. Observation pens may be used in addition to hospital pens should such areas become crowded. All medication programs are doomed to failure if the progression of disease has reached an end stage before treatment is offered.

Respiratory disease is the primary problem in the starting period, and digestive disorders rank a distant second. Classic clinical signs of respiratory disease in the feedyard include depression, anorexia, lethargy, and weakness. Ocular and nasal discharge are usually present. Respiratory rate is usually increased, and coughing may be present. There is no feasible clinical criterion that can be used to differentiate respiratory diseases in the pen; therefore, educate the pen checkers to recognize these general signs and have them pull the cattle for "not looking right." Allow the more knowledgeable doctoring crew members to make a tentative diagnosis and initiate therapy.

The veterinarian must evaluate the efficiency of pulling sick cattle, the quality of treatment, and the response to medication. Comprehensive record keeping is critical and essential to all facets of the feedyard.

FINISHING PHASE

The principles of cattle worker management and cattle management apply to the finishing phase, but the prevalence of disease conditions differs from the starting phase. The problems encountered in this period will again be primarily respiratory, but digestive, reproductive, locomotor, and nervous disorders will also be common.

Because of the different disease problems occurring in this period, train feedlot personnel to observe and pull sick animals that are affected with these disease problems.

Generally, "respiratory pulls" should peak and decline by day 25 in the feedyard. If respiratory problems continue on a large scale during this time, a comprehensive reevaluation of processing, medication, and pulling practices should be initiated along with a complete diagnostic work up of the problem.

MEDICATION

Treatment programs are designed to function in the feedyard according to the type and quality of cattle received, their condition, weight, point of origin, and time of year. The specific treatment schedule is also customized to the facilities and to the persons involved in the actual treatment of sick animals. A basic medication program will function in all yards but must be fine tuned to fit the situation and circumstances illustrated previously. A sound background in bovine medicine, a working knowledge of applied pharmacology, and a keen sense of cattle management are the ingredients needed by a veterinarian to develop a successful medication program.

In our practice, we have a treatment book written for the feedyard personnel that includes common feedlot diseases along with clinical signs and appropriate treatments. This book is intended simply as an outline and is added to as questions and problems arise. This method functions very well as a starting point for the feedyard's old and new employees. Also, a written, formalized, and individualized program is available at the yard should questions occur. The book is modified at each yard, as deemed necessary.

Medication in the feedyard can be divided into 3 uses: (1) mass treatment upon arrival, (2) mass treatment after arrival, and (3) individual treatment. When choosing antibiotics, sulfonamides, and other drugs for use in a feedlot medication program, one must use a good posttreatment evaluation system, constant monitoring, and ancillary laboratory tests in order to define usage. One must also have a functional and efficient system of identifying individually treated animals, not only for response evaluation but also for identifying animals' posttreatment withdrawal dates.

Mass medication upon arrival is done at the time of processing and initiated only after evaluating the clinical appearance, past history, and origin of the cattle. One must first set goals for a mass medication program. For example, will medication be used for elimination of incubatory stages of disease or will it be used for the treatment of clinically ill animals? The question sounds obvious but must be considered in achieving effective cost to benefit ratios in mass treatment programs.

Drugs for mass medication commonly used include (1) oxytetracycline, (2) long-acting oxytetracycline, (3) long-acting oxytetracycline in combination with a long-acting sulfa bolus, and (4) amoxicillin. Generally, vitamin B therapy is used as an adjunct to treatment in the form of a B-complex vitamin or vitamin B_{12}.

Initial mass treatment may be used on a single-day administration when the purpose is to curb those animals that are in a true incubatory disease stage. Two or 3 successive days of initial therapy are needed when large numbers of animals are showing signs of clinical illness upon receipt.

Mass medication after arrival is used on animals in those pens that are experiencing high morbidity sometime in the feeding period. The veterinarian must use morbidity, feed consumption, and treatment response data in deciding when to best employ a mass medication program. Treatment response to medication offered in the hospital pen is an important determining factor in choosing therapy. The criteria that are used in our practice for determination of mass treatment are (1) greater than 25 per cent morbidity in a short time (3 to 5 days), (2) an abrupt 10 to 25 per cent decrease in feed consumption, (3) a failure of adequate response with sick pulls in the hospital pen and, (4) past experience with the particular origin or type of cattle.

Mass medication may also be delivered in the feed or water. Some of the more common feeding procedures employ the use of oxytetracycline alone, oxytetracycline and sulfonamide, or neomycin and oxytetracycline. Medication in the feed should be given over a short period (5 to 7 days) at a high level, then tapered for 2 to 3 days. Feeding low levels of antibiotics over a long period can lead to chronic respiratory disease. Medication in the water is usually in the form of a single sulfonamide or a combination of 3 sulfonamides. Flavoring is usually needed in the water in order to ensure adequate consumption. Sulfa drugs administered in this fashion are used for only 3 days. Medication programs administered by oral routes are very time-sparing procedures, but response to medication may not make this procedure cost effective on a routine basis.

When individual animals are pulled for treatment at the hospital pen, doctoring crews must first make a tentative diagnosis. Treatment offered depends on time of year, type of cattle, historical data, and severity of disease. A common respiratory treatment schedule would include therapeutic agents, such as these, administered to provide 3 days of therapy.

1. Oxytetracycline, 1 gm/100 kg, IM or IV.
2. Intravenous sulfonamides followed by oral administration.

Also included would be supportive agents used to counteract the secondary changes associated with disease and concomitant use of antibiotics. Table 2 contains a list of commonly used supportive drugs and the rationale behind their use. B-complex vitamins and antihistamines are always used in our practice on the first 2 days of treatment and as needed thereafter.

Although oxytetracycline and sulfonamides are the hallmark of respiratory therapy, other combinations are routinely used. The key to successful therapeutic combinations is to use them knowledgeably. Pharmacology has given us certain rules to follow, but experience has dictated certain refinements in those rules. Commonly, a combination of 2 drugs is used, but occasionally a 3-drug combination may be needed for additional treatment response. Table 3 lists commonly used drug combinations.

Table 2. *Supportive Medications for Respiratory Disease*

Medication	Route of Administration	Rationale for Use
Antihistamine	SC	Opens air passages, dry mucosal surfaces
B-complex vitamin	IM or IV	Appetite stimulation, replaces vitamin loss
Electrolytes	IV or PO	Replaces ion loss
Fluid therapy	PO	Replaces volume loss
Microbials	PO	Repopulate GI tract flora, appetite stimulation
Steroids (dexamethasone)*	IM or IV	Reduce swelling

*May potentiate disease.

Again, management is the key to success in the treatment phase. Hospital and sick pens should be clean, dry, and uncrowded. A high energy ration and fresh attractive hay should be supplied to sick cattle. After treatment, convalescent time should be available for 2 to 3 days to allow for a nonstressful recovery and also for observation.

When formulating a medication program, veterinarians must be well informed of withdrawal dates for drugs used. They must also be aware of the need to follow FDA regulations and procedures when acquiring, supplying, and using drugs not labeled specifically for use in food animals. Through the proper use of management techniques and antibiotic combinations, a medication program has the potential for excellent results.

RECORD KEEPING SYSTEM

A record keeping system that is easy yet retains all necessary information is absolutely essential for a complete feedlot health program. Figure 1 is an example of a processing work order used in such a manner that an accounting of specific processing compounds and medications can be made. Figure 2 is an example of a record that will allow one to monitor sick animal pulls from the pen and other cattle movements during the feeding period. This record is kept by the cowhand crew and pen checkers. Figure 3 is an example of an individual treatment card that can be filled out by doctoring crew members. The basic information needed for this report is body temperature, clinical severity, diagnosis, and treatment offered. An example of a hospital report is shown in Figure 4 and is used as a daily accounting tool for each treatment or hospital area.

Table 3. *Feedlot Medications for Respiratory Disease*

Basic Treatment Group 1	Basic Treatment Group 2	Alternative Treatment Regimens
Oxytetracycline Sulfonamides	Procaine, penicillin G Erythromycin	Oxytetracycline Tylosin Sulfonamide
		Oxytetracycline Erythromycin
		Oxytetracycline Sulfonamide Erythromycin
		Procaine, penicillin G Tylosin Erythromycin
		Sulfonamide Tylosin Erythromycin

WORK ORDER

Lot no. _____   Date _____   Steers _____

Pen no. _____   Owner _____   Heifers _____

No. of head _____   Origin _____   Bulls _____

ITEM	✔	MANUFACTURER	MFG. LOT NO.	UNIT COST	TOTAL COST
IBR					
IBR = Pl₃					
IBR = Leptospirosis					
BVD					
Clostridium					
ADE					
Wormer					
Implant					
Dehorn					
Castrate					
Dip					
Lot Brand					
				TOTAL CHARGES	

Figure 1. Processing order. Completed on each lot of cattle as they have been processed. Emphasis on drug manufacturer and manufacturer lot number.

These 4 examples of records will supply the veterinarian with the necessary information needed to evaluate a health program. The other purpose of this detailed record keeping system is to allow for accounting of withdrawal dates following antibiotic therapy, which is critical for a food animal production facility. It also fulfills cattle accounting needs in the feedyard and is easy for the health crews to keep.

CATTLE MOVEMENTS   Date _____

No. head _____ From _____

Brand _____ To _____

Code _____ Remarks _____

DEATH LOSS

No. head _____ Pen _____

Brand _____ Place _____

Code _____ Tag no. _____

Remarks _____

_____

Signed _____

Figure 2. Cattle movements and death loss slips. Filled out by pen riders when an animal has been removed from its home pen, hospital pen, or both. First record of movement within the feedyard.

THE APPROACH TO PROBLEMS

When facing a problem in the feedyard or when evaluating a new feedlot, one must remember that the problem may stem from 6 interacting factors. These factors are (1) stress, (2) infectious agents, (3) nutrition, (4) management, (5) medication, (6) economics. The veterinarian must also realize and understand these interactions and initiate the diagnostic process accordingly.

This article divides feedlot health into 5 broad phases. Management is the underlying theme of this approach and should be realized in any problem evaluation. Often the answer to a problem will not be in medication.

The subjective, objective, assessment, plan (SOAP) approach is uniquely suited for the feedyard. By using this method and dividing the feeding period into the 5 phases discussed herein, one can organize the information and formulate a straightforward resolution.

Subjective data should contain an overall evaluation of the facility, including an evaluation of the type of cattle, quality of personnel, and capablity of management. Data such as morbidity, mortality, feed consumption, and treatment response are essential for a good history.

Objective data will include a good clinical examination of animals in the problem pen, complete gross pathologic examination of any dead animals, and ancillary laboratory procedures. To be a successful feedlot veterinarian, one must be an excellent diagnostician and gross pathologist. Laboratory tests should be used as an adjunct to clinical data and not as the sole diagnostic tool. The 3 most important laboratory tests performed by feedlot veterinarians are bacterial culture and sensitivity, virus isolation, and serology.

Bacterial cultures supply very important data for problematic analysis. Sensitivity test results can be obtained

	Tag no.	Lot no.	Pen no.	Hosp. no.	Temp.	Sev.	Diag.	Date	No. days	Disp.
Drug day		1	2	3	4	5	6	Total Units	Cost / Unit	Total Cost
Temp.										
B-com.	46									
Amino acid conc.	45									
Antihist.	60									
Terr.	38									
Albon SR	50									
Pen	42									
LA 200	40									
Tylan.	41									
Eryth.	39									
Probios.	58									
Individual Hospitalization Card								TOTAL		

Severity		Disposition	
1. No treatment 3. Subacute		1. Recovered 4. Sale	
2. Acute 4. Chronic		2. Chronic 5. Rail	
		3. Died _____ Loc. _____	

Figure 3. Individual treatment card. Filled out by the hospital crew for each animal treated. This record is in triplicate: one copy to the hospital for filing, one for the owner's lot folder, and one for the veterinarian's notebook.

Hospital Report

Hospital _____ Date _____

No. head	Lot no.	Pen no.	Hospital tag no. and reason

R—Respiratory C—Cocci B—Buller S—Scours
I—Injury N—Not Eating Bl—Bloat O—Other

Figure 4. Hospital report. Completed by hospital crew to show the number of animals pulled for treatment, the animal's individual ear tag number, and diagnosis. This record is turned in daily from each hospital area to the feedlot office, and a copy is retained for the veterinarian's notebook.

with 2 methods—agar disk sensitivity and Minimum Inhibitory Concentration (MIC). Agar disk sensitivity results are dependant upon disk antibiotic concentration and diffusibility of the antibiotic in the agar medium. Because of these problems and the subjectibility of the test, results are inconsistent. The results of drug sensitivity of virulent *Pasteurella haemolytica* infections in the Texas Panhandle are strikingly consistent *in vitro*, although *in vivo* response is markedly different. MIC data have a much higher correlation *in vitro* than *in vivo* and are more useful to the feedlot diagnostician.

Virus isolation should be employed in any tissues containing lesions with possible viral disease. Lung lesions are often obliterated by overgrowth of respiratory bacterial pathogens. Tracheal swabs or deep tracheal washes can be used for this test in live animals and yield consistent and usable results. Serology is another test often misused by veterinarians. Serology is a subjective test for virus particles and should be interpreted as positive or negative rather than at a specific level. Acute and convalescent titers are far superior to single testing. Keep in mind that a certain titer level does not correlate completely with protection to viral challenge.

Once subjective and objective data have been gathered, an assessment of this data must be made. Take into account all the factors mentioned earlier and formulate a diagnosis. Resolution of a problem will result from a combination of management, medication, and prevention. In food animal practice, a cost to benefit ratio must exist before treatment can be justified. Sale of the animal will sometimes realize more money than treatment. Upon assessment of data, formulate a comprehensive plan.

In order to have a workable plan, the feedlot veterinarian must be able to communicate his or her findings to management and feedlot personnel in such a way that no questions exist in anyone's mind. The best diagnostic and therapeutic regimens have been failures because of a lack of communication. Continued evaluation of the plan of action is necessary to be sure of adequate understanding by everyone involved.

In summary, a successful comprehensive feedlot health program is dependent on the use of sound medical practice. A feedlot veterinarian must have this knowledge as well as a working understanding of cattle management. The veterinarian must then communicate this knowledge to the feedlot personnel in a useful and straightforward fashion. Continued evaluation and refinement of the program is necessary for ongoing success and improvement. Confidence will be gained from this approach, and it will offer the producer a cost-effective preventive program rather than a costly, ineffectual emergency service.

Backgrounding and Stocker Calf Management

ROBERT A. SMITH, D.V.M., M.S.

Backgrounding describes a management system where cattle, generally recently weaned calves, are assembled from many sources with little or no knowledge of their history and are kept for a period of time before placing them in a feedlot. Stocker calves of similar ages are assembled and placed on forage, generally grass or small grain pastures. When they are grown to a suitable size, they will be sold to the feedlot. Heifers intended for future breeding can also be handled in stocker operations.

Health management of calves in backgrounding or stocker programs can be among the greatest challenges facing the food animal practitioner. Calves in these programs have often been extremely stressed under the current management and marketing systems. Most are recently weaned, moved through auction markets where they are exposed to many pathogens for the first time, and then transported long distances. At the backgrounding or stocker operation, the calves must establish a new social order, adapt to different feedstuffs, and frequently must acclimate to new weather conditions. The result is that the calves suffer from fatigue, dehydration, hunger, and psychological stress, making them quite susceptible to bovine respiratory disease and other stress-related diseases. Many calves have been given antibiotics before arrival. Often these are given at incorrect dosages, for too short a time, and often in combination with corticosteroids. Morbidity in newly received calves is frequently 40 to 50 per cent, and mortality is often 5 per cent or more.

MANAGEMENT ON ARRIVAL

Calves should be inspected as they are unloaded to determine health status and shipping injuries. If they are unacceptable, the seller or buyer should be contacted immediately to determine their disposition. Calves that have been trampled or seriously injured during transit should not be accepted and are the responsibility of the trucker. Calves should be weighed upon arrival to deter-

mine shrinkage. Shrinkage of 7 to 8 per cent or more is often associated with greater health problems, and affected calves will require more intensive management during the receiving period. Occasionally, newly received calves will have unusually low shrinkage or even weigh more on arrival than their purchase weight, suggesting nutritional mismanagement and possibly increased management problems during the receiving period.

Once the calves are accepted, they should be placed in drylots with free access to good quality grass hay and fresh water and allowed to rest overnight. Drylots offer several advantages over grass traps. Calves kept in drylots have lower morbidity and mortality rates, improved gains, and lower labor costs. Traps allow calves too much room to walk fences, causing more physical stress, and allow them to stray too far from feedbunks and water sources. Confining calves for up to 3 weeks before turning them out to pasture is often necessary to allow recovery from stress-related diseases occurring during the receiving period. Water tanks with water running from a hydrant will often encourage calves to drink, since many are not accustomed to drinking from automatic waterers. Calves are not usually very competitive at the feed bunk, so a minimum of 1.5 ft of bunk space per animal should be provided. A 0.5 to 1.0 kg per head of a palatable protein pellet should be offered in the feedbunk on arrival.

Nutrition

Newly received, stressed calves have special nutritional problems. Inadequate or stress-inducing nutrition practices compound health problems. Sick animals often eat too little to achieve nutrient levels that aid in recovery. With many feeds, animals initially eat too little and later eat too much, which can lead to digestive upset and other health problems.

As seen in Table 1, the percentage of calves eating daily is less than satisfactory during the first 10 days after arrival. Feed intake is also low, ranging from 0.5 to 1.5 per cent of their body weight on a dry matter basis during the first week. Feed intake increases through the third week and follows a plateau during the fourth week, indicating that normal feed intake is achieved during the third week. It is essential that a palatable ration be offered, and nutrient densities must be raised when feed intake is low. Pounds of nutrients consumed during the receiving period are of greater importance than percentages of nutrients in rations.

Silage is often included in the ration of recently weaned and newly received calves, but it is sometimes associated

Table 1. *The Percentage of Calves Eating During the First 10 Days**

Day	Calves Eating (%)	Range (%)
1	21.7	0–50
2	36.7	10–60
3	56.7	30–90
4	61.7	30–90
5	66.7	40–90
6	68.3	40–90
7	70.0	60–90
8	71.7	60–80
9	73.3	60–90
10	85.0	60–100

*From Hutcheson, D. P.: Observations on Receiving New Cattle. Eighth
*Annual Texas Beef Conference Proceedings, Amarillo, Texas, 1980.

Table 2. *A 75 Per Cent Concentrate Receiving Diet**

Ingredient	Amount (% as fed)
Steam-flaked milo	47.5
Yellow hominy feed	7.0
Soybean meal	7.2
Ground alfalfa hay	18.0
Cottonseed hulls	7.0
Fat	3.0
Molasses	7.0
Urea	.5
Limestone	1.0
Monosodium phosphate	.3
Trace mineralized salt	.5
Premix†	1.0
TOTAL	100.0

*From Lofgreen, G. P.: Nutrition and management of stressed beef calves. Symposium on Herd Health Management. Vet. Clin. North Am. 5:96, 1983.

†Premix supplies 1000 IU of vitamin A/lb and 8 gm of bacitracin/ton of finished feed.

with higher morbidity and mortality rates. When silage is used in the receiving ration, it is essential to supplement it with protein while feed intake is low. Alfalfa hay, although palatable and of good nutrient value, often causes increased bloat and contributes to loose stools. Moldy or poor quality hay lessens consumption. Feeding an antibiotic at excessive levels during the receiving period depresses rumen function.

Concentrate levels above 55 per cent during the receiving period are usually accompanied by higher morbidity and higher medication costs; however, average daily gain (ADG) and feed efficiency (FE) will be improved. Feeding good quality, long-stem hay, such as prairie or oat hay, results in the lowest morbidity and mortality rates. A balance of good health performance, ADG, and FE is obtained when native hay is limit-fed with a 75 per cent concentrate ration (Table 2) fed free-choice. Feeding prairie hay free-choice with up to 1 kg/day of a palatable 40 per cent protein pellet (Table 3) results in excellent health performance, and gains of 0.5 to 1.0 kg/day can be expected during a 28-day receiving period.

Coccidiostats in receiving rations provide effective control of both clinical and subclinical coccidiosis. Clinical coccidiosis in newly received calves is quite common and results in noticeable losses in production as well as higher medication costs and deaths. Subclinical infections cause more subtle losses but can be costly owing to reduced performance and increased incidence of other stress-related diseases. Decoquinate (Deccox)[1] for 28 days as a feed additive at a dosage of 22.7 mg/45 kg of body weight or amprolium (Corid)[2] crumbles at 5.06 mg/kg of body weight for 21 days are effective preventive agents. Am-

Table 3. *Per Cent Composition of Protein Pellets* Used in Receiving Program†*

Soybean-oil meal	90.87 %
Limestone	1.50
Cottonseed hulls	1.75
Salt	3.00
Dicalcium phosphate	2.75
Vitamin mineral premix	0.12

*3/16-inch pellet.

†From Gill, D. R., Armbruster, S., and Richet, E. J.: The Nutrition of Newly Received Stress Stocker Cattle. Proceedings of 1980 Oklahoma Beef Symposium, Stillwater, Oklahoma.

prolium is also available as a liquid for use in drinking water. Improved ADG and FE result from the use of a coccidiostat during the receiving period. Rumensin[3] or Bovatec[4] can be placed in the ration after the calves have begun consuming normal quantities of feed. These compounds aid in the control of coccidiosis, but their use during the early receiving period may reduce feed intake.

PROCESSING

Proper handling and management of cattle during processing is essential to minimize stress, to reduce the risk of injury, and to detect sick cattle as soon as possible. The veterinarian plays a vital role in the success of this phase of the receiving program by providing detailed instructions to employees of the backgrounding yard or stocker operation on proper techniques to be used when processing calves, on the procedures to be performed, and on sanitation and the proper use and handling of vaccines and other drugs. The consulting veterinarian should provide a written processing protocol to both managers and their employees.

Processing should not be delayed for more than 24 to 36 hr after arrival. Longer delays result in higher rates of morbidity and do not take full advantage of the protection offered by vaccines or preventive medications. Each day that processing is delayed results in a 1 per cent increase in morbidity. In many veterinary practices, facilities are available to process cattle before they are delivered to local backgrounding or stocker operations. This reduces the labor and facility requirements of the producer.

The following guidelines for procedures to be accomplished during processing may be modified to fulfill specific needs to meet local conditions.

1. Body temperature: Body temperature can reliably indicate sickness if a few simple rules are followed:
   a. Newly arrived cattle are rested overnight before processing. Body temperatures of cattle just unloaded from the truck are not reliable indicators of illness.
   b. Process small groups, so no animal is out of its pen or waiting to be processed for more than 30 minutes.
   c. Process early in the morning; temperature readings are seldom meaningful when taken in the afternoon.
   d. Take extra care to move cattle through processing with a minimum of excitement or stress.
   e. Take body temperature as soon as the animal enters the chute.
   f. An electronic thermometer is essential. Calves with a body temperature of 104°F (40°C) or greater or showing other signs of illness should be separated from the group, placed in a treatment program, and kept in a hospital pen until they recover.
2. Vaccinations:
   a. IBR and PI₃. Either the intramuscular or intranasal vaccine can be used. PI₃ vaccine may not be of benefit in older cattle but should be used in younger calves.
   b. BVD vaccine should be used in endemic areas. The killed BVD vaccine can be given to extremely stressed calves.
   c. *Pasteurella* bacterins have shown no value in controlled trials and are not recommended in receiving programs.

d. Four-way *Clostridium (C. chauvoei, C. septicum, C. sordellii, C. novyi)* bacterin.

e. *Leptospira pomona* bacterin in endemic areas.

3. Deworm: Products for internal parasite control are Ivomec[5] injectable, Panacur[6] suspension, Omnizole[7] paste, Tramisol[8] injectable or gel, and Levasole.[9] Plasma pepsinogen levels can be determined by the state's diagnostic laboratories to determine the incidence of Type II ostertagiosis. Infected cattle should be dewormed with Ivomec or Panacur at twice the usual dosage. Type II ostertagiosis is most prevalent in cattle originating in the southeast, particularly after long, dry periods or in winter.

4. External parasites: Calves should be dipped in GX–118[10] or Co-Ral,[11] poured with Spotton,[12] or injected with Ivomec. Grubicides should not be used after the cut-off date, as host-parasite reactions may occur, although they are not common in younger calves.

5. Vitamin A injection (1 million units).

6. Implant with growth stimulant: Products include Compudose,[13] Ralgro,[14] and Synovex-S[15] for steers and Synovex-H[15] or Ralgro for heifers. Periodically, observe implanting procedures to ensure that they are done properly, as improper technique will not result in maximum benefit. Synovex-S and Synovex-H should not be used in calves weighing less than 180 kg. Bulls or heifers intended for breeding should not be implanted.

7. Tip horns.

8. Castrate.

9. Mass medication: Sustained-release antibacterials, such as Liquamycin LA 200[16] or Albon SR[17] boluses at processing will reduce the incidence of respiratory disease during the receiving period; however, this will greatly add to cost. If fresh cattle are received, and if there is sufficient skilled labor available, this practice may not be cost-effective. When there is a shortage of labor or when employees are not highly skilled at detecting sick cattle early, mass medication may be a useful management tool. It is of greatest benefit when used on sale-barn cattle assembled from several sources or on extremely stressed calves.

After processing, all cattle, except those taken to the hospital pen, are moved to their home pen and offered a receiving ration. Sick cattle are placed on an appropriate treatment program.

DIAGNOSIS AND TREATMENT

The veterinarian should train the pen riders and doctoring crews to recognize the more common diseases affecting calves, especially respiratory diseases, in backgrounding or stocker operations. All cattle should be inspected daily, and pens or problem calves should be checked twice daily. Cattle with signs of illness should be removed from the pens to the hospital pen as quietly as possible to minimize stress. They should remain in the hospital pen until they recover and are able to compete with penmates for feed and water. Sick cattle left in the pens another day or two in hope of spontaneous recovery often are less responsive to treatment than those that are removed early and treated.

Once the cattle are in the hospital pen, the doctoring crews should take the body temperature, assign a degree of illness (severe, moderate, or slight), and begin a hospital treatment card (Figures 1 and 2). Treatment should be based on written guidelines provided by the veterinarian. Drugs and dosages for the treatment of respiratory diseases are discussed in Section 10. Drug selection should be based on culture results, sensitivity tests, and clinical response to treatment.

Sick cattle should be examined and evaluated daily to determine response to treatment. The degree of illness (severe, moderate, or slight) and body temperature should

Pen _____ Tag _____ Date	Temp	Severity of Illness	LA 200	Albon SR	Oxyject 100	Sulfa bolus	Erythro	Amoxicillin	Penicillin	Tylan	Thiamine	Neomycin	Corid				

Figure 1. Hospital card (side 1).

Pen _____Tag _____Date First Pulled _____Time of Day _____

Body Temperature _____ Weight _____

Symptoms on date first pulled as sick:

Nose	Dry _____	Crusted _____		Discharge _____		Clear _____
Eyes	Clear _____	Cloudy _____		Ulcer _____		Watery _____
Breathing	Heavy _____	Labored _____		Rapid _____		Cough _____
Diarrhea (feces)	Blood _____	Watery _____		Black _____		
Abdomen	Bloated _____	Drawn _____		Full _____		
Foot Rot	Yes _____	No _____				
Nervous System	Staggering _____	Convulsions _____		Muscle Twitch _____		
Depression	Slight _____	Moderate _____		Severe _____		
Other	_____					

Diagnosis: _____

Severity of Illness: _____

Remarks:

Figure 2. Hospital card (side 2).

be evaluated in order to judge response. Depression, appetite, respiratory difficulties, and stool consistency are important factors to consider when assigning a degree to the illness. Useful criteria to consider when deciding to continue with the same medication or to change are as follows:

1. A calf with a temperature of 104°F (40°C) or greater on the first day it was pulled must show a 2° reduction in fever or drop to less than 104°F (40°C) within 24 hr of treatment to be designated as improved.

2. A calf with a temperature of less than 104°F (40°C) on the first day must improve physically within 24 hr of treatment to be designated as improved.

3. If one of the above criteria is not fulfilled, the animal is given the second drug in the sequence outlined by the veterinarian.

4. The animal is evaluated 24 hr later, and the same criteria are used to determine the response.

5. This sequence is repeated until a positive clinical response or drop in temperature is noted.

Once a calf is responding to a drug, it should be treated for at least 2 more days while fever, inappetence, depression, and other clinical signs are absent. It is often wise to extend the treatment of severely ill cattle for 2 to 3 additional days. A rectal temperature of 103°F (39.5°C) may be normal for a calf that has been injected with antimicrobials for several days, especially when drugs such as erythromycin or tylosin are used. These drugs cause severe muscle irritation when injected in large quantities for several days.

Treated calves should remain in the hospital or convalescent pen until they eat well enough to compete with penmates. If the cattle in the home pen are on a high concentrate ration, one must allow the treated calf to adjust to the higher concentrate ration before being returned to the home pen in order to avoid serious digestive upsets.

All dead cattle should undergo necropsy to determine the type and extent of lesions present and the cause of death. Samples should be submitted to the laboratory for culturing, sensitivity testing, histopathologic examination, and virus isolation. The necropsy can be a useful instructional tool to show health crews why the animal failed to respond to therapy, the reason for the clinical signs, and the need for early detection of sick cattle before lesions advance.

Records

Complete, accurate health records are essential. They provide documentation of charges, processing procedures, therapeutic regimens, and dispositions of cattle. They are necesary for the veterinarian to periodically evaluate the overall health program effectiveness and to determine the type and incidence of various health problems. Although an accurate, detailed handwritten system is adequate, computerized health records allow the veterinarian and manager more flexibility in retrieving and evaluating data.

PRODUCT LIST AND SUPPLIER

1. Deccox. Rhône-Poulenc Inc., Atlanta, GA 30342.
2. Corid. Merck, Sharp & Dohme Agvet, Rahway, NJ 07065.
3. Rumensin. Elanco Products Co., Indianapolis, IN 46285.
4. Bovatec. Hoffman-LaRoche Inc., Nutley, NJ 07110.
5. Ivomec injectable. MSD Agvet, Rahway, NJ 07065.
6. Panacur suspension. American Hoechst Corp., Somerville, NJ 08876.
7. Omnizole paste. Merck, Sharp & Dohme Agvet, Rahway, NJ 07065.
8. Tramisol injectable or gel. American Cyanamid Co., Wayne, NJ 07470.

9. Levasole. Pitman-Moore, Inc., Washington Crossing, NJ 08560.

10. GX-118. Starbar, Dallas, TX 75234.

11. Co-Ral. Cutter Laboratories Inc., Shawnee Mission, KS 66201.

12. Spotton. Cutter Laboratories Inc., Shawnee Mission, KS 66201.

13. Compudose. Elanco Products Co., Indianapolis, IN 46285.

14. Ralgro. IMC Corporation, Terre Haute, IN 47808.

15. Synovex-H and Synovex-S. Syntex Agribusiness Inc., Des Moines, IA 50303.

16. LA 200. Pfizer, Inc., New York, NY 10017.

17. Albon SR. Hoffman-LaRoche Inc., Nutley, NJ 07110.

Supplemental Reading

Lofgreen, G. P.: Nutrition and management of stressed beef calves. Vet. Clin. North Am. 5:87–101, 1983.

Parks, T. D.: Receiving, processing and treating light cattle. 1982. Light Cattle Management Seminar, Ft. Collins, Colorado, 1982.

Richey, E. J.: A treatment program for sick newly arrived stocker cattle. Proceedings of 1980 Oklahoma Beef Symposium, Stillwater, Oklahoma.

Thompson, G. B., and O'Mary, C. C.: The Feedlot, 3rd ed. Philadelphia: Lea & Febiger, 1983.

Sheep Flock Health Management

DON E. BAILEY, D.V.M.

ENTEROTOXEMIA TYPE D

Enterotoxemia type D is an acute infectious but not contagious disease of sheep. This disease occurs in young lambs that are nursing and in feeder lambs that are in the feedlot. The condition is also discussed in the article on Lamb Feedlot Management. It is characterized by sudden death, convulsions, and hyperglycemia. Some of the predisposing factors are diets consisting of large quantities of milk and rich concentrates such as cereal grains; sudden changes in feed; ewes and lambs on improved pastures undergoing rapid growth; sheep and lambs in good condition; and lambs that are nursing ewes with abundant milk and are predisposed to enterotoxemia type D. Death is not confined to lambs and can occur in adult sheep experiencing the same conditions. Enterotoxemia type D is caused by *Clostridium perfringens* type D.

Clinical Signs and Postmortem Lesions

Death from enterotoxemia is sudden, with sheep exhibiting nervous symptoms. The head is drawn back, with convulsive movements and salivation. Death usually occurs within 30 to 90 minutes, but in lambs recently vaccinated and not yet immune, death will occur later. Postmortem lesions are important in the diagnosis of enterotoxemia because symptoms are rarely observed. The subendocardium of the left ventricle usually has "paintbrush" hemorrhages. The pericardial sac is often enlarged with yellow fluid and fibrin. The lungs are congested with edematous fluid and coagulated blood. Small petechial hemorrhages on the thymus are found. The abomasum contains milk curds with the rest of the

digestive tract full. The ileum may be reddened. Rapid putrefaction of the carcass occurs quickly after death. The kidneys of sheep and lambs that have died from enterotoxemia tend to soften and degenerate very rapidly. Thus, the common term "pulpy kidney" is used to describe the disease. Diagnosis is suggested by the sudden death of unvaccinated, fat sheep grazing on improved pasture or in a feedlot. Suckling lambs in good condition may die as early as 1 month after birth. The differential diagnosis requires consideration of blackleg, black disease, bloat, anthrax, and poisoning. The laboratory test results can help confirm the diagnosis by identification of epsilon toxin from the contents of the ileum and from the blood.

Treatment

There is no satisfactory treatment for affected animals. All emphasis should be placed on prevention. In rare cases lambs have been saved after symptoms began with the use of large doses of antitoxins and oral antibiotics.

Prevention

In farm flocks, yearly booster vaccinations of adult sheep is recommended. Lambs are vaccinated twice, with the first dose given 10 days after birth and the second dose given 2 weeks later. One vaccination does not confer sufficient immunity. In some cases a third booster vaccination is needed. If ewes receive a booster vaccination 2 to 4 weeks before lambing, lambs will receive protection from the colostrum. This protection lasts about 30 days or long enough for 2 vaccinations to be given. Some purebred-sheep owners give 3 ml of antitoxin at birth in addition to later administration of the vaccine. Creep feeds containing 22 mg/kg of oxytetracycline or 22 mg/kg of chlortetracycline will help prevent enterotoxemia. Lambs should be revaccinated at weaning or when they enter the feedlot.

HEMORRHAGIC ENTEROTOXEMIA IN YOUNG LAMBS

Hemorrhage enterotoxemia is an acute, highly fatal disease of young lambs caused by the beta toxin of *Clostridium perfringens* type C and, occasionally, type B. Enterotoxemia caused by type A toxin does occur, but it is very rare. The disease usually affects young lambs 1 day to 4 weeks of age. The most common age for infection is 12 to 72 hr after birth. This disease in young lambs normally occurs when sheep are kept in lambing sheds and barns. Vigorous lambs die suddenly. Diarrhea may occur along with signs of colic. Postmortem examination reveals hemorrhagic enteritis. The abomasum is full of milk. Hemorrhages of subendocardium and thymus are present.

Treatment

Lambs are usually found dead. If symptoms do appear, *Clostridium perfringens* type BCD antitoxin can be used in recommended therapeutic dosages.

Prevention

Since this disease appears early in life, the most effective means of prevention is the vaccination of ewes during pregnancy with *Clostridium perfringens* types C and D toxoids. Commercial toxoids normally contain the type B toxoid. In endemic areas where type B is found, the toxoid should contain all 3 types. During the first year of vaccinations, the ewes should receive 2 inoculations, with the last administered 2 to 4 weeks preceding lambing. After that, booster vaccination is sufficient. In response to an outbreak, antitoxins can be given soon after birth. Orphan lambs on substitute high-fat milk develop acute type C hemorrhagic enterotoxemia and must be vaccinated twice before 1 month of age. *Clostridium perfringens* type C does occur in adult sheep and commonly is called "struck." Multiple clostridial vaccine given during a flock health program prevents the condition. Sanitary management practices also help to avoid or to reduce the disease. The environment of the lamb should be kept clean and dry. Caretakers with contaminated hands or instruments should avoid handling the lambs' mouths. Relocating ewes just before lambing helps reduce exposure. Antibiotics in the creep feed will also help prevent the disease.

TETANUS

Tetanus is a disease affecting the nervous system. *Clostridium tetani* spores, along with pyogenic bacteria from soil and manure, enter tissues through injuries, such as foot puncture, castration, docking, shearing, and other wounds. The use of elastrators for docking has been a major cause of tetanus in lambs. Early symptoms are erect ears, extended head, prolapsing nictitating membranes, and difficulty walking. Finally, the animal cannot stand, respiration accelerates, and muscular rigidity increases.

Treatment and Prevention

Management rules are as follows: (1) keep all surgical instruments clean and in a disinfectant solution, (2) clean pens and sheds, and (3) dock and castrate in clean, grassy areas. When using an elastrator, keep rubber rings in a disinfectant and use iodine around the elastrator ring after applying the ring. Give 100 units of tetanus antitoxin when docking with the elastrator. In an endemic area, the ewe should be given 1 ml tetanus toxoid. A second toxoid injection should be given the following year, and this treatment usually gives lifetime immunity. Treatment with tetanus antitoxin, tranquilizers, and antibiotics and redocking are not very often successful. Strychnine poisoning resembles tetanus but is of much shorter duration. Lambs infected with tetanus may live as long as 1 week after symptoms appear.

ABORTION

Abortion may occur at different stages of pregnancy, depending on the cause. Injuries due to rough handling or equipment bruising can cause abortion. Nutritional deficiencies such as low selenium intake may do the same. Other infectious diseases of sheep that cause abortions are vibriosis, enzootic abortion of ewes (EAE), brucellosis, leptospirosis, toxoplasmosis, salmonellosis, listeriosis, and bluetongue.

Vibriosis

Vibriosis is caused by the bacterium *Vibrio fetus intestinalis* and is characterized by late abortions, stillbirths, and weak lambs. The disease is widespread, causing abortion storms that result in great economic losses. Large numbers of organisms are shed with the placenta and in the vaginal discharge. Sometimes a ewe will expel a decomposed fetus while giving birth to a normal lamb. Vibriosis is spread by carrier ewes through ingestion of contaminated feed and water. Diagnosis is based on isolation of the causative bacteria from the aborted fetus or placenta. Occasionally, the livers of aborted fetuses will have characteristic white necrotic areas. Aborted lambs show a swollen appearance of the abdomen with sanguineous fluids between the skin and muscle and in the abdominal cavity.

Treatment and Prevention

V. fetus vaccine is used to stop abortion storms. Administer 5 ml of vaccine subcutaneously. At the time of vaccination, the ewe should be given an intramuscular injection of a penicillin-streptomycin preparation. The antibotic should be given the following 2 days, and this will stop most abortions. To prevent vibriosis in a flock, all ewes should be given 2 annual vaccinations. The first vaccination is given at breeding time, and the second vaccination is given at the beginning of the last trimester. Another method of controlling vibriosis abortions is by the use of tetracycline in the feed. Doses vary from 100 mg to 300 mg/ewe/day. This method has the advantage of helping to control other infectious diseases at the same time. Aborting ewes should be kept isolated, and all aborted lambs and placentas should be burned.

Enzootic Abortion of Ewes (EAE)

Enzootic abortion of ewes (EAE) is widespread in the United States. Like vibriosis, it is characterized by premature births and abortions. Ewes appear sick for 2 to 3 days after abortions. The placental membranes are usually retained with a brownish vaginal discharge. The disease is caused by a chlamydial organism. Abortions in a flock may be as high as 30 per cent the first year, with a 5 per cent abortion rate in subsequent years. Diagnosis is made by demonstrating the presence of the organism and by positive findings of serologic tests. In foreign countries, a vaccine is available and is used successfully. One vaccination is effective from 3 years of life. Strict sanitation and isolation of aborted ewes is helpful. Ewes that abort once will be immune for life and should be kept. The use of tetracycline in the feed of pregnant ewes exposed to EAE helps to control the disease. From 100 mg to 300 mg/head daily of tetracycline given for 3 weeks at breeding time and again for 3 weeks preceding lambing has protected first-lambing ewes.

Brucellosis

Brucellosis in sheep is caused by *Brucella ovis*. This organism is thought to be the main cause of epididymitis in rams. It also causes abortion in the third trimester of pregnancy. Placentas are not retained and contain gross plaques of a yellow-white exudate on the cotyledons. Diagnosis is based on isolation of *B. ovis* from the placental cotyledons or aborted fetus. Prevention is based on fertility testing and physical examination of the rams along with blood tests on ewes and rams.

Leptospirosis

Leptospirosis in sheep is characterized by fever, anemia, hemoglobinuria, icterus, and abortion. The principal *Leptospira* species are *Leptospira pomona*, *L. hardjo*, and *L.*

grippotyphosa. The leptospires are transmitted by carrier animals. This disease often causes the death of yearling sheep, and postmortem observations are jaundice, dark kidneys, and hematuria. Isolation of leptospires is difficult. Serologic testing is the most reliable diagnostic aid. Sheep may be vaccinated with multivalent vaccines.

Toxoplasmosis

Toxoplasmosis is a subacute or chronic infection characterized by placentitis, fetal encephalitis, abortion, and stillbirths. The disease has occurred to some extent in the United States but is of considerable importance in some foreign countries. It is caused by *Toxoplasma gondii*. Clinical signs depend on what organ is most affected. With metritis and placentitis, ewes abort during the last month of pregnancy. Congenitally infected lambs are mentally dull, physically weak, muscularly incoordinated, and unable to nurse. Diagnosis is based on the finding of swollen cotyledons with gray foci 1 to 2 mm in diameter. There is no treatment or vaccination. Elimination of barn cats stops the spread of toxoplasmosis.

Salmonellosis

Salmonellosis is an acute disease of sheep. It is characterized by diarrhea and sudden death in feedlot lambs and metritis and abortion in adult ewes. Abortions are usually caused by *Salmonella typhimurium*, *S. abortusovis*, and *S. dublin*. The organisms are ingested, penetrate the intestinal wall, invade the blood stream, and are carried to the uterus and placenta. The disease is diagnosed on the basis of isolation of salmonella from the placenta or aborted fetus. Prevention of the disease is dependent on sanitary practices. *Salmonella* vaccines (bacterins) are available. Results following the use of injectable antibiotics are disappointing.

Listeriosis

Listeriosis is an acute noncontagious disease caused by a bacterium (*Listeria monocytogenes*) that resides in soil and silage. The organism usually invades the brain, resulting in neurologic signs such as circling. This bacterium can cause placentitis, with abortions usually occurring in the last trimester. An intestinal form of the disease can also occur, usually in feedlot lambs. Diagnosis of listeriosis is confirmed by isolation of the bacteria from the placenta or aborted fetus. Ewes in affected flocks will manifest the nervous symptoms as well as abortion, thus providing a clue to the cause of abortions.

Viral Diseases

Infectious viral diseases resulting in abortion in sheep are bluetongue, Rift Valley fever, Wesselsbron disease, and tick-borne fever.

PNEUMONIA

Pneumonia in sheep is found throughout the sheep-producing countries of the world. It causes economic losses owing to death, unthriftiness, and cost of treatment. The periods of highest susceptibility are the first month of life and the time of weaning and shipping. Starvation is the most common cause of death in lambs from birth to 2 weeks of age, and pneumonia is the second most common cause of death. The first symptom may be sudden death. Most patients show a drooping of the ear, dyspnea, coughing, anorexia, and a temperature of 41 to 42°C. Sheep with pneumonia show a purulent discharge from the nostrils and lacrimation. Morbidity ranges from 10 to 50 per cent, with mortality averaging 10 per cent. The infectious agents that are identified with sheep pneumonia are *Pasteurella* (*P. haemolytica* and *P. multocida*), chlamydial organisms, and mycoplasmic agents. Predisposing factors are adverse weather conditions, crowding, poor sanitation, poor nutrition, shipping, and shearing. Transmission occurs as sheep are crowded in pens and around barns. The overuse of heat in reviving lambs may cause pneumonia. Improper use of drench guns can cause throat damage and foreign-body pneumonia. Diagnosis is based on symptoms, evidence at autopsy, and recovery of the organism that causes pneumonia. Lungworms and nematodes (*Dictyocaulus filaria*, *Protostrongylus rufescens*, and *Müllerius capillaris*) all cause verminous pneumonia. Chronic progressive pneumonia is a contagious nonfebrile disease of adult sheep characterized by weakness, dyspnea, and emaciation. It is caused by a virus. Some veterinarians have found that *Pasteurella* bacterins given twice a year reduce deaths in ewes and lambs. Therapeutic doses of sulfonamides (1 mg/kg/day) can be given orally or in the drinking water for 4 to 6 days. Alternatively, oxytetracycline may be administered parenterally for 4 to 6 days in a dose of 12 mg/kg/day.

CONTAGIOUS ECTHYMA

Contagious ecthyma, or "sore mouth," is an infectious disease of sheep and goats that causes the formation of thick, dark scabs on the lips, face, ears, and udders of affected sheep. This disease is caused by a virus, a member of the poxvirus group. It is widespread throughout sheep-raising countries, and the total cost to the industry is high. Economic losses result from unthriftiness, loss of physical condition, death of young lambs that cannot nurse, and mastitis and deformed teats following infection in adults. Contagious ecthyma also occurs in goats, humans, and sometimes dogs and cats. The incubation period is 2 to 3 days followed by a recovery period of 2 to 4 weeks. Differential diagnosis includes ulcerative dermatosis, sheep pox, photosensitization, and facial eczema. Contagious ecthyma pustules form proliferative nodules that rise above the surface of the skin. Ulcerative dermatosis lesions are characterized by ulcers and crusts on the skin of the face, feet, and genitalia. Sheep pox causes elevated pustules over much of the body.

Treatment and Prevention

Healing will occur spontaneously, but weak animals should be given supportive treatment, e.g., antibiotics, fluids, and kerosene applied to the scabby lip to dry up the inflammation. Vaccination before and at the start of an outbreak controls the spread. All sheep in the herd and all herd replacements in subsequent years should be vaccinated. Owners should be warned to wear gloves when vaccinating and to burn containers and gloves following use.

FOOT DISEASES OF SHEEP AND GOATS

Foot Rot

Foot rot is a highly contagious disease of sheep and goats that can affect 75 per cent of a flock. It can be acute or chronic and is characterized by lameness and bidigital separation of the hoof corneum from the basal epithelium and derma. The disease is caused by the interaction of *Bacteroides funduliformis* (*Sphaerophorus necrophorus* or *Fusiformis necrophorus*) and *Fusiformis nodosus*. The disease affects all ages of sheep and is recurrent. Losses result from unthriftiness, poor production, and high cost of labor and materials for treatment and control. The infection within the horny hoof has a characteristically foul odor. Foot overgrowth, rolled underhooves, wet, muddy conditions, and mild temperatures provide an excellent environment for the causative organisms to multiply. Foot rot can be controlled by a rigorous program of hoof trimming and foot bathing, using solutions of formalin, arsenicals, copper sulfate, and a constant culling of chronically affected sheep. Parenterally administered antibiotics have been shown to be effective in treating foot rot. Also, subcutaneous injections of antibiotics between the toes have been beneficial. Foot baths commonly contain 5 or 10 per cent formalin: 5 per cent is used if the sheep are left standing in the chute and 10 per cent is used if they walk through. The sides of the chute must be ventilated to prevent lung damage to the sheep and operator. Tag wool can be placed in the foot trough along with the solution to stop splashing and to allow the sheep to go through easier. Copper sulfate (20 per cent) is also used in foot baths. Foot rot vaccines are being used experimentally and show promise.

Foot Abscess

Foot abscess is an acute or chronic suppurative laminitis of a single digit. It is characterized by severe lameness and pus discharge through a sinus above the hoof and near the coronet. Incidence does not exceed 10 per cent, with the course of the disease lasting weeks to months. Sometimes the area of the foot affected (i.e., toe or heel) is used to describe different conditions. Foot abscess above the coronary band, toe, or heel, or between the toes (scald) is associated with *Fusiformis necrophorus*. Foot abscess above the foot responds to surgical drainage and antibiotic injection. Irrigation with nitrofuran and intramuscular injection of penicillin at the rate of 70,000 IU/kg of body weight are therapeutically effective. Foot scald has a higher morbidity, particularly in lambs. Foot scald commences with inflammation of the skin between the toes and progresses to the rear portion of the heel, causing separation from the hoof. This condition is controlled and treated in the same manner as foot rot. Some natural immunity to foot rot exists in flocks. To date, vaccination programs have been conducted with limited success. Numerous strains of *F. nodosus* have been identified. Where isolation and quarantine of infected flocks has been practiced, control of foot rot has been successful.

OBSTETRICS IN SHEEP

Difficulties in lambing or kidding are usually due to 1 of 3 conditions: (1) the lamb or the kid is too large for the pelvis, (2) the contraction of the uterus is too feeble to expel the lamb, or (3) the presentation of the lamb is abnormal. Normal birth should occur within 30 to 45 minutes after rupture of the membranes. Assistance is difficult when the ewe becomes exhausted, the vagina becomes dry and swollen, or the lamb becomes swollen. It is important to insure cleanliness and use lubrication and a disinfectant solution. A plastic device called a "lamb puller"* is very helpful in assisting delivery once the position of the lamb is corrected inside the uterus. Lambs are subject to navel infection, so it is important to disinfect the navel. Antibiotic uterine tablets placed in the uterus are helpful in preventing infection. In some cases where delivery is impossible, a cesarean section is indicated. Sheep and goats withstand the surgery well, and in most cases live lambs or kids result. Surgical approach varies with the individual veterinarian. The ventral approach and lateral left or right flank approach are equally used. Anesthetics vary from general intravenous barbiturates and inhalation anesthetics to local anesthetic infiltration of the surgical area. Antibiotics and orally administered analgesics (such as aspirin) will prevent shock and depression following surgery.

Vaginal Prolapse

Vaginal prolapse occurs in ewes during the prelambing period. Overfeeding of roughage in the ewe near parturition can cause vaginal prolapse. Nerve injury following docking the tail too close is thought to be another cause. High estrogen levels in legumes are also a contributing factor. Treatment consists of cleaning the prolapsed vagina and lifting the prolapse to allow easy micturition, thus reducing the straining. Next the vaginal prolapse should be covered with sulfa-urea ointment and then should be placed within the vagina. After replacing the vagina, insert the plastic bearing retainer and tie into wool on either side of the ewe. The ewe will then lamb through the plastic retainer at lambing time.†

Rectal Prolapse

Rectal prolapses usually occur in feedlot lambs on high concentrate rations. Some of the causes of rectal prolapse are growth implants, internal parasites, dusty conditions, extreme close docking of the tail, and pneumonia. A prolapse of 15 to 20 cm may eventually expose the rectum. If lambs are in market condition, they should be slaughtered. Other cases are treated surgically. A plastic pipe of the proper size is inserted into the lumen of the bowel up to the rectal area. Then an elastrator band is placed over the prolapse to the rectum. The prolapse will slough in a few days, and the plastic pipe will be expelled.

Supplemental Reading

Jensen, R.: Diseases of Sheep. Philadelphia, Lea & Febiger, 1974.
Moule, G. R.: Handbook for Wool Growers. Denver, Colorado, Abegg Printing.
Sheep Industry Development and American Sheep Producers Council: The Sheepman's Production Handbook, Second Edition, May, 1975.

---

*Lamb and kid puller available from Hergert's Industries, Star Rt. 38, Box 16, Drain, OR 97435.
†Bearing retainer available from Hergert's Industries, Star Rt. 38, Box 16, Drain, OR 97435.

Sheep Flock Health Management

Farm Flocks

R. D. SCOGGINS, D.V.M.

Maintaining a healthy sheep flock can depend on a good working relationship between producer and veterinarian. The veterinarian's role is primarily one of diagnostician and adviser. The size, disposition, and individual monetary value of sheep result in many do-it-yourself approaches to veterinary procedures.

The sick or dead individual animal is best utilized as a sentinel, signaling a problem. An early postmortem examination should always be performed when any question of cause of death exists. Individual treatment of sick animals is not always economically justifiable. Procedures that minimize or prevent economic loss due to disease are far more effective.

Flock health programs need to be developed on an individual farm basis. The requirements of each farm will depend on the goals, facilities, acreage, sheep number, and experience of the producer. A sequential calendar approach can be a useful way to plan for supply needs and to schedule procedures in a logical and timely manner.

Veterinarians should emphasize their diagnostic and advisory capabilities. Postmortem examinations, serologic surveys, fecal examinations for parasitism, bacterial cultures and sensitivity tests, and interpretation of laboratory results are all professional services the veterinarian can utilize to monitor a flock's health needs. Clients appreciate useful scientific procedures that help confirm the diagnosis.

Sheep producers and veterinarians face a dilemma in that very few useful drugs are presently approved for use in sheep. Economic reality does not suggest this problem will change much in the immediate future.

Maintaining flock health revolves around a continual parasite control program plus an effective immunization program. Immunization and parasite control are individualized for each farm. The program to be presented here has been proven useful for midwestern United States farm flocks.

Producers should be encouraged to develop a set of working facilities. Head gate, foot bath, and a crowding chute should be included. These facilities help diminish the effort needed to regularly repeat tedious procedures.

Only those procedures useful to specific farms should be utilized. The veterinarian should sort out the useful procedures from the unnecessary procedures. Advising, implementing, and evaluating the results of health care for the producer are professional services that are deserving of remuneration.

PREBREEDING (EWE FLOCK)

A. Immunization procedures—repeat annually.
   1. Ovine *Vibrio* bacterin.
   2. Ovine *Chlamydia* vaccine—may be combined with *Vibrio* bacterin.
   3. Leptospirosis bacterin—serologic test results should identify necessary species.
   4. Ovine ecthyma—if there is a positive history or if there is anticipation of shows or sales. Use the inner ear, base of ear, underside of tail, or perineum in breeds without wool in these areas.
   5. Inactivated BVD—when border disease or "hairy shaker" disease has been a problem. Administer one half the recommended cattle dose.
B. Deworm with an effective anthelmintic.
   1. Levamisole in any of its available forms.
   2. Benzimidazoles.
      a. Fenbendazole (Panacur,* Cattle Guard*) at 5.1 mgm/kg. At 11 mgm/kg, it is effective against large tapeworms.
      b. Mebendazole (Telmin).†
      c. Thiabendazole.
   3. Morantel tartrate (Nematal,† Rumatal†) shows good efficacy and safety in sheep. Administer one-half bolus for each 100 lb of body weight. Safety allows its use in any normal adult sheep weighing more than 50 kg.
   4. Ivermectin.
      a. The equine product Equalan‡ has been used successfully orally in sheep. It should not be injected.
      b. The bovine formulation Ivomec‡ has been used in sheep in countries other than United States with considerable success. One ml/50 kg is injected subcutaneously in the rear flank skin fold.
      c. Ivomec is effective against roundworms, lungworms, nasal bots, lice, keds, and mange mites when given systemically.
      d. Some products have reportedly caused toxicity problems in the past. This includes Loxon,§ which causes neuromuscular weakness or paralysis. Phenothiazine may cause wool staining and photosensitivity. Cambendazole has created respiratory problems in sheep in the United Kingdom, and its usage has been discontinued there.
C. Trim the ewe's feet and place them in a foot bath. Allow them to maintain contact for 3 to 5 minutes. Use one of the following:
   1. 10% $CuSO_4$.
   2. 10 to 20% $ZnSO_4$.
   3. 5% formalin.
D. Flush ewes by increasing their energy intake to provide a steady, gradual weight gain.
E. Shear and evaluate rams for fertility plus overall soundness. Protect them from sunburn and excessive heat. Bailey Ejaculators¶ are useful for obtaining semen samples.
F. Check several farm cats serologically for toxoplasmosis. Protect feed from cat fecal contamination and reduce excessive cat population when appropriate.

*Available from Hoechst-Roussel Pharmaceuticals, Inc., Somerville, NJ 08876.
†Available from Pitman-Moore, Inc., Washington Crossing, NJ 08560.
‡Available from Merck & Co., Inc., West Point, PA 19486.
§Available from Burroughs Wellcome Co., Research Triangle Park, NC 27709.
¶Available from Western Serum Co., Phoenix, AZ 85011.

BREEDING

A. Using vasectomized teaser rams will help group ewes more closely in breeding, i.e., use 2 weeks before breeding rams.
B. Remove teasers. Turn in fertility-checked breeding rams.
   1. Ram lambs: 1/15 ewes.
   2. Mature rams: 1/35 to 50 ewes.

POSTBREEDING (PREGNANCY)

A. Remove rams (60-day breeding season).
B. Maintain diet to avoid weight loss.
C. Give ovine *Vibrio* booster.

PRELAMBING (30 DAYS)

A. Immunization procedures.
   1. Clostridial bacterins—type C and D and tetanus toxoid plus any additional bacterins if necessary.
   2. Respiratory Modified Live Virus (MLV) vaccine for the PI_3 component. Nasal spray at one half the cattle dose.
   3. Bivalent *Pasteurella* bacterin has been recommended to reduce the incidence of *Pasteurella* mastitis. Give an injection followed by boosters every 30 days until weaning at one half the recommended cattle dosage.
B. Selenium supplementation.
   1. Oral supplement—salt base.
   2. Injectable—5 mgm/ewe.
C. Clean barn. Add 4 to 6 inches limestone plus clean bedding.
D. Shear ewes—reduces humidity, increases space, and provides cleaner environment for the lambs.
E. Parasite control.
   1. Deworm with a larvacidal drug, such as Levamisole. Ivermectin, where approved.
   2. Coccidia control.
      a. Add 15 gm monensin/ton of feed.
      b. Provide 1 kg Deccox* (6% decoquinate)/25 kg salt. Give feed free-choice to ewes 30 days prelambing through weaning.
      c. One kg Deccox/ton of grain is also effective.
   3. External parasite control.
      a. Ivermectin (Ivomec).†
      b. Organophosphate pour-ons (Spotton,‡ Koral,‡ and so forth) at recommended cattle dosages.

LAMBING

A. Client education.
   1. Teach lamb delivery techniques.
   2. Newborn lamb care—review the following procedures with the producer: Colostrum, feeding, *Clostridium* (C and D) antitoxin administration, lamb milk replacement, vitamin E and selenium injec-

tion, proper docking and castrating techniques, sore-mouth vaccination when indicated, tetanus antitoxin administration (150 to 200 units), and application of iodine to navel stump.
   3. Give lambs MLV nasal spray vaccine (Nasalgen*) to control PI_3 pneumonia within first 24 hr.

POSTLAMBING (LAMBS)

A. Thirty days.
   1. *Clostridium perfringens* type D bacterin-toxoid injection.
   2. Second vitamin E and selenium injection.
B. Sixty days.
   1. Second *Clostridium perfringens* type D injection.
   2. Prepare for weaning.
      a. Creep feeding of lambs.
      b. Remove grain from ewes 7 days before weaning. Allow only hay and water.
   3. Implant wether lambs if economically feasible.
C. Weaning.
   1. Leave lambs in familiar surroundings while the ewes are removed.
   2. Ewes receive only water and grass hay for 7 days in a dry lot.
   3. Observe udders closely. Dry treat ewes with a history of mastitis.
D. Postweaning (lambs).
   1. Select ewe lambs for replacements, according to growth, multiple births, and soundness histories.
   2. Feed market lambs using the most economically efficient method available.
   3. Raise replacements on clean pasture with supplements, parasite control measures, and immunizations as indicated.
   4. Monitor copper levels in feed sources. Copper content should be less than 7 ppm for safety reasons, with normal molybdenum levels. Cases of copper toxicity may be respond to daily administration of 100 mg of ammonium molybdate and 1 gm of sodium sulfate in 20 ml of water daily as a drench. Treatment for a minimum of 21 days is necessary.
E. Postweaning (ewes)
   1. Give anthelmintics as needed.
   2. Flush ewes if rebreeding for fall lambs.
   3. Cull according to production standards and soundness.
F. Conditions frequently arise necessitating more specific therapy (see Supplemental Reading).
   Two frequent problems in farm flock practice are listeriosis and urinary calculi. Neither responds well to treatment, but both can be controlled.
   1. Listeriosis can be significantly reduced with proper silage preparation. The following steps can be quite effective.
      a. Finely chop silage.
      b. Feed 32 to 38% dry matter.
      c. Add the following supplements to each ton of silage:
         (1) 15 lb of urea.
         (2) 10 lb of limestone.

---

*Available from Rhodia, Inc. Ashland, OH
†Available from Merck & Co., Inc., West Point, PA 19486.
‡Available from Haver-Lockhart Laboratories, Shawnee, KS 66201

---

*Available from Jensen-Salsbery Laboratories, Kansas City, MO 64141.

(3) 4 lb of dicalcium phosphate.

(4) 1 lb equivalent of pure sulfa.

2. Urinary calculi are frequently seen when high levels of grain (more than 50 per cent of diet) are fed. Dietary supplements can help diminish this problem in male sheep. Ammonium chloride, salt, and limestone are the supplements used. Up to 3-per cent salt, 1-per cent limestone, and 1-per cent ammonium chloride, uniformally blended in the grain mix, will help control calculi if a suitable, fresh, clean water supply is made available ad lib.

Veterinarians are the ones best trained to prescribe the proper drugs and the proper dosages and withdrawal times in order to avoid residues in the red meat supply. However, sheep producers will use veterinary services only if those services are both available and cost effective.

Supplemental Reading

Jensen, R., and Swift, B. L.: Diseases of Sheep, 2nd ed. Philadelphia: Lea & Febiger, 1982.

Commercial Lamb Feedlot Management

ROBERT E. PIERSON, D.V.M.
and CLEON KIMBERLING, D.V.M., M.P.H.

In large feedlots, lambs weighing approximately 32 kg arrive daily and within 80 days are usually ready for market weighing 50 to 52 kg. Daily weight gains average around 0.2 to 0.3 kg. Annual death loss averages 1.5 to 3 per cent.

Tables 1 and 2 show a summary of diseases and times found at necropsy in 3 feedlots in northern Colorado, feeding a total of 300,000 lambs annually. Scheduled visits were made 1 or 2 days a week for the purpose of performing necropsies on lambs. Diseases of the digestive and respiratory systems accounted for the majority of deaths with 54 per cent and 15 per cent, respectively (Table 3). This summary also shows the seasonal relationships of diseases. The greatest seasonal death loss (56 per cent) occurred during September, October, November, and December (Fig. 1). Stress is probably the major contributing factor, as this is the period when most lambs are being fed, plus the weather conditions are unsettled with extreme changes in day to night temperatures.

Enterotoxemia (*Clostridium perfringens* type D) is the most common disease of feedlot lambs, followed by acidosis. Enterotoxemia accounts for 25 per cent of the deaths due to diseases of the digestive system and occurs in spite of vaccinating lambs once and even twice for this disease (Tables 1 and 4).

Rectal prolapse is a common problem in some feedlots. The cause is complex and animals may be predisposed to it by implants with anabolic agents, dusty corrals, coughs, pneumonia, and excessive abdominal fat. Early slaughter of affected lambs is the most practical method of handling.

Table 2 shows the relationship of important diseases of feedlot lambs to length of time in the feedlot. Notice that most diseases occur within the first 30 days on feed.

If a veterinarian is engaged in lamb feedlot practice, it would be appropriate to perform necropsies on as many lambs as possible to determine the most common causes for death. Disease problems are influenced greatly by management practices, weather, nutrition, and geographic location.

SUGGESTED HEALTH PROCESSING PROCEDURE

1. Forty-eight hours after arrival.
   a. Vaccinate with enterotoxemia type D toxoid.
   b. Worm lambs with injectable levamisole.
   c. Implant with Ralgro* (anabolic agent).
2. Two weeks after arrival, shear lambs.
3. Three to 4 weeks after arrival, administer booster dose of toxoid.

SUGGESTED DIET FOR FEEDLOT LAMBS

The basic ingredients are alfalfa, corn, alfalfa silage, whole or cracked corn, and minerals. The average lamb will consume 1.1 to 1.4 kg of concentrate daily plus roughage. Ration is usually fed either as pelleted feed or loose in the form of silage or chopped hay or both. Mineral mix is fed free-choice. One of 2 systems of feeding is employed. Feed is placed either at the perimeter of the corral on the ground or in self-feeders. Receiving rations consist mainly of hay or silage or both, plus about 15 per cent concentrate as corn. At 2- to 5-day intervals, lambs are raised to higher levels of concentrate so that by 14 to 21 days lambs are receiving a finishing ration containing 85 per cent concentrate and 15 per cent roughage. Adequate fresh water is provided daily.

ACIDOSIS (LACTIC ACIDOSIS, GRAIN OVERLOAD, ACUTE INDIGESTION, FOUNDER)

Acidosis is characterized by inappetence, depression, diarrhea, and weakness and is one of the most common causes of death in a lamb feedlot operation.

Etiology

Lambs entering a feedlot are suddenly exposed to diets high in concentrates as opposed to their accustomed high roughage diet. Many lamb feeders attempt to rush lambs onto a finishing ration within 2 weeks of entry. An 8-step ration is commonly used, starting with a receiving ration and progressing to a finishing ration, with intermediate changes in the ration at 2-day intervals. The receiving ration consists of a corn-plant pellet (90 per cent roughage, 10 per cent concentrate) plus hay. As the ration is changed every 2 days, the per cent of concentrate increases until the finishing ration is reached (90 per cent concentrate, 10 per cent roughage).

This sudden change to a concentrate diet or the sudden change of feed causes acute indigestion.

Pathogenesis

The ruminal microflora of lambs entering a feedlot consist mainly of cellulolytic gram-negative bacteria plus protozoa. High concentrate rations favor the production

*Available from International Minerals and Chemical Corporation, Box 207, Terre Haute, IN 47808.

Table 1. Summary of Diseases Found at Necropsy for Three Lamb Feedlots*

	Jan	Feb	Mar	Apr	May	Jun	Jul	Aug	Sep	Oct	Nov	Dec	Total	(%)
Respiratory System														
Pneumonia	7	2	3	2	7	13	34	29	28	41	25	18	209	
Pyothorax	—	1	—	1	1	—	—	—	—	—	—	1	3	
Pulmonary congestion	—	—	—	—	1	—	—	—	—	1	1	—	3	
TOTALS	7	3	3	3	8	13	34	29	28	42	26	19	215	(15%)
Digestive System														
Enterotoxemia D	11	30	6	10	26	12	36	10	29	28	52	61	311	
Enterotoxemia C	—	—	1	—	—	—	1	1	—	1	10	8	22	
Acidosis	11	—	2	1	9	10	4	5	17	24	15	13	111	
Salmonellosis	2	1	—	—	6	5	10	3	20	43	16	—	106	
Coccidiosis	—	—	—	—	1	—	1	—	1	2	7	2	14	
Prolapsed rectum	4	5	4	8	—	4	22	21	10	8	5	1	92	
Septicemic pasteurellosis	1	2	—	—	—	—	1	5	10	19	13	19	70	
Bloat	1	—	—	—	—	1	—	—	—	2	2	1	7	
Rumenitis	—	—	—	—	—	—	—	—	—	2	1	—	3	
Torsion	1	—	—	—	—	1	—	—	—	2	1	2	4	
Parasites	—	—	—	1	—	—	3	2	—	1	1	1	9	
Perforated ulcer	—	1	—	—	—	—	—	—	—	1	1	2	5	
Choke	1	1	—	—	—	—	—	—	—	1	1	—	3	
Enteritis	1	1	—	—	—	—	1	—	1	2	5	2	13	
TOTALS	33	41	13	20	42	34	79	47	88	134	128	111	770	(54%)
Nervous System														
Polioencephalomalacia	4	—	—	—	6	—	—	1	2	2	2	10	27	
FSE	1	—	—	—	1	—	—	—	—	—	2	1	5	
CNS	1	—	1	—	1	—	—	1	—	1	4	1	10	
Suppurative meningitis	—	—	—	—	1	1	1	—	—	—	1	1	5	
Tetanus	—	1	—	—	1	—	—	—	—	—	—	—	2	
TOTALS	6	1	1	—	10	1	1	2	2	3	9	13	49	(3.4%)
Urinary System														
Calculosis	11	11	6	8	—	2	3	2	4	5	8	8	68	
Pyelonephritis	—	—	—	—	—	—	—	—	—	—	1	1	2	
Cystic kidney	1	—	—	—	—	—	—	—	—	—	—	—	1	
TOTALS	12	11	6	8	—	2	3	2	4	5	9	9	71	(4.9%)
Metabolic Diseases														
Transport tetany	2	1	1	—	19	—	1	—	12	8	3	3	50	(3.5%)
Miscellaneous	20	25	10	10	15	12	13	22	22	43	49	40	281	(19.6%)
Monthly Total	80	82	34	41	94	62	131	102	156	235	224	195		(100%)
Total Lambs Necropsied													1436	

*Jan. 1, 1974 to Dec. 31, 1978. Pierson, R. E., Jensen, R., and Breen, H.

Table 2. *Diseases of Feedlot Lambs in Relationship to Time in Feedlot*

Disease	First 30 Days			Middle Period			Last 30 Days
	Week 1	Week 2	Week 3	Week 4	Weeks 5 and 6	Weeks 7 and 8	
Enterotexemia type D	+	+	+ + +	+ +	+	+	+
Enterotoxemia type C			+	+			
Acidosis	+	+ + +	+	+	+		
Salmonellosis	+ +	+					
Coccidiosis		+	+ +				
Rectal prolapse					+	+	+ + +
Septicemic pasteurellosis		+	+				
Pneumonia	+	+	+				
Polioencephalomalacia					+	+	+ +
Calculosis				+	+	+	+ +
Transport tetany	+ +						

Key
+ Occurs
+ + Occurs more commonly
+ + + Occurs most comonly

of amylolytic gram-positive *Streptococcus bovis* and lactobacilli. As these bacteria form lactic acid, the gram-negative bacteria and the protozoa are destroyed. The normal pH values of 7 to 7.4 of the rumen drop to 3.8 to 4.3. Increased osmolality of the rumen pulls fluid (plasma) from the blood into the rumen. Acidosis develops. The acidity in the rumen and abomasum irritates the linings of both. Dehydration, loss of electrolytes, hemoconcentration, and endotoxic shock all contribute to the death of the lamb. Less seriously affected lambs gradually return to feed and resume fattening.

Clinical Signs

Within 12 to 36 hr after engorgement of concentrate feed, lambs lose their appetite, become depressed, and develop diarrhea. Severely affected animals become recumbent. Abdominal pain develops as a result of distention due to excessive feed, fluid, and gas. Membranes become hyperemic from the toxemia, respirations and pulse become rapid, and the lamb becomes weak and incoordinated. Coma and death follow.

The blood levels of lactate are > mM/L, and the pH drops to <7.l.

Necropsy Findings

The rumen is full of liquid ingesta, consisting of large quantities of corn or other concentrate. An acid odor of the ingesta is obvious. Ruminal papillae are swollen and hemorrhagic. Hemorrhagic abomasitis, a result of multiple erosions of the mucosal surface, is an important finding.

Diagnosis

A diagnosis of acidosis is based on history, clinical signs, and necropsy findings. History indicates a sudden change in feed in cases occurring within the first 2 weeks of the feeding period. Clinical signs of a distended abdomen, recumbency, toxemia, and depression with signs of diarrhea cause suspicion. At necropsy, the presence of a grain-filled rumen, an acid odor, and hemorrhagic abomasitis almost verifies the diagnosis. Laboratory findings of elevated blood lactate levels and lowered blood pH levels confirm the diagnosis.

Differential Diagnosis

Enterotoxemia, acute septicemia pasteurellosis, and calculosis must be considered in a differential diagnosis. Enterotoxemic lambs have a full rumen, but a hydropericardium with a fibrous clot contained within the pericardial fluid is also evident. Glucosuria is also present. An animal with acute septicemic pasteurellosis shows focal lesions of enteritis and multiple pale emboli in the liver and lung. Calculosis is often characterized by a ruptured bladder, diffuse peritonitis, and elevated BUN levels.

Table 3. *Systems Summary of Diseases at Necropsy for Three Lamb Feedlots, 1974–1978**

Disease Site	Lambs Necropsied	Per Cent
Digestive system	770	54
Respiratory system	215	15
Urinary system	68	4.9
Nervous system	49	3.4
Metabolic disease	50	3.5
Miscellaneous	281	19.6
TOTAL	1433	

*Pierson, R. E., Jensen, R., and Breen, H.

Table 4. *Causes of Death Involving the Digestive System, 1974–1978, for Three Lamb Feedlots*

Disease	Lambs Necropsied	Per Cent
Enterotoxemia type D	311	40
Acidosis	111	14
Salmonellosis	106	14
Prolapsed rectum	92	12
Septicemic pasteurellosis	70	9
Enterotoxemia type C	22	2.8
Coccidiosis	14	1.8
Others	44	5.7
	770	

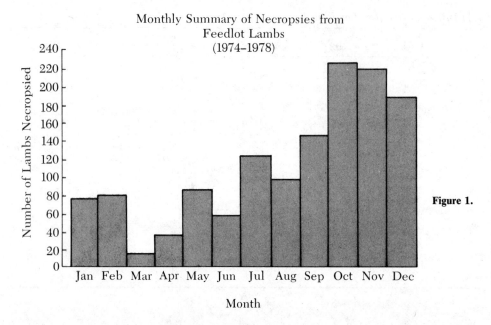

Figure 1.

Treatment

Treatment of acidosis is usually impractical. When a problem is encountered in a pen of lambs, it is prudent to remove all concentrate from the feed bunks or self-feeders and switch to good quality grass hay or alfalfa. After a period of 4 to 5 days on hay, the lambs can gradually be fed concentrate once again. Should individual treatment be attempted, it should be administered before signs of acidosis occur. Antibiotics, such as 0.3 to 1.0 gm of tetracycline or 500,000 units of penicillin, given orally will reduce the gram-positive microflora. Baking soda can be given orally or added to saline and given intravenously. Lambs can also be drenched with antacids. For individual treatment of sick lambs, add 83 gm of baking soda in 1 L of saline and administer intravenously.

Prevention

Allow more time for the lamb to adjust to the concentrate. Change levels of concentrate more gradually. If lambs are grazing corn fields, limit the time the lambs have access to the corn.

ENTEROTOXEMIA (TYPE D) (OVEREATING DISEASE)

Enterotoxemia, an acute infectious but noncontagious disease, is the most common cause of death in feedlot lambs. In spite of immunization programs, as many as 0.5 to 1.5 per cent of the lambs may die from enterotoxemia. Without immunization, a mortality of 8 to 10 per cent may be expected.

Losses from enterotoxemia may occur at any time during the feeding period but are most likely 2 to 3 weeks after fattening begins. Rations high in concentrate, especially barley or corn, are predisposing factors. Thrifty, healthy lambs are more likely to be affected.

Etiology

Enterotoxemia is caused by the epsilon toxin from the organism *Clostridium perfringens* type D. This organism is a gram-positive, anaerobic, spore-forming bacillus commonly found in the soil, manure, and alimentary tracts of animals.

Pathogenesis

Spores of *C. perfringens* type D enter the digestive tract through contaminated feed and water. Normally the spores and bacteria perish in the acid abomasum, but some bacteria survive and reach the small and large intestines. Even though some bacteria multiply and eventually produce epsilon toxin, normal peristaltic activity causes the bacteria and toxin to be excreted in the feces. However, when the lamb overeats concentrate, both bacteria and starch substrates reach the small intestine in large amounts. *C. perfringens* multiplies rapidly under these circumstances and produces a harmless prototoxin that is activated to a lethal toxin by trypsin. Feeds high in concentrates can cause stasis and damage to the lining and vasculature of the digestive tract. The combination of stasis and damage allows for absorption of toxin. Once absorbed, generalized toxemia results. Death is from injury to vital neurons and shock.

Clinical Signs

Sudden or unexpected death characterizes enterotoxemia. If signs are observed, they usually are those of a CNS disturbance and are characterized by convulsions, opisthotonos, salivation, jerking movements, impaired vision, coma, and death after a disease course of 30 to 90 minutes.

Necropsy Findings

At necropsy, the carcass is often found bloated. The rumen is full of feed, and subserosal hemorrhages may be found on portions of the intestinal tract. The most diagnostic lesions at necropsy are a hydropericardium and a fibrinous clot within the pericardial sac. Quantities of pale yellow fluid in the pericardial sac vary from a normal of 5 to 10 ml up to 125 ml. Congestion of the lung is a common finding. Other lesions include hemorrhages on the thymus, subepicardial hemorrhages, and subendocardial hemorrhages of the left ventricle. Blood sugar levels increase from a normal level of 40 to 65 mg per cent to as much as 360 mg per cent. Urine level will increase up to 6 per cent.

Diagnosis

Enterotoxemia diagnosis is based on history, typical signs, and lesions. Sudden death can occur at any time during the feeding period, particularly as the lambs are pushed on high concentrate feed or after the lambs experience a sudden change of feed.

Important lesions at necropsy are hydropericardium, fibrinous clot within the pericardial sac, congestion of the lung, hemorrhages on the thymus, and glucosuria.

Treatment

Since sheep die suddenly and are seldom observed to be sick, treatment is seldom possible or even attempted. If available, 40 to 50 ml of *C. perfringens* type D antiserum subcutaneously may be beneficial.

Prevention

C. perfringens type D toxoid should be administered within 2 to 3 days of arrival. The usual 2 ml dose is administered subcutaneously in the neck or axillary area. For best results, a booster dose is given 2 to 3 weeks later. Since type C enterotoxemia is also a problem in feedlot lambs, use of a bivalent vaccine is suggested.

HEMORRHAGIC ENTEROTOXEMIA (TYPE C)

Hemorrhagic enterotoxemia (type C) is an acute disease of lambs characterized by inflammation and hemorrhage of the digestive tract. The disease is most prevalent during the first 72 hr of life, but occasionally it causes deaths in feedlot lambs.

Etiology

The beta toxin of *C. perfringens* type C causes hemorrhagic enterotoxemia. The beta toxin produces a necrotizing effect on the intestinal tract.

It is hard to explain why feedlot lambs (4 to 8 months of age) would develop hemorrhagic enterotoxemia. Perhaps interaction of stress, concurrent diseases, and lack of natural immunity may account for some of the cases and subsequent deaths.

Clinical Signs

Sudden death is usually observed. Affected lambs show abdominal pain, bloat, shock, and normal to subnormal temperatures. Most affected lambs die after a disease course of a few hours.

At necropsy, lesions are limited to the digestive tract. Abomasitis may be present. The reddened and congested intestines, particularly the jejunum, ileum, cecum, and colon, are characteristic of hemorrhagic enteritis. The intestinal tract is bloated and contains bloody fluid. Mesenteric lymph nodes are swollen and hemorrhagic.

Differential diagnosis requires consideration of enterotoxemia type D, bloat, acidosis, volvulus, and torsion. Acute septicemic pasteurellosis may look like type C hemorrhagic enterotoxemia, on occasion. Diagnosis is based on signs and lesions. A positive diagnosis requires identifying the beta toxin by laboratory procedures.

Treatment

Since lambs die so suddenly from this disease, treatment is seldom attempted.

Prevention

Vaccinating lambs within 48 to 72 hr after arrival with the bivalent type C and D toxoid should be considered. A booster dose of vaccine 2 to 4 weeks later would enhance immunity.

SEPTICEMIC PASTEURELLOSIS

Septicemic pasteurellosis, an acute infectious disease of lambs, is characterized clinically by toxemia, shock, and sudden death. Pathologically, it is characterized by focal ulcerative and necrotic lesions in the stomachs or intestines or both and embolized infection in the liver and lungs. The etiologic agent is *Pasteurella haemolytica*. The widespread disease causes economic losses due to deaths, loss of live weight, and costly treatment.

Etiology and Pathogenesis

Septicemic pasteurellosis appears to begin as a gastrointestinal infection that ulcerates areas in the stomachs, small intestine, cecum, or colon. The causative agent, *P. haemolytica*, penetrates through the ulcers, enters the portal blod, and moves as emboli into the liver where it causes numerous foci of infection. Some emboli pass through the liver into the lungs.

Occurrence

Primarily a disease of late summer and fall, septicemic pasteurellosis commonly affects either pastured or feedlot lambs 1 to 3 weeks after arrival. As many as 2 to 3 per cent of a group of lambs can die within a few days. Losses often stop as quickly as they start, with or without treatment. On occasions, the disease course is protracted, with deaths spreading over several weeks.

Clinical Signs

Temperatures in affected lambs suddenly elevate to 41 to 42° C and quickly return to normal. Affected lambs separate from the flock, become severely depressed, and breathe rapidly, and visible membranes become congested. Death appears related to septicemia, toxemia, and shock.

Necropsy Findings

Lesions at necropsy are generalized and severe or mild and barely visible. Severe cases are characterized by subcutaneous, intramuscular, subpleural, and subserosal hemorrhages. Mild cases have minimal gross lesions.

Lymph nodes are swollen and hemorrhagic. The spleen may be grossly enlarged. Usually the omasum, abomasum, small intestines, and particularly the cecum and colon are edematous, ulcerated, hemorrhagic, and in some cases, necrotic. Intestinal contents may be bloody. Mesenteric lymph nodes are swollen and hemorrhagic.

Characteristic lesions are found in the liver and, to a lesser degree, in the lung. Within the liver and lung are pale foci (emboli) 0.2 to 1.0 mm in diameter that may be seen in the intact and cut surface. More emboli are seen in the liver than in the lung.

Diagnosis

Septicemic pasteurellosis is diagnosed from the history of sudden death in either pastured or feedlot lambs, from typical lesions on necropsy, and from cultures of *Pasteurella haemolytica* of feces, liver, lung, and mesenteric lymph nodes.

Differential Diagnosis

One must consider in a differential diagnosis all causes of sudden death (particularly enterotoxemia type C or D), acidosis, and salmonellosis. It is likely that some fatalities of septicemic pasteurellosis are caused by concurrent infections with enterotoxemia type C.

Treatment

The course of this disease is so short that treatment of the individual lamb would probably be useless. High levels of antibiotics given intravenously would probably be ineffective. Either chloretetracycline or oxytetracycline added to the feed at 11 mg per kg of body weight daily for 5 days could be used as prevention or treatment. Sulfathiazole added to the drinking water is an alternative method of prevention.

Prevention

The use of either antibiotics or sulfonamides in the drinking water for 5 days is indicated and helpful.

SALMONELLAL DYSENTERY (PARATYPHOID DYSENTERY, SALMONELLOSIS)

Salmonellosis, a serious disease of feedlot lambs, is characterized by gastroenteritis, diarrhea, septicemia, and high morbidity and mortality and is caused by *Salmonella typhimurium* and related species.

Although salmonellosis may occur at any time of the year among feedlot lambs, the disease is more common during summer and fall, usually within the first 10 days of arrival. In some shipments of lambs, morbidity varies between 50 and 70 per cent, while mortality of 10 per cent is common.

Predisposing factors are transportation from ranges to feedlots, which exposes lambs to stressful situations such as crowding, heat of confinement, and fasting. Placing feed in the corral often causes fecal contamination, resulting in oral ingestion of contaminated feed.

Clinical Signs

Signs often develop soon after arrival and consist of an elevated temperature of 41 to 41.6° C, anorexia, depression, and an arched back. Diarrhea, with feces frequently yellowish green in color and malodorous, develops and causes rapid dehydration. Death may occur after a disease course of 1 to 5 days.

Necropsy Findings

At necropsy, the wool around the perineal area is stained and soiled with feces. The digestive tract is virtually empty. Abomasitis and enteritis are present. Mesenteric lymph nodes are enlarged and hemorrhagic. The gallbladder is enlarged and edematous.

Diagnosis

Veterinarians diagnose salmonellal dysentery from typical history, signs, and necropsy findings. Confirmation is obtained by isolating *S. typhimurium* from bile, spleen, mesenteric nodes, feces, and blood of the heart. History usually indicates recent shipment and the occurrence of signs and death within 10 days of arrival. Signs are of greenish-yellow feces of diarrhea, pyrexia, and dehydration. At necropsy, gastroenteritis and enlarged hemorrhagic lymph nodes are found.

Differential diagnosis requires consideration of coccidiosis, acidosis, and acute septicemic pasteurellosis. Coccidiosis usually develops 2 to 3 weeks after lambs arrive in a feedlot. The feces, dark in color, contain blood and oocysts. Acidosis develops suddenly after a change of feed. Recumbent animals are full, sometimes bloated, and membranes are inflamed. Temperature is usually normal. Feces are loose and contain grain. Septicemic pasteurellosis is characterized by sudden death. At necropsy, lesions include focal areas of necrosis in the gastrointestinal tract, multiple septic emboli in the liver, and some metastatic septic emboli in the lung.

Treatment

Treatment of salmonellal dysentery in sheep is difficult and expensive. Since salmonellosis usually involves many lambs at one time, the entire pen of lambs is treated. Water is medicated because sick lambs are more likely to drink than eat. Although not too effective, water-soluble tetracycline and electrolytes may help. At least 1 gm of tetracycline per lamb per day for 7 to 10 days is the usual dosage. Oral sulfonamides plus electrolytes can be substituted for the antibiotic therapy.

COCCIDIOSIS (HEMORRHAGIC DIARRHEA, COCCIDIAL DYSENTERY)

Coccidiosis, an important disease of feedlot lambs, is characterized by diarrhea, dehydration, loss of weight, depression, weakness, and the presence of fecal oocysts. Most cases of feedlot coccidiosis occur within 2 to 3 weeks of entry into the feedlot, particularly during the late summer and autumn.

Etiology

Pathogenic species of coccidia in sheep and *Eimeria ninakohlyakimovae*, *E. arlsingi*, and *E. ahsata*. Coccidiosis is transmitted through ingestion of feed or water contaminated with large numbers of sporulated oocysts.

Clinical Signs

Soft feces turning to the watery feces of diarrhea is the first sign of the disease. Feces are dark and contain blood. Body temperatures rise to 40.5 to 41.1° C. A few days after diarrhea develops, lambs lose their appetite, and they become dehydrated, weak, and recumbent. Affected lambs strain, occasionally causing prolapsed rectums.

Morbidity ranges from 10 to 50 per cent with up to a 10 per cent mortality rate. (Recovered lambs become very inefficient.)

Necropsy Findings

Lesions of ovine coccidiosis are found in the ileum, cecum, and colon and are characterized by hyperemia, necrosis, and ulceration. Wool around the rectum becomes soiled, producing an environment for fly infestation. Mesenteric lymph nodes are swollen and edematous.

Diagnosis and Differential Diagnosis

Coccidiosis is diagnosed as based on history, signs, necropsy, and laboratory findings. Differential diagnosis requires consideration of acute salmonellosis, acidosis, and acute septicemic pasteurellosis.

Prevention and Treatment

Good management can help prevent coccidiosis by (1) avoiding overcrowding, (2) keeping pens dry, (3) cleaning pens regularly.

In some trials monensin, a coccidiostat, when mixed with the feed, significantly improved weight gains of lambs infected with *Eimeria*. In other trials with 6- to 11-week-old lambs, monensin prevented diarrhea, but these lambs gained less weight than did controls.

Sulfonamides plus electrolytes added to the drinking water is an effective treatment. As an example, Sulfa-Lite* (sulfathiazole, vitamins A and D, plus electrolytes) at the rate of 215 mg/kg initially followed by 107 mg/kg for the next 3 to 5 days, can be used.

PNEUMONIA (ENZOOTIC PNEUMONIA, PASTEURELLOSIS, SHIPPING FEVER, ENZOOTIC PNEUMONIA-PLEURISY COMPLEX)

Ovine feedlot pneumonia, second in importance to diseases of the digestive system as a cause for sickness and death, results in serious financial waste to the lamb feedlot industry. Economic losses are caused by death, delayed marketing, downgrading and condemning of carcasses at slaughter, and cost of treatments.

Occurrence

Ovine pneumonia, a broad term used for most types of pneumonia, is seen during July, August, September, and October. Pneumonia develops at any time in the feeding period but more commonly in the first 3 weeks and particularly after shearing in the autumn and winter.

Etiology

The cause of ovine pneumonia is complex, much like that of cattle, and probably is the result of an interaction of chlamydial organisms, *Pasteurella haemolytica* or *P. multocida* or both, *Mycoplasma* sp., and stresses. Parainfluenza virus type 3 may also interact with *P. haemolytica* to cause severe pneumonia. Important stresses are heat, dust, crowding, and prolonged confinement during shipment.

Clinical Signs

Some lambs die suddenly with pneumonia, and others die after a disease course of several days or even weeks. Affected lambs are depressed, segregate themselves, show elevated temperatures of 41 to 42° C, become anorexic, breathe rapidly, may cough, and lose body weight. Terminal cases are first recumbent. Membranes are injected and cyanotic. Nostrils accumulate exudate.

Treatment

Although sick lambs may be treated individually, ovine pneumonia is usually a pen problem, and all lambs are treated alike by either medicating feed or water. Various sulfonamides added to the drinking water will help. As an example, for drinking water, use one of the following:

1. Sulfaethoxypyridazine (SEZ)* is added to obtain a 6.25-per cent drinking water solution. Administer at the rate of 29.5 ml of solution per lamb per day for 4 consecutive days.
2. Electrosulf-3† (a combination of sodium sulfamethazine, sulfathiazole, sulfamerazine, and electrolytes) should be administered in drinking water for 3 to 4 days. Only 0.23 kg will treat approximately 1140 kg of body weight per day, or 33 lambs weighing 35 kg each.
3. Sulfa-Lite is given at the rate of 215 mg/kg for the first day, followed by 107 mg/kg for the next 3 to 5 days. Oxytetracycline in a dose of 11 mg/kg is given parenterally daily for 4 to 5 days.

POLIOENCEPHALOMALACIA

Polioencephalomalacia (PEM), a noninfectious disease of the brain, is characterized clinically by blindness, depression, and incoordination. Pathologically, it is characterized by focal necrosis in the cerebral cortex and thalamus. Of the 3 most common diseases involving the central nervous system—PEM, focal symmetrical encephalomalacia (FSE), and listeriosis—PEM is the most common. PEM can occur any time during the feeding period, any season of the year, and in animals on all types of feed, although it is more common when silage is being fed during winter.

Etiology

The disease probably is caused by a deficiency of metabolizable thiamine. Impaired thiamine metabolism might be due to thiaminase Type I activity or some other thiamine antagonism. Fecal thiaminase can be detected in normal as well as affected lambs. Cases of PEM are sometimes seen following administration of the anthelmintics Levamisol and thiabendazole.

Clinical Signs

The disease manifests itself either acutely or subacutely. In the acute form, affected lambs are found dead or prostrate. Even when comatose, lambs appear excitable and convulsive. Rectal temperatures are usually normal. In the subacute form, lambs are blind, incoordinated, and weak, and move more aimlessly and appear disoriented. Characteristic stances are lowering the head to ground level or staring along the horizon and extending the head over the back. Some affected lambs head press, others lose equilibrium and fall, while others remain in lateral recumbency without movement.

Necropsy Findings

Lesions are limited to the central nervous system and are often subtle. The cerebrum is often swollen, and meningeal vessels are congested. Fixing the brain in 10-per cent formalin allows for easier examination. The gray matter of the cerebral cortex contains foci of necrosis.

Examination of either the fixed or fresh brain under a Wood's lamp (ultraviolet light) may reveal fluorescence, particularly in chronic cases.

---

*Available from Bio-Ceutic Laboratories, Inc. A subsidiary of Phillips Roxane, Inc., St. Joseph, MO 64502.

*Available from American Cyanamid Co., P.O. Box 400, Princeton, NJ 08540.
†Available from Affiliated Laboratories, Myerstown, PA 17067.

Diagnosis

A diagnosis of PEM is based on signs and lesions. Blindness, normal temperature, depression, lateral recumbency, or abnormal position suggests polio. Histopathologic examination of the brain for evidence of cerebral cortical necrosis will confirm the diagnosis. Looking at the brain, either fresh or fixed, under a Wood's lamp for fluorescence is a rapid means of diagnosis. Differential diagnosis requires consideration of FSE, listeriosis, and enterotoxemia.

Treatment

Thiamine hydrochloride, 0.25 to 0.5 gm administered intramuscularly or intravenously for 3 to 5 days, is often effective for the average size feedlot lamb, unless brain damage is irreversible. Affected sheep should be isolated for easier handling and given easy access to feed and water.

FOCAL SYMMETRICAL ENCEPHALOMALACIA

FSE is a noncontagious disease of sheep caused by sublethal amounts of *Clostridium perfringens* type D toxin and is characterized clinically by blindness and incoordination. The disease is of minor importance to feedlot lambs. However, since the clinical signs of FSE look almost identical to PEM, it must be differentiated from this disease if preventive measures are to be undertaken.

Diagnosis

A positive diagnosis of FSE is based on (1) clinical signs similar to those of PEM, such as blindness, incoordination, and abnormal posture, (2) gross lesions, such as bilateral symmetrical lesions or hemorrhages and necrosis in the striatum, thalami, midbrain, and cerebellar peduncles, and (3) microscopic lesions of necrosis in the same areas. The use of a Wood's lamp may be helpful when examining either fresh or fixed brain to demonstrate fluorescence in the areas described.

Differential diagnosis requires consideration of PEM, brain abscesses, and tetanus.

Prevention and Treatment

Treatment is unlikely to produce results since brain damage is usually irreversible and fatal. Prevention consists of revaccinating the remaining lambs with *Clostridium perfringens* type D toxoid.

LISTERIOSIS (CIRCLING DISEASE)

Listeriosis, an infectious but noncontagious disease of sheep, is characterized by neurologic signs, such as fascial paralysis, circling, lateral recumbency, coma, and death. Once one of the most common neurologic diseases of feedlot lambs, it is seldom encountered now and has been replaced by PEM as the most common neurologic disease.

Occurrence

The encephalitic form is more common in feedlot lambs, and outbreaks frequently occur 3 to 4 weeks after feeding silage from a newly opened silo. Most cases of listeriosis develop during colder months of the year when lambs are closely confined. Whether the drop in incidence of this disease is due to the fact that ensilage is seldom fed in large lamb feedlot operations or to better methods of ensilage preparation is not known.

Etiology

The cause of listeriosis is the bacterium *Listeria monocytogenes*, which may be found in soil and silage as well as in milk, tears, and nasal secretions from infected sheep.

Clinical Signs

Early signs of listeriosis are depression, pyrexia, anorexia, and disorientation. Within 1 or 2 days a fascial paralysis develops followed by circling. Loss of the preservation reflex is observed in the eye on the paralyzed side. Sometimes blindness and opacity of the affected eye are present. The course is rapid and within a few days of onset, the lamb becomes recumbent and comatose and dies. On occasion, paralysis of one or more limbs is present.

Diagnosis and Differential Diagnosis

Listeric encephalitis is diagnosed using history, typical signs, and laboratory findings. History usually indicates a relationship to ensilage feeding in the winter. Circling movements and fascial paralysis suggest listeriosis. Confirmation requires isolation and identification of *L. monocytogenes* from the ground brain stem.

Both PEM and FSE must be considered in a differential diagnosis. Lambs with PEM are afebrile and blind, and have no fascial paralysis. Animals with FSE resemble those with PEM, are also afebrile, and show no fascial paralysis.

Treatment

Sheep with listeriosis seldom respond to treatment.

Prevention

Killinger (1968) has recommended the following preventive procedures:

1. Avoid feeding silage from the top layer of an upright silo.
2. Avoid feeding moldy and spoiled silage.
3. Start sheep on silage gradually.
4. Provide plenty of clean drinking water, with warm water during winter months to avoid freezing.
5. Prevent stress and overcrowding.
6. Isolate lambs with circling disease from the remainder of the flock.

UROLITHIASIS (CALCULOSIS, URINARY CALCULI, WATERBELLY)

Urolithiasis, a metabolic disease of sheep characterized by obstruction of the urinary tract with calculi, is one of the most common diseases of feedlot wether lambs. Although the disease occurs during all seasons of the year, the highest incidence is in the late fall, winter, and spring. Economic loss results from death of affected lambs and condemnation of carcasses at slaughter.

Etiology

With few exceptions, calculi formed under feedlot conditions are composed of phosphates, such as calcium, magnesium, and ammonium phosphate. The reasons for the formation of the calculi are better understood now, but the process is still complex.

Clinical Signs

Obstruction of the urinary tract in lambs is usually in the urethral process or in the sigmoid flexure. Irrespective of the location of the obstruction, the first sign of calculosis is usually discomfort, which is characterized by restlessness, tenesmus, anorexia, recumbency, and frequent attempts to urinate. Dribbling of urine from the prepuce may be noticed. Sooner or later, either the urethra or bladder ruptures. If the urethra ruptures, a large edematous-like swelling develops around the prepuce and may cover the entire ventral part of the abdomen and perineal area. If the bladder ruptures, the abdomen distends. Death follows within a few days.

Diagnosis

Urolithiasis is usually easily diagnosed from the typical signs. Diagnosis at necropsy is even simpler. In a suspected case, the penis can be exposed and the urethral process palpated for the presence of an obstruction. In other cases, a blood sample may be obtained for determination of BUN level.

Treatment

A feedlot lamb with urolithiasis is seldom treated because it is not economical. In cases where the obstruction involves the urethral process, it may be snipped off with scissors. It is far better to practice prevention than to treat.

Prevention

1. *Add salt (NaCl) to rations.* The purpose is to increase urine volume. Add up to 4 per cent NaCl to the ration. Make certain ample drinking water is available.

2. *Control phosphorus levels and calcium to phosphorus ratio.* This is one of the most important considerations in preventing calculosis. The calcium to phosphorus ratio should be close to 2:1. The use of ground limestone to provide a ratio of 2 to 2.5 parts of calcium to 1 part of phosphorus in high concentrate lamb rations has proved effective. Better results are obtained if the mineral is fed to the lambs rather than offered at free choice.

3. *Reduce the alkalinity of the urine.* Feed approximately 7.1 gm/head daily of ammonium chloride. Mix the ammonium chloride thoroughly in the feed to avoid a palatability problem.

In summary, follow these recommendations:

1. Purchase feeder lambs from areas with a low incidence of urolithiasis.
2. Provide plenty of vitamins A and D.
3. Feed a ration containing Ca and P in a ratio of 2 to 2.5:1.
4. Feed a protein supplement.
5. Add salt to the ration so that up to 2 to 4 per cent of the ration is salt.
6. Add up to 7.1 gm/head of ammonium chloride daily to the ration.
7. Have plenty of drinking water available.
8. Treat infections of the urinary tract.

POLYARTHRITIS (STIFF LAMB DISEASE)

Polyarthritis, a common nonfatal disease of feedlot lambs, is caused by a chlamydial organism and is characterized by pyrexia, lameness, conjunctivitis, and weight loss. This contagious disease may occur any time during the feeding period and can result in a 10 per cent reduction in live weight per affected lamb. On occasion, this disease may be related to a mineral imbalance compounded by rapid weight gain and high feed consumption.

Clinical Signs

Important signs are stiffness in all legs, reluctance to move, lateral or sternal recumbency, loss of body weight, and a rectal temperature of 40 to 42° C. Affected joints, although painful, are rarely enlarged. More severely affected lambs require assistance to get on their feet, but with effort soon "warm out" of the lameness. Severely involved lambs may remain in lateral recumbency and even show "central nervous system" signs, owing to involvement of the cervical vertebrae. Chlamydial conjunctivitis may or may not accompany the arthritic condition. When present, conjunctivitis is characterized by epiphora, conjunctival hyperemia, follicular hyperplasia, and some pannus formation.

Diagnosis

A diagnosis of polyarthritis is based on a high incidence of arthritis in a pen of lambs, characteristic ambulation, frequently associated conjunctivitis, and response to treatment. Differential diagnosis mmust consider arthritis caused by other agents, trauma, and laminitis.

Treatment

The chlamydial organism is susceptible to many of the broad-spectrum antibiotics. Oxytetracycline, 11 mg/kg, is administered intramuscularly daily for 3 to 5 days or procaine penicillin G is administered at a minimum dose of 2200 IU/kg BID for 3 to 5 days. When treating polyarthritis, it is advisable to isolate the lamb in a well-bedded open shed where feed and water are in easy reach. If more than 5 per cent of the lambs in a pen are affected at one time, treatment of all lambs is indicated. Feeding oxytetracycline at 500 mg to 1 gm per day per lamb for 1 week is helpful.

CONTAGIOUS ECTHYMA (CONTAGIOUS PUSTULAR DERMATITIS, SORE-MOUTH, SCABBY MOUTH, ORF)

Contagious ecthyma, an infectious dermatitis of sheep, is characterized clinically by proliferative, pustular encrustations that form on the lips and nostrils and on the mucous membranes of the oral and buccal cavities. It is caused by a member of the poxvirus group.

This disease is common in feedlot lambs during the autumn and early winter and usually occurs within the first 3 weeks of entry. Forty to 60 per cent morbidity is common in some pens of lambs, but the mortality is low. Economic losses result from unthriftiness, greater susceptibility to other diseases, and the occasional loss of a lamb. The disease may be contagious to humans.

Clinical Signs

The primary lesion develops on the skin of the lips, often at the commissure, and slowly extends so as to cover much or all of the lips. The lesions start as papules and progress through vesicular and pustular stages before encrusting and eventually turning into elevated scabs. Lip lesions, on occasion, may extend into the oral cavity and become painful. Sometimes the lesions continue into the esophagus and even into the rumen, particularly in young nursing lambs. At other times, the lesions may involve the nostril or eyelids. The disease runs its course in 1 to 3 weeks.

Diagnosis

Proliferative, scabby lesions on the lips are characteristic. Differential diagnosis includes ulcerative dermatosis and sheep pox. Ulcerative dermatosis is usually found in adult sheep and is characterized by well-defined, ulcerative lesions on the nostril or between the nostril and lips. Sheep pox is a foreign animal disease characterized by elevated papules over much of the skin surface and is generally fatal.

Treatment

Often, the disease runs its course and is treated only when severe cases result in difficulty eating. Those affected animals are isolated in a hospital pen and given soft, palatable feed. Workers wearing gloves remove lip scabs gently by rubbing them with cotton soaked in equal parts of iodine and glycerine. Nolvasan solution is also used. Following the removal of the scabs, the lips are gently rubbed with the same product once daily for 2 to 4 days.

Prevention

Lambs should be vaccinated at docking time with soremouth vaccine, a live product that is applied with a brush to a scarified portion of the skin in the ear or axillary region. This procedure could be followed in feedlot lambs if desired.

TRANSPORT TETANY

Transport tetany, a common metabolic disease of recently transported lambs, is caused by sudden hypocalcemia brought on by stress factors, such as fasting, warm weather, and transportation. Clinical signs are within 4 to 5 days after arrival of the lambs to the feedlot. Mortality seldom exceeds 1 to 2 per cent.

The serum calcium concentration in sheep can be depressed easily. Short periods of fasting induce marked depression of serum calcium levels. The absence of drinking water during fasting increases the adverse effects. Fasting and sultry weather enhance the likelihood of transport tetany, as does working the sheep directly off the trucks.

Clinical Signs

Early signs of the disease, often overlooked by the lamb feeder, are restlessness, incoordination, staggering gait, and partial paralysis of the hind limbs. It is not until the stage of lateral recumbency that the owner is suspicious something is wrong. By that time, 10 to 20 lambs may be found in lateral recumbency and another 3 to 4 may be found dead. Temperatures range from normal to 42° C. Hind legs are stiff and difficult to flex. Lambs become unconscious and die suddenly or within 1 to 2 days if untreated. Ballottement of the abdomen reveals splashing sounds in the rumen.

Clinicopathologic Findings

Serum calcium levels of affected lambs average 7.28 mg/100 ml of blood.

Necropsy Findings

Since this is a metabolic disease, no gross lesions are evident. The most characteristic change is found in the rumen. It is void of feed but contains a large volume of water.

Diagnosis

Diagnosis is based on history of recent shipment. Lambs are found in lateral recumbency, showing some stiffness of the hind legs. Splashing sounds on ballottement of the rumen and the absence of lesions on necropsy are observed. Differential diagnosis must include consideration of enterotoxemia and acidosis. Both of these diseases are characterized by a rumen full of ingesta. Enterotoxemia is characterized by hydropericardium and fibrinous clots within the pericardial fluid.

Treatment

Since transport tetany is related to hypocalcemia, the treatment of choice is to administer calcium. Intravenous or subcutaneous administration of 50 ml of calcium gluconate is effective in approximately 50 per cent of the cases. Some comatose lambs will respond to treatment only to relapse and die within a few hours.

Prevention

Avoid fasting and water deprivation prior to shipping. If lambs are to be transported for long periods, they should be unloaded during shipment and allowed a time for feeding, resting, and watering. Upon arrival, it is important that the lambs have access to clean water and palatable feed.

Supplemental Reading

Acidosis

Jensen, R., and Swift, B. L.: Diseases of Sheep, 2nd ed. Philadelphia, Lea & Febiger, 1982.

Enterotoxemia

Jensen, R., and Swift, B. L.: Diseases of Sheep, 2nd ed. Philadelphia, Lea & Febiger, 1982.
Pierson, R. E.: A survey of lamb health in feedlots. J. Am. Vet. Med. Assoc. *150*:293–302, 1967.
Pierson, R. E.: Immunization of feedlot lambs with enterotoxemia toxoid and bacterin. J. Am. Vet. Med. Assoc. *152*:380–381, 1968.

Hemorrhagic Enterotoxemia

Jensen, R., and Swift, B. L.: Diseases of Sheep, 2nd ed. Philadelphia, Lea & Febiger, 1982.

Septicemic Pasteurellosis

Biberstein, E. L., and Kennedy, P. C.: Septicemic pasteurellosis in lambs. Am. J. Vet. Res. *20*:94–101, 1959.
Carter, G. R.: *Pasteurella haemolytica:* An important pathogen of sheep and cattle. Vet. Med. *59*:722–724, 1964.
Jensen, R.: Diseases of Sheep. Philadelphia, Lea & Febiger, 176–178, 1974.
Jubb, K. V. F., and Kennedy, P. C.: Pathology of Domestic Animals, vol. 1. New York, Academic Press, 231–232, 1970.

Salmonellal Dysentery

Jensen, R., and Swift, B. L.: Diseases of Sheep. Philadelphia, Lea & Febiger, 1982.
Pierson, R. E., Poduska, P. J., Cholas, G., and Brown, G.: Relationship of management and nutrition to salmonellosis in feedlot lambs. J. Am. Vet. Med. Assoc. *161*:1217–1220, 1972.

Coccidiosis

Baker, N. F., Walter, G. T., and Fisk, R. A.: Amprolium for control of coccidiosis in feedlot lambs. Am. J. Vet. Res. *33*:83–85, 1972.
Bergstrom, R. C., and Moki, L. R.: Coccidiostatic action of monensin fed to lambs: body weight gains and feed conversion efficacy. Am. J. Vet. Res. *37*:79–81, 1976.

Fitzgerald, P. R., and Mansfield, M. C.: Ovine coccidiosis: effect of the antibiotic monensin against *Eimeria ninakohlyakimovae* and other naturally occurring coccidia of sheep. Am. J. Vet. Res. *39*:7–10, 1978.

Leek, R. G., Fayer, R., and McLoughlin, D. K.: Effect of monensin on experimental infections of *Eimeria ninakohlyakimovae* in lambs. Am. J. Vet. Res. *37*:339–341, 1976.

Pneumonia

Biberstein, E. L., Shreeve, B. J., Argus, K. W., and Thompson, D. A.: Experimental pneumonia of sheep: Clinical microbiological and pathological responses to infection with myxovirus parainfluenza 3 and *Pasteurella haemolytica*. J. Comp. Pathol. *81*:339–351, 1971.

Davies, D. H., Dungworth, D. L., Humphreys, S., and Johnson, A. J.: Concurrent infection of lambs with parainfluenza virus type 3 and *Pasteurella haemolytica*. N. Z. Vet. J. *25*:263–265, 1976.

McGowan, B., Thurley, D. C., McSporan, K. D., and Pfeffer, A. T.: Enzootic pneumonia-pleurisy complex in sheep and lambs. N. Z. Vet. J. *26*:169–172, 1977.

Thurley, D. C., Boyes, B. W., Davies, D. H., et al.: Subclinical pneumonia in lambs. N. Z. Vet. J. *25*:173–176, 1976.

Polioencephalomalacia

Linlsloter, K. A., Dyson, D. A., and Morgan, K. T.: Foecal thiaminase in clinically normal sheep associated with outbreaks of polioencephalomalacia. Res. Vet. Sci. *22*:308–312, 1977.

Pierson, R. E., and Jensen, R.: Polioencephalomalacia in feedlot lambs. J. Am. Vet. Med. Assoc. *166*:257–259, 1975.

Focal Symmetrical Encephalomalacia

Gay, C. C., Blood, D. C., and Wilkinson, J. S.: Clinical observations of sheep with focal symmetrical encephalomalacia. Aust. Vet. J. *51*:266–269, 1975.

Listeriosis

Gates, G. A., Blenden, D. C., and Kitner, L. D.: Listeric myelitis in sheep. J. Am. Vet. Med. Assoc. *150*:200–204, 1967.

Jensen, R., and Swift, B. L.: Diseases of Sheep, 2nd ed. Philadelphia, Lea & Febiger, 1982.

Killinger, A. H.: Problems associated with the prevention and control of listeriosis in sheep. Symposium on Sheep Diseases and Health, Davis, California, September 10 and 11, 1968.

Killinger, A. H., and Mansfield, M. E.: Epizootiology of listeric infection in sheep. J. Am. Vet. Med. Assoc. *157*:1318–1324, 1970.

Urolithiasis

Jensen, R., and Swift, B. L.: Diseases of Sheep, 2nd ed. Philadelphia, Lea & Febiger, 1982.

Polyarthritis

Pierson, R. E.: Polyarthritis in Colorado feedlot lambs. J. Am. Vet. Med. Assoc. *150*:1487–1492, 1967.

Storz, J., Pierson, R. E., Morriott, M. E., and Chow, T. L.: Isolation of psittacosis agents from follicular conjunctivitis of sheep. Proc. Soc. Exp. Biol. Med. *125*:857–860, 1967.

Contagious Ecthyma

Jensen, R., and Swift B. L.: Diseases of Sheep, 2nd ed. Philadelphia, Lea & Febiger, 1982.

Transport Tetany

Pierson, R. E., and Jensen, R.: Transport tetany of feedlot lambs. J. Am. Vet. Med. Assoc. *166*:260–261, 1975.

Dairy Goat Herd Health Management

CHRISTINE S. F. WILLIAMS, B.V.Sc., M.R.C.V.S.

Herd health programs have to be tailor-made to fit individual herds and will depend on the herd size, purpose, area, and attitude of the owner. There are relatively few large commercial goat dairies, but there are many small herds. Purebred sales, shows, 4-H projects, and production of milk and meat for home use are some of the reasons for these small herds. Few of these small herd owners sell milk legally, because most do not have Grade-A licenses.

Large herds have the usual problems associated with the high density of animals and the continual turnover. Small herds tend to have high nonproductive to productive ratios. Small herd owners often keep animals that would normally be culled from commercial dairy herds. Some of the reasons for this are sentimental, but often there is a desire to maintain certain blood lines. Often, the net result is the maintenance of animals with chronic illnesses that may serve as reservoirs of disease. Management practices contribute significantly to disease problems, and this makes it difficult for a practitioner who sees animals only in the office to get to the root of the problem. Occasional farm visits can be very rewarding in terms of disease and control. For example, if all the goats in a herd have untrimmed hooves, this tends to indicate a lack of available time and consequent difficulties in maintaining recommended herd health practices. Goat dairying is a very labor-intensive operation, and many herds are maintained by persons who earn their living from the farm.

In small hobby herds, there is sometimes a tendency to feed adult animals as if they were nonruminants. Excessive amounts of high energy and high protein grain feeds lead to digestive problems, enterotoxemia, polioencephalomalacia, urinary calculi, and fat goats with associated pregnancy ketosis. Young kids are often fed milk for several months at levels much higher than the recommended 10 per cent of body weight fed to calves. It is quite feasible to raise kids on 1.0 L of goats' milk per day for 6 to 7 weeks. There is considerable resistance to weaning kids early, although it has been done at 4 to 5 weeks in commercial herds in France. In herds being raised for show and sale, the kids may receive as much as 2.0 L of milk per day for several months. As a result, the kid pens are usually soaking wet. Many owners put all the kids in a small pen under a heat lamp, with the doors and windows closed. These conditions are a perfect environment for the develpment of pneumonia, enteritis, joint ill, coccidiosis, and other diseases.

KID CARE

Newborn kids should be dried and their navels should be dipped in 7-per cent tincture of iodine. Only in extremely cold weather is it advisable to use a heat lamp and then only for a few hours to fluff up the hair on the ears and feet to prevent frostbite. In regions where nutritional muscular dystrophy is a common problem, kids should receive vitamin E and selenium injections. Kids should be examined for congenital defects, such as cleft palate, undershot or overshot jaw, anal atresia, supernumerary teats, fishtail teats, fused double teats, hermaphroditism, and so forth. Hermaphroditism results from breeding polled bucks to polled does. Homozygous polled female kids will develop into hermaphrodites in utero. During the first week of life, kids should be dehorned with thermocautery. Caustic dehorning products are not advisable because the caustic material may get into the eyes or rub off the kid's head onto the dam's udder. Buck kids should be disbudded as early as possible to avoid growth of scurs. A small size calf dehorner works well but the large size calf dehorner may cause an excessive scar and raises the goat's eyebrows when the scar contracts.

In areas where tetanus is endemic, it may be advisable to inject at least 150 units of tetanus antitoxin at the time of disbudding. Tetanus is uncommon in goats, and only a few goat owners will refuse to initiate prophylaxis once a case has occurred in their small herd. In large dairy herds, tetanus vaccination is not a routine procedure, but it is advisable for the small family herds. Enterotoxemia vaccination is recommended. A convenient product is Clostroid D-T,* which contains both tetanus toxoid and enterotoxemia type D toxoid. The occurrence of type C enterotoxemia is poorly documented, but if it is diagnosed in a particular area and if other clostridial diseases are a problem, then a multiple clostridial vaccine should be used with the dose rate and schedule recommended for sheep.

Sore-mouth vaccination is not recommended, except under specific circumstances. Goat breeders who show animals extensively and who attend many stock sales may wish to vaccinate the animals early in life in order that the vaccine lesions will develop and heal prior to the show season or the anticipated date of sale. Both the natural disease and the vaccine-induced lesions last 2 to 4 weeks. Sore-mouth is an unpredictable disease, and even if endemic in a herd, it may not appear every year. Generally, once an animal has had the disease or the vaccine, it is immune. However, there is a benign goat poxvirus that causes scabby lesions scattered over the body. There is no vaccine for this virus disease, and there is no cross protection with sore-mouth.

Kids will acquire lice very early if the adults are infected. All animals in the herd should be treated at the same time. Adults should be sprayed or dusted with preparations suitable for lactating dairy cows, and young kids should be treated with flea powders suitable for cats. Kids may acquire ear mites in the first few weeks of life and will flap their ears and scratch them. Clients rarely request treatment because they are not aware of the disease. Remedies suitable for dog ear mites can be used, but the whole herd should be treated at the same time. It is very difficult to restrain goats (especially Nubians) to put liquid in their ears.

GROWING KIDS

Coccidiosis is a common problem in kids 3 weeks of age or older. It is the major cause of poor growth rate and frail looking kids. They acquire the oocysts from adults or older kids who have shed the parasites in their feces. Kids suckling their dams with plenty of clean dry space to run rarely show clinical signs. The communal kid pen in a dark corner of a barn, where new kids are added to the group and manure builds up, is a good place to develop clinical coccidiosis. Bloody diarrhea or greenish-gray pasty feces are observed. Occasionally, peracute cases occur in which the animal collapses and dies in less than 24 hr. On postmortem examination, the intestines will be full of blood, and coccidial lesions will be grossly visible, but only a few oocysts are in the feces. Grossly, the feces look normal. Amprolium,† a cattle coccidiostat used orally at 2.0 ml per 15 kg for 5 days, is effective in

some situations. In others, sulfonamides give better results. Feeding monensin* at 20 gm/ton of complete feed or lasalocid† at 20 to 30 gm/ton of complete feed (0.5 to 1 mg/lb/day) should give some protection to growing kids but neither of these products is licensed for dairy goats. Little or nothing can be done for peracute cases. Every effort should be made to analyze management practices and change those that are conducive to the development of coccidiosis. It is better to prevent this disease than to treat it.

Newborn kids born into a wet, dirty environment, where other kids have been running, are especially susceptible to joint ill. In early cases, animals may respond to penicillin injections. Chronic cases are difficult to resolve if there is permanent joint damage.

Growing kids are highly susceptible to pneumonia when raised in barns with poor ventilation. They would be better outside, with some protection from rain and wind. Many owners like to "keep the kids warm at night" and shut the barn doors and windows. Additionally, kids may be shown and are, therefore, trucked back and forth in either a poorly ventilated pick-up camper or a drafty trailer. They come in contact with other kids at the show and are put back in the herd at home. Tylosin and tetracyclines may be helpful, but again, preventing is better than curing.

Sick kids get well more easily if given goat's milk rather than ewe or cow milk replacer.

BUCKS

It is preferable to house bucks individually because of fighting. Dominant goats will guard feed troughs and prevent other goats from eating. Most bucks will lose condition during the breeding season, especially if they are housed next to does that are in estrus. Loss of libido can ocur if bucks are in very poor condition, parasitized, too fat, arthritic, or suffering from painful overgrown feet. Urinary calculi can be a problem when bucks are fed too much grain and not enough calcium. To help prevent urinary calculi, be sure the water supply is fresh and clean and that the bucks have access to loose trace mineral salt. A contaminated water supply will reduce water intake and will contribute significantly to urinary calculi. Warm fresh water will be tolerated better than icy water in winter.

Because of their odor and their habit of urinating on themselves, the bucks are often neglected in routine foot trimming, delousing, worming, and other herd maintenance activities. Many bucks die before they reach 5 or 6 years of age.

Descenting a buck by removing the scent gland on the top of the head, does not remove all of the odor. The bucks will still have an odor of dried urine. This odor problem can be improved by clipping and washing them occasionally. Urine scalds on the back of the front legs may be a problem.

There is very little documented evidence to demonstrate that bucks are the significant carriers of genital diseases.

---

*Available from Fort Dodge Laboratories, Fort Dodge, IA 50501.
†Available as Corid from Merck & Co., Rahway, NJ 07065.

*Available as Rumensin from Elanco, Division of Eli Lilly, Indianapolis, IN 46285.
†Available as Bovatec from Hoffmann-La Roche, Inc., Nutley, NJ 07110.

Although bulls are the carriers of cattle trichomoniasis, there are no reports of trichomoniasis in goats. However, bucks may pick up other diseases as they travel from one herd to another or stand at stud and breed all the neighborhood goats. Quarantine and closed herds are not general rules in the goat business.

Artificial insemination is in its infancy, and there are no data on disease transmission via frozen semen.

LACTATING DOES

Commercial dairymen are likely to consider the restricted breeding season and the lack of an economical pregnancy detection system more important than disease in a large goat herd. In small herds, there is no emphasis on the year-round fluid milk market but there is emphasis on stock sales. Pregnancy diagnosis can be accomplished with real-time ultrasonography, which is used externally from mid- to late gestation to count fetuses. The rectal Doppler machine can be used as early as 30 days to detect the fetal heart beat. Echoscanners are useful in midgestation but cannot assist in distinguishing between true and false pregnancy (cloudburst). Progesterone evaluation has the same limitations in goats as it does in dairy cattle. A low progesterone level indicates she's not pregnant. A high progesterone level means she has a functional corpus luteum only. The estrone sulfate test, performed on milk or urine starting at 40 to 50 days post-breeding, gives a strong indication of true pregnancy and continued fetal viability.

Mastitis in dairy goats is most likely to be caused by *Staphylococcus* spp. Acute gangrenous mastitis is often fatal or will cause half the udder to slough. Less acute cases end in fibrosis. In herds where *Staphylococcus* spp. are problems, dry goat treatment should be used. One half of a cow's single-dose mastitis tube should be infused into each half of the goat udder, using strict sanitary precautions. Nonhemolytic *Staphylococcus* spp. in association with firm, tender udders are accorded more significance in goats than they are in cows. The CMT (California Mastitis Test) in goats should not be considered indicative of mastitis unless a 2+ or 3+ is demonstrated. Somatic cell counts in goats may rise sharply to several million at the end of lactation without any increase in incidence of mastitis. If the majority of goats finish their lactation at the same time, which is likely because of the seasonal breeding, the bulk somatic cell count may be above the legal limit for fluid milk sales. Caprine arthritis encephalitis virus can cause accumulations of lymphoid cells in the udder tissue, and this is thought to be a major cause of the hard udder syndrome at parturition. This condition is known as congested udder or udder edema, but it is not analogous to dairy cattle edema, and it does not respond to diuretics.

Respiratory disease in adult goats can generally be traced to management problems. Compounding the problem is the tendency to keep a goat with chronic pneumonia for another pregnancy. Owners sometimes use cattle vaccines in an attempt to control "shipping fever," but there is little evidence to show that they work.

Johne's disease should always be considered when a cachectic goat is encountered. Diarrhea is not a consistent finding. The fecal culture is the only diagnostic test that does not give false-positive results. A disadvantage of this test is that it requires several months to obtain results. The AGID (Agar Gel Immuno Diffusion) test is the best serologic test for Johne's disease in goats and gives an early warning of the impending development of clinical signs. However, it cannot be used as a prepurchase screen. A negative result does not always indicate freedom from infection. There are no commercial vaccines available, and the only method of control is management. Keep the kids and growing stock away from adult goat manure as long as possible. The kids should be removed as soon as they are born and raised elsewhere using colostrum from known Johne's disease–free herds or from carefully sanitized udders.

Caseous lymphadenitis is another chronic disease to consider in cachectic goats. *Corynebacterium pseudotuberculosis* is the most common bacterium involved. It causes chronic abscesses in the regional lymph nodes, especially in the head region. *Staphylococcus aureus* and *C. pyogenes* occasionally cause abscesses, but are generally more rapid in onset and do not necessarily occur in the lymph nodes. Caseous lymphadenitis is a contagious disease and is thought to be transmitted by pus that contaminates the environment, the hay feeders, and so forth. Experimentally, the organisms can invade the intact shaved skin. Surgical removal of the intact abscessed lymph node offers the best hope of control in small herds in the early stages of infection. This is not economically feasible in most large herds. Abscesses in the lungs and liver obviously cannot be removed and are usually found postmortem. Autogenous vaccines have been used, but there are no published reports of their effectiveness. There is experimental evidence of some protection in goats vaccinated with an Australian sheep *C. pseudotuberculosis* product. Antibiotic treatment of chronic abscesses is useless. Antibiotics in the feed are sometimes suggested as a preventive, but there is no evidence regarding efficacy.

If abscesses have been allowed to rupture, a serious effort should be made to clean up the environment. All wood should be scrubbed with hot washing soda to remove the goat grease and then sprayed with a disinfectant. Contaminated hay feeders with cracks and crevices are better replaced. Goats with enlarged external lymph nodes should be culled or undergo surgery. Caseous lymphadenitis cannot be cured by drug therapy, but it can be controlled by intelligent measures designed to reduce contamination.

Tuberculosis and caprine brucellosis are not naturally occurring diseases in the United States. Many states require testing of out-of-state goats prior to entry. Also, testing is required for legal milk sales. The incidence of these 2 diseases is practically nil, as a result of the eradication programs. Goats occasionally react to the tuberculin test and then have to be tested by the double intradermal test using avian tuberculin as well. Goats may become sensitized to avian tuberculin by being housed with chickens affected by avian tuberculosis. Goat brucellosis is caused by *Brucella melitensis*. The same blood test as that for brucellosis is applicable. There has not been a natural case of goat brucellosis in the United States for many years.

There are a number of diseases that cause locomotor problems in goats. Arthritis is a widespread problem. Many yearling goats can be found with enlarged knees and stifle joints, and as they get older the disease gets worse, and the animals lose weight and productivity. Several *Myoplasma* spp. have been isolated from goats in the United States. Outbreaks of acute arthritis with high fever may occur in young kids, and an occasional adult may die of peracute infection following the stress of parturition. *Mycoplasma mycoides mycoides* (large-colony type) is the organism most commonly associated with this syndrome, and control programs involve culling all does that shed the organism in the colostrum and pasteurizing all milk fed to the kids. There is little that can be done to effect a cure in goats with chronic arthritis. A viral disease, caprine arthritis encephalomyelitis, will cause chronic arthritis in adults or rarely a demyelinating encephalomyelitis in young animals. There is no cure for this disease, and current control programs involve removing the kids immediately after they are born and raising them on pasteurized goat milk and goat colostrum that has been heat treated at 135°F for 1 hr, or cow colostrum. Animals raised in this manner should be isolated from seropositive animals. Serologic testing and culling of those that react positively can be used on a herd basis. The test cannot be used definitively as a prepurchase screen, since some infected animals give a negative reaction. The majority of goats that react positively do not develop clinical signs of the disease. However, the presence of a titer indicates the continued presence of the retrovirus. Listeriosis in the goat is usually sporadic and will cause encephalitis with a fever of 40 to 41°C, incoordination, circling, and collapse. Tetracycline administered intravenously can be attempted, but the prognosis is poor, and the goats usually die in less than 5 days. Polioencephalomalacia, rabies, and lead poisoning are other diseases to consider in the differential diagnosis. *Parelaphostrongylus* spp. will cause incoordination in goats that graze pastures inhabited by white tailed deer. The parasite migrates to the spinal cord. There is no specific treatment that will kill these parasites. Anthelmintic treatment of goats with haloxon results occasionally in permanent demyelination and posterior paralysis. This may occur days or weeks after the drug treatment. Polioencephalomalacia due to thiamine deficiency can occur, and it is wise to give any goat with abnormal neurologic signs 3 to 5 mg/lb of thiamine intravenously.

Infectious abortions in goats are generally due to *Chlamydia*. Vibriosis is extremely rare. *Listeria*-induced abortions are sporadic. Q fever is diagnosed occasionally and so is toxoplasmosis. Chlamydial abortions are usually late and in first fresheners or new additions to the herd. Older goats in endemic herds may abort again several years later as their immunity wanes. Goats may be vaccinated with the sheep vaccine, prior to breeding. Tetracycline may be used prophylactically at 150 to 200 mg/head/day for 3 weeks before breeding or used therapeutically during an abortion storm. Use 150 mg/head/day in feed or use slow release formulation at 9 mg/kg once or twice weekly.

Parasitism in dairy goats is a major factor in reducing milk yields and increasing mortality in adult goats. Coccidiosis does not usually affect adults clinically, although many adults shed oocysts. *Haemonchus contortus* is the major blood sucking nematode in the abomasum. This parasite will cause a coarse hair coat, weight loss, and a precipitous drop in hematocrit value. However, when this type of parasitism occurs, the whole herd health program should be evaluated. Many owners deworm their goats once a year and feel that this action will be satisfactory. Some deworm using organic materials, such as tobacco stems, diatomaceous earth, or garlic tablets. This type of treatment is often used in the first years of goat keeping, when goat numbers are low, pasture contamination minimal, and clinical parasitism extremely unlikely. However, after several more years of goat keeping, with increasing populations of both goats and worms, clinical parasitism appears. There is no specific deworming program that will work for every situation. Programs must be designed to fit individual farms and should be based on clinical experience, accurate records, and postmortem examinations.

Tapeworms in young animals cause more problems for the owners than for the goats, and in most cases treatment is not worthwhile. However, niclosamide* at dog dose rates has been used as have mebendazole† and fenbendazole.‡ None of these products are licensed for use in goats. Lungworms can be a problem, particularly since there are no licensed drugs that are effective. Levamisole is effective but is not licensed for use in goats in the United States. Lice can be a considerable problem in late winter and can debilitate goats.

Foot problems in the adult goat are usually the result of overgrown hooves and lack of foot care. Occasionally, foot abscesses or interdigital granulomas occur. Foot rot is not a significant problem.

Pinkeye in goats can be a most frustrating problem. There are varied causes, including *Mycoplasma* spp. There are several clinical syndromes, such as severe eyelid swelling, follicular conjunctivitis, and unilateral or bilateral corneal opacity. The course of the disease is entirely unpredictable, and the choice of a therapeutic agent is difficult. Sometimes, nothing seems to help, and the disease spreads through a herd. Corneal opacity is quite spectacular and will temporarily blind a goat. When the disease finally starts to resolve, the opacity often disappears rapidly.

Metabolic diseases, such as lactation ketosis, hypocalcemia (milk fever), and hypomagnesemia, are very uncommon. Pregnancy ketosis is much more likely to occur, especially in the overweight, underexercised goat carrying multiple fetuses. Goats tend to store fat internally, which leads the owner to think that the goat is never overweight. A goat that is carrying too much fat internally will have wads of fat behind each elbow on the rib cage. Clients should be advised to examine some of the "skinny" goats at slaughter or necropsy to see how much fat is stored internally.

Pregnant goats should not be allowed to get fat nor should they be allowed to be inactive. Fat goats with pregnancy toxemia respond poorly to the traditional remedies, such as propylene glycol and intravenous glucose. The condition can be avoided by proper management.

---

*Available as Yomesan from Haver-Lockhart, Shawnee, KS 66201

†Available as Telmin from Pitman-Moore, Inc., Washington Crossing, NJ 08560

‡Available as Panacur from American Hoechst Corp., North Somerville, NJ 08876.

Swine Herd Health Management

LeROY G. BIEHL, D.V.M., M.S.

Modifications in pork production techniques and changes in disease patterns have transformed the veterinary services sought by modern swine producers. Prior to the eradication of hog cholera, the veterinary practitioner made visits to the farm at least twice a year to vaccinate pigs and to offer disease management advice. Diseases were treated with medication either via injections administered by the veterinarian or via water. The arrival of confinement, medicated complete feed, and hog cholera eradication in a short span of years created a need for new and different health management programs. With only 5 per cent of the swine producers producing 50 per cent of the pork in the United States, the industrialization of pork production has evolved. Larger swine units have brought on new health challenges requiring constant surveillance. Owners of these large units are requesting professional consultation in the areas of health, reproduction, genetics, nutrition, environment, and economics. Since these areas are all interrelated in the herd health management scheme, the veterinarian also must have knowledge and ready access to appropriate specialists. The goal of the swine enterprise is profit, and the recommendations of the veterinarian serving the swine unit must be not only medically and scientifically sound but financially sound. The cost of the preventive measure or treatment should not exceed the expected yield in return. These decisions will vary from producer to producer, depending on the type, size, and location of operation and the capabilities of the staff and the goals of the owner.

Good communication by the veterinarian with the owner, manager, and employees is necessary for a herd health program to function successfully. Production goals should be established, and continuous positive discussions with the various employees who influence the production goals need to take place. Some owners use financial incentives for their employees, such as extra pay for each pig weaned over an established average. It is extremely important to have each employee consider himself or herself a part of the production team. The manager must have the willingness to accept changes in management programs and the ability to implement these changes into new programs.

Following the establishment of production targets for the unit, accurate records are a necessity. The records should be simple, practical, and usable. If the data collected are not going to be used for decision making at a later date, do not expend the effort to produce the data. Analysis of useful data, however, will frequently allow the veterinarian to pinpoint areas where disease is causing problems, and remedial action can be taken.

Computers have made the computation of data and the analysis of records a much simpler task, but useful, accurate information must be entered into the data bank if useful, accurate information is expected in return. The computer may provide the owner with the incentive and the required discipline to collect and record the accurate data desired for a large swine farm. Many software programs are available for personal computers that can be utilized by employees of most swine units unless the units are extremely large.

Basically, record keeping is required for the production areas: reproduction, farrowing, nursery, and growing-finishing. Information from the reproductive performance records should indicate conception rates, interval to weaning times, infertile animals, abortions, and farrowing rates. A record of boar performance will identify inferior boars. A sow and litter record in the farrowing area should contain farrowing date, number of pigs born alive and dead, number of mummies, number weaned, weight, and date of weaning (Fig. 1). Mortality records with cause of death should be included on the farrowing card. A pig identification system is necessary to monitor performance of the litter. Pigs can be individually notched. Commercial producers frequently notch the ears to indicate the week of the year the pig was born so the age at marketing is known.

Records of the nursery and growing-finishing area should indicate death loss, cause of death, and time to market (Figs. 2 and 3). Feed efficiency records and slaughter records in these production areas are important to the measurement of feed efficiency (Figs. 4 and 5). Declining feed efficiency performance may indicate nutritional imbalance, feed wastage, genetic decline, or the introduction of a disease agent into the herd.

The establishment of production goals or targets originally proposed by Muirhead of England allows management to measure programs.[1] If the goals are not attained, management and the veterinary practitioner can discuss why the targets were not achieved and what managerial steps need to be taken to improve the situation.

Tables 1, 2, and 3 present examples of production targets that may be applied to confinement herds.[2]

When initiating a herd health program, both the veterinarian and producer must be aware of each other's expectations. Frequency of visits to the farm, amount of time spent per visit, cost of medications, cost of emergency calls, and cost of the total service are points that should be agreed upon at the onset.

Fees will depend upon how much time the veterinarian spends on the farm and what drugs are furnished. Some fees are set as a predetermined amount for each pig weaned or marketed. This provides an incentive for the veterinarian, but the owner may not believe the veterinarian is spending enough time on the farm, especially during problem periods. Some veterinarians prefer charging by the hour, which is probably more fair to both parties, but some owners may feel veterinarians are not as efficient with their time as they could be. Whatever type of fee scheduling is chosen, a mutual trust between the owner, manager, and veterinarian is necessary if the herd health program is to be successful.

No single herd health program can be written to adequately cover all herds. The outline given here is only a reference point to build from. Modifications of the program will have to be made when the individual requirements of the herd, owner, and veterinarian make it necessary.

LITTER RECORD

Farrowing Date _____

Sow ID _____

Boar ID _____

Crate Location _____

Litter Notch _____

Parity 1 2 3 4 5 6 7 8 9

FARROWING	MORTALITY	WEANING
Alive G_____ P _____	Laid on _____	Date _____
Stillborn _____	Scour loss _____	Pigs weaned _____
Mummies _____	Weak and small loss _____	Weaning wt. _____
Birth wt. _____	Starvation _____	SPI _____
No. after trans. _____	Lame and arthritic _____	Boar M_____ T _____
Sow med. _____	Spraddle _____	
_____	Misc. _____	
_____	Liter med. _____	

(Back of card—only one copy)

	1	2	3	4	5	6
Date bred						
Boar ID						
No. farrowed						
No. weaned						

Figure 1. Sow and litter record. (*Note:* Card has a carbon with original and 1 copy.)

HERD HEALTH PROGRAM

I. Pregestation Period
  A. Gilt selection
    1. Select gilts 5 to 6 months of age, weighing 220 to 240 lb (100 to 110 kg).
    2. Select gilts with at least 12 well-spaced, prominent nipples from sows that
      a. wean a litter of at least 8 pigs.
      b. are sound on their feet and legs.
      c. have good milk production ability.
      d. have pigs without genetic defects.
  B. Boar selection and introduction of new breeding stock
    1. Purchase young boars tested for brucellosis, leptospirosis, and pseudorabies from a herd with a known health record at least 60 days before expected use.
    2. Isolate for 30 days and retest.
    3. Do not place the boar on any medication and observe for illness.
    4. Three or 4 sentinel animals may be placed in the pen on arrival of the boar, and they are observed for illness. They may be tested at the time of the boar test.
    5. Expose the boar to the sows and gilts 30 days prior to breeding by either feeding manure from the sows or placing 1 or 2 cull sows in the pen or both.
    6. Test the boar's mating ability and fertility by mating him with gilts. Semen evaluation can identify the infertile boar.
    7. The selected boar should also have at least 12 nipples, and none should be blind or inverted.
    8. Treat for mange.

NURSERY RECORD

	Mortality
Period _____ Date in ____	
Room no. ____ Date out ____	Scour loss _____
No. of pigs in nursery _____	Pneumonia loss _____
No. of pigs out of nursery ____	Lameness and joint loss _____
Wt. of pigs in nursery _____	Starvation loss _____
Wt. of pigs out of nursery ____	Runt loss _____
Notes:	Misc. loss _____

Figure 2. Nursery record. (*Note:* Card has a carbon with original and 1 copy.)

GROWING-FINISHING RECORD

	Mortality
Period farrowed _____	
No. pigs in _____	Scour loss _____
No. pigs sold _____	Pneumonia loss _____
No. sold <6 mo. of age ____	Lameness and arthritis loss ___
	Junk hogs _____
	Misc. loss _____

Figure 3. Growing-finishing record. (*Note:* Card has a carbon with original and 1 copy.)

SLAUGHTER RECORD

Month _____

No. finisher hogs sold	Total lb sold, finisher hogs	No. sows and boars sold	Total lb sold, sows and boars	No. feeder pigs sold	Total lb sold, feeder pigs

Figure 4. Slaughter record.

9. Examine feces for parasite eggs and treat accordingly.
C. Immunizations
 1. Parvovirus, leptospirosis (5-way), and erysipelas vaccines.
 2. Expose gilts to older animals (sows and boars) by feeding manure or by commingling at least 30 days prior to breeding to control SMEDI viruses.
D. Parasite control
 1. Deworm with broad-spectrum anthelmintics.
 2. Spray boars, gilts, and sows thoroughly for control of lice and mange. Repeat twice at weekly intervals. In countries where approved, Ivermectin may be given orally or as an injection.
E. Nutrition
 1. Boars, developing gilts.
  a. Protein (14–16 %).
  b. Calcium (0.85 %).
  c. Phosphorus (0.65 %).
  d. Total feed intake 4 to 6 lb (2 to 3 kg).
II. Breeding Period
 A. Move gilts to a different location and allow fenceline contact with boars.
 B. Flush gilts by increasing energy intake to 6 to 9 lb/day (3 to 4 kg/day).
 C. Breed during second or third estrus (7 to 8 months of age).
 D. Do not use boars that are less than 8 to 9 months of age.
 E. Use 1 boar for each 6 females to be bred in a 3-week period plus an extra boar in case of injury or sickness.
 F. Double mating at 12 and 24 hr after onset of estrus using different boars is preferable, but this may hinder identification of the poor boar.
 G. Hand mating requires fewer boars but more labor than pen mating.
 H. Reduce daily feed intake of gilt or sow immediately following breeding.

FEED EFFICIENCY RECORD

Period beginning_____ Period ending _____

Hogs marketed (lb) ÷ number sold = Average selling weight _____

CWT feed ground ÷ number marketed = CWT feed/head marketed _____

CWT feed ground ÷ CWT hogs sold = feed/CWT _____

Figure 5. Feed efficiency record.

III. Gestation Period
 A. Nutrition
  1. Maintain reduced feed intake until last trimester of pregnancy. Gilts should gain between 35 and 50 kg, and sows should gain between 25 and 30 kg during gestation.
  2. Ration
   a. Gilt
    (1) Protein (14 %)
    (2) Calcium (0.85 %, 15 gm/day)
    (3) Phosphorus (0.65 %, 12 gm/day)
    (4) Feed intake (2 to 3 kg/day)
   b. Sow
    (1) Protein (12 to 14 %)
    (2) Calcium (0.85 %, 15 gm/day)
    (3) Phosphorus (0.65, 12 gm/day)
    (4) Feed intake (2 to 3 kg/day)
  3. Increase feed to 3 kg in last trimester of pregnancy.
  4. Heavy-milking white sows may require more feed.
  5. Increase energy intake during winter.
 B. Immunization
  1. *Clostridium perfringens* type C toxoid, when necessary, 6 and 3 weeks prior to farrowing.
  2. *Escherischia coli* bacterin, when necessary, 5 and 3 weeks prior to farrowing or live oral milk vaccine.
  3. TGE vaccine if necessary.
   a. Injectable, 5 and 3 weeks prefarrowing.
   b. Oral, 5, 3, and 1 week prefarrowing.
  4. Atrophic rhinitis bacterin, when necessary, 5 and 3 weeks prefarrowing.
  5. Erysipelas vaccine 3 weeks prior to farrowing, when necessary, if not done prior to breeding.
 C. Retreat for mange 2 weeks prior to farrowing.
 D. Deworm 7 to 10 days prior to farrowing if needed

Table 1. *Production Targets: Reproductive Performance*

Reproductive Performance	Target
Parity of sows	
1st	20 %
2nd	20 %
3rd or more	60 %
Weaning to service interval	10 days
Lactation length	24–28 days
First breeding conception rate	
Sows	90 %
Gilts	80 %
Abortions	<1 %
Sows not in pig	<2 %
Farrowing rate	80 %
Sows mortality/yr	<3 %
Sow cull rate (disease)	<2 %
Litters/sow/yr	2.2 %

Table 2. *Production Targets: Production Performance*

Production Performance	Target
Pigs born alive/litter	10.0
Stillborn	7.0 %
Mummified	0.5 %
Suckling pig deaths	
0–7 days	7.0 %
8–14 days	1.5 %
15–21 days	1.0 %
>22 days	0.5 %
Total suckling pig deaths	10.0 %
No. pigs weaned/litter	9.0
Average weight at weaning—21 days	14 lbs.
Average weight at weaning — 28 days	18 lbs.
Litters/sow/yr	2.2
Pigs born/sow/yr	22.0
Pigs weaned/sow/yr	19.8
Total feed efficiency	3.6

(biannual fecal examinations of breeding herd will determine need and anthelmintic). Do not deworm with dichlorvos and treat with insecticide for mange simultaneously.

   E. Keep gestating sows isolated from new additions to prevent infection with viruses or bacteria that may cause abortions or mummies.

   F. Antibiotics are usually not added to gestation ration unless attempting to control a specific disease, such as atrophic rhinitis or colibacillosis.

   G. House animals on a clean, dry surface to prevent MMA (Metritis, Mastitis, Agalactia syndrome).

IV. Farrowing Period: Gilts or Sows

   A. Thoroughly clean and disinfect the farrowing house.

   B. Wash and use mild disinfectant on gilts and sows to rid them of parasite eggs and dirt before placing in farrowing crate or stall.

   C. Feed a bulky ration that will reduce constipation. If constipation is a problem, use 3.5 kg potassium chloride or 10 kg magnesium sulfate per ton of feed.

   D. Be present at farrowing to increase the number of pigs saved.

   E. Treat sows early that show evidence of agalactia.

   F. Observe feed intake of sows closely. Keeping farrowing room temperature below 23°C (80°F) will help increase intake.

   G. Do not allow manure buildup in pen or behind sows in the crate.

V. Farrowing to Weaning: Pig

   A. Environment

      1. Supply adequate heat with lamp or mats to avoid chilling at birth.

Table 3. *Production Targets: Boar Performance*

Boar Performance	Target
Total boar:sow ratio	1:15
Working boar:sow ratio	1:20
Matings/week	
Young boars	2
Mature boars	4
Rest between double matings	
Young boars	4 days
Mature boars	3 days
Total boars replaced/yr	50 %

      2. Farrowing boxes or hovers provide draft-free heat for the pig and allow a lower farrowing house temperature for the sow.

      3. Temperature for pig sleeping area should be 32 to 35°C (90 to 95°F).

   B. Administer dextrose plus electrolytes orally to weak pigs.

   C. Process pigs 12 to 24 hr after birth.

      1. Clip needle teeth.

      2. Dock tails.

      3. Notch ear to identify litter and week of birth.

      4. Castrate.

      5. Inject 100 to 150 mg iron into the neck muscle.

      6. Treat with antibiotic if necessary to control diarrhea or navel ill. Use sensitivity test results to determine best antibiotic.

      7. Identify litters with genetic defects.

   D. If several sows are farrowing simultaneously, adjust litters to equal size and number for each litter.

   E. Immunizations

      1. Inject *Clostridium perfringens* antitoxin, when necessary, immediately after birth.

      2. Administer atrophic rhinitis bacterin, if needed, at 7 and 28 days.

   F. Nutrition

      1. Provide water as a creep from day 1.

      2. Palatable creep feed provided at 10 to 14 days. Feed small amounts daily.

      3. Give second iron injection or oral iron at 2 weeks.

   G. Wean pigs at 3 to 4 weeks.

VI. Weaning Period

   A. Environment

      1. Place pigs in clean, warm 30°C (85°F) nursery, preferably with woven wire flooring or similar impervious perforated flooring.

      2. "All-in, all-out" farrowing and nursery will aid considerably in controlling disease.

   B. Nutrition

      1. Starter recommendations

         a. 5 to 10 kg (10 to 20 lb)

            (1) Protein (20 %)

            (2) Lysine (1.15 %)

            (3) Calcium (0.80 %)

            (4) Phosphorus (0.60 %)

         b. 7 to 15 kg (15 to 30 lb)

            (1) Protein (18 %)

            (2) Lysine (0.96 %)

            (3) Calcium (0.75 %)

            (4) Phosphorus (0.60 %)

      2. Diets need to be kept fresh, and pigs need to be fed once or twice a day.

      3. Add antibiotics to the ration.

   C. Immunization

      1. Atrophic rhinitis bacterin, when needed, second injection at 28 days.

      2. Erysipelas vaccination if necessary at 5 to 6 weeks.

      3. *Hemophilus pleuropneumonia* bacterin, when necessary, at 8 to 12 weeks.

   D. Parasites

      1. Treat for lice and mange if needed.

      2. Fecal samples should be collected after 10

weeks of age from a group of untreated pigs to determine infections. Deworm at 6 to 8 weeks when needed.

E. Monitor for postweaning diarrhea
1. Make definitive diagnosis and treat accordingly.
2. Medicate water if needed.

F. Postmortem examination of pigs if disease outbreak occurs.

VII. Growing-Finishing Period
A. Nutrition
1. Recommendations
a. 15 to 60 kg (30 to 120 lb)
(1) Protein (16 %)
(2) Lysine (0.75 %)
(3) Calcium (0.65 %)
(4) Phosphorus (0.55 %)
b. 120 to market
(1) Protein (14 %)
(2) Lysine (0.60 %)
(3) Calcium (0.60 %)
(4) Phosphorus (0.50 %)
2. Provide adequate feeder and water space.
3. Observe feed intake and adjust feeders to control waste.
4. Remove antibiotics from diet at 60 kg (120 lb) of body weight.
B. Immunization
1. Second or third *Hemophilus pleuropneumonia* bacterin, if needed, at 12 and 16 weeks of age.
C. Parasites
1. Monitor fecal examination results twice a year and treat accordingly.
2. Spray or treat for lice and mange if needed.
D. Check 20 pigs at slaughter at least twice a year to monitor incidence of disease problems.
E. Conduct postmortem examinations of pigs if needed.

As previously stated, the Herd Health Program outlined here is only a reference, and each farm should develop its own set of specific guidelines. Many of the vaccinations will not be used on all farms, since they are not necessary in all herds. The present trend is to eliminate as many vaccinations as possible from the program and to rely on strict isolation and sanitation for disease prevention.

GUIDELINES FOR BREEDING STOCK REPLACEMENTS

Most swine enterprises must eventually add new genetic material to the herd, and introducing replacement breeding stock into the herd is a critical management decision. The potential disease losses associated with the purchase of new breeding stock are enormous. Frequently the boar is replaced at breeding time, which compounds the risk of introducing and spreading a new disease on the farm.

Diseases can be brought onto the farm by carrier animals that show no clinical signs of external and internal parasites, brucellosis, leptospirosis, eperythrozoonosis, erysipelas, dysentery, salmonellosis, colibacillosis, rhinitis, mycoplasma pneumonia, arthritis, and possibly MMA. The list of virus diseases includes transmissible gastroenteritis, pseudorabies, influenza, and viruses of the SMEDI syndrome. It is virtually impossible to test or to ascertain that any animal is free of all these diseases.

Producers need to monitor their own herds before they establish the health requirements of additions. If the herd is currently infected with mycoplasma or parvovirus, it is not necessary to require the additions to be free of these diseases. The new additions should not show clinical signs of any diseases at the time of purchase.

The programs discussed next will substantially reduce the risk of disease when adding new genetic material to the farm.

Specific Pathogen Free (SPF). Purchasing from SPF herds should eliminate the risk of parasites, brucellosis, leptospirosis, dysentery, mycoplasma pneumonia, and atrophic rhinitis.

Artificial Insemination (AI). New genetic material can be introduced into the herd by AI, which keeps the boar, and any disease he may be carrying, off the farm. Although it is unlikely, several viruses may be transmitted through the semen.

Embryo Transfer. Swine embryos can be transferred from a seed stock herd to a recipient sow from the purchaser's farm. The pigs are born on the same farm on which they wil be raised. Although transmission of viruses is possible with embryo transfer, it is highly unlikely.

Purchase of a Pregnant Sow. Only 1 animal is brought into the herd, but the litter can provide several new genetic additions.

Purchase of Individual Herd Replacements. Buying boars or replacement gilts may be the most practical method of integrating genetic material into an otherwise closed herd. The herd history should be discussed thoroughly with the breeder. An identifiable health plan, including testing records and slaughter checks, should be available. In addition to examination of serologic testing results and other health records, production records of the seed stock producer should be viewed. Feed efficiency, litter size, farrowing rate, and death loss provide valuable information.

Discuss any guarantee offered by the breeder regarding the health status and reproductive performance. Breeders who accept the return of nonbreeder animals rather than sending them to slaughter are exposing their herds to new diseases. The answers to the next questions need to be considered before buying. Does the breeder provide or require visitors to wear boots or coveralls? Does the breeder have isolation facilities?

Both the purchaser and the seller have a responsibility to prevent transfer of disease from one herd to another. Sellers should monitor their seed stock herds and advise buyers of the disease status of the herds. Since no breeding animals are completely free of microorganisms, it is the buyer's responsibility to isolate and condition the purchased animals. Following the 30 day isolation period, the buyer should expose the purchased breeding animals and resident animals to each other by manure feeding or commingling or both as outlined earlier. A common herd immunity should be developed prior to breeding to prevent reproductive failure at the first breeding.

References

1. Muirhead, M. R.: Veterinary problems of intensive pig husbandry. Vet. Rec. *101*:177–180, 1977.
2. Johnson, Rodney G.: Records and Targets for Group Breeding Programs. Proc. Univ. of Minnesota Swine Herd Health Programming Conference: 129a–129f, 1983.

DIETARY MANAGEMENT

JIMMY L. HOWARD, D.V.M.
Consulting Editor

Nutritional Management of Stressed and Morbid Calves*

N. ANDY COLE, Ph.D.

Cattle encounter numerous periods of physiologic stress during their lifetime. When stress is severe and accompanied by infectious agents, the health and performance of the animal can be severely impaired.

During severe stress, nutrient requirements may increase owing to a hypermetabolic effect caused by increased secretions of adrenocorticoid hormones. Body protein is degraded more rapidly, and the excretion of some minerals is increased. Concurrently, various aspects of the animal's immune response may be reduced, leaving the animal more susceptible to infection. These adverse effects on metabolism and immunity may be accentuated by a reduction in feed consumption. In addition, the digestibility of the feed consumed may be reduced by an increased rumen turnover rate and a reduced rumen fermentative capacity. Although proper nutrition cannot alleviate stress, it can assist the animal in preparing for and recovering from stressful periods.

In beef cattle, severe stress is most often encountered during marketing, when cattle are moved from one production point to another, i.e., from the farm of origin to the feedyard. Calves may pass through several marketing channels and encounter lengthy periods of transport over a span of one to ten days. Feed and water may be limited or unavailable during this time.

The deprivation of feed and water has a detrimental effect on rumen function and subsequent feed intake of cattle. The volume of the ruminant's gastrointestinal tract may serve to buffer some of the effects of a short feed and water deprivation period (48 hours or less), since nutrients may be absorbed for two to four days after a meal is consumed. The extent of this buffering effect, however, is directly proportional to the calf's plane of nutrition before the deprivation period. Whereas the nonruminant will return to normal feed intake in 1 to 2 days after a feed and water deprivation period, the ruminant may require 7 to 14 days for feed intake to return to normal. The length of this recovery period is partly dependent upon the diet fed before and after the deprivation period as well as on the severity of the stress.

The nutrition of the calf before, during, and after the stresses of marketing and transport, therefore, can have a significant effect on the subsequent feed consumption, health, and performance.

DIETARY MANAGEMENT

Ideally, the diet fed to the calf prior to marketing and transport should be similar to the diet it will receive after marketing and transport. Since this is usually not practical, a good rule of thumb is that the calf should be accustomed to some grain in the diet before it leaves the farm of origin. Weaning and feeding calves for about 30 days before sale is expensive, time consuming, and of questionable economic benefit to the calf producer or feeder. Creep feeding calves for an extended period is also seldom of economic benefit to the producer and feeder. Short-term (24 days) creep feeding prior to sale, however, has yielded good results in preliminary studies.

The diet fed while a calf is in the marketing channel can also affect his subsequent health and performance. Calves fed an antibiotic-fortified, 50 per cent concentrate diet at the auction and orderbuyer barn will usually have fewer health problems than calves fed only hay. Since some calves will be unfamiliar with a milled diet, it may be more beneficial to provide the calf with a choice of hay and the milled diet. Yearlings will usually eat a milled diet more readily than calves; therefore, they should be provided hay along with a milled diet to avoid digestive disturbances.

Feeder calves normally have low feed consumption during the first few weeks in the feedyard. Many factors, such as reduced rumen fermentative capacity, reduced rumen contractions, fever, unfamiliarity with the diet, and other stress-related factors, may cause low feed consumption. When feed consumption is low, deficiencies of protein, vitamins, and minerals can be corrected by simply increasing the concentrations of these nutrients in the diet (Table 1). Energy, however, is usually the first limiting nutrient in calves with low feed consumption, and the lack of energy is the major reason for poor performance. The receiving diet and diet of morbid calves should be formulated to (1) replenish lost body stores of nutrients, (2) return feed intake to normal as rapidly as possible, and (3) avoid digestive disturbances. A variety of diets will meet these criteria; however, the following is a list of general rules for feeding the stressed or morbid calf:

1. If calves are going to the feedlot, a good quality long-grass hay or medium quality alfalfa hay should be

*Contribution from USDA, Agricultural Research Service, Bushland, TX 79012.

Table 1. Feed Dry Matter Intake of 200-kg Steer Calves After Arrival at the Feedlot

Item	Week After Arrival		
	1	2	3–4
Average intake, kg	2.0	4.0	6.0
Intake, % of body wt	1.0	2.0	3.0
Expected daily gain, kg/day*	−0.13	0.50	1.07
Required nutrient levels, %			
Crude protein	15.0	14.2	10.5
Calcium	0.30	0.35	0.45
Phosphorus	0.30	0.33	0.33

*Assumes NE_m of 1.7 Mcal/kg and NE_g of 0.95 Mcal/kg is ration.

provided *ad libitum* with a milled diet for at least three days after arrival and at all times in the hospital pens.

2. If calves are going to pasture, the calves should be fed a good quality grass hay along with 0.5 to 1.0 kg/day of a vitamin- and mineral-fortified, 40 per cent protein, pelleted supplement.

3. If calves are being adjusted to a high-concentrate diet, the milled portion of the receiving diet should contain the following concentrate levels: 100-kg calves: 70 per cent concentrate; 200-kg calves: 60 per cent concentrate; 300-kg yearlings: 50 per cent concentrate.

4. The complete diet (hay + milled portion) should contain 13 to 14 per cent protein, 1.0 to 1.4 per cent potassium, and adequate levels of calcium (about 0.45 per cent), phosphorus (about 0.4 per cent), and trace minerals.

5. High-moisture or fermented roughages should be restricted for 7 to 14 days.

6. Urea consumption should be restricted to less than 25 gm/head/day for 7 to 14 days.

7. Supplementation of B vitamins, especially niacin (250 ppm) and thiamine (1 gm/head/day), may be beneficial.

8. The feeding of 40 to 100 gm sodium bicarbonate/head/day may be beneficial.

SUPPORTIVE NUTRITION

Many stressed and morbid calves refuse to eat any diet offered to them. Under these circumstances, intensive intervention may be required to keep them alive. In the morbid calf, a reduction in body temperature may be adequate to start the animal eating. The use of some probiotics containing living *Lactobacillus acidophilus* cultures may also stimulate feed consumption in some animals. When other methods do not succeed, more strenuous measures, such as intraruminal or intraperitoneal (IP) infusion, may be warranted.

Research indicates that the stress of routinely infusing solutions intraruminally may be greater than the benefits received. When a calf refuses to eat and is in a depleted condition, however, the use of an intraruminal infusate may be warranted. Any infusate should supply supportive nutrition as well as assist in restarting rumen fermentation. Since the anorectic calf is in a severe energy deficiency, the energy source should be readily available to the animal. Glucose, sucrose (table sugar), and/or propylene glycol is a good energy source for intraruminal infusates. Because the level of infusate is normally limited to less than 0.5 kg/day, the risk of causing lactic acidosis is

remote even with highly degradable energy sources. Because the rumen pH of anorectic calves may exceed 7.5, the infusate should be slightly acidic (5.5 to 6.5) to help lower the rumen pH to a favorable level for the rumen microbes. The addition of acetic acid (vinegar) will lower the pH of the infusate as well as provide an additional energy source. The addition of small amounts of branched-chain volatile fatty acids (isobutyric and isovaleric) may aid in stimulating microbial growth. The infusate nitrogen source should contain a readily available nitrogen source such as casein or soybean meal. Urea and other non-protein nitrogen sources should not be used. The use of slowly degraded protein source (alfalfa dehy, blood meal, corn gluten meal), which will pass to the small intestine, may be of benefit, but its use is limited owing to its low solubility.

The use of B vitamins, trace minerals, and potassium in the infusate is recommended. Theoretically, the use of fresh rumen fluid from a donor animal should be beneficial to the anorectic calf. Practically, however, massive quantities are usually required to see any appreciable benefit. Rumen fluid, however, can be a partial source for the branched-chain volatile fatty acids, B vitamins, and trace minerals.

Some research has shown a stimulation in feed intake following IP infusion of 500 ml of hypertonic electrolyte and/or amino acid solutions. Owing to the risk of peritonitis, the use of IP infusions should be limited to only severe cases.

Supplemental Reading

Cole, N. A.: Nutrition-health interactions of newly arrived feeder cattle. Proceedings of Symposium on Management of Food Producing Animals. Purdue University. May, 1982.
Cole, N. A: A critical evaluation of preconditioning. Proceedings of North American Symposium on Bovine Respiratory Disease. Texas A&M University. September, 1983.
Cole, N. A., and Hutcheson, D. P.: Influence on beef steers of two sequential short periods of feed and water deprivation. J. Anim. Sci. *53*:907. 1981.
National Dairy Council: Nutritional demands imposed by stress. Dairy Council Digest *51*: No. 6, Nov.–Dec., 1980.

Growth Stimulants and Feed Additives for Beef Cattle

JACK G. RILEY, Ph.D.

Cattle producers have found it necessary to increase production and efficiency so that they can profit from their business. Improved rate of growth and reduced feed requirements have resulted in part, from the acceptance and use of commercially available growth-stimulating implants and feed additives.

The growth promotants approved for use in beef cattle are shown in Table 1. The ability of antibiotics and anabolic compounds to stimulate growth was first recognized in the late 1940s. In 1948, the synthetic estrogen diethylstilbestrol was reported to improve daily gain in heifers. A year later, the antibiotic chlortetracycline was found to increase growth in poultry. Commercial development of prospective products to improve growth continues, and second generation ingredients await approval. Even though the growth-promoting aspects of antibiotics

Table 1. *Growth Promotants Approved for Beef Cattle*

Feed Additives	Implants
Bacitracin	Compudose*
Bacitracin, zinc	Ralgro†
Chlortetracycline	STEER-oid‡
Erythromycin	HEIFER-oid‡
Lasalocid	Synovex-S§
Melengestrol acetate	Synovex-H§
Monensin	
Oxytetracycline	

*Compudose is a registered trademark product of Elanco Products Co., Indianapolis, IN.

†Ralgro is a registered trademark product of International Mineral and Chemical Corp. Terre Haute, IN.

‡STEER-oid and HEIFER-oid are registered trademark products of Anchor Laboratories, Inc., St. Joseph, MO.

§Synovex-S and -H are registered trademark products of Syntex Agribusiness Inc., Des Moines, IA.

and anabolic compounds are well documented, the apparent mode of action is not clearly understood.

GROWTH STIMULANTS: IMPLANTS

Implants are frequently referred to as anabolic agents. An anabolic compound is one that promotes constructive metabolism, i.e., one that increases protein (lean meat) deposition. Estrogens and androgens are two types of anabolic steroids that cause growth promotion. Estrogens are primarily produced by the female gonad and androgens by the male gonad.

There are currently six FDA-approved commercial implants available to cattle producers in the United States (see Table 1). Each of these products is recommended for subcutaneous implantation under the skin on top of the ear.

Ralgro is a nonhormonal anabolic agent, a resorcylic acid lactone otherwise known as zeranol, that directly stimulates the pituitary gland to produce greater amounts of natural growth hormone, somatotrophin. Prolactin and cortisol production is also stimulated, which gives the animal a sense of well-being. In association with a decrease in thyroxin production, the animal will be more tranquil.

Research has also indicated that anabolic agents lower blood urea nitrogen (BUN), which means that there is less nitrogen in the blood because it is being metabolized in the muscles. There is a decrease in insulin because of the release of glucose into the circulatory system by the liver. The blood glucose level is not affected, but there is an increase in the entrance and exit of glucose into the circulatory system, indicating that the muscles are utilizing the glucose more rapidly. Blood levels of naturally occurring hormones will vary from animal to animal. In spite of this, the increase of growth hormone has been very consistent in zeranol-implanted cattle.

Zeranol has been proven to be less toxic than aspirin when used in laboratory animals, and even when given to monkeys for ten years at 27,000 times the cattle dosage there has been no indication of toxicity or carcinogenicity. Dogs have been given 14,000 times the cattle dose for seven years with no problems observed.

Zeranol is approved as an implant for calves starting as early as birth but no later than 65 days prior to slaughter.

Duration of activity is probably 100 to 120 days, and additional benefits can be obtained from re-implanting at regular intervals of approximately 100 days. The approved dosage is 36 mg per animal (three pellets). Implants should not be used in bulls or heifers that are kept for breeding.

The recognition and development of naturally occurring steroids as growth promotants paralleled the development of the synthetic estrogen diethylstilbestrol (DES). The U. S. Food and Drug Administration (FDA) approved the original Synovex implant for steers in 1956. The first product contained 20 mg of estradiol and 1000 mg of progesterone. The implant site was in the head between the poll and left eye. Synovex was modified in 1956 to substitute estradiol benzoate for pure estradiol. An additional modification of the product resulted in the reduction of progesterone from 1000 to 200 mg per dose. The product was renamed Synovex-S Finishing Implants and is approved for use in steers weighing more than 400 pounds. Synovex-H implants are approved for use in heifers weighing more than 400 pounds and contains 20 mg of estradiol benzoate and 200 mg of testosterone propionate. There is *no withdrawal* period for Synovex-S or -H prior to slaughter. Each implant contains eight individual pellets per cartridge, and the recommended implant site is in the center third of the ear. The mode of action of Synovex implants is not fully understood. However, research suggests that a combination of estrogens, androgens, and progesterins has both direct and indirect effects on muscle synthesis, resulting in a greater accumulation of muscle protein.

Generic equivalents to Synovex-S and Synovex-H are implants with the trademark names of STEER-oid and HEIFER-oid. Composition of the implants and recommendations for most effective utilization are similar for all four products.

The final implant to be discussed is Compudose. The active ingredient in Compudose is estradiol-17B, a naturally occurring steroid hormone found in all mammalian species. However, the unique feature of the implant is its physical construction and attendant *uniform* release of drug. The implant consists of an inert, cylindrical core of silicone rubber surrounded by a thin layer of silicone rubber impregnated with 24 mg of estradiol-17B. This unusual design keeps the surface area of the implant constant, which, combined with the uniform chemical diffusion of estradiol out of the silicone rubber coating, results in a slow sustained release of growth stimulant over time. The 3/16-inch diameter and 1-inch length were chosen as the optimum dimensions and were designed to provide optimum daily release of hormone for a minimum of 200 days. In addition, the rubber construction prevents crushing of the implant during handling and administration. The original development of the implant included the requirement of a sufficient size to enable removal if regulations dictated. The FDA *does not* require removal, at least not at the present time. Compudose is only approved for use in steers. A special implanting tool is required, which holds a clip containing ten implants. Recommended implant location is under the skin in the middle third on the back of the ear. The implants are dusted with antibiotic after manufacturing to aid in preventing infection at the implant site. Compudose and Ralgro are the only implants currently approved for use in suckling steer calves.

Response to Implants

An excellent review article summarizing research on implants was prepared by Ward (1977). Calves that received implants during the nursing phase showed an average increase of 8.8 per cent in daily weight gain (range 4 to 14 per cent). The calves were implanted at various times from birth to 100 days of age with a positive response in each trial. Steers tended to have a greater response than heifers.

Cattle receiving implants during the growth phase from weaning until they were placed on a finishing ration exhibited an average response in daily weight gain of 15.1 per cent (range 8 to 28 per cent). Indications are that implantation during the initial growing phase did not decrease response to re-implantation during the following growing phase.

Implants have been most widely used during the finishing segment. Data from 10 experiment stations indicated an average response of 10.8 per cent (range 7 to 19 per cent) in daily weight gain. In addition to the growth response, the efficiency of feed utilization is improved by approximately 10 per cent.

Numerous research trials have been conducted with Compudose in suckling, growing, and finishing cattle. In a series of early trials, daily gains of suckling steers showed an 8.9 per cent response to Compudose, and weight gains of grazing steers were increased an average of 13.1 per cent in two trials conducted at Kansas State University. Results of early feedlot trials indicated gain to be improved by 13.2 per cent on 7.3 per cent less feed. No side effects or adverse influence on carcass quality was observed in any of the trials.

Additional Considerations

Cattle will continue to respond even when re-implanted as frequently as every 100–120 days; however, the magnitude of the response will probably diminish. One of the major theoretical advantages of the Compudose implant is the 200-day duration. The other four implants have an apparent active period of 100 days. Many segments of beef production, such as the 150-day grazing season or the 140-day feedlot period, exceed the optimum 100-day lifespan. Therefore, producers are encouraged to implant at 100-day intervals (200 days if Compudose is the product of choice). There also appears to be a carry-over effect from one segment of growth to the next if implanting is discontinued.

Implants are not approved for cattle intended to be used for breeding purposes. Heifers and bulls will respond to the implants, but potential side effects such as udder development and testicular degeneration should be sufficient to discourage the use of implants in replacement heifers or breeding bulls.

When used in conjunction with feed additives, implants have been observed to give a synergistic response. This added improvement in growth and efficiency is sufficient to recommend the routine implanting of cattle regardless of what oral additives are being fed.

Implant Usage

Survey results representing over 800 Kansas cow-calf producers indicated that 58 per cent were implanting calves at least once between birth and weaning. Approximately 43 per cent of those same producers were implanting more than once.

An extensive survey representing 60 per cent of the cattle being fed for slaughter in Kansas showed that implanting was done in 100 per cent of the feedlots with over 2000 head capacity, and 94.5 per cent of the smaller feedlots were implanting.

FEED ADDITIVES

A feed additive is defined as a drug or compound of a nonnutritive nature that will stimulate growth, improve feed utilization, or benefit the health of the animal. The mode of action by which additives improve animal performance is not a simple process. Of the theories proposed, those most frequently mentioned are the nutrient sparing effect, the metabolic effect, and the disease control effect.

The nutrient sparing mode of action can be explained by an additive that stimulates microorganisms to produce more favorable ratios for volatile fatty acids, and this is at least a partial explanation for the improved feed efficiency that results from feeding monensin sodium and lasalocid sodium. Microbial populations in the rumen could also influence (1) nutrient synthesis or degradation, (2) rate and extent of digestion, (3) rumen turnover, and (4) acid-base relationships.

The metabolic effect has been theorized to account for the bacteriostatic or bactericidal properties of antibiotics and certain other feed additives. The beneficial effects

Table 2. *Low-Level Feeding of Antibiotics to Beef Cattle**

	Growing-Wintering Cattle		Finishing Cattle		Finishing Cattle Fed Stilbestrol	
	Control	Antibiotic Supplemented†	Control	Antibiotic Supplemented†	Control	Antibiotic Supplemented†
Daily gain, kg	0.56	0.61	1.16	1.24	1.24	1.29
Feed per unit gain	12.70	12.02	9.85	9.37	9.33	8.94
Number animals	5352		2354		3007	
Av. initial wt, kg	228		310		330	
Av. number days on trial	112		117		124	
Per cent gain response	8.9		6.7		3.7	
Per cent feed conversion response	5.4		4.9		4.2	

*Adapted from the report by Bertrand, J. D.: West. Fla. Exp. Sta. Mimeo. Rep. pp. 68–73, 1968.
†Continuous low level (mostly 70 mg/head daily); the antibiotics involved were chlortetracycline, oxytetracycline, and bacitracin.

Table 3. *Monensin for Feedlot Cattle (19-Trial Summary)*

Monensin (gm/ton complete feed)	No. Pens	Feed Efficiency (lbs feed/lbs gain)*	Per Cent Improvement in Feed Efficiency	Average Daily Gain* (lbs)	Average Daily Feed* (lbs)
0	63	9.46	—	2.29	21.46
5	31	8.80	6.98	2.39	20.77
10	56	8.83	6.66	2.37	20.77
20	61	8.57	9.41	2.33	19.85
30	60	8.46	10.57	2.28	19.17

*Adjusted treatment means.

appear to be derived indirectly by influencing the metabolism of digestive tract microflora.

The disease control effect is largely suggestive, since in most cases the specific disease or disease incidence has not been well defined. Support of this theory is generated when healthy, disease-free animals fed in carefully cleaned and sterilized quarters do not respond to antibacterial additives.

Generally speaking, feed additives are included in rations at very low levels, such as 5 to 50 gm/ton of complete feed, when being used to promote growth, improve feed efficiency, or improve health status. Higher doses may be appropriate for therapeutic treatment of various diseases or metabolic disorders. Feed additives include a wide range of products, some of which are regulated by the FDA and others that are designated as "generally recognized as safe" (GRAS) compounds. The primary difference is that the FDA-regulated products were approved for use after extensive research investigation and make specific claims on their labels, including increased daily weight gain, improved efficiency, and liver abscess control. It is these compounds that are regulated by law and must be used appropriately. For that reason, the only additives summarized in this article are those that are FDA regulated.

Antibiotics for Beef Cattle

Antibiotics are the most widely used group of feed additives and by definition are compounds produced by one microorganism that inhibit the growth of another organism. Those that have been used extensively in cattle include chlortetracycline, oxytetracycline, bacitracin, tylosin, monensin, and lasalocid.

Burroughs summarized the results of 112 trials involving the feeding of low-level antibiotics (chlortetracycline and oxytetracycline) to feedlot cattle (1959). Growth rate was improved an average of 4 per cent and feeding efficiency an average of 3 per cent. Wallace adapted data by Bertrand, and his findings are shown in Table 2. In finishing studies involving 2,354 cattle, gains were improved by 6.7 per cent and feed efficiency by 4.7 per cent. Data derived from 5,352 growing-wintering cattle indicated gains were improved 8.9 per cent with a 5.4 per cent feed savings. These results suggest that growing-wintering cattle respond more to low-level continuous feeding of antibiotics than do finishing cattle.

Melengestrol Acetate (MGA)

Melengestrol acetate is a synthetic progestogen that has been shown to be effective in promoting growth, improving feed utilization, and suppressing estrus in heifers. It is approved for use only in heifers being fed for slaughter and is not effective in spayed heifers or steers. The approved daily dose range is 0.25 to 0.50 mg/head. The drug must be removed from the feed at least 48 hours prior to slaughter.

Results of 25 MGA feedlot trials by Upjohn and those supervised by University Experiment Stations showed that MGA improved weight gain by 11.2 per cent and feed efficiency by 7.6 per cent.

Monensin (Rumensin)

Monensin sodium was originally cleared as a coccidiosis drug for poultry but in 1975 was shown to be extremely effective in reducing the amount of feed required per unit of gain in growing-finishing cattle. Monensin alters rumen fermentation (VFA production), increasing the proportion of propionic acid produced while simultaneously decreasing acetic and butyric acid production, thereby making rumen fermentation and feed utilization more efficient. Additional factors, such as reduced methane production and slower rumen turnover, may be influencing the improved efficiency observed when monensin is fed. A 19-trial feedlot summary in 1976 found the optimum improvement in feed efficiency to be 10.6 per cent when cattle fed monensin-added feed (30 gm/ton) were compared with cattle not fed monensin. Each feedlot animal must receive not less than 50 nor more than 360 mg/head/day. The results of the 19-trial summary are shown in Table 3.

Clearance was granted in 1978 to feed monensin to cattle on pasture or range. The daily feed intake of cattle fed low-energy rations, including most pastures, is thought to be limited to bulk of the diet (i.e., the physical capacity of the animal). Monensin enables such cattle to obtain more energy from the daily consumption of feed. This increase in available energy enables the animal to gain weight at a faster rate. A 24-trial summary shown in Table 4 indicates that the feeding of 200 mg of monensin daily to supplemented cattle grazing pasture increased average daily weight gain from 1.23 to 1.43 lb. The 0.20-lb daily improvement represents a 16.3 per cent increase in rate of gain.

Lasalocid (Bovatec)

Lasalocid, the first ionophore, was first isolated and identified in 1951. By 1982, the total number of identified ionophores had expanded to 72. FDA cattle clearance for lasalocid was received in 1982, and the initial label ap-

Table 4. *Monensin for Pasture or Range Cattle (24-Trial Summary)*

Monensin (mg/hd/day)	Average Daily Gain*		Improvement	
	No. Pastures	Lbs	Lbs	Per Cent
0	41	1.23	—	—
200	41	1.43	+ 0.20	+ 16.3

*Adjusted treatment means.

Table 5. *Lasalocid for Feedlot Cattle (16-Trial Summary)*

Bovatec (gm/ton)	No. Pens	Average Daily Gain (lbs)	Per Cent Difference	Average Daily Feed Intake* (90% DM)	Per Cent Difference	Feed Conversion (feed/gain)	Per Cent Difference
0	52	2.67	—	22.27	—	8.62	—
10	22	2.69	+0.75	21.91	−1.62	0.23	−4.52
20	19	2.76	+3.37	21.77	−2.24	8.20	−4.87
30	40	2.81	+5.24	21.72	−2.47	7.92	−8.12

*Adjusted means.

proval was for growing-finishing beef cattle to improve rate of gain and feed efficiency.

A summary of 16 beef finishing trials (Table 5) indicated a 5.2 per cent increase in gain for cattle fed 30 gm lasalocid/ton as compared with the nonmedicated controls. Feed required per unit of gain was decreased by 8.1 per cent when lasalocid was fed at a rate of 30 gm/ton. Research continues to be conducted in anticipation of additional clearances and, in particular, approval for grazing beef cattle. There appear to be similarities in modes of action for the various ionophores, and comparative feeding trials will need to be conducted before preferential recommendations can be documented.

Requirements for Approval of Feed Additives

Products must meet the following requirements before they can be cleared by the FDA for use in cattle rations:

1. Research must establish that the additive will be safe to use.

2. No additive will be considered safe if it is found to induce cancer when ingested by man or animal.

3. No residue of additives in animal tissue will be allowed.

4. It must be proved effective for the requested use.

5. Levels of use, conditions of usage, and tolerances must be established.

6. Labels must give appropriate precautions and withdrawal statements.

7. A practical assay method must be available to monitor for residues.

Nonregulated Feed Additives

Producers of compounds such as buffers, enzymes, selected fermentation products, and certain B vitamins often make claims of improved cattle performance. However, since these compounds are not under the same FDA restrictions as those specified previously, there are only limited data to suggest that they will stimulate growth or improve feed efficiency. As more research data become available, one or more of the nonregulated products may be shown worthy of use.

Prospects for New Additives

The recent success of monensin, lasalocid, and Compudose has encouraged a renewed interest in research development of additional cattle feed additives and implants. Tremendous cost and time are required to get a new product approved through the regulatory structure. Presently, the most active areas of development appear to be involved with new antibiotics, bacterial fermentation products, rumen microorganisms, appetite stimulants, methane inhibitors, and hormone or hormonelike compounds.

Supplemental Reading

Bertrand, J. D.: Low-level use of antibiotics in beef cattle rations. West. Fla. Exp. Sta. Mimeo Rep. 68–73, 1968.

Brandt, W. E.: Bovatec for improved feed efficiency and increased rate of weight gain in beef cattle fed in confinement for slaughter. Proc. Bovatec Symposium, Scottsdale, AZ. 69–84. 1982.

Brown, R. G.: Safety of Ralgro. Terre Haute, IN, International Minerals and Chemical Corp, 1983.

Burroughs, W. C.: Five-year summary of more than 400 experimental comparisons of feed additives in beef cattle rations at college experiment stations. Am. Soc. Anim. Prod. Ext. Sect. Mgt., 1959.

Church, D. C.: Feed additives and growth stimulators. *In* Digestive Physiology and Nutrition of Ruminants, Vol. 3, Practical Nutrition. Corvallis, Oregon. O and B Books. 77, 1972.

Cravens, W. W., and Holck, G. I.: Economic benefits to the livestock producer and to the consumer from the use of feed additives. J. Anim. Sci. *31*:1102, 1970.

Raun, A. P.: Use of rumensin in feedlot cattle. 31st Kansas Formula Feed Conference, 1976.

Riley, J. G.: Rumensin in grazing programs. 33rd Kansas Formula Feed Conference, 1978.

Schilt, H.: Obtaining clearance for additive use. *In* Feed Additive Compendium. Minneapolis, The Miller Publishing Co., 1977.

Synovex Technical Manual. Des Moines, IA, Syntex Agribusiness Inc., 1983.

Thomas, O. O.: The relative value of growth promotives in beef cattle feeding. *In* Great Plains Beef Cattle Handbook. Cooperative Extension Service, USDA. 1603.1, 1978.

Wallace, H. D.: Biological responses to antibacterial feed additives in diets of meat producing animals. J. Anim. Sci. *31*:1118, 1970.

Ward, J. K.: Growth stimulants for beef cattle. Proceedings of the Range Beef Cow Symposium V. 69, 1977.

White, D. R.: Compudose Technical Manual. Indianapolis, IN, Elanco Products Co., 1982.

Developing Maximum Profit Feedlot Diets

DONALD R. GILL, Ph.D.

Formulation of finishing rations for beef cattle has developed into a complex science in which feed ingredients are combined considering all known variables to maximize feedlot profits. This means that balanced or even least cost balanced rations will not necessarily lead to profitable feeding programs. The degree to which this concept is understood is highly correlated with the success of any given feedlot operation.

Balancing a ration for maximum profit requires additional steps beyond those normally considered in "nutritional" balance. New formats are being developed to pinpoint nutritional requirements of feedlot cattle. These formats make it possible to balance rations for least cost production. These formats recognize the fact that requirements are based on at least three factors: (1) the sex and

Table 1. *Protein and Energy Requirements of Feedlot Cattle**

Daily Gain (lbs)	Body Weight = 400 lbs NE$_m$ 3.85 Mcal Steers NE$_g$†	Heifers NE$_g$	Crude Protein‡	Daily Gain (lbs)	Body Weight = 500 lbs NE$_m$ 4.55 Mcal Steers NE$_g$	Heifers NE$_g$	Crude Protein
1.0	1.25	1.39	1.00	1.0	1.48	1.64	1.10
1.2	1.52	1.69	1.07	1.2	1.80	2.00	1.18
1.4	1.79	2.01	1.14	1.4	2.12	2.38	1.25
1.6	2.07	2.34	1.22	1.6	2.45	2.77	1.33
1.8	2.35	2.68	1.30	1.8	2.78	3.17	1.41
2.0	2.64	3.03	1.37	2.0	3.12	3.58	1.48
2.2	2.94	3.39	1.45	2.2	3.47	4.01	1.56
2.4	3.24	3.76	1.52	2.4	3.83	4.44	1.64
2.6	3.54	4.14	1.60	2.6	4.19	4.89	1.71
2.8	3.86	4.53	1.68	2.8	4.56	5.35	1.79
3.0	4.17	4.93	1.75	3.0	4.93	5.82	1.86
3.2	4.49	5.34	1.83	3.2	5.31	6.31	1.94
3.4	4.82	5.76	1.90	3.4	5.70	6.81	2.02

Daily Gain (lbs)	Body Weight = 600 lbs NE$_m$ 5.21 Mcal Steers NE$_g$	Heifers NE$_g$	Crude Protein	Daily Gain (lbs)	Body Weight = 700 lbs NE$_m$ 5.85 Mcal Steers NE$_g$	Heifers NE$_g$	Crude Protein
1.0	1.70	1.88	1.21	1.0	1.91	2.11	1.31
1.2	2.06	2.30	1.29	1.2	2.31	2.58	1.39
1.4	2.43	2.73	1.36	1.4	2.73	3.06	1.46
1.6	2.81	3.17	1.44	1.6	3.15	3.56	1.54
1.8	3.19	3.63	1.51	1.8	3.58	4.08	1.62
2.0	3.58	4.11	1.59	2.0	4.02	4.61	1.69
2.2	3.98	4.59	1.67	2.2	4.47	5.16	1.77
2.4	4.39	5.09	1.74	2.4	4.93	5.72	1.84
2.6	4.80	5.61	1.82	2.6	5.39	6.30	1.92
2.8	5.22	6.14	1.89	2.8	5.87	6.89	2.00
3.0	5.65	6.68	1.97	3.0	6.35	7.50	2.07
3.2	6.09	7.23	2.05	3.2	6.84	8.12	2.15
3.4	6.54	7.80	2.12	3.4	7.24	8.76	2.22

Daily Gain (lbs)	Body Weight = 800 lbs NE$_m$ 6.47 Mcal Steers NE$_g$	Heifers NE$_g$	Crude Protein	Daily Gain (lbs)	Body Weight = 900 lbs NE$_m$ 7.06 Mcal Steers NE$_g$	Heifers NE$_g$	Crude Protein
1.0	2.11	2.33	1.41	1.0	2.30	2.55	1.51
1.2	2.56	2.85	1.49	1.2	2.79	3.11	1.58
1.4	3.01	3.39	1.56	1.4	3.29	3.70	1.66
1.6	3.48	3.94	1.64	1.6	3.80	4.30	1.73
1.8	3.96	4.51	1.71	1.8	4.33	4.92	1.81
2.0	4.45	5.09	1.79	2.0	4.86	5.57	1.89
2.2	4.94	5.70	1.87	2.2	5.40	6.23	1.96
2.4	5.45	6.32	1.94	2.4	5.95	6.90	2.04
2.6	5.96	6.96	2.02	2.6	6.51	7.60	2.11
2.8	6.48	7.61	2.09	2.8	7.08	8.32	2.19
3.0	7.02	8.29	2.17	3.0	7.67	9.05	2.27
3.2	7.56	8.98	2.25	3.2	8.26	9.81	2.34
3.4	8.11	9.68	2.32	3.4	8.86	10.58	2.42

Daily Gain (lbs)	Body Weight = 1000 lbs NE$_m$ 7.65 Mcal Steers NE$_g$	Heifers NE$_g$	Crude Protein	Daily Gain (lbs)	Body Weight = 1100 lbs NE$_m$ 8.21 Mcal Steers NE$_g$	Heifers NE$_g$	Crude Protein
1.0	2.49	2.76	1.60	1.0	2.68	—	1.69
1.2	3.02	3.37	1.67	1.2	3.25	—	1.76
1.4	3.56	4.00	1.75	1.4	3.83	—	1.84
1.6	4.12	4.66	1.83	1.6	4.42	—	1.92
1.8	4.68	5.33	1.90	1.8	5.03	—	1.99
2.0	5.26	6.02	1.98	2.0	5.65	—	2.07
2.2	5.84	6.74	2.05	2.2	6.28	—	2.14
2.4	6.44	7.47	2.13	2.4	6.92	—	2.22
2.6	7.05	8.23	2.21	2.6	7.57	—	2.30
2.8	7.67	9.00	2.28	2.8	8.23	—	2.37
3.0	8.30	9.80	2.36	3.0	8.91	—	2.45
3.2	8.94	10.61	2.43	3.2	9.60	—	2.52
3.4	9.59	11.45	2.51	3.4	10.30	—	2.60

*Daily requirements for maintenance.
†Meals per day.
‡Pounds per day.

Table 2. *Estimate of Optimum Mineral Levels for Cattle*

Percentage in 100% DM Ration		PPM in 100 Per Cent DM Ration	
Salt	0.2–0.3	Copper	10
Calcium	0.4–0.6	Iron	100
Phosphorus	0.3–0.45	Manganese	30
Magnesium	0.1	Zinc	60
Potassium	0.4–0.7	Cobalt	0.05–0.2
Sulfur	0.15	Iodine	0.2

Note: Vitamin A: 20,000 to 25,000 I.U./head/day.

size (weight) of the animal, (2) the level of production (daily gain), and (3) nutrient intake.

It is usually wasteful to feed more of any nutrient than is necessary for utilization of the most limiting nutrient in the diet. Because of the relationships among nutrients, it is no longer possible to state that the ideal ration will have a certain percentage of nutrients, since intakes differ. It instead appears more desirable to state the nutrient requirements in terms of daily requirements based on the sex, size (weight of the animal), and level of gain desired.

The nutrient requirements in terms of energy (Table 1), protein (see Table 1), and minerals and vitamins (Table 2) are presented. The reader will note that the protein and energy tables are based on the factors listed previously.

Why Change Ration Formulating Systems?

The reason for considering a change in formulating rations can best be demonstrated by two well-established feeding programs. The first is based on all-corn silage plus a minimum amount of protein supplement. The second is based on a 90 per cent concentrate ration. Numerous tests and claims have been made for the merits of both of these programs; however, an analysis of the projected gains and economics may be made using Drs. Lofgreen's and Garrett's net energy system for feedlot cattle.

Tables 3 and 4 show the two typical high silage and high grain programs, respectively, with fairly typical costs. Tables 5 and 6 show the projected gains based on energy alone for 800-lb. steers at various levels of feed intake.

Considerable experience has demonstrated the accuracy of these projections. Projected gains will be obtained only if all other nutrients (excluding energy) are adequate for level of gain indicated.

In the case of the high silage ration, an 800-lb steer must eat 22 lbs of dry matter to gain 2.55 lbs. Table 1 shows that for an 800-lb steer to gain 2.6 lbs, it would require 2.02 lbs of protein daily. Using these tables, it is possible to conclude that the high silage ration should contain 2.02/22 lbs of feed = 9.18 per cent protein to allow full utilization of the energy in the ration. In the

case of the high concentrate ration, the 800-lb steer would only need to eat 16 lbs to gain approximately 2.6 lbs. Again, the animal's daily protein requirements are the same at 2.02 lbs per day, but the ration should contain 2.02/16 lbs of feed, or 12.65 per cent protein.

Protein and energy make up the bulk of the cost of nutrients in cattle finishing rations, with energy being the most costly. In terms of total pounds, either of the two rations is needed to supply in excess of 10 lbs of usable energy components, about 2 lbs of crude protein, and less than 0.50 lb daily of all minerals and other nutrients to meet the nutrient requirements of 800-lb steers.

Thus, ration balancing systems designed for maximum profit must tie all other nutrients to energy, the largest component. Then, all other nutrients can be adjusted to make maximum utilization of energy. Developing a ration for finishing cattle, therefore, becomes primarily a function of energy and fixed cost economics.

Tables 5 and 6 provide an interesting comparison of all-corn silage and 90 per cent corn rations referred to previously. The gains possible on the high silage programs are lower than those possible on the high grain ration because the animals will only be able to eat between 18 and 26 lbs of dry matter per day. At 22 lbs intake (66.5 lbs as fed with 68 per cent moisture silage), gains of about 2.55 lbs should result in cattle of this weight. Feed cost per pound of gain should run about 43 cents using the prices shown in Table 3. Similar animals on the high grain ration (see Table 6) would probably eat about 20 lbs of dry matter (27 lbs as fed as in Table 4) and would gain about 3.54 lbs. Feed cost per pound of gain would run about 38 cents.

A feeder using the price relationships in Tables 3 and 4 and feed cost as the only consideration in ration formulation would use the 90 per cent concentrate program.

Energy Density

Some other factors should also be considered in ration formulation. Research indicates that cost of ownership of 800-lb cattle, including interest, labor, equipment, drugs, veterinary expenses, death losses, and taxes, is about 45 cents per head per day. If this 45 cents overhead cost per day is charged, the cost per pound of gain of the silage program then becomes 61 cents compared with 51 cents on the high grain program.

If rations are formulated to provide adequate protein, minerals, and vitamins to allow full utilization of the energy in the ration, then energy density in the ration becomes very important. Obviously, better gains cannot be obtained on the high corn silage ration illustrated in Tables 3 and 5 simply because the animals can seldom eat enough to reach their full gain potential. Most feeders think of energy density in terms of roughage:concentrate

Table 3. *High Silage Program*

	Ration DM (%)	As Fed Dry Matter (%)	Lbs to Make 100 lb DM	As Fed Composition (%)	Purchase Basis (% DM)	Cost ($)
Corn silage	94.90	32.00	296.56	98.13	32.00	1.50
44 per cent supl.	5.00	90.00	5.55	1.84	90.00	9.00
Additives	0.10	90.00	0.1111	0.04	90.00	16.00
TOTALS			302.21	100.00		

Notes: Calculated dry matter content of ration 33.09 per cent.
Cost per CWT of DM ration = $4.97
Cost per CWT of as fed ration = $1.64

Table 4. *High Grain Program*

	Ration Dry Matter (%)	As Fed Dry Matter (%)	Lb to Make 100 lb DM	As Fed Composition (%)	Purchase Basis (% DM)	Cost ($)
Corn	85.00	84.50	100.59	74.41	84.50	5.71
Soy meal	5.00	90.00	5.55	4.11	90.00	10.00
Additives	0.10	90.00	0.11	0.08	90.00	11.00
Corn silage	8.90	32.00	27.81	20.57	32.00	1.50
Mineral	1.00	90.00	1.11	0.82	90.00	4.00
TOTALS			135.17	100.00		

Notes: Calculated dry matter content of ration 73.97 per cent.
Cost per CWT of DM ration = $6.76
Cost per CWT of as fed ration = $5.00
Note that these rations are formulated on a dry matter basis to avoid confusion.

ratio. If nutritionally adequate rations were formulated at various energy levels ranging from very low (level of wheat straw) to very high (level of shelled corn), the relationship in Figure 1 would become apparent.

When energy density is very low, animals simply cannot eat enough feed to make gains; as energy density increases, gain increases. Maximum gain usually occurs on rations of about 50 to 70 per cent concentrate if the roughage portion of the ration is equivalent to good quality alfalfa hay. Higher or lower energy roughages will tend to move the relationship in the appropriate direction. A slight depression in gains is frequently observed on very high concentrate rations.

Figure 2 shows feed conversion (pounds of feed dry matter per pound of gain) superimposed on the diagram shown in Figure 1. Note that as energy density increases, the conversion ratio will similarly show an improvement in balanced rations.

Rate of gain and feed conversion ratio are very important factors in ration formulation because of their effect on cost of gain. However, neither maximum rate of gain nor the most efficient conversion ratio ensures economical gains. Feed prices are important in determining the cost of gain.

Figure 3 illustrates a hypothetical cost of gain curve superimposed on Figure 2.

Cost of Gain

The objective in the formulation of beef cattle finishing rations is to feed at the low point on the cost of gain curve. *It is probably true that more feeders experience high cost gains because they are far from optimum on the cost curve than because of a ration imbalance.*

The cost of gain curve is affected by the factors shown on both the rate and efficiency curves; however, feed price and overhead costs can move this curve to either the right or the left. If, for example, a feeder had good quality alfalfa at a price of $10 per ton delivered to the

cattle, then he might achieve maximum profit on a total ration made up of alfalfa providing he could achieve very low nonfeed fixed costs. Rate of gain and feed efficiency for cattle on this ration would most likely be less than maximum, yet this ration would produce maximum net profit. For most feeders, concentrates such as milo, corn, or barley may actually cost less per pound than any available roughage. For these feeders, a high concentrate ration will usually lead to lower cost gains.

All cattle feeders are affected by the relationships that affect the cost of gain curve. In areas where both corn and corn silage are available, the cost relationship of silage to grain frequently changes enough so that one year the high silage program may be better than the grain program and vice versa the next year. The steps necessary to approximate the low point on the cost gain curve (see Figure 3) are easy to follow and should be an essential part of balancing any feedlot ration.

Using the net energy values of common feeds (Table 7) and requirement tables (see Table 1), it is possible to project the cost of gain on any ration. By formulating and projecting higher or lower energy rations, the feeder can test to see if an improvement may be made in terms of cost of gain.

The examples shown in Table 8 are intended to illustrate extremes. The protein supplement is assumed to contain 0.60 Mcal NE_m and 0.40 Mcal NE_g per pound. Feeds are priced in the first ration and remain the same in all rations.

Following is the procedure for calculating projected gains and costs for a particular ration.
1. Calculate net energy for maintenance and net energy gain of the ration (use values of 0.54 Mcal NE_m/lb and 0.215 Mcal NE_g/lb for this example.
2. Estimate feed consumption (an 800-lb steer would probably eat about 24 lbs of DM).

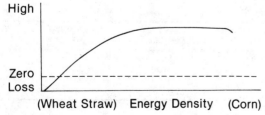

Figure 1. Effect of energy density on rate of gain.

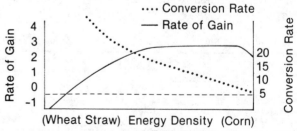

Figure 2. Effect of energy density on rate and efficiency of gain.

Table 5. *Estimated Daily Gain for Feed Containing 74 Mcal/CWT of Energy for Maintenance and 44 Mcal/CWT of Energy for Production with a Cost of $0.45/CWT*

Body Weight (lbs)	Daily Feed Intake (lbs)	Feed Required for Maintenance (lb)	Steers				Heifers					
			Daily Gain (lb)	Feed Conversion (lb)	Feed Cost/lb ($)	Total Cost/lb Gain ($)	Daily Gain (lb)	Feed Conversion (lb)	Feed Cost/lb ($)	Total Cost/lb Gain ($)	Feed Cost/Day ($)	Total Cost/Day ($)
800	17	8.74	1.66	10.22	0.51	0.78	1.47	11.56	0.57	0.88	0.84	1.29
800	18	8.74	1.85	9.74	0.48	0.73	1.63	11.07	0.55	0.83	0.89	1.34
800	19	8.74	2.03	9.37	0.47	0.69	1.78	10.68	0.53	0.78	0.94	1.39
800	20	8.74	2.20	9.07	0.45	0.66	1.93	10.38	0.52	0.75	0.99	1.44
800	21	8.74	2.38	8.83	0.44	0.63	2.07	10.13	0.50	0.72	1.04	1.49
800	22	8.74	2.55	8.63	0.43	0.61	2.21	9.93	0.49	0.70	1.09	1.54
800	23	8.74	2.72	8.46	0.42	0.59	2.35	9.77	0.49	0.68	1.14	1.59
800	24	8.74	2.89	8.32	0.41	0.57	2.49	9.63	0.48	0.66	1.19	1.64
800	25	8.74	3.05	8.20	0.41	0.56	2.63	9.52	0.47	0.64	1.24	1.69
800	26	8.74	3.21	8.10	0.40	0.54	2.76	9.43	0.47	0.63	1.29	1.74

Table 6. *Estimated Daily Gains for Feed Containing 98 Mcal/CWT of Energy for Maintenance and 63.5 Mcal/CWT for Gain with a Feed Cost of $6.76 per CWT (Nonfeed Fixed Cost $0.45)*

Body Weight (lbs)	Daily Feed Intake (lbs)	Feed Required for Maintenance (lb)	Steers				Heifers					
			Daily Gain (lb)	Feed Conversion (lb)	Feed Cost/lb ($)	Total Cost/lb Gain ($)	Daily Gain (lb)	Feed Conversion (lb)	Feed Cost/lb ($)	Total Cost/lb Gain ($)	Feed Cost/Day ($)	Total Cost/Day ($)
800	15	6.60	2.36	6.37	0.43	0.62	2.05	7.31	0.49	0.71	1.01	1.46
800	16	6.60	2.60	6.15	0.42	0.59	2.26	7.09	0.48	0.68	1.08	1.53
800	17	6.60	2.84	5.98	0.40	0.56	2.46	6.92	0.47	0.65	1.15	1.60
800	18	6.60	3.08	5.84	0.39	0.54	2.65	6.79	0.46	0.63	1.22	1.67
800	19	6.60	3.31	5.74	0.39	0.52	2.84	6.69	0.45	0.61	1.28	1.73
800	20	6.60	3.54	5.65	0.38	0.51	3.03	6.61	0.45	0.60	1.35	1.80
800	21	6.60	3.76	5.58	0.38	0.50	3.21	6.55	0.44	0.58	1.42	1.87
800	22	6.60	3.98	5.52	0.37	0.49	3.38	6.50	0.44	0.57	1.49	1.94
800	23	6.60	4.20	5.48	0.37	0.48	3.56	6.47	0.44	0.56	1.55	2.00
800	24	6.60	4.41	5.44	0.37	0.47	3.72	6.44	0.44	0.56	1.62	2.07

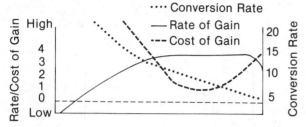

Figure 3. Effect of energy density of rate, efficiency, and cost of gain.

3. Calculate gain from net energy requirement tables and Step 1.
   a. NE required for maintenance = 6.47 (see Table 1).
   b. Feed required for maintenance = 6.47/0.54 = 11.98 lbs.
   c. Feed available for gain = 24 − 11.98 lbs = 12 lbs.
   d. NE_g available for gain = 12 × 0.215 = 2.58.
   e. Expected gain (See Table 1) = 1.20 lbs.
4. Cost projection.
   a. Ration cost per CWT = $4.32.
   b. Daily feed cost = 0.0432 × 24 = $1.04.
   c. Feed only cost per pound of gain = $1.04/1.2 lb/day = $0.8667 per pound.
   d. Total cost of gain = ($1.04 feed cost + $0.45 overhead)/lb gain = $1.24/lb of gain.

It is apparent that this ration will not give economical gains because of its low energy density. The formulator should follow the steps to project the performance of Ration 2 (see Table 8). In this case, a feed intake of about 22 lbs appears reasonable.

The calculated NE_m of the ration is 0.744 Mcal/lb, and the NE_g is 0.41 Mcal/lb. With an 800-lb steer consuming 22 lbs/day, 8.7 lbs will be used for maintenance, leaving 15.3 lbs for gain. 15.3 lbs × 0.41 Mcal/lb NE_g = Mcal NE_g daily for gain. Using Table 1, this level of energy would allow gains of about 2.7 lbs/day. Feed cost would run $1.26/2.7, or 46.6 cents/lb. However, total cost would run approximately 63.33 cents/lb.

Ration 3 (see Table 8) is a high nutrient density ration. Expected feed intake on 800-lb steers would be about 20 lbs/day. Using the procedure, 20 lbs of this ration would give gains at between 3.3 and 3.4 lbs/day. Feed only cost of gain is 36.78 cents. When 45 cents/day overhead is added, total gain costs would be 50.20 cents/lb of gain.

Nutritionists should test rations with different energy densities around the 90 per cent concentrate level to see if even more reduction in feed cost might be afforded. After selecting a ration, a comparison should be made of estimated and actual feed consumption. It may be necessary to make additional adjustments because of errors made in estimating feed intake or the abilities of the cattle.

Optimum Rations

It should be apparent from the three examples in Table 8 that recommendations cannot be made in terms of optimum energy levels that a cattle feeder should feed. Price relationships differ greatly among individual cattle feeding operations and within areas of the United States, so that an optimum ration for one feeder is frequently impractical for another. One fact is readily appear-

Table 7. *Net Energy and Protein Content of Common Feeds**

	NE_m (Mcal/lb)	NE_g (Mcal/lb)	Crude Protein (%)
Roughages			
Alfalfa hay, excellent	0.71	0.40	22.0
Alfalfa hay, good	0.57	0.27	20.6
Alfalfa hay, fair	0.51	0.18	17.1
Alfalfa hay, poor	0.47	0.09	13.7
Barley straw	0.46	0.07	4.1
Bermuda hay	0.48	0.13	7.9
Bermuda hay, good	0.54	0.24	10.2
Corn stover	0.56	0.26	6.5
Cottonseed hulls	0.47	0.10	4.3
Milo stover	0.41	0.13	3.6
Oat hay	0.52	0.18	9.9
Prairie hay, early cut	0.52	0.18	8.6
Prairie hay, average	0.49	0.13	8.1
Prairie hay, mature	0.49	0.11	5.5
Wheat straw	0.16	0.07	4.3
Silages			
Alfalfa silage, good	0.60	0.30	17.5
Alfalfa silage, average	0.54	0.24	17.7
Corn silage, excellent	0.73	0.46	8.4
Corn silage, average	0.73	0.43	8.0
Corn silage, fair	0.66	0.40	7.2
Sorghum silage	0.67	0.30	7.9
By-Product Feeds			
Alfalfa De Hy 15%	0.59	0.27	16.4
Alfalfa De Hy 17%	0.60	0.31	19.2
Beet pulp	0.73	0.47	9.6
Beet pulp MD	0.92	0.61	9.9
Beet molasses	0.92	0.62	8.5
Cane molasses	1.03	0.67	3.8
Cottonseed meal OP	0.82	0.54	44.7
Cottonseed meal sol.	0.77	0.50	45.6
Cottonseed, whole	0.91	0.54	25.6
Fat, animal	2.08	1.27	—
Guar meal	0.83	0.56	41.1
Hominy feed	1.04	0.68	11.8
Meat meal	0.71	0.48	55.2
Rice bran	0.75	0.50	14.2
Rice mill feed	0.38	0.20	6.4
Soybean meal, solvent	0.87	0.59	48.9
Soybeans, whole	1.08	0.70	42.1
Wheat middlings	0.87	0.49	17.2
Barley 48–50#	0.97	0.64	13.0
Barley 44–46#	0.80	0.53	13.3
Barley 38–42#	0.73	0.46	11.7
Corn, Dent No. 2	1.02	0.67	10.0
Milo, minimum process†	0.80	0.53	10.0
Milo, semi process‡	0.90	0.60	10.0
Milo, extreme process§	0.97	0.64	10.0
Oats 38# BU test	0.83	0.57	12.2
Oats 36# BU test	0.79	0.52	13.5
Oats 32# BU test	0.74	0.47	13.8
Oats 28# BU test	0.66	0.44	13.8
Wheat	1.00	0.65	14.3
Minerals			
Ammonium chloride	—	—	163
Bone meal	—	—	5.5
Dicalcium phosphate	—	—	—
Ground limestone	—	—	—
Monosodium phosphate	—	—	—
Oyster shell flour	—	—	—
Potassium chloride	—	—	—
Rock phosphate	—	—	—
Sodium tripoly phosphate	—	—	—
Urea	—	—	281

*All feeds expressed on a dry matter basis.

†Coarse, ground, or rolled.

‡Very fine grind, excellent dry roll, high-volume steam flaker, less than optimum high-moisture harvest, or reconstitution.

§Excellent quality milo with good job of steam flaking (24–26# BU test weight), optimum high-moisture harvest.

Table 8. Sample Rations

Commodity	Per Cent	Cost/CWT. ($)
Ration 1		
Alfalfa hay, fair	90	4.00
Corn Dent. No. 2	5	6.30
Supplement	5	8.00
		Cost 4.32
Ration 2		
Alfalfa hay, fair	50	4.00
Corn Dent. No. 2	45	6.30
Supplement	5	8.00
		Cost 5.24
Ration 3		
Alfalfa hay, 28% fiber	10	4.00
Corn Dent. No. 2	85	6.30
Supplement	5	8.00
		Cost 6.16

ent—regardless of area and feed prices, gains of very low orders are impractical because of the high fixed overhead costs in cattle feeding.

High interest rates, high labor costs, and increased cost of death loss resulting from high-priced feeders have, in many cases, doubled the fixed nonfeed costs associated with cattle ownership. These costs will add 40 to 50 cents/lb to the cost of low order gains, i.e., 0.75 to 1.25 lbs/day. Even with gains at 3 lbs/head/day, few of the most efficient cattle feeders have overhead costs per pound of gain of less than 15 or 16 cents.

Corn silage has in the past consistently proven to be the best roughage available for finishing cattle. Feeders who do not have good corn silage should be cautious not to conclude that the high roughage levels shown in Tables 3 and 5 are always desirable. For example, alfalfa hay (fair) has 39 per cent of the gain potential per pound of dry matter after maintenance as good corn silage. Substitution of fair alfalfa hay for corn silage in the ration shown in Table 3 would result in gains of less than $1.00/lb/day, and if the hay cost $60/ton, feed cost alone would run 72 cents per pound of gain, making the total cost approximately $1.17/lb.

The net energy system developed by Drs. Lofgreen and Garrett was a major breakthrough in beef cattle nutrition. By using this system, progressive cattle feeders can calculate rations that can be formulated to give the least cost gains. Computer programs are already developed* that can formulate any number of least cost rations, project these rations in terms of performance and cost, and then allow the feeder or nutritionist to select the ration most likely to produce least cost gains. Tables 3 through 6 are examples of these outputs.

As illustrated by the rations in Tables 3 and 4, feedlot cattle are capable of handling extremely wide ranges of energy levels. It is up to those men responsible for cattle feeding to select the optimum program for their situations.

NUTRITIONAL RECOMMENDATIONS

Energy Levels

Optimum energy levels vary with feed costs, cattle cost, overhead costs, and cattle type.

*Oklahoma State University "Feedmix."

Protein Levels

Beef cattle nutritionists now recognize the relationship between protein and energy. It is suggested that the tentative protein allowance tables (see Table 2) be used.

Feeding excessive levels of protein is usually costly. Protein requirements are much higher for young cattle and animals whose growth consists mostly of muscle tissue than for older cattle. A general review of recent research on protein requirements indicates a trend toward recommending higher protein levels than were believed necessary in recent years, especially on high concentrate rations.

Urea

The use of urea in finishing rations for feedlot cattle is well accepted. Excessive levels usually reduce rate and efficiency of gains. Including urea in rations at a rate of 0 to 0.45 per cent of the ration has given excellent results with most but not all types of rations. If natural proteins are expensive, sometimes it may be more economical to go to levels of up to 0.80 per cent of the ration as urea. In most cases gains and efficiency will be reduced somewhat from the more conservative levels. In formulating rations, feeders should note that some natural protein supplements are much lower than others in energy. Substitution of urea plus grain for cottonseed meal may be much more desirable than the same substitution for soybean oil, because soybean oil meal is much higher in energy for gain than cottonseed meal.

Phosphorus

Levels of phosphorus in the ration dry matter of between 0.30 and 0.50 per cent (higher level with very light cattle) seem to be accepted.

Calcium

Levels of 0.40 to 0.60 per cent in the ration dry matter are apparently adequate. Calcium to phosphorus ratios of 1:1 to 2:1 seem to be indicated; little problem is encountered, however, if higher amounts of calcium are in the ration as a result of feeding high calcium roughages such as alfalfa hay. The addition of calcium sources such as calcium carbonate at levels in excess of 1 per cent of the ration dry matter does not seem to be beneficial and frequently depresses performance.

Potassium

Potassium level is of little concern in high to moderate roughage rations. In high concentrate rations potassium levels probably should be brought up to at least 0.4 per cent, but little evidence supports going higher than 0.7 per cent of the ration dry matter. When feed intakes are very low, higher levels may improve performance.

Salt

If cattle feeders wish to sell or use feedlot manure as fertilizer they should give serious consideration to reducing salt levels of finishing rations to 0.2 to 0.3 per cent of the ration. These levels are adequate and do not contribute to the salt pollution problem to the extent that the generally accepted, but excessive, levels do.

Trace Minerals

It has been very difficult to demonstrate trace mineral deficiencies in feedlot rations. Optimum levels of the minor elements are suggested in Table 3. In most rations these are met with no additional elements. When careful chemical analysis does indicate a shortage of a trace element, care should be taken to add the element in an available form. Many trace minerals today are added to rations in poorly available forms, generally oxides, which tend to support university research showing that these elements are usually unnecessary. Many dollars are wasted nationally each year on unnecessary trace minerals, and a number of deficiencies are produced by the unskilled addition of trace elements that actually interfere with the availability of other elements.

Roughage Factor

It appears that the ruminant animal requires a minimum amount of roughage factor for normal rumen function. All concentrate rations show a response to small amounts of roughage factor. As little as 1 lb/day of some low-quality roughage such as alfalfa stems, rice hulls, or sorghum straw has improved efficiency ranging up to 15 per cent on all concentrate rations based on well-processed grains. Five pounds of "as fed" corn silage daily is an excellent roughage. In recent years there has been a trend toward greatly reduced roughage levels in feedlot diets. This has been brought about by the high handling and processing costs of bulky feeds. Even more important has been the near universal inclusion of an ionophore into the diet. Monensin or lasalocid appears to reduce the need for roughage, as these compounds help by reducing acidosis, founder, bloat, and feedlot sudden death associated with high grain diets.

Many cattle are finished on diets of whole corn and no roughage after they are worked up on feed. If there is a roughage requirement for feedlot cattle, whole corn seems to fill the need. Rumen walls and livers of cattle fed whole corn diets are shown to be much less damaged (rumenitis or liver abscess) than those of cattle fed processed grains with moderate amounts of conventional roughage.

General recommendations would state that finishing rations for cattle should contain at least 7 per cent "high roughage factor" roughages for optimum results or up to 95 per cent whole corn.

Vitamins

Only the addition of vitamin A at a rate of 20,000 to 30,000 IU per head per day is universally accepted for cattle finished in open lots. There is little evidence to support the need for other vitamin fortification of rations.

Feed Intake

The greatest practical problem in preventing nutritional deficiencies or waste of expensive nutrients is the ability to predict feed intake of feedlot cattle. All nutritional requirements are based on two primary factors: the maintenance of the metabolic mass, and an additional amount for production (including weight gain, work, growth of hair, and so on). The maintenance requirement as stated in the NRC tables is increased any time the animal is not in its thermal neutral environment. Cattle recently shipped to a new location often have two factors working against them. Recently received cattle often are not adapted to the environment and are often in poor flesh, which may also increase their maintenance requirements. Stressed animals frequently do not consume normal amounts of feed.

The percentage ration concept often causes problems for both cattle and nutritionists when animals eat abnormal amounts of feed. A stressed calf requiring 0.7 lb of protein a day for maintenance does not help itself much if it only eats 5 lbs of a 10 per cent protein feed. Thus, receiving diets should be designed based on expected feed intake. If intake is going to change greatly over a few days, a feeding system providing a fixed amount of protein-mineral-vitamin supplement per head per day may be helpful; as the animals increase their feed intake they can eat more of the grain-roughage portion of the diet.

The following equation is offered as an aid in predicting feed intake (dry matter) of feedlot cattle on moderate to high concentrate diets.

$$K = 0.21 + \frac{\text{In Weight} - 300}{10,000} + \frac{FG}{100}$$

$$\text{Consumption} = K \times \frac{\text{Current Weight}^{0.75}}{2.2}$$

$$- \frac{\text{Weight} - 500^2}{200} \times 0.90$$

When designing these equations we tried to tie how much feed an animal would consume to its frame score (i.e., 1 for the smallest frame type cattle and 5 for large frame cattle). On this scale, 2.5 is supposed to be average. This concept works well with calves, except that the average body type found in feedlot cattle is about 3.5 today (with very young cattle). Yearling cattle eat more feed, and feeder grades (FG) of 4.5 to 7.5 should be used with them. For healthy yearlings the following are suggested starting points: 600, 4.2; 650, 4.8; 700, 5.5; and 700, 6.0. When using this equation be sure and enter "In Weight" as the weight of the animal when it entered the feedlot (in the case of cattle transferred from a growing program, the weight that they were when they were started on the growing ration). Current weight is the weight today (the two are only the same on the first day on feed). If you feel the cattle should eat more feed, increase FG; each numerical unit will increase peak feed intake by about 1 lb.

Note the importance of the initial weight of the animal in the feedlot (In Weight) on the feed intake predicted. Feedlot in weight is a significant factor determining how much feed cattle consume. For example, if one steer entered the feedlot at 350 lbs and another at 700 lbs, when both cattle weigh 800 lbs you could expect the first steer to eat much less at the same weight. An example of the effect of in weight is shown with the same feeder grade of 4.

In Weight	500	Current Wt	500	600	700	800	900	1000
		Feed DM	14.22	16.08	17.40	18.20	18.50	18.29
In Weight	700	Current Wt			700	800	900	1000
		Feed DM			18.76	19.70	20.14	20.06

Skillful management of feedlot cattle to obtain maximum sustainable feed intake is the goal of every successful cattle feeder. The feed additives such as monensin or lasalocid have helped reduce problems associated with high intakes of high grain rations.

All cattle feeders should periodically review their rations and calculate how much they are spending on unnecessary feed nutrients and additives; energy cost will be the major cost in feeding cattle. The other nutrients and proven feed additives should be adjusted to levels to allow maximum use of the energy in the ration. Once this is accomplished, little more may be gained.

Field Calculations for Ration Formulation in Food Animals

JOHN C. SIMONS, D.V.M.
and MICHAEL S. HAND, D.V.M., Ph.D.

Any practical approach to food animal nutrition involves mathematical computation. Recently, methods and instruments have evolved that enable us to calculate these nutrition formulae rapidly. In many cases, equations and tables have been derived and formulated that enable one to compute with significant accuracy the nutrient requirements for maintenance, weight gain, and lactation. Educated guesses based on empirical data are still used to calculate requirements for gestation and work.

A balanced ration has acceptable palatability and contains, within the limits of daily consumption, all of the nutrients necessary for daily maintenance and production. The entities commonly measured include various categories of energy, protein, minerals, and vitamins. Water needs are generally expected to be met by offering potable water in unlimited quantities.

To balance rations we need to know (1) the daily nutrient requirements according to species, body weight, and physiologic state and (2) the nutrient concentrations in specific feeds. The primary sources of information about requirements and nutrient concentrations are the publications of the National Research Council.* Current NRC-NAS publications concerning food animals include the following:

Nutrient Requirements of Swine, 1979,
0–309–02870–1
Nutrient Requirements of Sheep, 1975,
0–309–02212–6
Nutrient Requirements of Beef Cattle, 1984,
0–309–03447–7
Nutrient Requirements of Dairy Cattle, 1978,
0–309–02749–7
Nutrient Requirements of Poultry, 1977,
0–309–02725–X
Nutrient Requirements of Rabbits, 1977,
0–309–026707–5
Nutrient Requirements of Cold Water Fishes, 1981,
0–309–03187–7
Nutrient Requirements of Warm Water Fishes and
Shell Fishes, 1983, 0–309–03428–0

*These publications are available from Printing and Publishing Office, National Academy of Sciences, 2101 Constitution Ave., N. W., Washington, D. C. 20418.

Nutrient requirements are expressed in heat units, weight units, or international units per animal per day. Nutrient concentrations are expressed as heat units, weight units, or international units per weight unit of feed. Table 1 demonstrates the mode of expression in the metric system.

The nutrient requirements for a given species are not strictly linear according to body weight for all physiologic states. Energy and protein requirements for maintaining and energy requirements for gain vary logarithmically according to body weight to about the 0.7 power (as weight doubles the requirement increases about 70 per cent). Energy needs are calculated according to $(BW)^{0.75}$ (in kg). (Metabolizable protein is often calculated according to $[BW]^{0.734}$ [in kg] from an equation derived by Smuts.)

The formulation of balanced rations requires considerable mathematical computation involving arithmetic and algebraic functions. Practical application requires electronic calculation. Calculators having exponential, logarithmic, and storage capability modes in addition to ordinary arithmetic functions are essential. The process is expedited significantly by the use of programmable calculators and computers. Within the last five years computer hardware has become both economically feasible and convenient. Usable programs have been produced by universities, commercial agricultural enterprises, computer manufacturers, and private enterprises interested in selling information. Access to microcomputers and to networks using centrally located mini and main frame computers is available to all.

This article is not concerned with computer literacy or programming, but the material presented is essential to such programming, and the understanding of this material should be valuable in evaluating computer hardware and programs.

ENERGY REQUIREMENTS (GENERAL)

Energy is the most important, the most critical, and the most expensive item to be considered in animal nutrition. It has no measurable dimensions or mass and is measured as heat in kilocalories (kcal) or megacalories (Mcal).

Energy is defined as the capacity to do work, and work is accomplished by matter in motion. When matter is organized, it contains potential energy. When organized matter becomes disorganized, it releases kinetic energy and work may be accomplished. The energy involved in nutrition is chemical energy, which is stored or released

Table 1. Metric Expressions of Nutrient Requirements of Animals and Nutrient Concentrations in DM Feeds

Nutrient	Daily Requirement Expressed as	Nutrient Concentration Expressed as
Energy	kcal or Mcal/animal/day	kcal or Mcal/kg of feed
Protein	g or kg/animal/day or % DM	g/kg of feed or % DM
Urea potential	Not applicable	g urea equivalent/kg DM (+ or −)
Macrominerals	g/animal/day or % ration	g/kg of feed
Microminerals	mg/animal/day	mg/kg of feed or ppm
Vitamin A	I.U./animal/day	mg B carotene/kg of feed
Vitamins (general)	I.U./animal/day	I.U./kg of feed

by chemical reactions. Endergonic reactions absorb and store energy. Examples include photosynthesis, growth, fat deposition, gestation, and lactation. Exergonic reactions release kinetic energy. Examples include glycolysis, the Krebs cycle, and electron transport. Kinetic energy released by exergonic reactions may be used to make muscles contract or glands secrete or to supply energy to be stored by endergonic reactions.

The kinetic energy released by exergonic reactions of energy nutrient metabolism contains free energy available for work and energy dissipated as heat. Some of the potential energy contained in feeds is lost in feces, combustible gases, and urine. Thus it is necessary to define a number of energy categories and understand their interrelationships.

1. Gross energy (GE), or heat of combustion, is the quantity of heat resulting from complete oxidation of a unit of feed.
2. Fecal energy (FE) is the quantity of heat resulting from complete oxidation of the fecal matter resulting from the digestion of a unit of feed. It includes energy contained in:
   a. undigested feed,
   b. enteric microbes and their products,
   c. excretions from the gastrointestinal tract, and
   d. cellular debris from the gastrointestinal tract.
3. Energy from combustible gases (CGE) is the quantity of heat resulting from the complete oxidation of nonabsorbable gases, which results from digestion of a unit of feed (primarily methane).
4. Digestible energy (DE) is GE minus FE.
5. Urinary energy (UE) is the heat resulting from the complete oxidation of the urine produced by the metabolism of a unit of feed.
6. Metabolizable energy (ME) is DE minus UE plus CGE.
7. Net energy is ME minus the heat increment (H_i) that results from the utilization of a unit of feed: $NE = ME - H_i$. Net energy is divided into two categories:
   a. net energy for maintenance (NE_m), which includes the heat produced by basal metabolism (H_b) plus the heat produced by basal activity (H_a), and
   b. net energy for production (NE_p), which includes energy deposited in growth and storage (NE_g), energy deposited in the products of gestation (NE_r), energy deposited in milk (NE_{lact}), and energy used to perform work (NE_w).

The interrelationships among the energy categories can be demonstrated schematically (Fig. 1).

One of the implications of the second law of thermo-

dynamics is that the total energy in any system is divided into two portions: (1) "bound energy" unavailable for work, called entropy, and (2) "free energy" available for work.

$$\Delta H = \Delta F + \Delta S$$

where ΔH is total energy in the system, ΔF is free energy, and ΔS is bound energy or entropy. In nutrition, ME corresponds to total energy change in a system, H_i corresponds to the bound energy, or entropy, and NE corresponds to free energy available for work. Thus,

$$\Delta H = \Delta F + \Delta S \text{ (thermodynamics)}$$

and

$$ME = NE + H_i \text{ (nutrition).}$$

For most species, the energy requirements and concentrations in feeds are measured as digestible energy (DE) or metabolizable energy (ME). It is generally accepted that each gram of total digestible nutrients (TDN) contains 4.409 kcal of DE. The mathematical relationships between DE and ME vary according to species and type of diet as follows.

For swine $ME = DE \times 0.96$
For sheep $ME = DE \times 0.82$
For beef cattle $ME = DE \times 0.82$
For dairy cattle $ME \text{ (Mcal/kg DM)} = -0.45 + 1.01$
                         $DE \text{ (Mcal/kg DM)}$

For swine, sheep, and beef cattle ME is computed as a direct linear function of DE and TDN. In these cases, any of these categories may be used without loss of accuracy. In the dairy cattle equation, ME as a percentage of DE varies linearly from 80 per cent at 50 per cent digestibility to 88 per cent at 80 per cent digestibility. In this case, the use of ME as a standard should give a more accurate prediction than will DE or TDN.

For ruminant animals, metabolizable energy is still not a satisfactory measurement. The heat increment (H_i) that results from the metabolism of roughages is significantly greater than that for concentrates, and the ME system tends to overrate roughages as an energy source, especially in the production area. For this reason, Lofgreen and Garrett in the late 1960's developed what is now known as the "California Net Energy System." This work was published in 1968 and has since been accepted by the feeding industry. The NRC publications for beef cattle have utilized the system in their requirement and concentration tables since 1972. The development of the system is of more than passing interest.

To tabulate energy requirements, there must be a way

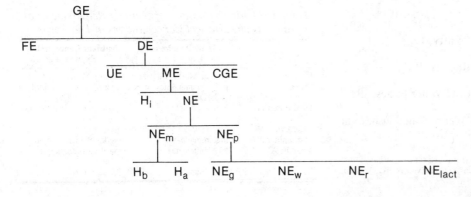

Figure 1. Schematic representation of the interrelationships among the energy categories (see text).

to measure heat production. The pioneers in the field used respiration calorimeters, but only three of these were ever built. It is obvious, then, why there was so little information about net energy. Lofgreen and Garrett used a different system based on the use of simple algebra. It has been stated that in nutrition

$$ME = NE + H_i.$$

If $ME = NE + H_i$, then

$$NE = ME - H_i$$

and

$$NE = NE_m + NE_p.$$

Therefore

$$NE_m + NE_p = ME - H_i$$

and

$$NE_m + H_i = ME - NE_p.$$

Since NE_m = heat of basal metabolism (H_b) plus heat of necessary activity (H_a), then

$$H_b + H_a + H_i = ME - NE_p$$

or

$$\text{Total heat } (H_b + H_a + H_i) = ME - NE_p.$$

Therefore, if we can measure ME and the energy deposited in a product, we can measure total heat production resulting from the use of a unit of feed without a respiration calorimeter. ME is obtained by subtracting FE, CGE, and UE from GE. Lofgreen and Garrett measured NE_p by the "Comparative Slaughter Technique" as follows:

1. A large number of animals are selected for uniformity.
2. A portion of these animals are weighed, slaughtered, and measured for carcass specific gravity (CSG).
   a. The dead carcass is weighed in air.
   b. The dead carcass is reweighed in water.
   c. The CSG is measured mathematically and used to calculate body composition.
3. The remaining animals are fed for a prescribed period.
   a. A valid sample of animals is chosen, and the animals are slaughtered.
   b. CSG for these animals is measured.
   c. Carcass composition is calculated from CSG.
   d. Energy in the final sampling minus energy in the initial sampling equals NE_p (in this case NE_g).

Validity of the specific gravity technique has been established by comparative quantitative and qualitative chemical analyses.

Modern nutritionists have access to combustion (bomb) calorimeters. These are standardized by the use of specifically purified benzoic acid. The caloric value of the benzoic acid has been determined by electrical units and computed in terms of joules/gram mole. The calorie has been standardized to equal 4.184 joules (Moore, 1977).

Net Energy for Maintenance and Gain in Cattle

The big problem in predicting gain from ME is the discrepancy in heat production between roughage and concentrate feed components. An experiment performed in California illustrates the point (Table 2). The results demonstrate that metabolizable energy is not a good way to predict what the production will be from a unit of feed. This is particularly true in ruminant rations where mix-

Table 2. *Relative Heat Production*

Ration 1: Free-Choice Alfalfa 19.45 lbs		Ration 2: 98 Per Cent Concentrate to Yield Gain Equal to Ration 1
20.714 Mcal	ME intake	13.919 Mcal
2.810 Mcal	NE_g	2.827 Mcal
17.904 Mcal	Heat produced	11.092 Mcal
(86% of intake)	% intake as heat	(80% of intake)

tures of roughages and concentrates are used to provide the energy requirement. The same is true of TDN or DE. If a valid prediction is to be made, net energy must be the unit of measurement. This principle is of less importance for monogastric animals, whose production rations are largely composed of concentrates.

The California Net Energy System provides a method of determining heat production in a large number of animals. It is now possible to measure heat production at different levels of intake and, by extrapolation, the net energy required for maintenance. Such measurements tell us that at moderate temperatures, the NE_m requirement for cattle in feedlot conditions is 77 kcal/kg $\times$ $(BW)^{0.75}$ (in kg):

$$NE_m \text{ (in Mcal)} = 0.077 \times (BW)^{0.75}.$$

The NE_m requirement is modified by weather. The NAS-NRC Manual for Beef Cattle, 1984, defines a thermoneutral zone of between 15 and 25°C. High temperatures and humidity may depress intake up to 30 per cent. Low humidity and comfortable nighttime conditions tend to moderate the effect. Relatively high roughage diets tend to be affected more severely than high concentrate diets. Conversely, intakes may be increased up to 30 per cent by low temperatures, particularly if the cattle remain dry. Extensive precipitation and muddy conditions can depress intake in both the thermoneutral zone and at lower temperatures. Intake can also be severely depressed for beef cows on winter range. Forage intake may be decreased up to 50 per cent during and following storms that produce low temperatures and snow cover.

The availability of nutrients from roughages may be altered by environmental temperature. DE, ME, and NE values may be modified by the following formula:

$$A = B + B (0.0010[T - 20])$$

where A is the adjusted value for environmental temperature, B is the unadjusted value, and T is the effective ambient temperature (°C). Thus, if the NE_m value of a feed is 1.6 Mcal/kg and the ambient temperature is 10° below the thermoneutral zone (5°C), the adjusted NE_m value of the feed is

$$1.6 + 1.6 (0.001[5 - 20]) = 1.585 \text{ Mcal/kg.}$$

The NE_m requirement should be adjusted for exposure to temperature outside the thermoneutral zone. Requirements for adapted animals should be modified to allow for changes in the basal metabolic rate and, possibly, for acute exposure to heat or cold. Requirements for unadapted animals should be modified for acute exposure to heat or cold only. For adapted animals, energy expenditure is inversely proportional to temperature unless normal respiration is affected by high temperature. The following equation expresses the NE_m requirement:

$$\text{Mcal } NE_m = (a) \text{ W/kg}^{0.75}$$

Table 3. *Determination of NE_m Concentration in Alfalfa Hay**

Feeding Level	Feed Eaten g/(BW†)$^{0.75}$	ME Intake kcal/(BW†)$^{0.75}$	Heat Produced kcal/(BW)$^{0.75}$	Energy Gain kcal/(BW†)$^{0.75}$
1. Fasting	0	0	77	−77
2. At maintenance‡	64	131	131	0
Difference	64	131	54	77

*Level in fasting.
†BW in kg.
‡Level 2 is equilibrium.

For animals acclimated to the thermoneutral zone, the factor (a) is taken as 0.077, and W/kg$^{0.75}$ is body weight in kilograms to the 0.75 power. For each degree Celsius above or below the thermoneutral zone, 0.0007 should be subtracted or added to (a) in this equation. Thus, for cattle exposed to temperatures of 30°C, (a) = 0.077 − (10 × 0.0007) = 0.070. For cattle exposed to a temperature of 0°C, (a) = 0.077 + (15 × 0.0007) = 0.088. For acute heat stress where the animals are showing rapid shallow breathing, add 7 per cent to (a). If the animals are showing open-mouthed panting, add 11 to 25 per cent to (a).

For acute cold stress, NE_m expenditures are increased according to exposures to temperatures below the lower critical temperature (LCT). The LCT for a specific animal depends on the animal's insulation and heat production. Wind velocity influences insulation and is an important environmental factor. Handley at Colorado State University proposed the use of a term, Temperature Wind Index (TWI), in which a wind velocity of 1 mph was equal to a decrease in temperature of 1°F. This would especially apply at temperatures below the thermoneutral zone. It would seem reasonable to use a figure of −0.06°C for each mph of wind velocity below the thermoneutral zone. Thus, if the temperature was 5°C and the wind velocity was 10 mph, the TWI would equal 5°C − (10°C × 0.6) = −1°C. The (a) value in the formula NE_m = a. W/kg$^{0.75}$ would be 0.077 plus 0.0007 × 16 = 0.088 Mcal/kg$^{0.75}$.

The LCT value varies widely for different cattle. For a one-week-old calf exposed to a low dry wind, the LCT is estimated to be +7.7°C. For a yearling steer gaining 1.1 kg/day and exposed to a low dry wind, the LCT is estimated to be −34.1°C. The increase in ME required per degree C below the LCT is from 1 to 3 per cent. For details on calculation of the energy requirements of acute cold exposure, see NRC report "Effect of Environment on Nutrient Requirements of Domestic Animals."

The energy concentrations in specific feeds have been determined by difference trials and by equations derived from data acquired from difference trials. Table 3 illustrates a difference trial to determine the NE_m concentration in alfalfa. 64 g of feed yields 77 kcal retention.

Therefore,

$$NE_m \text{ conc} = \frac{77}{64} = 1.2 \text{ kcal/g of feed,}$$

or

$$NE_m = 1.2 \text{ Mcal/kg.}$$

Some NE_g values in feed have been established by difference trials. Such values must be evaluated on a sample of feed used above the maintenance level as shown in Table 4. 82 g of feed yields 42 kcal NE_g. Therefore,

$$NE_g \text{ conc} = \frac{42}{82} = 0.51 \text{ kcal/g,}$$

or

$NE_g = 0.51$ Mcal/kg.

Interconversions between DE, ME, and NE values of feedstuffs are possible. The following relationships have been estimated. All units are Mcal/kg DM.

$$ME = 0.82 \text{ DE (NRC, 1976; ARC, 1965)}$$
$$NE_m = 1.37 \text{ ME} - 0.138 \text{ ME}^2 + 0.0105 \text{ ME}^3 - 1.12$$
$$NE_g = 1.43 \text{ ME} - 0.174 \text{ ME}^2 + 0.0122 \text{ ME}^3 - 1.65$$

The NE requirements for growth are estimated as the amount of energy deposited as nonfat organic matter (mostly protein) plus the energy deposited as fat. Relative caloric values include 9.4 kcal/g of fat and 5.6 kcal/g of nonfat organic matter. The relative quantities of fat and protein being deposited are dependent on two factors: (1) the intake of energy above the maintenance requirement (assuming all other nutrient requirements are satisfied) and (2) the phase of growth. For most conditions the energy content of a unit of weight gain will be between 1.2 (energy content of fat free body) and 8 Mcal/kg gain (energy content of adipose tissue). All relationships to estimate the caloric value of weight gain have been determined for some particular breeds and sex classes. These relationships may have to be adjusted for more precise use for other breeds and conditions (ARC, 1980). The observed weight gain is also influenced by the contents of the digestive tract. The weight of these contents

Table 4. *Determination of NE_g Concentration in Alfalfa Hay**

Feeding Level	Feed Eaten g/(BW†)$^{0.75}$	ME Intake kcal/(BW†)$^{0.75}$	Heat Produced kcal/(BW†)$^{0.75}$	Energy Gain kcal/(BW†)$^{0.75}$
1. At maintenance	64	131	131	0
2. Above maintenance‡	146	298	256	42
Difference	82	167	125	42

*Level 1 is at maintenance.
†BW in kg.
‡Level 2 is *ad libitum*.

can vary from less than 5 to 21 per cent of the shrunk weight of cattle depending on the diet and the weighing conditions.

The primary relationships used in the NRC-NAS Manual for Beef Cattle, 1984, to calculate the net energy values of empty body weight gain are taken from data furnished by Garrett. In these equations, RE (retained energy) is equivalent to NE_g. RE requirements for medium-frame British breed steers and heifers receiving hormonal adjuvants include

For steers: $RE = (0.0635 \ W^{0.75}) \ (EBG^{1.097})$
For heifers: $RE = (0.0783 \ W^{0.75}) \ (EBG^{1.119})$

Equivalent relationships in logarithmic form are as follows:

For steers:
$Log(RE/W^{0.75}) = 1.097 \ Log \ EBG - 1.197$
For heifers:
$Log(RE/W^{0.75}) = 1.119 \ Log \ EBG - 1.106$

In these equations EBG (empty body weight gain) and W (body weight) are in kilograms. RE is in Mcal/day and is equal to NE_g.

These basic relationships are easily modified for application to specific practical conditions. Examples follow.

1. Data summarized by Garrett (1980a) indicate that cattle not receiving hormonal adjuvants require a 5 per cent increase in energy per unit of gain. Thus, the equation for steers not implanted becomes:

$RE = 1.05 \ (0.0635 \ W^{0.75}) \ (EBG^{1.097})$,

or

$(0.0667 \ W^{0.75}) \ (EBG^{1.097})$.

2. Other modifications can be used to estimate RE or NE_g requirements for cattle with different frame sizies or sex classes.

   a. It is assumed that energy retention in a large-frame steer or medium-frame bull will be 15 per cent lower per unit of gain relative to that of a medium-frame steer. In this case the steer equation becomes:

   $RE = (0.0635[0.85 \ W]^{0.75}) \ (EBG^{1.097})$,

   or

   $RE = (0.0562 \ W^{0.75}) \ (EBG^{1.097})$

   b. Other modifications of the primary equations have been made to estimate the energy requirements of large-frame bulls and heifers (see NAS-NRC Manual for Beef Cattle, 1984, pp. 38–39).

The primary equations are based on empty body weight (EBW) and empty body weight gain (EBG). Under practical conditions these do not exist. The equations in Table 5 from the NAS-NRC Manual for Beef Cattle, 1984, are based on shrunk body weights (overnight without feed or water) and shrunk weight gains. The approach is simple and is based on a number of general assumptions:

1. Shrunk weight and shrunk weight gains are called live weight (LW) and live weight gains (LWG), respectively.
2. The assumed relationships include:
   a. empty body weight (EBW) = 0.891 LW, and
   b. empty body gain (EBW) = 0.0956 LW gain.

For further information see ARC, 1980, p. 38 and/or the NAS-NRC Manual for Beef Cattle, 1984, p. 4.

For an example we will calculate the RE needs for a 450-kg LW, medium-frame steer being fed in a thermoneutral environment to gain 1.2 kg/day.

$RE = 0.0635 \ ([450 \times 0.891]^{0.75}) \ ([0.956 \times 1.2]^{1.097})$
$\ \ \ = 6.61 \ Mcal/day$.

The relationship used to estimate NE_m requirements (0.77 Mcal/$W^{0.75}$) is not adjusted for EBW. Thus, in this example the NE_m requirement is assumed to be $450^{0.75} \times 0.077 = 7.52$ Mcal.

Current information is inadequate to modify the general system describing the energy values of feeds and the energy requirements of all cattle in all production situations. Users are encouraged to adjust the primary equations if a consistent over- or underestimation of animal performances appears.

Other procedures for adjusting generally determined energy requirements to specific conditions have been suggested by Garrett (1976), Webster (1978), ARC (1980), and Fox and Black (1984).

The primary equations to predict energy requirements have been re-arranged to estimate daily gain when animal weight and feed consumption are known.

For steers: $EBG = 12.341(RE/W^{0.75})^{0.9116}$, or
$EBG = 12.341 \ W^{-0.6837} \ RE^{0.9116}$.
For heifers: $EBG = 9.741(RE/W^{0.75})^{0.8936}$, or
$EBG = 9.741 \ W^{-0.6702} \ RE^{0.8936}$.

Equivalent relationships in logarithmic form include:
For steers:
$Log \ EBG = 0.9116 \ Log(RE/W^{0.75}) + 1.091$
For heifers:
$Log \ EBG = 0.8936 \ Log(RE/W^{0.75}) + 0.9884$

In these equations RE is the net energy available for gain.

Net Energy for Gestation and Lactation

Energy deposition in the products of conception of female beef cattle has been determined by Ferrell and colleagues (1976) and can be calculated from the data of Prior and Laster (1979). The gross efficiency of ME use for the products of conception has been estimated as 11 to 15 per cent for cattle (Ferrell et al.) and 12 to 13 per cent for sheep (Rattray et al., 1974). The average figure (13 per cent) is used to estimate the ME requirement. The ME requirement is converted into equivalent NE_m units. The relationship used to estimate the pregnancy requirement (kcal/day of NE_m equivalent) is based on expected birth weight of the calf and the day of gestation (t). It is assumed that the diet consists of averge roughage (ME = 2 Mcal/kg DM). The formula is as follows:

*calf birth weight $(0.0149 - 0.0000407t)e^{0.05883t-0.0000804t^2}$
$= Mcal \ NE_m/day$.

Thus, if the expected birth weight is 40 kg and t = day 235, then the NE_m requirement in Mcal would be

$40 \ kg \ (0.0149 - [0.0000407 \times 235])$

$(2.72^{[0.05883 \times 235] - [0.0000824 \times 235^2]}) = 2557 \ kcal = 2.56 \ Mcal$.

The energy requirements for milk production have been estimated from the information available for the dairy cow (NRC, 1978). The requirement can be calculated and expressed in NE_m units, as ME is utilized for lactation and maintenance at similar levels of efficiency. The NAS-

---

*e is the antilog of the natural log of 1 and is roughly equal to 2.72.

Table 5. *Prediction Equations for Estimating Nutrient Requirements and Feed Intake of Beef Cattle**

Energy

A. Maintenance requirements (Mcal/day) of steers, heifers, bulls, and cows:

$$NE_m = 0.077^{0.75}.$$

B. NE_g (Mcal/day) required (equivalent to RE) for empty body weight gain (EBG):

Medium-frame steer calves:

$$NE_g = 0.0635 \ W^{0.75} \ (EBG)^{1.097}.$$

Large-frame steer calves, compensating medium-frame yearling steers, and medium-frame bull calves:

$$NE_g = 0.0562 \ W^{0.75} \ (EBG)^{1.097}.$$

Large-frame bull calves and compensating large-frame yearling steers:

$$NE_g = 0.0498 \ W^{0.75} \ (EBG)^{1.097}.$$

Medium-frame heifer calves:

$$NE_g = 0.0783 \ W^{0.75} \ (EBG)^{1.119}.$$

Large-frame heifer calves and compensating yearling heifers:

$$NE_g = 0.0693 \ W^{0.75} \ (EBG)^{1.119}.$$

Mature thin cows:

$$NE_g = 6.5 \ Mcal/kg \ gain.$$

C. NE_g required for live weight gain (LWG):

Medium-frame steer calves:

$$NE_g = 0.0557 \ W^{0.75} \ (LWG)^{1.097}.$$

Large-frame steer calves, compensating medium-frame yearling steers, and medium-frame bull calves:

$$NE_g = 0.0493 \ W^{0.75} \ (LWG)^{1.097}.$$

Large-frame bull calves and compensating large-frame yearling steers:

$$NE_g = 0.0437 \ W^{0.75} \ (LWG)^{1.097}.$$

Medium-frame heifer calves:

$$NE_g = 0.0686 \ W^{0.75} \ (LWG)^{1.119}.$$

Large-frame heifer calves and compensating yearling heifers:

$$NE_g = 0.0608 \ W^{0.75} \ (LWG)^{1.119}.$$

Mature thin cows:

$$6.2 \ Mcal/kg \ gain.$$

D. Energy required for pregnancy (expressed as kcal NE_m/day):

$$NE_g = calf \ birth \ weight \ (0.0149 - 10.0000407t)e^{0.05883t \ - \ 0.0000.804t^2}.$$

E. Energy required for lactation (expressed as NE_m, Mcal/kg milk):

$$NE_m = 0.1 \ (\% \ fat) + 0.35.$$

F. Estimation of empty body weight gain (EBG) from NE_g available for gain:

Medium-frame steer calves:

$$EBG = 12.34 \ NE_g^{0.9116} \ W^{-0.6837}.$$

Large-frame steer calves, compensating medium-frame yearling steers, and medium-frame bull calves:

$$EBG = 13.80 \ NE_g^{0.9116} \ W^{-0.6837}.$$

Large-frame bull calves and compensating large-frame yearling steers:

$$EBG = 15.40 \ NE_g^{0.9116} \ W^{-0.6837}.$$

Medium-frame heifer calves:

$$EBG = 9.74 \ NE_g^{0.8936} \ W^{-0.6702}.$$

Large-frame heifer calves and compensating yearling heifers:

$$EBG = 10.86 \ NE_g^{0.8936} \ W^{-0.6702}.$$

G. Estimation of live weight gain (LWG) from NE_g available for gain:

Medium-frame steer calves:

$$LWG = 13.91 \ NE_g^{0.9116} \ W^{-0.6837}.$$

Large-frame steer calves, compensating medium-frame yearling steers, and medium-frame bulls:

$$LWG = 15.54 \ NE_g^{0.9116 \ W^{-0.6837}}.$$

Large-frame bull calves and compensating large-frame yearling steers:

$$LWG = 17.35 \ NE_g^{0.9116} \ W^{-0.6837}.$$

Medium-frame heifer calves:

$$LWG = 10.96 \ ME_g^{0.8936} \ W^{-0.6702}.$$

Large-frame heifer calves and compensating yearling heifers:

$$LWG = 12.21 \ NE_g^{0.8936} \ W^{-0.6702}.$$

Protein

Factorialized Protein Requirement:

$$CP = \frac{F + U + S + G + C + M}{D \times BV \times CE}$$

CP, Crude protein, g/day
F, Metabolic fecal protein loss = 3.34% dry matter intake
U, Endogenous urinary protein loss = $2.75W^{0.5}$
S, Scurf protein loss = $0.2W^{0.6}$
G, Tissue protein deposition (in grams) = $(268 - 29.4 \times$ energy content of gain, Mcal/kg) daily gain in kg
C, Conceptus, 55 g/day, last third of pregnancy
M, Milk protein production (in grams) = $33.5 \times$ milk production in kg
D, True protein digestibility = 0.90
BV, Biologic value = 0.66
CE, Conversion of dietary to postruminal protein = 1.0

Urea Potential:
g/kg dry feed = $11.78 \ NE_m + 6.85 - 0.0357 \ CP \times DEG$†
g/kg dry feed = $31.64 - 3.558 \ CP + ([945 \ NE_m - 887 - 179 \ NE_m^2])^{0.5}$‡
CP, Crude protein (%)
NE, Net energy maintenance (Mcal/kg)
DEG, Ruminal degradation of protein (%)

Calcium and Phosphorus:
Calcium, g/day = $((0.0154 \ (W_{kg}) + 0.071$ (protein gain, g/day) + 1.23 (milk/day, kg) + 0.0137 (fetal growth, g/day)) ÷ 0.5
Phosphorus, g/day = $((0.0280 \ (W_{kg}) + 0.039$ (protein gain g/day) + 0.95 (milk/day, kg) + 0.0076 (fetal growth, g/day)) ÷ 0.85

Feed Intake

Breeding Females:
Daily feed intake (kg dry matter) = $W^{0.75} \ (0.1462 \ NE_m - 0.0517 \ NE_m^2 - 0.0074)$.

Growing and Finishing Cattle:
Daily feed intake (kg dry matter) = $W^{0.75} \ (.1493 \ NE_m - 0.0460 \ NE_m^2 - 0.0196)$.
NE_m, net energy maintenance (Mcal/kg diet)

Adjustments for Frame Size:
None: Medium-frame steer calf, large-frame heifer, and medium-frame bull.
+ 10%: Large frame steer calf and medium-frame yearling steer.
+ 5%: Large-frame bulls.
−10%: Medium-frame heifers.

*Reprinted from National Research Council: Nutrient Requirements of Beef Cattle, 6th Rev. Ed. National Academy of Sciencies: Washington, D.C., 1984.

†From Burroughs, W., Nelson, D. K., and Mertens, D. R.: Protein physiology and its application in the lactating cow: the metabolizable protein feeding standard. J. Anim. Sci. *41*:933, 1975.

‡From Satter, L. D., and Roffler, R. E.: Nitrogen requirements and utilization in dairy cattle. J. Dairy Sci. *58*:1219, 1975.

NRC publication for dairy cattle (1978) uses one energy value (NE_{lact}) to express requirements for maintenance, gestation, lactation, and body weight change.

Because the methods of derivation of the values for NE_m and NE_{lact} were substantially different, there are some differences in individual values in the nutrient concentration tables. For beef cattle, energy requirements for lactation are estimated using the following formula:

NE_m in Mcal/kg milk = 0.1 (per cent fat + 0.35).

Thus, if a cow produces 5 kg of 3.5 per cent fat milk/day, her NE_m requirement would be

$$(0.1 [3.5] + 0.35) (5) = 3.5 \text{ Mcal.}$$

For dairy cows, the NE_{lact} requirements for maintenance plus gestation in the last two months of pregnancy are computed as

$$(0.104 \text{ Mcal } NE_{lact}) (BW^*)^{0.75}.$$

The NE_{lact} requirement for maintenance only at moderate temperatures is $(0.08 \text{ Mcal } NE_{lact}) (BW^*)^{0.75}$. The net NE_{lact} requirement for gestation equals $0.104 - 0.08 = 0.024 \text{ Mcal} \times (BW^*)^{0.75}$. Thus, the NE_{lact} requirement for pregnancy in the last two months for a 600-kg cow is $600^{0.75} \times 0.24 = 2.91 \text{ Mcal } NE_{lact}$. Requirements for lactation are tabulated according to butterfat content and range from 0.59 Mcal per kg of 2.5 per cent fat milk to 0.93 Mcal per kg of 6 per cent fat milk.

Sheep utilize ME at 12 to 14 per cent efficiency for conceptus development and at 16 to 18 per cent efficiency for uterine and mammary development (as determined by Rattray and associates, 1974). The research was done with diets containing 2.4 to 2.6 Mcal ME/kg DM. The NE requirements for pregnancy are listed as NE_{preg} in the NAS-NRC publication for sheep. NE pregnancy requirements above those for maintenance and growth are tabulated for ewes carrying single, twin, and triplet fetuses at different stages of late pregnancy. It has been shown by Rattray and co-workers (1974) that the efficiency of utilization of ME for maintenance and gain is not altered by pregnancy. Fetal growth and pregnancy requirements are subtantial in the last six weeks of gestation. The total maintenance and pregnancy requirements in this period average about 1.5 times maintenance levels for single–fetus bearing ewes and two times maintenance levels for ewes bearing twins. Few estimates of ME utilization for lactation in sheep are available. The lactation period is short, and the composition and quantity of milk produced by lactating ewes are difficult to determine. It has been estimated that from 65 per cent of ME for ewes suckling single lambs to 83 per cent of ME for ewes suckling twins is converted to milk energy during 12 weeks of lactation. The average value is slightly above that calculated for cattle. The same workers have also estimated that NE for lactation is 1.3 to 1.4 times maintenance levels for ewes suckling singles and 1.7 to 1.9 times maintenance levels for ewes suckling twins. The NE values (Mcal/kg DM) of feeds commonly used can be closely related to the ME value of the feed (Mcal/kg DM). The relationships are as follows:

$$NE_m = 0.80 \text{ ME} - 0.41 \text{ (r = 0.996, CV = 2.9)}$$
$$NE_g = 0.67 \text{ ME} - 0.68 \text{ (r = 0.95, CV = 15.5)}$$

---

*BW in kg.

Energy for Swine

The energy requirements for swine (NRC, 1979) are expressed as DE and ME values. Relative values are expressed in the following formula (NRC, 1979):

$$ME = DE \left(\frac{96 - [0.202 \times \text{crude protein \%}]}{100} \right)$$

Growing and finishing rations for swine ordinarily contain about 97 per cent grain and protein concentrates. Corn and soybean meal comprise the most popular combination. DE and ME values are probably the most practical units for ration formulation.

Energy consumed in excess of maintenance, growth, gestation, and lactation needs is deposited in body lipid. The lean to fat ratio of the pig may be controlled by the daily energy intake. The potential for fat deposition increases with maturity. If pregnant sows are fed a corn-soybean diet *ad libitum*, they will deposit excess body lipid. Therefore, the energy intake of gestating sows must be limited. Lactating sows should be fed at a level to support maintenance plus the requirements for milk production. ME intake can be adjusted in relation to litter size.

Research supports the view that optimum energy efficiency is achieved with moderate weight gains in gestation and moderate weight losses in lactation.

PROTEIN REQUIREMENT

Dietary protein supplies the animal with amino acids essential to vital synthetic processes in the body. Amino acids are the building units of all animal cells and tissues. In addition, all protein secretions, including enzymes, hormones, mucin, and milk, require specific assortments of amino acids. In ruminant animals, all of the required amino acids may be obtained from dietary protein, non-protein nitrogen (NPN) compounds, and fermentation products of microbial metabolism if all of the required elements are present. Monogastric animals and very young ruminant animals are unable to endogenously synthesize all of the amino acids that compose their specific proteins. The amino acids that cannot be synthesized by monogastric animals include arginine, histidine, isoleucine, leucine, lysine, methionine, phenylalanine, threonine, tryptophan, and valine. For swine, cystine can meet 50 per cent of the methionine requirement and tyrosine can meet 30 per cent of the requirement for phenylalanine.

Crude protein (CP) values for all species are calculated from nitrogen content. Protein averages 16 per cent nitrogen; therefore,

$$CP = N \times \frac{100}{16}$$
$$= N \times 6.25$$

Protein for Swine

The NRC publications for the various species differ somewhat in their approach to protein computation.

For swine, optimum performance requires that each essential amino acid be fed at the proper level at the proper time and with the proper level of all other essential amino acids. The nonessential amino acids are obtained from ordinary dietary components or can be synthesized

Table 6. *Lysine and Crude Protein Values for Corn and Soybean Meal*

Feed	Lysine (%)	Crude Protein (%)
Corn	0.24	10
Soybean meal	2.93	44

by using amino groups derived from excess amino acids in the diet. The amino acid requirements of growing swine increase as energy concentrations in the diet increase. In the NRC publication for swine the amino acid requirements are extrapolated for growing pigs (20 to 35 kg) on the basis of percentages of amino acids in a 16 per cent protein diet.

In corn-soybean diets lysine is the limiting amino acid. If the corn-soybean mixture is adjusted to furnish the recommended percentage of lysine, all other essential amino acids will be furnished in adequate amounts. Table 6 illustrates a satisfactory procedure. The recommended percentage of lysine for growing finishing swine weighing 20 to 35 kg is 0.7 per cent. It is assumed that corn and soybean meal will comprise 97 per cent of the dry matter. So, the lysine content of the corn-urea portion of the ration is

$$\frac{100}{97} \times 0.7 = 0.72 \text{ per cent.}$$

Use a Pearson's square to mix the corn and soybean meal:

1. The number in the left corner that is smaller than the recommendation is subtracted from the recommendation, and the difference is recorded in the opposite corner (0.72 − 0.24 = 0.48).
2. The recommendation is subtracted from the number in the left corner that is larger than the recommendation, and the difference is recorded in the opposite corner.
3. The recorded numbers in the right corners are the proportional parts of the ingredients (corn = 2.21 parts, soybean meal = 0.48 parts).
4. The proportional parts are added together and converted to fractions and percentages.

The requirements for pregnant gilts and sows are based on amounts required for satisfactory nitrogen retention in late pregnancy. The requirements for lactation have been extrapolated from published maintenance requirements for adult female swine plus amounts calculated to support the production of 6 kg of milk daily. Recommended percentages of crude protein vary from 27 per cent for growing pigs under 5 kg BW to 13 per cent for finishing pigs over 60 kg BW. Lactating gilts and sows require 13 per cent and gestating sows and gilts 12 per cent of crude protein in the air dry diet (DM content = 90 per cent).

Best results are obtained when concentrate mixtures are used in which the protein biologic values complement each other (maximum nitrogen retention). Corn and soybean meal present the classic example. By using these feeds, optimum percentages of both total protein and amino acid balance can be achieved.

Protein for Sheep

Protein requirements listed in the NAS-NRC publication Nutrient Requirements for Sheep are based on digestible crude protein percentages and digestible energy/digestible protein ratios. A ratio of about 20 g digestible protein per Mcal DE is adequate for mature nonlactating ewes. Higher levels of digestible protein per Mcal are required to support lactation, growth, and fat deposition.

Total crude protein requirements are calculated from digestible protein requirements by the following regression:

$$Y = 0.929 X - 3.48$$

where Y = digestible protein (% DM) and X = crude protein (% DM). The requirement for crude protein thus derived is probably high if concentrates form a significant part of the ration.

Apparent co-efficients of digestibility vary from 0 to 80 per cent, but in practical situations true digestibility generally approaches the maximum value. High crude fiber and low crude protein concentrations of low quality roughage result in lower digestibility.

Tables presenting protein requirements cannot be precisely accurate. Inaccuracies result from differences in breed, weight, condition, and physiologic state. Rounding off data for use in tables also results in a small degree of error.

Recent developments indicate that ruminal synthesis of microbial protein does not supply all of the essential amino acids in optimum amounts. Methionine is the first limiting amino acid for both growth of wool and gain. Lysine and threonine are also produced in short supply. Cystine can apparently replace methionine for growth of wool.

Urea and other sources of NPN have limited value in supplying supplemental nitrogen for protein synthesis. Maximal utilization requires readily available energy and essential minerals. Additions of sulfur enhance urea supplementation. Wool contains a high percentage of sulfur-containing amino acids, and a nitrogen-sulfur ratio of 10:1 in the diet is recommended for optimum wool production. Safest and best results from utilization of NPN are obtained when the diet contains less than 1 per cent of urea or equivalent.

Protein for Beef Cattle

The preruminant calf (less than eight weeks) has negligible rumen function. Amino acid requirements are met through milk or milk replacers. Supplementing with specific amino acids may be beneficial, but urea usefulness is quite limited. After the rumen becomes functional (six to eight weeks depending on diet), the crude protein needs for two systems must be met: (1) nitrogen for microbial fermentation in the reticulorumen, and (2) amino acids for post-ruminal absorption that will supply the tissue of the host ruminant.

A wide variety of microbial types thrive in the rumen. Many species of anaerobic bacteria, protozoa, and even fungi are included. Ultimately the microbes are swept out of the rumen into the abomasum and small intestine, where they are digested. These microbes typically furnish about half of the amino acids utilized by the ruminant animal.

Ruminal microbes can use various sources of nitrogen for amino acid and protein synthesis, including ammonia, some amino acids, and some peptides. Energy derived from fermentation and minerals are also required for growth. The requirements are interrelated, and any of these factors can limit microbial growth. The supply of ammonia can be inadequate when the intake of protein or the ruminal degradation of protein is low. Ammonia deficiency in the rumen reduces the efficiency of microbial growth and may reduce the rate and extent of digestion of organic matter in the rumen. Feed intake may also decrease as digestion efficiency is impaired. The minimal concentration of ammonia-nitrogen needed for microbial growth and digestion has been estimated by a variety of procedures (Satter and Slyter, 1974; Mehrez et al., 1977; Edwards and Bartley, 1979; Hespell, 1979; Slyter et al., 1979). There has been little consensus. Following are widely accepted generalities.

1. Ammonia-nitrogen is the primary supply of nitrogen for microbial protein synthesis.
2. Concentrations of ammonia in rumen fluid above 5 mg/100 ml do not increase microbial production.
3. Ammonia is derived from degradation of protein or nonprotein nitrogen (NPN) in the rumen.
4. Although most microbial species can survive using ammonia as their sole supply of nitrogen, added natural protein may stimulate microbial growth by providing amino acids, essential branched-chain fatty acids, and unidentified factors that enhance microbial growth.
5. Typically the least expensive dietary source of rumenal ammonia is some form of NPN. The most common source is urea.
6. Utilization of NPN for incorporation into microbial protein is limited by the energy supply. Best results are obtained using high energy–low crude protein rations.
7. Ammonia not used in microbial synthesis is absorbed from the rumen and circulated to the liver, where it is combined with carbon dioxide to form urea. Most of this urea is eliminated in urine, but a portion is recycled to the digestive tract in saliva and urine secretions. It is possible in some situations for the outflow of protein from the rumen to exceed the dietary intake of crude protein.
8. NPN is added to a diet only when the rumenal concentration of ammonia is inadequate for optimum microbial action to digest organic matter or supply ammonia for microbial protein synthesis. Theoretically, the amount of urea that can be used in a specific diet can be calculated. The calculations are based on the amount of protein degraded to ammonia in the rumen and microbial protein synthesis. Microbial protein synthesis is generally dependent on energy available in the rumen. Two formulas are recommended (NRC, 1984) to calculate the potential for using urea as a CP source.
   a. Urea potential = $11.78 \, NE_m + 6.85 - 0.0357 \, CP \times DEG$ (Burroughs et al., 1975), and
   b. Urea potential = $31.64 - 3.558 \, CP + ([945 \, NE_m - 887 - 179 \, NE_m^2])^{0.5}$ (Satter and Roffler, 1975).

The crude protein (CP) requirement of cattle can be subdivided into specific metabolic factors. These include metabolic fecal loss (F), endogenous urinary loss (U), scurf loss (S), tissue growth (G), fetal growth (C), and milk production (M). The factorial equation (NRC, 1984) is

$$CP = F + U + S + G + C + M/D \times BV \times CE.$$

D, BV, and CE are decimal figures that represent (1) digestion efficiency (per cent absorbed), (2) amount of absorbed protein that is retained in the body, and (3) the efficiency of converting dietary protein to ruminal protein output (75 to 120 per cent).

Equations to estimate the various crude protein factors (6.25 N) in grams include the following:
1. $F = 3.34\%$ dry matter intake
2. $U = 2.75 \, W^{0.5}$
3. $S = 0.2 \, W^{0.6}$
4. $G = 268 - (29.4 \times$ energy content of gain, Mcal/kg) (kg daily gain)
5. $C = 55$ gm/day, last third of pregnancy
6. $M = 33.5 \times$ milk production in kg

The factors in the divisors of the factorial equation are assumed to include D = 0.9, B.V. = 0.66, and CE = 1.0.

Net energy content of gain is estimated from prediction equations listed in Table 5. For example,

A medium frame steer calf whose shrunk weight equals 250 kg and the daily gain = 1.2 kg will deposit $\dfrac{0.5557 \times 250^{0.75} \times 1.2^{1.097}}{1.2} = 3.56$ Mcal NEg per kg of gain.

Thus, the crude protein requirement for a 400 kg medium frame steer calf consuming 8.3 kg DM and gaining 1.2 kg/day will be

$$F = 8300 \times .0334 = 277 \text{ gm}$$
$$U = 2.75 \times 400^{0.5} = 55 \text{ gm}$$
$$S = .2 \times 400^{0.6} = 7 \text{ gm}$$
$$G = 268 - (29.4 \times 5.07/1.2) \times (1.2) = 173 \text{ gm}$$

$$\frac{F + U + S + G}{0.9 \times 0.66 \times 1.0} = 853 \text{ gm}$$

$$NE_g = \frac{0.0557 \times 400^{0.75} \times 1.2^{1.097}}{1.2} = 5.07 \text{ Mcal/kg gain}$$

Protein for Dairy Cattle

The current NRC Manual for Dairy Cattle (1978) omits the use of digestible protein as a measure of required protein. Total or crude protein requirements are computed as follows.

Total crude protein (TCP) is

$$\frac{U + F + S + G + C}{E_p} + \frac{L}{E_p}$$

U is 6.25 times the amount of urinary nitrogen that would be lost on a nitrogen-free diet calculated according to $(BW^*)^{0.5}$, or

$$U = 2.75 \, (BW^*)^{0.5}.$$

F is 6.25 times the amount of fecal metabolic nitrogen that would be lost on a nitrogen-free diet for ruminating cattle calculated according to fecal dry matter (FDM), or

$$F = 0.068 \text{ FDM}$$

---

*BW in kg.

F is sometimes calculated with slightly less accuracy as 3 per cent of dry matter intake (DMI). Liquid milk diets for preruminating calves result in a high nitrogen content in feces. The protein equivalent value for milk-fed calves is

$$F = 0.0125 \text{ DMI (NRC Dairy Cattle, 1978).}$$

S is protein lost in skin secretions, scurf, and hair calculated according to $(BW^*)^{0.6}$.

$$S = 0.2 \ (BW^*)^{0.6}.$$

G is protein deposited in or associated with growth. Using animals containing less than 29 per cent fat, it was found that G decreases from 19 per cent of gain for newborn animals to 16 per cent of gain for animals approaching mature size.

C is protein deposited in the products of conception including fetus, fluids, membranes, and increased uterine size. C is calculated as $1.136 \ (BW^*)^{0.7}$.

L is net protein required for synthesis of milk protein. L equals total milk protein plus F losses (0.068 FDM) that result from increased feed allowances for lactating cattle. Milk protein percentage is predictable according to milk fat concentration. Milk protein per cent = 1.9 + 0.4 milk fat per cent.

E_p represents the factors necessary to convert the various net protein requirements to dietary crude protein. The efficiency factors are based upon (a) the percentage of dietary protein that may be absorbed as amino acids and (b) the efficiency of conversion of the absorbed amino acids to body protein. The E_p factors adopted to calculate total crude protein (TCP) for various classes include:

1. Baby calves fed only liquid milk (a.b.: 0.91 × 0.77 = 0.7),
2. 50-kg calves fed milk and concentrates (a.b.: 0.87 × 0.75 = 0.65),
3. 75-kg calves fed mainly concentrates (a.b.: 0.80 × 0.70 = 0.56),
4. 100-kg calves fed forages and concentrates (a.b.: 0.75 × 0.67 = 0.50),
5. 150-kg cattle fed forages and concentrates (a.b.: 0.75 × 0.63 = 0.47),
6. Cattle over 200 kg for maintenance and growth (a.b.: 0.75 × 0.60 = 0.45), and
7. Lactation (a.b.: 0.75 × 0.70 = 0.52).

If there are protein deficiencies in the basic energy ration, the required amount of protein will be added into the complete supplement.

COMPUTATION OF THE MINERAL REQUIREMENT

Calcium, phosphorus, magnesium, potassium, sodium, chlorine, sulfur, iodine, copper, cobalt, manganese, zinc, selenium, molybdenum, fluorine, chromium, silicon, vanadium, and probably nickel and tin have been established as essential minerals in the diet of one or more animal species. The mineral requirement tables listed in the NAS-NRC manuals are generally based on the data acquired by factorial computation or are experimentally established minimal amounts required to support maintenance plus

*BW in kg.

acceptable production objectives. Daily requirements per animal are listed in tables as grams or milligrams or as recommended percentages of rations (generally dry or air dry). Concentrations of minerals in feedstuffs are listed as grams or milligrams per kg of dry matter or as ppm of dry matter.

Rations are first balanced for energy and protein and then analyzed for mineral content. The mineral content is compared with requirement tables, and supplements are added where deficiencies are indicated. The common mineral supplements are listed in the nutrient concentration tables in the NAS-NRC manuals.

The minerals are listed in the tables as specific percentages of the supplement dry matter (dicalcium phosphate contains 19.3 per cent phosphorus and 22 per cent calcium as listed in the NAS-NRC Manual for Beef Cattle). The amount of supplement required equals the grams of nutrient required divided by the per cent of nutrient present in the supplement expressed as a decimal. If the deficiency is 20g of calcium, it will require $\dfrac{20}{0.22}$ g of dicalcium phosphate $\left(\dfrac{20}{0.22} = 90.9 \text{g} \right)$.

For most species it is recommended that 0.25 per cent of iodized salt be fed in the DM ration to supply the sodium, chlorine, and iodine requirements.

For practical ration formulation only those minerals that are likely to be in short supply or in balance are given consideration. A specific amount of a premixed trace mineral supplement may be added to a ration to ensure against deficiences of zinc, iron, copper, cobalt, and so on. Generally, for ruminant food animals consideration is given to calcium, phosphorus, sodium, potassium, and, in some rations, magnesium and sulfur. Chlorine and iodine are supplied in the sodium supplement. Trace minerals are given more consideration in swine and poultry relative to ruminants. In any case, mixing the minute amounts presents a problem. Most feeders rely on a preformed trace mineral supplement and incorporate a specific amount of that supplement in the daily ration as part of the complete supplement.

COMPUTATION OF THE VITAMIN REQUIREMENT

Food animals have a need for both fat- and water-soluble vitamins. Consideration in practical ration formulation is usually limited to those vitamins not expected to be adequately supplied by natural feeds, rumen synthesis, or tissue synthesis.

For ruminants, vitamins A, D, and E are usually present in significant amounts in high quality roughage. Members of the B vitamin group and vitamin K are synthesized in the rumen, and vitamin C is synthesized in the tissues. There are conditions under which the natural supply may be deficient. Forage may be fed in limited amounts or may be of low quality. Sun-cured hay or exposure to sunlight may be limiting for vitamin A. Calves exclusively fed milk replacers may develop some B vitamin deficiencies. Normally, vitamin A is most likely to be limiting. Concentrations of beta carotene are listed in the NAS-NRC tables. For cattle, 1 mg carotene = 400 I.U. of vitamin A. Vitamin A palmitate and vitamin A acetate provide practical and inexpensive supplementary sources. These products may be stored for significant periods of time in the tissues. They may be ingested in feed or water or may be injected parenterally.

As mentioned previously, rations are first balanced for energy and protein and then analyzed for vitamin content. If there are deficiencies, the specific vitamins are incorporated into the complete supplement.

For swine, the NAS-NRC tables list requirements for vitamins A, D, E, K, C, biotin, choline, folacin, niacin, pantothenic acid, riboflavin, thiamine, pyridoxine, and B_{12}. Because of micromixing problems, vitamin deficiencies of the basic ration are usually met by feeding complete commercial supplements. When energy-protein needs are supplied and balanced by the use of these supplements, the vitamin and mineral needs will be met also.

FORMULATING RATIONS

Ration formulation requires the following steps.
1. Assess the nutritional needs based on the requirements for maintenance and production.
2. Choose the least expensive ingredients for the basic energy ration and the complete supplement. Basic ingredients will include the least expensive sources for energy, fiber, protein, the limiting bulk minerals, vitamin A, and a premix of trace minerals. The NAS-NRC manual contains a table that lists the feeds and the concentrations of the necessary nutrients in these feeds. It may be necessary to include more than one feed for a specific category. Examples include the situation in which wheat is the least expensive energy feed for cattle and the one in which urea is the least expensive crude protein supplement. In these cases some people would recommend that wheat not be used to supply more than 50 per cent of the energy concentrate. It is widely accepted that urea should not be used to furnish more than 25 to 33 per cent of total nitrogen in cattle rations. Consideration must also be given to palatability, nutrient concentration, and transportation costs.
3. Balance the ration for energy.
4. Analyze the energy ration for deficiencies of protein, minerals, and vitamins.
5. Formulate the least expensive supplement to provide for deficiencies of protein, minerals, or vitamins in the energy ration. There are a number of viable approaches:
   a. Formulate a complete supplement and incorporate it into the energy ration.

   b. Incorporate the protein supplement in the energy ration and feed the mineral and vitamin supplements in a free-choice mixture either loose or in block form.
   c. Formulate a complete supplement using molasses as a carrier and feed in a licker. This is often a viable approach if NPN is used as a crude protein source.
   d. Use a prescribed amount of a preformulated commercial supplement. The recommended amount is generally 1 lb/animal/day. Such supplements supply recommended amounts of ionophores and chemotherapeutic agents. Crude protein, salt, and calcium will often be supplied in excess. Total requirements of vitamins A and D and trace minerals are generally supplied. Phosphorus and sometimes potassium contents may be marginal.
6. Formulate the ration to comply with available delivery systems. Blocks, cubes, or loose hay may be fed on the ground. Mangers or bunks with adequate space are necessary if ground, rolled, or pelleted feeds are used.

For example, we will formulate a ration for 250-kg (550-lb) medium-frame steer calves expected to gain 1 kg (2.2 lbs) per day in January. The daily NE_m requirement in Mcal = $0.093 \times BW/kg^{0.75}$.
1. Nutritional needs assessments (daily):
   a. $NE_m = 250^{0.75} \times 0.093 = 5.85$ Mcal.
   b. $NE_g = ([0.891 \times 250]^{0.75} \times 0.0635)([1 \times 0.956]^{1.097})$ = 3.48 Mcal.
   c. Consumption DM (assume NE_m of ration = 1.65 Mcal/kg DM). DM intake = $(0.1493 \times 1.65) - (0.046 \times 1.65^2) - (0.0196) \times (250^{0.75}) = 6.38$ kg
   d. Crude protein requirement,

   $F = 6380 \times 0.0334 = 213.1$
   $U = 2.75 \times 250^{0.5} = 43.5$
   $S = 0.2 \times 250^{0.5} = 5.5$
   $G = 268 - (29.4 \times 3.5/1) \times 1 = 165.1$

   $$\frac{F + U + S + G}{0.9 \times 0.66 \times 1.0} = 712 \text{ gm}$$

   e. Calcium requirement (from Table 1, NRC Manual for Beef Cattle, 1984) = 29 g.
   f. Phosphorus requirement (from Table 1, NRC Manual for Beef Cattle, 1984) = 16 g.
   g. Trace mineral salt = 0.5 per cent of DM ration = $0.005 \times 6070 = 30$ g.
   h. Potassium requirement = 0.7 per cent of DM ration = $0.007 \times 6070 = 42$ g.
   i. Vitamin A requirement = 2200 I.U. $\times 6.07$ kg = 13.354 I.U. (NRC Manual for Beef Cattle, 1984, p. 25).
2. Choice of least expensive ration ingredients (Table 7):

Table 7. *Analysis of Least Expensive Ingredients*

Ingredient	DM(%)	NE_m	NE_g	CP(%)	Ca(%)	P(%)	K(%)	Carotene (mg/kg DM)
Corn	89	2.15	1.42	10	0.03	0.31	0.35	1
Wheat	89	2.15	1.42	14	0.06	0.41	0.46	—
Cottonseed meal	93	1.69	1.11	44	0.17	1.31	1.53	—
Alfalfa silage	30	1.20	0.55	17	1.40	0.32	2.36	37
Corn silage	30	1.56	0.99	8	0.28	0.21	0.95	—
Dicalcium PO_4	100	—	—	—	23.13	18.65	—	—
Limestone	100	—	—	—	33.84	0.02	—	—
Salt	100	—	—	—	—	—	—	—
Trace mineral mix	100	—	—	—	—	—	—	—

Table 8. *Average Net Energies of Warm-Up Rations*

Feed	NE$_m^*$	NE$_g^*$	Average Energy Mcal/kg	Mcal/lb	Mcal/CWT
Corn	2.15	1.42	$(0.5 \times 2.15) + (0.5 \times 1.42) = 1.79$	0.81	81
Wheat	2.15	1.42	$(0.5 \times 2.15) + (0.5 \times 1.42) = 1.79$	0.81	81
Barley	1.93	1.29	$(0.5 \times 1.93) + (0.5 \times 1.29) = 1.61$	0.73	73
Sorghum	1.86	1.24	$(0.5 \times 1.86) + (0.5 \times 1.24) = 1.55$	0.70	70

*Mcal/kg DM.

a. Energy concentrate:

When daily gain is expected to be more than 2 lbs per day, an energy concentrate (TDN > 70 per cent) is necessary. Choices may include wheat, corn, barley, and sorghum. Using Table 4, NAS-NRC Requirements for Dairy Cattle, 1978, wheat and corn have very similar energy concentrations, but wheat is a superior protein source. Energy concentrations in barley and sorghum grains are also very similar (about 20 per cent lower than those of corn or wheat). Crude protein concentration in barley is similar to that of wheat. These concentrations are about 20 to 25 per cent higher than are the crude protein concentrations in corn and sorghum grains. Other considerations include palatability and toxicity. Sorghums are low in palatability, and wheat is relatively toxic. It is generally recommended that wheat be restricted to less than 50 per cent of the concentrate portion of the ration dry matter. To evaluate energy concentrate feeds it is necessary to compute the cost per Mcal of average net energy. Average net energy of a feed or ration depends on the relative percentages of the ration used for maintenance and gain. For example, in a high energy finishing ration, about 38 per cent of the ration is used for maintenance and 62 per cent is used for gain. In a warm-up ration, up to 50 per cent of the ration may be used for maintenance, and in a maintenance ration nearly all of the ration will be used for maintenance. Net energy is used more efficiently for maintenance than for gain. Therefore, the higher the percentage of the ration used for maintenance, the higher the average energy value for a feed or ration. It is necessary to evaluate all feeds according to the same criteria. Our example is a warm-up ration. We will assume that 50 per cent will be used for maintenance and 50 per cent for gain. Average energies for the four feeds we are considering are listed in Table 8. Table 9 contains the costs as fed. Using these prices, wheat is the cheapest energy source, but we are limited to half of the total energy concentrate. Corn is the second best energy choice, so our energy concentrate will include 50 per cent wheat and 50 per cent corn.

b. Crude protein:

Light cattle making substantial gains will probably require a protein supplement. Nonprotein nitrogen (NPN) sources are almost always the least cost. Use of NPN carries some restrictions. It is generally recommended that NPN not be fed to cattle under 600 lbs, especially if alfalfa is used as a substantial part of the roughage component. Large operations will design complete supplements incorporating protein supplements (CP > 20 per cent of DM) with bulk and trace mineral supplements. The complete supplement is tailored to the specific situation. Many farmers like to harvest their forage crops by warming up cattle. They handle relatively small numbers and do not own equipment capable of the intricate mixing required to formulate a complete supplement. These feeders will generally buy a commercial complete supplement from a feed company. Precise information about these supplements is generally lacking. The ingredients are not required to be listed in the order of their concentrations, and the general categories (salt, calcium, crude protein, and so forth) are listed as not less than or not more than (e.g., not > 10% salt, not < 40% CP, not > 30% from NPN). We should be aware that the 30% is 30% out of 40% and not 30% of 40%. The carrier ingredients are generally by products of the milling industry (middlings, millrun, short, and so forth) and alfalfa meal. About one half of the ingredients will be energy nutrients. NE$_m$ concentrations in these commercial supplements probably vary between 0.5 and 1.0 Mcal/kg DM and NE$_g$ concentrations probably vary between 0.3 and 0.5 Mcal/kg DM. The disadvantages include lack of information and the complications of NPN. These supplements should be viewed with caution if substantial amounts of alfalfa hay or ensilage (> 20 per cent) are used in the dry ration. For our ration we will formulate a complete supplement. If we have a protein deficiency in the basic energy ration, we will use either soybean meal or cottonseed meal in the supplement. The cost analysis of these two feeds will decide our choice (Table 10).

Cottonseed meal appears to be the least cost protein source, but before deciding we should look at relative energy values. We will value average net energy at $0.078/Mcal (Table 11). The difference in Net energy per CWT = $(0.716 - 0.636) \times 100$

Table 9. *Specific Feed Costs as Fed*

Feed	DM(%)	Cost/CWT	Cost/CWT DM	Cost/Mcal
Corn	89	5.75	5.75/0.89 = 6.46	6.46/81 = 0.0797
Wheat	89	5.50	5.50/0.89 = 6.18	6.18/81 = 0.0763
Barley	89	5.25	5.25/0.89 = 5.70	5.90/73 = 0.081
Sorghum	89	5.00	5.00/0.89 = 5.62	5.62/70 = 0.080

Table 10. *Crude Protein Cost Analysis*

Feed	CP in DM (%)	Cost/CWT as Fed	Cost CP/CWT
Soybean meal*	51.8	11.50	11.50/51.8 = 22.20
Cottonseed meal*	44.8	9.25	9.25/44.8 = 20.60

*Solvent extracted.

Table 11. *Relative Energy Values*

Feed	NE_m	NE_g	Average Energy (Mcal/lb)
Soybean meal	1.89	1.26	$\dfrac{(0.5 \times 1.89) + (0.5 \times 1.26)}{2.2} = 0.716$
Cottonseed meal	1.69	1.11	$\dfrac{(0.5 \times 1.69) + (0.5 \times 1.11)}{2.2} = 0.636$

lb = 8 Mcal. In value this difference = 8×0.078 = \$0.62/CWT in favor of soybean meal. The difference in protein values (CP = \$0.21/lb) per CWT = 22.20 − 20.60 = \$1.60 per CWT. Cottonseed meal is the least cost protein source.

c. Roughage:

There are a number of limitations on the choice of the roughage component. For large operations it is necessary to store several months of supply in the harvest season. Local availability is essential if ensilages are to be used. If corn ensilage is available, it will almost always be the least expensive roughage. This is particularly true when high concentrate finishing rations are used and NPN will provide an adequate crude protein source. Limitations on the use of corn silage include the following: (1) it requires substantial storage space and precise facilities, (2) it cannot be produced in many feeding areas, and (3) there is only one short harvest season; if weather disasters occur, availability may be a problem.

Alfalfa may be a viable alternative to corn silage. Advantages include the following: (1) ordinarily, alfalfa is harvested three to four times per season and weather problems are minimized, and (2) alfalfa has high crude protein concentrations and in maintenance and warm-up situations may provide enough crude protein to eliminate the need for supplement protein. Calcium concentrations are also high in alfalfa.

Small grain crops are often harvested in the vegetative growth stages for hay, and various types of tame and native grasses are often the obvious choices. For an example, we will compare alfalfa hay to corn ensilage on a least cost basis. We will assume that 50 per cent of the ration will be utilized for maintenance. Table 12 lists the values. In this case alfalfa is the least cost roughage source. For our ration we will use a roughage the dry matter of which is composed of 50 per cent alfalfa ensilage and 50 per cent corn ensilage.

d. Minerals:

For sodium chlorine and trace minerals we will use a commercial mix containing 50 per cent NaCl and 50 per cent of a trace mineral (TM) mixture containing magnesium sulfate, potassium sulfate, ferrous carbonate, manganous oxide, cobalt carbonate, calcium iodate, copper sulfate, and zinc sulfate. The TM mix will also contain monensin sodium (rumensin). It is intended that 0.25 per cent of the TM mix in the dry ration will furnish 25 g rumensin/ton DM. Limestone, dicalcium phosphate, and potassium chloride will be used as sources of Ca, P, and K, respectively, if the ration is deficient in these nutrients. If phosphorus is the limiting nutrient, dicalcium phosphate will furnish any necessary calcium as it meets the phosphorus needs.

e. Vitamins:

In general, ruminant animals are expected to synthesize the B vitamins via rumenal microbes. Vitamin C is synthesized in the tissues. Vitamin K is synthesized by microbes in the digestive system. Vitamin D is synthesized endogenously in animals exposed to sunlight. Vitamin A can be limiting if substantial amounts of green forage are not fed. This occurs in high concentrate finishing rations. Vitamin A supplementation may be economically provided by injection or by supplementing drinking water. Vitamin A palmitate is also stable if incorporated in the complete supplement. The metabolic role of vitamin E is linked to that of selenium. White muscle disease in calves and lambs often responds to vitamin E–selenium therapy. It is expected that natural feed stuffs contain adequate vitamin E to supply the requirements of adult cattle.

3. Balancing the ration for energy:

a. Concentrate component DM composed of 50 per cent corn and 50 per cent wheat.

$$NE_m = (0.5 \times 2.15) + (0.5 \times 2.15)$$
$$= 2.15 \text{ Mcal/kg}$$
$$NE_g = (0.5 \times 1.42) + (0.5 \times 1.42)$$
$$= 1.42 \text{ Mcal/kg}$$

Table 12. *Comparison of Alfalfa Hay and Corn Silage on Least Cost Basis*

Feed	DM(%)	NE_m^*	NE_g^*	CP(%)	Cost as Fed/CWT	Cost DM/CWT
Alfalfa hay	89	1.20	0.55	17.0	3.00	3.37
Corn ensilage	30	1.56	0.99	8.5	1.25	4.17

*Mcal/kg DM.

Notes: Average net energy values include:

For alfalfa: $\dfrac{(0.5 \times 1.2) + (0.5 \times 0.55)}{2.2} \times 100 = 40$ Mcal/CWT.

For corn silage: $\dfrac{(0.5 \times 1.56) + (0.5 \times 0.99)}{2.2} \times 100 = 58$ Mcal/CWT.

Crude protein values/CWT include:
For alfalfa: 17 lbs.
For corn silage: 8 lbs.
Comparative values include:
Average energy per Mcal = \$0.078.
Crude protein per lb = \$0.21.
For alfalfa comparative value equals:
$(40 \text{ Mcal} \times 0.078) + (17 \text{ lbs} \times 0.21) = \$6.69$.
For corn silage comparative value equals:
$(58 \text{ Mcal} \times 0.078) + (8.5 \text{ lbs} \times 0.21) = \$6.31$.

Table 13. *Balanced Energy DM Ration*

Feed	DM (kg/day)
Corn	$0.66/2 \times 6 = 1.98$
Wheat	$0.66/2 \times 6 = 1.98$
Alfalfa ensilage	$0.34/2 \times 6 = 1.02$
Corn ensilage	$0.34/2 \times 6 = 1.02$

Table 15. *Deficiencies of DH Energy Ration**

Nutrient	Requirement	Ration Value	Deficiency
Crude protein	0.72 kg	0.728 kg	None
Calcium	29 g	15.11 g	13.89 g
Phosphorus	16 g	20.1 g	None
Potassium	42 g	43.8 g	None
Vitamin A	14,000 I.U.	15,680 I.U.	None

*Computed by comparing the nutritional needs assessment with the nutrient values in the DM ration.

b. Roughage component DM composed of 50 per cent alfalfa ensilage and 50 per cent corn ensilage.

$$NE_m = (0.5 \times 1.56) + (0.5 \times 1.2)$$
$$= 1.38 \text{ Mcal/kg}$$
$$NE_g = (0.5 \times 0.99) + (0.5 \times 0.55)$$
$$= 0.77 \text{ Mcal/kg}$$

c. The desired gain is 1 kg/day. The total DM is estimated as 6.07 kg. We will possibly have to include some supplement, so we will begin our formulation using 6 kg of concentrate plus roughage.

(1) Compute gain using 6 kg of concentrate.

$$\left(RE = 6 \text{ kg} - \frac{5.85 \text{ Mcal}}{2.15 \text{ Mcal/kg}} \right)$$
$$\times 1.42 \text{ Mcal/kg} = 4.67 \text{ Mcal}$$

Live Weight Gain (LWG) = $(13.91 \times 4.67^{0.9116}) (250^{-0.6837}) = 1.3$ kg/day

(2) Compute gain using 6 kg of roughage:

$$RE = \left(6 \text{ kg} - \frac{5.85}{1.38} \right) (0.77) = 1.36 \text{ Mcal}$$

Live Weight Gain (LWG) = $(13.91 \times 1.36^{0.9116}) (250^{-0.6837}) = 0.42$ kg/day

(3) Use the gain rates of the concentrate and roughage components and the desired rate of gain in a Pearson's square to compute the proper mixture of concentrate and roughage needed to balance the ration for energy:

LWG Concentrate 1.3 — $\dfrac{0.58}{0.88} = .66 = 66\%$

(square with 1 in center)

LWG Roughage 0.42 — $\dfrac{0.30}{0.88} = .34 = 34\%$

d. The balanced energy DM ration appears in Table 13.

4. Analyze the DM energy ration for deficiencies of protein, minerals, and vitamins (Tables 14 and 15).

5. Formation of the complete supplement:

a. It is assumed that salt and trace minerals will be required. Salt (0.25 per cent of DM) and a commercial trace mineral mix (0.25 per cent of DM) will be incorporated.

b. The only other deficiency is calcium equal to 13.89 g/animal/day. The least expensive source is limestone. It will require $\dfrac{13.89}{0.3384} = 41$ g of limestone to supply the deficiency.

c. The complete supplement will include:

Salt	$0.0025 \times 6 \text{ kg} \times 1000 \text{ g} =$	15 g
Trace minerals	$0.0025 \times 6 \text{ kg} \times 1000 \text{ g} =$	15 g
Limestone	=	41 g
TOTAL		71 g

Salt = 15/71 = 21 per cent of supplement
TM = 15/71 = 21 per cent of supplement
Limestone = 41/71 = 58 per cent of supplement

The total supplement is

$$\frac{0.071}{6} = 0.0092 = 0.012 \text{ of DM or}$$

1.2 per cent of DM.

6. The complete as fed ration appears in Table 16. It is assumed that implantation of a growth stimulant (Ralgro) will be used in these animals.

Explanation of changes in the revision.

1. In the last five years the availability and economy of computers to analyze and formulate rations have multiplied beyond expectation. For people who wish to get into ration formulation, programmable calculators have been largely superseded. Many people will continue to use these calculators and the programs involved, but ultimately they will change to computers and computer software. These will continue to evolve as both information and technology continue to improve.

2. In 1984, a new NAS-NRC manual, Nutrient Requirements of Beef Cattle, Sixth Revised Edition, was published. Formulas for computing net energy for production were simplified. A number of classes of cattle were added and considered according to frame size. Nutrient concentrations in feeds have been recalculated from an enlarged data base. Some significant changes are apparent. For our example ration we have used feed

Table 14. *Analysis of DM Energy Ration**

Feed	DM(kg)	CP†(kg)	Ca(g)	P(g)	K(g)	Vit. A (I.U.)
Corn	1.98	0.198	0.40	6.14	6.93	792
Wheat	1.98	0.277	1.19	8.12	9.11	—
Alfalfa silage	1.02	0.173	14.28	3.26	34.07	15,096
Corn silage	1.02	0.082	2.75	2.14	9.69	—
	6.00	0.73	18.62	19.66	59.80	15,888

*Values are computed from Table 7.
†CP = Crude protein.

Table 16. *Complete As Fed Ration*

Feed	kg DM	kg as Fed	Per Cent as Fed	1 Ton Formulation *lbs/ton*	*lbs*
Corn	2.22	2.22/0.89 = 2.494	24.3	2000 × 0.243	486
Wheat	2.22	2.22/0.89 = 2.494	24.3	2000 × 0.243	486
Alfalfa ensilage	0.78	0.78/0.3 = 2.6	25.35	2000 × 0.2535	507
Corn ensilage	0.78	0.78/0.3 = 2.6	25.35	2000 × 0.2535	507
Complete supplement	0.071	0.071	0.7	2000 × 0.006	14
	6.071	10.259	100		2000

Feed	kg DM	kg as Fed	Per Cent as Fed	1 Ton Formulation *lbs/ton*	*lbs*
Corn	1.98	1.98 /0.89 = 2.225	19.67	2000 × 0.1967	393.4
Wheat	1.98	1.98 /0.89 = 2.225	19.67	2000 × 0.1967	393.4
Alfalfa ensilage	1.02	1.02 /0.30 = 3.40	30.01	2000 × 0.3001	600.2
Corn ensilage	1.02	1.02 /0.30 = 3.40	30.01	2000 × 0.3001	600.2
Complete supplement	0.071	0.071/1 = 0.071	0.64	2000 × 0.0064	12.8
	6.071	11.321	100.00		2000.0

concentrations listed in NRC Manual for Dairy Cattle, 1978. This part of the revision was completed before NRC Manual for Beef Cattle, 1984, was available, and the concept has not changed. In this revision we are not using the Iowa State metabolizable protein system (Burroughs et al., 1975). We are using the concepts and computations recommended (NRC, 1984). The CP requirements are factorial computations for protein lost in feces, urine, and scurf plus protein deposited in gain, products of conception, and milk. The sum of these factors is divided by the product of digestion efficiency, biologic value, and conversion efficiency (protein intake/outflow of protein from the rumen). The Iowa State metabolizable protein system and other models proposed to evaluate net protein utility are discussed in the last article of this section. This article also considers current concepts of protein metabolism including microbial protein synthesis, digestion, and absorption.

References

1. Agricultural Research Council: The Nutrient Requirements of Ruminant Livestock. Commonwealth Agricultural Bureaux. Surrey, The Gresham Press, 1980.
2. Bartley, E. E., Davidovich, A., Barr, G. W., et al.: Ammonia toxicity in cattle. I. Rumen and blood changes associated with toxicity and treatment methods. J. Anim. Sci. 43:835, 1976.
3. Burroughs, W., Nelson, D. K., and Mertens, D. R.: Protein physiology and its application in the lactating cow: the metabolizable protein feeding standard. J. Anim. Sci. 41:933, 1975.
4. Brody, S.: Bioenergetics and Growth with Special Reference to the Efficiency Complex in Domestic Animals. New York, Reinhold Publishing Corp., 1945.
5. Byers, F. M., and Rompala, R. E.: Rate of protein deposition in beef cattle as a function of mature size, weight and rate of empty body growth. Ohio Beef Cattle Research Report, Animal Science Series 79-1, 1979.
6. Edwards, J. J., and Bartley, E. E.: Soybean meal or starea for microbial protein synthesis or milk production with rations above thirteen percent natural protein. J. Dairy Sci. 62:732, 1979.
7. Ferrell, C. L., Garrett, W. N., Hinman, N., and Grichting, G.: Energy utilization by pregnant and non-pregnant heifers. J. Anim. Sci. 42:937, 1976.
8. Fox, D. G., and Black, J. R.: A system for predicting body composition and performance of growing cattle. J. Anim. Sci. 58:725–730, 1984.
9. Garrett, W. N.: Energetic efficiency of beef and dairy steers. J. Anim. Sci. 32:451, 1971.
10. Garrett, W. N.: Influence of roughage quality on the performance of feedlot cattle. Calif. Feeders' Day Rep. 13:51, 1974.
11. Garrett, W. N.: Energy gain in mature, non-pregnant beef cows. J. Anim. Sci. 34:238 (Abstr.), 1974.
12. Garrett, W. N., and Hinman, N.: Reevaluation of the relationship

between carcass density and body composition of beef steers. J. Anim. Sci. 28:1, 1969.
13. Garrett, W. N.: Least cost gain and profit projection. 1. Estimating nutrient requirements. Calif. Feeders' Day Rep. 15:68, 1976.
14. Garrett, W. N.: Energy utilization of growing cattle as determined in seventy-two comparative slaughter experiments. 3. In Energy Metabolism, Mount, L. E. (ed.). EAAP publ. no. 26. London, Butterworths, 1980.
15. Garrett, W. N.: Factors influencing energetic efficiency of beef production. J. Anim. Sci. 51:1434, 1980.
16. Hespell, R. B.: Efficiency of growth by ruminal bacteria. Fed. Proc. 38:2707, 1979.
17. Johnson, D. E., and Crownover, J. C.: Energy requirements of feedlot cattle in North Central Colorado: variation in maintenance requirements by the month. Research Highlights of the Animal Science Dept., Colorado State University, Experimental Station General Series 948, 1975.
18. Lofgreen, G.: Ruminant energy nutrition. Preconvention Seminar II, Eleventh Annual Conference of the American Association of Bovine Practitioners. Baltimore, 1978.
19. Lofgreen, G. P., and Garrett, W. N.: A system for expressing net energy requirements and feeding values for growing and finishing beef cattle. J. Anim. Sci. 27:793–806, 1968.
20. Mehrez, A. Z., Orskov, E. R., and McDonald, I.: Rates of rumen fermentation in relation to ammonia concentration. Brit. J. Nutr. 38:447, 1977.
21. Moe, P. W., Flatt, W. P., and Tyrell, H. F.: Net energy value of feeds for lactation. J. Dairy Sci., 55:945, 1972.
22. Moore, T.: The calorie as the unit of nutritional energy. World Rev. Nutr. Diet. 26:1–25, 1977.
23. National Research Council: Nutrient Requirements of Beef Cattle, 6th rev. ed. National Academy of Sciences, Washington, D.C., 1984.
24. National Research Council: Nutrient Requirements of Dairy Cattle, 5th rev. ed. National Academy of Sciences, Washington, D.C., 1978.
25. National Research Council: Nutrient Requirements of Sheep, 5th rev. ed. National Academy of Sciences, Washington, D.C., 1975.
26. National Research Council: Effect of Environment on Nutrient Requirements of Domestic Animals. Washington, D.C., National Academy Press, 1981.
27. National Research Council: Nutrient Requirements of Swine, 8th rev. ed. National Academy of Sciences, Washington, D.C., 1979.
28. Owens, F. N. (ed.): Protein Requirements for Cattle: Symposium. Oklahoma State University. MP-109, 1982.
29. Owens, F. N., and Bergen, W. G.: Nitrogen metabolism of ruminant animals: Historical perspective, current understanding and future implications. J. Anim. Sci. 57:498, 1983.
30. Price, W. D., Brown, J. A., Menvielle, E. E., and Smith, W. H.: Effect of high levels of urea in purified diets for lambs: growth and metabolism. J. Anim. Sci. 35:848, 1972.
31. Prior, R. L., and Laster, D. B.: 1979. Development of the bovine fetus. J. Anim. Sci. 48:1546, 1979.
32. Rattray, P. V., Garrett, W. N., Hinman, N., et al.: A system for expressing the net energy requirements and net energy content of feeds for young sheep. J. Anim. Sci. 36:115–122, 1973.
33. Rattray, P. V., Garrett, W. N., East, N. E., and Hinman, N.: Net energy requirements for ewe lambs for maintenance gain and pregnancy and net energy values of feedstuffs for lambs. J. Anim. Sci. 37:853–857, 1973.

34. Rattray, P. V., Garrett, W. N., Meyer, H. H., et al.: Net energy requirements for growth of lambs age three to five months. J. Anim. Sci. *37*:1386–1389, 1973.

35. Rattray, P. V., Garrett, W. N., East, N. E., and Hinman, N.: Efficiency of utilization of metabolizable energy during pregnancy and energy requirements for pregnancy in sheep. J. Anim. Sci. *38*:383–393, 1974.

36. Satter, L. D., and Slyter, L. L.: Effect of ammonia concentration on rumen microbial protein production in vitro. Brit. J. Nutr., *32*:199, 1974.

37. Satter, L. D., and Roffler, R. E.: Nitrogen requirements and utilization in dairy cattle. J. Dairy Sci., *58*:1219, 1975.

38. Satter, L. D., Whitlow, L. W., and Beardsley, G. L.: Resistance of protein to rumen degradation and its significance to the dairy cow. Des Moines, Dist. Feed Res. Counc. Proc. *32*:63, 1977.

39. Slyter, L. L., Satter, L. D. and Dinius, D. A.: Effect of ruminal ammonia concentration on nitrogen utilization by steers. J. Anim. Sci. *48*:906, 1979.

40. Smuts, D. B.: The relation between the basal metabolism and the endogenous nitrogen metabolism with particular reference to the maintenance requirement of protein. J. Nutr. *9*:403, 1935.

41. Virtanen, A. I.: Milk production of cows on protein free feed. Science *153*:1603, 1966.

42. Webster, A. J. F.: Prediction of energy requirements for growth in beef cattle. World Rev. Nutr. Diet. *30*:189–226, 1978.

Special Dietary Management in Lactation and Gestation

JOHN C. SIMONS, D.V.M.
and MICHAEL S. HAND, D.V.M., Ph.D.

The total nutritional requirement of any animal is the sum of the individual requirements for maintenance, body weight change, the products of conception, and milk production. The needs for maintenance are related to environmental temperature and wind velocity. The energy and protein requirements per unit of body weight are inversely related to size. The requirements for weight change in any species vary according to rate of gain, age, and sex. Normal weight increase resulting from growth requires a diet that is high in protein and low in energy relative to the diet required for weight increase in excess of normal growth. Weight gain in females requires a diet that is high in fat (and thus energy) relative to that of males of the same species and comparable age, size, breed, and type.

Specific needs for the products of conception are practically negligible in the first two trimesters of gestation. In the third trimester there is a significant increase in the requirement for all nutrients. The deposition of nutrients in the products of conception increases daily. For convenience, we use average deposition over a period of time in nutrient requirement tables, but the actual situation is a dynamic one in which the need for nutrients is steadily increasing. Average gestation requirements for energy, protein, and minerals vary considerably among species.

The nutrient requirements for lactation are substantial and may exceed three times the maintenance requirement for sows nursing large litters or high-producing dairy cows. The efficiency of feed conversion for milk production is comparable to that of maintenance. Lactating animals may lose weight on what would appear to be maximum amounts of optimum rations.

This article deals with problems encountered in meeting the needs of gestating and lactating females of the food animal species and the consequences of nutritional deficiencies in these animals. In the interest of simplicity, we are using tables and figures derived from the equations and explanations documented in Article 4. Reference to these equations may be necessary for more complete understanding.

BEEF CATTLE

The beef cow is preserved and propagated in the interest of converting plants containing large amounts of cellulose into highly palatable foods that have efficient utility for man. In addition to plants, grains, oil meals, and by-products of food and brewing industries are often fed to beef cattle. The production entities, including growth, gestation, and lactation, can be sustained only after maintenance needs are met. The maintenance ration is the base line of cow-calf nutrition. The objective is to provide least cost rations that are adequate to maintain the cow and, in addition, that allow her to produce one calf every 12 months that will, at weaning time, weigh 40 per cent or more of the cow's normal weight. It is expected that the cow will be able to maintain this level of production until she is eight to ten years old (total lifetime production equals six to eight calves). It is important that we use the feeds that are not otherwise available for consumption by humans or monogastric food animals that are more efficient in the conversion of concentrate foods than are beef animals.

Of special interest is the utilization of roughages that are not of sufficient quality and/or concentration for practical milk production or for high-priced horse forage. Such roughages include the following:

1. Native pastures in mountain, plains, desert, forest, and swamp areas.

2. Crop residues including cornstalks, beet tops, straw, stubbles, and cannery wastes.

3. Medium to low quality hay and ensilage, especially between weaning and late gestation.

Concentrates and high quality roughages are used in beef cow rations in several situations:

1. When transportation costs prohibit exportation to favorable markets.

2. When the market price of high quality feed is low enough to consider in least cost formulations.

3. When supplementation of low quality feeds is necessary to meet practical production objectives.

Nonprotein nitrogen can be used as a protein supplement when the UFP (urea fermentation potential) of the basic ration is positive.

The normal, well-managed beef cow is either gestating, lactating, or both 100 per cent of the time. The heifers are bred as yearlings or two-year-olds (13 to 27 months), and many heifers produce two calves before they stop growing.

The primary considerations in beef cow nutrition include:

1. A nutritional needs assessment of the maintenance and production requirements.

2. A mathematical analysis of the basic forage ration in terms of consumption and nutrient concentration.

3. The deficiencies of the basic forage ration in meeting the maintenance and production requirements.

4. The most economical sources of the necessary supplements.

5. The most practical delivery system.

Ordinarily, beef cows will be offered a free-choice forage ration. This daily intake of forage may include all of the necessary nutrients in excess of maintenance and production objectives (dry cows will gain about 0.45 kg per day on good cornstalks or beet tops).

Most forage rations vary in quality and quantity with season and weather conditions. Cows on high quality free-choice forage may gain weight in the late lactation and post-weaning periods. Overweight cows may lose weight on sub-maintenance rations in mid-gestation without harm to the cow or fetus. The quality of late fall and early winter forage is relatively high and decreases in value and availability as the cow's needs increase in late winter. In late gestation and early lactation, the basic forage ration is often deficient, and knowledge of what is needed, available, and economical is essential in these periods. Cows should be in good condition at parturition and gaining in the breeding season. Quite naturally, native pastures are at their best in the time of greatest need.

The Need Assessment

The California Net Energy System most accurately describes the energy requirements for maintenance (NE_m) and gain (NE_g). At moderate temperatures, the daily requirement for NE_m in megacalories equals $0.077 \times (BW^*)^{0.75}$. This requirement is modified by weather. The Handley formula and/or the table devised by Johnson and Crownover can be used to evaluate the effect of the temperature wind index (TWI).[†]

Net energy for gain must be considered in the case of growing heifers. Table 1 is a reprint of Table 7 in the NAS-NRC publication for beef cattle (1984) and lists net energy requirements for maintenance and gain in 25-kg increments of body weight and varying increments of daily gain.

Net energy requirements for the products of conception can be determined from the following formula:

$$NE_m = \text{calf birth weight (kg)} (0.0149 - 0.0000407t) \times e^{0.05883t - 0.0000804t^2}$$

where NE_m is kcal/day, t is day of gestation, e is the antilog of the natural log of 1 and is approximately equal to 2.72, and a diet of average quality forage (ME of 2.00 Mcal/kg) is assumed. Thus, for a 34-kg anticipated calf birth weight on day 240 of the gestation period, 2300 kcal or 2.3 Mcal of NE_m are required for the conceptus. However, total net energy as well as metabolizable energy and TDN requirements for pregnancy can more readily and practically be obtained from Table 1.

The net energy requirement for lactation is also expressed in Mcal of NE_m. This requirement for dairy cows (NAS-NRC, 1978) is assumed to be 0.6 Mcal NE_m per kg of milk produced. Beef cows produce milk less efficiently. Their requirement is 0.75 Mcal NE_m per kg of milk produced (0.34 Mcal/lb milk). Therefore, a cow producing 4.54 kg (10 lb) of milk per day requires $4.54 \times 0.75 = 3.4$ Mcal NE_m per day for milk production. Total energy requirements for lactation are listed in Table 1.

The gross energy of feed minus fecal energy is termed digestible energy (DE). An approximately equivalent term, total digestible nutrients (TDN) measures DE in weight units. TDN can be converted to DE by the relationship 1 kg TDN = 4.4 Mcal DE (or 1 lb TDN = 2 Mcal DE). TDN and DE are easier to measure than NE_m and NE_g. Therefore, feed analysis laboratories more commonly represent the energy content of a feed in their reports in terms of TDN and DE rather than NE_m and NE_g. The major weakness of the TDN/DE system is that it overestimates the energy available in roughages and underestimates the energy available in concentrates. The system does adequately model energy metabolism in the beef cow. See Table 1 for TDN requirements at various stages of maturity, gestation, and lactation.

Lack of sufficient energy is probably the most common deficiency in cow-calf nutrition. When feed is limited on farms or overstocked ranges, low energy intake occurs. The results include reduction or cessation of growth, weight loss, failure to conceive, and increased mortality. Range animals on deficient rations are more prone to eat toxic plants and are more susceptible to internal parasites. Usually energy deficiency is accompanied by deficiencies of protein and other nutrients. In spite of these shortcomings, rations deficient in energy are sometimes economically acceptable. Desert and semi-desert ranges may be too sparse to supply intake sufficient for optimum production. Supplementation of such rations may be too expensive and inconvenient to justify. Such ranges may support conception and birth rates of 50 to 70 per cent without significant supplementation. Vast acreages of marginal rangeland are controlled by state and federal governments in the western United States. Grazing lease costs for these lands are relatively modest. Generally, cattle operations in these areas have been successful when operating costs have been kept at a minimum and below average production objectives have been accepted.

The crude protein (CP) requirement of breeding cattle is due to several physiologic expenditures. These include metabolic fecal loss (F), endogenous urinary loss (U), scurf loss (S), tissue growth (G), growth of the conceptus (C), and milk production (M). These are represented in a factorial equation for determining crude protein requirement:

$$CP = (F + U + S + G + C + M) \div (D \times BV \times CE)$$

where D is the percentage of dietary protein that may be absorbed as amino acids, BV is the efficiency of conversion of the absorbed amino acids to body protein (maintenance, gain, or milk), and CE is the efficiency of converting dietary protein to ruminal protein output.

Equations to estimate these various crude protein expenditures (grams) include the following:

1. F = 3 per cent of DM intake or 6.8 per cent of fecal DM.

2. $U = 2.75 \, W^{0.5}$.

3. $S = 0.2 \, W^{0.6}$.

4. G = daily gain in kg $\times$ (268 − 29.4 $\times$ energy content of gain in Mcal/kg). The net energy content of the gain = $0.0608 \, W/kg^{0.75}$ (LWG).[1.119] (W is weight in kilograms, and LWG is live weight gain.)

5. C = 55 g/day for the last trimester.

6. M = kg milk/day $\times$ 0.0335.

The factors in the divisors of the factorial equation are

---

*Table 1. Nutrient Requirements of Breeding Cattle**

Weight† (kg)	Daily Gain‡ (kg)	Daily DM§ (kg)	Energy Daily ME (Mcal)	TDN (kg)	NE_m (Mcal)	NE_g (Mcal)	In Diet DM ME (Mcal/kg)	TDN (%)	NE_m (Mcal/kg)	NE_g (Mcal/kg)	Total Protein Daily (g)	In Diet DM (%)	Calcium Daily (g)	In Diet DM (%)	Phosphorus Daily (g)	In Diet DM (%)	Vitamin A Daily (1000's I.U.)
Pregnant yearling heifers—Last third of pregnancy																		
325	0.4	7.1	14.2	3.9	8.04	NA**	2.00	55.2	1.15	NA**	591	8.4	19	0.27	14	0.20	20
325	0.6	7.3	15.7	4.3	8.04	0.77	2.15	59.3	1.29	0.72	649	8.9	23	0.32	15	0.21	20
325	0.8	7.3	17.2	4.8	8.04	1.67	2.35	64.9	1.47	0.88	697	9.5	27	0.37	16	0.22	20
350	0.4	7.5	14.8	4.1	8.38	NA	1.99	55.0	1.14	NA	616	8.3	20	0.27	15	0.21	21
350	0.6	7.7	16.5	4.6	8.38	0.81	2.14	59.1	1.28	0.71	674	8.8	24	0.32	16	0.21	22
350	0.8	7.8	18.1	5.0	8.38	1.76	2.34	64.6	1.46	0.88	720	9.3	27	0.35	17	0.22	22
375	0.4	7.8	15.5	4.3	8.71	NA	1.98	54.7	1.13	NA	641	8.2	21	0.27	15	0.19	22
375	0.6	8.1	17.2	4.8	8.71	0.86	2.13	58.8	1.27	0.70	697	8.6	25	0.31	17	0.21	23
375	0.8	8.2	19.0	5.2	8.71	1.86	2.32	64.1	1.45	0.86	743	9.1	27	0.33	18	0.22	23
400	0.5	8.2	16.1	4.5	9.04	NA	1.97	54.4	1.12	NA	664	8.1	22	0.27	16	0.20	23
400	0.6	8.5	18.0	5.0	9.04	0.90	2.12	58.6	1.26	0.69	721	8.5	25	0.30	18	0.21	24
400	0.8	8.6	19.8	5.5	9.04	1.95	2.31	63.8	1.44	0.85	764	8.9	28	0.33	18	0.20	24
425	0.4	8.6	16.8	4.6	9.36	NA	1.96	54.1	1.11	NA	687	8.0	23	0.27	17	0.20	24
425	0.6	8.9	18.7	5.2	9.36	0.94	2.11	58.3	1.25	0.69	743	8.4	26	0.30	18	0.20	25
425	0.8	9.0	20.7	5.7	9.36	2.04	2.30	63.5	1.43	0.84	786	8.8	28	0.31	19	0.21	25
450	0.4	8.9	17.3	4.8	9.67	NA	1.95	53.9	1.10	NA	710	8.0	23	0.26	18	0.20	25
450	0.6	9.2	19.4	5.4	9.67	0.98	2.10	58.0	1.25	0.68	765	8.3	26	0.29	19	0.21	26
450	0.8	9.4	21.5	5.9	9.67	2.13	2.29	63.3	1.42	0.84	807	8.6	28	0.30	20	0.21	26
Dry pregnant mature cows—Middle third of pregnancy																		
350	0.0	6.8	11.9	3.3	6.23	NA	1.76	48.6	0.92	NA	478	7.1	12	0.16	12	0.18	19
400	0.0	7.5	13.1	3.6	6.89	NA	1.76	48.6	0.92	NA	525	7.0	13	0.17	13	0.17	21
450	0.0	8.2	14.3	4.0	7.52	NA	1.76	48.6	0.92	NA	570	7.0	15	0.17	15	0.18	23
500	0.0	8.8	15.5	4.3	8.14	NA	1.76	48.6	0.92	NA	614	7.0	17	0.19	17	0.19	25
550	0.0	9.5	16.7	4.6	8.75	NA	1.76	48.6	0.92	NA	657	6.9	18	0.19	18	0.19	27
600	0.0	10.1	17.8	4.9	9.33	NA	1.76	48.6	0.92	NA	698	6.9	20	0.20	20	0.20	28
650	0.0	10.7	18.9	5.2	9.91	NA	1.76	48.6	0.92	NA	739	6.9	22	0.21	22	0.21	30
Dry pregnant mature cows—Last third of pregnancy																		
350	0.4	7.4	14.7	4.1	8.38	NA	1.98	54.7	1.13	NA	609	8.2	20	0.27	15	0.20	21
400	0.4	8.2	16.0	4.4	9.04	NA	1.96	54.1	1.11	NA	657	8.0	22	0.27	16	0.20	23
450	0.4	8.9	17.2	4.8	9.67	NA	1.94	53.6	1.10	NA	703	7.9	23	0.26	18	0.21	24
500	0.4	9.5	18.3	5.1	10.29	NA	1.92	53.1	1.08	NA	746	7.8	25	0.26	20	0.21	27
550	0.4	10.2	19.5	5.4	10.90	NA	1.91	52.8	1.07	NA	790	7.8	26	0.25	21	0.21	29
600	0.4	10.8	20.6	5.7	11.48	NA	1.90	52.5	1.06	NA	832	7.7	28	0.26	23	0.21	30
650	0.4	11.5	21.7	6.0	12.06	NA	1.89	52.2	1.05	NA	872	7.6	30	0.26	25	0.22	32

Two-year-old heifers nursing calves—First 3–4 months post partum—5.0 kg milk/day

300	0.2	6.9	16.6	4.6	9.30††	0.72	2.41	66.6	1.53	0.93	814‡‡	11.8	26	0.38	17	0.25	27
325	0.2	7.3	17.4	4.8	9.64††	0.77	2.37	65.5	1.49	0.90	841‡‡	11.5	27	0.37	18	0.25	28
350	0.2	7.8	18.1	5.0	9.98††	0.81	2.34	64.6	1.46	0.88	866‡‡	11.2	27	0.35	19	0.24	30
375	0.2	8.2	18.9	5.2	10.31††	0.86	2.31	63.8	1.44	0.85	892‡‡	10.9	28	0.34	19	0.23	32
400	0.2	8.6	19.7	5.4	10.64††	0.90	2.29	63.3	1.42	0.84	916‡‡	10.7	28	0.33	20	0.23	34
425	0.2	9.0	20.4	5.6	10.96††	0.94	2.27	62.7	1.40	0.82	939‡‡	10.5	29	0.32	21	0.23	35
450	0.2	9.4	21.1	5.8	11.27††	0.98	2.25	62.2	1.38	0.80	963‡‡	10.3	29	0.31	22	0.23	37

Cows nursing calves—Average milking ability—First 3–4 months post partum—5.0 kg milk/day

350	0.0	7.7	16.6	4.6	9.98††	NA	2.15	59.4	1.29	NA	814‡‡	10.6	23	0.30	18	0.23	30
400	0.0	8.5	17.9	4.9	10.64††	NA	2.11	58.3	1.25	NA	864‡‡	10.2	25	0.29	19	0.22	33
450	0.0	9.2	19.1	5.3	11.27††	NA	2.08	57.5	1.23	NA	911‡‡	9.9	26	0.28	21	0.23	36
500	0.0	9.9	20.3	5.6	11.89††	NA	2.05	56.6	1.20	NA	957‡‡	9.7	28	0.28	22	0.22	39
550	0.0	10.6	21.5	5.9	12.50††	NA	2.03	56.1	1.18	NA	1001‡‡	9.5	29	0.27	24	0.23	41
600	0.0	11.2	22.6	6.2	13.08††	NA	2.01	55.5	1.16	NA	1044‡‡	9.3	31	0.28	26	0.23	44
650	0.0	11.9	23.9	6.6	13.66††	NA	2.00	55.3	1.15	NA	1086‡‡	9.1	33	0.28	27	0.23	46

Cows nursing calves—Superior milking ability—First 3–4 months post partum—10.0 kg milk/day

350	0.0	6.2	18.5	5.1	13.73††	NA	3.00	82.9	2.03	NA	1009‡‡	16.4	36	0.58	24	0.39	24
400	0.0	7.6	21.4	5.9	14.39††	NA	2.80	77.4	1.86	NA	1099‡‡	14.4	37	0.49	25	0.33	30
450	0.0	9.1	23.2	6.4	15.02††	NA	2.56	70.7	1.66	NA	1186‡‡	13.1	39	0.43	26	0.29	35
500	0.0	10.0	24.6	6.8	15.64††	NA	2.45	67.7	1.56	NA	1246‡‡	12.4	40	0.40	28	0.28	39
550	0.0	10.9	25.8	7.1	16.25††	NA	2.38	65.8	1.50	NA	1299‡‡	12.0	42	0.39	30	0.27	42
600	0.0	11.6	27.0	7.5	16.83††	NA	2.32	64.1	1.45	NA	1348‡‡	11.6	43	0.37	31	0.27	45
650	0.0	12.4	28.2	7.8	17.41††	NA	2.28	63.0	1.14	NA	1394‡‡	11.3	45	0.36	33	0.26	48

*Expressed in metric units. (National Research Council, Committee on Animal Nutrition: Nutrient Requirements of Beef Cattle. NAS-NRC, Washington, D.C., 1984.)

†Average weight for feeding period.

‡Approximately 0.4 ± 0.1 kg of weight gain/day over the last third of pregnancy is accounted for by the products of conception. Daily 2.15 Mcal of NE_m and 55 g of protein are provided for this requirement for a calf with a birth weight of 36 kg.

§Dry matter consumption should vary depending on the energy concentration of the diet and environmental conditions. These intakes are based on the energy concentration shown in the table and assuming a thermoneutral environment without snow or mud conditions. If the energy concentrations of the diet to be fed exceed the tabular value, limited feeding may be required.

‖Vitamin A requirments per kilogram of diet are 2800 I.U. for pregnant heifers and cows and 3900 I.U. for lactating cows.

**Not applicable.

††Includes 0.75 Mcal NE_m/kg of milk produced.

‡‡Includes 33.5 g protein/kg of milk produced.

assumed to be: D = 0.9, BV = 0.66, and CE = 1.0. Thus, the daily crude protein requirement for a 364-kg (800-lb) two-year-old heifer consuming 8 kg (17.6 lb) of dry matter per day, gaining 0.23 kg (0.5 lb) per day, and nursing a 90-day-old calf (4.54 kg, or 10 lb milk per day) would be

$$CP = (8000 \times 0.0334) + (2.75 \times 364^{0.5}) + (0.2 \times 364^{0.6}) +$$
$$0.23 \times [268 - (29.4 \times 5.06)] + (4.54/0.01 \times 0.0335) = 843 \text{ g},$$
or 1.9 lb (see Table 1).

These calculations have been performed and tabulated for varying stages of maturity, gestation, and production (see Table 1). In nearly all instances, these listed values of crude protein requirement will suffice.

Depressed appetite is said to be the primary sign of protein deficiency in beef cattle diets. Diminished appetite for a ration that is complete and balanced at one level of intake will result in a deficiency of all nutrients when intake falls below that level. It is the authors' opinion that there is little chance for a protein level to fall below maintenance requirements if the animal is consuming enough energy to maintain body weight in any physiologic state. Irregular or delayed estrus is the primary sign of protein shortage in diets for breeding animals. This sign may result from energy deficiency resulting from a depressed appetite. What happens, in fact, is that many cows on rations deficient in protein and/or energy do not conceive while lactating. After weaning, such a cow will not be subject to the stress of either lactation or late gestation. Her requirement for energy and protein will be down, and she will probably be gaining in the following breeding season. Thus, there is a negative feedback mechanism that enables limited reproduction in marginal nutritive situations. Adequate supplementation of these cows may be frustrating. The cow may prefer to wait until tomorrow rather than work for the forage ration on a marginal pasture. Scattering the supplement over a wide area is very inconvenient, and there is some loss of efficiency. In some cases, below average production objectives, including fewer and smaller calves, may be the most practical answer.

Urea and certain other sources of nonprotein nitrogen may be used as supplemental protein and substituted for as much as 25 per cent of the total nitrogen in the diets of pregnant and lactating cows. Supplemental nonprotein nitrogen expressed as urea equivalents should not exceed 1 per cent of the diet. Nonprotein nitrogen is not as well utilized when fed as a supplement to low quality roughages. See Article 4 for methods of determining urea fermentation potential.

Minerals

In formulating mineral rations for beef cows, practical consideration needs to be given to salt, calcium, phosphorus, and magnesium. The specific requirement for some of these minerals may be affected by the potassium concentration in the diet, and sulfur should be considered if nonprotein nitrogen is used as a crude protein source. Iodine-deficient soils prevail in much of the northern United States. Supplementation of iodine is necessary for cattle grazing in deficient areas. Cobalt supplementation is necessary for cattle grazing in some areas of Florida, Michigan, Wisconsin, Massachusetts, New Hampshire, Pennsylvania, and New York. Both selenium-deficient and toxic areas exist in the United States.

The sodium and chlorine needs are expressed as the salt requirement. No special needs for gestation or lactation are apparent. Requirements for sodium and chlorine appear to be met by including 0.1 per cent salt in the dry matter ration. Salt is commonly self-fed free-choice. It is also commonly mixed with other ration ingredients. Intake varies considerably and often exceeds minimum requirements. Grazing cattle will voluntarily consume more salt than those fed dry feeds, and such consumption is increased if the forage is succulent. Salt is often used in beef cattle supplements to control intake of highly palatable supplements. Concentrations may vary from 10 to 50 per cent. Cattle should be gradually introduced to high salt intakes and should have free access to clean water. Salt deficiency produces an abnormal appetite for salt. Prolonged deficiency results in anorexia, unthrifty appearance, and decreased production.

The calcium requirement for beef cows will generally be exceeded by normal concentrations in the forage ration. The daily requirement varies between 12 g for small dry cows and 42 g for large lactating cows of superior milking ability (see Table 1 for specific requirements). Soils in arid and semi-arid climates are ordinarily low in phosphorus. Also, the phosphorus content of plants decreases with maturity. Deficiencies may occur in cattle subsisting on dry mature forage for long periods of time. The minimum for phosphorus (maintenance, gestation, lactation) is said to be 0.22 per cent of the dry diet (2.2 g/kg DM). This figure might possibly be high. Research workers at Utah State University have failed to produce deficiency symptoms in breeding beef cows over a five-year period using a straight forage ration (minimum P content 0.16 per cent). However, it is probably wise to supplement lactating cows grazing on less than excellent forage.

Specifically, the phosphorus requirements vary between 12 g daily for light cows and 31 g daily for heavy lactating cows of superior milking ability (NAS-NRC recommendation; see Table 1). If the phosphorus intake is adequate, wide Ca:P ratios are acceptable. Satisfactory performance has been achieved with Ca:P ratios as high as 7:1. Both calcium and phosphorus may be deficient in dry, mature range forage consisting mostly of grasses. Phosphorus deficiency causes decreased appetite and milk production. In extreme cases, bone changes, lameness, and stiffness may occur. Failure to cycle and conceive are likely consequences. Calcium deficiency is less common, and specific symptoms are not conspicuous. Bone changes will be apparent in advanced cases.

The magnesium requirement of the beef cow is between 7 and 9 g/day during gestation and 21, 22, and 18 g/day during early, mid, and late lactation, respectively. Most cattle feeds appear to contain adequate amounts of magnesium, but there are some complicating circumstances. Generally, magnesium in grains and other concentrates is more available to cattle than is magnesium contained in forages. Also, magnesium in preserved forages is more available relative to pasture forages. Net magnesium absorption is lowest from highly succulent pasture and, in contrast to most nutrients, increases with maturity.

The mean magnesium availability of pasture forage has been calculated to be about 17 per cent. Milk contains a relatively high magnesium level (about 0.08 per cent). Thus, the requirement is directly related to milk production. Under practical conditions two types of magnesium deficiency occur. The least prevalent results from feeding a magnesium-deficient diet for an extended period of time, e.g, calves on an all-milk diet. Young calves require 0.07 per cent magnesium in their diet. The second type (hypomagnesemia, or grass tetany) often occurs without any material depletion of body reserves. Grass tetany can be a major problem when lactating cows are grazing on lush, rapidly growing pastures. Absorption and/or mobilization deficiencies account for the symptoms. Nervousness, incoordination, convulsions, frothing, and sudden death comprise the common syndrome. Feeding high energy range blocks containing 2 to 3 per cent magnesium oxide and 10 to 20 per cent salt (intake control) is an effective preventive measure.

Potassium deficiencies are extremely rare in ordinary beef cattle rations. Lush, rapidly growing pasture may contain up to 3 per cent potassium in the dry matter. Under these conditions, potassium may interfere with magnesium absorption and may complicate the grass tetany problem.

Selenium deficiencies as well as toxicities may occur in the beef cow. Generally, soils (and therefore plants) in northwestern, northeastern, and Atlantic coastal states (including Florida) and in areas around the Great Lakes are deficient in selenium. Forages and grains grown on these soils may contain less selenium than the dietary requirement of 0.1 mg/kg. However, in isolated areas throughout the Rocky Mountain–Great Plains regions of the United States, some plants accumulate toxic amounts (>5 mg/kg) of selenium.

The signs of gross deficiency in cows grazing pastures deficient in selenium include the production of calves with nutritional muscular dystrophy (white muscle disease). Sub-clinical deficiencies of selenium are not easily determined and may limit performance. Infertility has been noted in ewes grazing in selenium-deficient pastures. Signs of toxicity include partial anorexia, loss of tail hair, and sloughing of hooves. Selenium supplementation is usually accomplished via drenches, injections, feed or salt additives, or selenium in fertilizers applied to pastures. Since selenium can be toxic, supplementation should be done carefully. For selenium toxic areas, utilize feeds from nonseleniferous areas and/or rotate cattle through nonseleniferous pastures.

When NPN (nonprotein nitrogen) is used in beef cow diets, sulfur supplements are probably a practical addition. Three grams of inorganic sulfur to 100 g urea is the recommended amount.

Table 2 lists common sources of supplementary minerals for beef cow rations.

Vitamins

Vitamin requirements will generally be met by the natural feeds plus microbial synthesis in the rumen. The exception is vitamin A when fresh forage or hay containing adequate concentrations of beta carotene is not available. The need for vitamin A in beef cows varies from 19,000 I.U. daily for light dry cows to 47,000 I.U. per day for heavy lactating cows of superior milking ability.

Vitamin A deficiency in breeding bulls may lead to a decline in sexual activity and semen quality. In breeding cows, estrus may not be impaired, but conception rates are decreased. Gestation periods may be shortened, and the incidence of retained placentas is increased. Under practical conditions, the following points should be considered: (1) in drought years with prolonged feeding of bleached grasses or hay or when replacement cattle of unknown history have an unthrifty appearance, the body stores of vitamin A may be low; (2) the carotene content of dried or sun-cured forages decreases upon storage in direct relation to temperature, exposure to air and sunlight, and length of storage; (3) vitamin A losses occur during the processing of feeds with steam and pressure or when feeds are mixed with certain oxidizing materials including some minerals or organic aids. In addition, it should be remembered that synthetic vitamin A supplements (vitamin A acetate or vitamin A palmitate) are generally more stable than vitamin A from natural sources. Vitamin A supplementation is relatively inexpensive. Practical administration procedures include feed supplements, addition to drinking water, and parenteral injection. The specific role of beta carotene in reproduction remains unclear.

Summary for Beef Cattle

Using data from NAS-NRC publications, laboratory analysis, and current weather information, requirements for maintenance, gain, late pregnancy, and lactation of beef cattle can be calculated. Use of the NAS-NRC publication *Nutrient Requirements of Dairy Cattle* (1978) to supplement information included in the NAS-NRC publication for beef cattle (1984) can be helpful.

1. Energy requirements for maintenance, late gestation, and lactation can all be calculated in terms of net energy for maintenance (NE_m).
   a. Maintenance needs are calculated from the equation $NE_m = 0.077 \times (BW^*)^{0.75}$ in moderate weather conditions. The effects of weather on the net energy requirements for maintenance can be calculated from the equation NE_m (kcal/kg) $(BW^*)^{0.75} = (116) - (0.8133 \times TWI)$ (temperature wind index). See Field Calculations for Ration Formulation in Food Animals.
   b. Late gestation needs may be assumed to equal maintenance needs plus 1.57 Mcal NE_m per day.
   c. Lactation needs = 0.75 Mcal NE_m/kg milk produced.
   d. Needs for gain in growing heifers and/or adult cows being flushed for breeding can be calculated by the following equations: for cows: $NE_g = 6.2$ Mcal/kg gain; for growing heifers: $NE_g = (0.0608 \times W^{0.75})(LWG)^{1.119}$.
2. Protein needs are calculated on the basis of crude protein.
   a. Crude protein concentrations in a wide variety of feeds are listed in Table 8 of the NAS-NRC publication *Nutrient Requirements of Beef Cattle* (1984).

Table 2. *Common Sources of Supplementary Minerals for Beef Cow Rations*

Mineral Deficiency	Source
Calcium and phosphorus	Dicalcium phosphate (23.13% Ca and 18.65% P)
Sodium, chlorine, and iodine	Iodized salt (40% Na, 60% Cl, and 0.01% I)
Magnesium	Magnesium oxide (50% Mg) or magnesium sulfate (20% Mg)
Sulfur	Magnesium sulfate (27% S) or calcium sulfate (24% S)
Selenium	Sodium selenite (45.6% Se)

*BW in kg.

b. Daily requirements of crude protein (CP) and digestible protein (DP) are listed in Table 1.
3. Daily requirements of calcium and phosphorus are listed in Table 1. Generally, salt is fed free-choice or at the rate of 0.1 per cent of the dry matter. Seven to nine grams of magnesium are required daily by the gestating cow, and 21, 22, and 18 g/day are needed during early, mid, and late lactation, respectively. The minimum requirement for selenium is 0.1 mg/kg dry matter, whereas over 5 mg/kg may be toxic.
4. Concentrations of vitamin A expressed as mg/kg of carotene per kg DM and the daily requirements for vitamin A (1 mg carotene = 400 I.U. vitamin A) are also listed in the NAS-NRC publication for beef cattle.
5. The requirements for vitamins D, E, and K and the B vitamins will usually be met by concentrations in the energy feeds or by microbial synthesis in the rumen.

A number of rules of thumb may be formulated from computation data. (1) Net energy requirements over maintenance increase about 25 per cent in late gestation, from 40 to 80 per cent at peak lactation, and from 15 to 20 per cent over maintenance plus lactation in the breeding season for growth and/or gain. (2) Protein requirements over maintenance increase 15 to 30 per cent in late gestation, 100 to 300 per cent in peak lactation, and 10 to 15 per cent over maintenance and lactation for growth and/or gain in the breeding season.

Calcium and phosphorus needs increase about 25 per cent in late gestation and from 100 to 375 per cent in peak lactation. Magnesium needs in gestating cows probably increase by 25 per cent. In lactation, these needs probably increase by 50 to 100 per cent. Magnesium absorption is decreased when the cows are eating succulent forage. Excess potassium and/or nitrogen may also interfere with absorption. In addition, magnesium deficiencies are more likely to manifest themselves if calcium is deficient. It is practical to feed a salt-controlled, high energy supplement containing 2 to 3 per cent magnesium oxide or 3 to 5 per cent magnesium sulfate when grass tetany is a problem. Vitamin A requirements increase by 15 to 25 per cent in late gestation and by up to 125 per cent in lactation (avg. 20 to 25 per cent).

Tall fescue is the major cool season grass grown in the southeast. Almost all of the tall fescue is infested by an endophyte fungus. This fungus (presumed to be present on fescue grazed during the high ambient temperatures of the summer months) has been incriminated in a number of conditions collectively referred to as the "summer syndrome." These conditions include unthriftiness and sometimes loss of body weight, rough hair coat, panting, and increased body temperature. Cattle being bred in the summer may experience poor reproductive performance (reduced conception rate) if grazing infested fescue. Also, cows grazing tall fescue in the summer produce less milk. Management procedures, which call for rotating cattle out of fescue pastures during the summer or planting clover with fescue, do much to control the problem. New fescue varieties being developed and certified fungus-free seed offer promise.

Example Ration Outline

I. Data
Location: Midwestern U.S.
Class: Conventional two-year-old heifers, breeding season

Body weight: 364 kg (800 lb)
Desired gain: 0.23 kg (0.5 lb) daily
Estimated milk production: 4.54 kg (10 lb daily)
Estimated DM consumption: 8 kg (17.6 lb) daily
Temperature wind index: 48 (NE_m reqmt = 0.077 × $[BW^*]^{0.75}$)

II. Daily requirements per heifer
   A. NE_m for maintenance plus lactation: 9.8 Mcal (from Table 1)
   NE_g for gain: 0.96 Mcal (from Table 1)
   TDN for maintenance and lactation: 5.1 kg (11.2 lb), or 63.8 per cent of the diet dry matter if consuming at least 2.3 per cent of body weight in DM (from Table 1).
   B. Crude protein requirement: 0.86 kg (1.9 lb), or 10.8 per cent of the diet dry matter if consuming at least 2.3 per cent of body weight in DM (from Table 1)
   C. Mineral requirement:
      1. Calcium: 17 g (from Table 1)
      2. Phosphorus: 19 g (from Table 1)
      3. Magnesium: 21 g (from text)
      4. Salt (0.5 per cent DM): 40 g (from text)
   D. Vitamin A: 31,000 I.U. (from Table 1)
III. Forage ration analysis: assume free-choice native short grass in an intermediate stage of maturity
   A. Nutrient concentration per kg DM:
   NE_m: 1.25 Mcal
   NE_g: 0.6 Mcal
   TDN: 650 g
   Crude protein: 110 g
   Calcium: 4.5 g
   Phosphorus: 1.6 g
   Magnesium: 1.4 g
   Salt: none
   B. Total nutrients in forage ration and requirements:
      1. NE_m for maintenance and lactation:
         Requirement: 9.8 Mcal
         Ration supplies 8 × 1.25 = 10 Mcal
         Ration available for gain $10 - \dfrac{9.8}{1.25} = 2.16$ kg
      2. NE_g for gain:
         Requirement for 0.23-kg gain = 1.13 Mcal
         Ration supplies 2.16 × 0.6 = 1.30 Mcal
      3. TDN:
         Requirement: 5.1 kg
         Ration supplies 8 × 650 g = 5.2 kg
      4. Crude protein:
         Requirement: 860 g
         Ration supplies 8 × 110 = 880 g
      5. Calcium:
         Requirement: 27 g
         Ration supplies 8 × 4.5 = 36 g
      6. Phosphorus:
         Requirement: 19 g
         Ration supplies 8 × 1.6 = 12.8 g
      7. Magnesium:
         Requirement: 21 g
         Ration supplies 8 × 1.4 = 11.2 g
      8. Salt:
         Requirement: 40 g
         Ration supplies 0

---

*BW in kg.

C. Deficiencies of the forage ration:
   Phosphorus 6.2 g
   Magnesium 9.8 g
D. Sources of supplements and required amounts:
   1. Phosphorus: 6.2-g deficiency
      Dicalcium phosphate (18.65 per cent P)

      $$\frac{6.2}{0.1865} = 33 \text{ g } (\sim 1 \text{ oz})$$

   2. Magnesium: 9.8-g deficiency
      Magnesium oxide (60 per cent Mg)

      $$\frac{9.8}{0.6} = 16 \text{ g } (\sim 0.5 \text{ oz})$$

   3. Salt: 40 g
   4. Total supplements per day: 89 g
E. Supplement delivery system:
   Supply a free-choice mixture containing:
   dicalcium phosphate 33/89 = 37 per cent
   magnesium oxide   16/89 = 18 per cent
   salt   40/89 = 45 per cent

THE DAIRY COW

The dry matter feed consumption of a lactating cow is equal to between 2 and 4 per cent of her body weight. The great variation is largely due to differences in milk production. An average-sized cow (600 kg or 1320 lb) producing 25 kg (55 lb) of 4 per cent fat-corrected milk (FCM 4 per cent) will consume about 3 per cent of her body weight (18 kg) in feed dry matter per day.

Energy

The NAS-NRC publication *Nutrient Requirements of Dairy Cattle* (1978) uses one value to express energy needs for maintenance, pregnancy, milk production, and body changes (Moe et al., 1972). This value is designated as net energy for lactation (NE_L).

The maintenance requirement of lactating cows was found to be 73 kcal NE_L/kg $(BW)^{0.75}$. An activity allowance of 10 per cent is added, so the maintenance requirement is computed as 80 kcal (0.080 Mcal) NE_L/kg $(BW)^{0.75}$. To support the activity of grazing, allowances for maintenance should be increased by 10 per cent on good quality pasture and 20 per cent on sparse.

The influence of cold is probably minimized by the normally high heat production of cows consuming large amounts of feed. When loose housing systems are used, it seems advisable to increase feed intake up to 8 per cent in severe winter conditions.

Few quantitative data are available for the energy requirements of gestation. Balance experiments (Flatt et al., 1969) indicated that the total energy requirements for pregnant cows increased markedly in the last four to eight weeks of gestation. It would appear that an additional 3 to 6 Mcal above maintenance are required to meet the need. The requirements for maintenance plus late gestation are currently calculated as 104 kcal (0.104 Mcal) NE_L/kg $(BW)^{0.75}$

The dry period of a dairy cow is relatively short (usually six to ten weeks). Liberal feeding in the last two to three months of gestation ensures proper fetal development and storage of energy that may be used in early lactation. Nevertheless, care should be taken to avoid overfattening, especially with corn ensilage–based diets. Cows in good condition should receive minimal amounts of concentrates throughout most of the dry period. Concentrate levels are increased in the last two to three weeks of pregnancy to adapt the rumen microorganisms to the high energy ratio that will be required for early lactation. Grain feeding does not significantly increase the severity of udder edema (Jensen et al., 1942; Schmidt and Schultz, 1959).

It is important to bring a cow to full feed as rapidly as possible following parturition to avoid excess weight loss and symptoms of ketosis. High-producing cows are often unable to consume enough feed in early lactation to prevent some loss of body energy, calcium, phosphorus, and perhaps protein. These losses are minimized by feeding maximum amounts, within safety limits, of a properly balanced ration during the first six to eight weeks of lactation. After the first two months of lactation, milk yields should be used to calculate the energy requirement. NE_L requirements for milk production are directly related to the fat content of the milk. The requirement for 4 per cent fat-corrected milk is 0.74 Mcal/kg of milk produced. Because the efficiency of milk production compares favorably with the efficiency of maintenance relative to energy consumption, energy deficiency will result in weight loss as well as decreased milk production. Consistent gradual weight loss acts as a negative feedback mechanism that interferes with the normal estrous cycle. It is difficult to maintain a calving interval of less than 380 days for adult cows and 400 days for growing heifers.

Energy utilization in ruminant animals depends to a large extent on microbial fermentation in the reticulorumen. The texture and content of ingested feedstuffs dictate the variety of microflora present in the rumen and, therefore, the nature and amounts of microbial metabolites available to the host animal. These metabolites in turn influence the way energy is used (i.e. milk synthesis vs. synthesis of body tissue). In general, rations with high roughage content result in higher acetate-propionate ratios and produce more milk fat than diets high in concentrates. Therefore, the roughage content (fiber) as well as the physical form are important considerations in a lactation ration. The roughage content of the dry cow ration can also have serious herd health ramifications. The feeding of high fiber rations during the dry period reduces the incidence of displaced abomasum and other postcalving disorders. Minimum crude fiber levels of 15 per cent of ration dry matter for heifers and bulls and 17 per cent for lactating and dry cows are recommended (NAS-NRC, 1978). The paradox most commonly encountered when feeding high-producing dairy cows is feeding enough energy *and* enough fiber.

Protein

The NAS-NRC publication for dairy cows uses a factorial method to compute the protein requirement. The factorial formula for adult female cattle is:

Total Crude Protein (TCP) =
$$\frac{(U + F + S + G + C)}{0.45} + \frac{(L)}{0.52}$$

In this formula:
U = Protein loss in urine,
F = Protein loss in fecal material,
S = Protein loss in skin secretions, scurf, and hair,
G = Protein deposited in growth or gain,

C = Protein deposited in the products of conception,

L = Protein deposited in milk

0.45 = Efficiency of crude protein utilization for processes other than lactation, and

0.52 = Efficiency of crude protein utilization for lactation.

Using Table 2, NAS-NRC, 1978, a 600-kg (1320-lb) cow requires daily: 489 g crude protein for maintenance, 931 g crude protein for maintenance plus the products of conception during the last two months of pregnancy, and 87 g crude protein per kg of 4 per cent FCM. Thus, a 600-kg cow producing 25 kg (55 lb) of 4 per cent milk requires (489) + (25 × 87) = 2664 grams of crude protein daily ($\frac{2664}{18,000}$ = 0.148, or 14.8 per cent of a dry diet of 18 kg).

The protein concentration in milk can be calculated from the fat concentration (per cent protein = 0.4 × per cent fat + 1.9). Thus, milk containing 4 per cent fat should contain 0.4 × 4 + 1.9 = 3.5 per cent protein.

Cows may store protein in blood, liver, and muscle tissue. These reserves will be rapidly depleted in late gestation or lactation if the diet is protein deficient. Chronic protein deficiency results in depressed appetite and, thus, concurrent deficiency of energy and other nutrients. The consequences include depressed milk production, loss of condition, and failure to cycle. The protein content of blood, liver, and muscle is decreased in protein-deficient animals. Protein concentration in blood serum can be used to diagnose the condition. Serum from animals having adequate protein nutrition normally contains 3 to 3.5 g of albumin, 4 to 5 g of globulins, and 10 to 20 mg of urea nitrogen per 100 ml. Serum concentrations of less than 2.5 g of albumin and 7 mg of urea nitrogen per 100 ml are indicative of protein-deficient diets. Pregnant cows on protein-deficient diets will have smaller than normal calves. Reduced transport and immune proteins and reduced hormone secretions may predispose animals to infections and metabolic diseases.

The use of urea and other nonprotein nitrogen substances in dairy cow rations is quite limited. It is feasible to use NPN to increase crude protein concentrations up to 12.6 per cent for an all-corn grain ration or up to 9.4 per cent for an all-corn silage ration.

If a 600-kg cow consumes 16.8 kg dry matter per day of an all-corn ration containing 33 per cent corn grain and 67 per cent corn silage and this ration is supplemented with urea to give a UFP value of 0, the nutrient analysis includes:

NE$_L$ = 29.1 Mcal (will support production of 25 kg 4 per cent FCM)*

CP = 10.5 per cent (will support production of 14.7 kg 4 per cent FCM)†

If milk production and, thus, energy intake are increased, the protein deficiencies of this ration become greater. Thus, it would appear that the use of NPN to supplement the rations of cows producing more than 24 kg (52.8 lb) of milk is not practical. If preformed protein supplements or alfalfa is used in significant amounts, the UFP of the total ration will be negative and NPN supplementation will be ineffective. Using Iowa State University

criteria, practical use of urea should not exceed 1.18 per cent of total dry matter for an all-corn grain ration and not more than 0.64 per cent of an all-corn silage ration. This recommendation is compatible with the NRC-NAS recommendation that urea should not exceed 1 per cent of the ration dry matter.

Minerals

Dairy cows are generally fed mixtures of high quality roughage and concentrates in amounts necessary to meet substantial production objectives. Deficiencies that are likely to occur include those of calcium when corn ensilage comprises the bulk of the forage ration; phosphorus when milk production exceeds about 25 kg of milk per cow per day; and magnesium when the cow is producing milk. The unsupplemented ration can probably be depended on to supply the maintenance need.

The maintenance requirement for calcium is assumed to be 1.6 g/100 kg BW (with adjustments for differences in metabolic size for mature animals). Calcium deposited during gestation is low until the last two months of pregnancy. About 75 per cent of total fetal calcium is deposited in this period. Each kilogram of 4 per cent FCM contains an average of 1.23 g of calcium. Assuming an availability of 45 per cent, the requirement for lactation is 2.7 g of calcium per kg of milk.

This NAS-NRC, 1978, recommendation recognizes some weaknesses in available data.

1. Endogenous and metabolic losses are not consistently measured by different experimental techniques.

2. True absorption (availability) is difficult to measure because dairy cattle maintain calcium reserves by increasing or decreasing the percentage of calcium absorbed.

3. Young animals absorb calcium more efficiently than do mature animals.

4. The absorption of calcium may also be affected by vitamin D, phosphorus intake, and acid-base balance. High fat diets increase calcium losses through the formation of soaps.

The calcium requirement values are consistent with results from many feeding trials and successful feeding practices.

Calcium deficiency in dairy cows is manifested by two well-known syndromes.

1. Depletion of calcium reserves in the skeleton results in weakened and fragile bones in mature animals and rickets in young animals. It is quite common for high-producing cows to lose calcium in early lactation and replace it as production decreases. It is only in extreme cases that significant fragility of bones and decreased milk production occur.

2. Parturient paresis (milk fever) is caused by a disturbance in calcium metabolism. The syndrome is manifested by a marked drop in blood serum calcium at or near parturition. Calcium intake during the dry period influences the problem. Experimental data indicate that high calcium intake in the dry period aggravates the condition and low calcium intake (8 g daily per 450-kg cow) in the last two weeks of gestation followed by a calcium-rich diet after parturition tends to prevent the problem. Some data indicate that the calcium-phosphorus ratio is critical, but other evidence suggests that the calcium level is more important.

The estimated phosphorus requirement is based on an apparent decline in true digestibility of phosphorus rela-

---

*NAS-NRC recommendation for energy.

†NAS-NRC recommendation for CP.

tive to age. Experimental data suggest a decline from about 99 per cent in calves to about 55 per cent in animals weighing over 400 kg. For gestation, the requirement is based on slaughter data (a 40-kg calf contains 298 g of phosphorus). About 75 per cent of this deposition takes place in the last two months of gestation. The phosphorus requirement for milk production is assumed to be the phosphorus content of the milk divided by 0.55. Phytate phosphorus appears to be utilized by ruminants with an efficiency comparable to that of phosphorus from inorganic sources.

The calcium-phosphorus ratio is apparently less critical in ruminants compared with nonruminants. Experimental data demonstrate satisfactory performance with ratios varying from 1:1 up to 8:1. In long-term experiments, better absorption occurred with a ratio of 2:1 than with a ratio of 1:1.

Relative to calcium, plasma phosphorus is not as closely regulated by homeostatic control mechanisms. Thus, when inadequate diets are fed, signs of deficiency become evident at an earlier stage than with calcium deficiency. Signs of phosphorus deficiency include increased fragility of bone and anorexia, and blood plasma inorganic phosphorus declines to subnormal levels (below 4 mg/100 ml). In chronic phosphorus deficiency, the animal sometimes becomes stiff in the joints. Anestrus and low conception rates may be manifested in breeding animals. The phosphorus content of milk does not decline.

The magnesium requirement for lactating cows is about 2 to 2.5 g of available magnesium daily plus 0.12 g per kg of milk produced. There are many factors that affect this requirement under practical conditions. It is difficult to select a dietary level that is adequate at all times without having more than is needed part of the time. Since cattle have a good homeostatic control mechanism for eliminating excess magnesium via the urine and relatively poor homeostatic control of mobilizing the skeletal reserves, in the face of deficiency, modest errors on the high side are tolerable. The suggested magnesium concentration in the dry diets of lactating cows is 0.2 per cent in cows fed substantially on preserved forages and/or concentrates. The concentration should be increased to 0.25 per cent in cows fed on lush pasture in cool seasons. Some supplemental magnesium in a readily available form (magnesium oxide) should be supplied in the concentrate or mineral mixture under these conditions. Magnesium toxicity is not known to be a practical problem in dairy cattle.

Magnesium deficiency produces the same syndrome in dairy as in beef cows. It is less likely to occur because substantially more concentrates are fed to dairy cows and conscientious supplementation is more likely to be carried out.

Potassium deficiency is not generally considered to be a practical problem in gestating or lactating cows. As a rule, the forage ration contains more than adequate amounts.

It is expected that the sodium, chlorine, and iodine needs will be met by feeding iodized sodium chloride equal to 0.5 per cent of the dry ration. The NAS-NRC, 1978, recommendation for iodine is 12 mg/day (0.6 to 0.8 ppm ration). Iodine toxicosis can occur when dietary intake exceeds 100 mg/day. Herd complaints associated with excessive iodine supplementation include decreased milk production and feed consumption and increased incidence of disease.

Sulfur may be beneficial when significant amounts of NPN are fed. For efficient utilization of urea, a nitrogen-sulfur ratio of 10:1 is suggested.

Vitamins

When high quality ingredients are fed to meet production objectives, all vitamin requirements are usually met without supplementation. However, there are exceptions.

1. Cows that are kept in the barn all of the time may develop symptoms of vitamin D deficiency.

2. Cows fed less than 3.6 to 4.5 kg (8 to 10 lb) of good quality alfalfa hay may require vitamin A supplementation.

3. There is growing evidence that niacin supplementation (6 g/day) is of value, particularly in stressed cows, as evidenced by increased feed intake and milk production. The effect may be on microbial protein synthesis and/or reduction of sub-clinical ketosis in early lactation (Kung et al., 1980).

Common Problems

A number of problems related to nutrition continue to plague the dairyman, and better solutions are still being sought.

1. Maintaining a 12- to 13-month calving interval is very difficult for high-producing dairy cows, especially for heifers that are still growing in the first lactation period.

2. The appetites of cows are ordinarily decreased for a short time after parturition. Hypoglycemia and ketosis present special problems. The problems are minimized by adjusting the rumen to concentrate feeds in the last two to three weeks of gestation,

3. High concentrate rations tend to propagate lactic acid–producing bacteria. Butter fat content may be lowered by such rations. Finely ground high quality roughage may cause similar problems. Sodium bicarbonate, magnesium oxide, and/or yeast is commonly fed to lactating cows to prevent the syndrome.

4. Hypocalcemia is a constant problem at or near parturition. Reducing the calcium level in the ration of dry cows in late gestation to deficiency levels (1.1 g per 50 kg body weight) while maintaining adequate phosphorus intake is an effective method of preventing milk fever in susceptible cows. This procedure should be undertaken during the last two to four weeks of gestation. Calcium-rich diets are begun in the immediate post-parturient period. The low intake of dietary calcium is believed to stimulate the secretion of parathormone, which catalyzes the formation of active vitamin D.

5. Grass tetany may occur in cattle grazing rapidly growing succulent pasture or being fed similar green chop. Feeding 28 to 85 g (1 to 3 oz) of magnesium oxide daily in grain or salt will prevent the condition.

Ration Formulation (Adult Lactating Cows)

I. Assumptions:

The energy requirement is based on net energy for lactating cows (NE_L). The protein requirement is based on data from the NAS-NRC publication *Nutrient Requirements of Dairy Cattle* (1978). The requirements for calcium, phosphorus, salt, and magnesium are computed from tables from this publication.

NE_L values for maintenance =

$$0.08 \text{ Mcal } NE_L/(BW)^{0.75}$$

Table 3. *Formulation of Energy-Protein Ration (Dry Matter)*

Ingredient	NE_Ld	CP	CF	Ca	P	NaCl	Mg	Vit. A
Ground corn	2.03	10.0	2	0.03	0.31	—	0.13	1
Soybean meal	1.86	49.6	7	0.36	0.75	0.31 (Na)	0.30	—
Corn ensilage	1.59	8.0	24	0.27	0.20	—	0.28	18
Alfalfa hay	1.25	16.0	33	1.35	0.22	—	0.29	26
Salt	—	—	—	—	—	100	—	—
Dicalcium phosphate	—	—	—	23.7	18.84	2.71	—	—
Magnesium oxide	—	—	—	—	—	—	60	—

Body weight: 600 kg

Milk production: 25 kg, 4 per cent FCM per cow per day

Dry matter consumption: 18 kg per cow per day

Least cost nutrients include:

    For energy: ground corn 89 per cent DM

    For protein: soybean meal (SBM) sol. ext. 89 per cent DM

    For roughage (fiber): 60 per cent corn ensilage, 35 per cent DM; 40 per cent alfalfa hay, 89 per cent DM

    For Ca and P: dicalcium phosphate

    For Na, Cl, and I: iodized No. 4 salt

    For Mg: magnesium oxide

Ingredient analysis of dry matter for:

    Net energy for lactating cows (NE_L): Mcal/kg

    Crude protein (CP): g/kg

    Crude fiber (CFG): per cent

    Urea fermentation potential (UFP): g/kg

    Ca, P, NaCl, and Mg: per cent of DM

    Vitamin A: 1000 I.U./kg

II. Needs assessment (daily requirements per cow):

  NE_L: $(600^{0.75} \times 0.08) + (0.74 \times 25) = 28.2$ Mcal

  28.2 Mcal ÷ 18 kg DMI = 1.57 Mcal/kg DM

  NE_L concentration in dry matter: 28.2/18 = 1.57 Mcal/kg DM

  CP: (489 g for maintenance) + (87 g/kg milk × 25 kg milk) = 2664 g

  CF: at least 15 per cent of the ration dry matter, preferably 17 per cent

  Ca: (21) + (2.7 × 25) = 88.5 g

  P: (17) + (1.8 × 25) = 62 g

  NaCl: 0.005 × 18,000 = 90 g

  Mg: 0.002 × 18,000 = 36 g

  Vitamin A: 50,000 I.U.

III. Formulation of energy-protein ration (dry matter): Table 3

  A. Energy (NE_L):

    NE_L concentration in the roughage component = (0.6 × 1.59) + (0.4 × 1.25) = 1.45 Mcal/kg

    NE_L concentration in the concentrate component is estimated to be 1.98 Mcal/kg

    The Pearson's square is used to determine the relative percentages of the roughage and concentrate components.

1.98 — 12 parts concentrate percentage = 23% of DM

      [1.57]

1.45 — 41 parts roughage percentage = 77% of DM

      53 parts

  B. Protein (CP):

    The total crude protein of the ration will exceed 13 per cent of the dry matter so the total ration UFP will be negative. All of the positive UFP of the corn and corn ensilage will be utilized to synthesize microbial protein.

    Total CP available from concentrate (corn):

    18 kg DMI × 23 per cent = 4.4 kg corn

    4.14 kg × 10 per cent CP = 414 g CP

    Total CP available from roughage (ensilage 60 per cent plus alfalfa 40 per cent):

    18 kg DMI × 77 per cent = 13.86 kg roughage

    13.86 kg × 60 per cent = 8.32 kg ensilage

    13.86 kg × 40 per cent = 5.54 kg alfalfa

    8.32 kg × 8 per cent CP = 666 g CP ensilage

    5.54 kg × 16 per cent CP = +886 g CP alfalfa

                         1552 g CP roughage

                        +414 g CP concentrate

                        1966 g CP total ration

    CP requirement = 2664 g

    ration CP = 1996 g

    CP deficit = 698 g

    Determine amount of SBM required to meet total ration CP requirement:

    698 g ÷ 49.6 per cent CP (SBM) = 1.4 kg SBM

    Subtract 1.4 kg corn and add 1.4 kg SBM to make up new concentrate mix that contains 34 per cent SBM and 66 per cent corn.

  C. Check crude fiber (CF):

    8.32 kg ensilage ÷ 18 kg 46 per cent ration DM × 24 per cent CF = 11 per cent

    5.54 kg alfalfa ÷ 18 kg = 31 per cent ration DM × 33 per cent CF = 10 per cent

    1.4 kg SBM ÷ 18 kg = 8 per cent ration DM × 7 per cent CF = 0.5 per cent

    2.74 kg corn ÷ 18 kg = 15 per cent ration DM × 2 per cent CF = 0.3 per cent

            Total ration CF = 21.8 per cent

IV. Formulating mineral–vitamin A ration: Table 4

  A. Minerals and vitamins available in energy-protein ration in grams and 1000s of I.U.

  B. Deficiencies:

    Calcium, magnesium, and vitamin A are present in amounts that exceed the requirements.

    Deficiency for P: 62 − 47.8 = 14.2 g

    Deficiency for salt: 90 − 10.9 = 79 g

  C. Supplements:

    Dicalcium phosphate: $\dfrac{14.2}{0.1884} = 75$ g

    Salt: 75 g

    Adequate supplementation will best be ensured by adding $\dfrac{75}{18,000} = 0.42$ per cent dicalcium phosphate and $\dfrac{79}{18,000} = 0.44$ per cent iodized salt to the concentrate component of the ration.

V. Final dry matter ration: Table 5.

Table 4. *Formulation of Mineral–Vitamin A Ration*

Ingredient	Ca	P	NaCl	Mg	Vit. A
Corn	0.0003 × 2740 = 0.8	0.0031 × 2740 = 8.5	—	0.0013 × 2740 = 3.6	2.74
Soybean meal	0.0036 × 1400 = 5.0	0.0075 × 1400 = 10.5	$\frac{0.0031 \times 1400}{0.4} = 10.9$	0.0031 × 1400 = 4.3	—
Corn silage	0.0027 × 8320 = 22.5	0.002 × 8320 = 16.6	—	0.0028 × 8320 = 23.3	150
Alfalfa	0.0135 × 5540 = 74.8	0.0022 × 5540 = 22.2	—	0.0029 × 5540 = 16.1	144
TOTALS	103.1	47.8	10.9 (equivalent)	47.3	297

SOWS AND GILTS

Nutrient requirements for breeding swine are listed in Tables 7 and 8 of the NAS-NRC publication, *Nutrient Requirements of Swine* (1979). Nutrient concentrations in various feeds are listed in Table 8 of this publication.

Energy

Energy values are expressed for digestible energy (DE) and metabolizable energy (ME) in kilocalories per kilogram of feed and as kilocalories required per animal per day for various classes and physiologic states. Much of published information on energy requirements for pigs is expressed in terms of TDN. To use the caloric system, it is necessary to convert TDN values to DE or ME. One kilogram of TDN = 4400 kcal. DE values approximate 96 per cent of ME values with some significant variations.

The estimation requirements for energy of the pregnant sow or gilt have been markedly reduced in recent years. Research has shown that efficiency of energy utilization improves if only moderate weight gains are allowed in the gestation period and if feed intake is increased during lactation.

Protein

The quality of the dietary protein is determined by its ability to supply all of the essential amino acids in adequate amounts and sufficient nitrogen for synthesis of nonessential amino acids. Optimum performance requires essential amino acid balance and feed levels. Some variation in crude protein levels is acceptable if these conditions are met.

The requirements for essential amino acids listed in *Nutrient Requirements of Swine* (1979) correspond to the requirements for the natural isomer (L) that normally occurs in feeds. Synthetic amino acids comprised of other isomers may be used according to their biologic value in relation to that of the natural isomer. DL-Methionine can replace L-methionine completely. D-Tryptophan has a biologic value of about 60 per cent of the L isomer. It is assumed that D-phenylalanine can replace to some extent phenylalanine + tyrosine, but the efficiency of the inversion is in question. D-Histidine may replace L-histidine to a small extent. Isoleucine, leucine, lysine, threonine, and valine are poorly invertible. Pigs can synthesize arginine to supply about 60 to 70 per cent of their needs. Cystine can supply 50 to 70 per cent of the total need for sulfur-containing amino acids (methionine and cystine), and methionine can supply the entire need in the absence of cystine. Phenylalanine can supply the entire need for phenylalanine and tyrosine.

The nonessential amino acids are either obtained from normal dietary sources or synthesized by using amino groups derived from amino acids supplied in the diet in excess of need.

The protein requirements for pregnant sows and gilts are based on amounts required for satisfactory retention of nitrogen during the late stages of pregnancy. Such amounts must be adequate to support development of a normal litter.

Protein requirements for lactation are based on maintenance needs plus amounts required to support the production of 6 kg of milk daily.

Practical swine diets contain between 0.03 and 0.22 per cent of linoleic acid to ensure normal skin condition.

Minerals

Calcium and phosphorus are elements of major importance, and vitamin D is essential for absorption and retention of calcium and for normal skeletal development. The phytic acid content of the diet and the level of magnesium intake affect the retention of both calcium and phosphorus. The calcium:phosphorus ratio is less emphasized than formerly, but the most favorable ratio appears to be between 1:1 and 1.5:1. Data on calcium and phosphorus requirements of gestating and lactating sows are limited. In pregnancy, the dietary requirement is proportional to the need for fetal growth, reaching maximum levels in the final week of gestation. At recommended levels of dry matter intake 0.75 per cent calcium in the diet is adequate for breeding swine. Current recommendations assume that Ca and P will be present in forms that are well utilized. In grains, one half to two thirds of the phosphorus is in the phytate form. Phytase enzymes in corn and other grains may affect utilization of phytate phosphorus. Values listed in *Nutrient Requirements of Swine* (1979) assume 0.3 per cent phosphorus from the plant ingredients. Allowances are made for incomplete utilization of phytate phosphorus in the grain and plant protein portion of the diet. Utilization of phytate phosphorus is influenced by the levels of calcium, vitamin D, zinc, and alimentary pH.

Sodium, chloride, and iodine requirements are met by feeding iodized salt at a level of 0.4 to 0.5 per cent in the dry diet or by free access to an adequate mineral mixture. Symptoms of salt poisoning occur when intake equals 6 to 8 per cent of the dry diet. As little as 1.0 per cent dietary sodium chloride has produced toxicity signs when water has been restricted.

Table 5. *Final Dry Matter Ration*

Ingredient	Per Cent of DM	DM	As Fed
Ground corn	15.20	2.74 kg	3.08 kg (6.8 lb)
Soybean meal	7.77	1.4 kg	1.57 kg (3.5 lb)
Corn ensilage	45.86	8.32 kg	23.8 kg (52.4 lb)
Alfalfa hay	30.53	5.54 kg	6.22 kg (13.7 lb)
Dicalcium phosphate	0.42	75 g	75 g
Salt	0.44	70 g	79 g

Cobalt may be a necessary supplement if vitamin B_{12} is limiting. Levels of 0.1 mg/kg of dry diet are often added to swine rations.

Beyond breeding age, natural feedstuffs ordinarily furnish adequate copper for hemopoiesis and other copper-related functions.

Natural feedstuffs usually provide enough iron to supply the needs of swine after the nursing period.

It is suggested that swine diets contain a minimum of 400 mg/kg dry diet of magnesium and a minimum of 10 mg/kg dry diet of manganese.

A deficiency of potassium has not been observed in swine fed natural diets.

Ordinary feeds vary in their content of vitamin E and selenium. Deficiencies may occur in swine fed feed that has been grown on low-selenium soils. Injections of 5 mg sodium selenite or barium selenite every 28 days will prevent symptoms of selenium deficiency. Levels above 5 to 8 mg selenium/kg dry diet are toxic for swine.

Zinc deficiency in swine results in parakeratosis or dermatosis. High levels of calcium increase the zinc requirement. The recommended level is 50 mg/kg dry diet with normal levels of calcium and 100 mg/kg dry diet when excessive calcium is fed.

Vitamins

Any or all of the fat-soluble vitamins may be deficient in natural feedstuffs for swine. Vitamin A requirements can be met by either beta carotene or vitamin A (1 mg beta carotene = 500 I.U. vitamin A). Bred gilts and sows require 4000 I.U. vitamin A/kg dry diet. Lactating sows and gilts require 2000 I.U./kg dry diet. Except for corn and alfalfa, natural feeds for swine are deficient in vitamin D. The need can be met by feeding vitamin D_2 (irradiated dehydrocholesterol). Unless the pigs are exposed to direct sunlight daily, the diet should be fortified with vitamin D. The listed requirement is 200 I.U./kg dry diet per day for gestating swine and 200 I.U./kg dry diet per day for lactating swine. Symptoms of vitamin E deficiency are more likely to develop in sows and gilts fed chiefly on grains grown on soil that is low in selenium. It is suggested that 10 I.U. of vitamin E/kg dry diet be added to practical swine rations. Symptoms of vitamin K deficiency have been produced by feeding moldy feeds. Symptoms can ordinarily be reversed by feeding 5 μg menadiol diphosphate per kg dry diet.

Swine require most of the water-soluble vitamins, but only a few are of practical importance in diets based on natural feedstuffs. Deficiencies of niacin, pantothenic acid, riboflavin, choline, vitamin B_{12}, and possibly biotin may occur in ordinary diets. In practice, identifiable symptoms of a specific deficiency are generally not apparent. The specific natural feeds included in the diet are important in determining whether a deficiency of one or more of these vitamins may occur. Specifics include the following:

1. Niacin occurs in cereal grains in bound form and may be largely unavailable to the pig. Conventional assays may be misleading. The amino acid tryptophan converts to niacin and is important in determining the need and providing a source.

2. Pantothenic acid occurs in practically all feedstuffs but may be present in less than adequate amounts. Calcium pantothenate is the common supplementary source and is frequently marketed as the racemic mixture (DL-calcium pantothenate). Only the D isomer has vitamin activity.

3. 3.5 to 5 mg of riboflavin per kg dry diet are necessary to prevent symptoms of deficiency.

4. The choline requirement is related to the presence of the amino acid methionine. The requirement for sows is said to be 20 mg/kg body weight per day.

5. Feedstuffs of animal origin contain substantial but highly variable amounts of vitamin B_{12}. Synthesis by intestinal bacteria probably supplements dietary sources. Vitamin B_{12} contains the mineral cobalt, and bacterial synthesis is dependent on the presence of this mineral in the diet. Under some conditions, the reproductive performance of sows has been improved by the inclusion of levels of vitamin B_{12} greater than those of the current recommendation. The response is manifested by an increase in the number and birth weight of pigs. The positive response is not a consistent finding. Biotin is ordinarily synthesized in adequate amounts by intestinal microbes. Vitamin C, thiamine, pyridoxine, and folic acid are generally furnished in adequate amounts by natural feedstuffs or by endogenous synthesis.

Feeding Pregnant Sows and Gilts

Nutrients must be provided for maintenance, normal activity, growth of first litter gilts and second litter sows, development of the litter (especially in the last trimester), and nominal gain in the dam (9 to 13.5 kg parity net gain and 23 to 32 kg total gain per gestation).

Feedstuffs commonly used in diets for pregnant sows and gilts include No. 2 yellow corn, ground ear corn, milo grain, oats, barley, solvent-extracted soybean meal, meat and bone meal, alfalfa meal (sun-cured or dehydrated), fish meal, linseed meal, and bulking agents such as ground corn cobs, ground oats, ground oat hulls, and fair to high quality alfalfa meal.

Hand feeding and *ad libitum* feeding are both acceptable practices in the case of gestating swine. The advantages of hand feeding include the possibility of reducing bulk and mixing procedures. Corn, barley, oats, or milo or mixtures of these can comprise the major portion of the ration if mixed with appropriate amounts of balanced proteins, minerals, and vitamins. The disadvantage of these mixtures is that sows and gilts must be fed individually to control intake. About 1.8 to 2.0 kg of air dry ration is sufficient for bred sows and gilts if properly concentrated and balanced.

If gestating swine are fed in groups, the concentrates must be diluted with bulking agents. Recommended amounts of bulking agents depend on the specific concentrate used: 50 to 60 per cent with ground or cracked corn, milo, or barley; 35 to 45 per cent with ground ear corn; and 25 to 35 per cent with oats.

Commonly used feeds vary widely in essential amino acid, mineral, and vitamin content. No. 2 corn is the basic energy feed. It is low in crude protein but provides a substantial amount of true protein. It provides some vitamin A potency but is practically devoid of calcium. Ground ear corn contains about 20 per cent cob and should be ground through a 6.5-mm (1/4-inch) screen. Milo is similar to corn but has no vitamin A potency. Oats are an excellent dietary component for pregnant swine. Oats can be used as the only grain in a self-fed ration and at levels of up to 15 per cent in hand-fed rations. Barley contains metabolizable energy equal to about 80 per cent of that of corn. It is relatively high in crude protein (12 to 14 per cent) and can supply all or nearly all of the amino acid requirement for pregnant sows and gilts. Barley is very low in calcium and devoid of vitamin A. Solvent-extracted soybean meal (44 or 48.5 per cent protein) is the major source of supplemental protein used to correct the amino acid deficiencies in basic cereal grains.

Meat and bone meal (also meat meal with 55 per cent protein and tankage with 60 per cent protein) is an excellent source of total protein, calcium, and phosphorus. It is variable in vitamin B_{12}, poor in riboflavin and pantothenic acid, excellent in niacin, devoid of fat-soluble vitamins, good to excellent in choline, a desirable, but not essential, component for diets of gestating swine. Meat and bone meal can supply much of the needed calcium and phosphorus to correct deficiencies existing in cereal grains and soybean meal. It may be used as the only source of supplemental protein to barley and as the major source of supplemental protein to corn in hand-fed diets.

Alfalfa meal (sun-cured 17 per cent protein) is a good to excellent source of vitamins except B_{12}. A high quality product provides significant protein, calcium, and vitamin D. Alfalfa meal may be used in hand-fed diets (10 to 15 per cent) and at levels of up to 45 per cent in self-feeding programs. Fish meal is an excellent source of good to high quality protein and provides a good to excellent source of calcium and phosphorus. The price, however, is usually prohibitive. Linseed meal may be used in small amounts (3.5 per cent of the dry diet). It improves the laxative nature of the diet but is deficient in lysine.

Feeding levels have some effect on the reproductive performance of sows and gilts. Heavy feeding (flushing just prior to breeding) increases ovulation rates. Heavy feeding just after breeding increases embryo mortality. Limiting of feed just prior to breeding decreases the ovulation rate, and limiting of feed just following breeding increases embryo survival.

Feeding Sows at Farrowing Time

Farrowing diets should contain at least 12 per cent protein, 0.75 per cent calcium, and 0.60 per cent phosphorus. Vitamin inclusions generally correspond to those used in diets for hand feeding pregnant sows and gilts.

Diets at farrowing time may be of moderate energy content or fairly concentrated. In either case, the diet should be somewhat laxative in nature. Wheat bran is a feed of choice for many producers. It contributes bulk to the diet, reduces energy content, and improves the laxative nature of the diet. It generally constitutes from 15 to 25 per cent of the total diet. Wheat bran is relatively high in some B vitamins and phosphorus. It is deficient in B_{12}, and the niacin content may not be fully available. Linseed meal may be used in lieu of bran to some extent. It provides significant protein and phosphorus. One kilogram of linseed meal provides laxative properties equal to 3 kg of wheat bran. The farrowing diet should be fed for four to six days pre-farrowing and five to ten days post-farrowing. Intake should be adjusted to the condition of the sow, milk flow, and litter size. If sows are confined to farrowing stalls for three weeks, it may be advantageous to feed 3 to 5 per cent linseed meal to avoid constipation.

Diets for Lactation

These diets are generally high in energy and contain at least 13 per cent protein, 0.75 per cent calcium, 0.5 per cent phosphorus, and 0.5 per cent salt. Vitamins are included in the same concentrations as in diets for pregnant swine (using the same vitamin premix).

Diets for lactating swine generally do not contain more than 10 per cent ground oats and do not include alfalfa meal, wheat bran, or meat and bone meal. Lactating sows and gilts are usually fed to appetite, but they may be fed to scale to provide adequate nutrients for maintenance and milk production required to support the number of pigs being nursed. Diets fed in the lactation period are often formulated to be acceptable for small pigs. This may be advantageous in training these pigs to consume feed other than milk at an early age.

Wheat middlings (shorts) can sometimes be purchased economically in terms of TDN and crude protein concentration. They may constitute up to 20 per cent of a total ration.

Common sources of calcium, phosphorus, and NaCl are used. It is probably advisable to feed a high zinc trace mineral salt and the same vitamin premix as that used in the gestation diet.

Lactation diets are generally fed from three to seven days post-farrowing to the end of the lactation period. Feed consumption in terms of energy, protein, minerals, and vitamins is expected to be two and one half to three times the requirement for gestation.

BREEDING EWES

Breeding ewes are kept in a variety of conditions to utilize feeds not readily available to man or other types of livestock. Small flocks (1 to 100 ewes) are often maintained to harvest water courses, fence corners, woodlots, and crop residues. Larger flocks are maintained on permanent pastures where rainfall is abundant and/or irrigated pastures where rainfall is less than adequate. Many purebred breeding sheep are grazed on such pastures, and cured forages (ensilage and hay) are used extensively in winter and early spring. Concentrates are often used on a least cost basis to provide supplementary energy, protein, essential minerals, and vitamins in late gestation and lactation and when stressful environmental conditions dictate. Large flocks of sheep are maintained on western ranges (mountain and desert) on a seasonal basis. Range management in these areas is a unique combination of art and science that has been and continues to be studied extensively and that is subjected to stringent regulation on the public lands. There are a number of advantages to sheep husbandry.

1. The stress conditions of late gestation and peak lactation are relatively short.

2. Sheep generally utilize the nutrients of browse more efficiently than do cattle.

3. Sheep are relatively efficient in their utilization of plants growing on rough terrain.

4. Dogs can be used to handle sheep efficiently. There are also some disadvantages.

1. Sheep are relatively susceptible to predators.

2. Sheep are relatively susceptible to oxalate poisoning, lupine poisoning, and photosensitization.

The best source of information is the NAS-NRC publication *Nutrient Requirements of Sheep* (1975). The major nutrient requirements are listed in Table 1 (amounts per animal per day), Table 2 (concentrations of nutrients in diet dry matter), and Table 3 (yearly dry matter requirements for energy and protein in a 60-kg ewe) in this publication.

Energy

Insufficient energy limits the productive performance of sheep more than any other nutritional entity. Such deficiency results from inadequate intake and overdependence on low quality feeds. The most important consequences include reproductive failure (particularly in the breeding season), reduced milk production, and short lactation periods. Wool production and quality may be reduced, and the sheep may become more susceptible to internal and external parasites including bacterial infections. Generally, energy deficiencies are complicated with deficiencies of protein, minerals, and vitamins. As with cattle, rations that provide adequate energy require only limited supplementation.

Some practical values extrapolated from the tables of the NAS-NRC publication include the following:
1. Metabolizable energy concentrations recommended in dry diets of farm sheep:
   a. For maintenance and first 15 weeks of gestation: 2 Mcal/kg
   b. For last six weeks of gestation and last eight weeks of lactation (suckling singles): 2.1 Mcal/kg
   c. For first eight weeks suckling singles and last eight weeks suckling twins: 2.4 Mcal/kg
   d. For first eight weeks suckling twins: 2.4 Mcal/kg

Table 13 of the NAS-NRC publication lists 1.466 Mcal/kg as the dry diet ME concentration requirement of 60-kg ewes grazing intermountain winter range in early and mid-pregnancy. Requirements for range ewes appear to differ slightly from those reported for farm sheep.
2. Dry matter consumption as per cent of body weight:
   a. For maintenance: 1.6 to 2.0
   b. For first 15 weeks of gestation: 1.9 to 2.2
   c. For last six weeks of gestation and last eight weeks of lactation (suckling singles): 2.8 to 3.3
   d. For first eight weeks of lactation (suckling singles) and last eight weeks of lactation (suckling twins): 3.2 to 4.2
   e. For first eight weeks of lactation (suckling twins): 3.7 to 4.8
3. Metabolizable energy requirements for breeding ewes include:
   a. For maintenance: 98 kcal/$(BW)^{0.75}$ (in kg)
   b. For maintenance plus pregnancy in last six weeks of gestation: 1.5 × maintenance for singles.
   c. For maintenance plus lactation: 1.3 to 1.4 × maintenance (for singles and for twins: 1.7 to 1.9 × maintenance)
4. ME concentrations in ordinary range diets (dry matter) include:
   a. 100 per cent browse: 1.22 Mcal/kg
   b. 100 per cent grass: 2.05 Mcal/kg
   c. 70 per cent browse, 30 per cent grass: 1.47 Mcal/kg
   d. 30 per cent browse, 70 per cent grass: 1.80 Mcal/kg
5. ME concentrations in the dry matter of some ordinary concentrates include:
   a. Corn: 3.31 Mcal/kg
   b. Barley: 3.11 Mcal/kg
   c. Oats: 2.71 Mcal/kg
   d. Soybean meal: 3.00 Mcal/kg
   e. Cottonseed meal: 3.00 Mcal/kg
6. ME concentrations in the dry matter of some ordinary cured forages include:
   a. Alfalfa hay, midbloom, sun-cured: 1.94 Mcal/kg
   b. Prairie hay, midbloom, sun-cured: 2.02 Mcal/kg
   c. Corn ensilage, well-eared: 2.49 Mcal/kg

The maintenance requirements of sheep on pasture or range are 10 to 100 per cent higher than those for sheep kept in confinement. The size of the increase depends on the availability of feed and water, the nature of the terrain, and the distance traveled daily.

Protein

Satisfactory production from pregnant ewes (40 to 55 kg) has been realized with a daily intake of 45 to 60 g of digestible crude protein (about 3.5 to 5 per cent of the dry diet). These values are probably minimal in the latter stages of pregnancy for ewes carrying twins. These values are also minimal for optimum wool production unless the diet is relatively high in sulfur-containing amino acids.

Digestible energy–digestible protein ratios were considered in formulating the NAS-NRC recommendations. A ratio of about 20 g of digestible protein per 1 Mcal of DE has been shown to be adequate for mature nonlactating ewes. Higher levels are recommended when growth and/or lactation is involved.

Recent research indicates that protein quality (level and balance of amino acids) is more important than previously thought. The sulfur-containing amino acid methionine is first limiting in microbial protein for both wool production and weight gain. Lysine and threonine may also be limiting. The amount of protein escaping microbial action in the rumen and entering the abomasum intact (bypass protein) can influence the quality of protein that reaches the tissues. Heat treatments and the use of tannic acid or one of several aldehydes to complex proteins and reduce degradation in the rumen have been shown to reduce rumen ammonia levels and increase lamb performance. Such treatments are not common practice in current sheep production.

Nonprotein nitrogen has limited value in the diets of breeding ewes. Ordinary forage carries enough protein to supply maintenance and pregnancy needs. All-grass winter range (DP about 1.6 per cent) is an exception. Lactating ewes generally have access to fresh vegetative forage that is adequate in protein for maximum milk production. NPN can be utilized in combination with low quality forage and high energy supplements that have positive urea fermentation potentials (molasses or corn) for ewes in gestation or lactation. It is recommended that urea comprise not more than 1 per cent of the dry diet.

Symptoms of protein deficiency include reduced appetite and feed intake. The efficiency of total feed utilization is decreased. Reproductive efficiency is impaired, and wool production is decreased in both quantity and quality.

Recommended digestible protein levels as a percent of dry diet include:
1. For maintenance: 4.8 per cent
2. For first 15 weeks of gestation: 4.9 per cent
3. For last six weeks of gestation or last eight weeks of lactation (singles): 5.2 per cent
4. For first eight weeks of lactation (singles) or last eight weeks of lactation (twins): 6.2 per cent

5. For first eight weeks of lactation (twins): 7.2 per cent

Minerals

Fifteen minerals have been demonstrated to be essential for sheep. Major mineral constituents include sodium, chlorine, calcium, phosphorus, magnesium, potassium, and sulfur. Trace minerals include iodine, iron, copper, molybdenum, cobalt, manganese, zinc, and selenium.

Salt is an almost universal supplement. Range operators commonly provide 220 to 340 g of salt per ewe per month. When adding salt to mixed feeds, it is customary to use 0.5 per cent of the dry diet or 1 per cent of the concentrate portion. Salt may be safely used to limit intake of free-choice supplements if adequate water is available. Mixtures containing 10 to 50 per cent salt are commonly used. Trace mineralized salt should not be used for this purpose. Iodized salt is ordinarily used to supply the iodine requirement, especially in iodine-deficient areas.

Most pasture and range forage contains adequate amounts of calcium. Areas where calcium supplementation is required on pasture have been reported in Florida, Louisiana, Nebraska, Virginia, and West Virginia.

Mature pasture and range forage in North America are commonly deficient in phosphorus. Sheep are efficient utilizers of phosphorus and recycle considerable amounts through saliva. The phosphorus concentrations of saliva, rumen fluid, and blood serum are related to dietary intake. In some cases sheep recycle more phosphorus per day through parotid saliva than is required in the diet to maintain the body pools. Phosphorus supplementation may be necessary on winter range and is ordinarily supplied by dicalcium phosphate mixed with salt.

Diets that are significantly lacking in calcium and/or phosphorus result in abnormal bone development (rickets and osteomalacia). Blood serum levels of calcium below 9 mg/dl and of phosphorus below 4 mg/dl are indicative of deficiencies.

Forage containing 0.06 per cent magnesium is considered to be adequate for sheep. Hypomagnesemia can be a problem in lactating ewes on fresh vegetative forage. Such hypomagnesemia may be accompanied by hypocalcemia and produces symptoms of grass tetany. The need for a continuous supply of magnesium is recognized. The use of intraruminal magnesium alloy pellets (bullets) weighing 30 g has effectively prevented hypomagnesemia tetany in lactating ewes.

Ordinary forage supplies the potassium requirement.

Mature ewes require 0.14 to 0.18 per cent sulfur in the dry diet. Practically all common feedstuffs contain more than 0.1 per cent sulfur, but mature grass and grass hays may not furnish enough for optimum performance. When forages are low in sulfur or when significant amounts of urea are being fed, a sulfur supplement should be fed. Sulfate sulfur, elemental sulfur, or sulfur-containing proteins may be used. Inorganic compounds are generally relatively economical and convenient.

There is no evidence that iron deficiency occurs normally in breeding sheep.

Interactions of copper, molybdenum, and sulfate may produce significant effects on sheep, but the mechanisms involved are obscure. A high molybdenum intake can induce a copper deficiency even when the copper content of forage is quite high. This effect can be prevented by increasing the copper intake. When the pasture provides low intakes of molybdenum, an excess of copper accumulates in the tissues even when the copper intake is moderate. The liver copper concentrations may become very high, and, under certain stress conditions, copper from the liver is mobilized rapidly, increasing the copper content of blood and precipitating a fatal hemolytic jaundice. The disease can be prevented by increasing the molybdenum intake of the animals. These contrasting situations complicate the definition of copper and molybdenum requirements. It is difficult to predict the reactions of animals in any given pastoral situation.

Sheep are very susceptible to copper poisoning relative to cattle, and cattle are much more severely affected than sheep by high molybdenum intake. The dietary concentration of copper should be 5 ppm of dry matter when molybdenum and sulfate intakes are normal. Merino sheep are less efficient in absorbing copper than are English breeds, and an additional 1 to 2 ppm are recommended. Nutritional copper is adequate in forages over most of the United States. Deficient areas have been reported in Florida and in the coastal plains area of the Southeast. Copper can conveniently be provided by adding 0.5 per cent copper sulfate to the salt ration.

There is some question concerning the role of molybdenum in the diets of livestock. It is believed that molybdenum complexes with copper in the intestine and that copper thus bound is biologically inactive. Research has shown that feeds containing small amounts of molybdenum are more effectively digested and produce more rapid weight gains than do diets not containing molybdenum. An excess of molybdenum in forage in areas of California, Nevada, and England causes a diarrhea in sheep. Symptoms become apparent a few days after the sheep are turned on pasture having a high molybdenum content (5 to 20 ppm in the dry diet). If dietary copper levels are below normal or if sulfate levels are high, molybdenum intakes as low as 1 to 2 ppm may be toxic. Such toxicity is controlled by increasing the dietary copper level by 5 ppm. Complete manufactured feeds in the United States may contain 25 to 35 ppm of copper in the dry matter. These levels of copper can be extremely harmful if the molybdenum levels of the diet are low. An effective treatment for lambs is to drench each lamb daily with 100 mg of ammonium molybdate and 1 g of sodium sulfate in 20 ml of water for a minimum of three weeks. The FDA prohibits the use of molybdenum as a feed additive. Prevention of copper poisoning can often be achieved by eliminating extraneous sources of copper from the diet.

Areas deficient in cobalt have been widely reported in the United States and Canada. Feed or forage containing more than 0.07 ppm in the dry diet has prevented symptoms of deficiency. The recommended intake is 0.1 ppm in the dry diet. A preventive measure suggested for deficient areas is to feed cobalt as cobalt chloride or cobalt sulfate to furnish 12 g of cobalt/100 kg salt. Cobalt in excess of 4.5 ppm may be toxic.

Research has shown that 17.4 ppm of zinc in the dry diet are necessary for normal growth of lambs, and 32.4 ppm are necessary for normal reproductive development in ram lambs. Toxic symptoms (reduced feed consumption and gain) are produced when lambs are fed 1 g/kg of diet.

In the northwestern, northeastern, and southeastern parts of the United States, there are extensive areas where the selenium content is below 0.1 ppm in dry forage. This is the level considered adequate for preventing deficiency in sheep. The area between the Mississippi River and the Rocky Mountains produces forage that is in the adequate but nontoxic range. Parts of Wyoming, South Dakota, and Utah produce forage that causes selenium toxicity in farm animals. Selenium deficiency produces serious consequences (reduced growth and white muscle disease) in lamb production. The addition of 26 ppm of selenium as sodium selenite to trace-mineralized salt fed free-choice to ewes prevents white muscle disease in lambs two to eight weeks of age.

Experimental methods of supplying selenium to sheep include an oral drench, intramuscular or subcutaneous injection, addition to feedstuffs, and application of selenium in the soil. One method is to incorporate selenium in pellets composed of finely divided metallic iron and selenium in a proportion of 10:1. A single pellet in the reticulum has enhanced blood and tissue selenium levels for up to 12 months. The most common method of supplying selenium to deficient lambs is to inject a commercial pharmacologic product containing selenium and vitamin E. Two injections are given: one at birth and one two weeks later. The first injection contains 0.25 mg selenium and 68 I.U. of vitamin E as d-α-tocopherol. The second injection contains 1 mg selenium and 68 I.U. of vitamin E.

Chronic selenium toxicity occurs when sheep consume seleniferous plants containing more than 3 ppm of selenium over a prolonged period. Toxicity signs include loss of wool, soreness, sloughing of hooves, and marked reduction in reproductive performance. The most practical way to prevent livestock losses from selenium poisoning is to alternate grazing between selenium-bearing and other areas.

Fluorine rarely occurs free in nature but combines chemically to form fluorides that are toxic in amounts exceeding 60 ppm of fluorine in the dry diet. Forages may be seriously contaminated when grown near manufacturing plants that process minerals containing fluorides. Rock phosphate may contain up to 3 to 4 per cent fluorides and must be defluorinated prior to use for livestock supplementation.

Vitamins

Vitamin deficiencies are not common in breeding sheep fed ordinary diets. Vitamin C is synthesized endogenously. The B vitamins are synthesized in adequate amounts by rumen microflora. Vitamin K_2 is synthesized in large amounts in the rumen. No evidence has been found relating vitamin E deficiency to reproductive failure in sheep. Vitamin D is seldom deficient in sheep on pasture, although the question of adequacy arises if the weather is cloudy for long periods or when sheep are fed indoors. Sheep convert the carotenes to vitamin A with efficiency comparable to that of cattle (1 mg beta carotene = 400 to 500 I.U. vitamin A). Vitamin A values for carotene are lower in the following conditions:

1. When xanthophylls and other carotenes are diluents of beta carotene.
2. When animals are vitamin A deficient.
3. When the diets are of low digestibility.
4. When oxidants are present in the feed, ingesta, or tissues.
5. When goitrogenic agents are present.
6. When the diets are high in phosphorus.

7. When the diets are low in vitamin E.
8. When dietary fat levels are low.

Vitamin A is fat soluble and is stored in the body. About 200 days is required to entirely deplete liver storage in ewe lambs previously pastured on green plants. It is expected that sheep will perform well on low vitamin A diets for four to six months if they have grazed on green forage in the normal growing season. Sheep that weigh 32 kg or more and are deficient in vitamin A should receive 100,000 I.U. by injection, and their diets should be supplemented to provide recommended levels of vitamin A or carotene. Ewes deficient in vitamin A should be given vitamin A orally or by injection prior to breeding. The greatest need is in late pregnancy. Vitamin A requirements (NAS-NRC recommendation) vary from 1391 I.U./kg DM for maintenance to 2684 I.U./kg DM for ewes in the last six weeks of pregnancy.

Water

Sheep get water from snow, dew, guttation in feed and metabolic water and by drinking. Voluntary water intake is adjusted to balance body water and is indicative of need. Voluntary water intake is affected by ambient temperature, rainfall, snow, dew coverage, age, breed, stage of gestation, wool covering, respiratory rate, frequency of watering, feed composition, and exercise. Sheep normally drink after consuming feed in a dry lot. In general, water consumption is two to three times DM feed consumption. The total water intake to dry matter feed intake ratio (TWI/DMI) increases significantly in late gestation, doubles in the fifth month, and is maintained through the lactation period. Sheep may consume as much as 12 times more water in summer than in winter. On western ranges, snow is often the only source of water in winter. No adverse syndromes result when ambient temperatures are below 21°C.

Frequent watering in summer is sometimes difficult. Watering on alternate days is an acceptable practice when the temperature is below 4°C. The protein and mineral content of the diet markedly influences water consumption. Sheep fed 2 per cent protein hay showed no decrease in feed consumption when watered every fourth day, whereas sheep fed 15 per cent protein hay showed a marked decrease in feed consumption when watered at this rate. Sheep grazing on sagebrush-grass desert range in Utah consumed 2.7 liters of water per head daily. When they were confined to range growing shadscale, winterfat, or salt brush, their water consumption tripled. The water requirement is increased greatly when sheep graze halogeton (oxalate containing). The increased water consumption enhances the excretion of oxalate and reduces death loss. Breeding ewes can tolerate bicarbonate water in which the total salt concentration is 5000 ppm (0.5 per cent) and chloride water in which the total salt content is 10,000 ppm (1 per cent). Salt concentrations above these levels produce toxicity.

Special Requirements for Range Sheep

A knowledge of the nutritive value of range plants in various stages of growth and the nutrient concentrations according to area is essential to the optimal production of range sheep. Feed intake can be estimated, and balance of nutrients can be evaluated by periodically weighing the animals and/or assessing the body condition. The cost of activity must also be considered, especially on sparse

Table 6. *Average Degree of Utilization, or Preference Indexes, Used in Calculating a Diet for a Particular Sheep Allotment**

(1) Plant	(2) Plant Composition (Per Cent)	(3) Preference Index	(4) Plant Composition × Preference Index	(5) Diet† (Per Cent)	(6) Mcal ME/kg of Plant‡	(7) Mcal ME§
Sagebrush, big (*Artemisia tridentata*)	15	40	600	19	1.27	0.241
Sagebrush, bud (*Artemisia spinescens*)	10	20	200	6	2.01	0.121
Saltbush, shad scale (*Atriplex canescens*)	25	20	500	15	0.88	0.132
Winter fat (*Eurotia* sp.)	24	40	960	30	1.19	0.357
BROWSE TOTAL	74	—	—	70	—	—
Wheatgrass (*Agropyron cristatum*)	14	40	560	17	2.39	0.406
Galleta (*Hilaria jamesii*)	3	25	75	2	1.31	0.026
Needle and thread grasses (*Stipa comata*)	9	40	360	11	1.65	0.182
GRASS TOTAL	26	—	—	30	—	—
GRAND TOTAL	100	—	3255	100	—	1.465‖

*National Academy of Sciences-National Research Council: Nutrient Requirements of Sheep, 5th ed. NAS-NRC, Washington, D.C., 1975. Modified from Cook, C. W., et al.: The nutritive value of winter range plants in the Great Basin as determined with digestion trials with sheep. Utah Agr. Exp. St. Bull. 372, 1954.

†Obtained by dividing each value in column 4 by the total of that column (3255).
‡Dry matter basis.
§Calculated as column 5 times column 6.
‖Mcal ME/kg diet.

ranges. Seasonal functions including breeding, gestation, and lactation all present special problems and requirements. Considerable knowledge and careful planning and management are essential to a successful operation.

Research in Utah has demonstrated that range sheep respond to protein, phosphorus, and energy supplements when grazing desert forage in winter. When sheep are required to subsist on forage low in carotene for more than six months without intermittent access to green feed, vitamin A supplements are recommended. The intermountain range is deficient in iodine (iodized salt is recommended), but other trace minerals are not known to be deficient. In formulating supplements for range ewes, it is necessary to:

1. Calculate the requirements for metabolizable energy (ME), digestible protein (DP), and phosphorus (P).

2. Determine the composition of the forage and estimate the dry matter intake.

3. Compute the deficiencies and formulate the supplement in terms of ME, DP, and P.

The NAS-NRC publication *Nutrient Requirements of Sheep* (1975) is the recommended source of information (Tables 12, 13, 14, and 16 are especially helpful). These

tables (except Table 16) are reproduced here as Tables 6, 7, and 8.

A useful working calculation of the diet can be obtained by weighing the percentage of each floral component of the range forage by an index of the animal's preference for each species of forage present. The preferences that have been worked out for sheep are listed in Table 6. This table and Table 16 (page 217) can be used to calculate the nutrient make-up of the diet. The calculations usually include only the estimated forage intake and the energy, protein, and phosphorus concentrations in the forage. When the forage diet has been evaluated, the results may be compared with the sheep's requirements, as illustrated in Table 7. In this table, line 1 states the proposed requirement for pregnant ewes under intermountain range conditions. Line 2 indicates that the diet shown in Table 6 is only slightly deficient in phosphorus. Lines 3, 4, and 5 illustrate two basic facts concerning the diets of sheep on intermountain ranges in winter: (1) browse plants are the best sources of protein and phosphorus and are low in metabolizable energy, and (2) the grasses are adequate in energy but are seriously deficient in protein and phosphorus.

Table 7. *Typical Requirement, Probable Intake, and Deficiencies for 60-kg Ewes in Early and Mid-Pregnancy Grazing Intermountain Winter Range (100 Per Cent Dry Matter Basis)**

Line No.		Daily Intake kg	Daily Intake lb	Digestible Protein (Per Cent)	Metabolizable Energy (Mcal/kg)	Phosphorus (Per Cent)
1	Requirement	1.63	3.59	4.4	1.466	0.18
2	If 70 per cent browse and 30 per cent grass as given in Table 6	—	—	5.0	1.47	0.14†
3	If 100 per cent browse	—	—	6.5	1.22‡	0.15†
4	If 100 per cent grass	—	—	1.6‡	2.05	0.12‡
5	If 70 per cent grass and 30 per cent browse	—	—	3.1‡	1.80	0.13‡

*National Academy of Sciences-National Research Council: Nutrient Requirements of Sheep, 5th ed. NAS-NRC, Washington, D.C., 1975. Modified from Cook, C. W., et al.: The nutritive value of winter range plants in the Great Basin as determined with digestion trials with sheep. Utah Agr. Exp. St. Bull. 372, 1954; and Harris, L. E., et al.: Feeding phosphorus, protein and energy supplements to ewes on winter ranges of Utah. Utah Agr. Exp. St. Bull. 398, 1956.

†Slightly deficient.
‡Deficient.

Table 8. *Formulas for Range Supplements for Sheep (100 Per Cent Dry Matter Basis)**

Feed†		Recommended Level of Protein (Per Cent)		
		High	Medium	Low
Barley, grain		—	33.0	67.0
Corn, dent yellow, grain, gr 2 US mn 54 lb per bushel		5.0	10.0	15.0
Beet, sugar, molasses, mn 48% invert sugar mn 79.5 degrees brix, or Sugarcane, molasses, mn 48% invert sugar mn 79.5 degrees brix		5.0	5.0	10.0
Cotton, seeds w some hulls, solv-extd grnd, mn 41% protein mx 14% fiber mn 0.5% fat (cottonseed meal)		62.5	32.0	—
Soybean, seeds, solv-extd grnd, mx 7% fiber (soybean meal)		10.0	10.0	—
Alfalfa, aerial part, dehy grnd, mn 17% protein or Alfalfa, hay, s-c, early bloom		12.5	6.0	5.0
Calcium phosphate dibasic, commercial		4.0	3.0	2.0
Salt or trace mineralized salt		1.0	1.0	1.0
TOTAL		100.0	100.0	100.0
Composition‡				
Protein (N × 6.25)	%	36.5	26.4	12.0
Digestible protein	%	29.6	21.4	9.1
Metabolizable energy	Mcal/kg	2.4	2.7	3.0
Phosphorus	%	1.7	1.3	0.8
Carotene	mg/kg	22.0	11.0	9.0
Rate of feeding (kg/day)§		0.1 to 0.2	0.1 to 0.2	0.1 to 0.2‖

*National Academy of Sciences-National Research Council: Nutrient Requirements of Sheep, 5th ed. NAS-NRC, Washington, D.C., 1975.
†Feeds to be mixed and fed in meal or pellet form.
‡Sugarcane, molasses, and alfalfa hay, sun-cured, early bloom not included.
§Listed as dry matter basis, calculate to as-fed basis for mixing and feeding.
‖In emergency situations, up to 0.45 kg may be fed.

Tables 6 and 7 illustrate a basis for intelligent selection of supplements. Examples of physical and chemical composition of supplements are given in Table 8 and are applicable to such corrective measures as are indicated by the forage evaluation, the estimated intake, and the calculated requirements of the sheep. The suggested supplements in Table 8 are only examples and may be modified by availability, costs, and requirements. Feeds listed in Table 8 (and in Table 16 of the NAS-NRC publication cited earlier) are listed on a 100 per cent dry basis, and it is necessary to adjust these values to as-fed values in the final computation.

Deficient nutrients may be supplied by increasing ration intake or by using supplements. The normal range of supplementation for breeding ewes is 0.1 to 0.2 kg per day. On a group feeding basis, a rate of 0.1 kg per day is necessary for a practical delivery operation. Rates above 0.2 kg per day will result in reduced intake of range forage.

Supplements to balance diets and provide nutrients during short-term emergencies are added in the form of small quantities of a nutrient or a combination of nutrients. Supplements may be required for energy when forage is covered with snow or to prevent sheep from consuming poisonous plants while being trailed. Except for emergencies, if it is necessary to supplement the sheep with more than 0.2 kg DM per day, the practical value of using the range is questionable. On some public lands, supplementation beyond salt, phosphorus, and trace minerals is prohibited except in emergency situations. There is some danger of seeding range with noxious weeds.

Exceptional skill is required to recognize the physical and nutritional state of the sheep, the range condition, and the need for supplements. Sheep may be divided into flocks on the basis of age, condition, or function to provide an even plane of nutrition according to need. McDonald (1968) speaks to the complexities of grazing as follows:

…attention has been drawn to many gaps in our present knowledge of the nutrition of grazing nutrients. It has become clear that a full understanding of the subject cannot be obtained from research on animals handfed in pens; it is necessary to study the many interactions between soil, plant, animal and climate so that the mechanism governing the animal's response within the ecosystem can be elucidated. Knowledge of these mechanisms is essential to permit the effective application of scientific findings to practical husbandry in the pastoral system.

Special Aspects of Sheep Nutrition

High quality forage is more palatable and digestible than low quality forage and passes through the digestive tract more quickly; hence, sheep will consume more high quality forage than low quality forage. When sheep are forced to sustain themselves on low quality forage (low protein, low metabolizable energy, and so on), intake and utilization can be enhanced by adding sources of natural protein or properly formulated NPN supplements.

There are some advantages to pelleting or cubing forage components of sheep rations, including decreased wastage and convenience in handling and transport. Care must be exercised; parakeratosis (a degeneration of the rumen papilla) may result from feeding pellets, particularly those with a high concentrate content. Breeding animals should not be fed for extended periods on pelleted diets without long or chopped forage.

Antibiotics may be of value in creep diets. Chlortetracycline or oxytetracycline is especially effective at levels of 15 to 25 mg/kg of feed.

Creep feeding is advantageous in some situations. Lambs will usually consume some creep ration at about two weeks of age. The amount of creep feed consumed is inversely proportional to the ewe's milk production. Twin lambs generally consume more than singles. Lambs will generally consume significant amounts of creep feed at six to eight weeks of age. Lambs may prefer lush pasture to the creep ration. Soybean meal is an important ingredient in creep rations because of its palatability. Molasses (5 per cent) may also be added to increase acceptability of a ground ration.

Flushing is the practice of increasing the nutrient intake of ewes prior to mating. Its purpose is to increase the ovulation rate. Flushing is usually accomplished by providing fresh pastures, supplemental cured forage, or up to 0.25 kg of grain per day. This special feeding begins two to three weeks prior to and continues into the breeding season. Ewes maintained in a high state of nutrition benefit only slightly or not at all from flushing, but thin ewes benefit considerably. Mature ewes respond better than yearlings. Also, flushing is probably more beneficial early and late in the breeding season than during the peak when ovulation rates are highest.

Early weaning of lambs has some advantages when forage for ewes is limited. Weaning lambs at five to eight weeks of age and feeding them a relatively high concentrate diet in a dry lot is common practice. Weaning ewes from the lambs gradually is a good practice. It is suggested that the protein content of the lamb rations be about 16 per cent and the Ca:P ratio be about 2:1.

Halogeton and greasewood are common poisonous plants that grow in the arid and semi-arid regions of the West. They are toxic because of their high content of soluble oxalate (up to 30 per cent). When the oxalate is consumed, it may (1) be degraded by microorganisms, (2) combine with calcium in the rumen, and (3) be absorbed into the bloodstream. Intoxication occurs when large amounts are absorbed. Oxalate produces its effect through interference with certain steps of energy metabolism, its affinity for calcium, and its mechanical damage to rumen and kidney tissues as a result of crystal formation. The toxic dose is much lower (about 60 per cent) in a fasted animal, and there is much greater chance that a fasted animal will consume a lethal amount. The lethal dose is increased by about 50 per cent after the animals have been grazing halogeton for two to three days. This is probably due to increased water intake. Sheep should have access to good feed and water before entering halogeton areas. Supplementing sheep with grain or alfalfa pellets during stress periods of trailing or trucking is a valuable part of management.

Pregnancy disease (ketosis, acetonemia, or pregnancy toxemia) is associated with undernourishment. It occurs in late pregnancy and is more common in ewes carrying twins or triplets. Early symptoms include sluggishness, anorexia, staggering, and nervousness. Advanced symptoms include impaired vision, partial paralysis, and prostration. Ewes that give birth in the early stages generally recover. Pregnancy disease results from a disturbance of carbohydrate metabolism, causing hypoglycemia and acetonemia. Prevention is achieved by assuring adequate feed intake in late pregnancy and avoiding stress. A drench of propylene glycol can be used as an energy source for ewes refusing to eat at the onset of symptoms.

Lupine poisoning occurs sporadically in sheep grazing on western ranges, particularly in late summer and fall. The seeds of the plants carry the greatest concentrations of the toxic alkaloids. It is common for sheep to graze on lupine-infested ranges without problems, but occasionally acute and drastic syndromes develop. Mortality rates as high as 50 per cent have been reported. Hungry sheep are particularly susceptible. Prevention is best accomplished by supplementing diets with grain or alfalfa pellets while trailing and avoiding lupine-infested range in late summer and fall, particularly if the range is in poor condition.

Supplemental Reading

Beef Cattle

Chalupa, W.: Problems in feeding urea to ruminants. J. Anim. Sci. 27:201, 1968.

Dunn, T. G., Ingalls, J. E., Zimmerman, D. R., and Wiltbank, J. N.: Reproductive performance of 2-year-old Hereford and Angus heifers as influenced by pre- and post-calving energy intake. J. Anim. Sci. 29:719, 1969.

Lewis, L., Geasler, M., Lofgreen, G., Horton, D., Simons, J., Braddy, P., and Flack, D.: Bovine nutrition. Preconvention Seminar II, Eleventh Annual Conference of A.A.B.P., Baltimore, Md, 1978.

Lofgreen, G. P., and Garrett, W. N.: A system for expressing net energy requirements and feed values for growing and finishing beef cattle. J. Anim. Sci. 27:793, 1968.

Moe, P. W., Flatt, W. P., and Tyrell, H. F.: Net energy values of feeds for lactation. J. Dairy Sci. 55:945, 1972.

National Research Council, Committee on Animal Nutrition: Feed Phosphorus Shortage. Levels and Sources of Phosphorus Recommended for Livestock and Poultry. National Academy of Sciences, Washington, D.C., 1974.

National Research Council, Committee on Animal Nutrition: Nutrient Requirements of Beef Cattle. NAS-NRC, Washington, D.C., 1984.

National Research Council, Committee on Animal Nutrition: Nutrient Requirements of Dairy Cattle. NAS-NRC, Washington, D.C., 1971.

National Research Council, Committee on Animal Nutrition: Nutrient Requirements of Dairy Cattle, 5th rev. ed. NAS-NRC, Washington, D.C., 1978.

O'Kelley, R. E., and Fontenot, J. P.: Effects of feeding different levels of magnesium to dry lot fed, lactating beef cows. J. Anim. Sci. 26:959, 1969.

Oltjen, R. R.: Effects of feeding ruminants nonprotein nitrogen as the only nitrogen source. J. Anim. Sci. 28:673, 1969.

Pinney, D. O., Stephens, D. F., and Pope, L. S.: Lifetime effects of winter supplement feed level and age at first parturition on range beef cows. J. Anim. Sci. 34:1067, 1972.

Stillings, B. R., Bratzler, J. W., Marriot, L. F., and Miller, R. C.: Utilization of magnesium and other minerals by ruminants consuming low and high nitrogen containing forages and Vitamin D. J. Anim. Sci. 23:1148, 1964.

Swanson, E. W., Martin, G. G., Pardue, F. E., and Gorman, G. M.: Milk production of cows fed diets deficient in vitamin A. J. Anim. Sci. 27:541, 1968.

Ullrey, D. E., Covert, R. L., Wellenreiter, R. H., Greathouse, T. R., and Magee, W. T.: Vitamin A injections for wintering beef cows. In Beef Cattle Forage. Res. Rep. 118, Michigan State Univ. p. 38, 1970.

Wiltbank, J. N.: Puberty: The effect of breed and feed. Soc. Theriogenol. J. VII;2nd ed., 1973 (1976 reprint).

Wiltbank, J. N.: Influence of nutrition on calf crop. Soc. Theriogenol. J. III;2nd ed. (reprint), 1976.

Wiltbank, J. N., Bond, J., Warwick, E. J., Davis, R. E., Cook, A. C., Raynolds, W. L., and Hazen, M. W.: Influence of total feed and protein intake on reproductive performance in the beef female through second calving. U.S.D.A. Tech. Bull. 1314, 1965.

Dairy Cattle

Clifford, A. J., Goodrich, R. D., and Tillman, A. D.: Effect of supplementing ruminant all concentrate and purified diets with vitamins of the B complex. J. Anim. Sci. 26:400, 1967.

Dobson, R. C., and Ward, G.: Vitamin D physiology and its importance in dairy cattle: a review. J. Dairy Sci. 57:985, 1974.

Flatt, W. P., Moe, P. W., and Moore, L. A.: Influence of pregnancy and ration composition on energy utilization by dairy cows. Proceedings Fourth Symposium Energy Metabolism, Jablonna near Warsaw, Poland. Eur. Assn. Anim. Prod. Publ. 12:123, 1969.

Gullickson, T. W., Palmer, L. S., Boyd, W. L., Nelson, J. W., Olsen, F. C., Calverly, C. E., and Boyer, P. D.: Vitamin E in the nutrition of cattle. I. Effect of feeding Vitamin E poor rations on reproduction, health, milk production and growth. J. Dairy Sci. 32:495, 1949.

Harris, L. E., Asplund, J. M., and Crampton, E. W.: An international feed nomenclature and methods for summarizing and using feed data to calculate diets. Utah Agric. Exp. Stn. Bull. 479, 1968.

Huber, J. T.: Protein and nonprotein nitrogen utilization in practical dairy rations. J. Anim. Sci. 41:954, 1975.

Jorgenson, N. A.: Combating milk fever. J. Dairy Sci. 57:933, 1974.

Kung, L., Sr., Gubert, K., and Huber, J. T.: Supplemental niacin for lactating cows fed diets of natural protein or nonprotein nitrogen. J. Dairy Sci. 63:2020, 1980.

Lofgreen, P. A., and Warner, R. G.: Influence of various fiber sources and fractions on milk fat percentage. J. Dairy Sci. 53:296, 1970.

McGillivray, J. J.: Biological availability of phosphorus in feed ingredients. Proc. Minn. Nut. Conf. 15–21, 1974.

Miller, W. J.: New concepts and developments in metabolism and homeostasis of inorganic elements in dairy cattle: a review. J. Dairy Sci. 58:1549, 1975.

Moe, P. W., Flatt, W. P., and Tyrell, H. F.: The net energy value of feeds for lactation. J. Dairy Sci. 55:945, 1972.

Moe, P. W., and Tyrell, H. F.: The metabolizable energy requirement of pregnant dairy cows. J. Dairy Sci. 55:480, 1972.

Moe, P. W., and Tyrell, H. F.: Observations on the efficiency of utilization of metabolizable energy for meat and milk production. Univ. Nottingham Nutr. Conf. Feed Manufact. 7:27, 1974.

Moe, P. W., and Tyrell, H. F.: Estimating metabolizable and net energy of feeds. Proceedings 1st International Symposium on Feed Composition. Animal Nutrient Requirements and Computerization of Diets. International Feedstuffs Institute, Logan, Utah, 1976.

National Research Council: Urea and Other Nonprotein Nitrogen Compounds in Animal Nutrition. National Academy of Sciences, Washington, D.C., 1976.

National Research Council, Committee on Animal Nutrition: Nutrient Requirements of Dairy Cattle, 5th rev. NAS-NRC, Washington, D.C., 1978.

O'Dell, G. D., King, W. A., and Cook, C. W.: Effect of grinding, pelleting and frequency of feeding of forage on fat percentage of milk and milk production of dairy cows. J. Dairy Sci. 51:50, 1968.

Owen, J. B., Miller, E. L., and Bridge, P. S.: A study of the voluntary intake of food and water and the lactation performance of cows given diets of varying roughage content ad libitum. J. Agric. Sci. 70:223, 1968.

Ronning, M., Berousek, E. R., Griffith, J. R., and Gallup, W. D.: Carotene requirements of dairy cattle. Okla. Agric. Exp. Stn. Tech. Bull. T-76, 1959.

Satter, L. D., and Roffler, R. E.: Nitrogen requirements and utilization in dairy cattle. J. Dairy Sci. 58:1219, 1975.

Schmidt, G. H., and Schultz, L. H.: Effect of three levels of grain feeding during the dry period on the incidence of ketosis, severity of udder edema and subsequent milk production of dairy cows. J. Dairy Sci. 42:170, 1959.

Swanson, E. W.: Factors for computing requirements of protein for maintenance of cattle. J. Dairy Sci. 60:1583, 1977.

Swanson, E. W., Martin, G. G., Pardue, F. E., and Gorman, G. M.: Milk production of cows fed diets deficient in vitamin A. J. Anim. Sci. 27:541, 1968.

Ward, G., Dobson, R. C., and Dunham, J. R.: Influences of calcium and phosphorus intakes, vitamin D supplement and lactation on calcium and phosphorus balances. J. Dairy Sci. 55:768, 1972.

Swine

Jurgens, M. H.: Swine feeding guides. In M. H. Jurgens: Applied Animal Feeding and Nutrition. Dubuque, Ia, Kendall/Hunt Publishing Co., 95–105, 1974.

Leman, A. D.: Feeding pregnant sows and gilts; feeding sows at farrowing time; diets for feeding during lactation. Soc. Theriogenol. J. VII, 2nd ed., 1976.

National Research Council, Committee on Animal Nutrition: The Nutrient Requirements of Swine. 8th rev. ed. NAS-NRC, Washington, D. C., 1979.

Sheep

Armstrong, D. G., and Annison, E. F.: Amino acid requirements and amino acid supply in the sheep. Proc. Nutr. Soc. 32:107, 1973.

Asplund, J. M., and Pfander, W. H.: Effects of water restriction on nutrient digestibility in sheep receiving fixed water rations. J. Anim. Sci. 35:1271, 1972.

Bailey, C. B., Hironaka, R., and Slen, S. B.: Effects of the temperature on the environment and the drinking water on the temperature and water consumption of sheep. Can. J. Anim. Sci. 42:1, 1962.

Beardsly, D. W.: Symposium on forage utilization: Nutritive value of forages as affected by physical form. Beef cattle and sheep studies. J. Anim. Sci. 23:239, 1964.

Bogazoglu, P. A., Jordan, R. M., and Meade, R. J.: Sulfur-selenium-vitamin E interrelations in ovine nutrition. J. Anim. Sci. 26:1390, 1967.

Bhattacharya, A. N., and Pervez, E.: Effect of urea supplementation on intake and utilization of diets containing low quality roughages in sheep. J. Anim. Sci. 36:976, 1973.

Binns, W.: Range and pasture plants poisonous to sheep. J. Am. Vet. Med. Assoc. 164:284, 1974.

Buck, W. B., and Sharma, R. M.: Copper toxicity in sheep. Iowa State Univ. Vet. 31:4, 1969.

Butcher, J. E.: Is snow adequate and economical as a water source for sheep? Nat. Wool Grow. 60:28, 1970.

Calder, F. W., Nickolson, J. W. G., and Cunningham, H. M.: Water restriction for sheep on pasture and rate of consumption with other feeds. Can. J. Anim. Sci. 44:266, 1964.

Clifford, A. J., Goodrich, R. D., and Tillman, A. D.: Effects of supplementing ruminants all concentrate and purified diets with vitamins of the B complex. J. Anim. Sci. 26:400, 1967.

Cook, C. W., Stoddart, L. A., and Harris, L. E.: The nutritive value of winter range plants in the Great Basin as determined with digestion trials with sheep. Utah Agr. Exp. Stn. Bull. 372, 1954.

Cook, C. W., Stoddart, L. A., and Harris, L. E.: Comparative nutritive value and palatability of some introduced and native forage plants for spring and winter grazing. Utah Agr. Exp. Stn. Bull. 385, 1956.

Coop, I. E.: The energy requirements of sheep for maintenance and gain. 2. Pen fed sheep. J. Agr. Sci. 58:179, 1962.

Coop, I. E., and Hill, M. K.: The energy requirements of sheep for maintenance and gain. II. Grazing sheep. J. Agr. Sci. 58:187, 1962.

Daniels, L. B., Muhrer, M. E., Campbell, J. R., and Martz, F. A.: Feeding heated urea-cellulose preparations to ruminants. J. Anim. Sci. 32:348, 1971.

Dewey, D. W., Lee, H. J., and Marston, H. R.: Efficacy of cobalt pellets for providing cobalt for penned sheep. Aust. J. Agr. Res. 20:1109, 1969.

Driedger, A., and Hatfield, E. F.: Influence of tannins on the nutritive value of soybean meal for ruminants. J. Anim. Sci. 34:456, 1972.

Egan, D. A.: Control of an outbreak of hypomagnesaemic tetany in nursing ewes. Ir. Vet. J. 23:8, 1969.

Garrett, W. N., Meyer, J. H., and Lofgreen, G. P.: The comparative energy requirements for sheep and cattle for maintenance and gain. J. Anim. Sci. 18:528, 1959.

Garrigus, U. S.: The need for sulfur in the diets of ruminants. In O. H. Muth, and J. F. Olds: Symposium: Sulfur in Nutrition. Westport, Ct., A.V.I. Publishing Company, Inc., 126–152, 1970.

Goodrich, R. D., and Tillman, A. D.: Copper sulfate and molybdenum interrelationships in sheep. J. Nutr. 90:76, 1966.

Harris, L. E., Asplund, J. M., and Crampton, E. W.: An international feed nomenclature and methods for summarizing and using feed data to calculate diets. Utah Agr. Stn. Bull. 479 Logan 392P, 1968.

Harris, L. E., Cook, C. W., and Stoddart, L. A.: Feeding phosphorus, protein and energy supplements to ewes on winter ranges of Utah. Utah Agr. Exp. Bull. 398, 1956.

Hedrich, M. F., Elliot, J. M., and Low, J. E.: Response in vitamin B_{12} production and absorption to increasing cobalt intake in sheep. J. Nutr. 103:1646, 1973.

Hinds, F. C., Mansfield, M. E., and Lewis, J. M.: Early weaning of spring lambs. Ill. Res. 3:6, 1961.

Hogue, D. E.: The nutritional requirements of lactating ewes. In Sheep Nutrition and Feeding (Proceedings of a Symposium). Ames, Ia., Iowa State Univ., 32–39, 1968.

Holter, J. A., and Reid, J. T.: Relationships between the concentrations of crude protein and apparently digestible protein in forages. J. Anim. Sci. 18:1339, 1959.

Hopkins, L. L., Jr., Pope, A. L., and Baumann, C. A.: Contrasting nutritional responses to vitamin E and selenium in lambs. J. Anim. Sci. 23:674, 1964.

Huisingh, J., Gomez, G. G., and Matrone, G.: Interactions of copper, molybdenum and sulfate in ruminant nutrition. Fed. Proc. 32:1921, 1973.

Hutchings, S. S.: Managing winter sheep range for greater profit. U.S.D.A. Leaflet 423. Washington, D.C.: U.S. Government Printing Office, 1958.

Investigation Committee Report: Toxemic jaundice of sheep. Phytogenous chronic copper poisoning. Aust. Vet. J. 32:229, 1956.

James, L. F., and Butcher, J. E.: Halogen poisoning of sheep. Effect of high level oxalate intake. J. Anim. Sci. 35:1233, 1972.

James, L. F., Butcher, J. E., and VanKampen, K. R.: Relationship between Halogeton glomeratus consumption and water intake by sheep. J. Range Manage. 23:123, 1970.

Jensen, E., Klein, J. W., Rauchenstein, E., et al.: Input-output relationships in milk production. U.S.D.A. Tech. Bull. 815, 1942.

Jensen, R.: Diseases of Sheep. Philadelphia, Lea & Febiger, 246–247, 1974.

Joyce, J. P., Blaxter, K. L., and Park, C.: The effect of natural outdoor environments on the energy requirements of sheep. Res. Vet. Sci. 7:342, 1966.

Klosterman, E. W., Bolin, D. W., Buchanan, M. L., and Dinusson, W. E.: Protein requirements of ewes during breeding and pregnancy. J. Anim. Sci. 12:451, 1953.

Kromann, R. P., Joyner, A. E., and Sharp, J. E.: Influence of certain nutritional and physiological factors on urea toxicity in sheep. J. Anim. Sci. 32:732, 1971.

Langlands, J. P., Corbett, J. L., McDonald, I., and Duller, J. D.: Estimates of the energy required for maintenance by adult sheep. 1. Housed sheep. Anim. Prod. 5:11, 1963.

Langlands, J. P., Corbett, J. L., McDonald, I., and Reid, G. W.: Estimates of the energy required for maintenance by adult sheep. 2. Grazing sheep. Anim. Prod. 5:11, 1963.

Lee, H. J., and Marston, H. R.: The requirement for cobalt of sheep grazed on cobalt deficient pastures. Aust. J. Res. 20:905, 1969.

LeRoy, R. S., Zelter, S. Z., and Francois, A. C.: Protection of protein in feeds against deamination in the rumen. Nutr. Abstr. Rev. 35:444, 1965.

Lillie, R. J.: Air pollutants affecting the performance of domestic animals. In: Agriculture Handbook 380. Agr. Res. Service, U.S.D.A., Washington, D.C., 1970.

Marcilese, N. A., Ammerman, C. B., Valsecchi, R. M., Dunavant, B. G., and Davis, G. K.: Effect of dietary molybdenum and sulfate upon copper metabolism in sheep. J. Nutr. 99:177, 1969.

McDonald, I. W.: The nutrition of grazing ruminants. Nutr. Abstr. Rev. 38:381–400, 1968.

Mitchell, H. H., and Edman, M.: The fluorine problem in livestock feeding. Nutr. Abstr. Rev. 21:787, 1952.

Moir, R. J., Somers, M., and Bray, A. C.: Utilization of dietary sulfur and nitrogen by ruminants. Sulfur Inst. J. 3:15, 1967–1968.

National Academy of Sciences-National Research Council: Nutrient Requirements of Sheep, 5th ed. NAS-NRC, Washington, D.C., 1975.

Oltjen, R. R.: Effects of feeding ruminants nonprotein nitrogen as the only nitrogen source. J. Anim. Sci. 29:673, 1969.

Pierson, R. E., and Aanes, W. A.: Treatment of chronic copper poisoning in sheep. J. Am. Vet. Med. Assoc. 133:307, 1958.

Purser, D. B.: Nitrogen metabolism in the rumen: Microorganisms as a source of protein for the ruminant animal. J. Anim. Sci. 30:988, 1970.

Ranhotra, G. S., and Jordan, R. M.: Protein and energy requirements of lambs weaned at six to eight weeks of age as determined by growth and digestion studies. J. Anim. Sci. 25:630, 1966.

Rattray, P. V., Garrett, W. N., East, N. E., and Hinman, N.: Efficiency of utilization of metabolizable energy during pregnancy and energy requirements for sheep. J. Anim. Sci. 38:383, 1974.

Reid, R. L.: The physiopathology of undernourishment in pregnant sheep with particular reference to pregnancy toxemia. In C. A. Brandly, and C. E. Cornelius (eds.): Advances in Veterinary Science. New York, Academic Press, 163–238, 1968.

Reis, P. J.: The growth and composition of wool. 4. The differential response of growth and sulfur content of wool to the level of sulfur containing amino acids given per abomasum. Aust. J. Biol. Sci. 20:809, 1967.

Ross, D. B.: The effect of oral ammonium molybdate and sodium sulfate given to lambs with high levels of copper concentration. Res. Vet. Sci. 11:295, 1970.

Sheepman's Production Handbook, Denver, Co., SID Inc., 1970.

Subcommittee on Feed Composition, Committee on Animal Nutrition, National Research Council: United States-Canadian Tables of Feed Composition. National Academy of Sciences, Washington, D. C., 1969.

Subcommittee on Fluorosis, Committee on Animal Nutrition, National Research Council: Effects of Fluorides in Animals. National Academy of Sciences, Washington, D.C., 1974.

Subcommittee on Selenium, Committee on Animal Nutrition, National Research Council: Selenium in Nutrition. National Academy of Sciences, Washington, D.C., 1971.

Tomas, F. M., Jones, G. B., Potter, B. J., and Langsford, G. L.: Influence of saline drinking water on mineral balances in sheep. Aust. J. Res. 24:377, 1973.

Torrell, D. T., Hume, I. D., and Weir, W. C.: Flushing of range ewes by supplementation, dry lot feeding or grazing of improved pasture. J. Range Manage. 25:357, 1972.

Underwood, E. J., and Somers, M.: Studies of zinc nutrition in sheep. 1. The relation of zinc to growth, testicular development and spermatogenesis in young rams. Aust. J. Agr. Res. 20:889, 1969.

VanSoest, P. J.: Symposium on factors influencing the voluntary intake of herbage by ruminants: Voluntary intake in relation to chemical composition and digestibility. J. Anim. Sci. 24:834, 1965.

Weir, W. C., and Torrell, D. T.: Supplemental feeding of sheep grazing on dry range. Calif. Agr. Exp. Stn. Bull. 832, 1967.

Wilson, A. D., and Dudzinski, M. L.: Influence of the concentration and volume of saline water on the food intake of sheep and their excretion of sodium and water in urine and faeces. Aust. J. Agr. Res. 24:245, 1973.

Wright, P. L., Pope, A. L., and Phillips, P. H.: Pelleted roughages for gestating and lactating ewes. Wis. Agr. Exp. Stn. Res. Bull. 239, 1962.

Young, B. A., and Corbett, J. L.: Maintenance energy requirements of grazing sheep in relation to herbage availability. I. Calorimetric estimates. Aust. J. Agr. Res. 23:57, 1972.

General Pediatric Feeding: Milk Replacers in Pediatric Feeding

LAVERNE M. SCHUGEL, D.V.M.

The nutrition of the pre-ruminant calf is most important to a successful dairy calf rearing program. Numerous surveys have shown that the loss due to death of the pre-ruminant calf in the United States is about 15 per cent. Good nutrition can aid the young calf in combating stress, thus lowering the risk of disease. Unfortunately, many of the nutritional requirements of the neonatal calf are not clearly defined.

DIGESTIVE SYSTEM AND DIGESTIVE ACTIVITY OF THE NEWBORN CALF

When considering the nutritional requirements of the neonatal calf, an important fact to remember is that the digestive system of the neonatal calf functions much differently than that of the adult bovine.

The newborn calf has a stomach with four parts like the adult bovine; however, the various parts are much different in comparative size. In the newborn calf, the abomasum has a capacity of more than twice that of the other compartments and is the only functional portion. In the adult bovine, the abomasum comprises only 8 per cent of the total capacity, whereas the rumen represents 80 per cent of the total.[1]

In the young calf, the liquid is shunted by the reticulorumen and is directed into the abomasum by flowing through a tube formed by the esophageal groove. The groove, which extends from the cardia to the reticuloomasal orifice, is closed by a reflex reaction that is stimulated by consumption of liquids.[2] Milk is the best stimulant; however, glucose and sodium bicarbonate solutions are usually effective stimulants. Water will effect closure of the groove in the very young calf but becomes less effective as the calf becomes older.

As milk is ingested, the first enzyme activity to start the digestive process is the salivary lipase. Minutes after the milk reaches the abomasum, it begins to clot owing to the action of the enzyme renin. Pepsin activity starts very early in life also.[3] As early as five minutes after feeding and continuing for three to four hours, whey is released from the clot and passes into the duodenum, followed thereafter by partially digested casein.[4]

The enzyme activity of the intestine is largely that of lactase. Until the calf is about seven or eight weeks of age, there is very little maltase, amylase, or sucrase activity.[5] This is why the neonatal calf can utilize only milk carbohydrates or simple sugars.

The age at which ruminal digestion begins is largely dependent upon the diet the calf receives. The earlier the calf is exposed to dry feed with a fiber source, the earlier ruminal development will start, and the faster it will progress. The longer the calf receives a plentiful milk supply, the less inclined the calf is to supplement its nutrient intake with dry food. However, if the liquid diet is limited, the calf will start to consume dry food at a few days of age.

NUTRIENT REQUIREMENTS OF THE CALF

Dry Matter Intake

The dry matter intake of the young calf depends somewhat on the form of the diet offered. Until the calf reaches 75 kg, the dry matter intake will be higher in liquid form than in dry form.[3] The concentration of the liquid diet will affect dry matter intake. The higher concentrated liquid feeds—up to 25 per cent dry matter—result in higher dry matter intake.[6] The maximum dry matter intake in the neonatal calf is just over 2 per cent of body weight and increases as the calf grows older.

The higher the digestible energy of the ration, the higher will be the dry matter intake. Thus, the importance of providing high quality feeds for the pre-ruminant calf becomes clear. Temperature will affect voluntary feed intake. High ambient temperatures will decrease feed intake.

Water

Adequate water supply is an important part of calf nutrition. Many factors affect water intake. High ambient temperatures, high dry matter intake, high levels of salt, and high protein levels will all increase water intake. When water is offered in unlimited amounts, dry matter intake increases.

Energy

The energy requirements for the calf are divided into maintenance requirements and growth requirements. The maintenance requirements consist of those for basal metabolism, plus a small loss in the urine, plus the production of heat from any voluntary activity. Blaxter and Wood found that the maintenance requirement for the pre-ruminant calf is 52.4 kcal digestible energy per kg per day and 307 kcal for 100 g of body weight gain.[7] Brisson and co-workers reported a growth requirement of 268 kcal digestible energy per 100 g of body weight gain and 44.7 kcal digestible energy per kg of body weight per day.[8] Considering that whole milk contains about 700 kcal per kg and a high quality milk replacer contains about 4400 kcal per kg of dry matter, the young calf needs about 3.2 kg of whole milk or 0.45 kg of dry, quality milk replacer daily for maintenance. An additional 4 to 5 kg of whole milk or 0.6 to 0.8 kg of milk replacer is necessary to put on 1 kg of weight.[9]

Protein

The protein requirements for the calf are determined by the body weight of the calf, plus the amount of weight gain per day plus the percentage of body weight gain per day. The amount of digestible protein required for maintenance is 0.5 g per kg of body weight, and the amount of digestible protein needed for growth is 22 g per 100 g of weight gain.[9]

The digestibility of the protein of whole milk and of a good quality milk replacer is about 97 per cent and 94 per cent, respectively.

Only a portion of the protein that is digested is actually retained in the body. This portion is termed "biologic value." The biologic value of milk is 80 to 90.[7, 8] Other protein sources will usually have a lower biologic value.

Minerals

The dietary mineral requirements of the pre-ruminant calf are incompletely defined in most cases. The requirements for calcium and phosphorus have been designated by the National Research Council.[10] The National Research Council states that a 40-kg calf requires 2.2 g of calcium and 1.7 g of phosphorus daily.[10] The true absorption of dietary calcium decreases with age, but it is markedly affected by the source of calcium. The absorption of calcium from milk is much higher than that from dry feed. This is also true of phosphorus. The presence of chronic diarrhea in the young calf markedly decreases absorption of calcium and phosphorus and also limits retention of calcium and phosphorus.[11]

Magnesium requirements are met as soon as the calf receives grain or roughage in the diet. If the calf's diet contains solely milk for several weeks, milk tetany may develop.[12]

The requirements for potassium, which is found largely in soft tissues, are not well defined. Normal diets usually are more than adequate in potassium. Potassium deficiencies occur only during diarrheal conditions. Thus, potassium should be part of any electrolyte therapy.

Unlike potassium, sodium is found largely in body fluids. When feeding a milk diet, the sodium and chloride requirements are met by the natural salts contained in the milk ingredients. Again, sodium deficiencies usually occur when diarrheal conditions exist.

Trace mineral nutrition of the young calf can be very complex. In most cases, a normally balanced nutritional diet will meet the calf's needs. However, particular deficiencies can occur in different geographic areas.

Vitamins

The calf is born with minimal reserves of vitamin A and is dependent upon colostrum as an immediate source. However, when the dam is deficient in vitamin A, the colostrum may also be low in vitamin A.

The National Research Council recommends about 42 I.U. units of vitamin A per kg of body weight.[10] Higher levels are usually recommended because of the problems incurred with deficiencies.

Vitamin D is important to the calf and is associated with calcium and phosphorus metabolism. The National Research Council recommends about 6.5 I.U. units per kg of body weight.[10] As with vitamin A, higher levels are usually recommended.

A deficiency of vitamin E will result in white muscle disease. Until the calf consumes cereal grains, vitamin E supplementation is usually necessary. Selenium is intimately linked with the function of vitamin E, and a shortage of either will affect the other. The ratio will determine how much vitamin E supplementation is necessary. It is usually in the range of 15 to 35 mg per kg of dry matter.[9]

Table 1. *Daily B Vitamin Requirement for 45-kg Calf*

Vitamin	Daily Requirement (mg)
Thiamine	2.9
Riboflavin	2.0
Niacin	11.7
Pyridoxine	2.9
Pantothenic acid	8.8
Biotin	0.9
Choline	1170.0
Folic acid	0.7
Inositol	234.0

The various B vitamins are essential for the calf. However, all B vitamins are usually in sufficient supply in milk products except for vitamin B_{12}. Once rumination starts, calves will synthesize their own B vitamins. Table 1 includes the suggested daily requirements for a 45-kg calf.[13]

Because vitamin B_{12} exists in low quantities in milk products, it is necessary to supplement the diet of the calf. The National Research Council suggests that the requirement of vitamin B_{12} per kg of live weight is 0.34 to 0.68 mg.[10]

NUTRIENT SOURCES

The first feed the calf usually receives is colostrum. Colostrum feeding continues for a minimum of three to four days.

After the first three or four days, the dairyman has three choices to provide milk:

1. Whole milk.
2. Excess colostrum.
3. Milk substitutes or milk replacers.

Whole milk is the most perfect food for the young calf. However, economics makes it almost mandatory that the dairyman select another source of milk nutrients for the calf.

Excess colostrum, or more correctly called fresh-cow milk, is an excellent food. However, it is extremely variable in composition. The solids content of colostrum, which is approximately 27.4 per cent at the time of parturition, drops to 12.8 per cent by 96 hours. The protein content will drop from 13.9 per cent to 2.7 per cent.[9] These variations must be considered when excess colostrum is used.

Excess colostrum may be used fresh, frozen, or fermented. If it is used fresh, it must all be used daily. Thus, only large herds can utilize this method. Freezing colostrum requires a considerable amount of time and effort. Fermented colostrum has become very popular. However, in warm weather, users of fermented colostrum have encountered some difficulties such as offensive odors, putrefaction, and calf refusal. Colostrum preservatives have been researched and reported effective.[14]

Surveys have shown that 70 per cent of the dairymen in the United States use milk replacers. However, it is important that quality milk replacers are used.

Schugel has classified milk replacers into four categories: (1) optimum, (2) acceptable, (3) passable, and (4) inferior.[9]

The optimum milk replacers contain protein only from milk sources. The protein level should be at least 20 per cent. The National Research Council recommends a protein level of 22 per cent. However, there is research evidence and field experience indicating that 20 per cent protein is sufficient if all of the protein is from quality milk ingredients.[15] The fat level should be at least 10 per cent, but higher levels—up to 20 per cent—will give better results. To be in the optimum range, all of the ingredients in a milk replacer must be of the highest quality.

The milk replacers in the acceptable range differ from those in the optimum range in that a portion of the protein may be derived from specially manufactured soy flours or soy concentrates. The protein level should be 22 per cent and the fat level at least 10 per cent. These milk replacers will give reasonably good performance but not as good as those in the optimum range.

The passable category contains those milk replacers in which a portion of the protein is from nonmilk sources and the milk ingredients are not all of high quality. The protein level should be at least 22 per cent and the fat level 10 per cent. Even under excellent conditions, the passable milk replacers will not give satisfactory results and should not be used.

In the last category are the inferior milk replacers. This category includes all milk replacers that do not fit any of the previous categories and should not be used under any circumstances.

Not only should calf starters be nutritionally sound, but they should be palatable as well. The calf starter should contain at least 16 per cent protein, all from natural sources.[10] If the calf is introduced to dry feed early, full ruminal development can occur at six to eight weeks of age.

Hay may be introduced by the second week. However, the introduction of hay can be delayed as long as two months with satisfactory results. For maximum efficiency, the hay used should be of the highest quality available.

Hay or corn silage is not recommended until the calf is at least two months of age. Because of limited digestive capacity, the younger calf cannot utilize these high moisture feeds.

References

1. Sisson, S.: The Anatomy of the Domestic Animals, 5th ed. Philadelphia, W. B. Saunders Company, 1975.
2. Comline, R. S., and Titcher, D. A.: Reflex contraction of the esophageal groove in young ruminants. J. Physiol. *115*:210–226, 1951.
3. Roy, J. H. B.: The Calf, 3rd ed. State College, Pa., Penn State University Press, 1970.
4. Mylrea, P. J.: Digestion of milk in young calves. Res. Vet. Sci. *7*:333–341, 1966.
5. Okamoto, M., Thomas, J. W., and Johnson, T. L.: Utilization of various carbohydrates by young calves. J. Dairy Sci. *42*:920, 1959.
6. Pettyjohn, J. S., Everett, J. P., Jr., and Mochrie, R. D.: Responses of dairy calves to milk replacers fed at various concentrations. J. Dairy Sci. *46*:710–714, 1963.
7. Blaxter, K. L., and Wood, W. A.: The nutrition of the young Ayrshire calf. Br. J. Nutr. *5*:55–67, 1951.
8. Brisson, G. J., Cunningham, H. M., and Haskell, S. R.: The protein and energy requirements of young dairy calves. Can. J. Anim. Sci. *37*:157–167, 1957.
9. Schugel, L. M.: Proceedings 6th Annual Convention American Association of Bovine Practitioners. Fort Worth, Texas, 82–89, 1973.
10. National Research Council: Nutrient Requirements of Dairy Cattle No. 3. National Academy of Science—National Research Council, Washington, D.C., 1978.
11. Raven, A. M., and Robinson, K. L.: Studies of the nutrition of the young calf. Br. J. Nutr. *12*:469–482, 1958.

12. Rook, J. A. F., and Storry, J. E.: Magnesium in the nutrition of farm animals. Nutr. Abstr. Rev. *32*:1055–1077, 1962.
13. Radostits, O. M., and Bell, J. M.: Nutrition of the pre-ruminant dairy calf with special reference to the digestion and absorption of nutrients. A review. Can. J. Anim. Sci. *50*:405–452, 1970.
14. Polzin, H. W., Otterby, D. E., and Johnson, D. J.: Performance of baby calves fed fermented or acidified colostrum. J. Dairy Sci. *58*:692, 1975.
15. Schugel, L. M., Friedrich, F. L., and Englestad, W.: Protein levels in milk replacers. J. Dairy Sci. *55*:703, 1972.

Protein Nutrition and Nonprotein Nitrogen

H. H. VAN HORN, Ph.D.

Next to energy, protein is required in larger magnitude than any other nutrient. Since protein is the principal constituent of the organs and soft structures of the animal body, a liberal and continuous supply is needed in food throughout life for growth and repair. Thus, transformation of food protein into body protein is a very important part of the nutrition process. In order to be utilized by an animal, protein first must be broken down by digestion into the amino acids from which it was made. Proteins from various sources have different combinations of amino acids. The generalized chemical structure of an amino acid is

where R represents different carbon chains with varying lengths, configurations, and combinations with other chemical elements. Some amino acids can be made within the body from other compounds, but others can be made only by plants and bacteria. For more than a century it has been known that not all proteins are of equal value. The variation has been shown to be due to amino acid content for nonruminants and to a combination of amino acid content and ability to escape degradation within the rumen for ruminants. Amino acids that cannot be manufactured by the animal's metabolism in adequate amounts are termed "essential amino acids." Simple-stomached animals all require dietary sources of these amino acids. Research has progressed to the point where we know requirements for most limiting amino acids for poultry and swine and is concerned now with whether or not amino acids delivered from the rumen to the lower intestine for digestion and absorption adequately meet optimum performance requirements for ruminant animals and, if not, how to get "by-pass" protein through the rumen most efficiently to meet these requirements.

Fortunately, a ruminant animal such as the cow has billions of microorganisms in its rumen that are capable of synthesizing proteins for themselves from amino acids and nonprotein nitrogen (NPN) derived from the cow's diet. These microbial proteins subsequently are digested and absorbed by the cow, giving her a source of all essential amino acids even though her diet may not have contained all of them in adequate amounts. Therefore, protein quality is not of as much importance to the cow as it is to simple-stomached animals because the rumen microorganisms alter dietary content. Cows eating purified diets with all of the nitrogen in the form of urea and ammonium salt not only have survived and maintained themselves but have produced as much as 4500 kg of milk in a year and reproduced normally. These experiments have demonstrated that ruminants can live without any preformed protein in their rations so long as nitrogen is available to ruminal microorganisms for protein synthesis. However, this level of milk production is not high by today's standards, thus indicating that rumen synthesis of amino acids cannot totally meet optimum performance needs of ruminants.

Of possible detriment to the ruminant animal is the degradation of much (60 per cent is common) dietary true protein to peptides, amino acids, and ammonia by microorganisms as they metabolize for the synthesis of more microbial cells. Ammonia is used extensively by many species of microorganisms; however, some require preformed peptides or amino acids. If these are not provided in the diet, some microorganisms may disappear from the rumen, changing the balance of species. The total quantity of protein synthesized may thus be altered. There may be a reduction in yield if ammonia concentration is low, i.e., less than 8 mg N/100 ml. This is a situation in which NPN is used as efficiently as protein nitrogen.

Protein deficiencies usually do not show up immediately to the extent observed with a decline in feed intake. However, over a period of a few weeks or more, growth and/or milk production will be subnormal from protein-deficient diets. Severe protein deficiencies will reduce growth rate in both the fetus (resulting in small animals at birth) and the young animal. With deficiencies of essential amino acids in the diet, animals will not grow at a normal rate even though there may be an excess of other amino acids available.

ANALYSIS OF FEEDS FOR PROTEIN

In common with fats and carbohydrates, proteins contain carbon, hydrogen, and oxygen. In addition, they contain a large and fairly constant percentage of nitrogen. Most of them also contain sulfur, and a few contain phosphorus and iron. Since proteins uniquely contain a large amount of nitrogen (about 16 per cent) whereas other major nutrients contain no nitrogen, protein can be estimated from nitrogen analysis. Crude protein is calculated by multiplying the nitrogen content of a feed by 6.25. This figure is derived from the fact that most proteins contain about 16 per cent nitrogen. (If one divides 100 by 16, the quotient is 6.25. Therefore, if the nitrogen content is multiplied by 6.25 the result will approximate the protein content of a feed.)

Not all of the nitrogen in feeds is in the form of protein. Some feeds, particularly green roughages, contain one third or more of their nitrogen as NPN substances, such as amides, ammonium salts, amino acids, alkaloids, and other nitrogenous compounds. Because of NPN, multiplication of nitrogen content by 6.25 does not give a value for true protein. Crude protein, therefore, represents a combination of true protein and NPN. For ruminant animals that can make use of some NPN, however, crude protein is quite useful and often is as good a measure for protein allowances as true protein. Nonruminants, however, cannot use crude protein from all sources equally because of the variation in NPN content.

Digestible protein is the amount of crude protein consumed minus the crude protein excreted in the feces. In actuality, this should be called apparent digestible protein rather than true digestible protein. This is because part of the nitrogen in feces is in the form of metabolic fecal nitrogen, which is independent of the protein consumed and arises from metabolic functions in the body, such as residues of bile and other digestive juices, epithelial cells from the alimentary tract, and undigested bacterial residues. It is very difficult to separate metabolic fecal nitrogen from truly undigested feed nitrogen, and since both represent losses to the animal, digestible protein has come to mean apparent digestible protein in practical usage.

Digestible protein has been the measure most commonly used in the past for listing protein allowances for many classes of livestock. Table values, which are digestibility estimates from experiments, exist for most feed ingredients. However, apparent digestibility of feed proteins is directly related to percentage of total crude protein in the ration. Metabolic fecal nitrogen, being independent of the amount of protein consumed, contributes a larger proportion of the total fecal nitrogen excreted when low-protein rations are fed compared with high-protein diets. Thus, digestibility coefficients are reduced further for low-protein feeds than for high-protein feeds by not accounting for metabolic fecal nitrogen. Crude protein, therefore, is a more accurate measure when calculating protein allowances in typical rations. Furthermore, crude protein is much simpler to determine. Both crude protein and digestible protein values must be tempered by knowledge of NPN levels in feeds and the ability of animals to utilize NPN.

DETERMINING PROTEIN REQUIREMENTS

Even though requirements may be generally known, costs for protein supplements of commonly available energy sources have been quite variable and at times extremely high. Thus, substitutions for traditional supplements and restriction of protein to the low side of the optimum protein range may give more profits. Also, rapid gains in livestock performance and continued research breakthroughs in the understanding of protein metabolism in ruminants and in the availability of amino acids in nonruminants continually stimulate re-evaluation of protein feeding standards. Since lactating animals require more than growing animals and much more than animals being fed maintenance rations only, a lactation example is used here to show typical variation in performance response to different dietary protein percentages. Since soybean meal is a widely used protein supplement and a high quality protein source, the example uses soybean meal as the supplement to other ingredients. Lactation responses of dairy cows to protein can be observed quite easily when higher protein from added soybean meal is compared with rations with crude protein of 11.0 per cent of the total ration dry matter or less. The graph in Figure 1 summarizes 13 experiments in which soybean meal was the protein source in complete rations for dairy cows. It

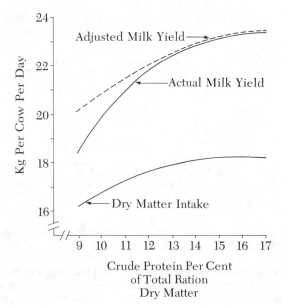

Figure 1. Milk yield and feed intake responses to increasing ration protein with soybean meal.

is obvious that the response follows a diminishing returns curve with particularly small returns above 14 per cent.

In most research showing a response to higher protein, cows ate more of high-protein diets. Figure 1 also shows a feed intake response curve to increasing protein and a milk yield curve adjusted for feed intake effect. In comparing actual milk yield with milk yield adjusted for feed intake, it can be seen that the effect of protein on feed intake disappears at about 13 per cent of ration dry matter. Other data indicate greater efficiency of energy utilization along with increasing feed intake.

Considering the data in Figure 1, establishing the optimum protein level for a diet with known protein quality is difficult because of the curvilinear nature of the response that shows less and less performance return for each increment of protein. Obviously, with response curves such as those in Figure 1, an economic decision must be made to select the optimum protein level.

Table 1 utilizes milk yield and feed intakes plotted in Figure 1 to make a choice of an optimum protein level. Changes in milk yield and intake for each 1 per cent increase in crude protein per cent of the dry matter are shown. The changes in kg per day are given so that actual increases in dollars returned and in dollars of extra feed cost can be calculated. Feed costs increase owing to extra feed consumption, increases in the cost of each unit of all that is fed, and the cost of increasing the percentage of protein. In this example, using $10 per hundredweight milk, $100 per ton for the total air-dry ration, and soybean meal costing $100 per ton more than corn, feed costs exceeded added value of milk in changing crude protein from 14 to 15 per cent of the total ration dry matter. Thus, 14 per cent protein is the optimum level. If $12 per hundredweight milk had been chosen, no financial loss would have been incurred in increasing to 15 per cent crude protein in the total ration dry matter. The data in Figure 1 and Table 2 are good examples of the kind of information needed to properly interpret performance responses to changing ration protein.

Table 1. *Marginal Changes in Milk, Dry Matter (DM) Intake, and Estimated Returns to Changing Ration Protein Per Cent with Soybean Meal*

Change in Protein Per Cent of DM from	Per Cent Increase in		KG/Day Increase in		Daily Increase in	
	Milk*	DM Intake*	Milk*	DM Intake*	Milk Value†	Feed Cost†
9 to 10%	7.9%	3.9%	1.46 kg	0.63 kg	$0.32	$0.12
10 to 11	5.6	2.9	1.12	0.49	0.25	0.11
11 to 12	4.0	2.1	0.83	0.36	0.18	0.10
12 to 13	2.7	1.6	0.60	0.26	0.13	0.09
13 to 14	1.8	0.8	0.40	0.16	0.09	0.08
14 to 15	1.2	0.6	0.28	0.10	0.06	0.07
15 to 16	0.9	0.3	0.20	0.05	0.04	0.06
16 to 17	0.7	0.1	0.17	0.02	0.04	0.06

*The base values for 9 per cent diets used in this example are 18.41 kg milk per day and 16.20 kg feed intake per day.
†Milk value for this estimate is assumed to be $10 per 100 pounds (22¢/kg) and feed cost of $100 per ton (11¢/kg) for 9 per cent crude protein ration. It is assumed also that soybean meal costs $100/ton (11¢/kg) more than corn.

Variation in amount and balance of absorbable amino acids may be brought about by factors other than level of protein, e.g., protein source, supplementation with limiting amino acids, heat treatment, or processing methods that affect digestibility of proteins. For example, cottonseed meal gives a different response curve than soybean meal, and most certainly the response curve would be varied further with post-ruminal supplementation of limiting amino acids. In all cases, diminishing returns curves such as those in Figure 1 exist, giving the opportunity for economic data to be applied before selecting optimum protein rations.

NONPROTEIN NITROGEN (NPN) UTILIZATION

For the most part, NPN utilization is of concern in protein metabolism in ruminant animals since it is only in ruminants that proteins and amino acids derived from microbial fermentation are made available in large quantities to the host animal. However, it is possible that NPN could be of some benefit for nonruminants if essential amino acids were available at adequate levels but nonessential amino acids were not. Then, with available ammonia and proper carbon structures for transamination, nonessential amino acids might be metabolized by the nonruminant in the absence of microbial intervention. However, NPN utilization relates primarily to ruminants.

Urea is by far the major feed additive used to supply NPN to rumen microorganisms for use in protein synthesis during microbial growth. The major justification for incorporation of NPN into rations is one of economics. Generally, reduced feed costs and increased profits have resulted from inclusion of as much NPN in ruminant rations as possible without depressing growth and milk

Table 2. *Response to Incremental Additions of Urea to Rations for Lactating Dairy Cows*

Ration	Urea (%)	Crude Protein (%)	Milk Yield (KG/Day)
Basal ration	1.1	11.4	16.9
Plus 1 increment urea	1.7	13.2	17.4
Plus 2 increments urea	2.3	15.0	17.0
Basal ration	0.4	11.2	17.6
Plus 1 increment urea	1.7	14.3	17.7
Plus 2 increments urea	3.0	18.8	16.4

yield or impairing the health of animals. In many rations, 3.2 kg of shelled corn and 0.45 kg of urea is equal in net energy and crude protein to 3.6 kg of soybean meal. The amount of savings possible depends directly on the price of soybean meal and corn in this kind of comparison. However, a savings of 7 to 10 cents per cow daily can be realized at feed prices of $2.50 to $3.50 per bushel for corn and about $160 per ton for soybean meal. Extrapolating these savings per day to large herds makes reductions in feed costs great enough to encourage use of NPN to the fullest extent possible without reduction in animal performance.

Complete substitution of NPN for protein in purified diets for ruminants has shown that animals do not perform as well as when some natural protein is provided. Growth and feed efficiency are reduced with these purified diets, and attempts at improving performance with amino acid supplementation either singly or in combination have been largely unsuccessful. Ruminants fed diets free of protein have depressed concentrations of branch chain volatile fatty acids. They also have depressed free blood plasma concentrations of essential amino acids and increased concentrations of glycine and serine. Ruminal synthesis of B vitamins is apparently normal, and cattle raised on purified diets from 84 days of age to 4 years of age have been fertile and reproduced normally. Also, moderate milk production (up to 4500 kg per cow yearly) has been obtained.

It has been shown *in vitro* that true protein from growing rumen microorganisms increases rapidly with diets up to 12 per cent crude protein of dry matter but does not increase further with added NPN.[1] Ammonia accumulates after microorganisms stop increasing their growth rate at 12 per cent crude protein. These data suggest that if higher levels of feed protein are needed for optimum performance in ruminants, the extra protein added to diets must be natural feed protein so that even after 60 per cent, or at least a large part, of feed protein is degraded in the rumen, some net gain will be achieved in the amount of protein leaving the rumen and being digested and absorbed. Although this model was developed mostly from fermentation studies in the laboratory, results are confirmed with direct feeding trials. For example, Table 2 shows no milk yield response in lactating cows receiving added urea as a source of NPN above basal rations that were either 11.4 or 11.2 per cent crude protein of total ration dry matter. Numerous other studies show the benefit of urea supplementation in bringing crude protein of rations up to approximately 12 per cent crude protein in total ration dry matter. Some experiments even show some benefit to adding urea slightly above 12 per cent protein levels.

It can be seen by this point that neither a model using digestible protein nor one using crude protein adequately describes the expected protein effects of a particular diet on animal performance with reference to comparative values of NPN and true protein. Recently, Iowa State University researchers described protein requirements for ruminant animals in terms of "metabolizable protein," which is the amount of protein (amino acids) absorbed from the gastrointestinal tract.[2] Metabolizable protein for ruminants represents *protein leaving the rumen* as feed or microbial protein *that is digested and absorbed*. This can be quite different from crude or true protein in the ration, since protein increases in the rumen with some high NPN diets and decreases in variable amounts with other rations depending on amount of protein degradation by rumen microorganisms. The advantage of this concept over a model using true protein or digestible protein is that it accounts for the effectiveness of NPN in substituting for true protein needs of cattle in some rations and for the ineffectiveness of NPN in other rations and for differences in rumen degradation of true protein of ration ingredients. Variation in energy value as it affects NPN conversion to bacterial protein is also considered.

Table 3 gives data supporting the metabolizable protein concept but indicates the need for further information before a shift can occur to this system as the standard for animal requirements and ration balancing. The table presents data from two experiments. In one animal, performance, as measured through milk yield, was compared with low-protein (basal) rations and rations that had the same NPN levels but were increased in protein by adding soybean meal (soy increment diets). The second experiment measured metabolism of true protein (tungstic acid precipitable protein) from these same diets in rumen-fistulated animals that were not lactating. Note that the basal diets were formulated to be as equal as possible in estimated metabolizable protein, using estimated metabolizable coefficients of various ration ingredients presented by Burroughs and associates.[2] They have estimated degradation of feedstuffs within the rumen and the amount of NPN that can be fermented to microbial protein (urea fermentation potential).

Although the 1.90 per cent urea diet was estimated to be equal to the other basal diets, milk yield data showed that it was not equal. The basal diet with no urea (supplemented with soybean meal) was not superior to the 0.95 per cent urea diet, thus indicating that 0.95 per cent urea could be satisfactorily substituted for some soybean meal. Metabolized true protein of these diets was distinctly higher for 0.95 per cent and nonurea diets compared with those containing 1.90 per cent urea. Note also that metabolized true protein closely parallels milk yield for all diets in the soy increment diets. Metabolizable protein, therefore, seems to be potentially a good feeding standard, as added research allows increased accuracy of estimating degradability and urea fermentation potential of various feed ingredients. Estimated metabolizable protein values of Burroughs and associates also appear to fit performance well except for the overestimation of urea utilization in the 1.90 per cent urea supplemented basal diet.[2]

Solubility of protein within the rumen is a major factor affecting protein degradability within the rumen and is considered in metabolizable protein. It is discussed here because some nutritionists have devised standards for soluble protein as an easy-to-determine and hopeful equivalent of metabolizable protein. For example, casein (milk protein) is readily soluble and highly degradable within the rumen. Thus, although it is a high-quality protein if delivered intact to the lower digestive tract, it would have very little additional value above urea in the rumen because of its degradation to constituent amino acids and on further to ammonia and volatile fatty acids. Conversely, less soluble proteins, such as zein (corn protein) may escape degradation to a large extent within the rumen and then be digested in the lower digestive system. The value of this protein then depends on its quality (amino acid balance and extent digested in lower digestive tract). If proteins escape degradation in the rumen but are really lower quality than microbial protein that might be made had they been broken down in the rumen, no gain is achieved. Until more definitive data are available to help in applied situations, the ruminant nutritionist should use crude protein feeding standards and good judgment regarding solubility and estimates of metabolizable protein to decide how much of the crude protein can be from NPN. Some helpful guidelines are:

1. Urea (or equivalent NPN from ammonia or other sources) is not likely to be beneficial in ruminant diets when used in excess of 1.0 per cent of the total ration dry matter. For dairy cows, which need at least 14 per cent protein, probably no more than 0.5 per cent urea can be effectively utilized.

2. Some natural protein will be beneficial in performance rations. For example, urea-supplemented corn silage

Table 3. *Evaluation of Metabolizable Protein (MP) as the Ruminant Protein Response Variable*

Ration	Urea (Per Cent)	Milk Yield (KG/Day)	Estimated MP Per Cent of Dry Ration*	Metabolized True Protein Per Cent of Air Dry Ration†
Basal Diets				
11.0%	1.90	15.0	5.9	3.8
11.9%	0.95	16.5	5.4	4.7
10.1%	0.00	16.4	5.9	4.6
Soy Increments Diets				
14.3%	1.90	18.0	5.5	5.2
14.2%	0.95	18.1	5.8	5.2
15.0%	0.00	18.9	6.7	5.8

*Metabolizable protein per cent (MP per cent) was estimated using rumen degradation and urea fermentation values of Burroughs et al.[2]
†Tungstic acid precipitable protein was the measure of true protein.

may be adequate without any natural protein supplementation for older animals on a finishing diet and animals on maintenance rations but will not be adequate for young, fast-growing animals. The usual level for supplementing urea is about 9.1 kg per ton, which usually brings the crude protein on the dry matter basis up to about 12 per cent.

3. Urea is less likely to be beneficial in diets that have a large amount of highly soluble protein as compared with low-protein diets that also contain some less soluble protein sources such as corn, soybean meal, or cottonseed meal. Some of these more soluble sources might include linseed meal, wheat middlings and wheat bran, and dried whey. If over 30 per cent of the crude protein nitrogen in ration ingredients is soluble and the total ration crude protein is to be over 12 per cent of dry matter, addition of urea will be of no benefit. One should either supplement with natural protein or feed a lower protein diet.

CONCERNS OVER NPN FEEDING

Palatability

Concentrates containing over 2 per cent urea result in depressed feed intakes, even though animals might be physically adapted to tolerate higher amounts. Even at lower urea levels (1 to 1.5 per cent), high-moisture concentrate (14 to 16 per cent) can cause feed intake problems, probably because of partial hydrolysis of urea to ammonia. This can present serious difficulty with urea feeds held in storage during warm, humid weather. Adding molasses to diets with higher levels of urea improves intake in some cases but not others. Addition of urea to corn silage effectively alleviates palatability problems, probably because partial breakdown to ammonia during ensiling results in part of the nitrogen being consumed as ammonium salts and also because silage acids effectively cover urea taste. Within the maximum levels recommended for addition to ruminant rations (approximately 1.0 per cent of total ration dry matter or 1.5 per cent for the concentrate mixture), urea should not present palatability problems.

Reproductive Performance

Some veterinarians and dairymen have suggested that feeding rations containing NPN lowers conception rates of cattle. This is not true. Implicating urea has usually been done only as a hopeful correction to an otherwise unexplainable reproduction problem. No research study that has reported reproduction information has shown any relation between urea and breeding efficiency. In a Michigan survey of over 600 dairy herds involving 85,281 individual cow lactations and 3157 herd-year observations, no reduction in calving interval was found in herds that were fed urea. Urea was fed in 1709 of the 3157 herd-years with an average intake per cow for the herds that were fed urea of 81 g per day. This extensive survey gives additional proof to many other studies stating that urea is not detrimental to reproduction.

Relationship to a Possible Nitrate Toxicity

Neither logic nor experimental evidence supports the notion that urea and nitrate are additive in their toxic effects on ruminants. Both are simple nitrogenous compounds but are quite different in physiologic action.

Nitrate accumulates in plants grown on soils high in nitrogen, mainly in hot weather or during drought. The possibility of nitrate enhancing urea toxicity is meager. This is because the nitrogen content of nitrates is relatively small and only a small proportion has potential for being reduced to ammonia. Conversely, oxidation of ammonia to nitrite, which would aggravate a nitrate toxicity, is highly unlikely because the rumen is a reducing environment.

Ammonia Toxicity

It is well known that dietary urea, if consumed in large quantities in a short time, can be toxic. In a Kansas experiment testing different urea-containing products, animals were dosed with 0.5 g urea per 1 kg body weight, which was added through a rumen fistula.[3] Approximately one half of the doses resulted in toxicity, most of which occurred within 60 minutes after dosing (average time 52.8 minutes). In toxic cases, blood ammonia was elevated (to 2.9 mg per 100 ml blood in 60 minutes) and rumen pH was elevated to 7.41 in 60 minutes, which was significantly higher than 7.16 for nontoxic cases.

Toxicity signs included uneasiness, dullness, muscle and skin tremors, excessive salivation, frequent urination and defecation, rapid respiration, incoordination, stiffening of the front legs, prostration, tetany, and death. Muscle tremors followed by muscle spasms were the most frequently observed symptom (all 125 toxic cases). Bloat was never observed. As tetany became severe, most animals lost muscular coordination, usually of the hind limbs, and became prostrate. When tetany became severe, any loud noise, such as talking, slamming doors, or dropping metal objects, caused a violent involuntary contraction of the muscles (convulsion), characterized by stiffening of the fore and hind legs.

A common recommendation for treatment has been acetic acid injected intraruminally. In this experiment cattle were given approximately 1 mole acetic acid (5 per cent v/v) per mole nitrogen administered to bring about the toxicity.[3] Acetic acid treatment was undependable but usually worked when it was administered prior to time of tetany. In this study emptying rumen contents of animals in severe tetany did bring about survival of all animals.[3] If left alone in a quiet place the animal would show signs of decreasing tetany that would usually cease about 30 minutes after rumen content removal. Respiration and heart rate would return to normal, and after about 30 additional minutes of quiescence the animals would stand and appear normal. For severe field cases, it is suggested the animal be stabbed in the paralumbar fossa area and an opening of sufficient size be made to evacuate the rumen contents rapidly. In their studies, Bartley and associates added about 4 liters of warm water to the rumen when the animal stood and appeared normal.[3] Recovery was dramatic, and rumen fermentation was good 48 hours after the experiment. Great precaution would need to be taken to prevent peritonitis with this treatment, but it is probably the only way of preventing mortality when animals have progressed to severe tetany.

Ammonia toxicity is covered last in relation to utilization of NPN because there is no danger of ammonia toxicity if recommendations are followed. In fact, large tolerances beyond recommendations exist. Toxicity is usually associated with consumption of high levels of urea (over 44 g per 100 kg body weight) in a short period by unadapted cattle. Mistakes such as animals breaking into urea supplies or areas where feed was inadvertently spilled or miscalculation of the intended feeding levels are sometimes found as causes of toxic situations.

References

1. Satter, L. D., and Roffler, R. E.: Nitrogen requirement and utilization in dairy cattle. J. Dairy Sci. 58:1219, 1975.
2. Burroughs, W., Nelson, D. K., and Mertens, D. R.: Protein physiology and its application in the lactating cow: The metabolizable protein feeding standard. J. Anim. Sci. 41:933, 1975.
3. Bartley, E. E., Davidovich, A. D., Barr, G. W., Griffel, G. W., Dayton, A. D., Deyoe, C. W., and Bechtel, R. M.: Ammonia toxicity in cattle. I. Rumen and blood changes associated with toxicity and treatment methods. J. Anim. Sci. 43:835, 1976.

Dietary Management of Dairy Cattle

J. T. HUBER, Ph.D.

Milk production in cows is highly dependent on reproduction and is largely controlled by the endocrine system. Exerting greatest control on reproduction and lactation are secretions from the pituitary, hypothalamus, and ovary glands, but other secretions have a direct or indirect influence, with 25 individual hormones that affect growth, reproduction, and lactation of dairy cows.[2]

For optimum milk production a cow must reproduce at least once per year. Endocrine stimulation during gestation prepares the mammary gland for milk synthesis. The normal lactation curve of the cow is largely a reflection of hormonal secretions. On the other hand, hormonal levels are influenced by dietary constituents; hence, nutrient deficiencies, excesses, or imbalances can affect endocrine output. Many hormone-diet interrelationships have been shown but most are not well understood and offer a fertile field for future investigations.

ENERGY MANAGEMENT OF THE LACTATING COW

Mismanagement of energy feeding in dairy rations is probably the most costly error made by dairymen. The problem manifests itself by undernutrition in early lactation when propensity for milk production is greatest and by overfeeding during the late lactation and dry periods resulting in excessive fattening and consequent metabolic embarrassment. Aside from quantity of energy, form of energy also profoundly affects milk yield and quality. This article will address problems of energy management of the dairy cow during the different phases of lactation and remedies.

Feeding In Early Lactation

For six to eight weeks immediately following parturition (after the cow has had a chance to recover), the milk synthesis machinery of the mammary gland is at optimum function. However, the cow's desire to consume nutrients to make milk is seriously limiting. Mean intakes for cows during the first few weeks of lactation seldom exceed 2.5 per cent of body weight even though highly palatable rations are provided.[13] For high-yielding cows this creates an energy deficit that must be compensated for by mobilization of body tissue. It has been well-documented that the early lactation cow has a great capacity for fat mobilization and conversion of that energy to milk.[12] Energy balance studies showed that a cow may incur an energy deficit of as high as 20 Mcal/day (roughly equal to 3 kg of body fat) for the first three weeks of lactation.[11] For a group of cows consuming all they would eat of a ration containing 40 per cent concentrate and 60 per cent alfalfa hay, the average loss of energy was 7 Mcal/day for the first 66 days of lactation. From 66 to 176 days the cows were essentially at energy equilibrium with a slight positive balance of 0.7 Mcal/day, which increased to 3.4 Mcal/day between 176 and 292 days.

Cows mobilizing fat at a fast rate in early lactation run a high risk of metabolic disorders, and the practice should be avoided. Solving the appetite problem during early lactation looms as one of the greatest challenges facing dairy nutritionists today.

There are several considerations for maintaining high intakes of cows in early lactation. (1) Rations should be adequately balanced for the necessary nutrients. (2) Sufficient fiber should be available to maintain optimal rumen function. This appears to be 17 to 19 per cent acid detergent fiber (on a dry matter basis). When corn silage is the main forage source, with limited hay, concentrate should not exceed 50 per cent of the total dry matter. When fiber is too low and concentrate too high, erratic consumption patterns and a high incidence of displaced abomasum will result. (3) Texture and sweetness of the concentrate mix are also important. Cows prefer a rough chewy texture (as with cracked or rolled grains or pellets) to one that is finely ground. They also respond favorably to molasses; generally 4 to 6 per cent in concentrate is sufficient.

On the day of calving, the cow has little desire to eat. Thereafter, feed (particularly concentrate) should be increased slowly. Overconsumption will cause digestive upsets. The type of ration received in early lactation should be similar to that received during the last two to three weeks of the dry period. One system suggested for building up energy intake of the fresh cow is to offer daily about 4 kg of concentrate just after calving and increase in increments of 0.7 to 1 kg per day up to a level commensurate with that cow's need for milk production. For most cows it will take 10 to 14 days to build up to the desired concentrate intake.

Body Conditioning of Dairy Cows

High-producing cows will lose weight during early lactation when milk yields are greatest and appetite lowest. As mentioned, too rapid a loss in weight causes metabolic disturbances that seriously impair the productivity and profitability of the cow for the entire lactation. However, a moderate amount of body fat available for mobilization and milk synthesis is desirable. Large cows can safely lose 100 kg body fat during the first 70 days of lactation. This would amount to about 15 per cent of their post-calving weight and should furnish enough energy for production of approximately 650 kg of milk. Smaller cows might lose a proportional amount. Body weights, however, do not always reflect tissue loss at this stage of lactation because of changes in gut fill and shifts in body composition (water-filling adipose space).

Table 1. *Disease Conditions and Losses from the "Fat Cow Syndrome" in a 600-Cow Holstein-Friesian Dairy Herd During a Four-Month Period Before and After Treatment and Preventive Procedures Were Initiated**

		Disease Condition			Losses		
Time	No.	Parturient Paresis (%)	Ketosis (%)	Retained Fetal Membranes (%)	Mastitis (%)	Sold (%)	Died (%)
Before prevention† (2/1–5/31)	120	5	38	62	6	3	25
After prevention† (6/1–9/30)	120	2	5	13	2	2	3

*Reprinted with permission from Morrow, D. A., Hillman, D., Dade, A. W., and Kitchen, H.: Clinical investigation of a dairy herd with the fat cow syndrome. J. Am. Vet. Med. Assoc. *174*:161, 1979.

†Prevention consisted of decreasing intakes of energy and other nutrients from about 150 per cent to 100 per cent of the recommended allowance.[36] The white blood cell count from eight cows diagnosed to have "fat cow syndrome" averaged just 2800 per mm³.

Restoration of body tissue should occur during mid- and late lactation. If allowed *ad libitum* consumption, intakes are usually maximized at 40 to 50 days post partum, and cows reach an energy equilibrium shortly thereafter. As milk production decreases, feeding excessive energy relative to needs allows for regaining lost tissues.

Extra allotment of energy should not usually continue into the dry period because fat accumulated by nonlactating cows is less efficiently converted to milk (about 70 per cent as efficient) than that gained during lactation.[33] Moreover, there is greater danger of excessive fattening if dry cows are allowed to overconsume energy. Extremely fat cows are more susceptible to ketosis, parturient paresis, mastitis, metritis, displaced abomasum, and poor appetite. The "fat cow syndrome," characterized by hyperlipemia and fatty livers and kidneys, results in decreased resistance to pathogenic challenges because of an impaired synthesis of white blood cells.[34] Table 1 lists metabolic diseases encountered in cows calving to one dairy herd over an eight-month period. Approximately one year previous to the recorded dates, a reproductive problem occurred in this herd that increased the nonlactating period of many cows. These cows, which were dry for long periods, had a tendency to become excessively fat. Also, energy furnished the herd prior to making ration adjustments on June 1 was about 50 per cent above that recommended by the NRC.[36] The mean white cell count from eight cows with "fat cow syndrome," sampled just before ration changes were made, was about 33 per cent of normal (2800 versus 8100 cells/mm³). For large breeds, maintenance of body weight when turned dry plus

about 70 kg for calf and placental growth appears desirable. Typical rations for dry cows are given in Table 2.

Accurate assessment of body condition of a cow is often difficult. Some cows that might not appear excessively fat may suffer from the "fat cow syndrome," and large amounts of internal fat surrounding vital organs might be present. As mentioned, body weight changes do not always indicate gain or loss in body fat because of possible changes in body composition or fill. It is my opinion that weight changes more accurately reflect fat accumulation than loss.

The experienced dairyman, however, who observes his cows day after day is often the best judge of when a cow is becoming "too fat." Animals that are so heavy that ribs are not visible and hipbones barely protrude above the plane of the back usually suffer post-parturient problems. Cows that are dry for long periods of time, because of a miscalculated breeding date or cessation of lactation, will often become excessively fat.

Grouping of Cows for Maximum Milk Production

Loose housing and group feeding of forages and concentrates have often caused problems in furnishing the individual cow her nutrient needs. Each cow has specific nutrient requirements related to milk production, body size, age, and stage of gestation. Because of imbalanced rations, social behavior, availability to feed, bunk space, and a variety of other reasons, it is doubtful that a large percentage of the cows in group feeding situations are receiving their most profitable ration.

The practice of grouping cows according to stage of lactation and milk production has worked successfully for many dairymen. Often unbred animals are placed in one group. This group will usually include all cows up to 90 days after calving. Other cows are divided according to milk production into two or three groups. Dry cows and springing heifers will usually comprise an additional group. Where facilities permit (in larger herds), first- and second-calf heifers would be separated from mature cows to feed for extra growth. Nutrients for the different groups are allotted according to the group needs. Generally, energy and protein will be supplied at about 10 per cent in excess of the group's average requirement to accommodate the needs of the higher producing cows in the group. Complete rations fed to cow groups will vary from 0 to 60 per cent concentrate to meet nutrient needs at the different stages of lactation. Feeding concentrate to late lactation and dry cows is often unprofitable. However, these rations should be balanced for protein, vitamins, and minerals.

Table 2. *Typical Rations for Dry Cows Based on Different Forages*

Requirement: 14 Mcal NE, 1 kg crude protein
Type of Ration*
Corn silage (25 kg at 33 per cent DM) plus 0.45 kg per cent 50 CP soybean meal
Corn silage—urea or ammonia treated (27 kg at 33 per cent DM)
Sorghum silage (29.5 kg at 33 per cent DM) plus 0.68 kg SBM
Sorghum silage—treated with ammonia or urea (32 kg at 33 per cent DM)
Alfalfa hay† (12 kg)—protein sufficient
Alfalfa hay (6 kg) plus corn silage (13.5 kg)
Grass hay† (13.5 kg)—may need supplemental protein depending on protein content of hay
Pasture—protein sufficient

*Mineral supplementation will vary with the ration fed, but all should include TM salt, and Ca:P ratio should be about 1.5:1.

†If forage quality is low, then a limited amount of grain is recommended.

Where facilities do not permit physical separation of cows, magnet feeders, electronic gates, or transponder feeding units have allowed consumption of extra concentrate by high producers. Magnet feeders are usually the simplest and most economical of the three and are widely used on dairy farms in the United States (Figure 1). Computerized feeding systems that electronically control quantity of feeds allowed each cow depending on her needs are available and are in use on some farms. One advantage of these systems over those methods mentioned previously is that release of feed is timed so that only the correct cow consumes her own feed. Large expansion of such practices might be expected in the future. Many dairymen have boosted milk yields and profits by systems that provide extra feed to high producers. However, if they are not well-managed by controlling cows that have access to them, they might prove quite unprofitable.

Milk Production as Related to Forage Quality

Forage quality often makes the difference between profit and loss in a dairy feeding program and is one variable over which the farmer can exert considerable control. Poorly managed, low quality forages are usually unpalatable and of reduced value in usable nutrients, principally in energy, protein, and minerals.[21]

Maturity at harvest greatly influences the quality of forages.[38] First-cut cool season grasses and legumes are highest in energy and protein at the young, vegetative state and decrease in digestible energy by 0.3 to 0.5 per cent per day for each day harvest is delayed. The nutritive value of subsequent cuttings (aftermath) generally decreases at a slower rate than that of first cutting. To achieve maximum crop energy yields and greatest animal productivity, alfalfa and other legumes should be harvested at about 10 per cent bloom and perennial grasses (orchard grass, timothy grass, ryegrass) just prior to budding. Summer annuals (such as Sudan grass and Sudax grass) usually grow at a very rapid rate (if moisture is available) and should be harvested between 90 and 130 cm in height.[21]

Because of starch accumulation in kernels with advanced maturity, the organic matter digestibility of most corn plant varieties changes very little between the tassel and hard dough stages, but nutrient yield is almost doubled during this time.[24] Thus, corn should be harvested for silage at approximately the time when starch deposition in the kernels is completed. An easy method for detection of this stage is appearance of a small black layer where the kernel is attached to the cob. Corn harvested at this maturity will possess 33 to 37 per cent dry matter, which is ideal for ensiling in most silo structures (Figure 2). Fortuitously, corn silage harvested at hard dough (about 35 per cent dry matter) is also more palatable for cattle compared with that harvested earlier (25 per cent

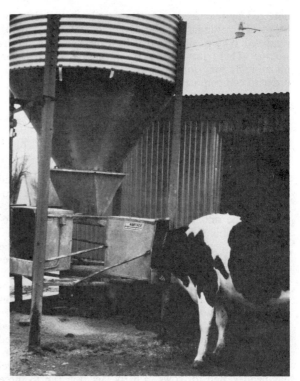

Figure 1. A dairy cow eating grain from a magnet feeder. The magnet attached to her neck chain activates the flow of grain into the feeder box.

dry matter) or later (45 per cent dry matter) and, as shown in Table 3, resulted in higher milk yields in controlled studies.[22] Another disadvantage of delaying harvest is high field loss, particularly in severe weather. Also, with the drier silage, exclusion of oxygen is more difficult, and heating and spoiling frequently occur.

The particle size of forages can exert a profound effect on utilization by cows.[20] Forages that are cut too fine (whether grasses, legumes, or grain silages) exit the rumen more rapidly, causing a shift in rumen fermentation toward increased propionate and decreased acetate-to-propionate ratio. They result in depressed butterfat and a higher incidence of displaced abomasums. An average size of about 7 mm for forage particles should avoid most problems, but minimums might be higher for the denser materials. Silages chopped to achieve a 7- to 12-mm particle size are desirable. On the other hand, silage particles that are too large result in poor packing and a greater chance of spoilage.

Silages inadequately packed or ensiled too dry will undergo excessive heating and a marked decrease in protein and energy availability. Extent of heat damage is

Table 3. *Influence of Maturity on the Feeding Value of Corn Silage*[*]

Maturity	Per Cent DM of Silage	Per Cent of Total DM as Ears	Milk Yield (kg/day)	Silage DM[†] Intake (Per Cent BW)	TDN in Silage (Per Cent DM)
Soft dough	25	37	17.2	1.95	68.2
Medium dough	30	47	18.4	2.13	68.4
Hard dough	33	51	19.1	2.30	68.0

*Reprinted with permission from Huber, J. T., Graf, G. C., and Engel, R. W.: Effect of maturity on the nutritive value of corn silage for lactating cows. J. Dairy Sci. *48*:1121, 1965.

†Cows were fed only corn silage *(ad libitum)* and soybean meal (1 kg/9.2 kg milk).

detected by increased acid detergent insoluble nitrogen. Moreover, vitamins A and E are heat labile and are rendered biologically inactive by excessive heat during storage. These factors should be considered when formulating rations for dairy cows fed heated forages in order to compensate for the lost nutrients.

MEETING THE PROTEIN NEEDS OF LACTATING COWS

Effect of Protein Level on Milk Yields

Protein allowances of milk production are expressed here as "total crude protein." The term "digestible protein" has little functional significance for ruminants because of the rumen microbial alteration of dietary nitrogen, the minimal value of ammonia nitrogen released from the rumen into blood (which would be considered totally digestible), and the high positive correlation between nitrogen intake and fecal nitrogen output.

Protein requirements for lactation vary with the level of milk production. National Research Council allowances for a 650-kg cow producing different amounts of milk are shown in Table 4.[36] Also, allowances have been calculated that the author feels are more realistic for commonly used rations in the midwestern United States.

Studies during the past ten years in which protein level has been varied for cows in early lactation (up to three months post partum) have generally shown increased milk production as per cent crude protein increased from 11 to about 17 per cent, but most reports have shown little boost above 16 to 17 per cent.[25] Usually when milk yields increased with higher protein, there was also an increase in the amount of feed eaten by cows. Response to higher protein seems mainly to be a stimulation in feed intake. In several studies in which intakes were not improved at ration crude proteins higher than 13 per cent, little increase in milk production was noted.[6, 13]

One reason for the higher intakes with increased protein appears to be an increase in the digestibility of the ration the cow is eating, which would increase turnover rate of feed in the digestive tract and allow more space for new feed.[27] Why digestibility is improved with increased protein is not clear, but up to about 14 per cent crude protein it appears related to a more active rumen fermentation. Increased buffering due to greater ammonia release has been proposed as another reason for the higher intakes.

A second important effect of increased protein has been

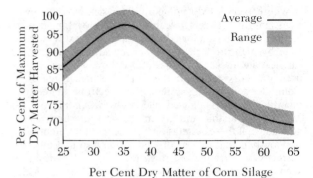

Figure 2. Effect of stage of maturity of corn silage on dry matter harvested per acre. (Summary of research conducted at Michigan, Indiana, and U.S.D.A.)

that as level of protein increased and more nearly approached the requirement for maximum milk, response in milk yields per unit protein decreased.[39] Table 5 presents milk yields and intakes of three recent studies in which protein levels were varied for early lactation cows and shows greater increase in both intakes and milk production when raising protein from 12 to 15 per cent than when raising protein from 15 to 17 or 18 per cent.

Special consideration of protein needs should be given to early lactation cows producing high levels of milk that appear to be losing large amounts of body weight. Owing to the normally diminished intakes in these cows, calculations show that as high as 19 to 20 per cent crude protein might be beneficial to avoid excessive depletion of body protein stores; however, the type of extra protein for these cows should be of low rumen degradability.

Economics of Protein Feeding

The law of diminishing returns in response to protein level is operative in lactating cows.[39] So as ration protein approaches the physiologic requirement, increased milk yields per unit protein decrease. Hence, the most profitable amount of protein to feed is often less than that which elicits maximum milk production. Table 6 shows that at low costs for protein supplements, more protein can be profitably added to a dairy ration than at higher costs. Considering present costs of protein supplements, it is doubtful that routine feeding of more than 15 to 16% crude protein would be profitable for most herds.

An additional factor not considered in Table 6 is the effect of added protein on peak milk production. For each

Table 4. *Suggested Protein Allowances for Lactating Dairy Cows of Varying Milk Yields (1400-lb, Mature Cow)*

	Feed Intake		Suggested Protein Required			
			NRC Allowance*		Author's Allowance†	
Milk Yield (lb/day)	(lb DM/day)	(% BW)	(lb/day)	(% Ration DM)	(lb/day)	(% Ration DM)
33	36	2.5	3.8	10.7	4.3‡	12.0‡
55	43	3.0	5.7	13.2	5.5	12.7
77	46	3.2	7.5	16.3	7.1	15.5
88§	39	2.8	8.4	21.6	7.9	20.4
100	49	3.4	9.3	19.0	8.3	17.0

*Maintenance = 515 g/day, milk (3.5 per cent fat) = 82 g/kg (based on NRC[36]).

†Maintenance = 636 g/day, milk (3.5 per cent fat) = 74 g/kg (based on author's calculations).

‡Feed this group at least 12 per cent crude protein to prevent depressed digestibility of dry matter and lowered intakes even though calculated needs are only 10.7 per cent.

§This calculation is for a cow in very early lactation that peaks in milk yields before intake is maximized. She is obviously using considerable body fat, but the available protein reserve is not known.

Table 5. *Milk Yields and Intakes in Response to Increasing Protein in Three Studies*

Location	Protein (% DM)	Milk Yield (lb/day)	Intake (lb DM/day)
Kansas State University[10]	13.0	54.7	40.5
(8 cows/trt, 1–21 weeks)	15.0	62.5	43.2
	17.0	61.4	41.9
Michigan State University[31]	11.3	69.5	36.4
(12 cows/trt, 3–13 weeks)	14.5	74.1	42.0
	17.5	76.3	47.0
New Hampshire University[17]	11.1	60.0	38.5
(8 cows/trt, 2–23 weeks)	13.7	67.4	40.2
	15.7	75.0	41.2
	19.2	73.4	41.7

additional 0.45-kg increase in peak production, it was proposed that total lactation yields are increased 90 kg. Hence, a protein level that might not show a profit in early lactation but that increases peak yields might be more profitable when the complete lactation is taken into consideration.[27]

Type of Protein to Feed

Amino acids absorbed from the small intestine are the end products of protein feeding and directly supply the cow's needs for milk synthesis and tissue replenishment. These amino acids come from microbial protein synthesized in the rumen or from feed protein that escapes rumen degradation. Because of its anaerobic nature, the rumen fermentation is inherently limited in the amount of protein it can supply. Estimates are that protein from microbes might be sufficient for the cow's maintenance and 10 to 12 kg of milk. Hence, a substantial amount of rumen undegraded protein must be available in high-producing cows for small intestinal digestion.[25, 40] Early studies that indicated a post-ruminal response to protein was that of direct infusion of casein into the abomasum and showed increased milk yields and milk protein production.[7] Analysis of blood of infused cows suggested that the amino acids in lowest supply for milk synthesis on typical dairy rations high in corn silage were methionine, lysine, phenylalanine, and threonine.[42] From infusion studies, Wisconsin workers[41] identified lysine and methionine as the amino acids giving the greatest increase in milk protein production after abomasal infusion.

Measures for increasing undegradable protein have often yielded positive results in rations fed during early lactation to high-producing cows. Mid- and late lactation feeding of protected protein has not usually been beneficial. Methods for decreasing rumen degradability of protein have included selection of certain protein supplements, heat and extrusion processing of proteins, and chemical treatment (as with formaldehyde).

The approach of formulating rations on the basis of selecting for protein low degradability is being commercially developed by a large farmer cooperative group in the United States. A patent was granted to Braund and associates[4] based on studies showing increased milk production of cows fed a dairy concentrate that was of reduced protein solubility (according to methods developed by Wohlt and co-workers[43]) compared with normal concentrate. Table 7 summarizes data from this study. The principal change in the supplements to achieve reduced solubility was an increase in brewers' grains and distillers' dried grains and a decrease in corn gluten feed. Future development in the area of rumen bypass protein for lactating cows is needed and should contribute to higher and more efficient milk yields.

Combining Undegraded Protein and NPN

The rumen microbes use ammonia for protein synthesis, which is furnished most economically from NPN (urea or ammonia). Ideally, the most profitable ration for high-producing cows would supply the rumen microbes with ammonia from NPN and the small intestine with rumen "bypass" protein to better meet the needs for milk synthesis. In a recent study (Table 8), we tested this idea and showed that feeding soybean meal heated to inhibit rumen degradation resulted in about 1.36 kg more milk per day than control soybean meal, but production was slightly higher and profit greatest when ammonia-treated corn silage and heat-treated soy were combined in the same ration.[31] The data clearly indicate that in feeding high-producing cows early in lactation, a dairyman can take advantage of the savings in feed costs by using NPN and also by feeding rumen undegraded protein to maximize milk production.

Overprotection of the protein from excessive heating or too much added chemical (such as formaldehyde) will result in poorer digestion of protein in the small intestine. Usually, marked increases in fiber-bound protein (ADIN)

Table 6. *Economics of Increasing Protein Fed**

	Change In			Feed Cost—SBM at		
Ration (%)	Milk Yield (lb/day)	Intake of DM (lb/day)	Milk Value (¢/day)	$200/ton (¢/day)	$250/ton (¢/day)	$300/ton (¢/day)
10–12	7.5	4.5	98	39	47	53
12–14	3.9	1.5	51	21	28	36
14–16	2.4	0.7	31	16	24	31
16–18	1.5	0.5	20	15	22	30

*Adapted from Satter, L. D., Whitlow, L. W., and Santos, K. A.: Supplementing protein to the dairy cow for maximum profit. Proc. Distillers Feed Research Council 34:77, 1979.

Note: Prices used were: milk = $13/cwt; grain = 6¢/lb.

Table 7. *Summary Data of Protein Solubility Experiment**

Treatment	Ration Characteristics		Milk Production (lb/day)
	Crude Protein (%)	Soluble Protein (% CP)	
Normal	17.8	38.2	64.2
Low solubility	18.5	21.3	70.2

*Reprinted with permission from Braund, D. G., Dolge, K. L., Goings, R. L., and Steele, R. L.: Method for formulating dairy rations. Pat. No. 4,188,513. Washington, D.C., U.S. Patent Office, 1978.

Note: 20 cows per treatment, from 5 to 15 weeks post partum.

indicate overheating. In one study (Table 9), we showed that heating soybean meal for two hours at 300° F (149° C) essentially maximized rumen undegradability and only slightly decreased dry matter digestibility estimates.[31] However, heating for four and six hours greatly increased the unavailable protein. Insufficient ammonia for optimum rumen function is another problem that might occur on rations too high in undegradable protein. The preferred source of nitrogen for 80 per cent of the bacteria in the rumen (particularly the fiber digestors) is ammonia, so a uniform supply of adequate ammonia is necessary for growth of these organisms. Some unfavorable results that have occurred from incorporation of bypass protein into dairy rations were attributed to a lack of ammonia in the rumen.

Nonprotein Nitrogen (NPN)

Ruminants possess the unique ability to meet a large percentage of their nitrogen requirements with simple nitrogenous compounds such as urea, ammonia, biuret, and others. It was recently estimated that an annual saving in feed costs of over $500 million is realized by United States livestock producers through feeding NPN to ruminants. In periods of high cost of oilseed meals, savings are greater. Increased profit available to dairy farmers feeding high-energy, low-protein rations who replace about 50 to 60 per cent of the supplemental natural protein fed lactating cows with NPN is about $70 per cow annually.[22]

However, a high level of management is necessary for successful incorporation of NPN into dairy cattle rations, and failure to follow recommended practices might reduce milk yields, making use of NPN unprofitable. Rations ideal for using maximum NPN are low in protein and high in energy, such as those that use liberal quantities of grain and grain silages, typical of those fed in the midwestern

and eastern United States. An adaptation period of about two weeks is advisable during which cattle rations are gradually raised in NPN level.

Limits for Feeding NPN

The maximum level at which NPN is profitable in a dairy ration depends largely on the feeding system used.[25] When added as urea to concentrate fed twice daily, intake should not exceed 200 to 220 g/day (as urea or urea equivalent). Adding NPN to complete rations, to silages, to grain being gelatinized (Starea), or to dehydrated alfalfa during pelletization (Dehy-100) better synchronized the ammonia release from NPN with rumen energy availability for microbial protein synthesis. These improved methods of NPN delivery have been shown to allow for greater quantities of NPN to be consumed without depressing milk yields or decreasing intakes. The approximate limit of adding urea to dairy concentrate is 1.7 per cent, to complete rations is 1.2 per cent (or equivalent as nitrogen), and to silage is 2 per cent of the silage dry matter. When feeding Starea or Dehy-100, the recommended limit is 300 g of urea equivalent daily per cow.

Response of High-Producing Cows to NPN

A common practice for feeding lactating cows in many dairy herds in the midwestern United States is to provide a basal ration of 11 to 12 per cent natural protein and add NPN to increase total crude protein to 14 to 15 per cent. There has been some controversy over feeding NPN-containing rations to high-producing cows, particularly in the early stages of lactation (up to four months). Satter and Roffler[40] suggested that NPN is contra-indicated when the crude protein requirement exceeds 11 to 12 per cent. However, recent experiments (Table 10) show milk yields of early lactation cows fed NPN rations of 15 to 17 per cent crude protein to be just as high as those of cows fed equal protein from all natural sources. These studies also showed an increase of 5.5 per cent in milk yields from adding urea to negative control rations containing 12 to 13 per cent crude protein, whereas the increase from natural protein was 6.5 per cent. A summary of milk yields of high-producing cows from several Michigan experiments[19] also showed NPN equal to soybean meal for supplementing rations up to 14 per cent crude protein.

In contrast, Illinois studies[44] showed that cows fed 14.5 per cent crude protein rations with 1.5 per cent urea in concentrate during the entire lactation produced less milk than those fed all natural protein at 14.5 per cent. Energy

Table 8. *Milk Production, Intake, and Economic Evaluation of Different Protein Regimens for Early Lactation Cows**

Corn Silage/Soybean Meal	Protein Type†		
	Normal/Normal	Normal/Heated	Ammoniated/Heated
Milk production (lb/day)	75.2	77.8	78.5
Dry matter intake (lb/day)	45.0	42.6	44.4
Cost of feed ($/day)‡	3.33	3.17	3.01
Milk income ($/day)§	9.85	10.11	10.26
Income over feed cost ($/day)	6.52	6.94	7.25

*Adapted from Kung, L., Jr., and Huber, J. T.: Performance of high producing cows in early lactation fed protein of varying amounts, sources and degradability. J. Dairy Sci. 66:227, 1983.

†Each protein type represents a mean of 24 cows: 12 on 14.5 per cent and 12 on 17.5 per cent CP. Treatments were from 3 to 13 weeks of lactation.

‡Feed costs ($/ton): hay, 60; corn silage-CS, 22; corn silage-AS, 24; high moisture ear corn (65 per cent DM), 85; soybean meal-NS, 300; soybean meal-HS, 400.

§Milk = 13¢/lb.

Table 9. *Selected Measurements for Soybean Meal Heated for Various Times**

Hours at 300° F	N Disappearance From Nylon Bags† (%)	N Solubility (%)	In Vitro Dry Matter Disappearance (%)	ADIN/N‡ (%)
0	76.9	26.5	92.1	1.9
2	36.3	3.9	89.0	4.6
4	38.0	3.8	86.5	8.9
6	37.9	4.1	82.3	19.7

*Adapted from Kung, L., Jr., and Huber, J. T.: Performance of high producing cows in early lactation fed protein of varying amounts, sources and degradability. J. Dairy Sci. 66:227, 1983.
†After 12 hours suspension in the rumen.
‡Acid detergent insoluble nitrogen as a per cent of total nitrogen (fiber bound protein).
Note: Means of 2 to 4 replicates.

consumption and initial yields were lower in the cows fed urea, accounting for a large part of the decreased production. This study conflicts with an earlier study by Holter and colleagues,[18] who showed no difference between milk yields of groups in a high-producing herd fed urea or soybean meal at levels similar to the ones used in the Illinois study.

In conclusion, present data do not warrant excluding NPN from rations for high-producing cows early in lactation. They suggest there is as efficient utilization of nitrogen from nonprotein as natural protein sources in rations containing up to 15 per cent crude protein. However, NPN should be used judiciously, and if lowered energy consumption results from feeding NPN at this critical time in lactation, it should be withdrawn from the ration.

Adding NPN to Silage

Urea. Studies have shown that one of the preferred methods of incorporating NPN into rations for lactating cows is its addition to grain silages.[27] Comparisons of isonitrogenous rations containing urea-treated and control silages have shown slightly higher milk yields for the urea silages (Table 11). Data clearly show that neither urea nor ammonia should be added to silages harvested in excess of 45 per cent dry matter.[26]

Ammonia. Addition of ammonia to grain silages has been extensively investigated[22] and is now commonly used for silage treatment in the United States and Canada. A key incentive for developing the ammonia treatment methods was that ammonia nitrogen usually costs about 60 per cent as much as urea nitrogen.

Unlike the bound ammonia in ammoniated industrial wastes, which was largely unavailable for microbial use, the animal receives most of the ammonia from ammonia-treated silage as the free ammonium salts of silage organic acids.[23] These acids also keep the ammonia from escaping into the atmosphere before feeding.

Ammonia treatment of silage inhibits initial plant respiration and proteolysis, thereby conserving silage energy and natural protein. This protein-sparing action of the

ammonia was confirmed in ^{15}N studies[23] and was probably responsible for superior results with ammonia-treated compared with urea-treated silage in which lactating cows were fed large quantities of NPN. Ammonia treatment also protects the silage from mold and yeast growth (with accompanying heating) after exposure to air while being fed to cattle. This prevention of secondary fermentation can be quite beneficial in warm weather and during feeding of silages with large exposed surfaces. A third benefit of treating silages with ammonia is preservation of ensiled energy.[25] Studies by Beltsville workers showed that 5 per cent more dry matter and 8 per cent more energy was saved by adding ammonia to corn silage compared with untreated silage.

SPECIAL PROBLEMS RELATED TO MINERAL AND VITAMIN FEEDING OF LACTATING COWS

There is much confusion regarding feeding minerals to dairy cattle. Farmers are continually bombarded by numerous mineral salesmen whose product is claimed (by that particular salesman) to be superior to all others. A problem often encountered in the field is that the same mineral is sold regardless of the type of ration the farmer is feeding. Need for supplemental minerals differs greatly depending on the other ration ingredients. Table 12 gives the mineral needs and concentrations for a 1400-lb cow producing 66 lb of milk as calculated from the NRC values.[36] The concentrations in the ration given would apply to all classes of dairy cattle, as would the problem allowance factor.

Calcium, Phosphorus, and Vitamin D Relationship to Milk Fever

There may not be one ideal ratio of Ca to P for dairy cows. The optimum ratio probably varies according to the function of the cow (whether milking or dry) and the type of feeds consumed. A ratio of 1.4:1 is calculated from NRC standards. This ratio is probably satisfactory for the

Table 10. *Response of High-Producing Cows in Early Lactation to NPN on Natural Protein**

Item	Basal Ration (12–13% CP)	Soybean Ration (15–17% CP)	Urea Ration (15–17% CP)
Milk yields (lb/day)	67.6	72.0	71.3
Dry matter intake (% BW)	3.22	3.18	3.23

*Pooled from four recent studies comparing 54 cows per treatment starting 0 to 5 weeks post partum and continuing to 9 to 20 weeks. Data from Kwan et al.[32]; Murdock and Hodgson[35]; Clay et al.[8]; Foldager and Huber.[13]

Table 11. *Response of Dairy Cows to Urea-Treated Corn Silage**

	Silage Treatment			
	Control	*Urea*	*Urea*	*Control*
CP in concentrate (per cent)	8.1	8.1	12.3	18.4
CP in total ration (per cent)	8.2	10.5	13.0	13.5
Milk yield (lb/day)	42.3[a]	52.2[b]	58.2[c]	56.4[c]
DM intake (per cent BW)	2.46[a]	2.65[b]	3.05[c]	2.81[bc]
DM digestibility (per cent)	56.4[a]	59.0[ab]	65.0[bc]	69.2[c]

*Adapted from Huber, J. T., and Thomas, J. W.: Urea-treated corn silage in low protein rations for lactating cows. J. Dairy Sci. *54*:224, 1971.
Note: Treatment comparisons not sharing a common letter are different (P < 0.05).

dry cow but too narrow for lactating animals. Research has shown that ratios narrower than 1:1 and wider than 2.5:1 tend to increase the incidence of milk fever.[14] High calcium diets just prior to calving stimulate secretion of the hormone thyrocalcitonin, which moves minerals from the blood to the bone, whereas the heavy drain of calcium for milk synthesis requires movement in the opposite direction, from the bone through the blood into milk.

Just as too high a level of calcium is detrimental to lactating cows, so is excessive phosphorus.[5] Primiparous Holstein cows fed phosphorus at 138 per cent of the NRC allowance for the first 12 weeks of lactation yielded an average of 5.9 lb less milk per day for the entire lactation (305 days) than similar cows fed 98 per cent of the suggested requirement. The reason for decreased milk production resulting from high phosphorus intake is not known, but these data illustrate the danger of feeding excessive phosphorus to lactating cows and should discourage the indiscriminate and uncontrolled addition of several phosphorus sources to dairy rations, as has been practiced on some farms.

Heavy supplementation of vitamin D on a routine basis is not desirable, but feeding massive doses (10 to 20 million I.U./day) for seven days before calving has alleviated milk fever, particularly in aged cows.[15] However, feeding for longer than seven days is dangerous, and it is often difficult to predict calving dates close enough for treatment to be effective but not excessive. Recent research has shown that more biologically active metabolites of vitamin D (hydroxylated cholecalciferols) effectively prevented milk fever in smaller doses (50 to 60,000 I.U. for three days).[28] Further studies should make their use commercially feasible.

Based on the current state of knowledge, with many questions relating to calcium and phosphorus feeding still unanswered, our current recommendation is that dairymen provide phosphorus at 90 to 100 per cent of the allowance recommended by the National Research Council standard (17 g for maintenance and 1.75 g/kg milk). Calcium would be calculated from phosphorus to provide a 1.7 to 2.0:1 ratio of Ca to P for milking cows and a 1.5:1 ratio for dry cows. In rations where corn silage constitutes the main forage, both calcium and phosphorus should be supplemented, whereas only phosphorus is needed when high levels of legumes are fed.

Sulfur

With increased supplementation of nonprotein nitrogen (urea, ammonia, biuret, and so on) in ruminant rations, there has been a decrease in natural protein supplements that contain sulfur amino acids. Also, heavier feeding of corn silage with less legume hay has decreased sulfur intake by animals.

The sulfur needs of cattle are often expressed in relation to the nitrogen content of the ration. Rations for lactating dairy cows containing about 14 per cent crude protein should have 0.2 per cent sulfur. When corn grain and corn silage are the main components, the sulfur level will not usually exceed 0.12 per cent, so supplemental sulfur is needed. Addition to about 2 kg/ton of calcium or sodium sulfate to dairy cattle concentrate should correct any possible sulfur deficiency of high corn and NPN rations. Precautions should be made not to exceed 0.35 per cent sulfur or ration intake might decrease.[3] When legume hay is fed in liberal amounts, supplemental sulfur is not needed.

Table 12. *Minerals Needed By the Lactating Cow Producing 66 lb Milk Daily (BW = 1400 lb)*

Mineral	Suggested Allowance per Day*	Ration Concentration (DM Basis)	Reported to Cause Problems (DM Basis)	Problem Allowance Factor
Calcium (Ca)†	142 g	0.7%	1.4%	2.0
Phosphorus (P)†, ‡	71 g	0.36%	0.6%	1.7
Magnesium (Mg)†, ‡	40 g	0.20%	2.0%	10.0
Potassium (K)†	150 g	0.75%	3.0%	4.0
Salt (NaCl)†	60 g	0.30%	5.0%	16.0
Sulfur (S)†	40 g	0.20%	0.35%	1.8
Iron (Fe)†, ‡	1 g	50 mg/kg	1000 mg/kg	20.0
Manganese (Mn)†, ‡	0.4 g	20 mg/kg	1000 mg/kg	50.0
Copper (Cu)†	0.16 g	8 mg/kg	100 mg/kg	12.0
Zinc (Zn)†, ‡	0.8 g	40 mg/kg	600 mg/kg	15.0
Cobalt (Co)†	2 mg	0.1 mg/kg	10 mg/kg	100.0
Iodine (I)†	8 mg	0.4 mg/kg	10 mg/kg	25.0
Selenium (Se)†	2 mg	0.1 mg/kg	3 mg/kg	30.0

*Adapted from National Research Council: Nutrient Requirements of Dairy Cattle, 5th rev. ed. Washington, D.C., National Academy of Sciences, 1978.
†May need supplementation on high corn silage rations.
‡May need supplementation on high alfalfa rations.

Selenium and Vitamin E

Selenium (Se) is an essential nutrient that is part of the enzyme glutathione peroxidase, which, in consort with vitamin E, prevents harmful biologic oxidations.[1] Excessive selenium accumulates in some plants in certain areas and has been shown to be toxic (at 5 ppm). Conversely, soils in large regions of the United States (in the Northwest and eastern Midwest) are deficient in selenium, so rations in those areas require supplementation up to a required level of 0.1 ppm. Recent approval by the FDA allows for adding selenium to dairy and beef cattle rations.

A problem related to low selenium intake on high corn rations is retained placentas in post-parturient cows. Julien and co-workers[29] found that injection of 50 mg sodium selenite and 680 mg vitamin E approximately 14 days before calving effectively reduced the per cent of placentas retained over 24 hours. Vitamin E–selenium injections before calving have effectively decreased retained placentas among herds fed borderline levels of selenium or vitamin E.

Fluoride

It was generally thought that most dairy cattle can tolerate up to 30 ppm fluoride (F) without adverse effects. However, recent data reported by Hillman and colleagues[16] showed damaged teeth (mottled and broken) and bone lesions when cattle consumed phosphates that furnished 15 to 20 ppm fluoride in the total ration. Cornell workers[30] also reported fluoride toxicity in cattle on Cornwall Island in animals exposed to less than 40 ppm fluoride for prolonged periods (three months of age to adult). Achieving a lower level of fluoride, now required in some states, often requires special processing of phosphate supplements, rendering them more expensive. Until research clearly establishes toxic levels, caution is recommended because bone damage from fluorosis is not reversible.

How to Feed Minerals

The feeding of minerals free choice has long been practiced by many dairymen. It was generally accepted that if the correct minerals were offered to cows, they would consume according to their needs. However, studies in New York[9] and Minnesota[37] showed no relationship between the amount of minerals needed by ruminants and free choice consumption.

Minerals should be force-fed by adding them to the concentrate or forage or both. These major feed ingredients are usually consumed in relation to the animals' needs; thus, problems of mineral shortages to individual cows would be less likely to occur with force-feeding than with free-choice feeding. Conversely, force-feeding of minerals should also prevent overconsumption by cows. Free-choice feeding often results in harmful excesses or deficiencies of certain minerals. Silages are ideal carriers of many of the minerals needed in dairy rations, and in some cases minerals exert a beneficial effect upon fermentation. When cattle are grazing, there is usually no way to force-feed minerals, so offering them free choice on pasture is still recommended.

NUTRIENT REQUIREMENTS FOR DAIRY CATTLE

Table 13 lists feed requirements for heifer calves and growing dairy heifers from birth to 24 months of age, the recommended time of calving. To calculate feed for a specific time, divide totals for two months by 60 and allot a little more if age is toward the end of the period. These quantities of feed are for large breeds (Holstein, Brown Swiss, and so on). For the smaller breeds, follow recommendations according to body weight, except for milk for the baby calf, which would be about 20 per cent less (mean of 2.75 to 3.0 versus 3.50 to 3.75 kg/day).

*Table 13. Approximate Feed Requirements for Holstein Heifers on Alfalfa Hay or Corn Silage**

Age (mo)	Weight (lb)	Liquid Ration (lb)	Grain† (lb)	Hay Systems‡ (lb)	Corn Silage Systems‡ (lb)
1 and 2	90–150	340§	80	45	—
3 and 4	150–230	0	190	200	—
5 and 6	230–340	0	180	425	995
7 and 8	340–450			600	1400
9 and 10	450–560			880	2060
11 and 12	560–670			1050	2460
Total to 1 year		340	450	3200	6915
13 and 14	679–780‖	0		1180	2760
15 and 16	780–870			1280	3000
17 and 18	870–950			1400	3275
19 and 20	950–1040			1500	3500
21 and 22	1040–1150			1590	3700
23 and 24	1130–1260**		300	1350	3160
Total 1 to 2 years		0	300	8300	19,395
Total: Birth to 2 years		340	750	11,500	26,310

*Partially adapted from Hillman, D., et al.: Raising calves. Mich. State Univ. Ext. Bull. 412, Nov. 1971.

†Grain fed to calves up to three to four months of age should be a high-energy calf starter containing approximately 16 per cent crude protein and balanced for vitamins and minerals. Feed about 3 lb per day from weaning to four months while offering high quality hay *ad libitum*.

‡Assume corn silage of 35 per cent dry matter supplemented with soybean meal or NPN (urea or ammonia) to contain at least 13.5 per cent crude protein. Feed according to hay system up to four months. If hay quality is low during any part of the growth period, grain feeding should be increased to maintain desired energy intake. Corn silage–fed heifers do not need grain during five and six months. Supplement corn silage with dicalcium phosphate and trace-mineralized (TM) salt. Hay systems usually only require TM salt addition.

§This can be diluted colostrum (2:1 with water), waste whole milk, whole milk, or milk replacer (reconstituted to about 12 per cent solids). Feed approximately 8 lb per day and wean at five to six weeks when calves are eating about 1½ lb/day of starter.

‖Breed at 14 to 15 months so heifers will calve by 24 months of age.

**Weight includes fetus and associative organs (or about 150 lb).

Note* Clean, fresh water should be available at all times.

Table 14. *Daily Nutrient Requirements of Lactating and Pregnant Cows**

Body Weight (kg)	Feed Energy				Total Crude Protein (g)	Calcium (g)	Phosphorus (g)	Vitamin A (1000 I.U.)
	NE_1 (Mcal)	ME (Mcal)	DE (Mcal)	TDN (kg)				
Maintenance of Mature Lactating Cows†								
350	6.47	10.76	12.54	2.85	341	14	11	27
400	7.16	11.90	13.86	3.15	373	15	13	30
450	7.82	12.99	15.14	3.44	403	17	14	34
500	8.46	14.06	16.39	3.72	432	18	15	38
550	9.09	15.11	17.60	4.00	461	20	16	42
600	9.70	16.12	18.79	4.27	489	21	17	46
650	10.30	17.12	19.95	4.53	515	22	18	50
700	10.89	18.10	21.09	4.79	542	24	19	53
750	11.47	19.06	22.21	5.04	567	25	20	57
800	12.03	20.01	23.32	5.29	592	27	21	61
Maintenance Plus Last Two Months of Gestation of Mature Dry Cows								
350	8.42	14.00	16.26	3.71	642	23	16	27
400	9.30	15.47	17.98	4.10	702	26	18	30
450	10.16	16.90	19.64	4.47	763	29	20	34
500	11.00	18.29	21.25	4.84	821	31	22	38
550	11.81	19.65	22.83	5.20	877	34	24	42
600	12.61	20.97	24.37	5.55	931	37	26	46
650	13.39	22.27	25.87	5.90	984	39	28	50
700	14.15	23.54	27.35	6.23	1035	42	30	53
750	14.90	24.79	28.81	6.56	1086	45	32	57
800	15.64	26.02	30.24	6.89	1136	47	34	61
Milk Production (Nutrients Per kg Milk of Different Fat Percentages)								
2.5	0.59	0.99	1.15	0.260	72	2.40	1.65	
3.0	0.64	1.07	1.24	0.282	77	2.50	1.70	
3.5	0.69	1.16	1.34	0.304	82	2.60	1.75	
4.0	0.74	1.24	1.44	0.326	87	2.70	1.80	
4.5	0.78	1.31	1.52	0.344	92	2.80	1.85	
5.0	0.83	1.39	1.61	0.365	98	2.90	1.90	
5.5	0.88	1.48	1.71	0.387	103	3.00	2.00	
6.0	0.93	1.56	1.81	0.410	108	3.10	2.05	
Body Weight Change During Lactation (Nutrients Per kg Weight Change)								
Weight loss	-4.92	-8.25	-9.55	-2.17	-320			
Weight gain	5.12	8.55	9.96	2.26	500			

*National Research Council: Nutrient Requirements of Dairy Cattle, 5th rev. ed. Washington, D.C., National Academy of Sciences, 1978.

†To allow for growth of young lactating cows, increase the maintenance allowances for all nutrients except vitamin A by 20 per cent during the first lactation and 10 per cent during the second lactation.

Table 15. Recommended Nutrient Content of Rations for Dairy Cattle*

Weight (kg) / Daily Milk Yields (kg) for Rations I–IV:

Weight (kg)	I	II	III	IV
≤400	<8	8–13	13–18	<18
500	<11	11–17	17–23	<23
600	<14	14–21	21–29	<29
≥700	<18	18–26	26–35	<35

Nutrients (Concentration in Feed DM)	I	II	III	IV	V Dry Pregnant Cows	VI Mature Bulls	VII Growing Heifers and Bulls	VIII Starter Concentrate Mix	IX Calf Milk Replacer	Max (Maximum Concentrations, All Classes)
Crude protein, %	13.0	14.0	15.0	16.0	11.0	8.5	12.0	16.0	22.0	—
Energy										
NE_1, Mcal/kg	1.42	1.52	1.62	1.72	1.35	—	—	—	—	—
NE_m, Mcal/kg	—	—	—	—	—	1.20	1.26	1.90	2.40	—
NE_g, Mcal/kg	—	—	—	—	—	—	0.60	1.20	1.55	—
ME, Mcal/kg	2.36	2.53	2.71	2.89	2.23	2.04	2.23	3.12	3.78	—
DE, Mcal/kg	2.78	2.95	3.13	3.31	2.65	2.47	2.65	3.53	4.19	—
TDN, %	63.0	67.0	71.0	75.0	60.0	56.0	60.0	80.0	95.0	—
Crude fiber, %	17.0	17.0	17.0	17.0†	17.0	—	15.0	—	—	—
Acid detergent fiber, %	21.0	21.0	21.0	21.0	21.0	19.0	19.0	—	—	—
Ether extract, %	2.0	2.0	2.0	2.0	2.0	2.0	2.0	2.0	10.0	—
Minerals‡										
Calcium, %	0.43	0.48	0.54	0.60	0.37	0.24	0.40	0.60	0.70	—
Phosphorus, %	0.31	0.34	0.38	0.40	0.26	0.18	0.26	0.42	0.50	—
Magnesium, %§	0.20	0.20	0.20	0.20	0.16	0.16	0.16	0.07	0.07	—
Potassium, %	0.80	0.80	0.80	0.80	0.80	0.80	0.80	0.80	0.80	—
Sodium, %	0.18	0.18	0.18	0.18	0.10	0.10	0.10	0.10	0.10	—
Sodium chloride, %‖	0.46	0.46	0.46	0.46	0.25	0.25	0.25	0.25	0.25	5
Sulfur, %‖	0.20	0.20	0.20	0.20	0.17	0.11	0.16	0.21	0.29	0.35
Iron, ppm‖,**	50.0	50.0	50.0	50.0	50.0	50.0	50.0	100.0	100.0	1,000
Cobalt, ppm	0.10	0.10	0.10	0.10	0.10	0.10	0.10	0.10	0.10	10
Copper, ppm‖,††	10.0	10.0	10.0	10.0	10.0	10.0	10.0	10.0	10.0	80
Manganese, ppm‖	40.0	40.0	40.0	40.0	40.0	40.0	40.0	40.0	40.0	1,000
Zinc, ppm‖,‡‡	40.0	40.0	40.0	40.0	40.0	40.0	40.0	40.0	40.0	500
Iodine, ppm‖,§§	0.50	0.50	0.50	0.50	0.50	0.25	0.25	0.25	0.25	50
Molybdenum, ppm‖,‖‖	—	—	—	—	—	—	—	—	—	6
Selenium, ppm	0.10	0.10	0.10	0.10	0.10	0.10	0.10	0.10	0.10	5
Fluorine, ppm***	—	—	—	—	—	—	—	—	—	30
Vitamins†††										
A, I.U./kg	3,200	3,200	3,200	3,200	3,200	3,200	2,200	2,200	3,800	—
D, I.U./kg	300	300	300	300	300	300	300	300	600	—
E, ppm	—	—	—	—	—	—	—	—	300	—

*National Research Council: Nutrient Requirements of Dairy Cattle, 5th rev. ed. Washington, D.C., National Academy of Sciences, 1978.

†It is difficult to formulate high-energy rations with a minimum of 17 per cent crude fiber. However, fat percentage depression may occur when rations with less than 17 per cent crude fiber or 21 per cent ADF are fed to lactating cows.

‡The mineral values presented in this table are intended as guidelines for use by professionals in ration formulation. Because of many factors affecting such values, they are not intended and should not be used as a legal or regulatory base.

§Under conditions conducive to grass tetany (see text), these values should be increased to 0.25 or higher.

‖The maximum safe levels for many of the mineral elements are not well defined; estimates given here, especially for sulfur, sodium chloride, iron, copper, zinc, and manganese, are based on very limited data; safe levels may be substantially affected by specific feeding conditions.

**The maximum safe level of supplemental iron in some forms is materially lower than 1000 ppm. As little as 400 ppm added iron as ferrous sulfate has reduced weight gains (Standish et al., 1969).

††High copper may increase the susceptibility of milk to oxidized flavor (see text).

‡‡Maximum safe level of zinc for mature dairy cattle is 1000 ppm.

§§If diet contains as much as 25 per cent goitrogenic feed on dry basis, iodine provided should be increased two times or more.

‖‖If diet contains sufficient copper, dairy cattle tolerate substantially more than 6 ppm molybdenum (see text).

***Maximum safe level of fluorine for growing heifers and bulls is lower than that for other dairy cattle. Somewhat higher levels are tolerated when the fluorine is from less available sources such as phosphates (see text). Minimum requirements for molybdenum and fluorine are not yet established.

†††The following minimum quantities of B complex vitamins are suggested per unit of milk replacer; niacin, 2.6 ppm; pantothenic acid, 13 ppm; riboflavin, 6.5 ppm; pyridoxine, 6.5 ppm; thiamine, 6.5 ppm; folic acid, 0.5 ppm; biotin, 0.1 ppm; vitamin B_{12}, 0.07 ppm; choline, 0.26 per cent. It appears that adequate amounts of these vitamins are furnished when calves have functional rumens (usually at 6 weeks of age) by a combination of rumen synthesis and natural feedstuffs.

Table 14 gives the recommended nutrient requirements for lactating and pregnant dairy cows as published by the National Research Council.[36] The NE_l system for feed energy is probably the most accurate of the four listed, but the others are probably satisfactory in any given feeding situation. It must be remembered that successful feeding for high-level milk production is an art as well as a science, and a great deal will depend on the daily observations and contact of the feeder with the cows. These are only suggested guides to be used in combination with sound judgment. As mentioned, crude protein allowances suggested by NRC[36] are probably too low for low-producing and dry cows and too high for cows yielding over 35 kg milk/day. Also, calcium to phosphorus ratios are lower than many nutritionists recommend for lactating cows (see Table 12).

Recommended nutrient content of dairy cattle rations is given in Table 15 with suggested concentrations for differing levels of milk production and other functions. Please read the footnotes of this table carefully, because they contain needed information for its successful application.

SUMMARY

The milk synthesizing machinery is at peak function in early lactation, but desire of the animal to consume nutrients lags behind her need for high milk production. Hence, large amounts of body tissue (principally fat) are mobilized for producing milk until the cow reaches an energy equilibrium (eight to ten weeks post partum). Caution should be exercised in building fat reserves in the cow that might be drawn upon just after calving so as to avoid "fat cow syndrome," ketosis, metritis, mastitis, and displaced abomasum. Restoration of body fat should be during mid- and late lactation rather than while dry because greater efficiency is realized from fat accumulated while milking.

Wise energy management of dairy cows also includes grouping cows according to milk production and, at times, reproduction. Harvesting forages at the correct maturity for optimizing nutrient quality and quantity as well as storing under conditions that prevent deterioration are extremely important for successful dairying. Profits are usually greatest from harvesting legumes at 10 per cent bloom, grasses just before the bud stage, corn for silage in hard dough or dent, and small grains for silage in soft dough.

Protein requirements for lactating cows vary with milk yields. National Research Council allowances appear too low in low-yielding cows (because efficiency of energy utilization decreases in rations lower than 12 per cent protein) and excessive at the higher production levels (above 35 kg milk/day) because of possible problems in handling excess rumen ammonia. Response in milk production to increased protein diminishes as the ration approaches the theoretical requirement of the cow. Under current prices of protein supplements, it is doubtful that rations that exceed 16 per cent crude protein will increase milk yields enough to pay for the higher protein. Feeding nonprotein nitrogen (NPN) can increase profits from dairy cattle. Improved methods of delivering NPN to dairy cattle to better synchronize release of ammonia with the fermentation of energy in the rumen include mixing NPN in complete rations, adding to corn silage (as urea or ammonia), and feeding modified forms of urea such as Starea or Dehy-100. Reports suggesting that high-producing cows early in lactation are not benefited by NPN were based mostly on rumen *in vitro* studies. Recent investigations showed NPN as beneficial as natural protein in rations fed high-producing cows that contained up to 16 per cent crude protein.

For prevention of milk fever, calcium to phosphorus ratios of 2:1 for lactating cows and 1.5:1 for dry cows are recommended. These are slightly higher than those calculated from NRC allowances of 1.4:1 recommended for both lactating and dry cows. Activated forms of vitamin D (hydroxycholecalciferols) effectively prevented milk fever in susceptible cows when administered three to five days before calving. This material is safer and more effective than massive doses of vitamin D.

Sulfur should be supplemented to dairy rations high in corn and corn silage that contain NPN. Selenium is also low in such rations and is now allowed to be added at up to 0.1 mg/kg ration dry matter. A re-evaluation of fluoride levels that are damaging to the lifetime performance of dairy cattle appears warranted.

References

1. Ammerman, C. B., and Miller, S. M.: Selenium in ruminant nutrition: a review. J. Dairy Sci. 58:1561, 1975.
2. Bath, D. L., Dickerson, F. N., Tucker, H. A., and Appleman, R. D.: Dairy Cattle: Principles, Practices, Problems, Profits, 2nd ed. Philadelphia, Lea & Febiger, 1978.
3. Bouchard, R., and Conrad, H. R.: Sulfur requirement of lactating dairy cows. I. Sulfur balances and dietary supplementation. J. Dairy Sci. 56:1276, 1973.
4. Braund, D. G., Dolge, K. L., Goings, R. L., and Steele, R. L.: Method for formulating dairy rations. Pat. No. 4,188,513. Washington, D.C., U.S. Patent Office, 1978.
5. Carstairs, J. A.: Postpartum reproductive and lactational performance of cows relative to energy phosphorus and hormonal status. Ph.D. thesis, Michigan State University, 1978.
6. Chandler, P. T., Brown, C. A., Johnston, R. P., Jr., Macleod, G. K., McCarthy, R. D., Moss, B. R., Rakes, A. H., and Satter, L. D.: Protein and methionine hydroxy analog for lactating cows. J. Dairy Sci. 59:1897, 1976.
7. Clark, J. H.: Lactational responses to postruminal administration of proteins and amino acids. J. Dairy Sci. 58:178, 1975.
8. Clay, A. B., Buckley, B. A., Hasbullah, M., and Satter, L. D.: Milk production response to either plant protein or NPN. J. Dairy Sci. 61(Suppl. 1):170, 1978.
9. Coppock, C. E., Everett, R. W., and Merrill, W. G.: Effect of ration on free choice consumption of calcium-phosphorus supplements for dairy cattle. J. Dairy Sci. 55:245, 1972.
10. Edwards, J. S., Bartley, E. E., and Dayton, A. D.: Effects of dietary protein concentrations on lactating cows. J. Dairy Sci. 63:243, 1980.
11. Flatt, W. P., Coppock, C. E., and Moore, L. A.: Energy balance studies with lactating non-pregnant dairy cows consuming rations with varying hay to grain ratios. Proc. 3rd Symp. Energy Metab., Eur. Assoc. Anim. Prod. Publ. 11:121, 1965.
12. Flatt, W. P.: Influence of pregnancy and ration composition on energy utilization by dairy cows. Proc. 4th Symp. Energy Metab., Eur. Assoc. Anim. Prod. Publ. 12:123, 1969.
13. Foldager, J., and Huber, J. T.: Influence of protein and source on cows in early lactation. J. Dairy Sci. 62:954, 1979.
14. Gardner, R. W., and Park, R. L.: Effects on prepartum energy intake and calcium to phosphorus ratios on lactation response and parturient paresis. J. Dairy Sci. 56:385, 1973.
15. Hibbs, J. W., and Conrad, H. R.: Studies on milk fever in dairy cows. VI. Effect of three prepartal dosage levels of vitamin D on milk fever incidence. J. Dairy Sci. 43:1124, 1960.
16. Hillman, D., Bolenbaugh, D., and Convey, E. M.: Fluorosis from phosphate mineral supplements in Michigan dairy cattle. Mich. State Univ. Farm Sci. Res. Rep. 365, 1978.

17. Holter, J. B., Byrne, J. A., and Schwab, C. G.: Crude protein for high milk production. J. Dairy Sci. 65:1175, 1982.
18. Holter, J. B., Colovos, N. R., and Urban, W. E., Jr.: Urea for lactating dairy cattle. IV. Effect of urea vs. no urea in concentrate on production performance in a high producing herd. J. Dairy Sci. 51:1403, 1968.
19. Huber, J. T.: Protein and nonprotein nitrogen utilization in practical dairy rations. J. Anim. Sci. 41:954, 1975.
20. Huber, J. T.: Feeding corn silage to ruminants. Proc. 11th Ann. Pacific Northwest Nutr. Conf., 1976.
21. Huber, J. T.: The effect of maturity on the digestibility of plant. In Handbook of Nutrition Series. Vol. 111. West Palm Beach. Fl., CRC Press, 1979.
22. Huber, J. T.: Nonprotein nitrogen in dairy cattle rations. In Large Dairy Herd Management, University Press of Florida, 1979.
23. Huber, J. T., Foldager, J., and Smith, N. E.: Nitrogen distribution in corn silage treated with varying levels of ammonia. J. Dairy Sci. 61:(Suppl. 1):138, 1978.
24. Huber, J. T., Graf, G. C., and Engel, R. W.: Effect of maturity on the nutritive value of corn silage for lactating cows. J. Dairy Sci. 48:1121, 1965.
25. Huber, J. T., and Kung, L., Jr.: Protein and nonprotein nitrogen utilization by dairy cattle. J. Dairy Sci. 64:1176, 1981.
26. Huber, J. T., Lichtenwalner, R. E., and Thomas, J. W.: Factors affecting response of lactating dairy cows to ammonia-treated corn silages. J. Dairy Sci. 56:1283, 1973.
27. Huber, J. T., and Thomas, J. W.: Urea treated corn silage in low protein rations for lactating cows. J. Dairy Sci. 54:224, 1971.
28. Jorgensen, N. A.: Combating milk fever. J. Dairy Sci. 57:933, 1974.
29. Julien, W. E., Conrad, H. R., and Moxon, A. L.: Selenium and vitamin E and incidence of retained placenta in parturient dairy cows. II. Prevention in commercial herds and prepartum treatment. J. Dairy Sci. 59:1960, 1976.
30. Krook, L., and Maylin, G. A.: Industrial fluoride pollution: chronic poisoning of cattle on Cornwall Island. Cornwall Vet. 6(Suppl. 8):1, 1979.
31. Kung, L., Jr., and Huber, J. T.: Performance of high producing cows in early lactation fed protein of varying amounts, sources and degradability. J. Dairy Sci. 66:227, 1983.
32. Kwan, K., Coppock, C. E., Lake, G. B., Fettman, M. J., Chase, L. E., and McDowell, R. E.: Use of urea by early postpartum Holstein cows. J. Dairy Sci. 60:1706, 1977.
33. Moe, P. W., Tyrrell, H. F., and Flatt, W. P.: Energetics of body tissue mobilization. J. Dairy Sci. 54:548, 1971.
34. Morrow, D. A., Hillman, D., Dade, A. W., and Kitchen, H.: Clinical investigation of a dairy herd with the fat cow syndrome. J. Am. Vet. Med. Assoc. 174:161, 1979.
35. Murdock, F. R., and Hodgson, A. S.: Effects of protein level and urea on milk production of high performance cows. J. Dairy Sci. 61(Suppl. 1):183, 1978.
36. National Research Council: Nutrient Requirements of Dairy Cattle, 5th rev. ed. Washington, D. C., National Academy of Sciences, 1978.
37. Pamp, D. E., Goodrich, R. D., and Meiski, J. C.: Free choice minerals for lambs fed calcium or phosphorus deficient rations. J. Anim. Sci. 45:1458, 1977.
38. Reid, J. T., Kennedy, W. K., Turk, K. L., Slack, S. T., Trimberger, G. W., and Murphy, R. P.: Effect of growth stage, chemical composition and physical properties upon the nutritive values of forages. J. Dairy Sci. 42:567, 1959.
39. Satter, L. D., Whitlow, L. W., and Santos, K. A.: Supplementing protein to the dairy cow for maximum profit. Proc. Distillers Feed Research Council 34:77, 1979.
40. Satter, L. D., and Roffler, R. E.: Nitrogen requirements and utilization in dairy cattle. J. Dairy Sci. 58:1219, 1975.
41. Schwab, C. G., Sutter, I. D., and Clay, A. B.: Response of lactating dairy cows to abomasal infusion of amino acids. J. Dairy Sci. 59:1254, 1976.
42. Standish, J. F., Ammerman, C. F., Simpson, F. C., et al.: Influence of graded levels of dietary iron as ferrous sulfate, on performance and tissue mineral composition of steers. J. Anim. Sci. 29:496–503, 1969.
43. Vik-Mo, L., Huber, J. T., Bergen, W. G., Lichtenwalner, R. E., and Emery, R. S.: Blood metabolites in cows abomasally infused with casein or glucose. J. Dairy Sci. 57:1024, 1974.
44. Wohlt, J. E., Sniffen, C. J., and Hoover, W. H.: Measurement of protein solubility in common feedstuffs. J. Dairy Sci. 56:1052, 1973.
45. Wohlt, J. E., and Clark, J. H.: Nutritional value of urea vs. performed protein for ruminants. I. Lactation of dairy cows fed corn based diets containing supplemental nitrogen from urea and/or soybean meal. J. Dairy Sci. 61:902, 1978.

Dietary Management in Sheep

F. C. HINDS, Ph.D.

Although traditional management systems of sheep impose conditions requiring attention be given to dietary management, today's intensive systems of production impose much greater stress on the need to properly formulate and manage the diet of sheep. Under traditional systems of management and production, sheep are allowed to graze more or less freely and thus exercise their skill at selective grazing. Often sheep have been found to consume diets much higher in nutritive value than the average quality of total forage available to them. This results from their ability to selectively consume the more nutritious parts of the available plants. This is not to imply that sheep have "nutritional wisdom"—the ability to properly balance their daily nutrient needs if provided an assortment of feeds. But the ability to be reasonably selective in choosing what to eat does aid the shepherd in meeting the sheep's needs.

As systems of management have reduced the opportunity for selective intake by sheep, the shepherd must use greater and greater control in dietary management. During the harvesting and processing of feedstuffs the particle size of feedstuffs is reduced. Generally, the greater the reduction in particle size, the less selectivity sheep can practice. This physical change in the feedstuff can influence several factors that will be discussed later. Also, today's production systems generally emphasize maximum growth rate of market animals, and this introduces diets high in feedgrains and other sources of concentrated nutrients. Diets high in concentrates present a very real challenge to proper dietary management and management in general, since the slightest error in judgment or execution can cause the death of a high percentage of the animals receiving a high-concentrate diet. Thus it can be seen that the degree and skill of dietary management necessary to successfully provide the nutrients for optimal productivity are dependent upon the system of management used.

When considering diets for sheep, it is important to realize that physical form as well as chemical composition and availability is important. Also, it is important to recognize that nutritionally the sheep is not a one component system. Under most conditions consumed feedstuff *first* is exposed to billions of anaerobic bacteria and millions of protozoa. These microorganisms have nutrient requirements just as do other biologic systems, and since they come in contact with the feedstuff first, they metabolize and utilize the nutrients to meet *their* needs. If there is a nutrient deficiency for an individual microbial species, a group of species, or the entire microbial population, their performance (i.e., cellulose degradation) is greatly or, in some cases, completely impaired. Thus, although it may not be realized, the microbial population's nutrient needs must be considered *first,* and if the nutrient needs of the microorganisms are met, very likely the needs of the animal will be met. Although this article will not deal with rumen microbiology and its interaction with nutrition of the ruminant, it is important that the reader recognize the very complex symbiotic relationship that exists. The nonmetabolized nutrients from the feedstuff, the by-products of the anaerobic fermentation, and the microbial tissue *per se* are the materials leaving the rumen and reaching the small intestine and thus are available for enzymatic digestion.

In the formulation of diets for sheep it must be recognized that under normal conditions the microbial populations in the reticulorumen are capable of synthesizing in sufficient quantities all of the water-soluble vitamins (B vitamins) in addition to vitamin K. Thus dietary sources of these vitamins need not be supplied except in unusual situations. Vitamins of importance as dietary additions are vitamin A and vitamin E. Vitamin D is rarely needed if animals have access to solar radiation or feedstuffs that have been irradiated during curing (i.e., sun-cured hays).

The microorganisms in the reticulorumen also synthesize as part of their own tissue all of the essential amino acids. These amino acids are made available to the animal as the result of enzymatic digestion of the synthesized microbial tissue in the abomasum and small intestine. Unfortunately, the quantity of protein synthesized by the microorganisms may not be large enough to meet the needs of rapidly growing lambs or heavy milking ewes during lactation. Thus diets for these two types of sheep will need to provide sufficient supplementary protein (not nonprotein nitrogen) to ensure that in addition to the microbial requirement the animal requirement is met.

Much of the energy made available to the animal is as a result of the fermentation occurring in the reticulorumen and is provided in the form of volatile fatty acids (largely acetic, propionic, and butyric acids) that are in large part absorbed from the four stomach compartments. Generally, 50 per cent or more of the energy available to the animal from feedstuffs consumed is in the form of volatile fatty acids. Because acetic and butyric acids are ketogenic and only propionic acid is glucogenic, animals with a high demand for glucose (late gestation and peak lactation) need special consideration in satisfying their demand for glucose.

With the foregoing as a general background, let's move to a more specific discussion of the life cycle dietary management of sheep.

DIETARY MANAGEMENT

Lambs

Nutrient Needs

The newborn arrives with very little nutrient reserve except for small amounts of fat (energy) and protein (energy and amino acids) and thus must be provided with a highly concentrated source of nutrients. Normal colostrum contains large quantities of vitamin A and vitamin E as well as fats and protein. Thus, not only is colostrum vital from an immunologic point of view but it also provides the newborn lamb with essential nutrients.

Vitamin A deficiencies in neonatal lambs are rare, but apparent vitamin E deficiencies (stiff lamb disease or white muscle disease) are not uncommon. Milk-fed lambs are generally more susceptible to vitamin E deficiencies than older lambs that have been weaned to dry feed because vitamin E functions in the body as an antioxidant, helping to prevent peroxide formation in tissues resulting from the oxidation of fats (unsaturated fats). Lambs consuming milk from the ewe receive over 50 per cent of their dietary energy in the form of fat in milk. This is a very high level of fat and thus there is need for high levels of vitamin E to prevent peroxide formation in tissues. As the lamb's digestive tract matures as a result of eating dry feed and its reticulorumen begins to function as that of a "mature ruminant," two things reduce the stress on dietary vitamin E. First, the dry feed consumed will contain far less (3 to 5 per cent) fat, and secondly, the microorganisms in the reticulorumen attack dietary fat and saturate it, thus removing the double bonds in the unsaturated fat that tend to readily form peroxides in the animal's tissues. As the lamb moves on to dry feed and begins to gain maximally, it is not uncommon to find the lambs doing best in terms of growth showing vitamin E deficiency symptoms such as stiff limbs and even heart failure during exercise. This situation likely represents the case in which a rapidly growing lamb simply outgrows its dietary supply of vitamin E and thus succumbs to the deficiency. Slow-growing lambs less often show the symptoms.

Not all vitamin E deficiencies are straightforward vitamin E deficiencies. Selenium (recently approved for addition to sheep supplements) is an essential element required in the protein that transports vitamin E in blood. Thus, any time selenium is deficient the gross symptoms will be those of vitamin E deficiency. Selenium deficiencies are fairly common and occur in areas with highly leached soils. Generally in affected geographic areas the occurrence is well known and preventative programs have been developed. Borderline areas exist where selenium levels of feedstuffs are almost deficient, and in these areas (Great Lakes states) sheepmen may have chronic problems.

Treatment is best handled for the milk-fed lamb as an injectable (IM) containing both vitamin E and selenium. Repeated treatments may be necessary. Lambs on dry feed can be treated initially using injectable products containing both vitamin E and selenium but also must receive a diet containing added vitamin E and selenium to prevent further occurrence of the problem. Whether the problem is only vitamin E or selenium deficiency can best be determined by using two different therapies on several animals—one of only vitamin E and the other of both vitamin E and selenium—and by differential response the cause of the deficiency is apparent.

Another dietary problem that may become more common is an iron deficiency in lambs less than one month of age. This will occur almost exclusively in confinement and especially where strict sanitation is practiced. Newborn lambs, as newborn piglets, obtain their iron as "contaminant iron" on their mother's udder. Within the first 21 to 28 days of life, fetal red blood cells are replaced by adult red blood cells, and unless sufficient iron is available for synthesis of the adult cells, anemia will result. Once lambs begin to consume dry feed (creep or with the ewes), iron nutrition is no problem, but milk is a very poor source of iron. Again the most rapidly gaining lambs will experience deficiencies and have gross symptoms of pneumonia—thumps. Closer observation will reveal anemia (pale vascular beds around the eyes similar to those found in older sheep with nematode infections). Serologic evaluation reveals very low hematocrit and hemaglobin levels. Treatment is best handled using injectable iron-dextran similar to that used for baby pigs. One injection at one or two days of age will prevent occurrence. If a deficiency is encountered in lambs 21 to 28 days of age, it is essential that iron be provided immediately, and this should be the injectable source previously mentioned. In addition, care must be taken to reduce stress—especially that associated with exercise, environment, and disease—that may increase the oxygen needs of the animal. Some lambs may recover spontaneously, but it is likely that performance will have been reduced.

Although not a common practice, it is not unusual to find lambs being weaned from their dams at 24 or so hours of age and artificially reared. This will likely become more common as reproductive rates in ewes continue to increase and more intensive management is used. Several nutrition considerations are very important. The milk replacer used should be designed for lambs because of the high levels and quality of fat and protein used in formulation. Using dairy calf replacers will not allow for maximum performance because of low levels and quality of fat and protein. The management of the feeding program requires that the lamb receive colostrum and, following weaning, must be trained to use a nipple and the milk dispensing system of choice. Untrained lambs should not be mixed with older trained lambs during the training period. The milk replacer should be fed cold (refrigerated) to avoid overconsumption and reduce the rate of spoilage. A small amount (1.1 ml per 4 liters of milk replacer) of formaldehyde can be added to milk replacer to further reduce the rate of spoilage. Once lambs are readily consuming milk replacer, provide them with a highly palatable preweaning feed. The preweaning feed can be specially formulated to meet all the young lamb's needs and should contain about 90 per cent concentrate and at least 20 per cent crude protein, all from intact protein. A baby pig preweaning feed can be used instead of a special diet. It is also advisable to place a flake of high quality alfalfa hay in the pen because some lambs prefer to pick at roughage. The goal is to start lambs eating dry feed as early in life as possible and thus hasten rumen development in preparation for weaning. Lambs are best abruptly weaned from milk replacer once they are eating dry feed (no earlier than 24 days and generally at 28 to 35 days of age). Upon weaning, the lambs may experience a setback or check in growth, but by market weight no difference in overall performance will be evident. Once the lambs are weaned, they should be maintained on a high-concentrate (80 to 90 per cent) diet high in crude protein (20 to 25 per cent) until they weigh 18 to 23 kg, at which time the protein level can be reduced to 15 to 17 per cent. From this point they are handled as any other weaned lamb.

Caution should be used in meeting a lamb's nutrient needs if an appropriate milk replacer is not available. Augmentation of cow's milk with table sugar or ingredients other than glucose or lactose may cause severe digestive upsets. The newborn lamb is equipped with digestive enzymes capable of degrading products commonly found only in milk, and thus carbohydrates other than glucose and lactose are not able to be digested until at least three weeks after birth. At that time the lamb's digestive tract experiences a major change to the production of "adult enzymes." After this time many oligosaccharides can be degraded by the enzymes produced in the abomasum, pancreas, and small intestine. Sucrose (table sugar), although readily fermented in the reticulorumen, cannot be digested by even "adult" enzymes in the small

intestine and thus is only useful to a lamb with an active fermentation in its reticulorumen.

The stomach of the newborn lamb must undergo major changes before it is able to assume adult function. The largest of the four compartments at birth is the abomasum. The development of "normal" compartment volumes (relative and absolute) and metabolic maturity of the tissues as well as musculature of the compartments are dependent upon the consumption of dry feed and the presence of an active fermentation. Early in life lambs learn to eat from their mothers, and although the amounts of food are relatively small, they may start to eat dry feed as early as several days of age. During normal grooming of the lamb by the ewe and the lamb's consuming feed previously mouthed by adult sheep, the young lamb's reticulorumen is inoculated with the necessary microorganisms to establish a "normal" fermentation. Once the lamb starts consuming dry feed and receives its inoculum, its stomach starts undergoing a major change that culminates in the rumen becoming by far the largest compartment. From a nutritional point of view the lamb raised with access to dry feed will be essentially nonruminant in its nutrient needs (intact protein, B vitamins, and relatively simple energy sources) from birth to three weeks of age. From three to eight weeks of age the lamb is in transition between its previous nonruminant and future ruminant states and thus must still be considered to be a nonruminant. After eight weeks of age lambs that have had access to dry feed have a sufficiently well-developed reticulorumen and omasum to be considered functional ruminants.

More common is the practice of rearing lambs on their dams and early weaning them at 42 to 90 days of age. Although some few sheepmen may wean lambs as early as 28 days of age, the more common age is 50 to 70 days. Because the lambs will be weaned onto dry feed at an early age, it is essential that a creep diet be provided. This diet should be available to lambs within the first week to ten days of life. Since lambs generally learn to eat with the ewes, the best physical form for the diet (whole, ground, pelleted, and so on) will depend on what the ewes receive. Most research on creep diet composition indicates it needs to be high in available energy (concentrates) and need not be high in protein or other nutrients. Apparently these other nutrients are not as limiting as energy; however, once the lambs are weaned, the level of crude protein must be 16 to 17 per cent for optimum performance. Nonprotein nitrogen (urea, ammonium salts, and other sources) should not be substituted for intact protein until the lambs are within three to four weeks of market weight and finish. If urea is used, it should not make up over 1 per cent of the diet or one third of the total dietary crude protein or over one half of the supplemental crude protein. Once early weaned lambs have gained two thirds of the weight from weaning to market weight, the crude protein level can be reduced to 14 to 15 per cent of the diet, and during the last three to four weeks of finishing 12 to 13 per cent crude protein is adequate.

The available energy level of diets for early weaned lambs must be high to ensure optimum performance. Although all-concentrate diets can be fed, slightly greater gains will be obtained if 10 per cent ground forage is included in the diet. As much as 25 per cent ground forage can be included in diets without a marked reduction in gain; however, levels of forage greater than 25 per cent will reduce gains. Diets high in available energy are specially important for lambs close to market weight and finish. Early weaned lambs should be vaccinated against enterotoxemia (type D), although with proper management losses to this disease should be able to be minimized. From both labor and nutritional points of view, self-feeding a complete diet should be recommended. Clean water must be available at all times, and environmental stresses should be minimized.

Mineral Needs

The mineral nutrition of early weaned lambs must be carefully controlled. Urinary calculi in males may occur because of excesses of several mineral elements. Most common in lambs fed high-concentrate diets are phosphatic calculi. Generally, a calcium to phosphorus ratio of 2:1 will prevent the occurrence of urinary calculi. If this does not prevent calculi, the addition of ammonium chloride as 0.5 per cent of the diet will give good results. Ammonium sulfate has been used to replace ammonium chloride but generally results favor use of the latter. If the foregoing do not prevent calculi, chemical analysis of the calculi *per se* as well as the feed and water should provide valuable information as to the type of calculi causing the problem.

Selenium, as mentioned previously, must be provided in adequate amounts to ensure optimal availability and use of vitamin E. In areas known to be selenium-deficient mineral mixtures containing selenium should be added to all diets. It is not recommended that individual producers prepare their own selenium supplements. Selenium is very toxic and small mixing errors could cause high death losses.

Although high dietary copper levels may not always cause a toxicity in market lambs, the improper supplementation of copper may ultimately cause death losses if ewes or rams are retained and used as replacements. Sheep are especially efficient at retaining absorbed copper and storing large quantities in their liver. Once copper in liver reaches "critical" levels, the liver releases the copper and a hemolytic crisis occurs resulting in hemolysis. Some, but few, sheep survive the hemolytic crisis. In most cases copper toxicity occurs because of the overfeeding of copper. Most commonly, trace mineral salt mixtures are fed free choice, or trace mineral mixtures (fed free choice or mixed in complete diets) that are used have been developed for use in swine or poultry diets and may contain four or more times as much copper as those developed for use in sheep diets. Copper levels of finished diets should not exceed 10 ppm.

In addition to overfeeding copper, too low levels of molybdenum and sulfate ion can cause normal copper levels to elicit a toxicity. Molybdenum can be used at low levels to increase the mobilization of copper from the liver and thus serve a therapeutic function. It should be emphasized that although molybdenum increases the rate of copper mobilization from the liver, the rate of reduction is relatively slow and thus if molybdenum is used once copper toxicity is a problem. Additionally, it does not rapidly reduce liver levels and losses subsequent to therapy are not uncommon. If a toxicity is encountered or suspected, it is important to minimize stress and exercise, since sheep not experiencing a hemolytic crisis very likely have elevated liver copper levels and could be forced into a crisis or the crisis could be exacerbated.

If early weaned lambs are to be retained as replacements, it is essential that growth and not fattening be encouraged. Ewe lambs should be removed from the fattening pen prior to reaching market weight and finish and placed on a diet containing half good quality forage and half concentrate. Crude protein levels should be 12 to 13 per cent of the diet. Ewes gaining about 0.10 kg a day, if past puberty, will have the highest productivity. Both high and low levels of available energy prebreeding will reduce reproductive performance.

Ram lambs kept as replacements can be fed diets containing 25 per cent roughage and 75 per cent concentrate until such time as their growth starts to slow down, at which time diets containing 50 to 60 per cent roughage should be fed. Again, overfeeding and underfeeding both may influence a ram's reproductive performance. Dietary crude protein levels should be 14 to 15 per cent until growth slows, at which time 12 to 13 per cent should be adequate. Again, copper nutrition must be watched or valuable animals can be lost.

Weaned Lambs

Conventionally reared lambs produced in the farm flock states may or may not receive creep feed while on pasture with the ewes. If creep is provided, it should be high concentrate and reasonably high (15 per cent) in crude protein. Often lambs are weaned once pasture becomes limiting, the ewes need to be prepared for rebreeding, or the lambs are ready for market. If not sent to market, or if sold to a feeder, such lambs are termed "feeder lambs." Dietary management for feeder lambs is, contrary to many people's beliefs, rather similar to that for early weaned lambs of comparable size. Levels of dietary roughage and protein should be similar to those for early weaned lambs of similar size. In cases where lambs have not received creep feed or feed other than pasture prior to weaning, it is essential to gradually introduce prepared feed to the lambs. Often hay is first fed on the ground and then in bunks, and finally small amounts of grain are introduced.

Caution must be used in changing levels and types of feeds, especially when introducing animals to new feeds. Both the animal and its digestive tract must adjust to dietary changes. All animals must have ready access to feed if hand feeding is practiced. If not, dominant animals may overconsume and experience lactic acidosis. Also changes in level of concentrate, if elevated too abruptly, can cause many lambs to experience lactic acidosis. Changes should be gradual, allowing two to three days at any new level of grain feeding before further changes are made. The amount of change should be on the order of 0.23 kg of grain per period of change. Larger amounts may cause problems. Dietary management is the key to prevention of lactic acidosis. Most lambs will experience slight "digestive upsets" often caused by lactic acidosis that results in a small depression in appetite and mild diarrhea. Often lamb feeders prefer to feed higher levels of roughage to reduce problems of enterotoxemia and lactic acidosis. The higher the level of concentrate in the diet, the greater the importance of proper dietary management.

Patience is required while introducing range lambs to fences, prepared feed, and tank water. Although preconditioning of lambs going to feedlots would be very helpful, this is not widely practiced; thus, problems arising from insufficient water and feed intake may be common. If dietary changes are made too abruptly, the time required for re-adaptation of the lambs to the feed will be greatly extended because not only is the time lost that the animal is "off-feed" but the lamb will start all over in increasing and adjusting its intake.

The adaptation of the microorganisms to specific feedstuffs is much like the animal's adjustment. Too rapid change causes rapid growth of specific types of microorganisms, creating conditions inhibiting to the growth of other organisms essential in maintaining normality within the reticulorumen. Usually eight to ten days are required for the microorganisms to completely adjust to a major change (introduction of grain) in feedstuff. As with the animal, a gradual change will assist the microbial population in adjustment without major problems.

Adult Sheep

Adult sheep moving from one productive function to another require the same care and attention in dietary management as lambs. Prior to the breeding season the ewe has a fairly low energy and crude protein requirement. Care must be taken on many native forages not to allow ewes to become too fat. As explained in discussing ewe lamb replacements, ewes that are too fat or too thin will not reproduce optimally. Stocking rate and grazing time both can be modified to influence ewe condition. Then ewes must be carefully evaluated to be certain their condition is related to plane of nutrition and not parasite load. The influence of parasites cannot be eliminated with adequate nutrients; one cannot feed around parasites.

Breeding

As the breeding season approaches, some sort of flushing program is valuable. Two to three weeks prior to turning the rams with the ewes, the ewes should either receive 0.23 to 0.34 kg of grain per head per day or be placed on fresh highly nutritious pasture saved for flushing. Specific types of pastures in specific areas are notorious for causing breeding problems. In Ohio it is not uncommon to find ladino clover, Dutch White clover, and birdsfoot trefoil reducing early season conception rates of ewes. Elsewhere, alfalfa, birdsfoot trefoil, ladino clover, and Dutch White clover among other legumes have been known to cause reduced reproductive performance largely because of estrogenic materials found associated with the plant. The practice of flushing causes an increase in number of eggs ovulated per ewe. As the breeding season progresses and natural levels of ovulation increase, the response to flushing decreases. Flushing is as effective late in the breeding as early. Flushing (improved plane of nutrition) should continue through the first heat cycle for maximum benefit. Ewes in fat condition do not respond to the same degree as ewes in average to thin condition.

During the first thirds of gestation ewes need to be in average condition and need not gain weight. Their nutrient requirements are low (the same as those for dry ewes). However, during the last third of gestation the available energy in the diet needs to be increased to the equivalent of 0.23 to 0.45 kg of grain per head per day. This is because of the rapid growth of fetal tissues and thus the increased demand for energy, largely glucose. In addition to the demand of the fetal tissues, the volume the fetal tissues occupy in the peritoneal cavity reduces the capacity of the stomach, making it impossible for the ewe to compensate for the increased nutrient demand by increasing feed intake if only roughage is fed. If the available energy level in the diet is not increased, ewes

carrying two or more lambs may develop ketosis or pregnancy disease. Ketosis is more likely to occur in fat than in thin ewes. Therapy will be discussed elsewhere, but needless to say unless attended the lambs and often the ewe die. Prevention through proper dietary management is by far the most effective treatment since therapy is often not overly successful.

At lambing, it is important not to overfeed ewes. For the first five to seven days do not increase grain over that fed during late gestation. After that period, ewes with single lambs should be grouped separate from ewes with twin lambs. Separation of ewe and lamb pairs from singles will permit more effective feeding of both types of ewes. Ewes with twins may produce as much as 40 per cent more milk than ewes with singles, thus the need for greater dietary crude protein and available energy. Large heavy milking ewes with twins may need as much as 1.1 to 1.4 kg of grain per day in addition to all the hay they can eat. Ewes with single lambs should be fed from 0.7 to 0.9 kg of grain per day.

If lambs are going to be weaned early, the ewes must be properly dried up to reduce the occurrence of mastitis. One week prior to weaning the lambs, remove all grain from the ewe's daily ration. One day prior to weaning, remove all feed and water, and a day after weaning, allow only water. Three to four days following weaning, provide some low-quality roughage (not pasture) and gradually increase to normal feed. This should dry up ewes with little trouble from mastitis. One further caution—*do not milk ewes once the lambs have been removed; this will only further complicate matters.*

Other Dietary Concerns

Not all concerns related to dietary management are associated with the chemical composition of feedstuffs. Physical form of the diet—long hay, chopped hay, ground hay, or pelleted hay, and similar descriptions for grains—has a major influence on animal performance and behavior. From the animal's point of view two factors are important. First, lambs and older sheep self-fed or hand-fed ground diets or feedstuffs (i.e., hay) often cough as a result of dustiness of the diet. Although coughing is not good for any type of sheep, it is often found to be a serious problem with lambs just prior to reaching market weight and condition. Coughing and thus dustiness of the diet are closely linked to rectal prolapse, especially in lambs confined to feedlots. Rapidly growing lambs consume large quantities of feed, and as they consume feed their respiratory system is often irritated by the dustiness of the feed and they cough. These coughs are often violent and prolonged. This entire situation puts undue stress on the anal sphincter and often causes eversions of the rectum. Unless attended to immediately, rectal prolapses will cause a sharp drop in lamb performance. Although much of the stimulus for prolapse is dietary and possibly environmental, there is clear evidence that a tendency to prolapse can be genetic. Thus, any offspring or relatives of a prolapsed sheep should be carefully considered as candidates for culling.

The second problem with the physical form of diets is small particle size. Sheep during their evolution have developed the process of regurgitation and rumination into a highly efficient and important process of reducing particle size of fibrous materials found in the reticulorumen. From 8 to 12 hours per day may be spent ruminating. When man, through chopping and grinding, reduces the particle size of feedstuffs to a very small size, sheep are unable to regurgitate and therefore do not ruminate. Because large amounts of time are normally spent ruminating, a sheep on feeds of small particle size that cannot ruminate has much "idle" time. This "idle" time is used in developing vices such as wool-picking, cribbing, and metal polishing. Wool-picking represents the most serious of the vices because it may seriously decrease the performance of several sheep within the group. This vice is thought to occur through inquisitiveness expressed as a picking at particles on fleeces of pen mates. Eventually and accidentally, wool, in addition to feed particles in the fleece, is plucked by the picking sheep. Picking is not an act of aggression, nor is it considered to be associated with mineral, vitamin, or protein deficiencies or imbalances. It occurs in all ages and classes of sheep once dry feed is consumed. It is of greatest concern in adult ewes, especially during the winter when a denuded sheep may not be able to survive the ensuing environmental stress. The proper treatment includes isolation of the picked sheep and an increase in both the fiber level and particle size of the diet to allow normal regurgitation and rumination.

Dietary Management in Goats

R. S. ADAMS, B.S., Ph.D.

The nutritional needs of goats have not been well established. More research must be conducted, and improved feeding standards and nutritional allowances must be developed. Current recommendations are based upon limited studies with goats, basic ruminant nutrition, and farm experiences.

Since interest in goats has increased greatly in recent years and many goat owners, husbandry people, and practitioners are not well informed on their feeding and management, considerable background information has been included in this article. Expected performance data for various classes and breeds of goats are given in Table 1.

Dairy goats and cows are quite similar in respect to basic nutritional needs and metabolic functions. The goat, however, has a higher metabolic rate. Thus a high-producing goat may eat about twice as much dry matter and produce more milk per unit of body weight than a dairy cow. Nevertheless, the net efficiency of utilization of metabolizable energy for maintenance and milk production is approximately 70 per cent for goats as well as sheep and dairy cows.

Differences exist in the transfer of milk precursors to the mammary gland. These are reflected in differences in milk composition. Goat milk generally contains less protein and lactose than cow's milk. Exceptionally high-producing goats may yield 1500 to 3000 kg of milk per lactation. The lactation curve for goats is similar to that of cows. Peak production usually occurs within four to six weeks postpartum.

ROUGHAGE FEEDING

Good quality forage or roughage should be provided in adequate amounts. Intensively managed goats do not need

to browse when good forage is available. Roughage must be fed at levels that allow the goats to select the most nutritious material. It should not only be relatively high in nutritive content but also relatively free from mustiness, mold, dust, weeds, and so on.

Types

Legumes and grasses in the form of pasture, green-chop, or hay are the primary roughage sources for goats. Good quality haylage and silages may be used. However, the relatively small amounts needed for most goat herds make silos and ensiling quite impractical. The use of ensiled materials also may increase the risk of acidosis and digestive disturbances as well as infections and metabolic disorders.

Straw may replace 25 per cent of the usual hay-equivalent fed to goats. During forage shortages or periods of extremely high forage prices, some by-product ingredients with a high content of effective fiber may be substituted for 25 per cent of the normal forage ration. Such ingredients include beet pulp, corncobs, cottonseed hulls, bagasse, soybran flakes, and cardboard waste. Extra care must be taken to balance rations containing forage substitutes to make certain proper amounts of protein, minerals, and fat-soluble vitamins are provided.

Legumes such as alfalfa, birdsfoot trefoil, and clover are the forage of choice for does in milk. Grasses are better suited for dry goats to avoid excessive calcium and protein intakes. Quaker comfrey is not superior to other legumes in most cases. Legume-grass mixtures and small grain forages also are satisfactory for goats. Apparently goats appreciate variety in their diet more than some ruminants. Thus it is preferable, but not essential, to feed several forages.

Fine-stemmed, pliable forage should be used for young kids. Grasses or mixtures containing largely grass should

Table 1. Performance Data for Goats

Milk Production

Bread	kg/Lactation	% Milkfat Test
Saanen	979	3.6
Alpine	970	3.5
Toggenburg	921	3.3
LaMancha	835	3.9
Nubian	817	4.5

Lactation length: 240 to 305 days (average 278 days)
Peak production: Within 4 to 6 weeks of kidding

Reproduction

Puberty: At 4 to 5 months of age
Breeding: At 30 to 34 kg or 8 to 10 months; hold most Angoras until second year
Re-breeding: About 180 days after kidding
Season: Late August to mid-March with most breedings in Sept. to Jan.
Estrus: 18- to 23-day cycle   Duration: 12 to 36 hours (average 18 hours)
Gestation: 145 to 155 days (average 149 days)
Kidding rate: Angoras 50 per cent, dairy goats 100 to 200 per cent
Some well-fed goats may have 3 kids per pregnancy
Average 2.0 to 2.3 kids/doe yearly

Growth

Birthweight: 2.0 to 4.0 kg (usually 2.6 to 3.5 kg)
Dependent upon breed and number of kids

Average daily gain (kg)	Male	Female
First 8 months	0.11–0.14	0.09–0.11
Fattening	0.18–0.23	0.18–0.20
Vealing at 20–40 days	0.20	0.18

be fed to male kids being raised for breeding purposes. This avoids excessive calcium intake, which may result in osteopetrosis and nutritional arthritis in males.

Stored forage or hay may be used as the sole source of forage year-round if it is properly supplemented with vitamins A, D, and E. However, it often may improve reproduction, health, and sometimes production to provide a minimum of 50 per cent of the forage ration as pasture or fresh green-chop for a period of at least 4 to 6 weeks each year. Fresh forage may replenish body stores of fat-soluble vitamins and increase hormonal intake. Grazing also may provide more exercise for goats.

The amount of stored forage to be fed on pasture depends on the quality and amounts of pasture available. Little or no hay may be needed with excellent pasture that is kept in an actively growing state. Some herd owners prefer to feed 25 to 50 per cent of the usual amounts of stored forage when goats are on pasture. Some dry hay fed before pasturing may help prevent bloat on legumes.

The value of browse for goats is questionable. When good browse is available goats have the uncanny ability to utilize its more nutritious portions. Some goat authorities feel that good browse may be beneficial for dry does that have been fed relatively heavy on concentrates owing to their high milk production.

When browse or brush is available to goats in nonintensive areas, over 50 per cent of their diet may consist of browse and mast as opposed to pasture or forage. Good browse consists of wood-like plants that are high in cellulose. Such plants as ground ivy, mixed forbs, and cinquefoil apparently are quite digestible. Foliage twigs and buds from some trees such as dogwood, red maple, elm, birch, rosewood, and belah may be less well utilized. Dead leaves are quite low in feeding value.

Controlled experiments indicate that such browse is not essential for dairy goats. Considerable research does indicate, however, that digestibility of low-quality roughage by goats is generally higher than that by sheep or cattle. This fact may be of considerable value in extensive farming systems and in areas requiring biologic brush control.

Physical Forms

Not all physical forms of forage are of equal value as a roughage source for ruminants. Hay baled in long form or *coarsely* chopped is superior to forage of smaller particle size. Cubed hay is superior to finely ground and pelleted forage. Preferably cubed hay should not furnish over 50 to 60 per cent of the forage ration, whereas pelleted forage should not provide over 25 per cent of the hay-equivalent intake. The average length of forage particles should be at least 3/8 to 3/4 inch to provide for normal rumen metabolism. By-product materials with smaller particle size must not be considered as normal roughage and should be limited to not over 25 per cent of the hay-equivalent intake.

Intake

Forage or roughage intake generally is expressed as hay-equivalent since items of widely varying moisture contents may be fed. It takes 4 to 4.5 kg of pasture at 78 to 80 per cent moisture to equal 1 kg of hay in dry matter content. Silage at 70 per cent moisture has a hay-equivalent factor of 3.0, whereas haylage at 45 per cent moisture has a factor of 2.0. The hay-equivalent factor at any moisture content may be calculated by dividing the con-

stant 90 by the dry matter content of the forage. Total hay-equivalent intake divided by the body weight times 100 results in rate of equivalent intake expressed as a per cent of body weight. For example, a doe weighing 54.5 kg eating 2.0 kg of hay has a hay-equivalent intake of 3.7 per cent ($2.0 \div 54.5 \times 100$).

Recommended hay-equivalent intakes for various classes of goats are presented in Table 2. Certain minimum amounts of roughage are needed to maintain normal rumen metabolism, milk composition, and health. The total ration should contain more roughage than concentrate dry matter if it is to be fed for extended periods. Minimum hay-equivalent intakes given in Table 2 for does should not be used for more than 90 to 120 days.

Excessive intakes of low-quality forage or roughage may restrict total dry matter intake and turnover or flow rates in the digestive tract. This may result in insufficient energy intake by goats producing at relatively high levels. Thus the forage or roughage ration fed to milking goats should contain the equivalent of at least 60 per cent TDN (total digestible nutrients) on a dry matter basis. Certain maximum roughage intakes also need to be considered in the feeding of high-producing dairy goats. These also may be found in Table 2 and may be necessary to maintain sufficient energy density in the total ration.

Usually hay-equivalent intake is greater for highly digestible forage and less for low-quality material. Hay-equivalent intake may vary by as much as 30 per cent between good and low-quality forages fed in a balanced ration.

Roughage is not essential for kids during the first one to two months of life. In most cases, however, roughage and a calf or kid starter should be provided within the first one to two weeks of life to encourage rumen development. Rumen function in kids fed dry feeds soon after birth may approach that in adult goats within four to eight weeks.

Table 2. *Recommended Hay-Equivalent Intakes for Goats**

Class	Per Cent of Body Weight Daily		
	Usual	Minimum†	Maximum‡
Milking does (av 55 kg)	3.6	3.2	4.0
Dry does (pregnant)			
1st lactation (av 40 kg)	3.8	3.5	4.1
2nd lactation (av 55 kg)	2.5	2.2	2.8
Bucks			
1st season (64 kg)			
Breeding	3.9	3.7	4.1
Nonbreeding	2.0	1.9	2.2
Mature			
Breeding	1.9	1.7	2.1
Nonbreeding	1.3	1.2	1.4
Kids			
40 kg (12 to 13 mo, open)	2.6	2.3	2.9
30 kg (10 mo)	3.0	2.7	3.3
14 kg (3 mo)	1.3	1.2	1.4
Fattening			
Starting	3.4	3.1	3.7
Intermediate	2.3	2.1	2.5
Finishing	1.4†	1.3†	1.6

*Refers to amount of hay or other forage adjusted to a 10 per cent moisture, 90 per cent dry matter basis. Up to 25 per cent of the hay-equivalent indicated may be replaced by certain high-fiber, coarse by-products and other ingredients as detailed in the text.

†Should not be used for periods to exceed 90 to 120 days.

‡Rough guide to maximum intake. Room must be left for adequate concentrate intake when necessary. Dependent upon quality of roughage available.

Frequency of roughage or forage feeding depends upon manger capacity, housing, ventilation, and other environmental conditions. Two or three feedings daily generally result in satisfactory hay-equivalent intakes. Forage kept before the animals should be relatively free from bedding, slobber, manure, or heavy barn odors. Roughage intake often increases during cooler weather and may be depressed in hot, humid weather. A moderate decrease in forage intake, coupled with improved forage quality and a modest increase in concentrate feeding, may aid performance under extremely hot, humid conditions.

In most cases forage or roughage should be full-fed to growing kids and milking does. This means that it should be fed to the point of about 5 per cent refusal daily. Roughage intake may need to be restricted for low producers, dry does, and bucks to avoid overconditioning.

CONCENTRATE FEEDING

The concentrate portion of the ration should provide the necessary nutrients lacking in the forage or roughage. Thus the amounts of concentrate and nutritional specifications for it depend largely on the type, quality, and amounts of roughage consumed. Preferably a mixture should be fed rather than grains and supplement separately. Minerals should be force-fed in a properly balanced concentrate rather than provided free-choice for most goats.

Type of Concentrate

Most goats prefer a coarse, relatively dust-free concentrate that is reasonably fresh. Many different ingredients and combinations may be used, provided nutritional specifications are reasonably met and care is taken to maintain palatability.

Concentrate mixtures may be fed in several physical forms. A coarse-textured, partially pelleted feed often is used. Corn in such feeds may be cracked, rolled, or flaked, whereas small grains may be rolled or crimped. The fines, which contain ingredients with a small particle size, may be pelleted. Such pelleted fines may consist of wheat by-products, oil meals, minerals, and vitamins.

All-pelleted feeds also may be fed satisfactorily. The ingredients in a pellet must be relatively fine before processing. Meals containing coarsely ground grains and/ or palatable by-product ingredients sometimes may be consumed in adequate amounts, especially if they contain 4 to 6 per cent molasses and are not dusty.

It is important to realize that the heat treatment of grains that occurs in flaking, steam rolling, and pelleting may alter the starch present. Milkfat test depression and more acidosis may result in milking does if the concentrate mixture contains over 35 per cent starchy grains that have been heat treated. Such processing, however, may improve growth and fattening through alterations in rumen

Table 4. *Proportion of Concentrate Dry Matter in the Total Ration of Goats*

Class	Usual (%)	Maximum (%)
Milking does kg milk daily		
2.0	15	20
3.3	33	38
4.6	45	50
7.3	60	60
Dry does, pregnant		
1st lactation	21	26
2nd lactation	23	28
Bucks		
1st season		
Breeding	23	28
Nonbreeding	26	31
Later seasons		
Breeding	25	30
Nonbreeding	25	30
Kids		
40 kg (open)	15	20
30 kg	17	22
14 kg	70	70
Fattening		
Starting	25	50
Intermediate	50	60
Finishing	70	75

Table 3. *Levels of Concentrate Intake for Goats*

Class	Per Cent of Body Weight	
	Minimum	*Maximum*
Milking does	0.35	5.0
Dry does, pregnant		
1st lactation	0.65	1.10
Later lactations	0.47	0.75
Bucks		
1st season		
Breeding	0.52	0.92
Nonbreeding	0.46*	0.81
Later seasons		
Breeding	0.48	0.78
Nonbreeding	0.28*	0.48
Kids		
14 kg	2.47	2.94
30 kg	0.45	0.75
40 kg (open)	0.38	0.58
Fattening		
Starting	0.90	1.35
Intermediate	1.80	2.75
Finishing	2.85†	3.55†

*Little or no concentrate would be necessary when good-quality pasture is abundant.

†Do not use for periods to exceed 90 to 120 days.

Table 5. *Expected Total Dry Matter Intakes by Goats**

Class	Usual (%)	Range (%)
Milking does (kg milk daily)		
2.0	3.8	3.6–4.0
3.3	4.8	4.6–5.0
4.6	5.8	5.6–6.0
7.3	8.0	7.7–8.3
Dry does		
40 kg (1st lactation)	4.3	4.1–4.5
55 kg (later lactations)	2.8	2.6–3.0
Bucks		
65 kg (1st season)		
Breeding	3.1	2.9–3.3
Nonbreeding	2.4	2.2–2.6
85 kg (later seasons)		
Breeding	2.2	2.4–2.6
Nonbreeding	1.5	1.4–1.6
Kids		
40 kg (12 to 13 mo, open)	2.7	2.5–2.9
30 kg (9 mo)	3.2	3.0–3.4
14 kg (3 mo)	4.0	3.8–4.2
Fattening		
Starting	4.0	3.7–4.3
Intermediate	4.0	3.8–4.2
Finishing	4.2	4.0–4.4

*Includes dry matter furnished by both roughage and concentrates.

Table 6. *Feeding Guide for Milking Does**

Milk Produced Daily		Concentrate to Feed Daily†	
kg	*(lb)*	*kg*	*(lb)*
0.9	(2)	0.17	(0.37)
1.4	(3)	0.25	(0.56)
1.8	(4)	0.34	(0.74)
2.3	(5)	0.70	(1.53)
2.7	(6)	0.83	(1.83)
3.2	(7)	0.97	(2.14)
3.6	(8)	1.31	(2.88)
4.1	(9)	1.47	(3.23)
4.5	(10)	1.64	(3.60)
5.0	(11)	2.03	(4.47)
5.5	(12)	2.21	(4.87)
5.9	(13)	2.45	(5.38)
6.4	(14)	2.58	(5.69)
6.8	(15)	2.77	(6.10)
7.3	(16)	2.95	(6.50)
over 7.3	(over 16)	‡¢	(‡¢)

*Assumes hay-equivalent intake to be 3.6 per cent of body weight daily (e.g., 1.5 and 2.0 kg for 41 and 55 kg does, respectively).

Important: Feed first-lactation does 0.30 kg extra concentrate daily to meet growth needs. Does nursing one, two, and three kids should be fed for 2.3, 2.7, and 3.2 kg of milk production, respectively.

†Use only as a guide. Adjustments of 5 to 10 per cent may be made for different hay-equivalent intakes, flesh needs, or energy levels in concentrates or roughage. Energy levels equivalent to 52 and 75 per cent TDN were assumed for hay and concentrate on an as-fed basis.

‡Limit concentrate intake to not over 5.0 per cent of body weight daily to avoid digestive upsets, other health disorders, and milkfat test depression. Restrict further if necessary.

metabolism. Starch in corn, milo, and barley appears to be more susceptible to heat treatment than that in oats or wheat. Buffers may be included in heat-treated concentrates containing over 35 per cent starchy grains to alleviate possible effects on milkfat test and/or production. Such mixtures may contain 1.0 to 1.5 per cent sodium bicarbonate, 0.5 to 0.8 per cent magnesium oxide, and 1.0 to 1.5 per cent limestone. Sometimes sodium bentonite also may be included at a 1 to 2 per cent level.

The fat content in the concentrate mixture is not critical if adequate energy is provided by the ingredients used. Low levels of added fat (1 to 2 per cent) may reduce dustiness in some formulas. It is preferable to use high-quality animal fats rather than vegetable oils in unsaturated form. The fiber content of concentrates fed also is not critical if stored forages are being fed at recommended levels and the energy content in the concentrate is maintained at a level equivalent to 70 to 80 per cent TDN. Nonprotein nitrogen sources such as urea may be used in feeding goats as a finished ration to a maximum of 1.5 per cent. They may, however, reduce palatability of concentrate mixtures.

Table 7. *Feeding Guide for Dry Does*

Hay-equivalent intake*
  1st lactation: 1.53 kg per head daily
  2nd lactation: 1.35 kg per head daily
Concentrate intake:
  1st lactation: (0.40 kg) per head daily
  Later lactations: (0.40 kg) per head daily
Crude protein content of concentrate mixture:
  With legume, mixed legume-grass (50:50) 10 per cent
  With grass, cereal grain forage 12 per cent
Dry period: 5 to 8 weeks minimum
  1st lactation does need more than older ones
Avoid both over- and underfleshing

*Preferably limit legume or mixed mainly legume forage to not over 30 to 50 per cent of the hay-equivalent intake by dry does to help avoid metabolic diseases.

Small herd owners generally may find it more convenient and practical to use commercial or manufactured feeds for their goats. Some concerns market specialized products for goats. Others may have lines of dairy or other feeds that may be satisfactorily used. Sometimes fewer problems with concentrate intake may occur with high-volume dairy feeds than with low-volume goat feeds. Freshness can be a factor. Avoid feeds with over 5 to 6 per cent molasses.

Levels of Concentrate

Concentrates should be fed in amounts that reasonably balance the forage ration in respect to the energy needs of the animals. Minimum levels may be needed to maintain a rumen microflora and lining that is adapted to a mixed ration of roughage and concentrates as well as to improve mineral utilization. Maximums must be placed on concentrate intake to avoid inadequate roughage consumption and adverse effects on milk composition and flavor. Suggested minimum and maximum concentrate intakes for various classes of goats may be found in Table 3. Note that these are expressed as a per cent of body weight. They assume that forage or roughage is being full-fed.

Recommended proportions of concentrate in the total ration dry matter for use in complete ration cubes or total mixed rations of roughage and concentrates are given in Table 4. These may also be used in trouble-shooting problems. Expected total dry matter intakes of roughage and concentrate combined are listed in Table 5. Within narrow limits, total dry matter intake may be somewhat higher with rations of reasonably lower energy density and somewhat less with those containing a higher proportion of concentrate or greater energy density.

Symptoms of overfeeding concentrates to goats include more off-feed problems, ketosis, milkfat test depression,

Table 8. *Feeding Guide for Bucks*

Class	Breeding	Nonbreeding
1st season		
Hay-equivalent intake,* kg per head daily	1.8	1.3
Concentrate intake, kg per head daily	0.55	0.45
Later seasons		
Hay-equivalent intake,* kg per head daily	1.6	1.0
Concentrate intake, kg per head daily	0.55	0.36
Crude protein in concentrate mixture for all seasons and breeding status:		
Legume, mixed legume-grass forage (50:50)	10 per cent	
Grass, cereal grain forage	12 per cent	

*Preferably limit legume or mixed mainly legume forage for bucks to 0.5 hay-equivalent per head daily to avoid osteopetrosis.

Table 9. *Feeding Guide for Kids: Birth Through Five Months*

Colostrum: birth through four days
Hand-feed 85 to 114 g (3 to 4 oz) as soon as kid will nurse from a nipple bottle, usually within minutes or a few hours of birth
Repeat with nursings or feedings of 85 to 114 g (3 to 4 oz) every 3 to 4 hours for a total of about 0.70 to 0.85 kg during the first day
Liquid feeding: days 5 through 60 to 90
Feed 0.75 to 1.0 kg per head daily, use one of the following:
Lamb or veal replacer reconstituted according to the manufacturer's directions
Sour colostrum diluted with water (2 to 3 parts colostrum: 1 part water)
Whole milk
Wean from liquid at 2 to 3 months
Should be eating at least 0.11 kg of concentrate mix daily and some roughage before weaning
Solid feeding:
Commercial calf or kid starter
Provide within 1st week through 5th month
With legume or mixed legume grass (50:50) forage
Use 10 to 11 per cent crude protein
With grass or cereal grain forage
Use 12 to 14 per cent crude protein
Self-feed up to 0.40 kg per head daily
Roughage feeding:
Provide within 1 to 2 weeks of age
Self-feed with no maximum
Hay-equivalent intake should approach or exceed 1.3 per cent of body weight daily within 1 to 2 months (e.g., 0.18 kg for 14-kg kid)
Use fresh, pliable hay of good quality
Water
Provide fresh, clean water by 2 to 3 weeks of age
Avoid overloading after liquid feeding or nursing is completed

Table 10. *Feeding Guide for Kids: Six Months Through Kidding*

Six through 10 months
Hay-equivalent intake
3.0 per cent of body weight daily (e.g., 0.81 kg for 27-kg kid)
Concentrate feeding
With legume or mixed legume-grass (50:50) forage
Use 10 per cent dairy or kid feed
With grass or cereal grain forage
Use 12 per cent dairy or kid feed
Feed about 0.2 to 0.3 kg per head daily
Eleven months to kidding
Hay-equivalent intake
2.6 per cent of body weight daily (e.g., 1.0 kg for a 40-kg kid)
Concentrate feeding
With legume or mixed legume-grass (50:50) forage
Use a dairy or kid feed with 10 per cent crude protein
With grass or cereal grain forage
Use a dairy or kid feed with 12 per cent crude protein
Amounts fed per head daily
To last 6 weeks of gestation: 0.20 to 0.30 kg per head daily
Last 6 weeks of gestation: 0.40 kg per head daily (increase to this level at a rate of 45 g daily)

Table 11. *Feeding Guide for Fattening Kids*

	% Body Weight Daily
Hay-equivalent intake	
Starting	3.4
Intermediate	2.3
Finishing*	1.4
Concentrate intake	
Starting	1.1
Intermediate	2.3
Finishing*	3.3

Crude protein content for concentrate mixture	Forage	
	Legume, Mixed 50:50 (%)	Grass, Cereal Grain (%)
Starting	12	15
Intermediate	11	13
Finishing*	10	11

*Do not feed finishing ration for periods to exceed 90 to 120 days.

sour and light-colored feces, diarrhea, bloat, founder, and sometimes death. Goats considerably overfed concentrate for extended periods, especially when dry, may be more susceptible to numerous metabolic and infectious problems at parturition. Reproduction also may be adversely affected. Obesity should be avoided in all goats from birth on. It may increase maintenance requirements, reduce milk production, increase health problems, and shorten life span.

Table 12. *Nutritional Specifications for Concentrates Fed to Does**

Component	Milking Does			Dry Does	
	Legume (%)	59:50† (%)	Grass (%)	Legume 50:50†	Grass, Cereal
Crude protein‡	10–11	12–13	14–15	10–11	12–13
Fat	1–7	1–7	1–7	1–7	1–7
Crude fiber	3–10	3–10	3–10	3–10	3–10
TDN, min	70	70	70	70	70
Calcium	0.25	0.40	0.60	0.25	0.50
Phosphorus	0.40	0.40	0.45	0.40	0.40
Magnesium	0.17	0.27	0.34	0.29	0.44
Potassium, min	0.40	0.40	0.40	0.40	0.40
Sulfur	0.15	0.23	0.30	0.22	0.38
Salt	1.00	1.00	1.00	1.00	1.00
Added (ppm):					
Manganese	21	21	21	11	11
Iron	16	16	16	16	16
Copper	15	15	15	21	21
Zinc	113	113	113	180	180
Iodine	0.53	0.53	0.53	0.85	0.85
Selenium§	1.32	1.32	1.32	2.12	2.12
Vitamin (I.U./kg)	0.26	0.26	0.26	0.43	0.43
A	5800	5800	5800	3000	3000
D	2900	2900	2900	1500	1500
E	66	66	66	60	60

*Use only as a guide. Feed programming based on forage testing should be obtained for specific recommendations.
†Mixed legume-grass (50:50).
‡Use lower level in most cases.
§Use only if cleared by governmental agencies and in selenium-deficient areas.

Table 13. *Nutritional Specifications for Concentrates Fed to Bucks**

Component	Legume 50:50† (%)	Grass Cereal (%)
Crude protein‡	10–11	12–13
Fat	1–7	1–7
Crude fiber	3–10	3–10
TDN, min	70	70
Calcium	0.25	0.34
Phosphorus	0.40	0.40
Magnesium	0.28	0.41
Potassium, min	0.40	0.40
Sulfur	0.23	0.36
Salt	1.00	1.00
Added (ppm):		
Manganese	21	21
Iron	16	16
Copper	15	15
Zinc	180	180
Cobalt	0.75	0.75
Iodine	1.87	1.87
Selenium§	0.35	0.35
Vitamin (I.U./kg)		
A	6500	6500
D	1300	1300
E	65	65

*Use only as a guide. Feed programming based on forage testing should be obtained for more specific recommendations.
†Mixed legume-grass (50:50).
‡Use lower level in most cases.
§Use only if cleared by governmental agencies and in selenium-deficient areas.

FEEDING PROGRAMS

A number of feeding guides are presented in Tables 6 through 11. These indicate the varying needs on several basic forage rations: legume, mixed legume-grass (50:50), and grass.

Nutritional specifications for the various concentrate and mineral mixtures indicated may be found in Tables 12 through 18. Some commercial dairy or even goat feeds may vary considerably from those recommended specifications and still produce satisfactory results. When prob-

Table 14. *Some Nutritional Specifications for Milk Replacers**

Crude protein, %	20–24
Fat, %	15–30
Crude fiber, %	0.25–0.50
Added:	
Selenium,† ppm	0.10†
Vitamin E, I.U./kg	44–66
Vitamin A, I.U./kg	55,000
Vitamin D, I.U./kg	11,000

*Preferably use a lamb replacer. If not available, use a veal replacer.
†Use only if cleared by governmental agencies and in selenium-deficient areas.

Table 15. *Nutritional Specifications for Concentrates Fed to Kids (0–11 Months)**

Component	Legume 50:50† (%)	Grass Cereal (%)
Crude protein‡	10–11	12–14
Fat	1–7	1–7
Crude fiber	3–10	3–10
TDN	70	70
Calcium	0.25	0.55
Phosphorus	0.40	0.40
Magnesium	0.33	0.40
Potassium, min	0.40	0.50
Sulfur	0.22	0.40
Salt	0.35	0.35
Added (ppm):		
Manganese	11	11
Iron	16	16
Copper	21	21
Zinc	180	180
Cobalt	1.1	1.1
Iodine	2.7	2.7
Selenium§	0.6	0.6
Vitamin (I.U./kg)		
A	4400	4400
D	2200	2200
E	44	44

*These should serve as a guide only. Feed programming based on forage testing should be obtained for specific recommendations.
†Mixed legume-grass (50:50).
‡Use lower level in most cases.
§Use only if cleared by governmental agencies and in selenium-deficient areas.

Table 16. *Nutritional Specifications for Concentrates Fed to Fattening Kids**

Component	Starting Legume 50:50† (%)	Starting Grass Cereal (%)	Intermediate Legume 50:50† (%)	Intermediate Grass Cereal (%)	Finishing Legume 50:50† (%)	Finishing Grass Cereal (%)
Crude protein‡	10–12	15–16	10–12	13–15	8–10	11–12
Fat	1–7	1–7	1–7	1–7	1–7	1–7
Crude fiber	2–7	2–7	2–7	2–7	2–7	2–7
TDN	75–80	75–80	75–80	75–80	75–80	75–80
Calcium	0.15	0.25	0.15	0.30	0.15	0.30
Phosphorus	0.62	0.40	0.20	0.29	0.30	0.30
Magnesium	0.13	0.30	0.18	0.24	0.20	0.21
Potassium, min	0.30	0.40	0.30	0.30	0.10	0.41
Sulfur	0.10	0.24	0.18	0.22	0.13	0.15
Salt	1.25	1.25	0.80	0.80	0.56	0.56
Added (ppm):						
Manganese	18	18	24	24	29	29
Iron	27	27	31	31	42	42
Copper	17	17	7	7	6	6
Zinc	140	140	68	68	53	53
Cobalt	3.5	3.5	1.7	1.7	1.2	1.2
Iodine	7.0	7.0	3.4	3.4	2.4	2.4
Selenium§	0.30	0.30	0.10	0.10	0.10	0.10
Vitamin (I.U./kg)						
A	5500	5500	2500	2500	2000	2000
D	1100	1100	500	500	400	400
E	55	55	25	25	20	20

*Use only as a guide. Feed programming based on forage testing should be obtained for specific recommendations.
†Mixed legume-grass (50:50).
‡Use lower level in most cases.
§Use only if cleared by FDA and in selenium-deficient areas.

Table 17. *Trace Mineral Salt for Goats*

Mineral	%
Salt	90 or more
Manganese	0.2080
Iron	0.1570
Copper	0.1450
Zinc	1.1310
Cobalt	0.0059
Iodine	0.0148
Selenium*	0.0026

*Use only when approved by governmental agencies and in selenium-deficient areas.

Table 18. *Nutritional Specifications for a General Purpose Mineral-Vitamin Mixture**

Component	%
Calcium	18.0
Phosphorus	1.20
Magnesium	4.0
Sulfur	3.0
Potassium	2.0
Manganese	0.100
Iron	0.125
Copper	0.075
Zinc	0.550
Cobalt	0.0025
Iodine	0.0075
Selenium†	0.0013
Vitamin (I.U./kg)	
A	220,000
D	110,000
E	1,760

*For free-choice feeding to animals, not force-fed minerals on range or pasture. Also provide salt free choice.

†Use only when permitted by governmental agencies and in selenium-deficient areas.

lems arise on feeds or products that vary widely from recommended levels, these specifications may be used to help alleviate related problems through extra supplementation or possibly a change in the concentrate fed to one that more reasonably approaches recommended nutrient content. Levels of protein and major minerals are of greater importance than vitamin content. An overage of 2 to 4 per cent in crude protein may be well tolerated under some conditions. Levels of sulfur in concentrates for Angora or other fiber-producing goats should be increased by approximately 0.25 per cent over those given in the tables. Wool production also requires extra energy and protein, as indicated in Table 21.

Specifications for a trace mineral salt to be used in feeding goats may be found in Table 17. Specifications for a general purpose mineral-vitamin mixture for free-choice feeding of goats on pasture or range are given in Table 18. This is designed for use when no minerals are

being force fed via a concentrate. When intakes are not adequate to prevent problems related to magnesium, selenium, or vitamin E, two parts of the mix may be blended with one part oil meal or ground grain to improve consumption.

Water is an important item in the diet that should not be overlooked. Goats may drink less water than sheep under similar conditions. Goats often will consume 2500 to 3000 ml daily. More digestive upsets, off-feed problems,

Table 19. *Daily Nutrient Allowances for Goats**

Body Weight (kg)	TDN (g)	Metabolizable Energy (Mcal)	Total Crude Protein (g)	Ca (g)	P (g)	Vitamin A (1000 I.U.)	Vitamin D (I.U.)	Est Dry Matter Intake (kg)
Maintenance only (stable or drylot conditions and early pregnancy)								
10	159	0.57	22	1.0	0.7	0.4	84	0.28
20	267	0.96	38	1.0	0.7	0.7	144	0.48
30	362	1.30	51	2.0	1.4	0.9	195	0.65
40	448	1.61	63	2.0	1.4	1.2	243	0.81
50	530	1.91	75	3.0	2.1	1.4	285	0.95
60	608	2.19	86	3.0	2.1	1.6	327	1.09
70	682	2.45	96	4.0	2.8	1.8	369	1.23
80	754	2.17	106	4.0	2.8	2.0	408	1.36
90	824	2.96	116	4.0	2.8	2.2	444	1.48
100	891	3.21	126	5.0	3.5	2.4	480	1.60
Gestation (additional needs for late pregnancy)								
	397	1.42	82	2.0	1.4	1.1	213	0.71
Growth (additional needs for growth at 100 g daily)								
	200	0.72	28	1.0	0.7	0.5	108	0.36
Additional needs for growth at 150 g daily								
	300	1.08	42	2.0	1.4	0.8	162	0.54

*Adapted from National Research Council: Nutrient Requirements of Goats. Washington, D.C., National Academy Press, 1981.

Table 20. *Additional Nutrient Allowances per kg of Milk Production by Goats**

Milk Fat (%)	TDN (g)	Metabolizable Energy (Mcal)	Total Crude Protein (g)	Ca (g)	P (g)	Vitamin A (1000 I.U.)	Vitamin D (I.U.)
2.5	333	1.20	59	2.0	1.4	3.8	760
3.0	337	1.21	64	2.0	1.4	3.8	760
3.5	342	1.23	68	2.0	1.4	3.8	760
4.0	346	1.25	72	3.0	2.1	3.8	760
4.5	351	1.26	77	3.0	2.1	3.8	760
5.0	356	1.28	82	3.0	2.1	3.8	760
5.5	360	1.29	86	3.0	2.1	3.8	760
6.0	365	1.31	90	3.0	2.1	3.8	760

*Adapted from National Research Council: Nutrient Requirements of Goats. Washington, D.C., National Academy Press, 1981.

Table 21. *Additional Nutrient Allowances Daily for Mohair**

Fleece Yield (kg)	TDN (g)	Metabolizable Energy (Mcal)	Total Crude Protein (g)
2	16	0.06	9
4	34	0.12	17
6	50	0.18	26
8	66	0.24	34

*Adapted from National Research Council: Nutrient Requirements of Goats. Washington, D.C., National Academy Press, 1981.

and ketosis may occur when the water source or supply contains high total bacteria or coliform counts. Preferably, water used for replacers or feeding young kids should not contain any fecal coliform count. Water with pH below 5.6 or over 8.4 may be suspect regarding metabolic disturbances. Water containing over 100 ppm of nitrate ion may increase usual reproductive problems or reduce growth. Over 3 ppm nitrite ion may be quite toxic.

A partial listing of the nutritional requirements for goats may be found in Tables 19, 20, and 21. Many of feeding recommendations in this material on dietary management are based on the 1981 NRC standards with the following exceptions: calcium needs have been set at 1.75 times phosphorus, and vitamin A levels used are 3 times NRC. It is generally assumed that 1 mg of beta carotene is equivalent to 400 I.U. of vitamin A for ruminants.

Supplemental Reading

Devendra, C., and Burns, M.: Goat Production in the Tropics. Bucks, England, Commonwealth Argicultural Bureau, Farnham Royal, 1970.
Guss, S. B.: Management and Diseases of Dairy Goats. Scottsdale, Az., Dairy Goat Journal Publishing Corporation, 1977.
Hanlein, G. F. W.: Dairy goat management. J. Dairy Sci. *61*:1011–1021, 1978.
Hanlein, G. F. W., and Ace, D. L.: Goat Extension Handbook. Newark, Delaware, Cooperative Extension Service, University of Delaware, 1983.
Huston, J. E.: Forage utilization and nutrient requirements of the goat. J. Dairy Sci. *61*:988–993, 1978.
National Research Council: Nutrient Requirements of Goats. Washington, D.C., National Academy Press, 1981.
Shelton, M.: Reproduction and breeding of goats. J. Dairy Sci. *61*:994–1010, 1978.

Dietary Management in Pigs

R. A. EASTER, Ph.D. and G. R. HOLLIS, Ph.D.

The ability of domestic swine to prosper under a wide array of feeding programs is legendary, as is the pig's reputation as a consumer of "scraps" from the human food supply. Obviously, the nutrient needs of the pig can be met with many different feed ingredients, but certain requirements *must* be provided if efficient growth and reproduction are to prevail.

Nutrients that must be present in swine diets are generally discussed in five broad categories: protein, minerals, vitamins, fat, and water. Energy, though essential, can be derived from the metabolism of protein, carbohydrates, or fat. Specific nutrients within the five categories are listed in Table 1.

NUTRITIONAL COMPONENTS OF SWINE DIETS

Protein

The pig does not require dietary protein *per se* but rather the individual amino acids that make up protein. Ten of the amino acids must be present in the diet at minimal levels for maximum growth. Arginine is not required during pregnancy; thus only nine are essential components of the gestation diet. In addition there is a requirement for nitrogen for the synthesis of the nonessential amino acids. This nitrogen is generally provided from the catabolism of the nonessential amino acids found in dietary protein.

Unfortunately, very few feed ingredients provide the essential amino acids in the exact proportions that the pig requires. Thus a major problem of diet formulation is to combine feed stuffs that will result in a diet that meets amino acid requirements with a minimum of excesses. This is typically achieved by a combination of cereal grain, an energy source deficient in amino acids, and a protein feed such as soybean meal or fish meal. Amino acid balance, or the relationship of dietary levels of amino acids to actual requirements, is an important consideration

Table 1. *Nutrients That Are Essential Dietary Components for the Pig*

Protein	Minerals*	Vitamins	Fat†	Water
Methionine	Calcium	Vitamin A	Linoleic acid	
Arginine	Phosphorus	Vitamin D		
Tryptophan	Sodium	Vitamin E		
Threonine	Chlorine	Vitamin K		
Histidine	Potassium	Riboflavin		
Isoleucine	Magnesium	Niacin		
Lysine	Iron	Pantothenic acid		
Leucine	Zinc	Vitamin B₁₂		
Phenylalanine	Manganese	Choline		
Valine	Copper	Thiamine		
Nitrogen‡	Iodine	Vitamin B₆		
	Selenium	Biotin		
		Folacin		

*The minerals listed here are clearly needed. Indirect evidence suggests that fluorine, tin, chromium, vanadium, silicon, and nickel may also be needed; however, these elements have never been shown to be deficient in practical swine diets.
†The essentiality of linoleic acid is questionable. Natural food ingredients provide a sufficient amount to meet the requirement.
‡In addition to the essential amino acids, a source of nitrogen, usually nonessential amino acid nitrogen, is required for the synthesis of nonessential amino acids.

in formulation, particularly when plant proteins that are extremely deficient in lysine relative to other amino acids are used in the formulation process. The point is illustrated by the data in Table 2. In this experiment a sorghum–peanut meal diet (diet 2) was formulated to 20.2 per cent crude protein, a level generally adequate for starter pigs. Poor growth resulted because the diet was lysine deficient compared with the sorghum–soybean meal control (diet 1). The lysine deficiency was overcome in diet 3 by the simple addition of synthetic lysine. In the fourth diet sorghum was replaced with peanut meal until the lysine level in the control diet (diet 1) was achieved. Note that this brought the protein level to 40.0 per cent. Although diets 3 and 4 contained equal amounts of lysine, pig performance was severely depressed with diet 4 as a result of the imbalance created by the tremendous amino acid excesses found in the 40 per cent crude protein diet.

Synthetically produced feed grade preparations of methionine and lysine are available for commercial use in swine feeds. The sulfur amino acid requirement is generally met by diets formulated with natural feedstuffs; hence the use of supplemental methionine is rare.

Most plant materials are deficient in lysine. Synthetic lysine can often be used to economic advantage either as a replacement for soybean meal lysine or to supplement lysine-deficient proteins such as cottonseed, sunflower, or safflower seed meal. In the specific case of soybean meal the crude protein level in starter, grower, and finisher diets can be reduced by 2 percentage units when soybean meal is replaced by lysine. Thus a 14 per cent crude protein diet plus lysine would yield performance equivalent to that seen with the 16 per cent diet used for growing pigs. The level of supplemental lysine is an important consideration. It is a fact that the requirement, expressed as a per cent of the diet, decreases by 0.02 percentage unit for each 1 percentage unit decrease in crude protein. Thus the 16 per cent growing pig diet would usually contain 0.77 per cent lysine, but the 14 per cent replacement of that diet need contain only 0.73 per cent lysine.

Commercial lysine is sold as a product containing 98 per cent lysine HCl or 78 per cent pure lysine. The 78 per cent value should be used in calculations. The pig can use only the L-isomer of lysine.

There is no advantage to exceeding the established protein requirements. Overconsumption of protein will not, however, result in "protein poisoning." Pigs have been fed pure soybean meal during the grower-finishing period with no effect on performance, and only a mild diarrhea resulted from fermentation of the indigestible oligosaccharide component of the soybean meal in the cecum and large intestine.

Clinical signs of a protein/amino acid deficiency include poor growth, rough hair coat, and impaired lactation.

Specific amino acid deficiencies cannot be diagnosed on the basis of signs alone.

Vitamins

Although required in multiple amounts, the omission of certain vitamin supplements from practical swine diets can have devastating consequences. Other vitamins, though essential for cellular function, are not required as supplement to practical diets because they are (1) present in sufficient quantity in natural feeds or (2) produced in sufficient quantity by the intestinal microflora to meet the requirement. It is generally accepted today that the grain–soybean meal diet should be supplemented with vitamins A, D, E, K, riboflavin, niacin, pantothenic acid, choline, and vitamin B_{12}.

Much attention has been given to the visible signs of vitamin deficiency, and this may have led to erroneous presumptive diagnoses of specific deficiencies. The signs should be considered in conjunction with a general knowledge of conditions likely to precipitate a deficiency in order to develop a working assessment of the problem. Clinical tests should always precede any recommendations of a major dietary change.

The following discussion concerns vitamins that are likely to be deficient in practical swine diets.

Vitamin A

Classically vitamin A has been associated with vision, but it is also important to the maintenance of the integrity of epithelial tissue. A deficiency may provide suitable conditions for respiratory infections and reproductive failure. Vitamin A deficiency during gestation results in multiple birth defects (malformed eyes, cleft palates, and misplaced kidneys).

Feedstuffs vary considerably in carotenoid concentrations. Carotenoids are the dietary precursors of vitamin A. Because of the variability and general instability of carotenoids in stored feeds, it is appropriate to supplement all swine diets with vitamin A. The pure vitamin is unstable; thus only stabilized forms such as vitamin A palmitate or vitamin A acetate should be used in feed. Vitamin A requirements are usually expressed as units of vitamin A activity since several natural and synthetic compounds can be used to meet requirements, each of which differs from the rest in potency. One international unit (I.U.) of vitamin A activity is equivalent to 0.30 µg of vitamin A acetate or 0.550 µg of vitamin A palmitate.

Excessive use of vitamin A should be avoided as this vitamin, when fed in great excess, is toxic to swine.

Vitamin D

This vitamin is rarely a problem when pigs receive ample exposure to sunlight. The vitamin D precursor,

Table 2. *Effect of Amino Acid Balance on Gain and Feed Efficiency of Pigs**

Type of Diet	Dietary Lysine (%)	Dietary Protein (%)	Daily Gain (lb)	Daily Feed (lb)	Gain/Feed
1. Sorghum-soybean meal	1.07	20.2	1.19	2.28	0.52
2. Sorghum-peanut meal	0.54	20.2	0.55	1.54	0.36
3. Sorghum-peanut meal + lysine	1.07	20.2	0.92	2.23	0.41
4. Sorghum-peanut meal	1.07	40.0	0.68	1.55	0.44

*Data from Tanksley, T. D., Jr., and Baker, D. H.: Protein and amino acids for swine. Pork Industry Handbook, Bull. No. 5. Cooperative Extension Service, Urbana, Ill., University of Illinois, 1977.

7-dehydrocholesterol, is activated by irradiation at the skin surface by the ultraviolet portion of sunlight. Since this does not always occur in confinement, vitamin D supplementation of practical diets is necessary. The pig can utilize both vitamin D_2 and vitamin D_3, the two forms of the vitamin that are commercially available.

Vitamin D deficiency results in impaired calcium absorption, the most obvious consequences of which are rickets in growing pigs and demineralization of bone in adult pigs. This problem may be particularly acute in sows following lactation when major bones weakened by demineralization fracture as the sow is subjected to the stress of moving.

Excess vitamin D is toxic, resulting in calcification of soft tissue. The toxicity is underscored by the fact that it is used as a rodenticide in some countries.

Vitamin E

In most cases the omission of vitamin E from cereal-based swine diets will not affect pig performance. Vitamin E is related in function to selenium, and "E" can provide antioxidant protection against cellular damage, muscular atrophy, and death when selenium is deficient. For this reason vitamin E should be added to swine diets as protection against a possible selenium deficiency.

There is no evidence that the reproductive performance of either sows or boars is enhanced by vitamin E supplementation of diets, contrary to the popular notion that vitamin E is a "fertility" vitamin.

Vitamin K

This vitamin functions in the blood clotting process. There is no need to add it to practical diets under most circumstances. However, the hemorrhagic syndrome produced by mycotoxicosis can be partially prevented by the inclusion of vitamin K (or the synthetic menadione) at the rate of 2 g/ton of diet. Thus, it is prudent to add vitamin K to feeds when a mold problem is likely. Menadione is sold in three commercial forms: menadione sodium bisulfite (50 per cent menadione), menadione dimethyl pyrimidinol bisulfite (45.5 per cent menadione), and the menadione sodium bisulfite complex (33 per cent menadione).

Riboflavin

Riboflavin-deficient pigs grow slowly and exhibit a form of dermatitis. The deficiency in females causes cessation of the estrus cycle and the farrowing of mummified and stillborn pigs. Riboflavin is destroyed by sunlight but is stable when protected. It should always be added to grain–soybean meal diets.

Niacin

A deficiency of this vitamin produces necrotic diarrhea with an attendant appetite and growth depression. Although the vitamin is present in appreciable quantities in cereal grains, it is largely unavailable from these sources. Swine diets should be supplemented with either crystalline niacin or niacinamide, another form of the vitamin.

Pantothenic Acid

Although this vitamin is ubiquitous in nature, it is only marginally adequate in most diets. Swine diets are supplemented with the D-isomer; the L-isomer of pantothenic acid is not utilized by the pig. A deficiency is characterized by poor appetite and growth and an unusual gait commonly referred to as "goose stepping."

Choline

This nutrient is not a vitamin by strict definition, but it is an important dietary constituent. There is good evidence that reproductive performance, i.e., litter size at birth and weaning, is improved when grain–soybean meal diets are supplemented with choline. There is no evidence of a benefit from choline supplementation of similar diets for growing-finishing pigs. The clinical signs of a deficiency are nonspecific: poor growth and reduced litter size.

Vitamin B_{12}

This vitamin is of microbial origin, and it is not present in diets based on plant material unless it is added. The effect of a B_{12} deficiency on pig growth is dramatic and underscores the importance of the supplementation of practical diets with this vitamin.

Other Vitamins

Several other vitamins (biotin, folacin, vitamin B_6, and thianine) must be present in swine diets; however, available evidence indicates that practical diets contain enough of these vitamins so that that supplementation is unwarranted.

Minerals

The mineral elements are generally classified as macroelements, those required in relatively large quantities, and micro- or trace elements, those required in very small amounts.

Sodium, chlorine, calcium, and phosphorus are the macroelements generally lacking in grain–soybean meal diets. The other macroelements—magnesium, potassium, and sulfur—are generally provided in abundance by the feed ingredients. Sodium and chlorine are provided as salt. Calcium and phosphorus come from a number of sources, some of which are listed in Table 3.

Salt

The actual amount of salt that should be added to the swine diet has been debated for many years. Like other species, pigs exhibit an adaptive ability to conserve sodium and chlorine when it is in short supply in the diet. Current data indicate that growing-finishing pigs fed *ad libitum* do well on as little as 0.2 per cent salt in the diet. The minimum requirement for limit-feed gestating sows and boars is higher as a per cent of the diet. To minimize confusion, 0.35 per cent has been adopted in recent years as a common level for all swine diets.

***Table 3.** Sources of Supplemental Calcium and Phosphorus for Swine**

Source	Nutrient Content (%)	
	Calcium	Phosphorus
Steamed bone meal	24.0	12.0
Limestone	36.0	trace
Oyster shell	38.0	trace
Dicalcium phosphate	20.0	18.5
Phosphoric acid (75%)	trace	23.8
Curacao phosphate	34.0	15.0
Defluorinated rock phosphate	32.0	18.0

*As-fed basis of expression.

Salt is toxic to swine. As little as 1.0 per cent dietary sodium chloride is toxic when water is restricted. This can become a problem when swine are fed improperly salt-preserved products such as fish meal. Mild salt toxicity is characterized by depressed growth, while in more severe cases staggering, seizures, paralysis, and death may occur.

Calcium and Phosphorus

Calcium and phosphorus are essential for bone formation and a host of metabolic reactions. The clinical signs of a deficiency are similar and much like those associated with vitamin D, i.e., rickets in growing pigs and demineralization of bone in adults. Calcium deficiency has little effect on growth, but a minimal phosphorus deficiency will cause a significant reduction in daily gain. Signs of a deficiency can be precipitated by a major deviation from a ratio of 1.0 to 1.5 parts calcium to 1.0 part phosphorus.

Controversy surrounds the current dietary calcium and phosphorus recommendations despite much research. This is largely because the levels of these elements required for maximal bone strength are in considerable excess of the levels required to produce "acceptable" bones. The values in Table 6 appear to be adequate for all known cases.

Calcium can be easily provided by calcium carbonate from several sources such as ground limestone and oyster shell. Plant phosphorus is largely present in the unavailable phytate form; some recent estimates place the availability of phosphorus in grain at only 15 to 30 per cent. No more than 30 per cent of plant phosphorus should be considered of value in meeting requirements for swine. Efforts to increase the availability of plant phosphorus by various methods (steam pelleting, high moisture storage of grain, and yeast addition) have not proved consistently beneficial.

Iron

Iron is not a general problem when pigs are reared on dirt but is a major nutritional concern when pigs are reared in total confinement. Pigs are considered anemic when blood hemoglobin drops below 8 g/100 ml. The initial effect of anemia is growth depression that in severe cases may be followed by death. The period just after birth is particularly critical. Iron stores at birth are quite low, and the great iron demand for hemoglobin synthesis during the post-natal period of rapid growth is not met by sow's milk that averages only 1 mg/L.

Supplemental iron can be administered in several ways: by swabbing the sow's udder with iron sulfate, by spreading iron sulfate enriched soil in the pigs' environment, by oral administration, or by intramuscular injection of iron dextrin or iron dextran. The last-named method is preferred for reasons of convenience and effectiveness. Current research suggests that oral iron has potential, though absorption after gut closure and the effect of an abundance of iron on intestinal pathogens are major unanswered questions.

A single injection shortly after birth (one to three days) of 150 to 200 mg of iron dextran or dextrin is sufficient to protect the pig against anemia during the suckling period. After weaning, iron should be provided in the diet. There is considerable variation in the availability of iron from different chemical forms, as may be seen in Table 4.

Table 4. *Biologic Value of Iron from Various Sources**

Iron Source	Relative Biologic Value (%)
Ferrous sulfate (mono- or hepta-hydrated)	100
Ferric ammonium citrate	107
Ferric choline citrate	102
Ferric glycero phosphate	93
Ferric citrate	73
Ferric pyrophosphate	45
Ferric orthophosphate	14
Ferric oxide	4
Ferric carbonate	2
Ferrous fumarate	95

*Data from Miller, E. R.: Biological availability of iron in iron supplements. Feedstuffs 50:35, 1978.

Zinc

A zinc deficiency may result from a dietary deficiency of the element, or it may be induced by excess dietary calcium. Zinc-deficient pigs exhibit a depressed appetite and poor gains, but the most definitive sign is a parakeratosis characterized by mild to severe cracking of the skin. Zinc, like phosphorus, forms an insoluble complex with phytic acid in plant material and may be considered poorly available. Grain–soybean meal diets should be supplemented with zinc.

Manganese

Manganese is commonly added to swine diets, though the requirement is not clearly established. Signs of a manganese deficiency include impairment of lactation, irregular estrus, resorption of fetuses, and abnormal skeletal development.

Copper

Copper is definitely required by pigs, though the actual requirement is probably met by dietary ingredients in most cases. Copper deficiency impairs hemoglobin formation and leads to anemia. Copper also has a role in keratinization, formation of the melanin pigment of skin, and maintenance of the integrity of the myelin sheath. Copper is toxic to swine at levels above 250 ppm and may result in reduced growth and, in severe cases, death. Copper, at levels below toxicity, is used extensively in many swine-producing countries as an effective growth promoter. This practice is not approved in the United States.

Cobalt

Cobalt is required only as a component of vitamin B_{12}. The pig cannot synthesize this vitamin; however, the microflora of the large intestine and cecum are capable of B_{12} synthesis. Because there is no clear evidence that B_{12} synthesized in the lower gut can be of benefit to the pig, the routine addition of cobalt to swine diets is unwarranted.

Selenium

Selenium gained early notoriety as the toxic factor in "alkali disease" prevalent on western ranges. It was not until 1967 that selenium deficiency was first linked to the "sudden death" syndrome in swine. Selenium deficiency is related to the vitamin E status of the pig. This relationship stems from the role that these two nutrients share in the protection of cell membranes against damage by cellular peroxides. Selenium functions as an essential component of glutathione peroxidase, the enzyme that breaks down peroxides.

A selenium–vitamin E deficiency in swine is characterized by sudden death of pigs, particularly after periods of exertion and environmental stress. On autopsy the liver is pale and swollen with focal lesions on the liver surface. Major skeletal muscles are often pale with evidence of deterioration. There may be a mottled appearance of the myocardium. Edema of the gastrointestinal tract is also found.

Selenium toxicity, on the other hand, results in loss of appetite accompanied by hair loss, fat accumulation in the liver, and kidney degeneration.

The incidence of diagnosed cases of vitamin E–selenium deficiency has increased significantly in recent years for several reasons: pigs reared in confinement lack access to selenium-rich pasture plants, there has been a decrease in the use of selenium sources such as fish meal and alfalfa meal in swine diets, and there is evidence that continuous cropping has resulted in a gradual depletion of selenium in the root zone of soils. The problem is regional in nature, as is indicated by the data in Table 5.

Approval to add 0.1 ppm to swine diets as sodium selenite or sodium selenate was reluctantly granted by the United States government in 1974 because selenium is carcinogenic. Field reports continue to suggest that 0.1 ppm may be inadequate in some cases. Experimental levels as high as 0.3 ppm have been necessary to prevent death loss due to selenium deficiency.

Iodine

Iodine has become a traditional component of the trace mineral salt in most swine-feeding programs. The iodine content of feedstuffs of plant origin is dependent on the iodine content of the soil on which the crop was grown. Thus, there is considerable variation, and the potential exists for a deficient condition to develop when supplemental iodine is not added to the diet, particularly when the diet contains goitrogens or excessive amounts of arsenic, fluoride, cobalt, calcium, or salt.

Iodine deficiency is most obvious in pigs born to sows fed a deficient diet. The piglets are hairless, have thickened skin, and are weak and die shortly after birth.

Other Mineral Elements

Potassium and magnesium are required by pigs but are not commonly added to diets as the requirements are met by the feedstuffs.

Table 5. *Selenium Content of Corn Produced at Different Locations in the United States**

State of Origin	No. of Samples	Average Selenium (ppm)
Illinois	31	0.05
Indiana	17	0.04
Iowa	25	0.05
Michigan	17	0.01–0.09
Minnesota	23	0.09
Missouri	4	0.05
Nebraska	6	0.35
South Dakota	9	0.40
North Dakota	5	0.19

*Data from Ullrey, D. E.: Selenium deficiency in swine production. Feedstuffs 45:47:30, 1973.

Water

The pig cannot be totally deprived of water for very long without severe consequences. Marginal water deprivation can result in reduced gain and feed efficiency without being obvious. The pig requires 2 to 2.5 kg of water per kg of feed consumed under most circumstances. Increases in environmental temperature, dietary mineral level, or dietary protein can result in an increased need for water. Water should be provided free-choice unless restriction is dictated by management.

LIFE CYCLE FEEDING OF SWINE

Nutrient Requirements

For most purposes swine-feeding programs can be divided into five phases: gestation, lactation, prestarter and starter, grower, and finisher. It is scientifically valid, but generally impractical, to further sub-divide the growth phases. The nutrient requirements of the pig for each phase of growth are summarized in Table 6. It should be noted that these requirements are expressed as a percentage of the diet on an as-fed basis. As-fed means that the diet generally contains about 90 per cent dry matter. Feed consumption is generally regulated by the pig's need for energy, i.e., pigs eat to meet energy needs. Thus the absolute amount of any nutrient consumed per day depends on (1) the concentration of that nutrient in the diet and (2) the quantity of feed consumed. It should be apparent that pigs fed a low-energy diet will eat more feed per day and thus consume more of each nutrient. Thus, when requirements are considered for formulation, one should consider the energy level of the diet and proportionally adjust the requirements as a percentage of the diet to avoid both excessive supplementation and deficiencies. A good example of this situation is found with high-moisture grain (75 to 80 per cent dry matter) wherein water in the grain serves as a dilutant. The pig will routinely consume more kilograms of a high-moisture diet per day; thus the percentage of nutrients in the diet can be reduced, while still maintaining the same absolute intake of nutrients per day.

Boars and Breeding Females

It is important that both boars and sows be in good condition but not overweight. Obese sows have lower conception rates and increased embryonic mortality, whereas obese boars experience difficulty in the physical act of breeding. Feed intake should be regulated for both boars and developing gilts to allow for maturation and maintenance but not for obesity. In a thermoneutral environment this can be achieved with 1.8 to 2.3 kg per day of a grain–soybean meal diet.

Much attention has been given to the practice of flushing or feeding double the daily ration for several days before breeding. Most research indicates that this practice is of no value when the gilt or sow is in "good" condition at breeding; there is, however, an increase in ovulation rate in some herds when gilts and sows are in poor nutritional status at breeding.

Gestation

Control of feed intake is a practical problem in gestation nutrition programs. The sow housed in a comfortable,

Table 6. *Suggested Nutrient Alllowances for Swine**

Nutrient	Starter 10–30 lb	Grower 30–120 lb	Finisher 120 lb to Mkt	Breeder Gestation†	Lactation
Amino Acids (% of diet)					
Lysine	1.00	0.74	0.60‡	0.42	0.60
Methionine§	0.60	0.50	0.30	0.28	0.36
Tryptophan	0.14	0.11	0.07	0.08	0.13
Arginine	0.37	0.25	0.16	— ‖	0.34
Histidine	0.34	0.23	0.14	0.13	0.26
Isoleucine	0.70	0.52	0.40	0.37	0.39
Leucine	0.84	0.67	0.45	0.40	0.79
Phenylalanine	0.63	0.50	0.40	0.37	0.40
Threonine	0.66	0.45	0.37	0.34	0.51
Valine	0.67	0.46	0.36	0.46	0.68
Protein**	0.20	0.16	0.14	0.12	0.14
Vitamins					
Vitamin A, I.U./lb	1500	1500	1500	2500	1500
Vitamin D, I.U./lb	300	150	75	150	150
Vitamin E, I.U./lb	5	5	5	5	5
Vitamin K, mg/lb	1	1	1	1	1
Riboflavin, mg/lb	1.5	1.0	0.8	1.0	1.0
Niacin, mg/lb	12	8	6	8	8
Pantothenic acid, mg/lb	6	5	5	5	5
Choline, mg/lb	600	400	350	400	400
Vitamin B_{12}, mcg/lb	9	6	4	6	6
Energy (kcal/lb g Dietary dry matter)					
Digestible	1680	1670	1670	1650	1670
Metabolizable	1560	1580	1590	1580	1580
Minerals					
Calcium (%)	0.80	0.60	0.60	0.75	0.75
Phosphorus (%)	0.60	0.50	0.50	0.50	0.50
NaCl (%)	0.35	0.35	0.25	0.35	0.35
Trace minerals (for all ages)	mg/lb or ppm				
Iron	36.0	80			
Copper	2.7	6			
Manganese	4.5	10			
Zinc	23.0	50			
Iodine	0.1	0.22			
Selenium	0.045	0.10			

*Data from Jensen, A. H.: Dietary nutrient allowances for swine. Feedstuffs *51*:29:41, 1979.

Note: Requirements expressed on "as-fed" basis. For greater detail the reader is referred to *Nutrient Requirements of Domestic Animals: Nutrient Requirements of Swine.* National Academy of Science/National Research Council publication.

†Nutrient levels adequate for the gestation gilt should be adequate for the mature boar.

‡This amount is required for maximum gain per unit of feed and lean tissue development. Maximum daily gain can be achieved with 0.52 per cent.

§Methionine + cystine; cystine can provide up to 56 per cent of the requirement.

‖Arginine is not essential for gestation.

**These values were determined with corn–soybean meal diets. Use of other grains and protein sources should be made on the basis of amino acid requirement.

i.e., thermoneutral, environment, requires from 5500 to 6300 kcal of metabolizable energy per day. If allowed to eat free choice the sow will consume as much as 15,000 kcal of energy per day. Inevitably she becomes overweight, experiences dystocia, and tends to kill pigs by overlay.

Intake is best restricted by hand-feeding sows. This provides an opportunity for maximum caretaker attention to the needs of individual sows but requires a major labor input, a limited resource on most farms.

There are four viable alternatives to hand-feeding. Sows can be fed individually with automatic devices. A bulky, low-energy diet can be fed free-choice with energy restriction accomplished by the sheer physical mass of the feed. Compounds that suppress appetite can be used to control intake. And, the pregnant gilt or sow can be allowed to eat a high-energy diet free-choice but for restricted time periods. This practice is often referred to as every-third-day feeding.

Gestation weight gain is probably the best indication of adequacy of the gestation feeding program. Gilts should gain 45 to 57 kg total weight (weight just prior to farrowing minus weight at breeding) during pregnancy, whereas mature sows need gain only 34 to 45 kg. Inadequate gestation weight gain is characterized by small piglet size at birth.

Satisfactory reproduction can be achieved with simple grain–soybean meal diets formulated to meet established nutrient requirements. There is no evidence of improved reproduction when fibrous material, such as alfalfa meal or beet pulp, is added to the gestation diet. Similarly, there is no reason to increase either the daily feed allotment or the crude protein level in late gestation. A diet inadequate in protein (i.e., grain fortified with vitamins and minerals) can be fed during early gestation providing a surfeit (i.e., 16 per cent crude protein) is provided in late gestation. Good quality pasture can be used as an effective nutrient source during gestation;

however, it may be necessary to supplement the pasture with a high-energy feed to maintain acceptable weight gains.

Protein or amino acid deprivation during gestation does not significantly affect piglet weight at birth or number of pigs born; however, both litter size and piglet weaning weights are depressed when amino acid requirements are not met during gestation. The gestation amino acid deficiencies appear to impair both lactation and the production and transfer of passive immunity to the piglet via the colostrum.

Lactation

The demand for energy and specific nutrients increases dramatically during lactation and exceeds the capacity for consumption in most cases. Mobilization of nutrients from maternal tissue occurs, and there is a net maternal weight loss during lactation. The sow should be allowed to eat *ad libitum* during lactation to minimize maternal weight loss.

Dilution of the energy in the lactation diet with fibrous material (e.g., bran, alfalfa meal, beet pulp) is counterproductive in that it reduces the metabolizable energy that the sow can consume when compared with a nonfibrous diet. The high-energy, low-fiber diet predisposes to constipation. Fecal passage can be facilitated by adding either 0.75 per cent potassium chloride or 1.0 per cent magnesium sulfate to the diet.

Inadequate feed intake during lactation is frequently related to high ambient temperature in the farrowing house, as indicated by the data in Table 7. This problem illustrates the importance of providing different environmental conditions for the sow and the pigs she nurses.

Addition of fat to the lactating sow's diet increases the fat content of milk and thus the energy density of milk. There is little advantage for normal pigs, but survival of pigs weighing less than 1 kg at birth is significantly increased. Other attempts to provide specific nutrients (e.g., iron) to the suckling pig by supplementation of the sow's diet have been ineffective.

Prestarter and Starter Diets

A supplement to sow's milk should be offered by at least two weeks of age. The practical value of both liquid and dry supplements before this time is questionable and should receive consideration only when milk production is inadequate to sustain maximum growth.

Prestarter diets generally contain appreciable quantities of milk products owing to the character of the digestive enzymes available to the pig prior to weaning. Numerous studies with starter diets show that gain in the first four to six weeks post weaning is greater when a complex diet

containing milk products (principally whey) and animal protein is fed; however, compensatory gain in later stages of growth negates this early advantage by the time market weight is reached.

Typically there is a period of minimal feed intake just after weaning, probably caused by the necessity for adaptation of the digestive system to a nonmilk diet. Nonpathogenic diarrhea that occurs during this period can be alleviated by the inclusion of 30 per cent ground whole oats in the diet. There have been numerous attempts to stimulate feed consumption during this period through the use of natural and artificial flavoring agents. If given a choice, the pig will exhibit an obvious dietary preference, but total daily consumption is unaffected by flavor.

Growing and Finishing Pigs

Growing and finishing pigs, almost without exception, are allowed to eat free-choice in the United States despite the fact that both carcass quality and feed efficiency can be improved by feed restriction during the growing-finishing period.

The ingredients in all swine diets should be ground prior to mixing to improve both feed efficiency and mixing characteristics. The advantage of grinding is proportional to particle size. Finely ground diets produce more efficient gains than coarsely ground diets, but finely ground diets are ulcerogenic. To avoid dietary induction of gastric ulcers, the dietary ingredients should be coarsely ground (6- to 13-mm screen openings in the hammermill). The advantage of grinding is greatest for older pigs; young pigs tend to masticate the diet thoroughly and benefit less from grinding feed.

Pigs fed pelleted diets gain 6 to 8 per cent more weight per ton of feed than pigs fed diets in a meal or ground form. Rate of gain is also increased but not as much. The cost of pelleting, however, generally exceeds the savings due to increased feed efficiency. Other processing methods, such as micronizing, steam flaking, and roasting, have not been shown to be of significant benefit for swine.

The increasing cost of energy for use in drying grain to normal storage moisture levels has caused interest in the potential for storage of grains with high (25 to 32 per cent) moisture content. The results of a number of experiments with high-moisture corn are summarized in Table 8. Two things are evident from these data. First, when compared on an equal dry matter basis, high-moisture grain is equal in feeding value to normal grain, and, secondly, high-moisture grain should always be fed with vitamin-mineral-protein supplements in a complete feed. If offered supplement and high-moisture corn in separate feeders, the pigs will not consume a nutritionally balanced diet.

Table 7. *Effect of Environmental Temperature on Sow and Litter*[*]

| | Temperature (°F) | | | |
| | Experiment 1 | | Experiment 2 | |
	81	*70*	*81*	*60*
No. sows	20	20	16	16
Sow feed/day (lb)	10.1	11.4	9.2	12.3
Pig wt, 28 days (lb)	13.6	15.4	14.1	16.1
Rectal temp in lactation (°F)	102.4	101.6	102.0	101.5

*Data from Lynch, P. B.: Environment and the breeding sow. Moorepark Pig Farming Conference. Dublin, Ireland: An Foras Taluntais, 1978, p. 18.

Table 8. *Performance of Growing-Finishing Pigs Fed Diets Containing High-Moisture Corn or Air-Dry Corn*

	Experimental Diets	
	Air-Dry Corn	High-Moisture Corn
*All Experiments**		
Average daily gain (lb)	1.51	1.50
Feed/pound of gain (lb)†	3.35	3.45
Only Experiments with Completely Mixed Diets‡		
Average daily gain (lb)	1.62	1.59
Feed/pound of gain (lb)†	3.38	3.40

*Summary of 15 experiments conducted with ensiled corn in Iowa, Illinois, and Indiana.

†Summary of six experiments in which the high-moisture corn was mixed with supplement to form a complete feed.

‡Feed efficiency data calculated with both diets on an equal moisture basis.

Antibiotics

There is clear evidence that the rate of gain and feed efficiency are improved when subtherapeutic antibiotics are added to swine diets. The gain response is consistently greater than the improvement in feed efficiency. Both responses are greatest in the starter period and least in the finishing period. There appears to be little value in rotating antibiotics (i.e., changing the antibiotic used frequently) during the growth period. The notion that once started, antibiotic feeding must continue until marketing, is false. Deletion of antibiotics at any point in growth will depress performance only to the performance level of pigs that had never received antibiotics.

Use of antibiotics in feed is carefully regulated, and the reader is referred to the *Feed Additive Compendium** for a detailed discussion of usage levels and withdrawal periods.

---

*Feed Additive Compendium. Minneapolis, Minn.: Miller Publishing Co., 1980.

References

1. Jensen, A. H.: Dietary nutrient allowances for swine. Feedstuffs 51:29:41, 1979.
2. Lynch, P. B.: Environment and the breeding sow. Moorepark Pig Farming Conference. Dublin, Ireland: An Foras Taluntais. 1978, p. 18.
3. Miller, E. R.: Biological availability of iron in iron supplements. Feedstuffs 50:35, 1978.
4. Tanksley, T. D., Jr., and Baker, D. H.: Protein and amino acids for swine. Pork Industry Handbook, Bull. No. 5. Cooperative Extension Service, Urbana, Ill., University of Illinois, 1977.
5. Ullrey, D. E.: Selenium deficiency in swine production. Feedstuffs 45:47:30, 1973.

Deficiencies of Mineral Nutrients

JAMES T. BAXTER, M.A., Ph.D., F.I.Biol., M.R.C.V.S.

Certain minerals are known to be essential for the good health, production, and reproduction of farm animals, and in practical situations their deficiency results in disease and depressed productivity. In the case of some other elements, deficiency diseases have only been induced experimentally and not necessarily even in food-producing animals. As husbandry systems become more intensive and the raw stuff of rations is altered to cut costs, deficiencies produced only experimentally at present may be diagnosed in practice in due course. For example, unidentified deficiencies of potassium or sulfur may already be occurring in some circumstances. In this article, however, the discussion will be confined to the deficiencies that are currently recognized in practical animal production.

Throughout the world, mineral deficiencies in livestock cause considerable financial losses, which are best appreciated when clinical signs are present. They are usually underestimated when milk or subclinical deficiency occurs. The latter invariably causes depression of growth and weight gain in young and fattening animals and, frequently, suboptimal fecundity and milk production in adults. Depending on the animals' functional state and the amount of mineral available, the effects of the deficiency may be transient, periodical, or persistent, severe, and progressive. Young stock and lactating animals have especially high requirements for minerals and are the most susceptible to deficiency. Breed variations in mineral metabolism and susceptibility to deficiency occur, and infectious and other diseases also increase the animals' requirements.

More than one mineral may be deficient at a time in a herd, and deficiencies may be simple or conditioned. In the former, the mineral is simply lacking in the diet, whereas in conditioned deficiency, although analysis may reveal the presence of the mineral in normal amounts, some other dietary factor inhibits its availability to the animal. Mineral interactions such as those of excessive calcium on zinc and iron and of excessive molybdenum and sulfur on copper are of this nature.

CALCIUM AND PHOSPHORUS DEFICIENCIES

Dietary calcium (Ca) and phosphorus (P) deficiencies and imbalances depress production and cause skeletal and dental defects in ruminants and pigs.

Occurrence and Etiology

Acute clinical disturbances of calcium, phosphorus, and magnesium metabolism are discussed elsewhere. This section deals with the depressed production and skeletal defects that are associated with dietary deficiency or imbalance of calcium and phosphorus and in which vitamin D is also frequently involved.

Herbage of low phosphorus content is widespread in dry tropical countries and elsewhere in areas of blanket bog and rain-leached hills. In temperate areas, dry mature unimproved pasture is low in phosphorus, and even improved pasture can become sporadically phosphorus deficient, especially during periods of drought. This causes unexpected problems in dairy cows and, less often, in sheep. Sheep grazing green cereals may become phosphorus deficient.

Although calcium deficiency is less likely than phosphorus deficiency in grazing animals, a conditioned or simple calcium deficiency can occur in pigs, intensively managed cattle, high-yielding dairy cows, and yard-fed sheep on a predominantly cereal diet rich in phosphorus and low in calcium and vitamin D. The deficiencies especially occur in rapidly growing and lactating animals. As well as the classical deficiency syndromes, there is considerable depression of fecundity, growth rate, weight gain, and feed conversion efficiency. The skeletal changes result from inadequate mineralization of bone, as in rickets, or excessive demineralization, as in the osteomalacia syndrome.

Rickets

Clinical Signs. In young growing animals, the epiphyses, especially of the long bones, and the costochondral junctions (rachitic rosary) become enlarged and painful. The animal is stiff, the forelegs become bowed or knock-kneed, and the back becomes arched. Teeth are mottled and poorly calcified, and their eruption is delayed. Appetite, growth rate, body condition, and feed utilization are all poor.

Clinical Pathology. Serum alkaline phosphatase values are elevated. Serum calcium and phosphorus levels are little affected.

Diagnosis. The appropriate clinical picture in young animals and response to treatment are strongly indicative of rickets, but definitive diagnosis requires analytical evidence of deficiency or imbalance in dietary calcium, phosphorus, or vitamin D. In normal bone, the ratio of ash:organic matter is 3:2, and in rickets it is 1:2 or even 1:3 in very severe cases. The differential diagnosis includes protein deficiency and all forms of arthritis in young animals and, in calves, copper deficiency and epiphysitis also. In chronic fluorosis, lesions occur in the permanent dentition.

Osteomalacia

Clinical Signs. In phosphorus-deficient areas, osteomalacia can affect grazing adult cattle, then sheep, and, rarely, goats. Pregnant and lactating animals are at greatest risk. In housed animals it results from calcium-deficient diets, and sows, after rearing a litter, may have excessive bone resorption. In some cases, the calcium deficiency is secondary, being induced by excessive dietary phosphorus.

In grazing cattle, poor milk yield, reduced appetite, and poor weight gains or loss of condition progress to pica, the "classic" sign of aphosphorosis. Other signs include lowered fertility, stiff and creaking joints, shifting lameness (e.g., milk lameness), and lengthening periods of recumbency. Fractures occur easily, especially of the hips (knocked-down hip) and ribs.

Clinical Pathology. In severe cases, serum alkaline phosphatase levels are elevated and in ruminants serum inorganic phosphate falls from the normal 1.3 to 1.6 mmol/L to 0.48 to 1.13 mmol/L. If ingestion of excessive phosphorus is the cause, serum phosphorus values are elevated. Radiologic examination reveals osteoporosis.

Diagnosis. The epidemiology, clinical picture, pathology, and response to treatment give good guidance. Definitive diagnosis is made on analysis of the diet and comparison with the recommended allowances for the class of animal affected. Cobalt deficiency and chronic fluorosis should be excluded.

Other Conditions

Other clinical conditions associated with abnormal calcium, phosphorus, and vitamin D nutrition include osteodystrophia fibrosa, recognized as calcium deficiency in pigs; degenerative joint disease of cattle; "bowie", a phosphorus-deficiency osteoporosis of young lambs on unimproved pasture in New Zealand; and a possibly similar condition, "double scalp" of Scottish hill sheep, in which softening of the frontal bones occurs. Calcium-deficient, phosphorus-excessive diets predispose to urolithiasis in sheep.

Treatment and Prevention

These depend on feeding sufficient calcium and phosphorus in the correct ratio. Vitamin D is also essential, and in minor Ca:P imbalances adequate vitamin D may rectify the problem. Severe structural changes are difficult to correct, but the other features of deficiency respond well to treatment. In calcium deficiency, any excess of dietary phosphorus should be reduced. When restoring the calcium intake, excess should be avoided, as this can induce deficiency of copper, magnesium, manganese, and zinc. Grazing cattle should have access to mineral mixes containing calcium (as powdered limestone), and dairy cows should have this in addition to the calcium incorporated in the ration. Also, where phosphorus is deficient, free-access salt mixes containing dicalcium or disodium phosphate 50:50 with common salt are indicated. Phosphorus can also be incorporated into the rations. Where it is economically feasible, top-dressing pasture with super-phosphate is indicated.

The requirements for calcium and phosphorus vary considerably depending on the species, breed, age, sex, and reproductive and lactating status of the animals. For details of the amounts to be fed, the relevant publications of the U.K. Agricultural Research Council and the U.S. National Academy of Sciences should be consulted (see Supplemental Reading).

COBALT DEFICIENCY

Cobalt (Co) deficiency causes depressed appetite and wasting in ruminants.

Occurrence and Etiology

Cobalt deficiency is important in many parts of the world and mainly affects ruminants grazing pasture of low cobalt content. Sheep are more susceptible than cattle and young stock more than adults, the most susceptible being recently weaned lambs. Goats are also affected. In certain circumstances, pigs may have cobalt-responsive conditions.

Soils of low cobalt status, high pH, and high manganese status produce cobalt-deficient pasture. When poor wet land is improved by draining, liming, and reseeding, the herbage uptake of cobalt is reduced. Herbage containing less than 0.11 mg Co/kg DM induces cobalt deficiency in grazing lambs and calves, and less than 0.07 mg/kg and 0.05 mg/kg DM causes deficiency in adult sheep and cattle, respectively. Feeds grown in cobalt-deficient areas or diets rich in sulfur can cause deficiency.

Pathogenesis

In adults, cobalt is the essential substrate for the formation of vitamin B_{12} by rumen microflora. Insufficient dietary cobalt causes vitamin B_{12} deficiency, which leads to a failure of enzyme systems including that which metabolizes propionate via methylmalonyl co-enzyme A to succinate.

Clinical Signs

There is no single characteristic sign, but loss of appetite is important. On farms where the lambs' growth rate is depressed, ewes and calves may be apparently unaffected. These mild and subclinical forms are more common than severe deficiency and are economically important. Severe deficiency causes inappetence, poor growth, weight loss, pale mucous membranes, lassitude, dyspnea, reduced fertility, increased neonatal mortality, depressed milk yields, and pica. Muscle wasting progresses to emaciation, and resistance to other diseases is reduced. In sheep, the fleece grows slowly and is poor and brittle. Profuse lacrimation stains the face. Cattle also have poor rough coats, with some loss of color. Depending on the animal's age and cobalt intake and reserves, the disease may run a course of from several weeks to over six months before death supervenes.

Autopsy Findings

Pathognomonic lesions are absent, but emaciation, bone marrow hypoplasia, and hemosiderin deposits in the spleen and liver are present.

Clinical Pathology

The levels of vitamin B_{12} and cobalt are depressed in the liver, blood, and ruminal contents. Over 0.19 μg vitamin B_{12}/g fresh (wet) liver is normal, and severe deficiency is present below 0.11 μg/g. Normal serum vitamin B_{12} levels are from 1.0 to 3.0 μg/L, levels below 0.8 μg/L indicating deficiency and clinical signs appearing at 0.2 μg/L. Normocytic normochromic anemia occurs. Plasma glucose, alkaline phosphatase, ascorbic acid, and thiamine levels are low, and aspartate aminotransferase and pyruvate levels are high.

In ruminants, abnormally high urinary concentrations of methylmalonic acid (MMA) occur owing to failure of propionate metabolism. Even in the early stages of vitamin B_{12} deficiency, formiminoglutamic acid (FIGLU) appears in the urine if the sheep is losing weight.

Diagnosis

Diagnosis takes into account causes of poor growth, loss of condition, and anemia and includes deficiencies of dietary energy, protein, copper, and selenium and parasitic gastro-enteritis, fascioliasis, Johne's disease, and chronic respiratory disease. In the field, improved appetite and weight gain following test therapy of part of the group with cobalt or vitamin B_{12} are regarded as diagnostic. Definitive diagnosis is made based on the low levels of vitamin B_{12} in serum or liver biopsy samples.

Urinary MMA and FIGLU can be assayed. Urinary FIGLU levels are inversely related to serum B_{12} levels and indicate the severity of the cobalt deficiency. The cobalt content of soil and herbage can also be estimated.

Treatment

The aim is to restore the animals' vitamin B_{12} status to normal by administering cobalt salts orally or B_{12} parenterally. Vitamin B_{12} *per os* is also effective but uneconomical, and cobalt salts parenterally are of little use. Injections of vitamin B_{12}, 100 and 300 μg for lambs and adult sheep, respectively, are repeated once weekly. Frequent oral dosing with cobalt is not generally adopted, but sheep require 1.0 mg cobalt daily and once weekly oral dosing with 7.0 mg is effective; oral dosing once a month with

300 mg cobalt produces only suboptimal growth. Cattle require ten times the dose of sheep. To supply 1.0 mg cobalt, it is necessary to give 5.0 mg cobalt chloride or cobalt sulfate dissolved in water.

Response to treatment is rapid. Serum vitamin B_{12} levels rise in 24 hours, the appetite returns in a few days, and bodily condition is seen to improve within a fortnight. The anemia responds more slowly. Cobalt treatment of pregnant and lactating mothers benefits the offspring, as it crosses the placenta and also enters the colostrum and milk as vitamin B_{12}.

Prevention

Stock require an adequate continuous supply of cobalt. The main preventive methods are dosing with cobalt bullets, applying cobaltized fertilizers to the land, providing cobalt-enriched salt licks (1 g Co/kg of lick), incorporating cobalt in the concentrate part of the rations (2 mg Co/kg DM), and supplying it in the drinking water.

Proprietary "bullets" containing cobalt oxide are given orally to cattle and sheep of ruminating age. The bullet lodges in the reticulum, releasing cobalt for months. Treatment is repeated every six months for cattle. The bullets may be effective for up to three years in sheep. As some bullets are lost by regurgitation, animals thriving less well than others should be redosed.

Cobalt-deficient grazings can be top-dressed with 2 to 3 kg hydrated cobalt sulfate/hectare. This should last for three or four years. Inaccessible areas can be treated from the air. The top-dressing need only be applied to a number of scattered plots onto which the stock are regularly and frequently herded. With soils of high pH and high manganese content, the use of cobaltized fertilizer is unreliable. Foliar application of cobalt sulfate or chloride, 15 g/ha, gives grazing stock immediate protection.

Water-degradable cobalt compound tablets yield an automatically regulated concentration of cobalt in the water troughs. Alternatively, metered quantities, e.g., 0.2 to 0.4 mg Co/L water, may be provided. These methods are not yet widely used. Their effectiveness depends on other water supplies not being available to the stock.

COPPER DEFICIENCY

Copper (Cu) deficiency occurs in ruminants and, occasionally, in pigs. It depresses production and causes coat and skeletal changes, diarrhea, and anemia. The offspring of copper-deficient dams may have central nervous system abnormalities.

Occurrence and Etiology

Copper deficiency occurs worldwide, and both subclinical and clinical forms are economically important. It can be primary or induced (the latter is discussed elsewhere). Primary deficiency occurs in stock grazing copper-deficient pasture growing on copper-deficient soil. Herbage containing less than 3.0 mg Cu/k DM causes clinical hypocuprosis and, at 3.0 to 5.0 mg/kg, hypocupremia, usually subclinical, occurs. Young animals are more susceptible than adults, and cattle are more susceptible than sheep. The requirements of calves, lambs, adult sheep, beef cattle and lactating cows, and pregnant cows are met by 1.2, 1.0 to 5.0, 5.0 to 9.0, 8.0 to 15.0, and 13.0 to 20 mg Cu/kg dietary DM, respectively. For pigs, 4.0 to 6.0 mg Cu/kg suffices.

Clinical Signs

Most of the signs reflect impaired tissue oxidation due to malfunctioning copper-related enzyme systems. Where clinical hypocuprosis occurs, subclinical deficiency usually exists in neighboring stock.

Cattle. Calves a few weeks old can be affected, but usually three or four months on a deficient diet are needed before signs appear. The coat is harsh, becoming yellow on red cattle and rusty brown on black cattle; this hypochromotrichia causes a "bespectacled" appearance. Poor growth, poor condition, intermittent diarrhea, and subestrus occur. In severe hypocuprosis, anemia eventually develops. After weeks or months, untreated animals become emaciated and die.

Calves pastured with suckler cows, which often remain clinically normal, may also develop skeletal changes such as hard epiphyseal swellings, bowed legs, and arched back. The calves walk on their toes owing to flexor tendon contraction. In Australia, acute heart failure in severely copper-deficient adult cattle causes "falling disease."

Sheep. Slow growth and, less commonly, anemia and diarrhea, occur. Economically important fleece abnormalities are reported. Severely deficient sheep become emaciated and die. Copper-deficient, but apparently healthy, pregnant ewes of any breed, age, and parity may give birth to swayback (enzootic ataxia) lambs. Up to half the flock may be affected, and it may be neonatal or delayed. In the commoner neonatal form, some lambs are born dead or die within a few days. Animals less severely affected have a staggering gait with swaying of the hindquarters and either become recumbent or recover. The delayed form first appears when the lambs are several weeks old, and they are likely to survive although are variably ataxic. Neonatal ataxia of kid goats, and, rarely, of calves also occurs.

Pigs. Copper-responsive anemia has been reported in young growing pigs, but practical diets usually contain enough copper to prevent deficiency.

Clinical Pathology

In normal adult cattle and neonatal calves, the liver contains 1.55 to 3.15 and 3.15 to 9.40 mmol Cu/kg DM, respectively. Clinically affected adults, yearlings, and calves have below 0.16, 0.32, and 0.79 mmol Cu/kg, respectively. Adult sheep normally have 0.8 to 9.4 mmol Cu/kg liver DM, are deficient at 0.32 to 0.47, and at levels below 0.24 mmol/kg are likely to produce swayback lambs. Swayback lambs and kids have 0.065 to 0.24 mmol Cu/kg liver DM.

In normal cattle and sheep, blood copper is 9.0 to 26.0 μmol/L. Levels below 9.0 indicate hypocupremia with subclinical effects, and clinical signs appear at 3.0 to 4.5 μmol/L. Anemia, when present, is hypochromic macrocytic in ewes and cattle and microcytic in lambs.

In pigs, normal blood copper is 10.0 to 29.0 μmol/L. Anemia develops below 3.0 μmol/L.

Autopsy Findings

Emaciation and, in young animals, osteoporosis are present, and calves may have epiphyseal enlargements. Some swayback cases have visible cerebral cavitation; microscopically, all have local absence of myelin and neuronal necrosis in the brain and spinal cord and degeneration of spinal nerve fibers. In "falling disease," venous congestion, a flabby fibrotic heart, and hemosiderosis are present.

Diagnosis

Diagnosis encompasses the history, clinical signs, and response to copper therapy confirmed by assay of blood and liver copper. Cytochrome oxidase activity (normal: over 7.0 μmol/g wet liver) and ceruloplasmin levels correlate directly with plasma copper levels and are easier to estimate. Estimating copper in the diet, pasture, and soil helps to establish the source of the deficiency.

Differential diagnosis of wasting includes parasitic gastro-enteritis, chronic fascioliasis and salmonellosis, and Johne's disease. The skeletal deformities should be distinguished from those caused by deficiency or imbalance of calcium, phosphorus, and vitamin D. Enzootic ataxia is differentiated from cerebellar agenesis, spinal abscesses, other CNS infections, white muscle disease, and tick bite pyemia. Histopathologic and microbiologic examinations are indicated.

Treatment

The oral administration of aqueous solutions containing 4.0 g copper sulfate to cattle and 1.5 g to adult sheep, repeated weekly, or the injection of copper preparations parenterally provides the copper immediately needed. Generally, response to treatment is good, but severe skeletal, nervous, and circulatory system lesions are irreversible.

Prevention

Choice of method depends on the number of animals, the terrain, the system of management, and costs.

1. Deficient pasture can be sprayed with copper salts or fertilized with copperized superphosphate. Except on badly leached and calcareous soils, one application of copper sulfate, 5 to 7 kg/ha, is sufficient for one to four years.

2. Salt licks can be used, providing 0.5 per cent copper sulfate (1.25 g Cu/kg salt) for cattle and sheep or up to 2 per cent copper sulfate (5.0 g Cu/kg) for cattle only. In Great Britain, the addition of copper to mineral licks or mixes for sheep requires a veterinary prescription.

3. The concentrate ration can be enriched with copper sulfate. In Great Britain, if copper in cattle feeds exceeds 50 mg/kg it must be declared.

4. Proprietary copper-containing tablets are available that, when placed in water troughs, maintain a constant concentration of the mineral. This is for cattle only.

5. Although proprietary copper-organic compound injections require individual handling of stock, they are convenient, permit accurate dosing, and ensure that every animal is treated. They provide a body store of copper for three to six months. Depending on the formulation, the dose is from 60 to 240 mg copper adult cattle and 15 to 50 mg copper for adult sheep and calves under ten weeks old. The manufacturer's recommendations about quantity, route, and frequency of treatment must be followed. Inflammatory reactions may occur at subcutaneous sites. If given intramuscularly, precautions against blackleg may be necessary. Because of toxicity risks, copper injections should not be given to animals receiving other copper supplements or to sheep with severe fascioliasis. Any regulations about withholding periods should be observed.

6. Recently, gelatin capsules containing 4 g cupric oxide needles have become available. They are administered orally, by balling gun, to ewes. They pass to the abomasum to provide copper over a period of some weeks.

To prevent swayback in lambs, their mothers are individually treated in early to mid-pregnancy orally with cupric oxide capsules or by parenteral injection with copper compound. In delayed swayback, all lambs in the flock receive 20 to 35 mg copper sulfate in water, orally, every three or four weeks until weaning. Only some of the parenteral injections of copper are safe for lambs. Where calves to be born in spring are at risk of hypocuprosis because of their mothers' hypocupremia and the low copper status of pasture, the cows should be injected with copper late in pregnancy. Sufficient copper passes to the fetus to protect it post-natally for most of the summer grazing period. Alternatively, injecting the calves when two months old protects them for the next four to five months.

IODINE DEFICIENCY

Iodine (I) deficiency results in hypothyroidism and goiter, especially affecting the unborn and neonatal offspring of deficient cows, ewes, goats, and sows.

Occurrence and Etiology

Although primary (simple) iodine deficiency occurs widely and results from ingesting crops, pasture, and water derived from iodine-deficient soils, it is generally well controlled. Conditioned iodine deficiency results from ingesting excess calcium or high levels of goitrogens in, for example, brassicas. Insufficiency of iodine reduces thyroid hormonogenesis, and the adenohypophysis responds by producing thyrotropic hormone. Goiter results.

Clinical Signs

Iodine-deficient cows have depressed reproductive function, including anovulatory estrus. Pregnant ruminants and sows may resorb their fetuses, abort, or produce stillborn or poorly viable offspring. Affected neonatal animals have complete or partial alopecia, piglets have some myxedema, lambs and calves may have patently enlarged thyroids, and death is common. Newborn animals that are less severely affected have dry skin and sparse coats. In growing pigs, a depression of weight gain that responds to iodine has been reported.

Clinical Pathology and Autopsy Findings

In adult ruminants, the normal range of serum protein bound iodine (PBI) is 190 to 320 nmol/L or more, and serum thyroxine (T_4) values range from 20 to 120 nmol/L. Lower circulating levels of thyroid hormones indicate either low iodine intake or other cause of dyshormonogenesis. Autopsy reveals enlarged thyroid glands and poor epiphyseal ossification. Normal fresh thyroids weight 6.5 to 11 g in full-term calves, over 13 g indicating goiter. Glands of normal lambs weigh 1.3 to 2.0 g, and 2.0 to 2.8 g suggests hypothyroidism, whereas greater weights are diagnostic. Normal thyroids of neonatal calves and lambs contain 15.6 to 39.0 mmol I/kg DM. The critical level is 9.5 mmol, and hyperplasia occurs at 7.9 mmol/kg DM.

Diagnosis

Diagnosis takes into account prolonged gestation, stillbirths, neonatal mortality, and alopecia; the size, weight, and iodine content of the thyroid; and the circulating thyroxine values. Assay of soil and pasture iodine is then indicated. Differential diagnosis includes goitrogen-induced hypothyroidism, the inherited defects of iodine metabolism recorded in ruminants, and causes of abortion, stillbirth, and perinatal mortality.

Treatment and Prevention

Iodine-deficient ewes are given 250 mg potassium iodide or 360 mg potassium iodate orally about 60 and 30 days pre-partum to protect their lambs. One ml poppyseed oil containing 40 per cent iodine, injected intramuscularly two months before lambing, is also effective and protects up to two crops of lambs against goiter. Supplementing concentrate feeds with iodine or providing free access to iodized salt licks reduces individual handling costs. Pregnant and lactating cows and ewes require 0.5 mg I/kg dietary DM, growing cattle need 0.25 mg/k, and other ruminants require 0.1 mg/kg. Four times as much is needed when goitrogenic diets are fed. Baby pigs and sows have higher iodine requirements than growers and finishers. Sows and growers receive 0.50 and 0.16 mg I/kg dietary DM, respectively, although much larger amounts are sometimes fed. For example, proprietary supplements contain sufficient iodine, when incorporated into the concentrate ration, to provide 1.0 to 10.0 mg I/kg. Free-access salt mixes containing 150 to 400 mg I/kg are also available, although 100 mg I/kg is adequate.

IRON DEFICIENCY

Nutritional iron (Fe) deficiency causes anemia and poor thriving in unweaned pigs.

Occurrence and Etiology

Baby pigs soon outgrow their iron reserves and the iron supplied by the sow's milk. At birth, the hemoglobin (Hb) level is 9.0 to 11.0 g/dl, falling to 4.0 to 5.0 g/dl by day 10. Hb deficiency causes reduced hemopoiesis and depressed oxygen transfer, and the iron-related enzyme systems become inefficient. Piglets on pasture or in dirty yards obtain sufficient iron from the environment, but unweaned pigs in very clean houses become iron deficient and do not eat enough creep feed in the first month of life to rectify this. Clinical signs start at seven to ten days and reach a peak at three weeks.

Clinical iron-deficiency anemia is uncommon in veal calves but occasionally follows errors in compounding the milk replacer.

Clinical Signs

Piglets and calves may have mild iron deficiency with asymptomatic anemia. Clinically affected pigs have pale skin and mucous membranes, reduced appetite, poor growth, lassitude, cardiac palpitations, dyspnea, slight diarrhea, and increased susceptibility to infections. A few develop subcutaneous edema, and some die. Survivors have hairy wrinkled skin. Spontaneous recovery ensues if they eat the sow's food. Clinically affected calves are lethargic and have poor appetites and weight gains.

Clinical Pathology and Autopsy Findings

When Hb levels are between 5.0 and 7.0 g/dl, the clinical effects may vary from very severe to poor appetite and depressed growth only. In animals with levels above 7.0 g/dl, the effects are marginal but iron responsive, whereas levels between 9.0 and 12.0 g/dl are normal. Iron-deficient piglets develop microcytic hypochromic anemia. When red cell counts (normal: 5.0 to 8.0 $\times$ 10^{12}/L) fall to 3.0 to 4.0 $\times$ 10^{12}/L or lower and Hb levels are 4.0 g/dl or less, deaths occur. Autopsy reveals pale edematous musculature, a flabby dilated heart, excessive fluid in the serous cavities, and a swollen mottled liver.

Diagnosis

Diagnosis is based on the clinical signs, hematology, response to iron therapy, and autopsy findings. Failure to respond to early iron therapy suggests infection or, less likely, copper deficiency. In differential diagnosis, enteric infections, isoimmune hemolytic disease, and eperythrozoonosis require consideration.

Treatment and Prevention

Earth put in the pen was a traditional source of iron for piglets. Another source is their mother's feces. Ten kg hydrated ferrous sulfate/tonne of sow feed (equivalent to 2 g Fe/kg) greatly increases the maternal fecal iron output. When piglets ingest the feces, they do not become anemic. More usually, individual piglets, at two to four days of age, are injected, deep in the thigh muscle, with 100 to 200 mg iron using one of the proprietary iron-polysaccharide complexes. This provides a three weeks' supply, and, where piglets also eat creep feeds containing 300 mg Fe/kg DM, clinical deficiency is usually avoided. The injection may be repeated in three weeks. Preparations for oral administration are also available. The very young progeny of selenium- or vitamin E–deficient sows may die within six hours following iron injection owing to hyperkalemia associated with severe coagulative myodegeneration.

When the milk substitute provides each veal calf with 30 to 40 mg iron and, later, 60 mg iron, daily, deficiency is prevented without increasing myoglobin levels sufficiently to darken muscle. Alternatively, 1.0 g iron as dextran or galactan can be given intramuscularly at one and six weeks of age.

Clinically evident anemia of calves and pigs is treated by deep intramuscular injection of 100 mg Fe/10 kg body weight, repeated at seven- to ten-day intervals.

MANGANESE DEFICIENCY

Manganese (Mn) deficiency occasionally causes impaired growth and reproduction in pigs. Levels considered to be adequate for growth in grazing ruminants have been associated with anestrus, subestrus, and reduced conception rates. Soil of low manganese status and high pH produces herbage low in manganese.

Diagnosis

There is no single specific diagnostic test for manganese-responsive infertility. More information is required about the diagnostic value of manganese levels in blood, hair, or fleece. Before the diagnosis is made, other causes of functional and infectious infertility should be excluded. Improved fecundity or weight gain following manganese supplementation of practical diets is diagnostically suggestive.

Treatment and Prevention

The recommended dietary allowance for cattle and sheep is 40 mg Mn/kg total diet. When manganese is incorporated into the concentrate part of the ration, 50 to 150 mg Mn/kg is adequate, even when dietary calcium and phosphorus levels are high. Alternatively, dairy cattle can be given free access to mineral mixtures containing up to 6.0 g Mn/kg salt. Pigs receive 20 mg MN/kg diet. These allowances are, as usual, greater than the estimated requirements to ensure that sufficient manganese is provided. Nonetheless, it has been suggested that pasture with less than 80 mg Mn/kg DM does not sustain optimum fertility in cattle.

SELENIUM DEFICIENCY

Insufficient dietary selenium (Se), sometimes with concurrent vitamin E deficiency and/or excessive polyunsaturated fatty acids, causes various syndromes, of which the best known in ruminants is nutritional myopathy or muscular dystrophy (NMD). However, in some parts of the world there are other selenium-responsive conditions, which, although less specific, appear to be of greater economic importance, and these are considered in this section.

Occurrence and Etiology

Selenium deficiency affects ruminants on deficient pasture and animals fed on crops harvested from deficient soils. Such soils are widely distributed, and the pasture uptake of selenium is readily altered by weather and by management factors, including the use of excessive amounts of phosphate fertilizer. Diets, including pasture, containing 0.16 to 0.17 mg Se/kg DM are optimal, and levels of up to 0.39 mg Se/kg are satisfactory for sheep. Marginally deficient diets contain 0.03 to 0.05 mg Se/kg, the latter being regarded as the minimal safe level. Selenium-responsive disorders may occur, however, even at 0.05 to 0.08 mg/kg if conditioned by concurrent dietary vitamin E deficiency. Herbage with less than 0.03 mg Se/kg DM is likely to produce clinical signs. Selenium deficiency results in lack of the selenium-containing enzyme glutathione peroxidase, and protection against oxidative degradation of tissue is thus impaired.

Clinical Signs

Sheep. The most important effect of selenium deficiency, apart from NMD, is subclinical or clinical depression of growth and weight gain (ill thrift) in growing sheep. In some areas, young animals die. Occasionally, adults also die in these areas, but, more often, the ewes have sub-optimal wool yields and develop periodontal disease. It is not yet clear whether failure of embryonic implantation is part of the selenium deficiency syndrome.

Cattle. Selenium deficiency is one cause of retained placenta, and it may be involved in the "downer cow" syndrome. It is associated with ill thrift and infertility in cattle; the birth of premature, weak, or dead calves; and sudden death syndrome in milk-fed calves up to four months of age. In the last-mentioned group, microscopic areas of peracute myocardial degeneration are found. Other young animals in the same herds have subclinical selenium deficiency. Increased susceptibility to infectious diseases, e.g., calf pneumonia, has been suggested.

Pigs. Neonatal losses, responsive to selenium administered to preparturient sows, occur in some piggeries. Hepatosis dietetica and mulberry heart disease (MHD) affect pigs from one month of age onward, some or all of the pigs in a litter exhibiting an acute but ill-defined afebrile fatal illness with inappetence, weakness, and recumbency. In animals with MHD, dyspnea, tachycardia, and cyanosis also occur.

Clinical Pathology

The normal values of selenium in whole blood are above 1.26, 0.63, and 0.60 μmol/L for sheep, cattle, and pigs, respectively, and for calves it is 1.14 μmol/L. In sheep, cattle, and pigs, values of 0.60, 0.40, and 0.20 μmol/L, respectively, indicate deficiency. Intermediate values are associated with suboptimal production, which responds to selenium. The values of erythrocyte glutathione peroxidase (GSH-Px) closely parallel those of selenium, and in selenium deficiency GSH-Px values decline. Liver and kidney cortex selenium values below 4.0 and 40.0 μmol/kg DM, respectively, in sheep and below 3.0 and 30.0 μmol/kg DM, respectively, in calves indicate deficiency. Pigs with hepatosis dietetica have less than 3.0 μmol Se/kg liver DM.

In hepatosis dietetica and MHD, the serum levels of the liver-specific enzyme ornithine carbamyl transferase, the muscle-specific enzyme creatinine phosphokinase, respectively, and of alanine and aspartate aminotransferase are elevated.

Autopsy Findings

Lambs and calves that die of the selenium-responsive disorders discussed here show emaciation, osteoporosis, and ceroid pigmentation of remaining fat, except that calves dying of peracute myocardial degeneration have not lost condition. In porcine MHD, there is extensive, severe myocardial hemorrhage, and in hepatosis dietetica the liver is enlarged and has necrotic foci. In both conditions, there may be some skeletal muscle degeneration, subcutaneous edema, and gastric ulceration.

Diagnosis

Diagnosis includes the clinical, biochemical, and post mortem findings and knowledge of the environment and diet. A presumptive diagnosis is made when selenium administration improves health and growth in young animals and the fecundity of adults. Definitive diagnosis is based on the selenium content of blood and, at autopsy, the liver and renal cortex. In ruminants, erythrocyte GSH-Px levels give the best guide to selenium status, but, as methods vary between laboratories, the results should be interpreted locally.

Differential diagnosis in young ruminants excludes other nutritional deficiencies, parasitic gastro-enteritis, and, in sudden death in calves, hypomagnesemic tetany; in ewes, other forms of infertility and chronic disorders depressing fleece growth; in cows, other causes of retained placenta; and in pigs, other causes of neonatal mortality and sudden death in growing pigs.

Treatment and Prevention

Proprietary preparations for parenteral or oral administration usually contain sodium selenite or sodium, potassium, or barium selenate. The doses stated here are of elemental selenium, and care should be taken because of the risk of toxicity. In very severely deficient areas, ewes are given 5 mg selenium parenterally or orally before mating, in mid-pregnancy, and three weeks before lambing, and the lambs receive 1 mg selenium at docking and 2 mg at weaning, repeated two and four months later. Less suffices in milder deficiency. Cattle receive 3 mg Se/45 kg body weight, repeated in three to four months as necessary. Selenium passes the placental barrier and also enters the milk.

Where selenium-deficient grains are fed, injecting sows with 1.5 mg Se/25 kg body weight at two- to four-week intervals increases the percentage of viable piglets born. When any pigs in a group have MHD or hepatosis dietetica, all should be treated with selenium–vitamin E injections. In all of these procedures the preparations used supply selenium for a few weeks after administration. Other preparations slowly release their selenium to the animal. For example, a proprietary barium selenate, containing 50 mg elemental Se/ml of injection, is given, subcutaneously only, as 1 ml of injection/50 kg body weight to adult cattle and sheep to create a depot that provides up to one year's supply of selenium. Another method consists of the oral administration to cattle and sheep of ruminating age of selenium-containing pellets, which lie in the ruminoreticulum, slowly releasing their selenium. Although sheep may retain the pellet for up to three years, it is considered that satisfactory health and body selenium levels are maintained for only a year or so. In some countries, subcutaneous implants containing slow-release selenium (45 mg selenium for ewes in mid-pregnancy, 15 mg selenium for newborn calves) are marketed.

When animals are treated individually, the veterinarian must advise his client about any statutory withholding period in respect of milk or of the animal itself if it is intended for human consumption. The regulations differ from country to country.

Selenium is also made available to livestock in free-access mineral mixes. In Great Britain, these mixes contain 2.5 to 8.0 mg Se/kg salt for ruminants. Higher concentrations, up to 20 and 30 mg/kg salt for cattle and sheep, respectively, are used elsewhere. Selenium can also be incorporated into the feed, the practical requirements of beef and dairy cattle being met by 0.05 and 0.1 mg Se/kg diet, respectively. In the U.S. and Great Britain, pigs get 0.1 mg selenium added/kg feed, and 0.15 mg/kg feed is permitted in New Zealand.

Proprietary pellets, available for immersion in the water of drinking troughs, are formulated to release selenium slowly to maintain a constant concentration. An alternative is the metered addition of selenium to the water. All of these methods are being continually re-assessed and refined.

Top-dressing of pasture with selenium is costly and potentially dangerous, and other methods of control are preferable. Selenium salts have been applied in phosphatic fertilizers. In New Zealand, the maximum permitted rate of application is 10 g Se/ha, and this prevents deficiency in grazing stock for one year.

SODIUM CHLORIDE DEFICIENCY

Sodium (Na) and chloride (Cl) are essential for body function. The diet usually supplies sufficient chlorine, but sodium deficiency can occur.

Occurrence and Etiology

In the tropics, cattle often show sodium deficiency, resulting from the loss of much sodium in sweat and from the grazing of stock on dry tropical pasture of low sodium status. In temperate zones sodium deficiency affects dairy cows, usually subclinically, on leys highly fertilized with potash (K), as sodium uptake by herbage is depressed by potash. Contributory factors include the sodium secreted in milk, insufficient sodium chloride in the concentrate ration, and lack of salt licks. It can affect other ruminants, especially rapidly growing young animals and pigs on cereal and vegetable diets, as these are relatively poor sodium sources.

Clinical Signs

Even subclinically deficient cows produce less milk than expected. Pica, including urine drinking after some weeks of deficiency, occurs. Ruminants and pigs, after a further period of very severe deficiency, have marked depression of activity, appetite, growth, and feed utilization, and they lose body weight.

Clinical Pathology

Bovine plasma sodium ranges from 135.0 to 150.0 mmol/L, with lower levels in severe deficiency. Both the parotid saliva and the urine contain less sodium and more potassium than normal.

Diagnosis

The animals' rapid improvement in appetite, production, and general health when enough sodium is provided gives the best practical diagnosis, as hyponatremia is measurable in very severe cases only. Food and water supplies can have their sodium content assayed. The pica should not be ascribed to aphosphorosis.

Treatment and Prevention

Grazing stock should have free access to common salt licks. Spraying salt solutions (16 kg NaCl/ha) on pasture is done less often. Common salt can be incorporated in the feed at the following rates: lactating cows and all pigs, 5 g NaCl/kg concentrate DM; nonlactating cattle, 2.5 g NaCl/kg feed DM; feedlot sheep, 5 g NaCl/kg complete ration or 10 g/kg concentrate diet. The water supply should be adequate, and salt should not be added to it.

ZINC DEFICIENCY

Zinc (Zn) deficiency causes depression of productivity and parakeratosis of pigs and, less frequently, of ruminants.

Occurrence and Etiology

Primary zinc deficiency occurs in pigs on rations containing less than 40 mg Zn/kg DM, especially when the diet is dry and on free access. Conditioned zinc deficiency stems from diets with excessive calcium (over 7 g/kg DM for growers). Subsidiary conditioning factors are proteins of vegetable origin, deficiency of unsaturated fatty acids, and high levels of copper. Fatalities are rare, and unprofitability results from poor feed conversion and growth rates.

Zinc deficiency is occasionally recognized in ruminants. In some parts of the world, grazing sheep may have suboptimal intake during mating and pregnancy. Sometimes the pastures grazed appear to have adequate zinc (over 40 mg/kg pasture DM), and the presence of conditioning factors has not always been established. Sheep kept in yards on conserved herbage and concentrates grown on deficient soil are at risk of becoming deficient. Malabsorption of zinc occurs in an inherited disease of calves.

Clinical Signs

Zinc deficiency ranges from subclinical to severe. Mild cases have reduced appetite, suboptimal weight gains, and poor feed utilization. Fertility may be subnormal in ruminants. Severe cases thrive badly and develop parakeratosis of the lower parts of the legs, within the thighs, and on the scrotum and face. In ruminants, the leg joints may swell and excessive salivation occurs; young animals are worse affected than adults.

Pigs. The belly, hams, and back are also affected. The lesions progress in two or three weeks from small red spots, through papules, to large dry patches with fissured crusts several millimeters deep. Mild diarrhea often occurs. Subclinical zinc deficiency in gilts has been associated with small litters, the individual piglets of which have low birth weights.

Cattle. Calves become rough coated. The affected skin is thick and wrinkled and may be painfully fissured. On cows, the lesions usually involve the udder; milk yield is depressed. Low zinc status is suspected to predispose to bovine infectious pododermatitis. A zinc-responsive subclinical depression of productivity occurs in feedlot cattle.

Sheep. The fleece loses its crimp and becomes thin, badly stained, and easily shed. The hooves soften and become distorted.

Clinical Pathology

Normal plasma zinc levels are 9.0 to 18.0 μmol/L in ruminants and in young pigs 9.0 μmol/L. At half the normal level, cattle show signs. On a very deficient diet the level falls to 3.0 to 4.5 μmol/L in seven to ten weeks. Serum albumin, alkaline phosphatase (a zinc metalloenzyme), and amylase levels decline, and serum globulin levels rise. Zinc-deficient piglets have a lymphocytopenia.

Diagnosis

The clinical findings, diet composition, and response to zinc therapy provide a diagnosis. Diagnostic reliability requires a series of low plasma zinc reading from animals in the group. Differential diagnosis in the pig includes sarcoptic mange, exudative epidermitis, and pityriasis rosea. In cattle it includes mange, other ectoparasitisms, ringworm, vitamin A deficiency, chronic seleniosis, mycotic dermatitis, photosensitization, and, also in sheep, contagious pustular dermatitis.

Treatment

In all species treatment consists of adding zinc to the diet, e.g., 200 g zinc carbonate/tonne of feed supplies about 100 mg Zn/kg diet. Alternatively, three-month-old calves and adult cattle can be given 0.5 g and 2.0 to 4.0 g zinc sulfate, respectively, in water *per os* once weekly. The calcium content of the diet should be corrected. Response to treatment is good, the appetite quickly improves, weight gains improve in a week or two, and the skin returns to normal in three to five weeks.

Prevention

When calcium is restricted to 5.0 g/kg DM, pig rations containing 50 to 60 mg Zn/kg DM give good results, although more may be needed when copper is used as a growth promotant. In the presence of a moderate excess of calcium, 100 mg Zn/kg is protective. Cattle and sheep are protected by providing free-access proprietary salt licks containing 2.5 to 5.0 g Zn/kg or by incorporating supplemental zinc into the diet at 50 mg/kg of total dietary DM. Pellets containing zinc can be given orally to ewes on zinc-deficient pasture, and a better lamb crop is obtained. In the rumen, the pellets liberate sufficient zinc to afford protection for six or seven weeks.

Supplemental Reading

Agricultural Research Council: The Nutrient Requirements of Ruminant Livestock. Farnham Royal, Commonwealth Agricultural Bureaux, 1980.

Agricultural Research Council: The Nutrient Requirements of Pigs. Farnham Royal, Commonwealth Agricultural Bureaux, 1981.

Blood, D. C., Radostits, O. M., and Henderson, J. A.: Veterinary Medicine, 6th ed. London, Bailliere Tindall, 1983.

National Research Council: Nutrient Requirements of Domestic Animals.
No. 2. Nutrient Requirements of Swine, 1979.
No. 3. Nutrient Requirements of Dairy Cattle, 1978.
No. 4. Nutrient Requirements of Beef Cattle, 1976.
No. 5. Nutrient Requirements of Sheep, 1975.
No. 15. Nutrient Requirements of Goats, 1981.
Washington, D.C., National Academy of Sciences.

Underwood, E.J.: The Mineral Nutrition of Livestock, 2nd ed. Farmham Royal, Commonwealth Agricultural Bureaux, 1981.

Vitamins in Food Animal Nutrition

ROBERT A. EASTER, Ph.D.

Vitamins are fundamental factors in cellular metabolism—the production losses that accompany deficiencies of individual vitamins are well-documented in the nutrition literature. Yet, vitamin deficiency diseases are often considered "unlikely" in the minds of many practitioners—and with good reason. Frank deficiencies are rare when properly fortified diets are used. Unexpected deficiencies do occur, however, and with some frequency in diets that would appear to be adequate. Mixing errors, loss of potency, poor availability, and a host of other factors can have severe economic consequences unless the feeder identifies the deficiency early and corrects the underlying problem in nutritional management.

On the other hand, vitamin therapy should not be viewed as a panacea for a host of real and imagined ills. Vitamins are required for specific, well-defined physiologic functions, and there is no improvement in these functions by exceeding the required amount. Megavitamin therapy should be avoided because it is economically wasteful and, more importantly, because it may actually be deleterious to the animal. For example, both vitamins A and D are lethal when fed at high levels for a prolonged period of time.

The vitamins are traditionally classified according to solubility characteristics, although the classification scheme is of limited value in practical nutrition. Vitamins A, D, E, and K are termed "fat-soluble" because of their solubility in organic solvents. The fat-soluble vitamins are stored in appreciable quantities in tissues. The B vitamins are water-soluble, as is vitamin C. Storage of B vitamins is limited in most species. The B vitamin numbering system—that is, B_1, B_2, B_6 and so on—is used extensively; however, there is a general trend to use the actual names—that is, thiamine, riboflavin, pyridoxine, and so on.

Although each vitamin may be present at the cellular level for normal metabolism, not all vitamins need be added to practical diets. Three factors are involved. First, some vitamins may be synthesized metabolically from dietary precursors to meet cellular needs. Second, some vitamins may be produced by the microflora of the digestive system in sufficient quantity. This is true for nonruminants as well as ruminants. Third, some vitamins are consistently provided in adequate amounts by the feedstuffs in the diet.

The clinical signs or visible indicators of vitamin deficiencies for the major food animal species have been summarized by the various committees of the National Research Council–National Academy of Sciences responsible for the development of nutrient requirements (Tables 1 and 2). Unfortunately, the clinically evident signs are rarely sufficient to establish a definitive diagnosis of a specific deficiency. The signs can be useful in the development of a presumptive diagnosis when considered in conjunction with other factors likely to precipitate a deficiency. Biochemical assessment of vitamin status in food animals generally follows the procedures outlined by Sauberlich and associates (1974) in *Laboratory Tests for the Assessment of Nutritional Status*.

CHARACTERISTICS AND FUNCTIONS OF THE VITAMINS

Fat-Soluble Vitamins

Vitamin A

The major source of vitamin A for most animals is β-carotene, though other carotenoids exhibit vitamin A activity. Carotene, often referred to as *provitamin A,* is either converted to vitamin A by mucosal enzymes or absorbed intact and converted to vitamin A by other tissue. Significant storage of vitamin A occurs principally in the liver, but there is some storage in adipose tissue as well. Because various carotenoids can contribute to the vitamin A nutrition of an animal, it is convenient to describe the nutritive value of feedstuffs in terms of International Units (I.U.) of vitamin A activity rather than as the amount of each of the carotenoids in the feed ingredient. Occasionally, United States Pharmacopeia units (U.S.P. units) are used in lieu of International Units. They are equal. One I.U. or U.S.P. unit has the activity of 0.300 microgram of crystalline retinol (vitamin A alcohol) or 0.344 and 0.550 microgram of vitamin A acetate and vitamin A palmitate, respectively. The conversion of carotene to vitamin A is 400 I.U. of A activity per mg of β-carotene for cattle and sheep. Swine derive 500 I.U. of A activity from 1 mg of β-carotene, whereas poultry obtain about 1560 I.U.

Vitamin A is absorbed as a lipid; thus, biliary obstruction or other pathologic conditions affecting lipid absorption will also affect vitamin A absorption.

Table 1. *Clinical Signs of Fat-Soluble Vitamin Deficiencies in Ruminant and Nonruminant Species*

Poultry*	Sheep†	Cattle‡	Swine§
Vitamin A			
Depressed weight gain	Keratinization of the respiratory, alimentary, reproductive, urinary, and ocular epithelia	Depressed feed intake and gains	Incoordination
Keratinization of epithelial tissue		Night blindness	Lordosis
Discharge from eye, lacrimation, and xerophthalmia		Muscular incoordination	Paralysis of rear limbs
		Staggering gait, convulsive seizures	Night blindness
		Excessive lacrimation, diarrhea	Congenital defects
		Impaired conception, birth defects	Atrophy of epithelial layers of genital tract
Vitamin C			
Not required by poultry	Not required by sheep	Not required by cattle	Not required by swine
Vitamin D			
Rickets	Rickets	Rickets	Rickets
Rubbery beak	Congenital malformations	Poor appetite	Osteomalacia
Beaded ribs		Locomotion difficulty	Low calcium tetany
Thin-shelled eggs		Weak, dead, or deformed calves	Rib and vertebra fracture (posterior paralysis)
Decreased egg production		Difficulty in breathing, irritability, weakness and occasionally tetany and convulsions	
Embryonic death			
Vitamin E (related to Se)			
Encephalomalacia (sudden prostration with head retraction)	White muscle disease characterized by stiffness in rear quarters	White muscle disease (muscular dystrophy) in calves characterized by heart failure and paralysis	Generalized edema, sudden death, liver necrosis, cardiac muscle degeneration, muscular dystrophy
Exudative diathesis	Muscles have white striations with bilateral lesions		
Muscular dystrophy			
Edema of heart and pericardium			
Myopathy			
Reproductive failure			
Vitamin K			
Delayed blood clotting, with subcutaneous, intramuscular, or intraperitoneal bleeding	No need for dietary supplementation has been established	Bleeding when fed moldy sweet clover rich in dicoumarol	Anemia, poor blood clotting, internal hemorrhage
			Pale newborn pigs with blood loss from umbilical cord

*Data from NRC No. 1, 1977.
†Data from NRC No. 5, 1975.
‡Data from NRC No. 4, 1970.
§Data from NRC No. 2, 1979.

The biochemical function of vitamin A in the visual cycle is well elucidated. Other functions are not clearly established; however, it is essential to bone development, maintenance of epithelial membranes, and proper functioning of the immune system. The loss of the integrity of membranes due to vitamin A deficiency establishes an opportune environment for pathogen invasion of the respiratory system. The deficiency is also consistently associated with reproductive failure. Excessive intake of vitamin A can lead to toxicosis, with bone failure and, in extreme cases, death.

The provitamin A content of feedstuffs declines rapidly in storage, and it is generally recommended that supplemental vitamin A be added to both ruminant and nonruminant diets. Pure vitamin A is subject to rapid oxidative loss and should not be used as a supplement to diets. Stabilized forms, such as vitamin A acetate and vitamin A palmitate, are acceptable substitutes. Vitamin A can be injected intramuscularly if dietary administration is impractical.

Vitamin D

Recent discoveries have greatly enhanced our understanding of the biochemical role of vitamin D in calcium metabolism. Beginning with either an irradiated plant sterol (ergocalciferol: vitamin D_2) or animal sterol (cholecalciferol: vitamin D_3), enzymes in the liver form 25-hydroxycholecalciferol (25-HCC). Subsequently, the 25-HCC is further hydroxylated to 1,25-dihydroxycholecalciferol (1,25-DHCC) by kidney tissue. This 1,25-DHCC, acting as a hormone at a mucosal receptor site, stimulates the synthesis of the calcium binding protein needed for the transport of calcium from the intestinal lumen into the cell. Vitamin D may have a role in metabolism of other mineral elements, particularly phosphorus.

Animals in environments that provide exposure to sunlight are able to form vitamin D by the natural process of irradiation of 7-dehydrocholesterol produced at the skin surface. When animals are housed in confinement with limited exposure to sunlight, it becomes necessary to provide vitamin D supplementation as either an injection or a dietary additive. Synthetic vitamin D is available as either D_2 (ergocalciferol) or D_3 (cholecalciferol). Swine can use both D_2 and D_3 effectively; poultry use D_3 well but use D_2 very poorly.

As with vitamin A, requirements for vitamin D are expressed in International Units. One International Unit of vitamin D is, by definition, the biologic activity of 0.025 μg of cholecalciferol.

Vitamin D is subject to perioxidative damage in feeds. Available data suggest that it is quite stable in the pure form. There is a loss of potency in both vitamin premixes and complete feeds that may be as much as 8 per cent per month.

Table 2. *Clinical Signs of B Vitamin Deficiencies in Swine and Poultry*

Vitamin	Swine*	Poultry†
Thiamine	Poor appetite and growth Sudden death Cardiac hypertrophy, bradycardia	Polyneuritis characterized early by lethargy and head tumors followed by retraction of the head over the back
Riboflavin	Slow growth, seborrhea Decreased conception and increased incidence of stillborn pigs with skeletal anomalies	Retarded growth and diarrhea Curled toe paralysis Decreased hatchability
Niacin	Anorexia with depressed growth Diarrhea and intestinal necrosis Hair loss and exfoliative dermatitis	"Black tongue" or inflammation of the tongue and mouth cavity Poor growth and feathering Perosis-like disorder in turkeys
Pantothenic acid	Poor appetite and growth Diarrhea and colonic inflammation Unusual gait (goose-stepping) Impaired reproduction	Poor growth and feathering Exudative eyelids Lesions at the corners of the mouth and on the feet Reduced hatchability and survival
Vitamin B_6	Poor growth Microcytic, hypochromic anemia Elevated urinary xanthurenic acid Seizures	Loss of appetite and poor growth Perosis Abormal behavior, constant cheeping, excitement, convulsions Reduced egg production and hatchability
Vitamin B_{12}	Decreased growth Reduced sow productivity	Reduced growth and egg hatchability High mortality in chicks from deficient dams Fatty heart, liver, and kidney may occur
Choline	Slow growth, fatty livers Poor conception rate and reduced litter size	Reduced growth rate Perosis
Biotin	Feet lesions Spasticity of hind legs	Dermatitis Feet lesions and mandibular lesions Reduced egg hatchability
Folacin	Poor growth and generalized weakness Normocytic anemia	Anemia Reduced egg production and hatchability Turkey poults are nervous and some exhibit cervical paralysis

*Data from NRC No. 2, 1979.
†Data from NRC No. 1, 1977.

Vitamin D–deficient growing animals develop rickets as a consequence of inadequate mineralization of bone. Mature animals may develop fractures due to demineralization of bone. Poultry are particularly sensitive to vitamin D deficiency because of the great demand for calcium used in the formation of egg shell.

Excessive vitamin D is toxic, characterized by calcification of soft tissue in the kidney and cardiovascular system. Death can result if the toxicity is severe.

Vitamin E

Despite its early reputation for antisterility activity, until recently vitamin E was characterized as a vitamin in search of a disease. Today, vitamin E is recognized as a fat-soluble cellular anti-oxidant. Its presence in the cell prevents the peroxidation of membrane lipids and thus helps to maintain membrane integrity. In this role, vitamin E has a very close relationship to selenium. If peroxides are allowed to form, they can be destroyed in the cytosol by the enzyme glutathione peroxidase before peroxidation of membrane lipids occurs. This enzyme requires selenium as an essential component of its molecular structure. In most cases, vitamin E can protect against a selenium deficiency, and selenium can afford protection in a vitamin E deficiency. This has become of practical interest in recent years with the occurrence of selenium-deficient corn, particularly in the Midwest. In some cases the legal level of selenium addition to diets may not completely protect the animal against selenium deficiency. For that reason it is generally a good practice to include a vitamin E supplement in the diet.

Vitamin E/selenium deficiency affects both heart and skeletal muscle function. The condition is referred to as white muscle disease in calves, stiff lamb disease in sheep, and mulberry heart disease in swine. Deficient pigs appear to be in good health, until they die suddenly when subjected to movement or mixing stress; thus another common name is sudden death syndrome.

Several benefits have been ascribed to vitamin E therapy of "normal" animals. Under very specific conditions of noise stress there does appear to be a benefit derived from supplementing diets with E. Other claims for vitamin E are not supported by sound research at present. In particular, there is no evidence that reproductive performance is enhanced when food animals in good nutritional status are given extra vitamin E.

Chemically, vitamin E belongs to a group of compounds called tocopherols, of which d-α-tocopherol exhibits the greatest amount of vitamin E activity. The requirement is defined in International Units, and one I.U. has the biologic activity of 1 mg of dl-α-tocopheryl acetate.

The vitamin E product used in diet supplementation, α-tocopheryl acetate, is commonly supplied in dry form on a cereal carrier. It is generally stable in premixes and complete diets. Naturally occurring tocopherols found in feedstuffs undergo loss of potency with time.

Vitamin K

This vitamin is found in both plant and animal materials. Several forms exist. Vitamin K_1, or phylloquinone, has been isolated from alfalfa, whereas K_2, menaquinone, is found in fish meal. The synthetic vitamin menadione is marketed in several forms, as shown in Table 3.

Vitamin K is essential to the blood clotting process, though the exact mechanism is unclear. Limited evidence indicates that K is a cofactor in the carboxylation reaction leading to the formation of the protein precursors for prothrombin. Animals deficient in the vitamin exhibit impaired blood clotting, and, if the deficiency goes uncorrected uncontrollable hemorrhage and death may result.

The vitamin is synthesized by rumen microbes and by the microbial inhabitants of the nonruminant digestive tract. A frank deficiency is unlikely to occur under normal conditions but can develop rapidly if K activity is depleted by an antimetabolite. The best-known antimetabolite is dicoumarol, found in sweet clover. Another common source of anti-K activity is found in moldy grain. Certain forms of mycotoxin-induced hemophilia can be alleviated by providing extra menadione in the diet. For this reason, swine and poultry diets are generally supplemented with menadione.

Pure vitamin K is a viscous liquid that is subject to decomposition by light, alkalies, halogens, and reducing agents. The different forms of menadione vary somewhat in stability, with moisture and temperature being two factors that affect stability.

Vitamin C

In vivo synthesis of this vitamin is adequate to meet cellular requirements of the major food animal species—swine, sheep, beef cattle, and poultry—without dietary supplementation.

B Vitamins

Vitamins in this category are required by both ruminant and nonruminant species. Synthesis by the rumen microflora is generally sufficient to meet the B vitamin requirements of both sheep and beef cattle. Signs of B vitamin deficiencies may become evident when rumen function is subnormal, as is the case with lambs and calves weaned before the rumen is fully functional or in a severe protein deficiency when microbial growth is limited.

Thiamine

Also called vitamin B_1, thiamine is phosphorylated in the liver to form thiamine pyrophosphate, which functions in the decarboxylation reactions of metabolism.

A thiamine deficiency can be easily demonstrated with experimental diets, but it rarely occurs in practical feed situations. Grains and grain by-products fed to nonruminants are relatively rich in this vitamin, thus supplementation of diets with thiamine is not generally recommended. There are naturally occurring compounds that

Table 3. *Sources of Menadione (Synthetic K)**

Source	Per Cent Menadione
Menadione sodium bisulfite	50
Menadione dimethyl pyrimidinol bisulfite	45.4
Menadione sodium bisulfite complex	33

*Also called vitamin K_3.

interfere with thiamine nutrition. Uncooked fish contains thiaminase, an enzyme that inactivates the vitamin. Bracken fern rhizomes contain an antithiamine substance of nonenzymatic nature.

Signs of a thiamine deficiency include depressed appetite and weight gain, which may progress to obvious nervous disorders. Polyneuritis in chicks is unique to a thiamine deficiency. Chicks with this condition retract the head to the point that it actually rests on the back.

Stability data for synthetic thiamine are lacking; however, it is rapidly destroyed when placed in an alkaline environment.

Riboflavin

Riboflavin, or vitamin B_2, has a vital role in energy metabolism as the flavin component of flavin mononucleotide (FMN) and flavin adenine dinucleotide (FAD). These coenzymes are important in a number of enzyme systems. This vitamin is marginal in practical diets, thus it should be routinely added as a supplement to prevent the deficiency. Early signs of a deficiency are reduced feed consumption and rate of gain. Chicks exhibit diarrhea and a curled-toe paralysis condition in which they squat on their hocks with the toes pointing inward. Swine develop mild dermatitis. There is cessation of the estrous cycle in open females; gravid sows give birth to dead pigs, of which about half are stillborn and the others are mummified pigs in various stages of resorption. Similar embryonic death has been noted in poultry as evidenced by reduced hatchability.

Crystalline riboflavin is a yellow, photolabile compound. No serious stability problems have been noted when riboflavin is mixed in complete diets.

Niacin

Also called nicotinic acid, niacin is present in abundance in feed grains, but the niacin in these sources is almost completely unavailable to nonruminants.

Nicotinic acid is a component of nicotinamide adenine dinucleotide (NAD) and nicotinamide adenine dinucleotide phosphate (NADP). These coenzymes operate as hydrogen and electron transfer agents in a host of reactions in lipid, carbohydrate, and protein metabolism.

Swine fed deficient diets develop anorexia, reduced weight gain, exfoliative dermatitis, and diarrhea. Chicks exhibit inflammation of the tongue and mouth cavity, retarded growth, and feathering. Poults exhibit a perosis-like hock disorder.

There is conversion of tryptophan to niacin in both swine and poultry, although the conversion is not quantitatively great. In swine each 50 mg of tryptophan yields 1 mg of niacin. As most nonruminant diets are marginal in tryptophan, this is not an important source of the vitamin.

Commercial nicotinic acid is a stable, white crystalline powder that forms acidic solutions in water. This can be a problem in certain vitamin premixes. For example, in a premix the reduction in pH can cause a significant loss in potency of calcium pantothenate. Niacin is also available as niacinamide, a product that does not form acid solutions and can be used when niacin compatibility would be a problem.

Pantothenic Acid

This vitamin is widely distributed in feedstuffs; in fact "panto" is derived from the ubiquitous forest god of mythology, Pan. The principal metabolic role of pantothenic acid is as a constituent of coenzyme A, a key participant in many reactions in lipid and carbohydrate metabolism. Many clinical signs are associated with the deficiency: skin disorders, gastritis and enteritis, and hemorrhage and necrosis of the adrenal cortex. In chickens the deficiency is noted as retarded growth, poor feather development, and reduced hatchability. In swine there is reduced gain and feed efficiency with a very characteristic "goose stepping" due to locomotive incoordination in the back legs. This ambulatory aberration should not be confused with a similar condition resulting from foot lesions.

It is generally recommended that pantothenic acid supplement be added to nonruminant diets. The likelihood of a deficiency is greatest when the diets of reproducing females are not supplemented. The D-isomer of pantothenic acid is well utilized; L-pantothenic acid is not. The free acid is an unstable, viscous oil, thus the calcium salt is the usual commercial product.

Vitamin B₁₂

This vitamin, also known as cyanocobalamin, is of microbial origin. It is almost completely absent from plant material but is present in animal tissue. Without synthetic B_{12} it is impossible to formulate diets that are nutritionally adequate for nonruminants unless animal protein sources are included. The discovery and production of synthetic B_{12} in the 1950's made the use of the grain–soybean meal diet possible. Cobalt is required for the synthesis of vitamin B_{12}, and this element is often deficient in feedstuffs fed to ruminant animals. Cobalt should be added to the trace mineral salt provided by both sheep and cattle to ensure that B_{12} synthesis by rumen microbes will be sufficient to meet needs. The addition of cobalt to nonruminant diets cannot be justified, since B_{12} produced by microbes in the lower gut is probably not absorbed and utilized by either swine or poultry.

A B_{12} and/or cobalt deficiency results in anemia and a general impairment of productive functions—i.e., wool production, growth, fertility, and milk synthesis.

Vitamin B_{12} is one of the most potent therapeutic substances known; biologic effects are seen with only 1 to 3 mcg/kg of diet. Commercial preparations of the vitamin are generally very stable, though there is some decomposition in the presence of reducing agents such as cysteine, ascorbic acid, and thiamine. Iron salts such as ferrous sulfate are destructive.

Choline

Choline does not fit the strict definition of a vitamin in that it is synthesized by the body, is a component of fat and nerve tissue, and is required in large quantities. Choline participates in a number of important functions: it is a constituent of acetylcholine, the major chemical in nerve transmission; it is an important source of methyl groups in one-carbon transfer reactions; and in the bound form it is a component of the structural phospholipids lecithin and sphingomyelin.

Most nonruminant diets contain significant quantities of choline, particularly diets that are formulated with soybean meal. There is some question about the value of choline supplementation of all nonruminant diets. There is clear evidence that the growing-finishing pig diet does not need added choline in most cases. There is, however, a significant increase in litter size when choline is added to swine gestation diets. The growing chick that is fed practical diets is likely to be choline deficient, but the laying hen appears to be able to meet cellular needs from dietary and metabolic sources.

Unthriftiness, depressed gain, and fatty infiltration of the liver characterize a choline deficiency in swine. Perosis and growth retardation are observed in chicks, poults, and ducklings.

Commercial choline is available in an aqueous solution or as a dry premix, usually on a cereal carrier. It is usually marketed as the salt, choline chloride, which is 86.7 per cent choline by weight. Choline chloride preparations are stable as liquid solutions or on dry cereal carriers. Choline chloride in the dry form is extremely hygroscopic. This property, along with the tendency to form acid in aqueous solution, can create stability problems for other vitamins when premixed with choline chloride.

Vitamin B₆

Three compounds, pyridoxine, pyridoxal, and pyridoxamine, possess vitamin B_6 activity in nature. The vitamin has several key roles in amino acid metabolism. As pyridoxal phosphate it is the prosthetic group of enzymes that decarboxylate tyrosine, arginine, glutamic acid, and other amino acids. It acts as a co-enzyme for serine and threonine dehydrase, is involved in transamination reactions, and in the case of methionine functions in transulfuration. The clinical test for B_6 status is based on the increased urinary excretion of xanthurenic acid caused by impairment of tryptophan metabolism in B_6 deficiency.

A deficiency of this vitamin causes a general depression in appetite, growth, and reproductive performance. Frequently there are nervous disorders characterized by abnormal excitement and convulsions. The deficiency may be accompanied by nonhemolytic anemia and, in some species, dermatitis.

Vitamin B_6 is widely distributed in natural feed ingredients, and spontaneous deficiencies are extremely rare. There is no good evidence that the supplementation of practical diets is justified.

Biotin

Biotin functions metabolically in carboxylation and decarboxylation reactions. In most cases the requirement is met by the biotin in feeds and that produced by microbial synthesis in the gastrointestinal tract. The deficiency has been studied in most species using either avidin (a protein found in raw egg white that binds biotin, rendering it unavailable) or sulfa drugs (antimicrobial agents that greatly reduce biotin synthesis by the gut microflora) to create the deficiency. The clinical signs of the deficiency are poor appetite, poor growth, and a form of dermatitis. These are signs typical of several B vitamin deficiencies and are of little diagnostic value. In addition, lesions of the footpads have been reported in both poultry and swine.

Considerable controversy surrounds the question of biotin supplementation for practical diets. There is limited evidence of a beneficial effect in both poultry and swine, particularly when diets are formulated with wheat or barley, cereals low in available biotin. The preponderance of work in swine shows an absence of any response to biotin. It may be that the deficiency observed with some practical diets is associated with moldy grain.

Table 4. *Vitamin Requirements of Swine (Amt/lb Diet)** *

Vitamin	Starter 10 to 30 Lb	Grower 30 to 120 Lb	Finisher 120 Lb to Mkt Wt	Gestation	Lactation
Vitamin A, I.U.	1500	1500	1500	2500	1500
Vitamin D, I.U.	300	150	75	150	150
Vitamin E, I.U.	5	5	5	5	5
Vitamin K, mg	1	1	1	1	1
Thiamine, mg	0.6	0.5	0.5	0.5	0.5
Riboflavin, mg	1.5	1.0	0.8	1.0	1.0
Pantothenic acid, mg	6	5	5	5	5
Nicotinic acid, mg	12	8	6	8	8
Vitamin B_6, mg	0.7	0.5	0.5	0.5	0.5
Choline, mg	600	400	350	400	400
Vitamin B_{12}, mcg	9	6	4	6	6
Biotin, mg	0.05	0.05	0.05	0.05	0.5
Folacin, mg	0.3	0.3	0.3	0.3	0.3

*Reprinted with permission from Jensen, A. H.: Dietary Nutrient Allowances for Swine. Feedstuffs Reference Issue *51*:29:41–44, 1979.
Note: For diets containing 1450 to 1550 kcal of ME/lb and fed *ad libitum* to pigs in all phases of production except gestation.

Folacin

Folacin is known chemically as pteroylglutamic acid. There are at least three nutritionally significant pteroylglutamates, which differ only in the number of glutamic acid residues in the molecule. The folic acid co-enzymes are concerned with the biochemical reactions involving one-carbon moieties.

Folacin deficiency results in poor feathering and anemia in chicks; nervousness, droopy wings, and, in some cases, cervical paralysis in poults; and reduced egg production and hatchability in breeder hens.

Folacin addition to diets formulated with common feedstuffs has been shown to be beneficial in turkey breeder and prestarter diets. It is often added to chicken starter and breeder diets. There is no evidence of any value from the addition of folacin to practical swine diets in any phase of production.

Commercially available folacin is stable in dry form, but it is sensitive to light and there is complete destruction when it is placed in solutions with pH values less than 6.

Inositol, Lipoic Acid, and Para-Aminobenzoic Acid

There are a number of compounds that are frequently included in a discussion of vitamins, although they are not vitamins in the traditional sense.

There are nine isomers of inositol; myoinositol is the only one that exhibits biologic activity. The nutritional significance of inositol is not clear. Rats exhibit alopecia, spectacled eye, and growth and lactation failure when inositol is omitted from the diet. Encephalomalacia and exudative diathesis have been reported for deficient chicks. Supplementation of practical diets is not necessary.

Lipoic acid is required for growth by several microbial species; however, it can be synthesized by higher animals. Lipoic acid functions in reactions involved in dehydrogenation and acyl group transfer. Lipoic acid is not needed in the diet of food animals.

Para-aminobenzoic acid, often called PABA, is not required in the diets of food animals. It is a growth factor for some microbes and appears to serve as a precursor in the synthesis of the vitamin folacin.

VITAMIN REQUIREMENTS

Since the advent of inexpensive, synthetic vitamins, there has been little interest in the precise quantitative determination of vitamin requirements. Published requirements in some cases rely heavily on data extrapolated from laboratory animals. The recommended levels shown in Tables 4 and 5 are known to be adequate; the actual requirements in some instances may be less. Note also

Table 5. *Vitamin Requirements of Chickens and Turkeys (Amt/lb Diet)** *

Vitamins	Chickens				Turkeys			
	Starting†	Growing†	Laying‡	Breeding‡	Starting	Growing	Finishing	Breeding
Vitamin A, I.U.	5000	3000	4000	5000	5000	3000	3000	5000
Vitamin D_3, I.U.	1000	1000	1000	1000	1500	1500	1000	1500
Vitamin E, I.U.	5	4	—	7.5	7.5	5	5	15
Vitamin K, mg	1	1	1	1	1	1	1	1
Thiamine, mg	1	1	1	1	1	1	1	1
Riboflavin, mg	2	2	2	2.5	2.5	2	2	2.5
Pantothenic acid, mg	6.5	6	2.5	7.5	8	6	6	10
Nicotinic acid, mg	15	15	12	15	35	30	20	20
Vitamin B_6, mg	2	1.5	1.5	2	2	1.5	1.5	2
Choline, mg	600	450	500	500	900	800	600	600
Vitamin B_{12}, mcg	4.5	2.5	4.5	5.0	6.0	5.0	3.0	6.0
Biotin, mg	0.06	0.05	0.05	0.08	0.15	0.12	0.1	0.15
Folacin, mg	0.6	0.18	0.18	0.4	0.8	0.45	0.4	0.5

*Reprinted with permission from Scott, M. L.: Dietary Nutrient Allowances for Chickens and Turkeys. Feedstuffs Reference Issue *51*:29:63–64, 1979.
†Diets contain 1400 kcal ME/lb.
‡Diets contain 1500 kcal ME/lb.

Table 6. *Vitamin Requirements of Beef Cattle (Amt/lb Dry Feed)**

	Growing and Finishing Steers and Heifers	Dry, Pregnant Cows	Breeding Bulls and Lactating Cows
Vitamin A I.U.	1000	1375	1775
Vitamin D I.U.	125	125	125
Vitamin E I.U.	7–28	—	7–28

*Data from NRC No. 4, 1970.

that the diets are based on diets formulated to specific energy levels and are thus indirectly related to daily feed consumption. It is wise to consider factors that may affect feed consumption in the evaluation of a potential deficiency. For example, if the caloric density of the diet is increased, the daily *ad libitum* intake will decrease. In order to sustain a constant level of vitamin intake on a daily basis, the vitamin concentration in the diet would have to be increased in proportion to the increase in energy level. Heat stress is another example of a factor that may affect feed intake.

The vitamin requirements of ruminant animals depend to an extent on the feeding level, weight, and age of the animal. The requirements for beef cattle shown in Table 6 are a general summary. The sheep requirements are not listed in tabular form but can be calculated on the following basis (NRC No. 5, 1975). Daily intakes of 44 to 55 I.U. of carotene per kg of body weight are required to prevent night blindness, whereas 220 to 275 I.U. per kg are required for reproduction and vitamin A storage. It is suggested that the minimums be multiplied by 5 for a recommended level for gestation, lactation, and early-weaned lambs. Similarly, the values for replacement lambs and yearlings can be multiplied by 2.5. During early gestation, ewes should receive about 1.5 times the minimum requirement. The vitamin D recommendation is 300 I.U. per 45.4 kg of body weight for early-weaned lambs and 250 I.U. per 45.4 kg of body weight for all other classifications. Vitamin E should be provided at the rate of approximately 75 mg per 45.4 kg of body weight per day.

Supplemental Reading

Jensen, A. H.: Dietary Nutrient Allowances for Swine. Feedstuffs Reference Issue *51*:29:41–44, 1979.

NRC: Nutrient Requirements of Domestic Animals, No. 1. Nutrient Requirements of Poultry, 7th ed. Washington, D.C., National Academy of Sciences–National Research Council, 1977.

NRC: Nutrient Requirements of Domestic Animals, No. 2. Nutrient Requirements of Swine, 8th ed. Washington, D.C., National Academy of Sciences–National Research Council, 1979.

NRC: Nutrient Requirements of Domestic Animals, No. 4. Nutrient Requirements of Beef Cattle, 4th ed. Washington, D.C., National Academy of Sciences–National Research Council, 1970.

NRC: Nutrient Requirements of Domestic Animals, No. 5. Nutrient Requirements of Sheep, 5th ed. Washington, D.C., National Academy of Sciences–National Research Council, 1975.

Sauberlich, H. E., Skala, J. H., and Dowdy, R. P.: Laboratory Tests for The Assessment of Nutritional Status. Cleveland, Ohio, CRC Press, 1974.

Scott, M. L.: Dietary Nutrient Allowances for Chickens and Turkeys. Feedstuffs Reference Issue *51*:29:63–64, 1979.

New Concepts for Measuring Proteins for Cattle

JOHN C. SIMONS, D.V.M.,
JIM FULLER, B.S., M.S.,
IVAN G. RUSH, Ph.D.,
and MICHAEL S. HAND., D.V.M., Ph.D.

Proteins are essential components of both plants and animals. They are necessary to the structure of all cells of all animals. They comprise basic portions of all enzyme systems, antibodies, and part of the hormones. Plasma proteins are necessary to maintain osmotic pressure and water balance. They also assist in the blood clotting process. There are vast numbers of different proteins. Each has a specific structure that permits a specific function.

Proteins are essential in the diets of all animals except those that harbor a microbial population in the digestive tract that is capable of synthesizing proteins from nonprotein nitrogen and energy nutrients.

The levels of dietary protein required by young growing animals are high relative to those of mature animals. The processes of gestation and lactation include protein deposition and thus increase the dietary requirements. If carbohydrates and fats are in short supply, proteins will be metabolized to produce energy. The amino acid components will be de-aminated, and the excess nitrogen will be incorporated into urea by the liver. The urea thus produced will be eliminated in urine or recycled to the digestive tract. When energy requirements are met by carbohydrate and fat, excess protein will be de-aminated and the energy-containing portions will be incorporated into fat.

Structurally, proteins are long polymers of alpha amino carboxylic acids combined by peptide linkages. Each alpha amino acid has a carboxyl group bound to an adjacent (alpha) carbon. The alpha carbon contains an amino group and a specific R group (Fig. 1). There are about 20 different R groups that occur naturally. The R groups differentiate and identify the individual amino acids. In protein molecules the amino group of one amino acid is combined with the carboxyl group of another amino acid to form a peptide bond (Fig. 2).

In synthesis one molecule of water is formed with each peptide linkage formed. Up to 300 amino acids may be linked together in a single molecule of protein. In addition, long polymers of amino acids may link together with hydrogen or disulfide bonds to make sheets and layers of fibrous protein. Also, the protein molecules may be coiled or folded by polar bonds between parts of the molecule. Lastly, several protein polymers may be linked to a common chemical entity to make a complex compound such as hemoglobin.

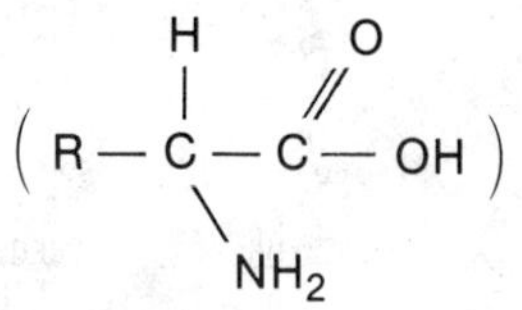

Figure 1. Structure of the alpha carbon.

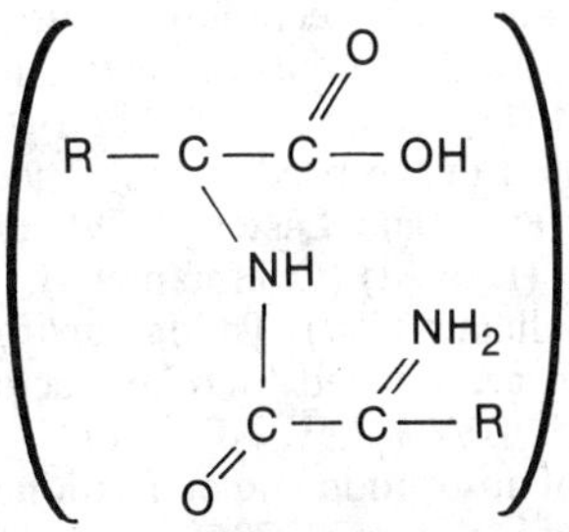

Figure 2. A peptide bond of a protein molecule.

Given access to amino nitrogen and energy nutrients, animals can synthesize most of the amino acids in the cells. Microbial populations maintained in the forestomachs of ruminant animals are capable of synthesizing all of the amino acids if all of the essential elements are available. The amino acids incorporated in the microbial protein are available for digestion and absorption in ruminant animals.

Nine specific alpha amino acids must be present in the diets of monogastric animals including the monogastric herbivores. These (essential) amino acids cannot be synthesized endogenously by monogastric carnivores or omnivores. Microbial populations in the lower digestive tracts of monogastric herbivores may synthesize all of the amino acids, but microbial protein is not significantly susceptible to digestion and absorption in these animals. These essential amino acids include methionine, threonine, tryptophan, isoleucine, leucine, lycine, valine, phenylalanine, and histidine. Three of the alpha amino acids contain sulfur in the R groups.

Complete protein rations contain all of the amino acids essential to animal nutrition in amounts adequate to meet the maintenance and production requirements of the animal being fed. High-quality food protein is not only complete but contains all of the essential amino acids in amounts proportional to the body's need for them. High quality also implies high digestibility, absorbability, and utility.

Food protein sources include both animal and plant proteins. Generally, the quality of animal protein (eggs, meat, dairy products) is relatively high. All plants contain some protein. Seeds, stems, leaves, and some roots are all potential sources. Combinations of plant proteins using two or more plant sources whose essential amino acid components compliment each other may approach animal protein quality.

Commonly used forages (pasture, hay, ensilage) and energy concentrates (grains and tubers) are often deficient in protein required to meet the maintenance and production objectives. Feeds classified as protein supplements are used to supply the deficiencies. These are generally high-energy feeds containing more than 20 per cent crude protein. Commonly used plant protein supplements include soybean meal, cottonseed meal, linseed meal, peanut meal, and low-quality beans. Animal-source protein supplements are not widely used in ruminant rations. They are, however, commonly used in poultry and swine rations when the market is favorable. Common animal-source protein supplements include meat meal, fish meal, tankage, and by-products of the diary industry. Protein

supplements formed by combining nonprotein nitrogen (NPN) compounds with a high-energy carrier (corn-urea) are often used to supplement ruminant rations.

PROTEIN DIGESTION AND ABSORPTION IN MONOGASTRIC ANIMALS

Digestion is the process whereby foodstuffs are taken into the digestive tract and the nutrients are prepared for absorption. The process of digestion begins when food enters the mouth. The food is ground and mixed with saliva. The saliva contains water, mucous, and a starch-splitting enzyme (salivary amylase), which begins to hydrolyze starch. In the stomach the food is mixed with hydrochloric acid, which acts to degrade and separate the nutrients. Also, a proteolytic enzyme precursor is secreted in the stomach. This pro-enzyme (pepsinogen) is converted by HCl into the proteolytic enzyme pepsin, which begins to hydrolyze the food protein into shorter fragments called peptides.

The food passes from the stomach to the small intestine, where it is subject to the pancreatic secretions. These secretions include bicarbonate to neutralize the gastric acid and a number of digestive enzymes including pancreatic lipase, pancreatic amylase, and three prominent proteolytic enzyme precursors—trypsinogen, chymotrypsinogen, and propolypeptidase. The trypsinogen is converted by an enteric enzyme, enterokinase, into trypsin. The trypsin converts chymotrysinogen to chymotrypsin and propolypeptidase to polypeptidase. These enzymes convert protein and peptides to simple dipeptide molecules. The absorptive cells of the small intestine contain enzymes called dipeptidases that hydrolyze dipeptides into individual alpha amino acids. The amino acids are actively transported or diffused across the absorptive cells into the capillaries that supply and drain the small intestine. The absorptive surface of the small intestine is multiplied by folds, villi, and the brush borders of the absorptive cells. These structures multiply the absorptive surface of the small intestine about 600 times.

PROTEIN DIGESTION AND ABSORPTION IN RUMINANTS

There are no digestive enzymes in the saliva of ruminant animals. The food is ingested, masticated, and swallowed before significant hydrolysis of complex nutrient molecules begins. The digestive process in the stomach of ruminants differs markedly from that of monogastric animals. The nonglandular portion of the ruminant stomach is very large and is divided into three different compartments including the rumen, the reticulum, and the omasum. The rumen and the reticulum communicate freely and can be thought of as a single functional entity. This reticulorumen comprises a large fermentation vat containing a vast and varied microbial population including bacteria, protozoa, and fungi. A unique symbiotic relationship between the ruminal microbes and the host animal has evolved.

The rumen is not fully developed and functional at birth. Neonate ruminants can be practically regarded as monogastric animals. The rumen becomes functional at six to eight weeks of age, depending on diet. After rumen function is established, the crude protein needs for two systems must be met: nitrogen (crude protein) for microbial protein synthesis in the reticulorumen, and post-ruminal amino acids for the host animal (NRC, 1984). The rumen microbes aid in the degradation of cellulytic compounds that are indigestible for monogastric animals These microbes are also capable of converting nonprotein nitrogen (NPN) into microbial protein. This microbial protein is utilized by the host animal and furnishes about one half of the protein requirements of ruminant animals (Owens and Bergen, 1983).

There is general agreement among current investigators regarding the principles involved in the digestion of proteins and proteinaceous materials by ruminants.

1. Degradation in the rumen of a substantial portion of true protein and NPN contained in feedstuffs. The nitrogen content of the degraded material is largely incorporated into ammonia.

2. Bypass or escape of some true protein contained in feedstuffs from the rumen into the lower digestive tract without degradation.

3. Incorporation of ammonia accumulated in the rumen into microbial protein (including synthesis of essential amino acids).

4. Absorption of ammonia not incorporated in microbial protein from the rumen and intestines.

5. Conversion of absorbed ammonia into urea by the liver. Most of this urea is eliminated in urine.

6. Recycling of a portion of the urea synthesized in the liver into the digestive tract via salivary and ruminal secretions.

7. Digestion of bypass and microbial protein in the abomasum and small intestine into alpha amino acids. The abomasum and small intestine of the ruminant are very similar in function to the stomachs and small intestines of monogastric animals.

8. Absorption of alpha amino acids from the small intestine.

ESTIMATING PROTEIN CONTENT IN FEEDS

Protein content in feeds is generally expressed as crude protein (CP). CP is determined by measuring the nitrogen content of the feed and multiplying by 6.25 or dividing by 0.16. Protein is generally considered to contain 16 per cent nitrogen. It is assumed that all nitrogen is incorporated in protein, so CP = N × 6.25 or N/0.16. The computation of apparently digestible protein has been eliminated from the NRC recommendations (Dairy Cattle, 1978; Beef Cattle, 1984). If a value for digestible protein of a diet is desired, it will be more accurate to calculate it from a prediction equation rather than to use weighted averages of component feed values (Preston, 1972). Glover and associates (1957) showed that the digestion co-efficient can be derived by the equation CPDC = (70 Log X) − 15, where X is the crude protein percentage in the feed. Thus, if the CP per cent is 11 per cent, CPDC = (70 × 1.0414) − 15 = 57.9 per cent, or 0.579. This formula is reputed to be valid for both forages and mixed diets (NRC, 1978).

Current NRC requirements for protein in dairy and beef animals (Dairy Cattle, 1978; Beef Cattle, 1984) are derived by factorial methods (Mitchell, 1929). The maintenance factors include protein lost in urine (U), fecal material (F), and skin secretions, scurf, and hair (S) (Swanson, 1977). The production factors include increase in body weight (G) (Reed and Robb, 1971; NRC 1984), protein deposited in the products of conception (C) (Jakobsen, 1957; Prior and Laster, 1979), and protein deposited in milk (L or M) (Overman et al., 1939; Lamond et al., 1969; Williams 1979). The factors for maintenance and production are divided by other factors (Ep: NRC, 1978; and D × BV × CE: NRC, 1984) to account for the efficiency of absorption and deposition (Brisson et al., 1957; Hogan and Weston, 1970; Satter and Roffler, 1975; Blaxter, 1964; Lofgreen et al., 1951; Reid, 1967; Roy, 1970; Stobo and Roy, 1973; Swanson and Herman, 1943; Van Es and Bockholt, 1976; NRC, 1984). The factors have been derived from empirical values established by experimentation.

In recent years the accuracy of the factorial methods has been called into question. Considerable effort has gone into deriving models and methods to measure metabolizable protein and using them in place of the empirical data that are still in current use.

In November 1980, an international symposium to consider the protein requirements for cattle was held at Oklahoma State University. Current findings concerning protein and nonprotein nitrogen utilization were discussed by a number of experts in the field. The discussions included the presentation of a number of models of nitrogen utilization in ruminants and proposed computations to estimate metabolizable protein requirements in beef and dairy animals.

In his summary of the conference, R. R. Johnson said that . . . *full appreciation of the topics and discussions will come only to those scholars who place the composite information from this conference in perspective with the problems of supplying food and particularly animal protein to a hungry world.* He also pointed out that *The role of the ruminant in food production has possibly been debated too often, but even the most casual student of world history and geography will quickly realize that the ruminant was likely one of the first, if not the first, producer of animal protein by domesticated animals and will unquestionably be the one food producing animal which survives the longest in the competition between animals and man for plant feedstuffs.*

It was generally expressed in the conference that "traditional systems for calculating ruminant protein requirements are recognized to be of limited value," and that . . . *it is clear that the traditional use of crude protein and digestible protein must be modified to reflect the intervention of rumen microbes in the digestive process and to recognize the contribution of endogenous nitrogen and microbial residues to fecal output.*

Our primary objective in this article is to illustrate the models and systems that are being designed, studied, and modified to enable a more practical approach to protein utilization. The objectives of these designs, studies, and modifications include:

1. Refinement of concepts of actual biologic happenings.

2. Provision to those associated with food production (producers, allied industries, and extension specialists) a more precise way to perform their tasks.

3. The end result: a system that adequately enables the formulation of ruminant rations before they are fed.

The models and systems outlined in the conference included:

1. Empirical Value of Crude Protein Systems for Feedlot Cattle, R. L. Preston, Washington State University.

*2. The Metabolizable Protein Feeding Standard, Allen Trenkle, Iowa State University.

†3. A Metabolizable Protein System Keyed to Ruminal Ammonia Concentration—The Wisconsin System, Larry D. Satter, University of Wisconsin.

‡4. A Net Protein System for Cattle: The Rumen Submodel for Nitrogen, P. J. Van Soest, C. J. Sniffen, D. R. Mertens, D. J. Fox, P. H. Robinson, and U. Krishna Moorthy, Cornell University.

5. Foreign Systems for Meeting the Requirements of Ruminants, D. R. Waldo and B. P. Glenn, U.S.D.A. and University of Maryland.

6. Nebraska Growth System, Terry Klopfenstein, Robert Britton, and Rick Stock, University of Nebraska.

7. Michigan Protein Systems, J. C. Waller, R. Black, and W. G. Bergen, Michigan State University, and D. E. Johnson, Colorado State University.

All of the systems are based on the common assumptions listed earlier. We have selected and outlined three of these systems: the Iowa State System, the Wisconsin System, and the Cornell System. We do not imply superiority for these systems, but they are representative of current thinking and we are limited by space.

The Iowa State System

The use of urea as a source of dietary nitrogen in cattle is extensive. There is a definite need for improving methods of expressing protein requirements of cattle. The Iowa State System (Burroughs et al., 1975) outlines a concept that expresses these protein requirements as metabolizable protein (MP). The system also expresses the capacity of a ration to benefit from urea supplementation as the urea fermentation potential (UFP).

Since microbial protein is formed from NPN and energy nutrients, utilization is dependent on (1) the amount of nitrogen in the feed that is reduced to ammonia in the rumen, and (2) the amount of digestible energy nutrients that are available in the rumen.

The relationship between the ammonia and the TDN in the rumen is expressed as the UFP in grams of urea per kilogram of dry matter feed. If the available energy nutrients in the rumen exceed the amount required to convert the entire rumen ammonia pool to microbial protein, the UFP is positive. If there is insufficient energy to convert the entire ammonia pool to microbial protein, the UFP is negative.

Definitions necessary to understand the concept include the following.

1. Degraded protein is that portion of protein or NPN in a feed from which all of the nitrogen (100 per cent) will be reduced to ammonia in the rumen.

2. Undegraded protein is that portion of protein in a feed that is not degraded or digested in the rumen. This portion of protein will not be affected by rumen fermentation but will be digested into amino acids in the abomasum and small intestine. It is sometimes called bypass protein.

3. Microbial protein is the dietary protein incorporated in the cells of the rumen microbes. For a specific feed, microbial protein equals 0.1044 TDN if the UFP is negative or 100 per cent of the degraded protein if the UFP is positive.

4. The urea fermentation potential (UFP) expressed in grams of urea/kg of dry matter $(11.78 \ NE_m + 6.85) - (0.0357 \ CP \times DEG)$ where NE_m = net energy for maintenance (Mcal/kg), CP = crude protein per cent in the DM, and DEG = degraded protein per cent. The UFP can also be expressed as

$$\frac{(0.1044 \text{ g TDN/kg DM}) - \text{g degraded protein/kg DM}}{2.8^*}$$

The Metabolizable Protein Model (Fig. 3)

By way of explanation:

1. Feeds vary in degradability from 52 to 95 per cent. Examples from the data include corn grain 62 per cent DEG and alfalfa 95 per cent DEG.

2. 10.44 per cent is the portion of TDN that will be available for microbial protein synthesis. It is the product of the assumed percentage of TDN digested in the rumen (52 per cent) multiplied by the percentage of TDN used in microbial synthesis (25 per cent) multiplied by the efficiency factor (80 per cent): $0.52 \times 0.25 \times 0.8 = 0.104$.

3. Escaped or bypass protein is assumed to be digested into amino acids and absorbed with an efficiency of 90 per cent.

4. 15 grams of fecal crude protein (2.4 g N) per kg DM feed is assumed to be lost from the total microbial protein production. 80 per cent of the remaining microbial protein is assumed to be digested into amino acids and absorbed.

5. Thus, metabolizable protein/kg DM feed is

$$(P_1 \times 0.9) + ([P_2\text{-}15] [0.8])$$

where P_1 = g bypass protein/kg DM feed, P_2 = g microbial protein produced/kg DM feed, and 15 = microbial protein lost in fecal material/kg DM feed.

6. Estimates of protein degradation and microbial protein passage from the rumen and the digestion co-efficients for bypass and microbial protein and fecal protein losses are based upon:

a. data published in the literature (various sources),

b. feeding trials with young growing cattle (Burroughs et al., 1975)

c. analysis of post-ruminal digesta by several laboratories,

d. average true digestion of undegraded feed protein in monogastric species (various sources), and

e. studies of protein digestibility in sheep (Mason and Fredericksen, 1979).

Feed Analysis

Data concerning feed concentration ingredients pertinent to metabolizable protein computations are listed in Table 1.

---

*The Iowa State System.
†The Wisconsin System.
‡The Cornell System.

---

*2.8 is the crude protein equivalent of urea. Protein contains 16 per cent nitrogen, and urea contains about 45 per cent nitrogen; thus 45/16 = 2.81

IN THE RUMEN

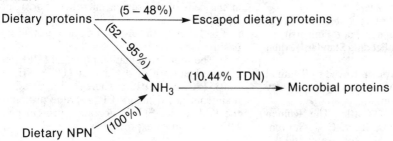

IN THE SMALL INTESTINE

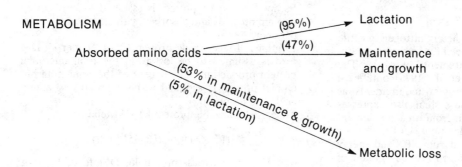

Figure 3. The metabolizable protein model.

Table 1. Metabolizable Protein Available for Body Purposes Plus Urea Fermentation of Feedstuffs*

Feed	TDN (% DM)	CP (% DM)	Abomasal Protein		Rumen		Met Prot (g/kg DM)	UFP (g/kg DM)
			UDG (g/kg DM)	MCB (g/kg DM)	Prot (% DM)	Deg (g/kg DM)		
Alfala (aerial part)	61	19.3	9.6	63.7	95	183	47.6	−42.8
Alfalfa	57	16.3	8.2	59.5	95	155	43	−34
Barley grain	83	13	39	86.6	70	91	92.4	−1.6
Beet aerial + crown	54	12.7	25	56.4	80	102	56	−16.1
Beet pulp	72	10	20	75.2	80	80	66.2	−1.7
Brome grass	68	20.3	10	71	95	193	53	−43.5
Brome grass	65	6.4	16	48	75	48	40.8	+7.1
Buffalo grass	59	9.2	13.8	62	85	78	49.7	−5.9
Corn (ears)	89	9.3	32.6	60	65	60	65.8	+11.6
Corn grain #2	91	10	38	62	62	62	71.8	+11.8
Corn (aerial ensiled)	70	8.1	26	55	68	55	55.4	+6.4
Cotton seed meal (sol. ext.)	75	44.8	112	78	75	336	151.4	−92
Oat grain	76	13.2	39.6	79	70	92	87	−4.7
Prairie grass	50	8.1	12	52	85	69	40.6	−6
Prairie grass	54	4.6	11.5	35	75	35	2.6	+7.8
Sorghum grain	80	12.4	59.5	65	52	65	93	+6.8
Soybean meal (sol. ext.)	81	51.5	129	85	75	386	171.6	−108
Urea	0	280	—	—	—	—	223	—
Wheat grain	88	14.3	42.9	92	70	100	100	−2.9

*Extrapolated from Metabolizable Protein (Amino Acid) Feeding Standard for Cattle and Sheep Fed Rations Containing Either Alpha Amino or Nonprotein Nitrogen. Iowa State University Agr. Station Leaflet R190, 1974, Table 6.

Note: TDN = Total digestible nutrients; CP = crude protein; UNG = undegraded; MCB = microbial protein; Prot = protein; DEG = degraded; Met Prot = metabolizable protein; UFP = urea fermentation potential.

The Metabolizable Protein Requirement

A factorial system is used to establish the requirements for growth and maintenance.

1. The net protein requirement for maintenance is computed from a formula developed by Smuts (1935). Protein (g/day) required for maintenance = $(0.0125) \times (70.4 \text{ W/kg}^{0.734})$.

2. The net protein requirements for growth are based on the quantity and composition of empty body weight gain. If the gain = 1 kg/day and contains 15 per cent protein, the net protein requirement for gain = 150 g/day.

3. The net protein requirements for lactation equals the protein deposited in milk. If daily milk production = 10 kg of milk containing 3.5 per cent protein, the requirement = $10 \times 0:035 = 0.35$ kg (350 g).

These requirements must be subjected to efficiency factors and added together to total the net protein requirement for a specific animal. The maintenance and growth factor = 47 per cent. The lactation factor = 95 per cent. The requirements for MP listed previously should be multiplied by a factor of 1.1 to 1.2 to account for the less than perfect amino acid balance presented for absorption.

The requirements for growth are based on the assumption that cattle of a given weight deposit gain having a constant composition. The per cent of protein in gain is inversely proportional to body weight. Table 2 lists the assumed protein deposition in the gain of cattle of various body weights.

The system is under constant surveillance at Iowa State University and the recommendations are subject to change. Considerations include the following.

1. Recent studies indicate that composition of gain for a given weight of cattle varies with the rate of gain.

2. Some feeding trials seem to indicate that the tabulated UFP values are too low (see the Wisconsin System).

3. There is some argument that the fecal protein computation is too low.

The system is flexible and susceptible to alteration, and we think it is based on practical concepts that will improve as research progresses.

The Practical Application

For an example we will use the Iowa State System to formulate an energy protein ration as follows:

1. Class: Medium-frame steers.
2. Live weight: 300 kg.
3. Metabolic weight $(300^{0.75})$: 72.08 kg.
4. Expected daily gain: 1 kg.
5. NE_m requirement (cold weather) (0.09×72.08): 6.48 Mcal.

Table 2. *Assumed Protein Deposition*

Body Weight (kg)	Protein Deposition in Gain (g/kg)
150	150
200	140
300	130
400	120
500	110

6. NE_g requirement (Table 1, NRC, 1984): 4.02 Mcal.

7. Metabolic protein requirement (Iowa model):

$$\left(300^{0.734} \times \frac{0.0125 \times 70.4 \times 1.2}{0.47}\right) + (130/0.47 \times 1.2) = 480 \text{ g}.$$

8. DM consumption (feed intake equation, NRC, 1984): 7.1 kg.

9. Least cost feed sources (Table 3).

10. Basic energy ration—Table 4 (25 per cent corn #2, 75 per cent corn silage).
$NE_m = (0.25 \times 2.24) + (0.75 \times 1.63) = 1.78$ Mcal/kg.
$NE_g = (0.25 \times 1.55) + (0.75 \times 1.03) = 1.16$ Mcal/kg.

Daily DM consumption $= \left(\frac{6.48}{1.78}\right) + \frac{4.02}{1.16} = 7.1$ kg.

The metabolizable protein deficiency = $480 - 422.5 = 57.5$ g. 122.5 g of MP equivalent from UFP is more than 57.5 g deficiency, so we will use corn-urea for an MP supplement.

11. Computation of substituting corn-urea for corn in the ration to maintain energy and supply the MP deficiency.

a. To maintain energy we need to put in 1 kg of corn-urea to replace 0.85 kg of corn.

b. When we substitute 1 kg corn-urea for 0.85 kg corn we gain $(75 + [143 \times 2.225]) - (0.85 \times 71.8) = 332$ g MP. (Assumes energy will be supplied to convert the negative UFP to microbial protein.)

c. We need $\frac{57.5}{332} = 0.173$ kg corn-urea to be added to the ration and $0.173 \text{ kg} \times 0.85 = 0.147$ kg corn removed from the ration.

12. The final DM energy protein ration (Table 5).
Total MP in energy-protein ration:

$$(1.653 \times 71.8) + (0.173 \times 75) + (0.173 \times 143 \times 2.225) + (5.32 \times 55.4) = 481.4 \text{ g}.$$

Table 3. *Least Cost Feed Sources*

Category	Feed	TDN %	DM %	NE_m	NE_g	MP	UFP	MP Equiv of UFP
Energy	Corn #2	90	88	2.24	1.55	71.8	+11.8	26.26
Fiber	Corn silage	70	30	1.63	1.03	55.4	+6.4	14.24
Protein*	Soybean meal	89	89	2.06	1.40	171.6	−107.7	238.1
Protein†	Corn-urea (85/15)	90	90	1.90	1.32	75	−143	318.2

*Use if MP deficiency >MP equivalent of UFP.

†Use if MP equivalent of UFP >MP deficiency.

Note: TDN = total digestible nutrients; DM = dry matter; Ne_m = net energy for maintenance (Mcal/kg DM); NE_g = net energy for gain (Mcal/kg DM); MP = metabolizable protein (g/kg DM); UFP = urea fermentation potential (g/kg DM); MP Equiv. of UFP = metabolizable protein equivalent of UFP (g/kg DM).

Table 4. *Basic Energy Ration*

Feed	DM (kg)	MP (g)	UFP (g)	MP Equiv of UFP (g)
Corn	1.78	$(71.8 \times 1.78) = 127.8$	$(11.8 \times 1.78) = 21$	$21 \times 2.225 = 46.7$
Corn silage	5.32	$(55.4 \times 5.32) = 294.7$	$(6.4 \times 5.32) = 34$	$34 \times 2.225 = 75.8$
TOTALS	7.10	422.5	55	122.5

The Wisconsin System (Satter and Roffler, 1975)

Most approaches used to estimate the metabolizable protein sources and requirements involve the summation of the rumen microbial protein synthesized and the dietary true protein that escapes degradation in the rumen. This is a logical way to proceed, but it is currently susceptible to error owing to lack of information on protein degradability of many feedstuffs and variations in estimates of microbial synthesis.

The approach used by Satter and Roffler (1975) is keyed to rumen ammonia concentration. When this concentration gets beyond a critical point, ammonia is absorbed from the digestive tract and does not contribute to microbial protein synthesis. The critical point is related to TDN and crude protein concentrations in the diet.

The amount of ammonia that can be utilized by the rumen microbes depends on the number of such microbes and how rapidly they are growing. The size of the microbial population and its rate of growth are determined by the amount of fermentable energy nutrients that are available to the microbes. Feeds high in TDN are generally more fermentable than those with lower TDN values. It follows that larger amounts of ammonia and dietary NPN can be utilized by high digestible feeds than by less digestible feeds.

It apparently makes little difference to the animal whether or not dietary true protein is degraded as long as the rumen microbes can utilize all of the available ammonia. In these cases both dietary and recycled nitrogen end up as protein presented to the intestine for digestion and absorption. When ammonia production exceeds the microbial requirement for protein synthesis, only dietary true protein that escapes degradation in the rumen can contribute to the intestinal amino acid pool. Ammonia produced beyond the capacity of microbial utilization results in ammonia overflow (absorption from the rumen and/or intestines). The ammonia overflow does not contribute to metabolizable protein and is useless to the animal.

The prediction of the point of ammonia overflow in the rumen is important in the determination of practical quantities of NPN that can be used in ruminant rations. Two pieces of information are essential for the prediction: (1) the concentration of ruminal ammonia necessary to support maximal microbial growth, and (2) the mean concentration of ruminal ammonia produced by specific rations and feeding conditions. The objective is to relate mean ruminal ammonia concentration to TDN and crude protein content. These are well-understood and readily measured characteristics, and the relationship is used to predict the point of ammonia overflow.

The question of optimal concentrations of ammonia in the rumen to support microbial growth is controversial. Several enzymes are known to be involved. Two of the more important ones are said to be glutamate dehydrogenase (low affinity for ammonia) and glutamine synthetase (high affinity for ammonia). Studies by Baldwin and Denham (1979) and Schaefer and co-workers (1980) have provided significant information.

The vast bulk of available evidence suggests that mixed populations of rumen microbes attain maximum yields of cell protein when the rumen fluid has a minimum average concentration of 5 mg ammonia nitrogen/100 ml. This concentration equals 3.6 mmol ammonia per liter (Roffler and Satter, 1975b; Satter and Slyter, 1974).

Roffler and Satter (1975a) studied the influence of ration composition on mean ruminal ammonia concentrations. They collected more than 1000 samples from 211 cattle. The cattle were fed in average groups of six. Thirty-five different rations were used. The rations varied from 8 to 24 per cent crude protein (N × 6.25) and from 53 to 85 per cent TDN. CP was established by Kjeldahl analysis, and TDN was established by NRC tables. Only natural protein resources were used. A multiple regression equation was formulated as follows:

Ammonia nitrogen (mg/100 ml) = $38.73 - (3.04 \times \% \text{ CP} + (0.171 \times \% \text{ CP}^2) - (0.49 \times \% \text{ TDN}) + (0.0024 \times \% \text{ TDN}^2)$, $R^2 = 0.92$

A less precise equation has been formulated to predict ruminal ammonia concentration in sheep:

*NH_3-N (mg/100 ml) = $5.2 + (1.25 \times \% \text{ CP}) - (0.18 \times \% \text{ DDM})$, $R^2 = 0.76$

Substituting NPN for true protein in the ruminant ration results in a decreasing percentage of true protein escape, and the fraction of dietary nitrogen contributing to the rumen ammonia pool increases. As the NPN content of the ration is increased, the point of zero utilization of NPN is reached at a corresponding lower protein concentration in the ration. Thus, the point of excessive ammonia accumulation in the rumen is affected by TDN, per cent

*DDM = digestible dry matter and is equal to TDN.

Table 5. *Final DM Energy Protein Ration*

Feed	kg DM	kg As Fed	% As Fed
Corn	$1.78 - 0.147 = 1.653$	$1.653/0.88 = 1.878$	9.5
Corn-urea	$= 0.173$	$0.173/0.9 = 0.192$	1.0
Corn silage	$= 5.32$	$5.32/0.3 = 17.733$	89.5
TOTALS	7.146	19.8	100

total protein in the unsupplemented ration, and the NPN added to the ration as a crude protein supplement.

Calculations using these criteria indicate that no benefit will result from NPN supplementation if the CP per cent of a ration is greater than 8 per cent and the TDN per cent is less than 60 per cent. NPN supplementation of rations containing more than 80 per cent TDN may be used to increase the utilizable CP per cent from 8 to 11.6 per cent and from 12 to 13.6 per cent. NPN supplementation will be of no benefit in rations containing more than 13.6 per cent CP. Nor will NPN supplementation benefit low TDN rations (less than 60 per cent) to produce CP content above 8 per cent. These estimates for limitation of NPN supplementation are comparable to those of Burroughs and colleagues at Iowa State University. The current NAS-NRC publication for beef cattle (1984) recommends usage of the Satter-Roffler (1975) data to establish a relationship that determines the practical limitation for the use of urea as a crude protein supplement.

Urea potential (g/kg dry feed) = $31.64 - (3.558 \text{ CP}) + [(945 \text{ NE}_m - 887 - 179 \text{ NE}_m^2)]^{0.5}$

Where CP = crude protein per cent and NE_m = Mcal/kg DM. Thus, in a ration containing 9 per cent CP and an NE_m concentration of 1.9 Mcal/kg, the urea potential is

$31.64 - \{(3.558 \times 9) + [(945 \times 1.9) - (887) - (179 \times 1.9^2)]^{0.5}\} = 14.48$ g/kg DM

The following assumptions form the basis for the Wisconsin system of estimating metabolizable protein (Fig. 4). Some of these assumptions are well documented, but others must be considered tentative. All values are averages associated with variance.

1. The amount of nitrogen recycled into the reticulo-rumen is equal to 12 per cent of dietary nitrogen intake.

2. 85 per cent of the dietary nitrogen intake with typical ruminant rations, including protein supplements, is in the form of true protein; 15 per cent is in the form of NPN.

3. An average of 40 per cent of the true dietary protein escapes degradation in the rumen and passes to the abomasum and small intestine intact. About 87 per cent of escaped protein will be absorbed from the small intestine as amino acids. All of the dietary NPN and recycled nitrogen passes through the ruminal ammonia pool.

4. 90 per cent of all ruminal ammonia produced is incorporated into microbial nitrogen when the ration fed does not exceed the upper limit value for crude protein (ruminal ammonia does not exceed 5 mg/100 ml).

5. None of the ruminal ammonia produced in excess of 5 mg/100 ml of rumen fluid is incorporated into microbial nitrogen.

6. 80 per cent of microbial nitrogen is in true protein form, and 20 per cent is in the form of NPN and is not available to the animal as an amino acid nitrogen.

7. 80 per cent of the microbial true protein will be absorbed as metabolizable protein.

Under conditions where ruminal ammonia does not exceed microbial use, 1 kg of dietary protein produces about 750 g metabolizable protein. Of this amount, 450 g is from microbial origin and 300 g is from bypass protein origin. For the sake of simplicity, all forms of dietary nitrogen are considered to be equal when dietary protein does not exceed the upper limit of microbial utilization.

When the rumen ammonia pool exceeds the upper limit of microbial utilization, the efficiency of amino acid absorption decreases significantly. In these cases only the escaped true protein (40 per cent of total CP) is available as a source of amino acids. The metabolizable protein will be limited to $0.75 \times 0.40 = 30$ per cent of the dietary crude protein. It is assumed that the efficiency of tissue deposition will remain the same. Thus, the prediction of efficiency for dietary protein utilization above the point

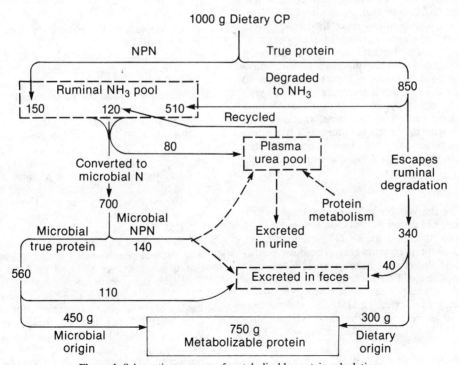

Figure 4. Schematic summary of metabolizable protein calculations.

where ruminal ammonia concentration exceeds 5 mg/100 ml of rumen fluid is $0.75 \times 0.4 \times 0.6 = 0.18$, or 18 per cent.

In summary, the efficiency of dietary protein utilization is $0.75 \times 0.6 = 0.45$, or 45 per cent, when the ruminal ammonia concentration is less than 5 mg/ml and decreases to 18 per cent when the ruminal ammonia concentration is more than 5 mg/100 ml of rumen fluid.

Crude protein concentrations in feeds are established by laboratory analysis (Kjeldahl) or by using tables from current NAS-NRC manuals. Perhaps a practical approach is to rely on the tables for concentrate analysis and use laboratory analysis to evaluate roughage.

The daily requirements for metabolizable protein include the following.

1. The maintenance requirement $= 2.4$ g/kg $BW^{0.75}$.
2. The requirement for body weight gain $= \dfrac{0.15 \text{ kg/kg gain}}{0.6}$. Such gain includes normal growth, fat deposition, and the products of conception.
3. The requirement for lactation $= \dfrac{CP \text{ in milk}}{0.6}$.

The protein requirement for dairy cows is complicated by the stage of milk production. Generally, high-producing cows will lose 30 to 70 kg of body weight in the first 40 days of lactation. This will be followed by a brief period of weight stabilization and then a gradual weight gain for the remainder of the lactation period. Lactation typically peaks about six weeks after parturition, and feed consumption peaks about 10 to 12 weeks after parturition. The ordinary diet for lactating dairy cows is high in protein (more than 13 per cent CP), also supplementary protein will be metabolized at low rates of efficiency. In early lactation when appetite is less than maximum and milk production is ascending, crude protein requirements in terms of per cent of dry diet are potentially high. Some compensation is achieved because of each kg of weight loss, 150 g metabolizable protein are made available for milk production. Undoubtedly some of the tissue protein is used for energy. The amino groups of energy contributing protein are converted to urea in the liver, and some of this urea is released into the digestive tract in saliva and rumen secretions. Such urea is probably useless to the animal owing to high rumen ammonia associated with high protein consumption typical of dairy rations. On the other hand, milk production is an efficient process relative to gestation, growth, and even maintenance. It is quite probable that a significant amount of amino acids liberated by the catabolism of body tissue is incorporated into milk protein.

Practical Application

Examples using the Wisconsin System to compute protein requirements and ration formulation follow.

1. The protein requirements for a 400-kg medium-frame steer being fed for maximum gain. The basic energy ration contains 90 per cent flaked corn ($NE_m = 2.38$ Mcal/kg DM, $Ne_g = 1.67$ Mcal/kg DM, CP = 11.2 per cent DM) and 10 per cent corn silage ($NE_m = 1.6$ Mcal/Kg, $NE_g = 1.03$ Mcal/kg DM, CP = 8 per cent DM). We will assume normal weather. NE_m requirements $= 0.077$ Mcal/kg $W^{0.75}$. DM intake $= 0.022$ W $= 8.8$ kg DM.

   a. Metabolic weight of steer: $400^{0.75} = 89.44$ kg.

   b. NE_m of basic energy ration: $(0.9 \times 2.38) + (0.1 \times 1.6) = 2.30$ Mcal/kg.

   c. NE_g of basic energy ration: $(0.9 \times 1.67) + (0.1 \times 1.03) = 1.61$ Mcal/kg.

   d. CP per cent of basic energy ration $= (0.9 \times 11.2) + (0.1 \times 8) = 10.88$ per cent.

   e. TDN per cent of basic energy ration: $(0.9 \times 95) + (0.1 \times 70) = 92.5$ per cent.

   f. NH_3 concentration in rumen fluid:

$$38.73 - (3.04 \times 10.88) + (0.171 \times 10.88^2) - (0.49 \times 92.5) + (0.0024 \times 92.5^2) = 1.11 \text{ mg/100 ml.}$$

   g. Urea potential:

$$31.64 - (3.558 \times 10.88) + ([945 \times 2.30] - 887 - 179 \times 2.30^2)^{0.5} = 11.4 \text{ g/kg DM.}$$

   We can use NPN to increase the CP per cent of the ration to more than 13 per cent without loss of metabolic efficiency.

   h. The NE_m requirement: $0.077 \times 400^{0.75} = 8.05$ Mcal.

   i. The NE_g available (RE):

$$8.8 \text{ kg} - \frac{8.05 \text{ Mcal}}{2.3} \times 1.61 \text{ Mcal} = 8.5 \text{ Mcal.}$$

   j. Estimated empty body weight gain:

$$12.341 \left(\frac{RE}{89.44}\right)^{0.9116} = 1.44 \text{ kg/day.}$$

   k. Estimated live weight gain:

$$\frac{1.44}{0.756} = 1.51 \text{ kg/day.}$$

   l. The CP requirement in grams:

$$\frac{(2.4 \times 89.44) + (1.51 \times 0.15 \times 1000)}{0.75 \times 0.6} = 981 \text{ g.}$$

   m. CP content in the basic energy ration: $0.1088 \times 8.8 = 957$ g.

   n. The CP deficiency: $981 - 957 = 24$ g. This deficiency is probably negligible, but our urea potential enables the use of urea as a CP supplement far beyond the requirement.

   One method of supplying the CP deficiency is to use a corn-urea mix (85 per cent corn, 15 per cent urea). The corn-urea mix contains about 51 per cent CP. To keep energy levels constant, it will require 100 g corn-urea mix to replace 85 g corn. Such an exchange would produce $51 - (0.112 \times 85) = 41$ g net CP gain. We need to use $24/41 \times 100 = 58.5$ g corn-urea mix to replace $24/41 \times 85 = 49.8$ g corn in the basic energy ration. The daily DM consumption is expected to increase from 8.8 to 8.809 kg.

2. The protein requirements for a 600-kg cow in mid-lactation, producing 30 kg of milk per day. The milk is assumed to contain 3.5 per cent fat and 3.3 per cent CP. We will assume a daily body weight gain of 0.2 kg/day and the NE_L requirement for maintenance of $0.08 \times BW^{0.75}$ per day. The basic energy ration dry matter contains 40 per cent ground corn ($NE_L = 2.03$ Mcal/kg, $NE_g = 1.42$ Mcal/kg, CP = 10 per cent); 30 per cent corn ensilage ($NE_L = 1.64$ Mcal/kg, $NE_g =$

1.03 Mcal/kg, CP = 8.8 per cent); and 30 per cent alfalfa hay (NE_L = 1.3 Mcal/kg, NE_g = 0.59 Mcal/kg, CP = 17.2 per cent).

a. Metabolic weight of the cow: $600^{0.75}$ = 121.23 kg.
b. NE_L of basic energy ration: 1.69 Mcal/kg DM.
c. NE_g of basic energy ration: 1.05 Mcal/kg DM.
d. CP per cent of basic energy ration: 11.8 per cent of DM.
e. TDN of basic energy ration: 74 per cent.
f. NH_3 concentration in rumen fluid:

$$38.73 - (3.04 \times 11.8) + (0.171 \times 11.8^2) - (0.49 \times 74) + (0.0024 \times 74^2) = 3.55 \text{ mg/100 ml.}$$

g. The urea potential of the ration:

$$31.64 - (3.558 \times 11.8) + ([945 \times 1.69 - 887 - 179 \times 1.69^2])^{0.5} = 3.76 \text{ g/kg DM.}$$

Urea can only be used to increase the CP per cent to about 12.6 per cent. The cow's requirement will be considerably higher, so NPN cannot be beneficially used in this ration.

h. The daily Ne_L requirement:

$$(0.08 \times 121.23) + (30 \times 0.69) = 30.4 \text{ Mcal.}$$

i. The NE_g requirement = 1.21 Mcal (NRC, 1984).
j. The estimated DM intake: $\dfrac{30.4}{1.69} + \dfrac{1.12}{1.05}$ = 19.14 kg.
k. Estimated DM intake per cent = 19.14/600 = 0.032 = 3.2 per cent BW.
l. The metabolic protein requirement:

$$(2.4 \times 121.23) + \frac{(0.033 \times 30 \times 1000)}{0.6} + \frac{(0.15 \times 0.2 \times 1000)}{0.6} = 1991 \text{ g } (1.991 \text{ kg}).$$

m. The CP requirement:
The cow will convert CP to metabolizable protein at about 75 per cent efficiency until the ruminal ammonia exceeds 5 mg/100ml of rumen fluid (CP > 12.6 per cent in DM). This means that the first 2.41 kg of CP in the diet will produce 1.81 kg metabolizable protein. It also means that 1.991 − 1.81 kg of metabolizable protein must come from escaped true protein. The crude protein necessary to increase metabolizable protein beyond 1.81 kg will be converted to metabolizable protein at 30 per cent efficiency. Thus, the total CP requirement will be $\dfrac{1.81 \text{ kg}}{0.75} + \dfrac{1.991 - 1.81}{0.30}$ = 3.02 kg.

n. The CP per cent in the final ration should be 3.20/19.14 = 15.8 per cent.
o. The basic energy ration contains 0.118×19.14 = 2.26 kg CP, which will convert to 2.26×0.75 = 1.69 kg metabolizable protein. We have a deficiency of 3.02 − 2.26 = 0.76 kg CP.

p. One method of supplying the deficiency is to substitute the least cost, high-energy, true protein supplement for corn. We will assume that soybean meal is that supplement. As most of the energy is used for maintenance and lactation, we can use NE_L to compare relative energy values: NE_L for corn = 2.03 Mcal/kg DM; NE_L for SBM = 1.86 Mcal/kg DM. Thus, it requires $2.03/1.86 \times 100$ = 109 g SBM to replace 100 g corn.

The crude protein gain = $(109 \times 0.518) - (100 \times 0.1)$ = 46.5 g for each 100 g corn replaced. The CP deficiency of our basic energy ration is 0.76 kg (760 g). We will need to replace $\dfrac{760}{46.5} \times 100$ = 1634 g (1.63 kg) of corn with 1634×1.09 = 1781 g (1.78 kg) of SBM to supply the CP deficiency and maintain the energy requirement. Our final dry matter ration will include:

Corn $(19.41 \times 0.4) - 1.63$	= 6.03 kg
SBM	= 1.78 kg
Corn silage 19.14×0.3	= 5.74 kg
Alfalfa 19.14×0.3	= 5.75 kg
	19.29 kg

The total CP =

$$(6.03 \times 0.1) + (1.78 \times 0.518) + (5.74 \times 0.088) + (5.74 \times 0.172) = 3.02 \text{ kg.}$$

The CP per cent = 3.02/19.29 = 15.6 per cent.

Comparing our two examples with NRC recommendations (NRC, 1978, 1984) we get the data that appears in Table 6.

Two tables have been designed for practical applications of the Wisconsin System (Satter and Roffler, 1976). We have summarized these tables (Tables 7 and 8).

In summary, the results obtained using the Wisconsin System are very similar to those obtained using the factorial systems recommended by the NAS-NRC publications (NRC, 1978, 1984). The advantage of the Wisconsin System is its simplicity. No tables to show degradability of individual or mixed feeds are necessary. The aim of the system is practical application in a variety of situations. From a critical standpoint, the estimation of recycled urea nitrogen (12 per cent) is quite high relative to other systems. Also, the Wisconsin System assumes a constant percentage of protein in gain and a constant percentage of degradability in all feeds and mixtures of feeds. These assumptions differ significantly from those of other systems.

The Cornell System

The Cornell System is possibly the most sophisticated and forward-looking of those reviewed. Other proposed systems are based on static models that assume fixed rates of protein degradation and microbial synthesis in the rumen. They also assume fixed rates of protein digestion

***Table 6.** Protein Requirements: NRC versus Wisconsin System*

Class	BW (kg)	Gain (kg/day)	Milk Prod (kg)	NRC Reqmt CP (kg)	Wisconsin System Reqmt CP (kg)
Beef steer	400	1.5	—	0.978	0.981
Dairy cow	600	0.2	30	3.37	3.02

$$*\text{NRC requirement} = \frac{(2.75 \times 600^{0.5})}{0.45} + \frac{(0.03 \times 19290)}{0.45} + \frac{(0.2 \times 600^{0.5})}{0.45} + \frac{(0.2 \times 160)}{0.45} + \frac{(30 \times 0.032)}{0.52} = 3374 \text{ g} = 3.37 \text{ kg.}$$

Table 7. *Upper Limit for NPN Utilization*

CP % in Basic DM Ration*	TDN % 55–60	TDN % 60–65	TDN % 65–70	TDN % 70–75	TDN % 75–80	TDN % 80–85
			(% CP after NPN Addition)			
8	NB*	10	10.5	10.9	11.2	11.4
9	NB	10.4	10.9	11.3	11.6	11.8
10	NB	10.8	11.3	11.7	12	12.2
11	NB	11.2	11.7	12.1	12.4	12.6
12	NB	NB	12.1	12.5	12.8	13.0

*No benefit.

and absorption in the small intestine. The Cornell System presents a dynamic model that assumes variations in these criteria caused by differences in feed intake, energy concentrations, diet mixtures, and rates of flow of ingesta through the digestive tract.

Rumen Dynamics

Plant cells are degraded (starch and cellulose → short chain fatty acids) in the forestomachs of ruminant animals. The rate and degree of this degradation are related to feed intake and digestibility (Mertens, 1973). The rate of cell wall degradation competes with passage from the rumen. Slow rates of degradation and rapid rates of flow from the rumen lead to depressions of digestibility and fecal losses (Van Soest, 1975). Depressions of digestibility are characteristic of high feed intake. These depressions appear to be the result of ruminal escape of plant cell wall without degradation.

In ruminants dietary protein is also affected by variable rates of degradation (proteins → volatile fatty acids and ammonia), but the consequences are quite different. Complex carbohydrates that escape degradation in the rumen have reduced chances of digestion and absorption from the small intestine. There are no pancreatic or enteric enzymes that can digest cellulose. In contrast, true protein that escapes ruminal degradation is utilized more efficiently than is microbial protein synthesized in the rumen from the degradation products of carbohydrate, dietary protein, and NPN.

The relative inefficiency of microbial protein utilization results because the rumen microbes may degrade true protein beyond their needs for cell synthesis. The products of excess degradation are ammonia and volatile fatty acids. These are not available to produce amino acids in the abomasum and intestines. In addition, more than 30 per cent of microbial crude protein is in the form of NPN. Such includes RNA, DNA, capsular peptides, and glyco proteins. This microbial NPN is not available for amino acid synthesis and thus is not a source of metabolizable protein for the animal. The chief benefit of rumen microbes is to convert dietary and recycled NPN into microbial protein in the rumen.

The relative efficiency of escaped protein has stimulated research aimed at increasing ruminal escape of dietary protein. It has been assumed that insoluble proteins are less likely to be degraded in the rumen. Heat or formaldehyde is sometimes used to reduce protein solubility in the rumen and thus increase the percentage of relatively efficient escape or bypass protein. This concept can be questioned in several respects (Pichard and Van Soest, 1977; Mahadevan et al., 1980).

1. Many feedstuffs contain NPN that is the most soluble crude protein fraction.

2. Most heat- or formaldehyde-treated feedstuffs contain increased amounts of bound unavailable nitrogen.

3. Both forages and concentrates contain buffer-insoluble proteins that have very fast rates of degradation in the rumen.

4. Feedstuffs also may contain soluble proteins that have slow rates of degradation.

Treatment to increase bypass protein will not likely have a positive effect if microbial protein synthesis is limited by the treatment.

Animal data suggest that microbial yields vary significantly. In general they are larger with high-quality forage–based diets as compared with high concentrate diets. Diets producing low microbial yields appear to be fermented or overprotected by heat or formaldehyde. The decreased utilization of fermented feeds may be related to increased percentages of unavailable nitrogen content. Microbial yields may also be limited by the lack of readily available carbohydrate. The capacity of microbes to increase protein quality (synthesize essential amino acids) is also worthy of consideration.

Feed Analysis

The Cornell System classifies feed nitrogen into three biological groups: soluble nitrogen (fraction A), available true proteins (fraction B), and bound unavailable nitrogen (fraction C).

The B fraction is subdivided into groups. These include (1) proteins that are rapidly degraded in the rumen (B_1), (2) proteins that are degraded in the rumen at intermediate rates (B_2), and (3) proteins that are degraded slowly in the rumen (B_3). The B fractions are the only feed nitrogen sources that are relevant to escape estimates.

The C fraction is composed of Maillard products, leather (tannin-protein condensates), and liquified nitro-

Table 8. *Dietary CP Where Ruminal Ammonia Equals 5 mg/100 ml Rumen Fluid*

Species	DDM %* 50–55	DDM % 55–60	DDM % 60–65	DDM % 65–70	DDM % 70–75	DDM % 75–80	DDM % 80–85
			Rumen NH₃-N/100 ml = 5 mg at				
Cattle	—	—	10.3% CP	11.8% CP	12.6% CP	13.2% CP	13.6%CP
Sheep	7.4% CP	8.1% CP	8.8% CP	.9.6% CP	10.3% CP	11.0% CP	11.7% CP

*DDM = digestible dry matter; DDM is practically synonymous with TDN.

gen. In fermented feeds the A and C fractions may be increased by depeletion of the B fraction. Use of crude protein values in ration formulation from feeds containing these damaged ingredients may cause underfeeding of usable nitrogen.

The Rumen Model

The rumen model used in the Cornell System (Fox et al., 1979) is based on the total disappearance of protein from the digestive tract by absorption and passage. Ruminal escape and microbial yield are treated as variables. Figure 5 outlines the rumen submodel. Figure 6 outlines the conceptual model of the net protein system for ration formulation.

Rumen Degradation Rates

The determination of protein degradation rates is complex. The generalities of the procedures include the following.

1. Total nitrogen is determined by the Kjeldahl method.

2. The A fraction is determined as NPN by means of tungstic acid precipitation.

3. Bound unavailable nitrogen (fraction C) is determined as acid detergent fiber nitrogen (ADFN) (Goering and Van Soest, 1970).

4. The B fraction is determined by subtracting the A and C fractions from total nitrogen. B = total N − (fraction A + fraction C). The B fraction is referred to as "residual available protein" (RAP).

The individual degradabilities of the various fractions are measured by the use of microbial proteases in a sterile system.

The partition of the available true protein (fraction B) into subfractions and their inherent rates of digestion are obtained from the mathematical analysis of time-sequence digestion measurements. The fractional rate for the NPN fraction (A) is considered to be infinite and is not used in any calculation. The B fractions show considerable variation among the various feedstuffs. For example, corn shows a single slow digesting pool (B_3); soybean meal shows two faster digesting fractions (B_1 and B_2); whereas timothy and brewers grain show B_1, B_2, and B_3 fractions. The heating of a feedstuff can have substantial effect on proteolytic rates and the distribution of the respective fractions.

Examples of digestion rates calculated from log plots of protease degradation measurements published in the Proceedings of the International Symposium on Protein Requirements for Cattle, 1980 (Van Soest) are shown in Table 9.

Potentially Digestible Organic Matter

To simplify the model, all fermentable organic matter constituents are aggregated into a single component called potentially digestible organic matter (PDOM). PDOM is calculated as:

$$PDOM = 100 - (2.4\ \text{lignin} + \text{ash}).$$

Lignin multiplied by 2.4 represents the indigestible organic matter associated with lignin (Mertens, 1973). The rates of digestion and lag times for PDOM are approximated from kinetic information for fiber digestion (Mertens, 1973; Van Soest and Robertson, unpublished) and nonstructural carbohydrate (Hungate, 1966).

Rates of passage (K_p) are estimated for each feed

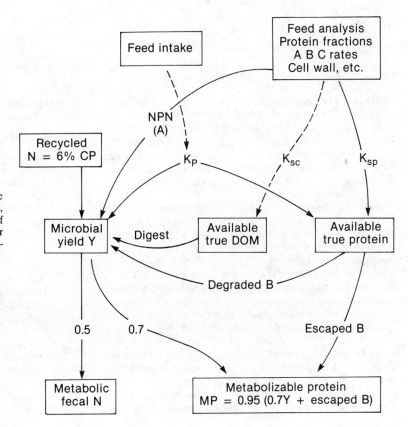

Figure 5. The rumen submodel. K_{sp} is the fractional rate of proteolysis for each protein, and K_{sc} is the fractional rate of digestion of carbohydrate. Dashed lines indicate features for which information is incomplete and more research is needed.

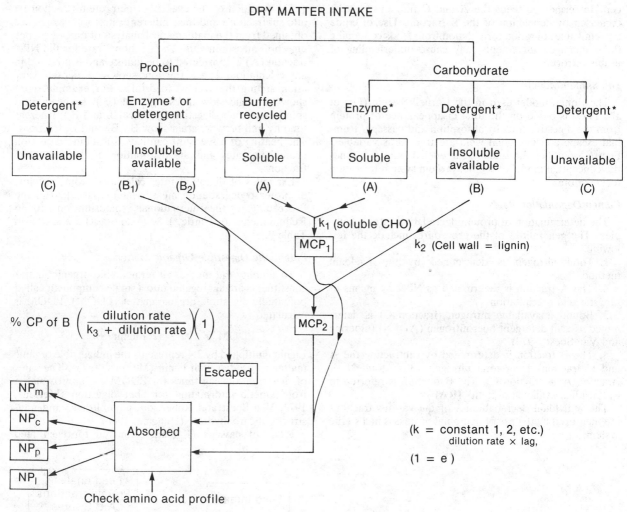

Figure 6. Net protein system for cattle. (Data from Fox, D. G., Sniffen, C. J., Van Soest, P. J., and Robinson, P. H. Proc. Okla. Protein Symposium, 1981.) *Van Soest system of feed analysis.

ingredient at each intake level (Hartnell and Satter, 1979; Colucci, 1979; Owens et al., 1979). Rates were estimated to be faster for feeds of small particle size and high density (concentrates faster than forages) and for high feed intakes. Liquid turnover rates are estimated from literature values for lactating cows and beef cattle. Rates of passage of liquids vary according to levels of productivity and frame size of the animal.

Rates of passage for liquids are important variables. They are used to estimate microbial protein yield per unit of fermented organic matter. There is significant variability among and within experiments designed to analyze liquid turnover (Hartnell and Satter, 1979; Colucci, 1979; Owens et al., 1979). It does not seem probable that a predictive relationship between liquid turnover and body weight, forage, concentrate, or DM intake can be developed, but some general conclusions can be made.

There appear to be two distinct groups of liquid rates of passage. Animals restricted to DM intakes of less than 2 per cent of body weight had low rates of liquid passage. Animals fed *ad libitum* with DM intakes of more than 2 per cent of body weight showed more variation in rates of liquid passage. There was a trend toward increase of passage with increased intake, but the r² values were low.

It is probable that factors other than body weight and intake influence rates of liquid passage.

Mathematical Considerations

1. PDOM = 100 (2.4 lignin + ash).
2. Fractional escapes:
   a. Digestion and passage rates are proportional to substrate concentration (Mertens, 1973; Waldo et al., 1972), leading to the general differential equation

   $$\frac{-ds}{dt} = S(K_s + K_p)$$

   where K_s and K_p are rates of digestion and passage, respectively, and S is substrate concentration in the rumen. The proportion of substrate (S) escaping rumen fermentation is a function of the competition between digestion and passage. Theoretically, S is a constant for any given feeding situation.
   b. Each escape function applies only to uniform feed fractions that have similar digestion and passage rates. $E = \dfrac{K_p}{K_p + K_s}$.

Table 9. *Digestion Rates*

Feed	% Total Crude Protein	Fraction	% DM	% B
Corn	9.93	A	1.1	—
		B_3	8.3	100
		C	0.5	—
Soybean meal	54.8	A	11.15	—
		B_1	33.6	81
		B_2	7.9	19
		C	2.2	—
Brewers grains	31.73	A	2.6	—
		B_1	18.3	71
		B_2	7.5	29
		C	3.3	—
Timothy	8.09	A	2.1	—
		B_1	1.5	27
		B_2	1.2	22
		B_3	2.7	51
		C	0.6	—
Wheat middlings	19.07	A	11.54	—
		B_1	4.42	59
		B_2	1.05	14
		B_3	2.03	27
		C	0.63	—

c. The protein fractions (B_1, B_2, B_3) in the diet will have different digestion rates but possibly similar passage co-efficients. Dairy cattle on mixed diets appear to have three main passage pools: liquids, concentrate fiber (may include insoluble proteins and starch), and coarse fiber. The rate of passage decreases in that order. The total escape of protein, then, will be the sum of the respective component feed fractions classified according to their particular digestion and passage rates. To calculate total escape of true protein (TPE), all escape fractions must be multiplied by their respective protein substrate concentrations in the feed (B_1) and the DM intake (A). The total escape is described by the following equation:

$$TPE = \sum_{i=1}^{n} B_i A \left(\frac{K_{pi}}{K_{si} + K_{pi}} \right)$$

3. Lag effects:
The primary objective of biochemical analysis of feedstuffs is to characterize the limitation of the substrate. Therefore, protease measurements must be operated under conditions of limiting substrate (excess enzyme). However, evidence indicates that the rumen may not be substrate, limited especially during fermentation periods when microbial numbers are low. For this reason a lag function has been introduced into the model (Mertens, 1977):

$$P_i = e^{K_{pi} L_i} \text{ and } FE_i = L - e^{K_{pi} L_i}$$

where P_i is the proportion of protein remaining when digestion begins, K_{pi} is rate of passage, L_i is the lag time in hours, and FE_i is the fraction that escapes

during the digestion lag. These lag functions are incorporated into the TPE equation as follows:

$$TPEL = \sum_{i=1}^{n} (B_i) (A) \left[\left(\frac{K_{pi}}{K_{si} + K_{pi}} \right) (P_i) + FE_i \right]$$

where TPEL = total true protein escaped with lag effect.

Comparison of protease degradation rates with proteolytic activity suggests that adding the lag effect brings the estimate of protein escape into reasonable approximation with *in vivo* results. The concentration of enzyme used in the protease procedure is the amount required to saturate soybean meal (about 6 mg/ml). About 80 per cent of the soybean protein is hydrolyzed in one hour. These rates are much faster than those reported for the rumen using the azocasein technique (Mahadaven et al., 1979)

Assay of rumen fluid meaures only the free proteolytic activity in the rumen. If maximum proteolysis occurs when microbes are in close proximity to protein, then it is likely that there is a lag in proteolysis when microbial numbers are low or microbes are not in close association with protein particles.

4. Microbial protein output from the rumen:
In order to calculate the amount of microbial protein that can be produced during fermentation in the rumen, the amount of potentially digestible organic matter that is fermented in the rumen must be estimated. An equation to measure true fermented organic matter (TFOM) has been derived (Mertens, 1977) as follows:

$$TFOM = (A) \frac{(PDOM)}{100} \left(\frac{K_s}{K_s + K_p} \right) (e^{\kappa} p^L)$$

where TFOM = true fermented organic matter, A = DM feed intake, and K_s, K_p, and L = digestion rate, passage rate, and lag time of PDOM, respectively. Microbial protein output (MICP) from rumen fermentation is calculated by multiplying microbial yield (MY) by the amount of TFOM.

MY in g protein/100 g TFOM =

$$(6.25) \left(\frac{1}{0.14 + 0.015\ K_{Liq}} \right)$$

Where K_{Liq} is the fractional rate of liquid passage from the rumen. Microbial protein output is calculated by the equation MICP = (TFOM) (MY). Fecal metabolic nitrogen loss is calculated as indigestible microbial matter according to Mason (1979) and Mason and Fredricksen (1979).

Model Simulation Results

Model simulations predict the following.

1. Milk yields greater than 33 kg/day can be better predicted by dynamic microbial yield and dietary escape estimates than by conventional methods.

2. Microbial yield and rumen escape are confounded in animal responses obtained at higher feed intakes.

3. Animal response to increased metabolizable protein depends on the animal's requirement for amino acid nitrogen being greater than the nitrogen requirement of rumen microbes.

4. The requirements for metabolizable protein of most ruminants are probably lower than the nitrogen required by rumen microbes. Exceptions include very rapidly growing young ruminants and perhaps high-producing dairy cattle (Orskov, 1976).

5. Ruminants with metabolizable protein requirements lower than those required by rumen microbes are energy limited and will respond to monensin or other methanogenic inhibitors that reduce microbial yields (Poos et al., 1979). Response to antimethanogens is not expected when animal protein requirements exceed the nitrogen required by rumen microbes.

6. The response to NPN is variable depending on microbial requirements and nitrogen supply. Overprotection of dietary nitrogen will cause rumen fermentation to become nitrogen limiting and theoretically responsive to any level of urea addition. It has been observed that milk production decreases when higher levels of insoluble protein are included in the diet (Davis, 1978). The exact value for the dietary NPN equivalent for recycled nitrogen is not known. This value is probably reduced when digestible nitrogen sources are lacking, and the basal value is probably about 6 per cent of crude protein equivalent (the level at which digestibility and intake are reduced in low-protein diets) (Milford and Minson, 1965; Ellis and Lippke, 1976).

Alternate Nitrogen Fractionization Systems

Fractionization of protein is an important input to the rumen submodel. There is an alternative to using proteases to measure protein degradation. True protein can be divided into soluble and insoluble parts in acid detergent (AD) and neutral detergent (ND). This scheme avoids the technical expertise and standardization needed for biologic systems. Classifications include the following.

1. Protein soluble in ND is a constituent of cell solubles and would have a fast rate of digestion (B_1).

2. Protein insoluble in ND but soluble in AD is completely available but is digested at a slower rate than the ND soluble fraction and corresponds to the B_2 fraction. This fraction is markedly affected by heating and processing (Pichard and Van Soest, 1977). Protein insoluble in AD is unavailable and represents the C fraction. The ND-AD method of measuring protein degradation in the rumen is based on the large range in ND-insoluble nitrogen that is observed in feedstuffs. Also, feedstuffs contain a variable mixture of protein types with differing solubility characteristics. The analysis is simpler than the protease procedure but has less accuracy and theoretical meaning. Also, knowledge is lacking about the proteins that are insoluble in ND. Whatever system is used, the quantitative partition of the nitrogen fraction into A, B_1, B_2, and C portions is required. The estimation of kinetic digestion rates is only applicable to the B fractions. The rate for A (NPN) is not relevant since it can only be converted into microbial protein and rumen escape of A has no meaning. The rate for fraction C is assumed to be zero.

Summary

The Cornell submodel dynamically models protein digestion based on rates of passage and digestion. The operation of the system requires a more precise definition of nitrogen fractions than can be obtained from solubility measurements. The model offers the possibility of a more flexible method of predicting responses of ruminants to various diets. However, it generates the need for requisite dietary feed information.

The people at Cornell have taken a stepwise approach to develop a net protein system that (1) accurately describes the actual net protein needs for maintenance, weight gain, pregnancy, and milk production; (2) allows accurate calculation of the net protein value of individual feedstuffs in a specific diet; and (3) determines supplemental protein needs from chemical analysis of individual feedstuffs in the diet. The developmental steps include:

1. To develop a conceptually correct model that is closely related to physiologic function. Also, the model must lend itself to laboratory analysis to adjust feed values for various field conditions.

2. To develop a computer program for purposes of sensitivity analysis to determine which estimates of physiologic function have the greatest impact and to identify those that need more refinement.

3. To validate the program with field experimentation.

4. To develop a program for microcomputers that can be used over a wide array of conditions.

ANIMAL REQUIREMENTS

The protein content of tissue or milk determines the dietary protein requirements of each animal. These requirements are met by combining feeds to meet microbial protein needs and provide escaped protein as needed to supplement microbial protein. Amounts and forms of energy consumed and dilution rates of energy substrates in the rumen determine maximum rates of microbial synthesis and growth.

Determining the protein requirement for a specific situation is a stepwise procedure.

1. The first step is to ensure that adequate protein is provided to optimize energy utilization for microbial protein synthesis.

2. Then feed sources high in escape protein are substituted into the diet for highly degraded protein sources if:
   a. microbial protein output is maximal, and
   b. tissue or milk requirements are not met.
3. When microbial and tissue needs are met, an amino acid profile can be calculated to check for any deficiencies or inbalances.

The equation of Smuts (1935) is used to estimate metabolizable protein required for maintenance (NP_m): $NP_m = (70.4 \text{ wt/kg}^{0.735}) (0.0125)$.

The requirements for microbial protein synthesis are assumed to be equal to the maximum microbial protein that can be synthesized each day. The protein available to meet this requirement is dietary NPN, recycled nitrogen (assumed to be equal to NP_m), and degraded B fraction protein. The following input information is required to calculate microbial protein synthesis and feed protein escaping degradation in the rumen.

1. Dry matter intake.
2. Concentrations of the protein subfractions including nonprotein nitrogen (NPN) and protein rapidly available (B_1), intermediate in availability (B_2), slowly available (B_3), and unavailable (C).
3. Concentrations of the energy fractions (available and unavailable fiber, fat, and rapidly available and unavailable carbohydrates).
4. Rates of digestion for each protein and energy fraction.
5. Rates of passage for liquids and solids (see mathematical considerations).

Determination of net protein required for weight gain (NP_g) is a two-step procedure as follows:

1. Determine energy allowable gain.

The system described by Fox and Black (1984) is used to predict daily gain allowable by the dietary energy intake. This predicted gain becomes the daily gain used to calculate the NP_g requirement. In this system the NRC NE_m requirement equation (NRC, 1976) is adjusted for environmental and breed effects. The weight used in the modified equation is called the animal's equivalent weight. The weight of various frame sizes and sexes is multiplied by an adjustment factor to determine the weight of an average-frame steer having the same body composition. This equivalent weight is then used in the NE_g equation to determine the daily NE_g requirement. Use of this procedure eliminates the need for separate equations for each cattle type.

Dry matter intake is assumed to be 100 g/wt $kg^{0.75}$. Actual intake declines linearly after animals achieve about 22 per cent body fat and as net energy concentration in the diet increases above 1.27 Mcal/kg DM feed. Adjustment is made for use of growth stimulants, feed additives, body condition, and environment (Fox and Black, 1984).

2. Determine protein allowable gain.

The net dietary protein available for weight gain is a summation of absorbed microbial and escaped protein adjusted for metabolic losses. Those who formulated the Cornell System say that "further study is still required to determine if these values are appropriate for all ages and physiological states." Net protein requirements are calculated by the equation $(0.235 - 0.00026 \text{ W}) (\text{DG})$ where DG = kg

expected daily gain and W = equivalent weight in kg (Fox et al., 1977). This expression was developed from the body composition equation of Simpfendorfer (1974) $Y = 0.235 \text{ X} - 0.00013 \text{ X}^2 - 2.418$ where Y = protein per cent expressed as a decimal and X = body weight in kg.

Validation trials have shown that energy concentrations in the diet influence protein requirements. For example, trials on 144 steer calves showed that protein composition of the gain was 14.2 per cent when ration grain content was less than 50 per cent of DM, 13.1 per cent when ration grain content was 50 to 80 per cent of DM, and 12.8 per cent when ration grain content was more than 80 per cent of DM.

The Cornell net protein system was accurate in predicting protein content of the gain when high-silage diets were fed (predicted = 14 to 14.5 per cent; actual = 14.2 per cent). The system overestimated protein gain when cattle were fed high-grain diets continually from weaning (predicted = 14 to 14.5 per cent; actual = 13 per cent). This difference would result in an increase of 0.5 per cent in the crude protein requirements. Thus, it would seem that the error in not adjusting body protein gain for feeding high-grain rations is small.

APPLICATION USING A MICROCOMPUTER

The following shows the input/output of computer programs that are being developed at Cornell University to evaluate and test the net protein system described. Field application is also demonstrated. Data from two forms of soybeans were compared (raw versus 135° C heat treatment) when fed to young calves. Alternate runs of the program were used to demonstrate the program operation and how it can be used to evaluate diets. Actual performance is listed next to predicted performance.

1. Enter profile of animal characteristics:
   a. Age (1 = calf; 2 = yearling): 1
   b. Sex (1 = steer; 2 = heifer; 3 = bull): 1
   c. Breed (1 = beef; 2 = Holstein cross; 3 = Holstein): 3
   d. Frame size (1 = small; 5 = average; 9 = large): 9
   e. No of feeding periods (1 to 6): 1
   f. Quality of animals' environment: 7
      (1) = no shelter, extended period of mud/cold
      (5) = no shelter, lot well drained
      (7) = no stress
   g. Body condition (1 = fleshy; 5 = average; 9 = thin): 5
   h. Average weight = 330 lb
   i. Per cent of standard intake: 104 first treatment, 110 second treatment
   j. Feed additives and growth stimulants:
      (1) = none
      (2) = antibiotics
      (3) = estrogens (heifers)
      (4) = estrogens or Ralgro (steers); Ralgro (heifers)
      (5) = rumensin
      (6) = rumensin plus antibiotics
      (7) = rumensin plus estrogens (heifers)
      (8) = rumensin + estrogens or Ralgro (steers): 4

Table 10. Protein Profile for Soybeans

Fraction	% DM	K_s	Lag time (hr)
Raw			
Soluble	18	99	0.3
B_1	5	2.55	0.5
B_2	15.5	0.12	1.5
B_3	0	0	0
Bound	3.5	0	99
Roasted			
Soluble	3.5	99	0.3
B_1	0	0	0
B_2	16.6	0.12	1.5
B_3	2	0	99
Bound	2	0	99

Note: K_s = degradation rate, % hr.
Lag time = hours before degradation begins.

2. Enter feedstuff descriptions:
This section is for feed data entry. Data for feeds typically used can be stored. Only minor changes are necessary as diets are reformulated. The user can also call in a feed from a feed dictionary that includes average values for NE_m, NE_g, ADF, Ca, P, Mg, K, Na, Cl, S, Zn, Fe, Cu, Mn, Se, and vitamins A, D, and E. The various energy and protein fraction values outlined previously are included. The user can adjust only the values that can be obtained from feed analysis. The protein profile for two types of soybeans (raw and roasted) is listed in Table 10.
3. Enter ration description (Table 11):
Feeding management for protein supplement: 3
(1) = once/day
(2) = twice/day
(3) = total mixed ration
4. Results of computer analysis:
a. Growth and intake predictions (Table 12).
b. Comparable gain predictions and actual gains (Table 13).
c. Protein classification analysis (Table 14).
d. Daily gains of Holstein calves as influenced by weight, dietary energy, and supplemental protein source (Table 15).
As shown in the protein profile (Table 10), predicted energy allowable gain was about 9 per cent less on the raw soybean–supplemented ration. This results from a 6 per cent lower daily intake. The predicted protein allowable gain was 29 per cent less with the raw soybean ration. In the raw soybean–supplemented ration actual daily gain was limited by available protein. In the roasted soybean–supplemented ration the protein allowable gain was similar to the energy allowable gain, indicating that neither protein nor energy would be wasted. The object of the program is to analyze the key factors known to affect performance and then supplement at a level that is neither limiting or wasted.

Table 11. Ration Description

Ingredient	% of Ration Dry Matter	
	1st Analysis	*2nd Analysis*
Corn silage	72	72
Supplement 380	3.8	3.8
Raw soybeans	23.2	—
Roasted soybeans	—	23.2
Calcium carbonate	1.0	1.0

Table 12. Growth and Intake Predictions

Statistic	1st Analysis Raw Soybeans	2nd Analysis Roasted Soybeans
Animal body weight (lb)	330	330
Energy allowable gain (lb/day)	2.84	3.09
Actual feed DMH (lb/day)		
Corn silage	6.99	7.4
Supplement 380	0.37	0.39
Raw soybeans	2.25	—
Roasted soybeans	—	2.38
Calcium carbonate	0.10	0.10
TOTALS	9.71	10.27

The protein profile helps identify some of the dietary factors involved in the lower availability of net protein from the raw soybeans. Both diets contained 16 per cent crude protein, but the actual crude protein intake was 5.8 per cent higher with the roasted soybeans because of increased dry matter intake. In addition, net protein intake was 24.8 per cent higher with the roasted soybean–supplemented diet because a higher proportion of the roasted beans escaped degradation in the rumen. One gram of escape protein yields 0.54 g net protein, whereas 1 g microbial protein yields only 0.39 g net protein. However, caution must be taken that the amount of degraded protein available in the rumen is adequate to support the microbial growth that is predicted to be synthesized from the predicted digestible organic matter. The available degraded protein should be equal to or exceed that needed to support microbial growth. Otherwise, fiber digestion would be depressed and performance would be reduced.

MODEL EVALUATION

Development and refinement of the protein model continue to be ongoing processes. The biologic systems being described are very complex, and there is a need for more complete data in many areas. Nevertheless, a number of general observations can be made based on simulations with the model and evaluations to date.
1. Reducing dietary protein rumen degradability to meet animal protein requirements will have the greatest affect in calves under 270 kg equivalent weight and in dairy cows producing over 33 kg milk per day. This is especially true if the diet contains a high proportion of fermented forage. Table 15 summarizes the results of a series of experiments (unpublished data, D. G. Fox, Cornell Univ.) with young light Holstein steers fed a wide range of diets. Light calves fed all corn silage diets were very responsive to the provision of dietary escape protein. The corn silage–based diet is high in protein fractions that will be degraded in the rumen. Those fed the dry shelled corn diet were more sensitive to reduced ruminal nitrogen when both basal and

Table 13. Comparable Gain Predictions and Actual Gains

Statistics	1st Analysis Raw Soybeans	2nd Analysis Roasted Soybeans
Energy allowable gain (lb/day)	2.84	3.09
Protein allowable gain (lb/day)	2.3	2.96
Actual daily gain (270–440 lb)	(2.28)	(3.04)

Table 14. *Protein Classification Analysis*

| | 1st Analysis | | 2nd Analysis | |
| | Raw Soybeans | | Roasted Soybeans | |
Category	Required	Avail	Required	Avail
Net protein (g)	296	246	319	307
Crude protein (g)	?	711	?	752
Rapidly degraded (g)	?	340	?	172
Slowly degraded (g)	?	85	?	96
Total microbial (g)	?	425	?	286
Feed escaped (g)	?	145	?	373

supplemental protein sources were low in rumen degradability. It is apparent that protein fractions must be balanced to meet both microbial and animal requirements. It is also apparent that a dynamic model that can take into account variation in protein fractions between and within individual feedstuffs and changes in dry matter intake is also essential. The data of Thomas and associates (1983) demonstrate the impact of variation in protein fractions in corn silage on performance.

2. The metabolic protein requirements of cattle at later stages of growth or lower levels of milk production will often be met or exceeded if nitrogen requirements of rumen microorganisms are met.
3. Minimum dietary protein concentration needed to maximize rumen fermentation and thus dry matter intake will vary with the diet. For example, model predictions indicate that dietary protein must equal at least 9 per cent in high corn silage diets but only 6 to 7 per cent in hay diets. These predictions agree with protein levels at which dry matter intake is maximized (Lomas et al., 1982; Milford and Minson, 1965).
4. Cattle should be grouped for feeding according to their stage of growth and level of production. Such grouping is necessary to match both total dietary protein and protein sources required to properly meet both microbial and animal requirements.
5. A complex dynamic biologic model can be applied in

the field because of the availability and acceptance of powerful microcomputers by livestock producers.
6. The major area still needing refinement before this model can be directly applied on a wide basis is the rumen submodel. Improved methods are needed to:
   a. Identify protein and carbohydrate fractions with routine laboratory analysis.
   b. Predict degradation rates and turnover rates for liquids and solids. These are key components necessary to accurate prediction of microbial yield and escaped true dietary protein.
   c. Determine if and how efficiency of use of absorbed nitrogen varies with physiologic state (growth, pregnancy, lactation).

Supplemental Reading

Baldwin, R. L., and Denham, S. C.: Quantitative and dynamic aspects of nitrogen metabolism in the rumen: A modeling analysis. J. Anim. Sci. 49:1631, 1979.

Brisson, G. J., Cunningham, H. M., and Haskell, S. R.: The protein and energy requirements of young dairy calves. J. Anim. Sci. 37:157, 1957.

Blaxter, K. L.: Protein metabolism and requirements in pregnancy and lactation. In Munro, H. N. (ed): Mammalian Protein Metabolism, Vol. 2. New York, Academic Press, 173–223, 1964.

Burroughs, W., Nelson, D. K., and Mertens, D. R.: Protein physiology and its application in the lactating cow: The metabolizable protein feeding standard. J. Anim. Sci. 41:933, 1975.

Burroughs, W., Trenkle, W. A., and Vetter, R.: Metabolizable Protein (Amino Acid) Feeding Standard for Cattle and Sheep Fed Rations Containing Either Alpha Amino or Nonprotein Nitrogen. Iowa State Univ. Coop Ext. Serv. A. S. Leaflet R190, 1974.

Colucci, R. D.: Rate of passage of digesta through the gastrointestinal tract of cattle. M. S. Thesis, Cornell University, 1979.

Davis, R. F.: Response of dairy cattle to ration protein of different solubilities. Proc. MD Nutr. Conf., 116–120, 1978.

Ellis, W. C., and Lippke, H.: Nutritional value of forages. In Grasses and Legumes in Texas—Development, Production and Utilization. Texas Agr. Exp. Sta. Res. Monog., 26–66, 1976.

Fox, D. G., and Black, J. R.: A system to predict body composition and performance of growing cattle. J. Anim. Sci. 58:725–730, 1984.

Fox, D. G., Crickenberger, R. G., Bergen, W. G., and Black, J. R.: A net protein system for predicting protein requirements and feed protein values for growing cattle. Mich. Agri. Exp. Sta. Rpt. 328:141, 1977.

Fox, D. G., Sniffen, C. J., Van Soest, P. J., and Robinson, P. H.: A net protein system for formulating beef and dairy rations. Proc. Cornell Nutr. Conf., 57, 62, 1979.

Table 15. *Daily Gains of Holstein Calves as Influenced by Weight, Dietary Energy, and Supplemental Protein Source***

| | Supplemental Protein Source‡ | | | |
Growth Price† (kg)	Urea	Raw SB	50:50	High Roast
Experiment 1 (corn-silage–based diet)				
124–242 kg	—	0.99	1.02	1.15
242–548 kg	—	0.97	0.96	0.96
Experiment 2 (corn silage–based diet)				
96–251 kg	0.97	1.07	1.2	1.23
251–423 kg	1.04	1.05	0.97	1.01
Experiment 3 (corn silage–based diet)				
92–275 kg	0.85	1.05	—	1.15
Experiment 4 (high-moisture cor–based diet)				
167–243 kg	1.30	1.29	1.35	1.45
243–390 kg	0.91	0.88	0.83	0.90
Experiment 5 (dry shelled corn–based diet)				
102–245 kg	1.15	1.06	—	1.18
245–335 kg	1.35	1.29	—	1.23

*From unpublished data, D. G. Fox, Cornell University.

†Each value represents the mean of three pens of four Holstein steer calves each.

‡Raw or high roast = form of whole soybeans; high roast = heated to 135°C; 50:50 = one half raw and one half heated soybeans.

Fox, D. G., Sniffen, C. J., Van Soest, P. J., and Robinson, P. H.: Net protein system for cattle. Proc. Okla. Protein Symposium, 1981.

Fox, D. G., Sniffen, C. J., and Van Soest, P. J.: Proc. Georgia Nutr. Conf., 1984.

Goering, H. K., and Van Soest, P. J.: Forage Fiber Analyses (Apparatus, Reagents, Procedures and Some Applications). Agric. Handbook No. 379. Washington, D.C., Agr. Res. Ser. USDA, 1970.

Glover, J., Duthie, D. W., and French, M. H.: The apparent digestibility of crude protein by the ruminant I.A. Synthesis of the results of digestibility trials with herbage and mixed feeds. J. Agric. Sci. 48:373, 1957.

Hartnell, G. F., and Satter, L. D.: Determination of rumen fill, retention time and ruminal turnover rates of ingesta at different stages of lactation in dairy cows. J. Anim. Sci. 48:381, 1979.

Hogan, J. P., and Weston, R. H.: Quantitative aspects of microbial protein synthesis in the rumen. In Phillipson, A. T. (ed.): Physiology of Digestion and Metabolism in the Ruminant. Newcastle-upon-Tyne, England, Oriel Press Ltd., 474–485, 1970.

Hungate, R. E.: The Rumen and Its Microbes. New York, Academic Press, 1966.

Jakopsen, P. E., Sorensen, P. H., and Larsen, H.: Energy investigations as related to fetus formation in cattle. Acta Agri. Scand. 7:103–112, 1957.

Lamond, D. R., Holmes, J. H. G., and Haydock, K. P.: Estimation of yield and composition of milk produced by grazing beef cows. J. Anim. Sci. 29:606, 1969.

Lofgreen, G. P., Loosli, J. K., and Maynard, L. A.: Comparative study of conventional protein allowances and theoretical requirements of growing Holstein heifers. J. Anim. Sci. 10:171, 1951.

Lomas, L. W., and Fox, D. G.: Ammonia treatment of corn silage. I. Feedlot performances of growing and finishing steers. J. Anim. Sci. 55:924, 1982.

Mahadevan, S., Erfle, J. D., and Sauer, F. D.: A colormetric method for the determination of proteolytic degradation of feed proteins by rumen microorganisms. J. Anim. Sci. 48:947, 1979.

Mahadevan, S., Erfle, J. D., and Sauer, F. D.: Degradation of soluble and insoluble proteins by Bacteroides amylophylus protease and by rumen microorganisms. J. Anim. Sci. 50:723, 1980.

Mason, V. C.: The quantitative importance of bacterial residues in the nondietary faecal nitrogen of sheep. Z. Tierphyseol., Tievernahrg. u. Futtermittelkde. 41:140, 1979.

Mason, V., and Fredricksen, J. H.: Partition of the nitrogen metabolism in the hindgut and nitrogen excretion. Proc. 2nd Int. Symp. Prot. Metab. and Nutr., 61, 1979.

Mertens, D. R.: Application of theoretical mathematical models to cell wall digestion and forage intake in ruminants. Ph.D. Thesis, Cornell University, 1973.

Mertens, D. R.: Dietary fiber components, relationship to the rate and extent of ruminal digestion. Fed. Proc. 36:187, 1977.

Milford, R., and Minson, D. J.: The relation between crude protein content and the digestible crude protein of tropical pasture plants. J. Br. Grass L. Soc. 18:177, 1965.

Mitchell, H. H.: The minimum protein requirements of cattle. Nat. Res. Council Bull. 67, 1929.

National Research Council: Nutrient Requirements of Dairy Cattle. Washington, D.C., National Academy of Sciences, 1978.

National Research Council: Nutrient Requirements of Beef Cattle. Washington, D.C., National Academy of Sciences, 1978.

National Research Council: Nutrient Requirements of Beef Cattle. Washington, D.C., National Academy of Sciences, 1984.

Orskov, E. R.: Factors influencing protein and nonprotein nitrogen utilization in young ruminants. In Cole, D. J. A., Boorman, K. N., Buttery, P. J., Lewis, D., Neale, R. J., Swann, L. L. (eds.): Proc. 1st Int. Symp. Protein Metabolism and Nutrition. EAFA P. P. No. 16. London, Butterworths, 457–476, 1976.

Overman, O. R., Garrett, O. F., Wright, K. E., and Sanmann, F. P.: Composition of milk of brown Swiss cows with summary of data on the composition of milk from cows of other dairy breeds. Ill. Agric. Exp. Sta. Bull. 457:575, 1939.

Owens, F. N., and Bergen, W. G.: Nitrogen metabolism of ruminant animals: Historical perspective, current understanding and future implications. J. Anim. Sci. 57(Suppl. 2):498, 1983.

Owens, F. N., Kazema, M., Galveen, M. L., Mizwicky, K. L., and Solaiman, S. G.: Ruminal turnover rate. Influence of feed additives, feed intake and roughage level. Okla. Anim. Sci. Res. Rpts., 27, 1979.

Pichard, G., and Van Soest, P. J.: Protein solubility of ruminant feeds. Proc. Cornell Nutr. Conf., 91, 1977.

Poos, M. I., Hanson, T. L., and Klopfenstein, T. J.: Monensin effects on diet digestibility, ruminal protein bypass and microbial protein synthesis. J. Anim. Sci. 48:1516, 1979.

Preston, R. L.: Empirical value of crude protein systems for feedlot cattle, 1980. Proc. Int. Symp. Protein Requirements for Cattle. Oklahoma, Okla State Univ., 1980.

Roffler, R. E., and Satter, L. D.: Relationship between ruminal ammonia and nonprotein nitrogen utilization by cattle. I. Development of a model for predicting nonprotein nitrogen utilization by cattle. J. Dairy Sci. 58:1880, 1975.

Roffler, R. E., and Satter, L. D.: Relationship between ruminal ammonia and nonprotein nitrogen utilization by cattle. II. Application of published evidence to the development of a theoretical model for predicting nonprotein nitrogen utilization. J. Dairy Sci. 58:1889, 1975b.

Roy, J. H., Balch, C. C., Miller, E. L., Orskov, E. R., and Smith, R. H.: Calculation of the N-requirement for ruminants from nitrogen metabolism studies. In Protein Metabolism and Nutrition Proc. Second Int. Symposium. The Netherlands. Eur. Assoc. Anim. Prod. Pub. No. 22 Centre for Agri. Pub. Documentation. Wageningen, 126, 1977.

Roy, J. H., Stobo, I. J. F., Gaston, H. J., and Greatorex, J. C.: Nutrition of the veal calf. 2. The effect of different levels of protein and fat in milk substitute diets. Brit. J. Nutr. 24:441–457, 1970.

Satter, L. D., and Roffler, R. E.: Nitrogen requirements and utilization in dairy cattle. J. Dairy Sci. 58:1219, 1975.

Satter, L. D., and Roffler, R. E.: Relationship between ruminal ammonia and nonprotein nitrogen utilization by ruminants. In Tracer Studies on Nonprotein Nitrogen for Ruminants III. Vienna, International Atomic Energy Agency, 1976.

Satter, L. D., and Slyter, L. L.: Effect of ammonia concentration on rumen microbial protein production in vitro. Br. J. Nutr. 32:199, 1974.

Schaefer, D. M., Davis, C. L., and Bryant, M. P.: Ammonia saturation constants for predominant species of rumen bacteria. J. Dairy Sci. 63:1248, 1980.

Sempindorfer, S.: Relationship of body type and size, sex and energy intake to the body composition of cattle. Ph.D. Thesis, Cornell University, 1974.

Smuts, B. B.: The relation between the basal metabolism and the endogenous nitrogen metabolism with particular reference to the maintenance requirement of protein. J. Nutri. 9:403, 1935.

Stobo, I. J. F., and Roy, J. H. B.: The protein requirement of the ruminant calf. 4. Nitrogen balance studies on rapidly growing calves given diets of different protein content. Brit. J. Nutr. 30:113–125, 1973.

Swanson, E. W., and Herman, H. A.: The nutritive value of Korean lespedeza proteins and the determination of biological value of proteins for growing dairy heifers. Mo. Agric. Exp. Stn. Bull. 372, 1943.

Swanson, E. W.: Factors for computing requirements for protein for maintenance of cattle. J. Dairy Sci. 60:1583–1593, 1977.

Thomas, E., Trenkle, A., and Burroughs, W.: Evaluation of protective agents applied to soybean meal and fed to cattle. II. Feedlot trials. J. Anim. Sci. 49:1346, 1979.

Trenkle, A., and Burroughs, W.: Supplemental protein requirements of finishing yearling heifers. Iowa State Univ. Coop. Ext. Serv. A. S. Leaflet R291, 1979.

Van Soest, P. J.: International Ruminant Conf. Univ. New England Publishing Unit, 1975.

Van Soest, P. J.: Nutritional Ecology of the Ruminant. Corvalis, Or., O and B Books, Inc., 1982.

Van Soest, P. J., and Mertens, D. R.: The use of neutral detergent fiber versus acid detergent fiber in balancing dairy rations. Monsanto Tech. Symp., Fresno, Ca., 1984.

Van Soest, P. J., and Sniffen, C. J.: Nitrogen Tractions in NDF and ADF, Vol. 39. Distillers Feed Conf., Cincinnati, Oh., 1984.

Van Es, A. J. H., and Bockholt, H. A.: Protein requirements in relation to the lactation cycle. In Protein Metabolism and Nutrition. Eur. Assoc. Anim. Prod. Publ. 16. London, Butterworths, 441–455, 1976.

Waldo, D. R., Smith, L. W., and Cox, E. L.: Model of cellulose disappearance from the rumen. J. Dairy Sci. 55:125, 1972.

Whitlow, L. W.: Rumen microbial degradation of feed protein. Ph.D. Thesis, University of Wisconsin, 1979.

Whitlow, L. W., and Satter, L. D.: Evaluation of models which predict amino acid flow to the intestine. Annales de Recherches Veterinaires 10:307, 1979.

Williams, J. H., Anderson, D. C., and Kress, D. D.: Milk production in Hereford cattle. I. Effects of separation interval on weigh-suckle-weigh milk production estimates. J. Dairy Sci. 49:1498, 1979.

Yu, Y., and Thomas, J. W.: Estimation of the extent of heat damage in alfalfa by laboratory damage. J. Anim. Sci. 42:766, 1976.

Refer to the first volume of Current Veterinary Therapy: Food Animal Practice for the following: Braddy, P. M. and Horton, D.: Feedlot Nutrition. Section 4, Dietary Management and Therapy.

METABOLIC DISORDERS

IVAN W. CAPLE, B.V.Sc., Ph.D.
Consulting Editor

Parturient Paresis (Milk Fever) and Hypocalcemia (Cows, Ewes, and Goats)

WILLIAM MAURICE ALLEN, Ph.D., M.Sc.,
B.V.Sc., M.R.C.V.S.
and BERNARD FREDERICK SANSOM, M.A.,
D.Phil.

Milk fever or parturient paresis is one of the most common metabolic disorders of food animals, and it has been given many alternative names, including paresis puerperalis, eclampsia, and parturient apoplexy. It occurs principally in cattle and to a lesser extent in sheep and goats. The disease is associated with hypocalcemia and occurs at or close to parturition, as a result of an acute imbalance between the output and input of calcium. In sheep, the disease associated with hypocalcemia is less related to parturition and is more common during late pregnancy, and it can also occur in early lactation.

OCCURRENCE

In cattle, milk fever is one of the most economically important diseases because it occurs widely and often leads to complications, such as the downer cow syndrome. The incidence of milk fever appears to increase as the average milk production increases. For example, in the United Kingdom in 1975 the annual milk fever incidence in dairy cattle was 9.0 per cent, whereas in 1960 it had been only 3.4 per cent. During the same period, average lactation yields had risen by approximately 30 per cent. In Finland, Sweden, and Norway, the annual rates have recently approximated 10 per cent, 8 per cent, and 7.5 per cent, respectively, whereas in Denmark during 1973, the incidence was only 4 per cent. On 64 farms in Australia (Southwest Victoria), the frequency of the disease in cows after their first lactation was reported to be more than 3 per cent. In these assessments of the national averages there has been no estimate of the "between-year" and "between-farm" variations. In the United Kingdom, the occurrence of the disease on different farms can vary in a single year from 0 to more than 60 per cent, and similarly the average incidence on 8 farms has been observed to change from 16 per cent in one year to 34 per cent in the next year.

Estimates of the cost of the disease must allow not only for the costs of treatment and prevention but also for the losses due to animals that fail to respond to treatment and become downer cows. The prognosis for these cows is poor, and they often die or have to be slaughtered. Estimates of the proportion of cows with milk fever that become downer cows have varied from 4 to 28 per cent, and estimates of the proportion of downer cows that subsequently die or have to be slaughtered vary from 20 to 70 per cent.

In the United Kingdom, a conservative estimate of the cost of the disease can be obtained by assuming an incidence of 9 per cent in the national herd of 3.5 million dairy cows and a death rate of 3 per cent in the affected cows. For approximately 315,000 cows affected annually the costs are as follows:

	$£ \times 10^3$
1. Treatment (or 1 bottle calcium borogluconate) £2/cow:	630
2. Deaths, 3 per cent of cases: 9500 cows at £600/cow	5700
3. Extra labor for nursing and veterinary services: £5/cow	1575
4. Loss of milk from surviving cases: approximately 20 L/cow at £0.15/L	945
5. Loss of milk from deaths: 9500 × margin over concentrates: £400	3800
*Total	12,650

Several important predisposing factors influence the occurrence of parturient paresis.

Age of Cow. As the age and parity of cows increases, the incidence of the disease rises. It is rare for parturient paresis to occur in heifers, but the frequency gradually increases with parity so that by the sixth lactation and onward it is common for more than 20 per cent of cows to succumb. This change is mainly due to the gradual decrease in the cow's ability to mobilize its own body stores of calcium when there are either sudden increases in the demand for calcium, such as occur at the onset of lactation, or decreases in the input of calcium, such as occur during transient starvation. In addition to this decreased ability to mobilize calcium, the milk yield of the cow also increases with parity, particularly up to the fourth lactation. Thus the cow's requirements for the output of calcium increase with age and tend to exacerbate the imbalance.

Breed of Cow. The particular susceptibility of the Jersey breed to parturient paresis is well known, but its physiologic basis is still unexplained. It may be related to the relatively high productivity of this small breed of cow.

---

*Or £3.6/cow/yr (approximately $5.00/cow/yr in United States currency).

Nutritional Factors. These include both long-term and short-term factors and are discussed in the section on prevention.

Seasonal Factors. It is important not to confuse apparent seasonal variations in the incidence of the disease with the effect of a seasonal calving pattern. There is nevertheless some evidence that the incidence of the disease is higher at the end of the grazing season. This effect may be due to the limitations on nutritional input from autumn grazing and particularly to the limitations on magnesium intake.

ETIOLOGY AND PATHOGENESIS

In all ruminants, milk fever is characterized by severe hypocalcemia. Some degree of hypocalcemia occurs normally in cows at and close to calving, but it is only when it becomes severe that disease occurs. Frequently, hypocalcemia is accompanied by hypophosphatemia and hypermagnesemia. Hyperglycemia is also often observed.

The normal concentration of calcium in plasma (and the extracellular fluid) lies within the range 2.2–2.6 mmol/L (8.8–10.4 mg/100 ml). This normal range of calcium concentration is maintained by balancing the rates at which calcium enters and leaves the plasma.

Entry or input into the plasma depends upon two processes: (1) the absorption of calcium across the intestinal wall from the diet and (2) the resorption or mobilization of the stores of calcium within the skeleton. The absorption of calcium from the diet varies with the animal's requirements and with the amount of calcium available in the diet. The provision of additional calcium to maintain a balance depends upon the mobilization of calcium from the skeletal stores. The processes of absorption and mobilization are subject to control mechanisms that are mediated through parathyroid hormone, calcitonin (produced in the thyroid C cells), and vitamin D and its metabolites.

The total rate of output of calcium from the plasma is the sum of the rates of output due to the following processes:

1. The endogenous (or obligatory) loss of calcium in the feces.
2. The smaller endogenous losses in the urine.
3. The calcium requirements for the growth of the fetal skeleton and the placenta during pregnancy.
4. The calcium secreted in the milk (approximately 1.2 gm/L) during lactation.
5. The calcium accreted into the skeleton of the cow.

Disease usually occurs when there are sudden changes in these requirements for output and when the input processes fail to adapt rapidly enough (Fig. 1). During the last stage of pregnancy the calcium requirements of the cow comprise approximately 10 gm Ca/day for the endogenous losses in feces and urine and up to 10 gm Ca/day for the growing fetus. Immediately after calving the endogenous loss of 10 gm Ca/day is maintained, but the demand for calcium for the production of colostrum increases to 30 gm/day. Thus, the total output of calcium rises at least 2-fold within a few hours. To maintain the homeostatic balance, the rate of absorption of calcium from the gut must be substantially increased or calcium stores must be mobilized from the skeleton or both. These

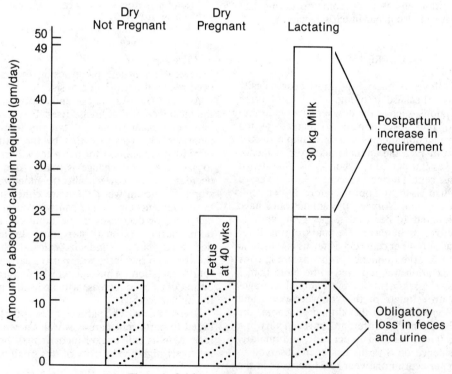

Calcium Requirement of the Cow (600 kg)

Figure 1. Calcium requirement of the cow.

adaptations must occur rapidly because the amount of calcium that can be mobilized very rapidly from body stores has been estimated to be only between 10 and 20 gm and thus may provide less than 50 per cent of 1 day's requirements. When the processes of adaptation fail, hypocalcemia becomes inevitable, and as it deepens, the concentration of calcium in tissues declines, and normal neuromuscular function is impaired.

In a healthy cow the processes of adaptation protect her against severe hypocalcemia. At the onset of hypocalcemia, the secretion of parathyroid hormone (PTH) is stimulated. In turn, PTH stimulates the production of a hydroxylase enzyme in the kidney that synthesizes the active form of vitamin D_3, 1,25 dihydroxycholecalciferol ($1,25(OH)_2D_3$) from 25-hydroxycholecalciferol ($25(OH)D_3$). The production of $25(OH)D_3$ from vitamin D_3 is not subject to a similar hormonal control mechanism. The $1,25(OH)_2D_3$ stimulates the absorption of calcium from the intestine through the synthesis of a calcium-binding protein. It can also mobilize calcium from the skeleton, in which it promotes osteoclast activity. At calving, the concentrations of both PTH and $1,25(OH)_2D_3$ increase in all cattle, and the increases are larger in cows with severe hypocalcemia. Thus, although the hormonal mechanisms for preventing hypocalcemia appear to be operating, in some cows disease still occurs. It has been suggested that one reason for this failure to prevent severe hypocalcemia is a rise in the rate of secretion of thyrocalcitonin. This hormone is secreted from the thyroid C cells in response to hypercalcemia and acts to decrease the rate of resorption of calcium from bone, thus reducing the rate of input of calcium into the plasma. However, there has been no recent evidence to support the role of calcitonin as a cause of milk fever. It seems more probable that the adaptation of the hormonal mechanisms and synthesis of $1,25(OH)_2D_3$ fails to stimulate the target organs of gut and bone rapidly enough to increase the rate of input of calcium.

Other factors may also influence the speed and extent of the response. Age has already been mentioned, older animals being less able to mobilize skeletal stores of calcium. Estrogens also inhibit calcium mobilization, and the concentration of estrogens increases at parturition and again, cyclically, later in lactation. The elevation of plasma estrogen concentrations associated with estrus may in part explain those few cases of milk fever that occur later in lactation. Another important factor that can reduce the mobilization of calcium is subclinical hypomagnesemia. Although at calving slight hypermagnesemia often occurs, the cow's diet during the last few weeks of pregnancy may have induced a sufficient degree of hypomagnesemia to prejudice the mobilization of calcium at parturition.

CLINICAL SIGNS

The clinical signs can be divided into 3 stages that are approximately related to the severity of the hypocalcemia. In the first stage, the cow loses her appetite and becomes dull and lethargic. She is afebrile and her ears may be cold. In some cases, the pupil of the eye is dilated even during this early stage. In the second stage, as the hypocalcemia becomes more severe, she stands with her hocks straight and paddles from one hind foot to the other. There may be tremors of the muscles, particularly of the

head and limbs. She sometimes grinds her teeth, and she eventually becomes incoordinated. Sometimes, she becomes very excitable and hypersensitive when approached and as a result she becomes difficult to restrain and sweats profusely. Finally, in the third stage, she is recumbent with a drowsy appearance and flaccid paralysis. At first, she lies on her sternum, often with a characteristic curvature of the neck, and may struggle to rise. Eventually, she lies on her side and becomes comatose, with dilated pupils and a dry muzzle. She does not pass urine or feces, and the anal reflex is lost. The rumen becomes tympanitic, and its contents may be regurgitated. Unless she is treated the cow will die of respiratory failure either as a result of the rumen tympany or as a result of the inhalation of rumen contents. As the third stage of the disease progresses, the body temperature tends to decrease, and the intensity of the heart sounds also decreases. The heart rate remains at about 60–80/min, and the respirations are shallow and slow. The pupillary reflex to light is absent, and the pupil is frequently dilated to the maximum. The stasis of the rumen and alimentary tract severely reduces the absorption of calcium from the intestine and so increases the severity of the hypocalcemia. As the hypocalcemia progresses to the terminal stage, the heart rate and breathing become more irregular, and respirations sometimes end with a forced expiratory grunt. The progress to the final stages may take 24 hr. At pasture, cows that have died of milk fever are often found trapped in a ditch or drowned in a stream.

An important consequence of the disease when it occurs before calving is the associated uterine inertia. The process of calving may stop, there is no straining of voluntary muscles, and dystocia may remain undetected. If calving does occur, a prolapse of the uterus is common in severely hypocalcemic cows.

CLINICAL PATHOLOGY

Measurement of the calcium concentration in plasma is the best method of confirming the disease. The normal range of calcium concentrations is between 2.2 and 2.6 mmol/L (8.8–10.4 mg/100 ml), but close to parturition the concentration almost always declines to some extent. However, clinical disease is rarely seen unless the concentration of calcium falls below 1.5 mmol/L (6 mg/100 ml). In some cows the calcium concentration may fall below this level without the cows showing clinical signs. In cows with the disease, the calcium concentration may be as low as 0.25 mmol/L.

Phosphorus concentrations also decrease. The normal range of concentrations is between 1.40 and 2.48 mmol/L (4.3–7.7 mg/100 ml), and in cows with milk fever the concentration may fall to 1.0 mmol/L or less. Magnesium concentrations usually increase to slightly above the upper limit of the normal range (0.85–1.25 mmol/L or 2–3 mg/100 ml), although occasionally they decrease. Hyperglycemia is usual during milk fever unless the cow is also ketotic, when the concentration of glucose in plasma is low.

There are changes in the white blood cell counts of all cows at parturition, including neutrophilia, lymphopenia, and eosinopenia. These changes resemble the response to stress or to adrenocortical hyperactivity or both.

In fatal cases of uncomplicated milk fever, there are no

characteristic postmortem gross or histologic lesions that can be ascribed specifically to the disease. There is often bruising of subcutaneous tissue and muscles due to the localized trauma associated with collapse, recumbency, and incoordinated struggling. There may also be gross lesions of the genital tract associated with calving. In some animals, the liver may be infiltrated with fat, and this infiltration may be gross, with yellow discoloration, and may affect other organs, including the kidney and heart.

DIAGNOSIS

Diagnosis of milk fever in the field is based on observation of the clinical signs as described—particularly paresis in cows close to calving. Quick, practical confirmation is often provided by a rapid response, sometimes within minutes, to treatment with calcium borogluconate solutions. Blood analysis can only confirm the diagnosis retrospectively.

The differential diagnosis of milk fever and other conditions that cause similar clinical signs must, however, be considered on every occasion. These conditions, which may arise as a sequel to milk fever, are discussed in detail next and include

1. The downer cow syndrome.
2. Severe toxemia.
3. Physical injury, e.g., obturatory paralysis, fracture of leg bones, pelvic rupture, and ruptured gastrocnemius tendon.
4. Hypomagnesemia.
5. Fat cow syndrome.

The Downer Cow Syndrome. A downer cow has been defined as a cow that has been in sternal recumbency for more than 24 hr. In the early stages, she appears bright, and she will usually eat, drink, defecate, and urinate normally. However, the condition may persist for 1 to 2 weeks, possibly resulting in damage due to pressure on the muscles, especially of the hind limbs. After only a few hours of recumbency, this damage can be so severe that muscles degenerate and ligaments rupture. At this stage, the damage becomes irreversible and results in mortality of up to 60 per cent.

The downer cow syndrome may arise because a cow fails to respond satisfactorily to the correct treatment for milk fever. However, it more often arises as a sequel to uncomplicated cases of milk fever that have either been treated too late or have been inadequately cared for during the period of incoordination and recumbency.

The condition can be diagnosed initially from the appearance of the clinical signs. The diagnosis can be confirmed by measuring the plasma concentration of those enzymes that are released from damaged muscle tissue. Two enzymes are suitable, creatine kinase (CK) and aspartate aminotransferase (AST). In downer cows the activity of these enzymes in plasma may be increased by several thousand-fold, and daily measurements may be used to assess the progress of the disease and its likely prognosis. If the activities of the enzymes continue to increase, the prognosis is very bad.

Severe Toxemia. Severe toxemia can easily be confused with the third stage of milk fever. The affected cow is drowsy, recumbent, and will not eat. She may lie with her head on her flank and make expiratory grunts. However, on clinical examination she may have acute mastitis

or metritis. In spite of this infection, the cow frequently does not show a febrile response, and her body temperature is normal, as in a cow with milk fever. There is usually an increase in the cow's heart rate, up to 120/min with a weak pulse, and she also has severe leucopenia.

Physical Injury. At calving a cow may suffer injuries, such as fracture of the pelvis or damage to the obturator nerve or sciatic plexus or both, which may make her recumbent. She may not have been provided with adequate bedding on slippery surfaces, and her legs may have been severely abducted or fractured by a serious slip. The animal will probably eat and drink normally, and her heart rate and gastrointestinal function will be normal. A careful physical examination of the recumbent animal is necessary in an attempt to define the site of the lesion. An assay of plasma CK or AST activities can be used to assess the approximate extent of the muscle damage.

Hypomagnesemia. Hypomagnesemia can affect cattle of all ages, and dairy cattle can be affected at any time during pregnancy and lactation. It can occur as a complication of milk fever. The clinical signs are a state of excitement and hypersensitivity followed by sudden collapse, frequently in tetanic spasms. The heart rate is generally increased, and the heart sounds are very loud.

A clinical diagnosis can be confirmed by measuring the concentration of magnesium in blood plasma. Concentrations below 0.8 mmol/L are abnormal, but in clinical cases the level may be much less.

Fat Cow Syndrome. In dairy cattle that are excessively fat during pregnancy, the incidence of milk fever and other periparturient diseases is higher. Some of these cows with milk fever fail to respond to treatment—the cow remains recumbent while subcutaneous fat is mobilized and then deposited in many tissues of the body, including the liver and skeletal muscle. The deposition of fat may be so great that the cow becomes severely ketotic and eventually dies.

The 5 conditions as discussed are some of the differential diagnoses that need to be considered during a clinical examination of a cow suspected of having milk fever.

TREATMENT

Treatment should be given as soon as possible after the clinical signs have been observed. The best treatment is to administer a solution of calcium borogluconate intravenously, and most cows with milk fever recover after a single intravenous dose of between 8 and 12 gm of calcium. A total of 12 gm of calcium can be administered in 400 ml of a 40-per cent solution of calcium borogluconate that should be infused over a 5–10 min period. The muscles of recumbent animals may twitch during treatment, and the animals may pass feces and urine and eructate rumen gases.

Treatment with solutions that contain magnesium and phosphorus as well as calcium has also been advocated. However, in uncomplicated cases there is no evidence of a higher rate of recovery among cows treated with solutions containing magnesium (1.03 gm) and phosphorus (2.6 gm) in addition to calcium (8 gm). When subclinical hypomagnesemia (plasma magnesium <0.85 mmol/L) is observed during the last month of pregnancy the addition of magnesium to the solution of calcium borogluconate is advisable. Similarly, when there is evidence either of hypophosphatemia (blood phosphorus <1.35 mmol/L) among cows in late pregnancy or of persistently low phosphorus among cows in relapse, the inclusion of phosphorus is advisable.

The administration of intravenous calcium rapidly increases the concentration of calcium in plasma and causes transient hypercalcemia. However, 8–12 gm of calcium is only a small amount, comparable with the pool of readily exchangeable calcium in the animal's body and considerably less than the amount excreted in the milk during 24 hr. The treatment cannot therefore be considered as substitution therapy. The short period during which plasma calcium concentrations are restored to normal or above normal appears to be sufficient to allow the re-establishment of the normal homeostatic mechanisms, and possibly the most important effects are to re-establish normal gut function and to stimulate the cow's appetite. Nevertheless, subclinical hypocalcemia persists in many cows for 24 hr or longer after they have been successfully treated for milk fever. If a cow does not recover within 5 to 8 hr of a single intravenous dose of calcium the cow should be re-examined and treated with calcium again, providing the diagnosis suggests that the problem remains an uncomplicated case of milk fever.

It is a common practice to administer calcium borogluconate subcutaneously at the same time as the single intravenous injection of calcium, and this subcutaneous injection can also contain magnesium and phosphorus. Although the total amount of calcium administered may then be as high as 18 gm, it has been demonstrated that these auxiliary subcutaneous injections do not reduce the likelihood of a cow relapsing after an initial recovery.

In addition to specific treatment with calcium, it is essential to provide the cow with adequate nursing and care. The calf should be removed, and the cow should not be milked out. If the cow is in lateral recumbency, she should be propped into the sternal position to prevent her from regurgitating rumen contents and running the risk of aspiration pneumonia. She should be turned from side to side at regular intervals and certainly not less than 4 to 5 times daily to prevent pressure damage to muscles. If she is lying on concrete or a similarly hard and slippery surface, it should be generously covered with sand, straw, or farmyard manure.

If a cow is recumbent for longer than 48 hr, it is advisable either to hoist her with a hip sling or to raise her on inflatable cushions so that she can stand for a short period and so that her ability to move her limbs can be assessed (Table 1).

PREVENTION

The ability to prevent milk fever depends upon a knowledge of the etiology of the disease. However, the etiology of individual cases of milk fever may vary because one or more of a variety of predisposing factors may be involved. As a result, preventive measures must be designed to reduce the adverse effects of as many of these predisposing factors as possible. They include age, breed, nutritional and husbandry systems, and body condition score at parturition.

Older cows, especially in certain breeds, are more susceptible to disease and need particular attention to avoid hypocalcemia.

Table 1. Equipment for Hypocalcemic Cows with Prolonged Recumbency

Equipment	Company and Address
Bagshaw Hoist (V713A)	Arnold's Veterinary Products Ltd., 14 Tessa Road, Richfield Avenue, Reading, Berkshire, RG1 8NF, UK.
The Downer Cow Air Cushion	Hamco Products, 68 Riverside Park, Otley, West Yorkshire, LS21 2RW, UK.

Several nutritional factors affect the likelihood of the occurrence of disease. They may be divided into those that are important in the long term—that is, during the dry period—and those that are particularly important in the short term—that is, between 48 hr before calving and 48 hr after calving. The long-term factors affect the cow's body condition at calving and also influence the way in which her vitamin D metabolism is primed to respond to the sudden increase in demand for calcium at calving. The short-term factors affect the ability of the cow to maintain a sufficient intake of calcium at the onset of lactation.

Long-term Factors. During the dry period it is important to maintain the concentration of magnesium in plasma above 0.85 mmol/L and if the concentration falls below this level, the cow can be considered to be subclinically hypomagnesemic. In the northern hemisphere, there are 2 periods in the year when dry cows at pasture are most likely to become hypomagnesemic: in the spring, when dry matter intake is likely to be low and the availability of magnesium in pastures (particularly if they have been heavily fertilized with potassium and nitrogen) is also low; and in the autumn, when similar constraints can affect the supply of magnesium. In the spring, the shortage of magnesium may be exacerbated because grasses contain less magnesium than clovers and other legumes, whose growth is relatively slower than grasses in spring. In the southern hemisphere, cows are likely to become hypomagnesemic in autumn or winter (see Ruminant Hypomagnesemic Tetanies).

Unfortunately, it is not easy to correct hypomagnesemia in dry cows. Cake or concentrate can be supplemented with calcined magnesite but even 50 gm/day of MgO does not always appear to provide the necessary intake of magnesium. The addition of magnesium acetate to the drinking water is effective provided that the cows have access only to a controlled water supply and provided that the weather is not so wet that the cows drink little water. Wet weather also reduces the effectiveness of dusting the pastures with magnesian limestone, because rain washes the powdered material off the leaves and into the soil.

The intake of calcium during the dry period is also important, and ideally the ration should contain as little calcium as possible. The optimum benefit of a low calcium diet occurs with diets supplying <20 gm Ca/day. Unfortunately, practical diets, especially those based on forage, rarely contain less than 50 gm Ca/day, and their protective effect is probably small. Nevertheless, the calcium content of the diet should be kept as low as is practicable. The beneficial effect of a low calcium intake is considered to be derived from the stimulation of $1,25(OH)_2D_3$ synthesis, which in turn increases the rates of mobilization and absorption of calcium at parturition. This process also probably explains the desirability of maintaining a low Ca:P ratio in the diet of dry cows, when the percentage of the calcium absorbed from the diet increases.

Short-term Factors. It is essential that the cow's appetite remain high at and around the time of parturition. If a cow has received a ration rich in concentrates during the dry period and if her body condition score is too high, her intake of dry matter will decline as parturition approaches, and the incidence of milk fever will be likely to increase. The effect of inappetance at this critical time, when increased supplies of calcium are needed, resembles temporary starvation. A similar mechanism may explain some of the increasing number of cases of a milk fever–like syndrome reported in higher yielding cows later on in lactation. These cows may become temporarily starved during transport or before the application of embryo-transfer techniques or through inappetance at estrus. Because the normal turnover of calcium from the diet to the milk is so large and so rapid even brief starvation may result in imbalance.

When parturition is imminent, calcium intake should be increased as rapidly as possible to provide for the cow's greater requirements for calcium. The use of readily absorbed calcium salts for this purpose is not easy. In one trial, this routine reduced the incidence of milk fever from 46 per cent to 23 per cent, but it is not easy to administer calcium chloride (150 gm/animal) by drenching on the day before calving and for 4 days after, and the method has not always proved effective. The beneficial increase in calcium absorption that occurs when the calcium content of the diet is increased has been demonstrated to persist for only a few days. This short-term response and the need to provide the dry cow with <20 gm Ca/day may explain the conflicting results obtained from different trials.

Another procedure that has been advocated and probably operates by raising the absorption of calcium from the diet in the short term is the alteration of the ionic balance of the diet (the acidity-alkalinity of the diet). The important determinants of acidity and alkalinity are considered to be $(SO_4^= + Cl^-)$ and $(Na^+ + K^+)$, respectively. The "acidity" of hay diets was increased by the addition of $CaCl_2$ and aluminum and magnesium sulfate, and these diets were fed for the last 4 weeks before calving. Such "acid" diets, and also diets based on silage preserved with mineral acids, may reduce the incidence of milk fever. However, it is again difficult to apply this system in practice.

There is more evidence that feeding either silage or hay alone during the last days of pregnancy can reduce the incidence of milk fever. Cows grazing lush grass pastures in late pregnancy commonly develop milk fever at parturition.

The administration of vitamin D in pharmacologic doses 5 to 10 days before calving can be beneficial. Recently acquired knowledge of the biochemical pathways of the vitamin, together with the chemical synthesis of its metabolites and their analogues, have provided opportunities for new prophylactic approaches to milk fever.

Feeding 20–30 × 10^6 IU of vitamin D_3 (cholecalciferol) daily for a maximum of 7 days starting 3 to 4 days prepartum has been claimed to reduce the incidence of milk fever. A single intramuscular injection of 10 × 10^6 IU (250 mg) vitamin D_3, approximately 10 days before calving, has also been said to lower the incidence of the disease, although its protective effect has been questioned.

Analogues of vitamin D_3 metabolites, including doses

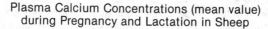

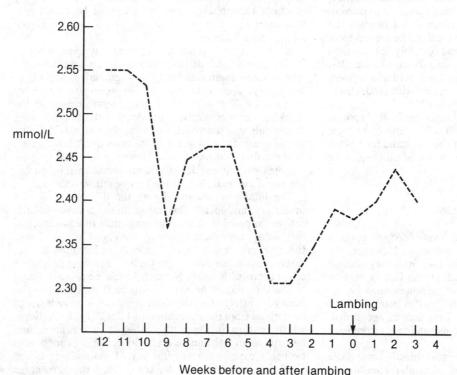

Figure 2. Plasma calcium concentrations (mean value) during pregnancy and lactation in sheep.

Table 2. Drug Therapy for Parturient Paresis and Hypocalcemia

Name of Drug*	Company and Address	Animal	Dose
Vitamin D Vitamin D₃	Duphar Veterinary Ltd., Southampton SO3 4QH, UK.	Cattle	10^7 IU between 8th and 2nd days before calving
Calcium borogluconate 20% wt/vol	Crown Chemical Co. Ltd., Lamberhurst, Kent, UK.	Cattle Sheep and Goats	Up to 800 ml IV or SC (12 gm Ca) 50–150 ml IV or SC
40% wt/vol	Willows Francis Veterinary, Horsham West Sussex, RH13 5QP, UK.	Cattle Sheep and Goats	Up to 400 ml IV or SC Up to 100 ml IV or SC
20% or 40% wt/vol +Mg 0.3–0.7% wt/vol +P 0.9–1.1% wt/vol	Dales Pharmaceuticals, Skipton, N. Yorks, BD23 2RW, UK.	Cattle Sheep	Up to 450 ml IV or SC Up to 100 ml IV or SC

*20% glucose and 5–20% dextrose may be added.

of 350–500 µg 1α-hydroxycholecalciferol (1αHCC) and 1,25(OH)₂D₃ (the active vitamin), have been used in trials to protect cows against milk fever. The results confirm that they can significantly lower the incidence of disease provided they are administered at least 24 hr and not more than 5 to 7 days before calving. The difficulty of predicting parturition in the cow has been overcome in some trials by combining the vitamin treatment with induction of parturition. However, this procedure can seriously increase the incidence of retained placenta. Thus, the use of 1αHCC has not become widespread, and it is at present available for prophylactic treatment only in Israel and the Netherlands.

HYPOCALCEMIA IN EWES

In sheep, hypocalcemia (and hypophosphatemia) are more likely to occur during the last month of pregnancy (Fig. 2) than at lambing, partly because the calcium requirement of the fetuses is proportionally higher in the sheep than in the cow, and partly because there is not such a rapid increase in the ewe's requirement for calcium at the beginning of lactation. Hypocalcemia is rare at lambing, but it can occur during lactation, most commonly during the first 6 weeks. The likelihood of clinical disease is increased by factors such as sudden inclement weather, strenuous exercise, and temporary starvation.

The clinical signs of disease are similar to those of cattle. Muscle tremors, however, are more common, and the clinical signs may easily be confused with those of hypomagnesemia.

The best method of treatment is by intravenous injection of 50 ml of a 40-per cent solution of calcium borogluconate, and more calcium can be provided subcutaneously. When hypomagnesemia is suspected, a mixture of calcium, magnesium, and phosphorus may be administered instead of calcium alone. The frequency of relapses after a single treatment is greater in sheep than in cattle, and repeated treatments may be necessary.

When nursing affected animals, it is as important with sheep as it is with cattle to maintain them in sternal recumbency, to avoid regurgitation of ruminal contents, and there is less danger of necrosis of muscles, presumably because of the sheep's lower body weight.

In order to prevent disease during the last 6 weeks of pregnancy, it is important to ensure that the ewe is receiving a continuously rising plane of nutrition. This will ensure that her greater requirement for calcium is provided by the increased intake of calcium from the diet.

During pregnancy and lactation, it is also important to maintain the ewe's feed intake, to provide her with shelter from inclement weather, and to avoid stressing her with severe or unaccustomed exercise.

HYPOCALCEMIA IN GOATS

The epidemiology of milk fever in goats is similar to that in cows. The disease is most common at the time close to parturition, and the principles for prevention, treatment, and care are similar.

Acute cases should be treated by the administration of 25 ml of 40-per cent calcium borogluconate intravenously, together with the administration of 75 ml of a 20-per cent solution subcutaneously. However, as 40-per cent solutions of calcium borogluconate can cause severe local reactions at the site of administration, it would be wise to administer solutions of no greater concentration than 20 per cent wt/vol.

Table 2 contains a synopsis of drug therapy for parturient paresis and hypocalcemia.

Acetonemia

IVAN W. CAPLE, B.V.Sc., Ph.D.
and J. G. McLEAN, B.V.Sc., Ph.D.

Acetonemia, or bovine ketosis, is a disease of lactating cows characterized by nervous signs, loss of body weight, reduced milk yield, and ketones in the urine and milk. Many of the biochemical changes are similar to those in other ketotic conditions of ruminants, including pregnancy toxemia of sheep, cows, and goats. There is no single specific metabolic lesion causing ketosis, and the biochemical changes include hypoglycemia, an accumulation of ketone bodies in body fluids, and increased plasma-free fatty acids and liver fat, together with decreased liver glycogen. These changes are associated with an inadequate supply of nutrients necessary for the normal carbohydrate and fat metabolism associated with high milk production usually seen in early lactation.

OCCURRENCE

Acetonemia may occur in dairy cows housed during the winter and also in dairy cows at pasture. Cows of any age including heifers may be affected, and ketosis is not confined to those in poor body condition. Where there is a high incidence of the disease, it becomes a major economic problem because of the loss of milk production and the failure to return to full production after recovery.

Acetonemia is most prevalent within 6 weeks after parturition when high-producing cows have difficulty adjusting their dietary intake to the production demand. Maximum milk yield usually occurs during the third week after parturition, but maximum intake of metabolizable energy may not be achieved until the seventh week. A cow can maintain a high yield for a limited period even when dietary intake is inadequate but loses weight because body reserves of protein and fat are utilized to overcome the energy deficit caused by the continuing synthesis of milk components. Subclinical acetonemia can occur when apparently normal cows continue in this state of negative energy balance, and these cows may excrete ketones in urine and milk but do not develop clinical signs. This delicate metabolic balance can rapidly deteriorate into a severe clinical ketosis, however, if any condition causes further reduction of the cow's dietary intake.

Primary spontaneous ketosis may still develop in cows being fed a high energy diet in early lactation. Factors considered to influence the occurrence of the disease are excessive feeding of silage containing a high content of butyric acid, inadequate exercise, excessive fatness at parturition, and digestive upsets.

Acetonemia can be found in cows grazing lush, rapidly growing grass pastures if they are unable to obtain sufficient nutrients because of the high water content of the diet. Specific dietary deficiencies of minerals, such as phosphorus, sodium, magnesium, and cobalt, in addition to a reduced food intake, may be associated with a high incidence of ketosis. Cobalt is required for rumen microbial synthesis of vitamin B_{12} and is also essential for adequate utilization of propionic acid.

Secondary ketosis can result from any disease causing a reduction in appetite during early lactation. Diseases frequently encountered are abomasal displacement, metritis, mastitis, and traumatic reticulitis.

ETIOLOGY AND PATHOGENESIS

The ruminant is always in a somewhat precarious position with respect to its carbohydrate metabolism. Very little glucose is obtained directly from the diet, as about 80 per cent of the ingested carbohydrates are fermented by the rumen microflora into volatile fatty acids—acetic, propionic, and butyric acids—which are then absorbed. Acetate may be oxidized by a variety of tissues or incorporated into milk fat by the mammary gland. Glucose, which is essential for function of the central nervous system, for maintenance of cellular osmotic environment, and for production of lactose in the mammary gland and of fructose in the fetus, is synthesized in the liver and renal cortex by way of the gluconeogenic pathway (Fig. 1). Approximately half of the glucose in the cow is normally derived from dietary propionic acid, which is incorporated into the tricarboxylic acid (TCA) cycle and then converted into glucose by gluconeogenesis. Glucogenic amino acids, lactic acid, and glycerol can also be converted into glucose by this process.

Any condition reducing the amount of propionic acid in the rumen can result in inadequate glucose production and a consequent lowering in blood glucose level. Hypo-

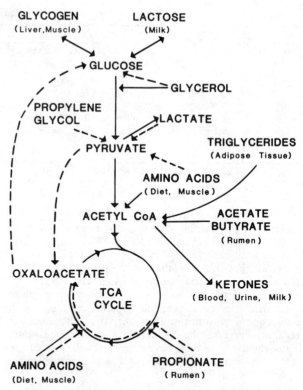

Figure 1. Pathways of glucose synthesis and ketone body production in ruminants. The gluconeogenic pathways are shown by the broken lines.

glycemia leads to a mobilization of free fatty acids and glycerol from fat stores. This mobilization is mediated by a number of factors, including the sympathetic nervous system and hormones such as epinephrine, glucagon, adrenocorticotropic hormone, glucocorticoids, and thyroid hormones. Tissues such as skeletal muscle and heart can utilize fatty acids for energy production when glucose is deficient. However, the liver has a limited ability to oxidize fatty acids because acetyl-CoA, which is the end-product of fatty acid oxidation, cannot be adequately incorporated into the TCA cycle because of low levels of oxaloacetate, resulting from active gluconeogenesis. The excess acetyl-CoA is converted into the ketone bodies acetoacetate and β-hydroxybutyrate and a smaller amount of acetone. Ketone bodies are readily oxidized by tissues other than liver, particularly muscle. If the production of ketone bodies by the liver exceeds the utilization by the peripheral tissues, they accumulate in the body, and pathologic ketosis results. Ketone bodies are excreted principally by way of the urine and milk. The total amount excreted usually never exceeds 10 per cent of the amount produced.

Because acetoacetate and β-hydroxybutyrate are strong acids, excessive accumulation in the body can produce acidosis, but this is not common in cows with acetonemia. Hypoglycemia is the major factor involved in the onset and development of the clinical signs.

CLINICAL SIGNS

Acetonemia in dairy cows is manifest by a range of syndromes in which loss of body condition is most common and variable nervous signs are present. There is a gradual but moderate decline in milk yield over 2 to 4 days. Cows may first refuse to eat grain, then silage, but continue to eat hay. The dairyworker may have noted that the cow has not eaten the concentrates provided during milking. Body weight is lost rapidly once appetite has decreased owing to utilization of body stores and dehydration. Cows often appear depressed and disinclined to move, their hair coat appears roughened, and their eyes appear "glazed" or "lackluster." Temperature and heart and respiratory rates are usually normal. The ruminal movements are commonly normal unless the condition is of long duration; then, they may be decreased or even absent. The odor of acetone may be detected on the breath. Some cows may stagger and may appear partially blind.

Other nervous signs that are seen in a small number of cows include excessive salivation, abnormal chewing movements, and exaggerated licking. Muscles, particularly in the shoulder and mid-flank regions show trembling, and cows have a staggering or swaying gait, appearing incoordinated and apparently blind. Hyperesthesia may be detected. Some cows may charge blindly if disturbed and can injure themselves during these recurrent nervous episodes.

CLINICAL PATHOLOGY

Field tests for ketosis are based on the qualitative detection of ketones in urine and milk by their reaction with sodium nitroprusside (Rothera's reaction) to form a pink to purple color (Acetest tablet, Ketostix and Labstix test strips*). The primary value of the urine test is the ability to rule out ketosis if the test is negative. Urine normally contains higher ketone levels than milk, and a positive urine test can be regarded as evidence of ketosis only when the milk is also positive.

Hypoglycemia, hyperketonemia, and excretion of ketones in urine and milk are characteristic of the disease, and plasma-free fatty acids and blood glycerol levels are elevated. The blood levels of glucose and ketones are the best measure of the severity of ketosis. Although quantitative chemical estimations of blood ketone levels is often impractical, plasma may react with Rothera's reagent. Blood glucose concentrations are reduced from normal levels of 40 to 50 mg/100 ml (2.2 to 2.8 mmol/L) to less than 25 mg/100 ml (1.4 mmol/L) and are usually lower in cases of primary ketosis than in cases of secondary ketosis. Total blood ketone levels are elevated from a normal value of <10 mg/100 ml (1.75 mmol/L) to more than 30 mg/100 ml (5.0 mmol/L). In herds with energy deficiency and subclinical ketosis, cows in the first 6 weeks of lactation often have serum β-hydroxybutyrate concentrations greater than 10 mg/100 ml (1.75 mmol/L). Blood urea nitrogen values may vary, but urinary ammonia concentration may be elevated.

Some cows have hypocalcemia with acetonemia, and cows with severe cases show an increase in serum aspartate aminotransferase (AST) activity that is related to the extent of anorexia and liver damage.

Although cows with acetonemia do not usually die, necrotic lesions consisting of fatty infiltration and degeneration of the liver and secondary changes in the anterior pituitary gland and adrenal cortex may be present.

DIAGNOSIS

Diagnosis of acetonemia is based on the presence of ketones in the urine and milk, the history related to the time of parturition, feeding program, signs associated with wasting and nervous dysfunction, together with elimination of other conditions that could lead to temporary reduction of appetite. Clinical indications of other diseases include increased temperature, increased heart and respiratory rates, and a rapid drop in or cessation of milk yield, as well as signs specific for conditions such as traumatic reticulitis, metritis, mastitis, abomasal displacement, indigestion, and constipation.

Acetonemia without complications is never fatal, and the nervous dysfunction is transient, which distinguishes it from listeriosis in which there is a fever. In comparison with acetonemia, rabies is characterized by mania and ascending paralysis, and is always fatal. With acetonemia there are no tetanic convulsions, and the condition responds rapidly to treatment. Cows that have ketosis and hypocalcemia concurrently may have a reeling staggering gait, hyperesthesia, and feeble paddling of the limbs when in lateral recumbency. These cows may show a clinical response to calcium therapy but usually have a poor appetite following treatment.

TREATMENT

The basis of treatment is as follows: (1) to immediately increase the glucose supply to organs where metabolic pathways are dependent on glucose availability, (2) to replenish the depleted intermediates of the TCA cycle in the liver so that fatty acids mobilized from fat stores are oxidized completely and the rate of ketone body formation is decreased, and (3) to increase the availability of dietary propionic acid and other glucogenic precursors (Table 1).

An intravenous injection of glucose (500 ml of 40-per cent solution) causes a transient hyperglycemia for about

Table 1. *Diagnostic Tests and Drug Therapy for Acetonemia*

Test* or Drug†	Species	Dose
Acetest tablets	Bovine	
Ketostix		
Glucose solution (40%)		500 ml (IV)
Propylene glycol (with		125–250 gm
mixtures containing cobalt		(orally twice daily)
available)		
Glucocorticoids		
Dexamethasone		5–20 mg
preparations		
Betamethasone		10–30 mg
Flumethasone		2.5–5 mg
Triamcinolone acetonide		2.5–10 mg
Anabolic steroids		
Trenbolone acetate		125–250 mg
Dehydrotestosterone		
undecyclenate		125–250 mg

*Division of Miles Laboratories, Inc., Mulgrave, Australia.

†These preparations are available under a variety of trade names. Consult Rossoff, I. S.: Handbook of Veterinary Drugs. Springer: New York, 1974.

*Available from Ames Company, Division of Miles Laboratories, Inc., Mulgrave, Australia.

2 hr and alleviates the clinical signs. Milk production is stimulated, but as lactose is lost in the milk, relapses commonly occur unless repeated or continuous infusions are given. The necessity for repeated injections of glucose can be overcome by the oral administration of glucose precursors, such as propylene glycol. The recommended dosage is 125–250 gm twice daily mixed with an equal volume of water. Propylene glycol is more effective than sodium propionate or glycerol, as it is not fermented in the rumen and provides a substrate for gluconeogenesis in the liver. High doses of propionate may cause digestive disturbances, and glycerol has the disadvantage of being converted to ketogenic acids as well as propionic acid in the rumen. Cobalt salts are added to propylene glycol to provide at least 100 mg cobalt/day in cases where there is cobalt deficiency.

Glucocorticoids are effective when used alone, when used with glucose therapy, or when followed by oral administration of glucose precursors. However, glucocorticoids may be contraindicated when infectious conditions predispose to secondary ketosis. Glucocorticoid treatment is accompanied by a reduction in ketone body formation due to greater utilization of the acetyl-CoA derived from fatty acid oxidation and an increase in blood glucose concentration due to a greater availability of glucose precursors in the liver. Most commercial preparations of synthetic glucocorticoids, such as dexamethasone and betamethasone, are effective, and a single dose is given (see Table 1). Excessive administration of glucocorticoids should be avoided, as it may reduce appetite and milk yield.

Anabolic steroids also produce a decrease in the levels of blood ketones and free fatty acids, and an increase in the concentrations of intermediates of the TCA cycle in the liver. Unlike glucocorticoids, anabolic steroids do not produce hyperglycemia in ketotic cows. Anabolic steroids stimulate appetite, which is beneficial in ensuring an increased supply of glucogenic precursors.

Chloral hydrate has long been used to treat the nervous form of acetonemia. The dosage is 28.5 gm in water or by capsule twice daily for 3 to 5 days.

It is important to ensure that the cow's food intake returns to normal as quickly as possible, and this is best achieved by the dairyworker who can entice the cow to eat by offering differing diets, such as hay and whole oats, until she consumes the full amount of her normal diet.

PREVENTION

Acetonemia in dairy cows occurs in housed cows in the northern hemisphere and in pastured cows in the southern hemisphere. The most successful control of the problem is through attention to feeding and management to ensure that cows have an adequate energy intake (see Dietary Management and Therapy, Section 4). Cows should not be in poor condition or excessively fat at calving. The ration to be used in lactation should be introduced at least 2 weeks before parturition to permit the rumen microflora to adapt to the change in diet. During the first 3 months of lactation, high-yielding cows should not be subjected to sudden changes in ration. The ration fed during early lactation should provide maximum glucose precursors with the minimum of ketogenic materials, such as hay crop or silage high in butyric acid, and at the same time give maximum energy without reducing food intake. Particular attention must be paid to providing good quality roughage that comprises a minimum of one third of the ration. A good practice is to include good quality alfalfa (lucerne) hay in the diet. If concentrates are used, the carbohydrate should be readily digestible (e.g., ground maize), and the ration should contain adequate amounts of vitamins and minerals. Cows that are housed should get some exercise each day. In problem herds, the prevalence of ketosis can be assessed from milk production records together with the monitoring of ketone levels in blood or milk. Blood glucose and β-hydroxybutyrate levels from metabolic profiles are useful in detecting subclinical cases, while other data may define the mineral and trace element status. The diet of susceptible cows should be supplemented with propylene glycol.

SUPPLEMENTAL READING

Hibbitt, K. G.: Bovine ketosis and its prevention. Vet. Rec. *105*:13–15, 1979.

Littledike, E. T., Young, J. W., and Beitz, D. D., et al.: Common metabolic diseases of cattle: ketosis, milk fever, grass tetany and downer cow complex. J. Dairy Sci. *64*:1465–1482, 1982.

Pregnancy Toxemia

IVAN W. CAPLE, B.V.Sc., Ph.D.
and J. G. McLEAN, B.V.Sc., Ph.D.

Pregnancy toxemia is primarily a metabolic disorder of ewes. A comparable condition is also seen in cows and goats. It is characterized principally by hypoglycemia and hyperketonemia, and is manifested clinically by nervous signs and recumbency. The disorder arises when synthesis of glucose by the liver is insufficient for metabolic requirements. This occurs when dietary intake is inadequate and utilization of glucogenic precursors from maternal reserves cannot compensate for the energy demands of the developing fetus. There is also a substantial mobilization of body fat reserves.

PREGNANCY TOXEMIA IN EWES

Occurrence

Pregnancy toxemia in ewes occurs during the last 6 weeks of pregnancy when there is a large demand for glucose by the developing fetus. The condition is seen in ewes with a single fetus, but ewes carrying multiple fetuses are most susceptible. It is very often a fatal disease and is usually seen as an outbreak when there is inadequate nutrition available or when there is a reduction in the voluntary food intake.

Inadequate nutrition arises when ewes are placed on low quality fibrous diets or on pastures that decline in nutritive value owing to seasonal or climatic conditions. The most variable factor in the nutrition of the pregnant ewe, however, is voluntary food intake. This declines in overfat ewes because intra-abdominal fat and the enlarging uterus decrease the capacity of the digestive tract. Transport of ewes to a new environment, change of diet such as introduction to grain feeding, and intercurrent diseases such as foot abscess, foot rot, and intestinal parasitism also diminish voluntary food intake. Starvation and hypocalcemia associated with management procedures, such as transport, yarding, shearing, and dipping, also contribute to many outbreaks.

Etiology and Pathogenesis

A gradual or sudden reduction in food intake is all that is required to produce pregnancy toxemia. The nutrient requirements of a ewe with twin fetuses rise to nearly twice the maintenance level during the last 2 months of pregnancy when the fetuses are growing rapidly. While inadequate energy and protein intake is the main predisposing factor, deficiencies of other nutritional factors, including choline and biotin, may contribute to the development of pregnancy toxemia.

The ewe cannot regulate the glucose demand of the fetus and must draw on body reserves to meet the demands that cannot be met by food intake alone. The ewe does not obtain the glucose essential for the fetus, the central nervous system, the eyes, the erythrocytes, and the mammary glands from its alimentary tract but must synthesize this glucose. Over half the glucose required is normally synthesized in the liver and in the kidney cortex from the propionic acid produced in the rumen by microbial fermentation of ingested carbohydrates. The remainder is obtained by gluconeogenesis from amino acids, lactic acid, and glycerol released from body fat stores.

In pregnancy toxemia, the propionic acid and glucogenic precursors derived from the diet and body reserves are unable to maintain glucose requirements. Hypoglycemia occurs, and this leads to depression of the central nervous system. Fatty acids, which are rapidly mobilized from fat stores under hormonal influence, enter the liver and are oxidized with the production of acetyl-CoA. When there is a deficiency of glucose precursors, there is a reduction in intermediates of the tricarboxylic acid (TCA) cycle, particularly oxaloacetate, which is required if acetyl-CoA is to be utilized by the TCA cycle. Acetyl-CoA accumulates and is diverted into the production of ketone bodies.

Excessive production of ketone bodies produces acidosis, because acetoacetate and β-hydroxybutyrate are strong acids, and prolonged urinary excretion results in loss of sodium and potassium ions and lowering of the plasma alkali reserve. Ketoacidosis leads to dyspnea and exacerbates the central nervous system depression, progressing to the irreversible stage in which there is dehydration, uremia, and loss of consciousness. The entry of fatty acids into the liver results in synthesis and accumulation of triglycerides, and this is responsible for the characteristic fatty liver.

Clinical Signs

In an affected flock the disease usually appears as a prolonged outbreak that may extend over several weeks, with a few ewes developing clinical signs each day. Although the course of the disease is as long as 7 days, affected ewes are frequently observed only in the latter stages. There is progressive development of clinical signs from an initial depression of consciousness through to muscular disturbances with abnormal posture, loss of muscle tone, balance, and locomotion, and then finally recumbency, coma, and death.

Initially affected ewes lag behind the flock when it moves. The ewes appear blind, and they can still hear and will face humans and dogs when approached but seldom move away. If forced to move they do so in an aimless manner with a staggering gait and will often lean awkwardly against obstacles. The pupillary light reflex is diminished, and the eye preservation reflex is absent. Temperature, heart rate, respiratory rate, and ruminal movements are mostly normal. As the condition progresses, ewes become more listless.

Neuromuscular disturbances appear as fine tremors of the muscles of the head with twitching of the ears and lips, and some ewes show convulsions. In the latter stages, ewes adopt abnormal postures and jaws are elevated —"stargazing." There may be grinding of the teeth and champing of the jaws. Ewes remain in sternal recumbency, with the head round near the flank, or in lateral recumbency. They become comatose, show labored breathing, and die after 3 to 4 days.

Occasionally, the fetus dies and the ewe experiences a transient recovery, but the ewe relapses as a result of toxemia if the fetus decomposes and is not aborted. Affected ewes commonly have difficulty during lambing. Some may pass a dead fetus and recover. Overfat ewes subjected to a period of acute starvation develop clinical signs more rapidly and die before the condition progresses to the comatose stage. These ewes usually have hypocalcemia as well as ketosis.

Clinical Pathology

In the early stages of pregnancy toxemia there is hypoglycemia, elevated plasma fatty acid and blood glycerol levels, and hyperketonemia, often with ketonuria. The presence of ketone bodies (acetoacetate and acetone) in the plasma and urine may be detected using sodium nitroprusside reagents (Rothera's test, Acetest tablets, and Ketostix test strips*). Plasma cortisol levels are increased. In animals with advanced cases of acidosis and renal failure, plasma bicarbonate concentration may be reduced by 50 per cent, and blood urea nitrogen level may be elevated. In the terminal stages, comatose ewes may even have hyperglycemia.

Necrotic lesions are often minimal. Usually twin fetuses or a large single fetus is present. The lambs may be dead, and a few may show varying stages of decomposition. The liver is enlarged, light yellow in color, friable, and the cut surface greasy. Fatty infiltration and degenerative changes may be seen in the adrenal glands, kidneys, and heart.

Diagnosis

Pregnancy toxemia is characterized by nervous signs and is often associated with a history of undernutrition or error of management. Ewes are affected in the last weeks of pregnancy and die in 3 to 5 days.

The disease has to be differentiated from hypocalcemia, which is characterized by paralysis and the "frog-leg" posture of recumbent ewes in which the hind limbs are extended. Hypocalcemia has a much shorter course (12 to 24 hr) than pregnancy toxemia and affects more ewes in the flock. Hypocalcemia is seen after sudden deprivation of food or after exertion and responds to treatment with calcium salts.

---

*Available from Ames Company, Division of Miles Laboratories, Inc., Mulgrave, Australia.

Treatment

Treatment is successful only in ewes that show initial signs of pregnancy toxemia and are able to stand. Recumbent or comatose ewes usually die despite treatment. Glucose administered as a hypertonic solution (40 per cent) parenterally is not usually effective, and it is impractical to administer to large numbers of ewes at frequent intervals. When intensive therapy can be given to a valuable animal, glucose should be incorporated into the electrolyte solutions given by intravenous infusion (see Fluid Therapy, Section 1). The object of treatment is to

1. Increase the availability of glucose precursors by increasing dietary intake, supplying glucogenic precursors, or causing their mobilization from body stores (Table 1).
   a. Supplementary feed should be provided. A 50-kg ewe with twin fetuses will require 2 kg of oats/day if no other pasture is available. When pregnancy toxemia occurs in flocks being fed grain as a supplement to pasture, it is often advisable to reduce the stocking rate as well as increase the supplementary feed.
   b. Affected ewes should be given 200 ml of a warm 50-per cent glycerol solution or propylene glycol orally twice daily until normal appetite returns completely.
   c. The anabolic steroid, trenbolone acetate (Finajet)* (30 mg intravenously or intramuscularly), stimulates appetite of affected ewes and reduces blood ketone and fatty acid concentrations.
2. Reduce the metabolic drain on the ewe by removal of the fetus by cesarean section or by induction of parturition. Cesarean section is a successful procedure for affected ewes that do not show severe acidosis and renal failure. Induction of parturition with 10 mg dexamethasone 21-isonicotinate (Voren)†, has resulted in higher survival rates of ewes and lambs in flocks predisposed to pregnancy toxemia by outbreaks of foot abscess or foot rot, which suddenly limit their ability to graze. Ewes subjected to prolonged undernutrition have had unreliable responses to glucocorticoids, and higher doses may be required.

Prevention

Ewes need to be watched closely during the last weeks of pregnancy. In flocks in which some ewes show pregnancy toxemia, other ewes may not be affected at the expense of growth and development of the fetus and mammary glands. This may lead to greater mortality in lambs with low birth weights, and poor growth of survivors because of reduced milk production by ewes.

Pregnancy testing may be used to determine those ewes potentially at risk in a flock. A blood glucose concentration profile obtained in mid-pregnancy can assist in selecting ewes that are at risk. An overnight fasting blood glucose concentration is determined in samples collected from ewes 90 days after mating, and those with levels below the median are considered to be at greater risk and should be managed accordingly. Plasma β-hydroxybuty-

*Available from Hoechst U.K. Ltd., Middlesex, U.K.
†Available from Div. of Boehringer Ingelheim, Sydney, Australia.

Table 1. *Diagnosis Tests and Drug Therapy for Pregnancy Toxemia*

Test* or Drug†	Species	Dose
Acetest tablets	Bovine	
Ketostix	Ovine	
Labstix		
Glycerol (50% solution)	Ovine	200 ml (orally twice daily)
Propylene glycol (50% solution)	Ovine	200 ml (orally twice daily)
Anabolic steroids		
Trenbolone acetate	Ovine	30 mg
Glucocorticoids		
Dexamethasone 21-isonicotinate	Ovine	10 mg
Glucose (40% solution)	Bovine	500 ml (IV)
Propylene glycol	Bovine	500 ml (daily)
Anabolic steroids	Bovine	
Trenbolone acetate		125–250 mg
Dehydrotestosterone undecyclenate		125–250 mg

*Ames Company, Division of Miles Laboratories, Inc., Mulgrave, Australia.
†Many of these preparations sold under a variety of tradenames. Consult Rossoff, I. S.: Handbook of Veterinary Drugs. Springer: New York, 1974.

rate concentration can be used as a guide to adjust supplementary feeding of flocks in the last few weeks of pregnancy. Ten per cent of the flock is sampled, and feeding is increased when the mean concentration of plasma β-hydroxybutyrate rises above 4.8 mg/100 ml (0.8 mmol/L).

If ewes are being fed a diet fulfilling all requirements during the last 3 months of pregnancy, they should gain at least 4 kg of body weight if carrying a single lamb and 7.5 kg of body weight if carrying twins.

When ewes are overfat at mating, their body weight should be decreased gradually by 20 per cent with restricted feeding in the first 2 months of pregnancy, and then the food supply should be increased for the next 3 months. Supplementary feed is given when necessary.

Ewes that are overfat in late pregnancy should be exercised by driving them slowly for about a mile each day. Concentrates can be given to increase energy intake. Shelter and additional feed should be provided during inclement weather. Intercurrent diseases such as parasitism and infections must be treated.

Under grazing or range conditions, lambing should be timed to coincide with maximum pasture growth. Aged ewes with incomplete dentition should be removed from the breeding flock.

PREGNANCY TOXEMIA IN BEEF COWS

Occurrence

Pregnancy toxemia, or ketosis, occurs in pastured and housed beef cows when nutrition is inadequate during the last 2 months of pregnancy. Cows of all ages are affected, and overfat animals and those bearing twin calves are particularly susceptible. Cows given unlimited access to spring pastures during the dry period become overfat, and they are predisposed to the toxemic condition when pastures decline in nutritive value during the summer or when they are placed on stubble pastures after cropping. The disease in beef cows has many similarities to pregnancy toxemia in ewes and to the fat cow syndrome in dairy cows. Pregnancy toxemia can be reproduced experimentally by not providing adequate nutrients for overfat cows during the last 6 weeks of pregnancy.

Clinical Signs

The clinical signs and the rates of progress of the condition are associated with the stage of pregnancy and the degree of nutritional stress.

Those cows that become affected between 7 and 9 months of pregnancy initially show lethargy and depression, stop foraging for food, and separate from the rest of the herd. Acetone can often be detected on the breath of most cows in an affected herd, but only a few cows have other clinical signs, such as reduced appetite, rapid deterioration of body condition, and eventual recumbency. Recumbent cows often have a forced expiratory grunt and increased respiratory rate, and there is usually a clear nasal discharge and muzzle epithelium flaking. Feces are sparse, hard, and dry in the early stages and are often covered with mucus that sometimes contains blood. Some cows have bloody diarrhea in the terminal stages. Rectal temperature ranges from 38 to 41°C. Affected cows become recumbent 3 to 14 days before they die, and while some remain in sternal recumbency, most fall into lateral recumbency after 2 days.

Cows affected within a few days before parturition show excitability, an incoordinated and high-stepping gait, and constipation. Experimentally, these signs can be produced in overfat cows with 2 days of starvation. Initially, they appear bright and alert, but they gradually become depressed, recumbent, unable to rise, and anorectic. Some cows may die during parturition, and others die within 30 days after calving. The condition in lactating beef cows is similar to the fatty liver syndrome in lactating dairy cows.

Clinical Pathology

In herds with clinical cases, cows with no obvious signs have hypoglycemia (blood glucose level <30 mg/100 ml), hyperketonemia, and ketonuria. In cows with clinical signs, blood ketone concentrations are more elevated (acetoacetate up to 16 mg/100 ml and β-hydroxybutyrate up to 125 mg/100 ml). Cows affected near parturition have hypocalcemia, and serum magnesium levels are either normal or low. Recumbent cows in the terminal stages have hyperphosphatemia (phosphate level up to 20 mg/100 ml) and hyperglycemia (blood glucose level up to 160 mg/100 ml). Serum aspartate aminotransferase (AST) activity is elevated. Urinalysis shows ketonuria, and in the terminal stages proteinuria and hematuria are evident. At necropsy, lesions consist of an enlarged, yellow fatty liver and fatty changes in the kidney and adrenal cortex. Histologic examination of the liver of cows with extreme cases shows gross fatty infiltration with an appearance resembling adipose tissue. Thrombi associated with infarcts are commonly present in the pulmonary, splenic, and portal veins.

Diagnosis

Usually only 1 or 2 cows show clinical signs before a veterinarian is consulted. General consideration of the history, stage of pregnancy, and nutritional status often enables a tentative diagnosis to be made on the basis of the clinical signs. Clinical pathologic tests will confirm elevated ketone and decreased calcium levels in urine and blood.

Differential diagnosis in individual animals includes traumatic reticulitis, pyelonephritis, ephemeral fever, and lead poisoning.

Treatment

Response to treatment depends on the duration and severity of the condition, and there is a high mortality rate.

Replacement therapy with intravenous solutions of glucose (500 ml of 40-per cent solution) or with combined solutions (500 ml of 20-per cent calcium borogluconate with phosphorus, magnesium, and 20-per cent glucose) is of value only in mild cases. Treatment with oral propylene glycol (500 ml daily) and fluids (see Fluid Therapy, Section 1) is aimed at supplying glucogenic precursors and correcting dehydration. Anabolic steroids (200–300 mg of 1-dehydrotestosterone undecyclenate (Vebonol)* and 125–250 mg of trenbolone acetate (Finajet)† are given to stimulate appetite in affected cows, and they also cause mobilization of glucogenic precursors that decrease ketone body production in the liver. Immediate removal of the calf by cesarean section decreases the metabolic drain on the cow and may save a valuable animal. Induction of parturition using glucocorticoids is not satisfactory in recumbent cows because of the delay in response.

Treatment of a herd is by provision of supplementary feed, such as good quality hay.

Prevention

Since fat cows are particularly susceptible, cows should not be in this condition in the later half of pregnancy, but neither should they be subjected to periods of starvation. Supplementary feed should be provided for cows when there is inadequate pasture available in the last 2 months of pregnancy. Changes in body weight of pregnant and lactating cows can be used as a guide to the need for supplementary feeding of the herd. When any pregnant cow shows a weight loss of 30 kg or more, or when a lactating cow shows a weight loss of 50 kg or more in 14 days, supplementary feed should be given.

Supplementary Reading

Pregnancy Toxemia in Ewes

Heitzman, R. J., Herriman, I. D., Austin, A. R., et al.: The response of sheep with pregnancy toxemia to trenbolone acetate. Vet. Rec. *100*:317–318, 1977.
Hunt, E. R.: Treatment of pregnancy toxemia in ewes by induction of parturition. Aust. Vet. J. *52*:338–339, 1976.
Reid, R. L.: The physiopathology of undernourishment in pregnant sheep, with particular reference to pregnancy toxemia. Adv. Vet. Sci. *12*:163–238, 1968.

Pregnancy Toxemia in Cows

Caple, I. W., Pemberton, D. H., Harrison, M. A., et al.: Starvation ketosis in pregnant beef cows. Aust. Vet. J. *53*:289–291, 1977.
Kingrey, B. W., Ludwing, V. D., Monlux, W. S., et al.: Pregnancy disease of cows. N. Am. Vet. *38*:321–322, 328, 1957.
Spence, A. B.: Pregnancy toxemia of beef cows in Orkney. Vet Rec. *102*:459–461, 1978.

---

*Available from Ciba-Geigy Ltd., Basel, Switzerland.
†Available from Hoechst U.K. Ltd., Middlesex, U.K.

Fat Cow Syndrome and Subclinical Fatty Liver

C. JEREMY ROBERTS, B.V.Sc., Ph.D., M.R.C.V.S.
and IAN M. REID, B.Sc., Ph.D., M.N.S.

In clinical dairy cattle practice in various countries, including the United States, Hungary, France, the Union of Soviet Socialist Republics, and the United Kingdom, fat cow syndrome (FCS) or fatty liver syndrome has been described in dairy cows after calving. The syndrome, as the name implies, occurs particularly in high-yielding dairy cows where overfeeding during the dry period results in overfat cows at calving. Depressed appetite and consequent energy deficit after calving result in a rapid loss of body weight and an accumulation of intracellular fat in various organs including the liver. The clinical syndrome is associated with a higher incidence of metabolic, infectious, and reproductive disorders, such as ketosis, milk fever, mastitis, and retained placenta.

FCS is a clinically recognizable entity that can be diagnosed by an experienced veterinarian. However, it is now known that FCS is only the "tip of an iceberg" (Fig. 1), and that a much larger number of cows may be affected by subclinical forms of the syndrome.

OCCURRENCE

FCS in its clinical and subclinical forms arises sporadically, as a result of faulty feeding in late lactation and the dry period. It is most frequently observed in loose housing where cattle in all stages of the reproductive cycle are fed and managed as one group. Cows with long dry periods due to infertility problems are particularly at risk of becoming overfat. Feeding high quality forage such as maize silage or lush grass ad lib in the dry period will also result in overfat cows.

The syndrome affects all breeds and all ages, though heifers are less at risk under most farming practices. FCS is most commonly seen in the first 2 weeks of lactation, but cases may occur before calving and as late as 1 month after calving.

INCIDENCE

FCS results from a herd feeding problem, and the incidence within the herd will depend to a large extent on the overall fatness of the herd and the severity of the postcalving energy deficit. Morbidity may be as high as

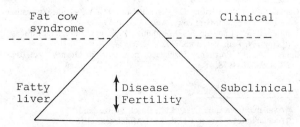

Figure 1. Fat cow syndrome and subclinical fatty liver.

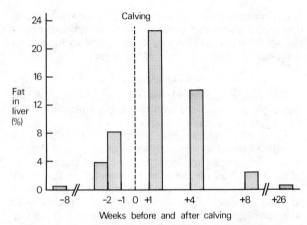

Figure 2. Average percentage of fat in the liver before and after calving.

50 to 90 per cent of newly calved cows, and mortality may reach 25 per cent.

The use of liver biopsy techniques in large numbers of cows in the United Kingdom has shown that the subclinical form of the syndrome is much more common than previously realized. About one third of dairy cows with milk yields greater than 5500 kg are affected, and the incidence in different herds ranges from 10 to 50 per cent.

PATHOGENESIS

A common feature of many cows in early lactation is the development of a negative energy balance because feed intake is insufficient to meet the nutritional demands for maintenance and lactation. As a result of this energy deficiency, cows mobilize body reserves of fat and muscle and so lose body weight and condition.

The mobilization of body reserves involves the release into the blood of free fatty acids from subcutaneous and internal fat depots and glucogenic amino acids from protein stores. The fatty acids are transported in the blood to various organs, such as liver, kidney, and muscle, where they are deposited as intracellular droplets of triglyceride. The greater mobilization of body reserves after calving is reflected in the high levels of fat in the liver at 1 and 4 weeks after calving (Fig. 2). Even before calving, fat is mobilized from body reserves as shown by the rise in liver fat per cent, which occurs 2 to 3 weeks before calving (see Fig. 2). This fat mobilization is probably brought about by the changing hormonal environment, as the cow approaches calving.

The extent of fat deposition in liver and other organs after calving is determined by a number of predisposing factors, including high milk yield potential, condition at calving, and loss of condition after calving.

At the biochemical level, 2 mechanisms appear to be responsible for the development of fatty liver. The first is greater hepatic uptake of fatty acids as a direct result of raised serum levels, resulting from fat mobilization. The second is inadequate hepatic secretion of triglycerides. This may be the result of suboptimal apolipoprotein production in the hepatocyte because of the inadequate supply of necessary amino acids. The extensive deposition of fat in tissues other than the liver suggests that failure of apolipoprotein production in the liver is important in the syndrome because other tissues depend on apolipoprotein synthesized in liver for construction of secretory lipoproteins.

CLINICAL SIGNS

The most useful signs are the presence of very fat cows in the dry cow group together with the presence of thin cows in the freshly calved group, indicating excessive loss of condition in the period immediately after calving. Other general signs in the herd may include evidence of decreased resistance to infection, such as an increase in mastitis, metritis, or salmonellosis, and evidence of increased incidence of metabolic diseases, such as ketosis and milk fever. Specific signs to be observed in individual animals include depression, anorexia, ketonuria, decrease in milk output, and extensive loss of condition. The enlarged liver may sometimes be palpated posterior to the last rib in the right sublumbar fossa.

Any combination of these conditions in the herd with an absence of overtly sick animals may indicate the presence of subclinical fatty liver. In particular, the poor response to treatment of cases that would normally be expected to respond well is a very useful aid in recognizing the presence of the syndrome.

CLINICAL PATHOLOGY

A number of blood constituents are significantly altered 1 week after calving in cows with fatty liver (Table 1). The changes in blood concentrations of albumin, bilirubin, and aspartate aminotransferase (AST) may all reflect alterations in liver function associated with hepatic fat accumulation. AST, however, is an enzyme that occurs not only in liver but also in muscle, kidney, small intestine, and brain. The elevation of AST in the blood of cows with fatty liver may indicate damage to other tissues, such as kidney and muscle as well as liver. Liver specific enzymes, such as ornithine carbamyl transferase (OCT) and glutamate dehydrogenase (GDH), do not appear to be reliable indicators of the presence of fatty liver.

The low blood magnesium concentrations in cows with fatty liver are probably related to the high free fatty acid concentrations and may be important in increasing the susceptibility of cows with fatty liver to milk fever, since hypomagnesemia reduces the ability to mobilize calcium in early lactation.

Table 1. *Alterations in Blood Constituents in Cows with Fatty Liver One Week after Calving*

Blood Constituent	Alteration
Free fatty acids Bilirubin Aspartate aminotransferase (AST) β-Hydroxybutyrate	Increased
Glucose* Cholesterol Albumin Magnesium Insulin White blood cell count	Decreased

*May be elevated in severe or terminal cases.

The white blood cell count is lowered in cows with fatty liver and may fall to as low as 3×10^9/L in cows with severe clinical FCS. The reduced count is largely due to reductions in neutrophils and lymphocytes.

PATHOLOGY

Postmortem findings depend on the degree of fat deposition, the presence or absence of other diseases, and any therapy received prior to death or slaughter. Most cows dying of FCS have large deposits of fat around the heart, kidney, pelvis, and in the omentum. These large deposits are usually present even if most subcutaneous fat depots have been depleted very quickly, and evidence of fat necrosis may be present, particularly in the perirenal adipose tissue.

The liver will show gross evidence of fat deposition by its large size, round edges, and pale color. Fat deposition is not easily detected macroscopically in other organs, although the kidney cortex and cardiac muscle may appear very pale and greasy. When making an assessment of the carcass, treatment of the animal prior to death should be borne in mind because certain agents such as choline and steroid hormones may have reduced the amount of fat in tissues without improving the underlying cause of the deposition.

Microscopically, the fat deposited in tissues may be detected most easily by the use of specific neutral fat stains (see Diagnosis). In the liver, the fat is deposited as globules of triglycerides within the hepatocyte cytoplasm. The extent of deposition may be as great as 70 per cent of the total hepatocyte volume. In addition, fatty cysts may occur, and evidence of damage to mitochondria and of diminished protein synthetic capacity exists. These changes, however, are all reversible in subclinical and nonfatal clinical cases with no evidence of long-term damage to the liver.

Fat also accumulates in the form of intracellular droplets of triglycerides in a number of other tissues, including proximal tubular cells of the kidney, cortical cells of the adrenal gland, Type I (slow, red, oxidative) skeletal muscle fibers, and cardiac muscle fibers. This highly specific distribution of the deposited fat suggests that in FCS, fat is deposited throughout the body in those cells that normally utilize fatty acids for energy metabolism.

It is important to recognize that some of the changes described here will be seen in animals that have been subjected to feed deprivation of more than 24 hr. Postmortem findings can only assist in a diagnosis of FCS or subclinical fatty liver when used in conjunction with the herd's history and clinical pathology.

DIAGNOSIS

There are 3 elements to be considered in the diagnosis of FCS or subclinical fatty liver: history, clinical pathology, and liver biopsy results. If the evidence from the history, including herd appraisal, is sufficiently strong, confirmatory evidence from blood sample test results or biopsy specimen findings may not be necessary. However, in cases of suspected subclinical fatty liver, diagnosis may only be possible by carrying out liver biopsy sample examinations on freshly calved cows.

Table 2. *Liver Fat Values for Diagnosis of Fatty Liver*

Method	Normal	Fatty
Chemical		
Total lipid (mg/gm)	≤ 100	> 100
Triglyceride (mg/gm)	≤ 50	> 50
Histologic		
Toluidine blue (% fat)	≤ 20	> 20
Oil red O (% fat)	≤ 24	> 24

History. Important diagnostic features are fat cows in the dry cow group, thin cows in early lactation, evidence of increased infectious and metabolic diseases with poor response to treatment, and reduced fertility.

Clinical Pathology. The major changes in blood chemistry profiles are shown in Table 1. Using an equation based on blood concentrations of nonesterified fatty acids (NEFA), glucose, and AST at 7 to 13 days after calving, it has been possible to correctly diagnose fatty liver in 3 out of 4 cows. The equation is as follows:

$$y = -0.51 - 0.0032 \text{ NEFA } (\mu\text{mol/L}) + 2.84 \text{ glucose} \\ (\text{mmol/L}) - 0.0528 \text{ AST (IU/L)}$$

If y <0, the cow has fatty liver.

The validity of this equation has been tested in a small number of herds in the United Kingdom and needs further testing before its routine use can be advised. It does, however, form a useful guideline for application in situations other than those in which the equation was formulated.

Liver Biopsy. Samples of liver can be obtained from cows by percutaneous needle biopsy under local anesthesia. The procedure is quick (with practice about 16/hr) and has no measurable effect on milk yield. Fat content of biopsy samples can then be estimated by one of a number of chemical and histologic methods.

CHEMICAL METHODS. These generally involve estimation of either hepatic total lipid or triglyceride content. In our view, triglyceride estimation is the chemical method of choice.

HISTOLOGIC METHODS. Histologic methods of estimating liver fat content may be more suitable for laboratories with routine histologic facilities. The percentage fat in the liver may be estimated by point-counting methods using plastic sections stained with toluidine blue or frozen sections stained with oil red O (ORO). In our view, fat estimation using frozen sections stained with ORO is the histologic method of choice for most routine purposes.

BUOYANCY AND NEEDLE BIOPSY. Another method suitable for estimating liver fat content in the field has been suggested. In the United States, liver fat content is based on buoyancy of needle biopsy samples in water or copper sulfate solutions.

Threshold values for the diagnosis of fatty liver, using the chemical and histologic methods described, are shown in Table 2.

TREATMENT

Various empirical treatments for fatty liver and FCS have been suggested, but there has been very little controlled research. Choline, at 50 gm/day for several days, has been used with limited success, indicating that methyl group donors may be of some value in this condition. Glucose by intravenous infusion at about 60 gm/hr has also been used but with little recorded evidence of success. We have examined the usefulness of niacin supplementation in feed, and although our experiment showed evidence of a reduction in lipolysis in treated animals, there was no reduction in the severity of fatty liver.

More promising results have been obtained with the use of hormones, particularly glucocorticoids and anabolic steroids. The use of these compounds is rational because the pathogenesis of fatty liver indicates that a shortage of gluconeogenic and protein synthetic capacities are major contributors to the syndrome. Increasing the glucose supply by administration of glucose, glycerol or propionate, and a short-acting glucocortocoid, followed by stimulation of protein synthesis by administration of an anabolic steroid appears to be the most logical way of restoring metabolic control.

At present, there is no evidence that "tonics," vitamins, or minerals will have a significant effect on the prognosis of the syndrome, except in those cases where blood levels of calcium or magnesium or both are severely depleted.

PREVENTION

Fatty liver is a problem of high producing cows that undergo substantial body weight losses in early lactation. We believe that the fatty liver is a *symptom* rather than a cause, i.e., it is a convenient measure of the success with which the cow's metabolism has adapted to the demands of lactation. The degree of success in that adaptation will be genetically determined in part but can, in considerable measure, be influenced by the feeding strategy adopted for late pregnancy and early lactation.

To reduce the incidence of fatty liver it is most important to prevent cows from being overfat at calving and to maximize their feed intake after calving. There are several ways of helping to achieve reduction of fatty liver incidence.

1. Cows calving in a lean condition have a higher potential for feed intake. If the feeding system and the feed quality help exploit this fact, then a minimum loss of body condition and less fatty liver need occur.

2. To reach high, dry matter intake rapidly after calving, forage of good quality should be available ad lib. Concentrates should be fed in small amounts and often, so that a rapid increase in intake can be achieved without disturbing the rumen.

3. It is important to supply adequate quantities of correctly balanced protein in the diet. Many diets for high producing cows in early lactation are deficient in undegradable protein. A protein supplement of low degradability will often improve production and may help to reduce the incidence of fatty liver.

Supplemental Reading

Morrow, D. A.: Fat cow syndrome. J. Dairy Sci. *59:*1625–1629, 1976.

Reid, I. M. and Roberts, C. J.: Fatty liver in dairy cows. *In* Practice. Supplement to Vet. Rec. *4:*164–168, 1982.

Reid, I. M. and Roberts, C. J.: Sub-clinical fatty liver in dairy cows—current research and future prospects: Ir. Vet. J. *37:*104–110, 1983.

Société Française de Buiatrie: Le syndrome de la vache grasse. Proceedings of a Symposium: Ecole Nationale Veterinaire de Nantes, 1980.

Downer Cow Syndrome

IVAN W. CAPLE, B.V.Sc., Ph.D.

The only clinical sign common in cows affected with the downer cow syndrome is the inability to rise. While this is the main criterion for diagnosis of the condition, there can be a number of other causes for prolonged recumbency. In practice, most downer cows are usually those that have failed to respond to treatment for hypocalcemia (see Parturient Paresis, Section 5), suggesting that some other complication is involved.

Every downer cow poses an immediate challenge to the diagnostic skills of the practitioner. Without an accurate initial diagnosis, satisfactory therapy and prognosis cannot be offered. Some conditions causing prolonged recumbency, such as bone fractures of pelvis and limbs, luxation of hip joints, and ruptures of major muscles, are hopeless in regard to recovery, and these, too, must be recognized.

OCCURRENCE

Although the syndrome is seen in cows at all stages of the production cycle, most are affected between 2 days before and 10 days after parturition. Downer cows are usually at their peak lactation age, are high producers, and many have a history of parturient paresis. Incidences vary according to the definitions of downers, but as many as 20 per cent of cows attended to by veterinarians for recumbency in the parturient period are affected.

ETIOLOGY AND PATHOGENESIS

There is no universal cause of the downer cow syndrome, but it is most frequently a sequela to parturient paresis. It appears that metabolic disorders, physical injuries during parturition, and traumatic muscular injuries associated with attempts to rise from prolonged recumbency contribute to the downer condition.

A number of risk factors can be associated with the development of the downer cow syndrome.

Parturient Paresis. Complications arise as a result of delayed or incomplete treatment for hypocalcemia, hypothermia, hyperthermia, bloat, and aspiration pneumonia. Prolonged recumbency commonly associated with this disorder may lead to ischemic muscle necrosis and nerve paralysis, particularly when the cow may be lying on 1 hind leg for 6 to 12 hr. Metabolic disorders secondary to parturient paresis, such as hypophosphatemia, hypomagnesemia, hypokalemia, hypoproteinemia, cerebral edema, and ketosis with liver failure, also have been suggested as factors but without direct evidence of their involvement.

Poor Housing Conditions. Poor housing conditions for cows during parturition, such as hard and slippery floors that predispose them to traumatic bone, joint, ligament, tendon, muscle, and nerve injuries when they attempt to stand following either parturition or treatment for hypocalcemia, are also risk factors. Seventy per cent of downer cows that are slaughtered have significant muscle and nerve damage.

Excess Fat. This may lead to traumatic nerve injury at parturition and muscle degeneration during prolonged recumbency. Obese cows are more susceptible to complex metabolic disturbances (hypocalcemia, hypomagnesemia, pregnancy toxemia, and fat cow syndrome). The feeding of excessive amounts of protein (15 per cent) to dry cows has been associated with higher incidences of downer cows in herds.

Septic Conditions. Examples of such conditions are mastitis, metritis, and traumatic pericarditis.

Malnutrition. During periods of prolonged starvation, malnutrition contributes to the development of the downer cow syndrome.

CLINICAL SIGNS

Cows with Downer cow syndrome may appear bright and alert, dull and depressed, or hyperexcited, depending upon the cause of recumbency and whether or not they have been treated with calcium and magnesium solutions.

Usually, cows first present with clinical signs similar to those of parturient paresis, but following treatment with calcium they are unable to rise or relapse after a partial recovery. No sign has been recognized at the initial clinical examination that can be used to forecast potential relapse. After treatment for hypocalcemia, the cows usually appear alert and normal in most respects but are weak in the hind limbs or make no effort to rise.

CLINICAL PATHOLOGY

Most cows that succumb to the downer cow syndrome initially have hypocalcemia (<8 mg Ca/100 ml or <2 mmol/L) and hypophosphatemia (<3 mg P/100 ml or <0.9 mmol/L), as do cows with uncomplicated parturient paresis. Serum calcium and phosphate levels normally rise when cows recover from parturient paresis following treatment with calcium, but in cows that remain downers phosphorus concentrations often remain low. Serum potassium levels have been reported to be low (<3.0 mmol/L) in "creeper" cows that are able to control their forelimbs following calcium therapy but are unable to use their hind limbs. Serum magnesium concentration may be low (<1.5 mg/100 ml or <0.65 mmol/L) in downer cows showing muscle tremors or excitability. Serum aspartate aminotransferase (AST) and creatine phosphokinase (CPK) levels are usually elevated and indicate muscle damage. Urinalysis may demonstrate proteinuria 2 or 3 days after extensive muscle damage, but the excretion of myoglobin is usually completed after this time and a negative test result does not exclude the possibility of muscle damage. In addition, myoglobinuria has to be distinguished from hemoglobinuria. Ketonuria and bilirubinuria may also be present in complicated cases. There are no specific lesions at necropsy but hemorrhage and degeneration can be found in the upper hind leg musculature and nerves of most downer cows, and some have myocarditis.

DIAGNOSIS

The clinical sign of persistent recumbency is the basis of diagnosis of downer cow syndrome. It is essential to conduct a systematic and thorough clinical examination to obtain an informed differential diagnosis. Special attention should be paid to the caudal part of the spine, including the tail, the pelvic ring, and the hind legs. Rectal

Table 1. *Drug Therapy for Downer Cow Syndrome*

Drug	Supplier	Species	Dose
Solution combining calcium magnesium phosphate and dextrose	Many		
Sodium acid phosphate			30 gm in 300 ml H$_2$O (IV)
Tonophosphan	Hoechst U.K. Ltd.	Bovine	20 ml (IV)
Vetibenzamine	Ciba-Geigy Ltd.	Bovine	0.5 mg/kg (IV)

examination is essential. Painful reactions to manipulation, abnormal mobility, lack of motor and sensory responses, or audible crepitation may reveal the site and nature of the physical injuries responsible for prolonged recumbency.

Cows that are recumbent for more than 2 days commonly develop degenerative changes in muscles of the hind limbs. An indication of the extent of muscle damage can be obtained from the activities of AST and CPK in serum and used as a guide for prognosis. Serum levels of AST greater than 200 mU/ml signify a guarded prognosis, and levels greater than 500 mU/ml signify a hopeless prognosis. Cows with severe parturient paresis often have hyperglycemia and proteinuria. Ketosis is usually present in cows that do not eat for 2 to 3 days.

TREATMENT

The basic aim of treatment is to get the cow onto her feet. Hoisting a cow with hip clamps is only of value if the cow will stand and if the clamps will take some weight off her hind legs. Therapy for hypocalcemia is outlined in an earlier article, Parturient Paresis. Cows that show relapses after treatment with calcium alone are given more calcium intravenously or are given solutions containing calcium, phosphorus, magnesium, glucose, and potassium. Phosphorus (30 gm sodium acid phosphate in 300 ml water given intravenously or Tonophosphan*) is used because downer cows have been shown to have persistent hypophosphatemia. Central nervous system stimulants, such as tripelennamine hydrochloride (Vetibenzamine†) given by slow intravenous injection (0.5 mg/ kg), are also used in conjunction with parenteral treatment with minerals (Table 1).

Serum potassium and skeletal muscle potassium concentrations have been found to be low in downer cows and "creeper" cows and have been thought to be associated with muscular weakness. Apparently, some cows have responded to potassium therapy. It is dangerous, however, to administer large amounts of hypertonic potassium solutions intravenously, since this may raise potassium levels rapidly and cause cardiac arrest. It is better to administer potassium by stomach tube to downer cows. Ten liters of water containing 80 gm sodium chloride and 20 gm potassium chloride are given by stomach tube, and a similar solution is provided in a bucket for the cow to drink. Another container is provided with fresh water.

Udder inflation has been recommended for cows with relapses of parturient paresis provided measures have been taken to ensure that glands to be inflated are not mastitic, and the technique does not introduce infection in healthy quarters.

Septic conditions such as mastitis and metritis are treated with broad-spectrum antibiotics administered in therapeutic daily doses.

Cows without obvious bone fractures and joint dislocations that do not rise following the described treatments should be persuaded to rise and provided with shelter, ample bedding, and food. Cows should be turned frequently (every 4 to 6 hr) from side to side. Some may eventually rise unaided after as long as 2 weeks.

PREVENTION

As there is no single cause of the downer cow syndrome, preventive measures are aimed at eliminating the risk factors that predispose cows to recumbency in the parturient period. Attention to nutrition to avoid excessively fat cows and to ensure a low calcium intake in the preparturient period in early lactation is most important. Early treatment of cows with parturient paresis is essential, and cows must be given sufficient calcium. The amount of calcium required to effect a recovery seems to vary, but at least 8 gm of calcium given intravenously may be requird to effect a cure. A solution of 25-per cent calcium borogluconate contains 10.4 gm Ca/500 ml. Cows should be observed closely after treatment in case there are relapses.

Provision of adequate bedding for cows housed during parturition and supervision of cows to minimize prolonged dystocia are important measures to prevent traumatic nerve and muscular damage.

Supplemental Reading

Cox, V. S.: Pathogenesis of the downer cow syndrome. Vet. Rec. *111*:67–69, 1982.

Dirksen, G.: Examination of cattle unable to rise. *In*: G. Rosenberger (ed.). Clinical Examination of Cattle. Philadelphia, W. B. Saunders Company, 388–390, 1979.

Kronfeld, D. S.: Management of downer cows. Mod. Vet. Pract. *57*:599–602, 1976.

Stober, M. and Dirksen, G.: The recumbent cow: differential diagnosis and differential therapy. Vet. Ann. *22*:81–94, 1982.

Ruminant Hypomagnesemic Tetanies

M. MERRALL, B.V.Sc., Ph.D, M.A.C.V.Sc.
and D. M. WEST, B.V.Sc., Ph.D., F.A.C.V.Sc.

The ruminant hypomagnesemic tetanies are a group of diseases occurring in both sexes and in a wide range of species, ages, and dietary, nutritional, and management conditions. At this time, the pathophysiology of the disease, while apparently following a similar course in each case, is not fully understood. The disease is charac-

---

*Available from Hoechst U.K. Ltd., Middlesex, U.K.
†Available from Ciba-Geigy Ltd., Basel, Switzerland.

terized by a fall in serum magnesium ion concentration, and other ions may fall in parallel fashion but do not appear to be an integral and essential feature of the disease.

OCCURRENCE

Grass Tetany. Grass tetany, lactation tetany, hypomagnesemia, hypomagnesemic tetany, and grass staggers all are part of the classic metabolic condition associated with tetanic convulsions observed most commonly in lactating cows feeding on lush, rapidly growing pasture, usually in the spring. Although most frequently seen in the lactating cows, it has been reported in calves and yearlings as well as in adult stock, bulls, steers, and nonlactating cows. It has also been known to occur in housed cattle inadvertently fed a diet low in magnesium.

Green-oat poisoning, barley poisoning, and wheat-pasture poisoning are terms applied to the tetany occurring in adult cattle that graze these growing cereals with low magnesium contents.

Grass tetany may occur in sheep and in ewes during lactation, and is less common in other classes. It has also been found in lactating goats in areas where the disease has been found in lactating cattle.

There is a wide variation in the morbidity of the disease in successive years on the same farm and on adjoining farms in the same year. Thus, variations of morbidity from 0 to 50 per cent have been recorded with variations of mortality reaching possibly 50 per cent in dairy stock even after appropriate therapy. Mortality of 100 per cent has occurred in affected herds of beef cattle, with no clinical signs preceding deaths.

ETIOLOGY AND PATHOGENESIS

A high physiologic demand for magnesium accompanied by a reduction in the amount of magnesium absorbed from the digestive tract are the main factors predisposing ruminants to grass tetany. Magnesium is lost from the body in feces, urine, and milk. The variable quantity lost in the feces is made up of an unabsorbed portion of the diet and the endogenous magnesium that enters the gastrointestinal tract via saliva and other gastrointestinal secretions. The endogenous loss has been estimated to be 2.0 gm/day in a cow. If excess magnesium is absorbed from the digestive tract this is excreted in the urine and the urinary magnesium output may rise to 5.0 gm/day. When magnesium absorption from the digestive tract falls to relatively low levels, then urinary magnesium also falls. It has been claimed that there is a correlation between serum and urinary magnesium levels, but urinary magnesium levels appear to drop more in response to lowered intestinal absorption than do serum magnesium levels. This fact is utilized in a urinary magnesium level assay kit used to assess individual or herd magnesium status.*

The amount of magnesium in milk varies among individuals, but for each individual it remains relatively constant. As much as 3.0 gm/day may be lost through the

milk, and this is often the factor that changes the magnesium balance from positive to negative.

To maintain magnesium homeostasis there must be a constant intake and absorption of magnesium. Feeds fluctuate widely in both content and availability of magnesium, and choice of pasture species is important because legumes, including clover and alfalfa, have a higher magnesium content than grasses. In some cases, the soil itself is important, as some soils have a low magnesium content. However, an absolute magnesium deficiency in soil is not necessary for the development of the problem in the ruminant. Plant magnesium content is related to the levels of exchangeable magnesium in the soil, although uptake may be modified by the levels of other exchangeable cations, e.g., calcium and potassium. Application of potassic fertilizer may therefore markedly alter the magnesium composition of grasses.

The availability of magnesium for absorption from the gastrointestinal tract is said to range from 4 to 35 per cent. Minerals and ions that are known to reduce the availability of magnesium in the bowel include Ca^{++}, K^+, and NH_4^+. More recently, it has been recorded that cattle dying from grass staggers had rumen aluminum levels more than 5 times the average of cattle on the same feed that were not affected. Other factors that have been claimed to affect magnesium intake and absorption are phosphate, sulfate, manganese, sodium, citrate, *trans*-aconitate, and lipid.

One important component in the disease is the energy balance of the animal. There is considerable evidence from starvation experiments and from energy supplementation experiments that alterations in the energy intake are associated with alterations in magnesium availability. It has been found that cold and inclement weather decreases the serum magnesium concentrations of both cattle and sheep, and one mechanism by which this is thought to occur is by reduced feed intake. A possibly more important feature in the regulation of serum magnesium level and in the relationship between low serum magnesium level and grass tetany is the role of intracellular magnesium, yet this has received little investigation.

The previous discussion is related to the maintenance of serum magnesium levels. It is quite possible for the animal to be severely hypomagnesemic, yet show little or no outward manifestation and recover normal serum magnesium levels after some interval. However, when the animal is hypomagnesemic or the serum magnesium level is falling rapidly, tetanic convulsions may occur. The critical factor for the initiation of tetany is the level of magnesium in the cerebrospinal fluid (CSF). Levels of magnesium in the CSF are held within strict limits despite wide variations in serum levels. Perfusion of the CSF space with low-magnesium CSF has demonstrated that initiation of tetany is more closely related to CSF magnesium than to serum magnesium, and this is also true in field cases when tetany develops only in hypomagnesemic cows that also have low CSF magnesium.

CLINICAL SIGNS

Affected animals tend to become restless, to separate themselves from the herd or flock, to stop grazing, and to suddenly walk or run for no apparent reason. Walking is often characterized by a high-stepping action of the

---

*Equipment: magnesium in bovine urine, no. 11005. E. Merck, Darmstadt, German Federal Republic.

forelimbs. The animal's legs become very stiff, and it falls when driven or subjected to stress, such as the introduction of a dog to the paddock. When recumbent, tetanic spasms are interspersed with bouts of clonic convulsions. Eyeballs are often distended, and eye movements are erratic and indicative of nystagmus. Fine muscle trembling is present with champing of the jaws and a fine frothy saliva round the mouth. The violence of the muscular activity causes a very rapid heart rate, and 150 beats/min and more are not uncommon. The force of the beats may make the heart sounds audible up to 2 meters away from the animal. Because of the extent of the muscular activity, the body temperature may reach 40.5° C. After bouts of convulsions the animal often relaxes in lateral recumbency, but stimulation such as the insertion of a hypodermic needle for therapy may trigger a further attack.

Chronic and subacute forms of hypomagnesemia have been described. The chronic form of the disease is associated with a vague change in temperament and a loss of appetite and body condition. The subacute form resembles the initial stages of the acute attack, and signs include nervous frequent urination and defecation and flinching around the head, with the animal acting as though it is going to be struck. Animals may be aggressive during this stage. There is a rapid pulse and respiratory rate but decreased appetite, ruminal movements, and milk production.

If the mean serum magnesium levels of 10 randomly selected cows from a herd is sufficiently low, then the herd is suffering from subclinical hypomagnesemia. There will be decreased milk fat production that is identifiable through the herd's response to therapy. The cause of this decline has not been fully identified, but it has been observed that hypomagnesemic cows tend to be less aggressive, and their subsequent access to better quality food is reduced. There is also a direct effect on rumen function, since production response to magnesium therapy only occurs following the oral route of administration.

The disease in sheep is almost identical to the disease in cattle, but in many cases hypomagnesemia has been associated with a more sustained undernutrition rather than with sudden exercise or change of diet. Older, twin-rearing ewes are most at risk.

In goats, signs are reported to be identical to those in cattle. Acute, subacute, and chronic forms of the disease have been recorded.

CLINICAL PATHOLOGY AND LESIONS

Estimations of the magnesium levels of serum and CSF are the most significant measurements. Healthy, normal animals generally have a serum magnesium level of 1.0 mmol/L. A herd mean level at which milk fat production is going to be depressed sufficiently that therapy is warranted is about 0.65 mmol/L. Animals with serum magnesium levels below 0.42 mmol/L are at risk for tetany, but levels as low as 0.05 mmol/L have been recorded when tetany was not present. Once magnesium levels in CSF fall below 0.60 mmol/L, tetany may be expected.

Hypocalcemia often accompanies hypomagnesemia, and hyperkalemia is often reported. Following tetany there is a transient rise in serum aspartate aminotransferase (AST) and creatine phosphokinase (CPK) levels, the latter to relatively high levels but returning to normal quite rapidly after recovery.

Necrotic lesions are few, nondiagnostic, and usually indicative only of violent antemortem activity. Thus, varying degrees of extravasation of blood would be seen as would regurgitation of rumen contents followed by aspiration and agonal emphysema. The magnesium level of heart muscle has been suggested as a means of confirming a diagnosis of hypomagnesemic tetany at necropsy. In a recently dead animal, a low CSF magnesium level would confirm a diagnosis, while a normal or high urinary magnesium level would eliminate hypomagnesemia as a possible diagnosis.

DIAGNOSIS

Grass tetany as a diagnosis must be considered on the basis of history and clinical signs of hyperesthesia and tetany. The important points in the history include time of year, stage of lactation, type of feed, weather, and type of pasture. Recovery following magnesium therapy may serve as confirmatory evidence. On a herd or flock basis, the mean serum magnesium levels of 10 randomly selected animals, possibly combined with urinary magnesium level estimations, would be the diagnostic criteria.

In cattle, acute lead poisoning produces similar clinical signs, but there is usually a history of access to lead, and there may be blindness and mania. Animals suffering with hypocalcemia may have limb rigidity and may show paddling but lack hyperesthesia and "pounding" heart. Rabies usually includes ascending paralysis, anesthesia, and absence of tetany. Nervous ketosis, lightning strike, plant poisoning, and meningitis need to be considered, but in the acute clinical case the disease is fairly easy to recognize. Paspalum staggers (*Claviceps paspali* poisoning) is a fairly important differential diagnosis but usually occurs at a different time of the year, and signs are more indicative of cerebellar ataxia. Diagnosis is therefore principally based on clinical findings supported by clinical, pathologic findings.

When a herd has suboptimal production, hypomagnesemia is one of the diseases that must be considered. Others would include parasitism, trace mineral deficiencies, such as of copper, cobalt, selenium, and iodine, and lack of balance in dietary composition. Results of laboratory analyses of appropriate samples are required to determine the actual cause of the condition.

TREATMENT

The treatment of hypomagnesemia changes according to the severity of the condition. The normal recommendation is to use solutions of magnesium salts and calcium salts separately or together. Available from a number of sources are sterile solutions of 10 per cent wt/vol magnesium sulfate, 20 per cent wt/vol magnesium sulfate, and combined solutions of calcium borogluconate (25 per cent wt/vol), dextrose (25 per cent wt/vol) with magnesium chloride (4 per cent wt/vol) or hypophosphite (5 per cent wt/vol), or calcium borogluconate (25 per cent wt/vol) and magnesium chloride (4 per cent). Other combinations include magnesium as the citrate, or varying the concentrations of the ingredients. Packaging is 100 ml for sheep and includes 200-, 300-, 350-, 500-, and 1000-ml sizes for cattle.

In most cases, the solutions are administered by slow

intravenous injection. When it is not a proprietary mixture, it is preferable to administer a calcium borogluconate solution first. The usual dose is 350 ml of 25 per cent wt/vol calcium borogluconate and 10 per cent wt/vol magnesium sulfate or 350 ml of a combined solution in cattle and 50 to 100 ml in sheep and goats. One important feature of the disease is that response to treatment is related to the interval between the onset of tetany and the onset of therapy—the longer the interval the less likely the therapy will be effective. Another important point is that serum magnesium levels following intravenous injection return to pre-injection levels in 6 hr, so relapses are almost the rule. The response in serum magnesium level is far more sustained after subcutaneous therapy, and it is common practice to inject 350 ml of 20 per cent magnesium sulfate solution subcutaneously. The use of magnesium lactate or gluconate has been suggested to provide a more sustained blood magnesium level.

Intravenous injection is not without its risks, and at higher magnesium concentrations cardiac embarrassment or medullary depression severe enough to cause respiratory failure or both have been recorded. The effects on these 2 areas exerted by calcium are almost opposite to the effects of magnesium. Alternating the intravenous administration of calcium borogluconate and magnesium sulfate solutions reduces the risk of untoward sequelae.

In cases where the animal is at risk of severe injury from continuous convulsions, the use of sedatives or tranquilizers has been recommended.

In all cases in which an individual has been treated for tetany, control measures should be instituted for the animal and should be continued for a minimum of 4 to 7 days to prevent relapse.

PREVENTION

The magnesium status of grazing animals may be improved by appropriate management of soil and pasture, and by direct supplementation of diet.

Soil. Soil management may play some part in altering the amount of magnesium available to the animal. If the pH of the soil is adjusted, this may favor the growth of legumes, which have a higher magnesium content. Top dressing with magnesium fertilizers can help. Levels of approximately 1 ton/ha magnesite have been suggested with the amount changing according to the magnesium content of the material. Care must be exercised, as excessive rates of fertilizer applications may reduce the yield of pasture dry matter. The extent and duration of the response is quite different in different soils, and trials should be carried out to assess the effectiveness in an individual area. Generally, the response is best in light sandy soils.

Other soil management factors are avoidance of excessive use of potassic fertilizers and avoidance of the use of nitrogen fertilizers at times of high risk of grass tetany.

Pasture. Little may be done in this regard. Pasture is managed to provide maximum dry matter yield. This often leads to supplying the stock a sward relatively deficient in magnesium. One method that may be used is the saving of some feed until mature. Coarse, relatively unimproved grasses may also be fed to stock during the nonlactation period. Alternatively, pasture species that have a higher magnesium content may be selected and encouraged in pasture development programs. Generally, these techniques do not favor maximum milk production.

Included at this point is the possibility of dusting pastures with magnesium compounds. This does not influence the plant content but does markedly affect the amount taken in by the grazing animal as part of the diet. The level as recommended is 0.5 to 0.75 kg/cow/week magnesium oxide. This is usually applied early in the morning when the grass is wet with dew. In the absence of adequate natural dew, these preparations may be applied as a solution of magnesium chloride or sulfate and as a watery or oily suspension of magnesium oxide to give comparable doses. Although re-application is necessary after heavy rain, the powder will adhere through rainfall of 40 to 50 mm once initial drying has occurred.

Diet Supplementation. To guarantee that each animal receives the optimum dose, individual drenching is recommended. The soluble salts of magnesium chloride and magnesium sulfate are very suitable for this purpose. At mixing ratios of 3:2 and 1:1 of the respective salts with water, a 120 ml dose supplies 10 gm and 8 gm respectively of elemental magnesium, the amount said to be required for optimum production response. Magnesium oxide is suitable and cheaper. The dosage is calculated at 28 gm/day/cow. The disadvantage of this preparation is that it is relatively insoluble and is suspended in water, so accurate dosing requires frequent agitation of the vessel. Microfined material (200–400 mesh) has eased this problem and also the problem of excessive wear on drenching equipment from silica particles in the material.

In many areas of the world where bloat is also a problem, bloat prophylaxis is being administered per os at the same time of the year as hypomagnesemia prophylaxis. Numerous attempts have been made to combine the 2 preparations for simpler administration. Some problems have been encountered when a reaction has occurred between the mixed ingredients. If products are diluted before mixing, in many cases a large dose volume results (e.g., 150 ml), which increases the risk of drench-gun injuries, occurring during administration.

Feeding of hay that has had supplemental magnesium added as a slurry of magnesium oxide or as a solution of soluble salts is also practiced. Dosages may be calculated to give the optimum dose and applied to the material immediately before feeding. Generally, approximately 50 per cent is added to the individual drenching dose to allow for losses and variations in intake.

Other forms of oral supplementation are the provision of magnesium-containing licks and the addition of magnesium salts to water supplies. Both suffer to some extent from the fact that palatability is not good. In the case of licks, it has been found that 35 per cent of the stock do not take in sufficient quantities to give protection. With treated water, cattle will reduce intake or drink untreated water in preference to the treated supply.

Magnesium bullets are composed of an alloy of 86 per cent magnesium, 12 per cent aluminium, and 2 per cent copper weighted with iron shot and may be given orally. The bullets remain within the rumen and provide a low level of continuing magnesium release for up to 35 days. Usually, 2 magnesium bullets are given to cows.

General. The saving and providing for the stock of a stand of mature pasture have been used as prophylaxis for grass tetany. Giving approximately half of the daily dry matter intake as hay has also been suggested. While these may aid in the prevention of grass tetany in beef cattle, they are not management systems suitable for high-producing dairy cows. In view of the relationship between inclement weather and grass tetany, shelter is considered a useful management practice. A change in calving date to a time of year when pasture magnesium is higher may also be considered.

Dosage figures given here include a number of regimens but most are for correction of a moderate dietary deficiency. Under severe tetany-prone conditions, dosages may not be adequate and an increase may be recommended. This practice is not without its hazards. Oral overdosing with any magnesium salt tends to induce osmotic diarrhea, and this may be difficult to detect on spring pasture. Overdosing by the parenteral route results in depression of consciousness, recumbency, and respiratory depression. This is reversed by the administration of calcium ions. The effect of long-term overdosing has been reported as a high incidence of osteoporosis and lameness.

The dosage regimens for prophylaxis in sheep and goats are proportionate to body weight. Where 60 gm daily of calcined magnesite may be needed in cattle, 7 gm daily is needed in sheep with lambs at foot, and 15 gm daily is needed in a heavily lactating dairy goat. Other compounds must be adjusted proportionately.

WHOLE MILK TETANY

Other disease conditions have been described as separate entities with hypomagnesemia as their primary cause. Whole milk tetany is one. Milk has a relatively low magnesium content but this is not a problem in the young calf, as absorption is very good. As the animal ages, its ability to absorb magnesium declines. In calves reared outdoors, however, greater intake of grass supplements the total magnesium intake, and no problems occur. In calves raised exclusively indoors on whole milk without additives, hypomagnesemia may develop at 2 to 4 months of age. Thus, the disease tends to occur in calves raised under these last conditions, especially those growing most rapidly.

Initial clinical signs are restless twitching of ears and of muscles around the face and hyperesthesia. There may be elevation of heart rate, respiratory rate, and temperature. The disease may resolve without treatment or may progress to a tetanic convulsion with tonic convulsions of the jaws and clonic convulsions of the limbs. Involuntary passage of urine and feces is observed. Respiratory movements cease during a convulsion, and death is often rapid.

During tetany, clinical pathology will reveal a low level of serum magnesium, often with a low level of serum calcium, a moderately elevated level of serum AST, and a markedly elevated level of serum CPK. A variety of lesions have been described on necropsy, none of which appear to be consistent or pathognomonic. Unlike adult cattle, bone magnesium is seriously depleted in the calf, and bone calcium:bone magnesium estimations may be a useful aid at necropsy. A ratio of 70:1 is regarded as normal, and 90:1 is indicative of severe depletion.

Differential diagnosis involves several conditions, such as acute lead poisoning, tetanus, strychnine poisoning, polioencephalomacia, and enterotoxemia caused by the toxin of *Clostridium perfringens*. Autopsy generally does not reveal differences between the diseases, and specimens must be taken to confirm or eliminate other diseases.

Response to magnesium treatment is only transitory. Doses of 100 ml of 10 per cent wt/vol $MgSO_4$ solution often relieve tetany, but follow-up oral magnesium therapy is essential to restore bone reserves and to sustain satisfactory intake. Suggested dosages are 1, 2, and 3 gm magnesium oxide daily for calves 0 to 5, 5 to 10, 10 to 15 weeks of age, respectively.

Post-parturient Hemoglobinuria

IVAN W. CAPLE, B.V.Sc., Ph.D.

Post-parturient hemoglobinuria of dairy cows is characterized by intravascular hemolysis, hemoglobinuria, and anemia. The disorder appears to be associated with a variety of factors and has been observed in many countries. It is not common and causes minor economic losses. Usually, only 1 or 2 cows in a herd are affected, although incidences of up to 40 per cent have been recorded, and up to 50 per cent of affected cows may die.

OCCURRENCE

The disease in mature cows usually occurs within 6 weeks after parturition when cows housed during the winter are turned out to graze on grass in spring and summer. When cows are kept at pasture, the disease occurs in the winter, especially if it is preceded by a dry summer and fall. Generally, affected cows have been fed hay and limited access to grass pasture in the dry period, then allowed unlimited access to grass pasture during early lactation.

Phosphorus deficiency has long been associated with the occurrence of the condition in cows, as has the ingestion of green oats, lush perennial rye grass, newly established subterranean clover, turnips, rape, kale, and other cruciferous plants. Anemia and hemoglobinemia may occur in sheep and cattle grazing cruciferous plants and may not be related to the post-parturient period. In New Zealand, predisposition of younger cows to the condition has been attributed to a copper deficiency associated with excessive application of molybdenum fertilizer and lime to pastures.

Etiology and Pathogenesis

The mechanisms operating to cause intravascular hemolysis are unknown and may be different, depending on the nature of the predisposing factors. Not all outbreaks can be associated with phosphorus deficiency, molybdenum-induced copper deficiency, or cruciferous plant feeding. It has been postulated that hemolytic factors present in some diets may produce oxidative damage to hemoglobin, whereas other diets may render the erythrocytes more susceptible to oxidant challenge. Protection against peroxidation in erythrocytes depends on adequate levels of NADPH and reduced glutathione, on the function of the pentose phosphate pathway, and on an adequate supply of glucose. The erythrocyte is also protected from oxidant injury by the actions of the copper-containing enzyme superoxide dismutase, the selenium-containing enzyme glutathione peroxidase, and vitamin E. Their activity in the erythrocytes is determined by the copper, selenium, and vitamin E intake of the cow. The importance of various nutritional factors in the pathogenesis of hemolysis and in the predisposition of cows to post-parturient hemoglobinuria remains to be defined.

The hemolytic anemia of kale poisoning is due to *S*-methylcysteine sulfoxide that is converted in the rumen to a secondary hemolysin, dimethyl disulfide. The onset of the hemolytic crisis is indicated by increased Heinz body counts and erythrocyte osmotic fragility and by decreased hemoglobin and blood glutathione. Heinz bodies are breakdown products formed as a result of oxidative damage to hemoglobin that bind to the erythrocyte membranes.

Other dietary oxidants suggested to be involved are nitrates yielding hydroxylamine, unsaturated fatty acids, aromatic amines, and hydropteridines.

Heinz body anemia is the main feature of post-parturient hemoglobinuria associated with molybdenum-induced copper deficiency in dairy cows in New Zealand. This disorder is not related to phosphorus deficiency, and there is no increase in erythrocyte osmotic fragility. Heinz bodies have not been a consistent finding in outbreaks associated with phosphorus deficiency elsewhere, or where cows have developed the disorder on rye grass or clover pastures.

CLINICAL SIGNS

The onset of clinical signs is usually rapid, and the disease runs an acute course of 3 to 5 days. Sickness is first indicated by weakness and staggering gait, lowered milk production, and hemoglobinuria characterized by dark red-brown to black urine, which is often moderately turbid. In less acute cases, appetite and milk yield may be unaffected for 24 hr after hemoglobinuria is observed. In severe cases, milk production ceases, and the cow may lose weight and become dehydrated. The heart rate is increased (50 to 130 beats/min), and the jugular pulse is more pronounced. Respiratory rate is greater, and rectal temperature is often slightly elevated (39 to 40°C) in the first stage of the disease, but usually it is normal or subnormal.

As the condition progresses, the visible mucous membranes are pale indicating anemia, and the cow becomes dehydrated, weaker, and recumbent. Jaundice is observed if the cow lives long enough. Gangrene and sloughing of the teats, of the tip of the tail, and of the digits has been observed occasionally, as has diarrhea. Intercurrent diseases such as mastitis and a history of forced exercise is often associated with fatal cases. In nonfatal cases, ketosis commonly occurs coincidentally, and convalescence takes from 3 weeks to 2 months. A number of other clinical signs is observed with the predisposing factors. Pica is common in phosphorus-deficient animals. Anemia is common in cows fed cruciferous plants and in cows in copper-deficient areas.

CLINICAL PATHOLOGY

The presence of hemoglobin in the urine can be determined by its reaction with reagent strips (Labstix)*, and absence of erythrocytes on microscopic examination of

*Available from Ames Company, Division of Miles Laboratories, Inc., Mulgrave, Australia.

urine confirms hemoglobinuria. Hematologic examination shows a low hemoglobin value (<8 gm/100 ml) and a low erythrocyte count (<5 × 10^6/μl) together with evidence of bone marrow response to anemia—anisocytosis, macrocytosis with polychromasia, basophilic stippling of erythrocytes, and higher numbers of nucleated erythrocytes. Heinz bodies may be demonstrated by mixing whole blood (or sedimented cells retrieved from a clotted sample) with 4 volumes of 0.5-per cent methyl violet in 0.85-per cent saline. The mixture is left to stand for 10 minutes, is centrifuged at low speed, and a film is made from the deposited cells. Heinz bodies are intensely purple-stained intracorpuscular structures near the edges of the erythrocytes in 3 to 50 per cent of cells.

In phosphorus-deficient areas, normally lactating cows have low serum concentrations of inorganic phosphate (2 to 3 mg/100 ml or 0.6 to 0.9 mmol/L), and affected cows have levels of 0.3 to 1 mg/100 ml (0.09 to 0.3 mmol/L). When copper deficiency exists, blood copper concentration is usually less than 30 μg/100 ml, and liver copper concentration is less than 5 mg/kg on a dry matter basis. Elevated serum bilirubin and blood urea nitrogen levels are found in cows during the advanced stages of the disorder.

At necropsy, lesions observed are a general jaundiced condition of the carcass, a pale swollen liver with centrilobular necrosis attributed to anemic anoxia, and hemoglobinuric nephrosis of the kidneys.

DIAGNOSIS

Laboratory examination is needed to confirm the diagnosis of post-parturient hemoglobinuria. An acute hemolytic anemia and hemoglobinuria in cows within 6 weeks of calving is only suggestive of this disease, and other diseases to be considered in the differential diagnosis are leptospirosis, babesiosis, bacillary hemoglobinuria, pyelonephritis, and copper poisoning. Some plants contain phenolic compounds that when eaten by cows lead to the formation of red, brown, or black urine.

TREATMENT

As the cause of the condition is unknown, supportive therapy is given to combat acute hemolytic anemia and dehydration, and the predisposing causes are eliminated. At least 5 to 10 L of whole blood should be given to severely affected cows, and additional fluids can be administered orally. When phosphorus deficiency is considered to be a predisposing cause, intravenous injection of 60 gm sodium acid phosphate in 300 ml of sterile distilled water and a similar subcutaneous dose are given, followed by further injections at 12-hr intervals for 3 treatments (Table 1). All cows are drenched with 30 gm sodium acid phosphate or 100 gm bone meal. In view of the importance of an adequate supply of glucose in preventing hemolysis of erythrocytes, glucose should be included in solutions given intravenously. Calcium hypophosphite (30 gm in 100 ml of 10-per cent glucose) has been used to treat affected cows. Glucocorticoids (20 mg dexamethasone intramuscularly) and oral treatments for ketosis are also beneficial.

Table 1. Tests and Drug Therapy for Post-parturient Hemoglobinuria

Test or Drug	Supplier	Species	Dose
Labstix*	Ames Company		
Sodium acid phosphate		Bovine	60 gm in 300 ml H_2O (IV)
Calcium hypophosphite		Bovine	30 gm in 100 ml 10-per cent glucose (IV)
Glucocorticoids Dexamethasone	Many	Bovine	5 mg/100 kg (IM)
Copper glycinate Cuprate	Burns-Biotec†	Bovine	2 ml containing 120 mg Cu (SC)

*Division of Miles Laboratories, Inc., Mulgrave, Australia.
†Division of Chromalloy Pharmaceuticals, Inc., Oakland, California.

In copper-deficient areas, cows are given copper glycinate subcutaneously to provide 120 mg available copper. Other cows should be treated within 48 hr of calving to prevent the condition. Cruciferous plants should be removed from the diet, and the cows should be fed good quality hay. Hematinics, including iron supplementation, folic acid, and vitamin B_{12}, have been given to affected cows, but their therapeutic value has not been evaluated. Any intercurrent disease must also be treated.

PREVENTION

An adequate dietary intake of phosphorus in early lactation is essential in phosphorus-deficient areas. This can be ensured by supplementation with sodium acid phosphate (30 gm/cow/day), bone meal (100 gm/cow/day), or bone-meal licks. In copper-deficient areas, pastures can be top dressed with copper, or cows can be given copper glycinate subcutaneously to provide 120 mg of available copper in the month before parturition. Restricting the intake of cruciferous plants to less than 15 kg/day, and restricting the intake of turnips and beet pulp during the first 2 months of lactation is advisable.

Supplemental Reading

Madsen, D. E. and Nielson, H. M.: Parturient hemoglobinemia of dairy cows. J. Am. Vet. Med. Assoc. 47:577–586, 1939.
MacWilliams, P. S., Searcy, G. P., and Bellamy, J. E. C.: Bovine post-parturient hemoglobinuria: a review of the literature. Can. Vet. J. 23:309–312, 1982.
Parkinson, B. and Sutherland, A. K.: Post-parturient haemoglobinuria of dairy cows. Aust. Vet. J. 30:232–236, 1954.
Smith, B.: The effects of copper supplementation on stock health and production. 1. Field investigations into the effects of copper supplementation on stock health in dairy herds with a history of post-parturient haemoglobinuria. N. Z. Vet. 23:73–77, 1975.
Smith, R. H.: S-methylcysteine sulphoxide, the brassica anaemia factor (A valuable dietary for man?) Vet. Sci. Comm. 2:47–61, 1978.

PHYSICAL AND CHEMICAL DISORDERS

WILLIAM B. BUCK, D.V.M., M.S.
Consulting Editor

Use of Diagnostic Laboratories

WILLIAM B. BUCK, D.V.M., M.S.

An accurate diagnosis is the single most important factor in dealing with animal toxicosis. Once the cause of a problem is known, specific treatment and preventive measures can be initiated. Prior to that, however, the veterinarian is limited to support and treatment of symptoms. The toxicologic diagnosis is based upon a knowledge of pertinent criteria in the case, qualified laboratory evaluation of proper specimens, and intelligent interpretation of laboratory results in light of the circumstances associated with the problem.

When the clinician consults with diagnostic laboratory personnel, certain fundamental information should be given, such as the veterinarian's name and address, the owner's name and address, and the species, breed, sex, age, and weight of the animal. When livestock and poultry are involved, additional facts should be included, such as the number of animals in the herd or flock, the number of animals affected, the number of animals that have died, the course of events in hours or days, the type of management, and feeding programs, history of past illnesses, and immunization records. Other factors that often guide the diagnostician include (1) the length of time animals have been given the last batch of prepared feed, (2) the type of pasture (if the animals are on pasture) and whether or not trash, rubbish, old motors, or farm machinery are accessible to the animal, (3) detailed description of clinical signs, (4) detailed description of postmortem findings, (5) the last time the animal was observed before its death and its condition at that time, (6) what medications were given, if any, when the medications were given, and the response, (7) a history regarding any spraying or treating for internal or external parasites.

CHEMICAL ANALYSES

Chemical evidence is often an indispensable aid in diagnosing toxicologic problems. Used properly and in the right perspective, chemical analyses provide the most important diagnostic criteria. There are limitations, however, to the value of chemical analyses. Rarely should results be used alone in making a diagnosis. Positive chemical data plus history, clinical signs, and postmortem findings may provide evidence enabling one to arrive at an accurate diagnosis. One should never request a chemistry laboratory to simply "analyze for poisons" because an animal died of unknown causes. There are thousands of toxic chemicals and plants, and analyses for all of them would be impossible not only because of the limited amount of sample available but also because of the cost. In addition, there are many toxic plants and even some chemical agents for which no chemical analytical procedures are available.

Although some toxicologic tests are suitable for the veterinary hospital or clinical laboratory, many procedures for toxicologic analyses are complicated, time consuming, and require expensive equipment. Unfortunately, many of the screening qualitative tests for toxicants are not worth the time it takes to perform them. An example is the Reinsch test for arsenic and mercury. When performed by an inexperienced individual, this test is worse than no test at all. Several metals such as arsenic, mercury, and antimony will give a positive reaction to this test. Sulfur and other elements found in biologic specimens will give false-positive results with the Reinsch test. Unless a laboratory is adequately staffed and equipped for analytical chemistry procedures, little significance can be placed on toxicologic screening tests. Perhaps a certain amount of screening and preliminary testing can be performed by a veterinary clinic for the sole purpose of aiding in treatment rationale, but the clinic should then rely upon subsequent chemical confirmation by a qualified toxicology laboratory.

SUBMITTING SPECIMENS FOR LABORATORY EVALUATION

When submitting specimens to a diagnostic laboratory, certain considerations should be made. The importance of supplying a complete account of history, signs, and lesions with the specimens cannot be overemphasized. Such information will enable the toxicologist to select toxicants intelligently for analysis. This is especially important when a test for the toxicant originally suspected proves negative. A chemist still has the opportunity to test for other poisons if adequate specimens have been submitted.

The choice of specimen is important in making a chemical analysis. Specimens should be free of chemical contamination and debris and should not be washed because of the possibility of removing residues of the toxic agent or of contaminating the specimen with the water. One is often dealing with trace amounts of a particular chemical, and even the slightest contamination may produce erroneous results. Tissue specimens should be frozen and packaged to arrive at the laboratory while still frozen. Serum and blood should not be frozen but refrigerated. Always package specimens of various organs separately. Use clean glass or plastic containers that can be tightly sealed. Always label each specimen with the owner's name, the animal's name or number, and the tissue or specimen in the container. Never add preservatives such as formalin to specimens unless there is a specific reason for doing so, and such information is included along with the specimen. Always send more material than you think is necessary. It is easier for the laboratory personnel to throw away excess specimen than for the veterinarian to obtain more specimen after the carcass has been discarded.

Serum cation and enzyme analyses may be very helpful in the diagnosis of certain toxic and metabolic conditions. To obtain meaningful results, several general rules for collection and preservation of serum should be followed. Always collect blood with clean equipment and transfer it to clean vials or tubes. Avoid excessive aspiration pressure, splashing, or time lag during collection to minimize hemolysis. Make every effort to avoid damaging the unclotted or clotted sample. Allow sufficient time for the blood to clot and to retract, usually about 1 hr. Remove serum from the clot within 2 hr. This may be done by carefully pouring off serum from the retracted clot or by centrifugation. After the serum is separated from the clot, it can be frozen and transported with ice.

Specimens that should be submitted from a live animal include (1) 5 ml of serum with clot removed, (2) 10 ml of whole blood, (3) 50 ml of urine, and (4) 200 gm of vomitus, stomach or rumen contents, or feces.

Specimens that should be submitted from a dead animal include (1) 5 and 10 ml of serum and whole blood, respectively, (2) 50 ml of urine, and 100 g each of liver, kidney, spleen, and body fat. The entire brain should be submitted. Many disorders resembling poisoning can be differentiated by examining brain lesions. If an infectious or inflammatory process is suspected, separate the brain longitudinally, fix half in 10–15 per cent buffered formalin and freeze the other half. Up to 500 gm of stomach contents should be submitted.

Table 1. *Specimens Required for Specific Tests*

Poison or Analysis	Specimen Required	Amount of Specimen	Comments
Ammonia	Whole blood or serum	5 ml	Frozen (1–2 drops of saturated $HgCl_2$ may be used instead of freezing rumen contents)
	Rumen contents (composite)	100 gm	
	Urine	5 ml	
ANTU	Stomach and intestinal contents	200 gm	Can be detected only within 12–24 hr after ingestion
	Liver	200 gm	
Antimony, arsenic, or selenium	Liver	50 gm	
	Kidney	50 gm	
	Feed	100 gm	
	Whole blood	15 ml	
	Stomach contents	100 gm	
	Rumen contents	100 gm	
	Urine	50 ml	
Calcium, magnesium, potassium, or sodium	Serum	2 ml	Serum must *not* be hemolyzed; separate clot before transit
	Feed	100 gm	
	Brain	50 gm	
	Spinal fluid	1 ml	
Carbon monoxide	Whole blood	15 ml	
Chloride	See calcium, magnesium, potassium, or sodium		
Chlorinated hydrocarbon insecticides	Brain (cerebrum)	Half of brain	Must not be contaminated with hairs or stomach contents; preferable to use chemically clean glass jars; avoid plastic containers; wrap specimens in clean aluminum foil
	Stomach contents	100 gm	
	Rumen contents	100 gm	
	Liver	50 gm	
	Body fat	100 gm	
	Kidney	50 gm	
Copper, nickel, iron, cobalt, or chromium	Kidney	50 gm	
	Liver	50 gm	
	Whole blood	10 ml	
	Feces	100 gm	
	Feed	100 gm	
Cyanide	Whole blood	10 ml	Freeze specimen promptly in air-tight container
	Liver	50 gm	
	Forage, silage	100 gm	
	Other materials	100 gm	

Table continued on the opposite page

Table 1. Specimens Required for Specific Tests (Continued)

Poison or Analysis	Specimen Required	Amount of Specimen	Comments
Ethylene glycol	Serum Kidney (in formalin) Urine	10 ml Whole organ 10 ml	One kidney in large animals, both kidneys in small animals
Fluoroacetate	Stomach contents Liver	All available 100 gm	Frozen Frozen
Fluorides	Bone Water Forage Soil Urine	5 gm 100 ml 100 gm 100 gm 50 ml	Representative of whole skeleton Representative sample
Herbicides (Diquat, Paraquat, 2,4D)	Weeds Urine Rumen contents Liver Kidney	100 gm 50 ml 200 gm 50 gm 50 gm	See also chlorinated hydrocarbons and organophosphorus insecticides Frozen Frozen
Lead, thallium, or mercury	Urine Kidney Liver	10 ml 50 gm 50 gm	
Nitrates or nitrites	Water Forage, silage Whole blood (methemoglobin) Aqueous humor (eye) Other materials	50 ml 100 gm 10 ml 10 ml 100 gm	Blood should be hemolyzed to prevent breakdown of methemoglobin (e.g., equal parts water)
Carbamates or organophosphorus insecticides	Feed Stomach contents (composite) Rumen contents (composite) Urine	100 gm 50 gm 50 gm 50 ml	Normal animals' blood, urine, stomach or rumen contents are very valuable references
Cholinesterase	Blood (heparinized) Brain (refrigerated or frozen)	10 ml Half of cerebrum	
Oxalates	Fresh forage Kidney (in formalin)	6–8 plants Whole organ	Do *not* chop plants; freeze promptly One kidney in large animals, both kidneys in small animals
Phenols	Stomach contents Rumen contents Other materials	500 gm 500 gm 200 gm	Pack in air-tight container
Strychnine	Liver Kidney Urine Stomach contents	50 gm Whole organ 50 ml 100 gm	
Sulfa drugs, antibiotics, arsenicals, or phenothiazines	Feed Other materials Serum Urine Liver Kidney	50 gm 50 gm 10 ml 50 ml 50 gm 50 gm	
Phosphates	Serum Bone Other materials	5 ml 25 gm 100 gm	
Urea	Feed Other materials See ammonia	100 gm 500 gm	All specimens should be frozen
Warfarin	Whole blood Feed Liver Other materials	5 ml 100 gm 100 gm 100 gm	
Zinc	Liver Kidney Other materials	50 gm 50 gm 100 gm	

Plastic bags, newspaper, bags or cans of ice, and cardboard are good materials for transporting specimens. Liquids such as blood, urine, stomach contents, and water should be shipped in a glass or heavy plastic container that can be sealed.

If one is in doubt about proper tissues for analysis or the availability of confirmatory tests, much time, effort, and confusion can be avoided by placing a telephone call to the laboratory staff.

SPECIMENS FOR DIAGNOSIS OF SPECIFIC TOXICANTS

The procedures for sending in specimens, as outlined previously, are suitable for the detection of most toxicants. There are instances, however, when special considerations regarding chemical analysis and pathologic evaluation are required. Some specific examples for specific toxicants are given in Table 1.

INTERPRETATION OF LABORATORY RESULTS

Interpretation of laboratory results should be done carefully, taking into consideration other evidence. Positive chemical findings are not always evidence of intoxication, nor are negative findings always evidence of the absence of intoxication. For example, chlorinated hydrocarbon insecticides in the fatty tissue of an animal indicates only that the animal was exposed to the insecticide, not that the insecticide produced toxicosis. On the other hand, failure to find certain organophosphorus insecticides in the body tissues would not guarantee that the animal had not been poisoned by such a chemical. In the case of most chlorinated hydrocarbon insecticides, an animal may store a considerable amount of them in its tissues without apparent harmful effects. With organophosphorus insecticides, the animal may metabolize them so rapidly that they are not detectable by chemical analysis.

LABORATORIES OFFERING TOXICOLOGY-CHEMICAL ANALYTIC SERVICE

In 1982, the Veterinary Services Laboratory, Animal and Plant Inspection Services, United States Department of Agriculture, Ames, Iowa, made a survey of public and private veterinary diagnostic laboratories in the United States. The following is a list of those laboratories reporting capabilities for general toxicology-chemical analyses. For a more complete listing, refer to the Directory of Animal Disease Diagnostic Laboratories, September, 1982, United States Government Printing Office, Washington, D.C.

National Animal Poison Control Center
2001 S. Lincoln Avenue
Urbana, Illinois 61801
Hotline (24 hr) (217)333–3611

Alaska

Alaska State-Federal Laboratory
P.O. Box 720
Palmer, Alaska 99654
(907)745–3236

Arizona

Arizona State Department of Health
1520 West Adams Street
Phoenix, Arizona 85007
(602)765–4551

Department of Veterinary Science
University of Arizona
Tucson, Arizona 85721
(602)884–2355

California

California Veterinary Diagnostic Laboratory, Toxicology Section
University of California
Davis, California 95616
(916)752–6322

County of Los Angeles, Department of Health Services Division
12824 Horton Avenue
Downey, California 90242
(213)923–0641

California Department of Agriculture Veterinary Laboratory Services
P.O. Box 255
San Gabriel, California 91778
(213)282–6127

California Department of Agriculture Veterinary Laboratory Services
P.O. Box 5579
San Bernardino, California 92412
(714)384–4287

Colorado

Colorado State University Diagnostic Laboratory
Fort Collins, Colorado 80521
(303)491–6128

Connecticut

Department of Pathobiology
Box U–89
University of Connecticut
Storrs, Connecticut 06268
(203)486–4000

Delaware

Eastern Shore Laboratories Inc.
P.O. Box 657
Laurel, Delaware 19956
(302)749–2284

Florida

Kissimee Animal Disease Diagnostic Laboratory
P.O. Box 460
Kissimee, Florida 32741
(305)847–3185

Jackson County Animal Disease Diagnostic Laboratory
P.O. Box 37
37 E. Hwy 90
Cottondale, Florida 32431
(904)352–4461

Fish Doctor Res. Center
P.O. Box 765
Brandon, Florida 33511
(813)626–1805 or 9551

Georgia

Diagnostic and Investigational Laboratories
Route 2, Brighton Road
Tifton, Georgia 31794
(912)386–3340

Diagnostic Assistance Laboratory
College of Veterinary Medicine
University of Georgia
Athens, Georgia 30601
(404)542–5568

Hawaii

Department of Agriculture Veterinary Laboratory Branch
1428 South King Street
Honolulu, Hawaii 96814
(808)941–3071 (Ext. 158)

Idaho

Livestock Disease Control Laboratory
P.O. Box 7249
Boise, Idaho 83707
(208)384–3111

Clear Springs Trout Co.
P.O. Box 712
Buhl, Idaho 83316
(208)543–4316

Illinois

Laboratories of Veterinary Diagnostic Medicine
University of Illinois
Urbana, Illinois 61801
(217)333–1620

Animal Disease Diagnostic Laboratory
235 North Walnut Street
Centralia, Illinois 62801
(618)532–6701

Indiana

Animal Disease Diagnostic Laboratory
School of Veterinary Medicine
Purdue University
West Lafayette, Indiana 47907
(317)749–2496

Iowa

Veterinary Diagnostic Laboratory
College of Veterinary Medicine
Iowa State University
Ames, Iowa 50010
(515)294–1950

Kansas

Veterinary Diagnostic Laboratory
College of Veterinary Medicine
Kansas State University
Manhattan, Kansas 66506
(913)532–5650

Kentucky

Livestock Disease Diagnostic Center
1429 Newton Pike
Lexington, Kentucky 40505
(606)253–0571

Murray State University Veterinary Diagnostic and Research
 Center
P.O. Box 2000
Hopkinsville, Kentucky 44240
(502)886–3959

Louisiana

Louisiana Veterinary Medical Diagnostic Laboratory
LSU–School of Veterinary Medicine
Baton Rouge, Louisiana
(504)346–3193

Northwest Louisiana Livestock Diagnostic and Research
 Laboratory
P.O. Box 2156
N.S.U.
Natchitoches, Louisiana 71457
(318)352–6272

Central Louisiana Livestock Diagnostic Laboratory
Route 2, Box 51–F
Lecompte, Louisiana 71346
(318)443–6993

Ruston Diagnostic Laboratory
P.O. Box 811
Ag. Drive
Ruston, Louisiana 71270
(318)255–1933

Maine

Maine Poultry Consultants
Box 788
Waterville, Maine 04901
(207)873–3405

Massachusetts

Large Animal Diagnostic Laboratory
Paige Laboratory
University of Massachusetts
Amherst, Massachusetts 01003
(413)545–2427

Michigan

Michigan Department of Agriculture Laboratory Division
1615 South Harrison Road
East Lansing, Michigan 48823
(517)373–6410

Animal Health Diagnostic Laboratory
Michigan State University
P.O. Box 30076
East Lansing, Michigan 48909
(517)353–1683

Wildlife Pathology Laboratory, Michigan Department of Natural
 Resources
8562 E. Stoll Road, R. 1
East Lansing, Michigan 48823
(517)339–8638

Minnesota

Veterinary Diagnostic Laboratories
E220 Diagnostic Research Bldg.
College of Veterinary Medicine
University of Minnesota
St. Paul, Minnesota 55101
(612)373–0774

Mississippi

Mississippi Veterinary Diagnostic Laboratory
P.O. Box 4389
Jackson, Mississippi 39216
(601)354–6091

Missouri

Bureau of Laboratory Services
Missouri Division of Health
Public Health Laboratory Bldg.
307 W. McCarthy
Jefferson City, Missouri 65101
(314)751–3334
(FTS)758–7212

Ralston Purina Veterinary Laboratories
Veterinary Service Department
Checkerboard Square
St. Louis, Missouri 63188
(314)982–2611

Veterinary Medical Diagnostic Laboratory
School of Veterinary Medicine
University of Missouri
Columbia, Missouri 65201
(314)882–6811 or 6695

Montana

State of Montana Animal Health Division Diagnostic Laboratory
P.O. Box 997
Bozeman, Montana 59715
(406)586–8558
(FTS)585–4339

Nebraska

Harris Laboratories Inc.
P.O. Box 80837
Lincoln, Nebraska 68501
(402)432–2811

Veterinary Science Laboratory
University of Nebraska
North Platte, Nebraska 69101
(308)532–3611

North Carolina

Rollins Animal Disease Diagnostic Laboratory
P.O. Box 12223 Cameron Village Station
Raleigh, North Carolina 27606
(919)733–3986

North Dakota

North Dakota State University Veterinary Diagnostic Laboratory
Fargo, North Dakota 58102
(701)237–7511

Oklahoma

Oklahoma Animal Disease Diagnostic Laboratory
College of Veterinary Medicine
Oklahoma State University
Stillwater, Oklahoma 74074
(405)624–6623

Pennsylvania

Pennsylvania Department of Agriculture
Bureau of Animal Industry Laboratory
Summerdale, Pennsylvania 17093
(717)637–8808
(FTS)637–8808

South Dakota

Animal Disease Research and Diagnostic Laboratory
South Dakota State University
Box 2175
Brookings, South Dakota 57007
(605)688–5171

Tennessee

C. E. Kord Animal Disease Laboratory
P.O. Box 40627 Mel. Station
Nashville, Tennessee 37204
(615)741–1506
(FTS)853–1506

Texas

Texas Veterinary Medical Diagnostic Laboratory
Drawer 3040
College Station, Texas 77840
(713)845–3414

Texas A. & M. Veterinary Medical Diagnostic Laboratory
P.O. Box 3200
Amarillo, Texas 79106
(806)353–7478

Utah

Veterinary Reference Laboratory
870E 7145 South
Midvale, Utah 84047
(801)561–2244
(800)453–4530

Branch Veterinary Laboratory, Utah Agricultural Experiment Station
P.O. Box 1068
Provo, Utah 84601
(801)373–6383

State Chemists Office and State-Federal Cooperative Laboratory
360 N. Redwood Rd.
Salt Lake City, Utah 84114
(801)533–5421

Utah State University Veterinary Diagnostic Laboratory
Logan, Utah 84321
(801)750–1880

Virginia

Division of Animal Health and Dairies Research Laboratory
116 Reservoir Street
Harrisonburg, Virginia 22801
(703)434–3897

Division of Animal Health and Dairies Regulatory Laboratory
Box 4191
Lynchburg, Virginia 24502
(804)528–6731

Division of Animal Health and Dairies Regulatory Laboratory
234 West Shirley Avenue
Warrenton, Virginia 22186
(703)347–3131

Washington

Washington Animal Disease Diagnostic Laboratory
P.O. Box 2037
College Station, WSU
Pullman, Washington 99163
(509)335–9696

National Fishery and Wildlife Research Center
Building 204, Sand Point
Naval Support Activity
Seattle, Washington 98115
(206)442–5960
(FTS)8–399–5960

Poultry Diagnostic Laboratory, Western Washington Research
  and Extension Center
Washington State University
Puyallup, Washington 98371
(206)593–8536

West Virginia

State Federal Cooperative Animal Health Laboratory
4720 Brinda Lane
Charleston, West Virginia 25315
(304)348–3418
(FTS)885–3418

Wisconsin

Central Animal Health Laboratory
6101 Mineral Point Road
Madison, Wisconsin 53705
(608)266–2465

Wyoming

Wyoming State Veterinary Laboratory
Box 950
Laramie, Wyoming 82070
(307)742–6638

Management and Treatment of Toxicosis in Cattle*

E. MURL BAILEY, Jr., D.V.M., Ph.D.

Intoxication of domestic livestock continues to confront veterinary practitioners with therapeutic and prophylactic problems. The current widespread and necessary use of pesticides for agricultural purposes in the United States continues to cause accidental intoxications in animals. Because of the constant likelihood of intoxications in animals, it is imperative that veterinarians maintain the attempt to educate their clients about the inherent dangers of pesticides and other toxicants and to urge their clients to use proper handling and storage techniques. When the

*Supported in part by Texas Agricultural Experiment Station, Project No. H–6255.

users and those who apply toxic chemicals control these chemicals properly, the number of intoxications will be lowered.

The greater incidence of domestic animal intoxications necessitates the present emphasis on treating diseases caused by such incidences. Consequently, the purposes of this article are to briefly identify some of the more common toxicants that cause intoxications in animals and to describe the therapeutic and management procedures that should be instituted to treat the resulting diseases.

BASIC CONCEPTS OF INTOXICATION THERAPY

The primary goals of therapy in cases of intoxication are
1. Providing emergency intervention and prevention of further exposure.
2. Establishing a tentative diagnosis upon which to base rational therapeutic measures.
3. Delaying further absorption.
4. Applying specific antidotes and remedial measures.
5. Hastening elimination of the absorbed toxicant.
6. Administering supportive therapy.
7. Determining the source of the toxicant.
8. Educating the client.

When initiating therapy for animal intoxications, veterinary clinicians should direct their efforts toward treating the signs exhibited by the affected animals, unless the correct diagnosis is obvious. Pre-existing conditions and the diagnosis should be determined following stabilization of the patient.

It is important that neither the client nor the clinician wastes time. The animal should be examined by the veterinarian as soon as possible. The owners should be instructed to bring suspected toxic materials or their containers with them to aid in the diagnosis. The client should be advised to place the specimens in clean, sealed glass jars or plastic containers and not to contaminate the material, because it may be important from a medico-legal aspect.

The most important aspect of treatment of intoxication is to ensure adequate physiologic function. This may include establishment of a patent airway, artificial respiration, cardiac massage, and perhaps the application of defibrillation. Following the stabilization of the animal's vital signs, the clinician may proceed with therapeutic measures discussed next, in any order.

Delaying Absorption

Preventing the animal from absorbing additional intoxicant is a major factor in treating cases of intoxication. In many instances, intoxication may be prevented if the animal was observed ingesting or being in contact with suspected material. Removal of the animal from the affected environment is a necessary first step to prevent further absorption. It is hoped that bringing the animal to the veterinary clinic or hospital will resolve this problem. Washing the animal's skin to remove the noxious agent, may also be necessary. If an external toxicant is involved, caution must be exercised to avoid the contamination of all persons handling the animal. Protective clothing, such as rubber aprons and gloves, is a necessity. In addition, the judicious use of adsorbents and cathartics will further aid in the prevention of further absorption of ingested toxic materials. Absorption may also be retarded by precipitation, inactivation, neutralization, oxidation, and chelation. Several of these mechanisms may be accomplished using carefully chosen locally acting chemical antidotes, as listed in Table 1.

Adsorbents

Activated charcoal is probably the best adsorbing agent available. Although it does not detoxify toxicants, it will effectively prevent absorption of a toxicant if properly utilized. Activated charcoal can be successfully combined with emetics or gastric lavage or used by itself.

The correct type of activated charcoal for treatment of intoxication is of petroleum or of vegetable origin and not of mineral or animal origin. There are several commercial types of activated charcoal available (Norit,* Nuchar C,† Darco G-60‡, and Superchar Vet§). The proper technique for employing activated charcoal is as follows: (1) make a slurry of the charcoal using water. The proper dose is 1–3 gm/kg; in a concentration 1 gm charcoal/3–5 ml of water. (2) Administer the charcoal by stomach tube. (3) During administration of the charcoal, a cathartic of sodium or magnesium sulfate should be given. The dose should be repeated within 8 to 12 hr in many instances.

Activated charcoal is highly adsorptive for many toxicants, including insecticides, herbicides, mercuric chloride and strychnine. Many other alkaloids including morphine, atropine, barbiturates, and ethylene glycol are adsorbed.

Cathartics

Sodium sulfate is a more efficient and preferable agent for evacuation of the bowel than magnesium sulfate, especially with activated charcoal. With magnesium sulfate, there is some danger of central nervous system (CNS) depression due to the magnesium ion. The dose of sodium or magnesium sulfate is 1 gm/kg. Either agent may be used in an emergency.

Elimination of Absorbed Toxicants

Absorbed toxicants are generally excreted via the kidneys. Some toxicants may be excreted by other routes (bile, feces, lung, other body secretions). Renal excretion can be manipulated in many instances. Urinary excretion of toxicants may be enhanced by the use of diuretics or by altering the pH of the urine.

The use of diuretics to enhance urinary excretion of toxicants requires adequate renal function and hydration of the affected animal. Once these conditions are established, diuretics are indicated. Monitoring of urinary output is essential, and a minimum urinary flow of 0.1 ml/kg/min is necessary. The diuretics of choice are mannitol and furosemide (Lasix‖). Both of these agents are very potent diuretics. The dosage of mannitol is 1 gm/lb/hr and of furosemide is 2 mg/kg.

Alteration of urinary pH to expedite the excretion of toxicants and foreign chemicals is a classic pharmacologic technique. The technique relies on the physiochemical

phenomenon that ionized compounds do not readily traverse cell membranes and hence are not reabsorbed by the renal tubules. Consequently, acid compounds such as acetylsalicylic acid (aspirin) and some barbiturates remain ionized in acidic urine. As a result, urinary excretion of many toxic compounds may be enhanced by modifying the urine pH. Sodium bicarbonate may be used as the alkalinizing agent.

Peritoneal dialysis is indicated in small animals, but is difficult to initiate in large animals when they exhibit oliguria or anuria. It is a rather time consuming but effective technique for many conditions. The procedure requires the use of 2 separate solutions, and the solutions should be exchanged every 30 to 60 min. Two dialyzing solutions that may be used are 5-per cent dextrose in 0.45-per cent NaCl with 15 mEq/L of potassium as potassium chloride and 5-per cent dextrose in water with 44.6 mEq of bicarbonate and 15 mEq of potassium. Other dialyzing solutions are also appropriate.

The process of peritoneal dialysis involves the infusion of 10 to 20 ml/kg of the first dialyzing solution into the peritoneal cavity, waiting, withdrawing the first dialyzing solution, and infusing the second dialyzing solution. The infusion and withdrawal cycles with alternating solutions should be maintained for 12 to 14 hr, or until normal renal function is restored. The pH of the dialyzing solutions may be altered to maintain the ionized state of the offending compound.

In cattle, a rumenotomy is an excellent way to rapidly empty the rumen.

SUPPORTIVE MEASURES

Supportive measures are very important in the treatment of intoxications. These measures are control of body temperature, maintenance of respiratory and cardiovascular functions, control of CNS signs, and control of pain.

Body Temperature Control

Hypothermia is controlled using blankets and keeping the animals in warm, draft-free stalls. Infrared lamps should be used with caution and constant observation.

Hyperthermia is treated with ice bags, cold water baths, cold water enemas, or cold peritoneal dialysis solutions.

Regardless of the type of temperature control required, it is vitally important that the animal's body temperature be constantly monitored to ensure that overcorrection does not occur.

Respiratory Support

Adequate respiratory support requires the presence of an adequate, patent airway. A patent airway may be obtained either with a cuffed endotracheal tube for an unconscious animal or with a tracheostomy using a local anesthetic for a conscious animal. An emergency tracheostomy tube may be made from a cuffed endotracheal tube, which has been shortened to reduce dead space.

A respirator is of great value in cases of respiratory depression; however, an anesthetic machine may be utilized with manual compression of the bag. A mixture of 50-per cent oxygen and 50-per cent room air is generally adequate unless the respiratory membrane is thickened, in which case 100-per cent oxygen is necessary.

---

*Available from American Norit, Jacksonville, Fla 32208.
†Available from West Virginia Pulp and Paper, Richard, W VA 23225.
‡Available from Atlas Chemical, Wilmington, Del 19899.
§Available from Gulf Biosystems, Dallas, Tex (telephone 214–386–0442).
‖Available from Hoechst-Roussel Pharmaceuticals, Inc., Somerville, NJ 08876.

Table 1. *Locally Acting Antidotes Against Unabsorbed Poisons*

Poisons	Antidotes, Doses, or Concentrations	Poisons	Antidotes, Doses, or Concentrations
Acids, Corrosive	Magnesium oxide solution: large animals, 20–30 gm	Lead*	Sodium or magnesium sulfate orally (500–1000 gm for large animals)
	Milk of magnesia: large animals, 30–300 ml		Tannic acid (see Alkaloids)
Alkali, Caustic	Weak acid: vinegar (diluted 1:4), 1% acetic acid or lemon juice orally		Albumin
Alkaloids and glycosides	Activated charcoal (1–3 gm/kg) plus sodium or magnesium sulfate (1gm/kg).	Mercury	Protein: milk, egg whites
			Magnesium oxide (see Acids, Corrosive)
	Potassium permanganate (1:5000 to 1:10,000) for lavage and/or oral administration.		Sodium formaldehyde sulfoxylate: 5-per cent solution for lavage
	Tannic acid or strong tea, except in cases of poisoning by cocaine, nicotine, physostigmine, atropine, or morphine: large animals, 5–25 gm in 0.5–1 gallon water (2–4 L)	Oak (Shin Oak)	Activated charcoal: large animals, 250–500 gm
			Prophylactic hydrated lime (calcium hydroxide): 1080 lb cottonseed meal, 600 lb dehydrated alfalfa, 120 lb vegetable oil, 200 lb hydrated lime, feed 4 lb/day
	Purgative should be used for prompt removal of tannates.		*Note:* Treatment is not effective for kidney damage
Arsenic*	Sodium thiosulfate: 10-per cent solution orally, large animals, 20–30 gm	Oxalic Acid (oxalates)*	Calcium hydroxide as 0.15-per cent solution. Other alkalies are contraindicated because their salts are more soluble than calcium hydroxide
	Protein: evaporated milk, egg whites, and so forth		Chalk or other calcium salts
	Tannic acid or strong tea		Magnesium sulfate as cathartic
Barium Salts	Sodium sulfate or magnesium sulfate: 20% solution orally, large animals, 250–1000 gm		Maintain diuresis to prevent calcium oxalate deposition in kidney
Bismuth Salts	Acacia or gum arabic as mucilage	Petroleum Distillates (Aliphatic Hydrocarbons)	Olive oil or other vegetable oil orally. After one-half hr, magnesium sulfate as cathartic
Carbon Tetrachloride	Empty rumen; high protein and carbohydrate diet; maintain fluid and electrolyte balance. Hemodialysis is indicated in anuria. Epinephrine is contraindicated (ventricular fibrillation).	Phenol and Cresols	Soap and water or alcohol washing of skin
			Sodium bicarbonate 0.5-per cent dressings
			Activated charcoal plus saline cathartic
Copper	Albumin	Phosphorus	Copper sulfate as 0.2–0.4-per cent solution or potassium permanganate 1:5000 solution for lavage
	Magnesium oxide solution (see Acids, Corrosive)		
Detergents, Cationic (Chlorides, iodides, and so forth)	Soap (e.g., Castile) dissolved in 4 times its bulk of hot water.		Turpentine (preferably old and oxidized) in gelatin capsules or floated on hot water. For small animals, give 2 ml, 4 times at 15 min intervals
			Activated charcoal plus saline cathartic
Detergents, Anionic (Na, K, NH⁺ salts)	Milk or water followed by demulcent (oil, acacia, gelatin, starch, egg white, and so forth)		Do not give vegetable oil cathartic
			Remove all fat from diet
		Silver Nitrate	Normal saline for lavage
Fluoride*	Calcium (milk, lime water or powdered chalk mixed with water) orally		Albumin
Formaldehyde	Ammonia water (9.2 per cent orally) or ammonium acetate (1 per cent lavage)	Urea	Acetic acid, 5-per cent solution in 20-per cent glucose, orally
	Starch: 1 part starch to 15 parts hot water added gradually.		For large animals, give 1–4 L
	Gelatin soaked in water for one-half hr		*Diluted vinegar* may be used for large cows
	Sodium thiosulfate (see Arsenic)		Give 1 gal orally and repeat in 1–2 hr
Iron*	Sodium bicarbonate: 1 per cent lavage	Unknown	Activated charcoal (replaces universal antidote): large animals, 1–3 gm/kg plus sodium or magnesium sulfate (1 gm/kg)
	Deferoxamine: 5-per cent solution orally (0.5–1.5 gm for dogs)		

*Systemic antidote also available (see Table 2).

The use of analeptic drugs in cases of severe respiratory depression or apnea is questionable owing to the short duration of their effects and other undesirable side effects. Positive pressure ventilatory support is of greater value than analeptic drugs. The uses and dosages of several analeptic drugs are presented in the section on CNS depression.

Cardiovascular Support

Cardiovascular support requires the presence of adequate circulating volume, cardiac function, tissue perfusion, and acid-base balance. Volume and cardiac activity are of immediate concern, while perfusion and acid-base balance, though of no lesser importance, are not.

In the presence of hypovolemia due to loss of both cells and volume, whole blood is needed. A good rule of thumb is to give a sufficient quantity of whole blood to raise the packed cell volume up to 75 per cent of the animal's estimated normal volume.

Cases of hypovolemia due to fluid loss alone can be treated with the administration of lactated Ringer's solution or plasma expanders. Central venous pressure should be monitored to prevent overloading the heart with too much volume, too rapidly.

Tissue perfusion should also be monitored periodically to determine the adequacy of the replacement therapy. In some cases it may be necessary to administer massive doses of corticosteroids intravenously to restore adequate tissue perfusion (dexamethasone, Azium,* 2 to 10 mg/kg).

Cardiac activity can be aided by the application of closed chest massage for immediate requirements, but the administration of pharmaceutic agents that can stimulate inotropic and chronotropic activities must also be undertaken in most instances. One of these agents is calcium gluconate that is infused very slowly. This agent is also reported as being a good nonspecific measure to take in

*Available from Schering Corporation, Kenilworth, NJ 07033.

many cases of toxicoses. Other agents are glucagon, 25 to 50 μg/kg and digoxin, 0.2 to 0.6 mg/kg, both intravenously. Care must be taken not to give overdoses of cardio-active agents, as they are highly toxic to the myocardium.

Acid-Base Balance

Control of acid-base balance problems consists primarily of physiologically maintaining an animal in a homeostatic condition. The most common acid-base disturbance in animals is acidosis mainly of metabolic origin. However, acidosis or alkalosis may occur in cases of intoxication.

In correcting acidosis not of respiratory origin, sodium bicarbonate administered intravenously at a dosage rate of 2 to 4 mEq/kg every 15 min is the treatment of choice. Other alkalinizing solutions are one-sixth molar sodium lactate, 16 to 32 ml/kg; lactated Ringer's solution, 120 ml/kg; and Tromethamine buffer, 300 mg/kg. Bicarbonate is generally the easiest to administer in regard to volume, and it requires no metabolic conversion. Caution must be exercised against the induction of alkalosis with all alkalinizing agents.

Alkalosis, unless drug-induced, does not generally occur in animals. However, if alkalosis is present, the intravenous administration of 0.9-per cent NaCl (physiologic saline), 10 ml/kg, is usually sufficient for initial therapy. This should be followed by the oral administration of ammonium chloride, 200 mg/kg/day in divided doses. As with acidosis, the clinician should be cautious about overtreatment of alkalosis.

Central Nervous System (CNS)

Management of CNS disorders, in cases of intoxication, is simple in appearance but complex in practice. The type of therapy depends upon the presence of depression or hyperactivity. Depression can easily be changed into hyperactivity or vice versa by overzealous therapeutic measures.

CNS Depression

CNS depression can be considered in the same way as respiratory depression because the management of the 2 conditions is very similar. Although analeptic agents, such as doxapram (Dopram*), 5 to 10 mg/kg, methetharimide (Mikedimide†), 10 to 20 mg/kg, or pentylenetetrazol (Metrazol‡), 6 to 10 mg/kg, are reported as efficacious when administered intravenously. Their actions are short-lived, and CNS depression can return if the animals are not continuously monitored. Another disadvantage is that analeptics induce convulsions. Artificial respiration or respiratory support is of greater value in animals exhibiting CNS depression and may be the treatment of choice.

CNS Hyperactivity

Cases of CNS hyperactivity and convulsions can be managed by the administration of CNS depressants or tranquilizers. Pentobarbital sodium is generally the agent of choice for cases of CNS hyperactivity and convulsions. Care must be taken since a respiratory-depressing dose may be required to alleviate the signs. In such cases, respiratory support is mandatory.

Inhalant anesthetics have been reported as excellent for long-term management of CNS hyperactivity, but this involves removing the inhalant equipment from the operating room for extended periods and may not be practical with large animals. Central acting skeletal muscle relaxants and minor tranquilizers have been reported for use in cases of convulsant intoxicants. Some of these drugs include methocarbamol (Robaxin*), 110 mg/kg, IV; glyceryl guaiacolate (Gecolate†), 110 mg/kg, IV; and diazepam (Valium‡), 0.5 to 1.5 mg/kg, IV or IM. In cases of CNS stimulation due to amphetamines and hallucinogens such as LSD and phencyclidine, phenothiazine tranquilizers have produced adequate control. Regardless of the regimen of therapy for CNS hyperactivity, the animals should be placed in a quiet, dark room or stall to prevent additional auditory or visual stimulation.

SYSTEMIC AND SPECIFIC ANTIDOTES

When a poison has been absorbed, use of a systemic antidote, if available, is indicated. In most situations, it is advisable to treat immediately with a systemic antidote, to promote elimination (excretion), and to apply supportive therapy. However, specific antidotes are available for only a few poisons.

Systemic and specific antidotes and the dosages for each are presented in Table 2. The dosages and durations of treatment given in the table are to serve only as guidelines and must be adjusted according to the severity of the poisoning and the condition of the animal.

Systemic antidotes possessing specific actions for their antidotal activities are classified by the following mechanisms

1. Complexing with a poison, rendering it inert (e.g., dimercaprol for arsenic poisoning).

2. Accelerating the metabolic conversion of a toxic product to a nontoxic product (e.g., thiosulfate for cyanide poisoning).

3. Blocking the metabolic formation of a poison from a nontoxic precursor.

4. Specifically accelerating the excretion of a poison (e.g., chloride for bromide poisoning).

5. Competing with a poison for essential receptors (e.g., vitamin K_1 for coumarin derivative poisoning).

6. Blocking receptors responsible for toxic effects (e.g., atropine sulfate for cholinesterase inhibition).

7. Restoring normal function by repairing or by-passing the effects of a poison (e.g., methylene blue for methemoglobinemia).

A number of drugs, poisons, and other chemicals can either cause a toxic reaction when used to inhibit drug (or poison) metabolism or cause a state of tolerance by stimulating the activity of the liver's microsomal drug metabolizing enzymes. Great species differences and genetic variations in drug or poison metabolism also exist.

A discussion of therapeutic measures for some of the more common intoxications in livestock is presented next.

---

*Available from A. H. Robins Co., Richmond, VA 23220.
†Available from Parlam Division, Ormont Drug, Englewood, NJ 07631.
‡Available from Knoll Pharmaceutical Co., Whippany, NJ 07981.

*Available from A. H. Robins Co., Richmond, VA 23220.
†Available from Summit Hill Laboratories, Avalon, NJ 08202.
‡Available from Hoffman-La Roche Inc., Nutley, NJ 07110.

Table 2. *Systemic and Specific Antidotes and Dosages*

Toxic Agents	Systemic and Specific Antidotes	Dosages and Treatment Methods
Amphetamines	Chlorpromazine	1 mg/kg IM, IP, IV; administer only half the dose if barbiturates have been given; blocks excitation
	Acetic acid*	2–5-per cent cold vinegar (12–20 L)
Ammonia (urea)	γ-Aminobutyric acid*	2-per cent solution; give large animals 1 ml/lb IV, repeat as needed. Protective effect observed in experimental ammonia intoxication of rats
Arsenic, mercury and other heavy metals except silver, selenium and thallium (not for organic compounds)	Dimercaprol (BAL)	10-per cent solution in oil; 2.5–5 mg/kg IM every 4 hr for 2 days, 3 times a day on third day and then twice a day for the next 10 days or until recovery. *Note:* 5 mg/kg dose should be given on the first day in severely acute poisoning
	Sodium thiosulfate (only for arsenic poisoning)	20-per cent solution; give large animals 30–40 mg/kg IV or PO (double the dose for PO) 2–3 times daily until recovery (usually 3–4 days)
	N-Acetyl-DL-penicillamine* (only for mercury poisoning)	Developed for chronic mercury poisoning, now a promising drug; no reports of dosages in animals. Human dosage is 250 mg orally, every 6 hr for 10 days
Atropine, belladonna alkaloids	Physostigmine salicylate	0.01–0.6 mg/kg
Barbiturates	Pentylenetetrazol	10-per cent solution; give 10–20 mg/kg IV or IM, repeat at 15- to 30-min intervals, as needed. Give large animals total dose of 1000–3000 mg IV
	Doxapram	2-per cent solution; give 3–5 mg/kg IV only; repeat as necessary.
	Bemegride	3-per cent solution; give 5–10 mg/kg IV only by slow infusion or by intermittent doses
	Amphetamine	5-per cent solution; give 0.5–1 mg/kg SC, IV or IP. Do not repeat within 60 min. Give large animals 100–300 mg SC. *Note:* Both doses are reliable only when depression is mild. For deeper levels of depression, artificial respiration and oxygen is preferred
Bromides	Chlorides (sodium or ammonium salts)	2.5–5 mg/kg orally for several days to hasten excretion
Bracken fern	DL-batyl alcohol	10-per cent solution in olive oil; give cows 10 ml SC daily for 5 days. Blood transfusion may be helpful.
	Protamine sulfate	0.2 mg/kg and blood transfusion.
Carbon monoxide	Oxygen	Pure oxygen at normal or high pressure or oxygen with 5-per cent carbon dioxide; artificial respiration, blood transfusion.
Cholinergic agents	Atropine sulfate	0.02–0.04 mg/kg as needed.
Cholinesterase inhibitors	Atropine sulfate	Dose for large animals is 0.2 mg/kg, repeated as needed for atropinization. Blocks only muscarinic effect. Atropine in oil may be injected for a prolonged effect during the night. If present, treat cyanosis first
Cholinesterase inhibitors (organophophates, some carbamates but not carbaryl, dimetilan, and so forth)	Pralidoxime chloride (2-Pam.)	10-per cent solution; for large animals (cows) give 25–50 mg/kg IV during a 6-min period; maximum dose is 100 mg/kg via drip. 2-Pam alleviates nicotinic effect and regenerates cholinesterase. Morphine, succinylcholine, and phenothiazine tranquilizers are contraindicated.
Copper	D-Penicillamine	Dose for animals not established. Human dosage is 1–4 gm daily in divided doses (250 mg tablets). Suggest 15–60 mg/kg daily.
	Ammonium or sodium molybdate	For chronic poisoning in sheep: 100 mg ammonium molybdate and 0.3–1 sodium sulfate orally daily for 3 weeks. Molybdenum salt for prevention.
Curare (tubocurarine)	Neostigmine methylsulfate	Solution of 1:2000 or 1:500 (1 ml = 0.5 mg or 2 mg). Dose for large animals is 1 mg/100 lb SC or IV; if given IV, administer very slowly and follow with IV injection of a 1-per cent solution of atropine (0.04 mg/kg)
	Edrophonium	1-per cent solution; give small animals 0.05–1 mg/kg IV
Coumarin, derivative anticoagulants	Vitamin K$_1$	5-per cent stable emulsion; give large animals 0.5–1 mg/kg IM or IV in 5-per cent solution of glucose at the rate of 10 mg vitamin K/min; maximum effect occurs within 50–60 min. Give 5 mg/kg IM for 3 days (longer if necessary)
	Whole blood or plasma	Blood transfusion for large animals at 2–4 L/500 kg
Cyanide	Sodium nitrite (to form methemoglobin)	1-per cent solution of sodium nitrite; 16 mg/kg IV for both large and small animals. Follow with 20-per cent solution of sodium thiosulfate at 30–40 mg/kg IV. If treatment is repeated, use only sodium thiosulfate.
	Sodium thiosulfate	*Note:* Both sodium nitrite and sodium thiosulfate may be given simultaneously as follows: 20 ml/50 kg combination consisting of 10 gm sodium nitrite, 15 gm sodium thiosulfate, and distilled water QS (250 ml) that may be repeated once. If further treatment is required, give only 20-per cent solution of sodium thiosulfate at 10–20 ml/50 kg IV

Table continued on following page

Table 2. *Systemic and Specific Antidotes and Dosages* (Continued)

Toxic Agents	Systemic and Specific Antidotes	Dosages and Treatment Methods
Digitalis glycosides	Potassium chloride	Give 0.5–2 gm orally in divided doses or as a diluted solution by slow IV drip (ECG monitor is essential)
	Propranolol (beta blocker)	0.5–1 mg/kg IV or IM as needed to control cardiac arrhythmias
	Atropine sulfate	0.02–0.04 mg/kg as needed for cholinergic control
Fluoroacetate (1080)	Glyceryl monoacetin*	0.1–0.5 mg/kg IM hourly for several hours (total 2–4 mg/kg) or diluted (0.5–1 per cent) IV (danger of hemolysis). Monoacetin is available only from chemical suppliers
	Acetamide*	Animal may be protected if acetamide is given prior to or simultaneously with 1080 (experimental)
Fluoride	Calcium borogluconate	23-per cent solution; give large animals: 250–500 ml IV at body temperature and by very slow injection (danger of heart block)
Heparin	Protamine sulfate	1-per cent solution; give 1–1.5 mg by slow IV injection to antagonize each 1 mg of heparin. Reduce dose of protamine sulfate as time increases between heparin injection and start of treatment (after 30 min, give only 0.5 mg)
	Hexadimethrine	1 mg hexadimethrine for each 1 mg heparin by slow IV injection. Hexadimethrine is a synthetic product that causes fewer side effects than protamine
Iron salts	Desferrioxamine (deferoxamine)	Dose for animals not yet established. Human dosage is 5 gm of 5-per cent solution given orally, then 20 mg/kg IM every 4 hr. In case of shock, dosage is 40 mg/kg by IV drip over 4-hr period and may be repeated in 6 hr. Following that, 20 mg/kg by drip every 12 hr
Lead	Calcium disodium edetate (EDTA), EDTA and BAL	Maximum safe dose is 75 mg/kg/24 hr (only for severe cases). EDTA is available in 6.6-per cent solution. For IV drip and for IM, add procaine to solution. BAL is given as 10-per cent solution in oil. In severe cases (CNS involvement or >100 mg Pb/100 gm whole blood) give 4 mg/kg BAL only as initial dose; follow after 4 hr and every 4 hr for 3 or 4 days with BAL and EDTA at separate IM sites; skip 2 or 3 days and then treat again for 3 to 4 days. In subacute cases or <100 mg Pb/100 gm whole blood, give 50 mg EDTA/kg/24 hr only for 3 to 5 days
Methanol and ethylene glycol	Ethanol	25-per cent solution; 0.75 mg/kg IV. Then give 0.5 mg/kg every 4 hr for 4 days. To prevent or correct acidosis, use sodium bicarbonate IV. Activated charcoal aids if within 4 hr of ingestion.
Methemoglobinemia-producing agents (nitrates, chlorates, and so forth)	Methylene blue	1-per cent solution (maximum concentration); give 8.8 mg/kg by slow IV injection, repeat if necessary. To prevent fall in blood pressure in cases of nitrite poisoning, use a sympathomimetic drug (ephedrine, epinephrine, and so forth)
Morphine and related drugs	Nalorphine hydrochloride	1–2.5 ml of solution containing 5 mg/ml IV. Do not repeat if respiration is not satisfactory
	Levallorphan tartrate	0.1–0.5 ml of solution containing 1 mg/ml IV
	Naloxone hydrochloride	0.04 mg/kg IV, IM, SC; repeat as necessary. *Note:* Use of the 3 antidotes for morphine intoxication is only for acute cases. Artificial respiration may be indicated.
Molybdenum	Copper sulfate	Prophylaxis; 1–5 per cent in salt or orally
	Cobalt	1 gm copper sulfate and 1 mg/100 lb of cobalt carbonate per cow, daily at weekly intervals for 4 to 6 weeks. Supplement ration with phosphorus
	Copper glycinate	Solution containing 60 mg/ml; inject into dewlap; 1 ml for calves and 2 ml for cows, repeat once or twice during a season
Oleander glycosides	Atropine sulfate	0.04 mg/kg IV or IM; repeat as needed. Controls cholinergic effects
	Propranolol	0.5 mg/kg IV or IM; repeat as needed. Controls cardiac arrhythmias (ECG monitor is necessary)
Oxalates	Calcium	23-per cent solution of calcium borogluconate IV; large animals 250–500 mg; small animals 3–20 ml (to control hypocalcemia) 25-per cent dicalcium phosphate as a prophylactic in salt ration or 10-per cent dicalcium phosphate in alfalfa cubes
Phenothiazine derivatives	Methylamphetamine	For horses, 0.1–0.2 mg/kg IV. Also blood transfusion
Phytotoxins and botulinus	Antitoxins	As indicated for specific antitoxins. Examples of phytotoxins include ricin, abrin, robin, curcin, and crotin
Red squill	Atropine sulfate, propranolol	See oleander glycosides
Selenium and its analog Selenocystathionine	Cystine,* methionine,* vitamin E*	Application is still experimental and dosages of these drugs have not been established.
	Arsenic	For alkali-type disease give large animals 25 ppm sodium arsenite in salt or 5 ppm sodium arsenite in drinking water. Arsanilic acid (0.02 per cent) in the ration of calves and pigs has protected against as much as 10 ppm of selenite in the body. Increasing the protein content of the ration seems to help detoxification
	Neostigmine	1–2 mg/100 lb IM with glucose IV, give daily for 3 to 4 days

Table continued on opposite page

Table 2. *Systemic and Specific Antidotes and Dosages* (Continued)

Toxic Agents	Systemic and Specific Antidotes	Dosages and Treatment Methods
Strychnine and brucine	Pentobarbital	Give IP or IV to effect. A higher dose than is required for anesthesia is usual. If necessary, repeat with a lower dose. Place animal in warm, dark, and quiet room
	Amytal	Give by slow IV injection to effect. Duration of sedation is usually 4–6 hr
	Methocarbamol	10-per cent solution; average first dose for dogs is 149 mg/kg IV (range of 40–300 mg) to effect; repeat half the dose as needed
	Chloral hydrate	Give dose common for large animals
	Glyceryl guaiacolate	110 mg/kg IV, repeat as necessary.
Strontium	Calcium salts	Usual dose of calcium borogluconate IV
	Ammonium chloride	0.2–0.5 gm orally in water, 3 to 4 times daily for small animals; 5–30 gm in divided doses for large animals
Thallium	Diphenylthiocarbazone*	70 mg/kg orally, 3 times a day for 6 days for dogs. Hastens elimination, but is potentially toxic
	Ferric cyanoferrate (Prussian blue)	0.2 mg/kg orally in divided doses
	Potassium chloride	Give simultaneously with thiocarbasone or Prussian blue. Daily dose is 2–6 gm orally, in divided doses

*Experimental drug, practical efficacy not well established.

SPECIFIC THERAPEUTIC MEASURES

Warfarin (Anticoagulant Rodenticides)

Transfusion of whole blood constitutes the single most effective treatment for warfarin poisoning, since it provides prothrombin as well as red blood cells and fluid lost by the patient. A citrated whole blood mixture consisting of 100 ml of an aqueous solution containing 2 gm sodium acid citrate and 2.5 gm dextrose, to which is added 300 ml whole blood, may be used. This mixture can be refrigerated for a maximum of 14 days. In cases of poisoning, a minimum volume of 9 ml/lb should be administered. Half the estimated volume should be given if the mucous membranes still appear pallid.

The administration of vitamin K_1 (Aquamephyton*) is indicated to promote the production of prothrombin and other clotting factors by the liver. The dosage is 0.5 to 2.5 mg/kg IV in 5-per cent dextrose at a rate of 10 mg/min. Subsequent doses of vitamin K_1 may be given SQ or IM. In cases involving new rodenticides (i.e., Diphacinone and Brodifacoum), 3 to 4 weeks of parenteral vitamin K_1 therapy may be required. The monitoring of blood clotting factors is requisite in these cases. One should not use synthetic vitamin K analogs in the initial therapy, as numerous studies have shown them to be clearly inferior to vitamin K_1 in decreasing blood clotting time.

Cyanide

Perhaps the most commonly used and most effective of the cyanide antidotes is the combination of nitrate and thiosulfate. Therapy is directed at splitting the cytochrome-cyanide bond and the subsequent rapid removal of the cyanide complex. The cyanide-cytochrome bond is broken by the addition of sodium nitrite with the formation of methemoglobin that competes with cytochrome oxidase for the cyanide ion, and cyanmethemoglobin is formed. Thiosulfate then reacts with cyanide under the influence of the enzyme rhodanese to form thiocyanate, which is readily excreted in the urine. A recommended therapeutic regimen is the intravenous administration of

a mixture of 1 ml of 20-per cent sodium nitrite and of 3 ml of 20-per cent sodium thiosulfate at 4 ml/45 kg. Commercial solutions for treatment of prussic acid poisoning are available.

$$MetHb:CN^- + S_2O_3^= \longrightarrow SCN^- + SO_3 + MetHb$$

Care must be taken in administration of the nitrite so as not to form too much methemoglobin and compromise oxygen carrying ability. Some benefits have been shown with cobalt salts when administered for cyanide poisoning. However, nitrite and thiosulfate therapy remains most effective.

Nitrate-Nitrite

Therapy is aimed at restoring the iron in the hemoglobin to the divalent state. To do this, methylene blue is added to the system. It is rapidly reduced to leukomethylene blue and then serves as the reducing agent to convert methemoglobin (Fe^{+3}) to hemoglobin (Fe^{+2}) as follows:

$$\text{NADPH} \rightarrow \left(\begin{array}{c} \text{Methylene Blue (oxidized)} \\ \text{Leukomethylene Blue (reduced)} \end{array} \right) \rightarrow \left(\begin{array}{c} \text{Hemoglobin } Fe^{+2} \\ \text{Methemoglobin } (Fe^{+3}) \end{array} \right)$$
$$\text{NADP}$$

Overpowering the system with methylene blue will also produce methemoglobinemia. The suggested dose is 8.8 mg/kg administered in a 1-per cent solution. This dose may be repeated, since absorption of nitrate-nitrate from a full rumen can continue. Mineral oil given via a stomach tube will counteract the caustic action of nitrate salts and help speed elimination. For nitrate poisoning from forage, purging with saline cathartics and controlling of bacterial nitrate reduction with intraruminal antibiotics and 3 to 5 gal (12 to 20 L) of cold water may be beneficial.

Urea and Ammonium Ion

The best treatment for urea and ammonium ion poisoning is to give several gallons of cold water orally. As much as 5 to 10 gal (20 to 40 L) should be given to a cow.

If 6-per cent acetic acid or vinegar is available, up to 3 gal should be given along with the cold water. The rationale is that water lowers the rumen temperature and

*Available from Merck, Sharp & Dohme Research Laboratories, Rahway, NJ 07065.

dilutes the reacting medium, while acetic acid lowers rumen pH (preventing ammonia absorption) and also supplies molecular carbon skeletons needed by rumen bacteria. Urea intoxicated animals should be watched closely for at least 14 hr after treatment or apparent recovery, since an occasional relapse may occur.

Lead

Prior to the advent of lead chelating agents, treatment consisted mainly of attempts to induce the deposition of lead in bone, such as the administration of large quantities of calcium phosphate and vitamin D. Dimercaprol (BAL) initially increases urinary excretion of lead quite markedly, but the effect wanes rapidly, and the amount of lead mobilized is negligible. Apparently, only the lead in the blood can be chelated by dimercaprol. The lead in bone and soft tissues is too firmly bound to be mobilized. In animals, dimercaprol gives unpredictable results and may add to the toxicity of the lead that is bound to it.

The discovery of the efficacy of calcium disodium edetate (EDTA) in the treatment of lead poisoning added greatly to the successful management of plumbism. Nevertheless, EDTA proved to have certain shortcomings in addition to its own toxic potential and the necessity for intravenous administration. In the treatment of lead encephalopathy, EDTA may exacerbate the syndrome during the first day of therapy. Attempts should be made to remove lead by saline purgatives, gastric lavage, and rumenotomy. Chemical antidotes in the form of soluble sulfates (sodium sulfate, magnesium sulfate), milk and egg white, and tannic acid are recommended to immobilize lead in the gut by precipitating it as insoluble sulfate, albuminate, or tannate, respectively. Sedatives may be used to control convulsions.

The treatment recommended for livestock consists of the slow, intravenous administration of a 6.6-per cent (wt/vol) solution of CaEDTA (Havidote*) at the rate of 1 ml/kg (67 mg/kg). This should be given twice daily for 2 days, withheld for 2 days, and given again for 2 more days. Success is best achieved when the blood lead is less than 1 ppm. Cattle require 10 to 14 days to recover and may require several series of treatments in severe cases. Supportive therapy of forced feeding and oral fluids is very important, since animals are frequently anorectic, emaciated, and dehydrated. Excessive quantities of fluids should not be given parenterally, since water loading will compound brain edema. Oral magnesium sulfate may be of some value in limiting further absorption of lead as well as serving as a purge. Animals with neurologic involvement are accorded a poor prognosis.

Chlorinated Hydrocarbon Insecticides

Treatment must control the violent seizures, remove the offending material, and maintain body fluid and electrolyte balance. The barbiturates, particularly pentobarbitol sodium, are the sedatives of choice. Care is required in selecting a dosage to prevent further depression of the respiratory system.

Since chlorinated hydrocarbon compounds are stored in the fat, the clinical course may be somewhat protracted. Maintenance of normal or nearly normal states of nutrition and hydration is mandatory. Maintaining adequate

urine formation is especially important, as the chlorinated hydrocarbons are excreted by the kidneys. Since cerebral edema has been described postmortem, dexamethasone (2 mg/kg) or mannitol (1 gm/kg) or both might be beneficial. Dietary fat should be avoided, as it encourages chlorinated hydrocarbon absorption. Calcium gluconate (2 to 4 ml/kg of a 10-per cent solution) has been recommended, but its efficacy is disputed. If the route of exposure was oral, activated charcoal (1–3 gm/kg) and sodium or magnesium sulfate (1 gm/kg) should be given orally in an aqueous slurry.

Organophosphate and Carbamate Insecticides

Atropine sulfate is the pharmacologic antidote for organosphosphate and carbamate insecticide poisonings. Although atropine sulfate is highly effective as an antidote, it is important to realize that it has no effect on the fundamental biochemical lesions. Atropine sulfate acts only to block or counteract some of the more important effects of acetylcholine accumulation. Animals poisoned by cholinesterase inhibitors have a higher tolerance to atropine, and the doses should be more than is usually recommended. For ruminants, an average of 0.5 mg/kg should be administered. About one fourth of the dosage should be given intravenously, and the remainder should be given subcutaneously or intramuscularly. Improvement in the animal's condition should take place within a few minutes. It may be necessary to repeat the dose every 3 to 4 hr for 1 to 2 days, depending upon the reoccurrence of signs. With each successive treatment, however, the response becomes less and less apparent.

The development of specific antidotes for organophosphorus poisonings shows promise with hydroximic acids and oximes. Compounds such as 2-Pam (pralidoxime) and TMB-4 act competitively breaking down the phosphorylated enzyme complex, freeing acetylcholinesterase, and at the same time tying up the organophosphate, making it available for hydrolysis and excretion. Doses of approximately 20 mg/kg have been effectively used in animals. The oximes may not be effective in the treatment of carbamate poisoning. In cases of massive oral exposure, especially in ruminants, the use of both atropine and the oximes may be ineffective because of the continued absorption of the insecticide from the rumen. Animals may make a transient recovery only to relapse into a condition characteristic of a more severe poisoning than was initially observed. For this reason, activated charcoal together with a saline cathartic should be given orally (1–3 gm/kg of charcoal and 1 gm/kg sodium or magnesium sulfate).

A number of drugs are contraindicated in treating organophosphorus poisonings. These are morphine, succinylcholine, and phenothiazine.

Herbicides and Fungicides

Treatment of most poisoning cases caused by herbicides and fungicides is symptomatic and supportive in nature because of the lack of specific antidotes. The introductory recommendations on treatment of poisonings should be followed in caring for animals poisoned by these agents. Activated charcoal (1–3 gm/kg) and a saline cathartic (1–3 gm/kg) mixture should be given if exposure has been oral.

Animals intoxicated with sodium chlorate, which forms methemoglobin, should be given a 1-per cent solution of methylene blue 8.8 mg/kg. The methylene blue must be

---

*Available from Haver-Lockhart Laboratories, Box 390, Shawnee, Kansas 66201.

given slowly, and the animal must be closely observed, because an overdose of methylene blue also causes methemoglobin formation. Because sodium chlorate is not rapidly biotransformed, a poisoned animal may have to be treated for several days to ensure proper recovery. Other supportive measures such as fluid and electrolyte therapy should also be instituted.

In poisonings caused by organic mercurial fungicides, signs may not become apparent until permanent nerve damage has occurred. BAL, when used for arsenical poisonings, may be of value along with other supportive measures.

ADVERSE DRUG REACTIONS

Drugs are developed for the beneficial effects that may be achieved with proper use. However, all drugs have side effects, and the therapeutic effects of drugs may be modified by many factors including gastrointestinal absorption (modification of microflora), feed, xenobiotics (insecticides, cleaning agents, cosmetics, inhalants, and so forth), genetic variations of individuals in drug metabolism (susceptibility, idiosyncrasy), species, sex (hormonal effect), age (difference in drug metabolizing ability), nutritional status, body temperature, dosage, route of administration, and pathophysiologic factors modifying drug response (enzyme deficiency, liver or kidney disease, and so forth). The decrease in drug effectiveness or increase in drug action up to the toxic level caused by these many factors has become a major concern in modern therapeutics.

Normal doses of a single drug tolerated by the majority of humans or animals (in any one species) may cause adverse reactions in some individuals. Many of these reactions are due to (1) hypersensitivity, (2) idiosyncrasy, (3) allergy, (4) drug resistance, (5) tolerance, tachyphylaxis, and physical dependence, and (6) drug and bioactive environmental chemical toxicity (acute or chronic effects, including mutagenesis, teratogenesis, and tumorigenesis).

Drug incompatibilities may properly be classified as iatrogenic drug interactions. There may be some justifiable reasons for extemporaneous mixtures of drugs, including economy of time, convenience, and avoiding multiple injection sites. However, the reasons for not mixing drugs *in vivo* should be given serious consideration. Certainly, an important reason for refraining from mixing drugs is the possibility of inactivating 1 or more of the active ingredients. Visible signs of *in vitro* incompatibility or inactivation are colloidal formation, color changes, or gas formation. Some reactions may occur that are not visible but nevertheless may render an ingredient inactive. For instances, certain sulfonamides and penicillins are incompatible because the high pH of the sulfonamides will inactivate the penicillins. Unfortunately, this interaction is not grossly observable in the vial. It would be advantageous to consult with a pharmacist before mixing drugs.

Allergic Drug Reactions

Hypersensitivity reactions or allergic drug reactions are those caused by immunologic responses and are the result of antigen-antibody reactions. Other types of adverse effects, such as direct toxicity, overdosages, side effects, or interactions between drugs are not caused by immune mechanisms.

Predispositions to Drug Reactions

Factors contributing most significantly to the incidence of side effects and interactions are as follows:

1. The great number of potent drugs available to practitioners.
2. The practice of administering more than 1 drug to a patient.
3. Availability of potent drugs without prescription.
4. Animal exposure to environmental pollutants (e.g., insecticides, pesticides, fertilizers, and so forth).
5. Lack of knowledge concerning the pharmacology, pharmacokinetics, and chemistry of the drug.
6. Failure to set a therapeutic end point, producing an overdose effect (e.g., digitalis therapy).
7. Lack of a precise diagnosis followed by administration of a useless drug.
8. Lack of knowledge of predisposing factors in both health and disease, which contributes to poor drug prescription practices.

Difficulties in Recognizing Drug Reactions

Frequently, a series of clinical accidents due to drug reactions has led to discovery of underlying toxicologic mechanisms. In many stituations, however, drug reactions are not recognized because of the following reasons:

1. Apparent proximate cause and effect of some drugs are lacking (e.g., phenothiazines concentrate in the retina and may cause later damage).
2. Use of multiple drugs that are not needed.
3. Poor documentation of drug reactions (minimizing some toxic effects).
4. Lack of concern about potential toxicity of many drugs, and reluctancy of practitioners to accept that treatment may aggravate the patient's condition.
5. Occult drug toxicity.
6. Emergency treatment that often contributes to the irrational use of drugs.

Minimizing Adverse Drug Reactions

1. When possible, avoid multiple drug therapy. The knowledgeable use of a single drug in pharmacotherapy is superior to the blind administration of a series of drugs with no regard to how they may influence one another.
2. Avoid combination products.
3. Avoid simultaneous use of drugs that may be antagonistic.
4. Minimize the personal formulary to the point of thorough familiarity with each drug. The danger of overtreatment is greater than of undertreatment in most cases.
5. Limit intravenous infusion solutions to only 1 drug additive to avoid incompatibility.
6. Always have on hand appropriate drugs with which to treat acute allergic reactions. If dispensing drugs for administration by the owner, explain how to recognize and treat an anaphylactic reaction. Penicillin allergy in cattle is more common today.
7. When in doubt about a drug, consult a local pharmacist. By training, he or she is an excellent source of information on drug incompatibilities, interactions, and adverse effects.
8. Finally, it may be concluded that some adverse reactions are inevitable. The number, however, can be reduced if a correct diagnosis is made initially, if only the proper drug administered, and if an old principle in therapy is always observed: *primum non nocere* (first of all—do no harm).

Prevention and Management of Drug and Chemical Residues in Meat and Milk

H. DWIGHT MERCER, D.V.M., Ph.D.

The use of drugs in food producing animals is an established and well recognized requirement in the production of essential foodstuffs for a growing world population. Inherent in the widespread use of drugs are the problems associated with the fact that most chemical substances administered to animals produce residual levels in various tissues and body fluids. Thus, drug withdrawal periods must be established that become criteria for drug usage.

Today, there are more than 1000 drug products approved by the Food and Drug Administration (FDA) for use by veterinarians and livestock and poultry producers. Considering drug combinations, this number of drugs expands to approximately 2600. These drugs are used in a variety of ways: to treat diseased animals by both laymen and veterinarians, to protect animals from infections as well as to aid them in growing to market weight faster on less feed, and a large percentage (>50 per cent) of antimicrobial agents manufactured and imported into the United States today are used to supplement feed.

DRUG USAGE PATTERNS

In general, the following uses are the most common for drugs that are fed to animals in large volumes.

Herd Health. Disease outbreak and transmission often involve an entire herd or flock. One of the quickest and safest means of treatment is via the feed or water, although individual animal therapy may be oral or parenteral use of a drug.

Disease Prevention. Animals may be exposed to a disease and may be in an incubation phase but may still be healthy. These animals receive drugs in feed or water to prevent an outbreak.

Growth Promotion and Improved Feed Efficiency. Drugs, mostly antimicrobials, administered at low levels (subtherapeutic) are used to increase weight gain and promote feed efficiency. Feed additives can help to conserve feed, particularly grain.

Control of Parasites. Anthelmintics may be added at various levels in feed to prevent low grade infestations and to avoid excessive handling and restraint of animals associated with individual treatment. Examples are coccidiostats in poultry and phenothiazine in range cattle.

Nutrient Supplementation. Vitamins and minerals, particularly essential minerals such as selenium, are common components of feedstuffs.

DRUG LEVELS IN FEEDS

It is necessary understand the rate of drug usage as well as the terminology often used by feed and drug representatives.

Therapeutic Levels. These are generally recognized as levels in feed that will give rise to therapeutic concentra-

tions in the blood stream. The dose depends upon the drug and the size of the animal. For example, 250 gm of drug per ton of feed will give the following calculated therapeutic concentration of an antibiotic in a 30-pound (13.6-kg) pig:

250 gm of drug/ton feed = 275 ppm = 275 mg/kg feed

A 30-lb (13.6-kg) pig eats 8 per cent of its body weight per day. Conversion to mg/kg is as follows:

$$\text{Dose} = \frac{(\text{ppm in feed}) \times (\text{kg feed eaten})}{\text{body weight (kg)}}$$

$$\text{Dose} = \frac{(275 \text{ mg/kg}) \times (2.4 \div 2.205 \text{ lbs/kg})}{(30 \div 2.205 \text{ lbs/kg})}$$

$$\text{Dose} = \frac{275 \times 1.09}{13.6} = \frac{299.8}{13.6} = 22.0 \text{ mg/kg}$$

Dose in 30-lb (13.6-kg) pig is 22.0 mg/kg.

In general, this dose rate of an absorbable antibiotic will yield a therapeutic concentration in the blood, and thus it is considered that 250 to 1000 gm/ton is therapeutic.

Disease Prevention Levels. There are 2 aspects that must be considered:

1. *A disease outbreak is imminent.* A few animals have a history of disease, and the diagnosis indicates that spread to other animals is likely. In this instance, the disease prevention level is the same as the therapeutic level, e.g., 250 to 1000 gm/ton. This represents the only scientifically valid disease prevention dose rate.

2. *A disease is endemic on the farm.* A previous history of a disease such as atrophic rhinitis in swines is an example. In this instance, subtherapeutic levels are used effectively to prevent recurrence. For example, 100 to 250 gm/ton of feed is often used. The classic example is ASP-250, which is therapeutic in young pigs but subtherapeutic in old pigs, and the rate of feed consumption is reduced. The concept of subtherapeutic use of antimicrobial drugs in animal feeds is considered by many to be unsound owing to the confirmed sequelae of mass antimicrobial resistance that develops and is transferable.

Growth Promotion (Feed Efficiency Levels). These doses range from 4 to 50 gm/ton.

There are several theories of mechanisms of action of growth-promoting antimicrobial additives. Briefly they are as follows:

1. *Nutrient-sparing effect.* This reduces dietary requirements for certain nutrients either by depressing microorganisms that compete with the animal for nutrients or by stimulating growth of those microorganisms that synthesize nutrients (vitamins and amino acids).

2. *Thinning of the gut wall.* This increases the absorptive capacities of the intestinal tract. The implication is that organisms cause damage to and thickening of the gut wall by direct invasion or liberation of toxins. Antibiotics suppress these undesirable organisms and improve absorption of essential nutrients.

3. *Metabolic effects.* Certain enzyme systems may be affected by antibiotics. There may be direct effects on systemic enzymes (chlortetracycline reduces metabolic rate in pigs) or effects on enzyme systems of microorganisms (urease).

The precise mechanism of action of antibiotics is still unknown even though they have been in use for over 20 years.

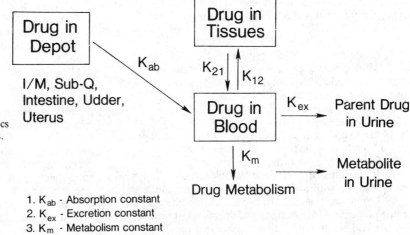

Figure 1. Conceptual model of drug kinetics as it relates to the problem of drug residues.

1. K_{ab} - Absorption constant
2. K_{ex} - Excretion constant
3. K_m - Metabolism constant
4. K_{12}/K_{21} - Rate of drug distribution into and out of tissue
(Relates to volume of distribution)

NEW DRUG DEVELOPMENT

The search for new drugs and their subsequent development follows a long and intense scientific pathway. Development of manufacturing methods, analytical procedures, formulations, stability, posology, toxicology, packaging, and marketing are only a few of the major endeavors required for new drugs. The FDA adds several additional requirements for use in food animals, including drug residue studies in target animals, metabolism studies, and potential human toxicity studies. The development of drug residue data is one of the most costly steps in drug development for food animals. The establishment of drug withdrawal requirements and setting of tolerances to ensure that the intended drug will not pose a threat to public health is the single most important aspect of the FDA's responsibilities in approving new drugs for use in food animals.[1]

Pharmacokinetics is the quantitative study of absorption, distribution, metabolism, and excretion of drugs and their pharmacologic, therapeutic, or toxic responses in animals and man.[2] In order to understand the problems of drug residues, it is necessary to have an appreciation of drug kinetics.

Conventional methods used to determine the residual nature of a drug in food animals may involve the following sequence of events:

1. Develop an analytical method for quantitative determination of the parent drug in biologic fluids and tissues.

2. Dose a series of animals via the intended route with the proposed formulation. Radiolabeled compounds are often used for this purpose.

3. At various intervals after dosing (i.e., at 0, 1, 3, 5, 7, 9, 12 days), slaughter at least 3 animals, collect a variety of tissues, including liver, muscle, fat, and kidney, and conduct assays to establish the necessary withdrawal interval.

4. Provide supporting toxicologic data for establishing tolerances.

5. Refinement and modification of the analytical procedures to the desired sensitivity level (parent drug and metabolites) may be necessary.

6. Establish withdrawal requirements. In many instances, the duration and extent of drug dosage for efficacy purposes may produce residue. In striving to develop a drug that maintains concentrations in serum and tissues for a lengthy time interval, it is often found that this desired characteristic is incompatible with a short withdrawal interval. In fact, this is the paradox of the drug residue problem for the practitioner.

Figure 1 represents a conceptual model for drug kinetics as it relates to the problem of drug residues. Based upon this model, it becomes apparent that the majority of drug residue problems are associated with the drug either in depot phase or in tissue phase. A group of characteristics has been developed that often helps explain why certain drugs cause residue problems. These characteristics have been grouped into 3 major types of drugs (I, II, and III). The following criteria provide the most realistic basis for understanding drug residue problems.

Criteria for Type I Drugs

1. Rapid absorption rate constant (k_{ab}).

2. High degree of absorption (>90 per cent). Absorption of drugs from aqueous solutions is rapid and almost complete.

3. Low volume of distribution (V_d), e.g., organic acids, <0.2–0.25 L/kg.

4. Short biologic half-life ($t_{1/2} \leq 1$ hr), e.g., penicillins and cephalosporins.[3]

5. One and 2 compartment model drugs, i.e., drug generally remains in the central blood compartment.

6. Low affinity for tissues.

Most drugs that meet these criteria will provide relatively high blood concentrations that are diminished at a rapid rate. The use of this type of drug requires repetitive dosing on a daily basis to maintain therapeutic concentrations in the blood.

These properties are highly desirable from the standpoint of drug residue when used in food animals. Classic examples include most of the penicillins, cephalosporins, sulfisoxazole, and sulfadiazine. It is often an objective with this class of drugs to lengthen the dosage interval. The formulation (e.g., less soluble salts and oil bases) required to lengthen the dosage interval often leads to type II drugs in this classification scheme.

Criteria for Type II Drugs

1. Moderate to rapid absorption rate constants.
2. Moderate degree of absorption (>70 per cent) as a result of vehicle effects, e.g., propylene glycol, polyvinylpyrrolidone, and certain oil type bases.
3. High volume of distribution (>1 L/kg), often true of organic bases.
4. Median biologic half-life (3 to 8 hr), e.g., sulfamethazine,[4] oxytetracycline,[5] and erythromycin.[2]
5. Two compartment model drugs.
6. Indications of drug depot problems, e.g., injection site problems with oxytetracycline[5] and sulfonamides.[6]
7. Drugs such as erythromycin lactobionate and procaine penicillin G are examples of drugs that are converted by the body from type I drug to type II drug.

A more extensive effort is required in the development of a drug residue profile for type II drugs. Subcutaneous or intravenous routes of administration might be chosen if intramuscular sites contain residues for long periods. The oral route may be the only acceptable route. Depot problems may be solved by route or vehicle modifications. This type of drug is considered a greater residue producing risk, and its use may be more closely monitored and controlled. Also, it is more costly to develop this type of drug because of the greater increase in residue studies required. Classic examples include intramuscularly administered oxytetracycline, benzathine penicillin, and certain sulfonamides.

Criteria for Type III Drugs

1. Slow absorption rate constant.
2. Incomplete absorption (<50 per cent).
3. High volume of distribution.
4. Long half-life (>12 hr).
5. Two or more compartment drugs.
6. Strong affinity for tissue depots and binding ability

(e.g., chlorinated hydrocarbons accumulate in fat and kidneys and aminoglycosides bind to kidney tissue).

Extreme caution must be taken, and extensive residue data are required for the development of this type of drug. Usage patterns should be strictly limited to therapeutic purposes, with stringent restrictions recommended to the practitioner. Marketing channels should be limited to professional use only. Several classic examples are parenteral streptomycin and neomycin,[1] long-acting sulfonamides (sulfadimethoxine),[7] and chlorinated hydrocarbons. While the goal of restricted use for this type of drug has not been realized, it is reasonable to expect that the practicing veterinarian will ultimately be given this responsibility. This should be particularly true if drug residue problems continue to occur, and other means fail to control the incidences of drug residues in food animals.

Figure 2 is used to illustrate the biologic half-life concept of a drug in the animal body. The absorption phase is a rate limiting phase. As indicated earlier, problems with absorption often translate into drug residue problems. It generally requires about 6 half-lives for a drug to be depleted below its therapeutic usefulness. This generally occurs within a matter of hours. After this point, the depletion pattern reflects the residual nature of the drug. Once depletion reaches ppm, ppb, or ppt levels, it is at these concentrations for which tolerances are established. Theoretically, once a drug has entered the system, it will require an infinite time for the last molecule to be eliminated. Thus, establishment of tolerances becomes a necessity. There are several types of tolerances as illustrated in Figure 2. A discussion of tolerances is available.[8]

DRUG RESIDUE SURVEILLANCE

Analytical methods for tissue residues are tested by the FDA and the USDA Animal and Plant Health Inspection Service (APHIS) for every new drug intended for use in food animals beore it is approved for marketing. The

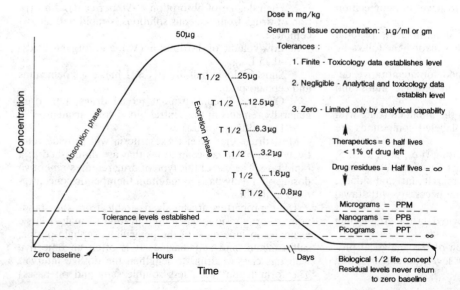

Figure 2. Biological half-life concept.

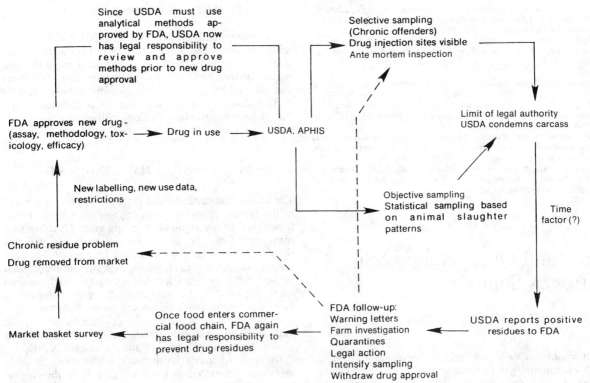

Figure 3. Drug residue surveillance.

purpose is to find methods that are specific for the compound tested, consistently accurate, reproducible by various laboratories, and sufficiently rapid so that they are useful for regulating control of the compounds tested.

The USDA regularly monitors tissue samples from slaughtered animals for between 30 and 40 agricultural and environmental chemical compounds. Classes and examples of compounds presently monitored include

Antimicrobials. Sulfonamides, penicillins, streptomycin, tetracyclines, erythromycin, and neomycin.

Other Drugs. Coccidiostats, growth promotants, and other special purpose drugs.

Pesticides. Chlorinated hydrocarbons, various industrial chemicals, hexachlorobenzene, and polychlorinated benzene.

Elements. Lead, cadmium, mercury, and arsenic.

The USDA's drug detection program consists of 2 parts: the monitoring phase and the surveillance phase.

The incidence of illegal drug residues reported by the National Monitoring Program was about 2.4 per cent in fiscal year 1973, about 1.9 per cent in fiscal year 1974, and has remained around 2.0 per cent during the past few years.

The following summary and Figure 3 illustrate the cooperative efforts of the regulatory agencies in the control of drug residues.

1. APHIS and the FDA agree on the effectiveness and feasibility of a drug firm's proposed residue detection method.

2. APHIS monitors food animals for tissue residues of drugs, pesticides, and environmental contaminants.

3. Violative drug residues detected by APHIS are reported to the FDA, the producer, and the state authorities.

4. Animals shipped by the producer who has a record of shipped animals with violative levels of residues are subject to certain restrictions until there is evidence that the producer's animals are in compliance.

5. FDA initiates an on site investigation of the suspect producer. If the evidence shows a flagrant violation of the law or if the case involves a repetition of an earlier illegal residue violation, the producer may face criminal charges.

6. The convicted producer can be fined and possibly imprisoned for this crime.

7. Animals with above tolerance residues are condemned by APHIS. Producers of these animals are subject to restrictions on the marketing of future shipments until they can prove their animals are in compliance with tolerances.

The practicing food animal veterinarian, while not always directly involved in the drug usage pattern, represents the individual in the community who has the training and experience to educate and advise producers on the problems of drug residues. As drugs become more potent, and their uses become more sophisticated, the role of the veterinarian will become more advisory. If the local feed store operator has the responsibility for providing the data and knowledge required for the proper use of drugs and the methods needed to prevent residues, it is apparent that illegal drug residues in the food chain will continue.

References

1. Mercer, H. D.: Antimicrobial drugs in food producing animals. Control mechanisms of government agencies. Vet. Clin. North Am. 5:3–33, 1975.
2. Baggot, J. D., and Gingerich, D. A.: Pharmacokinetic interpretation of erythromycin and tylosin activity in serum after intravenous administration of a single dose to cows. Res. Vet. Sci. 21:318–323, 1976.

3. Ziv, G., Shani, J., and Sulman, F. G.: Pharmacokinetic evaluation of penicillin and cephalosporin derivatives in serum and milk of lactating cows and ewes. Am. J. Vet. Res. *34*:1561–1565, 1973.
4. Food and Drug Administration: Contracts 70–204 and 71–69. Urbana, Illinois: Department of Veterinary Anatomy, Physiology and Pharmacology, College of Veterinary Medicine, University of Illinois, 1970–1974.
5. Pilloud, M.: Pharmacokinetics, plasma protein binding and dosage of oxytetracycline in cattle and horses. Res. Vet. Sci. *15*:224–230, 1973.
6. Boxenbaum, H. G., and Kaplan, S. A.: Potential source of error in absorption rate calculations. J. Pharmacokinet. Biopharm. *3*:257–264, 1975.
7. Rasmussen, F., and Svendsen, O.: Tissue damage and concentration at the injection site after intramuscular injection of chemotherapeutics and vehicles in pigs. Res. Vet. Sci. *20*:55–60, 1976.
8. Jones, L. M., Booth, N. H., and McDonald, L. E.: Veterinary Pharmacology and Therapeutics, 4th ed. Ames, Iowa, Iowa State University Press, Chapter 63, 1977.

Urea and Other Nonprotein Nitrogen Sources

W. EUGENE LLOYD, D.V.M., Ph.D.

Ruminant animals can utilize nonprotein nitrogen (NPN) compounds to provide up to 40 per cent of their protein nitrogen requirements. NPN compounds are commonly used in ruminant rations, depending on the relative costs of natural protein feedstuffs, grains, forages, and NPN compounds. NPN compounds are usually efficient and safe, but they frequently cause acute poisonings owing to misuse. Toxicoses occur when animals ingest compounds that release excessive quantities of ammonia (NH_3) into the gastrointestinal tract with a resultant hyperammonemia.

SOURCES

The most common NPN compounds are urea and ammonia or ammonium salts. These compounds are usually added to dry or liquid protein supplements and are frequently incorporated into protein concentrate blocks, ruminant complete rations, or grain concentrate mixtures. Biuret, a good NPN source with a low order of toxicity, is not being manufactured for commercial use. Dry and liquid fertilizers usually contain ammonia, ammonium salts, or urea and may be accidentally ingested by farm animals.

TOXICITY

All farm animals are susceptible to poisoning by ammonium salts, with doses of 0.3 to 0.5 gm/kg usually causing clinical signs of toxicoses, and doses of 0.5 to 1.5 gm/kg being the minimum lethal dose (MLD). The toxicity of urea in ruminant animals is similar to the toxicity of ammonium salts. Horses are moderately susceptible to urea toxicoses, with doses ≥4.0 gm/kg being the MLD. Monogastric animals, such as the pig and calf, are unaffected by oral ingestion of urea except for transient diuretic actions.

CONDITIONS CAUSING TOXICOSIS

NPN compounds furnish ammonia (NH_3), which rumen microorganisms use along with carbohydrates to synthesize amino acids and proteins. Toxicosis is likely to occur when ingested NPN compounds release more NH_3 than can be used by rumen microorganisms, or when soluble carbohydrate levels are low. Urea is hydrolyzed in less than 1 hr in the ruminoreticulum by the reaction

$$NH_2-\overset{\overset{\textstyle O}{\|}}{C}-NH_2 + H_2O \rightarrow 2NH_3 + CO_2$$

The urease that catalyzes this reaction is normally present in the rumen, probably because some urea in the blood is returned to the ruminal ammonia pool. Contrary to a common belief, the urease in raw soybeans will not significantly increase the toxicity of urea when the 2 are ingested concurrently. However, high protein feeds, such as soybeans, soybean meal, cottonseed meal, linseed meal, fish meal, and dried skim milk, may contribute to or produce ammonia toxicosis due to the fact that amino acids in these soluble proteins are deaminated to NH_3 and keto acids. A gelatinized starch-urea product is designed to slow the hydrolysis of urea and the release of NH_3.

Ruminal ammonia levels peak within minutes after ingestion of ammonium salts, within 1 hr in the case of urea and within 1 to 4 hrs in the case of high protein feedstuffs. Ammonia from forage reaches peak rumen levels within 4 to 12 hr, since soluble proteins are released after cellulose digestion. A relatively small amount of the protein in ruminant rations escapes hydrolysis and is digested in the abomasum and intestinal tract, along with the myriad numbers of bacteria and protozoa, in a manner conventional of monogastric animals. The toxicity of biuret is relatively low, since biuretase is not normally present in the ruminoreticulum and is induced only by feeding biuret.

The toxicity of the NH_3 in the ruminoreticulum pool, whether from ammonium salts and urea or protein feeds, is related to ammonia levels and rumen pH values. Only nonionized or free NH_3 diffuses from the rumen into the portal blood. At pH 8.4, approximately 1/10 of the total $NH_3:NH_4^+$ is present as NH_3, which favors toxicosis. At pH 6.4, 1/1000 of the $NH_3:NH_4^+$ is present as NH_3, and toxicosis may or may not occur, depending on total rumen NH_3 concentration. At pH 4.4, only 1/100,000 of the $NH_3:NH_4^+$ is present as NH_3, and toxicosis is virtually impossible.

Urea increases rumen pH, but ammonium salts may moderately increase or decrease pH, depending on whether the anion is weak or strong. Protein feeds raise or lower pH, according to the relative amounts of soluble proteins and carbohydrates. Carbohydrate feeds, such as corn, molasses, barley, and sorghum grain, depress ruminal pH, predominantly owing to the release of the volatile fatty acids (VFA):acetic, propionic, and butyric. During grain overloads, the VFA and lactic acid may depress the pH to 3.0 to 4.5. Corn silage lowers ruminal pH, but most hays and forages raise pH. Fasting ruminants have ruminal pH values between 6.5 and 7.2.

Ruminant microorganisms rapidly adapt to NPN feeding, and animals may tolerate daily doses of 0.5 to 1.0 gm/kg, and yet the same doses may poison animals after fasting for 24 hr. Circumstances that lead to NPN toxicosis in cattle, goats, and sheep are improper mixing or formulation of NPN rations and feeding NPN substances with low carbohydrate, high fiber diets, and feeding NPN substances to animals that are hungry and unadapted to NPN utilization.

Cattle are frequently poisoned when NPN-containing protein supplements are fed as top dressings over concentrates or are fed undiluted to wintered cattle. Protein blocks with NPN compounds frequently poison animals if they have been softened by moist climatic conditions. Liquid supplements can be lethal, despite the molasses content, if animals can rapidly ingest them. Lick tanks that are improperly adjusted may allow animals to ingest supplements too rapidly. Relatively large amounts of liquid supplements may be drunk after being diluted with rainwater. Poorly formulated liquids occasionally produce concentrations of urea in the bottom of tanks. Cattle and sheep have been poisoned by eating granular fertilizers that have been spilled, or by drinking liquid fertilizers. Animals consuming ammonium nitrate show signs of ammonia, not nitrate, toxicoses.

PATHOGENESIS AND CLINICAL SIGNS

Ammonia absorbed from the ruminoreticulum is normally detoxified by conversion to urea in the liver. When large amounts of NH_3 overwhelm the liver detoxifying mechanism, toxicosis results owing to hyperammonemia.

During toxicosis, there is a relative ruminal alkalosis and lactic acidemia, with blood pH values lowering to approximately 7.0 before death. There are significant elevations in the values of blood packed cell volume, glucose, potassium, phosphorus, SGOT, SGPT, and BUN. The BUN levels cannot be used to confirm a diagnosis of NH_3 toxicosis, however. Ammonia apparently inhibits the citrate cycle, and death is probably due to hyperkalemic cardiac shock and cessation of respiration.

Normal NH_3-N levels in blood or serum range from 0.1 to 0.2 mg/dl. Clinical signs first occur at levels of 1.0 mg/dl, and death may occur when values are 3.0 to 6.0 mg/dl. Following ingestion of urea, signs may occur within 20 to 60 min in cattle and within 30 to 90 min in sheep. Signs are muscle tremors of the face and ears, frothy salivation, grinding of teeth, abdominal pain, and other muscle tremors. Cattle often become violent and tetanic as toxicosis progresses, but sheep usually appear depressed. All animals are initially polyuric, but become anuric near death. Mild ruminal tympany usually exists but is not a primary cause of death. Near death, respiration becomes forced, body temperature becomes elevated, and after a terminal tonic spasm of body musculature death becomes inevitable. Death usually occurs within 40 min to 2 hr in cattle and within 60 min to 4 hr in sheep. Recovered animals appear normal within 12 hr. No studies have been published that show NPN feeding induces chronic untoward effects or exacerbates infectious diseases.

DIAGNOSIS

A diagnosis of NPN poisoning can be made after considering clinical signs and the history of feeding NPN compounds. A change in the feeding regimen or a change in weather that alters feeding habits may predispose animals to poisoning. Postmortem examination may not confirm a diagnosis. Sheep frequently vomit and inhale the rumen contents. No other changes are common. In some cases, the odor of NH_3 is present, but NH_3 toxicosis occurs without it. Ruminal pH values > 7.5 are indicative of urea toxicosis, but urea ammonia toxicosis may occur with pH values as low as 6.0, especially with high carbohydrate liquid supplements.

Fresh jugular blood or serum, if available, should be kept frozen until chemically analyzed. A composite sample of rumen fluid, composed of several subsamples from the rumen and reticulum, should be preserved by freezing or by addition of a few drops of a saturated solution of mercuric chloride to each 100 ml of fluid. NH_3-N levels of 2 to 6 mg/dl in blood and serum, and >80 mg/dl in rumen fluid are diagnostically significant. Autolysis of improperly preserved blood and rumen fluid samples will increase NH_3 levels, rendering blood samples diagnostically worthless. Autolysis of rumen contents may raise NH_3 levels 20 to 50 mg/dl above levels that existed at death. Analyses of biologic samples for urea is worthless. Feed samples can be analyzed for urea and ammonia levels, and if mixing errors are suspected, at least 2 samples should be analyzed.

One part of urea is equivalent to 2.92 parts of protein, conversely, 1 per cent of protein is equivalent to 0.34 per cent of urea. To calculate a toxic dose, urea and ammonium salts can be considered together.

Example: The feed tag states that the feed contains 64 per cent crude protein with 59 per cent of the protein equivalent from NPN sources.
59% × 0.34 = 20.0% urea content.
One kg (or 2.2 lb) would contain 200 gm urea, enough to intoxicate a 200- to 400-kg animal, if rapidly ingested.

Differential diagnoses should be designed to rule out toxicoses due to organophosphate and carbamate insecticides, chlorinated hydrocarbon insecticides, nitrate and cyanide poisonings, and grain overloads. Encephalitic diseases, such as thromboembolic meningoencephalitis, polioencephalomalacia, and pseudorabies, should also be excluded.

TREATMENT

Treatment is seldom possible, but a 5 per cent acetic acid solution or vinegar should be administered via ruminal infusions at doses of 0.5 to 1.0 L in sheep and goats and 2.0 to 6.0 L in cattle, followed by large infusions of cold water. Intravenous infusions of calcium and magnesium solutions are indicated to alleviate tetany, and normal saline solutions are used to correct dehydration. Animals that are down and in a moribund state are generally unresponsive to treatment. A rumenotomy with replacement of rumen contents may save a severely affected animal. Recovery is generally uneventful, but it may be necessary to repeat treatment in 6 to 8 hr.

BOVINE BONKERS SYNDROME

Bovine bonkers syndrome is caused by 4-methyl imidazole, a compound sometimes produced when high quality forages, such as sorghum, Sudan cereal grain, brome or fescue hays, are treated with ammonia. The same syndrome may result from feeding of ammoniated molasses.

The primary intent of ammoniation of forage is to increase quality, but the ammoniation of high quality forage is uneconomical and may be dangerous. Adult cattle and nonnursing and nursing calves may be poisoned. Metabolites of 4-methyl imidazole can be transmitted in the milk.

Clinical Signs

Clinical signs of toxicosis have a rapid onset after the feeding of treated hay for a few days to weeks. Hyperexcitability, wild running, circling, convulsive seizures, and death are common.

Treatment

Terminate exposure to ammoniated hay. The symptomatic control of seizures and hyperactivity may be accomplished with barbiturate or chloral hydrate administration to effect. Activated charcoal (1–3 gm/kg) with a saline cathartic (1 gm/kg) should be given orally.

Supplemental Reading

Bicknell, E. J.: Experimental ammonia toxicosis in the pig. Ph.D. Thesis. Lansing, Michigan, Michigan State University, 1965.

Buck, W. B., Osweiler, G. D., and Van Gelder, G. A.: Clinical and Diagnostic Veterinary Toxicology. Dubuque, Iowa, Kendall/Hunt Publishing Co., 1976.

Lloyd, W. E.: Chemical and metabolic aspects of urea-ammonia toxicosis in cattle and sheep. Ph.D. Thesis. Ames, Iowa, Iowa State University, 1970.

Singer, R. H.: Acute ammonium salt poisoning in sheep. M.S. Thesis. Ames, Iowa, Iowa State University, 1969.

Salt Poisoning—Water Deprivation

WILLIAM B. BUCK, D.V.M., M.S.

Salt poisoning—water deprivation primarily occurs in swine and poultry but occasionally occurs in ruminants under husbandry practices in which high concentrations of sodium are consumed without adequate consumption of water. In swine and poultry, any practice that results in limited water intake may cause the problem. Common reasons for reduced water intake include mechanical problems with automatic waterers, frozen water, neglect of hand watering, medication in water, overcrowding, and strange environments where the water may be difficult to find. All livestock and poultry are susceptible to the consequences of high sodium content of feed and water if adequate fresh water is not available. On the other hand, if adequate fresh water is consumed, most species can tolerate high concentrations of salt in the diet, but only low concentrations of salt in the water. Thus, swine have been poisoned on diets containing as little as 0.5 per cent salt when water was withheld, but have tolerated diets containing 13 per cent salt when fresh water was available. Brine or water containing 3.5 per cent salt, as found in the vicinity of oil drilling operations, is especially hazardous to cattle and other species of livestock and poultry. A salt concentration in water of 0.25 per cent is the maximum tolerated by poultry. Most species of livestock can tolerate no greater than 0.5 per cent in their water, although sheep have tolerated 1 per cent.

Cattle and occasionally sheep have been poisoned on the high concentrations of salt in concentrates or mineral and protein supplements. Salt usually constitutes 25 to 35 per cent of these preparations and is in sufficient concentration to prevent animals from overeating. Unfortunately, if adequate water is not available and animals are extremely hungry, they may consume enough of the mixtures to produce salt toxicoses.

The mechanism of salt poisoning—water deprivation is not thoroughly understood, however, it is well established that the sodium ion is the offending agent regardless of its source. A plausible explanation for the clinical signs that occur is as follows: sodium passes passively from the plasma to the cerebrospinal fluid (CSF), however, the transport from CSF to plasma requires energy and, therefore, is active transport. With limited water intake, dehydration occurs in the body, resulting in a rise in the sodium level of the blood compartment. Because of its concentration in the blood, sodium passively crosses into the CSF, resulting in concentrations of 155 to 185 mEq/L or greater (normal CSF concentrations range between 135 and 145 mEq/L). Sodium at the higher concentration inhibits anaerobic glycolysis, resulting in reduced energy production in the brain. Since there is reduced energy available for active transport of sodium from the CSF to the plasma, the high level of sodium in the brain prevents the sodium from going back into the blood. The high sodium concentration in the brain causes an osmotic gradient that results in fluid coming into the brain tissue, causing edema. Edema produces pressure, and this results in malacia.

CLINICAL SIGNS

In swine, the early signs of increased thirst, pruritus, and constipation are rarely recognized by the herder. Usually, the first signs that are noted occur from 1 to 5 days after water deprivation has commenced. Intermittent convulsive seizures become more and more frequent until they are continuous, and the animal becomes recumbent and comatose. Affected animals may be blind and oblivious to their surroundings. They usually will not eat, drink, or respond to external stimuli. They often wander aimlessly, push against objects, and circle or pivot around a front or rear limb. Convulsive seizures consist of the animal sitting on its haunches, drawing its head backwards and upwards in a jerking motion, finally falling over on its side in clonic-tonic seizures, and opisthotonos. Comatose swine, in a terminal state, usually lie on their side paddling.

Salt poisoning—water deprivation in poultry is manifested by excessive thirst, respiratory distress, discharge of fluid from the beak, wet feces, and paralysis of the limbs.

Cattle and sheep have both alimentary tract and central nervous system signs. There may be vomiting, diarrhea, abdominal pain, anorexia, and mucus in the feces. Constant polyuria and nasal discharge may be present. The neurologic signs include blindness and convulsive seizures followed by partial paralysis and knuckling of the fetlocks. Animals usually die within 12 to 24 hr of the appearance of clinical signs. Recovery normally takes several days, and during this time animals are depressed and lethargic.

A characteristic sequela to salt poisoning in cattle is the dragging of the rear feet while walking and, in more severe cases, knuckling of the fetlock joints. This occurs apparently without pain to the animal, although there may be severe damage to tendons, peripheral nerves, and tissues.

PATHOLOGY

Gross postmortem changes in both swine and cattle usually include some form of gastric inflammation and ulceration. In swine, pinpoint ulcers filled with blood are common in those receiving high levels of salt in the diet. There may be marked congestion of the gastric mucosa, however, this finding is frequently observed in apparently normal animals.

Microscopic changes are characteristic, especially in swine. The lesions occur in the deep layers of the cortex and the adjacent white matter. The initial change is an infiltration of the meningeal and cerebral blood vessels by eosinophils. This mysterious attraction of circulating eosinophils to the cerebral vascular and meningeal areas is observed only in swine and is referred to as eosinophilic meningoencephalitis. Another microscopic change that occurs in the brain of swine and other species is a greater vascularity of the deep layers of the cortex and adjacent white matter. In addition, there is often a higher number of histiocytes or gitter cells in the white matter adjacent to the deep layers of the cortex. If the animal survives, there is more vacuolization and breakup of the continuity of the tissue in the junction of the cortex and the white matter. This is a reflection of edema or early necrosis and malacia. In swine, the eosinophils disappear from the brain and reappear in the blood during the latter phases of the syndrome.

DIAGNOSIS

It is important to obtain a history. A history of limited water intake and high levels of sodium in the diet or water may be difficult to obtain, however, because animal caretakers may not be willing to admit deficient husbandry practices. Laboratory confirmation procedures are analysis of serum, CSF, and cerebral tissue for sodium concentrations. Levels above 160 mEq/L in both serum and CSF and 1800 ppm in cerebral tissue are sufficient for formation of a tentative diagnosis. Confirmation of a diagnosis is dependent upon finding the characteristic pathologic changes in the cerebral cortex. Necropsy specimens submitted to a laboratory should include refrigerated, nonfrozen CSF and blood serum, frozen cerebral tissue, and thin slices of cerebral cortex preserved in 10-per cent buffered formalin.

There are several conditions that appear similar to salt poisoning—water deprivation in swine: pseudorabies, nonspecific viral encephalomyelitic conditions, chlorinated hydrocarbon insecticide poisoning, and enterotoxemia.

TREATMENT

Treatment of salt poisoning—water deprivation is nonspecific and may be of little value. Affected animals should be given small amounts of fresh water at frequent inter-

vals. They should not be allowed to receive water *ad lib*, as such a practice may enhance brain edema and exacerbate the syndrome. It may take 4 to 5 days or longer for an affected animal to fully recover. Usually about 50 per cent of those affected die regardless of treatment. Diuretics and anticonvulsants have been recommended but have not produced outstanding results.

Supplemental Reading

Buck, W. B., Osweiler, G. D., and Van Gelder, G. A.: Clinical and Veterinary Diagnostic Toxicology. Dubuque, Iowa, Kendall/Hunt Publishing Co., 1976.

Dunn, H. W., and Leman, A. D. (eds.): Diseases of Swine, 4th ed. Ames, Iowa, Iowa State University Press, 854–860, 1975.

Iodine

WILLIAM B. BUCK, D.V.M., M.S.

Iodine is an essential element that has its entire functional significance via the thyroid hormones. Like other trace elements, deficiency syndromes in food animals associated with this element may be more frequently encountered than toxicoses. Manifestations of iodine deficiency are enlargement of the thyroid gland (goiter), dwarfism, stunted growth, mental sluggishness, nervous irritability, muscle tremors, subnormal sexual vigor, delayed maturation of genitalia, and reproductive failure. Fetal development may be arrested at any stage, leading to early death and reabsorption, to abortion and stillbirth, or to live birth of weak, hairless fetuses, which is often associated with prolonged gestation and retention of fetal membranes.

The minimum dietary requirements of iodine for food animals are given in Table 1.

Many different iodine containing compounds have been used in veterinary medicine. Salts of iodine such as potassium and sodium iodide have been given for the treatment of granulomatous infections and footrot for many years. An organic iodide, ethylenediaminedihydriodide (EDDI), is recommended as a feed additive for livestock and poultry but not for dairy cattle in production (Table 2).

In addition to its metabolic action, iodine appears to have other peculiar effects on the mammalian system that has enabled it to be used as a therapeutic agent. Salts of iodine, whether inorganic or organic (such as KI or EDDI), have an expectorant action via stimulation of the vagus nerve in the gastrointestinal tract. Thus, iodides are used as expectorants to aid in the treatment of mild respiratory infection.

Another reputed property of iodine is its specific anti-

Table 1. *Estimated Minimum Dietary Requirements of Iodine*

Food Animal	Body Weight (kg)	Iodine Requirement (µg/day)
Poultry	2.3	5–9
Swine	68.2	80–160
Sheep	50.0	50–100
Dairy cow (in production)	454.5	400–800

Table 2. *Recommended Oral Levels of EDDI**

Animal	Level	Use
Cattle	50 mg/head/day in feed or salt continuously	Prevent footrot and soft tissue lumpy jaw
	400 to 500 mg/head/day for 2 to 3 weeks (not to dairy cattle in production)	Treatment of footrot and soft tissue lumpy jaw
Sheep	12 mg/head/day continuously	Prevent soft tissue lumpy jaw
Swine	250 to 500 mg/day for 7 days	Aid in control of respiratory difficulties by loosening mucus and relieving congestion in the upper respiratory tract
Turkeys and chickens	0.11 kg/ton of feed (120 ppm) for 5 to 7 days	Aid in removal of mucus from the upper respiratory tract following treatment for chronic respiratory disease

*The FDA Center for Veterinary Medicine is considering the limited use of EDDI for nutritional purposes only. The FDA is also deciding whether or not any use of EDDI will be permitted without an approved new drug application (NDA).

fibrotic effect. KI and EDDI have been effective in the treatment of granulomatous conditions such as soft tissue lumpy jaw. This action is apparently due to iodine's capacity to penetrate fibrotic tissue. High levels of iodine may, however, enhance the inflammatory process.

TOXICITY

There is a wide range between the acute toxic dose and the minimum daily required dose of iodine in animals. For this reason, the toxicity of EDDI to livestock and poultry has not been systematically studied. In 1975, Buck and Rosiles fed EDDI to 227-kg beef steers in dosages ranging from 0 to 1000 mg/head/day for 21 days, after which all animals except the controls were given 50 mg/head/day for an additional 75 days. Although no signs of toxicoses were observed, all animals given 500 and 1000 mg/head/day manifested EDDI's expectorant action in the form of a translucent nasal discharge after 5 to 10 days. This was accompanied by a mild, intermittent nonproductive cough during the remainder of a 21-day high level feeding period. The signs described subsided significantly within 2 days after EDDI was reduced to 50 mg/head/day. Those animals given 50 mg/head/day exhibited slight nasal discharge, and there was an occasional animal with a mild cough beginning after 2 weeks of exposure throughout the feeding trial. Excessive lacrimation was not observed in any of the animals during the feeding period. There was no statistically significant difference in body temperatures and in mean body weight gains of any of the animals on the various levels of iodine. All animals gained an average of 0.77 kg/day. Total serum iodine concentrations were determined during the feeding trial. Although peak mean total serum iodine concentrations averaged 1600 μ/100 ml after 2 weeks of EDDI exposure to 1000 mg/head/day, the concentrations rapidly diminished when exposure was reduced to 50 $\geqq$/head/day. Also, statistically significant differences in parameters, such as complete blood count and serum transaminase, creatinine, plasma fibrinogen, and total serum protein levels were noted. It was concluded that except for signs reflecting the expectorant action of EDDI, no adverse effects occurred.

In summary, the nutritional requirement for iodine for most animals is in the general range of 1.1 to 2.2 μg/kg body weight. The recommended continuous feeding level for the prevention of diseases, such as soft tissue lumpy jaw and footrot, is about 50 to 100 times the nutritional requirement. Furthermore, the level that would be expected to produce clinical signs of excessive eposure when fed continuously is about 1000 times the nutritional requirements for cattle and for other livestock.

CLINICAL SIGNS

The initial clinical sign of iodism in most species is increased secretion of the respiratory tract fluid with an accompanying intermittent nonproductive cough. As the amount or time of exposure increases, the eyes, skin, joints, and the hematopoietic system and, ultimately, the reproductive system are involved.

The early sign of greater seromucoid nasal discharge with an accompanying intermittent cough is followed by lacrimation and skin changes. In cattle, the skin of the dorsum, neck, ear, brisket, shoulders, and head of the tail become scaly owing to sloughing of the epidermis. If animals are exposed to very high levels of iodine for a prolonged period of time, other signs may include lameness of the knee and hock joints. In chickens, very high levels of iodine in the diet (2500 ppm) have been associated with cessation of egg production.

Clinical signs of iodism disappear rapidly after exposure is discontinued. Also, a concomitant reduction in total serum iodine concentration occurs within 2 to 3 days following cessation of high doses of iodine.

DIAGNOSIS

The development of a syndrome manifested by a seromucoid nasal discharge, intermittent coughing, and perhaps excessive lacrimation together with a history of exposure to high concentrations of iodine is sufficient to warrant a tentative diagnosis of mild iodism. The serum levels of iodine may reach 1600 μg/100 ml in cattle with only increased nasal discharge and occasional cough. If clinical signs include lacrimations, scaling of the epidermis, and joint related lameness, one can expect to find the iodine exposure to be considerably higher than is recommended for therapeutic purposes. In such a case, the total serum iodine concentration may reach 4000 to 5000 μg/ml or greater. Background concentrations of total serum iodine in cattle usually range from 25 to 50 μg/100 ml.

TREATMENT

Since iodine is rapidly metabolized and excreted from body tissues, the best treatment is removal of the iodine source.

Supplemental Reading

Buck, W. B., Osweiler, G. D., and Van Gelder, G. A.: Clinical and Diagnostic Veterinary Toxicology, 2nd ed., Dubuque, Iowa, Kendall/Hunt Publishing Co., 69–75, 1976.

Feed Additive Compendium. Minneapolis, Minnesota, Miller Publishing Co., 1982.

Underwood, E. J.: Trace Elements in Human and Animal Nutrition, 3rd ed., New York, Academic Press, 281–322, 1971.

Ionophores: Monensin, Lasalocid, Salinomycin, Narasin

MELITON N. NOVILLA, D.V.M., M.S., Ph.D.
and THOMAS M. FOLKERTS, D.V.M.

Ionophores are compounds that form lipid soluble, dynamically reversible complexes with cations and by this means, facilitate specific ionic transport across biologic membranes. There are 2 major subclasses of ionophores, (1) neutral ionophores, which are highly toxic because they form charged cationic complexes that are capable of perturbing biologic membranes and action potentials, and (2) carboxylic ionophores, which form zwitterionic complexes with cations and promote electrically neutral cation exchange diffusion that is tolerated better in intact organisms.[23]

The carboxylic ionophore, monensin, has been used widely in the United States as Coban,* which was introduced in 1971 for the control of coccidiosis in chickens and as Rumensin,* which was introduced in 1975 to promote growth or increase feed conversion in cattle. Other potential benefits of monensin are (1) reduction of coccidial oocyst discharge in ruminants, (2) prevention of acute bovine pulmonary edema and emphysema, (3) decreased incidence of bloat, (4) prevention of ruminal lactic acidosis, and (5) amelioration of ketosis in lactating dairy cows.[22] The reduction of deaths in some cattle herds has been hypothetically related to the reduction of indigestion, metabolic stress, bloat, and enterotoxemia associated with monensin feeding.[4] In addition to monensin, other carboxylic ionophores are available. Lasalocid has been marketed as Avatec† for chickens since 1977 and was introduced in the marketplace as Bovatec† for cattle in 1982. The Food and Drug Administration recently approved salinomycin (Biocox‡) for avian coccidiosis, while a fourth member of this group, narasin, is currently under experimental investigation.

IONOPHORE TOXICITY

Carboxylic ionophores are known to form cationic (Na$^+$, K$^+$, Ca^{++}) complexes that enhance their transport across bimolecular lipid membranes.[23] This alteration in the transport of cations is the basis for the metabolic, organic, and functional disturbances that occur in relation to toxicity with this class of compounds.[29]

Adverse reactions in target animals result from consumption of higher than recommended levels in feed owing to either a mixing error in the ration or ingestion of a premix concentrate containing an unsafe amount of the compound. Overt toxicity may also result from misuse, either accidental or intentional, in nontarget animal species, such as horses, sheep, pigs, chickens, and turkeys. Toxicity also results from drug incompatibilities with compounds such as tiamulin and triacetyloleandomycin.[21]

The incidence of misuse of monensin has been relatively low.[2] A recent review of the commercial use of monensin in broiler chicken and beef cattle production in the United States also revealed a very low incidence of toxicity.[21] Most, if not all, cases of monensin toxicoses involving chickens and cattle have resulted from feed mixing errors. More information and reports of adverse reactions are available for monensin than the other ionophores because of monensin's long-standing and widespread use in the poultry and livestock industries. Other ionophores, such as lasalocid, salinomycin, and narasin, can produce a toxic syndrome similar to that of monensin following overdosage and misuse.[10, 11, 14]

Clinical Signs

Over the years, several studies of acute toxicity have been conducted with monensin in laboratory and domestic animals. Single oral median lethal doses (LD_{50}) have been determined for most species (Table 1). The LD_{50} of monensin varies from 200 mg/kg in broiler chickens to 2 to 3 mg/kg in horses, the most sensitive domestic animal species.

Physical signs of toxicosis attributed to monensin are the following: anorexia, diarrhea, depression, hypoactivity with stiffness and reluctance to move, dyspnea, leg weakness and ataxia, recumbency, attempts to rise and thrashing of limbs, uneasiness, sweating, polyuria, vomiting, and reduction in gut motility, jugular pulse, and egg production. Most of the first 7 signs occur in all animals tested. Variations of these and other signs have been observed in certain species. For instance, diarrhea is not

Table 1. *Acute Oral Toxicity of Monensin*[29]*

Animal Species	LD_{50} ± SE mg/kg
Mouse	
Male	70.0 ± 9.0
Female	96.0 ± 12.0
Rat	
Male	40.1 ± 3.0
Female	28.6 ± 3.8
Dog	
Male	>20.0
Female	>10.0
Rabbit	41.7 ± 3.6
Monkey	>160.0
Chicken	200.0
Cattle	26.4
Sheep	11.9 ± 1.2
Goat	26.4 ± 4
Swine	16.7 ± 3.57
Horse	2–3 (estimated)

*Single oral dose.

*Available from Elanco Products Co., Division of Eli Lilly & Co., Indianapolis, IN 46206.

†Available from Hoffman-La Roche Inc., Nutley, NJ 07110.

‡Available from A. H. Robins Co., Richmond, VA 23220.

present in dogs and horses. Sweating and polyuria were noted in horses, and myoglobinuria was noted in pigs and dogs.

The most consistent clinical sign in target animals that have ingested toxic levels of monensin is partial to complete anorexia. In chickens, anorexia is associated with diarrhea, drowsiness, extreme weakness, and sternal recumbency with legs extended posteriorly.[13, 16] Depression of growth and feed conversion as well as higher mortality occur in broilers fed 5 times the recommended level of monensin for 8 weeks. Poor feathering in broilers has been attributed to approved levels of monensin (90 to 110 gm/ton), but the cause and effect relationship has not been established. Broiler breeders exposed to high levels of monensin manifest severe drops in egg production, anorexia, depression, paralysis, and death in sternal recumbency.[3, 16] Similar signs were reported in adult turkeys exposed to feed contaminated with approved levels of monensin and salinomycin for broiler use. Mortality was variable, but high death losses (up to 96.7 per cent) were recorded with salinomycin.[11] In pigs, anorexia, diarrhea, lethargy, ataxia, dyspnea, and myoglobinuria were present prior to death from monensin toxicoses.[30, 31] Uneasiness, sweating, and polyuria along with anorexia, dyspnea, and progressive ataxia have been reported in horses intoxicated with monensin. Recumbency is followed by frequent attempts to rise with thrashing of the limbs. In 1981, Hanson and coworkers reported similar findings except for sweating in lasalocid-intoxicated horses.[14]

In cattle, clinical signs of monensin toxicosis include anorexia, dark-colored feces of diarrhea, ataxia, recumbency, depression, and nonresponsiveness to visual stimuli.[22, 33] There is a definite correlation between onset of clinical signs and amount of monensin consumed.[22] All intoxicated cattle manifest partial to complete anorexia. Severely intoxicated animals develop anorexia within 24 hr. Animals exposed to lower levels may take up to 48 hr to develop anorexia. Diarrhea usually is evident in 24 to 48 hr in animals receiving high doses of monensin. Exposure to low doses may result in a delay of up to 5 days in the onset of diarrhea. Onset of depression follows a similar pattern, being observed by day 3 in animals receiving excessive monensin overdoses while being observed after 1 week in animals receiving less than excessive overdoses. Rapid breathing and ataxia may be present only in animals that have consumed extremely high levels. In cattle, death occurs without any manifestations of struggle. Lambs have signs similar to cattle (anorexia, diarrhea, ataxia) but frequently exhibit labored breathing, frothing at the mouth, and kicking at the abdomen. Galitzer and coworkers in 1982 found that lasalocid-intoxicated cattle manifested early signs of forced watery feces of diarrhea, muscle tremors, greater cardiac and respiratory rates followed by or concurrent with anorexia. Delayed signs of cardiac insufficiency were evident 7 to 10 days after administration of the toxic dose.[10]

Postmortem Findings

At necropsy, hemorrhages and pale areas in the heart, pale areas in some limb muscles, pulmonary edema, and inflammation of the stomach and intestines may be present.[3, 7, 13, 29–33] Animals that die soon after exposure often will have no lesions either obvious or subtle. Those surviving longer than a week may have hydropericardium, pulmonary edema, hydrothorax, ascites, subcutaneous edema of the abdomen and limbs, and reddish-mottled liver at necropsy.

Histopathologic Findings

The most important change seen using light microscopy, is a toxic myopathy characterized by focal areas of degeneration, necrosis, and inflammation in cardiac and skeletal muscles. Lesions are similar to those described for compound A204, the first polyether antibiotic tested at Lilly Research Laboratories.[28] Doses and time factors influence the severity and distribution of lesions in monensin toxicoses. Generally, no significant lesions are seen by light microscopy in animals that die immediately, and animals that die after an acute course may have only a few scattered degenerated fibers in the heart and highly active muscles, e.g., the diaphragm. Lesions are most pronounced within 7 to 14 days following ingestion of a toxic dose and are accompanied by profound attempts at repair.[29, 32] Skeletal muscle fibers regenerate rapidly, and lesions are completely healed in about a month. Heart muscle fibers do not regenerate, but repair takes place by replacement fibrosis. Secondary lesions of congestive heart failure can be seen, depending upon the severity of heart damage.

Observations to date indicate that in horses, the heart suffers the greatest damage from monensin toxicoses with little or no involvement of skeletal muscles. This finding is in contrast to dogs and pigs in which the lesions are most pronounced in skeletal muscles.[29, 31] Chickens, cattle, and rodents have about equal predilection for cardiac and skeletal muscle lesions.

Other Laboratory Findings

Mitochondrial swelling, myelin figures, and lipid vesicles were observed ultrastructurally in cardiac and skeletal muscles of ponies given monensin at 4 mg/kg and observed for 79 hr.[20] Recently, Van Vleet and Ferrans (1983) described the myocardial ultrastructural alterations in cattle with monensin toxicosis.[32] Early degenerative changes were sarcoplasmic vacuolation from swollen mitochondria and accumulation of lipid. Severely injured mitochondria had marked swelling, disrupted cristae, and dense matrical granules. Scattered myelin figures were present in muscle cells with numerous disrupted mitochondria. Subsequently, necrosis occurred in degenerated myocytes and was characterized by dense fibers with intact sarcomeres or disrupted fibers with hypercontraction bands. Necrosis was followed rapidly by extensive macrophage infiltration with lysis of disrupted organelles and contractile material. Confer and coworkers in 1983 reported similar ultrastructural findings in hearts and skeletal muscles of sheep given monensin.[7] Regeneration as evidenced by myoblast proliferation was observed as early as 4 days post-treatment.

Hematologic parameters are not significantly affected by monensin toxicosis.[29] Elevation of serum enzymes, notably creatine phosphokinase, lactate dehydrogenase, and glutamic oxaloacetic transaminase, may indicate damage to cardiac and skeletal muscles.[1, 29, 31, 33] Alkaline phosphatase, inorganic phosphorus, and total bilirubin levels are also higher, while serum levels of calcium and potassium are lower. The progressive hypokalemia and attendant cardiac conduction disturbances demonstrated in ponies were considered the life-threatening events in early acute monensin toxicosis.[1]

DIAGNOSIS

The clinical signs and lesions induced by *toxic* levels of ionophores are *not pathognomonic.* However, a history of recent introduction of newly formulated feed or supplement to a flock or herd in which signs and lesions are present may cause one to suspect that acute intoxication has occurred. Some animals with substantive heart damage from very high levels of monensin and other ionophores may later develop congestive heart failure. Lesions are likely to be found in animals that survived longer than a week. The most active skeletal muscles may be involved when the heart is not affected or is only slightly affected. Because the lesions are focally distributed, tissue samples should include 1 section each of the atria, ventricles, interventricular septum, diaphragm, and abdominal and thigh muscles.

Although a presumptive diagnosis can be made based on history, clinical signs, and lesions compatible with ionophore toxicosis, specific assays are needed for confirmation. With the introduction of other ionophores, such as lasalocid and salinomycin, the need for confirmatory assays has become greater.[12] In monensin toxicosis, values greater than 5 times the recommended use level in the feed are usually confirmatory. Assays on stomach contents from peracute and acute cases of toxicity can prove exposure, but values obtained have been low. Only minimal residues of monensin (less than 0.021 ppm) have been detected in target tissues of cattle given the optimum dose of monensin.[8, 15] Further, blood levels of monensin are low or undetectable even in intoxicated animals, and accumulation in target tissues does not occur.[9]

Ionophore toxicosis may be confused with acute infectious diseases, deficiencies, and other intoxications.[3, 6, 21, 31, 33] In the differential diagnosis of monensin toxicosis, myopathic conditions should be considered first. In cattle, these would include (1) ionophore toxicosis, (2) vitamin E and selenium deficiencies, (3) poisonous plant ingestion, e.g., senna, coyotillo, white snakeroot, vetch, and (4) the common, yet puzzling, sudden death syndrome with myocardial necrosis. Ionophore toxicosis usually involves an accompanying history of feed supplementation or feed change and usually involves many animals. Clinical signs are anorexia, diarrhea, lethargy and ataxia, and the suggestion of damage to striated muscles. Vitamin E and selenium deficiency occurs sporadically and produces prominent degeneration and necrosis with calcification of cardiac and skeletal muscles. Plant poisonings are usually localized to areas where the toxic plants are indigenous.[6, 18] For instance, coffee senna (*Cassia occidentalis*) poisoning occurs in the southeastern United States. It may cause anorexia, diarrhea and the production of dark urine, but generally causes more pronounced lesions in skeletal muscles than in the heart. The coyotillo plant (*Karwinskia humboldtiana*) in southwest Texas and Mexico produces limberleg in sheep and goats characterized by progressive weakness of the legs, muscular incoordination, recumbency, respiratory distress, and death. Lesions are observed both in cardiac and skeletal muscles as well as peripheral nerves and the liver. White snakeroot (*Eupa-*

torium rugosum), a plant indigenous to much of eastern Canada and the United States, causes "trembles" in goats, sheep, cattle, horses, and swine. Cardiac and skeletal muscle lesions may be present in animals that ingested this plant.[17, 18, 25] However, in trembles there is constipation, blood in feces, an odor of acetone in the breath, and severe fatty degeneration in the liver and kidney that are not seen in ionophore toxicosis. Hairy vetch (*Vicia villosa*) also produces myocardial necrosis but, unlike monensin toxicosis, it produces dermatitis, conjunctivitis, and abortion as well as lesions in the kidneys, adrenal glands, lymph nodes, and thyroid gland. The syndrome of sudden death with myocardial necrosis in cattle, especially calves, is common but sporadic in occurrence and is associated with lesions in cardiac but not skeletal muscle.[5] Hence, clinical history and detailed pathologic studies will help distinguish among ionophore toxicosis, acute infectious diseases, deficiencies, and other intoxications.

From a clinical standpoint, respiratory diseases, particularly infectious bovine rhinotracheitis and the shipping fever complex, are considered in the differential diagnosis because of the respiratory difficulties that occur with monensin toxicosis. At necropsy, however, pneumonic lesions are consistent with these diseases. Animals with acute bovine pulmonary edema and emphysema or fog fever, nitrogen dioxide intoxication, or rape, turnip, or kale poisoning also exhibit respiratory difficulties but, in these conditions, gross lesions will include severe interstitial and interlobular emphysema or pneumonia or both rather than edema. The incoordination, stiff wobbly gait, and loss of visual reflexes may lead one to suspect polioencephalomalacia and thromboembolic meningoencephalitis but, in these conditions, histologic lesions present in the brain are confirmatory. Unequivocal central nervous system lesions have not been found in cases of monensin toxicosis. Salt poisoning will cause nervous signs, paralysis, and diarrhea, but knowledge that insufficient amounts of water were available to the animals will also point to this problem. Eosinophilic meningoencephalitis is pathognomonic for salt poisoning in pigs, but this lesion does not occur in other species. Laboratory procedures used to confirm a diagnosis include assays of serum, cerebrospinal fluid, and brain tissue for sodium concentrations.[6] In cattle, urea toxicosis must be considered when sudden collapse, bloat, violent convulsions, terminal tetanic spasms, and high death losses occur within 10 min to 4 hr from exposure to newly formulated feed.[6] Deaths occurring earlier than 72 hr have not been reported in cattle gavaged with toxic doses of monensin. Acute nitrate poisoning is indicated by coffee-brown colored blood, which is not seen in monensin toxicosis.[19]

In poultry, nutritional myopathy, coffee senna toxicity, botulism, and sodium chloride toxicosis should be considered in the differential diagnosis. Although no striated muscle lesions are produced in the last 2 conditions, clinical signs of limberneck and lesions of "water belly," may be confused with monensin toxicosis. Monensin per se does not produce "barebacks" in broilers, and downers among replacement birds may be suffering from viral arthritis. Therefore, this common reovirus infection must be excluded as a cause of the problem in flocks.

In pigs, vitamin E and selenium deficiency and porcine stress syndrome (PSS) should be considered in the differential diagnosis since skeletal and cardiac lesions may be found in these conditions.[31] In monensin toxicosis, the striated muscle lesions appear more frequently and are more severe in skeletal muscle than in cardiac muscle. Myoglobinuria may also be present. Widespread cardiac and skeletal muscle lesions, vascular damage, dietetic, hepatosis, and gastric ulceration may be found in vitamin E and selenium deficiency. With PSS, cardiac and skeletal muscle lesions may or may not be observed following a history of stress.

Colic, blister beetle intoxication, laminitis, exertional myopathy, and white snakeroot or coffee senna poisoning must be considered in the differential diagnosis of ionophore toxicosis in the horse.[1, 3, 25] Clinical examination, response to treatment, and necropsy findings may help exclude the above conditions as causes.

TREATMENT AND PREVENTION

At present, there is no antidote for ionophore toxicity, and therapeutic approaches are largely supportive. Fluid therapy and mineral oil and potassium supplementation have been recommended for monensin-intoxicated horses.[1] However, supportive therapy may not be practical for a herd or flock. Further studies are needed to determine mechanisms in ionophore toxicosis that are amenable to preventive and therapeutic intervention.

The primary action of all ionophores is to facilitate ion transport across biologic membranes, but ion proclivitis differ and evidence gathered in various laboratories indicates that carboxylic ionophores may have multiple effects at the cellular level.[23] Monensin acts as a Na^+ selective ionophore and produces higher cellular concentrations of Na^+ and Ca^{++} (Fig. 1). Lasalocid forms complexes with divalent cations, such as Ca^{++} and Mg^{++}, with a range of complexing and transport capabilities, including primary amines, e.g., catecholamines. Salinomycin and narasin preferentially complex K^+ over Na^+ at a ratio of 1:4. An ionophore-mediated rise in intracellular Na^+ is known to increase the intracellular levels of Ca^{++}. Excessive influxes of Na^+ and Ca^{++} could lead to degeneration and necrosis of cardiac and skeletal muscle cells. Monensin also causes release of catecholamines from cultured adrenal chromaffin cells, and salinomycin causes a multifold augmentation of plasma catecholamines in animals. Catecholamines and

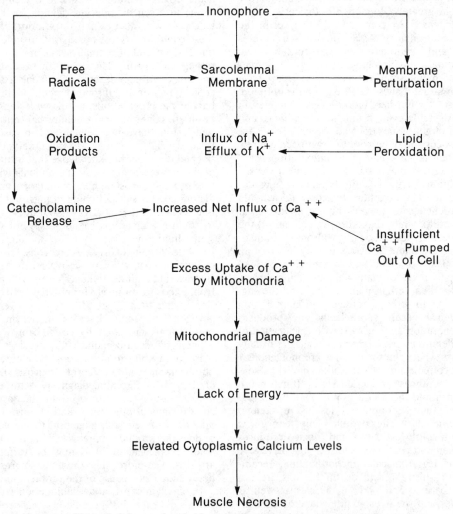

Figure 1. Scheme of probable events occurring in monensin toxicity.

toxic oxidation products have been implicated in myocardial necrosis through greater influx of Ca^{++} and formation of free radicals.[24, 26, 33]

There is no direct evidence for increased lipid peroxidation in ionophore toxicity. However, indirect support for lipid peroxidation as a factor in monensin toxicology was published recently.[30] Van Vleet and coworkers at Purdue University obtained protection against the development of *clinical* monensin toxicity in pigs treated with selenium and vitamin E (selenium as selenite at 0.25 mg/kg and vitamin E as α-tocopherol acetate at 17 IU/kg) prior to a single oral dose of 50 mg monensin/kg (LD_{50} 16.7 ± 3.57 mg/kg). The protection against monensin toxicity was theorized to be produced by stabilization of cellular membranes. Selenium and vitamin E are known to prevent and control peroxidation-mediated cellular injury.[27] Monensin, like all polyether carboxylic ionophores, is lipophilic and may produce dose-dependent membrane perturbations and increased lipid peroxidation, which then could lead to degradative processes as shown in Figure 1. If this sequence of events proves to be the common pathway for toxicity to develop, vitamin E and selenium administration may have an important role in the prevention and treatment of ionophore toxicosis.

Until proper and effective therapy is available, prevention of ionophore toxicity with proper use, appropriate dosing, and adherence to species recommendation is encouraged.

References

1. Amend, J. F., Mallon, F. M., Wren, W. B., and Ramos, A. S.: Equine monensin toxicosis: some experimental clinocopathologic observations. Comp. Cont. Ed. *11*:S173–S183, 1981.
2. Anonymous: Cattle reported killed in Missouri because of monensin misuse. Food Chemical News *36*:1981.
3. Beck, B. E., and Harries, W. N.: The diagnosis of monensin toxicity: a report on outbreaks in horses, cattle and chickens. Proc. Am. Assn. Vet. Lab. Diag. 269–282, 1979.
4. Black, B., and McQuilken, G.: A judgment against sudden death. Calf News *18*:28, 1980.
5. Bradley, R., Markson, L. M., and Bailey, J.: Sudden death and myocardial necrosis in cattle. J. Pathol. *135*:19–38, 1981.
6. Buck, W. B., Osweiller, G. D., and Van Gelder, G. A.: Clinical and Diagnostic Veterinary Toxicology, 2nd ed. Kendall/Hunt Publishing Co., Dubuque, Iowa, 1976.
7. Confer, A. W., Reavis, D. I., and Panciera, R. J.: Light and electron microscopic changes in cardiac and skeletal muscle of sheep with experimental monensin toxicosis. Vet. Pathol. *20*:590–602, 1983.
8. Donoho, A., Manthey, J., Occolowitz, J., and Jones, L.: Metabolism of monensin in the steer and rat. J. Agri. Food Chem. *26*:1090–1092, 1978.
9. Donoho, A. L.: Biochemical studies on the fate of monensin in animals and in the environment. J. Anim. Sci. *58*:1528–1539, 1984.
10. Galitzer, S. J., Bartley, E. E., and Oehme, F. W.: Preliminary studies on lasalocid toxicosis in cattle. Vet. Hum. Toxicol. *24*:406–409, 1982.
11. Halvorson, D. A., Van Dijk, C., and Brown, P.: Ionophore toxicity in turkey breeders. Avian Dis. *26*:634–639, 1982.
12. Handy, P. R.: Analysis and identification of monensin in feeds and tissues. Symposium on Veterinary Analytical Toxicology. 26th Annual Meeting, American Association of Laboratory Diagnosticians. Las Vegas, Nevada, October 16–18, 1983.
13. Hanrahan, L. A., Corrier, D. F., and Naqi, S. A.: Monensin toxicosis in broiler chickens. Vet. Pathol. *18*:665–671, 1981.
14. Hanson, L. J., Eisenbeis, H. G., and Givens, S. V.: Toxic effects of lasalocid in horses. Am. J. Vet. Res. *42*:456–461, 1981.
15. Herberg, R., Manthey, J., Richardson, L., et al.: Excretion and distribution of [14C]-monensin in cattle. J. Agri. Food Chem. *26*:1087–1089, 1978.
16. Howell, J., Hanson, J., Onderka, D., and Harries, W. N.: Monensin toxicity in chickens. Avian Dis. *24*:1050–1053, 1980.
17. Hubert, L. C., and Oehme, F. W.: Plants Poisonous to Livestock, 3rd ed. Manhattan, Kansas, Kansas State University Printing Service, 1968.
18. Kingsbury, J. M.: Poisonous plants of the United States and Canada. Englewood Cliffs, N.J., Prentice-Hall, Inc., 1964.
19. Malone, P.: Monensin sodium toxicity in cattle. Vet. Rec. *103*:477–478, 1978.
20. Mollenhauer, H. H., Rowe, L. D., Cysewski, S. J., and Witzel, D. A.: Ultrastructural observations in ponies after treatment with monensin. Am. J. Vet. Res. *42*:35–40, 1981.
21. Novilla, M. N.: An overview of monensin toxicity. Symposium on Veterinary Analytical Toxicology. 26th Annual Meeting, American Association of Veterinary Laboratory Diagnosticians, Las Vegas, Nevada, October 16–18, 1983.
22. Potter, E. L., Van Duyn, R. L., and Cooley, C. O.: Monensin toxicity in cattle. J. Anim. Sci. *58*:1499–1511, 1984.
23. Pressman, B. C., and Fahim, M.: Pharmacology and toxicology of the monovalent carboxylic ionophores. Ann. Rev. Pharmacol. Toxicol. *22*:465–490, 1982.
24. Reichenback, D. D., and Benditt, E. P.: Catecholamines and cardiomyopathy: the pathogenesis and potential importance of myofibrillar degeneration. Human Pathol. *1*:125–150, 1982.
25. Shivaprasad, H. L.: White snakeroot toxicosis in the horse. Fall Meeting, Midwest Association of Veterinary Pathologists. University of Illinois, Urbana, Illinois, October 21, 1983.
26. Singal, P. K., Yates, J. C., Beamish, R. E., and Dhalla, N. S.: Influence of reducing agents on adrenochrome-induced changes in the heart. Arch. Pathol. Lab. Med. *105*:664–669, 1981.
27. Tappel, A. L.: Vitamin E and selenium protection from *in vitro* lipid peroxidation. Ann. N.Y. Acad. Sci. *355*:18–31, 1981.
28. Todd, G. C., Meyers, D. B., Pierce, E. C., and Worth, H. M.: Acute reversible myopathy produced by compound A204. Antimicrob. Agri. Chemo. Ther. 361–365, 1970.
29. Todd, G. C., Novilla, M. N., and Howard, L. C.: Comparative toxicology of monensin sodium in laboratory animals. J. Anim. Sci. *58*:1512–1517, 1984.
30. Van Vleet, J. F., Amstutz, H. E., Weirich, W. E., et al.: Acute monensin toxicosis in swine: effect of graded doses of rumensin and protection of swine by pretreatment with selenium-vitamin E. Am. J. Vet. Res. *44*:1460–1468, 1983.
31. Van Vleet, J. F., Amstutz, H. E., Weirich, W. E., et al.: Clinical, clinicopathologic and pathologic alterations of monensin toxicosis in swine. Am. J. Vet. Res. *4*:1469–1475, 1983.
32. Van Vleet, J. F., and Ferrans, V. J.: Ultrastructural myocardial alterations in monensin toxicosis of cattle. Am. J. Vet. Res. *44*:1629–1636, 1983.
33. Van Vleet, J. F., Amstutz, H. E., Weirich, W. E., et al.: Clinical, clinicopathologic and pathologic alterations in acute monensin toxicosis in cattle. Am. J. Vet. Res. *44*:2133–2144, 1983.
34. Yates, J. C., Beamish, R. E., and Dhalla, N. S.: Ventricular dysfunction and necrosis produced by adrenochrome metabolite of epinephrine: relation to pathogenesis of catecholamine cardiomyopathy. Amer. Heart J. *102*:210–221, 1981.

Aflatoxins

R. W. COPPOCK, D.V.M., M.S., Ph.D.
and S. P. SWANSON, M.S.

Aflatoxins are a family of closely related bisfuranocoumarin compounds produced by *Aspergillus flavus* and *A. parasiticus*. Eighteen different aflatoxins have been identified, some of which are produced by fungi and others of which are produced by animals following ingestion. Of the aflatoxins, 4 are commonly identified in feed, i.e., B_1, B_2, G_1, and G_2. These 4 aflatoxins were named according to their fluorescent colors when viewed under ultraviolet light and according to their migration distances on thin layer chromatography (TLC) plates. Aflatoxins B_1 and B_2 fluoresce blue with B_1 migrating further than B_2, and aflatoxins G_1 and G_2 fluoresce blue-green with G_1 migrating further than G_2. Results of quantitative tests for aflatoxins are generally given as the sum of B_1, B_2, G_1, and G_2.

Aflatoxin B_1 is the most toxic and is generally the major toxin produced. *A. flavus* generally produces only B_1 and B_2 with B_1 predominant, whereas *A. parasiticus* may produce all 4 aflatoxins.

Domestic animals metabolize aflatoxins to a variety of metabolites. Aflatoxin B_1 can be converted to the metabolite M_1, which is also toxic, and both B_1 and M_1 may be secreted into the milk of animals ingesting aflatoxin-contaminated feed.

SOURCES OF AFLATOXINS

The formation of aflatoxins differs according to substrate, environmental conditions, and toxigenic fungi. *A. flavus* is found predominantly in corn, whereas *A. parasiticus* is found predominantly in peanuts. Of the animal feedstuffs, aflatoxins are most frequently found in corn, cottonseed, grain sorghums, peanuts, feed concentrates, and finished feeds. Conditions necessary for aflatoxin production are substrate moisture above 15 per cent and temperature above 25° C (77° F).

Seeds with the pericarp damaged by excessive moisture, inordinate or harsh handling, and insects are more susceptible to mold invasion. Toxic quantities of aflatoxin can be produced in 24 to 72 hr. Feedstuffs, such as ground high moisture corn, wet drought-damaged corn, and cottonseed, have the potential for "explosive" aflatoxin production. Careful handling and good storage practices are critical to prevent the production of aflatoxins. Rapid production of aflatoxins in feedstuffs accounts for a significant number of the field cases of acute aflatoxicosis.

PRODUCTION OF AFLATOXINS

Aflatoxins may be produced in feedstuffs before harvesting and during the transporting, drying, and storing operations. Under adverse growing conditions, significant quantities of aflatoxin may be found in corn, cottonseed, and peanuts before harvest. The most important factor in the post-harvest production of aflatoxins is the moisture content of the seeds. Virtually all dry feeds are safe from mold invasion when stored at a moisture content that is in equilibrium with a relative humidity of 60 per cent. This corresponds to a moisture content below 14.0 per cent for grains and soybeans and 8.0 to 9.0 per cent for protein supplements and finished feeds.

Specific areas of a storage facility may be more favorable to aflatoxin production. Localized areas of high moisture content and heating of the grain may result from condensation, intermittent drying, insects, trash, a leaking roof, and blowing snow. Alternating ambient temperatures may augment these conditions, especially condensation. Localized production of aflatoxins in a storage facility results in "hot spots" of the toxin.

Wet corn should not be placed in a bin with dry corn. Once bin drying operations are started, they should not be interrupted until the corn is dry.

STABILITY OF AFLATOXINS IN FEEDS

Aflatoxins are very stable compounds and are not destroyed by most feed processing practices, including silage fermentation. Corn standing in the field and intended for silage, if contaminated with aflatoxins, will have the toxins in the ears (kernels, cobs, silk, and husks). The mixing of the foliage with the cobs and kernels at harvest is a form of blending that reduces the total concentration of aflatoxins in the final silage. However, fermentation of high moisture corn in the silo will not destroy the aflatoxins. Aflatoxins are concentrated, on a dry weight basis, in the spent grains following alcohol fermentation. Very little, if any, aflatoxins are found in the alcohol. Drying grains generally increases the concentration of aflatoxins. Roasting aflatoxin-contaminated corn at a temperature sufficient to destroy aflatoxins reduces the nutrient value, and therefore roasting does not appear to be an economical practice, especially if the corn is intended for swine feed. Ammoniation of corn and cotton seed does significantly lower the concentration of aflatoxins. This is a moisture- and temperature-dependent reaction and may not be an economical practice in certain geographic locations.

Feedstuffs that have been processed to reduce aflatoxin concentration should be assayed. Clients should be advised that acceptance of these feeds suspected to contain aflatoxins should be contingent upon the purchaser's analysis for aflatoxins. Samples for analyses should be taken by the client, the veterinarian, or a trained assistant.

Collection of Samples for Laboratory Analysis

Useful laboratory analysis for aflatoxin must be done on representative samples. The more heterogeneously the aflatoxins are distributed in the feedstuff, the more difficult it is to obtain a representative feed sample. All locations of a feed storage unit must be sampled, especially the areas that are suspected to contain aflatoxins. A 10-lb sample is the absolute minimum that should be submitted for analysis. Feed representative of what the poisoned animals are eating or are suspected of eating (although at the time difficult to obtain) should be submitted for analysis.

Methods of Analysis

There are several methods of qualitative, semiquantitative, and quantitative analyses for aflatoxins. These methods are listed in Table 1. The black light method is a rapid screening method that is nonspecific for aflatoxins. In this method, corn samples are viewed under long-wave ultraviolet light (Wood's lamp) for a bright greenish-yellow fluorescence. The kernels should be cracked prior to observation. The fluorescing material is a metabolite of kojic acid, which is produced by several fungi including those that produce aflatoxins. Another screening method, which is a semiquantitative method, involves the use of a

Table 1. *Methods of Aflatoxin Analyses*

Test	Method
Screening	Black light
Semiquantitative	Minicolumn
Quantitative	TLC visual detection, and densitometric detection
	HPLC
	Ultraviolet absorption detection
	Fluorescence detection
Biologic	Ducklings
	Chick embryos

Table 2. *Relative Sensitivity of Livestock and Poultry to Aflatoxins in Order of Decreasing Susceptibility*

Livestock	Poultry
Young pigs	Ducklings
Pregnant sows	Turkey poults
Dogs, calves, horses, feeder pigs	Geese
Finishing hogs	Pheasants
Lambs	
Dairy cattle	
Feeder cattle	
Mature sheep	

minicolumn. Quantitative assays generally employ the use of TLC or high performance liquid chromatography (HPLC).

BIOLOGIC EFFECTS OF AFLATOXINS

Aflatoxin B_1 is the most biologically active of the known aflatoxins. It is approximately twice as toxic as G_1 and M_1, and about 4 and 8 times more toxic than B_2 and G_2, respectively.

Diets containing aflatoxin are palatable and have been observed to be hepatotoxic to mammals, poultry, and fish. Susceptibility to aflatoxin varies greatly according to species, age, and sex (Table 2). In all species, the young are more susceptible than the adults. Mature males are more susceptible than females, except pregnant females. The susceptibility of females to aflatoxins appears to be dependent on the state of the sex hormones and the stage of the reproductive cycle.

The liver and immune system are the primary targets for aflatoxins. Pyrrolizidine alkaloids and aflatoxins have similar hepatotoxic properties. In acute aflatoxicosis, liver necrosis is a common finding. Hepatic changes in chronic aflatoxicosis or in acute aflatoxicosis are biliary hyperplasia, hepatocytomegaly, keratomegaly of the hepatocytes, and hyperplastic nodules. Aflatoxins suppress immunity acquired from vaccines and shorten the incubation time for infectious diseases.

Aflatoxins are potent inducers of liver neoplasia. This aspect of aflatoxicosis has caused a great deal of concern among regulatory agencies, such as the Food and Drug Administration (FDA). At the present time, aflatoxin is one of the mycotoxins carefully monitored by the FDA.

In some species, aflatoxins decrease liver stores of vitamin A in essentially all species of livestock. This finding may be of significance to the clinician.

Diseases that damage the liver, such as parasitism by liver flukes and poisonings by cadmium and other toxicants, may potentiate aflatoxin toxicity. The interaction between commonly used drugs and aflatoxins has not been established.

Cattle

Clinical signs of aflatoxicosis in cattle generally are not readily identifiable. Unbalanced diets, parasitic infestations, and debilitating diseases may mimic aflatoxicosis. Aflatoxins and other mycotoxins exacerbate other herd health problems. The threshold level for clinical effects from aflatoxins appears to be 100 to 300 ppb for dairy cattle and 200 to 300 ppb for feeder cattle. The sensitivity of cattle to aflatoxins decreases with age. Bred cows are more sensitive to aflatoxins than open cows. Table 3 summarizes the effects of aflatoxin-amended diets on feeder cattle. The effects of aflatoxin-amended diets on dairy cattle is summarized in Table 4.

The most common clinical sign of aflatoxicosis in cattle is loss of production. Rough hair coat, depressed appetite, and intermittent diarrhea may be observed. In acute cases, depression, intermittent hyperpyrexia, and anorexia are sometimes present. Cattle exposed to aflatoxins for extended periods may appear to be acutely affected. These animals may die soon after clinical signs are observed.

Cattle exposed to aflatoxins may also have lowered native resistance to disease. This finding may not be apparent until they are stressed, or until "new" cattle are introduced into the herd. Reduced vaccination protection may be observed. Aflatoxins also may exacerbate mastitis.

Cattle receiving diets containing urea appear to have a higher susceptibility to urea intoxication. The threshold for hypervitaminosis A may be lowered. Aflatoxins do not appear to affect copper metabolism in cattle.

Clinical pathologic changes observed during acute aflatoxicosis are indicative of liver disease. Serum levels of ornithine carbamyl transferase, sorbitol dehydrogenase, and alkaline phosphatase are raised. Blood urea nitrogen concentration is decreased, and blood ammonia concentration may be increased. Serum albumin level is generally low, and globulin level is low. Total serum protein values may not change, however, the albumin:globulin ratio may be altered. Liver clearance of Bromsulphalein (BSP) is often decreased. Changes in the complete blood count are generally due to infectious diseases. Prothrombin time may be longer.

The best treatment of bovine aflatoxicosis is to remove all aflatoxins from the diet. The diet should be given a detailed review and balanced appropriately. Natural protein should replace urea. Supplementing the diet with choline (10 mg/kg/day) and vitamin A (20,000 IU/450 kg/day) appears to be beneficial. Steroids seem to enhance the immune suppression action of aflatoxins. Supportive care and palliative treatment is generally successful. Animals that recover may be chronic "poor doers," and culling of these animals may prevent further economic loss.

Because aflatoxins are carcinogens, the FDA has set the action level for M_1 at 0.5 ppb in milk. Clinicians may be asked to assist dairy farmers who have been stopped

Table 3. *Effects of Aflatoxins on 6- to 8-Month-Old Beef Cattle*

| Observation | Dietary Concentration of Aflatoxins in ppb | | | | |
	0	100	300	700	1000
Number of animals	10	10	10	10	10
Daily gain kg (lb)	1.130 (2.51)	1.190 (2.63)	1.090 (2.40)	0.860 (1.90)	0.860 (1.70)
Feed efficiency	0.175	0.164	0.159	0.155	0.152

Adapted from Wyllie, T. D. and Morehouse, L. D.: Mycotoxins and Mycotoxicosis: An Encyclopedia Handbook. New York, Dekker, 1977.

Table 4. *Effects of Aflatoxins on Milk Production of Holstein Friesian Cows*

Estimated Dietary Level (ppb)*	Daily Intake (mg/kg/day)	Milk Production kg(lb)/day Weekly Study						
		0†	1	2	3	4	5	6
0	0	21 (46)	21 (46)	20 (44)	20 (44)	20 (44)	20 (44)	—
396	5	21 (46)	20 (44)	20 (44)	21 (46)	18 (39)	17 (37)	16 (36)
854	10	20 (44)	15 (33)	13 (29)	12 (26)	12 (26)	13 (29)	12 (26)
1190	20	25 (54)	21 (46)	19 (43)	21 (46)	18 (39)	18 (39)	17 (37)
2324	40	20 (44)	19 (43)	18 (39)	13 (29)	11 (25)	‡	
4210	80	23 (50)	19 (43)	13 (29)	9 (20)	§		

*Estimates corrected for feed consumption and not proportional to mg/kg/day values.
†Control values.
‡Removed from the diet.
§ Cow died.
Adapted from Wyllie, T. D., and Morehouse, L. D.: Mycotoxins and Mycotoxicosis: An Encyclopedia Handbook. New York, Dekker, 1977.

from shipping aflatoxin-contaminated milk. In dealing with this problem, the clinician should quantify all dietary sources of aflatoxins. The concentrations of aflatoxins in the milk should be determined. The feed:milk ratio of aflatoxin should be calculated. The calculated diet to milk ratio can be used to determine the maximum amount of aflatoxin-contaminated feed that can be given without producing a residue problem. As a general rule, the feed to milk ratio is approximately 300:1. Once the dietary intake of aflatoxins is lowered, milk production may be raised. If essentially all aflatoxins are removed from the diet, time for aflatoxin residues to be cleared from the milk is approximately 72 hr.

The diet:skeletal muscle ratio of aflatoxins ($B_1 + M_1$) for cattle varies from 150:1 to 14,000:1. Of the edible tissues, liver and kidneys are the most likely to contain aflatoxins.

Swine

Aflatoxins, in certain areas of the United States, cause considerable losses to swine producers. These losses occur primarily from reduced feed conversion and resistance to infectious diseases. High death losses, although generally not documented in veterinary literature, do occur.

Acute aflatoxicosis in swine is generally associated with "explosive" production of aflatoxins in feedstuffs. Clinical signs of acute aflatoxicosis—depression, weakness, trembling, and ataxia—occur 6 to 24 hr after exposure. Diarrhea, often with bloody feces, is generally observed 12 to 30 hr following ingestion. As the disease progresses, twilight coma or stimuli-induced convulsive seizures may be observed. Liver enzyme levels, i.e., alkaline phosphatase, SGOT, ornithine carbamyl transferase, and isocitric dehydrogenase may be elevated in the serum. The time for BSP clearance from plasma is generally longer. Blood urea nitrogen level is usually decreased, and blood ammonia level is usually increased. Hyperpyrexia is observed 6 to 14 hr following exposure and may have a somewhat cyclic pattern. A white blood cell count of 30,000 accompanied by lymphopenia may be observed in the first 24 hr post-exposure. Icterus generally becomes visible 24 hr after initial exposure. Pigs, although affected, may continue to eat and drink. Those that survive acute intoxication develop rough hair coats, have poor feed conversion, and are generally uneconomical. Dietary concentrations of aflatoxin above 1000 ppb or daily doses above 1.0 mg/kg will result in acute aflatoxicosis.

Chronic aflatoxicosis is often difficult to recognize. The most common clinical sign, often unnoticed, is a reduction in feed conversion and the decline in native disease resistance may go undetected. Producers often complain, "This batch of pigs are poor doers." The dietary concentrations that cause chronic aflatoxicosis are variable. As a general rule, weanling pigs should not receive feed that exceeds 50 to 100 ppb aflatoxin. Older feeder pigs seem to have problems with dietary concentrations of aflatoxin of more than 200 to 350 ppb. Feeder pigs may consume diets containing 500 to 700 ppb aflatoxin for several weeks before signs of aflatoxicosis appear. Dietary concentrations of aflatoxin tolerated by pregnant sows are variable, however, dietary concentrations of 50 to 200 ppb appear safe.

Chronically exposed pigs develop rough hair coats. Clinical signs are similar to those of acutely exposed pigs. Hepatic enzymes, although variable, may be detected in the serum. Bile pigments are also often found in the serum. The half-life of BSP in plasma is generally longer.

The best treatment of swine aflatoxicosis is to remove all aflatoxins from the diet. Swine on a high protein diet appear to be more tolerant of aflatoxins. The addition of choline (3 mg/kg/day) to the diet seems beneficial. The addition of sodium bentonite (2.5 per cent of diet by weight)* to the diet as an adsorbent may be of benefit. Aflatoxins may increase the side effects of drugs, especially those detoxified by the liver. Injections of vitamin K_1 (0.5 to 2.5 mg/kg) may help restore blood clotting.

Supplemental Reading

Aller, W. W., Edds, G. T., and Asquith, R. L.: Effects of aflatoxins in young ponies. Am. J. Vet. Res. *42*:2162–2164, 1981.

Angsubhakorn, S., Poomvises, P., Romruen, K., and Newberne, P. M.: Aflatoxicosis in horses. J. Am. Vet. Med. Assoc. *178*:274–278, 1981.

Asquith, R. L., Edds, G. T., Aller, W. W., and Bortell, R.: Plasma concentrations of iditol dehydrogenase (Sorbitol Dehydrogenase) in ponies treated with aflatoxin B. Am. J. Vet. Res. *41*:925–927, 1980.

Brown, R. W., Pier, A. C., Richard, J. L., and Krogstad, R. E.: Effects of dietary aflatoxins on existing bacterial intramammary infections of dairy cows. Am. J. Vet. Res. *42*:927–933, 1981.

Cysewski, S. J., Pier, A. C., Engstron, G. W., et al.: Clinical pathologic features of acute aflatoxicosis of swine. Am. J. Vet. Res. *29*:1577–1590, 1968.

Cysewski, S. J., Pier, A. C., Baetz, A. L., and Cheville, N. F.: Experimental equine aflatoxicosis. Toxicol. Appl. Pharmacol. *65*:354–356, 1982.

Davis, N. D., Dickens, J. W., Fries, et al.: Protocol for surveys, sampling, post-collection handling and analysis of grain samples involved in mycotoxin problems. J. Assoc. Off. Anal. Chem. *63*:95–101, 1980.

---

*Should replace corn in a corn-soy diet.

Edds, J. T.: Aflatoxins. *In* Shimoda, W. (ed.). Conference on Mycotoxins in Animal Feed and Grains Related to Animal Health. Rockville, Maryland, United States Government, 1979.

Jones, L. A., Pier, A. C., and Cutlip, R. C.: Effects of aflatoxin consumption on the clinical course of swine dysentery. Am. J. Vet. Res. *42*:1770–1772, 1981.

Pier, A. C.: Mycotoxins and animal health. Adv. Vet. Sci. Comp. Med. *25*:185–243, 1981.

Rodricks, J. V., and Stoloff, L.: Aflatoxin Residues from Contaminated Feed in Edible Tissues of Food-Producing Animals. *In* Rodricks, J. V. (ed.). Mycotoxins in Human and Animal Health. Park Forest, Illinois, Pathox Publishers, Inc., 67–79, 1972.

Southern, L. L., and Clawson, A. J.: Effects of aflatoxins on finishing swine. J. Anim. Sci. *49*:1006–1011, 1979.

Stuart, B. P., and DuBois, P. R.: Aflatoxins. *In* Howard, J. L. Current Veterinary Therapy: Food Animal Practice. Philadelphia, W. B. Saunders Company, 1981.

Wogan, G.: Aflatoxin Carcinogenesis. *In* Methods in Cancer Research. New York, Academic Press, 309–344, 1973.

Wyllie, T. D., and Morehouse, L. D.: Mycotoxic Fungi. Mycotoxins and Mycotoxicosis: An Encyclopedia Handbook. New York, Dekker, 1977.

Citrinin

WILLIAM W. CARLTON, D.V.M., Ph.D.
and PALLE KROGH, D.V.M., Ph.D.

Citrinin, a nephrotoxic secondary fungal metabolite, was first isolated from a culture of *Penicillium citrinum* and since has been obtained from many other *Penicillium* spp. and from a few *Aspergillus* spp. Of the several fungal producers of citrinin, *P. viridicatum* may be of greatest significance in regard to contamination of grains with mycotoxin. In some cases, other mycotoxins including patulin, oxalic acid, and ochratoxin A occur with citrinin in the same culture. Occurrence of both citrinin and ochratoxin A has been demonstrated in naturally contaminated cereals as well.

Chemically, citrinin is a *p*-quinone methide and crystallizes from alcohol as yellow needles. It is very sparingly soluble in water but is soluble in dilute sodium hydroxide, sodium bicarbonate, and sodium acetate solutions and in many organic solvents.

NATURAL OCCURRENCE

Citrinin at concentrations of 0.07 to 80 ppm was found in samples of Canadian grains. Most of the samples were wheat. Concentrations in Danish grain samples were lower, ranging from 0.16 to 2 ppm. These concentrations are lower than those required to produce nephropathy in swine.

CLINICAL SIGNS AND PATHOLOGY

Naturally occurring mycotoxic disease of domestic animals due exclusively to citrinin contamination of feedstuffs has not been conclusively established. Citrinin may play some role in certain cases of Danish endemic porcine nephropathy (see Ochratoxin). In pigs, depression, weight loss, and glucosuria, along with elevation of blood urea nitrogen and creatinine levels, were produced experimentally by sublethal doses of citrinin given over a 6-week period. Lesions in swine due to citrinin toxicosis are restricted to the kidneys. Grossly, the kidneys are en-

larged, gray-yellow, and have small subcapsular cysts. Depending on the dose of citrinin, degenerative and necotic changes are present in the proximal renal tubules accompanied by dilatation of tubules, thickening of tubular basement membranes, and interstitial fibrosis.

DIAGNOSIS, TREATMENT, AND CONTROL

Citrinin mycotoxicosis may be included in the differential diagnosis of tubular nephrosis in swine and cattle, especially if lesions are absent from other tissues. Diagnosis would depend upon the chemical detection in feeds of citrinin at concentrations sufficient to produce renal disease in the species under consideration.

No specific antidotes are available. Treatment includes removing contaminated feedstuffs and supplying fresh, noncontaminated feedstuffs. Correction of dehydration would be indicated. After exposure is terminated, recovery is likely in those animals not acutely ill.

Control can be achieved by excluding contaminated grains from the diets of swine and cattle.

Supplemental Reading

Carlton, W. W., and Tuite, J.: Metabolites of *Penicillium viridicatum*: Toxicology. *In* Rodricks, J. V., Hesseltime, C. W., and Mahlman, M. A. (eds.): Mycotoxins in Human and Animal Health. Park Forest South, Illinois, Pathotox Publishers, Inc., 527–541, 1977.

Hald, B., and Krogh, P.: Analysis and chemical confirmation of citrinin in barley. J. Assoc. Off. Anal. Chem. *56*:1440–1443, 1973.

Krogh, P., Hald, B., and Pedersen, E. J.: Occurrence of ochratoxin A and citrinin in cereals associated with mycotoxic porcine nephropathy. Acta Pathol. Microbiol. *81*:689–695, 1973.

Scott, P. M.: Penicillium mycotoxins. *In* Wyllie, T. D., and Morehouse, L. G. (eds.): Mycotoxic Fungi, Mycotoxins and Mycotoxicoses. New York, Dekker, 291–296, 1978.

Scott, P. M., van Walbeek, W., Kennedy, B., and Angeti, D.: Mycotoxins (ochratoxin A, citrinin and sterigmatocystin) and toxigenic fungi in grains and other agricultural products. J. Agric. Fed. Chem. *20*:1103–1109, 1972.

Wilson, D. M., Tabor, W. H., and Trucksess, M. W.: Screening method for detection of aflatoxin, ochratoxin, zearalenone, penicillic acid and citrinin. J. Assoc. Off. Anal. Chem. *59*:125–127, 1976.

Ergot (Gangrenous)

GARY D. OSWEILER, D.V.M., M.S., Ph.D.

Gangrenous ergotism is a chronic disease affecting primarily cattle and occasionally swine. It is characterized by lameness followed by necrosis of the extremities with loss of hooves, tail, and ears in extreme cases. Swine are less commonly affected by gangrene, but lactating sows may have noninflammatory agalactia.

Ergotism is due to several alkaloids produced in the sclerotium (visible, vegetative part) of *Claviceps purpurea*, which invades more than 200 grasses and cultivated cereals. The infestation is most prevalent in rye but occurs to some extent in barley, oats, wheat, and common pasture grasses, resulting in potential exposure via overgrown pastures or contaminated small grains. The type and quantity of alkaloid may vary with season, region, year, and type of grain. Generally, alkaloid content increases as grain reaches maturity. Ergot sclerotia are commonly removed from cereal grains during cleaning procedures. The "screenings" from such grain may be mixed or milled into other feeds given to livestock. Once grinding or milling has occurred, ergot can only be recognized by microscopic examination or chemical analysis for ergot alkaloids. Ergotism is reported sporadically from many locations in North America. General morbidity within a herd is low, and unless exposure continues recovery or salvage of affected animals is possible.

The pathogenesis of gangrenous ergotism is reportedly due to the alkaloid-induced smooth muscle stimulation of arterioles. This results in congestion proximal to the lesion and ischemia distal to the arteriolar spasm. Endothelial swelling and degeneration in affected vascular beds often exist. The result is localized ischemia, resulting in pain, lameness, and eventual necrosis. The clinical effects appear to be accentuated by cold weather, and appendages (feet, ears, tail) are most prone to damage. Frostbite may occur more readily in affected animals.

In swine, a centrally mediated inhibition of prolactin secretion is believed to result in failure of mammary development and lactogenesis. Affected sows farrow normally, but udders do not develop, and milk secretion is diminished or absent. The lesion is noninflammatory, and sows appear healthy.

CLINICAL SIGNS

The toxicity of ergot alkaloids in feeds has often been expressed as the percentage of ergot sclerotia by weight in a given grain. This value is subject to wide variance, depending on the amount of grain consumed by different animals as well as the specific alkaloid content of ergot sclerotia. Based on limited studies, ergot alkaloid content in sclerotia may range from 0.2 to 0.6 per cent of total sclerotic weight. Approximately 0.5 per cent of ergot in cattle rations is associated with reduced weight gain, poor feed consumption, rough hair coat, and some nonspecific signs. Ergot dietary contamination of several weeks ranging between 0.3 per cent and 1 per cent has been associated with gangrenous ergotism.

Early typical signs of gangrenous ergotism in cattle are lameness or apparent pain or both. Hindlimbs are often affected first. Swelling may occur just above the coronary band and extend upward past the fetlock. Affected cattle appear nervous and may walk with an ataxic or abnormal gait. Temperature, pulse, and respiration are sometimes increased, and milk production or body weight may drop drastically. Feed grains containing ergot alkaloids may be unpalatable and hence are eaten poorly or refused by animals. A toxic dose of ergot is difficult to establish owing to variability of alkaloid content. Any diet containing in excess of 0.25 per cent ergot sclerotia should be considered suspect. On a body weight basis, 40 to 60 mg/kg has been considered toxic. In sheep, there are reports of salivation, nausea, and diarrhea. Abortion is infrequently reported as a consequence of ergot ingestion by ruminants. Field and experimental results are conflicting, but generally a strong case cannot be found for ergot-induced abortions.

In swine, feeding of ergot-containing grains often results in partial or complete feed refusal with decreased weight. Gangrene is infrequently reported, although I have seen several causes involving loss of margins of ears or tips of noses associated with ergot-containing grain and cold weather. A serious ergot related problem in swine occurs in late gestation and early lactation. Gestation may be shortened by 3 to 5 days, and newborn piglets are smaller than normal. Abortion rarely occurs. When ergot is fed in the last 2 to 4 weeks of gestation, udder development does not occur, and lactation is inhibited or absent. The resulting agalactia can generally be differentiated from the MMA (metritis-mastitis-agalactia) complex by general good health of sows, lack of fever, and absence of congestive or inflammatory lesions of the udder. If affected sows are removed from the ergot-containing diet within a few days, many will lactate within 5 to 7 days. Usually this is not soon enough to prevent losses from starvation in piglets. The agalactia syndrome has been induced by diets containing from 0.1 to 1.0 per cent ergot. Results vary greatly depending on alkaloid content.

CLINICAL PATHOLOGY AND LESIONS

There are no distinctive clinical pathologic lesions to confirm ergotism. Gross lesions of gangrenous ergotism may range from mild swelling, ischemia, and edema to severe ischemia, necrosis, and characteristic gangrene of the extremities that is sharply demarcated from unaffected tissue. The lesion is deep as well as superficial, and the entire appendage may slough. Microscopic lesions of necrosis, edema, endothelial damage, and thrombosis are seen.

DIAGNOSIS

Gangrenous ergotism should be differentiated from infectious pododermatitis (footrot), fescue toxicosis, frostbite, trauma, and perhaps the vesicular diseases. The lesion is distinctive and should alert one to inspect the feed and forage for ergot sclerotia. These are dark purple to black bodies, which are slightly larger than the grain or grass seed that they replace. They are elongated and roughly resemble a banana in shape. If grain has been milled, gross identification is nearly impossible. Representative feed samples should be submitted to a laboratory for microscopic or chemical analysis. Identification of ergot alkaloids or ricenoleic acid (in the absence of castor bean meal) is confirmatory of exposure to ergot. In swine, differentiation from mastitis or MMA syndrome is of most concern. Ergot poisoned sows probably will respond poorly or not at all to parenteral oxytocin.

TREATMENT

The only effective treatment for ergot poisoning is removal of the source. If agalactia is not advanced or if gangrene is not present, the prognosis is guarded to good. Animals with gangrenous ergotism should be protected from cold, damp conditions, and if circumstances allow, hot packs should be applied to enhance circulation. Since little is known of the absorption and excretion of ergot alkaloids, specific therapy to enhance excretion cannot be recommended. A broad-spectrum antibiotic such as oxytetracycline HCl (Liquamycin)* at 6 to 10 mg/kg or a long-acting penicillin such as benzathine penicillin G and procaine penicillin G (Longicil)† at 4000 units/kg should be used to control secondary infections.

---

*Available from Pfizer, Inc., New York, NY 10017.
†Available from Fort Dodge Laboratories, Fort Dodge, IA 50501.

PREVENTION AND MANAGEMENT

Ergot alkaloids do not appear to persist as a residue, and animals fully recovered from acute or gangrenous effects should be safe to market. Producers should be cautioned to examine growing or purchased grain or grasses for signs of ergot. Close grazing or clipping of pastures to prevent development of seed heads is recommended.

Supplemental Reading

Burfening, P. J.: Ergotism. J. Am. Vet. Med. Assoc. *163*:1288, 1973.
Mantle, P. G.: Ergotism in cattle. Ergotism in swine. *In* Wyllie, T. D., and Morehouse, L. G. (eds.): Mycotoxic Fungi, Mycotoxins, Mycotoxicoses. An Encyclopedic Handbook. New York, Dekker, 145, 273, 1977.

Nervous Form of Ergotism

WILLIAM B. BUCK, D.V.M., M.S.
and S. J. CYSEWSKI, D.V.M., M.S.*

The nervous ergotism syndrome has been associated with the ingestion of rye, wheat, or barley parasitized by the classic ergot fungus *Claviceps purpurea*, but the disease is rare from this source. It is common in cattle on pasture of Dallis grass (*Paspalum dilatatum*) parasitized with *C. paspali*, hence, the names Dallis grass and paspalum staggers. Nervous syndromes have also been associated with tobosa grass (*Hilaria mutica*) and galleta grass (*H. jamesii*) parasitized by *C. cinera*.

These fungi invade the flower of the host plant in early summer and proliferate in the ovary, producing spores in a sticky exudate, the "honeydew." This, the sphacelial stage, is enhanced by moist conditions. Early in August, if the weather is dry, the mass of fungal tissue enlarges and forms a dry compact mass called the sclerotium. *C. paspali* sclerotia are rough surfaced, nearly spherical, buff to brown, and 2 to 4 mm in diameter. The toxic fungal metabolites are found predominantly in the mature sclerotia.

The ergot fungi produce several alkaloids that stimulate smooth muscle, and this results in the majority of lesions of chronic ergotism. Recent reports indicate that the alkaloid components of *C. paspali* is not the cause of the signs of Dallis grass poisoning. Paspalum ergot, in addition to alkaloids, contains a group of tremorgenic substances with neurotoxic properties that are expressed as paspalum staggers in cattle. One tremorgen has been identified chemically and named paspalinine. Further work is needed to identify all the potential tremorgens in *C. paspali* and to establish their role in paspalum staggers. Paspaline is similar to some of the tremorgens isolated from various species of *Penicillium* and *Aspergillus* (see Tremorgenic Toxins).

CLINICAL SIGNS

The first signs of nervous ergotism are hyperexcitability and tremors that are intensified by excitement or forced movement. At rest the animals may stand with the rear

---

*Deceased.

legs extended and exhibit swaying motions. When made to run they exhibit exaggerated flexure of the forelegs and incoordination that often becomes severe enough to cause the animals to fall. Once down, cattle usually lie for a short time, the severity of the signs decreases, and they regain their upright position, and walk off slowly. In severely affected animals, extensor rigidity, opisthotonos, and clonic convulsions occur when they are down. When animals are left alone, the trembling and incoordination usually are minimal, and animals are able to move about slowly and graze.

PATHOLOGIC CHANGES

There are no reports of clinical pathologic alterations in paspalum staggers. Apparently no characteristic gross or microscopic changes are associated with the disease.

DIAGNOSIS

The diagnosis is based primarily upon observing typical signs in cattle grazing pastures where mature sclerotia are present in the flowers of the grass. The problem usually occurs in late summer or early fall. Rye grass staggers and bermuda grass tremors have similar clinical manifestations. Differentiation rests primarily on the type of pasture to which the animals have access.

TREATMENT AND PREVENTION

Treatment consists of removing animals from affected pastures. Since death is generally accidental, care should be taken to avoid undue excitement in handling and moving cattle.

The time of greatest risk is in late summer or early fall when the pasture grasses have developed seed heads. Cattle may selectively graze grass heads containing sclerotia, thus obtaining a concentrated amount of toxic material. Control can be effected by grazing forage before it reaches the seed head stage or by clipping the heads as they form. Hay made from such pastures is potentially toxic, but sclerotia usually drop out as the hay is handled.

Supplemental Reading

Cole, R. J., Dorner, J. W., Lansder, J. A., et al.: Paspalum staggers: isolation and identification of tremorgenic metabolites from sclerotia of *Claviceps paspali*. J. Agri. Food Chem. *25*:1197–1202, 1977.
Mantle, P. G., Mortimer, P. H., and White, E. P.: Mycotoxic tremorgens of *Claviceps paspali* and *Penicillium cyclopium*: a comparative study of effects on sheep and cattle in relation to natural staggers syndromes. Res. Vet. Sci. *24*:49–56, 1977.

Ochratoxin

PALLE KROGH, D.V.M., Ph.D.
and WILLIAM W. CARLTON, D.V.M., Ph.D.

Ochratoxin A, a nephrotoxic secondary fungal metabolite, was first isolated from a culture of *Aspergillus ochraceus*, and has since been obtained from 6 other members of the *A. ochraceus* group as well as from a number of *Penicillium* species. It appears that *P. viridi-*

catum and *P. cyclopium* are the main producers in natural products. Although other ochratoxins have been isolated from fungal cultures under laboratory conditions, only orchratoxin A (and very rarely ochratoxin B) occur in naturally contaminated products. Some strains of *P. viridicatum* produce citrinin and other mycotoxins in addition to ochratoxin, and co-occurrence of ochratoxin A and citrinin has been encountered in several grain lots.

Ochratoxin A, a dihydro-isocoumarin derivative linked through its 7-carboxy group to L-β-phenylalanine (a molecular weight of 403), is a colorless compound, soluble in polar organic solvents, slightly soluble in water, and soluble in dilute aqueous sodium bicarbonate.

NATURAL OCCURRENCE

Ochratoxin A has been found in a variety of plant products, including wheat, corn, barley, oats, rye, peanuts, and coffee beans. Frequencies of ochratoxin contamination from a few per cent to more than 50 per cent have been observed, with concentrations from 10 to 20 µg/kg up to 27.5 mg/kg. Tissue residues of ochratoxin A have been found in pigs and poultry fed ochratoxin-contaminated feed. The blood and the kidneys of these animals contained the highest concentrations of ochratoxin A.

CLINICAL SIGNS AND PATHOLOGY

At dietary concentrations of ochratoxin A below 5 to 10 mg/kg, the kidneys constitute the sole target tissue. At higher feed levels, rarely encountered in naturally contaminated products, extrarenal effects have been seen involving the liver, intestine, lymphoid tissue, spleen, and leukocytes.

Nephropathy has been induced experimentally by ochratoxin A in a variety of animals, including pigs, dogs, poultry, and fish. Naturally occurring cases of nephropathy causally associated with ochratoxin A have been observed in pigs and poultry in several countries of Europe. Most information on natural occurrence has been obtained on porcine nephropathy, and this disease is likely to occur in most countries.

The clinical signs are polyuria, glucosuria, and growth depression as well as increased levels of blood urea nitrogen and blood creatinine. Grossly, the kidneys are pale and enlarged and may have small subcapsular cysts. Microscopically, the changes include degeneration of the proximal tubules and interstitial formation of connective tissue. At later stages, atrophied and sclerotic glomerular tufts may develop.

Perirenal edema is a disease with high mortality in piglets and with renal changes similar to those just described (see Nephrotoxic Plants). Although pig weed (*Amaranthus retroflexus*) has been causally involved in a specific syndrome of perirenal edema in pigs, similar nephroses may have several causal determinants, one of which seems to be mycotoxins from *P. viridicatum*. Ochratoxin A may also be a possible cause, but proof has not yet been obtained.

EPIDEMIOLOGY

In countries where epidemiologic investigations have been conducted (Denmark, Sweden), the disease occurs endemically in all areas, but with differences in prevalence rates from area to area. Thus, rates from 0.6 to 65.9 per 10,000 pigs were observed in various areas of Denmark in 1971. In addition to the endemic occurrence, epidemic outbreaks of porcine nephropathy associated with such climatic conditions as high humidity at harvest have been observed. Not all pigs in a herd are affected by the disease, and the disease may be absent in a herd in subsequent years when noncontaminated feedstuffs are fed.

DIAGNOSIS, TREATMENT, AND CONTROL

Ochratoxin-induced nephropathy should be considered in the differential diagnosis of noninflammatory renal diseases in swine, poultry, and possibly horses.

Polyuria and glucosuria are suggestive signs, but the diagnosis would depend upon the chemical detection of ochratoxin A in feeds consumed the previous few weeks. The detection of ochratoxin residues in blood, kidney, liver, and other tissues would enhance the diagnosis.

No specific antidotes are available. Treatment includes removal of contaminated feedstuffs and supplying of feeds free of ochratoxin A. Treatment to correct dehydration would be indicated. After exposure is terminated, recovery is likely in animals not acutely ill. Several weeks are required to clear all tissues in pigs of ochratoxin residues after ending exposure. In Denmark, pigs with nephropathy are considered unsuitable at slaughter for human consumption if residues of ochratoxin A can be detected. Control is achieved by excluding contaminated feeds from the diets.

Supplemental Reading

Carlton, W. W., and Tuite, J.: Metabolites of *Penicillium viridicatum*: Toxicology. *In* Rodricks, J. V., Hesseltine, C. W., and Mahlman, M. A. (eds.): Mycotoxins in Human and Animal Health. Park Forest South, Illinois, Pathotox Publishers, Inc., 527–541, 1977.
Krogh, P.: Epidemiology of mycotoxic porcine nephropathy. Nord. Vet. Med. 28:452–458, 1976.
Krogh, P.: Causal association of mycotoxic nephropathy. Acta Pathol. Microbiol. Scand. Sect. A, suppl. no. 269, 1978.
Krogh, P., Hald, B., and Pedersen, E. J.: Occurrence of ochratoxin A and citrinin in cereals associated with mycotoxic porcine nephropathy. Acta Pathol. Microbiol. 81:689–695, 1973.
Nesheim, S., Hardin, N. F., Francis, O. J., and Langham, W. S.: Analysis of ochratoxin A and B and their esters in barley using partition and thin layer chromatography. I. Development of the method. J. Assoc. Off. Anal. Chem. 56:817–821, 1973.
Scott, P. M.: Penicillium mycotoxins. *In* Wyllie, T. D., and Morehouse, L. G. (eds.): Mycotoxic Fungi, Mycotoxins and Mycotoxicoses. New York, Dekker, 291–296, 1978.
Scott, P. M., van Walbeek, W., Kennedy, B., and Angeti, D.: Mycotoxins (orchratoxin A, citrinin and sterigmatocystin) and toxigenic fungi in grains and other agricultural products. J. Agric. Food Chem. 20:1103–1109, 1972.
Wilson, D. M., Tabot, W. H., and Trucksess, M. W.: Screening method for the detection of aflatoxin, ochratoxin, zearalenone, penicillic acid and citrinin. J. Assoc. Off. Anal. Chem. 59:125–127, 1976.

Rubratoxin

ALLAN C. PIER, D.V.M., Ph.D.

Rubratoxin is a mycotoxin created during the growth of toxigenic strains of *Penicillium rubrum* and *P. purpurogenum* on suitable substrates. Rubratoxin B ($C_{26}H_{30}O_{11}$), the toxic bisanhydride, is the principal toxin and is a hepatotoxic agent. Experimental intoxication has been demonstrated in cattle, poultry, dogs, and laboratory animals. Signs of intoxication are hepatitis and coagulopathy. Natural cases of intoxication have been suspected in cattle and swine, but definitive evidence for naturally occurring intoxication has not been reported.[1, 2]

CLINICAL SIGNS

Clinical signs of rubratoxicosis in cattle include moderate depression, inappetance, reduced rate of weight gain, hepatic failure, coagulopathy, hemorrhage of the gut mucosa, bloody feces, and death.[3, 4] Interaction between rubratoxin and aflatoxin greatly enhances their pathogenic effects as seen by depression in rate of weight gain, reduced liver function, hemorrhage, and death. Similar clinical signs have been reported in swine consuming corn heavily infested with *P. rubrum* and *Aspergillus flavus*, but definitive identification of specific mycotoxins was not accomplished.[5] Experimental intoxication of food-producing animals with rubratoxin has been limited to cattle and poultry. The clinical response in a number of animal species, i.e., cattle and laboratory animals appears to be biphasic. The clinical signs progress from mild to severe, at which time the animal either dies or the symptoms recede despite continued consumption of the toxin. Apparently, tolerance may develop in later stages of toxin intake. LD_{50} of rubratoxin for rats is 400 mg/kg and for chicks is 83 mg/kg. A daily dose of 16 mg/kg in a calf caused hepatic failure and death in 7 days. The toxin is inactivated at low pH, which may account for the high LD_{50} in animals with simple stomachs. Teratogenic studies have not been reported in large animals, but teratogenic effects have been reported in laboratory animals: prenatal mortality, exencephaly, and other malformations of the head.[3]

PATHOLOGIC CHANGES

Clinicopathologic changes with rubratoxicosis are the same as those associated with hepatitis and liver failure. Bromsulfophthalein clearance times are longer in calves that have consumed from 8 to 16 mg rubratoxin B/kg/day, which are very high doses. The minimal effective dose is not known. Calves consuming rubratoxin at 8 to 16 mg/kg/day developed mild to severe hepatic lesions with cloudy swelling and occasional areas of hepatic cell necrosis. Necrosis was not sufficient to cause elevation in SGOT activity. These calves did not have prolonged prothrombin times, but some blood was observed in the feces at the highest levels of consumption. It is probable that coagulopathy would follow prolonged consumption of high levels of toxin. When rubratoxin is consumed with relatively low doses of aflatoxin, more severe effects on liver function, pathologic condition, coagulopathy, and rate of weight gain have been reported.[2]

DIAGNOSIS

Positive diagnosis of rubratoxicosis, as with any mycotoxicosis, requires the demonstration of the mycotoxin in the feed or in animal tissue at sufficient quantity to cause the clinical and pathologic changes.[7] Current tests for rubratoxin B do not have the necessary degree of sensitivity. At the present time, the method of Hayes and McCain is recommended.[8] Major clinical signs and reduced rate of weight gain, coagulopathy, and discoloration (yellow, mottled) of the liver at necropsy. Suspect feed may show areas of red pigmentation from growth of *P. rubrum*.

TREATMENT AND PREVENTION

Treatment of rubratoxicosis, if it is recognized in the field, consists of removal of the feed source and provision of supportive care for hepatitis. No residual effects are known (other than teratogenic effects in laboratory animals). An early recovery from intoxication would be expected after removal of the contaminated feed. Surgical procedures (e.g., dehorning, castration, ear tagging) should not be done during intake of or immediately after a suspected period of consumption of this or other hepatotoxic mycotoxins.

Prevention of rubratoxicosis, as with other mycotoxicoses, is the primary line of defense. Do not recommend feeding of obviously mold-containing feeds unless they have been tested by an accredited laboratory that has personnel with expertise identifying a variety of mycotoxins. The first biologic sign of low level mycotoxic effect with most mycotoxins is a reduced rate of weight gain. Close observation by the clinician and livestock owner is necessary to detect the subtle changes of early intoxication. Whenever mycotoxicosis is suspected, have the feed checked at a reputable laboratory.

Mycotoxins may enter the feed supply from field crops following crop damage during maturation following excessive rain, drought, hail or insect damage, which encourages invasion by toxigenic fungi. Once harvested, if the grain is dried below 15 per cent moisture content and properly stored, there is little chance of additional mycotoxin formation. High-moisture corn, particularly if ground, is particularly susceptible to fungal invasion and toxin formation. Rapid and careful ensiling (anaerobic conditions prevent fungal growth and toxin formation) or the addition of adequate quantities of organic acid (e.g., propionic acid at approximately 1 per cent, depending on moisture and storage conditions) is recommended to prevent the formation of additional mycotoxin after the feed is treated. However, these procedures will not reduce levels of toxin that existed before grain was treated or ensiled. There is no known decontamination procedure.

References

1. Moss, M. O.: The rubratoxins, toxic metabolites of *Penicillium rubrum* (Stoll). *In* Ciegler, A., Kadis, S., and Ajl, S. (eds.): Microbial Toxins. New York, Academic Press, 381–407, 1971.
2. Pier, A. C., Cysewski, S. J., Richard, J. L., et al.: Experimental mycotoxicoses in calves with aflatoxin, ochratoxin, rubratoxin and T-2 toxin. Proc. U.S. Anim. Health Assoc. 130–145, 1976.
3. Wilson, B. J., and Harbison, R. D.: Rubratoxins. J. Am. Vet. Med. Assoc. *163*:1274–1276, 1973.
4. Wogan, G. N., Edwards, G. S., and Newberne, P. M.: Acute and chronic toxicity of rubratoxin B. Tox. Appl. Pharm. *19*:712–720, 1971.
5. Sippel, W. L., Burnside, J. E., and Atwood, M. B.: A disease of swine and cattle caused by eating moldy corn. Proc. 90th Ann. Meet. Am. Vet. Med. Assoc. 174–181, 1953.
6. Hayes, A. W.: Mycotoxin teratogenicity. *In* Rosenberg, P. (ed.): Toxins: Animal, Plant and Microbial. New York, Pergamon, 739–758, 1978.
7. Pier, A. C., Cysewski, S. J., and Richard, J. L.: Mycotoxicoses of

domestic animals and their diagnosis. Proc. Am. Assoc. Vet. Lab. Diag. 419–431, 1975.

8. Hayes, A. W., and McCain, H. W.: A procedure for the extraction and estimation of rubratoxin B from corn. Food Cosmet. Toxicol. *13*:221–229, 1975.

Trichothecenes

VAL R. BEASLEY, D.V.M., Ph.D.

Trichothecene mycotoxins, also known as 12, 13-epoxytrichothecenes, comprise a group of more than 50 compounds of widely varying toxicity. These toxins tend to form after the exposure of grain to wet weather and fluctuating temperature. Conditions favoring mycotoxin formation prevail in temperate climates during years in which wet weather delays harvest. Although the fungi producing the toxins may later be destroyed, the toxins are quite stable.

Members of this group of mycotoxins causing problems in farm animals are deoxynivalenol (vomitoxin), nivalenol, T-2 toxin, diacetoxyscirpenol (DAS), the macrocyclic trichothecenes, such as roridin A and verrucarin A, and others. Our present experience indicates that in the United States and Canada the most commonly encountered trichothecene is deoxynivalenol (Vesonder and Hesseltine, 1981). This toxin has also been the source of difficulty in France, Austria, and Japan.

T-2 toxin and DAS have occasionally been responsible for toxicity of grains in North America. T-2 toxin has also caused widespread epidemics in farm animals and humans in the Soviet Union and problems in horses in northern Japan. The macrocyclic trichothecenes are extremely potent and have been the source of serious outbreaks of toxicoses in horses of eastern Europe.

Trichothecenes are produced by several genera of fungi: *Myrothecium, Trichoderma, Trichothecium, Cephalosporium, Gliocladium, Stachybotrys*, and especially *Fusarium*. *F. roseum (Gibberella zeae) (F. graminearum)* is the principal producer of deoxynivalenol and may also produce zearalanol and zearalenone. The latter estrogen-like compounds may be found in the same grain as deoxynivalenol. None of these compounds may be produced in spite of fungal growth or any one of these compounds may be produced in the absence of detectable concentrations of the others. T-2 toxin especially is produced by *F. sporotrichoides* (frequently identified in the past as *F. tricinctum*). The detection of a given trichothecene mycotoxin should alert the clinician that other related (or unrelated) compounds may also be present. Generally, mycotoxin assays are directed only toward specific compounds, and toxins not looked for in the analytical screening procedure will be missed. Because of the unavailability of standards and the number of possible compounds, this situation is likely to continue. The diagnostic problem is further aggravated by wide variations among samples of the same feed, sensitivities of animals, and interactions between the toxins and other stresses on the animals. These factors also make it extremely difficult to recommend safe concentrations in feed.

Deoxynivalenol is not among the more acutely toxic trichothecenes, but neither is it innocuous. Its synonym, vomitoxin, is a misnomer since affected animals rarely vomit, although they sometimes do. In swine, the consumption of a sufficient amount of deoxynivalenol more often results in feed refusal and especially in reduced intake. Less often, soft stools and sometimes diarrhea occur. Individually or together, these effects may cause young animals to fail to thrive and may increase the effects of other sources of stress, such as infection, parasitism, and nutritional imbalance. In some instances, pigs may eventually overcome deoxynivalenol toxicoses and begin to catch up with nonexposed pigs in spite of continued deoxynivalenol consumption.

Although death has occurred in clinical outbreaks of deoxynivalenol-associated disease, this should not be expected in most cases. Furthermore, specific lesions may not be found, although mild thickening of the squamous (esophageal) mucosa of the stomach has been noted in the findings of feeding studies.

Swine are among the most sensitive species to deoxynivalenol, as they are to zearalenone. Experimentally, approximately 4 ppm deoxynivalenol in the feed causes a 20 per cent reduction in consumption and at 40 ppm, a 90 per cent reduction is recorded. Limited studies in cattle suggest that calves are considerably less sensitive to both of these *F. roseum* mycotoxins. Chickens are apparently somewhat more resistant.

In a recent survey based on submission of problem feeds and feed components to a regional diagnostic laboratory, far more instances of rectal and vaginal prolapses, abortions, and infertility were associated with the finding of deoxynivalenol than with the finding of zearalenone. This reflects the ubiquitousness of deoxynivalenol in some years and indicates that it may serve as a marker for other, possibly estrogenic toxins, which are presumably produced by *F. roseum*. Deoxynivalenol alone probably does not have estrogenic properties.

T-2 toxin, DAS, and the macrocyclic trichothecenes are far more toxic than deoxynivalenol. Feed refusal, reduced feed consumption, and "failure to thrive" are significant aspects of these toxicoses. Hemorrhages have been reported in field outbreaks in swine and cattle but have been difficult to reproduce experimentally except after injection of comparatively high doses in single or multiple administration. With massive oral exposure, swine may die after manifesting vomiting, abdominal rigidity, weakness, especially in the rear legs, and cardiovascular shock. Lesions in such animals may include extreme gastric hyperemia and severe congestion of the intestinal tract, which increases in the posterior jejunum and to the terminal ileum. The most striking histologic lesion is lymphoid necrosis. This syndrome is essentially identical to that which occurs after intravenous administration of lethal doses. Cattle are slightly more resistant, but massive oral doses also cause cardiovascular shock and weakness as well as extreme somnolence. These single massive dose effects in survivors tend to resolve by 48 hr. Acute clinical signs are not likely to be encountered in cases of subacute or chronic toxicoses.

Experimentally, swine and cattle have tended to refuse to eat lethal doses of T-2 toxin in feeds. The local cytotoxic effects of these compounds may be associated with lesions on the snout, muzzle, lips, tongue, and pharynx. In calves given T-2 toxin for up to 6 weeks, the most striking and consistent lesion was atrophy of the thymus. T-2 toxin in calves and swine causes defects in immune function. In calves, lowered clotting functions have been documented both after single and multiple doses of the toxin.

Reproductive effects of T-2 toxin at 12 ppm in sow rations were repeat breeding and small litter size.

DIAGNOSIS

The definitive diagnosis of trichothecene mycotoxicoses is based upon the results of tests for specific trichothecenes in feeds. T-2 toxin and DAS will not be found in tissues, although they may be detected in stomach contents. Deoxynivalenol may be found in stomach contents or urine, but diagnostic concentrations have not been established in these specimens. Clinicians or pathologists who encounter the problems of increased incidence of feed refusal and failure to thrive should include trichothecenes in the differential diagnosis, sample the feed, and rule out readily diagnosable alternative causes of these signs. Submission of the suspect feed to the laboratory allows assessment of the possible contribution of mycotoxins to the syndrome. Generally, 10 lb (4.5 kg) of feed collected as a composite from several areas of the feed bin and shipped to arrive without further mold growth is requested. Oral inflammatory or necrotic lesions may indicate the need to test for the more toxic trichothecenes. Reproductive, digestive, and immunosuppressive effects in most species, and possibly hemorrhage in cattle, may also warrant consideration of trichothecene toxicosis.

Cultural identification of offending fungi, while sometimes meaningful to the mycologist or toxicologist, cannot be relied upon by the diagnostician. A given fungal species known to produce trichothecenes may or may not produce significant toxin concentrations even when subjected to conditions that favor maximal toxin production. Skin irritation bioassays are nonspecific but may be used in screening for the more toxic compounds, provided that positive results are confirmed chemically before interpretation.

TREATMENT

There are no specific antidotes for trichothecene mycotoxicoses, therefore, supportive and symptomatic treatment in conjunction with a change of diet are indicated. Activated charcoal (1–3 gm/kg) readily adsorbs the trichothecene mycotoxins and is recommended along with a saline cathartic (1 gm/kg), such as sodium or magnesium sulfate (1 gm/kg). If animals have oral lesions, a nonirritating diet should be chosen. The feed to be used as replacement should obviously be free of mycotoxin contamination and should be of slightly elevated protein content. Stress should be minimized and contact with other groups of animals avoided.

PREVENTION

These mycotoxicoses are best avoided by proper grain handling so as to avoid enhanced fungal growth and toxin production in the first place. When this is not possible, extremely moldy feedstuffs should not be used. When necessary, analyses of the grain may be performed and a small test group of young animals may be fed the grain. If no toxic effects occur, the feed may be used, but it is probably best to avoid feeding it to breeding stock and to younger animals. Feeds containing comparatively low concentrations of trichothecene toxins can be fed to poultry with fewer toxic effects than would be anticipated in mammals. Although analytical testing of feeds for specific toxins is desirable, negative results do not guarantee safe feed.

Supplemental Reading

Beasley, V. R., Swanson, S. P., Reynolds, R. D., et al.: Current status of toxicokinetics and residue detection of trichothecene mycotoxins in swine, cattle and feedstuffs. Proceedings of the United States Animal Health Association, 1982.

Côté, L. M., Reynolds, J. D., Vesonder, R. F., et al.: Survey of vomitoxin-contaminated feed grains in midwestern United States, and associated health problems in swine. J. Am. Vet. Med. Assoc., 184:189–192, 1984.

Hamilton, Pat B.: Fallacies in our understanding of mycotoxins. J. Food Protect. 41:404–408, 1978.

Vesonder, R. F., and Hesseltine, C. W.: Metabolites of Fusarium. In Nelson, T. E., Toussoun, T. A., and Cook, R. J. (eds.). Fusarium: Diseases, Biology and Taxonomy. University Park, Pennsylvania State University Press, 350–364, 1981.

Weaver, G. A., Kurtz, H. J., Mirocha, C. J., et al.: Acute toxicity of the mycotoxin diacetoxyscirpenol in swine. Can. Vet. J. 19:267–271, 1978.

Weaver, G. A., Kurtz, H. J., Mirocha, C. J. et al.: Effect of T-2 toxin on porcine reproduction. Can. Vet. J. 19:310–314, 1978.

Slaframine (Slobber Factor)

EUGENE B. SMALLEY, Ph.D.
and JULIE M. SANDERSON, M.S.

The salivary syndrome, characterized by excessive salivation, results from the consumption of legume forages, particularly red clover (Trifolium pratense), parasitized by the fungus Rhizoctonia leguminicola.[1] Ingestion of a single nonlethal dose of infested forage causes salivary episodes lasting from 6 to 8 hr in small animals and to over 3 days in cattle.[1, 2] The parasympathomimetic piperidine alkaloid, slaframine (1-acetoxy-6-aminooctahydroindolizine), has been isolated and chemically characterized from pure cultures of R. leguminicola (Fig. 1).[3, 4, 5, 6] The alkaloid has also been isolated directly from toxic red clover hay.[7] When activated by liver microsomes to a ketoimine, it induces much of the natural disease syndrome in experimental animals and is considered the salivary factor.[8] Greater detail concerning various aspects of the salivary syndrome and slaframine can be found in several review articles.[1, 3, 4, 6, 8, 9, 10]

Swainsonine (1,2,8-trihydroxyoctahydroindolizine) is another indolizidine alkaloid produced by R. leguminicola (Fig. 2).[11, 12] This alkaloid was originally found in Darling pea (Swainsona canescens)[13] and has recently been found in spotted locoweed (Astragalus lentiginosus).[14] Ingestion

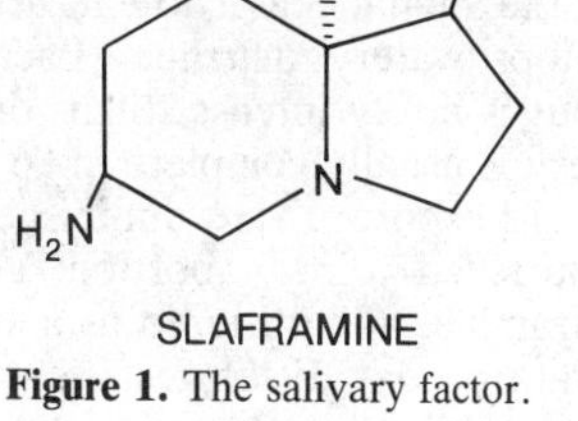

SLAFRAMINE
Figure 1. The salivary factor.

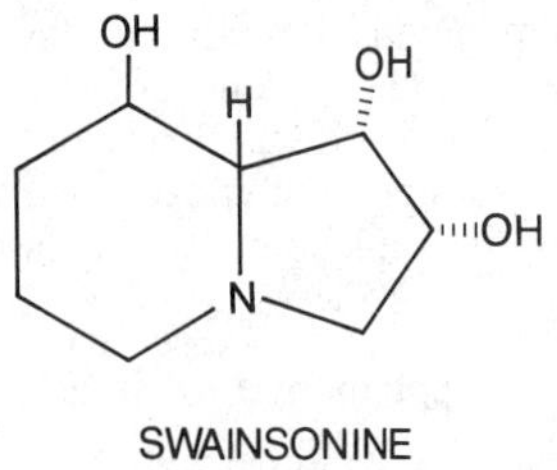

SWAINSONINE

Figure 2. Possible α-mannosidase inhibitor.

of *S. canescens* or *A. lentiginosus* induces *Swainsona* toxicosis or locoism, respectively.[13, 14] Symptoms that are common to both of these diseases are neurologic disturbances, loss of body weight, addiction to the plants, and vacuolation of tissue cells as a result of lysosomal storage of mannose-rich oligosaccharides.[13, 15] Mannosidosis, a genetic deficiency of α-mannosidase, is also characterized by neurologic disturbance and cell vacuolation.[13] Swainsonine is thought to act as an α-mannosidase inhibitor in both swainsonine toxicosis and locoism. Work is underway to assess the role of swainsonine in the salivary syndrome.[16]

OCCURRENCE

The salivary syndrome has been observed in cattle, sheep, goats, and horses in many parts of the eastern and central United States and in Japan.[1, 17, 18] The disease of red clover induced by *R. leguminicola,* black patch, is similarly distributed and has also been found in Alberta, Canada[19] and Japan.[17, 18] Although the syndrome cannot be considered a major mycotoxic problem, the potential for serious outbreaks is present whenever red clover is grown for forage. Although red clover is the major host of *R. leguminicola,* black patch disease has also been reported on other legumes: white clover, soybeans, kudzu, cowpea, blue lupine, alsike clover, alfalfa, Korean lespedeza, black medick, sainfoin, and cicer milk vetch, and these hosts are potential inducers of the salivation syndrome.[1] *R. leguminicola* overwinters on infested straw and survives at least 2 years on infected seed.[20] It develops most severely during periods of wet weather and high humidity, and farmers often confuse the development of dark-brown infected plant parts with normal plant maturation.[20] Because of this, red clover may be cut, dried, and baled as normally cured hay but still induce severe salivary episodes when fed to farm animals.[21, 22]

CLINICAL SIGNS

Cattle, the principal farm animals affected, begin salivating 30 min to 1 hr after eating infested hay.[2, 21] The response from a single exposure intensifies up to 24 hr, at which time the animal ceases to eat, urinates frequently, and develops watery diarrhea. Lacrimation occurs periodically but is rarely intense. Signs diminish after 48 hr and recovery is usually complete in 96 hr. Other signs after longer field exposures are diminished milk production, bloat, stiffened joints, abortion, and occasionally death.[2, 21] Slaframine, administered as a semipurified culture concentrate on day 19 of gestation, caused uterine hemorrhaging, abortion, and occasional death in pregnant rats and guinea pigs.[23]

In guinea pigs, swine, and in probably all animals that react to slaframine, mild to severe respiratory difficulties are associated with the salivary response (Fig. 3).[2] Suffocation, accompanied by severe emphysema, appears to be the most probable cause of death from lethal doses of slaframine.[2] The syndrome appears to be quite similar to that induced by acetylcholine, and studies indicate that activated slaframine binds to acetylcholine receptors.[10]

PHYSIOLOGY

A delay between the time of oral dosing and the onset of salivation (10 to 60 min) results because of the time necessary for the bioactivation of slaframine by liver microsomes.[8] Although slaframine causes specific stimulation of exocrine glands, particularly the salivary glands and the pancreas,[24] other effects are decreases in heart rate, respiration, and body temperature, and increases in peristalsis and uterine motility.[2, 23]

CLINICAL PATHOLOGY

Farm animals reacting to slaframine usually recover completely when the contaminated hay or toxin is withheld. A chronic 3-week exposure of guinea pigs to sublethal doses of slaframine failed to induce observable gross or histologic change.[2] Occasional deaths in cattle and abortions in horses have been reported, however, suggesting more complex pathologic changes. Postmortem examination of guinea pigs given lethal doses of slaframine

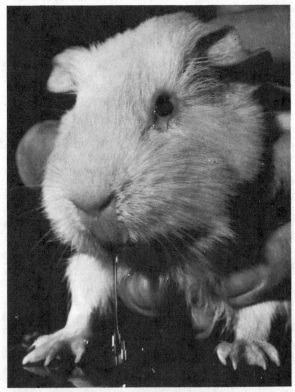

Figure 3. Salivation, lacrimation, and pilo-erection in guinea pigs force-fed blended mycelium of *Rhizoctonia leguminicola.* Reprinted from Crump et al., 1967, by courtesy of the American Veterinary Medical Association.

revealed that the blood vessels in the thoracic and abdominal cavities had become engorged with blood.[2] The lung surface was pale and dry, with many small hemorrhagic areas, and lung sections revealed large areas of emphysema. Both the liver and kidney were congested, and the submucosal glands of the trachea appeared extremely active, with many eosinophils in the submucosa.

DIAGNOSIS

Diagnosis of slaframine-induced excessive salivation can be based tentatively upon distinctive symptoms (e.g., extreme salivation, lacrimation, diarrhea, frequent urination, and anorexia) following ingestion of legume forage, usually second-cutting red clover hay. Confirmation can be made by identification of the fungus *R. leguminicola* in the suspect forage. The fungus survives for many months in infested dried hay and can readily be isolated in pure culture. Chemical assays for slaframine are not usually necessary for diagnostic purposes because of the unique nature of the clinical signs and obvious presence of the dark brown, coarse mycelium of the fungus in great abundance throughout the cured hay. However, a gas chromatographic method has been developed for direct identification of slaframine in toxic hay.[7]

TREATMENT

Although ruminants usually recover without treatment when the toxic legume forage is withheld, reactions can be expected to continue for a day or two after the toxic feed is withdrawn. In cases of severe intoxication, atropine therapy may be useful but will not be entirely effective.[2] In a trial using guinea pigs, simultaneous administration of atropine with a lethal dose of slaframine prevented signs of toxicosis for 5 hr, after which mild salivation appeared. When atropine was administered 2 or 4 hr after a lethal dose of slaframine, the salivation response was intense, but no fatalities occurred.[2]

PREVENTION

Control of the black patch disease of red clover could provide a major means for prevention of the salivary syndrome. However, fungicides applied before flowering did not reduce seed infection, and ground sprays at the time of renewed growth in the spring and immediately after the first cutting did not reduce foliar symptoms.[25] Chemical seed treatments to eradicate the seed-borne phase of the disease provide an excellent means of control in locations free of the disease. Careful use of red clover forage in ruminant feeding programs seems mandatory in areas of endemic black patch infection. Precautionary feeding of red clover forage to a few animals prior to general feeding is useful in preventing extensive outbreaks of salivary syndrome.

References

1. Smalley, E. B.: Salivary syndrome in cattle. In Wyllie, T. D., and Morehouse, L. G. (eds.). Mycotoxic Fungi, Mycotoxins, and Mycotoxicoses. New York, Dekker, 121–141, 1978.
2. Crump, M. H., Smalley, E. B., Nichols, R. E., and Rainey, D. P.: Pharmacologic properties of a slobber-inducing mycotoxin from *Rhizoctonia leguminicola*. Am. J. Vet. Res. 28:865–874, 1967.
3. Aust, S. D.: *Rhizoctonia leguminicola*—slaframine. In Purchase, I. F. H. (ed.). Mycotoxins. Amsterdam, Elsevier Science Publishing Co. Inc., 97–109, 1974.
4. Broquist, H. P., and Snyder, J. J.: *Rhizoctonia* toxin. In Kadis, S., Ciegler, A., and Aji, S. J. (eds.). Microbial Toxins, vol. 7. New York, Academic Press, 319–330, 1971.
5. Gardiner, R. A., Rinehart, Jr., K. I., Snyder, J. J., and Broquist, H. P.: Slaframine. Absolute stereochemistry and a revised structure. J. Am. Chem. Soc. 90:5639–5640, 1968.
6. Smalley, E. B.: Chemistry and physiology of slaframine. In Wyllie, T. D., and Morehouse, L. C., (eds.). Mycotoxic Fungi, Mycotoxins, and Mycotoxicoses. New York, Dekker, 449–458, 1977.
7. Hagler, W. M., and Behlow, R. F.: Salivary syndrome in horses: identification of slaframine in red clover hay. Appl. Environ. Microbiol. 42:1067–1073, 1981.
8. Guengerich, F. P., and Aust, S. D.: Activation of the parasympathomimetic alkaloid slaframine by microsomal and photochemical oxidation. Mol. Pharmacol. 13:185–195, 1977.
9. Crump, M. H.: Slaframine (slobber factor) toxicosis. J. Am. Vet. Med. Assoc. 163:1300–1302, 1973.
10. Guengerich, F. P., and Broquist, H. P.: Novel piperidine alkaloids from the fungus *Rhizoctonia leguminicola*: characterization, biosynthesis, bioactivation and related studies. Bioorg. Chem. 78:97–109, 1978.
11. Schneider, M. J., Ungenmach, F. S., Broquist, H. P., and Harris, T. M.: (1S, 2R, 8R, 8aR)-1,2,8-trihydroxyoctahydroindolizine (swainsonine), and α-mannosidase inhibitor from *Rhizoctonia leguminicola*. Tetrahedron 39:29–32, 1983.
12. Schneider, M. J., Ungenmach, F. S., Broquist, H. P., and Harris, T. M.: Biosynthesis of swainsonine in *Rhizoctonia leguminicola*. Epimerization at the ring fusion. J. Am. Chem. Soc. 104:6863–6864, 1982.
13. Colegate, S. M., Dorling, P. R., and Huxtable, C. R.: A spectroscopic investigation of swainsonine: an α-mannosidase inhibitor isolated from *Swainsona canescens*. Aust. J. Chem. 32:2257–2264, 1979.
14. Molyneux, R. J., and James, L. F.: Loco intoxication: indolizidine alkaloids of spotted locoweed (*Astragalus lentiginosus*). Science 216:190–191, 1982.
15. Dorling, P. R., Huxtable, C. R., and Vogel, P.: Lysosomal storage in *Swainsona* sp. toxicosis: and induced mannosidosis. Neuropath. Appl. Neurobiol. 4:285–296, 1978.
16. Broquist, H. P.: Personal communication, July 21, 1983.
17. Isawa, K.: The black patch infection of leguminous grasses by *Rhizoctonia leguminicola* causing excessive salivation in livestock. Anim. Husb. 27:63–66, 1973.
18. Isawa, K., Tajimi, A., and Nishihara, N.: The excessive salivation of goats caused by some Japanese isolates of black patch disease fungus (*Rhizoctonia leguminicola*) of leguminous forage. Bull. Nat. Inst. Animal Ind. 25:59–65, 1971 (in Japanese).
19. Berenkamp, B.: Black patch of forage legumes. Can. Plant Dis. Sur. 57:65–67, 1977.
20. Elliot, E. S.: Diseases, insects and other factors in relation to red clover failure in West Virginia. W. Va. Agric. Exp. Sta. Bull. 351T, April 1952.
21. Crump, M. H., Smalley, E. B., Henning, J. N., and Nichols, R. E.: Mycotoxicosis in animals fed legume hay with *Rhizoctonia leguminicola*. J. Am. Vet. Med. Assoc. 143:996–997, 1963.
22. Smalley, E. B.: Personal observations, 1959–1963.
23. Maseehuddin, H., and Nichols, R. E.: Some pharmacological effects on rats and mice of a mycotoxin produced by *Rhizoctonia leguminicola* from red clover forage. Refuah Veterinarith. 28:152–155, 1971.
24. Aust, S. D.: Evidence for bioactivation of slaframine. Biochem. Pharmacol. 18:929–932, 1969.
25. Gough, F. J., and Elliot, E. S.: Black patch of red clover and other legumes caused by *Rhizoctonia leguminicola*. W. Va. Agric. Exp. Sta. Bull. 387T, Nov. 1956.

Sporidesmins Facial Eczema and Pithomycotoxicosis

C. V. BAGLEY, D.V.M. and J. L. SHUPE, D.V.M.

Sporidesmin is a hepatotoxic mycotoxin produced only, as far as is known, by the fungal agent *Pithomyces chartarum* (formerly *Sporidesmium bakeri*). When ingested in excessive amounts, sporidesmin causes a hepatogenous photosensitivity that has long been recognized in New Zealand and more recently in Australia as facial eczema (FE) of sheep and cattle. Pithomycotoxicosis has been proposed as a more descriptive name for the disease syndrome caused by sporidesmin.

P. chartarum is a saprophyte and has been found on a wide variety of dead plant litter of grasses, legumes, and herbaceous weeds in both native and cultivated pastures. It is widely dispersed geographically and has been identified in New Zealand, Australia, South Africa, the United States, Japan, and Canada. Facial eczema has been correlated with sporidesmin ingestion by sheep and cattle in New Zealand and Australia and by sheep in South Africa. Outbreaks of photosensitization in cattle, which are described as being very similar to those of FE, have occurred in Texas, Oklahoma, Florida, and Utah and, although sporidesmin has not yet been proved as the cause in the United States, it is certainly a potential cause.

PATHOGENESIS

Outbreaks of FE occur in New Zealand only in certain geographic areas where temperature, humidity, and available plant litter favor the growth of *P. chartarum*. The presence of FE is sporadic, with 3- to 10-year intervals between major outbreaks. They usually are in late summer or early autumn, after a period of rain followed by several warm, humid days. The high risk period has been identified as 3 consecutive days of overcast skies with rain showers of 1 cm or more, relative humidity greater than 80 per cent, and air temperature continuously greater than 16°C. Maximum sporulation of *P. chartarum* takes place at close to 100-per cent relative humidity, and little if any sporulation takes place at less than 80-per cent humidity. The optimum temperature is 24°C (75°F). Sporidesmin is contained in the conidia and is not produced until cultures are producing spores. The conidia of *P. chartarum* are dark brown or black and form clusters in sooty patches. They are dry and are dispersed through the air.

After the spores are ingested by animals, sporidesmin is rapidly absorbed from the intestinal tract, enters the portal circulation, and penetrates the liver. It induces some early but reversible toxic damage to hepatocytes, but the major damaging effect is on the biliary tree. Early in the course of the disease, sporidesmin acts as an inflammatory agent, increases the permeability of the blood capillaries, and induces a marked swelling of the bile duct epithelium and edema of the portal tracts. This compresses the lumina of the small bile ducts and impedes bile flow. Later there is progressive obliterative cholangitis due to an exuberant reactive, granulation tissue repair process. In sheep, a single dose of 1 mg/kg of sporidesmin will result in almost complete cessation of bile flow in 10 to 14 days.

Sporidesmin is excreted primarily in the bile, with some appearing in the urine. The majority of sporidesmin that enters the general circulation is apparently detoxified rather rapidly.

Because of the sporidesmin-induced bile duct and liver damage, phylloerythrin accumulates in the body. It is a normal metabolic product of chlorophyll and an active photodynamic agent. In nonpigmented skin areas it reacts with sunlight and results in photosensitization. Surgical ligation of the bile duct induces a similar response.

Sporidesmin is classified chemically as an epipolythio-dioxopiperazine, and its biologic activity is related to its sulfur-containing ring. It is evidently derived biosynthetically from the amino acids tryptophan, alanine, and methionine. Sporidesmin metabolites have been identified and are named B,C,D,E,F,G, and H.

P. chartarum is only a minor component of the microflora present on plant litter, even under favorable conditions. During an outbreak of FE, its growth may be inapparent on the litter, and in some mycotic culture and isolation studies it has made up only 1 per cent of the fungal isolates. Not all isolates of *P. chartarum* produce sporidesmin when cultured. In South Africa, both toxigenic and nontoxigenic types were frequently isolated from the same plant litter, but the nontoxigenic types predominated. There may be toxigenic and nontoxigenic strains of *P. chartarum*, or some isolates may simply require different nutrients or conditions in order to produce sporidesmin. A strain of *P. chartarum* was isolated in Texas from a pasture in which cattle developed photosensitization while grazing, but this strain did not produce sporidesmin in the laboratory. Furthermore, the relative toxicity from various isolates has varied by more than 100-fold from the least to most toxic isolates.

Pastures remain toxic for a relatively short time because sporidesmin is soluble in and removed by water. Drying will also destroy it. Spores lose their toxin in heavy rain or in dew, and toxicity of hay or plant litter collections can only be maintained by freezing or rapidly drying with forced hot air.

Sheep and cattle of all ages are susceptible to sporidesmin, and horses have also been affected, but there is individual animal variation in which liver metabolic rate is apparently a factor. The morbidity rate is usually slightly lower in cattle than in sheep. There is little risk of FE in New Zealand unless spore numbers are high (i.e., 10^5/gm dry wt. of pasture). A young sheep would have to eat approximately 7 gm of spores in order to develop FE. The sensitivity of young laboratory rats is inversely related to the protein concentration of their food.

Two additional photosensitivity diseases in South Africa are apparently related to sporidesmin toxicity. These are "geeldikkop," which is associated with ingestion of the plant *Tribulus terrestris,* and "dikoor," which is associated with ingestion of the grasses *Panicum*. The 2 diseases are really indistinguishable, except that they occur in different geographic areas and dikoor is supposedly milder than geeldikkop. In addition to photosensitization and the usual liver lesions which occur with FE, both diseases induce an accumulation of crystals in the bile duct system and pigmentation of Kupffer cells. It has now been shown that although geeldikkop is a more complex disease and is not FE per se, it can be reproduced by simultaneous dosing of sporidesmin and *T. terrestris.*

CLINICAL SIGNS

The signs evident after sporidesmin ingestion are dose dependent and include photosensitization, weight loss, icterus, liver lesions, and death within 3 to 5 days. Icterus and photosensitive dermatitis are both variable and may or may not occur. In sheep given a 3 mg/kg total sporidesmin dose over a 3-day period, there was 100 per cent mortality after 4 days, but no evidence of photosensitization.

Table 1. *Species and Total Lethal Oral Dose of Sporidesmin*

Species	Lethal Oral Dose (mg/kg)
Sheep and cattle	1
Rabbits	1–2
Guinea pigs	2–4
Chickens	5–10
Rats	20–30
Mice	200–300

The relative species toxicities are indicated in Table 1 as the total lethal oral dose. Early signs are sudden lethargy, dullness, and anorexia. The signs of photosensitization include inflammation of the conjunctiva, nasal discharge, violent headshaking, pruritus of affected areas of skin, frequent urination, and shade-seeking behavior. Later, the light-colored skin of the ears, eyelids, face, muzzle, teats, or vulva becomes red, and "sunburnt" lesions appear along with serum exudation, scabbing, sloughing, and scarification. Still later, there may be icterus (individual variation), general debility, and finally death after several weeks. Some hepatic lesions often develop in the absence of photosensitization. After the early stages subside, some animals may suffer chronic ill health, poor condition, and susceptibility to stress and secondary complications. Even photosensitivity may recur if they are fed on lush green pasture.

In addition to the environmental conditions and to the doses that influence the clinical signs, there are various individual biologic responses that may be related: species, skin color, level of nutrition, and physiologic state.

PATHOLOGY

At necropsy, major gross changes are evident in the liver. In the early stages of the disease it becomes enlarged with rounded yellow-green borders. The bile duct walls are edematous, thick, and fibrous, and the lumina may be partially obstructed with bile and cellular debris. Advanced cases show hepatic fibrosis, fatty infiltration, and nodular regeneration. The kidneys may also be swollen with hemosiderosis.

Early histopathologic changes are degeneration of medium-sized bile ducts, periductal edema, and some infiltration of leukocytes into portal triads. Later the connective tissue proliferates around the bile ducts, which narrows the lumina and causes occlusion with bile and sloughed epithelial debris. This is followed by a proliferation of the bile ductules, and eventually the area is filled with fibrous tissue and bile ducts. There is very little effect on the parenchymal cells of the liver.

The liver damage is of greater importance than can be judged by just the cases of photosensitization that develop. Impaired production, susceptibility to other diseases, and stress must also be considered and may account for a greater economic loss than does the photosensitization.

DIAGNOSIS

Sporidesmin toxicosis should be suspected in any outbreak of photosensitization in sheep or cattle, and efforts should be made to make a definitive diagnosis. The presence of the characteristic liver lesions should assist in making a differential diagnosis.

Detection and estimation of the amount of sporidesmin present in forage has not been amenable to a rapid and practical test, but the technique would be of value in field investigations. A "beaker" test was used in New Zealand, but it did not detect sporidesmin directly, only another substance produced by *P. chartarum*. Later in the season this substance often remained after the pasture toxicity disappeared and resulted in false-positive tests.

Other laboratory methods that have been used to detect and quantify the amounts of sporidesmin produced by cultures of *P. chartarum* have been the sodium azide-potassium iodide spray, paper chromatography, thin layer chromatography, and high performance liquid chromatography.

A guinea pig toxicity test used to detect mycotoxin in pasture samples has been rather reliable. Weaned guinea pigs were fed 20 to 30 gm of dried pasture samples for 3 to 4 weeks. They were then killed, and the liver of each animal was examined histologically and graded on the character and degree of injury. The results were used to advise on the relative hazard of grazing those pastures. The pasture samples to be used for feed in this type of test should probably be frozen or quickly hot-air dried to preserve any sporidesmin present.

P. chartarum is best isolated from forage litter by transferring small pieces of dead leaf tissue directly onto 1.5-per cent malt extract agar with 110 mg of sodium novobiocin/L and incubating at 25°C. A number of cultures should be made since *P. chartarum* is usually not the dominant fungal organism present. Its colonies are usually confined to the plant material rather than having spread to the agar medium. Direct stereomicroscopic examination can be made for colonies of *P. chartarum*. It must be remembered that even if *P. chartarum* is isolated, it could still be a nontoxic producer.

The diagnosis is further complicated by the fact that clinical signs may not be evident for several days or weeks after exposure of a flock or herd to sporidesmin. The fungal microflora may change rapidly, and this results in the presence of organisms that were not present at the time of intoxication.

Hepatic function and serum enzyme test results can aid in determining the extent of liver involvement in cases of photosensitization. Those values that have been most helpful are higher serum bilirubin (both total and direct or conjugated), SGOT (serum glutamate oxaloacetic transaminase), GGT (gamma-glutamyl transpeptidase), and phylloerythrin.

It is necessary to differentiate the other causes of photosensitivity and hepatitis. Sporidesmin is the only mycotoxin to be extensively investigated as an agent of photosensitivity, but other mycotic agents may also be involved under certain conditions. *Periconia* spp. of the southern United States closely resembles *P. chartarum* and is believed to grow on dead forage. Xanthomegnin and related quinone metabolites have caused hepatic damage and photosensitization in laboratory animals, although they have not been implicated in any natural outbreaks. These mycotoxins are produced by *Penicillium* (spp.), *Aspergillus* (5 spp.), *Trichophyton* (3 spp.), and *Microsporum* (1 spp.).

Phomopsis leptostromiformis has been implicated in photosensitization but not studied extensively.

Chaetomin, a type of antibiotic produced by *Chaetomium cochliodes* and *C. globosum* is chemically related to and in the same family of compounds as sporidesmin. It has been implicated in an ovine ill thrift problem in Nova Scotia, but there is currently no evidence of photosensitization from chaetomin. Gliotoxin, an antibiotic produced by *Gliocladium virens* is also classified chemically in this same family of compounds.

TREATMENT AND CONTROL

Supportive treatment should be administered for hepatitis and photosensitization.

Control has been directed toward 4 main areas: prediction of high risk periods, grazing management, spraying pastures with fungicides, and zinc supplementation. Prediction methods have been based on meteorologic data and spore catches from high risk areas. With either warning system, the producers could remove their stock to other feed sources during high risk periods. The major problem has been one of false alarms, i.e., prediction of a problem period that did not occur.

Two grazing control systems have been used with reasonable success. One consists of irrigating the pastures during the dry part of summer to maintain growth along with intensive grazing to reduce leaf death from shading. The second is to control grazing with an electric fence and a back fence and then to allow very light grazing of the pasture in strips. The stock are moved on to a new strip before they graze down to the dead plant litter.

Both Thiabendazole and Benlate have been used as fungicides for pasture spraying in New Zealand. They have been effective at levels as low as 4 oz/acre. The chemical should be applied before the usual peak of spore production, with a second application made about a month later, before the usual second peak. These fungicides function by suppressing sporulation will not eliminate the sporidesmin already present.

It has been shown that liver damage due to sporidesmin can be prevented with a daily supplemental intake of zinc. The problem is how to get a consistent dose into the animals so as to protect and yet not to be toxic. Zinc at 20 mg/kg is protective, 40 mg/kg is potentially toxic, and 10 mg/kg is insufficient. Attempts to add zinc to the water have proved unsatisfactory owing to the many factors that influence the individual variations of water intake.

Supplemental Reading

Atherton, L. G., Brewer, D., and Taylor, A.: *Pithomyces chartarum*: a fungal parameter in the aetiology of some diseases of domestic animals. *In* Purchase, I.F.H. (ed.). Mycotoxins. New York, Elsevier Scientific Publishing Co. Inc., 29–68, 1974.

Brook, P. J.: *Pithomyces chartarum* in pasture and measures for prevention of facial eczema. J. Stored Prod. Res. *5*:203–209, 1969.

Dodd, D. C.: Facial eczema in ruminants. *In* Wogan, G. N. (ed.). Mycotoxins in Foodstuffs. Cambridge, Massachusetts, M.I.T. Press, 105–110, 1964.

Ford, E. J. H.: Activity of gamma-glutamyl transpeptidase and other enzymes in the serum of sheep with liver or kidney damage. J. Comp. Path. *84*:231–262, 1980.

Galitzen, S. J., and Oehme, F. W.: Photosensitization: a literature review. Vet. Sci. Comun. *2*:217–230, 1978.

Kellerman, T. S., Van Der Westhuizen, G. C. A., Coetzer, J. A. W., et al.: Photosensitivity in South Africa. II. The experimental production of the ovine hepatogenous photosensitivity disease geeldikkop (*Tribulosis ovis*) by the simultaneous ingestion of *Tribulus terrestris* plants and cultures of *Pithomyces chartarum* containing the mycotoxin sporidesmin. Onderstepoort J. Vet. Res. *47*:231–262, 1980.

Marasas, W. F. O., and Kellerman, T. S.: Pithomycotoxicosis "facial eczema" in cattle. *In* Wyllie, T. D. and Morehouse, L. G. (eds.). Mycotoxic Fungi, Mycotoxins and Mycotoxicoses. New York, Dekker, 63–72, 1978.

Mortimer, P. H., White, E. P., and di Menna, M. E.: Pithomycotoxicosis "facial eczema" in sheep. *In* Wyllie, T. D. and Morehouse, L. G. (eds.). Mycotoxic Fungi, Mycotoxins and Mycotoxicoses. New York, Dekker, 195–203, 1978.

Richard, J. L.: Mycotoxin photosensitivity. J. Am. Vet. Med. Assoc. *163*:1298–1299.

Taylor, A.: The Toxicology of Sporidesmins and other epipolythiodioxopiperazines. *In* Kadis, S., Ciegler, A., and Ajl, S. J. (eds.). Microbial Toxins. New York, Academic Press, 337–376, 1971.

White, E. P., Mortimer, P. H., and de Menna, M. E.: Chemistry of the Sporidesmins. *In* Wyllie, T. D. and Morehouse, L. G. (eds.): Mycotoxic Fungi, Mycotoxins and Mycotoxicoses. New York, Dekker, 427–447, 1977.

Tremorgenic Toxins

WILLIAM B. BUCK, D.V.M., M.S.
and S. J. CYSEWSKI, D.V.M., M.S.*

This article is concerned with neurologic diseases of cattle that are characterized by sustained tremors that may proceed to convulsions and death. Six tremorgenic mycotoxins have been chemically identified and assigned the trivial names penitrem, fumitremorgen, verruculogen, tryptoquivalone, tryptoquivaline, and paxilline. These tremorgens are produced by several different species of fungi belonging to the genera *Aspergillus* and *Penicillium*. Some isolates of the fungi may produce more than 1 tremorgen at the same time (e.g., fumitremorgen and tryptoquivalone).

The majority of studies on the effects of these tremorgens on animals has been concerned with a variety of laboratory animal species. All of these compounds produce very similar clinical signs. Although only penitrem has been administered to cattle, it is reasonable to suspect that other toxins besides penitrem would affect cattle also, because several species of laboratory animals are susceptible to these toxins.

The role of these fungal tremorgens in naturally occurring diseases of cattle is problematic. There is strong circumstantial evidence that at least some outbreaks of rye grass staggers are caused by tremorgenic *Penicillium* that produce the mycotoxin penitrem. Bermuda grass staggers is clinically similar to rye grass staggers; however, the cause of Bermuda grass staggers is unknown. Finally, a highly fatal mycotoxicosis of cattle caused by *A. clavatus* has been reported in Africa and France. The toxic principle is unknown, but it does not appear to be any of the known fungal tremorgens. In one case, animals were fed molded germinated wheat and in another case, molded sorghum beer residue, as part of the concentrate in their ration.

CLINICAL SIGNS

Signs observed in outbreaks of rye grass staggers are indistinguishable from those produced experimentally in cattle by penitrem. Most affected animals show no signs

---

*Deceased.

unless disturbed or excited. Signs vary from fine muscular tremors and swaying when animals are at rest to marked incoordination and falling when they move or are excited. When forced to run, animals develop an exaggerated high stepping action, making less and less progress and finally halting or falling. If left undisturbed, they usually recover and regain a standing position. More severely affected cattle stand with their limbs stiff and moderately adducted and sway rhythmically. Signs in the most severely affected animals are lateral recumbency with paddling motions of the feet, marked tremors, intermittent extensor rigidity, and opisthotonos, having the appearance of tonic-clonic convulsions. Occasionally, nystagmus and some excess salivation are observed.

Bermuda grass staggers is clinically very similar to rye grass staggers and penitrem intoxication.

Poisoning with *A. clavatus* tremorgen (ACT) is characterized by hypersensitivity, severe muscular tremors, ataxia, progressive paresis, and paralysis. Affected animals have a stifflegged gait and hold the hindquarters upright, sometimes knuckling over. When startled they assume a splaylegged stance with the hocks slightly bent and the neck held rigidly extended. When animals become recumbent, a progressive paresis develops. Survivors sometimes display lasting locomotor disturbances.

PATHOLOGY

Changes in the plasma levels of substances associated with carbohydrate metabolism and selected enzymes have been associated with penitrem intoxication. Plasma lactic acid, pyruvic acid, and creatinine phosphokinase activity rise markedly. Plasma levels of oxaloacetic transaminase, glutamic pyruvic transaminase, and lactic dehydrogenase have increased but to a lesser degree. Significant changes in plasma cholinesterase activity and electrolytes were not seen in calves intoxicated with penitrem.

There are no reports of clinical pathologic changes associated with rye grass or Bermuda grass staggers. Changes similar to those seen with penitrem intoxication would be expected.

An elevation of serum glutamic oxaloacetic transaminase activity was reported for some but not all animals poisoned with ACT. The most notable lesions were degenerative and necrotic changes in skeletal muscles, hemorrhages on serosal surfaces, and gastrointestinal stasis. Microscopically, there were cytopathologic changes in the central nervous system, consisting of degeneration of neurons in the ventral horns of the spinal cord and in numerous nuclei in the medulla oblongata, midbrain, and thalamus.

DIAGNOSIS

As with any case of mycotoxicosis, confirmation that 1 of the fungal tremorgens is the cause of a disease rests on finding the toxin in the feed at levels sufficient to have caused the problem. Isolation from the feed of a fungus that produces a tremorgenic toxin would only be presumptive; cultural conditions may not have been appropriate when it grew on the feed for the organism to elaborate the toxin.

Diagnosis of rye grass staggers would be based on observing appropriate signs in animals grazing a rye grass stubble pasture. If penitrem is the causative toxin, the producing fungi would probably be present in the soil.

Diagnosis of Bermuda grass staggers is also based upon observing signs in animals on pasture or on Bermuda grass hay. The causative toxin is unknown.

The principal condition to be differentiated is the nervous form of ergotism, in which case sclerotia of 1 of the ergot fungi would be present.

TREATMENT AND PREVENTION

In all cases, removal of toxic feed is the first step. Animals with mild to moderate signs of rye grass or Bermuda grass staggers will recover unaided when provided with a new feed source and water and left undisturbed. Animals that are unable to rise will require hand feeding and watering until they are able to get up. A few severely affected animals may never get up.

Prevention of rye grass staggers involves avoiding stubble fields, although not all are toxic. Adequate information is not available to permit the prediction of which Bermuda grass pastures are toxic, so no preventative action can be recommended.

Supplemental Reading

Cole, R. J.: Tremorgenic mycotoxins. *In* Rodricks, J. W., Hesseltine, C. W., and Mehlman, A. (eds.). Mycotoxins in Human and Animal Health. Park Forest South, Illinois, Pathotox Pubs., Inc., 583–597, 1977.

Cysewski, S. J.: The effects of tremorgenic mycotoxins in cattle. *In* Wyllie, T. D. and Morehouse, L. G. (eds.). Mycotoxic Fungi, Mycotoxins and Mycotoxicoses, An Encyclopedic Handbook. New York, Dekker, 142–145, 1978.

Kellerman, T. S., Pienaar, J. G., Van Der Westhuizen, G. C. A., et al.: A highly fatal tremorgenic cycotoxicosis of cattle caused by *Aspergillus clavatus*. Onderstepoort J. Vet. Res. *43*:147–154, 1976.

Mantle, P. G., Mortimer, P. H., and White, E. P.: Mycotoxin tremorgens of *Claviceps paspali* and *Penicillium cyclopium*: a comparative study of effects on sheep and cattle in relation to natural staggers syndromes, Res. Vet. Sci., *24*:49–56, 1977.

Stachybotryotoxicosis

WILLIAM W. CARLTON, D.V.M., Ph.D.
and PALLE KROGH, D.V.M., Ph.D.

Stachybotryotoxicosis is a mycotoxic disease of horses, cattle, sheep, zoo-confined ruminants, and swine that is due to the ingestion of toxins produced on hay and straw by the fungus *Stachybotrys alternans* (synonyms *S. atra* and *S. chartarum*). The fungus is a common saprophyte that grows well on moist hay and straw and produces a dark layer of sooty appearance on the straw or hay. The toxin responsible for the toxicity of the fungus has not been established, but may be a member (satratoxin) of the trichothecene group of fungal metabolites.

Stachybotryotoxicosis has been recorded from various regions of the world, but most reports have come from Russia and eastern Europe. Outbreaks of this mycotoxicosis have not been reported in North America. The disease has been observed more commonly during the indoor feeding period when animals are exposed to contaminated staw or hay.

CLINICAL SIGNS

The clinical signs and disease course depend on the amount and the time of toxin ingestion. The disease can be divided into acute and chronic forms. The acute form is due to ingestion of larger amounts of toxins over a short time period, and the chronic form is due to ingestion of smaller amounts of toxin over a long time period.

Poisoned cattle refuse feed, develop diarrhea, have reduced milk production, and develop petechial and ulcerative lesions of the lips, tongue, and buccal mucosae. Fever, conjunctivitis, and a serohemorrhagic nasal discharge are present in some cattle. In terminal cases, there is bloody diarrhea, emaciation, no lactation, and abortion in pregnant cows. The clinical syndrome of stachybotryotoxicosis in sheep is similar to that described in cattle: fever, reduced appetite, oral edema and erosions, salivation, decreased milk production, and diarrhea.

Stachybotryotoxicosis in swine may be manifested as necrotic dermatitis, as general toxicosis, and as abortion. The cutaneous form is found in piglets and sows and appears as focal necrotic ulcerative lesions of the nose and mouth of the piglets and of the udders of the sows. Beginning with swelling and hyperemia of the snout and corners of the mouth, erosions are followed by ulceration and by the development of brown crusts over affected areas. Ingestion of highly toxic feeds results in an acute, atypical toxicosis characterized by vomiting, salivation, marked depression, and muscular tremors. In the more typical form, feed intake is decreased, the animal is depressed, and blood dyscrasias, as described in the horse, develop. Such affected swine may also have lesions of the skin and oral mucosae.

PATHOLOGY

The principal gross findings in horses, cattle, sheep, and swine are similar and characteristically consist of hemorrhagic and necrotic lesions in many tissues. Hemorrhages varying from petechiae to extravasations occur in serous membranes, skeletal musculature, the gastrointestinal tract, lymph nodes, lungs, and the central nervous system. Foci of necrosis are found in the mucosae of most regions of the alimentary tract but are seen principally affecting the buccal structures, the stomach (abomasum), and the large intestine. Lymph nodes, especially the mesenteric and pharyngeal, are enlarged and hemorrhagic.

DIAGNOSIS, TREATMENT, AND CONTROL

The clinical signs and gross lesions of the typical form, while suggestive of stachybotryotoxicosis, are not diagnostic, and various symptoms can be confused with those of other diseases. This is especially true of certain mucosal diseases of cattle. Diagnosis is aided by demonstrating that animals were exposed to fungus-contaminated forage. The fungus grows particularly well on straws and hays, producing a black sooty layer. Microscopic examination of such materials will reveal the black mycelia and conidiospores and thus supports the clinical diagnosis. Producing the disease in laboratory animals by the feeding of suspect forages might be attempted as a part of diagnostic procedures. Because the toxic principle has not been firmly established, methods for clinical detection of the toxin are not presently available.

Specific antidotes are not available. Removal of suspect forages from the affected animals would be the first logical procedure. Broad-spectrum antibiotics combined with fluid therapy and blood transfusions might be recommended for especially valuable animals. Control is achieved by preventing exposure of animals to hays and straws with extensive growth of *S. alternans*.

Supplemental Reading

Eppley, R. M.: Chemistry of stachybotryotoxicosis. *In* Rodricks, J. V., Hesseltine, C. W., and Mehlman, M. A. (eds.). Mycotoxins in Human and Animal Health. Park Forest South, Illinois, Pathotox Publishers, Inc., 285–293, 1977.

Hintikka (nee Korpinen), E. L.: Stachybotryotoxicosis in cattle and captive animals. Stachybotryotoxicosis in horses. Stachybotryotoxicosis in sheep. Stachybotryotoxicosis in swine. *In* Wyllie, T. D., and Morehouse, L. G. (eds.). Mycotoxic Fungi, Mycotoxins and Mycotoxicoses. New York, Dekker, 152–161, 181–185, 203–207, 268–273, 1978.

Sarkisov, A. Kh. Koroleva, V. P., Kvashnina, E. S., and Grezin, V. F.: Stachybotryotoxicosis. *In* Diagnostic Procedures for Fungal-Induced Diseases in Animals (Mycoses and Mycotoxicoses). Moscow, Kolos, 84–91, 1971. (In Russian).

Schneider, D. J., Marasas, W. F. O., Dale Kuys, et al.: A field outbreak of suspected stachybotryotoxicosis in sheep. J. South Afri. Vet. Med. Assoc. 50:73–81, 1979.

Zearalenone (F-2)

LAWRENCE P. RUHR, D.V.M., Ph.D.

Zearalenone (F-2) is a mycotoxin produced by the fungus *Fusarium roseum (graminearum),* also known as *Gibberella zeae.* This mycotoxin is most often found in corn or feeds containing corn. However, zearalenone has been reported in small grains, such as wheat, barley, and maize as well as in hay. In the field, the fungus is commonly found as a saprophyte. Maximal fungal growth occurs when grain moisture content is greater than 23 per cent and the ambient temperature is near 27° C. The enzymes responsible for zearalenone production are induced at much lower temperatures (12 to 14° C). For maximal production of the mycotoxin, there should be alternating periods of these temperature extremes. Because of these requirements, zearalenone is often found in high moisture ear corn that has been stored over winter, especially in northern climates.

Zearalenone has estrogenic activity in many species, though chemically it is phenolic rather than steroidal. Swine are probably the most sensitive of the food-producing animals to the estrogenic effects of zearalenone. Well documented disease conditions associated with zearalenone are almost all seen in swine. However, estrogenic conditions have also been reported in dairy cattle when zearalenone was found in the hay.

As an estrogenic substance, zearalenone affects the organs normally receptive to estrogen. Specifically, the mammae, the ovaries, and the tubular organs of the female reproductive tract are affected.

CLINICAL SIGNS

The usual presenting clinical sign in gilts and sows is mammary and vulvar enlargement. Within the range of individual variation this occurs throughout the group of animals being fed zearalenone-contaminated feed. Other signs are rectal or vaginal prolapse, or both, abortion, small litters, stillbirths, and fetal mummification.

The gilts and sows may appear to be in prolonged estrus. This is not a "standing heat"; they are not receptive to the boar. Some mature cycling sows may become anestrous.

Barrows are reported to have mammary and preputial enlargement. Boars are reported to have mammary and preputial enlargement, testicular atrophy, and loss of libido. To date, these observations have not been confirmed, using purified zearalenone at naturally occurring levels.

These clinical signs and observations have been observed in field cases. The causal relationship of zearalenone has not always been well documented. Some other substances (e.g., deoxynivalenol (vomitoxin) as described in the article Trichothecenes) may have been present that actually produced some of the described signs.

PATHOLOGY

Though called vulvovaginitis, there is no primary inflammatory process. The changes best described are enlargement of the uterus with thickening of the endometrium, and hypoplastic ovaries, with atretic follicles and no corpora lutea.

Histologically, there is edema and proliferation of the mucosal epithelium of the vagina and cervix with metaplasia. The myometrium is also enlarged, with edema, hypertrophy, and hyperplasia. Mammary enlargement when present results from epithelial hyperplasia, with metaplasia in the ducts of the mammary gland. Some interstitial edema may also be present.

A common sequela of the "vulvovaginitis" is rectal or vaginal prolapse that may then become involved in an inflammatory process.

The pathologic condition of zearalenone exposure in boars has not been documented.

DIAGNOSIS

Zearalenone intoxication should be suspected when many sows and gilts in a herd develop what appears to be persistent estrus. Rectal and vaginal prolapse may be observed. Abortion, stillbirths, or other reproductive problems may also be part of the herd situation.

When presented with this picture, an estrogenic agent influencing the animals must be considered. It is necessary to identify the estrogenic substance and the source. Feed and feed components should be examined for zearalenone, zearalanol, and other estrogenic substances, such as diethylstilbestrol (DES). This requires toxicologic testing. A complete history should be submitted to an appropriate laboratory along with feed samples.

If the history and clinical signs are consistent, and zearalenone is identified in the feed, a diagnosis of zearalenone-induced intoxication can be made.

TREATMENT AND PREVENTION

Treatment of zearalenone intoxication is limited to the identification of the contaminated feed and its removal from the diet. Signs have usually been reported to regress within 2 weeks. No long-term effects have been documented.

Prevention is also limited to elimination of zearalenone-contaminated feeds from the diet of susceptible animals. This can be accomplished by toxicologic screening of the suspected feed. Screening must be done shortly before the feed or feed component is to be used, as zearalenone production can occur in storage. Identification of fungi, even fungi known to produce zearalenone, is not a sufficiently reliable screening method. The zearalenone can be present when no viable fungi are present. Also, the fungi that are present may not be toxigenic.

It is not possible to recommend any use for contaminated feeds. Dilution of contaminated feed with clean feed is not recommended because viable fungi may produce more zearalenone and contaminate the entire lot. Zearalenone may not be the only mycotoxin in the feed. Others may be present for which one cannot or does not test. There appear to be species differences in susceptibility to zearalenone; however, these are not well documented. The presence of other mycotoxins makes a recommendation of feeding the contaminated feed to other classes of livestock inadvisable.

Supplemental Reading

Kurtz, H. J., and Mirocha, C. J.: Zearalenone (F-2) induced estrogenic syndrome in swine. In Wyllie, T. D., and Morehouse, L. G. (eds.). Myotoxic Fungi, Mycotoxins, Mycotoxicoses. New York, Dekker, 256–268, 1978.
Mirocha, C. J., and Christensen, C. M.: Oestrogenic mycotoxins synthesized by fusarium. In Purchase, I. F. H. (ed.). Mycotoxins. New York, Elsevier Scientific Publishing Co., 129–148, 1974.
Nelson, G. H., Christensen, C. M., and Mirocha, C. J.: Fusarium and estrogenism in swine. J. Am. Vet. Med. Asoc. 163:1276–1277, 1973.

Water Quality for Livestock

T. L. CARSON, D.V.M., M.S., Ph.D.

The 1968 Water Resources Council estimated that 1.7 billion gallons of water were required per day by livestock in the United States. Sixty per cent of this water comes from wells, with the rest originating in streams, lakes, springs, and impoundments. With such a massive volume of water involved in the livestock industry, it is not difficult to appreciate the importance of good water quality. Increased physical concentrations of livestock, combined with heightened emphasis on nutrition and health, have raised the number of inquiries about water quality. The following discussion summarizes some of the major parameters of water quality for livestock.

PALATABILITY

Palatability directly affects water consumption. A restricted water intake is soon followed by reduced feed consumption and thus reduced productive efficiency. Water supplies with high salinities are less palatable than water supplies with low salinities. Likewise, odors, such as hydrogen sulfide, will reduce water palatability. The palatibility of water is enhanced by the presence of CO_2.

MICROBIOLOGIC STANDARDS

Microbiologic examination of water samples will reveal the general sanitary quality and the degree of contamination from human and animal sources.

In general, these examinations are not done to isolate pathogenic bacteria, but to detect the presence of indicator organisms. The coliform group of bacteria has traditionally been the indicator used to assess the degree of water pollution and thus the sanitary quality of the particular sample. A recent advance in the microbiologic examination of water, the differentiation of fecal coliforms as a subgroup within the general category of coliforms, is encouraging. The United States Environmental Protection Agency (EPA) proposed in 1973 that acceptable limitations for water to be used directly by livestock should not exceed 5000 coliforms/100 ml, and the monthly arithmetic density of fecal coliforms should not exceed 1000 coliforms/100 ml.[1] Many believe, however, that as long as animals are allowed to range freely and drink surface waters, these proposed limits would be unenforceable and of doubtful value.

The standard plate count, which enumerates the number of bacteria multiplying at 35°C, is of questionable significance in evaluating livestock water sources other than in helping to judge the efficiency of various water treatment processes.

HARDNESS

Water hardness has been understood to indicate the tendency of water to precipitate soap or to form scale on heated surfaces. Hardness is generally expressed as the sum of calcium and magnesium concentrations reported in equivalent amounts of calcium carbonate. Hardness is sometimes confused with salinity, but the two are not necessarily correlated. Waters containing high levels of sodium salts and therefore having high salinity can be very soft if they contain low levels of calcium and magnesium. Most ground waters generally have hardness values of less than 2000 mg/L, but in some arid regions these values may be higher. Hardness, sometimes reported as grains per gallon (1 grain per gallon = 17.1

mg/L), is in itself not a problem in livestock drinking water.

SALINITY

Salinity is defined as the total concentration of solids in water after all carbonates have been converted to oxides, all bromides and iodides have been replaced by chloride, and all organic matter has been oxidized. In more general terms, salinity is an expression of the amount of dissolved salts in a particular water sample. The ions most commonly involved in highly saline waters are calcium, magnesium, and sodium in the bicarbonate, chloride, or sulfate form.

The general recommendations for the use of saline water for livestock are presented in Table 1.

TOXIC ELEMENTS

A number of elements found in water seldom offer any problem to livestock because they do not occur at high levels in soluble form or because they are toxic only in excessive concentrations. Examples of these are iron, aluminum, beryllium, boron, chromium, cobalt, copper, iodide, manganese, molybdenum, and zinc. Also, these elements do not seem to accumulate in meat, milk, or eggs to the extent that they would constitute a problem in livestock drinking waters under any but the most unusual conditions. Proposed acceptable limits for these elements in livestock water are presented in Table 2.

Because arsenic, cadmium, fluorine, lead, mercury, and selenium may under some circumstances present a hazard to livestock, these elements should be evaluated on an individual case basis.

NITRATE AND NITRITE

The nitrate ion (NO_3^-) is both a product and a reactant in the chain of animal and plant nitrogen metabolism. The nitrate ion can be reduced to form the nitrite ion (NO_2^-). Decaying animal or plant protein, animal meta-

Table 1. *A Guide to the Use of Saline Waters for Livestock**

Total Soluble Salt Content of Water (mg/L)	Comments
Less than 1000	A relatively low level of salinity with no serious burden for any class of livestock.
1000–2999	Satisfactory for all classes of livestock. They may cause temporary and mild diarrhea in livestock not accustomed to them, but should not affect health or performance.
3000–4999	Satisfactory for livestock, although they might cause temporary diarrhea or refusal at first by animals not accustomed to them.
5000–6999	Reasonably safe for dairy and beef cattle, sheep, swine, and horses. It may be well to avoid the use of those with higher levels for pregnant or lactating animals.
7000–10,000	Probably unfit for swine. Considerable risk may exist in using them for pregnant or lactating cows, horses, sheep, the young of these species, or for any animals subjected to heavy heat stress or water loss. In general, their use should be avoided, although older ruminants, horses, and even swine may subsist on them for long periods under conditions of low stress.
More than 10,000	The risks with these highly saline waters are so great that they cannot be recommended for use under any conditions.

*Adapted from NAS Subcommittee on Nutrient and Toxic Elements in Water: Nutrients and toxic substances in water for livestock and poultry. Washington, D.C.: National Academy of Sciences, 1974.

Table 2. *Recommended Limits of Concentration of Some Potentially Toxic Substances in Drinking Water for Livestock*

	Safe Upper Limit of Concentration (mg/L)		
Element	U.S. EPA[9] (for humans)	U.S. EPA[1] (for livestock)	NAS[10] (for livestock)
Aluminum		5.0	
Arsenic	0.05	0.2	0.2
Barium	1.0		NE*
Beryllium		No limit*	
Boron		5.0	
Cadmium	0.01	0.05	0.05
Chromium	0.05	1.0	1.0
Cobalt		1.0	1.0
Copper		0.5	0.5
Fluoride		2.0	2.0
Iron		No limit	NE
Lead	0.05	0.1	0.1
Manganese		No limit	NE
Mercury	0.002	0.001	0.01
Molybdenum		No limit	NE
Nickel			1.0
Nitrate	45	100	440
Nitrite		33	33
Selenium	0.01	0.05	
Vanadium		0.1	0.1
Zinc		25.0	25.0

*Not established as no limit. Experimental data available are not sufficient to make definite recommendations.

bolic waste (urea and ammonia), nitrogen fertilizers, silage juices, and soil high in nitrogen-fixing bacteria may be sources of nitrates and nitrites. Nitrates and nitrites are water soluble and thus if added to soil may be leached away, moving with the ground water into the water table. The likelihood of high levels of nitrate contamination to a well or reservoir is much greater when the source of the nitrate is nearby. The most common source of contamination to wells is surface water runoff into shallow, poorly cased wells. Ponded water that collects feedlot or fertilizer runoff may contain toxic levels of nitrates.

Levels of nitrates in water may be expressed in a number of ways. Each of these expressions can be converted to the other (Table 3). One must be cognizant of these distinctions when evaluating laboratory data.

The nitrate ion itself is not particularly toxic. However, nitrite, the reduced form of nitrate, is readily absorbed and is quite toxic. Ruminants and herbivores can readily reduce nitrate to nitrite, and toxicosis may occur. The nitrite ion oxidizes the ferrous ion in hemoglobin to the ferric (trivalent) state, forming methemoglobin, which cannot accept molecular oxygen. The result is tissue hypoxia or anoxia due to poorly oxygenated blood.

Acute nitrate poisoning in animals may be expected when nitrates exceed 500 mg/L in the water or 1.0-per cent nitrate (dry weight basis) in the forage.[2] One report[3] indicates that water containing 2000 mg/L nitrate can be fed at 10-per cent of body weight to cattle for as long as 17 days with no indication of acute toxic effects. However, 3000 mg/L given to cattle for 3 days resulted in death from acute nitrate poisoning.

The effects of feed and water nitrate levels are additive, and both must therefore be considered when evaluating a potential nitrate problem.

The EPA maximum limit for nitrate in water that is to be used for preparation of human baby formula is 45 mg/L and is set to prevent the methemoglobinemia or "blue baby" syndrome. It has been suggested that neonatal swine are also quite susceptible to elevated levels of nitrates, but Emerick[4] and associates have concluded that pigs 1-week old are no more susceptible to nitrate-induced methemoglobinemia than older pigs.

The experimental reproduction of chronic or low level nitrate poisoning syndrome in animals has been extensively reviewed.[5–8] The bulk of the evidence indicates that sublethal or chronic effects are extremely rare and difficult to verify. When present, the clinical signs usually reflect a lowered degree of acute toxicosis. Even in view of these findings, however, moderate levels of nitrate in water continue to be incriminated in several animal health problems. Among these are poor growth rate, abortion, infertility, vitamin A deficiency, interference with iodine metabolism, and greater susceptibility to infection. Experimental evidence to substantiate many of these claims is lacking.

PESTICIDES

Pesticides enter water from soil runoff, drift, infall, direct application, accidental spills, or faulty waste disposal techniques. Concern is frequently raised regarding the effects of these waterborne pesticides on livestock. In general, however, there are not sufficient data available, considering the great number of pesticides, the variability of species response, and the dilution of factors usually present, to make hard and fast recommendations on allowable limits for livestock water.

The EPA[9] has, however, set maximum allowable concentrations of several pesticides in human drinking water (Table 4), but data are insufficient at this time to establish

Table 3. *Nitrate and Nitrite Expressions and Conversion Factors for Converting from One Expression to Another**

	Form B				
Form A	N	NO_2^-	NO_3^-	KNO_3	$NaNO_3$
Nitrate-nitrogen (N)	1.0	3.3	4.4	7.2	6.1
Nitrite-nitrogen (N)	1.0	3.3	4.4	7.2	6.1
Nitrate (NO_3^-)	0.23	0.74	1.0	1.63	1.37
Nitrite (NO_2^-)	0.3	1.0	1.34	2.2	1.85
Potassium nitrate (KNO_3)	0.14	0.64	0.61	1.0	0.84
Sodium nitrate ($NaNO_3$)	0.16	0.54	0.72	1.2	1.0

*To convert Form A to the equivalent amount of Form B, multiply A by the appropriate conversion factor: (Form A × Conversion Factor = Form B).

Table 4. *Maximum Allowable Concentrations of Pesticides in Human Drinking Water*

Pesticide	Maximum Concentration (mg/L)
Aldrin	0.001
DDT	0.05
Dieldrin	0.001
Chlordane	0.003
Endrin	0.0002
Heptachlor	0.0001
Heptachlor epoxide	0.0001
Lindane	0.004
Methoxychlor	0.1
Toxaphene	0.005
2,4–D	0.1
2,4,5–T	0.01

limits for organophosphorus insecticides in potable water.

In animal husbandry, it is sometimes easy to incriminate the water as the cause of poor performance and nonspecific disease conditions in livestock. It is imperative that attempts to evaluate water quality in the face of animal health problems include obtaining a thorough history, making astute observations, and asking intelligent questions. A thorough laboratory examination of animal specimens and water samples should be evaluated in view of existing standards for livestock water quality.

References

1. United States Environmental Protection Agency: Proposed criteria for water quality. I. Quality of water for livestock. Environ. Rep. 4:663, 1973.
2. Buck, W. B., Osweiler, G. D., and VanGelder, G. A.: Clinical and Diagnostic Veterinary Toxicology, 2nd ed. Dubuque, Iowa, Kendall/Hunt Publishing Co., 1976.
3. Dollahite, J. W., and Rowe, L. D.: Nitrate and nitrite intoxication in rabbits and cattle. Southwest.Vet. 27:246, 1974.
4. Emerick, R., Embry, L. B., and Seerly, R. W.: Rate of formation and reduction of nitrate induced methemogloblin in vitro and in vivo as influenced by diet of sheep and age of swine. J. Anim. Sci. 24:221–230, 1965.
5. Emerick, R. J.: Consequences of high nitrate levels in food and water supplies. Fed. Proc. 33:1183, 1974.
6. Murdock, F. R., Hodgson, A. S., and Baker, A. S.: Utilization of nitrates by dairy cows. J. Dairy Sci. 55:640, 1972.
7. Ridder, W. E. and Oehme, F. W.: Nitrates as an environmental, animal, and human hazard. Clin. Toxicol. 7:145, 1974.
8. Turner, C. A., and Kienholz, E. W.: Nitrate toxicity. Feedstuffs. 44:28–30, 1972.
9. United States Environmental Protection Agency: Primary drinking water proposed interim standards. Fed. Reg. 40:11990, 1975.
10. National Academy of Sciences Subcommittee on Nutrient and Toxic Elements in Water: Nutrients and toxic substances in water for livestock and poultry. Washington, D.C., National Academy of Sciences, 1974.
11. National Academy of Sciences Safe Drinking Water Committee, Advisory Center on Toxicology: Drinking water and health. Washington, D.C., National Academy of Sciences, 1977.

Toxicants in Geothermal Waters, Cooling Waters, and in Mine Tailings*

J. L. SHUPE, D.V.M.,
H.B. PETERSON, Ph.D.,
and A. E. OLSON, M.S.

Animals may be exposed to many naturally produced, artificially manufactured, and elusive toxic substances. Some so-called toxicants or pollutants (in proper amounts) are essential for animal health and growth. Major sources of these toxic or potentially toxic agents for animals, both domestic and wild, are water, soil, volcanic dusts, and vegetation. Toxins also exist in industrial wastes, rodenticides, insecticides, fungicides, herbicides, feed additives, fertilizers, biotoxins, emissions from internal combustion engines, and by-products from the commercial conversion and public use of energy.

As human populations grow, so do the numbers and complexities of toxicologic problems. These problems are

usually not induced by just one factor, but frequently by a representation of a combination of factors, sometimes from multiple sources. The nature of this complexity is illustrated in Figure 1. The potential additive or synergistic influence of a combination of toxicants from multiple sources is a major concern.

The health of animals in industralized societies is influenced by numerous interactions among the physical, chemical, biologic, and social components of their environment. One way to estimate and evaluate such interactions and their effects on animals consists of identifying the toxicants or pollutants and determining their environmental pathways, ecological aspects, and health effects. This is particularly important with the ever-increasing demand for new sources of energy (e.g., geothermal waters and coal-conversion plants), mining and smelting operations, and related industries.

COMPOSITION

Geothermal Waters

Geothermal waters are usually contaminated with some elements of underground origin. The concentrations of these elements may vary from a few hundred mg/L to many thousands mg/L. The most common elements or combinations of elements are sodium, potassium, lithium, calcium, magnesium, ammonium, silica, chloride, fluoride, borate, sulfate, carbonate, bicarbonate, hydrogen sulfide, and carbon dioxide. Other common elements of particular toxicologic concern include arsenic, molybdenum, selenium, and heavy metals. Of the potential toxicants, fluorides are the ones most often present in toxic concentrations.

These toxic or potentially toxic substances may occur as suspended solids, in solution, or in combination. These substances may be accessible to livestock in drinking water or after application to forage crops via irrigation water.

Cooling Waters

When electricity is generated by use of fossil fuels, it is necessary to utilize water for effluent cooling and cleaning. It is customary to repeatedly cycle the water through cooling and scrubbing towers. The recycling concentrates the soluble constituents. Any potential pollutant or toxic substance may thus be concentrated perhaps 5 to 20 times. For example, source water safe for consumption with 0.2 mg/L fluoride may contain 2 to 4 mg/L fluoride as effluent water. Animals may drink the effluent water or eat forage that has been contaminated by sprinkler-irrigated effluent water.

Tailings

Tailings are finely ground rock and minerals that have been processed to remove desirable ores. Tailings differ greatly in their physical and chemical characteristics. The variability may be influenced by the type of mining operation, composition of the ore body, amounts of pyrites present, type of milling process, and the composition of the water used to transport the tailings to the tailing pile. Excessive concentrations of soluble salts are often present in many tailings. The toxicants may be leached out of tailing piles into animal drinking water supplies.

*Published with the approval of the Utah State University Agricultural Experiment Station, Logan, Utah, as Journal Paper No. 2881.

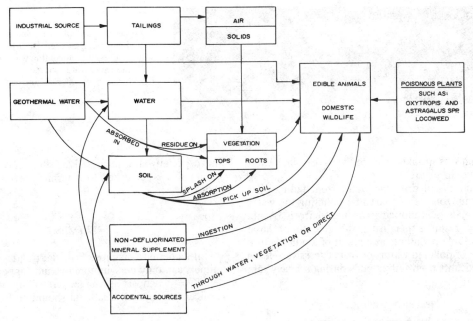

Figure 1. Possible routes of toxicants in geothermal waters and in mine tailings.

Tailing piles, which are poor sustainers of vegetation, do not act like normal agricultural soils. They are normally low in water-holding capacity, devoid of plant nutrients, and subject to wind erosion. The wind erosion of a tailing pile may contaminate nearby forage crops with particulate toxic materials.

Most mine tailing materials contain many kinds of sulfides that, when oxidized, form acids, lower the pH, and increase the amount of soluble heavy metals. The relation between pH and soluble heavy metals is illustrated by the data in Table 1. Drainage waters from waste piles having low pH values could pollute a water supply for animals. The hazard of pollution with heavy metals therefore is greater as the tailing waters age by oxidation. Molybdenum compounds, if present, are more soluble at near neutral pH. Drainage pollution is greater from waste piles of pH 6 to 8 than from acid piles. As illustrated in Figure 1, animals may obtain pollutants from routes other than directly from contaminated water.

COMPLEXITY OF PROBLEM

One only has to visualize the many variables and their possible interactions to realize the extreme complexity and potential hazards of utilizing for livestock geothermal waters, industrial cooling or effluent waters, or water exposed to mine tailings.

Little information has been obtained under rigid experimental conditions about the effects of the amounts of different combinations of chemical elements in drinking water and feed. Some elements may be either antagonistic or synergistic to the other elements present in feeds, water supplies, or even mineral supplements. All of these interrelationships need to be considered and determined insofar as possible when investigating an actual or potential toxicosis.

Digestion processes may markedly alter the availability of certain chemicals to an animal. Other factors that should also be evaluated are duration of intake (short-term compared to long-term), effects on young or healthy animals compared to effects on mature or unhealthy animals, rate of water consumption, composition of diet, physiologic demands, and how differences among species and other factors may be affecting potential toxicities.

Based on past experience and present knowledge, the many variables and possible interactions involved make it difficult—if not impossible—to determine exact critical toxic levels of many of these chemical combinations.

DIAGNOSIS

Clinical Signs

Every available means of obtaining an accurate differential diagnosis should be utilized. In many cases, much effort and laboratory assistance will be required to support or substantiate a tentative clinical diagnosis. A complete history, including changes in management, recent storms, recent access to new range areas or water sources, and other possible factors, is necessary; all factors should be considered and studied. Close observation of live animals may lead to a positive diagnosis. Bovine dental fluorosis induced by prolonged consumption of geothermal water

***Table 1.** Analysis of Water Extracts of Tailings Materials**

Sample Source	pH Extract	Concentration of Saturation Extract (mg/L)				
		Cu	Fe	Mn	Zn	Pb
Copper tailings						
New Mexico	2.2	>600	3000	21	21	< 5
Montana	7.6	< 1	< 0.5	0.6	0.2	< 5
Uranium tailings						
Utah	1.9	>600	>5000	1005	77	30
Colorado	8	< 1	< 0.5	< 0.2	0.2	< 5

*Each material was wet to saturation, and the water was extracted by suction. Determination of the content was made with a Jarrell-Ash Direct Reading Spectrophotometer.

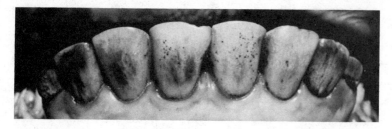

Figure 2. Permanent bovine incisor teeth with dental fluorosis induced by drinking geothermal water and eating forage that was sprinkle-irrigated with the same water source. Note chalkiness and discoloration of enamel and bilateral nature of lesions.

and forage that was sprinkle-irrigated with the same water source is shown in Figure 2.

Limited amounts of drainage water from tailing piles may be constant sources of toxicants, polluting the water supply of animals, and inducing chronic toxicosis. Acute toxicosis may result either from the release of large amounts of soluble pollutants as a result of a pond failure and discharge of polluted waters or from excessive release of soluble toxicants from tailing piles during a heavy rain or flood.

Necropsy Findings

If animals have died or have been sacrificed, a complete necropsy should be performed. If toxicoses of any specific type are suspected, lesions reflecting those toxicoses should certainly be sought. Any lesion should be noted, however, because of the many possibilities of lesion mimicry, toxicant interaction, or other causes of death. Tissues and specimens should be properly collected for chemical, microbiologic, and histologic evaluations. It is important to properly correlate the clinical signs and lesions prior to making a diagnosis. Assumptions should never be based merely upon casual observations. The animals themselves are the best indicators of their own state of health, and it behooves the clinician to accurately observe and evaluate each animal's clinical signs and lesions.

Laboratory Findings

Every possible effort should be made to have clinical and necropsy findings substantiated by reliable laboratory personnel.

Animal tissues, particularly those primarily involved in detoxification, such as liver and kidney, should be sampled and examined. Gastrointestinal contents and lesions may be most helpful in determining the presence or absence of many toxic elements and in diagnosing the causes. Lymph nodes are important as filters and should be examined. Body fluids, both blood and urine, should be examined as to color, physical characteristics, and chemical content.

Because of the expense involved in complete chemical analyses for some elements and chemicals, diligent efforts should be made, based on history, clinical signs, and lesions, to selectively limit the scope of the laboratory tests to those toxicants most likely involved in given cases. Some special cases, however, may warrant extensive chemical analysis and laboratory testing.

In addition to tests of animal tissues, all possible sources of toxic substances should be considered and checked when indicated. All possible drinking water supplies, forage or other feed sources, and mineral supplements should be analyzed for suspected toxicants. Soil samples, and especially any mine tailings that may be involved, should also be analyzed to determine levels of suspected toxicants.

TREATMENT

Until a definite diagnosis is made, treatment of affected animals can only be symptomatic and supportive. After a definitive diagnosis is made, prevailing recommended medical therapy and treatment should be followed.

PREVENTION

The most practical approach to preventing or alleviating future toxicologic problems may vary, depending on the situation's total perspective. The major objective is to prevent or limit the access of animals to the toxicant's source. Animals may be totally removed from the source or replaced with animal species less susceptible to the particular toxicant involved.

If animals must be exposed to environmental toxicants, then all possible effort should be made to eliminate other stresses on those animals. If animals must drink geothermal waters with high fluoride content, they should be fed roughage with low fluoride content. In areas of low temperatures, geothermal water should not be used even though the animals prefer it to cold water. There should be adequate feed of good quality to preclude overgrazing. This will be particularly helpful when the offending elements are in abundance in the soil or in the tailing piles. Overgrazing promotes ingestion of large quantities of soil with the feed. Also, the roots and crowns of the vegetation may hold particularly high concentrations of heavy metals.

Providing adequate and balanced mineral supplementation is important when either tailings or geothermal waters are involved. Either source may contain some of the essential mineral elements required for good health, but the hazards of also ingesting excessive detrimental amounts of other unwanted toxic elements are too great to risk. Depraved mineral appetites or salt hunger may induce animals to ingest toxic quantities of undesirable compounds.

Efforts should be made to cultivate tailing areas with vegetation to prevent wind or water erosion of these tailings into water supplies or onto forage crops. Vegetation planted on these areas, however, should be unpalatable to livestock. Such plant species should be left to flourish and thereby hold the tailings together, since animals will not be likely to graze in the hazardous areas.

It might also be wise to look at alternative land uses for areas where toxic elements in the soil create hazards for livestock. Other productive agricultural uses may be made of such land. The area, if properly managed, may have recreation potential with complete removal of livestock.

If the area in question is suited only for livestock grazing, then certain practices should be adopted. Animals should certainly be fenced away from known toxic sites and toxic water supplies. Avoid overgrazing and be aware of what sudden heavy rainfalls can do, especially in more arid areas, to normal soil conditions and to limited water supplies.

More knowledge and concern is needed relative to the possible effects of exposure of livestock to all the combinations of chemicals in their environment. Chronic toxicosis of a subtle insidious nature is often more difficult to diagnose and has greater economic importance than the more alarming and publicized acute toxicosis. The concerns and warnings that have been given here regarding potential toxicants in geothermal waters and mine tailings could also apply to many other toxicants that are not properly handled and managed. Today, there is an urgent need for proper interpretation of existing information, as well as the development of essential data regarding the effects of the combination or interaction of toxicants under conditions that would simulate (as closely as possible) field conditions. Preventive measures are more important than curative procedures in most cases of toxicoses induced by geothermal or industrial cooling waters and mine tailings.

Supplemental Reading

Biological implications of metals in the environment. Proceedings of the Fifteenth Annual Hanford Life Sciences Symposium, Richland, Washington, 1975.
Buck, W. B., Osweiler, G. D., and Van Gelder, G. A.: Clinical and Diagnostic Veterinary Toxicology, 2nd ed. Dubuque, Iowa, Kendall/Hunt Publishing Co., 1976.
Coles, E. H.: Veterinary Clinical Pathology, 2nd ed. Philadelphia, W. B. Saunders Company, 1974.
Geochemistry and the Environment, vol. 1. The Relation of Selected Trace Elements to Health and Disease. Washington, D.C.: National Academy of Sciences, 1974.
Hibbs, C. M., and Thilstead, J. P.: Toxicosis in cattle from contaminated well water. Vet. Hum. Toxicol. 23:253–254, 1983.
International Conference on Heavy Metals. vols 1, 2, 3. Toronto, Ontario, Canada, 1975.
Lead-airborne lead in perspective. In Biological Effects of Atmospheric Pollutants. Washington, D.C., National Academy of Sciences and National Research Council, 1972.
Oehme, F. W.: Toxicity of Heavy Metals in the Environment. parts 1 and 2. New York, Dekker, 1978–1979.
Peterson, H. B., and Nielson, R. F.: Toxicities and Deficiencies in Mine Tailings. Ecology and Reclamation of Devastated Land. vol 1. New York, Gordon and Beach Co., 15–25, 1973.
Peterson, H. B., and Shupe, J. L.: Problems of Managing Geothermal Waters for Irrigation. Proceedings of the International Salinity Conference, Lubbock, Texas, Texas Technical University, 211–219, 1976.
Peterson, H. B., and Nielson, R. F.: Heavy Metals in Relation to Plant Growth on Mine and Mill Wastes. Environmental Management of Mineral Wastes. Alphen aan den Rijn, The Netherlands, Sigthoff and Noordhoff, 297–309, 1978.
Principles for Evaluating Chemicals in the Environment. Washington, D.C., National Academy of Sciences, 1975.
Radeleff, R. D.: Veterinary Toxicology, 2nd ed. Philadelphia, Lea & Febiger, 1970.
Shupe, J. L.: Diagnosis of fluorosis in cattle. In Fourth International Meeting of the World Association for Buiatrics. publ. no. 4, Zurich, Switzerland, 15–30, 1967.
Shupe, J. L.: Fluorine toxicosis and industry. Am. Ind. Hyg. Assoc. J. 31:240–247, 1970.
Shupe, J. L., Peterson, H. B., and Olson, A. E.: Inorganic Toxicants and Poisonous Plants. Effects of Poisonous Plants on Livestock. New York, Academic Press, 35–36, 1978.
Smith, H. A., Hanes, T. C., and Hunt, R. D.: Veterinary Pathology, 4th ed. Philadelphia, Lea & Febiger, 1972.
The relation of selected trace elements to health and disease. In Geochemistry and the Environment. vol 1. Washington, D.C., National Academy of Sciences and National Research Council, 1974.
Trace Substances in Environmental Health—VII. Proceedings of University of Missouri's 7th Annual Conference on Trace Substances in Environmental Health. Columbia, Missouri, University of Missouri, 1973.
Underwood, E. J.: Trace Elements in Human and Animal Nutrition, 3rd ed. New York, Academic Press, 1971.

Poisonous Plants in Harvested or Prepared Feeds

MURRAY E. FOWLER, D.V.M.

Hundreds of plants are potentially toxic to cattle, sheep, goats, and swine. Only a few are likely to be found in harvested feeds. However, many livestock producers now buy feed from commercial growers, thus having minimal control over feed quality. With modern methods of feed preparation (grinding, pelleting, and cubing) it may be impossible to detect or prevent the inclusion of poisonous plants unless quality control is rigidly practiced from the field of forage to the feeding of the animal.

Agricultural regulations are designed to maintain quality standards for grains, hays, and mixed feeds entering into commercial trade. It is illegal to sell hay in California that is known to contain poisonous or deleterious substances. This is likely to be the case in most states. Yet hay has been sold in California containing as much as 80 per cent common groundsel, Senecio vulgaris, with a pyrrolizidine alkaloid content of approximately 0.08 per cent.

In spite of legal action, it has been extremely difficult for the livestock owners to realize compensation for losses. To date, the only protection an animal feeder has is to buy hay and other prepared feeds from a reliable source.

POISONOUS PLANTS FOUND IN PREPARED FEEDS

Table 1 lists some of the more important poisonous plants or biotoxins likely to be found in feeds in the United States. Many more plant species may be found in feed grown in a particular local area, so the list is far from exhaustive. A discussion of a few of these plants may serve to illustrate some of the types of problems that arise.

Table 1. *Plant Toxicants in Harvested or Prepared Feeds*

Nitrates (numerous species including sorghum)
Cyanides (*Sorghum* spp., *Triglochin martima*)
Pyrrolizidine alkaloids (*Senecio* spp., *Amsinckia* spp., *Crotalaria* spp.)
Mycotoxins
Oleander (*Nerium oleander*)
Milkweeds (*Asclepias* spp.)
Nightshades (*Solanum* spp.)
Tree tobacco (*Nicotiana glauca*)
Sweet peas (*Lathyrus* sp.)
Jimson weed seed (*Datura* spp.)

MYCOTOXINS

Diagnosis of mycotoxicosis is becoming more and more common as sophisticated diagnostic tests are developed. Mycotoxins are produced by molds that are most likely to develop maximally on improperly stored feeds. Feed producers and animal feeders must be continually alert to guard against mold contamination of feeds. Some states are now screening livestock feeds for the presence of mycotoxins. This trend is likely to continue.

NITRATE ACCUMULATOR PLANTS

Nitrite poisoning caused by the ingestion of excessive nitrates is a serious problem in ruminants, particularly cattle. Harvested and prepared feeds are a common source of excessive nitrates. From an economic viewpoint, nitrite poisoning may be the most important plant poisoning problem involving harvested forages. Unfortunately, some important forage crops tend to accumulate nitrates when pushed for maximal production with heavy fertilization.

Sudan grass (Sorghum vulgare var. sudanensis) may be involved with both cyanide and nitrite poisoning. Nitrite poisoning is the more likely to occur because of the amount of nitrogen applied to the soil in order to obtain maximum yields. Sudan grass is fed as green chop or as hay. In either form, accumulated nitrates may cause poisoning under certain conditions.

Stocker cattle and growing stock are frequently at risk. Generally, poor quality hays are fed to these animals, and supplements are rarely added. In 1 instance 18 of 20 heifers died from nitrite poisoning after being fed a weedy "hay" consisting of 90 per cent lambsquarter, Chemopodium album. The "hay" contained 6 per cent KNO_3.

In this regard it is important to recognize that well-nourished cattle can tolerate higher levels of nitrate in the diet than poorly nourished cattle. Healthy animals may consume 2 to 5 per cent nitrate for a short period without apparent ill effects if the ration is also high in carbohydrates and complete protein.

Truck-garden trimmings (lettuce, celery, broccoli) may contain high amounts of nitrates. Many forage crops and weeds are capable of accumulating nitrates under special circumstances.

CYANIDE POISONING

Cyanide toxicosis is generally seen in pastured ruminants. Cyanogenic glycosides are volatile, so that drying usually renders the forage nontoxic. There are, however, 2 situations in which cattle, sheep, or goats may be poisoned with cyanide in harvested feeds. The first is the feeding of green chop. If sudan grass or sorghum is fed as green chop in the fall after frost or early in the season before frost ends, the harvested feed may contain toxic levels of cyanide.

Arrow grass (Triglochin maritima) grows in wet meadows that may be harvested for hay. The glycoside in this plant is not detoxified during the drying process.

Differentiation between nitrate and cyanide toxicosis is crucial as antidotes for cyanide poisoning exacerbate nitrate toxicity. A venous blood sample provides a quick, accurate test. The venous blood from an animal with cyanide toxicity is bright red while that of an animal with nitrate toxicity is dark or even brownish in color.

PYRROLIZIDINE ALKALOIDS

Pyrrolizidine alkaloid toxicosis is described in the article on hepatotoxic plants. Pyrrolizidine alkaloids are produced by 5 or 6 plant species, but only 2 species occur frequently in harvested feeds: fiddleneck or fireweed (Amsinckia intermedia) and common groundsel (Senecio vulgaris). Both of these plants are weeds of hay fields, growing in California and possibly other states. New plantings of alfalfa may be overgrown with weeds. The first cutting may contain 10 to 50 per cent weeds. Alfalfa stands weakened by heavy infestations of weevils may may also allow weeds to take over. Oat hay may also be contaminated with these weeds.

Both plants are readily identifiable in baled hay, but it is virtually impossible to ascertain the presence of the poisonous plant in weedy hay that is cubed or pelleted (not an uncommon practice). The fact that the clinical signs of pyrrolizidine alkaloid poisoning do not appear until 2 to 8 months after ingestion complicates correlation of plant consumption and disease. This delay in effect again stresses the importance for the feeder to know the source of harvested feeds.

The seeds of fiddleneck and crotalaria (Crotalaria spp.) are a concentrated source of the alkaloid. Swine and poultry have been poisoned when fed screenings containing weed seeds.

OLEANDER POISONING

Oleander is a popular ornamental plant and may border hay fields. The plant is extremely toxic, and high mortality may occur when hay containing dropped leaves or plant trimmings is fed to livestock.

MILKWEED POISONING

Plants of the genus Asclepias contain toxic resins and glycosides. These plants may be found in harvested hays and are toxic in the fresh or dry state. Milkweeds are cosmopolitan in distribution throughout the United States. Different species have different habitats, but all must be considered to be potentially poisonous. The clinical syndrome associated with milkweed poisoning may involve the gastrointestinal system or the nervous system.

LATHYRISM

Lathyrism is a rare disease that is periodically reported in various areas of the United States. Lathyrism is caused by dipeptides in plants of the genus Lathyrus, resulting in posterior spinal cord neuronal degeneration. Lathyrism in humans was recognized before the birth of Christ and still occurs in areas of the world where pulses are the staple diet. Ornamental sweet peas, caley peas or rough peas are species of Lathyrus, which are leguminous plants closely related to and sometimes confused with vetch, Vicia sp.

In one instance, a field had been planted with what was assumed to be vetch. The plants grew and were cut and baled as vetch hay. Cattle and horses fed the "vetch" hay for 2 to 3 weeks developed neurolathyrism. The clinical syndrome approximates the "tying up" syndrome of horses. Animals have a stilted gait. The center of gravity is pushed forward over the front legs giving the appearance that the animal is balancing on the front legs and using the hind legs to move forward in short mincing steps. The muscles over the back, rump, and hind legs are *not* hot, swollen, or painful, differentiating this condition from "tying up" syndrome.

Animals removed from the hay soon after being affected may return to normal. Continued ingestion of *Lathyrus* results in permanent neuronal damage and posterior paresis. No specific treatment is known.

Fescue Toxicosis (Summer Syndrome)

DUANE MIKSCH, D.V.M., M.S.
and GARRY LACEFIELD, M.S., Ph.D.

Tall fescue (*Festuca arundinacea* Schreb.) is grown on approximately 35 million acres in the south central United States. It is a versatile plant used for livestock feed, lawn, turf, and conservation purposes. Tall fescue is a long-lived grass that is adapted to a wide range of soil and climatic conditions. It is relatively easy to establish and tolerant of poor grazing management. Tall fescue compares favorably to other transition zone grasses for chemical components that reflect forage quality. However, animal performance from grazing tall fescue has been erratic and frequently less than acceptable.

"Summer syndrome" and "fescue toxicosis" are terms that have been widely used to denote poor animal performance by cattle grazing tall fescue during summer. Characteristic of this condition are reduced feed intake, decreased rate of gain or milk production or both, rough hair coat, rapid breathing, increased body temperature, and general unthriftiness. This condition has been shown to be associated with an endophytic fungus.

THE ENDOPHYTE OF TALL FESCUE

Case History

In June 1973, Dr. Joe Robbins, USDA, Athens, Georgia, visited the farm of Mr. A. E. Hays, Mansfield, Georgia. The Hays farm consisted of fescue pastures being grazed by 2 separate herds of Angus cattle. One herd exhibited nearly all the signs associated with summer syndrome. The herd in an adjacent fescue pasture had no signs of the summer syndrome. Mr. Hays had kept the herds separated in their respective pastures for 10 years.

After making the observations at the Hays farm, Dr. Robbins and colleagues, Drs. C. W. Bacon and J. K. Porter, hypothesized that a fungus was involved in the toxic syndrome and began to examine the plants for fungi. Most of the research team's efforts were concentrated on external fungi until they became aware of work by J. C. Neil in New Zealand. Neil, in 1941, published results of his work showing that fescue is subject to infection

with an endophyte (a plant living within a plant). The endophyte of tall fescue is a fungus, *Acremonium coenophialum*.

Dr. Bacon examined fescue from the toxic areas of the Hays farm in 1976 and found it to be 100 per cent infected with the endophyte, whereas the nontoxic pasture was only 10 per cent infected. Samples of fescue from toxic and nontoxic pastures in Kentucky, Maryland, Missouri, and Virginia were collected and analyzed for the endophyte. Samples from toxic pastures were all infected while nontoxic samples had an infection rate of less than 50 per cent.

ANIMAL PERFORMANCE

Animals consuming fescue containing the endophyte have demonstrated lower feed intake, weight gain, and milk production. Higher respiration rate, rectal temperature, and water consumption are also indications of fescue consumption. Rough hair coat, more time spent in shade, more salivation, greater urine volume, reduced serum prolactin levels, lowered reproductive performance, and greater nervousness compared to animals consuming non-infected fescue are observed. Some or all of these responses have been present in dairy cattle, beef cattle, and sheep consuming endophyte-infected pasture, green chop, hay, and seed.

Research done at the University of Kentucky revealed a 39 per cent reduction in forage intake and a 37 per cent reduction in milk production during summer in lactating dairy cows consuming endophyte-infected fescue. Cows consuming endophyte-infected fescue lost weight while cows consuming noninfected fescue gained weight. Similar results have been found in grazing studies with beef cattle. Initial grazing studies at Auburn University showed an increase in beef production of 185 lb (84 kg)/acre with a 0.83 lb (0.377 kg) increase in average daily gain (ADG) with endophyte-free fescue. Trials at the University of Kentucky showed ADG for animals grazing fescue containing high levels of endophyte was 0.81 lb (0.368 kg)/day, while the ADG for animals consuming fescue containing low levels of endophyte was 1.37 lbs (0.623 kg)/day. Johnstone (a newly released low-endophyte variety) resulted in a 0.97 lbs (0.44 kg)/day increase in ADG over KY 31 (an endophyte-infected variety). Animals grazing endophyte-infected fescue showed typical "summer syndrome" symptoms, while animals consuming low-endophyte fescue remained healthy. Studies at Auburn University and the University of Kentucky have also shown higher intake and daily gains and lower body temperatures of steers consuming endophyte-free seed or hay when compared with endophyte-infected seed or hay. Preliminary work in Kentucky showed a 19 per cent increase in conception rate in beef cows grazing noninfected fescue compared with beef cows grazing highly infected fescue.

Fescue toxicosis symptoms are not obvious during winter. Animal performance, however, is reduced in cattle consuming infected forage. Endophyte-infected forage fed year round may have an accumulative effect.

CHARACTERISTICS OF THE ENDOPHYTE

A majority of established fescue is infected to some degree with the endophyte. Surveys in Kentucky and Alabama showed more than 95 per cent of tall fescue pastures were infected. Spread of the fungus occurs slowly.

The endophyte grows between the plant cells, overwintering in the perennial parts of the plant. In spring, fungus growth closely parallels tiller growth. Fungal hyphae have not been detected in roots or leaf blades but have been found in the leaf sheath. The primary method (and perhaps the only method) of transmitting the fungus is through infected seed.

A cause-effect relationship between the endophyte and a toxic component has not been proved conclusively. The endophyte has been shown to be associated with the occurrence of pyrrolizidine alkaloids in tall fescue. These alkaloids have been related to the summer syndrome condition.

Workers at the University of Missouri developed an ion-exchange chromotography method in which the chemical constituents of toxic fescue were separated into a fraction (anion) that produces fescue foot and a fraction (cation) that produces summer syndrome. The "anion fraction" contains plant and fungal organic acids, whereas the "cation fraction" contains plant and fungal alkaloids. Additional studies are needed to isolate a chemical or chemicals responsible for toxicity and to determine the interrelationships among host plant, endophyte, toxic compound, animal, and environment.

CONTROL OF THE ENDOPHYTE

Release of new varieties of tall fescue, along with selection within currently available varieties, is providing low-endophyte seed for new plantings. Johnstone, a new tall fescue variety, contains low alkaloid and low-endophyte. This variety has shown excellent results in grazing and performance trials. Other new varieties include AU Triumph, Forager, and MO–96. Selection within the Kenhy variety has resulted in low-endophyte seed.

A seed certification program has been implemented that provides testing, labeling, and tagging of seed with low endophyte content. Rather than take the word of a seller that the seed is low in endophyte, request proof of official laboratory test results when purchasing low-endophyte seed or look for the required official label on seed bags certified to contain low-endophyte seed. A new variety that is simply "low-endophyte" will be of little or no value if it is not adapted, does not produce well, or is susceptible to disease or other pests. When considering a new variety, attention should be given to adaptability, agronomic performance, animal performance, persistence, and pest resistance.

Negative effects on animal performance associated with the endophyte and alkaloids can be diluted substantially by the presence of legumes in the animal diet. In Alabama and Kentucky, even small amounts of birdsfoot trefoil, ladino clover, or red clover in endophyte-infected fescue pastures sharply increased cattle gains.

CONCLUSIONS

Knowledge of the association between the fungal endophyte *Acremonium coenophialum* and fescue toxicosis of cattle is a major breakthrough. Use of low-endophyte tall fescue forage greatly improves animal performance.

Evidence that the endophyte is transmitted only via infected seed is encouraging. Identification of a toxin produced either by the endophyte or by the fescue plant in response to the endophyte awaits discovery.

Supplemental Reading

Arkansas Agricultural Experimental Station: Utilization of Fescue by Cattle. Special Report 116. June, 1984.

Proceedings: Tall Fescue Toxicosis Workshop. Atlanta, Georgia, March, 1983.

Siegel, M. R., Varney, D. R., Johnson, M. C., et al.: A fungal endophyte in tall fescue: incidence and dissemination. Phytopathology 74:932–937, 1984.

Siegel, M. R. Varney, D. R., Johnson, M. C., et al.: A fungal endophyte in tall fescue: evaluation of control methods. Phytopathology 74:937–941, 1984.

Cyanogenic Plants

FREDERICK W. OEHME, D.V.M., Ph.D

Livestock poisoning from cyanide is almost always due to the ingestion of plants containing cyanogenic glycosides that liberate cyanide gas (HCN) upon hydrolysis in the rumen content or the acid media of the stomach. All species of farm animals may be affected with this acute toxicosis, although cattle, sheep, and horses are most often involved.

CYANIDE-CONTAINING PLANTS

Numerous plants contain cyanogenic glycosides at 1 or all stages of their growth process, but several are unique in having a characteristically high content early in their growth stage or in having the ability to accumulate high levels of glycoside under varying conditions of stress. The plants with cyanogenic potential are given in Table 1.

Of these, the ones most commonly involved with livestock poisoning are arrow grass (*Triglochin* spp.), Johnson grass (*Sorghum halepense*), Sudan grass (*S. vulgare* var. *sudanensis*), common sorghum (*S. vulgare*), wild black

Table 1. Plants with Cyanogenic Potential

Scientific Name	Common Name
Acacia greggii	Catclaw
Bahia oppositifolia	Bahia
Cerocarpus spp.	Mountain mahogany
Florestina tripteris	Florestina
Glyceria striata	Fowl mannagrass
Holcus lanatus	Velvet grass
Hydrangea spp.	Hydrangea
Linum spp.	Flax
Lotus corniculatus	Birdsfoot trefoil
Manihot esculenia	Cassava
Phaseolus lunatus	Lima bean
Prunus spp.	Cherries
Pyrus malus	Apple
Sorghum spp.	Sudan grass, Johnson grass, etc.
Stilligia treculeana	Queen's delight
Suckleya suckleyana	Poison suckleya
Trifolium repens	White clover
Triglochin spp.	Arrowgrass
Vicia sativa	Vetch seed
Zea mays	Maize, corn

cherry (*Prunus serotina),* choke cherry *(P. virginiana),* pin cherry *(P. pennsylvanica)*, and flax *(Linum usitatissimum)*. Johnson grass is the most toxic of the sorghums and commonly produces problems if under frost or drought conditions. The *Prunus* species (choke or black cherry) are often involved with toxicosis following cutting, when the branches and the leaves are allowed to wilt in pasture. This results in the enzymatic hydrolysis of the glycoside to the more readily available and toxic HCN. Freezing also produces a similar effect. Spraying of cyanogenic plants with a herbicide, resulting in their wilting, may also increase the hazard. Very young rapidly growing plants contain greater quantities of the actual cyanogenic glycoside, and feeding of these forages is best postponed until the plant is mature. The content of cyanogenic glycoside is also increased by heavy nitrate fertilization and by plant injury, as may result from trampling, plant diseases, or stunting due to adverse weather conditions.

CLINICAL SIGNS AND LESIONS

The enzymatic or acid hydrolysis of the cyanogenic glycoside in the digestive tract yields free HCN. The cyanide is rapidly absorbed into the blood and rapidly distributed throughout the body. At the cellular level, cyanide enters the mitochondria and blocks the terminal cytochrome oxidase enzyme of the electron transport system by reacting with the trivalent iron it contains. This effectively stops the intracellular oxidative process by preventing the transfer of oxygen from the blood to its place of molecular utilization in the mitochondria. Cellular hypoxia results. The most oxygen-sensitive cells in the body are the neurons in the brain. These cells sense the lack of available oxygen, trigger greater respiratory efforts, and the circulating blood becomes hyperoxygenated and bright red in color; however, the brain cells are still deficient in oxygen, triggering greater respiratory efforts and finally nervous signs and convulsions.

Because of the rapid hydrolysis and absorption of HCN, the clinical signs occur rapidly upon consumption of toxic quantities of the plant. The actual time interval will depend upon the concentration of cyanogenic glycoside in the plant and the time period over which the plant was consumed. If large doses are eaten rapidly, signs and death will occur within a few minutes. If smaller amounts are eaten, the clinical course is initiated by sudden onset of salivation and by greater respiratory effort. Within 5 to 10 minutes, marked dyspnea develops, muscle fasciculations occur, and the heart rate becomes rapid and weak. Most animals stagger and struggle before they become prostrate. Muscle fasciculations are present while animals are still standing and progress into generalized spasms immediately prior to death. Death results from respiratory paralysis during the severe terminal convulsions. While circulating blood is bright red, respiratory paralysis may produce cyanosis of the mucous membranes. Mucous membranes are bright red while the animal is still breathing. The heart continues to beat for several minutes after convulsions and breathing stop. The total course of the syndrome usually does not exceed 30 minutes from onset, and the animals that live 1½ to 2 hr after clinical signs begin usually recover.

On postmortem examination, the venous blood may be bright red owing to the high oxygen content, but if necropsy is delayed, loss of oxygen to the tissues from decomposition and from terminal respiratory paralysis will produce dark-colored blood that clots slowly. The tracheal mucosa may be hemorrhagic, and froth may be present in the respiratory passageways. Congestion of the lungs and liver is common with hemorrhage on many serosal surfaces. The rumen is distended with gas, and a bitter almond odor may be detected when the rumen is opened. No other significant changes are seen.

Recently, horses grazing hybrid strains of sorghum have been affected with a unique cyanogenic glycoside effect that has been named "sorghum cystitis-ataxia syndrome." Bladder paralysis and posterior ataxia are common and are related to lesions in the spinal cord. It has been suggested that the HCN released from the glycoside reacts with cystine and produces a precursor to the dipeptide that has been shown to produce a similar neuropathologic condition. Affected horses initially exhibit urinary incontinence with urinary burns on the hindquarters. Incoordination of the hindlegs also occurs, and pregnant mares may abort or give birth to foals with arthrogryposis. On necropsy, a fibrinopurulent cystitis or ulcerative cystitis is seen grossly. Microscopic examination reveals focal axonal degeneration and demyelination of the lumbar and sacral segments of the spinal cord.

DIAGNOSIS

A history of cyanogenic-containing plant consumption, clinical signs, and characteristic color of blood on postmortem examination should permit accurate diagnosis. Field tests may be performed on rumen content or forage to verify the presence of the toxic glycoside. Samples collected for this assay or for submission to a laboratory for analysis should be sealed in an air-tight container as soon as possible after the animal's death, then refrigerated and submitted promptly for analysis. Rumen contents may be tested with a reagent consisting of 5 gm of sodium bicarbonate and 0.5 gm of picric acid in 100 ml of distilled water. A large drop or more of reagent is placed on a white blotter or a piece of filter paper, and a drop or more of ruminal fluid is touched to the reagent. If HCN is present the color will change from yellow to red. If the color changes in less than 10 min, one may suspect that there is a fatal amount of HCN.

Cynanogenic plant materal may be tested as follows: Prepare "picrate paper" by wetting filter paper with a solution of 5.0 gm sodium bicarbonate and 0.5 gm of picric acid in 100 ml water. The solution keeps indefinitely, but dried papers keep only a few days. Crush suspected plant or rumen contents and place in water in a test tube or jar that can be corked. If possible, add a few drops of chloroform to hasten autolysis. Suspend strips in bottle with a cork after moistening it. Then heat to 29–35° C. A brick-red color on paper indictes HCN. Well-marked color appearing in a few minutes is significant, but a mild reaction in 1 to several hours is not of much concern.

TREATMENT AND PREVENTION

The treatment of HCN toxicosis is very specific and effective, and as long as heart action is present, intravenous therapy can result in prompt recovery. The cyanide must be removed from the cytochrome enzyme by creation of a subclinical level of methemoglobin. Methemoglobinemia is produced by the intravenous administration of sodium nitrite (20 per cent). Sodium thiosulfate (20 per cent) is given simultaneously to provide a sulfur donor. The sodium nitrite causes methemoglobin formation that pulls the cyanide radical from the blocked enzyme, forming cyanmethemoglobin. The thiosulfate releases sulfur and with the aid of the enzyme rhodanase combines with the HCN from the cyanmethemoglobin, or that in the tissues, to form the nontoxic hydrogen thiocyanate. The released methemoglobin is free to be used again for HCN capture, and the thiocyanate is excreted in the urine. Ten ml of the sodium nitrite are mixed with 30 ml of sodium thiosulfate, and the 40 ml mixture is given intravenously per 454 kg of body weight.

Sodium thiosulfate may also be given orally to detoxify any HCN in the rumen. The animal may also be given a laxative to remove any potential HCN material from the digestive tract, but because of the rapidity of HCN effects, those animals that do not show clinical signs shortly after consumption of the forage will likely not have effects from that consumption.

Methylene blue may also be used to form methemoglobin. It is given intravenously at the rate of 4 to 6 gm/454 kg of body weight. The resulting nontoxic cyanmethemoglobin is slowly excreted from the body, primarily by combining with endogenous sulfur through the action of rhodanase.

While there is little danger from feeding well-cured hay made from cyanogenic glycoside-containing plants, efforts must be directed toward managing animals to avoid their grazing these plants when the hazard is high. Plants should be tested for glycoside content in doubtful cases, and if increased cyanogenic glycoside levels are present, the forage should be mixed with other nontoxic plant material if used as feed. If the cyanogenic glycoside content is very great, the forage may have to be discarded rather than offered to animals on a high risk basis.

Nitrate Accumulators

LAWRENCE P. RUHR, D.V.M., Ph.D.
and GARY D. OSWEILER, D.V.M., Ph.D.

Nitrate poisoning occurs in ruminants grazing on pasture or ingesting hay that has accumulated elevated nitrate or nitrite levels. Many plants have been reported to accumulate nitrate under certain conditions (Table 1).

Many factors have been associated with nitrate accumulation. Those important to livestock management are discussed in this article. Nitrate accumulates in plants under conditions of excessive fertilization or under conditions of water stress from drought or rain after a drought. An enzyme in the plant, nitrate reductase, is necessary to prevent the accumulation of nitrate. This enzyme is light and temperature dependent. Nitrate tends to accumulate in plant tissues at night, on cloudy days, and when environmental temperatures are cool. Nitrate levels are highest in the roots and stems, lower in leaves, and almost no nitrate accumulates in the flower and seed. Herbicides have also been reported to modify the plant's metabolism, resulting in nitrate accumulation 3 to 5 days after application of the herbicide.

Table 1. *Nitrate-Containing Plants*

Range Plants	
Amaranthus spp.	Pigweed
Bromus spp.	Brome, rescue grass
Chenopodium spp.	Lamb's quarter
Datura sp.	Jimson weed
Helianthus spp.	Sunflower
Kochia sp.	Fireweed
Melilotus spp.	Sweetclover
Panicum spp.	Switchgrass, witchgrass
Rumex spp.	Dock
Solanum spp.	Nightshade
Solidago spp.	Goldenrod
Sorghum spp.	Johnson grass, sorghum
Crop Plants	
Avena sativa	Oat hay
Brassica spp.	Rape, kale, turnips
Hordeum vulgare	Barley
Triticum aestivum	Wheat
Zea mays	Corn

Nitrate (NO_3^-) when ingested by ruminants is reduced by microorganisms in the rumen to nitrite (NO_2^-), which is absorbed. The nitrite interacts with the ferrous iron (Fe^{+2}) in the hemoglobin, oxidizing it to ferric iron (Fe^{+3}). The resultant methemoglobin is unable to carry oxygen. Should nitrite be ingested the effect is the same, except microbial reduction is not required. As methemoglobin levels reach 30 to 40 per cent of total hemoglobin, oxygen-carrying capacity is reduced sufficiently for clinical signs to be seen. The condition progresses from distress, to prostration, and finally to coma. When methemoglobin levels reach 80 to 90 per cent, death occurs.

CLINICAL SIGNS

Nitrate poisoning in ruminants is an acute or subacute condition. Clinical signs generally are seen within 6 hr following ingestion of high nitrate forage, though as much as a week may pass. Signs are usually related to anoxia resulting from methemoglobinemia. Depression and a cyanotic or brown cast to mucous membranes along with a rapid, weak pulse are often present. Animals occasionally show behavioral changes, muscular tremors, ataxia, and weakness. Exercise may accentuate the clinical signs and often results in marked dyspnea or collapse or both. If not treated, animals may die within several hours to a day after onset of clinical signs. Abortions can result a few days after an episode of acute nitrate intoxication, even in animals that were not obviously affected.

Chronic nitrate intoxication has been reported. Most often this is associated with decreased weight gains and lactation, reproductive failure, and deranged vitamin A and thyroid metabolism. To date these reports are field observations. Controlled studies to document chronic effects from nitrate have not been reported.

DIAGNOSIS

Animals affected with nitrate intoxication have elevated methemoglobin levels. The per cent methemoglobin can be used to evaluate the condition of animals. Methemoglobin is not stable in refrigerated, heparinized blood for more than a few hours. Laboratory determination of methemoglobin must be done within this time or the methemoglobin must be preserved. One part blood may be mixed with 20 parts phosphate buffer (pH 6.6) to preserve the methemoglobin. A 1:20 dilution with distilled water has also been effective in preserving methemoglobin. This sample may then be refrigerated or frozen and delivered to the laboratory. High levels of methemoglobin result in the blood being a dark "chocolate" brown. This characteristic color of the blood is suggestive of the appropriate diagnosis.

The postmortem lesions are limited to the chocolate brown cast of the blood, mucous membranes, viscera, and muscles, especially if the postmortem investigation is conducted soon after death. Other findings such as pulmonary edema and emphysema, or agonal hemorrhages associated with respiratory distress, may occasionally be present.

Chemical confirmation of elevated nitrate or nitrite levels is required for a firm diagnosis, even if clinical signs, history, and successful treatment all are strongly suggestive of nitrate intoxication. Forage, hay, or feed samples should be analyzed for nitrate content. A field test using diphenylamine should be available to all practitioners. One-half gm of diphenylamine* is added to 20 ml of water, then brought to a volume of 100 ml with sulfuric acid. This stock solution should be stored in a brown glass bottle. The working solution is made by mixing equal parts of the stock solution and 80 per cent sulfuric acid. The working solution should also be stored in a brown glass bottle. Plant material may be tested by placing a drop of working solution on the inside of the split stem at a node or joint. Several plants from different locations should always be tested. A deep blue color will develop within about 10 seconds if 2 per cent or greater nitrate is present. Similar field tests are also available for nitrite, though they are not used as often. Most of the problems associated with plants are caused by nitrate rather than nitrite.

Nitrate has an acute oral toxicity of approximately 0.5 g/kg body weight for ruminants receiving a single bolus of soluble nitrate salt. Acute nitrate poisoning can occur when feed materials contain greater than 1 per cent nitrate on a dry weight basis. The diphenylamine test is not able to detect some potentially toxic feeds. Nitrate in water at levels in excess of 500 parts per million (ppm) has been associated with acute nitrate intoxication. The lower levels required in water to produce toxicosis reflect greater availability for microbial conversion and more rapid absorption from water. All sources of nitrate must be considered when evaluating the potential for nitrate intoxication. All sources of nitrate are additive.

Levels of nitrate in forage, hay, feed, and water are suggestive only, as under some conditions high levels will be tolerated by animals. Three major considerations affect the degree of intoxication associated with a given level of nitrate in feed or water. If a large bolus of nitrate is ingested and absorbed in a short time, the effect is greater than if nitrate is ingested over a longer period. A high carbohydrate grain ration fed simultaneously is protective for nitrate intoxication because it increases the amount of nitrate that can be converted to bacterial protein. In our experience, 1 kg grain/200 kg body weight has been helpful. Finally, acclimation to progressively higher nitrate

levels in feeds and water is possible, as the animals make physiologic adjustments in erythrocyte numbers and metabolic processes. The previous values have been given in parts per million or per cent nitrate. Care must be exercised when using laboratory values for nitrate since several systems of reporting exist. Other common systems are nitrate-nitrogen (NO_3–N) and nitrite-nitrogen (NO_2–N). These are converted to nitrate values when multiplied by 4.4 and 3.3, respectively.

Additional chemical confirmation can be attempted by examining body fluids, such as urine, plasma, serum, aqueous humor, and rumen contents for nitrate. These analyses may vary and can be helpful but not always definitive. Dry feed may be mailed as is. Water, fresh plant material, rumen contents, and other biologic samples, however, should be frozen and mailed in such a way as to arrive frozen.

DIFFERENTIAL DIAGNOSIS

Chlorates (desiccant herbicides) are another class of compounds producing methemoglobinemia in food-producing animals. Distinguishing between chlorate and nitrate poisoning is readily accomplished by analysis for nitrate in feed and water samples. No distinction need be made in treatment other than to be especially careful about relapses when chlorates are the etiologic agent. One other common plant toxin may be confused with nitrate. Cyanide is often suspected in nitrate intoxication. These 2 can be readily differentiated by observing the color of the blood. Nitrate intoxication results in a chocolate brown blood, while cyanide intoxication results in a bright cherry red blood.

TREATMENT

Methylene blue is the principal therapeutic agent. Methylene blue causes reduction of ferric iron in hemoglobin to the ferrous state so that hemoglobin can again accept and transport oxygen. The suggested dose is 4.4 mg/kg body weight administered intravenously in a 2- to 4-per cent solution. The treatment may be repeated if clinical signs recur. Mineral oil (1 L/400 kg) orally or saline cathartics (sodium sulfate 0.5 kg/400 kg) orally have been suggested for lessening the time the high nitrate material remains in the gastrointestinal tract and is available for conversion to nitrite. (See Table 2 for a summary of drug dosages.) Nitrate intoxication usually results from feed or water sources, and many animals in a herd will

Table 2. Common Drug Dosages

Name of Drug	Available From	Species	Dose
Methylene blue	Mallinckrodt Chemical Co. St. Louis, MO	Bovine	4.4 mg/kg IV (2 to 4 per cent solution)
Mineral oil	Standard Oil Company Chicago, IL	Bovine	1 L/400 kg orally
Sodium sulfate	Mallinckrodt Chemical Co. St. Louis, MO	Bovine	0.5 kg/400 kg orally

*Available from Sigma Chemical Company, St. Louis, MO 63166.

be exposed. As initially affected animals are treated, others may be developing signs.

Removal of the suspected source of nitrate should also be undertaken. Chemical confirmation of the nitrate source allows recommendations to be made for preventing recurrences.

If treatment is prompt and continues for sufficient time and the high nitrate source can be removed, the prognosis is good, though abortions may still occur within a few days.

PREVENTION

Prevention centers around eliminating the exposure to feed and water containing high levels of nitrate. Detection of high nitrate concentrations can be accomplished by using the diphenylamine test on forage and hay. If this is not practical, a few animals may be introduced to the suspected source and watched for the development of clinical signs. When this is not possible, the animals should be fed before being allowed access to the suspected feed. This will decrease the initial bolus of nitrate for the animals. Some accommodation to nitrate is possible. With these techniques it may also be advisable to feed a grain supplement as discussed earlier.

Forages with high nitrate concentrations may be dealt with in several ways. As the forage matures and sets seed, the nitrate levels will generally decrease. This may be enough to make the forage safe to feed. The ensiling process will usually convert the nitrate to bacterial protein and produce a safe feed. If the forage is to become hay, raising the cutter bar by 25 to 30 cm will lower the amount of nitrate by lowering the amount of stem in the hay (which contains the highest levels of nitrate). Finally, by cutting forage late in the day on a warm sunny day the nitrate reductase in the plant will have decreased the nitrate level. There is little that can be done with hay that contains high levels of nitrate, as it does not dissipate with time. If the hay must be salvaged, the only option is to dilute high nitrate hay with good hay in a complete ration. The nitrate levels should be determined quantitatively. The hay should be ground and mixed with other hay and feedstuff into a feed containing less than 0.5 per cent nitrate. Grinding or some other technique that allows complete mixing and prevents selective consumption of the high nitrate hay is necessary. This procedure, while salvaging high nitrate hay, is not without hazard.

When dealing with potentially toxic nitrate levels in forage, hay, or water, one or more of these recommendations may be necessary to minimize the impact of nitrate on the health of the animals.

Supplemental Reading

Buck, W. B., Osweiler, G. D., and Van Gelder, G. A.: Clinical and Diagnostic Veterinary Toxicology. Dubuque, Iowa, Kendall/Hunt Publishing Co., 1976.

Clay, B. R., Edwards, W. C., and Peterson, D. R.: Toxic nitrate accumulation in the sorghums. Bov. Pract. *11*:28–32, 1976.

Emerick, R. J.: Consequences of high nitrate levels in feed and water supplies. Fed. Proc. *33*:1183–1187, 1974.

Kingsbury, J. M.: Poisonous Plants of the United States and Canada. Englewood Cliffs, N. J., Prentice-Hall, Inc., 1964.

Selenium Accumulators

LYNN F. JAMES, Ph.D.
and J. L. SHUPE, D.V.M.

Selenium is present in certain soils at levels that may produce plants toxic to livestock. Plants that grow on seleniferous soils may accumulate selenium in quantities from less than 1 ppm to several thousand ppm. Plants capable of accumulating high levels of selenium ($>$ 1000 ppm) include some species of *Astragalus* (Fig. 1), *Stanleya*, *Haplopappus*, and *Machaeranthera*. These plants are often referred to as "selenium accumulator" or "indicator" plants because of their preference for seleniferous soils and their ability to accumulate high levels of selenium. Such plants normally have an unpleasant odor and are unpalatable to livestock. Animals are poisoned by the selenium in the plants when they are forced to graze on them because of a shortage of other plants.

Many species of *Aster*, *Atriplex*, *Castelleja*, and *Gutierrezia* accumulate less selenium than the major accumulator plants—rarely more than a few hundred ppm. Many weeds, most crop plants, and grasses can accumulate up to 50 ppm of selenium when grown on seleniferous soils. Pigs and chickens fed seleniferous small grains and grazing animals ingesting these selenium-accumulating forages can be poisoned.

The distribution of selenium, especially as selenate, throughout the soil profile is important because it relates to the selenium content of the plants. Selenium that has been leached into the deeper soil profiles is available to the deep-rooted plants. Many of the selenium indicator plants are deep rooted and therefore accumulate selenium at high levels.

Selenium in small grains is present in association with protein, whereas the selenium in the indicator plants is largely in water-soluble form that suggests its occurrence in some form other than protein.

Selenium accumulated in plants occurs in a variety of chemical forms. The comparative toxicity of these various compounds has not been elucidated; therefore, evaluation of the toxicity of these plants based on total selenium

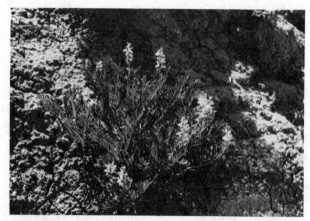

Figure 1. *Astragalus bisulcatus.* One of the principal selenium accumulating plants.

content can be misleading. Total selenium content should serve only as a guide to the toxicity of a plant.

CLINICAL SIGNS

Selenium poisoning in livestock can be either acute or chronic. Animals suffer acute poisoning when they ingest sufficient quantities of selenium accumulator plants to induce sudden death, usually in a short time. Because of the unpalatability of selenium accumulator plants, acute toxicosis is uncommon.

The signs of acute selenium-induced poisoning are either sudden death or severe distress, labored breathing, abnormal movement and posture, frequent urination, diarrhea, prostration, and then death. Sheep exhibit increased rate of respiration and sudden death. Animals may die within a few hours or not for several days with very few signs.

Two types of chronic intoxication have been described. These are "blind staggers" and "alkali disease." Chronic selenium intoxication of the blind staggers type is said to result from the consumption of accumulator plants in limited amounts over an extended period. The blind staggers type is characterized by inappetence, impairment of vision, wandering (often in circles), weakness, partial or entire paralysis of tongue and swallowing mechanism, abdominal pain, excessive salivation, and death. Although for many years blind staggers has been associated with selenium poisoning, some investigators now question this. The blind staggers type of selenium poisoning has not been verified through research. "Blind staggers" is a term used to describe animals that appear blind and show evidence of the previously listed signs of poisoning, but blind staggers is probably a complex of disease syndromes of unknown origin. In the past, many of these problems have probably been incorrectly diagnosed as selenium poisoning.

Chronic selenium poisoning of the alkali disease type results from ingesting forage containing from 5 to about 40 ppm of selenium for a prolonged period. The time and amount of selenium necessary for poisoning varies considerably with individual animals. Signs of poisoning in cattle and horses include lameness, hoof alterations, emaciation, and loss of long hair from the mane and tail. Sheep do not respond to chronic selenium poisoning as do cattle and horses in that they do not show hoof or wool effects.

Signs of poisoning vary with animal species. Pigs fed diets containing 25 ppm selenium or more have developed severe spinal cord lesions, which ultimately lead to varying degrees of paralysis. These lesions are preceded by loss of hair and hoof lesions (Fig. 2). Decreased hatchability of chicken eggs has been observed. A reduction in reproductive performance is probably the most significant economic effect of chronic selenium poisoning in livestock. Reproduction may be depressed rather severely without the animal's showing typical signs of poisoning.

Although selenium poisoning is classified according to severity, the toxic effects of selenium increase in severity as selenium intake increases, so that it may become difficult to differentiate between the forms. Young animals are more susceptible to selenium poisoning than older ones.

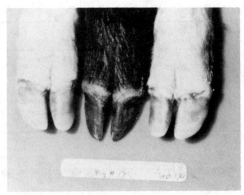

Figure 2. Feet of a pig poisoned by selenium. Note the separation of the hoof at the coronary border.

DIAGNOSIS

Diagnosis of selenium poisoning will be discussed under 2 headings, the acute and chronic (alkali disease syndrome). In view of the questionable status of the so-called "blind staggers disease," additional discussion of this problem should await further clarification.

Acute selenium poisoning is rare and associated with the grazing of plants, such as the selenium-accumulating *Astragalus* plants in which selenium levels can vary from a few hundred to several thousand ppm. If animals die from acute selenium poisoning, forage that is high in selenium is probably located in the general area where the animals have been grazing. Signs observed relate to the level of selenium in the plant and rate of consumption. Animals may die rather quickly with few signs, or when intake has been lower, they may linger for a few days. If animals linger, there may be abnormal posture, diarrhea, frequent urination, respiratory distress, prostration, and death. Postmortem examination reveals primarily a marked congestion of the lungs and hyperemia of the gastrointestinal tract. Microscopic examination of the tissues substantiates the gross lesions listed.

Chronic poisoning accompanies the grazing of seleniferous forage of 5 to 40 ppm over a prolonged period. Chemical analysis of vegetation in the area where the animals have been grazing or of forage fed to the animals should reflect such selenium intake levels. Not all vegetation in all the areas where animals have grazed will contain the same amounts of selenium.

Horses, cattle, and pigs show the adverse changes in hair coat and hoofs and emaciation as described. Reproductive performance declines in all species of farm animals exposed to excessive levels of selenium.

Anemia, cirrhosis and atrophy of the liver, and atrophy of the heart have been observed in cattle and horses with chronic selenium toxicosis. The only known chronic effect of selenium poisoning in sheep is a severely reduced rate of reproduction.

The guidelines in Table 1 have been set by the South Dakota Agricultural Experiment Station for the selenium content of blood and hair.

Some selenium-accumulator plants such as *Astragalus bisulcatus* may contain toxins other than selenium, and in

Table 1. *Toxic Levels of Selenium in Blood and Hair*

Blood (ppm)	Hair (ppm)	Comments
<1.0	<5.0	Chronic selenium poisoning not expected
1.0–2.0	5.0–10.0	Borderline problem
>2.0	>10.0	Selenium intake excessive and selenosis should be expected; animals at this level may not show signs of toxicosis

cases of chronic toxicosis involving these plants, toxins other than selenium may be involved.

TREATMENT

There is no known treatment for acute selenium poisoning. Chronically poisoned animals should be removed from seleniferous forage. The rate, extent, and incidence of recovery depend on the severity of toxicosis.

PREVENTION

The prevention of chronic selenium poisoning requires the limiting of selenium intake. Control measures should be based on management. Management procedures require, in the case of range animals, a mapping of the range area based on geology and plant analysis. On the basis of the selenium content of the vegetation from the various sites of a range, grazing procedures are established to regulate selenium intake within safe limits when both time and selenium content of the forage are considered.

Supplemental Reading

Anderson, M. S., Lakin, H. W., Beeson, K. C., et al.: Selenium in agriculture. United States Department of Agriculture Handbook 200, 1961.

Moxon, A. L.: Alkali diesase or selenium poisoning. S.D. St. Agric. Exp. Sta. Bull. 311, 1937.

National Research Council: Medical and biologic effects of environmental pollutants: selenium. Washington, D.C., National Academy of Sciences, 1976.

Olsen, O., Keeler, R. F., Van Kampen, K. R., and James, L. F. (eds.): Selenium: A cause of poisoning. *In* Effects of Poisonous Plants on Livestock. New York, Academic Press, 1978.

Rosenfeld, I. and Beath, O. A.: Selenium: Geobotany, Biochemistry, Toxicity, and Nutrition. New York, Academic Press, 1964.

Oxalate Accumulators

LYNN F. JAMES, Ph.D.
and A. EARL JOHNSON, M.S.

Oxalic-acid and oxalate poisonings are of considerable importance throughout the world. Not only are domestic animals affected, but so are household pets and humans affected. Oxalic acid, an organic dicarboxylic acid, has a great affinity for calcium and magnesium, and the resulting salts are virtually insoluble in water. This acid also forms soluble salts with sodium, potassium, and ammonium. These soluble salts—sodium, potassium, and ammonium oxalates—and oxalic acid itself are both corrosive and systemic poisons. Under natural conditions, oxalic acid or soluble oxalates are toxic primarily because of their chemical reaction within the body rather than because of their corrosive effects.

Oxalic acid occurs naturally in plants in the form of soluble and insoluble oxalates. Oxalate intoxication in livestock results primarily from the ingestion of plants containing the oxalates. Plants producing high levels of oxalates (generally considered to be 10 per cent or more anhydrous oxalic acid on a dry weight basis) are worldwide in distribution. Some plants may have in excess of 30 per cent oxalate on a dry weight basis. Examples of such plants are halogeton (*Halogeton glomeratus*) and greasewood (*Sarcobatus vermiculatus*) of the Chenopodiaceae family, soursob (*Oxalis pes-caprae*) and the sorrels of the Oxalidaceae family, and certain of the *Rumex* species of the Polygonaceae family.

Some plants with oxalate levels of less than 10 per cent, including some grasses consumed by cattle, can cause problems. The fungi *Aspergillus niger* and *A. flavus* can produce large amounts of oxalates on feeds and on moist straw. Livestock poisoning cases have been reported involving such feeds and straw.

The plants producing high oxalate levels can be divided into 2 groups.

1. Plants such as soursobs and some species of *Rumex* that have a sap pH of about 2. The oxalate anion is chiefly found as the acid oxalate ($HC_2O_4^-$).

2. Plants such as halogeton that have a sap pH of about 6. The oxalate anion is chiefly found as the oxalate ion ($C_2O_4^{2-}$).

The oxalate in group 1 is present chiefly as acid potassium oxalate, and the oxalate in group 2 is present chiefly as soluble sodium oxalate and insoluble calcium oxalate. One species of grass (*Setaria sphacelata*) in Australia produces oxalate at lower levels and has caused intoxication in horses and cattle. The grass species is thought to hold the oxalate as ammonium oxalate.

Two of the principal oxalate-producing plants of the world are soursob of Australia and halogeton of the western United States. Both of them are introduced plants.

Most oxalate-containing plants are palatable to livestock, therefore, livestock with access to this group of plants must be managed more carefully.

EFFECTS OF OXALATES IN THE DIETS OF RUMINANT LIVESTOCK

When a ruminant eats an oxalate-containing plant, 3 things can occur, (1) the soluble oxalates may be detoxified by the metabolic activity of the rumen bacteria, (2) the soluble oxalates may react with calcium in the digestive system to form insoluble calcium oxalate that is excreted in the feces, or (3) the soluble oxalates may be absorbed into the blood stream where they may react with calcium or other blood constituents.

Certain microorganisms in the rumen can detoxify the oxalate ion. Ingestion of sublethal levels of soluble oxalate may gradually increase the rate at which rumen microorganisms detoxify the oxalate. This change in rumen microflora can increase the amount of soluble oxalate a ruminant can safely ingest by about 75 per cent. Therefore, allowing ruminants to graze small amounts of oxalate-producing plants permits the rumen bacteria to become adjusted to the oxalate and thus increases protection against oxalate poisoning.

Soluble oxalates can combine with calcium in the rumen and can be excreted as insoluble calcium oxalate.

If the soluble oxalates are ingested rapidly, as when an animal is hungry, the microflora may not be able to detoxify them, and the soluble oxalates are absorbed into the blood stream. If absorption is in large enough amounts, the animal becomes intoxicated. The oxalate combines with tissue calcium and forms crystals that are deposited in the wall of the rumen and in the renal tubules. Hypocalcemia may result. Oxalate also interferes with the enzymes lactic dehydrogenase and succinic dehydrogenase, both of which are essential for energy metabolism. Thus, there is interference with energy metabolism.

Oxalate intoxication in an animal is a complex phenomenon influenced not only by the previously mentioned reactions, but by the following factors as well:

1. Amount of oxalate-containing plant ingested.
2. Rate of consumption.
3. Concentration of soluble oxalate in the plant.
4. Amount of other feed in the rumen (dilution factor).
5. Recent exposure to oxalate-containing plants.

A ruminant may consume large quantities of oxalate-containing plants without harmful effects if ingested slowly over the grazing period, whereas the same amount may prove lethal if ingested rapidly. Oxalate poisoning occurs primarily when hungry animals are allowed to graze on heavy stands of plants with a high oxalate content. A full rumen not only dilutes the oxalate and thus slows absorption, but it also discourages the animal from eating too much.

Oxalate-producing plants are high in soluble salts, thus, diets containing an abundance of these plants increase water consumption because water is needed to excrete the salts.

Water intake is influenced by dry matter consumption, salt intake, and ambient temperature. As any of these factors increase, water intake increases. If water is withheld, feed consumption is less so that an animal can become hungry by withholding feed or water. When water is withheld and an animal becomes hungry, it will eat after it has been given water. At such times, animals are much less discriminating about what they eat. If animals are hungry and are feeding on sites infested with oxalate-producing plants such as halogeton, the animals may become intoxicated. Oxalate poisoning often occurs in sheep after trucking or extensive handling.

Some grasses have been reported to contain low levels of oxalate. These have caused negative calcium balance and intoxication in cattle. There is 1 report of secondary nutritional hyperparathyroidism in horses grazing such plants.

DIAGNOSIS

Ruminants, primarily, are poisoned on oxalates, and more sheep than cattle have been poisoned, perhaps because of differences in management practices. Two clinically distinct conditions exist from oxalate ingestion—acute and subacute poisoning and chronic poisoning. In the United States, only acute oxalate poisoning has been described in sheep.

Signs of poisoning are rapid and labored respiration, depression, weakness, coma, and death. There is stasis of the gastrointestinal tract. Mild tetany may be observed in a few individuals. Gross pathologic conditions are hemorrhage and edema of the rumen wall, hyperemia of the abomasal wall and intestinal mucosa, and ascites. Histopathologic changes include hemorrhage and calcium oxalate crystal formation in the rumen wall and oxalate crystals and accompanying cellular damage in the renal tubules. The animals can die within 1 to 2 hr or as long as several days after eating a lethal dose of halogeton. When death is rapid, few lesions are observed. Serum calcium levels decrease and plasma urea nitrogen, serum glutamic oxaloacetic transaminase, and lactic dehydrogenase levels all increase. The extent of the changes is dependent on the acuteness of the intoxication.

Subacute and chronic poisonings in sheep grazing soursobs in Australia have been reported. These animals develop a stiffness of gait and eventually collapse. They usually remain bright, continue to feed, and may remain in this condition for weeks until they either die or recover gradually. The kidneys of these animals become fibrotic. The difference observed between soursob poisoning in Australia and halogeton poisoning in the United States is believed to be due to the difference in the chemical form of the oxalate in the halogeton plant.

In India, cattle have been reported to develop a negative calcium balance when fed paddy straw that contains low levels of oxalate. Horses develop secondary nutritional hyperparathyroidism when grazing the grass *Setaria sphacelata*, containing low levels of oxalate. Cattle have also been poisoned on this grass. Cattle grazing halogeton develop a stiffness of the limbs when driven. If pressed, these animals may become recumbent, but they will usually recover with proper treatment.

TREATMENT

The constant observation of hypocalcemia in animals poisoned on oxalate suggests that the appropriate treatment might be the intravenous administration of readily available calcium, such as calcium gluconate. A number of investigators have tried this approach, but it has not been effective.

PREVENTION

Prevention of oxalate poisoning lies principally with proper management. The following practices will help minimize losses in livestock due to oxalate poisoning:

1. Avoid overgrazing pastures and ranges to the extent that perennial vegetation is removed or depleted.
2. Develop a grazing program that will allow ranges and pastures to improve.
3. Supply adequate water and a good variety of forage.
4. Develop a grazing plan. Know what your animals are eating.
5. Allow livestock (ruminants) time to adapt to oxalate in the diet by grazing safe amounts of oxalate-producing plants. Introduce animals slowly into areas with heavy growth of oxalate plants.
6. Do not unload, drive, or bed livestock in areas with dense populations of oxalate-producing plants unless the animals have been well fed and watered.

7. Do not allow hungry animals to graze in dense stands of oxalate-producing plants.

Supplemental Reading

Cook, C. W., and Stoddard, L. A.: The halogeton problem in Utah. Utah Agri. Exp. Sta. Bull. 364, 1953.

Everist, S. L.: Poisonous Plants of Australia. Sydney, Australia, Angus and Robertson, 1974.

James, L. F.: Oxalate toxicosis. Clin. Toxicol. 25:231–243, 1972.

James, L. F., and Cronin, E. H.: Management practices to minimize death losses of sheep grazing halogeton-infested ranges. J. Range Manage. 27:424–426, 1974.

James, L. F., and Johnson, A. E.: Prevention of fatal *Halogeton glomeratus* poisoning in sheep. J. Am. Vet. Med. Assoc. 157:437–442, 1970.

Kingsbury, J. M.: Poisonous Plants of the United States and Canada. Englewood Cliffs, New Jersey, Prentice-Hall Inc., 1964.

Van Kampen, K. R., and James, L. F.: Acute halogeton poisoning in sheep: pathogenesis of lesions. Am. J. Vet. Res. 30:1779–1783, 1969.

Cardiotoxic Plants

MURRAY E. FOWLER, D.V.M.

Few species of plants contain toxic substances that primarily affect the cardiovascular system, but consumption of these few species of plants produces dramatic effects.

POISONOUS PRINCIPLES

Cardioactive glycosides are the principal agents producing cardiotoxicity. Many different cardioactive glycosides are found in plants. The concentration of glycosides within the plant varies with season, stage of maturity, part of the plant, and environmental conditions. The toxic effects of the various glycosides are generally similar, differing mostly in degree of severity and persistence of debility. All species of mammals and birds are susceptible to the toxic effects of cardioactive glycosides.

Some other chemicals may be cardiotoxic or may affect the autonomic nervous system and subsequently the heart (Table 1). Alkaloids found in yews have both direct and indirect cardiac effects.

PLANTS

Detailed taxonomic descriptions of cardiotoxic plants are not possible here. The reader is referred to a standard text for aid in plant identification.[1] Table 2 lists the cardiotoxic plants of North America.

Oleander

The plant most often responsible for cardiotoxicity is oleander *(Nerium oleander)*. Oleander, a shrub or a small

Table 1. *Plant-Derived Drugs Affecting Autonomic Nervous System*

Atropine	*Atropa belladonna, Datura* sp.
Muscarine	*Amanita muscaria*
Ephedrine	*Ephedra* sp.
Ergotamine	*Claviceps purpurea*
Nicotine	*Nicotiana* sp.

Table 2. *Cardiotoxic Plants*

Plant	Toxin
Oleander *(Nerium oleander)*	CAG*
Foxglove *(Digitalis purpurea)*	CAG
Indian hemp *(Apocynum cannabinum)*	CAG
Lily of the valley *(Convallaria majalis)*	CAG
Milkweed *(Asclepias* sp.)	CAG
Yew *(Taxus* sp.)	Alkaloid
False hellebore *(Veratrum* sp.)	Alkaloid

*CAG = cardioactive glycoside

tree, is grown as an ornamental in the southern United States and throughout much of California. It may be kept as a potted plant in more northern climates. Thus, oleander toxicity is a potential hazard almost anywhere in North America.

Oleander contains a potent cardioactive glycoside. All parts of the plant including leaves, roots, flowers, and bark, either dry or green, are dangerous. The glycoside is stable in boiling water. The lethal dose of oleander is approximately 110 mg of green or dry leaf/kg of body weight. Thus, 55 gm are fatal to a 500-kg animal.

Oleander leaves have a bitter taste and are unpalatable. If leaves fall from the shrub and wilt or dry, they are apparently more readily accepted by livestock, especially if they become mixed with grass clippings. Cattle housed in corrals surrounded by oleander plants seldom eat the shrub, but toxicity may result if cuttings of the shrub are left to wilt in a pasture or are placed in an area where cattle normally feed. Extremely hungry cattle, sheep, and goats have been poisoned when grazing a strange pasture containing little forage but oleander.

Hay may be a source of the plant. Cattle and sheep have died following ingestion of baled hay harvested from a field bordered by oleander shrubs.

Purple Foxglove

Digitalis purpurea is an ornamental grown in cool, moist climates in the United States. It has become a naturalized weed in north coastal California and Oregon.

Indian Hemp or Dogbane

Apocynum cannabinum is a short shrub of waste places (e.g., vacant lot, roadside, unused field, and so forth).

Lily of the Valley

Convallaria majalis is an ornamental ground cover.

Milkweed

A cardioactive glycoside is one component of the toxic agent of milkweed plants of the genus *Asclepias*. Although cardiac effects may accompany the clinical syndrome produced by consumption of milkweeds, other chemicals produce the major effects.

Yew

Taxus sp. is an ornamental evergreen shrub or small tree. In general appearance it resembles a conifer, but its fruit is a small fleshy berry instead of a cone. The poisonous principle is an alkaloid, affecting both the nervous system and the heart. The cardiac effects are bradycardia and cardiac arrest. Neural signs are depression, trembling, dyspnea, collapse, and sudden death. Subacute toxicity, as seen in cattle, is characterized additionally by gastroenteritis and diarrhea.

False Hellebore

The *Veratrum* sp. contains alkaloids that cause cardiac irregularities and potential death. Common syndromes associated with these plants are teratogenic effects of central nervous system derangement.

CLINICAL SIGNS

Cardioactive Glycoside Poisoning

Clinical signs of cardioactive glycoside poisoning develop 4 to 12 hr after ingestion of the plant. Ingestion of lethal quantities results in death within 12 to 24 hr. Clinical signs may persist for 2 or 3 days with ingestion of a sublethal dose. In cattle, continued release of glycosides in the rumen may prolong the syndrome or cause exacerbation after an apparent improvement. As the disease progresses, the animal becomes depressed and weak. Localized muscle fasciculation may occur, or generalized trembling can progress to terminal anoxic convulsions. Cattle commonly become weak and comatose.

Toxic doses of cardioactive glycosides exaggerate the therapeutic effects of these agents. During the course of a poisoning episode, a variety of cardiac conduction abnormalities are seen, such as bradycardia, tachycardia, dropped beats, heart block, auricular fibrillation, ventricular tachycardia, and ventricular fibrillation. There seems to be no set pattern to the sequence of development of irregularities except that fibrillation is usually a terminal sign. At any one moment, the heart rate and rhythm may sound normal. Auscultation over a period of minutes is necessary to detect cardiac irregularities.

Many clinical signs are a direct result of hypoxia caused by inability of the heart to circulate blood. Extremities are cold. Rectal temperature may be normal or slightly subnormal. The pulse is usually rapid and weak. Respiratory rate and depth are increased. Hemorrhagic nasal discharge and open-mouth breathing are seen in severely affected animals. Mucous membranes may be cyanotic.

Cardioactive glycosides (but not yew alkaloids) also produce gastrointestinal signs, such as colic and catarrhal or hemorrhagic diarrhea. In fact, signs of gastroenteritis may be the first symptoms noted. Swine may exhibit nausea and vomiting.

NECROPSY

The most consistent lesions are those of catarrhal or hemorrhagic gastroenteritis. Many organs are congested because of poor tissue perfusion. Petechial hemorrhages may be seen on serosal surfaces in the abdomen and the thoracic cavities. Blood-stained fluids are frequently found in body cavities. Usually no lesions are associated with yew poisoning.

DIAGNOSIS

Clinical signs are suggestive. Prolonged auscultation of the heart is a reliable diagnostic tool. Electrocardiographic examination is helpful but not required. A history of possible consumption of plants known to contain cardioactive glycosides is an aid and, in some cases, is necessary to make a definitive diagnosis. Necropsy lesions are not pathognomonic. Gastroenteric lesions are not easily differentiated from those caused by infectious agents.

Examination of rumen contents for plant segments may be very helpful. Oleander has characteristic leaves. Secondary veins branch from the main longitudinal vein in a parallel fashion. A diagnosis of oleander poisoning would be justified by the presence of any oleander plant segment in the rumen contents. Yew leaves are also distinctive but require close observation for distinguishing them from other forage materials in the rumen.

A differential diagnosis should include infectious enteritis and other toxicities, such as castor bean *(Ricinus communis)* or arsenic poisoning.

TREATMENT

The only effective treatment is to rid the gastrointestinal tract of residual plant material. In swine, an emetic should be administered followed by intubation and administration of activated charcoal (1–3 gm/kg) and sodium or magnesium sulfate (1 gm/kg). Ruminants are more difficult to treat. If an antemortem diagnosis has been made, a rumenotomy is indicated. All of the rumen contents must be extracted, and preferably the rumen should be washed. Any residual plant material is potentially lethal. A rumen content transplant from an animal with no possible exposure to the toxic substance may be required in order for proper rumen function to resume.

General nursing care is indicated. No specific antidotal agents are effective in food animals.

All access to continued ingestion of plants containing cardioactive glycosides must cease. In one case, lawn and garden clippings containing oleander had been dumped where cattle could reach them through a fence and consume them. The farmer was advised to remove the pile of leaves and grass. Losses continued. Finally it was ascertained that he had cleaned up the pile with a 4-tine pitchfork, leaving a few leaves at the site. With oleander, a few leaves can be lethal.

Reference

1. Kingsbury, J. M.: Poisonous Plants of the United States and Canada. Englewood Cliffs, New Jersey, Prentice-Hall, Inc., 1964.

Hepatotoxic Plants

MURRAY E. FOWLER, D.V.M.

Some plant toxins produce deleterious effects on the liver. The liver is a multiple function organ, and derangement may produce one or more malfunctions. The clinical syndrome produced by a particular toxin varies according to the function affected. Table 1 lists those plants of the United States and Canada that produce the hepatotoxicity as a major effect when ingested by livestock.

PLANT TOXINS

Pyrrolizidine Alkaloid Poisoning

Though over 100 pyrrolizidine alkaloids are known,[1] only a few are toxic. Plants containing the toxic alkaloids

Table 1. *Hepatotoxic Plants in the United States*

Plants containing pyrrolizidine alkaloids
  Senecio spp. (ragwort, groundsel, many other species)
  Amsinckia intermedia (fiddleneck, fireweed)
  Crotalaria sp. (rattlebox, rattleweed, wild pea)
Plants causing photosensitization
  Agave lechuguilla (century plant)
  Brassica napus (rape)
  Nolina texana (sacahiuste, bear grass)
  Tetradymia sp. (horse brush)
  Lantana sp. (lantana)
  Blue green algae (water bloom)
Others
  Aspergillus flavus (fungus)
  Amanita phalloides (death cap mushroom)

were recognized as hazardous to livestock as early as 1787. Pyrrolizidine alkaloid poisoning occurs worldwide, causing extensive livestock losses.

Lesion Pathogenesis

The precise metabolic derangement in the hepatocyte is not known, but much is known about the pathogenesis of the lesion produced.[1] The pyrrolizidine alkaloid is readily absorbed from the intestine and enters the portal circulation. The liver parenchyma is bathed with the alkaloid, and hepatocytes are diffusely affected. In high doses, necrosis of the hepatocyte occurs. More characteristically, the cell is affected by a metabolic lesion that prevents the hepatocyte from undergoing normal binary fission to regenerate hepatocytes. Unable to divide, the cell continues to grow. Both the nucleus and cytoplasm expand, sometimes as much as 10-fold (hepatocytomeglia, karyomeglia). Ultimately, the cell reaches a critical mass and dies. If a few cells die simultaneously, the histopathology will appear as parenchymal atrophy with hepatocytomeglia. If large numbers of cells die simultaneously (as might occur with a moderate dose), the necrotic cells will elicit a corrective tissue response, accompanied by bile duct proliferation. The 3 primary lesions of pyrrolizidine alkaloid poisoning (PAP) are hepatocytomeglia, fibrosis, and bile duct proliferation. Hepatocytomeglia is always present. The presence of the other 2 lesions is dependent upon the dose ingested and the rapidity of lesion maturation. A single dose of the alkaloid may elicit the response, or the liver may be continually exposed to the alkaloid over days, weeks, or months before eliciting the response.

Hepatocyte degeneration and loss cause decreased hepatic function. The liver has tremendous reserve capacity that enables an animal to continue to function normally for many weeks or months, even though the liver may be slowly degenerating. Ultimately, liver function collapses, and the animal suffers from a generalized hepatic insufficiency syndrome.

Discussion

Some unique characteristics of PAP must be understood by those dealing with the problem. First, development of the clinical syndrome occurs 2 to 8 months following ingestion of the alkaloid. The delay makes it extremely difficult to obtain feed samples to examine for presence of a suspect plant. Thus, obtaining a satisfactory history of ingestion becomes almost impossible. This fact seriously complicates attempts to adjudicate suspected losses in the courts. Secondly, pyrrolizidine alkaloids are rapidly excreted in body fluids such as urine and milk. Since certain pyrrolizidine alkaloids are considered to be carcinogens, this fact poses a potential public health problem.[2]

Young, growing animals are more susceptible to the hepatotoxic effects of the alkaloid than are adults. Furthermore, alkaloids can pass through the placenta and can affect the fetus. In one herd, calves were affected with PAP. The hay source was identified, but since no adult stock had been affected, the decision was made to continue feeding the hay to adult stock and to provide young stock with clean hay. Calf losses continued through the next year until it was recognized that fetuses were affected in utero.

PHOTOSENSITIZATION

Photosensitization is a disease caused by the presence of a photodynamic agent in the skin that sensitizes the epithelium to ultraviolet radiation. A lesion similar to that produced by sunburn results.

Three mechanisms may be involved. First, the photodynamic agent may be preformed in the plant ingested by an animal (primary photosensitization). A second mechanism is aberrant pigment synthesis by the animal. This tends to be a genetically controlled trait; congenital porphyria in cattle is an example. The third mechanism operates through hepatogenous photosensitization as a result of ingestion of certain plants containing toxins that damage the hepatic parenchyma (see Table 1).

One of the metabolites of chlorophyll metabolism is the photodynamic chemical phylloerythrin. Normally, the liver degrades phylloerythrin, keeping serum levels negligible. When the hepatic parenchyma is damaged, higher concentrations of phylloerythrin in the serum may cause photosensitization in light-skinned animals exposed to sunlight.

AFLATOXICOSIS

Toxins produced by the fungus *Aspergillus flavus* are highly hepatotoxic.

MUSHROOM TOXICITY

There are numerous species of poisonous mushrooms, but they are rarely consumed in sufficient quantity to produce clinical toxicity in livestock. One species, however, *Amanita phalloides* (death cap), contains alkaloids or polypeptides or both that are highly hepatotoxic. Consumption of 50 to 100 gm of these mushrooms may be sufficient to kill a calf, sheep, or pig.

The toxins in death cap mushrooms produce a massive diffuse necrosis of the hepatic parenchyma.

HEPATIC INSUFFICIENCY SYNDROME

This syndrome is not pathognomonic for any particular etiologic agent. Signs vary slightly from one species of animal to another.

Clinical Signs

An affected animal may experience some weight loss but need not be emaciated. Icterus is usually present. Light-skinned animals exposed to sunlight may develop photosensitization. Cattle characteristically show gastrointestinal signs consisting of colic, tenesmus, diarrhea, and rectal prolapse. Ascites may be due to hypoproteinemia or portal hypertension.

A hemogram may be normal or may indicate low grade anemia, leukocytosis, left-shift differential leukocyte count, and elevated icteric index.

Be cautious when evaluating serum chemistry parameters. Serum enzyme studies may be within normal limits in animals suffering from hepatic insufficiency caused by PAP because cellular necrosis is not necessarily taking place at the same time as the clinical disease. Plants such as *Lantana camara* and *Amanita phalloides,* which cause hepatic necrosis, produce markedly elevated serum enzyme levels.

Signs of acute hepatic insufficiency develop after a latent period of 6 to 24 hr following ingestion of the plant. Acute hepatic insufficiency caused by *A. phalloides* ingestion is characterized by vomiting, diarrhea, dehydration, muscle cramps, hypovolemic shock, hypoglycemia, hyponatremia, and leukocytosis with a left shift. Liver failure allows invasion of the host by enteric bacteria, with septicemia and fever resulting.

Hepatoencephalopathy

Signs of central nervous system depression are usually seen in hepatic insufficiency cases. The inability of the liver to detoxify nitrogenous waste products of the blood results in a plasma buildup, causing direct effects on the brain. Cattle become depressed. They may stand in awkward positions with legs crossed or fetlocks knuckled. If forced to move, they are incoordinated and may wander aimlessly or walk in circles. Occasionally, cattle will push against obstacles in their path, but this sign is much more common in horses than in cattle. The animal may be found in a comatose state and remain so for hours only to revive and appear normal for a time.

Livestock generally do not exhibit the aggressive signs seen in horses such as biting themselves, other animals, or the ground. Convulsions are also rare in cattle.

Diagnosis

Differential diagnosis must include infectious hepatitis, parasites, biliary obstruction, chemical hepatic necrosis (carbon tetrachloride, clay pigeon poisoning), rabies, other encephalomyelites, brain abscesses, tumors, and hemorrhages. Antemortem diagnosis of hepatopathies is based on clinical signs, clinical pathologic examination, and liver biopsy.

Necropsy

Grossly, the liver may be swollen, atrophic, fibrotic, yellowish, or mottled. One cannot evaluate hepatic insufficiency on the basis of gross lesions. Even with histologic examination, one cannot always make a diagnosis except in the case of pyrrolizidine alkaloid toxicosis or aflatoxicosis.

TREATMENT

When an animal shows clinical signs of PAP, the prognosis is grave and therapy is useless. For other hepatopathies, keep affected cattle out of direct sunlight to avoid photosensitization. Supporting treatment with broad-spectrum antibiotics, and administration of fluids (particularly 10-per cent glucose) and essential fatty acids are helpful. The prognosis is guarded in all cases of hepatopathy.

References

1. Bull, L. B., Culvenor, C. C. J., and Dick, A. T.: The Pyrrolizidine Alkaloids. Amsterdam, North-Holland Publishing Co., 1968.
2. Zimmerman, H. J.: Hepatotoxicity. New York, Appleton-Century-Crofts, 326, 1978.

Nephrotoxic Plants

GARY D. OSWEILER, D.V.M., M.S., Ph.D.

Plants with a primary toxic effect on the kidney are relatively few but in 2 instances cause severe and often widespread losses among food animals. The major nephrotoxic plants in North America are the oaks, *Quercus* spp., and the rough or redroot pigweed, *Amaranthus retroflexus*. Both of these plants are common throughout most of the United States except for the more arid and nonforested regions.[1]

Details of several other nephrotoxic plants are presented in Table 1. This article will not deal with oxalates as nephrotoxins.

OCCURRENCE OF POISONING

Occurrence of poisoning by both oak and pigweed is largely seasonal and species specific. Oak poisoning is found primarily in cattle as a subacute disease. It is confined in the southern states mainly to spring, when new buds and leaves of the shin oak, *Q. harvardi*, are consumed. In the central and upper midwest, poisoning commonly occurs from September through November, often when rain causes softening and sprouting of acorns, and many small oak seedlings are available. No particular oak is a proven cause, but the white oak group is suspected by many to be a major cause. Numbers of oak poisoning outbreaks are difficult to estimate, but it is a major problem in many areas from California to Texas, through the midwest, and into New England.

Pigweed toxicosis is generally confined to summer and fall (July through September), when pigweeds are actively growing and maturing. Most commonly affected animals are weanling or feeder swine given sudden access to pigweed. The plant is palatable and when consumed heavily for 2 to 3 days will cause toxicosis. Cattle may occasionally be poisoned by consuming pigweed, and the clinical and pathologic effects are similar to those for oak toxicosis.

POISONOUS PRINCIPLE

The toxic principle in oak buds and acorns is commonly considered to be a gallotannin. Tannin is present throughout the growing and fruiting seasons. No toxic principle has been identified in pigweed. Although nitrate and oxalate may occur in high concentrations, affected animals

Table 1. *Some Plants with Nephrotoxic Potential*

Scientific Name (Common Name)	Geographic Location	Circumstances	Major Clinical Effects	Systems Affected Secondarily	Comments
Quercus spp. (oak) *Amaranthus retroflexus* (redroot pigweed)	Entire USA except arid regions	Consumption of plant parts even when animals well nourished	Renal tubular nephrosis	Gastrointestinal tract (oak)	See text
Xanthocephalum spp. *Gutierrezia* spp. (broomweeds)	Arid regions of west and southwest USA	Consumption when desirable forage not available	Acute tubular nephrosis, uremia, and hematuria	Toxic hepatitis, abortion	Renal hemorrhages may be prominent
Vicia villosa (hairy vetch)	Primarily southern USA	Grazing freely on pastures containing hairy vetch	Dermatitis, hyperkeratosis, diarrhea, myocarditis, nephritis, thyroiditis, lymphadenopathy	Many systems	Renal lesion includes necrosis of tubules with replication of tubular cells and inflammatory cell infiltration
Agave lecheguilla (Lecheguilla)	Arid southwestern USA	Eaten when adequate forage is lacking	Acute toxic hepatitis and photosensitization	Renal tubules dilated; fatty change and albuminous casts present	High blood urea nitrogen level reported
Nolina texana (Sacahuiste)	Moderately arid southwest USA, mainly central and west Texas	Cattle and sheep eat the buds, blooms, and mature fruits	Toxic hepatitis with lesions of secondary photosensitization	Toxic tubular nephrosis characterized by fatty change and hydropic degeneration	Icterus, liver damage, and photosensitization most prominent
Xanthium spp. (cocklebur)	Entire USA, mainly in moist areas of Mississippi valley	Consumption of dicot stage seedlings in spring or moist autumn	Vomiting, weakness, muscle spasms, gastroenteritis, and toxic hepatitis	Kidneys affected by fatty change, tubular necrosis, and albuminous casts	Pig mostly commonly affected owing to eating habits; mature plant apparently not toxic

do not have signs of either oxalate or nitrate toxicosis. Other plants of minor importance in toxicology are listed in Table 1.

PATHOGENESIS

The exact mechanism of action of oak or pigweed toxins is not known. The tannins are commonly considered to be protein precipitants, but the importance of this to renal necrosis is not established. The toxins appear rather specific for renal tubules. There is early development of hyaline droplet degeneration, swelling of tubular epithelium, and finally coagulative necrosis of tubular cells. Necrotic cells slough into the tubular lumen and form eosinophilic granular casts. There may be rupture of the basement membrane with leakage of tubular fluid to the surface of the kidney. This results in perirenal edema and migration of fluids to other tissue spaces. As a result of tubular damage and swelling, acute disease is characterized by anuria or oliguria, elevated blood urea nitrogen (BUN) and serum creatinine levels, and hyperkalemia. In poisoning of several days' duration, there may be loss of phosphate and calcium control with hyperphosphatemia and hypocalcemia. Survival to a subacute or chronic stage is accompanied by formation of dilute, sometimes blood-tinged urine.

CLINICAL SIGNS

Oak poisoning most often occurs in cattle, less often in sheep. Both adults and calves are affected. Signs sometimes appear gradually. In other cases, dead animals are the first observed sign of nephrotoxicosis. In closely watched animals, early signs are anorexia, depression, and constipation. Dark dry fecal boluses covered with mucus or flecks of blood are passed. Occasionally, feces are dark and tarry. Auscultation and palpation reveal ruminal atony with contents of heavy doughy consistency.

Often there is tenesmus, and animals stand with persistent elevation of the lumbar area. Weakness progresses to prostration and death in 3 to 7 days. In advanced stages, there may be mild icterus and hematuria or, more commonly, polyuria with elimination of clear urine.

Swine poisoned by pigweed are usually affected 3 to 7 days after consuming the plant. Early signs are weakness, trembling, and incoordination followed by knuckling ataxia, paresis, and flaccid paralysis. Affected pigs generally lie in sternal recumbency. Temperature is normal, and appetite may be good until signs advance. Death can occur within 48 hr of onset or may be prolonged 5 to 15 days. Signs progress from those of acute renal failure to chronic renal failure characterized by passage of dilute urine, loss of weight, and distention of the abdomen. Kidneys of swine recovered from *A. retroflexus* poisoning may be white, scarred, and shrunken. These are occasionally noticed as incidental findings at a later necropsy or during slaughter inspection. Morbidity of pigweed poisoning ranges from 5 to 90 per cent in a herd, while mortality may exceed 75 per cent of those affected. The clinical signs of *A. retroflexus* toxicoses in cattle are essentially identical to the clinical signs of oak poisoning.

CLINICAL PATHOLOGY

Oak and pigweed poisoning have similar clinical pathologic features. There is elevation of BUN and serum creatinine levels accompanied by a moderate to marked hyperkalemia in acute cases. As chronicity develops, hyperphosphatemia and hypocalcemia may occur and serum sodium level is low. Glucosuria, proteinuria, and granular or hyaline casts are common. Urine specific gravity becomes low and urinary volume high.

Cardiovascular effects are consistent with hyperkalemia (bradycardia with increased QRS complex time and increased duration and amplitude of T wave) in swine, but these findings have not been verified in cattle.

Gross lesions of oak poisoning in cattle include ventral

edema, ascites, hydrothorax, perirenal edema (often blood-tinged), and enlarged, pale kidneys. The rumen contents are heavy and pasty and may contain acorns or oak leaves, although oak parts cannot consistently be found in the rumen. Often there is catarrhal enteritis and colitis with flecks of blood in the feces.

A. retroflexus toxicosis in swine results in hydrothorax, hydropericardium, ascites, ventral abdominal edema, perirenal edema, and infiltration of edema into the mesentery, mesometrium, or other spaces. The kidneys in acute poisoning cases are pale and swollen. In chronic cases, the kidneys may be enclosed in a cyst-like structure filled with blood and proteinaceous fluids.

The microscopic lesions of both oak and pigweed poisoning are nearly identical. Acute cases have numerous eosinophilic granular casts, hyaline casts, and coagulative necrosis of tubular epithelium. In advanced cases, there is loss of tubular epithelium, interstitial infiltration with mononuclear cells, and moderate to marked fibrosis. Many tubules appear dilated.

DIAGNOSIS

Tentative diagnosis is based on the clinical signs correlated with evidence of consumption of suspected plants. Characteristic clinical pathologic changes in blood, serum, and urine are helpful. Gross pathologic lesions are very characteristic, and demonstration of the microscopic lesion in fixed kidney tissue is considered confirmatory.

TREATMENT

There is no antidote for either oak or pigweed poisoning. Affected animals should be removed from the source as soon as possible. Supportive therapy is aimed at alleviating the effects of kidney failure. Fluids, especially those containing potassium, should be used cautiously unless urine flow is established. Proper supportive therapy will depend on laboratory evaluation of electrolyte and acid-base balance as well as renal function. I suggest the following therapeutic procedures for oak-poisoned cattle.

Detoxification by Elimination of Ingesta from the Gastrointestinal (GI) Tract. The prognosis for stimulating ruminal motility and effective GI emptying in ruminants is guarded. Harsh cathartics that depend on irritant principles or parasympathetic stimulation should be avoided. Cathartics recommended include mineral oil at 1 L/400 kg or sodium sulfate (Glauber's salt)* at 1 kg/400 kg (Table 2). Both products are given orally. Mineral oil should be given only by stomach tube to avoid potential aspiration. Use of sodium sulfate may exacerbate dehydration, so care should be taken to keep animals adequately hydrated.

Management and Support of Oliguric or Anuric Renal Failure. This phase of acute renal failure is difficult to manage even when specific laboratory findings are available. Proper therapy is also expensive and time consuming. If laboratory facilities are not available or are considered too expensive, some general suggestions for handling the oliguric or anuric animal are offered. Minimal considerations should include (1) state of hydration, (2) status

Table 2. Common Drug Dosages

Drug	Supplier	Species	Dose
Mannitol (IV 20%)	Abbott Laboratories North Chicago, IL	Cattle	1–2 gm/kg IV
Sodium sulfate	Fisher Scientific Springfield, NJ	Cattle and swine	1 kg/400 kg
Mineral oil	Fisher Scientific Springfield, NJ	Cattle and swine	1 L/400 kg
Calcium gluconate (Cal-Dextro special)	Fort Dodge Laboratories Fort Dodge, IA	Cattle	1 ml/kg of 23% solution
Calcium hydroxide (slaked lime; hydrated lime)	Available through local feed supplier	Cattle	0.5 gm/kg daily as a 15% supplement in feed

of urine formation, (3) bicarbonate requirement, and (4) hyperkalemia.

If an accurate means of weighing the animal is available, it can be used to monitor rehydration. Other means, such as skin pliability or retraction of the eyes into the orbit, depend on the clinical expertise and experience of the attending clinician. A common rule is that 6 per cent of body weight loss is considered moderate dehydration. Replacing 6 per cent of body weight in a 400 kg animal would require 24 L of fluids. In most oak-poisoned animals, a major amount of rehydration may be accomplished orally. This has the advantages of less stringent requirements for tonicity, volume, and asepsis. If diuresis has not been accomplished and the serum potassium level is not known, then isotonic saline should be used for any parenteral fluids given.

If plasma bicarbonate and blood pH values are unknown, a procedure for estimating bicarbonate needs in small animals has been reported by Low[2] when mild, moderate, and severe uremia are correlated with a bicarbonate requirement of 3, 6, and 9 mEq/kg body weight, respectively. Commonly available field kits for estimation of uremia may be helpful in estimating the degree of uremia. The procedure has apparently not been described in livestock, but is a rough guide to therapy for livestock.

After adequate hydration is accomplished, diuresis may be attempted with Mannitol* at 5 to 10 ml of a 20-per cent solution per kilogram of body weight administered intravenously. Urine formation may be monitored by catheterization of the urinary bladder or by palpation of the bladder per rectum.

Hyperkalemia induces cardiac arrhythmia and muscular weakness. If urine flow cannot be established, then potassium-containing fluids should be strictly avoided. If hyperkalemia is present, the effects can be countered temporarily by correction of bicarbonate deficit and administration of calcium. A dosage of calcium for this purpose has not been established for ruminants. Based on work in small animals, a similar dose in cattle would be 1 to 2 ml of a 23-per cent solution of calcium gluconate per kg body weight given slowly intravenously with careful monitoring of cardiac rate and rhythm.

Dealing With the Polyuric Phase of Tubular Necrosis. Many animals poisoned by oak or pigweed survive to a stage of polyuria commonly termed "high output failure,"

---

*Available from Fisher Scientific, Springfield, NJ 07081.

*Available from Abbott Laboratories, North Chicago, IL 60064.

Table 3. *Preventive Supplements*

Ingredient	Amount (kg)
Cottonseed meal	445
Dehydrated alfalfa	273
Vegetable oil	55
Hydrated lime, Ca(OH)$_2$	136

which indicates high urine output with reduced renal function. During this stage, there may be loss of water and sodium. In addition, phosphorus regulation is lost, and hyperphosphatemia develops. In large ruminants, it is probably impractical and uneconomical to continue therapy for prolonged periods in this phase. Sodium-containing solutions may be given parenterally, and the sodium content of the diet should be maintained, not restricted. The ration should contain minimal requirements for protein and phosphorus, with good quality legume hays and little or no grain. The polyuric phase may persist for 2 to 3 weeks with resolution either by tubular regeneration or by progressive failure with death due to dehydration, acidosis, and electrolyte imbalance. Clients should be advised that therapy is expensive, and the outcome is often doubtful. Recovered animals with chronic renal damage may never perform well.

PREVENTION

Owners should be aware of the season of most danger for oak or pigweed poisoning (spring in southern climates and fall in northern climates of the United States). Alternative pastures could be used during those seasons. If this is not possible, a preventive supplement for oak toxicosis (Table 3) has been devised by Dollahite and co-workers[3] consisting of 2 kg/day for cows and 1 kg/day for calves. Ca(OH)$_2$ is the active ingredient, and substitution of cottonseed meal with other feed grains has also been done. While this ration will reduce losses due to oak poisoning, it will not always prevent poisoning. Sometimes palatability of the mixture is a problem, but avoiding excessive Ca(OH)$_2$ usually prevents this.

Nephrotoxic plants pose serious problems, and animals generally respond poorly to therapy for overt toxicosis. Prevention and management of oak and pigweed infested areas is the only economical solution.

References

1. Buck, W. B., Osweiler, G. D., and Van Gelder, G. A.: Clinical and Diagnostic Veterinary Toxicology. 2nd ed. Dubuque, Iowa, Kendall/Hunt Publishing Co., 1976.
2. Low, D. G.: *In* Kirk, R. W. (ed.): Current Veterinary Therapy VI. Small Animal Practice. Philadelphia, W. B. Saunders Company, 1135, 1976.
3. Dollahite, J. W., Housholder, G. T., and Camp, B. J.: Effect of calcium hydroxide on the toxicity of post oak *(Quercus stellata)* in calves. J. Am. Vet. Med. Assoc. *148*:908, 1966.

Plants Affecting Blood Coagulation

GARY D. OSWEILER, D.V.M., M.S., Ph.D.
and LAWRENCE P. RUHR, D.V.M., Ph.D.

Defective blood coagulation may be induced by toxic agents in several ways. The coagulation system depends on a series of stepwise reactions involving coagulation factors each dependent on some other aspect of the series for its activity. Once a clot is formed, the stability of fibrin structure must be maintained, and if fibrinolysis occurs too early, hemorrhage may result. In addition to coagulation factors, thrombocytes (platelets) are the cellular component responsible for both mechanical and chemical initiation of coagulation. A complete discussion of coagulopathy is beyond the scope of this article, but the basic mechanisms involved are important to application of therapy. Not all hemorrhages are due to coagulopathies, since agents that severely damage vascular walls may also allow hemorrhage to occur.

Any toxin interfering with production or activation of clotting factors or both can result in coagulopathy. This attack may be direct (as with vitamin-K antagonists such as dicumarol) or indirect (e.g., severe liver damage from the plant *Hymenoxys odorata*, bitterweed). Platelet dysfunction or depletion is generally due to agents affecting production of these cells in the bone marrow, and often other cellular elements of the marrow are depleted as well. This article deals primarily with the 2 major plants that affect blood coagulation.

SWEET CLOVER (*Melitotus* sp.)

Sweet clover (*Melitotus* sp.) causes coagulopathy when its naturally occurring coumarin is dimerized to dicumarol (3,3' methylenebis[4-hydroxycoumarin]) as a result of fungal spoilage during curing. The toxin persists in hay or moldy silage and is relatively palatable so that animals consume it readily. Dicumarol interferes with complete synthesis of the prothrombin complex clotting factors (II, VII, IX, and X), thus acting as a vitamin-K antagonist. Since sweet clover is rarely used in hay production, it is no longer a widespread problem for cattle producers, but occasional cases may be devastating for individual herds, with high morbidity and moderate to high mortality. From 2 to 7 days' ingestion of moldy sweet clover may be required to induce the condition, since coagulation factors already present are not destroyed.

Dicumarol fed continuously at 30 ppm in hay caused clinical signs in cattle after 132 to 139 days. Up to 20 ppm fed for 100 days had no clinical effect. Levels of 60 to 70 ppm shortened onset of signs to 17 to 23 days.[1]

Because the disease is due to coagulopathy, hemorrhage occurs in body regions most affected by trauma. Early signs include epistaxis, dark tarry feces, and mild anemia. As signs progress, or when exposure is heavy, subcutaneous and periarticular hemorrhages result in soft fluctuating swellings, but temperature remains normal. Often the visible swellings are located at points of trauma, such as the submandibular space, brisket, tuber coxae, or carpal pads. Hemorrhage into spaces, such as joint cavities, spinal canal, and peritoneal cavity may result in lameness, posterior paresis, and anemia, respectively. Affected animals may have dyspnea due either to anemia-anoxemia or pulmonary interference by alveolar hemorrhage or hemothorax.

Dicumarol poisoning results in prolongation of clotting time, prothrombin time, and activated partial thromboplastin time; platelet numbers and functions are normal, and liver damage does not occur except potentially as a result of severe anemia and anoxia. Lesions of dicumarol poisoning are hemorrhage of almost any organs or tissues, but notably in subcutaneous tissue, around joints, in the thorax or abdomen, and throughout the gastrointestinal tract. Hemorrhages are generally evident as suffusions or hematomas rather than as petechiae or ecchymoses. If large areas of impounded blood are present, icterus may result.

Dicumarol poisoning may have to be differentiated from bracken-fern poisoning, mycotoxicoses (aflatoxicosis, fusariotoxicosis), clostridial diseases (*Clostridium chauvoei, C. septicum, C. novyi, C. haemolyticum*), leptospirosis, septicemia, and liver failure caused by plants, such as *Hymenoxys odorata*. A disease characterized by hemorrhages with coagulopathy in the absence of fever and liver damage should prompt a vigorous search for moldy sweet clover as a strong causative agent. Chemical analysis of blood, liver, or forages can confirm the presence of dicumarol and aid in diagnosis. Recently developed assays for dicumarol should improve diagnostic verification.[1]

Treatment

Treatment of sweet clover disease requires restoration of coagulation factors as rapidly as possible. If animals are severely affected, administer 1 liter of blood per 100 kg body weight. This will supply coagulation factors and reverse the coagulopathy within minutes. Vitamin K_1* is effective therapy (Table 1) and should be given at 1 mg/kg body weight intramuscularly or intravenously. Repeat 2 or 3 times daily for 2 days. Synthetic vitamin K (Menadione)† is less rapid in its effect, so it should not be relied upon in serious cases. Fractious animals must be handled carefully and may be sedated to prevent traumatic hemorrhage.

Recovering animals should receive oral Menadione† (synthetic vitamin K) at 5 mg/kg body weight/day for 7 to 10 additional days. Keep affected animals warm and supply high quality forage and grain. Supplementation with protein, iron, copper, and B complex vitamins will aid in production of erythrocytes lost to hemorrhage. See Table 1 for dosage details.

This disease is readily prevented when producers are knowledgeable about the potential toxicity of improperly cured sweet clover hay or moldy silage.

BRACKEN FERN (*Pteridium* sp.)

Bracken fern is widely distributed throughout the United States wherever forested areas exist. This range includes nearly all states except the Great Plains. Toxicosis from bracken fern has been reported most often in the Pacific northwest and the north central midwest. The plant is large, 0.6 to 1.8 m high, growing in dense stands and spreading underground by rhizomes. All parts, including rhizomes, are toxic, and the toxin persists after drying of the plant. It is palatable, and poisoning occurs by prolonged ingestion of rhizomes (in swine), by grazing the plant, or by consuming contaminated hay. Several toxic factors are recognized including (1) cyanogenetic glycosides, (2) thiaminase, (3) an aplastic anemia factor, (4) a hematuria-causing factor, and (5) a carcinogen.[2] This article deals only with thiaminase and the aplastic anemia factor, but veterinarians and producers should be aware that in the bovine, long-term consumption of bracken

Table 1. *Common Drug Dosages*

Drug	Supplier	Species	Dosage
Vitamin K_1	Merck & Company, Inc. Animal Health Division Rahway, NJ 07065	Bovine and swine	1 mg/kg IV or IM
Menadione	Heterochemical Corporation 111 East Hawthorne Ave. Valley Stream, NY 11580	Bovine and swine	5 mg/kg orally for 5–7 days
D-L Batyl Alcohol	Sigma Chemical Co. P.O. Box 14508 St. Louis, MO 63178	Bovine	0.5–1.0 gm per animal given IV daily
Tween 20	Fisher Scientific 52 Fadem Rd. Springfield, NJ 07081	Bovine	5 gm in 100 ml Batyl Alcohol solution
Protamine sulfate		Bovine and swine	100 mg per animal

fern has resulted in hematuria as well as in neoplasm of the urinary bladder and intestinal mucosa.

Clinical Signs

Pathogenesis and effects of bracken toxicosis vary with species. In nonruminants such as swine, 7 to 10 weeks of ingestion of bracken as 25 per cent of the diet results in thiamine deficiency. There is depressed growth rate, dyspnea, weakness, recumbency, and death in experimental swine. Bracken-fern toxicosis in cattle is considered a radiomimetic disease that occurs after 1 to 3 months of bracken fern ingestion equivalent to approximately 100 per cent of body weight. Clinical signs may occur several weeks after access to bracken ferns has ceased. Disease develops as a result of bone marrow depression affecting leukocytes and platelets. There is greater capillary fragility, prolonged bleeding time, and defective clot retraction. Clinical signs are depression, anorexia, and hemorrhagic diarrhea. Often there are petechiae on the visible mucous membranes, and bleeding from nostrils and intestinal and urogenital tracts may occur. Some animals develop laryngeal edema with difficult breathing. Secondary infections occur as a result of leucopenia.

One clinical pathologic change in swine is elevated blood pyruvate level. In cattle, there is anemia with little evidence of regeneration, leucopenia, and low platelet numbers. Bleeding time and clot retraction time are prolonged.

Bracken-fern toxicosis in ruminants may resemble septicemia (which may indeed be a secondary problem), leptospirosis, an overdose of x-rays, and trichloroethylene solvent (formerly used to extract oilseed meals) toxicosis. There is no readily available chemical test for confirmation.

Treatment

Treatment has been attempted in cattle, using D-L Batyl Alcohol* (see Table 1) as a bone marrow stimulant. D-L Batyl Alcohol is not an approved drug for food animals in the United States. A suspension of 2 gm of Batyl Alcohol in 100 ml of 1 per cent saline can be prepared by adding 5 gm of Tween 20† and boiling to put the mixture in solution. Twenty-five to 50 ml of the solution is given intravenously daily. This treatment is apparently not consistently effective. Batyl Alcohol ther-

*Available from Merck & Company, Inc., Rahway, NJ 07065.
†Available from Heterochemical Corporation, Valley Stream, NY 11580.

*Available from Sigma Chemical Co., St. Louis, MO 63178.
†Available from Fisher Scientific, Springfield, NJ 07081.

apy may be helpful if circulating leukocytes and thrombocytes are not below 2000 and 50,000–100,000 per mm^3, respectively.[4] Tustin and associates found 27 of 30 cattle recovered when treated with 1 injection of 10 ml protamine sulfate (1 per cent concentration) and 2.25 L to 4.5 L of blood given intravenously. Protamine sulfate is a heparin antagonist, and since heparin may be increased in bracken-fern toxicosis, protamine sulfate is rational therapy. Successful therapy may be largely dependent on early detection, while bone narrow is still responsive. Adjunctive therapy of broad-spectrum antibiotics to control secondary bacterial infections and nutritional therapy to combat anemia are recommended. Prevention of bracken-fern toxicosis depends on blocking access to the fern, both fresh and as a contaminant of feed or hay.

References

1. Casper, H. H., Alstad, A. D., Monson, S. B., and Johnson, L. J.: Dicumarol levels in sweet clover toxic to cattle. Proc. Am. Assoc. Vet. Lab. Diag. 25:41–48, 1982.
2. Clarke, E. G. C., and Clarke, M. D.: Veterinary Toxicology. Baltimore, Md. Williams & Wilkins, 301, 307, 1975.
3. Tustin, R. C., Adelaar, T. F., and Medal-Johnsen, C. M.: Bracken poisoning in cattle in the Natal Medlands. J. South Afri. Vet. Med. Assoc. 39:91, 1969.
4. Evans, I. A., Thomas, A. J., Evans, W. C., and Edwards, C. M.: Studies on bracken poisoning in cattle. Part V. Br. Vet. J. 114:253, 1958.

Dermatotoxic Plants

A. EARL JOHNSON, M.S.

Dermatotoxic plants are those plants that either directly or indirectly injure the skin. Although a few plants damage the skin directly, the majority of plants that cause economically important dermatoses are those that are eaten by livestock and thus damage the skin indirectly. Few plant species cause direct skin injury since the outer of the 2 primary skin layers, the epidermis, is primarily protective in function. The epidermis provides a shield of dead epithelial cells, it is avascular and relatively nonreactive, it becomes thickened where stress and wear are greatest, it contains pigments for protection against light, and it restricts the passage of fluids through it, thus providing protection against soluble toxins. Sebum and hair provide additional mechanical barriers to harmful agents. The underlying skin layer, the dermis or corium, is the site of the primary physiologic activities of the skin and is more reactive and susceptible to toxic agents, but there are few plant toxins capable of penetrating the mechanical and physiologic barriers of the epidermis to reach this more sensitive area.

Numerous factors may influence the development of skin disorders. One should consider predisposing factors and their relationship to primary causative agents in the generation of dermatoses.[1] Age, sex, heredity, nutrition, and previous exposure may influence the toxicity of poisonous agents. A given dermatotoxin is not uniformly toxic under all conditions.

INJURIES CAUSED BY DERMATOTOXIC PLANTS

The actions of dermatotoxic plants on healthy or sensitized skin may be classed broadly into 3 categories, (1) mechanical skin injury, (2) external contact producing localized skin reactions, and (3) skin injury following ingestion of the toxic plant. Toxins in category 3 may reach the skin following normal digestive and circulatory processes to produce dermatosis, or dermatosis may result after the ingested plant has caused an internal organ to malfunction.

Plants Causing Mechanical Injury

Plants classified in this group have received little attention in veterinary literature, probably because they are usually classified with other objects that cause mechanical injury. Awns, spines, and thorns, or any other plant part that can penetrate the skin may cause obvious damage. A few plants are provided with means to penetrate skin to deliver contact toxins with which they are coated. Awn-producing grasses can be particularly troublesome. The damage most often affects the mouth, internal ear, or eyes of exposed animals rather than the skin. Representative irritating grasses are porcupine or needlegrasses (*Stipa* spp.) and field sandbur (*Cenchrus pauciflorus*). Needlegrass may cause severe irritation and can penetrate and permanently damage the hide. Sandbur and puncture vine (*Tribulus terrestris*) do not penetrate the deep layers of the skin but often cause troublesome irritation around the hooves of animals.

Generally, mechanical injury by plants to animals is only occasional. Diagnosis is relatively easy, and treatment usually involves the removal of the source of irritation and the use of a soothing antiseptic or antibiotic ointment.

Plants Causing Contact Dermatoses

There are apparently only a few plants that cause contact dermatoses in animals. However, there are probably more plants involved than are presently recognized, since skin reactions to these plants are likely to be transitory, and the signs may be obscure. Poison ivy (*Toxicodendron radicans*) and poison oak (*Rhus toxicodendron*) are classic plants containing contact dermatotoxins to humans, but they do not cause significant problems in livestock.

Stinging nettles (*Urtica urens, U. dioica*) may cause rashes and discomfort in pigs similar to that in humans.[1]

Hairs of bull nettle (*Cnidoscolus stimulosus*) or spurge nettle (*Jatropha stimulosa*) are covered with caustic irritants that cause pain in humans, but the effect of these irritants on the skin of livestock is not known.

Ingested Plants Causing Photosensitization

Cutaneous photosensitization is by far the most important dermatosis in livestock, resulting from ingestion of plants. Plants that contain photodynamic agents or plants that cause photodynamic agents to be deposited in the skin may cause photosensitization when sunlight or light of a given wavelength is allowed to reach these agents in the skin. The photosensitized areas are usually the light-colored and the unprotected areas of skin, since skin pigmentation or dense hair may screen out sunlight.

The complete reaction of photosensitization in skin is not fully understood, but the explanation of Blum[2] is generally accepted. Briefly, he states that the photodynamic agent in the skin absorbs light energy and has the ability to transfer this energy to activated molecules, which in turn are oxidized. This reaction causes cellular damage, and inflammatory substances are released that give rise to the typical signs of photosensitization. These signs, regardless of the causative phototoxic agent, are remarkably similar, usually differing only in degree. Erythema, swelling, and pruritus are first noted. Sometimes there is vesiculation. Edema may become severe, and there may be serous exudation with or without vesiculation. Necrosis may extend into the deeper layers of skin, and lips, eyelids, and ears may slough or be permanently deformed. In sheep, wool may be lost permanently, and large areas of light-colored skin may slough in hard, leather-like sheets. Few animals die from photosensitization itself; however, they may die from secondary infection or starvation.

In 1922 Clare[3] classified photosensitization into 3 types: (1) primary, the photodynamic agent in the plant is absorbed from the digestive tract and reaches the skin by peripheral blood circulation, (2) congenital, aberrant pigment synthesis is the cause, (3) hepatogenous or secondary, the photodynamic agent is phylloerythrin, a degradation product of chlorophyll. Plant-related photosensitizations are either primary or secondary.

Primary Photosensitization

St. Johnswort (*Hypericum perforatum*), also called Klamath weed and goat weed, is perhaps the most well known plant causing primary photosensitization in livestock. It contains a red fluorescent pigment named hypericin that is the photodynamic compound. St. Johnswort grows in many parts of the world and was introduced into the eastern United States. It may now be found throughout the United States except in some of the more arid areas of the west and southwest. Other *Hypericum* species cause photosensitization, but they are not recognized as causing important economic problems in this country. St. Johnswort has caused economic problems to owners of cattle, sheep, and horses. Particularly severe losses have occurred in the western coastal states, but losses have been reduced greatly since methods of controlling the weed have been developed.

Cattle are more susceptible than other livestock to hypericin and may react to such an extent that huge pieces of hard, leather-like skin in white or light-colored areas slough. Animals that are removed from the plant source, protected from sunlight, and treated according to symptoms will usually recover, although permanent damage to the hide or wool may often result.

Photosensitization as a result of sheep, cattle, goats, pigs, and horses eating buckwheat (*Fagopyrum esculentum*) is also well known as a primary type of photosensitization. Fagopyrism, as the syndrome has been labeled, has been known since the late 1800s. It is uncommon in cattle, but sheep and pigs may be affected under certain conditions. The fresh, green plant, especially that containing blossoms, is considered the most toxic. The straw, grain, bran, and chaff of buckwheat may also cause photosensitization if eaten in sufficient quantity.

Two compounds, fagopyrin and photofagopyrin, have been identified as the photosensitizing substances.[4] They are closely related to hypericin.

Fagopyrism, or buckwheat rash, most often appears on the face, ears, eyelids, and neck. The degree of skin damage is dependent on the amount of plant ingested and the amount of sunlight to which the animal is exposed. In mild cases, erythema, slight swelling, and pruritus may be evident. In more severe cases, vesicular lesions develop and these may rupture, giving rise to crusty areas on the affected skin. Necrosis may also develop.

Treatment for fagopyrism is the same as for any photosensitization: remove the toxic feed or causative agent, keep animals out of sunlight, and provide food and rest. Antiseptic or antibiotic ointments may be applied if needed.

Spring parsley (*Cymopterus watsonii*), a small perennial umbelliferous plant that grows in the desert areas of Nevada and southern Utah, causes a primary photosensitization in livestock, particularly in sheep.[5] Van Kampen and coworkers[6] in 1969 demonstrated experimentally that spring parsley causes photosensitization in chickens and that deformities can result from photosensitization. With the exception of *Cymopterus longipes* that causes phototoxicity in fowl, other species of *Cymopterus* are not known to be phototoxic in fowl. However, other *Cymopterus* species are suspected of causing serious photosensitization in cattle.

Ewes that graze *C. watsonii* in early spring, when there may be a scarcity of other forage, become photosensitized in areas of the body not covered by wool, i.e., lips, udder, and vulva. These areas become erythematous, swollen, and extremely sore. Further development of the condition results in the formation of vesicles and their subsequent rupture and crust formation. Ewes so affected will not allow their lambs to nurse because of udder tenderness. Deaths of lambs from starvation and dehydration may approach 25 per cent in some herds.

Two psoralen compounds, xanthotoxin and bergapten, have been isolated from spring parsley.[7]

Secondary or Hepatogenous Photosensitization

Secondary or hepatogenous photosensitization is caused by the presence of phylloerythrin in the skin. Phylloerythrin is formed during microbial degradation of chlorophyll in the rumen of normal ruminants. It is absorbed into the blood stream, removed from the circulation by the liver, and excreted in the bile. Livers incapable of performing this excretion allow phylloerythrin to reach the peripheral circulation, and there it is activated by sunlight on the skin.

The mechanism by which phylloerythrin is removed and excreted and factors that influence this excretion are not fully understood. However, Johnson[8] and Keeler and associates[9] have shown that the photosensitization caused in sheep by *Tetradymia* species can be potentiated by certain sagebrush species. Also, studies by Horsley[10] suggest that secondary factors can enhance the effects of photosensitizers, such as those in St. Johnswort. Other investigators have found the experimental production of some secondary photosensitizations difficult and unpredictable, indicating that unknown predisposing factors may be important.

Livestock owners find that exposure of their stock to secondary photosensitizing plants does not always result in the expected photosensitizations. Some producers have a false sense of security about photosensitization, so they become careless in managing their livestock in areas where photosensitizing plants are present. The result is often a sudden outbreak of photosensitization involving many animals.

Plants known to cause secondary photosensitizations are too numerous to discuss individually; however, Table

Table 1. *Plants Causing Secondary Photosensitization and Livestock Frequently Affected*

Scientific Name	Common Name	Livestock Frequently Affected
Agave lecheguilla	Lechuguilla	Sheep and goats
Brassica napus	Cultivated rape	Cattle
Lantana spp.	Lantana	Cattle and sheep
Nolina texana	Texas sacahuiste	Cattle, sheep, and goats
Panicum coloratum	Kleingrass	Lambs
Tetradymia glabrata	Littleleaf horsebrush, coal oil brush	Sheep
Tetradymia canescens	Spineless or grey horsebrush	Sheep
Tribulus terrestris	Puncture vine	Sheep

1 presents a list of plants compiled by Kingsbury,[11] with a list of animals most frequently affected.

Numerous other plants, including common livestock feeds, e.g., oats, alfalfa, and clovers, cause sporadic outbreaks of photosensitization. The occurrence of such outbreaks is probably dependent on predisposing factors.

Kingsbury[11] further lists spotted spurge (*Euphorbia maculata*), smartweeds (*Polygonum* spp.), kochia (*Kochia scoparia*), sudan grass (*Sorghum sudanense*), and vetches (*Vicia* spp.) as phototoxic plants. These plants and oats, alfalfa, and clovers must be listed as unclassified photosensitizers until more definitive work is done.

PLANT PRODUCTS CAUSING DERMATOSES

Dermatitis and eczema occasionally occur in livestock that are fed plant products. Rashes may occur in individuals or in groups, depending on the type of food, the amount of food, the nutritional state of the animal, and other unknown predisposing factors. Feeds such as potatoes and their waste products, malt, coconut cake, beet pulp, palm oil cake, rice bran, adulterated linseed meal, cottonseed cake, and corn cake all have been reported to cause skin rashes of varying severity in different classes of livestock.[1] These rashes may occur on almost any part of the animal's body.

Treatment for these rashes is the same as for other dermatoses caused by plants. Often, however, the most difficult part is to determine which feed contains the causative agent.

References

1. Kral, F., and Schwartzman, R. M.: Veterinary and Comparative Dermatology. Philadelphia, J. B. Lippincott, 95, 1964.
2. Blum, H. F.: Photodynamic Action and Diseases Caused by Light. New York, Reinhold, 82, 1941.
3. Clare, N. T.: Photosensitization in Diseases of Domestic Animals. Bucks, England, Commonwealth Agricultural Bureaux, 10, 1952.
4. Brockmann, H.: Photodynamically active plant pigments. Proc. Chem. Soc. 304–312, 1957.
5. Binns, W. and James, L. F.: *Cymopterus watsonii*: A photosensitizing plant for sheep. Vet. Med. Small Anim. Clin. 59:4, 1964.
6. Van Kampen, K. R., Williams, M. C., and Binns, W.: Deformities in chickens photosensitized by feeding spring parsley (*Cymopterus watsonii*). Am. J. Vet. Res. 30:9, 1969.
7. Williams, M. C.: Xanthotoxin and bergapten in spring parsley. Weed Sci. 18:4, 1970.
8. Johnson, A. E.: Predisposing influence of range plants on tetradymia-related photosensitization in sheep: Work of Drs. A. B. Clawson and W. T. Huffman. Am. J. Vet. Res. 35:12, 1974.
9. Keeler, R. F., Van Kampen, K. R., and James, L. F.: Effects of Poisonous Plants on Livestock. New York, Academic Press, 209, 1978.
10. Horsley, C. H.: Investigation into the action of St. Johnswort. J. Pharmacol. Exp. Ther. 50:310, 1934.
11. Kingsbury, J. M.: Poisonous Plants of the United States and Canada. Englewood Cliffs, New Jersey, Prentice-Hall, Inc., 56, 1964.

Effects of Plant Toxins on the Central Nervous System

LYNN F. JAMES, Ph.D.
and KENT R. VAN KAMPEN, D.V.M., Ph.D.

There are many plants that when ingested by animals have profound effects on the central nervous system (CNS). These effects may be manifested acutely, manifested chronically as a result of prolonged daily ingestion, or manifested as fetal toxicity. The toxic effect will vary with the level of toxin contained within the plant, the amount of toxin ingested, the duration of toxin ingestion, and the species of animal.

Plants inducing CNS signs in animals cause a variety of physiologic effects or a variety of morphologic lesions. The important plants producing CNS disease are described as follows.

NITRO-BEARING PLANTS (*Astragalus miser*) AND RELATED SPECIES[1]

Certain *Astragalus* species or varieties (a total of 263) contain aliphatic nitro-compounds that are catabolized to 3-nitro-1 propanol (3-NPOH) and 3-nitropropionic acid (3-NPA) in the digestive tract of ruminants. 3-NPOH is more toxic than 3-NPA per mg of NO_2 ingested because it is absorbed more readily from the digestive tract. Animals acutely poisoned after eating nitro-bearing *Astragalus* have incoordination of the hindquarters, general weakness, and labored breathing. They die from cardiac and respiratory failure 4 to 20 hr following poisoning. Acutely poisoned animals suffer up to 20 per cent methemoglobinemia, but the cause of death is associated with the absorption of 3-NPOH into the circulatory system, subsequently affecting the motor and autonomic responsive areas of the brain.

Chronic poisoning by nitro-bearing *Astragalus* results in impairment of locomotion in the hindquarters with knuckling of the fetlocks and interference of the hocks when the animals are made to move. James and coworkers[2] have described wallerian degeneration in the spinal cord and varying degrees of alveolar emphysema associated with this disease.

ANNUAL RYEGRASS (*Lolium rigidium*)[3]

Annual ryegrass (*Lolium rigidium*) or Wimmera ryegrass often becomes infested with a nematode, *Anguina colii*, that bores into the developing flower, carrying with it a bacterium (*Corynebacterium* sp.), resulting in improper development of the seed. The resulting gall is extremely toxic to sheep. Sheep grazing the toxic grass, if disturbed, develop a staggering, stiff-legged gait and collapse with convulsions.

A similar disease has been reported in Oregon sheep grazing *Festuca rubra commutata* infested by *Anguina agrostis* and a bacterium thought to be a *Corynebacterium*.

Lesions described in sheep poisoned with annual ryegrass include pale, friable liver, congestion of the lungs, and hemorrhage into various organs. Culvenor and associates[3] have reported isolation of a toxin from the seedheads of ryegrass. Although the toxin has not yet been completely characterized, it has many of the properties of a lipopolysaccharide peptide.

PERENNIAL RYEGRASS (*Lolium perenne*)[4]

Ryegrass staggers, a neuromuscular disorder primarily affecting sheep but also affecting cattle and horses, has been observed in New Zealand, Australia, England, and the United States. The clinical signs of this disease are head shaking, degrees of incoordination, abnormal staggering gait, eventual stumbling, and collapse to the ground. The sheep may then have severe muscular spasms followed by the animal righting itself and walking away. The onset of these clinical signs is always preceded by disturbance or excitement of the animal.

Lesions associated with this disease are not pathognomonic, but degeneration of Purkinje's cells and status spongiosis of the cerebellum have been reported. Prolonged recumbency of the animal may result in focal areas of muscular degeneration thought to be a secondary change.

Some investigators have suggested that the clinical syndrome is related to tremorgenic *Penicillium* inhabiting the soil beneath the ryegrass, while other investigators have suggested that it is related to parasitism of the seedheads with *Claviceps paspali* sclerotia. While both agents cause tremors, the exact neurotoxin in perennial ryegrass remains unknown.

CYCADS (*Cycas* spp., *Zamia* spp., and *Macrozamia* spp.)[5]

The cycads are palm-like plants found in the tropical and subtropical areas of the world within well defined geographic locations. The toxins from these plants cause hepatic and gastrointestinal disturbances, ataxia, and a radiomimetic or carcinogenic effect upon the liver or intestines.

Cattle, sheep, horses, and pigs have been affected by cycad-induced ataxia. The primary clinical sign is a loss of proper control over the movement of the hindlimbs. Early in the disease there is hyperextension of the rear limbs with a "goose-stepping" gait. Later, incomplete extension occurs, and the limbs "knuckle over" at the phalanges.

The morphologic lesions of the CNS described with this disease include bilateral symmetric degeneration of nerve fibers in the fasciculus gracilis up to the nucleus gracilis and the dorsal spinocerebellar tract and possibly degeneration of nerve fibers in the ventral spinocerebellar tract up to the cerebullum through the posterior cerebellar peduncle. Morphologic lesions have been compared to amyotrophic lateral sclerosis, a disease that occurs in people living in the tropics who consume cycad plants.

LOCOWEED AND DARLING PEA (*Astragalus* spp., *Oxytropis* spp., and *Swainsona* spp.)[2, 6]

The locoweeds (certain species of the genera *Astragalus* and *Oxytropis*) have worldwide distribution in the temperate zones, especially in mountainous arid and semi-arid areas. Poisonous *Astragalus* have been divided into 3 categories according to the clinical manifestation of their toxic properties. These categories are (1) nitro-bearing plants, (2) locoweeds, and (3) selenium accumulators. *Swainsona* spp. are confined to Australia. Recently, an indolizidine alkaloid, swainsonine, was isolated from *Swainsona* and also from locoweeds and is thought to be these plants' toxin. The toxin inhibits the enzyme mannosidase.

Locoweed and *Swainsona* poisonings affect primarily cattle, sheep, and horses, although there are some reports of wild ruminants and insects becoming poisoned on locoweed. The clinical signs include emaciation, visual impairment, neurologic abnormalities, habituation, birth defects, and abortion. The latter 2 have not been described in *Swainsona* poisoning. The most significant neurologic problems are exaggerated movement, hyperexcitability, and aggressiveness. Exaggerated movements of mastication may result in slobbering or loss of ruminated ingesta. Intoxicated horses become totally unreliable because of the neurologic signs.

The morphologic lesions are not confined to the CNS. They are described as neurovisceral vacuolation of the cellular cytoplasm. Neurons in the CNS and autonomic ganglia, glia cells, plus endothelial cells in the CNS may be affected by the vacuolar process. The vacuoles are bound by a single membrane and resemble enlarged lysosomes. These lysosomes become distended, coalesce, and may cause rupture of the cytoplasmic membranes, resulting in destruction of the cells. When neurons are affected, there may be permanent damage to the CNS, especially in horses.

Ruminants ingesting locoweed may recover when removed from locoweed-infested areas, but they will selectively seek out the plants if returned to the same area, resulting in further intoxication.

FALSE HELLEBORE (*Veratrum californicum*)

Ingestion of this plant on the fourteenth day of gestation by a pregnant ewe may result in neurologic damage to the embryo. The clinical manifestations of poisoning may be the return of estrus to the ewe due to death of the embryo, prolonged gestation, "monkey-faced" lambs, or an abnormal fetus born as a twin to a normal fetus.

The damage to the CNS of the embryo is caused by the circulation of steroidal alkaloids from the plant within the gravid uterus. Keeler[7] has isolated and identified 3 compounds, all of which induce teratogenesis, i.e., jervine, cyclopamine, and cycloposine. These compounds cause severe craniofacial malformations, including anencephaly, hydranencephaly, hydrocephalus, and fusion of the cerebral hemispheres.

References

1. Williams, M. C. and James, L. F.: Livestock poisoning from nitro-bearing *Astragalus*. *In* Keeler, R. F., VanKampen, K. R., James, L. F., et al (eds.). Effects of Poisonous Plants on Livestock. New York, Academic Press, 379, 1978.
2. James, L. F., Hartley, W. J., Williams, M. C., and Van Kampen, K. R.: Field and experimental studies in cattle and sheep poisoned by nitro-bearing *Astragalus* on their toxins. Amer. J. Vet. Res. *41*:377–382, 1980.
3. Culvenor, C. C. J., Frahn, J. L., Jago, M. V., and Lanigan, G. W.: The toxin of *Lolium rigidum* (annual ryegrass) seedheads associated with nematode-bacterium infection. *In* Keeler, R. F., VanKampen, K. R., James, L. F., et al (eds.). Effects of Poisonous Plants on Livestock. New York, Academic Press, 349–352, 1978.
4. Mortimer, P. H.: Perennial ryegrass staggers in New Zealand. *In* Keeler, R. F., VanKampen, K. R., James, L. F., et al (eds.). Effects of Poisonous Plants on Livestock. New York, Academic Press, 353–362, 1978.
5. Hooper, P. T.: Cycad poisoning in Australia—Etiology and Pathology. *In* Keeler, R. F., VanKampen, K. R., James, L. F., et al (eds.). Effects of Poisonous Plants on Livestock. New York, Academic Press, 337–348, 1978.
6. Van Kampen, K. R., Rhees, R. W., and James, L. F.: Locoweed poisoning in the United States. *In* Keeler, R. F., VanKampen, K. R., James, L. F., et al (eds.). Effects of Poisonous Plants on Livestock. New York, Academic Press, 465–474, 1978.
7. Keeler, R. F.: Alkaloid teratogens from *Lupinus, Conium, Veratrum*, and related genera. *In* Keeler, R. F., VanKampen, K. R., James, L. F., et al (eds.). Effects of Poisonous Plants on Livestock. New York, Academic Press, 397–408, 1978.

Teratogenic Plants of Livestock

RICHARD F. KEELER, Ph.D.
and J. L. SHUPE, D.V.M.

The range forage of grazing domestic livestock is variable in nutritional value, sporadic in distribution, and potentially toxic. Many of the commonly ingested range plants have a direct toxic effect on the ingesting animal. They are among the group of classic poisonous plants. Furthermore, some poisonous plants may be classified as teratogenic because they induce congenital deformities in the offspring when grazed by pregnant livestock. The appearance of these congenital deformities is delayed from the time of plant ingestion by the dam until the time of parturition, and the effects are, therefore, rather insidious even though they occur at an incidence of up to 30 per cent of the calf or lamb crop in some herds. Plant-induced congenital deformities represent possibly one third of all spontaneous deformities in range livestock, with the other two thirds induced primarily by infectious diseases or genetic causes.

The concepti of domestic livestock are subject to teratogenic insult for many reasons. Teratogens ingested by the dam are not necessarily detoxified immediately or excreted. Some teratogens pass through the placenta more readily than was once thought and thus enter the circulatory system of the conceptus.

PRINCIPLES OF TERATOLOGY

Certain factors determine if a teratogen will induce a congenital defect, regardless of whether the teratogen is from a plant or is from some other source. Wilson[5] detailed 6 Principles of Teratology that govern the induction of congenital defects by teratogens. Consideration of these principles suggests reasons for the variability in teratogenic effects induced in livestock by poisonous plants. The principles are as follows:

1. Conceptus genotype determines susceptibility.
2. The teratogen, or its influence, must reach the conceptus.
3. Deformities are dose dependent.
4. Teratogens at elevated doses can produce death rather than deformity.
5. The conceptus must be exposed when it is susceptible.
6. Teratogens exert their effects by specific mechanisms.

Thus, we can expect (1) variation in susceptibility among species, breeds, and strains of livestock; (2) variation in incidence due to different doses or to different types of metabolism in rumen or liver; (3) possible associated increases in abortions or resorptions demonstrated as decreases in lamb or calf crop; (4) variation in effect and incidence due to gestation age at the time of insult; and, finally, (5) conditions with similar clinical signs induced by unrelated plants containing different teratogens.

We cite here a few of the congenital defects known to be induced in livestock by plants. The signs, diagnosis, epidemiology, compounds responsible, factors that influence incidence, and strategies for prevention are also discussed.

TERATOGENIC PLANTS

Locoweeds

Some locoweed plants (*Astragalus lentiginosus* and *A. pubentissimus*) induce congenital deformities and abortions in addition to classic locoism. Deformed lambs have greater incidences of malpositioning, malalignment, or rigidity of joints, excessive carpal flexure, tendon contracture, anterior flexure and hypermobility of the hock, or a combination of these signs. Gestational susceptibility is broad. The conceptus can be deformed under natural and experimental conditions at almost any period of gestation. Results of experimental trials proved the plant to be the cause. Incidence on the range is sporadic because of variable plant abundance. In years of great abundance, the incidence of abortion may approach 60 per cent, and up to 30 per cent or more of the lambs born alive may be deformed. Teratogen identity is unknown. Seeds of some locoweed plants are viable in soil for many years. Plant abundance evidently is governed by the amount of moisture available to initiate germination and early growth and by subsequent seedling competition. Chaining of ranges to remove juniper and sagebrush has often allowed the abundance of locoweed for a period.

Cultivated Tobacco

A teratogenic effect occurs in offspring from sows that graze tobacco stalks (*Nicotiana tabacum*) during gestation. In some midwestern tobacco-raising areas, farmers allow pigs to graze the tobacco stalks discarded in the field after the leaves have been removed for curing. Twisting of the fore or hind limbs and dorsal flexure of the hind limb digits are common in the offspring. Breeding records were used to rule out heredity as the cause, and feeding trials have established that the plant is responsible. The active principle remains unknown. The susceptible period was believed to be between days 10 and 30 of gestation based on epidemiologic observations, but feeding trials have established that susceptibility extends well beyond day 30.

Wild Tobacco

N. glauca (wild tree tobacco) induces limb and palate defects in livestock. Cattle, sheep, and pigs tested during feeding trials are known to be susceptible. Susceptibility extends from about day 40 to 75 in cattle, day 30 to 60 in sheep, and day 30 to 60 in pigs. Experimental work with *N. glauca* was undertaken to help elucidate details of the deformity induced by common tobacco (*N. tabacum*) described earlier. Spontaneous congenital deformities in livestock from *N. glauca* have not been observed, probably because of the limited distribution of the plant and its impalatability.

Lupine

Ingestion by cows of certain lupine plants during pregnancy induces crooked calf disease. The disease is common. Up to 30 per cent or more of the calves in some areas are born with twisted or bowed limbs with malalignment, malpositioning, or rigidity of joints, spinal curvature, twisted neck, cleft palate, or a combination of these deformities, resulting from maternal lupine ingestion. The effects are induced by other causes as well, but the major outbreaks are usually induced by lupine. The principal susceptible period is between the 40th and 70th days of gestation. The condition has been caused experimentally by feeding a purified alkaloid fraction from the plant containing very high levels of the quinolizidine alkaloid, anagyrine, which is believed to be the cause. Among the many hundreds of lupines, a few contain the compound: *Lupinus sericeus*, *L. caudatus*, and *L. laxiflorus* are among them.

Concentration of all alkaloids including anagyrine is high during early plant growth and declines markedly during maturity. The amount is also elevated for a brief period while mature seeds remain in the pods.

Teratogenic hazard is minimal when lupine in early flower or postseed stage is grazed by pregnant cows whose average stage of gestation is either earlier than the 40th or later than the 70th day. The degree and incidence of malformations are not necessarily related to the severity of clinical signs in the dam because of the variable concentration of a number of toxic but not teratogenic alkaloids in lupine.

Poison Hemlock

Ingestion of poison hemlock (*Conium maculatum*) by pregnant cows or sows may induce congenital deformities in calves or piglets. Sheep are resistant. The deformities in calves are similar to those induced by lupine. Incidence of poison hemlock–induced deformities is much lower than of lupine-induced deformities, because poison hemlock is less abundant and less palatable than lupine. Twisted limbs and spinal curvature are the typical signs. In piglets, both limb deformities and cleft palates are caused by the plant. The hazardous period for cows is from the 40th to the 70th day of gestation, and for pigs is from the 30th to 60th day of gestation. The teratogenic compounds in the plant are simple piperidine alkaloids. Feeding trials have shown that coniine and probably γ-coniceine induce the conditions. Concentration of these alkaloids in the plant is highly variable. The plants usually grow in restricted areas, mainly along fences, in waste places, and in overgrazed pastures.

Veratrum

Epidemics of cyclopia and related facial deformities sometimes occur in newborn lambs. Incidence has exceeded 25 per cent of lambs from some ranches. The deformed offspring are often single- or double-globe cyclopics. Ewes may undergo prolonged gestation, and lambs become too large for normal delivery. Lambs are usually dead at birth or die shortly thereafter. Feeding trials showed that *Veratrum californicum* was responsible for the condition when it was ingested by pregnant ewes on the 14th day of gestation.

The main teratogenic compound in the plant is cyclopamine, a steroidal alkaloid. The concentration of cyclopamine in the above-ground or forage parts of the plant is lowered as the plant matures during the summer.

PREVENTION

Therapy is not available for these conditions, and total prevention is not practical because of the logistics of range grazing. However, incidences can be significantly reduced by certain management strategies. They are related to the Principles of Teratology as follows:

1. Use of genotypes low in susceptibility.
2. Reduction of dose by selective herding.
3. Grazing at periods when plant teratogen concentration is low.
4. Reduction of plant abundance.
5. Reduction of conceptus exposure during susceptible gestational periods.

Cows seem to be affected mainly by the *Lupinus* teratogen, while sheep seem to be mainly affected by the *Veratrum* teratogen.

Cyclopia in sheep due to *Veratrum* develops only by insult on the 14th day of gestation. Selective herding of sheep bands to keep them away from *Veratrum* patches until all ewes have passed the 14th day of gestation can eliminate cyclopia and other facial deformities induced by the plant. However, a much lower incidence of other *Veratrum*-induced deformities, such as limb bone shortening, may still be found from insult on other gestational days.

In *Lupine*-induced crooked calf disease, susceptibility is mainly between the 40th and 70th days of gestation. The plants are most hazardous before flowering or when mature seeds are present. During flowering and after seed drop, plants are less hazardous. Consequently, restricting access of cows during the 40th to 70th days to plants that are very young or to plants with mature seeds reduces incidence. Sometimes exposure to hazardous plants can be reduced simply by shifting herd-breeding periods.

Incidences of *Conium*-induced calf deformities have been lowered by controlling plant abundance with tillage. Similar results might be expected from herbicidal treatment. Both are feasible because *Conium* is most abundant on cultivated rather than on native grazing lands.

Sows can be provided with feed that does not include tobacco stalks to eliminate the deformity problem in pigs from maternal tobacco stalk ingestion.

Locoweed induced deformity problems seem to be

intractable. The conceptus is susceptible at almost any gestational period, so no grazing period is "safe." The dose cannot be reduced by assuring adequate supplemental feed because ewes become addicted to the locoweed and seek it out, and careful herding in locoweed-infested areas is not fruitful. In "bad" locoweed years, plants are abundant on thousands of square miles of native range. Tillage or herbicide treatment is impractical and inadequate because of seed viability.

References

1. Crowe, M. W.: Tobacco—A Cause of Congenital Arthrogryposis. *In* Keeler, R. F., Van Kampen, K. R., James, L. F., et al (eds.). Effects of Poisonous Plants on Livestock. New York, Academic Press, 419–427, 1978.
2. Keeler, R. F.: Toxins and teratogens of higher plants. Lloydia *38*:56–86, 1975.
3. Keeler, R. F.: Naturally occurring teratogens from plants. *In* Keeler, R. F., and Tu, A. T. (eds.). Handbook of Natural Toxins, vol. 1. New York, Dekker, 161–199, 1983.
4. Shupe, J. L., and Keeler, R. F.: Crooked calf syndrome. *In* Amstutz, H. E. (ed.). Bovine Medicine and Surgery, vol. 1, 2nd ed. Santa Barbara, California, Amer. Vet. Publ. Inc., 489–492, 1980.
5. Wilson, J. G.: Current Status of Teratology—General Principles and Mechanisms Derived from Animal Studies. *In* Wilson, J. G., and Fraser F. C. (eds.). Handbook of Teratology, vol. 1. New York, Plenum Publishing Corp., 47, 1977.

Principal Poisonous Plants in the Southwestern United States*

E. MURL BAILEY, Jr., D.V.M., Ph.D.

Animal agriculture plays an important role in the economics of the southwestern United States. Grazing of the rangelands by ruminants is one of the mainstays of this aspect of agriculture. The occurrence of toxic plants on the southwestern ranges causes a tremendous economic loss to livestock owners in the form of animal deaths; decreased production of wool, fiber, and milk; and reproductive problems. In some years, it has been estimated that in Texas alone, the loss due to animal deaths is as high as 100 million dollars and probably averages 10 to 30 million dollars per year.[1]

There are over 130 species of plants toxic to livestock in Texas, and many of these same species occur in adjacent states and northern Mexico. In addition, there are plant species that do not occur in Texas but may occur in New Mexico, Arizona, and southeastern California.[6] It would be difficult to acquaint the reader with all of the toxic plants of the southwestern range, therefore, the purpose of this article is to describe some of the more common toxic plants of the southwestern United States.

PLANTS CAUSING CLINICAL SIGNS OF CENTRAL NERVOUS SYSTEM SYNDROME

Acacia berlandiera (Guajillo)

Guajillo is a member of the legume family, which grows on the Edwards Plateau region of Texas and southward

*Supported in part by Texas Agricultural Experiment Station, Project No. H-6255.

into Mexico. Under most circumstances, the plant is a valuable browse plant, but during drought, sheep and goats may develop central nervous system (CNS) syndrome if they consume an exclusive diet of this plant for about 6 months or longer. The syndrome is characterized by locomotor incoordination and posterior paralysis. The animals exhibit a "rubbery" action of the legs, and the syndrome is called "limberleg" or "Guajillo wobbles." No lesions have been reported.

Animals should be removed from infested areas when signs appear, or the stocking rates should be reduced and supplemental feeding initiated. Cobalt chloride at a rate of 1 lb/ton of salt may prevent intoxication. Three sympathomimetic amines have been isolated from the plants, but the toxic agent is unknown.[7] Some *Acacia* spp. in the southwestern United States are associated with cyanide poisoning,[5] but this is not common in Texas.

Astragalus spp. (Locoweeds) and *Oxytropis* spp. (Poison Vetch)

Locoweeds are very common in the western United States and in northern Mexico. They are common from the rangelands of the middle-altitude to the high-altitude ranges of the western United States. The toxic principles are alkaloids and nitriles, and many of these compounds have been identified. Cattle are very susceptible to the diseases produced by ingesting these plants. However, to contract such diseases requires that an animal eat an equivalent of greater than 300 per cent of its body weight over 3 months or longer in some cases. Clinical signs are progressive sensory and motor derangements. Cattle show signs of impaired vision and proprioception, progressing to depression. Animals may die in convulsions. Lesions observed are hyperemia and edema throughout the CNS. Neuronal degeneration with vascularization has been reported in some cases. The signs may disappear after removal of the animals from the infested pastures but may reappear if the animals are stressed. Locoweeds cause many syndromes in cattle: habituation and emaciation, neurologic disturbances, posterior paralysis, abortion, teratogenesis, and selenium accumulation. Suppressed estrus and depressed spermatogenesis have also been reported with *Astragalus* spp.

Claviceps spp. (Ergots)

Ergots are parasites of many plant species worldwide. The various species of *Claviceps* grow selectively on seed heads of certain grasses. *C. purpurea* occurs on rye grass, *C. cinerea* on Tobosa grass, and *C. paspali* on Bahia grass and Dallis grass. The toxic principles of the ergot include various derivatives of lysergic acid. Cattle are primarily affected, although horses and sheep may be susceptible. There are 2 syndromes associated with *Claviceps* intoxication, a nervous syndrome and a gangrenous syndrome (see article on Ergot). In cattle, the signs are characterized by high excitability, by fear of humans, and by some belligerence. Trembling and incoordination, exaggerated flexing of forelimbs when running, and tachycardia are often present. In severe cases, the animals may die within 3 days in tetanic convulsions with opisthotonus. In cases of average severity, animals may die in about 1 month from thirst or starvation due to incoordination. Postmortem histopathologic examination may reveal degenerative changes in the CNS. Abnormally low levels of vitamin A have been detected. The disease can be prevented by mowing the grass that has infested seed heads.

Cynodon dactylon (Bermuda Grass)

Bermuda grass is a native of Africa that has been introduced to the warmer areas of the United States. It is widely cultivated and is a very adaptable plant where there is sufficient moisture. The toxic agent is unknown but it may be from a fungus that grows on the grass. Affected cattle show tremors or posterior paralysis or both. These signs may be precipitated by forced exercise. In some cases, icterus and photosensitization have been observed, otherwise, there have been no discernible lesions. Treatment is to remove the animals from the affected Bermuda grass area.

Hymenoxys odorata (Bitterweed) Annual and H. richardsonii (Pingue, Rubberweed) Perennial

H. odorata, more commonly known as bitterweed, is probably the single most important problem plant to the sheep industry in Texas. The plant occurs west of the 99th meridian in Texas. *H. richardsonii* is found from Kansas to Mexico and west to California. Both plants can affect goats and cattle, but sheep are the primary species affected. A toxic agent, hymenoxon, a sesquiterpene lactone, has been isolated and characterized by Kim.[2] The clinical signs of toxicity are anorexia, depression, rumen stasis, regurgitation of ingesta, abdominal pain, and death. Sheep can become habituated to the plants, as recovered animals appear to seek the bitterweed plant when returned to pastures with other forages and forbs available. Chronically affected animals become "poor-doers."[7]

Isocoma wrightii (Rayless Goldenrod)

I. wrightii (rayless goldenrod) occurs in the southwestern United States and Mexico. It is quite common in Texas, New Mexico, and Arizona. The plants grow in general proximity to water. The toxic agent in these plants is tremetol, an unsaturated alcohol. Most domestic species can be intoxicated, and the toxic agent is excreted in the milk and can become a public health problem. High-producing dairy cows are not as apt to be affected, because sufficient tremetol would be excreted in the milk to keep the blood concentrations low. Clinical signs are a result of ingestion of either plants or milk produced by an intoxicated animal. Signs may become most noticeable after forced exercise. Trembling is present especially in muscles around the nose, in the legs, and in the shoulders. Animals may stand in a "humped-up" posture and move stiffly. Debilitation that leads to ultimate recumbency often occurs. Other signs are constipation, vomiting, respiratory and cardiac difficulties, and urinary incontinence. Postmortem, congestion of the abomasum and intestines has been seen along with a pale liver. The gallbladder is generally distended, because these animals stop eating. The brain and spinal cord may be congested. Treatment would involve purgative stimulants and laxative feeds.

Kallstroemia spp. (Caltrops)

Caltrops are found from Kansas to Colorado, south to Texas, northern Mexico, southern New Mexico, and Arizona. The plants generally grow in heavily grazed pastures and other disturbed soils. The toxic principle is unknown; however, cattle are very susceptible to intoxication by ingestion of this plant. They develop rear-limb weakness with knuckling of the fetlocks. This condition progresses to posterior paralysis, and convulsions often precede death. Congestion and hemorrhage of the lungs, heart, kidneys, stomach, and intestines are often reported. Affected animals should be placed in the shade with feed and water. Handling should be minimized during the time of greatest illness.

Karwinskia humboldtiana (Coyotillo)

Coyotillo is a shrub indigenous to southern Texas and northern Mexico. It grows in arroyos and canyons, gravelly hills, and ridges. The toxic principle is unknown, but death can result when animals ingest as little as 0.2 per cent of their body weight in fruit. All domestic species of animals may be affected. The signs would be depression, debilitation, trembling, incoordination and posterior paralysis, dyspnea, and death. Affected animals have pulmonary edema, and histologic lesions involve degeneration of skeletal and cardiac muscle, mild toxic nephritis, and hepatitis. A demyelinating neuropathy often occurs when animals have progressed to this state, and there is no recovery. Less severely affected animals may be treated with adequate feed and water and placed in a pen.

Lobelia berlandiere

Lobelia grows along the Texas Gulf Coast. Animals that can be affected are cattle, sheep, and goats. The clinical syndrome proceeds to depression, coma, and death. Some animals remain recumbent and depressed for several weeks but will eat and drink if feed and water are placed in the mouth. Many of these animals survive. Lesions in animals with *Lobelia* intoxication are extensive subcutaneous hemorrhages, congested brain with subdural edema, and congestion. An abnormally soft spleen has also been reported.[4] *N*-methyl piperidine has been isolated from *Lobelia*.[7]

Peganum harmala (African Rue)

African rue is a native of northern Africa and eastern Asia, which was introduced into New Mexico and spread into Texas and Arizona. The plant continues to expand its range in Texas. *P. mexicanum* (Mexican rue) is a native species, which has also caused problems. The plants grow on disturbed soils and are difficult to eradicate. Several alkaloids have been isolated from both species, including vasicine, harmaline, harmine, and harmalol. Cattle, sheep, and probably horses are susceptible. Acutely, animals exhibit stiffness, trembling, incoordination, frequent urination, and hypersalivation. Chronically, animals exhibit depression, weakness of the hind limbs, and knuckling of the fetlock joints. Lesions in this disease syndrome are severe gastroenteritis, pulmonary and renal congestion, congestion of the liver, and subepicardial hemorrhages.

Solanum dimidiatum (Western Horse Nettle)

Solanum spp. are generally associated with gastroenteritis, local skin irritation, and some CNS problems. In Texas, in a fairly well defined geographic area, a disease syndrome called "crazy-cow syndrome" occurs. It is characterized by incoordination, and although the death loss is quite low, affected cows never recover. Females may give birth to normal but small calves.

Microscopically, the disease is characterized by a loss of Purkinje's cells in the cerebellum. The experimental feeding of *S. dimidiatum* to 6 calves caused the development of CNS signs in 3 calves and a loss of Purkinje's cells in 5 calves.[3] Similar lesions in cattle fed *S. kwebense* have been reported from South Africa.

Sophora secundiflora (Mountain Laurel, Mescal Bean)

S. secundiflora grows in the Edwards Plateau and Trans-Pecos regions of Texas, while *S. sericae* (silky sophora) grows in western Texas, north to Wyoming, and west to Arizona.[6, 7] The plants contain an alkaloid, cytisine. Cattle, sheep, goats, and humans are susceptible. The seeds are very toxic if crushed, but the hard seed coat may allow the seed to pass through the gastrointestinal (GI) tract if left intact. Forced exercise often precipitates a stiffening of the hind limbs and muscular tremors over the shoulders and rump. Affected animals may fall, becoming comatose. Cattle often die, but sheep may recover.

PLANTS AFFECTING THE GI TRACT

Sesbania drummondii (Rattlebox) and S. versicaria (Bagpod)

Sesbania spp. grow along the Gulf Coast from Florida to Texas and into Mexico. The plant species inhabit disturbed areas with adequate moisture. A water-soluble toxicant that will produce GI irritation and death in rats and rabbits has been isolated. Sheep, cattle, and goats are susceptible to the plant. Affected animals exhibit depression, diarrhea, and weakness. Animals may die from 1 to 2 days following ingestion of the plant material. The primary lesion is GI irritation, especially a very inflamed, edematous abomasal mucosa.[7]

Solanum spp. (Nightshades)

The solanums, known as potato weeds or nightshades, are common worldwide, with many species prevalent throughout the United States. Most species occur in waste places or overgrazed pastures. There are several toxic agents that have been identified in *Solanum* spp., including glycoalkaloids. Some plants in this genus contain belladonna-like alkaloids. Other alkaloids are nicotine-like in nature. There are also saponins that produce GI irritation, and toxic materials that might produce cutaneous irritation. Signs attributed to the solanum group's toxicity include dyspnea, hypersalivation, possibly normal to slightly elevated body temperature, weakness, ataxia, trembling of muscles of the hind limbs, tachycardia, and anemia. Bloating and other GI signs are often present. Postmortem lesions are congested liver, kidneys, and lungs with interstitial emphysema. Animals showing nervous signs after ingestion of *Solanum dimidiatum* have exhibited necrosis of Purkinje's cells in the cerebellum. There is no specific treatment.

Xanthium spp. (Cocklebur)

Cockleburs are ubiquitous plants throughout the world. Although swine are commonly poisoned by the *Xanthium* spp., cattle, sheep, chickens, and horses are susceptible. In Texas, calves appear to be frequently intoxicated by young cocklebur plants.[4] Clinical signs may appear soon after ingestion of the plant, and they include weakness, hypothermia, dyspnea, vomiting, and a weak, rapid pulse. Convulsions may ensue. An inflamed and edematous GI tract is common. Slight icterus and ascites may also occur.[7]

PLANTS CAUSING MYOPATHIES

Cassia occidentalis (Coffee Senna), C. obtusifolia (Sickle Pod Senna), C. romeriana (Twin-Leaf Senna), and C. lindheimeriana (Lindheimer Senna)

Cassia spp. are widespread throughout tropic and subtropic areas. Susceptible animals are cattle and sheep. Clinical signs may appear after the ingestion of 10 gm/kg of the plant material daily for 7 days, and they include anorexia, weakness, and diarrhea. Death usually occurs within 24 hr of the onset of signs. Creatine phosphokinase, aspartate aminotransferase, and lactate dehydrogenase levels are elevated. Grossly, animals exhibit pulmonary edema and pale areas in skeletal muscles. Microscopically, skeletal muscle degeneration, toxic nephritis, and hepatitis occur in varying degrees. *Cassia* intoxications are important diseases in Texas, and intoxicated animals do not respond to vitamin E and selenium therapy. In fact, such therapy exacerbates the condition.[7]

PLANTS CAUSING CARDIAC DISEASE

Nerium oleander

Oleander is a common ornamental in the southwestern United States. The plant, which contains cardioactive glycosides, periodically causes intoxication in domestic animals. The disease occurs when well-meaning individuals trim and prune oleander bushes and give the green material to cattle and horses. All mammals are probably susceptible to the oleander glycosides. The intoxication is manifested initially by a GI syndrome, but cardiac arrhythmias follow.[7]

Asclepias spp. (Milkweeds)

Milkweeds periodically cause problems in livestock in the southwestern United States. Most *Asclepias* spp. are quite toxic to most domestic species. The toxic doses range from 1 to 5 gm of dry plant material per kg of body weight.[6] Intoxicated animals may show signs of abdominal pain, excessive salivation, and labored respiration, and they may die suddenly without struggling. At necropsy, hemorrhagic enteritis with congestion of many organs is observed. Cardioactive glycosides have been isolated from many *Asclepias* spp.

PLANTS AFFECTING THE KIDNEYS

Quercus spp. (Oaks)

Oaks range in size from shrubs to large trees. The blossoms, buds, and young leaves are very palatable until the leaves become one half their normal size, after which animals will not generally eat them. Acorns are toxic in the fall and winter. Oak buds, young leaves, and acorns contain gallotannins, which play an important role in the pathogenesis of the disease syndrome. Oak poisoning is important in the southwestern United States in the spring and early summer, whereas acorn poisoning is more important in other parts of the country, including eastern Texas in the fall. Cattle are most frequently intoxicated, but sheep and goats are susceptible. The signs of oak poisoning are emaciation, edema, and constipation or diarrhea with mucus or blood or both in the feces. The animals appear drawn, have a rough hair coat, and a dry nose. A bloody discharge may come from the nostrils. Lesions are gastroenteritis, petechial hemorrhages on the kidney, perirenal edema, subcutaneous edema, and ascites. Oak poisoning cases can be managed in the spring.[7] Management procedures include removing the animals from infested pastures for up to 1 month and hand feeding all of the herd. Calcium hydroxide can be used as a prophylactic agent if fed to animals for approximately 1 week before the onset of new leaf development or budding. The formula for preparation of calcium hydroxide–containing feed is as follows:

1. Cottonseed meal: 1040 lbs.
2. Alfalfa leaf meal: 600 lbs.
3. Calcium hydroxide: 200 lbs.
4. Vegetable oil: 160 lbs.

This preparation should be made into cubes and fed at the rate of 4 lb/head/day during the danger period. Calves should be creep-fed the same mixture in a meal form.[7]

PLANTS AFFECTING REPRODUCTION

Xanthocephalum microcephalum (Perennial Broomweed) and Gutierrizia microcephalum

Broomweeds are also known as turpentine weeds or slinkweeds. Broomweeds occur in central and western Texas, south into Mexico, west to California, and north to Idaho. They grow on dry rangelands and on deserts and become abundant on overgrazed ranges. The toxic agent is a triterpenoid saponin, which may cause contractions of uterine muscle in pregnant cows. Cattle, sheep, and goats are susceptible along with several laboratory animals. Acutely, animals may exhibit anorexia, a rough hair coat, diarrhea or constipation, hematuria, and death. Abortion may occur in various stages of gestation along with the production of weak, underweight calves with retention of the placenta when the calves are born. In milder disease states, abortion may be the only sign. In some years, abortion rates of 40 to 50 per cent are common for intoxicated herds. The disease occurs primarily on the sandy soils of the high plains of Texas and New Mexico but may occur anywhere the plant is present. The toxic status of annual broomweed (X. texanum) has not been determined.[7]

Astragalus spp. (Locoweeds)

Locoweeds cause a large economic loss in livestock as a result of abortions and other reproductive problems in the southwestern United States.[4, 7] This will be discussed in greater depth in the article Principal Poisonous Plants in the Western United States.

PLANTS CAUSING NUTRITIONAL DISEASES

Prosopis glandulosa (Mesquite) and P. juliflora

Mesquite has a wide geographic distribution in the southwest, from Kansas to Texas, west to California, and south to northern South America. Cattle are primarily susceptible. After eating mesquite beans exclusively for 2 months, cattle show gradual emaciation, ruminal atony, profuse salivation, and continuous chewing behavior. The animals exhibit submandibular swelling of the salivary glands and persistent protrusion of the tongue. They develop nervousness, tremors of the head, and if the weather is hot, they will denude large areas of hair by persistent licking. On postmortem examination, emaciation, congestion of the brain, a small, fatty liver, atrophy of the masseter and lingual muscles, and atrophy of rumen papillae may be observed.[4] The rumen may be filled with mesquite beans, undigested grass, and in some instances, soil. Mesquite beans contain large quantities of a pentose, which may play a role in this disease syndrome that resembles vitamin-B complex deficiency.[7]

PLANTS AFFECTING THE LIVER

Senecio longilobus and S. ridellii

Senecio spp. are very common in the southwestern United States. These plants, which contain pyrrolizidine alkaloids, are very hepatotoxic. Cattle and horses are primarily affected; sheep and goats are apparently more resistant and require more plant material to become intoxicated. Some animals have developed hepatic insufficiency disease up to 6 months after removal from infested pastures. The clinical signs in early states are continuous walking, nervous disturbances, and tenesmus with frequent voiding of small amounts of bile-stained feces. As the disease progresses, weakness is prominent. On postmortem examination, ascites with icterus, diffuse hepatic fibrosis, distention of the gallbladder (in cattle) and areas of hepatic regeneration are evident.[7]

HEPATIC FATTY CIRRHOSIS (HARD YELLOW LIVER)

Hepatic fatty cirrhosis (HFC) or Hard Yellow Liver (HYL) is a disease that occurs sporadically in sheep, cattle, goats, antelope, and deer in a circumscribed area in western Texas, in 2 counties in southern Texas, and in northern Mexico. The disease occurs at 4- to 7-year intervals and usually affects practically all of the ruminants in a pasture. Efforts to transmit the disease have failed. The disease appears to be of toxic origin owing to an antilipotropic agent, which allows excessive accumulation of fat in the hepatocytes. The excessive fat causes rupture of the liver cells, followed by a gradual destruction of normal liver parenchyma with ensuing fibrosis. When the amount of functional liver is reduced below body requirements, the animal starts exhibiting signs of illness. Icterus and photosensitization are not parts of the HYL condition. Approximately 80 different plants from the areas where HYL occurs have been fed in varying amounts to sheep, but the typical HYL lesion has not been reproduced.

PRIMARY PHOTOSENSITIZATION

Ammi majus and A. visagne (Bishop's Weed)

A. majus has a worldwide distribution, including the United States. The plants grow in waste areas along the seacoasts of the southern United States and in some subtropical areas of the world. The plants contain furocoumarin, and consequently it can be the etiologic agent in primary photosensitization. Many mammals (cattle and sheep) and birds (geese and ducks) may be affected. The plant has been incriminated in so-called "sand burn" of horses in Texas.

Thamnosma texana (Dutchman's Breeches, Desert Rue)

T. texana is a potent photsensitizing plant of grazing ruminants in the ranges of the western Edwards Plateau region of Texas. Chemical investigations have shown that these plants also contain furocoumarins.

HEPATOGENIC PHOTOSENSITIZATION

Agave lecheguilla (Lechuguilla)

Lechuguilla occurs commonly in western Texas, the southwestern United States, and Mexico. The plant contains a hepatotoxic saponin. Sheep and goats are primarily affected, but cattle may become affected. Icterus is a common sequela, along with the development of photosensitization.[7]

Nolina texana (Sacahuista)

Sacahuista and related species inhabit the southwestern ranges of the United States. Cattle, sheep, and goats may be intoxicated by the hepatotoxic agent. The toxic constituent in sacahuista occurs primarily in the flowers and fruit, while little if any occurs in the leaves. The leaves may be grazed extensively with no problems. Animals ingesting the flowers and fruit must ingest other green plants before photosensitization occurs, since sacahuista is low in chlorophyll. Icterus is also frequently observed.[7]

Panicum coloratum (Kleingrass 75)

Kleingrass was introduced in Texas in the 1950s from South Africa, After more than 10 years of research and development, Kleingrass 75 was released as the desirable variety since it is very nutritious and drought-resistant. Photosensitization associated with Kleingrass 75 has only occurred in sheep, while horses and cattle grazing the same pastures have not been affected. Young, weaned, and feeder age lambs appear to be more susceptible. However, older sheep and goats also can develop the disease syndrome. Another variety, Kleingrass verde, has been recently released but has not been tested fully in animals.

References

1. Dollahite, J. W.: The need for training and research in toxicology. Southwest. Vet. *20*:10–11, 1966.
2. Kim, H. L., Rowe, L. D., Camp, B. J.: Hymenoxon, a poisonous sesquiterpene lactone from *Hymenoxys odorata* DC (Bitterweed). Res. Commun. Chem. Pathol. Pharmacol. *22*:647–650, 1975.
3. Menzies, J. S., Bridges, C. H., Bailey, E. M.: A neurological disease of cattle associated with *Solanum dimidiatum*. Southwest. Vet. *32*: 545–549, 1979.
4. Reager, J. C.: Personal Communication, 1976.
5. Rowell, C. M.: A Guide to the Identification of Plants Poisonous to Livestock of Central West Texas. Angelo State University, B-1, 1975.
6. Schmitz, E. M., Freeman, B. N., Reed, R. E.: Livestock Poisoning Plants of Arizona. Tucson, Arizona, University of Arizona Press, 1963.
7. Sperry, O. E., Dollahite, J. W., Hoffman, G. O., Camp, B. J.: Texas Plants Poisonous to Livestock. Texas, Texas Agri. Expt. Sta. Ext. Ser. B-1028, 1968.

Principal Poisonous Plants in the Western United States

LYNN F. JAMES, Ph.D., J. L. SHUPE, D.V.M., and A. EARL JOHNSON, M.S.

Approximately 835 million acres of rangeland are in the 48 contiguous states. Nearly 60 per cent of this rangeland is in the 11 western states and 22 per cent is in the 6 plains states. Thus, 82 per cent of the rangeland of the United States is located in 17 states. Rangelands are, and have been, of great economic importance since the West was first settled. They supply forage for 18 million breeding cows yearlong, and with proper management, this number could be increased to an estimated 39 million breeding cows. Poisonous plants are one of the serious impediments to the proper use and productivity of these ranges and many pastures.

From the beginning of grazing of livestock on western ranges, poisoning of livestock by plants has been an important cause of economic loss to the livestock industry. This is also true today. Such losses are caused by death, chronic illness and debilitation, photosensitization, abortions, and birth defects. In addition, poisonous plants increase costs to land managers and livestock owners, in that these costs are associated with management of rangelands and pastures. These costs are for fencing, lowered forage production and utilization, altered grazing programs, nonuse of some infested range areas, and, in some cases, supplemental feeding programs and added veterinary expenses.

Losses of livestock due to poisoning by plants vary greatly from year to year and from region to region. Some poisonous plants grow only in localized and well-defined areas, whereas others seem to be omnipresent, but they all may be affected by environmental factors such as temperature and moisture and, as a result, may be more abundant and hazardous in one year than in another. Other factors such as the previous year's grazing pressure may also affect their abundance. Also, some plants are only seasonally toxic. Therefore, in considering poisonous plants or in attempting to diagnose or predict a poisonous plant problem, one should be aware of these influences, and one should be familiar with the poisonous plants likely to be encountered. Often, livestock herders, even those knowing of the presence of poisonous plants on their range, become lax regarding preventive measures because their animals have not been poisoned recently. Then, when conditions and circumstances become ideal for poisonous plants, the owners may suffer huge losses. Losses of livestock due to a great variety of poisonous plants have had devastating effects in many sections of the western United States.

Management errors have contributed heavily to this problem. Indeed, management practices used by the range livestock industry in many cases are conducive to the poisoning of livestock by plants. For example, lupine is more toxic to cattle than to sheep on a weight basis, yet literally thousands of sheep, but few cattle, have died from eating this plant. Halogeton is equally poisonous to cattle and to sheep, however, many sheep have died from halogeton poisoning, yet it has clinically affected relatively few cattle. The differences observed may be due to the way cattle and sheep are managed. Range sheep are usually kept in large flocks and moved from place to place as deemed necessary by the sheep herder. Cattle, however, are left to move freely about a range, limited only by fences and natural barriers. Sheep are normally given water and provided with new forage only when allowed by the herder, but cattle are usually free to search out water and forage as needed. Often sheep that are hungry may be driven through, bedded in, or unloaded from trucks into heavy stands of poisonous plants, and thus are exposed to plants that they would not normally graze.

Many poisonous plants are not palatable to livestock and are eaten only in stressful situations. Plants eaten under these conditions are death camas, copperweeds, milkweeds, and rubberweeds. Other plants such as lupine, halogeton, and greasewood are more palatable and may form an important and beneficial part of a range animal's diet. We need to recognize that plants with toxic properties do not always kill or otherwise harm animals when eaten. Death or serious damage often occurs when excessive amounts of toxic plants are consumed over short periods of time.

The cost of eliminating poisonous range plants where infestation is widespread is usually economically prohibitive and nearly physically impossible. Furthermore, chemical or mechanical treatment may be undesirable because of the adverse effects on desirable plants, and often both methods are inadequate.

Medical treatment of livestock poisoned by plants is generally of little value because of the time interval between intoxication and treatment. In addition, the number of animals involved is usually large. Therefore, the most logical approach to prevention of livestock poisoning by plants is proper management—management concerned not only with health of the livestock but also with pasture and range resources. Resource people, such as veterinarians, county agents, and range managers, can render valuable assistance in the development of managerial procedures for the prevention of poisoning of livestock by plants.

POISONOUS PLANTS

Space does not allow a detailed discussion of all plants toxic to livestock. The plants discussed will be those considered to be of greatest importance in the western United States.

Lupine (*Lupinus* spp.)

Lupine (*Lupinus* spp.) has been one of the most devastating of the range plants poisonous to sheep. Poisoning results most often when hungry sheep are given access to lupine that is in the seed stage of growth. The signs of poisoning in sheep include nervousness, depression, stiffness and reluctance to move, difficulty in breathing, twitching of muscles, loss of muscular control, convulsions, coma, and death. No effective treatment for lupine poisoning is known. Affected animals should not be disturbed until signs of poisoning have subsided. There are no characteristic lesions.

Losses can be minimized by preventing hungry sheep from grazing in heavy stands of lupine, especially when the plant is in the seed stage. Lupine poisoning is most frequently associated with the handling of animals when trucking or trailing. A plan should be developed for grazing and handling animals so that they can avoid grazing lupine during these periods of stress.

The several species of lupines vary considerably in toxicity. Those concerned should be aware of this fact and be familiar with the toxicity of the species the animals are likely to encounter.

A congenital skeletal malformation ("crooked calf") has been associated with cows grazing lupine during the early part of pregnancy. This condition can be avoided by changing the grazing or breeding season or both, so as not to allow grazing of lupine during the 40th to 70th days of pregnancy.

Larkspur (*Delphinium* spp.)

Larkspur (*Delphinium* spp.) is one of the principal poisonous plants affecting cattle in the western range states. Cattle graze larkspur even when there is an abundance of good forage available.

All species of larkspur are poisonous. The 2 general types of larkspur are (1) tall, which grows in moist areas at the higher elevations, 1829 to 3353 m (6000 to 11,000 ft) and (2) low, which grows in dry foothills and plains areas. Toxicity of the larkspurs is high during the early vegetating stages and is lowered as the plant matures, except in the seed stage.

The animal may be poisoned when it eats a relatively small amount of larkspur in a short period of time. Signs of poisoning appear in a few hours and are nervousness, staggering and falling, apparent nausea, salivation, frequent swallowing, muscle twitching, bloating, rapid, irregular heartbeat, respiratory paralysis, and death. There are no significant characteristic gross or microscopic lesions. No specific treatment is known, except to relieve bloating. Affected animals should not be disturbed. Larkspur is relatively nontoxic to horses and sheep.

Management to prevent poisoning consists of keeping animals away from the larkspur.

Death Camas (*Zygadenus* spp.)

Death camas (*Zygadenus* spp.) is an herb with grasslike leaves and an underground bulb. Several species of death camas have various degrees of toxicity. This group of plants is found principally in the western range states.

Death camas is one of the first plants to begin growth in the spring. Animals are usually poisoned at this time, when there is a shortage of good, desirable forage. Poisoning often occurs when a spring snow covers other forage and the death camas protrudes above the snow.

Signs of poisoning are high respiration rates, excessive salivation, apparent nausea, weakness and staggering, convulsions, coma, and death. No treatment is known for death camas poisoning. Severely poisoned animals usually die, while those less affected may recover. Animals poisoned on death camas should not be disturbed.

Prevention lies in avoiding grazing areas infested with death camas in the early spring. As other forage becomes available, livestock are less likely to graze the death camas.

Hemlocks (*Cicuta* spp. and *Conium maculatum*)

Water hemlock and poison hemlock are common poisonous plants often confused because of their similar names and appearance.

Water hemlock (*Cicuta* spp.) grows only in areas that are wet at least part of the time, such as stream banks and swamps. Its main distinguishing features are fascicled tuberous roots and chambered and swollen rootstocks. It is toxic to all classes of livestock, and poisoning in humans is not uncommon.

Cicutoxin, the poisonous principle of water hemlock, is

one of the most toxic of all plant toxins. The toxin is concentrated, especially in the roots. The leaves and stems contain the toxin, but they decrease in toxicity as the plant matures. The toxin acts directly on the nervous system, causing convulsions.

The signs of poisoning are muscle twitching, higher pulse rate and respiration, tremors, convulsions, dilation of pupils, salivation, coma, and death. Affected animals usually die rapidly. No satisfactory treatment is known for water hemlock poisoning.

Prevention of poisoning involves either controlling plants with the appropriate herbicides or keeping animals from grazing it. Animals are most often poisoned in the spring when the plant is young, and they have been poisoned when the roots are exposed during the cleaning of ditches.

Poison hemlock *(Conium maculatum)* is less toxic than water hemlock but, nevertheless, is responsible for numerous livestock losses. One of the distinguishing features of poison hemlock is the purple spots on the lower part of the stem, and the root is an unbranched taproot. Poison hemlock has a mousey odor.

The toxic principle, coniine, a volatile alkaloid, is toxic to all livestock and to humans. Signs of poisoning are nervousness, trembling, ataxia, dilation of pupils, weak and slow heartbeat, coldness of extremities, coma, and death. Poison hemlock can induce skeletal birth defects in calves.

Poison hemlock intoxication is usually associated with heavily grazed pastures. Prevention involves controlling the plant and proper grazing practices.

Halogeton (*Halogeton glomeratus*)

Halogeton *(Halogeton glomeratus)* is an annual plant that grows on the colder, arid, saline ranges of the West. The toxic principle is an oxalate that has been responsible for the death of many sheep and some cattle, This plant competes poorly with other vegetation, so ranges infested with halogeton should be expected to respond quite well to good range management practices. See Oxalate Accumulators for a more complete discussion.

Greasewood (*Sarcobatus vermiculatus*)

Greasewood *(Sarcobatus vermiculatus)* is an oxalate-producing shrub that grows in the colder, saline, arid and semi-arid regions of the western United States. It has been responsible for the deaths of numerous cattle and sheep.

Prevention of losses consists primarily of proper management. The plant sprouts from the crown and does not respond well to herbicide control. Most of the area where it grows is not adapted to the use of herbicides or mechanical treatment.

Greasewood can form a useful part of the diet of sheep and cattle if properly managed.

Chokecherry (*Prunus virginiana*)

Chokecherry *(Prunus virginiana)* is a low-growing shrub or tree on the western ranges. It contains toxic amounts of hydrocyanic acid. When sheep or cattle graze considerable amounts of chokecherry, they may become poisoned.

Prevention of chokecherry poisoning in animals on western ranges involves proper management procedures. Chokecherry is difficult to eliminate from the ranges.

Arrowgrass (*Triglochin* spp.)

Arrowgrass *(Triglochin* spp.) produces hydrocyanic acid under stressful conditions. Arrowgrass grows on wet, heavy, alkaline soil. Prevention involves keeping livestock from grazing this plant after drought or frost.

Senecio, Amsinckia, and Crotalaria spp.

Certain species of *Senecio, Amsinckia,* and *Crotalaria* contain pyrrolizidine alkaloids. These alkaloids are primarily hepatotoxic. They may cause an acute toxicosis that results in rapid death, but they usually cause a chronic cirrhosis-like condition of the liver that may not be manifest until months after the plants have been ingested. Horses and cattle are most susceptible to these alkaloids. Pyrrolizidine alkaloid toxicosis is discussed more fully in the article on Hepatotoxic Plants.

Selenium-Accumulating Plants

Several species of plants that grow on seleniferous soils accumulate selenium in such amounts that they become toxic to livestock grazing them. These plants are discussed in the article Selenium Accumulators.

Ponderosa Pine (*Pinus ponderosa*)

Ponderosa pine *(Pinus ponderosa),* when grazed by cows during the last trimester of gestation, can cause abortions. Ponderosa pine grows in all states west of the plains area and in western Canada. There are some abortions in those cattle that ingest pine needles in all of these states, and there are larger numbers of abortions in cattle of Arizona, Colorado, Idaho, Montana, New Mexico, Oregon, South Dakota, Washington, Wyoming, and western Canada.

Abortions can result when pregnant cows eat dried, wilted, or green ponderosa pine needles. Cattle in areas where the ponderosa pine grows generally have year-round access to the needles; however, the animals usually abort during the late fall, winter, and early spring. Several factors apparently cause the cattle to eat pine needles: sudden weather changes, such as cold winds and snow storms, hunger, changes in feed, and other stressful conditions. They will eat ponderosa pine needles even when good forage is available.

Some animals may abort within 48 hr after they ingest pine needles, and other animals may abort as long as 2 weeks after they are removed from access to the needles.

There are generally few signs of impending abortion. The abortion is characterized by weak parturition contractions, excessive uterine hemorrhage, and incomplete dilation of the cervix. A calf that is delivered near term when the needles are eaten generally survives.

Persistent retained placentas are a constant finding, regardless of stage of gestation of the abortion. Septic metritis often follows the abortion, and unless the animal is properly treated, generalized septicemia may follow. In acute cases, the cow appears to have toxemia and may die before or soon after she aborts. In such cases, there may be ecchymotic hemorrhages on the peritoneum, pleura, and viscera. There are no specific characteristic lesions in the aborted calves as a result of pine needle ingestions.

Prevention involves keeping the cows from grazing pine needles during the last trimester of gestation. Although cattle may graze in areas with ponderosa pine during the critical stage of gestation and not eat the needles, there is always the risk that they may.

Milkweeds (*Asclepias* spp.)

Milkweeds (*Asclepias* spp.) are widespread on many ranges of the western United States. They are perennial herbs that contain milky juice, stand erect, and have opposite or whorled leaf arrangements. The milkweeds are divided into 2 groups, the narrow-leaf milkweeds and the broad-leaf milkweeds. Not all species of milkweeds are toxic. The principal poisonous species in the West are *A. labriformis, A. subverticillata, A. eriocarpa,* and *A. fascicularis. A. labriformis* is among the most toxic of range plants. Milkweeds are unpalatable and usually eaten by hungry animals only. They may also be harvested with hay or green chop and thus cause poisoning as a forage contaminant.

The signs of poisoning include muscular incoordination, spasms, bloat, rapid weak pulse, respiratory difficulty, and death..

No treatment is known for animals poisoned on milkweed. Losses from milkweed can be reduced by maintaining ranges and pastures in good condition. Livestock that are hungry should not be allowed to graze in milkweed-infested areas. Milkweed should not be harvested with hay and other forages.

Horsebrush (*Tetradymia* spp.)

Horsebrush (*Tetradymia* spp.) is a shrub growing in the drier range areas of the West. These plants are principally a problem to sheep in the early spring. This plant is discussed in more detail in the article Dermatotoxic Plants.

Oak (*Quercus* spp.)

Oak (*Quercus* spp.) is poisonous primarily to cattle. Oaks of the West are low growing shrubs or small trees. Oak grows in dense stands, and growth starts early in the spring before most other range plants. It is most toxic during the bud and early leaf stage. As the leaves mature, they decrease in toxicity. Large amounts of oak must be eaten to poison cattle.

The signs of poisoning are rough hair coat, gaunt appearance, emaciation, edema, constipation or diarrhea, mucus or blood (or both) in the feces, dark brown urine, and death.

Lesions include gastroenteritis and edema of the intestinal walls. The kidney may have petechia, subcutaneous edema, and ascites.

Prevention consists of keeping cattle away from the oak brush during the period when oak is in the early bud stage, especially during times of feed shortage. This treatment may involve the development of a range or pasture free of oak brush.

Locoweed (*Astragalus* and *Oxytropis* spp.)

Locoweed (*Astragalus* and *Oxytropis* spp.) can affect all classes of livestock. Species of these plants grow throughout most of the range states and have the potential of poisoning animals where conditions favor their growth. More than 350 species of *Astragalus* grow in North America. About 18 of these cause classic locoism in livestock.

Locoweed poisoning is a chronic type of intoxication. An animal must graze the plant for about 30 days before signs of poisoning appear. The length of time between ingestion and appearance of signs is dependent on the rate of consumption and, to a lesser extent, on the species of plant.

The signs of locoweed poisoning are rough hair coat, dull eyes, emaciation, depression, and irregular gait. High incidences of abortions and birth defects have been associated with locoweed poisoning.

There are no specific or characteristic gross postmortem lesions. Microscopic lesions are general neurovisceral cytoplasmic vacuolations.

Animals that have become poisoned on locoweed may recover to varying degrees with proper care. However, locoweed can induce permanent damage, so an animal may show signs of poisoning throughout ,its lifetime. Locoweed is also habit forming. Once an animal starts to graze locoweed, it will continue to do so at the exclusion of other forage. If removed from and then exposed to locoweed at a later date, it may start grazing the plant again.

Prevention consists of keeping animals away from areas heavily infested with locoweed. If livestock must graze in such areas, they should be observed closely, and those starting to graze locoweed should be removed immediately. Dried locoweed plant is also toxic, and in several instances, livestock ranchers have sustained heavy losses when their livestock grazed dried locoweed plant.

Timber Milkvetch (*Astragalus miser*)

Timber milkvetch (*Astragalus miser*) and other *Astragalus* plants, such as *A. emoryanus, A. pterocarpus,* and *A. canadensis* that contain 3-nitro-1-propanol or 3-nitro-1-proprionic acid as a toxic constituent, grow in most of the 11 western states and Canada.

Depending on the rate at which it is eaten by livestock, this group of plants may induce acute or chronic poisoning. Acute intoxication is characterized by nervousness, irregular gait, general body weakness, rapid weak pulse, coma, and death. There are no significant lesions.

Chronic intoxication is characterized by dullness, incoordination of the hind legs when walking, and goose stepping. The animals may have cocked ankles and may fall when they run. There may be respiratory distress and posterior paralysis if the condition progresses to advanced stages. With proper care, poisoned animals may recover. However, animals grazing the plant usually die if they are not removed from the plant.

The postmortem lesions are not pathognomonic. The liver may be swollen, the pericardial fluid may be increased, and varying degrees of pulmonary emphysema are regularly observed.

Poisoning can best be prevented by not allowing animals to graze this plant over extended periods of time. Intoxication in areas where this plant is a problem seems to be more severe in periods of drought. Nursing cows are more often affected than dry cows. Cows poisoned on this plant should be handled carefully and should not be exposed to stressful conditions.

Rayless Goldenrod (*Haplopappus heterophyllus*)

Rayless goldenrod (*Haplopappus heterophyllus*) is common in the dry rangelands of the Southwest. It is an erect, unbranched perennial shrub with yellow flowers that grows from 61 to 122 cm (2 to 4 ft) tall. The poisonous principal is tremetol, a higher alcohol. It is toxic to all classes of range livestock. If animals that are grazing this plant are not removed from it, they will die.

The signs of poisoning are lassitude and depression, a humped-up posture, and stiff gait. The body may tremble, especially about the head and shoulders. Signs of poisoning may be accentuated by forced exercise. Postmortem findings are not characteristic. The liver may be pale, and the abomasum and intestines may be congested.

Prevention consists of eradication of the plants or of not allowing livestock to graze them.

Sneezeweed (*Helenium hoopesii*)

Sneezeweed *(Helenium hoopesii)* grows on moist slopes and well-drained meadows at elevations from 1524 to 3048 (5000 to 10,000 ft) throughout most of the 11 western states. Sneezeweed is a herbaceous perennial with yellow flowers, and it grows from 30 to 90 cm (1 to 3 ft) tall. It is primarily a problem in range sheep. Animals are poisoned after grazing the plant for about 10 days, most often in the late summer and early fall when better forage is gone or dried up. Signs of poisoning are depression, weakness, coughing, chronic vomiting (which leaves the area around the mouth stained green), and bloating. If the animals continue to graze the plant until vomiting starts, they usually die.

The principal lesions of sneezeweed poisoning are gastroenteritis, edema of the stomach walls, excessive fluid in the pericardial cavity, and ascites.

Prevention consists of control of the plants or removing the sheep from sneezeweed-infested ranges at frequent intervals.

Rubberweed (*Hymenoxys richardsonii*)

Rubber or pingue *(Hymenoxys richardsonii)* is a perennial herb with yellow flowers that grows from 15 to 46 cm (6 to 18 in) tall. It grows principally on dry foothill areas from 1220 to 3048 (4000 to 10,000 ft) of elevation. Rubberweed is principally a problem in range sheep. Heavy infestation of rubberweed indicates overgrazing. Signs of poisoning are salivation, anorexia, rumen stasis, apparent abdominal pain, uneasiness, weakness, and prostration. Lesions are associated with gastrointestinal irritation and hepatic degeneration.

Rubberweed is distasteful, therefore, the animal is poisoned primarily during trailing and during grazing of ranges heavily infested with the plant.

Prevention and Management

Poisoning of livestock by plants that are part of their normal diet is uncommon. Livestock poisoning on the range usually becomes a problem because of a shortage of nonpoisonous plants or because of an increase in poisonous plants, which results when the more desirable plants have been completely grazed. In general, the prevention of loss from poisonous plants is largely a problem of proper animal and range management. Most poisonous plants are distasteful to livestock. Exceptions are plants such as larkspur and, under some conditions, locoweeds.

Some general rules for preventing livestock poisoning by plants are as follows:

1. Know the poisonous plants, especially those of local significance.

2. Know how poisonous plants affect livestock and the conditions under which they are toxic.

3. Avoid areas infested with poisonous plants during holding, trailing, or unloading of animals. If these situations cannot be avoided, special preventive procedures should be considered.

4. Avoid grazing hungry animals in areas infested with poisonous plants. Animals may become hungry by withholding feed or water and by overgrazing. Provide animals with water and adequate forage of good quality.

5. Provide adequate salt and mineral supplements.

6. Where possible, control or eradicate poisonous plants, especially from problem areas.

7. Develop and practice proper grazing plans.

8. Keep the range in good condition. Avoid overgrazing.

9. Good management practices will prevent most cases of plant poisoning in livestock.

Supplemental Reading

James, L. F.: Symposium on poisonous plants. J. Range Manage. *31*:324–360, 1978.

James, L. F., and Johnson, A. E.: Some major plant toxicities of the western United States. J. Range Manage. *29*:356–363, 1976.

Keeler, R. F.: Toxins and teratogens of higher plants. Lloydia *38*:56–86, 1975.

Keeler, R. F., Van Kampen, K. R., and James, L. F. (eds.): Effects of Poisonous Plants on Livestock. New York, Academic Press, 1978.

Kingsbury, J. M.: Poisonous Plants of the United States and Canada. Englewood Cliffs, New Jersey, Prentice-Hall, Inc., 1964.

Principal Plant Problems in the Midwestern and Eastern United States

ARTHUR A. CASE, M.S., D.V.M.

The nondefinitive nature of the syndrome caused by poisonous plant intoxication, with a few exceptions, makes it difficult to define the importance of toxic plant principles in animal health. Many instances of gastrointestinal disorders are due to unknown factors, and toxic plants could be the cause of a considerable number of them. Many acute cases go undiagnosed.

Intoxications in farm animals may be due to natural environmental influences or to artificially induced influences. The conditions may be acute and dramatic, as in cyanide, nitrite, or yew poisoning, or the conditions may be chronic and insidious, as in seneciosis, fescue poisoning, or other conditions associated with progressive hepatosis or nephrosis. Some instances of intoxication are avoided by careful management practices and judicious operation of such equipment as harvester threshers and forage choppers. Forages and grains must be properly prepared and stored to avoid inclusion of known poisonous plants or toxic seeds and to avoid conditions leading to damage from molds or insect infestations.

Natural disasters which damage feed, such as hailstorms, tornados, floods, or droughts, and storage elevator explosions and fires, may create situations in which ruminants and swine will be subjected to calculated risks taken in an effort to salvage possibly toxic materials for feed.

Table 1. *Toxic Shrubs and Forbs*

Plant and Toxic Part	Habitat	Syndrome Observed and Toxin	Management
Family Taxaceae *Taxus* spp. All parts toxic.	Widely planted ornamental shrubs	Taxine causes cardiac arrest and sudden death.	Keep animals of all species away from yew ornamentals and yew trimmings.
Family Asclepiadaceae *Asclepias* spp. (milkweeds)	Grain fields; pastures; well-drained roadsides	Resinoid galoidotoxin and depressant alkaloids cause loss of body control, colic, spasms, tachycardia with weakness and very rapid respiration, prostration, coma, and death.	Avoid dense stands of milkweed or dogbane in hay fields. Keep animals off milkweed infected areas or adequately supplement ration. Milkweeds are readily eaten by both sheep and cattle if hungry.
Family Umbelliferae (parsley family) *Cicuta* spp. (water hemlock) Tubers most toxic.	Moist meadows; flood plains; marshes	Cicutoxin, a complex alkaloidal resinoid principle, produces violent convulsions, usually terminating in death. Ruminants most susceptible. Swine less susceptible.	Avoid areas where *Cicuta* spp. grow. Eradicate the plant where practical. Control convulsions and give supportive treatment. Evacuate digestive tract.
Conium maculatun (poison hemlock) All parts toxic.	Rich, well-drained soil nearly anywhere; pastures, roadsides, farm fields, barnyards	Coniine, an alkaloid with general depressive action, causes general anesthesia.	Give supportive treatment to correct CNS depression. Avoid pastures with dense stands of *Conium*. Eradicate plant where practical.
Pteridium spp. (bracken fern) Horsetail or scouring rush.	Woodland areas over most of northern midwest and eastern and southeastern states	Toxic principle unknown or possibly thiaminase. Cattle show hemorrhagic diathesis, elevated temperature.	Limit grazing time to 3 weeks and remove access to bracken fern or horsetail rush. Feed forage free of fern or rush.

Weather determines in many ways whether or not there will be plant-related problems with farm or ranch animals in any given season or year. This is the case with wild native or introduced plants as well as with field and forage crops, vegetable plants, and ornamental and forest shrubs and trees. Intensive farming areas no longer have many of the native toxic plants, but aggressive weeds, such as cocklebur (*Xanthuim* spp.), amaranths (pigweeds), milkweeds and dogbane, several species of the solanaceous plants, morning glory, and bindweeds, still invade the crop fields. Many such weeds are poisonous, have poisonous seeds, or concentrate such minerals as oxalate, nitrate and nitrite and, perhaps, other potentially toxic minerals. Valuable field crops such as corn (*Zea mays*), sorghum, and clover may also become toxic because of stress during growth. Some of those possibilities are discussed at length in other articles. The emphasis here will be on the toxic plants that can produce trauma but that may not be discussed elsewhere (Tables 1 to 5).

TOXIC PLANTS

The seasonal incidence of many toxic plants is shown in Figure 1. Some of the toxic evergreen shrubs may present a hazard to animals at any time of the year. Examples are yew (*Taxus* spp.), oleander (*Nerium* spp.), box (*Buxus* spp.), black locust (*Robinia pseudoacacia*), and other shrubs, trees, or vines likely to be present throughout the year, especially in the southeastern and gulf coastal plains. In the more northern areas, the seasonal incidence of the toxic plants likely to be present is much more definite, particularly in the native hardwood forest areas, such as the sharply rolling country immedi-

Table 2. *Shrubs and Trees of the Forest and Flood Plain*

Plant and Toxic Part	Habitat	Syndrome Observed and Toxin	Management
Oaks (*Quercus* spp.) Green foliage and possibly immature acorns.	Widely distributed east of the Great Plains with hardwood forest. Also grown as ornamentals.	Progressive nephrotoxicosis with ascites.	Avoid diets of 40% or more of oak foliage or green acorns. Give a calcium supplement plus supplemental feeding of calves or remove from access to oak.
Black locust (*Robinia pseudoacacia*) Cambium and green growth, seeds.	An important post, timber, and windbreak tree planted and naturalized in many areas.	Weakness, depression, hemorrhagic gastroenteritis in calves and swine. Lethal amount for ruminants about 400 gm/250 kg. Robin is a phytotoxin.	Avoid grazing cut locust stands or allowing access to bark strippings from lumber.
Fruit trees: plum, cherry, peach, almonds (both domestic and wild). Leaf and twig.	Orchards, forests, homesteads, and roadsides.	Prussic acid poisoning (see Cyanogenic Plants).	See Cyanogenic Plants. Avoid exposure to green growth. Antidotes are effective.
Elderberry (*Sanbucus canadensis*)	Roadsides, field margins, woods, and valleys near streams.	Prussic acid poisoning, especially after a freeze in the fall.	See Cyanogenic Plants.
Bittersweet (*Celastrus scandens*) Green growth.	Climbing vines in woods and forests or along fence rows, especially in eastern United States.	CNS disturbances, gastroenteritis. Sheep and goats more than cattle.	Bittersweet, euonymus, and moonseeds are climbing ornamental or wild vines with toxic foliage and fruit. Avoid heavy growth on fences and do not discard trimmings where farm animals have access.
Moonseed (*Menispermum canadense*)	Climbing vines in fence rows.		

Table 3. *Toxic Plants of Gardens, Fields, and Forests*

Plant and Toxic Part	Habitat	Toxin and Syndrome Observed	Management
Rhubarb (*Rheum* spp.) Leaves	Garden vegetable.	Oxalic acid poisoning (see Oxalate Accumulators).	Never discard rhubarb leaves where any animals have access.
Wild docks (*Rumex* spp.)	Common weeds of fields and pasture lots.	Oxalic acid poisoning.	Avoid heavily concentrated pasture areas of docks, especially with cattle and sheep.
Family Solanaceae Domestic and wild nightshades Tomato, greened, potato and sprouts, eggplant, ground cherry, and peppers. All parts except ripe fruit and potato tubers.	Garden vegetables or wild plants growing as weeds in fields, pastures, barnlots, waste areas. Roadsides over most of eastern and southeastern US.	Nightshades have saponins as well as solanine alkaloids. Gastroenteritis, CNS disturbances (convulsions), progressive weakness, coma, and death.	Do not allow farm animals of any species to have access to garden refuse (tomato, potato, eggplant forage). Do not include wild nightshades in hay or silage. Do not allow farm animals to have access to any nightshades when conditions are likely to encourage eating of the toxic vegetable.
Prickly nightshade (*Solanum rostatum*) All parts	The most common weed in most barnlots.	Solanine alkaloids. Syndrome the same as for nightshades plus trauma from spines.	Do not allow animals to have access to infested areas and do not include the prickly nightshade in hay or other feedstuffs.
Horsenettle or bullnettle, Carolina nightshade All parts	Pastures, fields, roadsides, prairies, woodlands. Common nearly everywhere.	Solanine steroids	Hungry and thirsty animals will readily eat the wild nightshades if given access.
Tobacco (both domestic and wild species) All parts	Crop fields, pastures.	Severe poisoning if eaten.	Do not bed swine with tobacco stalks nor discard green or sprouted potato tubers where hogs can eat them.
Jimson weed All parts	Crop fields, barnlots, pastures.	Severe poisoning if eaten.	Do not put hungry animals in pens with Jimson weed patches. Do not include Jimson weed in hay or silage.
Lima bean Vine and wilted leaf	Garden vegetable and field crop.	Prussic acid poisoning (see Cyanogenic Plants).	Do not discard lima bean vines where ruminants can eat them.

Table 4. *Toxic Ornamental Shrubs and Trees*

Plant and Toxic Part	Habitat	Toxin and Syndrome Observed	Management
Azalea, rhododendron, and laurel, especially *Kalmia* spp. All parts toxic.	Both ornamental and wild in mountain areas of eastern and southeastern US.	Excitement followed by depression, coma, and death from respiratory arrest. Extreme prostration in severe poisoning. Toxin—andromedotoxin.	Avoid the exposure of all farm animals to trimmings of ornamentals. Avoid forested mountain areas where native plants of the laurel family are abundant.
Daphne mezereum (Spurge laurel) All parts are toxic, but fruit is very toxic.	Widely planted ornamental of lawns and college campuses.	Colic, hemorrhagic diarrhea, convulsions, weakness, coma, and death. Toxin—daphnin.	Protect animals from access to ornamental plantings or trimmings of *Daphne*.
Laburnum anagyroides (golden chain tree, golden rain tree) Green growth and fruit.	Widely planted ornamentals of lawns, college campuses, and floral gardens.	Excitement followed by depression, prostration, coma, and death. Toxin—nicotine-like action.	Avoid the exposure of animals to ornamentals and their trimmings.
Gymnocladus diocia (Kentucky coffee tree)	Native forest and shade tree.	Severe colic, gastroenteritis, purging, and tenesmus. Toxin—cytisine alkaloid.	Avoid seed pods in water tanks. Keep fruit pods, trimmings, and green growth away from hungry cattle, sheep, and goats.
Yellow jessamine, Carolina jessamine (a climbing vine) All parts toxic.	Eastern and southeastern forested areas. Wild and domestic ornamentals.	Excitement followed by depression, prostration, coma, and death.	Do not allow animals access to mestic or wild jessamine, *Wisteria*, and similar plants.
Wisteria spp. Especially fruit pods and seeds.	Climbing vine, southeast and north to Missouri.	Toxin—unknown.	Avoid exposure of farm animals to ornamental *Wisteria*.

Table 5. *Poisonous Seeds in Hay and Grains*

Toxic Species	Adulterated Feedstuff	Susceptible Animals
Crotalaria spp.	Cereal grains and sorghums (milo).	All species, especially swine.
Corn cockle, cow cockle (*Agrostemma* spp., *Saponaria* spp.)	Cereal grains, especially spring planted, late harvested. Occasionally hay.	All species, especially swine. LD is about 0.02 gm/kg of the powerful sapotoxins.
Cocklebur (*Xanthium* spp.)	Corn, soybeans, late-cut hay, silage, or fresh chop.	All species. If cocklebur is milled, cocklebur nutlet is very toxic in small amounts.
Ergots (*Claviceps* spp.)	Ergot sclerotia are often found in rye, wheat, oats, triticale, and grass hays harvested in the seed stage or later.	All species are susceptible to ergotism. Acute from large amounts over a short time. Chronic from small amounts over a long time.
Morning glories (*Ipomoea* spp.)	Corn, soybeans, and occasionally milo or other fall harvested grains. Silage and green chop.	Swine are at greatest risk, but cattle, sheep, and goats are also sensitive to lysergic acid.
Solanaceae Jimson weed (*Datura*) Nightshades (*Solanum*)	Seed and fruit are often included in corn, soybeans, fresh chop, silage, or hay.	The powerful solanaceus toxins will poison any animal eating enough of them. Swine are most often affected. Calves and lambs as well as kids are susceptible.
Mustard Family (*Brassica* spp.) (*Thlaspi arvense*)	Mustard seeds contain isoallyl thiocynates and other toxic principals. In threshed grain or first cut hay.	All species are susceptible, but swine, lambs, and calves are most likely to be poisoned by mustard seeds.
Sneezeweeds (*Helenium* spp.) (*Senecio* spp.)	Seed heads of sneezeweeds or bitterweeds contaminate grain, hay, and fresh chop.	All species with swine, calves, lambs, and kids being most susceptible, especially over time.

Figure 1. Types of plant poisoning by seasons in the west northcentral United States based on information from the University of Missouri Veterinary Clinic records, reports from diagnostic laboratories of other states, and personal correspondence with veterinarians, extension personnel, producers, and other sources over a period of more than 30 years. Illustrated is the usual and quite limited time during the year that any particular toxic plant, forage, or feedstuff may be expected to produce intoxication in farm animals. Because intoxications are not considered reportable conditions in most states, it is nearly impossible to make any definite statements concerning the incidence and importance of poisonous plants except as based upon personal knowledge and the reports from those who do recognize and report such intoxications. (Modified from Case, A. A.: Toxicologic problems in large animals. J. Am. Vet. Med. Assoc. *149*(12):1714–1719, 1966.)

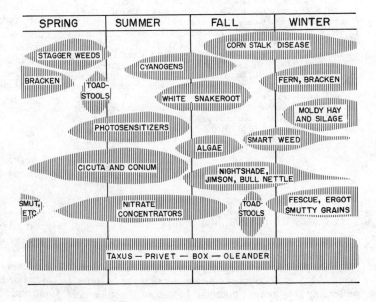

ately adjacent to the large rivers of the Ohio-Wabash-Tennessee-Illinois-Mississippi-Missouri territory between the Great Plains and the Appalachian mountains. Mountains and valleys that are part of the Appalachian system above the coastal plains have many toxic genera and species, which include the laurels, white snakeroot, death camas, many species of nightshades, and many other plants poisonous to farm animals, pets, and humans. The poisonous plant bulletins from Kentucky, Pennsylvania, Virginia, Maryland, North Carolina, Alabama, Georgia, and Florida are recommended for anyone interested in the poisonous plants of those areas. The native plants of the forested areas are likely to be as prevalent as ever, especially where the flood plain meets the river-hill forests. Such areas have always been possible hazards to humans and animals because of the toxic plants that grow there. Some, such as white snakeroot *(Eupatorium rugosum),* have made American history because of lethal effects on animals (trembles) and humans (milk-sickness or vomiting disease, the "pukes"). The toxic plants are still present but more persons are aware of their potential for harm and avoid them except for "city persons" moving to housing developments in the country.

Supplemental Reading

Case, A. A.: Toxicologic problems in large animals. J. Am. Vet. Med. Assoc. *149*:1714–1719, 1966.

Cole, R. J., Stuart, B. P., Lansden, J. A., and Cox, R. H.: Isolation and redefinition of the toxic agent from cocklebur *(Xanthium strumarium).* J. Agric. Food Chem., *28*:1330–1332, 1980.

Evers, R. A. and Link, R. P.: Poisonous Plants of the Midwest. Special Public, no. 24, College of Agriculture, University of Illinois, Urbana-Champaign, 1972.

Freeman, J. D. and Moore, H. D.: Livestock Poisoning by Vascular Plants of Alabama. Bulletin 460. Agriculture Experimental Stations, Auburn, Alabama, 1974.

Gress, E. M.: Poisonous Plants of Pennsylvania. Department of Agriculture. Bulletin 531. Pennsylvania Department of Agriculture, 1935.

Hulbert, L. C. and Dehme, F. W.: Plants Poisonous to Livestock, 3rd ed. Manhattan, Kansas, Kansas State University Printing Service, 1968.

Keeler, R. F., Van Kampen, K. R. and James, L.: Effects of Poisonous Plants on Livestock. New York, Academic Press, 1978.

Kingsbury, J. M.: Poisonous Plants of the United States and Canada. Englewood Cliffs, New Jersey, Prentice-Hall Inc., 1964.

Miller, J. F., Kates, A. H., Davis, D. E., and McCormach, J.: Poisonous Plants of the Southern United States, Cooperative Extension Service, University of Georgia College of Agriculture, Athens, Georgia, 1980.

Radeleff, R. D.: Veterinary Toxicology, Poisonous Plants, 2nd ed. Philadelphia, Pennsylvania, Lea and Febiger, 42–157, 1970.

Sigmond, O. H., Fraser, C. M., Archibald, J., et al.: Poisonous Plants of Temperate North America. *In* The Merck Veterinary Manual, 5th ed. Rahway, N. J., Merck & Co., Inc., 1020–1033, 1979.

Insecticides

T. L. CARSON, D.V.M., M.S., Ph.D.

The production of both livestock and crops on the same premises provides a unique opportunity for exposure of livestock to agricultural chemicals. Among the chemicals presenting the greatest potential hazard of livestock poisoning are the organophosphorous (OP), carbamate, and chlorinated hydrocarbon insecticides.

Poisoning often occurs when insecticides are accidentally incorporated into livestock feed. Discarded or unlabeled portions of granular insecticides can be mistaken for dry feed ingredients and mixed into animal feeds. When farm equipment used for feed handling is also used for insecticide transportation, contamination of this equipment may result in insecticides being inadvertently mixed into animal feeds. In addition, animals may have accidental access to insecticides where they are stored, discarded, or spilled on the farm premises. Improperly operating back rubbers and oilers may provide an additional source of these insecticides for livestock.

Miscalculation of insecticide concentration in spraying, dipping, and pour-on procedures may also result in toxicosis. Retreating animals with OP or carbamate preparations within a few days may cause poisoning.

Differences in susceptibility to insecticides, because of breed or sex or both, used for external parasite control have resulted in restricted use of famphur (Warbex)* on Brahman or Brahman-cross cattle and chlorpyrifos (Dursban)† on exotic breed beef cattle and mature bulls. Very young or stressed livestock generally should not be treated with insecticides.

ORGANOPHOSPHORUS AND CARBAMATE INSECTICIDES

The OP and carbamate insecticides will be discussed together because of their similar mechanism of action. Several of these insecticides are highly toxic to livestock with the capability of producing lethal effects at oral doses of less than 10 mg/kg. Therefore, in many instances, ingestion of only a few grams of commercial material may result in toxicosis.

Mechanism of Action

Cholinergic nerves utilize acetylcholine as a neurotransmitter. Under normal conditions, acetylcholine released at the synapses of parasympathetic nerves and myoneural junctions is quickly hydrolyzed by cholinesterase. When the hydrolyzing enzymes are inhibited, the continued presence of acetylcholine maintains a state of nerve stimulation and accounts for the clinical signs observed with poisoning from these insecticides. In general, inhibition of these enzymes by the OP insecticides tends to be irreversible, while inhibition of the enzymes by the carbamates tends to be reversible.

Clinical Signs

The clinical syndrome produced by OP and carbamate insecticides is similar in all species of animals and in general is characterized by overstimulation of the parasympathetic nervous system and skeletal muscles. Earliest clinical signs of acute poisoning frequently include mild progression to profuse salivation, frequent defecation, and urination, emesis, a stiff-legged or "saw horse" gait, and general uneasiness. As the syndrome progresses, profuse salivation, gastrointestinal hypermotility resulting in severe colic and abdominal cramps, diarrhea, excessive lacrimation, sweating miosis, dyspnea, cyanosis, urinary incontinence, and muscle tremors of the face, eyelids, and general body musculature can be observed. Hyperactivity of the skeletal muscles is generally followed by muscular paralysis, as the muscles are unable to respond to continued stimulation.

---

*Available from American Cyanamid Co., Princeton, NJ 08540.
†Available from Ft. Dodge Laboratories, Fort Dodge, IA 50501.

Cattle, sheep, and swine may exhibit increased central nervous system stimulation but rarely, if ever, exhibit convulsive seizures. More commonly, central nervous system depression occurs.

Death usually results from hypoxia due to excessive respiratory tract secretions, bronchoconstriction, and erratic slow heartbeat. The onset of clinical signs in cases of acute poisoning may be as short as a few minutes to several hours after exposure. In severe poisoning, death can occur from a few minutes to several hours after the first clinical signs are observed.

Postmortem Lesions

Postmortem lesions associated with acute OP or carbamate toxicosis are usually nonspecific. Excessive fluids in the mouth and respiratory tract as well as pulmonary edema may be observed.

Diagnosis

A history of exposure to OP or carbamate insecticides associated with clinical signs of parasympathetic stimulation warrants a tentative diagnosis of poisoning.

Chemical analyses of animal tissues for the presence of insecticides are usually unrewarding because of the rapid degradation of the OP and carbamate insecticides, resulting in low tissue residue levels. However, finding the insecticide in the stomach or rumen contents in addition to finding the insecticide in a sample of feed or suspect material can be quite valuable in establishing a diagnosis.

The best method of confirming a diagnosis is to assess the degree of inhibition of cholinesterase enzyme activity in the whole blood and tissue of the animal. A reduction of whole blood cholinesterase activity to less than 25 per cent of normal is indicative of excessive exposure to these insecticides. The cholinesterase activity level in the brain tissue of animals dying from these insecticides will generally be less than 10 per cent of normal cholinesterase activity level in the brain tissue. It must be remembered, however, that depletion of whole blood cholinesterase activity may not necessarily correlate with inhibition of cholinesterase at the parasympathetic synapses and myoneural junctions. Therefore, whole blood cholinesterase activity should be viewed as only an indication of the status of the cholinesterase enzymes in the body.

Whole blood and brain samples should be well chilled but not frozen for obtaining best laboratory results. Samples of rumen or stomach contents as well as the feed or suspect material should be submitted to a laboratory for chemical analyses.

The acute syndrome of OP and carbamate insecticide poisoning must be differentiated from acute urea or other nonprotein nitrogen toxicosis and acute grain overload. In addition, hypomagnesemia (grass tetany), nitrate toxicosis, cyanide poisoning, and acute bloat may be clinically similar to insecticide poisoning.

Treatment

The treatment of animals poisoned by these compounds should be considered on an emergency basis because of the rapid progression of the clinical syndrome.

Initial treatment for poisoned animals should be the use of atropine sulfate at approximately 0.5 mg/kg of body weight. This initial dose should be divided with about one fourth of the dose administered intravenously, and the balance administered subcutaneously or intra-muscularly. Atropine sulfate does not counteract the insecticide-enzyme bond but rather blocks the effects of accumulated acetylcholine at the nerve endings. Although a dramatic cessation of parasympathetic signs is generally observed within a few minutes after administration of atropine, it will not affect the skeletal muscle tremors. Repeated doses of atropine at approximately one half the initial dose may be required but should be used only to counteract parasympathetic signs. Caution should be observed with continued atropine therapy as rumen atony may be a complicating side effect in cattle and sheep. Oral activated charcoal is very beneficial for treatment of any ingested insecticide. The early use of activated charcoal (Superchar-Vet*) to adsorb OP or carbamate insecticides in the gastrointestinal tract is especially important in ruminants that continue to absorb insecticide from the rumen contents. The effective dose of activated charcoal ranges from 0.5 kg for sheep to 0.9 kg for adult cattle.

A water-charcoal slurry mixed with sodium or magnesium sulfate (1 gm/kg) should be given and repeated 8 to 12 hr later; or commercially prepared charcoal-kaolin (Toxiban)† may be pumped intraruminally with a stomach tube after initial respiratory distress has been alleviated with atropine.

Dermally exposed animals should be washed with soap and water to prevent continued absorption.

The oximes, such as TMB-4, 2-PAM, and pralidoxime chloride, are drugs that act specifically on the organophosphorus-enzyme complex, freeing the enzyme. The use of the oximes in large animals, though efficacious, may be economically unfeasible. Pralidoxime chloride is recommended at a dose of 20 mg/kg in small animals and at a dose of 10 mg/kg in large animals. The oximes are of no benefit or harm in treating carbamate toxicoses.

Morphine, succinylcholine, and phenothiazine tranquilizers should be avoided in treating OP poisoning.

CHLORINATED HYDROCARBON INSECTICIDE TOXICOSIS

The syndrome of acute chlorinated hydrocarbon insecticide toxicosis involves hyperexcitability, hyperesthesia, tonic-clonic convulsive seizures, and often periods of depression.

Mechanism of Action

Although the exact mechanism of action of these insecticides, other than DDT, is unknown, they appear to be diffuse stimulants of the central nervous system. DDT increases the firing rate of nerve fibers.

Clinical Signs

Initially, animals may appear apprehensive. A period of hyperexcitability characterized by exaggerated responses to stimuli and spontaneous muscle spasms are usually observed. The spontaneous tremors and fasciculations usually begin in the facial region to involve the lips, muscle, eyelids, and ears and progress caudally to involve the heavy muscles of the shoulder, back, and rear quarters. These spasms may progress into a tonic-clonic seizure. The seizure may start with the animal standing,

---

*Available from Gulf Biosystems Inc., Dallas, TX 75221.
†Available from Vet-A-Mix, Shenandoah, IA 51601.

followed by collapse into lateral recumbency. Abnormal posturing, elevation of the head, and chewing movements may be observed. Cattle often walk backward at the start of a seizure. Varying degrees of respiratory paralysis occur during the seizures, which are usually intermittent, with periods of depression and inactivity occurring between successive seizures.

The rapidity of onset and the severity of clinical signs provide a poor index of the prognosis for the animal. Occasionally, animals will die during seizures, while other animals may completely recover following several seizures.

Postmortem Lesions

Specific lesions other than those from the physical trauma of the seizures are generally not observed.

Diagnosis

Clinical signs of hyperexcitability and tonic-clonic convulsive seizures with a known exposure to chlorinated hydrocarbon insecticide should yield a tentative diagnosis of chlorinated hydrocarbon insecticide toxicosis.

The presence of significant levels of chlorinated hydrocarbon insecticide in liver and brain tissues is essential for confirming a diagnosis. Samples of these tissues, as well as stomach or rumen contents, and suspect material, such as feed or spray, should be submitted to a laboratory for analyses. Avoid contamination of specimens with hair or gut contents to avoid erroneous results.

Laboratory examination is usually required to differentiate this toxicosis from pseudorabies, water deprivation and gut edema in swine. In cattle, polioencephalomalacia, thromboembolic meningoencephalitis, pseudorabies, listeriosis, nervous coccidiosis, and lead poisoning must be differentiated from this toxicosis.

Treatment

Treatment is essentially of symptoms, since there are no specific antidotes for chlorinated hydrocarbon insecticides. Animals should be sedated with barbiturates, tranquilizers, or chloral hydrate to control convulsive seizures. Animals with dermal exposure should be washed with warm, soapy water to remove the chemical and to prevent continued exposure. If the chemical is orally ingested, activated charcoal (1 to 3 gm/kg) plus sodium or magnesium sulfate (1 gm/kg) may be used to prevent further absorption. Oil-based cathartics should be avoided, as they may hasten absorption of the chemicals. Intravenous fluids plus glucose may be needed in protracted cases.

Residues

Because of the persistence of these chemicals, the carcasses of animals that died of chlorinated hydrocarbon insecticide toxicosis are a source of contamination for feed ingredients, such as tankage, meat and bone meal, and fat. Therefore, proper disposal of contaminated carcasses is vitally important.

In addition, animals surviving an episode of insecticide exposure may contain significant residues in the adipose tissue. These residues have particular economic impact in market animals and in lactating dairy cows or goats.

Supplemental Reading

Buck, W., Osweiler, G. D., and Van Gelder, G. A.: Clinical and Diagnostic Veterinary Toxicology. 2nd ed. Dubuque, Iowa, Kendall Hunt Publishing Co., 1976.

Haas, P. J., Buck, W. B., Hixon, J. E., et al.: Effect of chlorpyrifos on Holstein steers and testosterone-treated Holstein bulls. Am. J. Vet. Res. 44:879–881, 1983.

Palmer, J. S.: Toxicity of famphur to young Brahman heifers and bulls. J. Amer Vet. Med. Assoc. 159:1263–1265, 1971.

Radeleff, R. D.: Veterinary Toxicology, 2nd ed. Philadelphia, Lea and Febiger, 1970.

Rodenticides

GARY D. OSWEILER, D.V.M., M.S., Ph.D.
and BARBARA S. HOOK, B.A., D.V.M.

Poisoning of food-producing animals by rodenticides has been reported only rarely. Verified instances of toxicosis in farm animals have occurred from exposure to strychnine, fluoroacetate, warfarin, and zinc phosphide. The low frequency of rodenticide toxicosis is due in part to several factors. The rodenticides are recognized as toxic agents by most livestock producers and are generally handled accordingly. Many commercial rodenticides are packaged in such a way that a large animal consuming a small package of bait receives a relatively low dose of rodenticide. The commonly used anticoagulant rodenticides require several days of exposure to cause poisoning if dosage is low. Unless feed contamination with a highly toxic rodenticide occurs, it is unlikely that more than 1 or 2 animals in a herd would be affected, since access is limited to available commercial packages. Strychnine, for example, is commonly formulated in bait at 0.3 per cent. This supplies 3 mg strychnine/gm bait. Toxicity of strychnine to cattle is 0.5 mg/kg, so that 250 mg would poison a 500-kg animal. Thus, as little as 83 gm (approximately 3 oz) of bait could poison a cow. Normally, this amount of bait would not be placed in one spot for rodent control. If 10 kg of bait were accidentally incorporated in 907 kg (1 ton) of feed (e.g., bait was mistaken for a premix), the result would be feed containing 10 kg × 3000 mg/kg × 1/907 kg strychnine, for a final concentration of approximately 33 mg/kg feed. Assuming a 500-kg animal eats 10 kg of feed, the body weight dose of strychnine received would be 10 kg × 33 mg/kg × 1/500 kg or 0.66 mg strychnine/kg body weight. Thus, highly toxic rodenticides if improperly used could result in acute poisoning.

The toxic principles and pathogenesis for various rodenticide toxicoses are as varied as the products. Information in Table 1 covers the toxicity, action, organs, major clinical and pathologic effects, and primary diagnostic features of toxicosis by rodenticides in livestock. Where applicable, therapy is outlined. The rodenticides of greatest hazard are discussed fully elsewhere. When access is given to rodenticides, the bait or carrier, which consists usually of grains or cereals, generally would be attractive and palatable to livestock. Except for thallium and warfarin or other anticoagulants, clinical signs appear rapidly after ingestion of rodenticides, and signs are acute and often dramatic. Various organ systems are affected, depending on the rodenticide involved. Once clinical signs develop, prognosis is guarded in all cases except anticoagulant toxicosis, where the outlook is slightly better. Clinical pathologic results are helpful in diagnosis of anticoagulant rodenticide poisoning, but other toxicants in the rodenticide category cause only vague or nonspecific changes. Analyses of tissues or baits for the suspected

Table 1. *Characteristics of Toxicosis by Rodenticides in Livestock*

Rodenticide	Toxicity	Mechanism of Action	Major Organs or Systems Involved	Clinical and Pathologic Effects	Diagnostic Features
ANTU (alpha-napthyl thio urea)	Varies with particle size, small particles less toxic; lethal dose pig: 25–50 mg/kg	Increased permeability of lung capillaries with development of edema	Lung	Vomiting, dyspnea, moist rales, weakness, hydrothorax, pulmonary edema, cyanosis	Analysis must be done within 24 hr after death; this product is rarely used now
Fluoroacetate and fluoroacetamide	Oral LD_{50} mg/kg Cattle: 0.39 Calves: 0.22 Sheep: 0.25–0.50 Swine: 0.4–1.0	Converted to fluoro-citrate, which enters Krebs cycle and inhibits aconitase; this stops Krebs cycle and results in accumulation of citrate	Cardiovascular in herbivores; cardiovascular and brain in swine	Cardiac arrhythmia, rapid weak pulse, ventricular fibrillation; sudden collapse and death. Swine may also show seizures and vomiting	Blood glucose, lactate and citrate levels are elevated; analyze for fluoroacetate in bait, liver, and stomach contents
Phosphorus	Toxic dose, per animal, in gm Cattle: 0.5–2 Swine: 0.05–0.3	Toxic forms are white and yellow phosphorus; hepatotoxic via disturbed lipid and protein metabolism	Liver, gastrointestinal, kidney	Early signs are vomiting, abdominal pain; hemorrhagic diarrhea. Later, icterus, depression, hepatorenal failure develop after several days	Vomitus may smell like garlic, fume and "glow in the dark"; chemical analysis of gastrointestinal contents
Strychnine	Oral lethal dose in mg/kg Cattle: 0.5 Swine: 0.5–1.0	Antagonizes spinal inhibitory neurons and transmitters, allowing overpowering effects of spinal reflex arc	Central nervous system	Acute onset of tetanic seizures; hyperesthesia and hyperreflexia aggravated by touch, noise, full stomach in monogastrics, rapid onset of rigor mortis	Seizures are characteristic; no significant lesions; analyze for strychnine in stomach contents, liver, or urine
Thallium	Toxic dose in mg/kg Cattle: 12–16 Sheep: 9–20	General cellular poison; probable inactivator of sulfhydryl-containing enzymes	Almost all body systems affected; most severe in gastrointestinal, respiratory, cutaneous, and nervous	Onset is delayed 2–3 days after ingestion, longer in chronic cases; gastroenteritis, sometimes hemorrhagic; dyspnea, fever, conjunctivitis, gingivitis; acute to chronic dermatitis and hair loss; may be tremors or seizures	Necrosis of many tissues, including GI, heart, skeletal muscles; lymphadenopathy; neutrophilia; analyze for thallium in urine, kidney, and liver
Warfarin and other anticoagulants	Toxic dose in mg/kg (warfarin) Cattle: 200 for 12 days Swine: 0.05 for 3–5 days	Competitive antagonism of vitamin K by interfering with final steps in hepatic synthesis of prothrombin complex; toxicity influenced by other drugs, vitamin K, and liver status	Coagulation system, factors II, VII, IX, and X; secondary lesions in the vascular system	Mild to massive hemorrhages; hemorrhagic diarrhea; epistaxis, subcutaneous hematoma, anemia	Numerous hemorrhages or coagulopathy in absence of liver disease or thrombocytopenia; elevated prothrombin time; analyze for anticoagulant in blood, liver, or urine
Vacor	Oral LD_{50} in calves and pigs 300 mg/kg	Antagonism of nicotine adenine dinucleotide (NAD) thus affects biologic oxidation-reduction reactions	General metabolic toxicant; gastrointestinal tract and nervous system, including visual system	Signs are vague: nausea, vomiting, colic, mental confusion; long-term signs *may* include autonomic dysfunction, diabetic-type ketoacidosis, visual defects	History of exposure; toxicosis unlikely unless exposure is large; chemical analysis of bait or stomach contents
Zinc phosphide	Lethal dose for cattle, sheep, goats, and swine: 20–40 mg/kg; toxicity greater when stomach is full	Zinc phosphide releases phosphine at acid pH, result is cardiovascular collapse along with direct irritation of GI tract	Cardiovascular, gastrointestinal, nervous	Vomiting, depression, dyspnea, colic, occasional animals with convulsive seizures	Breath, stomach contents, or bait *may* have odor of acetylene; analyze stomach contents or liver, preserve specimens by freezing

Table 2. *Suggested Therapy for Rodenticide Toxicoses*

Rodenticide	Detoxification and Supportive Measures	Antidotal Measures
ANTU (alpha-napthyl thio urea)	Keep animal quiet to reduce tissue oxygen demand, sedate if necessary; oxygen administration may be necessary; administration of osmotic diuretic (e.g., 50% glucose or 50% mannitol) and atropine (0.02–0.05 mg/kg) have been suggested to aid in control of pulmonary edema	No specific antidote Dimercaprol (BAL, BAL in oil*) has been suggested to compete for SH inactivating sites on ANTU; efficacy is not established
Fluoroacetate and fluoroacetamide	Control seizures with short-acting barbiturates given to effect; administer activated charcoal at 250 gm/100 kg body weight mixed as a slurry with a saline cathartic (1 gm/kg)	Glycerol monoacetate (Monoacetin)† at 0.1–0.5 mg/kg IM hourly for several hours; effective only if given before signs develop
Phosphorus	Administer 0.4% copper sulfate solution orally (2–4 L); saline cathartic may be used at 0.5–1.0 kg/500 kg animal; glucose and lipotropic agents (e.g., methionine) may aid in hepatotoxic states	No antidote
Strychnine	Control seizures with pentobarbital q.s., chloral hydrate, magnesium sulfate, and pentobarbital (Chloropent)‡ combination available commercially may be used at 20–50 ml/100 lb body weight IV; may need to be repeated at hourly intervals; glyceryl quiacolate 5% solution IV at 212 ml/kg is effective, but is *not approved for food animals*; give activated charcoal orally at 250 g/100 kg body weight mixed as a slurry with a saline cathartic (1 gm/kg)	No specific antidote
Thallium	Evacuate GI tract with a saline cathartic; use glucose, antibiotics, and parenteral vitamins as general supportive therapy	Dithizone has been recommended in small animals. Success is variable. Not evaluated in food animals and not approved for use in USA
Warfarin and other anticoagulants	If ingestion is recent (<1 day) give saline cathartic and activated charcoal; administer whole blood to anemic animals; evaluate for possible hemothorax and do thoracentesis if necessary	Vitamin K_1 (Aquamephyton)§ should be used at 1 mg/kg body weight in acute cases; blood or plasma (1–2 L) will also supply coagulation factors; follow with menadione (Hetrazeen)‖ (synthetic vitamin K) orally at 5 mg/kg for 3–4 weeks (see text).
Vacor	Empty the GI tract with lavage or saline cathartics; supportive therapy to replace fluid loss and control seizures may be indicated	Nicotinamide† (100 mg) is recommended for small animals; dosage for therapy in food animals not established; suggested dose is 1000 mg every 4 hr up to 36 hr; oral nicotinamide 1 gm/day should be used for 7 additional days
Zinc phosphide	Evaluate GI tract and give 2–4 L 5% sodium bicarbonate orally to neutralize stomach acidity; control acidosis with sodium bicarbonate at approximately 2 mEq/kg repeated as needed	No specific antidote

*Available from Hynson, Wescott & Dunning, Baltimore, Md. 21201
†Available from Fisher Scientific, Springfield, N.J. 07081
‡Available from Fort Dodge Laboratories, Fort Dodge, Ia. 50501
§Available from Merck & Co., Inc., Rahway, N.J. 07065
‖Available from Heterochemical Corporation, Valley Stream, N.Y. 11580

Table 3. *Common Drug Dosages*

Drug	Supplier	Species	Dose
Dimercaprol (BAL in oil)	Hynson, Westcott & Dunning Baltimore, Md. 21201	Bovine and swine	3 mg/kg qid, IM
Glycerol monoacetate (Monoacetin)	Fisher Scientific Springfield, N.J. 07081		0.1–0.5 mg/kg IV based on small animal dose recommendation
Chloral hydrate-magnesium sulfate-pentobarbital (Chloropent)	Fort Dodge Laboratories Fort Dodge, Ia. 50501	Bovine	20–50 ml/45 kg body weight
Vitamin K_1 (Aquamephyton)	Merck & Co., Inc. Rahway, N.J. 07065	Bovine and swine	1 mg/kg body weight IV or IM
Menadione dimethyl pyrimidinol bisulfite (Hetrazeen)	Heterochemical Corporation Valley Stream, N.Y. 11580	Bovine and swine	5 mg/kg orally for 5–7 days
Nicotinamide	Fisher Scientific Springfield, N.J. 07081		2–3 mg/kg every 4 hr up to 36 hr based on human dose recommendation

chemical may aid in diagnosis, but some toxicants (e.g., phosphorus, zinc phosphide, fluoroacetate) may be difficult to determine owing to lack of stability or absence of a suitable chemical analysis.

Treatment for selected rodenticide poisoning is outlined briefly in Table 2. In most instances of oral exposure, activated charcoal (1 to 3 gm/kg) mixed in a slurry with sodium or magnesium sulfate (1 gm/kg) should be given twice orally, 8 to 12 hr apart. Table 3 lists the common drug dosages and sources for the treatment of rodenticide toxicoses. Generally, only anticoagulant poisoning and strychnine toxicosis can be adequately treated once signs develop.

Supportive and symptomatic measures are best left to the judgment and expertise of individual clinicians in specific cases.

Supplemental Reading

Beasley, V. R., and Buck, W. B.: Warfarin and Other Anticoagulant Poisonings. In Current Veterinary Therapy, 7th ed. Philadelphia, W. B. Saunders Company, 101–106, 1983.

Clark, E. G. C., and Clark, M. L.: Veterinary Toxicology. Baltimore, Williams & Wilkins, 1975.

Hatch, R. C.: Veterinary Toxicology. In Jones, L. M., Booth, N. H., and McDonald, L. E. (eds.). Veterinary Pharmacology and Therapeutics, 4th ed. Ames, Iowa, Iowa State University Press, 1977.

Osweiler, G. D., Carson, T. L., Buck, W. B., and Van Gelder, G. A.: Clinical and Diagnostic Veterinary Toxicology, 2nd ed. Dubuque, Iowa, Kendall & Hunt Publishing Co., 1976.

Organic Herbicides

LOYD D. ROWE, D.V.M.,
and J. S. PALMER, D.V.M., M.P.H.*

Ingestion of herbicides by farm animals may involve a concentrated form, a diluted form in water or feed, or contaminated forage. During grazing, the likelihood of poisoning depends upon whether or not enough herbicide has been applied to forage to allow sufficient intake for toxicosis. Most herbicides are of low toxicity, and the majority of toxic cases are associated with human error or accident. Poisoning is not likely to result if proper herbicide applications and withholding times are observed. In food animals, poisoning from herbicides occurs much less frequently than does poisoning from insecticides. The minimum reported toxicity of some organic herbicides in cattle and sheep is presented in Table 1. These data and the signs and lesions of poisoning described next are primarily the results of experiments in which each herbicide was given to cattle and sheep as a single daily dose for several days.

ALIPHATICS

Sodium trichloroacetate and dalapon are herbicides of relatively low toxicity. Signs of poisoning in cattle and sheep include weight loss, anorexia, lethargy, depression, dull hair coat, diarrhea, and ataxia. Recovery should be rapid and uneventful once exposure is terminated.

*Deceased.

AMIDES

These materials are relatively toxic. All herbicides in this group listed in Table 1 produced anorexia. Loss of body weight was observed in some animals given naptalam without an obvious decrease in food intake, and diphenamid produced rumen dysfunction, as evidenced by the presence of undigested rumen contents at necropsy. Diarrhea was present in animals given diphenamid, naptalam, and propachlor. Depression was observed with CDAA and propachlor. Severe poisoning with CDAA, diphenamid, and naptalam resulted in prostration. Other signs of toxicosis produced by these herbicides include ataxia (diphenamid, propachlor), salivation (CDAA), lameness (diphenamid), muscular spasms (diphenamid), and bloat (naptalam plus dinoseb).

Postmortem findings in cattle and sheep poisoned with amide herbicides are enlargement of the liver (diphenamid), kidneys (CDAA), and adrenal glands (diphenamid, naptalam plus dinoseb). The liver was friable in animals given propachlor or naptalam plus dinoseb and pale in color in animals given diphenamid and naptalam plus dinoseb. Other observations are congestion of the kidneys (CDAA, diphenamid, naptalam, naptalam plus dinoseb), liver (naptalam, propachlor), lungs (CDAA, naptalam plus dinoseb) and respiratory mucosa (CDAA), and reddening of the intestinal mucosa (naptalam, propachlor). Gastrointestinal hemorrhage and petechial hemorrhages in the mucosa of the bladder were seen in poisoning with CDAA. Brown-tinged urine and a subcutaneous yellow gelatinous material were observed in a sheep poisoned by diphenamid.

ARSENICALS

The clinical effects and postmortem findings of these herbicides are similar to those described for inorganic arsenic poisoning. Consumption of forage treated with arsenical herbicides should always be considered hazardous. The persistence of arsenical compounds in the soil and their tendency to accumulate in plants present potential problems where repeated application is practiced.

BENZOICS

Dicamba is relatively nontoxic. Signs of poisoning in cattle and sheep include convulsions, bloat, and prostration. At necropsy of sheep poisoned with dicamba, lymph nodes throughout the body were enlarged and hemorrhagic. Subepicardial hemorrhages, congestion of the liver and kidneys, and enlargement of the spleen and intestinal mucosa were also reported.

BIPYRIDILIUMS

Diquat and paraquat are highly toxic to cattle and sheep; however, it is generally considered unlikely that these herbicides produce serious harm with proper use. The relatively low hazard of these materials to grazing stock despite high toxicity under laboratory conditions may be due to such factors as decomposition by UV light, rapid inactivation by soil, and reduced absorption when

Table 1. *Minimum Reported Toxicity of Some Organic Herbicides in Cattle (9 to 16 mo) and Sheep (mature)*

| Common Name | Chemical Name | Minimum Reported Toxicity* | | Estimate of Corresponding Application Rate† (kg AI/acre) |
		C(cattle) and S(sheep) (mg/kg/day)	(days)	
Aliphatics				
TCA	Trichloracetic acid, sodium salt	C 375	3	24.3
		S 175	2	11.3
Dalapon	2,2-Dichloropropionic acid, sodium salt	C 1000	5	64.8‡
		S 500	7	32.4‡
Amides				
CDAA	N,N-Diallyl-2-chloroacetamide	C 25	1	1.6
		S 25	4	1.6
CDAA and TCBC	N,N-Diallyl-2-chloroacetamide (30 %) and trichlorobenzyl chloride (70 %)	C 50	2	3.2
		S 25	5	1.6
Diphenamid	N,N-Dimethyl-2,2-diphenylacetamide	C 250	3	16.2‡
		S 250	7	16.2‡
Naptalam	N-1-Naphthylphthalamic acid, sodium salt	C 175	6	11.3‡
		S 100	3	6.5‡
Naptalam and Dinoseb	N-1-Naphthylphthalamic acid (66 %) and 2-sec-butyl-4,6-dinitrophenol (34 %)	C 25	8	1.6
		S 25	10	1.6
Propachlor	2-Chloro-N-isopropylacetanilide	C 25	3	1.6
		S 10	9	0.6
Propanil	3′,4′-Dichloropropionanilide	C 250	1	16.2‡
		S 100	10	6.5‡
Arsenicals				
Cacodylic Acid	Hydroxydimethylarsine oxide	C 25	8	1.6
		S 25	10	1.6
DSMA	Disodium methanearsonate	C 25	2	1.6
		S 25	5	1.6
MSMA	Monosodium methanearsonate	C 10	2	0.6
		S 50	3	3.2
Benzoics				
Dicamba	2-Methoxy-3,6-dichlorobenzoic acid, dimethylamine salt	C 250	2	16.2‡
		S 500	1	32.4‡
Bipyridiliums				
Diquat	6,7-Dihydrodipyrido[1,2-a:2′,1′-c] pyrazinediium ion, dibromide salt	C 5	8	0.3
		S 25	3	1.6
Paraquat	1,1′-Dimethyl-4,4′-bipyridium ion, methyl sulfate salt	C 10	10	0.6
		S 10	10	0.6
Carbamates				
Barban	4-Chloro-2-butynyl-m-chlorocarbanilate	C 25	1	1.6‡
		S 10	2	0.6
Chlorpropham	Isopropyl-m-chlorocarbanilate	C 100	2	6.5‡
		S 100	10	6.5‡
Dinitroanilines				
Benefin	N-Butyl-N-ethyl-α,α,α-trifluoro-2,6-dinitro-p-toluidine	C 25	6	1.6‡
		S 50	2	3.2‡
Trifluralin	α,α,α-Trifluoro-2,6-dinitro-N,N-dipropyl-p-toluidine	C 175	2	11.3‡
		S 175	2	11.3‡
Nitriles				
Dichlobenil	2,6-Dichlorobenzonitrile	C 50	1	3.2
		S 25	4	1.6
Phenols				
Nitrofen	2,4-Dichlorophenyl p-nitrophenyl ether	C 100	3	6.5‡
		S 100	3	6.5‡
Phenoxys				
2,4-D	(2,4-Dichlorophenoxy)acetic acid, dimethyl amine salt	C 100 Calves (6 to 8 weeks of age)	1	6.5‡
		C 100	10	6.5‡
		S 175	2	11.3‡

Table 1. *Minimum Reported Toxicity of Some Organic Herbicides in Cattle (9 to 16 mo) and Sheep (mature)* (Continued)

Common Name	Chemical Name	Minimum Reported Toxicity* C(cattle) and S(sheep) (mg/kg/day)	(days)	Estimate of Corresponding Application Rate† (kg AI/acre)
Phenoxys 2,4-D *(Continued)*	(2,4-Dichlorophenoxy)acetic acid, ethanol amine and isopropanolamine salts	C 250 S 100	15 8	16.2‡ 6.5‡
	(2,4-Dichlorophenoxy)acetic acid, propylene glycol butyl ether ester	C 250 S 250	3 2	16.2‡ 16.2‡
	(2,4-Dichlorophenoxy)acetic acid, 2-ethyl hexyl ester	C 250 S 50	6 10	16.2‡ 3.2‡
2,4-DB	4-(2,4-Dichlorophenoxy)butyric acid, dimethylamine salt	C 100 S 50	2 5	6.5‡ 3.2‡
MCPA	2-Methyl-4-chlorophenoxyacetic acid, sodium salt	C 175 S 100	3 5	11.2‡ 6.5‡
	2-Methyl-4-chlorophenoxyacetic acid, dimethylamine salt	C 175 S 100	10 10	11.3‡ 6.5‡
	2-Methyl-4-chlorophenoxyacetic acid, ethanolamine and isopropanolamine salts	C 500 S 100	8 4	32.4‡ 6.5‡
MCPB	4-(4-Chloro-2-methylphenoxy)butanoic acid, sodium salt	C 100 S 50	1 5	6.5‡ 3.2‡
Mecoprop	2-(2-Methyl-4-chlorophenoxy)propionic acid, diethanolamine salt	C 175 S 250	5 2	11.3‡ 16.2‡
Silvex	2-(2,4,5-Trichlorophenoxy)propionic acid, propylene glycol butyl ether ester	C 100 S 100	19 9	6.5‡ 6.5‡
2,4,5-T	(2,4,5-Trichlorophenoxy)acetic acid, triethylamine salt	C 100 S 50	10 5	6.5‡ 3.2‡
	(2,4,5-Trichlorophenoxy)acetic acid, propylene glycol butyl ether ester	C 250 S 100	4 3	16.2‡ 6.5‡
	(2,4,5-Trichlorophenoxy)acetic acid, 2-ethyl hexyl ester	C 100 S 50	10 10	6.5‡ 3.2‡
Thiocarbamates Diallate	S-(2,3-Dichloroallyl)diisopropylthiocarbamate	C 25 S 25	1 1	1.6 1.6
EPTC	*S*-Ethyl dipropylthiocarbamate	C 50 S 100	1 2	3.2 6.5‡
EPTC and 2,4-D	*S*-Ethyl dipropylthiocarbamate (57 %) and 2,4-D iso-octyl ester (43 %)	C 25 S 100	10 4	1.6 6.5‡
Molinate	*S*-Ethyl hexahydro-IH-azepine-1-carbothioate	C 50 S 75	1 1	3.2‡ 4.9‡
Pebulate	S-Propyl butylethylthiocarbamate	C 50 S 175	1 3	3.2 11.3‡
Triallate	S-(2,3,3-Trichloroallyl)diisopropylthiocarbamate	C 25 S 50	5 2	1.6‡ 3.2‡
Vernolate	S-Propyl dipropylthiocarbamate	C 100 S 250	3 8	6.5‡ 16.2‡
Triazines Atrazine	2-Chloro-4-ethylamino-6-isopropylamine-s-triazine	C 25 S 25	2 10	1.6 0.3
Prometone	2,4-*bis*(Isopropylamino)-6-methoxy-s-triazine	C 10 S 25	8 4	0.6 1.6
Prometryne	2,4-*bis*(Isopropylamino)-6-(methylthio)-s-triazine	C 50 S 100	2 6	3.2‡ 6.5‡
Propazine	2-Chloro-4,6-*bis*(isopropylamino)-s-triazine	C 25 S 25	3 5	1.6 1.6
Simazine	2-Chloro-4,6-*bis*(ethylamino)-s-triazine	C 25 S 50	3 10	1.6 3.2
Triazoles Amitrole	3-Amino-1H-1,2,4,-triazole	C 25 S 10	3 10	1.6 0.6
Uracils Bromacil	5-Bromo-3-sec-butyl-6-methyluracil	C 250 S 50	1 10	16.2‡ 3.2
Isocil	5-Bromo-3-isopropyl-6-methyluracil	C 50 S 100	7 1	3.2 6.5

Table continued on following page

Table 1. *Minimum Reported Toxicity of Some Organic Herbicides in Cattle (9 to 16 mo) and Sheep (mature)*
(Continued)

Common Name	Chemical Name	Minimum Reported Toxicity*		Estimate of Corresponding Application Rate† (kg AI/acre)
		C(cattle) and S(sheep) (mg/kg/day)	(days)	
Ureas				
Chloroxuron	3-[p-(p-Chlorophenoxy)phenyl]-1,1-dimethylurea	C 25	5	1.6
		S 25	8	1.6
Diuron	3-(3,4-Dichlorophenyl)-1,1-dimethylurea	C 100	10	6.5
		S 100	2	6.5
Fluometuron	1,1-Dimethyl-3-(α,α,α-trifluoro-m-tolyl) urea	C 100	2	6.5‡
		S 50	6	3.2‡
Linuron	N'-(3,4-Dichlorophenyl)-N-methoxy-N-methylurea	C 50	10	3.2‡
		S 50	1	3.2‡
Norea	3-(Hexahydro-4,7-methanoindan-5-yl)-1,1-dimethylurea	C 175	2	11.3‡
		S 250	5	16.2‡
Unclassified Herbicides				
Bensulide	0,0-Diisopropyl phosphorodithioate-S-ester with N-(2-mercaptoethyl)benzenesulfonamide	C 50	2	3.2
		S 100	3	6.5
DCPA	2,3,5,6 Tetrachloroterephthalic acid, dimethyl ester	C 250	5	16.2‡
		S >500	10	>32.5‡
Endothall	7-Oxabicyclo[2.2.1]heptane-2,3-dicarboxylic acid, potassium salt	C 25	2	1.6
		S 10	10	0.6
Fenac	2,3,6-Trichlorophenylacetic acid, sodium salt	C 50	1	3.2
		S 175	2	11.3
Glyphosate	N-(Phosphonomethyl)glycine, isopropylamine salt	C 206	5	13.3‡
		S —	—	—
Picloram	4-Amino-3,5,6-trichloropicolinic acid, potassium salt	C 500	8	32.4‡
		S 250	9	16.2‡
Pyrazon	5-Amino-4-chloro-2-phenyl-3(2H)-pyridazinone	C 100	3	6.5‡
		S 25	10	1.6
Triclopyr	[(3,5,6-Trichloro-2-pyridinyl)oxylacetic acid, triethylamine salt or ethylene glycol butyl ether ester	C 75 Steers (2 years of age) S —	3	4.9

*Least number of doses causing 5 % or greater weight loss or signs of poisoning for experimental oral exposures of less than 20 days.
†Application rate directly on forage theoretically capable of providing a daily dosage equivalent to the minimum reported toxicity (see text for method of estimation).
‡Sufficiently above the usual maximum application rate to consider normal usage of herbicide nonhazardous.

ingested on herbage vs. direct administration alone, as a single daily dose. Signs of acute poisoning are anorexia, depression, ataxia, diarrhea, accelerated and labored breathing, recumbency, convulsions, and coma. Diarrhea and mortality were the principal manifestations in sheep poisoned by accidental contamination of pasture by diquat. Necropsy findings were abomasitis, hemorrhage in the intestinal mucosa, heart, adrenals, and thyroid, and congestion of the lungs, liver, and kidneys. Fibrosing pneumonitis as occurs in humans and other species apparently has not been reported in sheep and cattle.

CARBAMATES

Anorexia was the most prominent sign of poisoning with these materials. Salivation was observed in sheep poisoned with barban, and death without forewarning signs was seen in an animal given chlorpropham. Postmortem findings were congestion of lungs, liver, kidneys, spleen, and gastrointestinal mucosa. Hemorrhage on the surface of the liver and kidney with hardening and light coloration of the liver was found with barban intoxication.

DINITROANILINES

Few, if any, cases of poisoning of livestock by these herbicides have been reported. Poisoning of cattle and sheep with benefin or trifluralin produced anorexia and weight loss. Trifluralin also produced diarrhea. Sheep severely poisoned with benefin exhibited bloating, depression, and prostration before death. Resolution of clinical signs and attainment of original body weight required about 1 month for animals poisoned with trifluralin. Postmortem findings in sheep poisoned with benefin were congestion of the abomasum and of the intestine. Lymph nodes associated with the gastrointestinal tract were swollen, and the liver was enlarged and friable.

NITRILES

Dichlobenil is applied directly to soil for prevention of seed germination and control of shallow-rooted weeds. Translocation takes place from the roots into aerial parts where the herbicide is metabolized or evaporates. Signs of toxicosis in cattle and sheep are increased salivation, anorexia, and depression. Convulsions were observed before death in some instances. At necropsy, lesions in cattle and sheep were extensive as in generalized toxemia. There were swollen, hemorrhagic lymph nodes throughout the body and hemorrhages in muscles, chiefly in the thoracic and cervical areas. Epicardial hemorrhages (petechiae) were also observed. Congestion of the lungs and upper respiratory tract were common, and the liver was swollen and congested in acute poisoning but often pale and friable in prolonged or chronic poisoning. The kidneys were congested and swollen but were found to be firm and reduced in size in a sheep that died 30 days after the last dose. The mucosa of the abomasum and intestinal tract was congested to markedly inflamed, depending on the acuteness of poisoning.

PHENOLS

Signs of poisoning by nitrofen in cattle and sheep included anorexia, diarrhea, hematuria, depression, and ataxia. At necropsy, the kidneys were congested, and the spleen was enlarged. Epicardial hemorrhages were present with clotted blood and edema fluid in the pericardial sac. The upper respiratory tract contained edema fluid and froth.

PHENOXYS

These herbicides are comparatively harmless and present little hazard to livestock except by way of accidental ingestion of concentrates or sprays. The danger of chronic toxicity is very low, and continuous high dosage over a period of months is required to produce severe signs of poisoning. These herbicides may, however, increase the palatability of poisonous plants to livestock or increase nitrate or cyanide content of forage. To avoid problems associated with these effects, it is recommended that treated areas not be used for pasture for at least a week after spraying with these herbicides. Signs of toxicity are anorexia, depression, rumen atony, and weakness (especially in the hind limbs). Animals may gradually become emaciated and moribund. Less frequently observed signs are diarrhea and bloating. Postmortem findings are congestion and enlargement of the liver and kidneys, greater friability of the liver, reddening of the intestinal and abomasal mucosa, bright undigested feed in the rumen, and enlarged, hyperemic lymph nodes.

THIOCARBAMATES

These herbicides are considered to be moderately toxic to cattle and sheep. Signs of poisoning are anorexia, weight loss, diarrhea, depression, ataxia, muscle spasms, and prostration. In addition, molinate and pebulate produced salivation and, occasionally, bloating. Anorexia was the only sign of poisoning in most animals poisoned with EPTC and vernolate. Signs produced by triallate poisoning were generally limited to significant weight loss followed by a long recuperative period. Partial to complete alopecia occurred up to 60 days following nonfatal poisoning by diallate. Lesions at necropsy were congestion of the lungs, kidneys, and thyroid. The liver was often enlarged, friable and pale, and the gastrointestinal mucosa was reddened or hemorrhagic.

TRIAZINES

Among the organic herbicides, this group is considered relatively toxic to cattle and sheep; however, little evidence of poisoning has resulted from their use. Experiments in which atrazine or prometone was ingested on treated forage for 27 days produced neither signs of poisoning nor gross or histopathologic lesions. Daily herbicide intake peaked during the second week of feeding at 68 mg/kg atrazine and 75 mg/kg prometone for calves and 69 mg/kg atrazine and 75 mg/kg prometone for sheep. The low toxicities of atrazine and prometone in these experiments when compared with data in Table 1 is likely due to differences in the mode of administration (eaten on forage vs. direct doses). In contrast, clinical signs consistent with triazine herbicide poisoning and 20 per cent mortality have been reported in sheep grazing nonpoisonous weeds during and soon after spraying with a mixture of simazine (1.2 kg/acre) and amitrole (0.4 kg/acre). Accidental poisoning of dairy animals following access to a bag of atrazine formulation produced hyperesthesia, moderate hypersalivation, muscle tremors, ataxia, recumbency, and death. Signs of poisoning from direct dosing with triazine herbicides are anorexia, depression, muscle spasms, uncoordinated gait, and weakness. Muscle spasms produced by atrazine varied in intensity and apparently were restricted to the hindquarters. The clinical condition of some animals moderately poisoned with atrazine seemed to improve despite continued dosing with the herbicide. These animals then died unexpectedly. Increasing dyspnea was an additional observation with simazine poisoning. Signs reported for prometone poisoning are somewhat different and consist of anorexia, increased salivation, and diarrhea. Necropsy lesions consisted of congested lungs, liver, and kidneys, pale, friable, and sometimes enlarged livers, enlarged adrenals and subepicardial petechial hemorrhages. Pulmonary edema and excessive amounts of fluid in the thoracic and abdominal cavities were seen in sheep chronically poisoned with propazine.

TRIAZOLES

Amitrole is relatively toxic to cattle and sheep, producing anorexia, ataxia, weakness, and loss of weight. Loss of body weight was the only sign of poisoning in some sheep given the herbicide at low dosage (10 to 25 mg/kg/day) for 10 days. At necropsy, there was congestion of the lungs and kidneys, an enlarged friable liver, and hemorrhages of the abomasal and intestinal mucosa.

URACILS

Cattle and sheep poisoned with bromacil or isocil exhibit anorexia, depression, loss of body weight, and occasionally ataxia and bloat. Enlarged hemorrhagic lymph nodes, congested lungs, and subepicardial hemorrhage are seen at necropsy.

UREAS

These materials are not considered highly hazardous to cattle or to sheep. Signs of poisoning, some of which appear suddenly, include ataxia, depression, prostration, anorexia, dyspnea, and weight loss. Additional signs seen in linuron poisoning are hypersalivation, marked weakness (cattle), and hematuria (sheep). Vomiting and diarrhea are additional signs in cattle poisoned with norea. Mild poisoning of cattle and sheep with fluometuron produced only anorexia and diarrhea. Necropsy findings included congestion of various internal organs. Most commonly involved were the kidneys, intestinal mucosa, and meninges. Animals poisoned with fluometuron and linuron had friable and sometimes pale livers. Excessive amounts of pericardial fluid and hemorrhages associated with the epicardium, bladder mucosa, and muscle fascia were found in sheep poisoned with linuron. Enlarged lymph nodes were observed in sheep poisoned with fluometuron.

UNCLASSIFIED HERBICIDES

The only signs of illness in sheep poisoned with bensulide were anorexia and death, but in cattle the signs were salivation, diarrhea, prostration, and ataxia. Congestion of the lungs, kidneys, pancreas, and intestinal mucosa was observed in bensulide-poisoned sheep at necropsy. DCPA produced anorexia and weight loss in cattle at a daily dosage of 250 mg/kg for 10 days. Sheep given DCPA for the same period of time remained clinically unaffected at daily doses of 500 mg/kg. Endothall, fenac, and glyphosate produced similar signs of intoxication: weight loss, anorexia, diarrhea, and ataxia. Dyspnea was seen in sheep and cattle poisoned with fenac and glyphosate. One sheep developed alopecia 30 days following the last dose of fenac. Necropsy of animals poisoned with endothall revealed congestion of the kidneys and adrenal glands, enlargement of the liver and adrenal glands, excessive peritoneal fluid, and gastrointestinal hemorrhage. Sheep poisoned with fenac had congestion of the liver, kidneys, and meninges, enlargement of the spleen, and petechial hemorrhages subcutaneously. No lesions were observed at necropsy of cattle poisoned with a formulation of glyphosate; however, mild to marked renal tubular vacuolization was seen microscopically. Prominent signs observed in cattle and sheep poisoned with picloram were weakness, depression, and anorexia. Fatally affected animals died 6 to 7 days after signs of poisoning appeared. Postmortem lesions in these animals included congestion of the lungs, liver, kidneys, adrenal glands, and intestinal mucosa. Lymph nodes of the anterior half of the body were swollen and hemorrhagic. The liver and adrenal glands were enlarged, and the rumen was filled with undigested feed. Pyrazon intoxication produced weight loss, lethargy, and convulsions in both cattle and sheep. Convulsions and death were observed in 1 sheep 90 days after the last dose of pyrazon had been given. Prominent lesions in acutely poisoned animals were congestion of the kidneys and meninges, hemorrhage of the intestinal mucosa, and a pale friable liver. Cattle poisoned with tryclopyr exhibited anorexia, depression, weakness, unsteady gait, tremors, and dyspnea. Constipation, sometimes followed by diarrhea, was a prominent feature of poisoning. Findings at necropsy were enlargement of the kidney, adrenal glands, and spleen. The liver was enlarged, pale, and friable, and the colon was congested or hemorrhagic. Mild toxic tubular nephrosis and hepatosis were seen microscopically.

DIAGNOSIS

Clinical signs and lesions produced by many of the organic herbicides are nonspecific, requiring that other evidence be considered. Diagnosis usually depends on quantitative evidence of exposure (how much for how long) with the presence of compatible clinical effects. An estimate of the degree of exposure should be made and compared with known toxicity data (Table 1) to establish the likelihood of poisoning.

The most commonly used method of assessing potential hazard involves the experimental determination of the minimum toxic dosage by direct oral administration of herbicide to cattle and sheep and comparing it to the dosage obtainable from treated forage. Several assumptions are used to estimate the daily dosage of a herbicide obtained by animals grazing treated forage. An arbitrary, although realistic, yield of 0.1 lb/ft^2 of air-dried forage is selected. This value would represent a high-quality, improved pasture yielding approximately 2 tons/acre of forage. Adjustments may be necessary for local conditions. A sparse cover of vegetation would allow more of the herbicide to reach the ground and to be unavailable to animals, whereas a lush cover of vegetation would tend to hold more of the herbicide and to be available to animals. In the latter case, however, less of the total forage of the area would be consumed in any 1 day. In these calculations, neither the influence of environmental factors nor the rate of decomposition of herbicides is considered. Further assumptions are (1) an animal would consume, as dry forage, 3 per cent of its body weight each day and (2) all the chemical formulation applied would adhere to the vegetation. Although the latter is never actually the case, this assumption gives the maximum exposure to be expected. An application of 1 lb/acre (1.12 kg/ha) active ingredient provides 10.4 mg/ft^2 and, therefore, a daily dose of 7 mg/kg of body weight to a grazing animal under the assumed conditions.

In addition to the minimum reported toxicity of a number of herbicides to cattle and sheep, Table 1 presents an estimate (using the approach described earlier) of the application rate necessary to provide an equivalent daily dose from grazing treated forage. Information in this table can be applied to cases of suspected herbicide poisonings as an aid in deciding if a condition of potentially hazardous exposure exists. It should be noted that most of these data are the result of direct oral administration of herbicides to a limited number of animals and calculations based on several conservative assumptions and, therefore, may or may not tend to magnify the actual hazard of a particular herbicide.

Analytical confirmation for many herbicides is expensive and time consuming; therefore, the clinician should have a reasonable level of suspicion that poisoning by a herbicide could have occurred before requesting chemical analysis. Samples to be submitted for analysis should include suspected forage, feed or water, liver, kidney, stomach, or rumen contents, urine and feces. The mere presence of herbicide residues in animal tissues and ingesta will confirm that exposure has occurred but may not necessarily be indicative of poisoning. Since many herbicides are rapidly eliminated from the body, the absence of residues may not exclude the possibility that poisoning has occurred, especially if death is delayed. Interpretation of the results of chemical analysis may be difficult in the absence of data concerning the levels and persistence of residues that can be expected in cases of poisoning.

TREATMENT

Animals with excessive oral exposure to most organic herbicides should be treated with activated charcoal (1 to 3 gm/kg) mixed in a slurry with sodium or magnesium sulfate (1 gm/kg). Poisoning by the arsenical herbicides should be treated in the same manner as inorganic arsenic poisoning. No specific antidotes are available for treatment of poisonings by other organic herbicides. Removal of intestinal contents, administration of activated charcoal (450 to 900 gm/100 kg body weight), forced diuresis, and supportive therapy for hepatic and renal functions may be useful.

PREVENTION

Prevention involves controlling or eliminating sources of exposure. Following label instructions with regard to application rates and grazing of treated forage will avoid poisoning as well as illegal residues in animal products. Grazing of treated areas should be discontinued at least until weeds are dead and no longer palatable. Care should be taken to prevent exposure of animals to concentrated chemicals from containers, spillage, and contaminated feed or water.

Supplemental Reading

Bovey, R. W., and Young, A. L.: Toxicology of Phenoxy Herbicides in Animals and Man. In Metcalf, R. L., Stumm, W. (eds.). The Science of 2–4,5–T and Associated Herbicides. New York, John Wiley & Sons, 71–132, 1980.

Buck, W. B., Osweiler, G. D., and Van Gelder, G. A.: Clinical and Diagnostic Veterinary Toxicology. 2nd ed. Dubuque, Iowa, Kendall Hunt Publishing Co., 1976.

Egyed, M. N., and Shlosberg, A.: Some considerations in the evaluation of a herbicide (simazine-aminotriazole) poisoning in sheep and horses. Vet. Tox. 19:83–84, 1977.

Johnson, A. E., Van Kampen, K. R., and Binns, W.: Effects on cattle and sheep of eating hay treated with triazine herbicides, atrazine and prometone. Am. J. Vet. Res. 33:1433–1438, 1972.

Palmer, J. S., and Radeleff, R. D.: The Toxicity of Some Organic Herbicides to Cattle, Sheep, and Chickens. United States Department of Agriculture Production Research Report, no. 106:26, 1969.

Palmer, J. S.: The Toxicity of 45 Organic Herbicides to Cattle, Sheep, and Chickens, United States Department of Agriculture Production Research Report, no. 137, 1972.

Arsenic

ALLAN FURR, D.V.M., M.S.
and WILLIAM B. BUCK, D.V.M., M.S.

Arsenicals are classified chemically as either inorganic or organic. In describing the toxic syndromes, it is better to distinguish the inorganic and organic arsenicals (pesticides) from the phenylarsonics (feed additives) agents. The combination of confirmed cases from both syndromes

makes arsenic one of the major causes of toxicoses in domestic animals.

INORGANIC AND ORGANIC ARSENICALS

The inorganic arsenicals, such as arsenic trioxide, arsenic acid, copper acetoarsenite (Paris Green), and other arsenic salts, cause a toxic syndrome that is similar to that caused by the organic arsenical pesticide group. This group includes compounds such as MAMA (monoammonium methanearsonate), DSMA (disodium methanearsonate), cacodylic acid, and MSMA (monosodium methanearsonate). Arsenical compounds are readily absorbed from the gastrointestinal tract, the lungs, and the skin. The major route of exposure is ingestion of contaminated feed stuffs. Cattle, horses, and sheep are most commonly affected.

Exposure occurs in many ways, including accidental incorporation of arsenicals into feed stuffs from improperly labeled containers, refuse in junk piles, old supplies in buildings, feeding crop residue such as "gin trash" from cotton that had been treated with an arsenic desiccant; improper treatment with arsenic medicaments, and eating of soil contaminated with arsenic.

Clinical Signs

The toxicity of arsenic is quite variable depending upon the solubility, the particle size, the oxidation state, the route of exposure, and the general condition of the exposed animal. This group of arsenicals primarily inhibits the sulfhydryl enzymes, resulting in rapid cell damage. They have a profound deleterious effect on the integrity of the capillaries, resulting in transudation of plasma and loss in blood volume with an accompanying loss in blood pressure. The resulting shock syndrome is consistently observed in the affected animal. The clinical signs in the acute episode are severe with a rapid onset. The affected animal is observed to progress quite rapidly through a syndrome of weakness, incoordination, trembling, and intense abdominal pain to collapse and death. The clinical signs in subacute episodes are not as rapid. The animal may linger for several days and is severely depressed, anorectic, and has watery diarrhea. Rapid dehydration and emaciation occur. The rumen is atonic, the temperature generally is subnormal, and the animal progressively becomes weaker with eventual collapse and death.

Necropsy Observations

The postmortem observations are characterized by foul-smelling, very fluid intestinal contents. The gastric and intestinal mucosa are intensely hyperemic with patchy hemorrhagic areas. The mucosa is often necrotic with shreds sloughing into the intestinal contents. In very acute cases excessive fluid in the gastrointestinal tract may be the only abnormal change observed.

Microscopic lesions are characterized by hemorrhage and necrosis of the intestinal mucosa, fatty change in the liver, and degeneration of the kidney tubules.

Diagnosis

Diagnosis is based on the objective evaluation of the history, clinical signs, postmortem observations, and chemical analyses. Arsenic tends to concentrate transiently in the kidney and liver in fulminating episodes. Liver and kidney levels of arsenic above 5 ppm (usually above 10 ppm) on a wet-weight basis are generally encountered. Levels less than 5 ppm can be considered diagnostically significant when evaluated with the entire syndrome.

Treatment

Treatment is not often attempted, as in most cases the affected animals are found dead with no observable illness. Treatment, when attempted, must be started without delay and with heroics. Under the best of circumstances, the results are often very disappointing. Treatment is based on removing or inactivating the unabsorbed arsenic from the intestinal tract by activated charcoal (2 gm) and by inactivation of the absorbed arsenic with sulfur-containing agents, such as sodium thiosulfate and dimercaprol.

Sodium thiosulfate is basically nontoxic; thus large, repeated doses can be given both intravenously and orally. It is recommended that 15 to 30 gm of sodium thiosulfate be given intravenously in a 10 to 20 per cent aqueous solution to the average adult horse or cow. In addition, 30 to 60 gm given orally and repeated at 6-hr intervals for 3 to 4 days is recommended. BAL* (dimercaprol) is recommended to be administered intramuscularly at 4 to 5 mg/kg and then repeated every 4 to 6 hr at 2 to 3 mg/kg the first day and at 1 mg/kg for at least 2 more days. BAL is suspended in arachis oil and intramuscular injections are quite painful. BAL appears to have some beneficial effect in treating animals poisoned with inorganic arsenicals but it has doubtful benefits in treating animals poisoned with organic arsenicals.

Recent work by Hatch and associates using thiotic acid at 50 mg/kg administered intramuscularly at 8-hr intervals to treat an inorganic arsenical toxicosis had some beneficial effect. The exposure level of 25 mg/kg of sodium arsenite evidently exceeded a favorable prognosis with any method of treatment. Dimercaptosuccinate (DMSA) and dimercaptopropanesulfonate (DMPS, Unithiol) at 20 mg/kg parenterally may also be effective antidotes according to studies by Aposhian, 1983.

The treatment regimen should also include symptomatic fluid therapy to counteract dehydration and oral demulcents to relieve abdominal distress.

PHENYLARSONICS

The phenylarsonic compounds are used extensively in swine and poultry feeds to control certain diseases, improve feed efficiency, and increase rate of weight gain.

The most commonly used phenylarsonic swine feed additives are arsanilic acid or sodium arsanilate and 3-nitro-4-hydroxy phenylarsonic acid ("3-Nitro").

Arsanilic acid and sodium arsanilate are used prophylactically at 0.005 to·0.01 per cent (45 to 90 gm/ton) and therapeutically to control swine dysentery at 0.025 to 0.04 per cent (225 to 360 gm/ton) for 5 to 6 days. "3-Nitro" is recommended prophylactically at 0.0025 to 0.0075 per cent (23 to 68 gm/ton) and therapeutically at 0.02 per cent (182 gm/ton) for 5 to 6 days. These compounds have a withdrawal period of 5 days before slaughter to avoid

tissue levels above the action threshold. For swine this is 2.0 ppm wet-weight in liver and 0.5 ppm in muscle tissue.

The phenylarsonic compounds are much less toxic than the other arsenicals. They also result in a different toxic syndrome from that produced by other arsenicals with characteristic clinical signs and pathologic lesions.

Toxicoses from phenylarsonic feed additives are invariably the result of human error: (1) adding excessive levels to the feed, (2) feeding for a prolonged period of time, (3) limiting water supply with decreased excretion, (4) mixing up feed formulations, and (5) feeding high levels to debilitated animals, especially those with a severe diarrhea.

The exact mechanism of action is not known, but the primary effect is observed in the peripheral nerves, notably the sciatic, brachial, and optic nerves.

Clinical Signs

The clinical signs may appear as early as 3 days after a high exposure, but generally there is a variable interval, depending upon the exposure level and general condition of the animals. The early clinical signs are typically incoordination, swaying body movements (drunken hog syndrome), and ataxia. The animals are alert, bright, and will still eat and drink. Blindness is an inconsistent finding partly due to its difficulty to diagnose. Continued ingestion can result in total paralysis and some deaths, but early observation and diagnosis should prevent deaths.

Necropsy Observations

Gross postmortem lesions are not specific for phenylarsonics. Downer pigs may have muscle atrophy as a result of nerve damage. Longitudinal sections of sciatic, brachial, and optic nerves typically have microscopic lesions indicating demyelination of the nerve tracts. The nerve degeneration results in erratic impulse transmission that is exemplified by the clinical signs. Microscopic lesions are not apparent until at least 2 weeks after the first exposure to excessive arsenical preparations.

Diagnosis

Diagnosis is based tentatively on the history and typical clinical signs. Confirmatory information is obtained from the chemical analysis of kidney and tissue levels plus the suspected feed. Tissue levels above 3 ppm wet-weight are diagnostically significant. Low tissue levels can be misleading if the affected animals have not been eating the arsenic-containing feed for just a few days, as domestic animals can excrete the arsenicals quite rapidly. Histopathologic changes in the peripheral nerves may have diagnostic significance, i.e., demyelination and gliosis. A diagnosis is based on objective evaluation of all the information obtained on the case.

Treatment

Treatment is quite simple and effective. Satisfactory recovery will generally occur spontaneously following complete removal of all phenylarsonic feed additives. If lesions of the nerves are extensive, complete paralysis may develop, while some animals may only partially recover and retain an altered gait with variable degrees of flaccid paralysis. Some animals will remain blind but do not appear handicapped under confinement conditions.

Arsenic compounds are all toxic and should be handled

---

*Available from Hynsan, Wescott & Dunning, Inc., Baltimore, MD. 21201.

carefully. Proper labeling, strict adherence to recommended uses and precautions, plus safe storage and proper disposal of old or excess materials, can prevent most cases of arsenic poisoning.

Supplemental Reading

Aposhian, H. V.: DMSA and DMPS—water soluble antidotes for heavy metal poisoning. Ann. Rev. Pharmacol. 23:193–215, 1983.

Blood, D. C., and Henderson, J. A.: Veterinary Medicine, 4th ed. Baltimore, Williams & Wilkins, 1974.

Buck, W. B., Osweiler, G. D., and Van Gelder, G. A.: Clinical and Diagnostic Veterinary Toxicology, 2nd ed. Dubuque, Iowa, Kendall/Hunt Publishing Co., 1976.

Buck, W. B., et al.: Feed Additives Compendium. Minneapolis, Minnesota, Miller Publishing Co., 1979.

Farm Chemicals Handbook. Willoughby, Ohio, Meister Publishing Co., 1978.

Hatch, R. C., Clark, J. D., and Jain, A. V.: Use of thiols and thiosulfate for treatment of experimentally induced acute arsenite toxicosis in cattle. Am. J. Vet. Res. 39:1411–1414, 1978.

Copper—Molybdenum

WILLIAM B. BUCK, D.V.M., M.S.

Copper is essential to life in all species of plants and animals. Molybdenum is essential to plant life, but an uncomplicated molybdenum deficiency has not been reproduced in humans or farm animals. The metabolism of copper, molybdenum, and the sulfate ion SO^{-2} is complex and interrelated, especially in ruminant species. Other elements including zinc and iron also interact with copper, especially in nonruminant species, such as swine, poultry, and laboratory animals.

The mechanisms responsible for copper-molybdenum-sulfate interaction are not entirely understood. It is likely that a copper-molybdenum complex inhibits copper and perhaps molybdenum utilization in animal tissues, especially the liver, resulting in a disturbance in synthesis of copper-protein compounds, including ceruloplasmin. Regardless of the mechanism, this phenomenon is dependent upon the presence of inorganic sulfate. The copper-molybdenum-sulfate interactions also strongly affect urinary excretion of these elements.

Zinc and iron have a profound effect upon copper metabolism in nonruminant animals, especially swine. Both zinc and iron have been shown to protect swine from the adverse effects of high levels of dietary copper. Similarly, zinc and iron deficiencies tend to exacerbate copper toxicity in swine.

COPPER DEFICIENCY (EXCESS MOLYBDENUM)

A variety of disorders in animals have been associated with copper deficiencies. When discussing the deficiency of copper, however, one should keep in mind that an important consideration is the relative concentration of copper in relation to other elements and molecules, such as molybdenum, zinc, iron, and sulfate. The ratio of copper to these dietary factors is just as important as the actual level of copper in the diet. For example, one is hard pressed to distinguish between clinical signs of copper deficiency and of molybdenum toxicosis, especially in ruminants.

Disorders that have been associated with a *relative* copper deficiency in various animal species are anemia, depressed growth, bone disorders, depigmentation of hair and wool, abnormal wool growth, neonatal ataxia, impaired reproductive performance, heart failure, cardiovascular defects, and gastrointestinal disturbances. Many factors influence the severity of these functions, such as species, age, dietary interrelationships, environment, sex, and even breed or strain characteristics. Anemia associated with copper deficiency occurs in most species and is characteristic of the anemia associated with iron deficiency. Bone abnormalities associated with copper deficiency have been reported in rabbits, mice, chicks, dogs, pigs, foals, sheep, and cattle. In ruminants, osteoporosis and spontaneous bone fractures are usually associated with excess dietary molybdenum and thus a relative copper deficiency. Sheep suffering from simple copper deficiency or excess molybdenum or both also develop depigmentation of dark wool together with loss of crimp and quality of their fine wool. In Australia a syndrome called "enzootic ataxia" and in the United Kingdom a condition called "swayback" are thought to be due to copper deficiency. Ewes become anemic with stringy wool, which corresponds with neurologic signs in their lambs in enzootic ataxia. The typical case of swayback is more acute in lambs, and the ewes' wool is normal. These diseases are noted in lambs under 1 month of age. Lambs are severely incoordinated, ataxic, and usually blind. Death is the result of starvation, exposure, or pneumonia. Swayback has been reported in California. Lesions associated with enzootic ataxis and swayback in lambs are characterized by lysis of the white matter of the cerebrum and degeneration of motor tracts of the spinal cord.

Falling Disease

A cardiovascular disorder in cattle known as falling disease is associated with a relative copper deficiency. The primary lesion is progressive atrophy of the myocardium with replacement fibrosis. Sudden death is characteristic of the disease, which has been attributed to heart failure usually after exercise or excitement. This condition has not been reported in sheep or horses but has occurred in pigs and chickens. Cattle apparently are more susceptible than sheep to excess molybdenum and deficient copper in their diet. When the ratio of copper to molybdenum in feed drops below 2:1, toxicosis can be expected in cattle. This syndrome is manifested by emaciation, liquid diarrhea full of gas bubbles, swollen genitalia, anemia, and achromotrichia. Poor weight gains and death from prolonged purgation usually occur. Osteoporosis and bone fractures have been reported in prolonged cases. Copper deficiency-like syndromes have resulted from feeding of forages and grains grown on soils naturally high in molybdenum or low in copper or both. In the United States such soils have been found in California, Oregon, Nevada, and Florida. Cattle grazing pastures on muck or shale soils in England, Ireland, New Zealand, and Holland have suffered severe molybdenosis.

When the copper levels of feed or forages are in the normal range of 8 to 11 ppm, cattle can be poisoned on molybdenum levels above 5 to 6 ppm, and sheep can be poisoned on levels above 10 to 12 ppm. When the dietary copper level falls below 8 to 11 ppm or when the sulfate ion level is high, even 1 to 2 ppm molybdenum may be toxic to cattle.

TREATMENT

Copper sulfate may be added to a salt-mineral mixture at 1 to 5 per cent, depending upon molybdenum levels in the diet. Other formulations have been recommended to provide approximately 1 gm of copper sulfate for an adult cow daily: 28 gm $CuSO_4$ to 95 L water, 0.23 to 0.45 kg of $CuSO_3$ to 45 kg salt, 45 kg of protein concentrate, 45 kg of fine salt, and 1.1 kg of $CuSO_4$ mixture given at a rate of 75.5 gm per day per cow. Copper glycinate can be given subcutaneously at a rate of 60 mg for calves and 120 mg for mature cattle. This treatment may need to be repeated during a season. Response to copper therapy is usually good.

COPPER TOXICOSIS (DEFICIENT MOLYBDENUM, IRON, ZINC)

The interaction of copper, molybdenum, and the sulfate ion in ruminants makes it impossible to delineate between the toxicity of one and the deficiency of the other. Thus, copper deficiency is manifested by the same syndrome as chronic molybdenum poisoning, and chronic copper poisoning, especially in sheep, results when the dietary ratio of copper to molybdenum increases above 6 to 10:1. Similarly, copper toxicosis in swine and other nonruminant species is accentuated by iron and zinc deficiency. These syndromes have occurred most frequently in sheep and swine.

Acute copper poisoning may occur in any species associated with the use of copper compounds for therapeutic and pesticidal purposes. Cattle may be poisoned by 200 to 800 mg $CuSO_4$/kg body weight, and sheep may be poisoned by 20 to 100 mg single dose. Copper chloride ($CuCl_2$) is 2 to 4 times more toxic than $CuSO_4$. Clinical signs associated with large oral doses of copper formulations include vomiting, excessive salivation, abdominal pain, diarrhea (greenish tinged), collapse, and death within 24 to 48 hr.

The most common form of copper toxicosis (molybdenum, zinc, or iron imbalance) results from chronic exposure to diets containing either excess copper or diets containing imbalanced ratios of copper, molybdenum, zinc, and iron.

Various conditions under which copper toxicosis (molybdenum deficiency) may occur, especially in sheep, include the following:

1. Consumption of forages contaminated by copper-containing pesticides.
2. Copper sulfate for the control of heliminthiasis and footrot.
3. Contamination of the pasture in the vicinity of copper mines.
4. Consumption of pasture forages containing an imbalance of copper and molybdenum (e.g., *Trifolium subteranium* in Australia).
5. Consumption of forages containing pyrrolizidine alkaloids that cause hepatic necrosis, resulting in inability to metabolize and excrete normal dietary levels of copper (e.g., *Heliotropium*, *Echium*, and *Senecio*).
6. Feeding of sheep under confinement conditions, usually associated with the supplementation of copper without molybdenum.
7. Providing mineral mixtures to sheep and cattle with improper ratios of copper and other elements.

8. Feeding complete feed with a copper imbalance. Copper is recognized as a feed ingredient, whereas molybdenum is not. Feeds to which copper has been added may be adequate for cattle but toxic for sheep.

Copper has been used as a feed additive for swine because of its growth promotant effects. If adequate zinc and iron levels are present in the diet, 250 ppm $CuSO_4$ may be beneficial. On the other hand, if iron and zinc concentrations are low in the diet, 250 ppm $CuSO_4$ may result in chronic toxicosis in swine.

Clinical signs of chronic toxicosis occur suddenly even when animals have consumed small but excessive amounts of copper over a period of weeks or months. The syndrome is that of an acute hemolytic crisis with death occurring within 24 to 48 hr. The animals become anorectic and weak. Hemoglobinuria, hemoglobinemia, and icterus are usually present. Occasionally, an animal may have only pale mucous membranes without icterus and hemoglobinemia. Affected animals may chew their wool. Although the morbidity is usually less than 5 per cent, the mortality is usually over 75 per cent.

Diagnosis of chronic copper poisoning or deficiency may be confirmed using chemical analysis of tissues and blood of affected animals, correlated with copper and molybdenum (iron and zinc in swine) concentrations in the ration, clinical signs, and necropsy findings, which are icterus, swollen, gun-metal colored kidneys, and pale or yellow liver. Normal concentrations of copper in serum and whole blood in most species range from 0.7 to 2 ppm. Concentrations above this are often associated with copper poisoning. Liver concentrations associated with copper poisoning are usually greater than 150 ppm on a wet-weight basis, whereas kidney concentrations are usually greater than 15 ppm. When the dietary copper to molybdenum ratio becomes greater than 6 to 10:1, toxicoses in sheep may begin to occur. Copper concentrations in swine diets associated with toxicosis will usually be greater than 100 ppm and associated with low levels of iron or zinc.

Diseases that should be differentiated from copper poisoning-molybdenum deficiency are as follows: leptospirosis, postparturient hemoglobinemia, bacillary hemoglobinuria, rape (brassica) poisoning, hepatitis, phenothiazine poisoning, onion poisoning, babesiosis, and anaplasmosis. Poisoning by metals such as arsenic, mercury, lead, and thallium may mimic the gastrointestinal effect of acute massive copper poisoning.

TREATMENT

The maintenance of proper copper to molybdenum, and copper to zinc and iron, ratios in the diet of sheep and swine is imperative for the prevention of feed-related copper toxicoses. The most common cause of copper toxicosis in sheep results from feeding complete feeds or mineral mixtures formulated for cattle. Such practices should be discontinued.

Molybdenum incorporated into phosphate fertilizer (114 gm/acre) can be used to increase the molybdenum content of pasture and reduce the retention of copper. Molybdenum-containing licks or mineral mixtures may also be used for preventive purposes (86 kg salt, 64 kg gypsum, and 0.45 kg sodium molybdate). Swine diets containing excessive copper should be fortified with zinc and iron.

Animals suffering from the acute hemolytic crisis of

copper toxicosis have a poor prognosis. Oral administration of 50 to 500 mg/day of ammonium or sodium molybdate and 0.3 to 1 gm/day thiosulfate for up to 3 weeks may have beneficial effects. Whole blood transfusions may be indicated in certain situations.

Supplemental Reading

Buck, W. B., Osweiler, G. D., and Van Gelder, G. A. (eds.): Clinical and Diagnostic Veterinary Toxicology, 2nd ed. Dubuque, Iowa, Kendall/Hunt Publishing Co., 1976.

Copper: Medical and Biologic Effects of Environmental Pollutants. Washington, D.C., National Academy of Sciences, 1977.

Underwood, E. J.: Trace Elements in Human and Animal Nutrition, 3rd ed. New York, Associated Press, 1971.

Lead

J. W. SEXTON, D.V.M., M.S.
and WILLIAM B. BUCK, D.V.M., M.S.

Lead is one of the most common causes of poisoning in farm animals, particularly in cattle, horses, and sheep. Each year in the United States 600,000 tons of lead are mined and another 600,000 tons are reclaimed; thus, the opportunity for exposure of animals and humans is very possible.

In livestock, the source of lead ingested is usually from storage batteries, used motor oil, grease, caulking compounds, lead-based paints, linoleum, and putty. Lead water pipes and lead connections can also be a source. Grass near heavily traveled highways may contain 500 ppm lead from engine exhaust systems. Pastures of poor quality cause animals to forage in unusual places, such as trash dumps, which increases the possibility of animals finding lead-laden materials. Mineral deficiencies and boredom caused by overcrowding of young animals often result in pica.

Lead accumulates in the body so that chronic exposure may result in toxicosis. Silage containing 140 ppm lead has poisoned cattle, and herbage grown on lead-contaminated soil may contain 260 to 914 ppm lead and cause death in calves. Normal herbage contains 3 to 7 ppm lead.

Swine are quite resistant to lead poisoning while cattle, horses, and sheep are more susceptible. Young animals are more susceptible than adults. The reason ruminants are more commonly affected may be due in part to the tendency of lead to settle in the reticulum and be converted to soluble lead by the action of the fluid of the forestomachs. In addition, cattle in particular seem to be attracted to lead paint and lead products, and if given the opportunity will drink crankcase oil and lick machinery grease.

Lethal doses of lead vary with species, ranging from 500 gm in horses, to 50 gm in cattle, to 30 gm in sheep. Death in cattle has occurred with doses as low as 4.8 mg/kg body weight. Pigs have been fed 33 to 66 mg/kg body weight for up to 14 weeks before toxic effects were seen. In calves single oral doses of lead acetate at a concentration of 0.2 to 0.4 gm/kg body weight have been fatal. Acute lethal single exposures are usually considered to be in the magnitude of 400 to 600 mg/kg in calves and 600 to 800 mg/kg in adult cattle.

Lead is relatively insoluble and even soluble forms such as lead acetate form insoluble compounds, such as lead sulfate, in the gastrointestinal tract. There are 2 forms of lead toxicosis: encephalopathic and gastrointestinal. In general, the ingestion of large doses of lead by susceptible animals such as calves produces central nervous system signs. Moderate doses produce gastroenteritis. The mechanism of brain damage is thought to be due to edema resulting from capillary degeneration. Neuronal degeneration and encephalomalacia have been associated with subacute lead poisoning in cattle. Lead can pass the placental barrier causing abortion.

CLINICAL SIGNS

Lead poisoning in animals produces 2 distinct manifestations, neurologic and abdominal, with the neurologic syndrome the most common in cattle, although most animals have both syndromes concomitantly. Both acute and subacute syndromes occur. The acute syndrome may result in animals being found dead before signs of illness have been noted. Clinical signs often include staggering, muscle tremors (especially of the head and neck), snapping of the eyelids, head bobbing, champing of the jaws, excessive salivation, bellowing, rolling of the eyes, apparent blindness, and clonic-tonic convulsions. Affected animals tend to go forward through fences, brush, or other obstacles. Animals usually die during seizures of respiratory failure.

In subacute cases animals have anorexia, blindness, incoordination, staggering, excessive salivation, grinding of the teeth, kicking at the abdomen (indicating abdominal pain), and rumen atony, causing constipation followed by a fetid diarrhea. The animal may also wander aimlessly and become depressed and lethargic.

The subacute syndrome is usual in sheep. Anorexia, constipation initially followed by a dark, foul smelling diarrhea, weakness, ataxia, and abdominal pain are common signs. Seldom is there excitement, tetany, or convulsions. Abortions are common.

Natural cases of lead poisoning have not been documented in swine.

PATHOLOGY

Death may occur without visible gross lesions. Depending on the source of lead exposure, pieces of lead may be found in the digestive tract, especially the rumen and reticulum. If the source is grease or used crankcase oil, this will be readily detected in the stomach contents. Lesions commonly seen following acute lead poisoning are mild gastritis (especially abomasitis), hemorrhages on both surfaces of the heart, increased cerebrospinal fluid pressure, brain edema, and possibly pale liver, kidneys, and skeletal muscle. Histologically, acid-fast intranuclear inclusion bodies may be present in renal tubular cells and hepatocytes. There may be both hepatic and renal epithelial cell degeneration. Basophilic stippling of red blood cells may be present if lead exposure has occurred over a period of several days or weeks.

Some workers have observed the following brain changes in bovine lead poisoning: edema, congestion of the cerebral cortex, prominent capillaries and endothelial swelling, petechial hemorrhage, and laminar neuronal necrosis. Others have observed more severe changes in protracted cases of lead poisoning in the bovine, including laminar cortical necrosis, endothelial and astrocytic proliferation, microglial accumulation, and eosinophilic infiltration of leptomeninges.

DIAGNOSIS

In the living animal, ingested lead can be recovered from feces, urine, milk, and blood. Because of the variability of lead levels in urine, feces, and milk owing to the time lapse between ingestion and illness and the difficulty of routinely obtaining satisfactory specimens, the blood analysis is by far the most reliable source of information. A heparinized blood sample having a lead concentration of 0.35 ppm or higher is considered indicative of lead toxicosis in cattle; however, it is imperative that clinical signs, history, and circumstantial evidence be consistent with lead poisoning. Lead levels of 1.0 ppm or higher dictate a guarded prognosis; however, recovering animals may have blood levels over 0.35 ppm and still improve with adequate medication. Liver and kidneys usually have 10 ppm lead or greater on a wet-weight basis, and stomach contents have variable concentrations.

Basophilic stippling of the red blood cells of cattle is not a consistent finding and when found must be evaluated by a hematologist to rule out some of the other causes of stippling. Lead poisoning can mimic many other diseases, some of which are hypomagnesemic tetany, malignant bovine catarrh, tetanus, brain abscesses, the nervous form of acetonemia, hypovitaminosis A, mercury poisoning, organic insecticide poisoning, polioencephalomalacia, pseudorabies, nervous coccidiosis, and rabies. The presence of nervous signs in cattle brings to mind 5 common and likely possibilities; rabies, polioencephalomalacia, thromboembolic meningoencephalitis, listeriosis, and lead poisoning. At the risk of sounding too cautious, it should be reemphasized that all cattle showing nervous signs should be regarded as rabid until proved otherwise.

TREATMENT

Although most cattle die of acute lead poisoning because of the nature of the material consumed and the susceptibility of the species, many animals can be saved if a correct diagnosis is made and treatment is started early. Magnesium sulfate given orally may aid in precipitating the soluble salts and in preventing some of the absorption in addition to its action as a purgative. One of the most effective drugs used in lead poisoning is calcium disodium EDTA (anhydrous) in a 6.6-per cent solution. This is administered by slow intravenous injection at the rate of 1 ml/0.9 kg of body weight daily and is best given in divided doses 2 or 3 times daily for 3 to 5 days. If additional treatment is indicated, a 2-day rest period is recommended that may be followed by another 5-day period of therapy. This solution increases lead excretion by 20 to 50 times. Good results depend heavily upon following directions closely and upon continuing treatment even when improvement is minimal. BAL (2,3-dimercapto-l-propanol) and d-penicillamine (B,B-dimethylcystein, a monothiol degradation product of penicillin F,G,K, and X) may also be used.

Recently there has been some clinical and experimental data strongly indicating that thiamin may be effective in treating and preventing lead intoxication in ruminants. Thiamin should be used with caution as its use is not entirely without risk. The intramuscular route is recommended. Dosages vary from 250 mg to 1000 mg twice daily for 4 to 5 days.

EDTA. In the event one does not have enough commercial Ca EDTA on hand, it can be prepared by using Na_4EDTA and adding it to a commercial calcium injection solution at the rate of 9.5 gm tetrasodium EDTA to each gm of calcium in solution.

Example: Cal-Dextrose #2 R solution contains 16.84 mg Ca/ml or 8.42 g Ca/500 ml. Add $9.5 \times 8.42 = 80$ gm tetrasodium EDTA to each 500 ml bottle of calcium solution. This solution will contain 60.96 gm $CaNa_2EDTA$ or 121.9 mg/ml. Administer 1 ml for each 3.0 to 3.5 kg body weight, 3 times daily IV for 5 days.

Blindness and anorexia may persist for days, and good nursing care and supportive treatment should be given. Feeding via stomach tube or helping blind animals have easy access to feed will save many animals that would otherwise die.

PREVENTION

Most cases of lead poisoning result from the thoughtless or careless handling of lead-containing materials. Disposing of old lead paint containers and batteries in dumps in pasture areas, leaving used motor oil or machinery with grease-exposed parts where cattle have access to it, and allowing animals to chew on boards painted with lead paint are the most common causes of lead poisoning in livestock and, therefore, should be prevented.

Supplemental Reading

Buck, W. B., Osweiler, G. D., and Van Gelder, G. A.: Clinical and Diagnostic Veterinary Toxicology, 2nd ed. Dubuque, Iowa, Kendall/Hunt Publishing Co., 1976.

Blood, D. C., and Henderson, J. A.: Veterinary Medicine, 3rd ed. Baltimore, Williams & Wilkins, 1971.

Bratton, G. R., Zmudzki, J., Kincaid, N., and Joyce, J.: Thiamin as treatment of lead poisoning in ruminants. Mod. Vet. Pract. 62:441–446, 1981.

Mercury

GARY D. OSWEILER, D.V.M., M.S., Ph.D.
and BARBARA S. HOOK, B.A., D.V.M.

Mercury poisoning of food animals has occurred sporadically in the past, usually as a result of feeding seed grains treated with organomercurial fungicides. However, use of mercurial seed dressings was banned in 1970. Since that time mercury poisoning in livestock has become much less common. Other causes of mercury toxicosis reported in the past have included ingestion of mercurial ointments, batteries, and pharmaceuticals. Recent concern for mercury reflects its persistence in the environment and the tendency of some forms to accumulate in the food chain of animals or humans. Mercury in whatever form may be taken up by aquatic organisms and accumulated as methyl or ethyl mercury. Other potential sources of residue accumulation include industrial effluents, ocean waters, bottom sludge from contaminated lakes, sewage sludge, and certain marine fish or shrimp.

PATHOGENESIS AND ETIOLOGIC AGENTS

To understand toxicosis by mercurial compounds, the form of compound must be considered. Inorganic mercury compounds (e.g., mercuric oxide) are absorbed readily from the gastrointestinal and respiratory tracts but are absorbed poorly through the skin. Inorganic mercury is found in highest concentration in liver and kidney. Organic mercury of the phenylmercury and methoxyethyl mercury types are metabolized to the inorganic form and then are handled by the animal as inorganic mercury.

Organic mercury of the alkyl type (methyl and ethyl mercury) is initially bound to erythrocytes, distributed throughout the body, and eventually accumulates primarily in brain and to some extent in kidney and muscle. The background distribution of mercury compounds in mammals is generally as follows: brain <0.1 ppm, liver <0.30 ppm, muscle <0.15 ppm, and kidney <2.75 ppm. Alkyl mercurials (methyl and ethyl mercury) are the most toxic of the various mercurials. Residues of these compounds in food animals also make them a public health risk. Their effects in livestock are cumulative and delayed.

Organic aryl materials (e.g., phenyl mercury) are metabolized rapidly, and their toxicity is roughly equivalent to that of the inorganic mercury compounds. Furthermore, clinical effects and speed of onset are different for alkyl mercury than for aryl and inorganic mercury. The toxicity of various mercury compounds is summarized in Table 1.

CLINICAL SIGNS

Clinical signs exhibited in food animals poisoned by mercury depend on the form of mercury ingested. Inorganic, aryl, and methoxyethyl mercury produces mainly gastrointestinal and urinary system signs. Toxicosis is characterized by acute to subacute signs of stomatitis, salivation, vomiting (swine), catarrhal to hemorrhagic or necrotic enteritis, anorexia, weakness, and hematuria. Skin changes may occur if clinical signs are prolonged for several days. In white pigs there is erythema. Other skin lesions are pustular dermatitis, hyperkeratinization, and loss of hair.

Exposure to an alkyl organomercury (e.g., methylmercury) results in chronic cumulative and progressive neurologic damage. Both swine and cattle are affected with ataxia, stumbling, weakness, occasional hyperesthesia, and convulsions followed generally by terminal prostration, coma, and death. Blindness often occurs. Swine poisoned by alkyl mercurials may develop postural abnormalities suggestive of proprioceptive or vestibular damage. The onset of clinical signs is quicker when large doses of methylmercury are received. Generally, several weeks may pass after consumption of treated grain before clinical signs appear.

Morbidity for mercury poisoning in livestock may be low or high, depending on the source and frequency of exposure to mercury. Mortality among affected animals is generally high and prognosis is always guarded or grave.

CLINICAL PATHOLOGY AND NECROPSY LESIONS

Inorganic and phenylmercury compounds cause lesions generally in the alimentary tract and kidneys. Acute hyperemic to necrotic and hemorrhagic gastroenteritis may be observed. Lesions can extend into the large intestine. Kidneys are pale and swollen. Histologically, there is epithelial necrosis of alimentary mucosa and renal tubules. Clinical pathologic changes related to renal damage may be seen, but laboratory findings vary with the severity and course of toxicosis.

Lesions of alkyl mercury toxicosis are mainly neurologic and are detected by microscopic examination. Focal malacia of cerebral cortex, demyelination, astrogliosis, microgliosis, loss of granular cells in the cerebellum, and fibrinoid degeneration of CNS arterioles are relatively general and consistent lesions of mercury toxicosis cases in swine and cattle.

DIAGNOSIS

Demonstration of a source of mercury is important in diagnosis since the availability of this toxicant is limited. Tissues from affected animals can be analyzed for mercury content. Residues from inorganic mercury poisoning are highest in kidney, while both brain and kidney accumulate high concentrations when alkyl mercury toxicosis occurs. In acute cases, kidney cortex and liver would be expected

Table 1. *Toxicity of Some Selected Mercury Compounds for Livestock*

Species	Compound	Toxicity
Cattle	Ethylmercury-*p*-toluene Sulfonanilide (1.5 % Hg) Ceresan M	1 mg Hg/kg daily for 8 days produces anorexia. CNS depression, fever, and diarrhea
Cattle	Methyl mercury dicyandiamide	0.23 mg Hg/kg for 56 days yields mild clinical signs
Swine	Methyl mercury dicyandiamide	One dose LD_{50} is 13.4 mg Hg/kg
Swine	Methyl mercury dicyandiamide	0.76 mg/kg for 44 days induces progressive cerebral dysfunction
Swine	Ethylmercuric chloride	0.76 mg/kg for 22 to 30 days induces progressive cerebral dysfunction
Chicken	Methyl mercury dicyandiamide	0.42 to 0.46 mg/kg/day for 40 to 44 days produces no clinical signs. Muscle and liver contained 10 ppm and 40 ppm Hg, respectively

Table 2. *Common Drug Dosages*

Name of Drug	Supplier	Species	Dose (mg/kg)
Sodium thiosulfate 10 % (Scarlet Drench Powder)	Haver-Lockhart Laboratories Shawnee, Kan. 66201	Bovine	30 gm total per adult bovine
Dimercaprol (BAL in oil)	Hynson, Wescott & Dunning Baltimore, Md. 21201	Bovine and swine	3 mg/kg QID given IM
Penicillamine (Cupramine)	Merck & Co., Inc. Rahway, N.J. 07065	Bovine and swine	15 to 50 mg/kg: dosage based on humans; not established in food animals

to contain in excess of 10 μg/gm mercury on a wet-weight basis. Brain tissue should be collected if alkyl mercury poisoning is suspected, since both chemical analysis and microscopic lesions are helpful in diagnosis. In the past, mercury poisoning has been confused with hog cholera, salmonellosis, swine erysipelas, organic arsenic poisoning in swine, and lead or arsenic poisoning in cattle.

TREATMENT

Treatment of either inorganic or organic mercury toxicosis in livestock is often unsuccessful. Removal of the animal from all sources of toxicant should be accomplished followed by administration of a saline cathartic (sodium sulfate) orally at the rate of 3 gm/kg body weight. Oral administration of sodium thiosulfate has been advocated, since mercurials may be complexed with the sulfhydryl radical. The dosage recommended for adult cattle is 30 gm orally in a 10-per cent solution. See Table 2 for details of common drug dosages. A commercial laxative containing 10 per cent sodium thiosulfate is available (Scarlet Drench Powder).* Dimercaprol (British Anti Lewisite or BAL)† is recommended as an antidote for mercury toxicosis. It is given at 3 mg/kg body weight 4 times daily for 3 days then twice daily for 10 days. It is an oil solution and should be given intramuscularly. An alternative therapy suggested for mercury toxicosis has been N-acetyl-DL-penicillamine (Cupramine).‡ No animal dosage has been established, but the human oral dose has ranged from 15 to 50 mg/kg. Both BAL and penicillamine are sulfhydryl compounds that chelate mercury and aid in excretion. Neither are very effective in cases of clinical poisonings with well developed signs.

2,3-Dimercaptosuccinic acid has been used experimentally for mercury toxicosis. It is less toxic than BAL, but a dosage has not been established for animals. It may prove to be a useful heavy metal antidote in the future.

PREVENTION

Positive diagnosis of mercury poisoning should be followed by a thorough search for and elimination of all potential sources. Meat, eggs, or milk from poisoned animals should not be used for human or livestock food. Fungicide-treated grains, especially if treatment method is unknown, should never be used for animal feed. Since antagonism between selenium and mercury has been demonstrated, adequate selenium in the diet should reduce the susceptibility of animals to mercury toxicosis.

Poisoning from mercury should no longer be a significant threat to livestock in well-managed production units. If toxicosis or contamination occurs, carelessness or neglect is usually involved and should be corrected as soon as possible.

Supplemental Reading

Buck, W. G., Osweiler, G. D., and Van Gelder, G. A.: Clinical and Diagnostic Veterinary Toxicology, 2nd ed. Dubuque, Iowa, Kendall/Hunt Publishing Co., 1976.

Cassidy, D. K., and Furr, A. A.: Toxicity of Inorganic and Organic Mercury Compounds in Animals. *In* Oehme, F. W. (ed.) Toxicity of Heavy Metals in the Environment. New York, Dekker, 303, 1978.

Jones, L. M., Booth, N. H., and McDonald, L. E.: Veterinary Pharmacology and Therapeutics, 4th ed. Ames, Iowa, Iowa State University Press, 1977.

Neatherly, M. W., and Miller, W. J.: Metabolism and toxicity of cadmium, mercury and lead: A review. J. Dairy Sci. 58:1767, 1975.

Fluorides*

J. L. SHUPE, D.V.M., A. E. OLSON, M.S., and H. B. PETERSON, Ph.D.

Fluoride toxicosis, often called fluorosis, results from the intake of excessive amounts of fluorides. Animals are exposed to fluorides, in various forms and concentrations, by ingestion of certain foods and waters, with only minimal amounts being absorbed from the atmosphere. Gaseous or particulate fluorides in the air breathed by animals are generally of little consequence to their health. Livestock normally consume variable, low level amounts of fluoride with no known adverse effects. Actually, ingestion of fluorides in proper amounts has been proved to exert beneficial effects on some tissues and physiologic processes in humans and some animals.

SOURCES

Forage crops usually constitute the most widespread source of excessive fluorides for livestock. These crops may be contaminated by fluoride-laden industrial effluents, by wind blown or rain splashed soil of high fluoride content, or by sprinkler irrigation water high in fluoride. In addition, some drinking water supplies contain appre-

---

*Available from Haver-Lockhart Laboratories, Shawnee, KS 66201.

†Available from Hynson, Wescott and Dunning, Inc., Baltimore, MD 21201.

‡Available from Merck & Company, Rahway, NJ 07065.

---

*Published with the approval of the Utah State University Agricultural Experiment Station, Logan, Utah as Journal Paper no. 2880.

ciable amounts of fluorides and contribute to the total fluoride intake. Improperly defluorinated inorganic phosphates, when used to provide supplementary dietary phosphorus, may be a major fluoride source in the diets of many domestic animals. The Association of American Feed Control Officials recommends a P to F ratio of at least 100:1 for defluorinated phosphate. Properly used, such phosphates are safe for livestock supplementation.

All possible sources of fluoride should be analyzed to ascertain their contribution to the total intake of the animals in question.

INFLUENCING FACTORS

The expression or severity of fluoride toxicosis may be altered or influenced by several factors. They are (1) amount of fluoride ingested, (2) duration of fluoride ingestion period, (3) bioavailability of ingested fluorides, (4) variations in fluoride ingestion levels (intermittent exposure), (5) species of animal, (6) age of animal at time of ingestion, (7) nutritional status, (8) exposure to other substances (with synergistic or alleviating effects), (9) general state of health of the animal, (10) stress, and (11) individual biologic response.

CLINICAL SIGNS

Acute Fluoride Toxicosis

Fluoride toxicosis may be either acute or chronic. Fortunately, acute fluoride toxicosis is relatively rare. It most often results from ingestion of organic and inorganic fluoride compounds and inorganic compounds, such as sodium fluorosilicate, sodium fluoride, sodium fluoroacetate, and methyl fluoroacetate. Some plants metabolize inorganic fluoride into various organic fluoride compounds, especially fluoroacetate. Fluoroacetate may accumulate in such plants to concentrations that are extremely toxic to herbivorous animals.

The rapidity with which signs appear and the exact nature of the signs depend on the amount and type of fluoride ingested. Clinical signs may include restlessness, stiffness, anorexia, excessive salivation, nausea, vomiting, incontinence of urine and feces, reduced milk production in lactating animals, clonic convulsions, weakness, severe depression, and cardiac failure. Chemical analyses of blood and urine from affected animals characteristically reveal high fluoride contents. Necropsy findings vary, but there is most often severe gastric and intestinal inflammation, degenerative changes in kidney tubular epithelium, epicardial and endocardial petechiae and ecchymoses, myocardial lesions, pulmonary congestion, and edema.

Chronic Fluoride Toxicosis

The much more common chronic fluoride toxicosis develops gradually and insidiously. Months or even years may intervene between the beginning of excess fluoride ingestion and the onset of readily observable clinical signs. Some manifestations of fluoride toxicosis may be confused with other toxicoses or certain debilitating or degenerative diseases. The following symptoms and lesions are of particular importance: (1) mottling and abrasion of permanent teeth, (2) degree of osteofluorosis, (3) amount of fluorine in the urine, and (4) intermittent lameness.

Dental Fluorosis

Fluorides have a great affinity for developing and mineralizing teeth. Such teeth are extremely sensitive to excessive fluoride. Some of the primary and most distinctive lesions induced by excessive fluoride ingestion are found in the teeth. Because of the nature and complexity of the disease, however, such dental lesions should not be the sole criterion on which a diagnosis is based. Once the teeth have formed, mineralized, and erupted into the oral cavity, fluoride ingestion will have little or no effect on them. Thus, young animals are most susceptible to dental fluorosis.

Fluoride-induced dental lesions are influenced by the 11 factors previously mentioned. The gross lesions may best be described by one or more of the following terms:

Mottling. White, chalk-like opaque areas or horizontal striations in the enamel.

Chalkiness. Dull white to pale yellow-chalk-like appearance.

Hypoplasia. Defective formation and structure.

Hypomineralization. Defective mineralization.

Discoloration. Pale white, creamy yellow, brown or black.

Attrition. Excessive abnormal wear.

Severely affected teeth are discolored (chalky-white or creamy yellow to brownish black), usually subject to increased attrition rate, and may also have lost enamel, with exposure of the dentine.

Clinical dental fluorosis is usually classified using numerical values (Fig. 1). The incisor teeth are evaluated for enamel quality, defects, and abrasion pattern (Fig. 2).

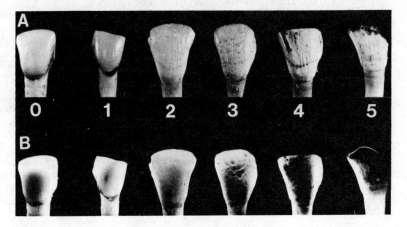

Figure 1. Classification of representative incisor teeth from cattle is from 0 to 5, reading from left to right in both *A* and *B*. *A* is with direct light; *B* is with transmitted light. (From Shupe, J. L., Minor, M. L., Greenwood, D. A., Harris, L. E., and Stoddard, G. E.: Am. J. Vet. Res. *24*:964–984, 1963.)

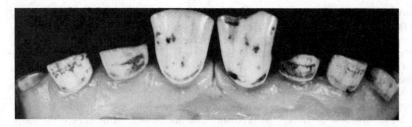

Figure 2. Permanent bovine incisor teeth. Note the chalkiness and discoloration of the enamel, hypoplasia, and excessive bilateral abrasion.

The usual classification system ranges from 0 (normal) to 5 (severe fluoride effects). The more difficult to examine cheek (premolar and molar) teeth are classified 0 to 5 based on attrition patterns only.

Osteofluorosis

Fluorides have great affinity for bone as well as for developing and mineralizing teeth. Excessive fluoride may affect bones at any time during an animal's life. Bones of young animals are more responsive to excessive fluoride levels than are those of mature animals. Osteofluorosis has been seen in animals with normal teeth, which accents the age-effect factor.

The amount of fluoride stored in bone normally increases over time without inducing any demonstrable changes in bone structure and function. If the amounts of fluoride ingested are significantly higher than normal over an appreciable length of time, structural bone changes occur.

In livestock, clinically palpable bone lesions usually first appear on the mandible, ribs, and medial portions of the metatarsal and metacarpal bones. The lesions are generally bilateral and somewhat symmetric. Characteristic histologic changes are associated with the various degrees of osteofluorosis. The type of bone changes seen depends on the previously listed factors that influence fluoride toxicosis.

DIAGNOSIS

Urinalysis

Urine samples, if properly collected, analyzed for fluoride, and interpreted, can provide supportive assistance for the diagnosis and evaluation of fluoride toxicosis. Individual random samples may be too variable to provide reliable information. Adequate numbers of uncontaminated samples should be collected at various intervals to provide accurate, representative values. The time of day that samples are taken and total urinary output also affect results. To counteract, insofar as possible, variations in volume of urine output, specific gravity is corrected to 1.040.

Urine serves as one of the major means of fluoride elimination from the body. On a low level fluoride diet, the urinary fluoride content of animals rises slightly as the animals age, and as the fluoride content of their bones rises. Urinary fluoride levels may remain high for some time after animals are changed from a high- to a low-fluoride diet, i.e., urine values may not reflect current levels of fluoride intake. There is a relationship among fluorine level in the urine, amount of fluoride consumed, age of animal, and amount of fluoride previously consumed. Under most circumstances, however, specific grav-

ity corrected urine values of less than 6 ppm fluoride are considered normal.

CLINICAL SIGNS

Animals with moderate to severe osteofluorosis sometimes exhibit an intermittent nonspecific atypical stiffness that may be associated with periods of stress, periosteal overgrowths, and calcification of periarticular structures and tendon insertions. While this stiffness or "lameness" is often transitory and intermittent in nature, its effect limits grazing or feeding time and leads to impaired animal performance. The type of stiffness is not definitive for fluoride toxicosis.

Other generalized but nonspecific symptoms sometimes associated with chronic fluoride toxicosis are unthriftiness, thickened, dry, unpliable skin, and other signs of poor performance.

In addition to noting clinical signs, analyses should be made of blood and urine, and of water and all dietary components ingested by animals suspected of having fluoride toxicosis so that the cause may be elucidated.

NECROPSY FINDINGS

If clinical examinations and chemical analyses indicate the need for more specific information, necropsies should be performed on selected, representative animals. For economic reasons, some animals may be sacrificed at a commercial abattoir and, after appropriate tissues are taken for detailed study and evaluation, the carcasses can be used for meat. There is no significant accumulation of fluorides in soft tissue. Ninety-six per cent or more of the fluoride in an animal's body is located in the bones and teeth.

Dental Lesions

The teeth should be carefully examined for evidence of fluoride-induced dental lesions. Incisor lesions (if present) should be carefully examined and correlated with any cheek tooth lesions developed during a chronologically similar time span of the animal's life.

Skeletal Lesions

Grossly, bones that are severely affected by fluoride appear chalky white, have a roughened irregular periosteal surface and are larger in diameter and heavier than normal (Fig. 3). The major bone changes are located on the periosteal surface. If the lesions are severe enough or of long enough duration, then some secondary peri- and intra-articular changes may be found. The exact nature of the bone changes varies according to the level and duration of fluoride intake, plus the other influencing factors previously mentioned. One or more of the following conditions may occur: osteosclerosis, osteoporosis, hyperostosis, osteophytosis, and osteomalacia.

The changes (such as increased density, porosity, hyperostosis, and osteophytosis) may be demonstrated radiographically as well as grossly. The usefulness of the radiographic evidence will depend on the degree and severity of osteofluorosis.

Microscopic evaluation of fluoride-affected bones gives additional insight into the described changes. Excessive periosteal, and at times endosteal, bone formation occurs. Porous areas, with excessive bone resorption or accelerated remodeling, appear when bone formation fails to keep a proper balance between bone removal and bone replacement. Osteones formed under the influence of excessive fluorides often vary in size and shape, with the osteocytes often being clumped or irregularly located near the periphery of the osteone, rather than evenly distributed throughout the osteone. Abnormal canaliculi are associated with the clumped abnormal cells.

The precise pathogenesis of osteofluorosis is not fully understood. There appear to be 3 phases associated with osteofluorosis: (1) elevated fluoride levels in the bone without detectable structural changes, (2) microscopic and radiographic bone changes without known alterations of function, and (3) sequential and progressive structural bone changes that result in abnormal bone structure and function with resultant alterations of mechanical properties. The abnormal bone appears to result from an acceleration of the remodeling rate in existing bone accompanied by compensatory periosteal and, at times, endosteal proliferation of abnormal bone. The osteoblasts are adversely affected and produce a defective organic matrix that in turn is irregularly and defectively mineralized.

Other valuable information may be provided by chemical analyses of bone for fluoride content, especially if certain precautions are taken in sampling. Sampling sites should be standardized and consistent as to location so that test results will be representative, and results can be properly interpreted. Medial or lateral aspects of some long bones (even at the same proximal or distal levels) may vary in their degree of change and amount of fluoride. Fluoride content of bones normally increases with age even if the animal is on a life-long low fluoride intake level.

Fluorides do not accumulate in soft tissues or in visceral organs in sufficient quantities to provide reliable, accurate, and consistent diagnostic information. Neither have fluorides been shown to induce characteristic, consistent, demonstrable changes in the visceral organs or soft tissues.

Diagnosis of Chronic Fluoride Toxicosis

Information accumulated from the examinations and procedures discussed previously should be carefully evaluated and correlated before a definitive diagnosis of chronic fluoride toxicosis is made. Results of clinical examinations should be compared with necropsy findings. Chemical analyses, especially of bone, reflect past exposure to fluoride.

All feed sources, including mineral supplements, should be analyzed for fluoride content. Likewise, all drinking water supplies should be analyzed. Sampling and analytical techniques should be standardized to insure reliable data.

In regard to forage crop sampling, intensive efforts should be made to accurately sample what the animals

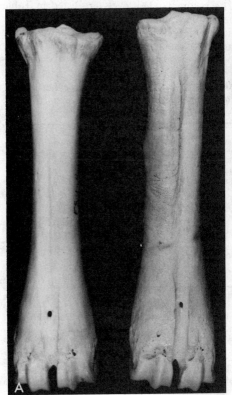
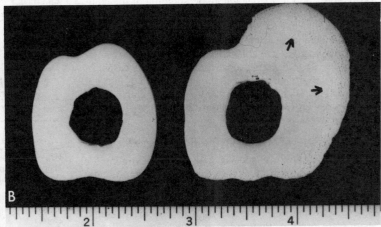

Figure 3. *A,* Metatarsal bones from two cows of the same breed, size, and age. The bone on the left is normal, while the bone on the right shows severe osteofluorosis. *B,* Cross-section of the two metatarsal bones shown above. The section of bone from arrow points outward is fluoride-induced abnormal bone.

have actually been ingesting. Fluorides accumulate on, as well as in, the plant structure, and therefore forage samples should not be washed before being analyzed. In areas of infrequent rainfall, sampling just after a rainfall will produce results significantly different from sampling just before a rainfall. Vegetation that has survived a long growing season will also have accumulated a higher fluoride content than lush vegetation that has grown rapidly.

There is considerable experimental information on the tolerances of animals to fluoride in feed when animals are housed and managed under ideal experimental conditions. There is a paucity of information, however, on tolerances of animals under field conditions when they may not be properly sheltered and managed. Data are also lacking on tolerances of some animals to waterborne fluoride. Responses of animals to waterborne fluoride vary, as ambient air temperature influences the amount of water consumed. Because of seasonal and physiologic differences in water requirements of animals, large variations occur in their water consumption and influence the expression of fluoride toxicosis.

Overall husbandry or management practices may also affect the expression of fluoride toxicosis. A complete clinical history of each animal should be obtained. Such things as seasonal changes in rangeland grazing patterns and variable feed sources may produce intermittent excessive fluoride exposure in animals.

Every effort should be made to delineate or differentially diagnose fluoride toxicosis. Other trace-element toxicoses or deficiencies may, in some ways, alter or mimic some aspects of chronic fluoride toxicosis. Some debilitating diseases such as degenerative joint disease (osteoarthritis) may also mimic certain aspects of clinical fluoride toxicosis.

All available clinical and analytical data, coupled with a complete and knowledgeable understanding of the complexity of chronic fluoride toxicosis, should be utilized in unequivocally diagnosing the condition. No single criterion is sufficient when making a definitive diagnosis. It is imperative to correlate clinical signs with laboratory analyses and with detailed necropsy findings in some cases. In making a definite diagnosis and final evaluation of fluoride toxicosis, the signs and lesions that the animals show should take precedence over fluoride analyses of current feed and water supplies.

Treatment of Chronic Fluoride Toxicosis

There is no known specific, successful treatment for chronic fluoride toxicosis. Supportive and symptomatic treatment based on the degree and extent of signs and lesions may be given. Complete reversal of lesions induced by excessive fluoride ingestion does not occur. If dental lesions are present, they are irreversible. In fact, if such lesions are severe enough to hasten dental abrasion, the accelerated wear will continue, especially if rough, abrasive feeds are utilized.

Osteofluorotic lesions may be prevented by reducing the total fluoride intake to normal levels. Animals with extensive bone lesions do not live long enough to have the bone remodeled to normal. After animals stop ingesting excessive fluoride levels, normal bone is laid down over previously induced osteofluorotic bones.

Animals already adversely affected by fluoride toxicosis may be assisted by providing adequate nutrition and by avoiding all possible physiologic stresses. The diet should be nutritionally well balanced, of good quality, and in sufficient amounts to promote desirable performance and growth. It is recommended that herbivorous animals be given as much good quality roughage as possible while poor quality abrasive roughage is minimized or eliminated. Succulent grains may be advisable in some cases.

If economic or logistic realities dictate that animals may not be removed from toxic sources of fluorides, some preventive relief may be obtained by feeding alleviating compounds. Beneficial effects have been observed after feeding of adequate mineral supplements and after adding of calcium carbonate, magnesium or aluminum compounds to the diet. Cattle, fed aluminum sulfate as 1 per cent of their total dry matter intake for 4 years, had 30 to 42 per cent less fluoride deposited in their ribs than did control animals that consumed equally high dietary levels of fluoride. Inclusion of some aluminum (most often aluminum sulfate) or calcium (calcium carbonate) compounds in the diet have lessened the effects of a given amount of fluoride. Some researchers have reported reduced dental lesions or reduced bone storage of fluorides, or both, when calcium or aluminum compounds were included in the diet. A nutritionally correct balance of other minerals, particularly phosphorus, should be maintained to obtain maximum benefits from aluminum and calcium additions. This may necessitate utilization of phosphate supplements.

SPECIES TOLERANCES

Tolerance levels for various livestock species have been determined. Where applicable, different levels for long-term production and reproduction animals, as compared to short-term fattening and slaughter animals, have been calculated. The recommended levels are listed in Table 1. It must be emphasized that the values given are for sodium fluoride or for compounds of similar bioavailability (toxicity) in the total dietary intake. Less soluble fluoride compounds, such as calcium fluoride, are less toxic. Fluor-

Table 1. *Recommended Fluoride Tolerance Levels in Feed and Water for Domestic Animals Based on Clinical Signs and Lesions**

Species	Feed† mg/kg(ppm)	Water‡ (mg/L)
Heifers, dairy and beef	30	2.5–4
Dairy cattle, mature	40	3–6
Beef cattle, mature	50	4–8
Finishing cattle	100	12–15
Breeding ewes	60	5–8
Feeder lambs	150	12–15
Horses	60	4–8
Swine, growing	70	5–8
Turkeys, growing	100	10–12
Chickens, growing	150	10–13
Dogs	50	3–8
Mink	45	3–8

*Biologic availability depends on chemical composition. Dissolved F in water appears to be more readily assimilated. The values must be reduced proportionally when both water and feed contain appreciable amounts of fluorides.

†This is a suggested guide when F in the feed is essentially the sole source of fluoride.

‡The average ambient air temperature and the physical and biologic activity of the animals influence the amount of water consumed and hence, the wide range of tolerance levels suggested. For active animals in a warm climate, the lower values should be used as critical level indicators.

ides in water are more bioavailable and thus more toxic than those in dietary dry matter intake. The variations in relative toxicities of the different fluoride forms or sources must also be taken into consideration when evaluating fluoride toxicosis.

PREVENTION

Caution must be exercised by livestock owners, animal feed processors, and industrialists to prevent the occurrence of fluoride toxicosis. Because fluorides accumulate in mineralizing tissues of the body, the total amount of feed, including mineral supplements, should not contain fluoride in excess of normal recommended levels. All sources of drinking water should be analyzed. Naturally warm spring waters frequently contain excessive amounts of fluorides. Soils that are high in fluoride content may also be a problem. The high-fluoride containing soils are primarily involved when they are naturally carried by wind or rain onto forage plants, not by translocation from the roots into the leaves and stems. Also, on high-fluoride containing soils, it is very important to avoid overgrazing by livestock so that chances of ingesting soil because of forced close grazing of vegetation are lessened.

One must also be aware of potential pollution from new industries in an area or from established industries that change methods of operation. Cases of fluoride toxicosis have been observed near some long established operations that had no history of excessive fluoride pollution. Such companies may have obtained a new source of raw materials, or may have altered their processing procedures, and only then started releasing excessive amounts of fluorides. Historically, phosphate smelters, aluminum, steel, and brick plants, and some coal-fired electricity generating plants have been emitters of fluorides. Another area of modern concern is the rapid expansion of sprinkler irrigation using geothermal or other high-fluoride containing waters. Some of these waters are safe for use in flood irrigation, but unpublished data indicate a high fluoride content in forage sprinkled with water containing high levels of fluoride (5 to 10 mg/L).

Livestock owners should routinely monitor all phases of animal health and should be aware of problems that may occur with infectious agents, nutritional imbalances, and now, more than ever, with toxicoses of all kinds, including fluoride toxicosis. Prevention and control of fluoride toxicosis in animals can be achieved when the complexity of the disease is realized, when it is properly diagnosed, and when the source of excessive fluorides is eliminated.

Supplemental Reading

AAFCO (Association of American Feed Control Officials Inc.): Official publication. Charleston, West Virginia, 1983.

Garlick, N. L.: The teeth of the ox in clinical diagnosis. IV. Dental fluorosis. Am. J. Vet. Res. 16:38–44, 1955.

Johnson, L. C.: Histogenesis and mechanisms in the development of osteofluorosis. In J. H. Simons (ed.). Fluorine Chemistry, vol. 4. New York, Academic Press. 424–441, 1965.

Miller, G. W., and Shupe, J. L.: Alkaline bone phosphatase activity as related to fluoride ingestion by dairy cattle. Am. J. Vet. Res. 23:24–31, 1962.

Neeley, K. L., and Harbaugh, F. G.: Effects of fluoride ingestion on a herd of dairy cattle in the Lubbock, Texas, area. J. Am. Vet. Med. Assoc. 124:344–350, 1954.

Peterson, H. B., and Shupe, J. L.: Problems of managing geothermal waters for irrigation. Proceedings of the International Salinity Conference. Texas Tech. University, Lubbock, Texas, 211–219, 1976.

Roholm, K.: Fluorine intoxication: A clinical-hygienic study with a review of the literature and some experimental investigations. London, H. K. Lewis & Co., Ltd., 1937.

Schmidt, H. J., Newell, G. W., and Rand, W. E.: The controlled feeding of fluorine, as sodium fluoride, to dairy cattle, Am. J. Vet. Res. 15:232–239, 1954.

Shupe, J. L.: Clinicopathologic features of fluoride toxicosis in cattle. J. Anim. Sci. 51:746–758, 1980.

Shupe, J. L.: Diagnosis of Fluorosis in Cattle. In IVth International Meeting of the World Association for Buiatrics. no. 4, Zurich, Switzerland, 15–30, 1976.

Shupe, J. L.: Clinical and pathological effects of fluoride toxicity in animals. In CIBA Foundation: Carbon-Fluorine Compounds: Chemistry, Biochemistry and Biological Activities. New York, American Elsevier, 357–388, 1972.

Shupe, J. L., Ammerman, C. B., Peeler, H. T., et al.: Effects of Fluorides in Animals. Washington, D.C., National Academy of Sciences and National Research Council, 1–70, 1974.

Shupe, J. L., Miner, M. L., Greenwood, D. A., et al.: The effect of fluorine on dairy cattle. II. Clinical and pathologic effects. Am. J. Vet. Res. 24:964–984, 1963.

Shupe, J. L., and Olson, A. E.: Clinical aspects of fluorosis in horses. J. Am. Vet. Med. Assoc. 158:167–174, 1971.

Shupe, J. L., Olson, A. E., and Sharma, R. P.: Fluoride toxicity in domestic and wild animals. Clin. Toxicol. 5:195–213, 1972.

Suttie, J. W., Carlson, J. R., and Faltin, E. C.: Effects of alternating periods of high- and low-fluoride ingestion on dairy cattle. J. Dairy Sci. 55:790–804, 1972.

Hexachlorobenzene

RICHARD H. TESKE, D.V.M., M.S.

Hexachlorobenzene (HCB) is registered for use as a fungicidal agent for treatment of seeds and occurs as a by-product of a number of industrial processes, including those for the manufacture of chlorine gas, perchlorethylene, carbon tetrachloride, and a variety of agricultural chemicals. Thus, HCB contamination of the environment is widespread. This is confirmed by the fact that the United States Department of Agriculture (USDA) in its residue surveillance program has reported positive (though generally "nonviolative") findings in virtually all types of food-producing animals and poultry from all areas of the United States.

HCB is a stable and persistent chemical. Like other chlorinated hydrocarbons, HCB is highly lipophilic and is selectively deposited in the body fat. Metabolites include pentachlorophenol and pentachlorothiophenol; however, the metabolites do not tend to accumulate in tissues other than the liver. Significant contamination incidents include contamination of cattle in Louisiana, thought to have resulted from airborne emissions and waste disposal from manufacturing plants, and contamination of sheep in western Texas and eastern California associated with use of pesticides that were contaminated with HCB.

PATHOGENESIS

Booth and McDowell[1] reviewed the toxicity of HCB in humans and animals. In an episode of HCB toxicosis in humans in Turkey, a diagnosis of porphyria cutanea tarda was made following consumption of HCB-treated wheat. This syndrome consists of blistering and epidermolysis causing the skin to be unusually sensitive to sunlight and to minor trauma. Hypertrichosis is also common in porphyria cutanea tarda. Lesions heal poorly and form pigmented scars. Signs of HCB intoxication during and after prolonged exposure in laboratory animals are tremors, ataxia, weakness, paralysis, porphyria, and weight loss. Pathologic changes reported were blood cell disorders, neurologic abnormalities, and hepatomegaly.

Weanling gilts receiving diets containing 100 ppm HCB for 90 days did not gain weight as well as controls, developed hepatomegaly, and became lymphopenic.[2] Reproduction was impaired in sows fed diets containing 20 ppm HCB during breeding, gestation, and lactation.[3] Other toxic and pathologic signs were neutrophilia and gastritis.

TREATMENT

There is no specific treatment available. Sources of HCB should be eliminated. Animals exhibiting porphyria should be closely observed for signs of photosensitization. Animals showing clinical signs of illness should be treated according to symptoms.

Residues of HCB in food products derived from animals are of primary concern. Although no finite tolerances have been established, the Environmental Protection Agency has, in response to specific contamination incidents, set an interim tolerance for HCB in cattle, sheep, goats, and horses at 0.5 ppm. Biomagnification of HCB has been shown to occur in the body fat of animals at concentrations 6 to 50 times the dietary level during long-term exposure.[4] Therefore, concentrations in finished feeds should not exceed 0.02 to 0.05 ppm (depending on duration of exposure).

Since HCB residue levels that would occur coincident with clinical HCB toxicosis would be exceptionally high and since the elimination rate of residues is very slow, during which time the animal would represent a source of contamination of premises and facilities, destruction of such animals and burial in a location selected to preclude contamination of premises and water is generally advisable.

References

1. Booth, N. H., and McDowell, J. R.: Toxicity of hexachlorobenzene and associated residues in edible animal tissues. J. Am. Vet. Med. Assoc. 166:591–595, 1975.
2. Hansen, L. G., Wilson, D. W., Byerly, C. S., et al.: Effects and residues of dietary hexachlorobenzene in growing swine. J. Toxicol. Environ. Health 2:557–567, 1977.
3. Hansen, L. G., Simon, J., Dorn, S. B., and Teske, R. H.: Hexachlorobenzene distribution in tissues of swine. Toxicol. Appl. Pharmacol. 51:1–7, 1979.
4. Reed, D. L., Bush, P. B., Booth, N. H., et al.: Tissue residues from feeding pentachloronitrobenzene to broiler chickens. Toxicol. Appl. Pharmacol. 42:433–441, 1977.

Polybrominated Biphenyls

RICHARD H. TESKE, D.V.M., M.S.

Polybrominated biphenyl (PBB) is an extremely stable industrial chemical sold from 1970–1975 under the tradename FireMaster for use as a fire retardant. During May, 1973, an unknown quantity of PBB (FireMaster) was accidentally included in a shipment of magnesium oxide (a feed additive sold under the tradename NutriMaster) to a commerical feed mill in Battle Creek, Michigan. What followed has been characterized as the most serious feed contamination incident in the history of United States agriculture.

At the Battle Creek mill some of the PBB was inadvertently added to animal feeds instead of magnesium oxide. The remainder was distributed to satellite mills where it also was unintentionally added to animal feeds in place of magnesium oxide. As a result of this accident, high level contamination of a number of production lots of livestock rations, particularly dairy rations, occurred. Because the causative agent (PBB) was not identified until approximately 9 months later, accurate determination of the incidence of clinical toxicosis resulting from consumption of contaminated feeds was difficult. However, the initial accident also resulted in widespread contamination of feedmills, feed storage facilities, and farm premises in Michigan. By mid-1977, 35,000 to 40,000 head of cattle, 4000 swine, 1375 sheep, 1,500,000 chickens, 865 tons of feed, 18,000 pounds of butter, 34,000 pounds of dried milk, and 404,000 dozen eggs in Michigan had been destroyed because of contamination with PBB residues. In spite of what were in many cases very extensive efforts to "clean up" mills and "decontaminate" premises, low level exposure of livestock to PBB has continued.

CLINICAL TOXICOSIS

The toxic syndrome associated with feeding a ration contaminated with PBB to dairy cattle was first characterized by Jackson and Halbert.[1] They reported on clinical toxicosis in a 400-cow dairy herd that had received rations containing PBB at concentrations up to 3000 ppm. The clinical course of toxicosis was divided into 2 phases. Phase I included anorexia, decreased milk production, increased frequency of urination and lacrimation, and some lameness. Rectal temperatures were normal, as were results of the Wisconsin mastitis test conducted on bulk milk samples. The udders of cows that had recently freshened began to shrink during the second through the fourth week of the course of toxicosis. Two weeks after the onset of toxicosis, cows that had been bred 4 to 6 weeks earlier began coming back into estrus and over the next 8 weeks 100 were rebred. Removal of the contaminated feed after approximately 16 days resulted in an immediate improvement in appetite and stabilization of milk production at about 60 per cent of the pre-PBB level.

Phase 2 began about 1 month after the onset of decreased milk production. Hematomas, which later became abscesses, developed in approximately 40 cows. High-producing cows continued to lose weight even though the ration had been changed and appetites were normal. There was abnormal hoof growth, hair became matted and fell out, and skin on the neck, shoulder, and thorax became thickened and wrinkled. Gestation was prolonged by 2 to 4 weeks in cows that had received the contaminated feeds during the first trimester. Dystocias in cows occurred as a result of large calves and the failure of pelvic ligaments to relax. Udders of these cows did not develop, and often the calf was delivered dead or died soon after birth. Development of metritis was common following parturition.

Clinical findings in experimentally induced PBB toxicosis were reported by Durst and coworkers.[2, 3] Toxicosis was induced in pregnant heifers by feeding 25,000 mg PBB/head/day. Dry matter intake was reduced by approximately 50 per cent after 4 days exposure. Clinical signs observed were anorexia, dehydration, diarrhea, excessive salivation and lacrimation, fetal death, abortion, and general depression, as evidenced by depressed heart and respiratory rates. All animals died or were sacrificed in a moribund state after exposure for 33 to 60 days. Clinicopathologic changes included elevated aspartate aminotransferase, lactate dehydrogenase, blood urea nitrogen, and bilirubin levels and depressed serum calcium and albumin levels. Concentrations of PBB in body fat of moribund animals ranged from 1100 to 6000 ppm.[4]

PATHOLOGY

Pathologic observations reported by Jackson and Halbert[1] were somewhat limited but included hemorrhagic necrotic hepatitis, fatty metamorphosis, amyloidosis of the liver, nephrosis, and acute, subacute, and chronic interstitial nephritis. Gross findings were hematomas and abscesses in the peritoneal and thoracic cavities.

Moorhead and associates[5, 6] described the pathologic conditions occurring in pregnant heifers in which clinical toxicosis had been induced by feeding PBB at a dosage rate of 25,000 mg/head for 33 to 60 days. Gross findings were emaciation, dehydration, subcutaneous emphysema and hemorhage, atrophy of the thymus, fetal death with concomitant necrosis of cotyledons, thickened wall of the gallbladder, inspissated bile, edema of abomasal folds, mucoid enteritis, and linear hemorrhage and edema of the rectal mucosa. The kidneys were greatly enlarged. Perirenal lymph nodes were enlarged and edematous. The most significant microscopic changes involved the kidneys, gallbladder, and eye lids. The kidneys exhibited extreme dilatation of collecting ducts and convoluted tubules with degenerative changes of epithelium including cloudy swelling, hydropic degeneration, and separation from the basement membrane. Sections from the eyelids exhibited hyperkeratosis of the epidermis with keratin accumulations in the hair follicles and squamous metaplasia with keratin cysts in the tarsal glands. Common changes in the gallbladder with hyperplasia and cystic dilatation of the mucous glands in the lamina propria. The similarity of these lesions with those of bovine hyperkeratosis (x disease) was noted.

TREATMENT

There is no specific treatment available for PBB toxicosis. Sources of PBB should be eliminated, and animals exhibiting clinical signs of illness should be treated according to symptoms.

Of special concern are residues of PBB in food products derived from animals exposed to PBB. The tolerance set by the Food and Drug Administration for PBB in milk and meat is 0.3 ppm, and for PBB in eggs and finished feeds is 0.05 ppm. Surprisingly high concentrations of PBB can be accumulated in tissues of cows without apparent signs of toxicity.[4] Therefore, since PBB residue levels that would occur coincident with clinical PBB toxicosis are exceptionally high, and since the elimination rate of residues is very slow during which time the animal would represent a source of contamination of premises and facilities, destruction of such animals and burial in a location selected to preclude contamination of premises and water is generally advisable. Attempts to stimulate the elimination of PBB from the body have been generally ineffective.

References

1. Jackson, T. F., and Halbert, F. L.: A toxic syndrome associated with the feeding of polybrominated biphenyl-contaminated protein concentrate to dairy cattle. J. Am. Vet. Med. Assoc. 165:437–438, 1974.
2. Durst, H. I., Willett, L. B., Brumm, C. J., and Mercer, H. D.: Effects of polybrominated biphenyls on health and performance of pregnant holstein heifers. J. Dairy Sci. 60:1294–1300, 1977.
3. Durst, H. I., Willett, L. B., Schanbacher, F. L., and Moorhead, P. D.: Effects of PBBs on Cattle. I. Clinical evaluations and clinical chemistry. Environ. Health Perspect. 23:83–89, 1978.
4. Willett, L. B., and Drust, H. I.: Effects of PBBs on Cattle. IV. Distribution and clearance of components of FireMaster BP-6. Environ. Health Perspect. 23:67–74, 1978.
5. Moorhead, P. D., Willett, L. B., Brumm, C. J., and Mercer, H. D.: Pathology of experimentally induced polybrominated biphenyl toxicosis in pregnant heifers. J. Am. Vet. Med. Assoc. 170:307–313, 1977.
6. Moorhead, P. D., Willett, L. B., and Schanbacher, F. L.: Effects of PBB on Cattle. II. Gross pathology and histopathology. Environ. Health Perspect. 23:111–118, 1978.

Polychlorinated Biphenyls

RICHARD H. TESKE, D.V.M., M.S.

Because of their superior cooling, insulating, and dielectric properties, polychlorinated biphenyls (PCBs) are widely used in the electrical industry. There is also a wide range of miscellaneous uses, such as plasticizers, components of carbonless duplicating paper, and additities to petroleum products, paints, sealants, printing inks, and pesticides.

PCBs are extremely stable chemicals, and, as a general rule, resistance to degradation or metabolic transformation increases with the level of chlorination. Like other chlorinated hydrocarbons, PCBs are highly lipophilic and are selectively deposited in body fat. Fish and aquatic invertebrates have been shown to accumulate PCBs to levels as high as 75,000 times that present in the water.[1]

Although considerable research has been conducted on the toxicology of PCBs in experimental animals,[2] definitive data on their toxicity in domestic animals is generally lacking. Hansen and coworkers[3] studied the effects of feeding a diet containing Aroclor 1242 at a concentration of 20 ppm to sows throughout gestation and nursing. The number of live pigs farrowed by treated sows was significantly lower than the number farrowed by control sows. However, performance of the pigs produced by treated sows was not affected. Feeding Aroclor 1242 or Aroclor 1254 to growing swine and sheep at levels of 20 ppm throughout the growing and finishing period did result in reduction of feed efficiency and rate of weight gain.[4]

Although incidents of clinical toxicosis in poultry,[5] mink,[6] and humans[7] have occurred, the major impact of PCBs relative to veterinary medicine has been PCB residues in animal products produced for human consumption. Incidents in which significant contamination of food products of animal origin have occurred generally resulted from direct contamination of animal feeds either accidentally (as during processing) or through the ill-advised use of PCBs or PCB-containing materials leading to contamination of animal feeds. For example, fishmeal used as a poultry ration supplement was contaminated by PCB heat transfer fluid leaking from a heat exchanger during pasteurization, resulting in excessive PCB residues in millions of chickens in the southeastern United States. Milk has become contaminated by PCB residues following the feeding of silage from concrete silos, the inside surfaces of which has been painted with a sealant containing PCB.[8]

PATHOGENESIS

The investigation and characterization of the toxicity associated with exposure to PCBs is complicated by the wide variation in PCB compounds. Commercial PCB products are known to contain 10 to 18 or more distinct isomers and congeners varying in number and location of chlorine atoms. Toxicity differs not only with the animal species involved but also with the particular isomers and congeners present in a given PCB product. Contamination by highly toxic impurities, including polychlorinated dibenzofurans is also a factor. Pathologic changes in mammals are follicular pyodermatitis (chloracne) and liver atrophy and necrosis. The dibenzofurans are strong hepatotoxic and acnegenic compounds, and tetra- and pentachloro-dibenzofuran impurities are considered to be the primary cause of chloracne, edema, hydropericardium, and liver necrosis.[9] Mink appear to be uniquely sensitive to PCB toxicosis with dietary levels of only a few ppm causing reproductive failure and mortality.[6]

TREATMENT

There is no specific treatment available. Sources of PCB should be eliminated. Animals exhibiting clinical signs of illness should be treated according to symptoms.

Residues of PCBs in food products derived from animals are of primary concern. The temporary tolerance set by the Food and Drug Administration for PCBs in finished animal feed for food-producing animals is 0.2 ppm. For animal feed components of animal origin, including fishmeal and finished animal feed concentrates, supplements, and premixes, the temporary tolerance is 2.0 ppm. Since PCB residue levels coincident with clinical PCB toxicosis would be exceptionally high, and since the very slow elimination rate of residues would leave time during which the animal would represent a source of contamination of premises and facilities, destruction of such animals and burial in a location selected to preclude contamination of premises and water is generally desirable.

References

1. Van Gelder, G. A., and Teske, R. H.: Biological impact of polychlorinated biphenyls with emphasis on veterinary aspects. Vet. Toxicol., 16:109, 1974.
2. Kimbrough, R., Buckley, J., Fishbein, L., et al.: Animal toxicology. Environ. Health Perspectives 24:173–184, 1978.
3. Hansen, L. G., Byerly, C. S., Metcalf, R. L., and Bevill, R. F.: Effect of a polychlorinated biphenyl mixture on swine reproduction and tissue residues. Am. J. Vet. Res. 36:23–26, 1975.
4. Hansen, L. G., Wilson, D. W., and Byerly, C. S.: Effects on growing swine and sheep of two polychlorinated biphenyls. Am. J. Vet. Res. 37:1021–1024, 1976.
5. Harris, J. R., and Rose, L.: Toxicity of polychlorinated biphenyls in poultry. J. Am. Vet. Med. Assoc. 161:1584–1586, 1972.
6. McCann, J.: High PCBs cause of mink decline. Biomedical News, Oct. 1972.
7. Kuratsune, M., Yoshimura, T., Matsuzaka, J., and Yamaguchi, A.: Epidemiologic study on Yusho, a poisoning caused by ingestion of rice oil contaminated with a commercial brand of polychlorinated biphenyls. Environ. Health Perspectives 1:119–128, 1972.
8. Willett, L. B., and Hess, J. F.: Polychlorinated biphenyl residues in silos in the United Statess. Residue Reviews 55:135–147, 1975.
9. Vos, J. G.: Toxicology of PCBs for mammals and for birds. Environ. Health Perspectives 1:105–117, 1972.

Trichloroethylene Extracted Soybean Oil Meal Poisoning*

E. MURL BAILEY, JR., D.V.M., Ph.D.

Trichloroethylene extracted soybean oil meal (TCESOM) poisoning is a disease condition in cattle manifested by fatal hemorrhage syndrome or by aplastic anemia. The disease occurs only with the feeding of soybean meal extracted by trichloroethylene and has not occurred with any other solvent extraction system. The disease was first reported by Stockman in 1916 and was a problem, especially in the midwest, until the middle 1950s.

Commercially prepared TCESOM has varied widely in its degree of toxicity to cattle under controlled conditions. The toxicity associated with the consumption of these meals is cumulative, and the times of death may vary from 30 to 270 days after feeding. It has been observed that young cattle appear to be more susceptible to toxic meals than old cattle. Animals may manifest the typical terminal symptoms at somewhat extended periods after ceasing to consume the toxic meal. Cattle that have consumed appreciable amounts of meal may appear quite normal when turned out to pasture, but may develop the disease several months later. The toxic material is apparently not passed in the milk of lactating cows.

CLINICAL SIGNS

The clinical syndrome is characterized by sudden onset of the disease, generally in 1 or 2 animals with the remainder of the herd apparently normal. The nature of the toxicity, which may take from 1 to 6 months to appear, is not often appreciated on first appraisal.

The typical syndrome in cattle is aplastic anemia with characteristic clinical hematologic signs. Many of the affected animals show marked salivation. Feces may appear normal at first, but one soon detects mixtures of blood and finally blood clots. In the acute stages, the animals exhibit a marked decline in condition, elevated body temperature, discharge of blood from natural body openings, occasional visible subcutaneous hemorrhage, collapse, and finally death.

Abdominal pain is present, and subcutaneous swellings may be seen over the protruding bones of the body. Few animals that develop signs recover. Death usually occurs within 4 to 5 days after the onset of the clinical signs.

*Supported in part by Texas Agricultural Experiment Station, Project no. H-6255.

Some animals may die as suddenly as the second day while others may live 12 to 15 days. The majority of animal deaths in a herd generally occur within 30 days following the first animal deaths.

Hematologic abnormalities of diagnostic significance are a gradual and finally a precipitous decline in white blood cell counts with a relative degree of lymphocytosis. Toward the end of the terminal clinical stage, leukopenia becomes severe with white blood cell counts ranging from 1000 to 2000/mm^3. Early in the course of the clinical syndrome, there is marked thrombocytopenia. In cases where profuse internal bleeding has occurred, anemia may be present.

Other animal species have not shown a susceptibility to toxic soybean meal as have cattle and young calves. Horses have developed fatal aplastic anemia in a manner similar to cows. The clinical signs take 200 to 300 days of daily feeding of TCESOM to develop.

The disease condition has also been produced in sheep. The hematologic changes observed in sheep are not always consistent with those associated with aplastic anemia. Sheep appear to be much more resistant to the toxic effect of TCESOM than cattle or horses. Mice, rats, hamsters, guinea pigs, rabbits, and dogs have been fed toxic TCESOM, and none showed any evidence of aplastic anemia or marked blood dyscrasia. Feeding this meal to guinea pigs and dogs produced a syndrome of generalized debilitation.

LESIONS

The basic lesions found at necropsy of cattle that have died as a result of this condition consist of petechiae, ecchymoses, and linear or diffuse hemorrhages. Various types of hemorrhages and ulcers are also noted in the gastrointestinal tract. Hemorrhages may be present in the subcutaneous tissues, muscles, tendons, and joints. The serosal surfaces of the thoracic and abdominal cavities are characterized by extensive hemorrhages. Free blood may be present in the abdominal cavity. Various hemorrhages may be seen on the brain when it is removed, giving rise to the likelihood of abnormal neurologic signs in the animals prior to death.

DIAGNOSIS

The occurrence of a disease syndrome of this nature must be differentiated from diseases such as bracken fern poisoning and warfarin-sweet clover poisoning in cattle. The clinical syndromes are quite similar and must be considered when making the diagnosis. In addition, gamma radiation could produce a disease syndrome of this nature. However, it is highly unlikely that this would happen under normal field conditions. The establishment of a diagnosis of TCESOM poisoning is very difficult since there has never been a toxic entity isolated from TCESOM. The practitioner should make every effort to get a complete history along with the source of the suspected toxic meal before making the conclusive diagnosis on the basis of clinical signs. Signs similar to TCESOM poisoning have been produced by the feeding of S-dichlorovinyl-L-cysteine, and it is thought that this compound might be closely related to the toxic agent that occurs in the extracted meal. However, neither this particular toxic agent nor any other toxic agent has ever been found in the toxic meal.

TREATMENT

There is no effective treatment for this condition; however, the early diagnosis of animals in the field can help avert or alleviate some of the disease signs in other animals. Immediate removal of the offending meal from the rations may result in the saving of some asymptomatic animals. Another type of protein meal should be substituted for the suspected toxic meal. Treatments in the past have not been successful; however, the administration of large quantities of whole blood with vitamin K$_1$ and massive antibiotic therapy may assist in combating the possible secondary invaders that often cause disease syndromes.

It is hoped that this disease is of historical significance only. However, with the constant search for new and more efficient ways of extracting protein from any source, this disease may arise in some other types of protein meal. Consequently, practitioners should be on the lookout for disease conditions of this nature.

Supplemental Reading

McKinney, L. L., Picken, J. C., Weakley, F. B., et al.: Possible toxic factor of trichloroethylene-extracted soybean oil meal. J. Am. Chem. Soc. 81:909–915, 1959.
Picken, J. C., Jr., Biester, H. E. and Covalt, C. H.: Trichloroethylene extracted soybean oil meal poisoning. Iowa State Vet. 16:137–141, 1952.
Picken, J. C., Jr., Jacobson, N. L., Allen, R. S., et al.: Toxicity of trichloroethylene-extracted soybean oil meal. Agri. Food Chem. 3:420–424, 1955.
Pritchard, W. R., Rehfeld, C. E., Mizuno, N. S., et al.: Studies on trichloro-extracted feeds. Am. J. Vet. Res. 17:425–454, 1956.

Crude Oils, Fuel Oils, and Kerosene

LOYD D. ROWE, D.V.M., M.S.
and WILLIAM C. EDWARDS, D.V.M., M.S.

The ingestion of crude oil or various petroleum distillates is occasionally the cause of illness or death in domestic ruminants. Cattle are usually the species affected. Carelessness in allowing ruminants free access to open containers of gasoline, kerosene, tractor fuel, or waste crankcase oil has resulted in poisonings by these materials. Cattle have been known to consume up to several gallons of crude oil at one time. The circumstances under which these animals ingest crude oil and other petroleum products are varied. It appears that ruminants ingest crude oil and petroleum products when they are thirsty and water is not readily available, when food or water is contaminated with petroleum, when seeking salt, or when grazing on poor quality pasture. Cattle are curious, and feeder calves seemingly ingest petroleum in an attempt to provide variety to their diets.

Potential hazards to livestock exist in many aspects of the oil industry: (1) during exploration, discarded chemicals are potential hazards, (2) during drilling operations, drilling muds, salt water, crude oil, caustic chemicals, acids, and heavy metals may constitute a hazard to livestock in the vicinity, (3) during production, crude oil, condensates, salt water, and slushpit materials have all been incriminated as causes of poisoning, (4) during transportation, hazards exist from pipeline breaks and chemicals used to maintain pipelines, (5) during the refinery phase, although closely regulated, contamination of land and water from various effluents and emissions through accident or carelessness may result. In certain areas of the United States, pollution of rangeland with petroleum hydrocarbons has been commonly associated with oil exploration and production activities. Livestock owners often suspect crude oil poisoning when sick or dead animals have a history of exposure to areas contaminated with crude oil.

Crude oil is a mixture of several hundred different chemical compounds. The composition of crude oil varies with the reserve from which it is produced, with weathering, and with other factors. Weathering may remove the more volatile and water soluble components. This variation in crude oil composition may explain some of the differences seen clinically, since acute signs seem to be related to the more volatile forms.

The potential for litigation exists whenever cattle in close proximity to drilling and production sites become ill or die. Many of these cases could have been avoided if livestock had been prevented access to such sites by fencing or by other means.

Cases of oil poisoning related to oil field pollution usually result from leaks in oil gathering or transportation systems. Ruptured pipelines can release large quantities of oil, gasoline, or other petroleum products in a short period of time. Significant pollution of pastures and streams by petroleum materials can also result from railroad and truck tank car accidents. Owners sometimes use kerosene or other petroleum products for treating a variety of disease conditions in their animals.

Petroleum hydrocarbon poisoning in ruminants generally involves the respiratory, digestive, and central nervous systems. The most serious consequence of crude oil or petroleum distillate ingestion by domestic ruminants is aspiration pneumonia due to aspiration of oil into the lungs. Acute bloat may quickly cause death in some animals when petroleum fractions more volatile than kerosene (primarily the naphtha and gasoline fractions) are present in large quantities. The mechanisms involved in the production of bloat are presumably the vaporization and rapid expansion of highly volatile hydrocarbons in the rumen following ingestion.

The acute toxicity of a particular hydrocarbon mixture is determined primarily by its aspiration hazard and its irritant activity on pulmonary tissue. For crude oils, this correlates with the relative content of volatile components, such as gasoline, naphtha, and kerosene. Hydrocarbon mixtures of high volatility and low viscosity are apparently more readily aspirated than their less volatile, more viscous counterparts. Aspiration may occur during ingestion, or abnormal eructation may inadvertently introduce oil from the rumen into an open glottis. The ability of an oil to induce vomiting or bloating may contribute to the likelihood that oil from the rumen will be aspirated. When aspirated, gasoline, naphtha, and kerosene produce tracheitis, bronchitis, and bronchopneumonia that is often fatal. Heavy petroleum hydrocarbons are less irritating to pulmonary tissues and produce a less severe lipoid pneumonia. Microorganisms in the respiratory tract that are carried into the lungs by the aspirated oil may be important to the final outcome. Animals aspirating small amounts of oil may develop pulmonary abscesses with death occurring after several weeks or months, during which a progressive decline in condition takes place.

The more volatile straight chain and aromatic hydrocarbons may have anesthetic-like action if absorbed systemically. Signs of central nervous system derangement have occurred in some cattle intoxicated with crude oil, condensate, diesel fuel, or kerosene. In some cases, development of abnormal nervous system signs seems to be associated with the development of pneumonia, suggesting that systemic absorption of low molecular weight hydrocarbons takes place from the lungs.

In cases in which aspiration does not occur, anorexia, decreased rumen motility, mild depression, and weight loss for a period of 1 to 2 weeks may be the only adverse effects produced after ingestion of large quantities (up to 40 mg/kg) of crude oil or petroleum distillates, such as kerosene or diesel oil. Single oral doses as low as 200 ml of odorless kerosene or light petroleum solvents given to cattle have caused no harm other than reduction of 40 to 90 per cent in feed intake over a 3 to 4 day period.

Petroleum distillates applied to the skin may cause irritation, thickening, and fissuring. Gasoline, kerosene, and naphtha dry and defat the skin and are moderate irritants; gas oil, diesel oil, and fuel oil fractions are intermediate, while lubricating oils have only slight irritant properties. All, however, may be irritating to damaged or inflamed skin.

CLINICAL SIGNS

Clinical signs in animals known to have ingested crude oil, condensate, and other petroleum hydrocarbons may vary from sudden death to no observable effects. Sudden death from peracute bloat following consumption of fresh, highly volatile crudes, naphtha, or gasoline usually occurs immediately after ingestion.

Abnormal nervous system signs are less common but may include excitability, depression, shivering, head tremors, confusion, decreased visual acuity, incoordination, mydriasis, prostration, and clonic-tonic convulsions.

Anorexia and mild depression, beginning in about 24 hr and lasting up to 10 days depending on the amount consumed, occur following ingestion of crude oil or distillates, such as gasoline, kerosene, or diesel fuel. These signs, along with a corresponding loss of weight, may be the only manifestation of toxicosis in animals that do not develop bloat or aspirate oil. Regurgitation of oil is common, and oil may be seen on the lips and muzzle. Vomited oily ingesta may be observed after consumption of highly volatile crude oil but is less likely after consumption of kerosene.

Gross evidence of oil in the feces may not appear for several days after ingestion of oil. At this time, the feces may become somewhat dry and formed if gasoline, naphtha, or kerosene is involved. In contrast, consumption of a crude oil high in lubricating (heavy) distillates may result in catharsis.

Aspiration pneumonia may be characterized by anorexia, loss of weight, progressive deterioration of health, weakness, and death after several days or weeks. Clinical signs of pneumonia and possibly pleuritis may be seen in cattle that aspirate fresh, highly volatile crude oil or volatile distillates. Signs in affected animals may be coughing, rapid shallow respiration, increased heart rate, reluctance to move, holding the head in a low attitude, weakness, an oil-stained mucous nasal discharge, and a dehydrated appearance, with death usually occurring several days after ingestion. Abnormal respiratory signs following aspiration of less volatile crude oil may be limited to dyspnea shortly before death. Animals developing pulmonary abscesses may gradually lose condition and may walk stiffly with an arched back and die after periods of up to several months.

CLINICAL BIOCHEMISTRY AND HEMATOLOGY

Cattle suffering from crude oil or kerosene toxicosis may after 4 or more days develop low blood glucose levels that are probably due to prolonged anorexia or disruption of normal rumen function or both. Other blood biochemical and hematologic changes should generally be associated with the development of pneumonia. These include increases in packed cell volume, hemoglobin, and blood urea nitrogen levels, indicating mild to moderate hemoconcentration. The leukocyte response may be characterized by initial leukopenia (neutropenia, lymphopenia, and eosinopenia) followed over the next 2 to 3 days by a relative increase in neutrophils. The total white blood cell count may remain depressed, return to normal, or become moderately elevated.

NECROPSY LESIONS

Lesions of foreign body pneumonia are the most usual necropsy findings. These may be accompanied by localized pleuritis and even hydrothorax if materials such as gasoline or naphtha or crude oils high in these components have been aspirated. The distribution of pulmonary lesions are usually bilateral and include the caudoventral apical, cardiac, cranioventral diaphragmatic, and intermediate lobes. The affected portions are usually dark purple, consolidated, and, in animals surviving several days after aspiration, may contain multiple abscesses. Oil may or may not be grossly visible in pulmonary tissue. Large encapsulated pulmonary abscesses may be found in cattle surviving up to several months following aspiration of oil. Oil may not be visible in the rumen of cattle that die more than 4 days after ingestion of oil. Specimens may be examined under ultraviolet light, as many petroleum hydrocarbons produce a yellow to yellow-green fluorescence under these conditions. However, it should be noted that many compounds, including some drugs, also produce such fluorescence.

DIAGNOSIS

One of the most difficult problems confronting the practicing veterinarian is the diagnosis of poisoning from oil field wastes particularly from crude oil, condensates, and other petroleum hydrocarbons. A diagnosis cannot be made on the basis of circumstantial evidence alone. Many cases where oil field wastes are suspected as a cause of illness or death turn out to be caused by other disease or management problems. This emphasizes the need for a complete postmortem examination and diagnostic work-up.

A thorough clinical examination of the animals must be done along with a careful postmortem examination of animals that have died. In recently exposed animals, oil in lung, rumen contents, or fecal material may be detectable by its odor and, if necessary, can be visualized by placing these materials in warm water, which will cause the oil to separate and float on the surface. Specimens to be collected for laboratory study should include rumen contents, feces, and a complete set of tissues for microscopic, bacteriologic, virologic, and toxicologic examinations. It is especially important to collect ample quantities of rumen contents, feces, and lung tissue for chemical analysis. These samples must be carefully protected from cross contamination during necropsy as well as from damage during shipment to the laboratory. Careful documentation of all observations is important due to the possibility of subsequent legal action. It is recommended that sick, moribund, or dead animals be submitted to a veterinary diagnostic laboratory accompanied by a complete history, tentative diagnosis, and known treatment.

The source of the toxicant should be identified. An intensive inspection of the premises should be accompanied by careful sampling of any spilled oil and contaminated water or forage for chemical analysis. In investigating animal health problems associated with petroleum exploration drilling and production activities, it is well to keep in mind that many hazardous materials are used. Some of these are explosives, lead from grease and "pipe dope," arsenicals, organophosphate esters, caustic acids, and alkali. Salt water is a common cause of poisoning in the oil field. Salt poisoning is often suspected when cattle are thought to have consumed oil and brine from slush pits. Cattle with an adequate supply of fresh water will not usually be poisoned by slush pit brine unless it contains very unusual ingredients. If only salt water is available, animals may limit their intake to the point of water deprivation.

Waste oils, including used crankcase oil, may be hazardous to livestock owing more to the presence of toxic contaminants than to natural petroleum hydrocarbons. Waste oil may contain toxic combustion products, heavy metals (especially lead), and perhaps other deleterious substances. On occasion, waste oils have been found to contain such highly toxic materials as tetrachlorodibenzodioxin (TCDD). Detection of petroleum in solvent extracts of rumen and intestinal contents, liver, lungs, and kidney by laboratory analysis is helpful. Attempts should be made to match the identity of the petroleum in the ingesta and tissue extracts with that of the suspected source. It should be emphasized that the finding of oil in the gastrointestinal tract does not necessarily justify a diagnosis of oil poisoning. Many oils are nontoxic if not aspirated into the lungs. Positive correlation of chemical findings with appropriate clinical signs and necropsy findings would confirm a field diagnosis of petroleum intoxication.

Prognosis hinges primarily upon whether or not aspiration occurred. Since aspiration pneumonia does not usually respond well to treatment, prognosis is grave.

Signs of aspiration may not appear for several days; therefore, prognosis based on initial clinical findings may be misleading.

TREATMENT

The primary objective of treatment is to remove the oil from the rumen as soon as possible to prevent aspiration of oil into the lungs, to mitigate gastrointestinal dysfunction, and to limit the possibility of systemic absorption. The safest and most efficient means of doing this is by the complete removal of rumen contents following rumenotomy and replacement with rumen material from healthy animals. Long-standing cases involving only prolonged anorexia and digestive hypofunction may also respond well to this procedure. These animals are generally hypoglycemic and should be treated with glucose intravenously prior to surgery. Intravenous fluids and electrolytes may be needed if animals have become dehydrated. Ruminal lavage via stomach tube is contraindicated because of the greater danger of aspiration.

In cases where rumenotomy is not feasible, the careful administration of vegetable oil (500 to 1000 ml) by nasogastric tube may be given in an attempt to reduce the hazard of aspiration by increasing the viscosity of the oil mixture in the rumen. This should be followed by administration of a saline cathartic to hasten evacuation of the gastrointestinal tract.

Treatment of aspiration pneumonia is rarely effective. Treatment with a broad-spectrum antibiotic or sulfonamide at the time of or soon after aspiration may prevent or reduce the severity of infection in the lung. For this reason, antimicrobial therapy should be used for at least 7 days in all animals known to or suspected to have consumed oil before signs of pneumonia appear. Anti-inflammatory agents, such as prednisone and dexamethasone, may be of benefit in reducing chemical pneumonitis. Such anti-inflammatory agents should be used only if antimicrobial therapy is used concurrently. Any antimicrobial or anti-inflammatory drugs should be administered parenterally if the rumen has not been evacuated.

Animals developing potentially lethal bloat should be treated by passing a stomach tube and allowing the hydrocarbon vapors to escape. Following this, treat the animal as described earlier. If damage to the skin has resulted from topical application of oil, the oil may be removed using mild detergents.

Prevention of oil poisoning can be accomplished only by assuring that animals do not gain access to oil. Adequate fencing of animals away from oil field operations is not usually done but is highly recommended.

Supplemental Reading

Edwards, W. C., Coppock, R. W., and Zinn, L. L.: Toxicosis related to the petroleum industry. Vet. and Human Toxicol. *21*:328–337, 1979.

Gleason, M. N., Gosselin, R. E., Hodge, H. C., and Smith, R. P.: Clinical Toxicology of Commercial Products, Acute Poisoning, 3rd ed. Baltimore, Williams & Wilkins Co., 132–137, 1969.

Ranger, S. F.: A case of diesel oil poisoning in a ewe. Vet. Rec. *99*:508–509, 1976.

Rowe, L. D., Dollahite, J. W., and Camp, B. J.: Toxicity of two crude oils and of kerosene to cattle. J. Am. Vet. Med. Assoc. *162*:61–66, 1973.

Coal Tar and Phenols

FREDERICK W. OEHME, D.V.M., Ph.D.

Phenolic chemicals are very useful due to their antimicrobial properties, their environmental stability, and their solubility and mixability with numerous other organic chemicals. Although the original form of pure phenol was an excellent disinfectant, it was proved too toxic for routine environmental and animal applications. Derivatives of phenol have been prepared that reduce this toxicity but retain its germicidal properties. Chlorine and other radicals have been added to the benzene ring of phenol to develop useful commercial materials, such as disinfectants and fungicides, chemical additives to insulation materials, plastics and disposable products, and components of multimixture materials that are likely to be disposed of and made inadvertently available to grazing animals.

Toxicoses are most commonly caused in food animals by coal tar and its derivatives, wood preservatives (such as pentachlorophenol), and a variety of other derivative phenols (such as o-phenylphenol) used as active ingredients in disinfectant mixtures.

COAL TAR POISONING

Coal tar poisoning is an acute, highly fatal disease that most often affects swine. It produces characteristic liver lesions that may be undetected until death.

Toxicosis most commonly results from swine consuming fragments of "clay pigeons" that have contaminated pastures at an earlier time. Death from this toxicosis may occur even several decades after the last known pasture contamination with clay pigeons, since the toxic compounds are environmentally stable. Tar paper, tarred building boards and roofing materials, and plumber's pitch also contain a variety of phenols and coal tar. Phenol, cresols, and a variety of aromatic hydrocarbons (naphthalene, naphthalene derivatives, anthracene, and anthracene oils) are the toxic agents found in pitch and tar paper materials. Pigs, especially those 6 to 20 weeks of age, that root the soil and chew on flooring, boards, and hard materials found in sheds and pasture, are most commonly affected, although ruminants may occasionally be exposed owing to inherent curiosity, contact with a new environment, or accidentally contaminated rations.

CLINICAL SIGNS

The most common syndrome is one of a rapid clinical course and sudden death without the presence of signs of diagnostic significance. This course develops from the progressive destructive properties of the coal tar-pitch compounds to the liver, which result in thoracic and abdominal fluid increase and sudden death often associated with exertion. Occasionally, a more chronic illness is observed. Anorexia, depression, weakness, a rough haircoat, and anemia with icterus may affect several animals in the herd for 1 or more days before death. In this instance, the animal may have an increased respiratory rate, incoordination and eventual recumbency with a tendency to assume the sternal position, difficulty in breathing, coma, and death. Almost all swine that exhibit this chronic syndrome die. Because of the pronounced liver involvement, vitamin A storage is reduced and abortions and stillbirths may occur. It is reasonable to assume that some pigs would be affected subclinically and would have liver damage and reduced growth efficiency, but would not have sufficient lesions to develop overt clinical signs. Those individuals are "poor doers" and may never develop the toxic syndrome except for visible pathologic changes at slaughter. Other animals in this category may not show signs until liver function becomes deficient as the animal's body weight increases.

The characteristic lesion of coal tar poisoning is a markedly swollen liver with a mottled appearance. The liver lobules are clearly outlined by a light-colored zone, and the centers often contain deep red foci. In chronic cases, the liver damage may be replaced by fibrosis. The carcass is icteric with large quantities of fluid present in the peritoneal and, usually, the pleural and pericardial cavities. Microscopically, the liver lobules contain central hemorrhages that extend to the periphery. Central lobular necrosis of liver cells is also present. These characteristic changes usually involve the entire liver, but in those animals that survive for several days or in those animals with subclinical effects, the lesions may be confined to local or peripheral areas.

PENTACHLOROPHENOL POISONING

Lumber used in the construction of farm buildings is often treated with wood preservatives, such as pentachlorophenol, creosote, and other related phenolic compounds. The chlorinated phenols are also used as bactericidal agents, herbicides, fungicides, and in some cases, insecticides. Exposure occurs in livestock through skin contact with treated lumber, through licking or chewing on treated portions of stabling, through consumption of contaminated feeds, or through erroneous topical application of these chlorinated compounds to the skin. In unusual circumstances, respiratory exposure may occur through the housing of animals in poorly ventilated barns that have been heavily treated with pentachlorophenol.

Other Phenolic Chemicals

Other phenolic chemicals may be found around livestock environments, and animals may be exposed via accidental application or via direct exposure through the carelessness of an uninformed owner. Dietary contamination can occur through sprays applied in feeding areas. Accidental dietary contamination is sometimes due to mistaken chemical identity.

CLINICAL SIGNS

Phenolics are rapidly absorbed from the intact skin or from the digestive tract. Early signs include incoordination, mild muscular fasciculation, depression leading to coma, and deepening coma with terminal respiratory failure. If phenolics are absorbed slowly, such as from skin application, increased red blood cell fragility and intravascular hemolysis may occur. Progressive icterus is then observed prior to death. Application of concentrated solutions of phenolic chemicals may be corrosive to membranes, skin, or the digestive tract. Mild poisoning may result in clinical signs occurring and regressing within 24 hr; more severe poisoning may produce death in 24 to 36 hr.

Necropsy lesions are consistent with the protein-coagulation properties of phenolic chemicals. Surface tissues may be irritated with coagulation necrosis present. Congestion of internal organs occurs, and generalized icterus may occur. The skin or digestive tract content may have a characteristic phenol odor. Microscopic lesions are coagulation necrosis of epithelial cells, moderate hepatocyte degeneration, and nonspecific nephrotoxic changes.

DIAGNOSIS

History and evidence of contact with phenolic-containing materials are invaluable for the diagnosis of coal tar or phenolic poisoning. The clinical signs are not sufficiently specific to allow diagnosis on that basis alone. The presence of one or more animals with progressively deepening coma, mild muscular fasciculation, and icterus should suggest the possibility of phenol toxicity. A rapidly performed presumptive screening test for phenolic compounds may be utilized on urine from animals suspected of this toxicosis. Two simple tests are available, and the combination of both giving positive results is presumptive evidence of poisoning. In the first procedure, 1 ml of a 20 per cent aqueous solution of ferric chloride is added to 10 ml of urine. A resulting purple color is positive. In the second test, 10 ml of suspected urine is boiled with 1 to 2 ml of Millon's reagent. Millon's reagent is made by dissolving 10 gm of mercury in 20 ml of nitric acid, diluting with an equal amount of distilled water, allowing the mixture to stand for 2 hr, and decanting the excess water. A positive reaction with urine results in a red color.

TREATMENT AND PREVENTION

Specific treatment for phenolic intoxications is not available. Washing of the exposed skin of animals will reduce the topical absorption, while administration of activated charcoal is effective in binding unabsorbed phenolic chemicals in the digestive tract. Removal of the animals from environments containing the phenolic chemicals prevents further exposure. Supportive therapy, including the maintenance of normal body temperature and respiration, and the administration of fluids should be included. Glucose may have some benefit in reducing liver damage and maintaining renal function. Recovery from phenolic poisoning is still largely determined by the total dose absorbed and the animal's ability to detoxify and excrete the offending chemical.

Supplemental Reading

Osweiler, G. D., Carson, T. L., Buck, W. B., and Van Gelder, G. A. (eds.): Clinical and Diagnostic Veterinary Toxicology, 3rd ed. Dubuque, Iowa, Kendall/Hunt Publishing Co., 1985.

Toxic Gases

STANLEY E. CURTIS, M.S., Ph.D.

The air breathed by food animals is frequently polluted with potentially toxic gases. Some gases have industrial origins, but most often they arise within the animal facilities themselves. Symptoms of chronic gas intoxication are commonly subtle and causes of acute cases are often obscure.

Ammonia, hydrogen sulfide, carbon dioxide, and methane from excreta and respiratory waste products enter the air continuously in animal houses. NH_3 and H_2S are important toxicants. CO_2 and CH_4 are asphyxiants but are generally present in innocuous concentrations. Several dozen volatile organic compounds, many containing nitrogen or sulfur, are given off in smaller amounts; they are the odorants characteristic of animal facilities but apparently not ordinarily present in toxic quantities. CO from improperly adjusted or vented fuel-burning heaters also can be toxic in closed houses. Another toxic gas sometimes encountered in food animal operations is NO_2 from fermenting plant material in silos.

Confinement of animals to enclosed structures increases the frequency of aerial toxicoses. Even at the relatively low ventilation rates recommended during cold weather, concentrations of NH_3 and H_2S usually remain below toxic levels. Accidents, power outages, and improper design or operation of ventilation systems can result in inadequate air exchange, and the air's content of noxious gases can rise to dangerous levels. Also, gases are released rapidly and in large quantities when anerobic waste slurry is agitated; then, especialy at low ventilation rates, gas concentrations can reach acutely toxic levels quickly.

In acute episodes, many exposed animals die, some suddenly. Treatment of survivors is straightforward, i.e., adequate ventilation rate for the facility is restored immediately. The problem tends to be transitory, so data on aerial gas concentrations at such times are meager. Once adequate ventilation has been reestablished, the crisis is over. Still, there may be residual effects on survivors.

Chronic cases have more varied signs, such as lethargy, dyspnea, anorexia, depressed growth, excessive lacrimation and salivation, a low incidence of sudden deaths over weeks or months, and a high incidence of stillbirths. Decreased resistance to certain infectious diseases and increased growth-depressant effects from other diseases are additional manifestations of chronic stress from any toxic gas.

Concentrations of noxious gases can be measured with colorimetric indicator reagents available in tubes, through which a precise volume of air is drawn by a special syringe. Gases taken up by aerial dust may be filtered out of the air along with the dust before reaching the indicator chemical, thus this system sometimes underestimates gas concentration.

Effective exposure dose of most air pollutants is calculated as average pollutant concentration multiplied by exposure duration. This is important to remember when air pollutant concentrations in animal houses are compared with threshold limit values set for occupation of industrial environments. Workers occupy their environments for only 40 hours weekly; animals occupy their environments all the time.

AMMONIA

Ammonia is the toxic air pollutant most often encountered in high concentration in animal houses, especially where excreta can decompose on a solid floor. It has a characteristic pungent odor detectable by humans at 10 ppm or lower. Being less dense than air, NH_3 moves readily throughout an enclosure. It is a chronic stressor. While NH_3 concentration usually remains below 30 ppm even with low ventilation rates, it can reach 50 ppm or higher during long periods of normal facility operation.

Aerial NH_3 iritates mucous membranes of the eyes and of the respiratory passages. Excessive lacrimation, shallow breathing, and discharge of clear or purulent nasal mucus are common signs of aerial NH_3 toxicosis. Lethargy is another symptom.

Growth rate and feed intake in food animals may be reduced 10 per cent or more by aerial NH_3 at concentrations as low as 50 ppm. As concentrations rise within the normal range the reduced growth rate and feed intake are even less in the presence of infectious diseases. Aerial NH_3 at concentrations around 50 ppm also may impair animals' defenses against respiratory and digestive tract infections.

Uncomplicated aerial NH_3 toxicosis produces no consistent gross or histopathologic changes. When lesions are found, they tend to be minor and confined to the upper respiratory passages. NH_3 is readily soluble in aqueous fluids, and so it may be absorbed completely from inspired air in the upper respiratory tract, where it may irritate the lining. In swine, aerial NH_3 can alter the pathogenesis of nasal turbinate infections.

CARBON DIOXIDE

CO_2, an odorless gas present in normal atmospheric air at 300 ppm, is given off by the animals and by improperly vented (though properly adjusted) fuel burning heaters. It is also the gas evolved in greatest quantity by decomposing excreta. Nevertheless, its concentration in closed houses rarely approaches levels that endanger an animal's well-being.

CO_2 at 50,000 ppm causes an animal to breathe faster and deeper but has no other significant effects. In extreme situations where CO_2, which is denser than air, collects in part of a facility, animals may exhibit anxiety followed by staggering, coma, and finally death, as the concentration rises to 400,000 ppm.

At one time, animal quarter ventilation standards were based on aerial CO_2 concentrations. If ventilation during cold weather maintains the proper water-vapor concentration inside the house and during hot weather the proper temperature, CO_2 concentration will be kept below 2000 ppm, and the air's oxygen content will be more than sufficient. Thus, ventilation recommendations are now based on moisture and heat balance.

Clinical findings in sublethal aerial CO_2 toxicosis are limited to changes in breathing pattern and high CO_2 levels in the blood, reflected by "dark" blood and tissues at necropsy.

CARBON MONOXIDE

CO is odorless and slightly less dense than air. It usually arises in animal houses from incomplete combustion of fuel (due to faulty heater adjustment) coupled with improper venting of the heater. When atmospheric CO concentration exceeds the normal background level of 5 ppm, the cause ought to be identified and corrected.

CO competes with oxygen for binding sites on a variety of proteins, including hemoglobin (Hb), with which most of the body's CO is associated. The affinity of Hb for CO is 250 times that for oxygen. When CO becomes bonded to a heme group, forming carboxyhemoglobin, that Hb molecule's oxygen-carrying capacity is reduced, and its hold on the oxygen molecules already bonded to it becomes more tenacious. As a result, CO toxicosis leads to hypoxia.

When the percentage of Hb in the blood in the form of HbCO reaches 20 per cent, the animal loses some locomotor control. At 30 per cent, other chemical changes occur throughout the body and lethargy ensues. Effects of sublethal CO toxicosis can be significant. Adult animals die when the percentage exceeds 60.

The amount of HbCO present depends on rates of formation (directly proportional to aerial CO concentration) and disappearance (half-life around 2 hr) and on duration of CO exposure. Thirty per cent HbCO is reached in adult animals after exposure to 1200 ppm CO for 1 hr or 400 ppm CO for 4 hr. Degradation is so rapid in relation to formation in an atmosphere of 200 ppm CO that the percentage of Hb present as HbCO never reaches 30.

Fetal Hb has a greater affinity for oxygen and CO than does adult Hb. In ruminants, this is because fetal Hb per se has the greater affinity. In swine, fetal and adult Hb are identical, but perinatal piglet erythrocytes contain less 2,3-diphosphoglycerate, which lowers Hb's affinity for oxygen and CO. This age difference starts to diminish at birth. Thus, HbCO percentage in a perinate is often several times higher than in an adult in the same environment. Furthermore, death can occur in perinatal animals at blood HbCO values even lower than 60 per cent saturation. CO toxicosis probably contributes to the death of fetal and neonatal animals in closed houses more often than is generally recognized.

Some signs of CO toxicosis mimic those of hypoxia, ranging from lethargy and incoordinated movements to coma and death. However, HbCO imparts a "bright cherry red" color to the blood, and tissues are bright pink or red at necropsy. Bronchodilation and nonspecific brain lesions are often seen. Recovery from CO intoxication can be hastened by administering oxygen mixed with enough CO_2 (around 5 per cent) to stimulate breathing.

HYDROGEN SULFIDE

With the probable exception of CO, acute H_2S poisoning is directly responsible for more deaths in closed animal houses than any other toxic gas. Many humans have died in H_2S accidents in and around animal houses. H_2S is formed continuously during anaerobic decomposition of excreta. It is denser than air and has the odor of "rotten eggs." The usual concentration of H_2S in animal quarters (less than 10 ppm) is not toxic. However, when waste slurry is agitated to resuspend solids prior to being pumped out, it rapidly releases much of its H_2S. It may pollute the air the animals breathe at levels of 1000 ppm and higher at such times.

H_2S irritates the conjunctiva and respiratory tract mucosa at low aerial concentrations. Increased sensitivity to light and a variety of infectious and noninfectious respiratory tract lesions have been found in animals exposed chronically to moderately high concentrations of H_2S. As concentration increases, signs of acute H_2S toxicosis appear: lethargy, incoordinated locomotion, depressed respiratory center, and generalized cyanosis. Spasms and coma may appear first, but death often occurs without warning after abrupt exposure to concentrations of 400 ppm or higher. Attempts at resuscitation are usually futile.

At necropsy, cyanosis, pulmonary edema and congestion, and emphysema are frequently observed.

NITROGEN DIOXIDE

NO_2 is an intermediate product of nitrate degradation during plant fermentation. It is a yellowish-brownish component of silo gas that can cause profound disease and even death—instantly or hours, days, or months later—in humans and animals alike. In humans, the toxicosis is called "silo filler's disease." Animals fed silage exposed to NO_2 often develop the same symptoms as if they had breathed NO_2.

Clinical findings are dyspnea, excessive lacrimation and salivation, low blood pressure, and methemoglobinemia. At necropsy, the pathologic changes commonly include "dark red" kidneys, pulmonary edema and hemorrhage, bronchiolitis, and emphysema.

Toxic concentrations of NO_2 have not been established for food animals. Exposure to NO_2 at concentrations as low as 5 ppm has caused respiratory tract lesions in laboratory animals. Its concentration in silo gas may exceed 100 ppm.

DUST

Particulate air pollutants, either alone or in combination with gases, are also of concern. For example, gaseous NH_3 rarely penetrates the respiratory tract to the lungs. However, aerial dust absorbs and carries certain gases, thus NH_3 may be transported to the lungs by dust particles small enough ($< 5 \mu m$ in diameter) to be carried into the lungs. When particles containing toxic compounds such as NH_3 deposit on respiratory linings, they serve to increase the absorbed compounds' concentrations at that point. If particle sizes are such that dust penetration exceeds gas penetration, the gas's effective toxicity is exacerbated.

Supplemental Reading

Buck, W. B., Osweiler, G. D., Van Gelder, G. A. (eds.): Clinical and Diagnostic Veterinary Toxicology, 2nd ed. Dubuque, Iowa, Kendall/Hunt Publishing Co., 1976.

Curtis, S. E.: Environmental Management in Animal Agriculture. Ames, Iowa, Iowa State University Press, 1983.

Donham, K. J., Carson, T. L., Adrian, B. R.: Carboxyhemoglobin values in swine relative to carbon monoxide exposure: guidelines for monitoring animal and human health hazards in swine confinement buildings. Amer. J. Vet. Res. 43:813, 1982.

Lillie, R. J.: Air Pollutants Affecting the Performance of Domestic Animals. Washington, D.C., United States Department of Agriculture, 1970.

Lightning Strike and Electrocution

F. K. RAMSEY, D.V.M., Ph.D.
and J. R. HOWARD, D.V.M., Ph.D.

Our 3-year study from 1962 to 1965 clearly indicated that gross lesions caused by lightning in some cases are minimal or not apparent. We have repeatedly stated that veterinarians should carefully evaluate other causes of death before they conclude that it is definitely lightning. At times it is difficult to say that the specific cause of death is lightning. The veterinary profession must not use the lack of macroscopic lesions of the thoracic and abdominal viscera as an alibi for a diagnosis of lightning, as *the lesions of some clostridial diseases may be in skeletal muscle tissues,* or *the etiologic agent may be in the central nervous system, thus making diagnosis difficult.*

DIAGNOSIS

History

In cases of lightning strike and electrocution, the history is sometimes of little value. Necropsy findings must be relied upon for an accurate diagnosis. The incidence of recent storms may confuse the issue and lead to unwarranted conclusions. The same can be said for losses occurring in the same field in prior years. Carcass position is not reliable as a diagnostic aid. Location of the carcass under a tree or next to a fence has positive value only when recent disruption of the bark, welding of wire, splitting of posts, or singeing of hair are encountered. Occasionally, groups of animals are killed. This is significant and usually is accompanied by evidence of lightning damage to surroundings and singeing of the hair of some animals.

Skin

Singe marks occur on about 30 per cent of the animals. They are more frequently found on the medial side of the legs. The individual hairs have a brownish discoloration and a distinctly abnormal kinking. Denuded areas have not been found.

Membranes lining the mouth, nostrils, and vagina are usually cyanotic with a blue discoloration and darkening.

Underneath the skin there may be congestion of small blood vessels causing it to appear slightly more pink than normal. Two to 3 per cent of the animals involved have hemorrhages in discrete areas, 5 to 8 cm or more in diameter, that do not involve the underlying muscle tissue. Usually, postmortem changes have caused gas to be collected under the skin. This finding may be indistinguishable from black leg.

Respiratory System

Consistently there is hemorrhage (or postmortem extravasation of blood) in the trachea. Hemorrhages vary from a dozen or so areas about the size of the head of a pin in the lining membrane to so many of them that the blood has broken through the membrane and is lying free in the lumen, perhaps mixed with froth. This gives the appearance of a rope of blood. The muscles of the larynx may be darker than normal from hemorrhage and congestion. The lungs are usually normal without hemorrhages and may be collapsed or distended with air. In a few cases there have been diffuse subpleural hemorrhages of both lungs, extending into lobular septae.

Cardiovascular System

About 20 per cent of the affected animals will have small hemorrhages on the surface of the heart. In 30 per cent of those affected (before postmortem decomposition becomes too advanced, about 6 hr), the left ventricle will be very much lighter in color than normal because of a reduced amount of blood in its veins and capillaries. The right ventricle will be darker than normal because of greater amounts of blood in the capillaries and veins. The blood is normal.

Hematopoietic System

Hemorrhage and hyperemia are common in the superficial lymph nodes, notably the prescapular and cervical. (We now realize that this so-called hyperemia and hemorrhage often are postmortem phenomena. Blood often does not clot immediately after death, and rapid gas formation in abdominal viscera forces the blood to the heart. From the heart the blood is forced into the anterior vena cava and travels in a retrograde manner to the superficial lymph nodes, subcutaneous tissues, and other tissues where there is less pressure. Here it causes congestion and postmortem extravasation, indistinguishable from that of antemortem hyperemia and hemorrhage.) Hemorrhage and hyperemia may consist of a few areas of redness in these nodes, but usually there is an outstanding red to black discoloration of the entire tissue. Internal lymph nodes are usually normal. The spleen of an occasional animal may be enlarged 2 to 3 times. Small hemorrhages occur in the tonsils and thymus.

Digestive System

It is emphasized that the digestive system should be carefully evaluated. *The contents of the alimentary canal are normal in lightning death.* Abnormal ingesta in the forestomachs or anywhere else in the digestive tract and the presence of gastroenteritis would indicate some other cause of death. Frequently, peristalsis continues after lightning death, and often a stool of normal feces is found.

Postmortem bloat is very common and may be very extensive. The muscle of the diaphagm or body wall may be separated by the force of the rumen.

In a healthy bovine the gallbladder should not be distended. A greatly enlarged gallbladder suggests that a bovine probably has not been eating of late as a result of some illness. Therefore, in a suspected case of lightning strike, one must consider other causes of death if a bovine is observed to have a greatly distended gallbladder.

Musculoskeletal System

Small pinpoint hemorrhages may be seen in the fascia in the connective tissue between the muscles, especially of the neck and shoulder. Fractures of the skull, vertebrae (especially lumbar and sacral), pelvis, femurs, and other bones often occur. This is noted in many of the injury cases.

Urogenital System

Lesions are rarely found.

Nervous System

Hemorrhages are occasionally found, and they are primary lesions of the central nervous system.

Endocrine System

We have not noted any pathologic alterations in this system.

DIFFERENTIAL DIAGNOSIS

It is often difficult to differentiate antemortem from postmortem bloat. In both instances, the membranes lining the mouth and nostrils are cyanotic, and gas may collect under the skin as decomposition advances. The extensive lymph node hemorrhages and the atelectatic lungs are the lesions that differentiate antemortem bloat from bloat occurring as a result of lightning strike.

The injury case is a problem that deserves consideration. In general, we can state that in no field case or experimental case have we encountered central nervous system symptoms that could be attributed to the direct effects of electricity on the brain or spinal cord. Crushed or fractured skull, vertebrae, and pelvis may cause hemorrhage and an impingement on the central nervous system that may indirectly affect the function of the brain and spinal cord. In steers, we have noted damage to ear mechanisms. Hogs have made eventual recoveries from broken pelves. If lightning injures an animal, its effects are instantaneous and not delayed.

Veterinarians, insurance personnel, and livestock owners must be aware that many other infectious diseases and noninfectious diseases may also cause rapid death. Therefore, etiologic factors other than lightning must always be kept in mind, and hence it follows that a complete necropsy should be done in every case. Circumstantial evidence may indicate that the brain and spinal cord should be removed in order to determine if the animal died of a central nervous disorder, such as polioencephalomalacia, *Hemophilus somnus* infection, or some other disease. It may be necessary for a diagnostic laboratory to perform bacteriologic, virologic, and histopathologic examinations.

Insurance personnel and livestock owners must realize that it may take a lot of time in *some lightning claims* to determine the specific cause of death. We are convinced that the cause of death in almost all lightning claims can be established by following the procedures presented in this article.

Heat Prostration*

E. MURL BAILEY, JR., D.V.M., Ph.D.

Overheating (heat prostration, heat stroke) is a sporadically encountered condition in livestock characterized by hyperthermia and sometimes complicated by alterations in acid-base balance, dehydration, intravascular clotting, and cerebral edema. High humidity contributes to the likelihood of heat stroke because water evaporation from

*Supported in part by Texas Agricultural Experiment Station, Project no. H-6255.

the oral and nasal cavities is decreased, in spite of rapid panting. Other predisposing factors are lack of available water, obesity, and depressed heat tolerance associated with young or old age. Heat is the essential causative factor. Lack of oxygen (poor circulation of air) and exercise are contributing factors. Fatigue and insufficient water and salt intake play significant, secondary roles. Procedures that result in crowding, excitement, and forced exercise during hot weather produce most of the cases.

TEMPERATURE REGULATION

Heat is lost from the body by radiation, conduction, and convection. The latter involves evaporation of water from the skin and respiratory passages. Considerable heat is also lost in feces and urine. When body temperature rises, whether from fever or from failure of heat dissipation to keep pace with heat production, the rate of metabolism is accelerated, and this aggravates hyperthermia.

The principal mechanisms of heat dissipation involve cutaneous vasodilation, evaporation of water, and avoidance of excessively hot environments. Cutaneous vasodilation serves to bring deep body heat to the surface with greater efficiency. Heat loss by this method depends upon the physical processes of radiation and convection and requires an environment that is cooler than body surface temperatures. At an environmental temperature of about 31°C (88°F) or greater, skin vasodilation no longer increases heat dissipation, and a rise in body temperature will result unless heat loss can be enhanced by other means.

Sweating is an efficient mechanism for heat dissipation in cattle. Thermoregulatory sweating is elicited in 2 ways, (1) reflexly by stimulation of warmth receptors in the skin and (2) by a rise of the hypothalamic temperature. Although reflex sweating may occur in the absence of elevated central temperature, a high skin temperature cannot elicit full-scale sweating without simultaneous hypothalamic facilitation. In many domestic animals, apocrine sweat glands are of importance for evaporative heat loss. In the cow, sweat gland activity rises in relation to the rise in temperature. The apocrine sweat glands of sheep and goats are under direct nervous control. In sheep, sweat secretion is of lesser importance than in the cow, therefore evaporative heat loss via the respiratory passages is more important in the sheep than in the cow.

Panting is an important heat regulatory device in cattle and sheep. Panting or polynea often occurs at rectal temperatures above 40°C (104°F) and may be initiated at lower temperatures. It is usually accompanied by more salivary secretion and may cause a considerable rise in respiratory evaporative cooling if the humidity of the inspired air is not too high. Studies of the panting mechanism in cattle have shown that evaporative cooling occurs in the upper respiratory passages and not in the lungs. In livestock, panting, in response to a higher environmental temperature, may start before there is an increase in the temperature of the blood supplying the brain.

Control of heat dissipation activities is associated with the areas around the preoptic and supraoptic nuclei in the hypothalamus above the optic chiasma and between that structure and the anterior commissure. Control of heat generating and conserving activities is located in the caudal hypothalamic areas. Heat dissipation mechanisms are superimposed on the primary heat conservation mechanisms. The stimulus that appears to activate either of the areas is the temperature of the perfusing blood.

Destructive lesions of the anterior hypothalamus often result in excessively high body temperatures. Such lesions may be caused by trauma and local pressure or direct impact, penetrating injuries that terminate activity of the heat dissipation centers. In these cases, heat generation and conservation centers operate unopposed. A similar situation may occur in central nervous system infections, and the high temperatures that accompany many types of encephalitis or meningitis can probably be explained by failure of the heat dissipating mechanism.

Cattle appear to have no special water conservation mechanisms, but there is an important difference between European cattle and Indian cattle (Zebu or Brahman cattle). Zebu cattle are better able to regulate body temperature when exposed to heat stress because they are capable of dissipating larger quantities of heat by evaporation of larger quantities of water from their body surface. Furthermore, Indian cattle have more and larger sweat glands over most of their body surface. This heat resistance, however, depends upon an ample supply of water.

In the sheep, the rectal temperature starts to rise above normal at an environmental temperature of 32°C (90°F), and open-mouth panting begins at a rectal temperature of 41°C (106°F). Unless the relative humidity is high (> 65 per cent), sheep are able to withstand an external temperature as high as 43°C (110°F) for hours.

The rectal temperature of the pig begins to rise above normal at an environmental temperature of 30 to 32°C (86 to 90°F). If the relative humidity is 65 per cent or more, the pig cannot tolerate a prolonged exposure to temperatures of 35°C (95°F) or greater. At 40°C (104°F), the pig is unable to withstand any humidity in the atmosphere.

CLINICAL SIGNS

The signs of overheating may develop suddenly and depend upon the environmental conditions and health status of the livestock. Some animals manifest restlessness, excitement, forced movement, and spasms of certain muscles. However, other animals may be dull and depressed. Respiration rate is rapid, and breathing is through the open mouth. A protruding tongue may be covered with frothy saliva, and frothy mucus is discharged from the nostrils. The conjunctiva is congested, and the pupils are dilated early but later may be constricted. Palpitation of the heart is present, and the pulse may be rapid and weak. The rectal temperatures in overheated cattle have ranged from 41.6 to 46.1°C (107 to 115°F). At first, the respiration rate is accelerated but may slow down. Death may occur during convulsions, but usually the terminal signs reflect progressive paralysis of the respiratory and vasomotor centers. A rectal temperature of 41°C (105.8°F) is near the danger point, and collapse will easily occur in swine.

Dehydration or hemoconcentration is commonly found during overheating, and high packed cell volumes (> 60 per cent) may occur. The first sign of dehydration is a tendency by the animal to seek water. Concomitantly,

there is a decline in urine volume. The degree of hemoconcentration in heat stroke may be severe. Signs attributed to dehydration can be observed when 5 per cent of the body weight has been lost as water. Dehydration to the extent of 10 per cent of the body weight is considered severe. The immediate source of water lost from the body is the extracellular fluid (ECF), and if the rate of loss is very rapid, ECF volume may be severely reduced. In slow dehydration, however, there will be a shift of water from the cells into the ECF. In early dehydration, greater quantities of sodium chloride appear in the urine as ECF is reduced. As cellular water shifts to the extracellular compartment, intracellular potassium also is excreted in the urine. This may produce a systemic hypokalemia even though serum potassium levels may be normal. Thus, after a long period of dehydration, the animal will be depleted of both water and primary electrolytes.

Disseminated intravascular coagulation is known to result from heat stroke in humans and dogs. Another complication of heat stroke is cerebral edema, although the mechanism by which heat stroke or hyperthermia induces cerebral edema is unknown.

LESIONS

The meninges and brain are greatly congested and contain numerous hemorrhages. Sometimes there is an accumulation of sanguineous fluid in the intermeningeal space, and the brain may be edematous. Putrefaction develops rapidly, and the large veins are distended with partially clotted blood. The lungs are intensely congested, and the visceral organs are degenerated.

TREATMENT

The first objective of therapy is to lower body temperature. Immediately after or immediately before submersion in cold water, dexamethasone should be administered intravenously in a dose (1 to 2 mg/kg) to counteract edema. Intravenous fluids are indicated if hemoconcentration is documented or if peripheral circulation failure is suspected. The patient should be allowed to drink cold water freely. Shade and free circulation of air should be provided if at all possible.

Special problems in fluid and electrolyte management for all species are produced by overheating syndromes. Heat exhaustion is due to an excessive loss of Na$^+$. The compensatory reaction of the body is to pass K$^+$ from the intracellular fluid (ICF) to the ECF to replace the lost Na$^+$. Renal excretion of Na$^+$ ceases, but water excretion continues. Heat prostration, on the other hand, involves the loss of both Na$^+$ and Cl$^-$. There is usually an associated respiratory alkalosis due to hyperventilation. In these conditions, the clinician must contunuously monitor the patient, using the appropriate laboratory test results as a guide.

Unless arterial blood gas determinations are done, decisions regarding acid-base therapy are impossible. In the absence of specific information, fluids that have little effect on acid-base balance, such as 5 per cent dextrose, should be administered.

Overheating in cattle can be prevented under most management conditions. Allowing animals access to water and mineral supplements ad lib with restrictions on strenuous handling techniques during hotter portions of the day will alleviate the condition. In addition, if animals have limited access to water under stressful situations, such as shipping by truck or train, they should be allowed access to water prior to further stressful situations.

Supplemental Reading

Andersson, B. E.: Temperature Regulation and Environmental Physiology. *In* Swenson, M. J. (ed.): Duke's Physiology of Domestic Animals, 9th ed. Ithaca, New York, Cornell University Press, 1977.

Gross, D. R.: General Concepts on Fluid Therapy. *In* Jones, L. M., Booth, N. H., and McDonald, L. E. (eds.): Veterinary Pharmacology and Therapeutics, 5th ed. Ames, Iowa, The Iowa State University Press, 1982.

Schall, W. D.: Heat Stroke (Heat Stress, Hyperpyrexia). *In* Kirk, R. W., (ed.): Current Veterinary Therapy, 8th ed. Philadelphia, W. B. Saunders, 1983.

Cold Stress

DAVID ROBERTSHAW, M.R.C.V.S., Ph.D.

This article reviews the mechanisms whereby low environmental temperature can reduce the efficiency of animal production. Efficiency is defined as the ratio between food intake and weight gain. If this ratio rises, i.e., an increase in food is required for an increase in body weight not associated with water retention, efficiency is said to be reduced.

The energy value of the food ingested is the gross energy intake. The difference between energy intake and energy lost in the feces is the digestible energy and, when expressed as a percentage, is known as the digestibility. Thus, any factor that decreases digestibility will also decrease the efficiency of food conversion. Of the total energy absorbed, i.e., digestible energy, some energy is lost in the urine, and the remainder is available to the animal for utilization. The difference between the digestible energy and the energy lost in the urine (and that lost as methane from the ruminants) is known as the metabolizable energy. There are very few factors that can reduce the efficiency of conversion of digestible energy to metabolizable energy. The metabolizable energy available to the animal is used, first of all, to maintain the metabolic processes of the body and thus, represents the maintenance requirements of the animal. Any surplus energy available beyond the maintenance requirement of the animal is available for production. The way in which this energy is used for productive purposes will vary: in a growing animal it will be retained largely as protein, in an adult largely as fat, in a lactating animal as milk, and in a pregnant animal as the fetus itself. A simple measurement of body weight gain does not tell us the nature of the weight gain and therefore, it is impossible to estimate the caloric value and the quantity of energy retained. Any process that increases the maintenance requirement of an animal will thus divert energy away from productive processes, and thus reduce the efficiency of food conversion of the animal.

To summarize, there appear to be 2 ways in which the climate may interact with an animal to reduce its feed conversion efficiency, by reducing the digestibility of the gross energy intake and by increasing the maintenance requirements.

An animal will respond to reductions in efficiency of feed conversion by increased appetite in order to maintain or elevate body weight. As a result, there is an economic impact on the producer.

PHYSIOLOGIC RESPONSE TO COLD ENVIRONMENT

Figure 1 shows the relationship between environmental temperature and the various avenues of heat exchange. The unique characteristics of birds and mammals are that they maintain a constant body temperature and possess physiologic mechanisms that ensure, except under extreme conditions, that the deep body temperature will remain constant. This is reflected in Figure 1. Within the zone represented by CD, an animal is able to maintain body temperature simply by adjusting blood flow to the skin and thereby altering the temperature gradient between the skin and the air. At temperatures above D, this is no longer sufficient, and the animal utilizes the latent heat of vaporization to increase heat loss. This is manifest as a rise in respiratory (panting) or cutaneous (sweating) heat loss. As the environmental temperature rises, the heat is lost by convection, i.e., nonevaporative heat loss declines, and at temperatures above deep body temperature, heat is actually gained from the environment. Below temperature C, the heat produced by the animal is less than the heat lost both by convection and evaporation. Temperature C is known as the *lower critical temperature* and at temperatures below C, heat production has to be increased in order to maintain a constant body temperature. At temperatures defined by B, heat production reaches a maximum known as the *summit metabolism,* and body temperature can no longer be maintained and falls. This fall in body temperature, i.e., hypothermia, is an unstable condition and will eventually lead to death unless some form of supportive treatment is instituted. Heat production is elevated by 2 main mechanisms, an intermittent contraction of muscles known as shivering and an increase in metabolism of brown fat. Brown fat oxidation is the strategy used largely by newborn animals, and the quantity of heat that can be produced by brown fat oxidation declines with age. This is more important in sheep and goats and is of minimal significance in cattle. The slope of the heat-production line below C gives an indication of the rate of heat flow away from the animal and is a measure of conductance. This is shown by the parallel slope of the nonevaporative heat-loss line. The difference in vertical distance between the lines is equivalent to the evaporative heat loss. The reciprocal of conductance is a measure of the resistance to heat loss known as the insulation. Greater insulation is one of the major means of cold acclimation in animals and will lower the slope of the nonevaporative heat-loss line and, likewise, lower the magnitude of the heat-production response.

EFFECT OF COLD ON MAINTENANCE REQUIREMENTS

It is readily apparent from Figure 1 that animals exposed to environmental temperatures below C require an increase in their rate of metabolism in order to maintain a constant body temperature. The higher rate of metabolism

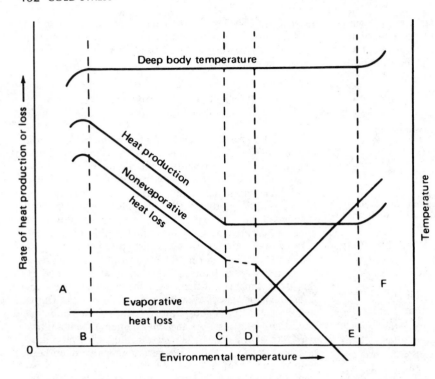

Figure 1. Diagram of relationship between heat production, nonevaporative and evaporative heat loss, and deep body temperature in a homeothermic animal. (From Ingram, D. L., and Mount, L. E.: Man and Animals in Hot Environments. Heidelberg, Springer-Verlag, 1975.)

means that the maintenance requirements of the animal are greater and, therefore, less of the metabolized energy is available for productive purposes. If this rise in maintenance requirements is not met by the food intake, the animal oxidizes its own body tissues to generate heat and literally starves. Figure 2 is a simplified diagram taken from Figure 1 relating to metabolism, to environmental temperature, and to heat load. It is obvious that for maximum efficiency an animal should be at an environmental heat load above the *lower critical temperature* (C in Fig, 1 and C_1 in Fig. 2). This point of minimal metabolic rate or heat production is also known as the thermoneutral or thermal-comfort zone. The hatched area in Figure 2 indicates the areas at which efficiency will be reduced. It will be apparent, therefore, that if animals can remain at a heat load in excess of C_1 (see Fig. 2) or between C and D (see Fig. 1), then climate will not affect energy retention and will not reduce feed efficiency.

This theoretical hypothesis was tested in 2 steers by Blaxter and Wainman (1961), and Figure 3 is taken from their results. They showed that at temperatures below 10 to 15°C, energy retention is reduced in an approximately linear fashion.

It can be seen that the *lower critical temperature* is thus an important consideration in determining the efficiency of an animal. More insulation will not only decrease the slope of the line below the *lower critical temperature*, thereby reducing the magnitude of the hatched area, but it will also decrease the *lower critical temperature*. Most domestic animals show a rise in insulation during the winter, which allows them to acclimate to declining environmental temperatures.

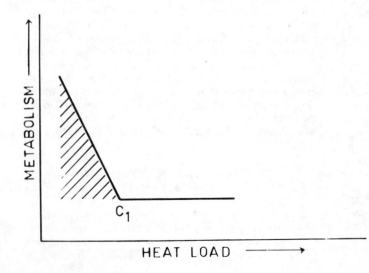

Figure 2. Diagram of the relationship between heat load and metabolism. The hatched area indicates the increment in maintenance requirement caused by exposure to heat loads below the lower critical temperature (C_1).

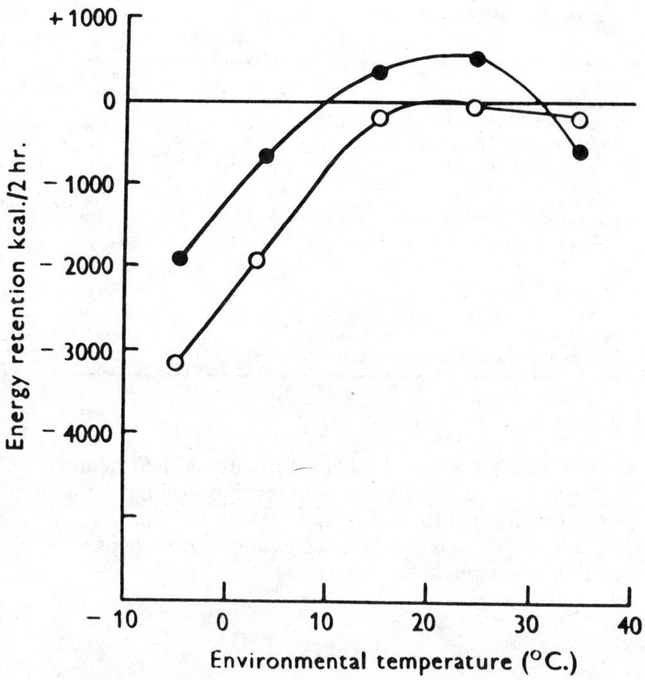

Figure 3. The effect of environmental temperature on energy retention of two steers. (From Blaxter, K. L., and Wainman, F. W.: Environmental temperature and the energy metabolism and heat emission of steers. J. Agric. Sci. 56:81–90, 1961.)

COLD EXPOSURE AND DIGESTIBILITY

It is apparent from the foregoing discussion if the *lower critical temperature* of an animal is known, then the reduction in food efficiency can be readily calculated. Using this information, workers in Canada attempted to determine the food consumption necessary for maintenance and productivity during the Canadian winter. In all cases, they found that their estimates were wrong and that efficiency was reduced more than they predicted. They investigated further and made 2 important observations that explained the greater than predicted reduction in efficiency.

1. Cold exposure itself is a stimulus to appetite. However, sudden exposure to cold by an animal that is not cold acclimated results in a physiologic stress response and a reduction in food intake rather than an increase in food intake. Thus, until the animals become acclimated, which takes 9 to 12 days, there will be a marked reduction in productivity.

2. Cold exposure has also been noted to elevate the rate of passage of food through the alimentary tract. In herbivorous animals, an increase in rate of passage is often associated with a decrease in digestibility, since retention of food is an essential feature for effective microbial degradation. Thus, there is a reduction in digestibility and thereby a reduction in feed efficiency.

SUMMARY

It can be seen from this presentation that as long as animals are maintained at temperatures within their thermoneutral zone, there is no impact of temperature on energy retention. However, at temperatures below the thermoneutral zone, efficiency is reduced in 3 ways: (1) the increase in metabolic rate necessary to maintain body temperature raises the maintenance requirements of the animal, (2) the increase in appetite induced by cold exposure raises the rate of passage and lowers digestibility, and (3) a transient reduction in food intake owing to exposure of a nonacclimated animal to sudden cold stress occurs. It is, therefore, essential for maximum economic return that owners of food-producing animals ensure adequate protection from low ambient temperatures, i.e., contented cows produce more milk.

Supplemental Reading

Blaxter, K. L., and Wainman, F. W.: Environmental temperature and the energy metabolism and heat emission of steers. J. Agri. Sci. 56:81–90, 1961.

Ingram, D. L., and Mount, L. E.: Man and Animals in Hot Enivronments. Heidelberg, Springer-Verlag, 1975.

Zootoxins

MURRAY E. FOWLER, D.V.M.

Zootoxicosis is a disease condition caused by the bite or sting of a venomous animal. Many species of snakes, arachnids, and insects have venomous bites or stings. Most lack sufficient potency to cause more than transient discomfort to livestock. Generally, the incidence of toxicity is very low in food animals, though in certain local geographic areas, the density of venomous snakes or insects may result in considerable loss.

Those species listed in Table 1 are capable of causing disease or death or both in livestock animals in the United States.

Venoms are complex organic substances composed of a wide variety of chemicals, including enzymes, peptides, polypeptides, amines, glycoside anticoagulants, and, in the case of ants, formic acid. Venoms may act locally,

Table 1. *Venomous Animals Causing Zootoxicosis of Food Animals in North America*

Snakes
 Rattlesnake (*Crotalus* sp.)
 Copperhead (*Agkistrodon contortrix*)
 Cottonmouth (*Agkistrodon piscivorus*)
 Coral snake (*Micrurus* sp., *Micruroides enryxanthus*)

Arachnids
 Black widow spider (*Lactrodectus mactans*)
 Scorpion (*Centuroides* sp.)

Insects
 Honey bee (*Apis mellifera*)
 Hornet (*Vespula* sp.)
 Wasp (*Polistes* sp.)
 Imported fire ant (*Solenopsis saevissima richteri*)

causing tissue necrosis, vascular thrombosis, and hemorrhage or may be transported to other sites throughout the body, causing neurotoxicity and hemolysis. Venoms are also allergenic, making previously sensitized animals susceptible to anaphylactic shock.

SNAKES

It is impossible to describe the clinical signs of poisonings from all the myriad types of venomous snakes found worldwide. The reader is directed to the literature for specific information on the exotic species in a particular area of the world.[1, 2] Unfortunately, it is not outside the realm of possibility for an animal to suffer a bite from a cobra in the United States, as cobras have escaped from captivity or have been deliberately released into the wild.

Coral snakes are small and secretive and rarely bite livestock. Bites from copperheads and water moccasins are usually innocuous in livestock. Therefore, this discussion is confined to the effects of rattlesnake bite.

Clinical Signs

Bites on the limbs cause erythema and marked edema at the injection site. Necrosis may result from the cytotoxic effects of venom, particularly that of the larger rattlesnakes. Based on reports of similar bites in humans, intense pain is associated with the swelling. Animals wince on palpation or manipulation of a swollen limb, a good clue to differentiate between snake bite and edema caused by venous stasis. Locomotion may be stiff and painful.

The exact site of envenomation is rarely visible. Shortly after the time of the bite, pronounced swelling will obliterate the marks of penetration. Bites on the head produce similar signs, with the added hazard of impaired breathing if swelling closes the nostrils. A bloodstained frothy discharge from the nostrils is common in bites on the muzzle. Death can result from occlusion of the airways. One or both eyes may be swollen shut, resulting in temporary blindness and inability to locate food.

Most North American rattlesnake venoms produce minimal neural signs. The Mojave green rattlesnake, *Crotalus scutulatus*, is an exception, injecting a potent neurotoxic venom. Cattle and sheep are grazed in the deserts inhabited by this snake, and bites may occur. Paralysis, convulsions, and death may ensue before local reactions become prominent. Diagnosis of such a bite would be extremely difficult without a satisfactory history.

Swine are not totally resistant to snake bite, but injection of the venom into subcutaneous fat diminishes absorption and severity of toxicity.[3]

Diagnosis

Differential diagnosis must include contusions and fractures of the head or limbs. Radiographs may be required. Abscess of the pharyngeal or parotid regions may cause venous stasis and edema of the head. Cellulitis from clostridial infections may mimic limb bites. Rattlesnakes are active only during warm seasons, so bites would likely be precluded during cold winter months.

Treatment

Rattlesnake bite in livestock is treated according to symptoms. Immediate cool hydrotherapy minimizes edema of an affected limb. Once the swelling has formed, warm hydrotherapy may effectively stimulate circulation and removal of tissue fluids. Bites on the head and neck require more intensive therapy. Be prepared to perform a tracheotomy if airways become obstructed.

Antihistamines are contraindicated because their hypotensive action may be additive with that of the venom. Corticosteroids may be beneficial in reducing inflammation but are not required for successful management of a bite.

Antivenin administration to livestock victims of snake bite in the western and northern sections of the country is rarely warranted except for calves, lambs, or piglets. In most cases, specific diagnosis is rarely made early enough for antivenin administration to be beneficial.

Bites of the large eastern diamondback rattlesnake, *Crotalus adamanteus*, may be lethal to cattle, sheep, and goats. If an animal is observed being bitten by such a snake, it is advisable to administer specific antivenin* intravenously within 2 hr. From 2 to 4 vials should be given, and the patient should be monitored for 8 to 10 hr to determine if additional antivenin is needed.

If necrosis and sloughing of tissue begins, débride the necrotic tissue and provide routine wound care. Parenteral antibiotics may be indicated if vital tissues, joints, tendons, or nerves are exposed.

SPIDERS AND SCORPIONS

Although animals are susceptible to the effects of spider and scorpion venoms, documented bites in livestock are rare.

INSECTS

Damage to livestock from poisonous insect bites is uncommon, but the hazard should be recognized. Stings from bees, wasps, hornets, and ants cause the same discomfort in animals as in humans.

Insect venoms are allergenic, so that multiple stings can be serious, especially if days or weeks elapse between envenomations. Sensitized animals may suffer anaphylaxis. Diagnosis is difficult if not impossible unless the sting and subsequent clinical signs are observed.

*Antivenin (Crotalidae) Polyvalent available from Wyeth Laboratories, Marietta, PA 17547.

Occasionally, an animal will become entrapped in an area where bees, wasps, or ants become enraged and descend upon the victim in large numbers, inflicting hundreds or thousands of stings. Such massive injections of venom may elicit a shock response and death within minutes to hours, or a delayed response similar to serum sickness may develop in 2 to 12 days.

The African honey bee, *Apis mellifera adansonii,* has spread to South America, and is called the killer bee. In Brazil, 300 to 400 human deaths a year are attributed to stinging by masses of this bee. Numerous livestock are also killed. Livestock handlers are fearful that this bee could gain a foothold in the United States as well.[4] Multiple stings by a colony of enraged bees can kill large animals. In India, giant Indian bees, *A. dorsata,* have killed water buffalo and even an elephant.[1] In the United States, individuals of all livestock species are potential victims of colonial wasp and bee attacks if an animal harasses the colony.

The fire ant, *Solenopsis saevissima richteri,* is a serious imported pest in the southeastern United States.[5] Adult livestock may be repeatedly stung and killed if they are unable to escape from a colony of fire ants.

Diagnosis

Single insect bites or stings produce local transient erythema, swelling, and pain. Without an adequate history, differential diagnosis must include contusions, foreign body penetration, localized cellulitis, and urticaria. Differentiation of systemic effects include drug reactions and other shock-inducing conditions.

Treatment

Local treatment of insect bites or stings is similar to that used for snake bites.

Injections of corticosteroids are indicated. Dexamethasone, 4 mg/kg every 4 hr intramuscularly or intravenously will aid in diminishing inflammatory and allergic response. If shock or anaphylaxis occurs, quick administration of epinephrine 1:1000 in doses of 1 ml/50 kg of body weight is indicated.

References

1. Caras, R.: Venomous Animals of the World. Englewood Cliffs, New Jersey, Prentice-Hall, Inc., 1974.
2. Moore, G. M. (ed.): Poisonous Snakes of the World, NAVMED P-5099. Washington, D.C.: United States Government Printing Office, 1966.
3. Oehme, F. W., Brown, J. F., and Fowler, M. E.: Toxins of Animal Origin. *In* Casarett, L. J., and Doull, J. (eds.): Toxicology. New York, Macmillan Publishing Co., 1975.
4. Rathmayer, W.: Hymenoptera: The Aculeate Wasps, Ants and Bees. *In* Grzimek, B. (ed.): Grzimek's Animal Life Encyclopedia, vol. 2: Insects. New York, Van Nostrand-Reinhold, 1975.
5. James, M. T., and Harwood, R. F.: Herm's Medical Entomology, 6th ed. New York, Macmillan Publishing Co., 1969.

Refer to the first volume of Current Veterinary Therapy: Food Animal Practice for the following:

Oehme, F. W.: Potential Sources of Poisoning in Food Animals. Section 6, Physical and Chemical Disorders.

Sorensen, D. K.: Chlorinated Naphthalenes. Section 6, Physical and Chemical Disorders.

Van Gelder, G. A.: Fungicides. Section 6, Physical and Chemical Disorders.

Van Gelder, G. A.: Fumigants. Section 6, Physical and Chemical Disorders.

Van Gelder, G. A.: Iron. Section 6, Physical and Chemical Disorders.

VIRUS, CHLAMYDIAE, AND MYCOPLASMA (BOVINE, SHEEP, GOAT, AND SWINE)

A. KONRAD EUGSTER, D.V.M., Ph.D.
Consulting Editor

Diagnosis of Viral Diseases

ROBERT A. CRANDELL, B.S., D.V.M., M.P.H.

A laboratory diagnosis of a viral disease may not influence the course of treatment. However, an accurate diagnosis of disease is important for reasons other than therapy. The demonstration of a virus as the etiologic agent may provide the information necessary to introduce control measures to prevent the recurrence or spread of the disease. This is especially true for those virus diseases for which specific vaccines are available. The discovery of new viral entities and the early recognition of foreign animal diseases are two very important reasons for establishing a definitive diagnosis. It is true that a diagnosis is retrospective; the diagnostic report often reaches the clinician after the animal has either died or recovered. However, the constant vigil in the search for causes of new disease entities is paramount to the livestock industry. This fact was most vividly demonstrated recently with the introduction of African swine fever into the Western Hemisphere. It is essential that the clinician notify the appropriate veterinary authorities whenever he suspects a reportable or exotic disease.

There are three basic approaches for obtaining a laboratory diagnosis of a viral infection: (1) examination of biologic material by microscopic techniques, (2) isolation and identification of the causative agent, and (3) demonstration of the appearance of or rise in serum titer to a specific antigen during a recent disease.

Microscopic Examination

Microscopic methods employing biologic specimens include the examination of impression smears and histologic sections, immunofluorescence, and electron microscopy. In these procedures, the tissues are examined for pathologic changes or presence of viral antigen.

The observation of characteristic pathologic lesions or the demonstration of typical inclusion bodies is of diagnostic value in some viral diseases. Some examples in which inclusion bodies are helpful in arriving at a diagnosis are canine distemper, rabies, herpesvirus, and animal and fowl pox infections. In conditions such as cytomegalic inclusion disease (inclusion body rhinitis [IBR]) of swine, the diagnosis is generally dependent upon the finding of large intranuclear inclusions. Bovine abortions due to IBR infection are often recognized by their characteristic histopathologic lesions.

The technique of "smear diagnosis" is sometimes helpful in virus diseases associated with inclusion bodies. It has been advocated for diseases such as canine hepatitis (adenovirus) and avian laryngotracheitis. However, it has limited usefulness and is not routinely used. Since many inclusion bodies are transient in nature, they are either absent or sparse during the later stages of illness and will not be found. The recognition of specific viral inclusions in tissue smears is difficult and requires experience.

In certain virus diseases in which these methods are applied, it is desirable to confirm the findings by some other procedure. It is always advisable in doubtful cases to freeze some tissue at the time of necropsy for further use. If inclusions or lesions suggestive of a virus infection are found on histologic examination, the frozen tissue may be used for isolation or fluorescent antibody studies. On the other hand, if the diagnosis is obviously of nonviral origin, the material can be discarded.

Since the demonstration of rabies antigen in tissues by fluorescent staining, the technique has become widely used in veterinary diagnostic medicine. The fluorescent antibody (FA) test for rabies diagnosis is more sensitive than the smear technique, and its results compare very well with those obtained by mouse inoculation. The antigen-antibody reaction is highly specific. The test is a visual observation of the localization of virus antigen in the tissues by its combination (reaction) with specific serum antibody labeled (conjugated) with fluorescein isothiocyanate.

Specific examples of other viral diseases in which the fluorescent antibody test is useful for detection of virus in clinical and necropsy material are calf rotavirus, infectious bovine rhinotracheitis, pseudorabies, and transmissible gastro-enteritis (TGE).

The application of the electron microscope to the diagnosis of virus infections has advanced the art of diagnostic medicine. The visualization of virus particles in clinical and necropsy specimens has contributed greatly to the recognition of new disease entities and the identification of many of the old ones. A diagnosis of pox infections can be made within an hour by electron microscopic examination of preparations of crusts from the lesions, whereas days are required by cell culture methods.

Isolation and Identification

The isolation and identification of viruses is the most costly approach to diagnosis in terms of resources and time. However, it is the method of choice under the following circumstances: (1) in undescribed disease conditions in which the etiologic agent has not been demonstrated and grown in the laboratory, (2) in highly acute illness with early death, (3) in those diseases involving viruses of multiple antigenic subtypes, and (4) in all suspect cases of an exotic or foreign disease.

In the first situation, the initial isolation and propagation of the viral agent from a new disease entity is necessary before any serologic test is possible. Without the antigen (causative agent) and efficient means of producing it, a serologic procedure cannot be developed. In those illnesses resulting in an early death, there may be insufficient time for the development of a demonstrable specific antibody response. Therefore, the recovery of the agent from tissue or body fluids is the only means of making a diagnosis.

Picornaviruses have been shown to exist in a multiplicity of antigenic types or subtypes in some species of animals (bovine and porcine). In these species, it is desirable at times to attempt virus isolation rather than perform serologic tests against so many viruses. Also, it must be remembered that there is a limit to the number of serologic procedures that can be performed on one serum sample. This is particularly true in cases involving smaller animals, where the quantity of serum is sometimes limited.

It is also advisable periodically to isolate viruses from animals with the more commonly known diseases. This offers an opportunity to conduct laboratory studies on the viruses in search of any biologic or antigenic alteration in current field strains. This knowledge is important, particularly if vaccines are used in their control.

When clinical material is submitted for virus isolation, it is recommended that paired (acute and convalescent) serum be included if available. If a virus is recovered, the sera can then be tested for specific antibodies against the isolate. This is important in determining the role that the virus played in the disease. Animals, like man, harbor many viruses that at times do not cause illness. The mere isolation of a virus from a clinical or pathologic specimen does not always constitute a definitive diagnosis.

Serology

Serologic procedures offer far greater usefulness in diagnostic medicine than the other two approaches. Generally, serologic methods provide laboratory information faster and are less expensive. However, serologic methods do not give the same degree of assurance of etiologic involvement. As stated earlier, serologic tests are limited to those diseases in which the causative agent has been isolated and can be successfully propagated. Serologic methods are not applicable in fatal infections where there has been insufficient time for the development of specific antibody. Isolation of the etiologic agent is then the only means of obtaining a diagnosis.

Serum specimens must be paired, since only a rise in specific antibody titer is positive evidence of current infection. The first sample should be collected as early as possible in the illness and the second from two to four weeks later during convalescence. Serologic tests now employed routinely for the diagnosis of common virus diseases are the serum neutralization, complement-fixation, hemagglutination-inhibition and immunodiffusion, and the indirect fluorescent antibody test. More recently, an enzyme-linked immunosorbent assay (ELISA) is being used.

The demonstration of antibodies in a single serum specimen is of little diagnostic value. It may be only an expression of the vaccination status of the animal or prior experience with the virus at an undetermined time. The occurrence of IBR antibody in many bovine populations is reported to be very common. With a high prevalence of positive animals, it is mandatory that paired serum be required if meaningful laboratory results are to be obtained. Serologic data on single serum specimens are useful in providing information on disease incidence and distribution if interpreted with caution.

COLLECTION AND PREPARATION OF SPECIMENS

Specimens for Virus Isolation

Materials for isolation should be obtained in the early acute, febrile stage of illness. The choice of specimen is obviously the material that is most likely to contain the virus. Therefore, the source of material will depend upon the nature of the clinical disease. For example, if the disease syndrome involves the respiratory system, nasal secretions would be the clinical specimen of choice. Since many animal viruses manifest themselves by producing diseases with varied clinical signs, it is necessary to obtain material according to the type of illness. This is particularly true with some enteroviruses and the viruses belonging to the herpesvirus group. Clinical and necropsy specimens should be collected with aseptic precautions, and sterile containers should be used. The usual clinical materials submitted include nasal, ocular, and vaginal swabs, blood, skin lesions, and feces.

A diagnosis for some virus diseases is best achieved by performing several diagnostic procedures. The recommended clinical and necropsy specimens for virus isolation, electron microscopy, and fluorescent staining are listed in Table 1. The table is intended to serve as a guide for the selection of specimens for virus diagnosis. The clinician should consult the diagnostic laboratory for more detailed information. It is also recommended that more than one animal be examined from an outbreak.

Swabs are obtained by using a sterile dry cotton swab to absorb the secretions from the conjunctiva or nasal, oropharyngeal, or vaginal mucosa. Preferably swabs should be immersed immediately into a tube containing about 1 to 2 ml of transport medium. The swab is rinsed in the medium and the fluid pressed out against the side

Table 1. Recommended Specimens for Virus Isolation, Electron Microscopy, and Fluorescent Antibody Test*

Anatomic Site or Type of Illness	Associated Virus	Clinical Specimen	Necropsy Specimen
Respiratory infections	Adenovirus	Nasal and ocular secretions, feces	Lung, feces
	Bovine virus diarrhea	Nasal secretions	Lung, spleen
	Infectious bovine rhinotracheitis	Nasal and ocular secretions	Lung, tracheal swab
	Influenza	Nasal and ocular secretions	Lung, tracheal swab
	Parainfluenza	Nasal and ocular secretions	Lung, tracheal swab
	Pseudorabies (Aujeszky's)	Nasal secretions	Tonsil, lung, brain
Infections of mucous membranes and skin	Pox viruses	Lesion scrapings, biopsy	Lesions
	Mammillitis (herpesvirus)	Lesion scrapings, biopsy	Lesions
	Foot-and-mouth Vesicular stomatitis Vesicular exanthema Swine vesicular disease	Vesicular fluid, epithelial covering of lesion	Vesicular fluid, epithelial covering of lesion
Infections of central nervous system	Enteroviruses	Nasal swab, feces	Tonsil, brain (swine); feces (cattle and swine)
	Infectious bovine rhinotracheitis	Nasal secretions	Brain, lung, tracheal swab
	Pseudorabies (Aujeszky's)	Nasal secretions, tonsillar swab	Brain, spinal cord (sheep and cattle); brain, tonsil, liver, spleen (swine)
	Rabies	Consult with laboratory personnel	Brain
Enteric infections	Bovine virus diarrhea	Blood, oral lesions, feces	Spleen, mesenteric nodes, intestinal mucosa, feces
	Enterovirus	Feces, oropharyngeal swab	Feces, tonsils
	Rinderpest	Blood	Spleen, mesenteric lymph nodes
	Transmissible gastroenteritis (TGE)	Feces, nasal secretions	Tonsils, jejunum, ileum, feces
	Rotaviruses	Feces	Feces
	Parvovirus	Feces	Feces
	Coronavirus	Feces	Feces
Hemorrhagic syndrome (viremia)	African swine fever	Blood	Spleen, liver, tonsil, lymph nodes, blood
	Hog cholera	Tonsil biopsy	Tonsil, spleen, liver, brain
	Bluetongue	Blood (heparinized)	Heart blood, spleen
Genital infections and abortions	Infectious bovine rhinotracheitis Enteroviruses Bovine virus diarrhea Pseudorabies (Aujeszky's) Parvovirus (swine) Bluetongue	Vaginal secretions, serum from dam or sow	Tissue from aborted fetus: liver spleen, lung, brain, kidney Body fluids for serology Lung (mummified fetus) Fetal heart blood, spleen, bone marrow

*Serum should be collected at the same time clinical specimens are obtained and again in two to three weeks for serologic testing.

of the collecting vessel. The fluid should be a balanced salt solution (BSS) buffered near neutral pH and should contain a protein that helps preserve the stability of the virus. Suggested transport fluid is Hanks' balanced salt solution with either 0.5 per cent gelatin, bovine serum albumin, or skim milk. If a transport medium is unavailable, place the cotton swab into a sterile blood collecting tube and close with the rubber stopper. Material from skin lesions is also collected in a similar manner.

Feces (10 to 15 g) and necropsy specimens should be placed in a small wide-mouthed glass jar or in a carton made of plastic or heavy waxed paper (Dixie cup) with a tight-sealing lid. Although rectal swabs are not as effective as feces, they may be collected with a moist cotton swab and handled like the nasal swabs.

All specimens for virus isolation should be frozen if it takes more than a few hours to get them to the laboratory. When delivered immediately, they should be kept in wet ice. For longer periods of time, dry ice is recommended. The specimens must be in an airtight container because dry ice releases CO_2 gas, which is deleterious to most viruses.

Leak-proof stoppers or caps should be used on all jars and tubes. Cork stoppers should not be used unless they are paraffin-treated. Always secure the tops in place with several turns of a high-quality adhesive tape.

No preservatives or fixatives should be added to specimens for virus isolation.

Serum for Serologic Tests

Blood should be collected in a clean, sterile, dry tube or syringe without an anticoagulant. An adequate amount of serum can be obtained from 10 to 15 ml of whole blood. The larger quantity of serum is desirable to allow for multiple tests, confirmation, or repetition of equivocal results. If bleeding is accomplished with a syringe, the needle should be removed before the blood is transferred to a sterile, dry tube. This precaution will reduce hemolysis. Rubber-stoppered vacutainer tubes without an anticoagulant are recommended for large animals. The tube should stand at room temperature for at least 30 minutes (more time may be desired) to allow the clot to form. The specimen is then refrigerated at 4°C (household refrigerator) to accelerate the contraction of the clot. The clot is separated by centrifugation at 1500 rpm for 10 minutes. The serum is carefully withdrawn from the clot with a sterile pipette. A rubber bulb attached to a Pasteur pipette is a very convenient means of removing the serum. The serum is transferred, preferably to a sterile, rubber-stoppered tube. Screw-capped tubes are not recommended because leakage frequently occurs. If screw-capped tubes are used, the cap should be secured with adhesive tape. When a centrifuge and pipettes are not available, the clear serum can be removed from the clot by pouring it into another sterile tube. It is recommended that the serum be separated from the clot before it is shipped to the laboratory.

The sterility and condition of serum for serodiagnosis cannot be overemphasized. Serum specimens with a microbial contamination or hemolysis are unsatisfactory for testing. Since living cell cultures or animals are used in serum neutralization tests, any contamination of the serum will result in death of the host employed. Hemolysis of red blood cells in serum interferes with the complement-fixation test and should be avoided. Preservatives such as phenol or Merthiolate should not be added, since they

are toxic to cell cultures. Whole blood intended for serologic testing *should never* be frozen.

PACKAGING AND SHIPPING OF SPECIMENS

Identification

Each individual specimen tube or jar should be clearly identified with the animal's number, date of collection, and type of specimen. It is recommended that adhesive tape be used to label each container. All information should be either typewritten or printed with a lead pencil. Fountain pens, ball-point pens, wax or indelible pencils, and markers should not be used to identify specimens. Markings made by these items become illegible through handling.

Packaging

Proper packaging not only ensures the safety of the specimens but also protects the mails and the personnel handling them.

Frozen specimens for virus isolation should be individually wrapped with an absorbent material such as cotton or paper towels. The wrapped specimens are then packed in a small cylindrical shipping container or can or any sturdy carton. The specimen package is then placed in the center of a larger insulated box next to dry ice. The specimen and dry ice are surrounded with about 15 cm of shock-resistant material (cotton, crumpled newspaper). It is important to have sufficient packing material to compensate for the loss of dry ice by evaporation. This will prevent the specimen from rattling freely in the package. *Never* ship dry ice in an air-tight container.

It is recommended that serum samples for serologic tests be shipped under refrigeration. The tubes must be packed adequately to protect them against leakage or breakage. The specimens should be shipped by the most rapid means.

Shipping

If long distances are involved, the specimens should be sent by *air mail*. In cases of virus isolation specimens, it is recommended that the diagnostic laboratory be notified by telephone of the contents, carrier, and estimated time of arrival. Frozen specimens should never be shipped over weekends or holidays. It is desirable to have specimens arrive at the laboratory during the working day.

All specimens should be accompanied by the standard laboratory submission form. The history should be as complete as possible. Additional information such as the vaccination status of an animal is necessary in interpreting serologic results.

The laboratory should be consulted by telephone if any doubt exists as to the type of specimen to collect or method of shipment.

Shipments should be identified (e.g., "Perishable," "Biologic Material," "Packed in Dry Ice," "Protect from Extreme Heat," "Fragile," or any other suitable designation) to help safeguard the contents and exposed persons.

When in doubt as to the mailability of any material, consult your local postmaster.

In addition to the mails, specimens may be shipped by United Parcel Service or bus transportation. If air transportation is used, the shipper must follow appropriate regulations.

Infectious Bovine Rhinotracheitis

ROBERT A. CRANDELL, B.S., D.V.M., M.P.H.

Infectious bovine rhinotracheitis (IBR) was first recognized in the United States as an acute, febrile, highly contagious respiratory illness of cattle. The causative agent is a virus that is now known to be the cause of a variety of clinical syndromes. The respiratory disease produced by this virus is often called necrotic rhinitis and red nose. The genital infections are referred to as coital vesicular exanthema, Bläschenausschlag, infectious pustular vulvovaginitis, and infectious pustular balanoposthitis. The virus is responsible for severe economic losses to the cattle industry, and it has worldwide distribution.

ETIOLOGY

IBR is caused by a herpesvirus. Because the virus is also the cause of infectious pustular vulvovaginitis (IPV), it is sometimes referred to as IBR/IPV. All isolated IBR viruses belong to one serotype. Although they are serologically indistinguishable, the viruses produce a variety of clinical manifestations. IBR virus is sensitive to lipid solvents, heat, and acid but persists for several days at 4°C and remains viable for years when frozen. The virus grows well in a large number of cell cultures and, with the exception of rabbits, does not produce illness in the common laboratory animals and embryonating eggs.

EPIZOOTIOLOGY

IBR virus is recognized as having a worldwide distribution and is the cause of two different diseases within two population groups of cattle. In areas where there is a high concentration of cattle, the most important disease involves the respiratory system, whereas in the less populated areas the diseases of the reproductive system are more common.

IBR was first recognized in the United States as a respiratory disease of cattle in 1950. The disease occurred sporadically in feedlots, where it became known as "red nose," "dust pneumonia," and necrotic rhinotracheitis. The upper respiratory disease also occurred in dairy herds in epizootic proportions. Infections of the respiratory tract continue to be prevalent where large concentrations of dairy and beef cattle are assembled.

Clinical signs usually appear in feeder cattle seven days to two weeks after entering the feedlot. Virus shed from the ocular and nasal secretions is transmitted to susceptible cattle by direct contact. Feeder calves usually enter the feedlot at an age when they have lost their maternal (passive) antibody and are susceptible to infection. Additional insults from shipment, exposure to multiple infectious agents, and other stresses reduce their resistance to infection.

The reproductive form of the disease is transmitted primarily by coitus. Genital infections are more common in the conventionally managed European dairy and beef herds. The virus is shed in secretions of the reproductive organs.

After introduction into the Western feedlots, the virus adapted to the new host-environmental relationship by acquiring an affinity for the respiratory tract. Since the animal population of the feedlots is mostly steers and heifers that are reproductively inactive, the virus was probably unable to maintain itself as a genital infection. Explosive outbreaks of infections of the genitalia have occurred by using IBR virus–contaminated semen for artificial insemination.

Although cattle are considered to be the major reservoir of infection, virus isolations have been reported in goats, pigs, water buffalo, antelope, and wildebeest. Antibodies have been demonstrated in several wildlife species, including deer. The significance of these observations in relation to the spread of the IBR is unknown.

The virus can persist in the animal for years following an infection. These latent infections are potential sources for new outbreaks. Latent virus is re-activated with injections of corticosteroids, resulting in active shedding of infectious virus.

It is believed that stress from a number of causes may induce re-activation of the virus. New outbreaks in feedlots and closed herds may result from excretion of virus from a latent carrier. All serologic-positive animals should be considered as potential carriers. The feature of latency in IBR infections presents a problem with the shipment and export of cattle to IBR-free areas.

CLINICAL FORMS AND SIGNS

IBR infections are manifested in a variety of clinical forms. The clinical diseases caused by the IBR virus can be grouped as (1) respiratory tract infections, (2) conjunctivitis, (3) genital tract infections and abortions, (4) central nervous system infections, (5) fatal generalized disease of neonatal calves, and (6) miscellaneous infections.

Respiratory Tract Infections

The respiratory disease was the first clinical manifestation of the IBR infection recognized in the United States and is the most common form of the disease. The respiratory illness has a sudden onset and is characterized by fever of 40.0 to 41.5°C, salivation, rhinitis, loss of appetite, rapid and shallow respiration, and dyspnea. Dairy cattle experience an abrupt drop in milk production.

The nasal secretions are serous at first, and the nasal mucosa is hyperemic. In severe cases the exudate becomes copious and fibrinopurulent and is loosely attached to the mucosal surface. Beneath the exudate the mucosa is reddened and may contain necrotic foci. In advanced cases, the airways become blocked, resulting in respiratory distress with open-mouth breathing.

Generally, auscultation reveals nothing more than the sounds due to obstruction of upper air passages. In field cases, pneumonia is a common complication, and rales become audible.

Conjunctivitis is not a consistent sign in the respiratory disease. When present, the ocular discharges become copious and purulent as the disease progresses.

The acute stage of illness lasts from 5 to 10 days, and most animals will recover in 10 to 14 days. The mortality rate is higher in the more stressed animal, and death is usually the result of a bacterial bronchopneumonia.

Conjunctivitis

Although a severe conjunctivitis with profuse lacrimation is common in the typical respiratory form of IBR infection, it may also occur as the primary clinical feature in some infections. The conjunctiva is inflamed and edematous, and the condition is usually bilateral. The ocular discharge is clear initially but becomes mucopurulent following bacterial involvement. The hair on the side of the face below the eyes becomes wet and soiled. Corneal opacities may occur and are often confused with other conditions such as infectious keratitis.

Genital Tract Infections and Abortions

Infectious pustular vulvovaginitis is the name given to the infection of the vaginal and vulvar mucosa. This disease has been known in Europe since the mid-nineteenth century as "Blaschenausschlag." The infection in bulls is called balanoposthitis. Genital infection has occurred concurrently in herds with the respiratory form of the disease.

The acute infection develops within one to three days after coitus. The disease may be mild and unnoticed; however, in severe infections animals exhibit pain, dysuria, and frequent urination, and tail swishing is common. The vulva is edematous and hyperemic, and the mucosal surface is covered with small pustules. These coalesce, forming white necrotic plaques that leave ulcers when removed from the mucosal surface. These changes extend into the vagina and are accompanied by a mucopurulent exudate. The lesions may heal in 10 to 14 days, but a vaginal discharge may persist in some animals for several weeks.

Lesions similar to those described for pustular vulvovaginitis develop on the mucosa of the penis and prepuce of infected bulls. Secondary infections are common with a mucopurulent discharge present at the preputial orifice. Semen becomes contaminated with virus from these lesions. In severe cases, extensive adhesions and penile distortion may occur.

Central Nervous System Infections

IBR virus has been isolated from the brains of fatal cases of nonpurulent meningo-encephalitis in young calves. The disease has been described in both dairy and beef calves. The animals refuse to eat and exhibit intermittent generalized tremors with periods of excitement characterized by incoordinated movements, running, circling, and stumbling. These are followed by depression, recumbency, coma, and death.

Generalized Disease of Neonatal Calves

A fatal generalized infection occurs in neonatal calves that become infected *in utero* or early after birth. The temperature may exceed 40°C and is accompanied by complete anorexia, depression, and respiratory distress. A serous ocular discharge and diarrhea may be present. The condition is often associated with a herd experiencing abortions.

Miscellaneous Infections

Infections of the udder and intestinal tract have been reported but seldom appear as a distinct clinical entity.

DIAGNOSIS

The clinical and pathologic features of the disease are helpful in obtaining a presumptive diagnosis. IBR should be considered in any sudden outbreak of an upper respiratory infection and in cases of vaginitis and abortions. The presence of white plaques on the mucosal surface of the nasal cavity and vagina are suggestive of IBR infection. A typical finding at necropsy is an inflamed trachea with a fibropurulent exudate loosely attached to the mucosal surface. Although intranuclear inclusion bodies are a characteristic feature of the herpesvirus infections, they are not a common histologic finding.

A definitive diagnosis can be obtained by laboratory procedures. The virus is easily isolated from a number of infected tissues by cell culture techniques. Clinical specimens selected for virus isolation should be collected during the febrile stage of illness. The type of specimen to collect is determined by the form of disease. Swabs containing ocular and nasal secretions are recommended in cases of conjunctivitis and respiratory forms of the disease. Vaginal and preputial swabs are the specimens of choice for diagnosing genital infections.

The fluorescent antibody technique is used to detect IBR virus in tissue from aborted fetuses and neonatal calves succumbing to a generalized infection. The liver, spleen, kidney, lung, and adrenals are the preferred tissues and are also used for virus isolation. Histopathologic examination of the fetal liver often reveals intranuclear inclusion bodies in epithelial cells surrounding areas of necrosis.

The central nervous system infections must be differentiated from other infectious diseases such as pseudorabies, rabies, *Haemophilus somnus* septicemia, and listeriosis.

The serum neutralization test is the serologic procedure used to measure the specific IBR antibodies in the blood serum. Since a rise in the antibody titer is evidence of a recent infection, it is necessary to test paired serum samples. The first sample should be obtained during the acute stage of illness, and the second is collected two to three weeks later. Titers on single serum specimens are of no diagnostic significance.

A complete history is necessary for a meaningful interpretation of laboratory results.

TREATMENT

Since IBR is a virus infection, the therapy is directed toward controlling the secondary bacterial complications. The early administration of antibiotics with supportive therapy is recommended. Good husbandry practices should be instituted to reduce and minimize stress. Sick animals should be isolated and provided shelter, food, and water. Results of recent studies indicate that the use of corticosteroids is contraindicated in the treatment of bronchopneumonia in cattle. *The administration of corticosteroids will re-activate latent IBR virus infections in cattle.*

PREVENTION AND CONTROL

Vaccines have played a major role in the prevention and control of IBR infections. Good management practices without vaccination have been relatively ineffective in preventing the spread of the virus to susceptible herds. The development of latent infections in recovered animals with virus shedding has contributed to the difficulty in preventing the introduction of the virus into clean herds. The isolation of severely infected cattle during an outbreak will, however, tend to limit the spread and severity of the disease within a herd.

Several types of effective vaccines are marketed. The parenteral modified live virus (MLV) is not recommended for use in pregnant animals. The intranasal MLV vaccines are reported to be safe for use in pregnant animals. Parenteral vaccines are considered by some to be easier to administer than the intranasal vaccines because less animal restraint is required. The parenteral vaccines are available in combination with bovine virus diarrhea (BVD) and parainfluenza-3 (PI-3) viruses. Some IBR intranasal vaccines contain PI-3 virus.

An inactivated IBR vaccine is available as a single virus vaccine or in combination with other agents.

The vaccination program, selection of vaccine, and frequency of vaccination are usually determined by the local circumstances and the practitioner's experience. Although a few general recommendations concerning vaccinations have been made, the recommendations of the manufacturer on the package insert should be followed. It has been suggested that all breeding females be vaccinated one or more times before their first breeding. Calves should be vaccinated between five and six months of age. If calves are vaccinated earlier, they should be revaccinated after five months but at least one month before breeding. Colostral acquired antibodies persist for about five months and will interfere with the effectiveness of the vaccine. Some preconditioning programs recommend that feeder calves be vaccinated at the time of weaning and at least one month before shipment. Unconditioned feeder calves are often vaccinated at the time of arrival at the feedlot. Although the practice of vaccinating cattle in the face of an outbreak is common, it can be hazardous. Vaccines are recommended for use in healthy animals. Vaccination of sick animals against IBR is an additional stress on the animals, particularly if the present illness is caused by another agent or is combined with the IBR virus.

PUBLIC HEALTH CONSIDERATIONS

There is no known direct health hazard of IBR virus to man.

Supplemental Reading

Kahrs, R. F.: Infectious bovine rhinotracheitis: a review and update. J. Am. Vet. Med. Assoc. 171:1055, 1977.

Kahrs, R. F.: Infectious bovine rhinotracheitis. In Viral Diseases of Cattle, 1st ed. Ames, Iowa, Iowa State University Press, 135, 1981.

Pastoret, P. P., Thiry, E., Brochier, B., and Derboven, G.: Bovid herpesvirus 1 infection of cattle: Pathogenesis, latency, consequences of latency. Ann. Rech. Vet. 13:211, 1982.

Bovine Mammillitis

W. B. MARTIN, Ph.D., M.R.C.V.S., D.V.S.M., F.R.S.E.

Bovine mammillitis (bovine herpes or ulcerative mammillitis) is a disease of lactating cows caused by bovine herpesvirus 2 (BHV2). Lesions caused by this virus usually occur as ulcers on the skin of the teats and udders of lactating cows. Sometimes scattered skin nodules occur (pseudo-lumpy skin disease). Ulcers have been described on the nose and in the mouth of calves in affected herds.

EPIZOOTIOLOGY

Evidence of infection has been found in Europe, Africa, Australia, and the United States. In temperate regions, recognizable disease occurs only in the autumn and early winter. The prevalence is generally low, although occasionally outbreaks occur on a number of farms within one area. The means of spread between farms is not known, but it is possible that biting flies mechanically carry infection between herds. Latent infection has been demonstrated[1] and has given rise to the suggestion that susceptible pregnant cows get infected before but do not develop recognizable lesions until parturition. Changes in the hormonal and immune mechanisms at calving may allow the virus to replicate with the development of overt disease.

Useful review articles have been written on this disease.[2, 3]

CLINICAL SIGNS AND LESIONS

First affected are often the primiparous heifers, which develop lesions within a few days of calving. A succession of such cases may occur, and subsequently infection can spread to other cows in the herd.

Signs of generalized illness are usually absent. One or more teats may be affected, and, because of the sudden onset and severe ulceration, traumatic injury may be suspected. Lesions (Fig. 1) may start in several ways but frequently appear as thickened, raised, oval plaques 1 to 2 cm in diameter in the wall of the teat. Another type of developing lesion may involve a large part of the teat, over which the skin becomes discolored, hard and inflexible. Vesicles, which are generally single and large, occur rarely.

Lesions progress rapidly to ulcers, which on the teats are deep, ragged, and painful, and on the udder and perineum are more extensive but superficial. Dark brown or black scabs composed of serous exudate, blood, and necrotic skin usually rapidly cover the ulcers, and healing occurs by granulation and regrowth of the epithelium. Damage caused by milking slows down this process so that healing may take several weeks. In some cows mastitis

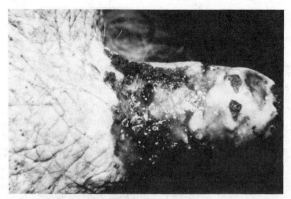

Figure 1. Severe teat lesions caused by bovine mammillitis virus.

develops, which may lead to permanent loss of one or more quarters.

In pseudo-lumpy skin disease, hard nodules develop on the skin and over the neck, thorax, and perineum.[4] This syndrome is most frequently seen in tropical and subtropical regions. These nodules separate slowly to leave a hairless patch that persists for months.

The main histologic changes that accompany infection with BHV2 are inflammation, hydropic degeneration, edema, and necrosis of the epidermis. Acidophilic or lightly basophilic intranuclear inclusion bodies and syncytia are present in the early lesions.

DIAGNOSIS

Herpetic lesions on the teats may be mistaken for traumatic injuries or other infections such as foot-and-mouth disease or cowpox. The association with recent calving in those first affected and the seasonal incidence are helpful diagnostic factors. Confirmation of the viral cause can best be obtained by collecting into transport medium the fluid that exudes or can be expressed from a lesion. Scab material is generally unsatisfactory for virus isolation, and tissue for histology is seldom readily obtained.

Serum samples may help to establish that infection is present in the herd.

TREATMENT, PREVENTION, AND CONTROL

Treatment is generally palliative. To date no specific anti-herpesvirus drugs have been shown to be of value in treating BHV2 infections.

Spread of infection between cows should be avoided by milking affected cows last and by general hygienic measures; e.g., dipping milking machine teat clusters in a suitable disinfectant after each cow has been milked is helpful as the virus is rapidly destroyed, particularly by iodophore solutions. Dipping teats in an iodophore solution after milking is also to be recommended.

As the epidemiology of BHV2 infection is not completely understood, no means of prevention can be convincingly recommended. As flies possibly transport virus, dry cows and heifers should be kept away from wooded or other areas where flies abound and sprayed periodically with one of the modern insecticidal preparations such as permethrin.

References

1. Martin, W. B., and Scott, F. M. M.: Latent infection of cattle with bovid herpesvirus 2. Arch. Virol. 6:51–58, 1979.
2. Cilli, V., and Castrucci, G.: Infection of cattle with bovid herpesvirus 2. Folia Vet. Latina 6:1–44, 1976.
3. Gibbs, E. P. J., and Rweyemamu, M. M.: Bovine herpesvirus. Part II. Bovine herpesvirus 2 and 3. Vet. Bull. 47: 411–425, 1977.
4. Weiss, K. E.: Lumpy skin disease. In Emerging Diseases of Animals, FAO Agricultural Studies No. 61. Rome, Food and Agric. Organization of the United Nations, 1963.

Malignant Catarrhal Fever

ANTHONY E. CASTRO, D.V.M., Ph.D.

Malignant catarrhal fever (MCF) has been described as a sporadic but highly fatal clinicopathologic condition of cattle. This viral disease of domesticated and exotic ruminant species has been characterized as a sheep-associated (European or American) form and as a wildebeest-derived (African) form. Recognition of the sheep-associated form of MCF has occurred worldwide; however, the African form of MCF has been limited to the African continent until recently.

ETIOLOGY

The wildebeest-derived MCF is caused by a herpesvirus (Bovid herpesvirus, type 3). This herpesvirus was isolated from a blue wildebeest in Africa by Plowright and associates. The herpesvirus of MCF has cubic symmetry (icosahedral) and is 100 to 240 nm in diameter, and the nucleocapsid is contained within an envelope. The herpesvirus is highly cell-associated and induces syncytia (i.e., multinucleated giant cells) with intranuclear (Cowdry, type A) inclusion bodies. Only 1 serotype is known. The prototype strain of MCF (WC11) is different from other bovine herpesviruses as determined by restriction-endonuclease fingerprinting of its DNA. MCF virus is extremely susceptible to freezing, although it can remain viable in cells at 4 to 5°C for periods ranging to 30 days. Cell-free MCF virus is infectious; however, it is known to be shed in this form only by newborn wildebeest calves for a three-month period. The MCF virus can be propagated in cells of other nonruminant species following adaptation. An etiologic agent has not yet been identified for the sheep-associated form of MCF. However, there is serologic evidence that certain sheep flocks and individual cattle contain antibodies to the African strain of MCF virus.

EPIZOOTIOLOGY

Worldwide, domestic cattle, buffaloes, bison, gaurs, greater kudus, deer, and antelope species have been reported to be affected by MCF. The incidence is generally sporadic, although epizootics of MCF have occurred. Mortality is usually 95 to 100 per cent following onset of clinical signs. In clinically ill animals, death usually occurs between 2 to 12 days after onset of pyrexia. The disease has no reference to age, sex, or breeds of cattle. MCF virus has been experimentally adapted to rabbits. Wildebeest, hartebeest, and topi are known carriers of the African strain of MCF, but no apparent disease occurs in these species. In these alcelaphine species, induction of virus excretion has occurred following betamethasone injections. Sheep inoculated with the herpesvirus of MCF have developed tumor-like masses, and malignant transformation of cells *in vivo* and *in vitro* may occur since MCF is a lymphoproliferative disease.

MCF virus occurs in nasal and ocular secretions of young wildebeest in a cell-free state. Cattle, however, have cell-associated virus, but not cell-free virus, in secretions, and this may explain the noncontagious nature of MCF when contact occurs with MCF-affected cattle. The association of virus with whole blood has led to the experimental reproduction of MCF in cattle by intravenous inoculation of blood obtained from clinically ill ruminants. However, the means by which MCF virus is transmitted in nature is not completely understood. The method of transmission of sheep-associated MCF has not been determined since the etiologic agent is unknown.

CLINICAL SIGNS (Fig. 1)

Of the herpesviruses of cattle, only MCF virus is known to persist in a viremic stage for prolonged intervals. Clinical forms of MCF have been characterized as (1) peracute with generalized disease, (2) intestinal, (3) head and eye (most common), and (4) a catarrhal form with mild symptoms of catarrh. The clinical signs of MCF include a high fever of 41 to 41.6°C, an encrusted muzzle, a mucopurulent catarrh, inflammatory and degenerative lesions of the respiratory and alimentary tract, ophthalmia with corneal opacity commencing at the limbus with eventual blindness, enlargement of lymph nodes, and diarrhea. The incubation period for African MCF is between two and eight weeks; however, the sheep-associated form may be longer.

DIAGNOSIS

The diagnosis of MCF is based on characteristic pathologic findings, ability to transmit disease by inoculation of blood into susceptible species, serologic conversion, and histopathologic evidence of a necrotizing vasculitis. Basic pathology includes a lymphoreticular cell proliferation in blood vessels of brain, kidney, and liver; angitis and cell infiltration; necrosis in paracortical areas of the lymph nodes; and a progressive destruction and associated dysfunction of thymic T cells.

Virus isolation can be accomplished from fresh buffy coat cells collected in heparinized blood and co-cultivated with cell cultures of fetal bovine kidney or thyroid cells. Identification of isolates of MCF virus can be made by immunofluorescent procedures or by serum-virus neutralization.

Differential diagnoses should include the mucosal disease complex, BVD-IBR, bluetongue, rinderpest, vesicular disease (FMD, VS), Borna disease, salmonellosis, certain toxicoses, and a wide variety of encephalitides of cattle. Because of the atypical cases that have been reported, laboratory diagnoses should be used for confir-

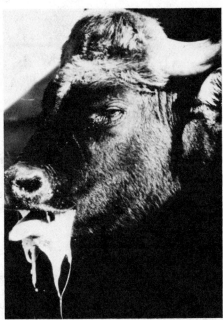

Figure 1. Mucopurulent catarrh associated with clinical MCF in an Indian gaur *(Bos gaurus)*. (Photographed by Dr. P. McCoy at the Oklahoma City Zoo.)

mation. An enzyme-linked immunosorbent assay (ELISA) for MCF that identifies seropositive ruminants has been reported recently.

TREATMENT

An effective treatment for MCF has not been developed. Treatment with corticosteroids, although palliative, is contra-indicated because of exacerbation of the clinical disease and possible abortion. Antibiotics and fluid therapy may prevent secondary clinical problems but will not prolong the life of a clinically ill animal.

PREVENTION AND CONTROL

Presently, control procedures are not available except for the isolation of clinical cases (usually these are fatal). Although arthropod vectors could provide a mechanical transfer, there is no evidence that this is a mode of transmission. If sheep that are lambing are present, segregation from cattle should be considered. An experimental vaccine for MCF has had limited success. Reports of tumor-like lesions in experimentally infected sheep, the fulminating septicemia-like disease, and the highly cell-associated nature of MCF virus indicate that clinically ill animals are unsuited for human or animal consumption.

Supplemental Reading

Castro, A. E., Daley, G. G., Zimmer, M. A., Whitenack, D. L., and Jensen, J.: Malignant catarrhal fever in an Indian gaur and greater kudu: Experimental transmission, isolation and identification of a herpesvirus. Am. J. Vet. Res. *43*:5–11, 1982.

Kahrs, R. F.: Malignant catarrhal fever. *In* Viral Diseases of Cattle, 1st ed. Ames, Iowa, Iowa State University Press, 157–163, 1981.

Mushi, E. Z., and Rurangirwa, F. R.: Epidemiology of bovine malignant catarrhal fevers, a review. Vet. Res. Comm. *5*:127–142, 1981.

Plowright, W., Ferris, R. D., and Scott, G. R.: Blue wildebeest and the aetiological agent of bovine malignant catarrhal fever. Nature *188*:1167–1169, 1960.

Other Bovine Herpesviruses

PAUL C. SMITH, D.V.M., M.S., Ph.D.

Isolations of bovine herpesviruses serologically unrelated to IBR/IPV, bovine herpes mammillitis (BVM), or the virus of the antelope-associated form of malignant catarrhal fever (MCF) from tissues of diseased and apparently healthy cattle are frequent.[1] Their size and morphology are consistent with classification in the family Herpetoviridae. The common biologic properties among these viral isolates include slow cytopathic effects and induction of small plaques in selected cell cultures, maturation and envelopment of virions on nuclear and endoplasmic membranes of infected cells, and antigens differing from other bovine herpesviruses.[2] The DNA genomes of these viral isolates have virtually identical restriction enzyme patterns, which differ from those of bovid herpesvirus-1 (BHV-1), BHV-2, and BHV-6.[3] All isolates studied so far fall into a group of herpesviruses with characteristics typical of cytomegaloviruses, and they are also referred to as bovid herpesvirus 4 (BVH-4).

Several of these viruses[3] (Movar 33/63; FTC-2; DN599) have been isolated from cattle with conjunctivitis and respiratory distress. A careful review of experiments designed to determine the pathogenicity of these viruses for the bovine respiratory system indicate that at best these viruses are of relatively low virulence.[1] Other isolations have been made from uterine exudates of a cow with metritis or from aborted fetuses as well as from lymphoid tissues of clinically normal cattle and cattle affected with MCF.[2, 3]

EPIZOOTIOLOGY

Infections with these herpesviruses in populations of cattle in North America and Europe appear to be widespread and are of a chronic nature. Transmission is suspected to be primarily by direct contact.

CLINICAL SIGNS

The appearance of clinical signs and lesions in infected cattle are ill-defined and nonspecific. In instances where clinical signs and lesions have been associated with virus isolations, the etiologic relationship between disease and virus has been difficult to establish. Recognition of the cytomegalic nature of these viruses may help to assess their pathogenic role, which appears to be characterized by persistent infection and expression by cattle that are immunologically compromised.

DIAGNOSIS

Diagnosis can only be made by isolation and identification of the virus and by indirect fluorescent antibody techniques.

The development of vaccines and treatments for these infections appear at present not to be warranted.

References

1. Smith, P. C.: The bovine herpesviruses: An overview. U.S. Anim. Health Assoc. 80th Ann. Mt., 1976.
2. Todd, W. J., and Storz, J.: Morphogenesis of a cytomegalovirus from an American bison affected with malignant catarrhal fever. J. Gen. Virol. 64:1025–1030, 1983.
3. Ludwig, H.: Bovine herpesviruses. In Roizman, B.: The Herpesviruses, 2nd ed. In Fraenkel-Conrad, H., and Wagner, R. R.: The Viruses. New York, Plenum Press, 1983, 135–428.

Pseudorabies (Aujeszky's Disease, "Mad Itch")

ROBERT A. CRANDELL, B.S., D.V.M., M.P.H.

Pseudorabies (PR) is an infectious disease affecting many animal species including the domestic ruminants. In cattle, sheep, and goats the disease is acute and is characterized by a severe local pruritus with a high mortality. The infected pig is the source of infection for ruminants.

ETIOLOGY

Pseudorabies is caused by a virus belonging to the herpesvirus group. The virus is relatively stable but is inactivated by 5 per cent phenol, sodium hypochlorite, 2 per cent sodium hydroxide, and quaternary ammonia.

EPIZOOTIOLOGY

The virus is transmitted to cattle through the nasal secretions and saliva of infected pigs. In the past it was thought that infections in cattle and sheep were the result of direct contact with the pigs; however, recent observations of natural infections indicate that these species can become infected through the respiratory tract. The virus has been recovered from the nasal mucosa, lungs, brain, and spinal cord of cattle. Infections in cattle and other species have always been considered fatal. However, recent serologic evidence suggests that some cattle have survived a pseudorabies infection.

CLINICAL SIGNS

Intense pruritus is the characteristic sign of illness in cattle. Recent observations indicate that all cattle exposed by the respiratory route may not exhibit pruritus. Some cattle will bloat and die acutely. Body temperatures of 40.5 to 41.5°C have been recorded. The duration of illness is usually short, lasting only one to two days. Infected animals will lick, bite, or rub the site of intense pruritus. Localized areas are frequently found on the head, chest, flank, perineum, and hind legs. The animal often rubs the affected part so as to inflict an open wound (Fig. 1). Infected cattle may not eat and often bellow and stomp their feet. The animals may show aggressiveness, a staggering gait, and partial paralysis of the hindquarters. Cattle, sheep, and goats of both sexes and of all ages and breeds are susceptible to infection. With a few exceptions, most infections in cattle are fatal.

The clinical syndrome in sheep and goats is similar to that observed in cattle.

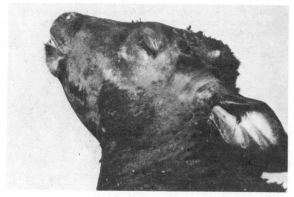

Figure 1. Pseudorabies in a calf. Note swelling and hair loss about the left orbital region and the base of the ear.

DIAGNOSIS

Clinical PR infection in cattle is usually recognized by the intense localized pruritus. However, in some cattle infected by the oral and nasal route, pruritus is not a major clinical feature. If pruritus is present in the anterior portion of the animal, brain stem and spinal cord specimens from the thoracic area should be collected for virus isolation. Brain and spinal cord specimens from the lumbar region are preferred when pruritus and paralysis occur in the posterior part of the body. Lung and brain stem specimens should also be submitted from those acute fatal cases without pruritus.

TREATMENT

There is no treatment that will reverse the course of illness after clinical signs appear.

CONTROL AND PREVENTION

Vaccination of cattle against PR has been reported in Europe; however, there are no vaccines available for cattle in the United States. To prevent the spread of PR infection to domestic ruminants, they should be removed from all contact with swine.

Supplemental Reading

Baker, J. C., Esser, M. B., and Larson, V. L: Pseudorabies in a goat. J. Am. Vet. Med. Assoc. *181*:607, 1982.
Beasley, V. R., Crandell, R. A., Buck, W. B., Ely, R. W., and Thilsted, J., Jr.: A clinical episode demonstrating variable characteristics of pseudorabies infection in cattle. Vet. Res. Commun. *4*:125, 1980.
Bitsch, V.: A study of outbreaks of Aujeszky's disease in cattle. 1. Virological and epidemiological findings. Acta Vet. Scand. *16*:420, 1975.

Cowpox and Bovine Vaccinia Mammillitis

E. PAUL J. GIBBS, B.V.Sc., Ph.D., F.R.C.V.S.

Whereas cowpox was once regarded as an etiologic entity, a clinically indistinguishable teat infection can be caused by both cowpox and vaccinia viruses. Whether vaccinia virus developed from cowpox virus following Jenner's use of the virus as described in 1798 to protect man against smallpox has long been a source of controversy. Whatever the provenance of vaccinia virus, the two viruses can now be easily differentiated by laboratory techniques. Although the mammillitis caused by these two viruses is identical, the different epidemiology of the two infections has necessitated a more exact taxonomy. The term *cowpox* is now used to denote an infection of the bovine teat skin by cowpox virus, and *bovine vaccinia mammillitis* refers to an infection with vaccinia virus.

EPIZOOTIOLOGY

Cowpox is only infrequently recorded and then only in western Europe.[1] The epidemiology of the disease is unknown. Cowpox virus is occasionally isolated from skin infections in man and carnivores, including domestic cats, where no direct contact with cattle can be established. In view of these observations it has been suggested that a rodent or similar animal reservoir exists in which cowpox infection is probably subclinical.[2] Outbreaks of mammillitis associated with vaccinia virus have occurred throughout the world.[1] The source of infection of these outbreaks has invariably been the smallpox vaccination site of the farmer or a member of his family.*

The method of transmission of vaccinia and cowpox viruses between cows has not been studied. The skin of the teats is normally resistant to infection unless abrasions or small wounds exist. These are, however, common in most herds, and the viruses are probably spread by the milking machine and the hands of attendants. Mechanical transmission of virus by biting insects has also been suggested.

CLINICAL SIGNS AND LESIONS (Fig. 1)

The incubation period is approximately five days, after which tenderness of the affected teats is noticed. Erythema with localized edema occurs at the site of future pock development, leading within 48 hours to the formation of a multiloculated vesicle. The vesicle rapidly progresses to a pustule that subsequently ruptures and suppurates. A thick red scab classically follows, but in milking cows ulceration is common. Healing is complete within four weeks. Lesions often affect all four teats and may extend to the skin of the udder.

DIAGNOSIS (Table 1)

The following points should be remembered.[3]

1. Examine the whole herd, not only severely affected stock presented by the farmer. A comparison of the developmental stages helps considerably in the differentiation of the condition, and mature lesions are often similar regardless of cause. A close examination of herds obviously affected with bovine herpes mammillitis or cowpox often reveals pseudocowpox as a second virus infection. Teat warts are also present in most herds.

2. If vesicles are noticed on the teats consider foot-and-mouth disease, vesicular stomatitis, and other reportable diseases.

---

*Readers will note the subtle irony; they should also remember that the root for "vaccination" and "vaccinia" is "vacca"—Latin for cow.

Table 1. *A Summary of the Differential Diagnoses of Cowpox/Bovine Vaccinia Mammillitis, Pseudocowpox, and Bovine Herpes Mammillitis*

Feature	Cowpox/Bovine Vaccinia Mammillitis	Pseudocowpox	Bovine Herpes Mammillitis
Geographical distribution	W. Europe/worldwide	Worldwide	Worldwide
Seasonal incidence	None	None, but outbreaks more common in fall and spring	Summer and fall
Characteristic clinical appearance	Moderate edema; vesicles soon form pustules that subsequently rupture and scab or remain as large ulcers; lesions are essentially proliferative	No vesication; papules progress to small scabs that are shed, leaving the pathognomonic lesions; lesions are essentially proliferative	Extensive edema and vesication giving rise to extensive ulcers that later scab; lesions are essentially ulcerative
Course of infection in the individual animal (uncomplicated)	3 to 4 weeks	6 weeks	3 to 4 weeks
Immunity	Probably lifelong	3 to 4 months, though some cows may be chronically infected	Probably lifelong; cattle may become virus carriers
Human infection	May give severe localized or generalized skin lesions	Localized skin lesions (milker's nodule)	Not recognized

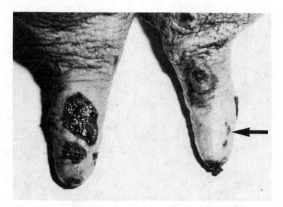

Figure 1. Ulcerated and scabbed lesions of cowpox approximately 1 week after onset of clinical signs. The arrow indicates a pseudocowpox lesion present as a second infection.

3. Calves sucking cows affected with bovine herpes mammillitis, pseudocowpox, or cowpox may show similar muzzle and/or oral lesions. The infection associated with pseudocowpox is indistinguishable from bovine papular stomatitis. Note generalized skin disease can be caused by the virus of bovine herpes mammillitis.

4. A history of recent smallpox vaccination of the farmer or the farmer's family may support the diagnosis of bovine vaccinia mammillitis. This is now unusual since in the United States only military personnel are vaccinated against smallpox.

Laboratory confirmation of the clinical diagnosis is advised for cowpox and bovine vaccinia mammillitis because these infections constitute a danger to public health.

The collection and examination of samples for the laboratory diagnosis is discussed in the literature.[3]

In susceptible herds infected with cowpox or bovine vaccinia mammillitis, it may be up to three months before the herd is free of disease. Several animals may need to be slaughtered because of subsequent bacterial mastitis.

TREATMENT

There are no specific antiviral drugs readily available for treating skin infections of the teat. Topical corticosteroids—in some cases combined with a local anesthetic and antibiotics—have been used to alleviate the pain associated with the early lesions of mammillitis, but their effectiveness has not been evaluated.

Once a teat lesion has become established it is very difficult to avoid secondary bacterial infection. Response to treatment is often slow owing to repeated infection and the trauma of milking or suckling a calf.

Antibiotic creams often prove too expensive for herd use. Teat dipping as discussed hereafter is simpler and probably as effective.

PREVENTION AND CONTROL

1. Quarantine and examine newly purchased cattle for 14 days before introduction to the milking herd.

2. Isolate infected cows or, if not possible, milk last.

3. Minimize risk of disease transmission by flies. Reduce fly population by improved husbandry and use of insecticides. Apply insect repellants to cattle, and incorporate teat dipping (after milking) into milking regimen. (Note that most teat dips are viricidal, particularly those that have a low pH; they are also repellant to insects).

4. Minimize risk of infection by ensuring cattle have teats free of minor abrasions. Improve husbandry, e.g., avoid gateways that are excessively muddy; use teat dips that incorporate an emollient such as lanolin or glycerol to promote a supple teat skin.

5. Minimize transmission of virus by fomites. Disinfect the teat cups of the milking machine between cows. Make attendants wear rubber gloves; the latter should be disinfected regularly. Do not allow attendants to visit other herds.

6. Although vaccinia virus could be used for protection of cattle against cowpox and bovine vaccinia mammillitis, the infrequency of these infections precludes prophylactic use.

References

1. Gibbs, E. P. J., Johnson, R. H., and Collings, D. F.: Cowpox in a dairy herd in the United Kingdom. Vet. Rec. *92*:56–64, 1973.
2. Baxby, D.: Poxvirus hosts and reservoirs. Arch. Virol. *55*:169–179, 1977.
3. Gibbs, E. P. J., Johnson, R. H., and Osborne, A. D.: The differential diagnosis of viral skin infections of the bovine teat. Vet. Rec. *87*:602–609, 1970.

Pseudocowpox

E. PAUL J. GIBBS, B.V.Sc., Ph.D., F.R.C.V.S.

Pseudocowpox is caused by a pox virus that is morphologically and serologically different from cowpox and vaccinia viruses. The virus is classified in the genus parapox with the viruses of contagious pustular dermatitis (synonyms are "orf" and "contagious ecthyma") and bovine papular stomatitis.

EPIZOOTIOLOGY

The disease, which has in the past been referred to as false or spurious cowpox, varicella, waterpox, udderpox, and natural cowpox, occurs commonly in most countries of the world.[1]

Jenner[2] recognized the disease, but it was not until the 1960's that it was demonstrated to be distinct from cowpox.[3]

Lesions of pseudocowpox may be seen in herds at any time of the year, and there seems to be only a temporary immunity to re-infection (approximately four to six months).[1] In many herds pseudocowpox is a chronic problem, and lesions are usually seen as relatively mild scabbing that causes little inconvenience. Cyclical waves of re-infection occur in these herds, often coinciding with inclement weather or calving of the majority of the herd. In completely susceptible herds, initial introduction of the virus may result in an acute infection that rapidly involves the majority of the herd. Severe lesions can also occur in susceptible stock introduced into chronically infected herds. Pseudocowpox also occurs in beef herds.

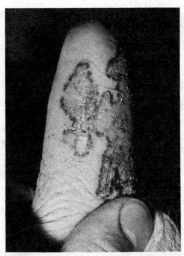

Figure 1. Extensive confluent "ring" scabs of pseudocowpox approximately 10 days after onset of clinical signs. This type of lesion appears to be pathognomonic for pseudocowpox.

CLINICAL SIGNS AND LESIONS (Fig. 1)

The clinical appearance of pseudocowpox is extremely variable, possibly owing to the generally mild nature of the infection, the susceptibility of cattle to re-infection, and the influence of the environment. Initial acute lesions in a susceptible animal are associated with a painful localized edema and erythema with a thin film of exudate over the edematous area; vesicle formation is uncommon. Within 48 hours of onset of signs a small papule develops, shortly followed by the formation of an elevated, small, dark-red scab. The edges of the lesion then extend, and the center becomes umbilicated; at one week the lesion measures approximately 1 cm in diameter. By ten days the central scab tends to desquamate, leaving a slightly raised scab commonly termed a "ring" or "horseshoe" scab that is pathognomonic for the disease. One teat may have several such lesions that coalesce to form linear scabs. The majority of lesions desquamate by six weeks without leaving scars, although occasionally cattle develop chronic infection. Only rarely is ulceration noted.

DIAGNOSIS

The differentiation of pseudocowpox from other diseases of the skin of the teat has been discussed in the previous article on cowpox. Pseudocowpox causes a mild skin lesion in man commonly called milker's nodule.[4]

Pseudocowpox is a chronic problem in most herds as mentioned previously. Good management will reduce the severity of the problem but will rarely eliminate it.

TREATMENT, PREVENTION, AND CONTROL

As discussed for cowpox in the previous article.

References

1. Gibbs, E. P. J., and Osborne, A. D.: Observations on the epidemiology of pseudocowpox in South West England and South Wales. Br. Vet. J. *130*:150–159, 1974.
2. Jenner, E.: "An enquiry into the causes and effects of *Variolae vaccinae*, a disease discovered in some of the western counties of England particularly Gloucestershire and known by the name of cowpox." London, Sampson Low, 1798.
3. Moscovici, C., Cohen, E. P., Sanders, J., and Delong, S. S.: Isolation of a viral agent from pseudocowpox disease. Science *141*:915–916, 1963.
4. Nagington, J., Lauder, I. M., and Smith, J. S.: Bovine papular stomatitis, pseudocowpox and milker's nodules. Vet. Rec. *81*: 306–313, 1967.

Bovine Papular Stomatitis

ROBERT A. CRANDELL, B.S., D.V.M., M.P.H.

The disease bovine papular stomatitis (BPS) has been described throughout the world. It is caused by a virus that affects cattle of all ages and both sexes. Although this virus has been considered to be of little economic importance, significant economic losses have occurred in individual outbreaks. The disease is important in the differential diagnosis of any bovine disease causing mouth lesions.

ETIOLOGY

The virus belongs to the genus *Parapoxvirus*, a large DNA-containing virus that is inactivated by lipid solvents. Although its relationship to other bovine poxviruses is not clear, some evidence suggests antigenic similarity. The virus has a limited host range. The common laboratory animals, such as mice, rabbits, and embryonating eggs, are resistant to infection.

EPIZOOTIOLOGY

Bovine papular stomatitis is a ubiquitous disease, and the virus appears to remain in the host as a latent infection. It is believed that the natural host is limited to the bovine species; however, human infections do occur. The virus is shed in the nasal secretions and saliva, and it spreads from animal to animal by contact. The lesions contain infective virus and, when inoculated into susceptible calves, produce the disease.

Generally, this is a disease of high morbidity and low mortality. The severity of the illness and mortality are influenced by the presence of certain predisposing factors. Chemical toxicity, parasitism, nutritional deficiencies, and other infectious agents in combination with BPS have been associated with animal losses. The stress associated with movement of animals is also a predisposing factor. Clinical outbreaks of BPS have occurred in feeder animals following shipment to feedlots and in young animals following importation by air. In well-managed herds without predisposing factors, the disease may go unnoticed. Mild infections are often found only by careful examination of the animals.

The incidence of lesions in young cattle in infected herds ranges from 10 to 100 per cent. The disease occurs throughout the year without any particular relationship to season. Both dairy and beef cattle are affected, and there are no known differences in breed susceptibility. However, most reported cases have involved beef cattle. The disease occurs in all ages of cattle but is more severe in the very young calf.

The occurrence of clinical BPS following stress from shipment or other factors suggests that latent infections exist. Since the disease is seen predominantly in younger animals, the cows are probably the source of infection.

CLINICAL FEATURES

BPS generally occurs as a mild disease without systemic signs. The disease may go undetected in many cases if the mouth is not examined. In the very young and in old, debilitated animals with complications, there may be a loss of appetite and excessive salivation. Clinical signs caused by other agents often confuse the clinical diagnosis of BPS.

The number and location of lesions vary considerably. The number of lesions in an animal may range from a single focus in one area to multiple lesions in different anatomic sites. The lesions are found chiefly on the muzzle, nostrils, lip, buccal papillae, dental pad, hard palate, soft palate, and lateral and ventral surfaces of the tongue. Although not common, lesions described as "wart-like" have occurred on the side, the abdomen, rear legs, scrotum, and prepuce of bulls. The pox lesions become infected with bacteria and have an offensive odor. At necropsy, lesions may be found on the mucosa of the esophagus (Fig. 1) and in the omasum, rumen, and reticulum, particularly in young animals. The most common lesion appears as a reddened focus that develops rapidly into a raised papule. The papule is either circular or oblong and hyperemic. The papule increases in size, and central necrosis occurs (Fig. 2). The center becomes white and roughened, and the lesion is surrounded by a hyperemic border. The lesions persist from a few days to several weeks. The lesions finally regress, leaving a red-brown discoloration of the tissue. The lesions of the hard palate follow the palatine ridges. Large circular lesions characterized by raised edges and necrotic centers surrounded by concentric colored rings are common on the soft palate. Vesiculation is not a feature of the lesion.

The course of the disease runs from a few days to

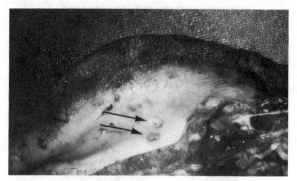

Figure 2. Lesions (arrows) on the tongue of a cow with bovine papular stomatitis.

several months, and the outcome varies. Recurrence of lesions is a common feature of this disease and suggests that latent infections occur. The immune response measured by the serum neutralization test is low.

DIAGNOSIS

Virus isolation, histopathology, and electron microscopy are useful laboratory procedures in diagnosing this disease. The virus has been isolated in cell culture from oral secretions and biopsy and necropsy specimens. The virus has been demonstrated in skin scrapings of bovine lesions and from necropsy material by electron microscopy techniques. The characteristic feature observed during histopathologic examination is the presence of cytoplasmic inclusion bodies in the cytoplasm in areas of hydropic degeneration.

The presence of systemic lesions with oral lesions may confuse the clinical diagnosis. Several infectious diseases that exhibit oral lesions need to be considered in the differential diagnosis. They are malignant catarrhal fever, bovine virus diarrhea, foot-and-mouth disease, rinderpest, vesicular stomatitis, and mycotic stomatitis.

PREVENTION AND CONTROL

There are no vaccines available for preventive measures. Although the disease occurs in well-managed herds, the losses are minimal. Good nutrition and freedom from parasites and unnecessary stress factors are recommended.

TREATMENT

The lesions in calves with mild infections will regress spontaneously without treatment. In the more severe cases where mixed infections are common, good husbandry is important. Antibiotic therapy is recommended to reduce secondary infections.

PUBLIC HEALTH CONSIDERATIONS

Cattlemen, veterinarians, and veterinary students acquire the infection by handling infected cattle. The virus from the oral lesions contaminates the nasal and oral

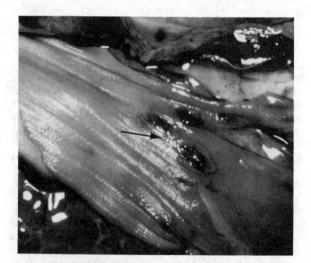

Figure 1. Erosions (arrow) on the mucosal surface of the esophagus of a calf with bovine papular stomatitis.

secretions. The most common sites of infection for man are on the arms and hands. The virus enters the exposed skin through a cut, bite, or scratch. Lesions appear at the site of entrance within three to six days after exposure. The lesion in man follows a course similar to that in cattle, and histologically the lesions are identical. Regression is complete within three to four weeks without treatment.

Supplemental Reading

Carson, C. A., and Kerr, K. M.: Bovine papular stomatitis with apparent transmission to man. J. Am. Vet. Med. Assoc. *151*:183, 1967.

Crandell, R. A., and Gosser, H. S.: Ulcerative esophagitis associated with poxvirus infection in a calf. J. Am. Vet. Med. Assoc. *165*:282, 1974.

Griesemer, R. A., and Cole, C. R.: Bovine papular stomatitis. 1. Recognition in the United States. J. Am. Vet. Med. Assoc. *137*:404, 1960.

Lumpy Skin Disease

CELESTINE O. NJOKU, D.V.M., Ph.D., F.R.V.C.S.

Lumpy skin disease (LSD), a highly infectious viral disease of cattle, is characterized by pox-like intracutaneous firm nodules varying in size from 0.5 to 10.0 cm in diameter, edema of the limbs, superficial lymph node swelling, and lymphangitis.

ETIOLOGY

LSD is caused by a virus immunologically related to sheep pox virus. By means of tissue culture techniques, three distinct groups of cytopathic agents associated with LSD have been isolated.

Group I (BZD) viruses, or "orphan viruses," isolated from the skin of normal cattle and from the suspensions of skin nodules or lymph nodes of LSD cattle, apparently produce no signs of the disease.

Group II (Allerton) virus, recovered from skin nodules, saliva, nasal secretions, and semen of affected cattle, produces a mild form of LSD. This virus is pathogenic for cattle by the intradermal, intravenous, and subcutaneous routes of inoculation of lesion suspensions or infected tissue culture fluids.

Group III (Neethling) virus, isolated from the blood, saliva, semen, and nasal mucus (but not from the urine or feces) of infected cattle, is the cause of LSD in cattle. It persists in the skin nodules for about 33 days.

EPIZOOTIOLOGY

LSD is mainly a disease of cattle and seems to be restricted to the African continent, although a similar disease was observed in herds of cattle in Iowa. Since LSD was first reported in Northern Rhodesia in 1929, it has spread to many other African countries including Botswana (1943), Republic of South Africa (1944), Southern Rhodesia (1945), Swaziland, Basutoland, and Mozambique (1946), Malagasy Republic (1954), Zaire (1955), Kenya (1957), Uganda (1958), Ruanda (1960), Burundi Angola, Cameroun, and South West Africa (1960), Sudan (1971), Niger (1973), and Nigeria (1974).

The mode of transmission is still under controversy because the disease had been reported to spread where direct or indirect contact between the infected and susceptible animals could be excluded. Even quarantine measures have failed to prevent the disease. Its rapid spread and the ease with which it traverses long distances suggest insect vectors, such as mosquitoes, arthropods, birds, and fomites.

The concept of insect transmission has been buttressed by the isolation of the virus from *Biomyia fasciata* and *Stomoxys calcitrans* caught on cattle with LSD. Other suggested means of transmission include ingestion of feed contaminated with saliva from LSD cattle and suckling of milk from infected cows.

Experimentally the disease has been transmitted by injection of infective blood (collected before the eruption of nodules) or emulsified nodules into susceptible cattle.

CLINICAL SIGNS AND LESIONS

The appearance of nodules in the skin and other body systems like the digestive, respiratory, and reproductive occurs after an initial viremia and fever.

The incubation period is from 2 to 5 weeks in natural infection and 4 to 14 days in experimentally induced infection. Morbidity rates range between 80 and 90 per cent, and mortality rates are usually less than 2 per cent. Higher mortality rates are usually due to secondary bacterial infection.

The first clinical sign observed is a diphasic fever reaching 41°C. The cutaneous eruption follows the second phase in about 7 to 10 days. These nodules measure about 0.5 to 10 cm in diameter and may affect the entire surface or any part of the body, especially the neck, brisket, back, thighs, legs, perineum, udder, and scrotum. In long-haired animals or in hairy parts of the body the smaller nodules may not be very obvious. On the other hand, the hair over the large nodules stands erect, thereby exaggerating their size and appearance. Nodules on the muzzle, vulva, prepuce, nostrils, eyes, and mouth tend to be softer and rupture easily, leaving erosions and ulcers. Oral lesions cause increased salivation, and those in the respiratory tract cause dyspnea due to occlusion. Conjunctivitis and keratitis are observed at times.

Induration of the skin nodules, which may persist for years, can occur, but usually these lesions undergo necrosis. A narrow (2 to 4 mm wide) groove or "moat" forms around the lesion, separating the lesion from the normal skin. This forms a "sit fast" that is eventually shed, leaving craters of varying depths and sizes (Fig. 1). These could serve as portals for secondary bacterial infection, resulting in metastatic abscesses in the regional lymph nodes, lungs, and other organs. In other cases scar formation is evident.

Palpable swelling of the superficial lymph nodes, especially the prescapular, precrural, and parotid, and thickening of the lymphatics may occur. In some cases, slight or marked edematous swellings of the limbs, dewlap, udder, vulva, scrotum, and prepuce may occur.

Apart from the cutaneous lesions already described, those of the alimentary and respiratory systems are usually covered by necrotic or ulcerated epithelium. The pulmonary lesions lead to edema and purulent pneumonia. Extensive granulation and cicatrization follow the development of the lesions in the trachea. A generalized

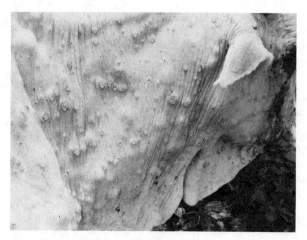

Figure 1. Lumpy skin disease. Cow with skin nodules of varying sizes and necrotic surfaces ("sit fasts"), resulting in craters following shedding.

lymphadenitis characterized by swelling and edema of the glands is a constant feature.

The microscopic changes in the disease involve the mesodermal tissues of the stratum papillaris, reticularis, and subcutis and secondly the surface epithelia, hair follicles, and associated glands. Below the epidermis, the early lesions include varying degrees of edema, fibroplasia, and perivascular cuffing with mononuclear cells (histiocytes, lymphocytes, and plasma cells) and some neutrophils and eosinophils. These cuffed vessels are usually thrombosed, possibly resulting in the overlying necrotic "sit fast" (Fig. 2).

DIAGNOSIS

Diagnosis of LSD can be made based on the appearance of characteristic skin lesions. However, it may be confused with urticaria, streptotrichosis, besnoitiosis, severe tick and insect bites, or demodectic mange.

For final diagnosis, histopathologic examination of skin nodule biopsies for characteristic changes, animal (cattle) inoculation, and viral isolation and identification (by tissue culture) are imperative. Electron microscopy and serology may be used too.

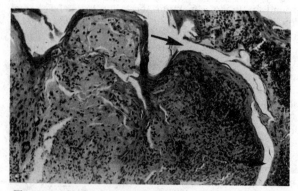

Figure 2. "Sit fast" or sequestrum. Notice line of separation (arrows) of necrotic tissue. Phloxine tartrazine sulfate stain. ×56.6.

TREATMENT

Specific treatment for LSD is not available, but prevention and control of secondary infection are necessary.

PREVENTION

Attempts to confine the disease by quarantine measures have failed, whereas slaughter of animals with very active cases, restriction of stock movement, and insect eradication have helped in checking the disease.

In enzootic areas, prophylactic immunization with sheep pox virus propagated in tissue culture and the egg-adapted, attenuated vaccine developed in South Africa have proved satisfactory and effective.

Recovery from natural infection confers a short-lived (about 11 months) immunity.

Supplemental Reading

Bida, S. A.: Confirmation by histopathology of the probable wide spread of Lumpy Skin Disease (LSD) in Nigeria. Bull. Anim. Health Prod. 25:317–324, 1977.
Emerging Diseases of Animals. FAO Agric. Studies No. 61. Rome, FAO/U.N., 1963, 177–201.
Jubb, K. V. F., and Kennedy, P. C.: Pathology of Domestic Animals, 2nd ed. New York, Academic Press, 1970.

Bovine Adenoviruses*

DONALD MATTSON, D.V.M., Ph.D.

Bovine adenovirus (BAV) possesses certain physico-chemical properties in common with other members of the Adenoviridae family. There are at least nine antigenic types of BAV. Additional isolates have been described but have not yet been accepted.

The bovine adenovirus group has been divided into two subgroups, subgroup 1 and subgroup 2. Major criteria for this division are based on replication ability in specific cell cultures, antigenic differences, and certain other characteristics.

BAV types 3 and 6 have been shown to resist inactivation by 70 per cent alcohol, alkyl benzyldimethylammonium chloride, chlorhexidine, dilute concentrations of sodium hypochlorite, and synthetic detergents with iodine. Other BAV types have not been tested with these chemicals.

EPIZOOTIOLOGY

BAV is distributed worldwide. These viruses are infectious, and over 70 per cent of adults may be serologically positive to viruses present in a specific herd.

BAV type 3 has been studied in more detail in the U.S., and it may serve as a model of other subgroup 1 members. BAV type 3 is probably endemic in most large open dairy and beef cattle herds. Calves usually become infected between two and six months of age. Infection may be enzootic in dairy calves, or the virus may spread in an epizootic fashion when calves are first placed in

*Oregon Agricultural Experiment Station Technical Paper No. 7018.

close confinement. By the time calves are six to eight months old, 40 to 60 per cent may be serologically positive. If calves are placed in a feedlot, the infection rate during the first six to eight weeks in the feeding period may be 20 per cent or higher.

Epizootiologic studies with members of the subgroup 2 BAV have not been conducted in the U.S. Three members of this subgroup (types 4, 6, and 7) have been isolated in this country. Epizootiologic studies conducted in Europe indicate that all types are widely distributed. Infection rate is highest when calves are two to six months old.

All BAV types are probably transmitted by direct animal contact or by aerosol transmission. The viruses are shed in lacrimal and nasal secretions as well as feces.

CLINICAL SIGNS AND LESIONS

Most infections with BAV are not clinically apparent. When clinical signs of disease are present, they are similar to those caused by other agents. The expression of clinical disease is believed to be determined by a variety of factors related to the virulence of the virus strain, concurrent infection with other microorganisms, stress, environmental conditions, and management practices.

Calves infected naturally or experimentally with BAV may show signs of an upper and lower respiratory tract infection. BAV type 3 has been associated with this disease more frequently than other types. Clinical signs in young calves may include conjunctivitis, pyrexia, cough, hyperpnea, and dyspnea. Pathologic changes may include areas of lung collapse, emphysema, and edema. Histopathologic changes may include evidence of bronchitis, bronchiolitis, and alveolar wall infiltration.

Pneumo-enteritis and enteritis have been associated more frequently with infection by the subgroup 2 BAV, i.e., types 4 through 8. Clinical signs of disease may include an excessive conjunctival and nasal discharge, pyrexia, hyperpnea, dyspnea, cough, and diarrhea. Infection with the subgroup 2 viruses may result in a viremia allowing the virus to localize in a number of organs.

Bovine adenovirus type 7 has been isolated from cases of the so-called weak calf syndrome. This disease is characterized by birth of calves that are listless and that have polyarthritis, subcutaneous hemorrhage over the joints, and bloody and fibrinous synovial fluid. Areas most often affected include the hock and metatarsal and metacarpal joints.

BAV has been isolated from cattle with conjunctivitis and keratoconjunctivitis in Australia. Invasion of the bacteria *Neisseria catarrhalis* and *Moraxella bovis* was sometimes associated with the production of keratoconjunctivitis. The specific virus strains that were recovered in Australia from cases of this disease have not been isolated in the U.S. However, BAV type 3 and other types have been isolated from cases of conjunctivitis in the U.S.

DIAGNOSIS

Inoculation of samples in several cell culture types and prolonged incubation of specimens are required to isolate all types of BAV. Most types of the virus replicate in a low concentration in the intestine, and detection of virus in feces may not be possible by routine electron microscopy examination. Samples for viral isolation must be taken early in the disease. Virus-infected cells can be detected by the fluorescent antibody technique.

Samples for serologic testing should be taken in the traditional manner. An agar gel precipitation test has been developed, and serum can be tested for a group-specific antibody titer increase for subgroup 1 viruses. Subgroup 2 viruses do not possess sufficient group-specific antigen to invoke this type of serologic response. The serum-viral neutralization test must be used for type-specific testing. Most diagnostic laboratories in the U.S. do not offer these services.

TREATMENT

There is no specific treatment for adenoviral infection in cattle.

PREVENTION AND CONTROL

There are no vaccines currently available in the U.S. for prevention of bovine adenoviral infection.

Supplemental Reading

Kahrs, R. F.: Adenoviruses. *In* Viral Diseases of Cattle. Ames, Iowa, Iowa State University Press, 1981, 61–70.
McFerran, J. B.: Adenoviruses of vertebrate animals. *In* Kurstak, E., and Kurstak, C. (eds.): Comparative Diagnosis of Viral Diseases. III. Vertebrate Animal and Related Viruses. Part A: DNA Viruses. New York, Academic Press, 1981, 118–123.

Papillomatosis in Cattle

CARL OLSON, D.V.M., Ph.D.

Cutaneous papillomatosis occurs in cattle, sheep, goats, horses, rabbits, fish, and humans. An oral papillomatosis occurs in dogs and rabbits. These warts, infectious verrucae, or papillomas are usually regarded as benign epithelial tumors. Viruses causing these tumors are similar in morphology but different in their other characteristics. The bovine papilloma virus (BPV), the ovine papilloma virus, and the deer fibroma virus will cause a fibroblastic tumor in the hamster. Otherwise, the known papilloma viruses are oncogenic only for their own species of origin. In addition, BPV will cause a fibroblastic tumor in horses, and evidence of the BPV genome is found in naturally occurring equine sarcoids.

EPIZOOTIOLOGY

Bovine papillomatosis is worldwide in distribution and is more common in cattle younger than two years of age that are housed in close contact with each other. The skin surfaces of the neck, legs, back, and abdomen are the more usual sites, since these locations are probably more subject to abrasions and wounds through which the virus may infect the tissues. Cutaneous papillomas in cattle can be of various size, depending on the area infected, and have a cauliflower-like appearance and a fibroma base in the dermis. Fibropapillomas of the penis and vulvovaginal mucosa have a smooth surface with less epithelial proliferation. The infective virus is concentrated in the outer keratinized epithelium of the papilloma and when shed can readily contaminate fomites such as fences, stanchions, and boards of the stable. These fomites with virus readily transmit the disease to susceptible cattle by causing skin wounds. Immunity develops in a few weeks after exposure to the virus, and older animals are more resistant than very young animals, probably because of prior inapparent exposure. The incubation period for cutaneous warts produced by BPV is approximately 30 days, and the duration of both naturally and experimentally produced fibropapillomas ranges from 1 to 12 months before regression.

CLINICAL SIGNS AND LESIONS

BPV causes fibroplasia or fibroblastic tumors of the dermis in addition to the epithelial hyperplasia. These are more properly called fibropapillomas. Progressively growing fibroblastic tumors of the brain can be experimentally produced in cattle and hamsters. Polypoid tumors of the urinary bladder can be produced with BPV in calves. In certain areas of the world, such as northern Japan, parts of Brazil, Scotland, Colombia, and Turkey, enzootic bovine hematuria is associated with the bracken fern grown in certain soils as well as BPV. A plant carcinogen seems to operate together with the BPV in causing these tumors. On bracken farms of the west coast of Scotland, papillomas and carcinomas are found on the tongue, pharynx, esophagus, esophageal groove, rumen, and intestine. A virus morphologically similar to BPV exists in these lesions, and extracts of the tumor have produced typical papillomas in the esophagus, palate, and skin. BPV is a DNA virus, and by molecular hybridization there are nine distinct types and indications of more types. Although two of these types (1 and 2) can be differentiated, they do have partial immunologic relationships.

BPV and the other papilloma viruses multiply only in epithelial cells. Morphologic evidence of infectious BPV cannot be found in the fibroblast that has been stimulated to neoplasia, but genome DNA sequences of BPV can be demonstrated by molecular hybridization.

The potential for BPV to produce tumors of the intestinal tract or the urinary bladder in concert with a carcinogen from bracken fern and its ability to transform fibroblasts into a neoplastic state may mean that BPV has a broader and more serious potential for neoplasia than thus far recognized. Therefore, other types of tumors could be considered as possibly involved with the virus.

Troublesome papilloma-like lesions not infrequently develop on teats and at the teat meatus of milking cows. This is a proliferation of epithelium as in a papilloma, but it lacks the fibroplasia of the underlying dermis as seen in the typical fibropapilloma of BPV. The etiology of this condition is a papilloma virus.

An atypical wart problem in cattle lacks the dermal fibroma component of the typical BPV-induced cutaneous fibropapilloma. The atypical tumors tended to persist rather than regress and involve adult animals as well as young stock. The atypical papillomas contain a virus morphologically identical to the typical BPV. Experimental transmission of the atypical wart virus has been par-

tially successful. A three-year herd vaccination program using atypical wart homogenates failed to influence the natural incidence of the disease.

PREVENTION AND CONTROL

Antibodies (precipitin, complement fixing, or hemagglutination inhibiting) can readily be found after exposure to BPV or commercial bovine wart vaccines. Formalized suspension of bovine warts with inactivated virus provides a vaccine for prophylactic immunization when cutaneous warts are a problem in a herd of cattle. Such problems can exist in cattle used for show, those being sent to slaughter where ante mortem inspection may cause a reduced price, and, particularly, in bull studs where young bulls can develop fibropapilloma of the penis, which may render them of no value as a bull stud. Such penile lesions tend to recur after surgery with eventual deformation. Therapeutic use of vaccine has been rather extensive in the past with variable but usually poor results. A controlled test of vaccine in an experimental trial of its therapeutic effect indicated that it was of no value.

Cryosurgery with liquid nitrogen has recently come into use and should be very effective when the cutaneous papillomas are not too large. In the absence of liquid nitrogen with its instrumentation, it should be possible, with care to protect the operator, to freeze the fibropapilloma in a similar manner with dry ice.

Supplemental Reading

Barthold, S. W., Koller, L. D., Olson, C., Studer, E., and Holtan, A.: Atypical warts in cattle. J. Am. Vet. Med. Assoc. 165:276, 1974.
Barthold, S. W., Olson, C., and Larson, L. L.: Precipitin response of cattle to commercial wart vaccine. Am. J. Vet. Res. 37:449, 1976.
Jarrett, W. F. H., McNeil, P. E., Grimshaw, W. T. R., Selman, I. E., and McIntyre, W. I. M.: High incidence area of cattle cancer with a possible interaction between an environmental carcinogen and a papilloma virus. Nature 274:215, 1978.
Koller, L. D., and Olson, C.: Attempted transmission of warts from man, cattle, and horses and of deer fibroma, to selected hosts. J. Invest. Dermatol. 58:366, 1972.
Lancaster, W. D., and Olson, C.: Animal papilloma viruses. Microbiol. Rev. 46:191, 1982.
Olson, C., Gordon, D. E., Robl, M. G., and Lee, K. P.: Oncogenicity of bovine papilloma virus. Arch. Environ. Health 19:827, 1969.
Olson, R. O., Olson, C., and Easterday, B. C.: Papillomatosis of the bovine teat. Am. J. Vet. Res. 43:2250, 1982.
Spradbrow, P.: Papilloma viruses, papillomas, and ocular cutaneous carcinomas in ruminant animals. Cold Spring Harbor Conf. Papilloma Viruses, 1982, 73.

Bovine Parvoviruses

J. STORZ, D.V.M., Ph.D.

Bovine parvoviruses (BPVs) are icosahedral viruses with a diameter of 20 to 22 nm. Four structural polypeptides with approximate molecular weights of 80,000, 72,000, 62,000, and 60,000 daltons comprise the capsid, which surrounds a single-stranded DNA genome of about 5,550 nucleotides. Parvoviruses are extremely resistant to chemical and physical inactivating factors. The most reliable disinfection is achieved with 0.5 per cent chlorox or ethylene oxide in the form of a nonexplosive mixture of 10 per cent ethylene oxide and 90 per cent carbon dioxide. All bovine parvoviral isolates agglutinate guinea pig and human type O erythrocytes. The isolates from cattle are antigenically related or identical to BPV 1. One BPV strain isolated in Japan appears to differ and is separated as BPV 2. Bovine parvoviruses differ antigenically from parvoviruses isolated from man, pigs, cats, dogs, rats, and rabbits.[1, 2]

BPV replicate to similar titers in bovine fetal testicle, spleen (BFS), and adrenal cells, but replication is less efficient in bovine fetal kidney cells and several cell lines. The host cell range is virtually restricted to bovine cells. The cytopathic effect resulting from bovine parvovirus replication in actively dividing BFS cells is distinctive and reproducible. Intranuclear inclusions with unique morphology are formed in infected cells and can be detected following Giemsa or acridine orange staining.[2]

EPIZOOTIOLOGY

Evidence for parvovirus infection of cattle through detection of antibodies was found in the United States, Algiers, Japan, England, and Austria. The incidence of cattle with antibodies ranged from 46 to 86 per cent. The majority of the serum samples involved newborn calves and cattle to 12 months of age. The highest percentage of positive calves was found in February in Austria, where the only attempt was made to analyze seasonal distribution. The infectious chain consisting of intestinal shedding and oral or oropharyngeal exposure is maintained within the cattle population.[1, 2] Vertical transmission of BPV was proven through detection of significant antibody titers in fetal serum and through isolation of parvovirus from tissues of fetuses from naturally occurring abortions. This pathogenic potential of BPV was confirmed through experimental inoculations of pregnant cows or direct fetal inoculations.[3]

CLINICAL SIGNS

Most parvoviral isolates described were made from fecal specimens of calves suffering from enteritis, combined occasionally with febrile respiratory illness and conjunctivitis. In several instances parvoviruses were isolated from feces of young cattle that were clinically normal. The diarrhea was mild to moderately severe in orally inoculated calves. Calves given the inoculum intravenously developed a more severe, watery diarrhea and became prostrate. The body temperatures reached 41°C two days after exposure.[2]

Pregnant cows did not develop adverse clinical signs immediately following inoculation. Their temperature and behavior remained normal. Abortions occurred in the first and early second trimesters. The aborted fetuses were edematous, and the placentas were edematous and had necrotic cotyledons.[3] A serologic survey in 12 commercial dairy herds indicated that BPV may be involved in other reproductive problems. The BPV seroreactor cows experienced higher rates of embryonic mortality and required more services per conception than did nonreactor cattle.[4]

LABORATORY DIAGNOSIS

Considering the high incidence of cattle with antibody titers, it is apparent that isolation of parvovirus from natural infections was relatively sporadic and inefficient with the various methods used. A cell-associated virus technique employing parasynchronous BFS cells was most reliable and recovered parvovirus from 82.5 per cent of FA positive tissue specimens. Serum free of antibodies against BPV or inhibitors of their hemagglutination must be used for successful isolation attempts and virus propagation.[2]

An efficient method to detect antibodies against BPV is the hemagglutination inhibition (HI) test employing guinea pig or human type O red blood cells. The HI antibody titers corresponded well with results obtained through infectivity neutralization tests and other methods for the detection of antibodies.[1, 2]

PREVENTION AND VACCINATION

A high percentage of cattle in the United States and other parts of the world have antibodies resulting from natural infections. There are herds of cattle that do not have antibodies, and they are thus without experience with this infection. Attempts to vaccinate cattle have not been described. As we learn more about the nature of this infection in cattle and the pathogenic potential of BPV, efforts to develop means of vaccination may be warranted, particularly for the prevention of reproductive disease problems.

References

1. Abinanti, F. R., and Warfield, M. S.: Recovery of a hemadsorbing virus (HADEN) from the gastrointestinal tract of calves. Virology 14:288–289, 1961.
2. Storz, J., Leary, J. J., Carlson, J. H., and Bates, R. C.: Parvoviruses associated with diarrhea in calves. Proceedings, Colloquium on Selected Diarrheal Diseases of Young Animals and Humans. J. Am. Vet. Med. Assoc. 173:624–627, 1978.
3. Storz, J., Young, S., Carroll, E. J., Bates, R. C., Bowen, R. A., and Keney, D. A.: Parvovirus infection of the bovine fetus: Distribution of infection, antibody response and age-related susceptibility. Am. J. Vet. Res. 39:1099–1102, 1978.
4. Barnes, M. A., Wright, R. E., Bodine, A. B., and Alberty, C. F.: Frequency of bluetongue and bovine parvovirus infection in cattle in South Carolina dairy herds. Am. J. Vet. Res. 43:1078–1080, 1982.

Bovine Viral Diarrhea-Mucosal Disease

WERNER P. HEUSCHELE, D.V.M., Ph.D.

Bovine viral diarrhea-mucosal disease (BVD) is a contagious viral disease of cattle and other ruminants first seen in 1946 in New York as a gastroenteritis with severe diarrhea, ulcerations of the muzzle and nasal and oral cavities, fever, leukopenia, reduction in milk secretion, cessation of rumination, and abortions. A similar disease exhibiting the same signs and lesions (only more severe, resembling rinderpest) occurred in Iowa in 1953. This disease was named mucosal disease. It is now recognized that both disease entities were caused by the same virus. A large proportion of BVD infections are subclinical.

ETIOLOGY

The causative RNA virus is a member of the family Togaviridae and the genus *Pestivirus,* which also includes hog cholera virus and the virus of Border disease of sheep. The three viruses are antigenically closely related and cross react serologically by virus neutralization, immunoprecipitation, and immunofluorescence. All are enveloped, ranging in size from 20 to 65 nm.

There is minor antigenic variation among BVD virus strains or isolates, but all cross neutralize.

The virus is readily inactivated by heat, low and high pH, and most disinfectants but is stable at low temperatures. It grows readily in cell cultures of bovine, ovine, or porcine origin. Although several cytopathogenic strains have been isolated, a larger proportion of BVD virus field isolates are noncytopathogenic in cell cultures.

EPIZOOTIOLOGY

Cattle are commonly infected with BVD virus throughout the world. In the U.S., infection prevalence ranges between 60 and 80 per cent as revealed by serologic surveys. Natural infection with BVD virus also occurs in sheep, goats, swine, and many wild ruminant species including deer, antelope, buffaloes, and so on in which clinical disease of varying severity is occasionally seen.

Domestic cattle are considered the principal reservoir of BVD virus. It is believed that latent persistent infections are common in cattle. Clinical BVD occurs most frequently in cattle six months to two years of age.

The virus of BVD is shed in feces and nasopharyngeal secretions. It is readily transmitted by aerosol droplets and direct and indirect contact. Fecal contamination of food and water sources is undoubtedly an important means of infection spread, with the oral route being the most probable route of entry. Entry via the respiratory tract by inhalation of infectious aerosols may also occur. It is possible that flies and other flying arthropods may serve as vectors of BVD virus from one premise to another. Mechanical transmission on contaminated clothing, footwear, equipment, utensils, and vehicles is also possible. Vertical transmission is considered common, as evidenced by the presence of BVD antibodies and/or virus in 10 to 20 per cent of bovine fetuses examined at abattoirs in the U.S.

CLINICAL SIGNS AND LESIONS

A majority of BVD infections are subclinical, involving only a biphasic fever and leukopenia followed by an immune response if uncomplicated by a concurrent infection. The wide range of clinical responses to BVD virus infection is very likely due to several factors: difference in the pathogenicity of virus strains, susceptibility of exposed herds, concurrent infections, stress conditions, and management factors. BVD virus is associated with many episodes of bovine respiratory disease (BRD) and is therefore a major component of the BRD complex. Usually other infectious agents are concurrently involved with BRD. The BVD virus may increase the pathogenicity of other infectious agents because of its suppressive effects on the host cellular and humoral defense mechanisms.

Clinical signs and lesions may therefore often be referrable to the co-infecting agents.

A typical outbreak of acute BVD will usually have the following features: a gradual build-up of cases beginning one to three weeks after the introduction of new animals, onset of fever, depression, anorexia, tachypnea, tachycardia, nasal discharge progressing from serous to mucopurulent, cough, hyperemia of nasal and sometimes oral mucosa, and encrustation around the nares and on the muzzle. Diarrhea is observed two to three days after the initial onset of fever, progressing from loose watery stools to bloody stools with considerable mucus. Oral erosions appear in the mouth accompanied by hypersalivation from three to seven days after the first fever. Laminitis may be observed in some animals. Pregnant cows may abort during or following the clinical episode or may produce calves with congenital abnormalities, especially cerebellar hypoplasia and ocular dysgenesis.

In some cases or herd outbreaks, diarrhea and typical erosive lesions may be minimal or absent, and respiratory signs are the only manifestations of BVD infection.

Chronic BVD may occur as a sequela to acute BVD or subclinical infections and is often manifested by intermittent diarrhea and nasal discharge and persistent ocular discharge. Chronic lameness due to laminitis and interdigital necrosis may be seen. Chronic patients often fail to develop circulating BVD antibodies and may have persistent viral infection. Areas of alopecia and reddening or hyperkeratosis of the skin, especially on the neck, may occur. Chronically infected animals usually appear unthrifty, often emaciated.

Although BVD virus primarily attacks the digestive tract, it also has a strong affinity for the lymphoreticular tissues, causing necrosis of lymphocytes and macrophages. Phagocytic functions of macrophages and neutrophils are impaired, and both B and T lymphocytes are suppressed. The result is immunosuppression and diminution of nonspecific cellular defense mechanisms as well. This can result in enhanced pathogenicity of other co-infecting organisms such as *Pasteurella* spp., coronavirus, rotavirus, *Cryptosporidia* spp., and so on.

In addition to erosions of the muzzle and all surfaces of the oral cavity, lesions of BVD may include linear esophageal erosions and erosions on the ruminal pillars, omasum, and abomasum. The pyloric portion of the abomasum may be edematous and hemorrhagic. Catarrhal enteritis may progress to include hemorrhage, erosions, and ulcers of the intestinal mucosa. There is swelling of Peyer's patches, often accompanied by necrosis and hemorrhage.

Histologically, there are varying degrees of necrosis of the germinal centers in lymph nodes and the spleen. In younger animals there may be marked atrophy of the thymus. Edema and inflammatory cell infiltration of the intestinal mucosa occur in varying degrees of severity throughout the digestive tract.

When BVD infection is associated with BRD complex, lesions are usually related to associated organisms such as *Pasteurella* spp. and the major respiratory viruses.

DIAGNOSIS

Clinical diagnosis of BVD in a herd must be based upon examination of several animals. A combination of clinical signs, lesions, and epizootiologic features of an outbreak is usually a reasonable basis for a provisional diagnosis of BVD. When fever, leukopenia (a total leukocyte count of 4000 or less per cmm of blood), respiratory signs, diarrhea, depression, and oral erosions are present. BVD should be strongly suspected.

BVD resembles several other diseases that cause erosive and ulcerative lesions in the digestive tract. Rinderpest produces clinical signs and lesions very similar to the severe acute mucosal disease form of BVD. In general, rinderpest has a higher morbidity and mortality than BVD. Malignant catarrhal fever (MCF) also strongly resembles BVD, presenting pronounced respiratory signs, erosions in the digestive tract, leukopenia, and occasionally diarrhea. Ocular involvement (ophthalmitis) is common in MCF and less so in BVD, and MCF episodes usually involve a lower morbidity, i.e., sporadic cases.

The differential diagnosis should also include bluetongue, vesicular diseases, infectious bovine rhinotracheitis, papular and ulcerative stomatitis, ingestion of caustic substances, and other causes of diarrhea such as salmonellosis, coccidiosis, and enteric viruses.

Definitive diagnosis requires laboratory procedures such as virus isolation, identification of viral antigens in tissue sections by immunofluorescence or enzyme immunoassay, and demonstration of rising antibody titers between acute and convalescent serum samples. Serologic methods used to demonstrate BVD serum antibodies include complement fixation, indirect immunofluorescence, enzyme immunoassay, immunodiffusion precipitation, and virus neutralization, the last-named being preferred by most laboratories.

Appropriate specimens for laboratory examination should include (1) paired sera, i.e., an acute phase sample and a sample collected two to four weeks later, (2) nasal swabs in Stewart's transport medium, which are available commercially, (3) feces or rectal swabs, and (4) unclotted blood with anticoagulants such as heparin or EDTA from clinically ill animals. Tissues from fresh necropsy cases for virus examination and histopathology should include tonsil, spleen, mesenteric lymph nodes, lung, and a section of ileum containing Peyer's patches (tied off and unopened).

The demonstration of a fourfold or greater rise in virus-neutralizing antibody titers between acute and convalescent serum samples provides a sound basis for the diagnosis of BVD infection. Isolation of BVD virus or demonstration of BVD antigens from specimens add further confirmation.

Because of the relatively high incidence of BVD infection in bovine fetuses, the isolation of BVD viruses or the demonstration of BVD antibodies in serum from an aborted late term fetus may not necessarily be diagnostic; i.e., BVD should not be considered the cause of the abortion unless BVD lesions are present or cases of BVD have recently occurred in the herd.

TREATMENT

Treatment of animals with clinical BVD is largely symptomatic and aimed at controlling diarrhea, respiratory signs, and secondary bacterial invaders. Antidiarrheals, antimicrobials such as antibiotics and sulfonamides, expectorants, and fluid and electrolyte therapy are used but in cases of severe acute mucosal disease are seldom of much benefit. Corticosteroids are contraindicated since they produce immunosuppression, which is additive to that produced by the BVD viral infection.

Sick animals should be separated from the rest of the herd.

PREVENTION AND CONTROL

Vaccination of susceptible cattle has been the principal approach to the prevention and control of BVD. The use of modified live virus BVD vaccines has been a subject of controversy. Some modified live virus (MLV) vaccines appear to be less attenuated than others and have been associated with post-vaccinal disease complications, especially when used in stressed, recently shipped cattle. Recent reports suggest that some MLV BVD vaccines cause some immunosuppression. However, post-vaccinal BVD disease can also be attributed to circumstances in which animals were in incubative stages of BVD at the time of vaccination. Contamination of MLV vaccines with adventitious virulent BVD virus also may occur occasionally. It would therefore appear that killed virus vaccines would be preferable to live ones. It is doubtful that current killed virus BVD vaccines confer immunity of as high a degree, quality, or duration as do the MLV vaccines. They have the advantage of being safe in pregnant cows and carry no risk of inducing post-vaccinal disease.

Immunity conferred by BVD vaccines has also been a controversial topic. It is questionable if vaccine prepared with a single BVD virus strain will provide lifelong protection against all BVD viral strains as was once believed. Field experience suggests that immunity against heterologous BVD strains may be of relatively short duration, i.e., 8 to 12 months. It is therefore recommended that animals be revaccinated annually in dairy or breeder stock. Beef cattle destined for feedlots should be vaccinated at four to six months of age, preferably before weaning stress.

In areas of high BVD endemicity, earlier vaccination at two to four weeks of age is advised, but this should be followed by a booster vaccination at six to eight months of age, since persisting maternal passive antibodies may reduce the magnitude of the immune response to vaccine in the young animal.

Although current vaccines for BVD have their limitations, they have proved to be of considerable value in reducing the impact of this costly disease. Undoubtedly, newer technologies of genetically engineered subunit vaccines for BVD will provide safer, more efficacious vaccines in the near future.

Supplemental Reading

Heuschele, W. P.: Preventive medicine for some economically important bovine viral diseases. Vet. Clin. North Am. *3*:403–408, 1981.

Kahrs, R. F.: Viral Diseases of Cattle. Ames, Iowa, Iowa State University Press, 1981, 89–105.

Karrar, A. E. R.: Comparative studies between cytopathogenic and non-cytopathogenic bovine viral diarrhea virus strains. Ph.D. dissertation. The Ohio State University, 1983.

Bovine Reoviruses

SASHI B. MOHANTY, B.V.Sc., A.H., Ph.D.

Reoviruses are of special interest in comparative virology because the agents of animal origin are indistinguishable from those of human origin. Antibodies against these viruses have been found in a wide range of domestic and wild animals. They have been isolated from both the respiratory and intestinal tracts of apparently healthy cattle and are antigenically identical to human serotypes. Three mammalian serotypes are recognized, and the existence of four subtypes of type 2 has been reported. Reoviruses, members of the genus *Reovirus* in the virus family Reoviridae, are 60 to 80 nm in diameter with icosahedral symmetry and a double protein shell. They have a double-stranded segmented RNA genome and are resistant to pH 3, ether, and chloroform, and they agglutinate human O red blood cells (RBC). Type 3 also agglutinates bovine RBC.

Reoviruses do not grow well in cell cultures of bovine origin, and they produce little or no cytopathic effects (CPE) in bovine kidney (BK) cells. However, they produce good CPE and eosinophilic intracytoplasmic inclusions in monkey kidney, in mouse fibroblast (L-929) cells, and in various human cell lines.

EPIZOOTIOLOGY

Antibodies to all three types of reoviruses are widespread in cattle populations. The virus enters via the fecal-oral and respiratory routes. Infected cattle shed reoviruses in the feces and nasal and conjunctival discharges for up to one month. Susceptible cattle may become infected through contact with these sources. Although interspecies infection can occur, it does not appear to be significant under natural conditions. Cattle could harbor reoviruses and transmit them to man or vice versa.

CLINICAL SIGNS AND LESIONS

The role of bovine reoviruses in the respiratory syndrome is not clear, and it appears that they cause an inapparent infection in nature. In one study, calves experimentally infected with reovirus type 1 had mild clinical signs characterized by a mild fever, anorexia, hyperpnea, nasal discharge, and coughing. Young calves were more susceptible than older ones. In other studies, types 1 and 2 induced no clinical illness in colostrum-deprived calves, but these calves had pneumonia at necropsy. *Pasteurella* spp. may not enhance reovirus infection, and maternal antibodies do not protect calves from these viral infections.

Gross lesions are confined to the lungs particularly at the roots. Histologic changes are mainly exudative. Interstitial pneumonia along with epithelialization of alveoli are common features.

DIAGNOSIS

Bovine reoviral infection may not be detected clinically. Pneumonia at necropsy has been found in cattle infected with bovine parainfluenza-3 and rhinoviruses that had no clinical signs. This possibility should be considered in the diagnosis of reovirus infections. Virus isolation from clinical specimens and seroconversion are considered adequate for diagnosis. Virus neutralization or hemagglutination-inhibition test can be used for demonstrating a rising antibody titer (fourfold or greater) in acute and convalescent serum samples.

TREATMENT, PREVENTION, AND CONTROL

Antibiotics are given only for secondary bacterial infections. There is no vaccine available.

Supplemental Reading

Lamont, P. H.: Reoviruses. J. Am. Vet. Med. Assoc. *152*:870, 1968.
Mohanty, S. B., and Dutta, S. K.: Veterinary Virology. Philadelphia, Lea & Febiger, 1981, 129–131.
Trainor, P. D., et al.: Experimental infection of calves with reovirus type 1. Am. J. Epidemiol. *83*:217, 1966.

Bluetongue in Cattle

MICHAEL M. JOCHIM, D.V.M., Ph.D.

Bluetongue (BT) is an infectious, noncontagious, arthropod-borne virus disease of domestic and wild ruminants. The infection is usually acute in sheep and inapparent in cattle, with only occasional reports of clinical signs in cattle. Goats appear to be less susceptible than sheep to BT. Infected cattle are important in the epizootiology of BT because cattle often are reservoirs of the virus. In the United States, bluetongue virus (BTV) has been isolated from cattle, sheep, or wild ruminants in 32 states, and serologic evidence has been reported in 48 states. Bluetongue is seasonal in areas in which vector activity is interrupted by freezing weather but may become enzootic in areas with yearlong vector populations. Though BTV causes direct losses in sheep production, its economic importance in cattle is associated with losses from embargos and restriction of export markets for cattle and cattle semen. Losses due to reproductive problems, abortions, congenital anomalies, and weak calves are less well defined but may also be significant.

Culicoides variipennis, a small biting gnat, has been proved to be the principal vector of BT in the United States. After *C. variipennis* was shown to be a biologic vector of BT, the virus was experimentally transmitted from infected sheep to susceptible cattle and vice versa. *Culicoides* spp. appear to be more attracted to cattle than to sheep, and this may be a significant factor for the role of cattle in the epizootiology of the disease. The vector is believed to remain infected for life after ingestion of BTV-infected blood.

Vertical transmission of BTV from infected dams to offspring has been shown. Infection of the fetus may result in early or late abortion and fetal malformation, and the calves may be chronically infected. Vertical transmission of BTV in cattle appears to play a role in the perpetuation of the disease, especially in areas where the vector appears only seasonally. Because prolonged viremia has been described in infected cattle, the probability of transmission of BTV from dam to fetus is greatly enhanced. Also, BTV has been isolated from the semen of infected bulls, and susceptible heifers have been infected after natural service. Experimental BTV infection of pre-implantation embryos from cattle was shown to cause rapid cytolysis of the developing embryos and suggested that persistently infected calves were unlikely to result from such early exposure.

CLINICAL SIGNS AND LESIONS

The clinical manifestations of BTV infection of cattle are unlike the typical field cases of BT in sheep. Bluetongue in cattle is best described as a subclinical infection; only a small percentage of cattle show acute signs. The morbidity is variable, usually under 10 per cent, and mortality is rare. A higher percentage of cattle develop serum antibodies to BTV than are ever observed to be clinically sick. Serologic studies have shown the prevalence of antibody to be well over 50 per cent in some areas of the West and Southwest. Clinical signs are more pronounced in naturally infected cattle than those experimentally infected with BTV; in fact the inoculation of susceptible cattle with virus recovered from acute cases of BT has failed to reproduce the very acute signs most often associated with field cases. Febrile responses are transient in naturally infected cattle and range from 40.0 to 41.0°C. Rapid, shallow respiration often accompanies the fever. Early in the infection, there may be stiffness or lameness that the animals tend to "warm out of." This is often the most frequent sign reported. Increased salivation and lacrimation may precede the inflammatory and ulcerative lesions of the oral mucosa. Drooling is often associated with swelling of the lips, gums, and tongue. Ulcers develop on the dental pad, lips, gums, and anterior part of the tongue; in severe cases there may be extensive necrosis of the dental pad. The skin over the muzzle may have a burned appearance and may be dry, cracked, and peeling. The skin over the neck, back, flanks, and perineal area is also affected in severe cases, and large patches of skin may slough. Skin lesions are accompanied by alopecia and an overall loss of condition. The udder and teats of dairy cows and nursing beef cows may be swollen; ulcers have been seen on teats of some cows. As the disease progresses, coronitis, lameness, and sloughing of the horny laminae may occur.

Abortion and congenital deformities occur in both sheep and cattle naturally infected with BTV. Hydranencephaly has been reported in the offspring of BTV-infected sheep and cattle. Also, calves infected experimentally *in utero* developed gingival hyperplasia, arthrogryposis (crooked legs), agnathia (tilted mandibles), prognathia, and hydrocephalus (domed cranium).

DIAGNOSIS

Clinical signs of BT in cattle are similar to those of epizootic hemorrhagic disease, vesicular stomatitis, bovine viral diarrhea, infectious rhinotracheitis, and mycotic stomatitis. Exotic diseases such as rinderpest and foot-and-mouth disease should also be considered in the differential diagnosis. In cattle BT is difficult to diagnose accurately without subsequent virus isolation. The BTV can be isolated from infective blood by inoculation of embryonating chicken eggs, cell cultures, or susceptible sheep.

The infection of animals with BTV can be confirmed by serologic tests. The BT immunodiffusion (BTID) and modified direct complement fixation (MDCF) tests are group-specific tests; both tests detect antibodies to any of the five BTV serotypes known to be present in the United States.

TREATMENT AND PREVENTION

Antibiotics are frequently used to treat animals infected with BTV in an effort to control secondary bacterial infections. Localized lesions on the muzzle and teats of infected cattle can be treated topically to minimize infection and promote healing. If pityriasis and alopecia are extensive, the animals should be protected from the sun. When mouth lesions are present on the lips and dental pad, good management is necessary to maintain body weight. Infected animals should be separated from the herd and fed less rough forage to minimize trauma to the oral mucosa.

An attenuated vaccine is licensed in the United States for control of BT in sheep; the vaccine contains BTV serotype 10, only one of five serotypes known to be active in the United States. At least 20 serotypes are known to exist worldwide. There is no licensed vaccine for use in cattle.

The control of BT within an infected cattle herd is difficult because subclinical infections and healthy carriers may be present. The single most important control measure for cattle appears to be vector control. Good water management is a primary step in vector control; the larvae of *C. variipennis* are found in the soft, silty, polluted mud in overflow areas around stock tanks or leaky septic tanks and along the edges of ponds, ditches, and streams. Providing good drainage and eliminating sources of animal and human pollution often reduce the number of potential vectors.

Good herd management may help control the spread of the disease. Moving animals from low-lying areas in which breeding sites of vectors predominate to a higher elevation is sometimes used to limit the spread of BT in sheep, but its usefulness with cattle is not known.

Supplemental Reading

Bowne, J. G.: Bluetongue disease. Adv. Vet. Sci. Comp. Med. *15*:1–46, 1971.
Howell, P. G.: Bluetongue. Emerg. Dis. Anim. *61*:111–153, 1963.
Metcalf, H. E., and Luedke, A. J.: Bluetongue and related diseases. Bovine Pract. *15*:188–193, 1980.

Bovine Enteroviruses

STEWART McCONNELL, D.V.M., M.Sc.

The family Picornaviridae comprises a group of viruses that are icosahedral in symmetry, 20 to 30 nm in diameter, and that contain RNA as their genetic component. The Picornaviridae are separated into four distinct genera: *Enterovirus, Cardiovirus, Rhinovirus,* and *Aphthovirus.* Enteroviruses are resistant to chloroform, ether, and acid medium (ph 3.0). They are readily isolated from nasopharyngeal secretions and feces.

Enteroviruses are subdivided according to the animal

species from which virus isolation occurred. To date over 60 strains of bovine enteroviruses (BEV) have been isolated. All BEV replicate readily in cell culture and are readily identified by their rapidly developing cytopathic effect (CPE). Serum neutralization and plaque reduction tests provide a basis for serologic classification of these viruses. Current classification by the World Health Organization and Food and Agricultural Organization (WHO/FAO) Comparative Virology Working Team shows seven serotypes to occur. These serotypes are designated BEV 1 through BEV 7.

Bovine enteroviruses have been isolated from apparently healthy cattle as well as from cattle suffering from clinical disease such as abortion, enteritis, and respiratory tract disease and from infertile bulls. Some investigators have isolated BEV from calves and pregnant cows with cough, fever, nasal discharges, enteritis, and so-called shipping fever. Others report that infection *in utero* may contribute to early death or lack of resistance of the newborn calf to bacterial infection.

Bovine enteroviruses have a worldwide distribution and appear to be ubiquitous among cattle populations. The frequent isolation of BEV from respiratory and enteric tracts of cattle suggests that these viruses are normal flora of the gastrointestinal tract. They are transient in nature and are not normally considered to be pathogenetic. Survival may depend on viral persistence; however, the mechanism of persistence is unknown. Infection with BEV is diagnosed by isolation of virus. There is a high prevalence of neutralizing antibodies in cattle.

Recently, a considerable cross reactivity among BEV strains has been observed, using cross neutralization and fluorescent antibody tests. This high prevalence of neutralizing antibodies in healthy cattle, a multiplicity of serotypes, and cross reactivity among bovine enteroviruses make serologic diagnosis of BEV infection impractical.

Since most BEV infections are subclinical and thus unrecognized, prevention and control are difficult. No vaccines have been developed to date and there are no specific prevention measures for bovine enterovirus infections.

Supplemental Reading

Bruner, D. W., and Gillespie, J. H.: Hagan's Infectious Diseases of Domestic Animals. Ithaca, Cornell University Press, 1973.

Kahrs, R. F.: Viral Diseases of Cattle. Ames, Iowa, Iowa State University Press, 1981, 115–120.

Mohanty, S. B., and Dutta, S. K.: Veterinary Virology. Philadelphia, Lea & Febiger, 1981, 120–122.

Bovine Rhinoviruses

BRUCE D. ROSENQUIST, D.V.M., Ph.D.

Although more than 113 serotypes of human rhinoviruses (RV) have been described, only 2 serotypes of bovine RV are officially recognized. With one exception, all isolates have been characterized as bovine RV type 1. A third serotype or a serologic variant may exist (Rosenquist, unpublished information). These serotypes are members of the Picornaviridae family.

EPIZOOTIOLOGY

Human RV do not cause infection in cattle and vice versa. Infection is no doubt worldwide and has been documented in England, Europe, Japan, Africa, and the United States. Exposure of calves is widespread. Approximately 95 per cent of Missouri beef and dairy calves less than one year of age that have been tested are seropositive to type 1 RV; virtually 100 per cent of those tested are seropositive by 10 to 12 months.

CLINICAL SIGNS AND LESIONS

Rhinoviruses, the most common cause of human colds, also cause respiratory infections in cattle. Opinions vary as to the pathogenicity of bovine RV. The author's personal prejudice, based on human RV literature and personal bovine RV experience, is that these viruses are important agents in the multifactorial etiology of bovine respiratory disease. In some cases, these have been the only viruses demonstrable in calves with respiratory disease. This does not rule out other agents or complicating factors. Clinical signs ascribed to RV infection include fever, lachrymation, nasal discharge, coughing, and increased respiratory rate. There may be no clinical signs observed.

DIAGNOSIS

Diagnosis requires laboratory confirmation of clinical suspicions by virus isolation in appropriate cell cultures or demonstration of a significant rise in neutralizing antibody titer between acute and convalescent phase sera. At present, laboratory diagnosis is confined to specialized laboratories.

TREATMENT

There is no specific treatment for RV. Treatment consists of supportive therapy and control of secondary infections.

PREVENTION AND CONTROL

Vaccines are not available.

Foot-and-Mouth Disease in Cattle

JERRY CALLIS, D.V.M., M.S., D.Sc.

Foot-and-mouth disease (FMD) is an acute, highly communicable disease caused by a virus of the Aphthovirus genus of the family Picornaviridae. There are seven distinct immunologic types, and immunity to one serotype does not confer protection against the other six. The virus is antigenically labile, resulting in numerous subtypes within each serotype. Subtypes may complicate control. Vaccination with some subtypes will not necessarily protect animals against other strains of the virus within the same serotype.

Infectivity of FMDV may be destroyed by chemicals such as acids, alkalis, formalin, and aziridines and by physical means such as high temperature, UV light, and x rays. Under natural conditions, the virus has been shown to survive for 14 days in a stall and for as long as 20 weeks on sacks and hay. A shift in the pH in either direction below 6 and above 9 makes conditions for survival less favorable. The most commonly used disinfectants are 2 per cent caustic soda, 4 per cent soda ash, and 2 per cent acetic acid.

EPIZOOTIOLOGY

Foot-and-mouth disease virus infects domesticated and wild cloven-hoofed animals, armadillos, rats, nutria, grizzly bears, and elephants. Dogs, cats, rabbits, chinchilla, mice, guinea pigs, and chickens are susceptible to experimental infection. Man can also be infected but only rarely; thus, FMD is not a public health problem. The disease occurs in livestock in all of the large land masses of the world where livestock are raised except Australia, New Zealand, North and Central America, and Greenland. The incidence in western Europe is low because of systematic application of well-produced and tested vaccines, control of movement of animals, and eradication efforts including decontamination when the disease occurs. The virus is spread by contact between infected and susceptible animals, by contaminated animal products such as meat and milk, by the airborne route, and by mechanical transfer. Cattle, sheep, goats, and cape buffalo have become carriers following recovery and are thought to serve as reservoirs between outbreaks. Contaminated products also serve to transmit the virus from one continent to another.

CLINICAL SIGNS AND LESIONS

FMD virus causes blisters or vesicles in the mouth, including the tongue, lips, gums, pharynx, teats, and palate and on the feet. There is also a sharp rise in body temperature of 1 to 3°C. Infected animals salivate, smack their lips, and are reluctant to move because of the pain caused by the blisters. These blisters rupture and leave eroded areas (Figs. 1 and 2).

DIAGNOSIS

There are other infections of the bovine that can be confused with FMD. Some of these are vesicular stomatitis, bovine papular stomatitis, infectious bovine rhinotracheitis, rinderpest, bluetongue, and malignant catarrhal fever. For this reason, a diagnosis of FMD based on clinical signs should be avoided, especially when it is the first occurrence of such a disease in the area. Specimens from the infected animal should be referred to an official laboratory with experienced staff and biocontainment facilities for containing the virus. There it can be diagnosed by isolation of the virus and identification by

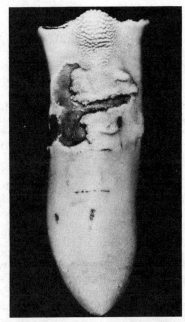

Figure 1. Ruptured vesicles caused by FMDV on bovine tongue.

complement-fixation, virus neutralization, enzyme-linked immunosorbent assay, and inoculation tests in livestock including the horse, which is not susceptible to FMD but is susceptible to vesicular stomatitis.

TREATMENT

There is no known specific cure for the infection, but palliative treatment may alleviate the signs.

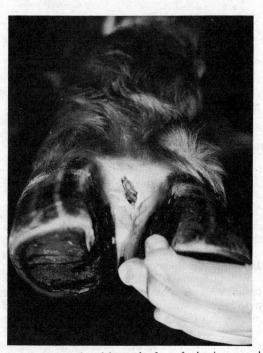

Figure 2. Ruptured vesicle on the foot of a bovine caused by FMDV.

PREVENTION AND CONTROL

In countries that are free from the disease, there are strict prohibitions on importation of animals or animal products from infected countries. Products that have been processed to assure their freedom from the virus, such as by cooking or drying, may be permitted entry. When FMD occurs, the disease-free countries eradicate it by slaughtering the infected animals, destroying the carcass by burning or burying, and decontaminating the premises. These procedures are practiced in several countries in Europe and North America.

Vaccines have been available since the 1930's and are used to control the incidence of infection in countries where FMD is enzootic or where eradication is impractical because of costs. In western Europe the judicious application of well-produced and tested vaccines is generally considered to be responsible for the low incidence of the disease. Vaccination alone has never been responsible for eradication of the disease. In endemic areas, vaccination is used to control the incidence of infection, and it has been used to lower the incidence to such levels that slaughter is economically feasible in eradication campaigns.

Supplemental Reading

Bachrach, H. L.: Foot-and-mouth disease. Ann. Rev. Microbiol. 22:201, 1968.

Callis, J. J., Cottral, G. E., and McKercher, P. D.: Foot-and-mouth disease. In CRC Handbook Series in Zoonoses: Viral Zoonoses, Volume II. CRC Press Inc., Boca Raton, Florida, 1981, 168–176.

Cottral, G. E., Shahan, M. S., and Seibold, H. R.: Foot-and-mouth disease. In Gibbons, W. J., Catcott, E. J., and Smithcors, J. F. (eds.): Bovine Medicine and Surgery. Wheaton, Ill., Amer. Vet. Pub., 1970, 47.

Bovine Rotavirus

CHARLES A. MEBUS, D.V.M., Ph.D.

Rotavirus is the name proposed for a new genus in the family Reoviridae. Thus far in cattle there is one serotype. Rotavirus is quite resistant; it remained viable for six months in fecal material held in a jar at room temperature. Resistance to disinfectants is most likely similar to that given for ovine rotavirus.

EPIZOOTOLOGY

Rotavirus infects a wide variety of domestic and wild ruminant and nonruminant species and man. To date, there is no evidence that cross-species infection is important under field conditions. Rotavirus diarrhea in cattle occurs worldwide. Infection is by ingestion through contact with teats, feed, bedding, equipment, or people contaminated with infected feces. Outbreaks of diarrhea have followed introduction into the herd of clinically normal animals from a salebarn and adult animals from a herd having a history of neonatal diarrhea. This circumstantial evidence suggests that clinically normal animals can be carriers.

CLINICAL SIGNS AND LESIONS

Rotavirus diarrhea in farm and ranch cattle most commonly occurs in calves from one day to three weeks old. The severity of clinical signs among calves varies; some calves become more depressed and have a more severe diarrhea than others. In general, onset of clinical signs is rapid. Within two to three hours, signs of illness will develop as follows: mild anorexia, depression to the degree that the calf may not stand, a few strings of thick saliva hanging from the lips, refusal to nurse, and diarrhea. In gnotobiotic calves, the diarrheal period lasts five or six hours. In natural infection, diarrhea may be more severe and may persist for several days, and animals may die. Calf mortality varies from herd to herd. Duration of the illness and mortality appear to be related to the type of secondary infection and to the quantity and type of passively acquired antibody.

Necropsy findings in natural infections may consist of some milk and thick fluid (saliva) in the abomasum and fluid contents in the large intestine. The color of the intestinal mucosa can vary from normal to reddened or even to areas of hemorrhage, depending upon the severity of secondary bacterial infection.

DIAGNOSIS

Diagnosis of rotavirus infections requires the demonstration of a large quantity of virus or virus-specific antigen in diarrheal feces. Methods used to detect rotavirus are negative-staining electron microscopy, immunofluorescent techniques, solid-phase radioimmunoassay, and enzyme-linked immunosorbent assay (ELISA).

TREATMENT

Diarrhea in very young calves with secondary bacterial complication will require immediate and careful treatment, but three-week-old calves with no secondary complications may recover rapidly with no treatment. When practical, milk feeding should be stopped. Calves with 5 per cent or less loss of body weight due to dehydration should be given fluids orally. Calves with 5 to 10 per cent dehydration should be given fluids orally and parenterally. Calves with greater than 10 per cent dehydration should be given fluids intravenously. To combat secondary bacterial infection, antibiotics should be given parenterally. In some cases, orally administered antibiotics are beneficial.

PREVENTION

Rotavirus can be introduced into a herd by the addition of infected cows or calves and by contaminated clothing and equipment. Therefore, management practices to minimize exposure are recommended.

Attenuated virus administered orally to newborn calves will protect against challenge inoculation. Efficacy of oral vaccination is affected by the level of rotavirus antibody in the colostrum and the timing of vaccine administration in relation to the first nursing. The vaccine appears to be most effective in herds in which rotavirus diarrhea is found in the very young calf. Vaccine administered to cows during gestation has also been shown to decrease the incidence of diarrhea in their calves.

Supplemental Reading

Lewis, L. D.: Calf diarrhea: Part III. Management, prevention and treatment of diarrhea. Norden News 53:22, 1978.

Mebus, C. A., and Newman, L. E.: Scanning electron, light and fluorescent microscopy of intestine of gnotobiotic calf infected with reovirus-like agent. Am. J. Vet. Res. 38:553, 1977.

Phillips, R. W., and Lewis, L. D.: Viral-induced changes in intestinal transport and resultant body fluid alterations in neonatal calves. Ann. Rech. Vet. 4:87, 1973.

Calf Coronavirus Diarrhea

CHARLES A. MEBUS, D.V.M., Ph.D.

As the name applies, this calf diarrhea is due to a coronavirus. To date there is one known serotype. Even though this virus is in the same genus as the virus of transmissible gastroenteritis of swine, these two viruses are serologically unrelated and do not cross infect.

EPIZOOTIOLOGY

Calf coronavirus infects only the bovine species. The disease has been diagnosed in North America and Europe but probably occurs worldwide. Route of infection is by ingestion through contact with teats, feed, or equipment contaminated with infected feces. The viral titer in feces passed during the first few hours of diarrhea is about 10^{10} particles/ml and decreases over the next five to seven days.

CLINICAL SIGNS

Coronavirus diarrhea occurs in farm and ranch calves one day to three or more weeks old. The incubation time in experimental calves varies from 20 to about 36 hours. The signs associated with appearance of the initial diarrhea are similar to those of rotavirus diarrhea; the feces are liquid and yellow, and the volume depends upon the amount of milk consumed before diarrhea. The clinical picture of coronavirus infection differs from that of rotavirus infections in that after the anorexia accompanying the initial diarrhea, noncomplicated coronavirus-infected calves will be hungry and, if fed milk, will continue to have diarrhea for five to six days. The feces will contain some curd and mucus, and the volume will depend upon the amount of milk fed. Bacteria-free calves fed a normal quantity of milk have died with signs of severe dehydration 48 to 62 hours after onset of diarrhea.

Necropsy findings in uncomplicated, natural infections are not dramatic. There may be milk in the abomasum and liquid contents in the colon. Reddening of the intestinal mucosa is due to secondary infection.

DIAGNOSIS

The preferred method of confirming a diagnosis of coronavirus enteritis is immunofluorescent staining of frozen sections of the spiral colon collected from a calf killed one to four days after onset of diarrhea.

TREATMENT

Treatment as described for rotavirus infection in ruminants is also applicable to bovine coronavirus infection. However, therapy may have to be continued for a longer period because of the more prolonged alteration of the small intestinal mucosa in coronavirus infection.

PREVENTION

Coronavirus can be introduced into a herd by a calf incubating the virus. Nothing is known about the carrier state of coronavirus infection. Good management practices to minimize exposure include avoiding introducing new animals immediately before or during calving and using only clean clothing, instruments, and equipment when working with calves.

Circulating immunoglobulin G coronavirus antibody will not protect a calf against coronavirus infection. Colostral immunoglobulin A in the intestinal lumen and that which is absorbed and resecreted will protect the calf for a limited time. Ideally, the calf should become infected when some antibody is still present, develop a subclinical infection, and thus become immunized.

Coronavirus vaccine administered orally to newborn calves induces resistance to challenge infection and production of local antibody within 72 hours. Efficacy of oral vaccinations is affected by the level of antibody in the colostrum and timing of vaccine administration in relation to the first nursing. Vaccine administered to the dam during gestation has also been shown to decrease the incidence of diarrhea in the newborn calf.

Supplemental Reading

Lewis, L. D., and Phillips, R. W.: Pathophysiologic changes due to coronavirus-induced diarrhea in the calf. J. Am. Vet. Med. Assoc. 173:636, 1978.

Mebus, C. A., Newman, L. E., and Stair, E. L., Jr.: Scanning electron, light and immunofluorescent microscopy of intestine of gnotobiotic calf infected with diarrhea coronavirus. Am. J. Vet. Res. 36:1, 1975.

Mebus, C. A., Torres-Medina, A., Twiehaus, M. J., and Bass, E.: Immune response to orally administered calf reovirus-like agent and coronavirus vaccine. Develop. Biol. Stand. 33:393, 1976.

Rift Valley Fever in Cattle

R. J. YEDLOUTSCHNIG, D.V.M.
and J. S. WALKER, D.V.M., M.S.

Rift Valley fever (RVF) is an acute, febrile, arthropod-borne viral disease primarily affecting sheep, goats, and cattle. The disease is caused by a mosquito-borne, pantropic, RNA virus of the family Bunyaviridae, genus *Phlebovirus*. The reference strains Entebbe, Smithburn,

Table 1. *Host Range of Rift Valley Fever Virus*

4+	3+	2+	1+	—
aLamb	Man Sheep	Goat Camel Buffalo Cattle	Cat	Swine
aKid	Calf (more than 1 week old)	Monkey (Indian and S. American)	Dog Horse	Chicken Guinea pig Rabbit
aCalf	Rat (some species)		Monkey (African)	
aPuppies				Hedgehog
aKittens		Rat (some species)		Tortoise Frog
White mice Hamster Field mice Dormouse Field vole		Gray squirrel		Canary Pigeon Parakeet

Key: 4+ = nearly 100 per cent fatal.
  3+ = severe illness with some mortality.
  2+ = severe illness, abortion in animals, and viremia.
  1+ = abortion, viremia, some illness to no overt signs of disease.
  − = refractive to natural disease and in those species tested to laboratory infection.
  aLess than one week old.
  Note: It is likely that with extensive laboratory testing the very young of several species noted above would fall into the 4+ classification. Also, based upon recent data from the epizootics of the 1970's, man has been placed under the 3+ column.

and Lunyo and several current strains are all serologically indistinguishable. The RVF virus (RVFV) is stable indefinitely at −70°C or lower, and there is little loss in virus titer at 4° to −40°C after one year of storage. The virus in infective lamb serum has remained viable at 37°C for up to three weeks and for four months at 25°C. The optimal stability of the virus is within a pH range of 7.0 to 8.0; it is inactivated rapidly below pH 6.2, even when frozen at −60°C. Some of the chemical inactivants include sodium deoxycholate, formalin, methylene blue in the presence of light, and 2 per cent acetic acid.

EPIZOOTIOLOGY

Rift Valley fever virus naturally affects sheep, cattle, buffalo, camels, and goats, causing high mortality in young lambs and calves and abortion in adults. Humans also become infected, especially by contact with infected animals and carcasses; clinical signs include an acute influenza-like illness with severe headache and generalized myalgia, sometimes culminating in death. As seen in Table 1, a variety of other animals are susceptible to RVFV in varying degrees. The disease occurs naturally only on the African continent; accidental infections have been confined to nonvaccinated laboratory workers in the United States, England, and Japan. Rift Valley fever was first described in 1931 in the Rift Valley of Kenya. A major epizootic occurred in 1950 to 1951 and another in 1975. In October and November 1977 an outbreak of RVF occurred for the first time in Egypt. In some severely affected areas, about 70 per cent of the human population was infected.

Several species of mosquitoes transmit RVF, including *Aedes, Eretmapodites,* and *Culex.* The spread of RVF in Egypt was attributed almost exclusively to *Culex pipiens.* Direct transmission from blood or other infected tissues via aerosol to other animals and to man and via aerosol in laboratories is common. Virus is shed from 24 hours before illness to the time of death. The major method of natural transmission is by mosquito bites after replication of the virus in the vector. Mechanical transmission by biting arthropods is also possible.

Aedes mosquitoes may maintain RVFV by transovarial transmission and thus serve as a possible reservoir host. RVFV may also be maintained for short periods by cyclic transmission between domestic animals and arthropods. A long-term carrier state in animals is not known. Birds, wild bovidae, rodents, and domestic cattle do not account for interepidemic maintenance of RVFV.

CLINICAL SIGNS

The initial clinical signs observed are a mortality rate of 90 to 100 per cent in newborn calves and a high rate of abortion in pregnant cows. The clinical signs in adult cattle include a high temperature of 40 to 41.6°C, leukopenia, salivation, anorexia, general weakness, fetid diarrhea, a rapid decrease in lactation, abortion, and a mortality rate of less than 10 per cent, which may be higher if the infected cattle are in a poor state of health or nutrition.

Gross pathologic changes are most consistently observed in the liver, which becomes enlarged, soft, and friable and has a yellowish-brown discoloration and frequent numerous 1- to 2-mm greyish-white necrotic foci. Hemorrhages are seen infrequently in the abomasum and intestinal tract.

DIAGNOSIS

Diagnostic features indicative of an outbreak of RVF include (1) high mortality rate in lambs, calves, and kids, but a lower mortality rate in adults; (2) high abortion rate among cows and ewes; (3) liver lesions at necropsy; (4) an influenza-like viral illness in humans, especially after handling infective material; and (5) suitable conditions for mosquitoes.

Characteristic hepatic lesions provide presumptive evidence, but virus isolation and various serologic techniques are necessary for a positive diagnosis. Tissues for virus isolation should include liver, spleen, brain, and whole blood or serum taken at the peak febrile response. Samples should be maintained at 4°C or frozen; if dry ice is used, the specimens must be protected from exposure to CO_2.

The standard method for diagnosis of RFV is virus isolation in inoculated baby or adult mice or hamsters, cell culture, or lambs and then serologic identification of the virus.

TREATMENT

The RVFV is sensitive to several antiviral agents and interferon *in vitro*; however, chemotherapy for the disease in animals has not been successful.

PREVENTION AND CONTROL

Passive antibody has produced inconsistent protection and is not practical in an epizootic. Mass vaccination is the method of choice in controlling RVF during an epizootic. Virus attenuated by serial intracerebral passage in mice has been used to produce vaccines. However, attenuated or modified live virus vaccines have caused abortions in pregnant animals. Immunity lasts several years, and there is no significant decrease in antibody levels in cattle and sheep 30 to 36 months after vaccination. The World Health Organization (WHO) recommends that the current live virus vaccines be used only in enzootic areas of Africa.

Because of the abortion problems with the attenuated vaccine, a killed vaccine produced in BHK cells has not been developed for animal use. Two doses of the vaccine are required for adequate protection. These killed vaccines are the only ones recommended by WHO for use outside of enzootic areas of Africa.

Virus grown in rhesus monkey kidney cell cultures and inactivated with formalin stimulates excellent immunity in humans and sheep without any side effects.

Reduction of exposure to mosquitoes by moving the animals to an altitude where mosquitoes are absent or application of residual insecticides to animals and their pens and barns will decrease the number of new cases.

Supplemental Reading

Shope, R. E., Peters, C. J., and Davies, F. G.: The spread of Rift Valley fever and approaches to its control. Bull. WHO 60:229–304, 1982.
Swartz, T. A., Klingberg, M. A., and Goldman, N. (eds.): Rift Valley Fever, Contributions to Epidemiology and Biostatistics, Vol. 3. Basel, S. Karger, 1981, 1–196.
Walker, J. S.: Rift Valley Fever. Foreign Animal Diseases. Richmond, Virginia, U.S. Animal Health Assoc., 1975, 209–221.

Akabane Disease in Cattle

A. J. DELLA-PORTA, B.Sc., Ph.D.

Akabane disease is a congenital disease of cattle, sheep, and goats characterized by hydranencephaly (HE), arthrogryposis (AG), micrencephaly, and porencephaly. It usually occurs as localized epizootics and less frequently as sporadic cases. There may also be an increased incidence of abortion and stillbirth in the months preceding the epizootic of congenital AG/HE.

The disease is caused by Akabane virus, an insect-transmitted virus (arbovirus) belonging to the family Bunyaviridae, that occurs as an inapparent infection in nonimmune animals. If infection occurs during early pregnancy (principally during the early stages of brain development in the fetus), the virus may cross the placenta, and the resulting infection of the fetus may cause deformities. It has been reported in Australia, Japan, Israel, and Turkey, and the virus has also been isolated in Kenya and South Africa. Akabane disease has occurred every few years as localized epizootics in Australia for at least the last 40 years and in Japan for at least the last 30 years.

In an area where the suspect insect vector is endemic, most animals become infected early in their life, and only isolated, sporadic cases of Akabane disease are seen. Epizootics are thought to occur when extended, warm, humid summers favor the extension of virus-infected insects beyond their normal geographic distribution to areas populated by susceptible pregnant animals.

CLINICAL SIGNS

Infection in the pregnant animal is inapparent. In some instances the first sign of disease is an increase in abortions. In calves, the apparent sequence of principal clinical signs appears to be mild incoordination, then arthrogryposis ("curly calves," fixed flexion, and sometimes extension of one or more limbs), and then hydranencephaly ("dummy calves," blind, with large portions of their brains replaced by fluid). These syndromes can overlap in sequence, and animals can be seen exhibiting more than one of these signs.

The central nervous system lesions can vary from mild to very severe, with absence of most of the cerebrum. When arthrogryposis is present, the gross appearance of the brain and spinal cord is often normal, but microscopically there is a severe, diffuse loss of myelinated fibers from the lateral and ventral horn neurons and loss of nerve fibers from ventral spinal nerves. There is also severe atrophy of the skeletal muscles. In the hydranencephaly seen toward the end of the epizootic both cerebral hemispheres of the majority of affected animals are almost completely replaced by fluid. Several of the pathologic changes can occur simultaneously and should not be considered as clearly defined, separate stages in Akabane disease.

DIAGNOSIS

As Akabane virus has not been isolated from congenitally affected offspring born at term and only occasionally from aborted fetuses, proof of infection must be based on serologic and pathologic evidence. In an outbreak the most important specimens for diagnosis are a sample of serum from the mother and a precolostrum sample from its affected offspring. Samples of brain and cervical, thoracic, and lumbar regions of the spinal cord should be preserved in 10 per cent neutral formalin for histologic examination.

Serologic diagnosis of infection is based on a neutralization test in African green monkey kidney Vero cells. If both the serum from the dam and the *precolostrum* serum from the offspring contain neutralizing antibodies against Akabane virus, then this virus probably caused the *in utero* damage to the fetus.

Similar congenital deformities in calves may be caused by bluetongue virus infection, may be of genetic or environmental origin, or may be associated with teratogenic chemicals. The deformities may also be of some unknown origin. The detection of elevated levels of specific immunoglobulin (IgG_1) in precolostrum serum samples from the affected calf would indicate whether an infectious agent was involved.

PREVENTION

As only susceptible pregnant animals can be involved in Akabane disease, prevention involves ensuring that either immunity to Akabane virus infection is developed early in life or in a nonbreeding period, or that animals are not pregnant when virus-infected insects are likely to be present in the area. An inactivated vaccine is available in Japan and may prove useful in preventing Akabane disease.

Supplemental Reading

Hartley, W. J., De Sarum, W. G., Della-Porta, A. J., Snowdon, W. A., and Shepherd, N. C.: Pathology of congenital bovine epizootic arthrogryposis and hydranencephaly and its relationship to Akabane virus. Aust. Vet. J. *53:*319–325, 1977.

Kurogi, H., Inaba, Y., Takahashi, E., Sato, K., Satoda, K., Goto, Y., Omori, T., and Matumoto, M.: Congenital abnormalities in newborn calves after inoculation of pregnant cows with Akabane virus. Infect. Immunol. *17:*338–343, 1977.

Porterfield, J. S., and Della-Porta, A. J.: Bunyaviridae: Infections and diagnosis. *In* Kurstak, E., and Kurstak, C. (eds.): Comparative Diagnosis of Viral Diseases, Vol. 4, Part B. New York, Academic Press, 1981, 479–508.

Parainfluenza-3 Virus

GLYNN H. FRANK, D.V.M., M.S., Ph.D.

Parainfluenza-3 (PI-3) virus is a paramyxovirus, and, thus far, all bovine and ovine isolates fall into one serologic group. The virus hemagglutinates the red blood cells (RBC) of many species and grows on primary cells and established cell lines of a number of species. The cytopathic effect (CPE) usually includes syncytia formation and intracytoplasmic inclusions and sometimes intranuclear inclusions. Reported strain markers have included hemagglutination patterns, neuraminidase content, and CPE type, but the stability of the markers is in question.

EPIZOOTIOLOGY

PI-3 virus has been isolated from cattle and sheep with respiratory disease and is one of the most common viruses involved in the "shipping fever complex" of cattle. The virus is found worldwide and seems to be, from numerous serologic surveys, ubiquitous in cattle and sheep. Seronegative cattle are relatively rare and are highly susceptible to the virus.

CLINICAL SIGNS

Uncomplicated PI-3 viral infections are mild, and the majority are probably asymptomatic. Young calves often seroconvert with no history of respiratory disease. The economic importance of the virus lies in its ability to predispose cattle to *Pasteurella haemolytica* pneumonia, the most common form of acute respiratory disease in feedlot cattle.

This respiratory disease is most likely to occur in calves that have been subjected to the stresses of the marketing procedure and transportation. It is most likely to occur within one to two weeks after calves arrive at the feedyard. Lung lesions of experimental uncomplicated PI-3 viral infections are quickly resolved, but the virus can persist in the alveolar macrophages, and the natural clearance of *P. haemolytica* from the lungs is impaired. Naturally occurring PI-3 virus infection, if severe, is part of a respiratory disease complex involving other agents. Viral lesions will usually be overshadowed by those of bacterial pneumonia. The role of PI-3 virus in respiratory disease of sheep is much the same as in cattle.

DIAGNOSIS

PI-3 virus is readily isolated from the nasal passages during the acute phase of respiratory disease but usually not from recovering animals. At necropsy, the virus can be isolated from several tissues of the respiratory tract but from the lungs for a longer time than from other tissues. Besides virus isolation and identification, the involvement of PI-3 virus in a respiratory disease outbreak is detected by serologic evidence. In the diagnostic laboratory, the virus is easily identified by standard procedures.

TREATMENT

Treatment would be necessary only in complicated infections. These would be evident as acute cases of respiratory disease, and treatment would consist of treating for bacterial pneumonia.

PREVENTION

Vaccines are available for cattle, and some advocate using the vaccines in sheep. A wide variety of vaccines, both killed and attenuated, are available. They all consist of PI-3 virus in combination with other agents. Vaccines have been shown to lessen the severity of experimental

PI-3 virus infection. Their effectiveness under field conditions is difficult to determine because of the large variety of etiologic agents involved in the bovine respiratory disease complex.

Supplemental Reading

Frank, G. H., and Marshall, R. G.: Parainfluenza-3 virus infection of cattle. J. Am. Vet. Med. Assoc. *163*:858, 1973.
Kahrs, R. F.: Parainfluenza-3. *In* Kahrs, R. F. (ed.): Viral Diseases of Cattle, 1st ed. Ames, Ia.: Iowa State University Press, 1981, 171–181.

Rinderpest

A. H. DARDIRI, D.V.M., M.V.Sc., M.Sc., Ph.D.

Rinderpest (RP), also known as cattle plague, is an acute, febrile, highly contagious, and usually fatal disease of ruminants, especially cattle and buffalo. It occurs also in sheep, goats, and wild ruminants. During the height of febrile reaction, the virus is found in all body tissues.

ETIOLOGY

Rinderpest virus (RPV) is a member of the Paramyxoviridae family and the genus *Morbillivirus*, as are the viruses causing measles, canine distemper, and peste des petits ruminants (PPR). It is spherical or ovoid with a maximum diameter of 120 to 300 nm.

Rinderpest virus will remain viable in frozen tissues for at least one year; its infectivity is maintained by storage at −70°C and lyophilization. Direct sunlight inactivates the virus in thin layers of blood after two hours of exposure. It is also inactivated by frequent freezing and thawing of blood and tissues samples. Furthermore, the virus loses infectivity at pH 12.0 and at pH 2.0 when exposed for 10 minutes. The changes associated with putrefaction of meat and lactic acid fermentation also inactivate the virus. Heparin or EDTA should be used as anticoagulant.

Rinderpest virus has an affinity to attack the leukocytes, the mucosa of the gastrointestinal tract, and lymphatic tissues. Strains of rinderpest are immunologically homologous; a vaccine prepared from one strain protects against all. Strains of RP from cattle are closely related serologically and immunologically to PPR virus. The virus of RP has been cultivated in several cell culture systems. There is only one immunologic type of RPV. Cattle that recover from RPV acquire a lifelong immunity.

EPIZOOTIOLOGY

Cattle and water buffalo are the most susceptible natural hosts of RPV. Camels can become infected when in close proximity with rinderpest-infected cattle. Domestic swine in Southeast Asia are susceptible. Several wildlife ruminants and pigs in Far-eastern Asia are naturally infected with RP, and domestic European pigs acquire an inapparent infection. The white-tailed deer and the white-colored peccaries, both native to the United States, were infected experimentally. Innate resistance does exist but varies widely within and between species and breeds of cattle.

In the 1960's, RP outbreaks were brought under control in Africa as a result of an international vaccine campaign; however, a significant resurgence of the disease occurred on that continent in 1980. In central Africa, the disease extends from the Sahelien countries to Ethiopia, and outbreaks have been reported in Chad, Egypt, and Tanzania. Additionally, in 1983, serious outbreaks were reported from the countries of the Near and Middle East.

Rinderpest is an airborne contagion and spreads rapidly by direct contact between sick and healthy animals. The disease is contagious from two days before the onset of fever to the start of convalescence or death. The virus enters through the mucosa of the respiratory tract. All discharges from sick animals contain the virus, and the two dominant routes of excretion are the nasal secretions and the feces.

CLINICAL SIGNS

The incubation period in domestic cattle ranges from 3 to 15 days and is longest in animals with high innate resistance. The incubation period is followed by sudden fever, depression, restlessness, and rapid shallow breathing. The muzzle is dry, visible mucosa are congested, and the appetite is impaired. As the disease progresses, necrotic mucosal foci appear in the oral cavity; the mucosa sloughs off, leaving punched-out erosions, and lacrimation is purulent. As the fever falls, diarrhea begins and the feces contain blood. Dehydration, emaciation, and prostration precede death.

Gross lesions are seen in the alimentary tract and lymphoid tissues. The mucosa of the mouth is eroded. The mucosa of the abomasum is usually edematous, congested, and sometimes ulcerated. In the small intestine, the Peyer's patches are swollen, hemorrhagic, and necrotic. The cecal and abomasal mucosa are often ulcerated and bleeding. In the large intestine, congested capillaries in the longitudinal folds of the mucosa produce a striped effect, called zebra stripes, that extends to the rectum. In animals that live longer, the lungs have alveolar and interstitial emphysema. Animals that die early may show subendocardial hemorrhage.

Rinderpest virus has an affinity to lymphocytes and the epithelial cells of the gastrointestinal mucosa. The lymphocytes are destroyed in the germinal centers of the lymph follicles; similar destruction of the lymphoid tissue occurs in the tonsils, Peyer's patches, cecal tonsils, and the splenic corpuscles.

DIAGNOSIS

Cases of RP conforming to the classical description are found when there are outbreaks in areas that had been free of the disease; however, laboratory diagnosis is essential.

Laboratory confirmation of RP diagnosis can be achieved by several tests: (1) virus isolation from sick and dead animals, (2) detection of virus-specific antigen by CF, AGDP, and FA tests, (3) demonstration of antibody development, and (4) histopathology showing virus-specific alterations. Successful isolation of the virus is from blood and tissues collected during the thermal response and the first four days before the onset of diarrhea. The

CF, AGAP, and direct FA tests give a rapid presumptive diagnosis; virus isolation and serologic identification provide a definitive diagnosis.

Diseases that have clinical features common with RP are bovine virus diarrhea, infectious bovine rhinotracheitis, acute gastro-enteritis, and conditions such as arsenic poisoning and acute coccidiosis. In small ruminants it must be differentiated from Nairobi sheep disease, bluetongue, and PPR.

Blood in EDTA or heparin, lymph nodes, and spleen are required for detection of the virus and its antigens. Tissues must be sent to the laboratory in sterile, sealed containers on wet or dry ice. Blood should not be sent frozen. It is preferable to collect the samples during the febrile stage of the disease, no longer than four days after the peak of temperature. Lymph node biopsies could be obtained from living animals for detection of precipitinogen.

PREVENTION AND CONTROL

Recently, the virulent Kabete "O" strain of RPV was attenuated by passage in calf kidney cell culture monolayers. This is the vaccine of choice. It is relatively inexpensive, produces solid immunity, does not produce clinical reaction, and has a long shelf life.

Control of virgin epizootics is achieved by slaughter of infected animals, contact ruminants, and swine together with disinfection of the premises and application of strict quarantine measures in areas of disease outbreaks. In enzootic areas, vaccination is practiced regularly.

Supplemental Reading

Dardiri, A. H., Yedloutschnig, R. J., and Taylor, W. D.: Clinical and serologic response of American white-colored peccaries to ASF, FMD, VS, VES, HC and rinderpest virus. Proc. U.S.A.H.A. 73rd meeting, 1969, 437–452.

Fenner, F.: Classification and nomenclature of viruses. Second report of international committee on taxonomy of viruses. Intervirology 7:59, 1976.

Hamdy, F. M., Dardiri, A. H., Ferris, D. H., and Breese, S. S., Jr.: Experimental infection of white-tailed deer with rinderpest virus. J. Wildlife Dis. 11:508, 1975.

Bovine Respiratory Syncytial Virus

M. H. SMITH, D.V.M., Ph.D.

Bovine respiratory syncytial virus (BRSV) was first recognized as causing disease in cattle in 1970. Since that time it has been recognized worldwide as being associated with bovine respiratory disease (BRD) of varying severity. BRSV is a pleomorphic virus of the family Paramyxoviridae, genus *Pneumovirus,* and only one serotype has been recognized. The virus does not survive for any appreciable time outside the host and is readily inactivated.

EPIZOOTIOLOGY

BRSV will infect cattle of all ages. Disease has been noted in calves and adult cows, both dairy and beef.

Respiratory syncytial (RS) viruses from a variety of species (man, bovine, caprine, ovine) are very closely related antigenically, and little difference has been found in viral polypeptides between RS viruses of man and bovine. Transmission of the disease occurs by droplet and aerosol.

CLINICAL SIGNS AND LESIONS

The spectrum of clinical signs extends from subclinical to mild to life-threatening. The high incidence of antibody in cattle populations is indicative of widespread subclinical infection.

Clinical signs include elevated temperature, hyperpnea, increased harshness in respiratory sounds, and spontaneous coughing that can vary from dry and nonproductive to moist. Coughing can often be easily induced. Nasal discharge in varying degrees is often present. Conjunctivitis is rarely seen. Most cases recover spontaneously. Severe cases often progress to death in spite of treatment.

Most efforts at experimentally infecting calves have resulted in only mild or subclinical manifestations of disease, whereas others have succeeded in producing severe disease. Speculation would have to be that there are differences in pathogenicity among virus isolates. Additional work needs to be done to ascertain this. Experimental infection consistently produces high temperatures (up to 107 to 108°F or 41 to 42°C), often without concurrent signs of disease.

Field cases of BRSV-induced respiratory disease often involve *Pasteurella* as a secondary invader. However, there is evidence that severe bronchopneumonia can result from a pure infection of BRSV. There is also mounting evidence that a mild BRSV infection can be followed a short time later by a severe pneumonia with emphysema resembling atypical interstitial pneumonia and is often fatal. Examination of affected lungs often reveals consolidation of cranioventral lobes with varying degrees of emphysema. There is usually no pleuritis or abscess formation unless secondary infection is obvious.

Lungs examined microscopically often exhibit bronchopneumonia with varying degrees of bronchiolitis obliterans and proliferation of bronchiolar epithelium. Syncytia with or without inclusions are frequently observed.

DIAGNOSIS

Serologic studies indicate that 40 to 50 per cent of respiratory disease outbreaks in feeder calves involve BRSV. However, there are few salient features that would assist a clinician in making a presumptive diagnosis of BRSV-induced disease. A diagnosis is often made only by virus isolation and/or a demonstration of a rise in antibody to the virus. BRSV is difficult to isolate because of its lability and because nasal swab material is usually taken too late. Samples taken early in the clinical course, when high temperatures exist and before signs of severe respiratory disease appear, are most likely to be successful in yielding the virus. Many cell types support replication of BRSV.

Immunofluorescent techniques, both direct and indirect, and serum neutralization tests are used to detect antibody to BRSV. Recently a hemagglutination inhibition test has been described. Enzyme-linked immunosorbent assay tests have been used with varying degrees of success. By the time severe signs of respiratory disease are noted, the antibody titer may already be quite elevated and the acute and convalescent serum titers may be inverted. A number of animals in an outbreak should be sampled for meaningful serologic studies.

TREATMENT, PREVENTION, AND CONTROL

Conventional treatment with antibiotics and supportive therapy to combat secondary infections is usually successful. Where severe clinical manifestations exist with emphysema and death occurs within the infected herd, more vigorous therapy with antihistamines and corticosteroids in addition to antibiotics and supportive therapy may be necessary.

Conventional management practices, such as preconditioning to lessen the stress coincident with weaning, are often helpful in disease prevention. Vaccines have been developed in countries such as Belgium. A vaccine has been developed and field tested in the U.S. and is awaiting licensing for marketing. Widespread use of the vaccine will determine its efficacy.

Supplemental Reading

Bohlender, R. E.: Bovine respiratory syncytial virus infection. Mod. Vet. Pract. 63:613–618, 1982.
Brugere-Picoux, I.: Le virus respiratoire synctial bovine—une revue: Rec. Med. Vet. 157:875–882, 1981.
Bryson, D. G., McNulty, M. S., Logan, E. F., and Cush, P. F.: Respiratory syncytial virus pneumonia in young calves: Clinical and pathologic findings: Am. J. Vet. Res. 44:1648–1655, 1983.
Hibbs, C. M., Frey, M. L., and Bohlender, R.: Pulmonary edema and emphysema in feeder calves. Mod. Vet. Pract. 62:381–383, 1981.
Martin, H. T.: Indirect hemagglutination test for the detection and assay of antibody to bovine respiratory syncytial virus: Vet. Rec. 113:290–293, 1983.
Smith, M. H., Frey, M. L., and Dierks, R. E.: Isolation, characterization, and pathogenicity studies of a bovine respiratory syncytial virus. Arch. Virol. 47:237–247, 1975.

Sporadic Bovine Encephalomyelitis (SBE)

PETER A. BACHMANN, D.V.M.

Sporadic bovine encephalomyelitis (SBE) is an acute to subacute disease of the central nervous system. Usually only single cases are observed, predominantly in cattle between one and three years of age, at a time when they have reached breeding age. About 65 to 75 per cent of all confirmed cases of SBE fall into this age group.

ETIOLOGY

Although the neurohistologic picture indicates that SBE is a virus-induced disease, the precise nature of the etiologic agent is not quite clear. From one of these cases a morbillivirus (Paramyxoviridae) was isolated by co-cultivating brain material with bovine and monkey cell cultures. The agent (PMV-107) is highly cell-associated and antigenically not related to any of the known viruses. But experimental inoculation of calves and heifers via

different routes did not result in the reproduction of clinical symptoms nor did histologic alterations occur in the CNS. Out of 21 experimentally infected cattle, 12 developed antibodies to PMV-107. The agent is widespread; and limited serologic surveys demonstrated fluorescing antibodies in titers of 1:10 in 54 out of 105 bovine sera from the U.S., 19 out of 32 sera from Australia, and 105 out of 157 sera from Germany. In addition, in 8 of 15 human sera from SSPE patients tested, antibody to PMV-107 was present with significantly lower titers than those against homologous viruses.

EPIZOOTIOLOGY

The clinical disease was first recognized in Switzerland and later in southern Germany. Because it is extremely rare, it probably has not been given much attention. In Switzerland, 18 cases of SBE were reported in one area during a ten year period. Epizootiologic investigations of 104 cases in southern Germany showed that between 0.5 and 1.5 cases per 100,000 head of cattle occurred each year. From this data it appears that sporadic bovine encephalitis is only of minor economic importance. However, since there are a number of more important bovine diseases with clinical symptoms similar to sporadic encephalomyelitis, their clinical symptoms must also be taken into account when considering differential diagnosis. Furthermore, the neurohistologic changes of these cases resemble those of experimentally induced encephalitis in calves with SSPE virus from man. SSPE virus is a measles virus variant that causes subacute sclerosing encephalitis in children, and there is some discussion that animals are involved in the epidemiology of SSPE because of its rural predominance.

The older literature refers to a chlamydial encephalomyelitis also as sporadic bovine encephalomyelitis (SBE). These are, however, two distinctly different disease entities.

CLINICAL SIGNS

The onset of clinical illness is sometimes sudden. The first general symptom is anorexia, and lactating animals show a reduction in milk production. Acutely sick animals rapidly lose weight and deteriorate. In some cases temperatures of up to 40°C are recorded.

The duration of the illness in the majority of cases varies between two and five days, after which time death occurs. Usually these animals are killed within two to four days after onset of clinical symptoms. Some animals have a more protracted course of the disease, which can last for weeks.

The specific symptoms vary. The majority of animals show psychic abnormalities such as depressed reactivity, somnolence, stubborn behavior, nonphysiologic eating behavior, and yawning. But also timidity, aggressiveness, raving madness during which animals run against fixed objects, and howling are observed. Attempts to excite the animals by trying to give them water, as can be done in the case of rabid cattle, however, are always negative. In all cases motor symptoms are quite pronounced. The animals sway, dot, and stagger, and sometimes circular movements by the animals are observed. Abnormal po-

Table 1. *Differential Diagnosis of Sporadic Bovine Encephalomyelitis*

Disease	Cause	Occurrence	Age Prevalence	Seasonality	Cardinal Signs of Disease
Sporadic bovine encephalomyelitis (SBE)	Not known, possible virus (paramyxovirus 107?)	Sporadic	1- to 3-year-old cattle	No	Depressed reactivity, somnolence, incoordination, abnormal positioning of head, asymmetric functional disorders
Rabies	Virus infection through bite	Sporadic	All ages except calves	Yes (fall/winter)	Hydrophobia, salivation, altered behavior, howling, excitation, death within 3 to 6 days
Pseudorabies	Virus infection	Sporadic, multiple cases	All ages	No	Irritation, rapid onset, death within 2 to 3 days
Listeriosis	*Listeria monocytogenes*	Sporadic	Adult cattle	Yes (winter)	Asymmetric functional disorders, circular movements, death within 4 to 14 days
Septicemic thrombosing meningoencephalitis (ISTME)	*Haemophilus somnus*	Multiple cases in herd	Young cattle	Yes (winter)	Somnolence, incoordination, extended neck
Botulism	*Clostridium botulinum* toxin	Multiple cases in herd	All ages	No	Paralysis of muscles
Tetanus	*Clostridium tetani* wound infection	Sporadic	All ages	No	"Sawing threstle" position, trismus
Lead intoxication	Ingestion of lead	Sporadic; or multiple cases in herd	All ages	No	Blindness, incoordination, pushing forward, teeth grinding, salivation, pareses

sitioning of the head; paralysis of the face, tongue, and pharynx; nonphysiologic positioning of limbs ("sawing threstle" position and split-position); and incoordination are frequent occurrences. With progressing paralysis, the inward bending of carpal and tarsal joints, falling down, and eventually complete paralysis of the hind limbs can be observed. Opisthotonus and nonphysiologic positioning of the head are frequent occurrences in the animals that become prostrate. Salivation, teeth grinding, difficulties in swallowing, tympany of the rumen, occasional diarrhea, and tenesmus are accompanying signs. The expression of the eyes alters, and slight miosis and ptosis occur. The animals become very weak, and dyspnea occurs before they die.

NECROPSY FINDINGS

Macroscopic alterations are missing or nonspecific: increased amount of liquor and more or less strong injection of meningeal vessels. Histologic alterations generally spread over all parts of the brain and stem, showing individual variations with respect to topography. They consist of perivascular infiltration, proliferation of glia, and parenchymal damage. The infiltration of blood vessels is comprised of lymphocytic and histiocytic cells and also of plasma cells along the smaller vessels. Proliferation of glia occurs diffusely or as small, round, and irregular foci. They occur in association with blood vessel alterations and are spread through white and gray matter. Parenchymal damage is more discrete when compared with the infiltration and proliferative changes.

DIAGNOSIS

Clinical diagnosis is difficult. All infections in which CNS symptoms predominate have to be taken into consideration. Sporadic encephalomyelitis occurs only in single cases with an age preference. Symptoms are mostly asymmetric. Particularly rabies, pseudorabies, listeriosis, tetanus, *Haemophilus somnus* infections, and lead intoxication must be considered in clinical differential diagnosis (Table 1).

Precise diagnosis can only be made by histologic investigation of the brain, demonstration of perivascular cuffing, proliferation of glia, and parenchymal damage in the absence of any other changes.

PREVENTION AND CONTROL

Therapy is not possible. Since the etiology of SBE is still uncertain and the importance of antibodies to PMV 107-virus in cattle and man is not known, it should be kept in mind that the causative agent of SBE is a potential hazard to man.

Supplemental Reading

Bachmann, P. A., ter Meulen, V., Jentsch, G., Appel, M., Iwasaki, Y., Meyermann, R., Koprowski, H., and Mayr, A.: Sporadic bovine meningo-encephalitis-isolation of a paramyxovirus. Arch. Virol. *48*:107–120, 1975.
Fanghauser, R.: Sporadische Meningo-Encephalitis beim Rind. Schw. Arch. Tierhlkd. *103*:225–235, 1967.

Thein, P., Mayr, A., ter Meulen, V., Koprowski, H., Kaeckell, M. Y., Muker, D., and Meyermann, R.: Subacute sclerosing panencephalitis. Transmission of the virus to calves and lambs. Arch. Neurol. *27*:540–548, 1972.

Rabies in Cattle

GEORGE M. BAER, D.V.M., M.P.H.

In recent years in the United States more cases of rabies have been reported in cattle than in either dogs or cats (Table 1). This situation has come about through the reduction of cases in dogs and cats rather than in a dramatic increase in bovine cases. In earlier years there were many more rabid dogs than cattle; in 1953, for instance, 5,688 rabid dogs and 842 rabid cattle were reported. The cattle cases are found in those states with the most skunk rabies (Figs. 1 and 2); in 1979 these were Iowa (39 cases), Texas (34), Minnesota (21), Missouri (18), South Dakota (17), Wisconsin (15), Illinois (12), North Dakota (9), Arkansas (8), and Kansas (6). Rabies cases in cattle are directly responsible for the relatively high number of persons exposed to these animals, mostly farmers, ranchers, and veterinarians.

CLINICAL SIGNS

The signs of rabies in cattle vary, but some of the following will be found in virtually all animals:

1. Straining with repeated efforts to urinate or defecate; the signs may be confused with the typical straining seen at parturition.

2. Paralysis, often starting in the hindquarters, very often in one leg only, with a typical knuckling at the fetlock joint.

3. Anorexia and the abrupt cessation of lactation, often confused with some intestinal disturbance such as impaction of the rumen or rectum.

4. Altered facial expression, a very tense alert appearance (Fig. 3), and the bells of the ears thrown forward. The eyes are wide open and follow any moving object with a fixed stare.

5. Bellowing is common. The head is extended, the back arched, the flanks tucked in, and a hoarse, sometimes high-pitched bellow is emitted. Sometimes observed is continuous bellowing for variable periods of time or attempts to bellow without any sound being produced.

6. Salivation occurs in less than half the animals affected and is usually seen as a drooling from the mouth rather than profuse salivation.

Table 1. *Reported Cases of Rabies*

	Cattle	Dogs	Cats
1977	186	120	108
1978	205	119	96
1979	228	196	156
1980	403	247	214
1981	465	216	285
1982	296	153	209

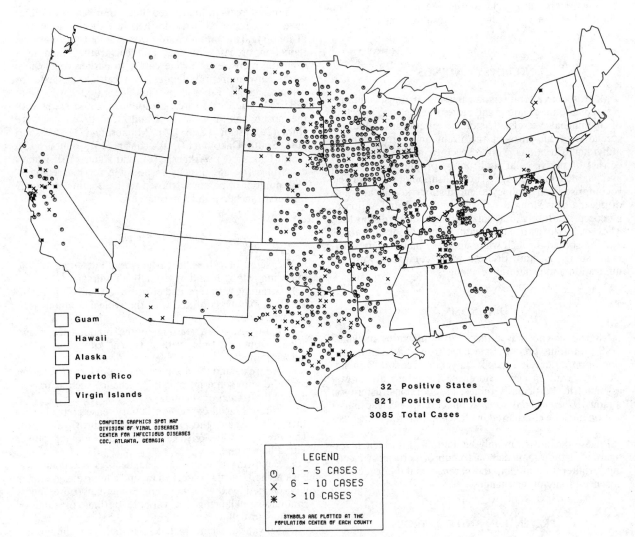

Guam

Hawaii

Alaska

Puerto Rico

Virgin Islands

COMPUTER GRAPHICS SPOT MAP
DIVISION OF VIRAL DISEASES
CENTER FOR INFECTIOUS DISEASES
CDC, ATLANTA, GEORGIA

32 Positive States

821 Positive Counties

3085 Total Cases

LEGEND
⊕ 1 - 5 CASES
× 6 - 10 CASES
✳ > 10 CASES

SYMBOLS ARE PLOTTED AT THE
POPULATION CENTER OF EACH COUNTY

Figure 1. Counties in the United States reporting skunk rabies (1982).

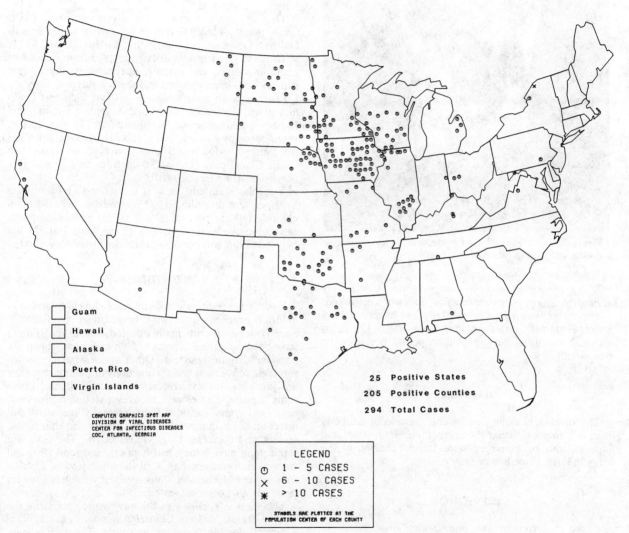

Figure 2. Counties in the Unites States reporting cattle rabies (1982).

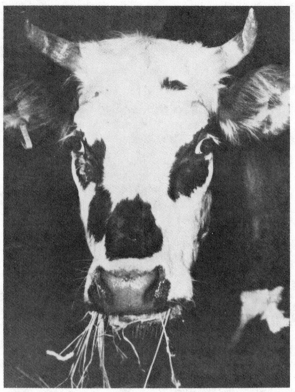

Figure 3. Facial expression of cattle with rabies: very tense and alert and bells of ears thrown forward.

7. Aggressiveness only on provocation. Cattle may attempt to charge people or other animals when provoked.

The incubation period in naturally and experimentally infected animals varies greatly, from 20 to 150 days, although the usual field incubation period is said to be one month or so.

DIAGNOSIS

The disease is diagnosed by the fluorescent antibody test; it is important that the cerebellum, brain stem, and hippocampus be examined since the distribution of the virus in large animals may vary greatly.

PREVENTION

There is currently only one vaccine (inactivated) licensed for use in cattle in the United States, although various products are used in other countries, including two attenuated vaccines (ERA and HEP Flury) and at least two inactivated vaccines (suckling mouse brain vaccine and Semple vaccine).

Supplemental Reading

Brückner, G. K., Hurter, L. R., and Boshoff, J. N.: Field observations on the occurrence of rabies in cattle in the magisterial districts of Soutpansberg and Messina. J. South African Vet. Assoc. 49:33–36, 1978.

Martell, M. A., Batalla C. D., Baer, G. M., and Acuña, J. B.: Experimental bovine paralytic rabies—"Derriengue." Vet. Rec. 95:527–530, 1974.

Starr, L. E.: Rabies prophylaxis in cattle. J. Am. Vet. Med. Assoc. 134:78–81, 1959.

Vesicular Stomatitis Virus in Cattle

ALVIN W. SMITH, D.V.M., Ph.D.

Vesicular stomatitis viruses (VSV) belongs to the family Rhabdoviridae and the genus *Vesiculovirus*. They are bullet-shaped, 65 by 185 nanometers in size, with a helically arranged single-stranded RNA genome, and their surface envelope is covered with spikes 10 nanometers long.

They are inactivated by lipid solvents and heat (58°C for 30 minutes) but will survive for several weeks in soils at 4 to 6°C and are resistant within a pH range of 2 to 11.

The first VS virus was isolated in 1925 from vesicles of cattle in Indiana and is the prototype virus. Subsequent isolates have been grouped into three serotypes. They are (1) Indiana with three strains as follows: Indiana 1 (Indiana strain), Indiana 2 (Cocal and Argentina strains), and Indiana 3 (Alagoas and Brazil strains); (2) New Jersey, represented by a single strain; and (3) Isfahan, which has three strains as follows: Isfahan (*Phlebotomus* strain from Iran), Chandipura (human strain from India), and Piry (opossum strain from Brazil).

Vesicular stomatitis virus is inactivated in 10 minutes by 1 per cent formalin, 1:200 Wescodyne, benzalkonium chloride (10 per cent at 1:200), 1:1000 Roccal, and 1:50 hexachlorophene septisol. Lye (2 per cent NaOH) has been used but will not de-activate the virus in two hours.

EPIZOOTIOLOGY

Vesicular stomatitis virus will cause clinical infection in naturally exposed cattle, swine, horses, deer, and humans. Sheep can be experimentally infected, and although there have been occasional reports of field infections, sheep are considered quite resistant. Other species having shown serologic conversion under conditions of natural exposure are javelinas, turkeys, raccoons, bobcats, skunks, opossums, squirrels, antelopes, monkeys, sloths, porcupines, bats, and some rodents. Experimentally the virus will infect all the common laboratory rodents and chinchillas, ferrets, and chickens. Dogs are refractive. The virus will replicate in mosquitoes, leaf hoppers, and sand flies, and transovarian passage has been demonstrated in *Phlebotomus* flies. Mechanical transmission by nonbiting insect pests has also been suggested.

The virus is confined to the new world, primarily the United States, Mexico, Central America, Panama, Venezuela, Colombia, Ecuador, and Peru. The disease stays endemic in the more tropical zones, which include the Gulf Coast, Georgia, and the Carolinas, then extends into Vera Cruz, Mexico, and Colombia. During the spring and summer, under favorable conditions, every ten years or so, VS will spread in epizootic fashion into the temperate zones of the United States, Brazil, and Argentina. Alaska, western Canada, New England, and eastern Canada have not experienced epizootics of VS. When epizootics do occur in the United States they move northward up the river valleys of the Appalachian chain, upper Mississippi, and Rocky Mountains as the summer progresses and occasionally extend north into central Canada. Epizootic spread is favored when environmental temperatures are above 20°C, lush vegetation occurs in river valleys, and some shade is present. Deserts, high mountains, and open planes act as barriers to spread. The epizootic form of the disease primarily affects cattle and horses, and the movement of infected animals can readily spread the disease.

The precise mechanisms of transmission and reasons for occasional epizootic spread out of endemic areas are not understood. Two important aspects of past epizootics have been that the incubation period is less than seven days and the disease dies out with the first killing frost in the autumn. The extensive and costly epizootic of 1982 did not follow this pattern: one dairy broke with the disease in a way that suggested a 30-day incubation period, and other outbreaks in dairies of the central valley of California occurred through the winter on into March of the following year.

CLINICAL SIGNS

The most important aspect of this disease is that the clinical disease in cattle mimics that in swine and must be rapidly differentiated from foot-and-mouth disease. Once animals become infected, vesicular lesions will occur on the tongue, lips, gums, teats, and coronary bands. If there are oral lesions, these will be accompanied by profuse salivation and a reluctance to eat. The incubation period is usually two to four days, and older animals will be more frequently affected. Economic losses in dairy and swine herds can be considerable, especially if there is secondary mycotic or bacterial invasion of lesions. Uncomplicated cases will fully recover in two weeks.

DIAGNOSIS

If horses have lesions, a presumptive diagnosis of VS can be made on clinical evidence because there are no other virus diseases that mimic the signs and lesions seen in horses. Laboratory diagnosis in cattle and swine is absolutely essential for differentiation from foot-and-mouth disease and must be made on the basis of virus isolation and the presence of specific antibodies. Appropriate laboratory specimens are epithelial tissues covering the vesicle and the vesicular fluid. These should be placed in buffered glycerol or frozen for shipment. Paired acute and convalescent serum samples are useful for compliment fixation and serum neutralization tests. One of the newer rapid diagnostic tests is a tissue microtitration complement-fixation test (TMCF), which can be performed in three hours at any time of the day or night. Although it has not been described for field cases, direct electron microscopic examination of lesion material could, in appropriate samples, rapidly and easily differentiate the rhabdovirus of VS from the enterovirus of foot-and-mouth disease and the calicivirus of vesicular exanthema of swine.

TREATMENT

There is no specific treatment except supportive therapy, e.g., feeding soft foods, providing rest and an abundance of water, and ensuring early treatment of secondary infections.

PREVENTION AND CONTROL

During epizootics livestock movements and other common mechanisms for contact transmission should be avoided; however, severely restrictive control measures within epizootic areas may not be warranted because of the sporadic nature of the disease. Live virus vaccines have been tested. They do show some efficacy and may be of use in endemic areas or during epizootics. Newer vaccines incorporating novel methods of viral inactivation and genetic manipulation are currently being developed but have not yet been released for field testing.

Supplemental Reading

Callis, J. J., Dardiri, A. H., Ferris, D. H., et al.: Illustrated Manual for the Recognition and Diagnosis of Certain Animal Diseases. Mexico-United States Commission for the Prevention of Foot and Mouth Disease, Plum Island Animal Disease Center. 1982, 17–19.
Jenney, E. W.: Vesicular stomatitis in the United States during the last 5 years (1963–1967). Proc. 71th Ann. Mtg. U.S. Livestock San. Assoc. 1967, 371–385.
Snyder, M. L., Jenney, E. W., Erickson, G. A., and Carbrey, E. A.: The 1982 resurgence of vesicular stomatitis in the United States: A summary of laboratory diagnostic findings. Am. Assoc. Vet. Lab. Diagnosticians, 25th Ann. Proc. 1983, 221–228.

Bovine Ephemeral Fever

P. B. SPRADBROW, B.V.Sc., Ph.D., D.V.Sc.

Bovine ephemeral fever virus is a vector-transmitted rhabdovirus. The insect vectors have not been specifically identified, but they are believed to include species of *Culicoides* and possibly mosquitoes. Only a single serologic type of bovine ephemeral fever virus is known. However, in Australia other rhabdoviruses with a distant serologic relationship to bovine ephemeral fever virus have been isolated. The presence of these viruses complicates the interpretation of serologic surveys.

EPIZOOTIOLOGY

Bovine ephemeral fever is a viral disease of cattle and possibly water buffaloes. Other species of domestic animals are apparently insusceptible, and reservoirs of infection among feral animals or birds have not been identified. Bovine ephemeral fever occurs in Australia, Asia, and Africa. Sporadic cases occur in endemic areas, and there are occasional extensive epizootics. The mortality rate is usually low, possibly less than 1 per cent.

Bovine ephemeral fever virus does not spread between cattle by contact. There is a brief period of viremia at the time when the animal is clinically ill, and blood-sucking vectors are presumably infected at this time. Some infected animals develop viremia but show no obvious clinical signs. Recovered carriers are not recognized. The seasonal incidence of the disease is related to periods of vector activity.

Bovine ephemeral fever is not a killing disease. It is important because it results in a great reduction in milk yield and because it immobilizes animals, making normal husbandry and marketing procedures impossible.

CLINICAL SIGNS

The early clinical signs of bovine ephemeral fever are inappetence and pyrexia. The fever is biphasic, and the temperature is normal or nearly normal between the two peaks. Stiffness or lameness is the most obvious sign in cattle in the field. This symptom usually develops a little after the febrile response commences, but it does not occur in all animals. Lameness usually affects more than one leg, and animals often become recumbent. There is a sudden and severe drop in milk production in lactating cows. Many animals experience difficulty in swallowing and salivate excessively.

Other inconstant clinical signs are shivering, nasal and ocular discharge, edema affecting the area around joints, and subcutaneous emphysema. Fever and lameness usually abate after three or four days. A few animals remain recumbent for long periods after the temperature returns to normal. Pregnant animals do not abort, but a reduction in semen quality occurs in some bulls.

The blood picture is one of leukocytosis and neutrophilia, returning to normal within a few days of recovery. Necropsy changes are usually slight and include edema of lymph nodes, congestion of abomasal mucous membranes, and variable inflammatory changes on serosal surfaces.

The pathogenesis of bovine ephemeral fever has not been fully explained. The basic lesion appears to be a serofibrinous polyserositis, presumably resulting from capillary damage to serosal surfaces in the body cavity and joints.

DIAGNOSIS

Bovine ephemeral fever is usually diagnosed on clinical grounds, especially during an epizootic. Isolated cases need to be differentiated from bovine chlamydiosis.

The laboratory diagnosis depends on the demonstration of viremia or of rising levels of neutralizing antibody. Bovine ephemeral fever virus can be isolated by serial, intracerebral passage in suckling mice or in Vero or BHK cell cultures. Diagnosis is also possible by fluorescent-antibody staining of blood smears prepared during viremia. Neutralizing antibodies are most conveniently detected in cell cultures.

The prognosis is usually favorable unless recumbency has been prolonged. Animals that have been down for long periods may die or they may be permanently ataxic.

TREATMENT

There is no specific treatment for this viral disease. Recumbent animals should be provided with shade and water. Nonspecific therapy aims at reducing fever and alleviating joint pain. Oral medication with liquids should be avoided because many animals have difficulty in swallowing.

Acetylsalicylic acid (Acetobols*) is given orally as a bolus or in a gelatin capsule to control fever. The dose for mature cattle is 60 to 120 g every 12 hours. Phenylbutazone, which has antipyretic action similar to that of acetylsalicylic acid, has additional anti-inflammatory ac-

tion. This drug can be given intravenously, an advantage in animals that will not readily take oral medication. Phenylbutazone is obtainable in combination with isopyrin (Tomanol*). Tomanol contains 120 mg phenylbutazone and 240 mg isopyrin per ml and is given by slow intravenous drip or by intramuscular injection. The dose for a mature animal is 20 to 30 ml.

PREVENTION

Vector control is not usually a practical remedy. Bovine ephemeral fever virus vaccines are used in South Africa and Japan. Experimental vaccines produced in Australia use living virus grown in cultures of Vero cells and mixed with adjuvants (aluminum hydroxide or saponin) immediately before use. Immunity following natural infection is long lasting.

Supplemental Reading

Bryden, D. I.: Ephemeral fever. In The Post-Graduate Committee in Veterinary Science: The Therapeutic Jungle. Proceedings No. 39. University of Sydney, Sydney, Australia, 1978, 312–314.
Burgess, G. W.: Bovine ephemeral fever: A review. Vet. Bull. 41:887, 1971.
Spradbrow, P. B.: Vaccines against bovine ephemeral fever. Aust. Vet. J. 53:351, 1977.

Bovine Leukemia Virus

JANICE M. MILLER, B.S., D.V.M., M.S., Ph.D.

Cancer of lymphatic tissue in cattle is known by several terms, including leukemia, leukosis, lymphosarcoma, and malignant lymphoma. The earliest descriptions of the disease appeared in eastern Europe about 1900. As case reports accumulated, it became clear there were four different clinicopathologic forms of lymphoid neoplasia: calf, thymic, skin, and adult. Epidemiologic studies indicated that the adult form was contagious, so it was called enzootic bovine leukosis (EBL). The other three forms were called sporadic because there was no evidence that they were infectious. The accuracy of this classification was finally proven in the 1970's when it was shown that a retrovirus, bovine leukemia virus (BLV), causes adult type leukosis but is not involved in the pathogenesis of any sporadic form. No etiology has been identified for the latter malignancies.

ETIOLOGY

BLV is a horizontally transmitted oncogenic virus that is antigenically unique. Although there are some minor differences between various isolates, immunologic tests have not identified more than one strain of the agent. The mode of replication in infected cells is characteristic of viruses belonging to the retrovirus family. The genetic information, which exists as RNA, is copied with the aid of a specific viral enzyme into a "mirror image" DNA molecule. This DNA, called provirus, is then integrated into chromosomal DNA and becomes a permanent part of the infected cell's genetic information, even in the

---

*Available from Parnell Laboratories Pty. Ltd., Peakhurst, N.S.W. 2210, Australia.

*Available from Intervet Pty. Ltd., Artarmon, N.S.W. 2064, Australia.

absence of further virus replication and in the presence of viral specific antibody. Thereafter, the provirus is perpetuated and multiplied coincidentally at each subsequent cell division.

All current evidence suggests that BLV-infected cattle do not produce significant amounts of cell-free virus in their tissues, secretions, or excretions. Therefore, environmental or chemical inactivation of the agent itself is not a pertinent consideration. Infection is apparently transmitted by the introduction of viable lymphocytes into a susceptible animal. After this transfer occurs, the lymphocytes become activated to produce complete virus particles that are infectious for the new host.

Because BLV transmission is strictly cell-associated, environmental and chemical inactivation of blood or other lymphocyte-rich secretions and excretions is an important consideration. It has been shown that freezing, drying, and temperatures above 50°C are lethal to lymphocytes, but the cells can survive in blood at 4°C for at least two weeks and in serum even longer. The use of chemicals to inactivate infective lymphocytes has not been studied, but any solvent or nonisotonic liquid would be expected to cause lysis.

EPIZOOTIOLOGY

Cattle are the primary natural hosts of BLV. Sheep can be infected experimentally and there are a few reports of natural infections in this species but the source and mode of transmission were not determined. The distribution of BLV is worldwide, although prevalence of infection varies greatly from one geographic region to another. Many European countries, through long-standing efforts to control the spread of leukosis, have succeeded in reducing virus prevalence to very low levels, and in some regions the infection has been totally eliminated. In the United States, BLV prevalence in dairy cattle ranges from 10 to 50 per cent in various parts of the country. In the same areas, infection in beef cattle is less common, ranging from 1 to 20 per cent. Regardless of production type, BLV prevalence in an individual herd can be very high, sometimes involving virtually all adult animals. Transmission of BLV apparently requires close, prolonged contact, and it is believed that most infections result from blood transfer into the skin of a susceptible animal. The most likely mechanisms for this type of transfer appear to be insects (over short distances) and traumatic, surgical, or other similar events that lead to blood contamination. There seems to be little or no risk of transmission by semen from infected bulls if artificial insemination is used; however, the close contact involved in natural service would present a greater potential for spreading virus. Calves can carry BLV at birth as a result of *in utero* exposure, but in most herds this involves less than 10 per cent of the calves from infected dams. Although milk from infected cows contains cells with provirus, oral transmission to nursing calves is a rare event, probably because most of them receive enough colostral antibody to neutralize virus particles produced in the gut.

CLINICAL SIGNS

The lymphosarcoma produced by BLV occurs in adult cattle, usually between four and eight years of age. The location of tumors is unpredictable, but tissues frequently involved include lymph nodes, heart, abomasum, kidney, spleen, uterus, lumbar spinal cord, and retrobulbar lymphatic tissue. Clinical symptoms vary, depending on the organ or tissues affected, but weight loss and decreased milk production are frequent nonspecific signs that accompany tumor development. When there is heart involvement a marked jugular pulse and ventral edema in the neck may be present. Abomasal tumors often lead to ulcers that are detected by the appearance of dark blood in the feces. Splenic lesions are generally not recognized clinically unless the organ becomes so large that it ruptures. Uterine and pelvic lymph node tumors may cause breeding problems and are often detected by rectal palpation. Posterior paresis or paralysis is the typical symptom associated with tumor in the spinal canal. The most obvious clinical signs of lymphosarcoma are enlargement of peripheral lymph nodes and exophthalmos due to tumor in the posterior orbit.

It is not unusual for cattle with EBL to have elevated lymphocyte counts in peripheral blood, but this usually is not a manifestation of the lymphoid cancer. Infection with BLV causes some animals (approximately one third) to develop persistent lymphocytosis, a condition that can be present for many years in the absence of other clinical signs. A few lymphocytotic cattle eventually develop tumor, but the situation is unpredictable and it is dangerous to use the blood profile as a prognostic or diagnostic indicator of disease.

For the purpose of comparison to EBL, a brief summary of the clinical findings in sporadic (non-BLV related) forms of bovine leukosis is presented here.

The *calf* form usually appears when animals are less than six months old. The hallmark of this form is tumor involvement of virtually all hematopoietic tissues and other organ systems as well. High blood lymphocyte counts are common.

An animal with *thymic* form is typically between six months and two years of age. The common clinical presentation is diffuse, firm swelling in the ventral neck, sometimes accompanied by enlargement of prescapular lymph nodes. Leukocyte counts are usually within normal limits.

Skin leukosis, the rarest form, is most frequently seen in young adults. Tumors occur only in the skin and usually regress after a few weeks. There may be a subsequent recurrence of generalized lymphosarcoma, which is fatal.

DIAGNOSIS

In considering the diagnosis of EBL, it is important to recognize that there are two different problems. One is the diagnosis of *disease* (tumor) and the other is diagnosis of BLV *infection*. Only a very few infected cattle (less than 1 per cent annually) will develop lymphoid cancer. The environmental, immunologic, genetic, or other factors that may play a role in determining which animals become clinically affected are unknown.

A conclusive diagnosis of lymphosarcoma requires histopathologic examination of affected tissue. The presumptive diagnosis is usually accurate, however, if the clinical history and physical examination suggest a noninflammatory, proliferative condition with lymphatic tissue involvement. Histopathologic confirmation rules out a granulomatous disease or other type of neoplasm that could produce similar gross tissue changes. Specimens for study should be submitted to the diagnostic laboratory in 10 per cent formalin.

The establishment of an etiologic diagnosis requires identification of BLV-infected cattle. Because the virus establishes a persistent infection, there is constant production of antigen and a consequent antibody response. This reaction can be detected by a number of serologic tests, the most sensitive of which is radioimmunoassay. Application of this technique has been limited because of its relatively high cost and requirement for sophisticated technology. The most widely used test is agar gel immunodiffusion (AGID). It has been shown that BLV infection can be detected by AGID within two to three months after virus exposure; thereafter the antibody titer rarely falls below a detectable level. The only time a positive AGID test is inconclusive is in the case of calves less than six months old. Because colostral antibody may persist for that length of time, a serologic test cannot determine if calves have active infection or just passive antibody. In this situation virus isolation is the only diagnostic test possible and, because it is technically very difficult, few laboratories provide the service.

TREATMENT

There is no treatment for animals with tumor. BLV infection is always persistent and cannot be eliminated by any drug currently available.

PREVENTION AND CONTROL

The only way to prevent EBL is to prevent BLV infection. Because the virus spreads primarily by contact, control must be instituted at the herd level unless the animals to be protected can be isolated. Eradication of the virus from a herd is accomplished by repeated serologic testing of animals over six months of age, followed by rapid removal of all infected cattle. The best interval for testing is three months, and with this method the virus is usually eliminated from the herd after the second or third test. A few European countries have used such procedures to eradicate BLV; several others have instituted programs designed to reduce the spread of infection. For this reason, serologic testing is now almost universally incorporated into international trade regulations. The resulting economic impact on sales of cattle, semen, and embryos has been the most serious national problem associated with BLV. Vaccination against infection appears to be feasible, but the protective antigen would seroconvert animals and make them ineligible for export certification. In some herds, tumor incidence is high enough to create substantial economic loss; however, demand for a vaccine has not been sufficient to stimulate a commercial interest in the necessary research and development to prove safety and efficacy.

Supplemental Reading

Miller, J. M., and Van Der Maaten, M. J.: Bovine leukosis—Its importance to the dairy industry in the United States. J. Dairy Sci. 65:2194–2203, 1982.

Stober, M.: The clinical picture of the enzootic and sporadic forms of bovine leukosis. Bov. Pract. 16:119–129, 1981.

Thurmond, M. C., and Burridge, M. J.: Application of research to control of bovine leukemia virus infection and to exportation of bovine leukemia virus-free cattle and semen. J. Am. Vet. Med. Assoc. 181:1531–1534, 1982.

Bovine Astroviruses

JANICE C. BRIDGER, B.Sc., Ph.D.

As are astroviruses from other animal species, bovine astroviruses are characterized by the presence of a five- or six-pointed star on a proportion of the smooth-edged, 28-nm particles. By immunofluorescence of infected cell cultures, they are related antigenically. There is insufficient knowledge to allow bovine astroviruses to be assigned to a particular virus group.

EPIZOOTIOLOGY

Astroviruses appear widespread in the British bovine population, but so far they have not been reported outside the United Kingdom. They are found in both normal and diarrheic calves, and serum antibody was found in 50 per cent of cows from 22 herds. It is possible that astroviruses are species-specific, as human and bovine astroviruses failed to infect experimental piglets, and cross-immunofluorescence between astroviruses from humans, cattle, and lambs does not occur.

CLINICAL SIGNS

The two strains studied to date did not produce disease after oral infection of gnotobiotic calves, aged 3 to 49 days, with fecal preparations, although virus was excreted in the feces for several days. With one of the strains a reduction in the ratio of villus height:crypt depth was found in one area of the small intestine five days after inoculation of a 19-day-old calf. The exact site of virus replication is unknown.

DIAGNOSIS

Bovine astroviruses can be identified by electron microscopy or by inoculation of primary calf kidney or testicular cells with fecal preparations. After 24 to 72 hours incubation, individual infected cells are detected by immunofluorescence with astrovirus-specific antisera. To date, bovine astroviruses have not been passaged serially in cell cultures.

TREATMENT, PREVENTION, AND CONTROL

As there is little evidence that bovine astroviruses are pathogens, no control is indicated.

Supplemental Reading

Bridger, J. C., Hall, G. A., and Brown, J. F.: Characterization of a calici-like virus (Newbury agent) found in association with astrovirus in bovine diarrhea. Infection and Immunity 43:133–138, 1984.

Woode, G. N., and Bridger, J. C.: Isolation of small viruses resembling astrovirus and caliciviruses from acute enteritis of calves. J. Med. Microbiol. *11*:441–452, 1978.

Woode, G. N., and Bridger, J. C.: Isolation of small viruses resembling astrovirus and calicivirus from acute enteritis of calves. J. Med. Microbiol. *11*:441–452, 1978.

Bovine Calici-like Viruses

JANICE C. BRIDGER, B.Sc., Ph.D.

Calici-like viruses resemble accepted caliciviruses in their size (diameter approximately 33 nm) and in the surface morphology of their particles, although the strains studied to date have not shown the clear "one-plus-six" pattern characteristic of caliciviruses and have not been propagated in cell culture. At least two, and possibly three, "types" occur that are not cross-protective.

EPIZOOTIOLOGY

The viruses have been commonly identified in outbreaks of calf diarrhea in the United Kingdom, and a virus cross-reacting with the SRV-1 strain has been identified in the United States (L. J. Saif, personal communication). They have been found either in association with other known enteric pathogens or alone. Little is known about inter-species infectivity: similar viruses occur in gastroenteritis of humans but the relationship, if any, to the bovine viruses remains to be elucidated.

CLINICAL SIGNS

Oral inoculation of gnotobiotic calves up to eight weeks of age produces anorexia, diarrhea, and xylose malabsorption although anorexia may not always occur. Feces become lighter in color, often yellow, and the volume excreted increases two- to tenfold. With the SRV-1 strain, small intestinal damage is restricted to the anterior half of the small intestine where desquamation of degenerate enterocytes results in stunted villi.

DIAGNOSIS

The only available method is electron microscopic examination of feces after differential centrifugation and negative staining. The number of particles tends to be lower than that usually found with rotaviruses and enteric coronaviruses.

TREATMENT, PREVENTION, AND CONTROL

No specific therapeutic studies have been performed and there are no available vaccines but oral rehydration therapy may be of value. If calici-like viruses are widespread in the cattle population, colostrum and early milk may contain protective levels of antibody.

Supplemental Reading

Bridger, J. C., Hall, G. A., and Brown, J. F.: Characterization of a calici-like virus (Newbury agent) found in association with astrovirus in bovine diarrhea. Infection and Immunity *43*:133–138, 1984.

Bovine Chlamydiosis

A. KONRAD EUGSTER, D.V.M., Ph.D.

Chlamydial agents are obligate intracellular bacteria susceptible to certain antibiotics, in particular, tetracyclines. The genus *Chlamydia* consists of two well-defined species, *Chlamydia trachomatis* and *Chlamydia psittaci*. Two major serotypes have been identified in cattle: type one includes all isolates from abortion and enteric infections and type two includes isolates recovered from cases of polyarthritis and encephalomyelitis.

ABORTION AND GENITAL INFECTIONS

Chlamydial Abortion

Chlamydiae have been identified as a cause of abortion in cattle in North America, Europe, Africa, and certain Asian countries. Generally no clinical signs are evident in cows prior to abortion. Cows of all ages are susceptible, and abortion can occur as early as the fifth month of gestation; however, most abortions occur during the last trimester of pregnancy; stillborn and weak calves can also be born. Placentas are frequently retained, and rebreeding problems are encountered. Chlamydial abortions are usually sporadic, but as high as 20 per cent of the cows have been reported to abort in a given herd.

A separate disease entity known as epizootic bovine abortion, or "foothill" abortion, exists in California. Although chlamydiae were isolated from some of these aborted fetuses, it appears now that this disease is vector-transmitted (*Ornithodoros coriaceus,* Koch ticks); however, the infective principal within these ticks has not yet been positively identified. Chlamydiae were not isolated from these ticks, although chlamydiae have been recovered from other ticks, and involvement of vectors in transmission of chlamydiae requires further studies.

The pathogenic events leading to abortion are not clearly understood. A most likely route is via the intestinal tract. Intestinal infections (clinically inapparent or overt) are relatively common, and abortions have been induced experimentally with enteric isolates. A venereal transmission may also be possible, inasmuch as heifers inseminated with chlamydia-containing semen did not conceive.

Clinical Signs

Abortions usually occur without any prior clinical signs. Reduction of milk production, retained placentas, metritis, and rebreeding problems can be present post partum. Placentitis is a consistent lesion. The trophoblastic epithelium is necrotic, especially in the inter- and periplacentomal areas. Fibrinopurulent exudate may be present between the endometrium and chorion. The intercotyledonary chorion may be of gelatinous (edematous) or leathery consistency.

Lesions in the fetus vary considerably depending on the stage of infection. Fetal lesions may be minimal in cases where the infection remained localized in the placenta and the abortion occurred prior to a fetal chlamydemia. Fetuses may show petechiae in the subcutis, thymus, and mucous/serosal surfaces; ascites; swollen livers with a mottled surface; and enlarged lymph nodes. Necrotic foci, vasculitis, and other inflammatory reactions may be seen in various somatic organs of the fetus, including the brain.

Diagnosis

None of the fetal or placental lesions are characteristic enough for a positive diagnosis without laboratory confirmation. Intracytoplasmic chlamydial inclusions are most abundant in the chorionic placental epithelial cells. Gimenez stain is preferred over Giemsa and H&E. Chlamydia can also be isolated in chick embryos or tissue culture from the placenta or various fetal tissues. The complement fixation test is a group-specific test, and a positive serologic diagnosis for chlamydial abortion is difficult to achieve. A rise in antibody titer between the time of abortion and 14 days post partum would be a good indicator for a causative chlamydial involvement in the abortion.

Treatment and Prevention

Since cows do not show any signs prior to abortion, it is difficult to prevent abortions. Two to five g of chlortetracycline daily per cow incorporated in pelleted alfalfa or protein molasses blocks did reduce the abortion rate in a field trial. This, however, is an expensive prophylactic regimen and is not practical except in special circumstances where a severe confirmed chlamydial abortion problem exists in a given herd. No chlamydial vaccines are available for use in cattle.

Seminal Vesiculitis Syndrome

This condition of primarily young bulls is characterized by a chronic inflammation of the epididymis, testicles, and accessory sex glands. The ejaculate usually contains large numbers of leukocytes and low numbers of spermatozoa with poor motility and primary and secondary sperm abnormalities. There are several causes for this syndrome; chlamydiae have been isolated from some affected bulls. Infertility is obviously a problem in herds with affected bulls; however, chlamydial abortions have not been reported in such herds. Seminal vesiculitis syndrome is diagnosed clinically during breeding soundness examinations. An etiologic diagnosis can only be made by isolation of chlamydiae or other pathogens from the ejaculate.

Chlamydial Endometritis

A report from Europe attributes Chlamydia as a cause of sterility. Chlamydial elementary bodies were demonstrated in the vaginal discharge. Endometritis has also been experimentally induced by directly placing chlamydiae into the uterus.

A similar condition has so far not been reported in the Americas.

ENTERIC CHLAMYDIAL INFECTIONS

Chlamydial infections of the intestine, particularly of the ileum, are not uncommon; they are clinically inapparent in adult cattle but can cause diarrhea in young calves. The most severe signs are observed in newborn calves, especially in those that do not receive colostrum or receive inadequate amounts.

In experimentally inoculated, colostrum-deprived calves, Chlamydia caused a severe diarrhea as well as pneumonia and polyarthritis and, in some cases, death.

Diagnosis

A laboratory diagnosis (isolation of Chlamydia in tissue culture or chick embryos) is essential to differentiate this condition from the many other causes of neonatal diarrhea.

Treatment

Fluid therapy and chlortetracycline (2.2 to 4.4 mg/kg body weight for seven days) are indicated if a positive diagnosis has been established.

RESPIRATORY CHLAMYDIAL INFECTION

Cattle affected by an uncomplicated chlamydial pneumonia have fever, serous or mucopurulent nasal discharge, cough, and dyspnea. All ages of cattle are susceptible. Infections with Mycoplasma, Pasteurella, Corynebacterium, and Streptococcus can occur simultaneously or secondarily, obviously adding to the severity of the disease.

Affected parts of the lung are well demarcated, firm, and located in the ventral parts of the anterior lobes. Bronchitis, bronchiolitis, peribronchitis with lymphocytic cuffing, and alveolitis are observed on histologic examination.

Diagnosis

Neither clinical signs nor lesions are characteristic enough to allow a diagnosis of Chlamydia-induced pneumonia. Isolation of the organism from lung, nasal secretions, or mediastinal lymph nodes has been used successfully to substantiate a diagnosis.

Treatment

Sick animals should be treated daily with either 11 mg/kg tetracycline or 135 to 200 mg/kg sulfamethazine until they recover.

Prevention

No vaccine is available. Sulfamethazine or sulfathiazole (135 mg/kg) in the drinking water may be indicated as a preventative.

CHLAMYDIAL POLYARTHRITIS

This condition occurs only in young calves. It follows a systemic chlamydial infection and other signs such as inappetence, fever, and diarrhea. The infection in some cases may also start in utero, as calves may be born weak and are reluctant to move.

Clinical Signs and Lesions

The joints are usually enlarged and painful on palpation. Calves frequently die despite various antibiotic treatments. Radiologic examinations are generally unrevealing. All joints can be affected, but usually weight-bearing joints of the extremities and the atlanto-occipital joint are more severely involved. There is excessive turbid yellow synovial fluid present, frequently containing fibrin plaques. The articular cartilage usually does not show any lesions. The periarticular area and especially the tendon sheaths are edematous, hyperemic, and hemorrhagic (petechiae as well as ecchymosis). The reactive changes in the synovial membranes and periarticular tissues are inflammatory and proliferative.

Diagnosis

Synovial cells and inflammatory cells may contain chlamydial inclusions when stained with Giemsa or Gimenez. Isolation of *Chlamydia* from synovial fluid is achieved early in the disease course. A rise in antibody titer (CF test) to *Chlamydia* between acute and convalescent samples is also of diagnostic aid.

Treatment and Prevention

Treatment of affected calves with tetracyclines or penicillin has generally not been beneficial.

CHLAMYDIAL CONJUNCTIVITIS

Chlamydial conjunctivitis is a well-recognized disease entity in guinea pigs, sheep, and man. In cattle, only one report from Czechoslovakia describes the isolation of *Chlamydia* from cattle with keratoconjunctivitis and the experimental reproduction of the disease in calves. Conjunctivitis has also been observed concurrently with polyarthritis in experimentally inoculated calves.

CHLAMYDIAL ENCEPHALOMYELITIS

This disease, also known as sporadic bovine encephalomyelitis (SBE), has been confirmed in various parts of the world in predominantly six-month- to three-year-old calves. This disease is not to be confused with SBE of viral origin (see page 499).

Clinical Signs

A marked fever is observed about 14 days after exposure. Inappetence, excessive salivation, and a diarrhea are also frequent early signs. Some cattle recover at this stage, whereas some develop nervous signs leading to stiff gait, circling, staggering, and paralysis. All parts of the brain and cord may show perivascular cuffs consisting of mononuclear cells.

Diagnosis

Isolation of *Chlamydia* from the brain along with the histologic changes is diagnostic.

Treatment and Prevention

Tetracyclines at therapeutic levels are effective if given early in the disease course before extensive chlamydial replication in the brain occurs.

Supplemental Reading

Pienaar, J. G., and Schutte, A. P.: The occurrence and pathology of chlamydiosis in domestic and laboratory animals: A review. Onderstepoort J. Vet. Res. *42*:77–90, 1975.

Storz, J.: Chlamydia and Chlamydia-Induced Diseases. Springfield, Ill., Charles C. Thomas, 1971.
Storz, J., and Whiteman, C. E.: Bovine chlamydial abortions. Bovine Pract. *16*:71–75, 1981.

Bovine Mycoplasmosis

MERWIN L. FREY, D.V.M., Ph.D.

The name "mycoplasma" is frequently applied to all agents of the order Mycoplasmatales. Members of the family Acholeplasmataceae are isolated from disease conditions in cattle but are considered to be relatively nonpathogenic. The recognized bovine pathogens are in the genera *Mycoplasma* and *Ureaplasma,* family Mycoplasmataceae, within which about 20 species have been isolated from cattle. The Mycoplasmatales possess most of the biologic characteristics of bacteria, but they are much smaller than most bacteria and they lack the relatively rigid bacterial cell wall. Thus they have the filterable characteristics of viruses and are fastidious because their small genome limits the number of enzyme systems. They are very susceptible to environmental and chemical factors, yet they flourish in the presence of specific hosts.

EPIZOOTIOLOGY

Mycoplasmas generally cause insidious diseases that spread from animal to animal relatively slowly. Direct and droplet contact between nasal, oral, ocular, and genital orifices are the most likely means of spread. It is known that infective aerosols can be created when mycoplasmas are present in splattered urine or milk or in coughed bronchial secretions. Infections with some pathogenic mycoplasmas are known to initiate in the respiratory tract and then spread elsewhere to the primary target organ. Many infections become chronic or perhaps latent, thus facilitating later spread to new susceptible animals.

CLINICAL SIGNS

Bovine Respiratory Mycoplasmosis

Mycoplasma mycoides subspecies *mycoides* causes contagious bovine pleuropneumonia (CBPP), a severe fibrinous pneumonia that was eradicated from the U.S. over a century ago. Mycoplasma species endemic to North America cause less severe cuffing pneumonias or alveolitis rather than fibrinous pneumonia. Mycoplasmal infection in bovine respiratory disease (BRD) is not often diagnosed, but widespread serologic studies and observed efficacy of antimycoplasmal antibiotics in many BRD outbreaks have led to a presumption of widespread infection. *Mycoplasma bovis* is the species most often associated with BRD in North America. It can cause or aggravate respiratory disease directly, but it also is important in its potential for spreading to other tissues to cause arthritis, mastitis, and possibly immunosuppression. *Mycoplasma dispar* and *Ureaplasma* spp. are associated with respiratory disease of calves probably as frequently as *M. bovis.* They are harder to isolate than *M. bovis* and thus are less well recognized as respiratory pathogens. Like

M. bovis, they are present in a large percentage of freshly collected and thoroughly tested diseased lungs from calves.

Certain clinical observations suggest mycoplasmal involvement in respiratory disease. A protracted course of respiratory disease with considerable coughing, followed by lameness in some animals or mastitis in lactating cows, is suggestive of mycoplasmal infection, as would be a response to an antibiotic such as tylosin that is more effective against mycoplasmas than the bacteria associated with BRD. Respiratory mycoplasmosis may be of very slow onset and thus may smolder in a herd for a long period of time. In addition it remains as an inapparent infection between times of exposure to physiologic or infectious stressors.

Mycoplasmal Mastitis

Many of the mycoplasma species that infect cattle can cause mastitis in lactating animals, but *M. bovis* is the one most frequently isolated from severe outbreaks. The first sign of mastitis caused by *M. bovis* is a sudden drop in milk flow, usually affecting all quarters. A painless mammary swelling often signals the onset, but occasionally there simply is a cessation of lactation. The milk is thicker than normal at first and usually goes through several changes in appearance to an increasingly yellow or tan color and then becomes purulent, watery, and fibrin-filled. Recovery of normal appearance usually occurs within about two weeks, although milk flow may remain well below normal for the duration of the lactation. Less frequent clinical signs include febrile response and sometimes arthritis, anorexia, and respiratory disease. There is usually a marked eosinophilic response in the mycoplasma-infected udder. *Mycoplasma bovigenitalium, M. alkalescens, M. californicum, M. canadense,* bovine serogroup 7, and *Ureaplasma* spp. may at times cause mastitis. Mycoplasmal mastitis is more of a problem in large herds, and its presence frequently leads to a higher culling rate.

Mycoplasmal Arthritis

Arthritis is a fairly common clinical sign in mycoplasma-infected cattle. It may be the only sign in young calves affected with CBPP. Among calves infected with mycoplasmas indigenous to North America, it usually appears secondary to respiratory disease or in milk-fed dairy calves following ingestion of milk from a herd affected with mycoplasmal mastitis. Although isolations of a number of species have been made from arthritic joints, the two species most often isolated are *M. bovis* and *M. bovigenitalium.* Bovine serogroup 7 and *M. alkalescens* also have been isolated from severe outbreaks of arthritis and have caused arthritis in experimentally infected calves.

In natural infections one or two joints in one limb may be affected, or more than one limb may be involved. Sometimes the lameness may shift from one limb to another. There is mild or no febrile response, but severely affected joints themselves feel quite warm to the touch. Mycoplasmal arthritis following a respiratory disease outbreak typically affects up to 5 or 10 per cent of the animals showing signs of BRD, but occasionally a considerably higher percentage is lame. Swelling usually becomes marked in affected joints after a day or two. A considerable increase in joint fluid is present, and it is usually somewhat cloudy. Pure cultures of the causative myco-

plasma can be cultured from the fluid early in untreated cases. After a week or two it becomes much harder to isolate the organisms as there is a high concentration of specific antibodies in the synovia. Experimentally, *M. bovis* has been shown to cause severe arthritis in the cervical spine. Such lesions may contribute to the severe depression sometimes seen in calves with respiratory disease.

Genital Tract Mycoplasmosis

Many bovine mycoplasmas have been isolated from various parts of normal and diseased male and female genital tracts. *Mycoplasma bovis* is most often associated causally with genital tract disease, and it causes endometritis, salpingitis, salpingoperitonitis, and infertility in experimental infections in cows. It causes seminal vesiculitis, epididymitis, and orchitis in bulls, and it frequently is isolated from semen, where it seems to cause decreased motility of spermatozoa. Other species, especially *M. bovigenitalium,* are thought to cause some of the same conditions, although less frequently. At least three species, *M. bovis, M. bovigenitalium,* and *M. canadense,* are thought to cause occasional abortions. *Ureaplasma* spp. are known to cause granular vulvovaginitis. They and *M. canadense* also are frequently present in bull semen.

Keratoconjunctivitis

Mycoplasma bovoculi, Acholeplasma oculi, and *Ureaplasma* spp. frequently are isolated from infectious bovine keratoconjunctivitis (IBK) but also from normal eyes as well. Experimentally *M. bovoculi* may cause a mild keratitis by itself, but, more important, it has been shown to be one of several predisposing insults leading to development of IBK when there is concomitant infection with the bacterium *Moraxella bovis.*

DIAGNOSIS

Methods of diagnosis of mycoplasma infections are difficult, costly, and frequently unavailable. Consequently, clinicians and pathologists usually must make presumptive diagnoses on the basis of clinical signs, lesions, and histopathology, and treatment must be empirical.

Some diagnostic laboratories that work with large numbers of milk samples are able to provide isolation and identification services for the common mastitis-causing mycoplasmas. Reports indicate that testing of bulk tank samples for pathogenic mycoplasmas is an effective way of detecting a very low percentage of infected cows. Routine checks would be very desirable in those areas of intensive milk production where mycoplasmal mastitis is known to be a problem.

TREATMENT AND CONTROL

Tetracyclines, tylosin, lincomycin, and spectinomycin (or the last two combined) are the antibiotics most frequently used successfully against the mycoplasmas. Based on their effectiveness *in vitro* and in experimental infections, tiamulin and two tetracycline derivatives, doxycycline and minocycline, would appear to be good choices where approved for use. High-side dosages are recommended for mycoplasmal infections, as the organisms often are sequestered where antibiotics do not penetrate readily. Oral antibiotic therapy started early against respiratory mycoplasmosis may prevent further progression of the disease. Oxytetracycline or chlortetracycline at about 16.5 mg per kg body weight has been suggested as an effective daily oral dose rate.

The control of mycoplasmal mastitis is difficult, and antibiotics are of little help. Early diagnosis is essential in preventing spread of infection to additional cows, as segregation or culling of infected animals is necessary. Unfortunately, shedding of mycoplasmas begins one to several days before onset of clinical signs. The best control is containment by bulk tank sampling, stringent milking hygiene, and avoidance of creation of aerosols during stripping and other milking procedures.

Effective CBPP vaccines are available in areas where the disease is endemic. Vaccines for other bovine mycoplasmas are not likely to be marketed until newer methods of vaccine production are developed and until a better understanding is gained of the importance of mycoplasmas.

Supplemental Reading

Gourley, R. N., and Howard, C. J.: Respiratory mycoplasmosis. Adv. Vet. Sci. Comp. Med. 26:289–332, 1982.
Jasper, D. E.: Mycoplasma and mycoplasmal mastitis. J. Am. Vet. Med. Assoc. 170:1167–1172, 1977.
Stalheim, O. H. V.: Mycoplasmal respiratory diseases of ruminants: A review and update. J. Am. Vet. Med. Assoc. 182:403–406, 1983.

Caprine Herpesvirus

D. G. McKERCHER, D.V.M., Ph.D.

The caprine herpesvirus is among the most recent of the herpesviruses of the domestic animals to be isolated. The original isolate was recovered from young kids undergoing a severe generalized infection in a small goat herd located in the coastal foothills of Monterey County in California. Abortions occurred concurrently in the affected herd. The virus was isolated in cultures of either ovine or bovine embryo kidney cells from the liver, kidney, spleen, lung, and bone marrow of kids that had died or were killed while moribund.[1]

ETIOLOGY

The virus is of the DNA type, sensitive to the action of lipid solvents and trypsin, and unable to agglutinate bovine erythrocytes. Morphologically it assumes the shape of a double membrane icosahedron, measuring 135 nanometers in diameter. It produces eosinophilic intranuclear inclusion bodies. These and other features identify it as a *Herpesvirus*. Serologically it is distinct from the IBR *(Bovine herpesvirus-1)* virus, although a slight non-reciprocating overlap exists between the two.[2] Immunologically, however, the two viruses are distinct.

The caprine isolate infects a wide range of cell types but lacks pathogenicity for chicken embryos, small laboratory animals, lambs, and calves. Thus far it is the only isolate of its kind to be reported from the United States. However, the isolation of a caprine herpesvirus has been reported from New Zealand[3] and Switzerland.[4] The Swiss isolate, classified as BHV-6, is closely related serologically to the California virus. The New Zealand isolate produces a vulvovaginitis in goats very similar to that caused in cattle by the IBR virus.

EPIZOOTIOLOGY

Although only limited studies of the epizootiology of the disease have been made, serologic evidence reveals that the infection is relatively widespread in California. Since the original isolate was recovered from kids in a herd to which additions were made prior to the outbreak, it would appear that the virus is carried latently in clinically recovered individuals. Once established in a flock, the virus is apparently transmitted by contact.

CLINICAL SIGNS

The naturally occurring infection is manifested in two forms in caprine dairy herds, i.e., by abortion in the adults and by a severe generalized infection in the young, accompanied by relatively mild respiratory tract signs. In the case of adult goats the infection is asymptomatic other than when abortion occurs. On experimental inoculation the adults become febrile and the white cell counts are elevated but the animals remain clinically normal until the intervention of abortion, which occurs between four and six weeks after exposure.

The infection in kids develops shortly after birth. It is characterized by fever, weakness, cyanosis of the oral mucosa, and signs of abdominal pain and depression. Although diarrhea is absent, palpation usually reveals an increased fluid content of the intestines and induces the passage of a small amount of watery, blood-tinged feces. The respiratory rate is accelerated (80/min) and the heart beat rapid (180/min). Infected animals are weak but remain in relatively good condition, especially those that survive. In severely affected kids the course of the disease is rapid and is characterized by depression and respiratory tract involvement, with death usually ensuing within a week of the appearance of clinical signs. The mortality rate ranges from 40 to 60 per cent. Kids inoculated intravenously with the virus display signs very similar to those associated with the naturally occurring infection.

Gross pathologic changes in infected kids include necrosis and ulceration of the rumen, cecum, and colon. Intranuclear inclusion bodies are present in the tissues of such animals.

DIAGNOSIS

The occurrence of abortion in a herd, accompanied by a severe enteritis in the kids, provides a presumptive diagnosis of caprine herpesvirus infection. It can be differentiated from chlamydial abortion by the absence of disease in the young and by the demonstration of elementary bodies in impression smears of the aborted placentas. In outbreaks of caprine herpesvirus infection, isolation and identification of the virus from tissues of sick kids is relatively easy to accomplish and provides a reliable diagnosis. A vaccine is not available. The usual recommendation is to treat the sick kids, following a therapeutic regimen for neonatal diarrhea of bacterial origin.

PREVENTION

No vaccine is available at this time.

References

1. Saito, J. K., Gribble, D. H., Berrios, P. E., Knight, H. D., and McKercher, D. G.: A new herpesvirus isolate from goats: Preliminary report. Am. J. Vet. Res. 35:847–848, 1974.
2. Berrios, P. E., and McKercher, D. G.: Characterization of a caprine *Herpesvirus*. Am. J. Vet. Res. 36:1755–1762, 1975.
3. Horner, G. W., Hunter, R., and Day, A. M.: An outbreak of vulvovaginitis in goats caused by a caprine *Herpesvirus*. N.Z. Vet. J. 30:150–152, 1982.
4. Mettler, F., Engels, M., Wild, P., and Bivetti, A.: Herpesvirus-infektion bei Zicklein in der Schweiz. Schweizer Archiv. fuer Tierheilkunde 121:655–662, 1979.

Ovine Herpesvirus

D. G. McKERCHER, D.V.M., Ph.D.

A herpesvirus was isolated from tumor tissues of sheep affected with pulmonary adenomatosis (PA). Antibodies to this virus are commonly present in sheep whether or not they are affected with PA. The current consensus is that this herpesvirus plays no role in the etiology of PA of sheep. There is evidence that a retrovirus is causatively involved in PA.

A HERPESVIRUS ASSOCIATED WITH ABORTION IN SHEEP

A virus was isolated from the tissues of a stillborn lamb from a flock in which abortion was occurring at the time. It was propagated in monolayers of either bovine or ovine embryonic kidney cells for further study. The isolate was subsequently shown to possess the biologic and morphologic properties of the herpesvirus group.

Ewes at approximately the 85th day of gestation and devoid of antibody to the virus were exposed to this isolation by either intravenous injection or nasal spray. Thirty-six hours later the IV inoculees became febrile but after 24 hours the temperatures became erratic for several days. However, the temperatures of the nasal inoculees remained within the normal range.

The virus was recovered from the buffy coat of the IV inoculees but not from that of the nasally exposed animals. Sixty days post inoculation the IV inoculees delivered weak lambs that died soon after birth. Virus was not recovered from their tissues, but antibody to the virus was demonstrated in the sera. The remaining inoculees lambed at term.

All sheep exposed to the virus developed neutralizing antibody except those exposed nasally. Reciprocal cross-neutralization tests with rabbit antiserum indicated that the ovine herpesvirus and the caprine isolate are closely related, if not identical, but are quite distinct from the IBR *(Bovine herpesvirus-1)* virus. Unfortunately pregnant goats were unavailable for pathogenicity studies when this study was conducted. To date, no further studies of the ovine isolate have been made.

Sheep and Goat Pox

E. PAUL J. GIBBS, B.V.Sc., Ph.D., F.R.C.V.S.

Sheep/goat pox virus is classified in the genus *Capripox,* which includes the virus of lumpy skin disease of cattle. Sheep/goat pox virus protects cattle from infection with lumpy skin disease virus but the viruses are not identical. Lumpy skin disease exists in geographic areas where sheep/goat pox is absent. Sheep and goat pox are often considered host specific; however, in areas of the world, particularly Africa, where sheep and goats are herded together, nonhost-dependent strains exist. For the present it should be accepted that sheep and goat pox are caused by the same virus.

The virus is transmitted by aerosol and by direct contact with sick animals or fomites.

Sheep/goat pox is the most important pox disease of domesticated animals and can cause extensive epidemics in which a large number of sheep and goats may die. The disease is common in the Middle East, the Indian subcontinent, and Africa mostly north of the equator; it has been eradicated from most of Europe and has not been reported from the Americas or Australia.

CLINICAL SIGNS (Figs. 1 and 2)

Sheep and goats of all ages can be affected. However, the disease is more severe in young animals. The first signs of disease are rhinitis, conjunctivitis, and pyrexia. Animals tend to stand with an arched back, have a poor coat, and lose their appetite. One to two days later cutaneous nodules develop (0.5 to 1.5 cm diameter) often accompanied by lesions on the external nares, lips, and within the mouth. The extent of nodule formation is variable; they are most obvious in the areas of skin where the wool/hair is shortest, such as the head, neck, ears, axillae, groin, perineum, and under the tail. The nodules mostly scab—although some regress without scab development—and these persist for three to four weeks.

Lesions within the mouth may be present on the tongue and gums; they tend to ulcerate. High mortality rates occur when lesions develop in the respiratory and alimentary tracts. Postmortem observations show these lesions in the lungs as multiple consolidated areas (0.5 to 2.0 cm diameter) beneath the pleural surface. Secondary bacterial pneumonia is the common cause of death. Similar lesions may be seen in the liver, kidneys, abomasum, and other organs.

DIAGNOSIS

Sheep/goat pox is a reportable disease in most countries of the world, and any clinical suspicion of disease should be reported to the appropriate authorities. Classical sheep/goat pox represents little difficulty in diagnosis but on occasion disease may be mild and complicated by the presence of contagious pustular dermatitis (synonyms are orf and contagious ecthyma) and dermatophilosis in the affected flock. In such cases laboratory confirmation is advised.

In the laboratory, sheep/goat pox virus can easily be differentiated from contagious pustular dermatitis virus

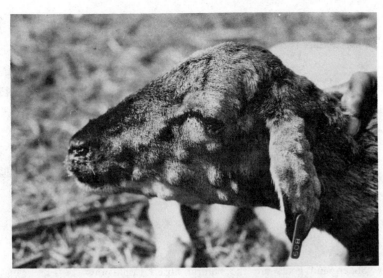

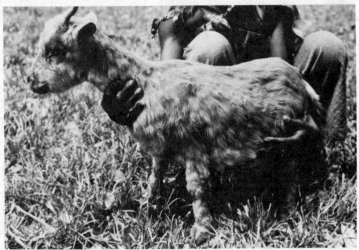

Figures 1 and 2. Sheep and goat pox. (Courtesy of M. A. Bonniwell.)

by examination of clinical material by electron microscopy or by isolation of the virus in tissue culture.

Morbidity can be as high as 75 per cent, with case mortality rates of 80 per cent. Some breeds, especially European, are said to be more susceptible, and heat stress is reported to influence the severity of disease.

TREATMENT

There is no specific treatment, but severely affected animals should be housed and given antibiotics. In some countries affected animals/flocks must be slaughtered.

PREVENTION AND CONTROL

Live attenuated sheep pox vaccines produced by growing the virus in cell cultures have been developed in Iran and Turkey,[1, 2, 3] and vaccines made from tissue culture virus adsorbed onto aluminum hydroxide and treated with formalin are in use in East Africa.[4]

References

1. Agyun, S. T.: The propagation of variola ovina virus in sheep embryonic tissue cultures and its usefulness as a vaccine against this disease. Archiv. Exp. Veterinaermed. 9:415–441, 1955.
2. Ramyar, H., and Hessami, M.: Development of an attenuated live virus vaccine against sheep pox. Zentralbl. Veterinaermed. 14:516–519, 1967.
3. Martin, W. B., Ergin, H., and Köylü, A.: Tests in sheep of attenuated sheep pox vaccines. Res. Vet. Sci. 14:53–61, 1973.
4. Davies, F. G.: Characteristics of a virus causing a pox disease in sheep and goats in Kenya, with observations on the epidemiology and control. J. Hyg. 76:163–171, 1976.

Contagious Ecthyma

ROBERT A. CRANDELL, B.S., D.V.M., M.P.H.

Contagious ecthyma (CE) is an acute infection primarily of young sheep and goats. The lesions located principally on the lips are characterized by vesiculopapular eruptions followed by development of pustules and scabs. Economical loss is usually in the reduction of weight gains and death of feedlot lambs. The disease in animals is commonly known as sore mouth, scabby mouth, lip and leg ulceration, and contagious pustular dermatitis, and the human disease is referred to as orf.

ETIOLOGY

The virus causing CE belongs to the genus *Parapoxvirus* and is inactivated by chloroform. There is only one serotype but biologic differences exist among strains. The virus survives for long periods of time outside the body in dried scabs. Exposure to heat at 60°C for 30 minutes destroys the infectivity of the virus. Contagious ecthyma virus propagates in a variety of cell cultures of caprine, ovine, and bovine tissues.

EPIZOOTIOLOGY

Sheep and goats are the natural hosts. Contagious ecthyma infections have been reported in musk-oxen *(Ovibos moschatus),* Dall sheep *(Ovis dalli),* Rocky Mountain bighorn sheep *(Ovis e. canadensis),* mountain goats *(Oreamnus moschatus),* chamois *(Rupicapra rupicapra),* tahr *(Hemitragus jemlahicus),* steinbok *(Raphicerus campestris)* and reindeer *(Rangifer tarandus).* Human infections are occupation-related.

Contagious ecthyma is worldwide wherever sheep are raised. There is a seasonal incidence, with most cases occurring during the lambing season and within two weeks after lambs enter feedlots. The disease is more prevalent in the young animals, and both sexes and all breeds are susceptible. Morbidity is high in infected flocks but the mortality is low. Cases complicated by bacterial infections may result in death.

Infection is spread among animals by direct and indirect methods. The disease is perpetuated under crowded conditions by animal-to-animal contact. Lambs become infected by nursing ewes with active lesions on their teats and udder. The virus is transmitted by fomites contaminated by virus-containing scabs and saliva.

CLINICAL SIGNS

The characteristic feature of this disease is the occurrence of epidermal lesions, particularly on the lips and face of the infected animal. Naturally infected young animals usually develop lesions within four to seven days after exposure to the virus. The lesion begins as a red, raised macule and progresses through papule, vesicle, and pustule stages. The vesicles increase in size, advance to the pustular stage, rupture, and release a yellowish exudate. Yellow-brown crusts or scabs form, covering the affected area. The epithelial cells proliferate, forming nodules that may coalesce into larger masses. The lesions may extend to the mucous membrane of the buccal cavity and spread to other parts of the body. Usually they occur at the commissure of the lips and extend along the lip affecting the gum (Fig. 1) and may involve both sides of the mouth. In the southwestern United States, gum lesions are not a feature of the disease in sheep and goats. Occasionally, lesions develop on the eyelids, nares, feet, and teats and udder of ewes. Infections also occur at the site of docking, forming dark crusty scabs along the

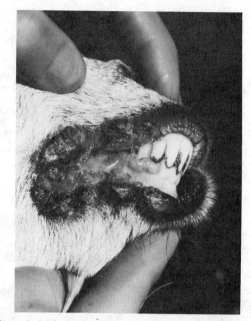

Figure 1. Lesions of contagious ecthyma on the lips and gum of doe. (Ott, R. S., and Nelson, D. R.: Contagious ecthyma in goats. J. Am. Vet. Med. Assoc. 173:81–82, 1978, with permission.)

incision. Extensive lesions on the face and in the mouth are painful to the animal and may lead to anorexia and loss of weight. The course of the illness varies between one and four weeks. In severe cases, the animals are overcome by secondary bacterial infections.

Recovery from clinical disease does not result in lifelong immunity, and animals may become re-infected within a year. In older, partially immune sheep, small dark, hard epithelial tags may occur at the commissure of the lips and go unnoticed. These are a source of infection to handlers. It is because of this short-lived immunity and the addition of susceptible animals to flocks that sporadic outbreaks recur within the same flocks. The persistence of the virus in flocks suggests that latent infections do occur.

DIAGNOSIS

A diagnosis is most often made based on the clinical appearance of the lesions. A history of previous outbreaks in the flock should be considered in the diagnosis-making process. The presence of oral and foot lesions may confuse the clinical diagnosis with other diseases. Several infectious diseases that should be considered in a differential diagnosis are bluetongue, sheep pox, ulcerative dermatosis, and foot-and-mouth disease. Scabs, scrapings, and lesion biopsies should be submitted to the diagnostic laboratory.

Virus isolation, histopathology, and fluorescent and electron microscopy are useful laboratory procedures to make a definitive diagnosis of this disease. The virus can be isolated in cell culture from scabs and scrapings of the lesion. Specific antigen is demonstrable in frozen sections of the lesion by fluorescent microscopy. Contagious ecthyma virus is readily detected in affected tissue by electron microscopy. The characteristic feature of the histopathology is the ballooning degeneration of the epithelial cells. Eosinophilic intracytoplasmic inclusion bodies have been described but are not a consistent finding.

CONTROL AND TREATMENT

There are licensed live, dried ecthyma virus vaccines available to prevent this disease in sheep and goats. Vaccination is recommended for each lamb and kid crop in infected flocks because the virus is resistant to environmental conditions. Range lambs should be vaccinated at least ten days before shipment to the feedlot. The vaccine is administered to scarified skin of wool-free areas such as the inside surface of the thigh and flank or the underside of the tail. Although the vaccine is recommended only for healthy animals, the course of illness has been shortened in some outbreaks after vaccination.

The live virus vaccines should not be used within 24 hours of dipping or spraying. People vaccinating the animals should take the proper precaution against infecting themselves with the vaccine virus. All vaccination instruments should be properly discarded.

Lesions may be softened with an antibiotic ointment. Removal of scabs causes bleeding and delays healing.

PUBLIC HEALTH CONSIDERATIONS

Veterinarians, veterinary students, ranchers, and sheep shearers acquire the infection by handling infected animals. The virus from the mouth lesions contaminates the saliva and wool and enters open lesions on the skin and arms of the handler. The disease in man is generally benign and self-limiting.

Occasionally, human infections become generalized.

Supplemental Reading

Dieterich, R. A., Spencer, G. R., Burger, D., Gallina, A. M., and VanderSchalie, J.: Contagious ecthyma in Alaska musk-oxen and Dall sheep. J. Am. Vet. Med. Assoc. *179*:1140–1143, 1981.

Jensen, R., and Swift, B. L.: Contagious ecthyma. *In* Diseases of Sheep. Lea & Febiger, Philadelphia, 1982, 109–111.

Moore, R. M. Jr.: Human orf in the United States, 1972. J. Infect. Dis. *127*:731–732, 1973.

Ulcerative Dermatosis of Sheep

BRINTON L. SWIFT, D.V.M.

The etiologic agent of ulcerative dermatosis (UD) is unclassified but probably is a member of the family Poxviridae. The virus is transmitted by direct and indirect contact. Skin abrasions facilitate growth of the virus in epithelial cells. Bacteria inhabiting the skin surface such as *Staphylococcus* spp. and *Fusobacterium necrophorum* contaminate the primary viral lesions.

EPIZOOTIOLOGY

UD affects all breeds and sexes of sheep and occurs most commonly during fall and winter. Geographically the disease is observed in Great Britain, South Africa,

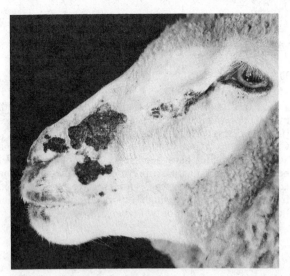

Figure 1. Ulcers on facial skin from ulcerative dermatosis. (Jensen, R., and Swift, B. L.: Diseases of Sheep, 2nd ed. Lea & Febiger: Philadelphia, 14–17, 1982, with permission.).

and the western intermountain region of the United States.

CLINICAL SIGNS

The lesions form on the face (Fig. 1), feet, or genitalia in two to five days following experimental inoculation. A pustule forms, followed by ulceration as a result of necrosis of surrounding tissue. The lesions frequently develop in only one anatomic location, but combinations of locations may exist. The morbidity of the facial form averages 20 per cent; the pedal form, 25 per cent; and the genital form, 80 per cent of breeding ewes and rams. The mortality is low.

DIAGNOSIS

UD is diagnosed on the basis of typical lesions. Confirmation of clinical diagnosis is based on histopathologic examination of skin lesions.

TREATMENT

There is no specific treatment for UD. Topical applications of antibiotic ointments are used to control bacterial complications and soften scabs.

PREVENTION AND CONTROL

No vaccine has been developed. Sheep vaccinated with commercial vaccines for contagious ecthyma are not protected from UD.

Supplemental Reading

Jensen, R., and Swift, B. L.: Ulcerative dermatosis. *In* Diseases of Sheep, 2nd ed. Philadelphia, Lea & Febiger, 14–17, 1982.

Ovine and Caprine Adenoviruses*

DONALD MATTSON, D.V.M., Ph.D.

Like all members of the family Adenoviridae, both ovine adenoviruses (OAV) and caprine adenoviruses (CAV) possess certain similar physicochemical properties. Currently, six types of OAV are recognized. Several additional isolates have been reported but have not yet been typed. Adenoviruses, previously classified as bovine adenoviruses (BAV types 2 and 7), have been isolated from sheep. There is a single report describing the isolation and identification of two types of CAV.

EPIZOOTIOLOGY

Few reports have been published concerning the distribution and incidence of infection from various types of OAV. In a serologic survey conducted in Scotland, the incidence of infection with selected OAV types varied from 21 to 68 per cent. In a similar survey with two untyped OAV recovered in Oregon, the incidence of infection was 21 and 60 per cent, respectively. With the same two Oregon OAV isolates, antibodies were found in 24 and 57 per cent, respectively, of normal adult goats.

The only report concerning the isolation of CAV was based on samples taken from goats in Nigeria. Antibodies to these two viruses were shown to be widespread in goats, sheep, and cattle in both Nigeria and England.

These data do not provide sufficient information to make an accurate conclusion regarding the distribution and incidence of OAV or CAV infection. These viruses are probably widespread. The possible role of interspecies transmission of virus among sheep, goats, and cattle has not been investigated.

Ovine adenoviruses are probably transmitted by direct contact or by aerosol droplet. In infected animals, the virus is shed in nasal and lacrimal secretions, feces, and, in some cases, urine.

CLINICAL SIGNS

Most isolations of OAV have been from normal lambs. Other isolations have been made from normal lambs in flocks that had a past history of respiratory and/or enteric disease. There have been some reports that have directly implicated these viruses as etiologic agents of enteric and respiratory disease in neonatal lambs. Lambs experimentally infected with various OAV or BAV isolates usually show mild clinical signs of disease and pathologic changes. Clinical signs of disease may include pyrexia, anorexia, hyperpnea, dyspnea, conjunctivitis, cough, and diarrhea. Lungs may have variable degrees of atelectasis and edema. Microscopic lesions include swelling, proliferation and necrosis of the bronchiolar epithelial cells, and an increased proliferation of cells in the alveolar septa. Infection may localize in the alimentary tract and produce a catarrhal enteritis. Virus may also replicate in the kidneys and produce swelling and proliferation of the endothelial cells.

DIAGNOSIS

For viral isolation, samples should be taken early in the disease from the conjunctiva, nasal cavity, and/or feces. Samples at necropsy should be taken from the affected portions of the respiratory or enteric tract and their regional lymphatic tissue. In early stages of the disease, virus-infected cells can be detected by the fluorescent antibody technique.

An agar gel precipitation test has been developed and serum can be tested for a group-specific antibody titer increase. For type-specific testing, the serum-viral neutralization test must be used.

TREATMENT

Treatment should be symptomatic and directed toward controlling infection by secondary microorganisms.

PREVENTION AND CONTROL

There are no vaccines available in the United States for the prevention of ovine or caprine adenoviral infection.

Supplemental Reading

Davies, D. H., Herceg, M., and Thurley, D. C.: Experimental infection of lambs with an adenovirus followed by *Pasturella haemolytica*. Vet. Microbiol. 7:369–381, 1982.

Lehmkuhl, H. D., and Cutlip, C.: Experimental infection of lambs with ovine adenovirus isolate RTS-151: Clinical, microbiological and serological response. Am. J. Vet. Res. 45:260–262, 1984.

Papillomatosis in Sheep and Goats

CARL OLSON, D.V.M., Ph.D.

Naturally occurring warts with virus were found on the legs and muzzle of sheep in two different outbreaks. The ovine papilloma virus produced warts in experimental sheep and fibromas in hamsters, but no lesions were produced in cattle or goats. Cutaneous papillomas have been reported in goats and in one instance these apparently progressed to carcinoma. The infrequent observation or reports of papillomas in sheep and goats may be due to the masking of such lesions by wool and hair or to the fact that the condition is rare in these animals. Papilloma virus and carcinoma have been associated in cattle and sheep of Australia. Sunlight and longevity of animals seem to be additional factors.

For further information on papilloma viruses, refer to article Papillomatosis in Cattle (page 483).

Supplemental Reading

Gibbs, E. P. J., Smale, C. J., and Lawman, M. J. P.: Warts in sheep. J. Comp. Path. 85:327, 1975.

---

*Oregon Agricultural Experiment Station Technical Paper No. 7017.

Moulton, J. E.: Cutaneous papillomas on the udders of milk goats. North Am. Vet. 35:29, 1954.

Theilen, G. H., Wheeldon, E. B., East, N., et al.: Goat papillomatosis. Cold Spring Harbor Conference. Papilloma Viruses. 73, 1982.

Border Disease

BENNIE I. OSBURN, D.V.M., Ph.D.

Border disease (BD) is a congenital infectious disease of sheep. Infection of embryos and fetuses results in embryonic death with resorption, fetal death, and birth of lambs with developmental abnormalities of the skin, nervous system, and bones. BD was first reported in sheep along the Welsh border of the United Kingdom; since then it has been observed in New Zealand, Australia, Europe, United States, and Canada. In New Zealand affected lambs are called "hairy shakers," whereas in western United States they are known as "fuzzies." The disease has been observed in most of the sheep-raising areas of the United States.

ETIOLOGY

The etiologic agent of BD is a pestivirus of the Togaviridae family. The noncytopathogenic agent is closely related to bovine virus, diarrhea virus, and hog cholera virus.

BD virus readily passes through the placenta of ewes infected between 16 and 80 days' gestation. Embryos and fetuses infected from 20 to 45 days after conception undergo embryonic or fetal death with resorption or abortion. Infection of the fetus between 45 and 80 days' gestation causes abnormalities of those organs undergoing major development including the skin, nervous, lymphoid, and skeletal systems and possibly others. Lambs infected through 80 days' gestation become persistently infected and immunologically compromised. The persistent infection lasts for the duration of the animal's life, serving as a reservoir of infection for others. There is no evidence that the virus infection is associated with clinical disease in the post-natal period other than abortion in susceptible ewes.

INCIDENCE

Clinical evidence of BD is most apparent at lambing time when as many as 50 per cent of the flock may be affected. Ewes are nonpregnant, abort, or deliver weak and/or malformed lambs. Serologic studies reveal that close to 90 per cent or more of the ewes in a flock may be affected; however clinical expression of disease occurs only in those lambs whose ewes were infected between 16 and 80 days' gestation.

TRANSMISSION

Natural transmission apparently occurs through contact with secretions and excretions of body fluids and tissues from infected animals. Urine, saliva, and placental fluids and tissues contain infective virus, and these serve as an important source for susceptible sheep. Appearance of the disease in a flock is usually associated with introduction of persistently infected animals that have minimal or no clinical evidence of disease. Persistently infected animals have been known to be viremic for over two years.

CLINICAL SYNDROME

BD is a disease of the embryo and fetus. The various forms of disease expression are related to the particular time during embryonic and fetal development that infection occurs. There are three major effects of infection.

1. *Embryonic and fetal death.* Infection during the embryonic and early fetal period (16 to 45 days' gestation) often leads to death and resorption of the embryo or fetus. The principal manifestation in flocks where this occurs is a small lamb crop because of many open ewes.

2. *Abnormal lambs.* The classical picture of BD is the birth of small, weak, lambs with hairy fleece and congenital tremors. Infection of fetal lambs between 45 and 80 days' gestation leads to dysplastic development of the hair follicles and nervous system and possible dysfunction in other organs. Lambs are usually small in stature with a preponderance of hairy fleece rather than wool. Often there is a dark pigmented area on the dorsal aspect of the neck. Tonic-clonic tremors may be so severe in some cases that lambs are unable to stand or suckle. Most of these lambs die within the first few days of birth.

3. *Weak lambs.* Birth of small, weak lambs with minimal neurologic and fleece abnormalities occurs in a small per cent of outbreaks. These lambs may survive with appropriate husbandry; however, they become the principle carriers of infection since they are persistently infected with BD virus.

The usual clinical history includes all three of these syndromes. The percentage of affected lambs with typical signs of hairy fleece and congenital tremors will vary and depends on the gestation period when infection occurred. The birth of these abnormal lambs usually prompts the livestock man to seek veterinary service. A critical review of past breeding records and of the current lamb crop will reveal a number of open, dry ewes and an unusually large number of neonatal deaths leading to a reduced lamb crop. If infection occurs in one year, the ewes appear to recover from infection and develop sufficient immunity so that cases of BD are minimal the following year.

PATHOLOGY

The principal gross findings consist of a hairy fleece in place of wool, hyperpigmentation over the dorsal cervical area, and a small undernourished lamb. Radiographs of long bones reveal dense bands around growth plates suggesting arrested growth during fetal development. The cranium is domed in severely affected individuals. Microscopic changes are in the nervous system and consist of dysmyelinogenesis and hypercellularity of the white matter. Special myelin stains are required to detect the lack of myelin in the cerebellum and spinal cord.

IMMUNOLOGY

The increased susceptibility to other infections and the poor viability due to intercurrent infectious have been attributed to immune deficits. There is evidence of depressed cell-mediated immune responsiveness. Antibody responses to BD virus are negligible, further suggesting that affected lambs are immunocompromised. The failure of the immune system to overcome BD virus and eliminate the virus from the system is probably the result of immunomodulation resulting from the fetal viral infection.

DIAGNOSIS

An impression of BD can be gained by obtaining a flock history consisting of a combination of reduced lamb crop, abortions, weak lambs with poor viability, and lambs with hairy fleece and congenital tremors. Submission of a single specimen does not allow a definitive diagnosis unless BD virus is isolated. A definitive diagnosis can be made upon isolation of virus from heparinized peripheral blood or brain, spinal cord, spleen, and bone marrow from affected lambs. Frozen tissues can be examined for evidence of BD viral antigens with fluorescent tagged hyperimmune bovine viral diarrhea antiserum. Nervous tissue fixed in formalin can be examined for hypercellularity and decreased myelin staining of white matter.

Serologic evaluation of ewe and affected lamb sera for evidence of antibodies to pestiviruses such as BD and BVD may assist diagnosis.

PREVENTION

The usual history associated with outbreaks of BD is that if it occurs one year, it is an insignificant cause of losses in the succeeding year. Infection usually spreads through a flock, resulting in subclinical viral infection and recovery with good immunity. Precautions need to be taken in flocks where BD carriers are introduced to susceptible populations with no previous history of BD infection. This must be considered as well in ewes and flocks where flock immunity to BD has declined.

Recently there have been reports suggesting that BVD vaccines prescribed for cattle when given to sheep may provide sufficient immunity for sheep flocks at risk. Inactivated or killed BVD vaccines should be used on sheep until an appropriate licensed product for sheep immunity is available.

Supplemental Reading

Barlow, R. M., and Gardiner, A. C.: Experiments in Border disease. 1. Transmission, pathology and some serological aspects of the experimental disease. J. Comp. Path. 79:397–405, 1969.

Osburn, B. I., Crenshaw, G. L., and Jackson, T. A.: Unthriftiness, hairy fleece, and tremors in newborn lambs. J. Am. Vet. Med. Assoc. 160:442–445, 1972.

Terlecki, S.: Border disease: A viral teratogen of farm animals. Vet. Ann. 17:74–79, 1977.

Wesselsbron Disease

B. J. H. BARNARD, B.V. Sc., M. Med. Vet.

Wesselsbron (WSL) virus is 1 of more than 40 distinct flaviviruses. The flaviviruses share certain basic physical and chemical properties and are distinguished from each other by serologic tests. WSL virus has a particle diameter of 45 nm and an electron dense core of approximately 25 nm.

EPIZOOTIOLOGY

WSL disease usually manifests itself after abundant rains and consequent increase in the arthropod vector population. It has been shown that *Aedes caballus* and *Aedes circumluteolus* transmit WSL virus. Contact and/or airborne transmission to sheep and man has been described. WSL virus has a wide host range including cattle, sheep, goats, pigs, horses, guinea pigs, rabbits, dogs, donkeys, wild birds, wild mammals, and man. Serologic evidence indicates the widespread occurrence of the virus in South Africa, Zimbabwe, Zambia, Malawi, Maputu, Kenya, Gabon, Namibia, and the Malagazy Republic. Despite its widespread occurrence the disease has a low incidence and appears to exist in an enzootic form over greater parts of Africa.

Only three outbreaks and some sporadic cases have been recorded in South Africa since 1956.

CLINICAL SIGNS

Sheep of all ages, cattle, horses, and pigs are susceptible to experimental infection with WSL virus. After an incubation period of from 24 to 120 hours a febrile reaction occurs that lasts for approximately 48 hours. No other symptoms are observed in nonpregnant adult sheep, cattle, horses, or pigs. The most prominent effect in pregnant ewes is abortion. Hydranencephaly and arthrogryposis associated with *hydrops amnii* are occasionally observed. In newborn and 4-week-old lambs, weakness, loss of appetite, and an increased respiratory rate are noticed. In some cases the perineum is soiled with bright yellow feces. The mortality rate in newborn lambs is relatively high (approximately 30 per cent). Although WSL virus has been isolated from bovine fetuses and calves, the significance of WSL disease in species other than the sheep has not yet been determined.

Lambs that recover show a leukopenia, whereas those that succumb reveal a neutrophilic leukocytosis before they die. Lymphopenia is a constant finding during the early stages of WSL disease. At necropsy moderate to severe icterus and a slight to moderate, yellow to orangebrown liver with a soft friable consistency are the most consistent lesions. Petechial and ecchymotic hemorrhages of the mucosa of the abomasum, serosal surface of the entire gut, capsule of the spleen, lymph nodes, and kidneys have been described in some cases.

In humans, influenza-like symptoms develop after an incubation period of three to four days. A sudden onset of fever, which lasts from 10 to 25 hours, is accompanied by rigors and acute muscular pains. Other symptoms, such as hyperesthesia of the skin and a mild rash on the back and abdomen, may occur.

DIAGNOSIS

WSL virus can be isolated by intracerebral inoculation of infant mice with brain and liver suspensions prepared from tissues of dead animals or from blood collected during the febrile reaction. The mice usually die within five to seven days. The virus can be identified by means of specific serum neutralization tests.

All animals and humans that become infected develop neutralizing antibodies demonstrable in their sera. The distribution, epizootiology, and pathologic manifestations of WSL disease are very similar to those exhibited by Rift Valley fever. On account of this similarity, confirmation of a clinical diagnosis is essential.

TREATMENT AND PREVENTION

Since there is no known therapeutic treatment for the disease, control measures are purely prophylactic in nature. An attenuated virus strain is used for the production of a live virus vaccine in infant mice or in cell cultures. The progeny of immune animals must not be vaccinated before they are at least six months old, whereas those of susceptible animals can be vaccinated with safety at any age. As the vaccine may cause abortion, pregnant animals should not be immunized. A good, usually lifelong immunity develops about three weeks after vaccination. Since no vaccine is 100 per cent effective, other preventive measures, such as mosquito control, the avoidance of low lying areas, and stabling of valuable animals, should also be undertaken.

Supplemental Reading

Coetzer, J. A. W., Theodoridis, A., and Van Heerden, A.: Wesselsbron disease. Pathological, haematological and clinical studies in natural cases and experimentally infected new-born lambs. Onderstepoort J. Vet. Res. 45:93–106, 1978.

Weiss, K. E.: Wesselsbron virus disease. Bull. Epizoot. Dis. Afr. 5:459–46,1957.

Foot-and-Mouth Disease in Sheep and in Goats

JERRY CALLIS, D.V.M. M.S., D.Sc.

Foot-and-mouth disease (FMD) is caused by a picornavirus. There are seven distinct immunologic types and numerous subtypes within each. The virus is antigenically labile, and to protect by vaccination it is necessary to produce vaccines homologous with the virus in the field.

EPIZOOTIOLOGY

Foot-and-mouth disease occurs in all species of cloven-hoofed animals. The disease is generally less severe in sheep and goats than in cattle and swine. The virus has a tendency to become species-adapted and in such instances the infection in sheep and goats may be severe. FMD virus occurs worldwide except in Australia, New Zealand, North and Central America, and Greenland. The virus is transmitted by infected animals and animal products. It can also be airborne. Recovered sheep and goats become carriers of the virus; although it has not been proven, they are thought to be responsible for spreading the virus to susceptible animals.

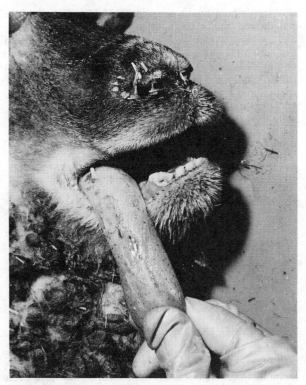

Figure 1. Ruptured vesicles on tongue of sheep infected with FMDV.

CLINICAL SIGNS

Sheep and goats suffer less than cattle and swine. In some instances clinical signs are not readily evident. The most pronounced sign is lameness. Careful examination is necessary to notice the usually small vesicles or erosions on the dental pad and tongue and between the claws (Fig. 1). In severe infections, pregnant sheep and goats may abort.

DIAGNOSIS

Sheep and goats are also susceptible to vesicular stomatitis, bluetongue, and contagious ecthyma. The lesions of FMD and these diseases show common features; therefore, laboratory tests are essential for differential diagnosis. FMD is diagnosed by isolation of the virus or tests such as complement fixation, virus neutralization, agar-gel precipitin, and enzyme-linked immunosorbent assays.

TREATMENT

There is no specific cure for FMD. Palliative treatment may make the animal more comfortable.

PREVENTION AND CONTROL

Prevention is the best policy. Animals should be isolated from infected animals or animal products. In FMD-free countries when the disease appears, infected animals are slaughtered, the carcass is destroyed by burial or burning, and the premises are decontaminated. Vaccines have been available since the 1930's but are not widely used in sheep and goats because these species are less susceptible than cattle. The insidious nature of the infection in these species makes it particularly dangerous during outbreaks and signs of infection may go unnoticed.

Supplemental Reading

Bachrach, H. L.: Foot-and-mouth disease. Ann. Rev. Microbiol. *22*:201, 1968.

Callis, J. J., and McKercher, P. D.: Foot-and-Mouth Disease: *In* Dunne, H. W., and Leman, A. D. (eds.) Diseases of Swine, 5th ed. Ames, Ia.: Iowa State University Press, 1981, 278–287.

McVicar, J. W., and Sutmoller, P.: Sheep and goats as foot-and-mouth disease carriers. Proc. Ann. Mtg., U.S. Livestock Sanit. Assoc. 72:400, 1969.

St. George, N.: The epizootiology and epidemiology of foot-and-mouth disease. Adv. Vet. Sci. Comp. Med. *14*:261, 307, 1970.

Ovine and Caprine Reoviruses

SASHI B. MOHANTY, B.V.Sc.&A.H., Ph.D.

All three types of reoviruses, similar to those found in humans, have been isolated from sheep. They have been isolated from nasal and rectal swabs of lambs with respiratory signs and diarrhea and from the nasal secretions and feces of clinically normal lambs. These viruses replicate in embryonic lamb kidney cells and produce cytopathic effects. A survey of reovirus antibody in sheep sera showed that antibody to type 3 reovirus was present in 46 per cent of sera tested. There is no report of caprine reoviral isolation.

CLINICAL SIGNS

The role of reoviruses in diseases of sheep is not clear, and further investigations are required to elucidate their role. Ovine reovirus type 1 induced mild respiratory illness and diarrhea in 2- to 4-week-old lambs. One strain of type 3 reovirus, however, induced no clinical signs in experimentally infected sheep. Focal consolidation of lungs, interstitial pneumonia, and catarrh of the mucous membranes of the upper respiratory and intestinal tracts were seen with type 1 reoviral infection.

DIAGNOSIS, PREVENTION, AND CONTROL

Virus isolation and seroconversion are considered adequate for diagnosis. There is no vaccine available.

Supplemental Reading

Belak, S., and Palfi, V.: Isolation of reovirus type 1 from lambs showing respiratory and intestinal symptoms. Arch. Ges. Virusforsch. *44*:177, 1974.

McFerran, J. B., et al.: Isolation and characterization of reoviruses isolated from sheep. Arch. Ges. Virusforsch. *40*:72, 1973.

Snodgrass, D. R., et al.: Isolation of reovirus type 2 from respiratory tract of sheep. Arch. Virol. *52*:143, 1976.

Bluetongue Infection in Sheep and Goats

STEWART McCONNELL, D.V.M., Mc.S.

Bluetongue (BT) is a viral arthropod-borne disease primarily affecting sheep but also occurring in other ruminant species. BT infection must be distinguished from BT disease because many animals, especially cattle, are infected with BT but exhibit no overt clinical signs of disease. The severity of BT disease is related to breed, individual animal susceptibility, environmental conditions, stress, and pathogenicity of the bluetongue virus (BTV) strain.

ETIOLOGY

Bluetongue virus (BTV) is a member of the orbivirus subgroup in the Reoviridae family. The virus has a segmented double-stranded genome in a core particle with 32 surface capsomeres arranged in icosahedral symmetry. The virus genome contains ten segments that code for ten polypeptides. The core particle is surrounded by an outer capsid protein layer containing two major virus-specific polypeptides.

The bluetongue virus serogroup contains 22 or possibly 23 different serotypes. All BTV serotypes share a common antigenic component detected by complement fixation, immunofluorescence, and immunodiffusion tests. However, serum neutralization tests must be utilized to detect the different serotypes. Only five serotypes, BTV 2, BTV 10, BTV 11, BTV 13, and BTV 17, have been isolated and identified in the United States. The distribution and occurrence of each serotype may vary periodically, and the cyclic activity suggests that widespread immunity to one serotype may cause another to be more prevalent the following year.

EPIZOOTIOLOGY

The host range of BTV includes sheep, goats, cattle, and various species of artiodactyls. Clinical illness commonly occurs in infected sheep and wild ruminants and rarely occurs in cattle and goats. BTV has been isolated from sheep, cattle, goats, and wild ruminants in at least 32 states, with serologic evidence reported from 48 states.

The established natural transmission of BTV is by the small, night-flying blood-feeding gnats of the genus *Culicoides*. Epizootics among sheep are seen when the gnat population reaches peak numbers, usually late summer and early fall. Intra- and transpecies transmission between sheep and cattle via the biologic vector *Culicoides variipennis* has been reported.

Vertical transmission has been demonstrated in both sheep and cattle. In sheep transplacental infection of the fetus in early gestation may result in abortion and fetal malformation. Cattle, because of prolonged viremias, vertical transmission, and isolation of BTV from semen of infected bulls, are believed to be a principal reservoir of BTV.

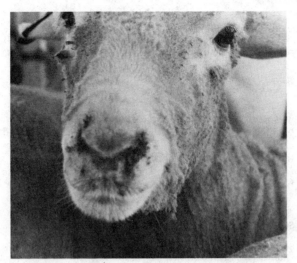

Figure 1. BTV infection showing crusted muzzle.

CLINICAL SIGNS

BT infection in sheep produces subclinical, mild, or severe infection with morbidity of 50 per cent in some flocks. Mortality is much lower (0.5 to 10 per cent) but is influenced by the virulence of the strain involved, care and management of the flock, and environmental factors such as high ambient temperatures.

The incubation period in sheep experimentally is 6 to 14 days. Signs of illness include fever, catarrhal nasal discharge, and edema and congestion of the lips, ears, and oral mucosa. Fever occurs four to eight days post-inoculation and may peak at 41.5°C, accompanied by a marked leukopenia and a detectable viremia. Virus can first be recovered two or three days after infection with peak viremias on day 7 or 8 post-inoculation. Virus may be isolated for a variable period up to approximately 30 days in sheep.

Inflammation of lips, muzzle, and oral mucosa are associated with excessive nasal discharge forming a hard crust over the muzzle (Fig. 1). Shallow ulcers (Fig. 2)

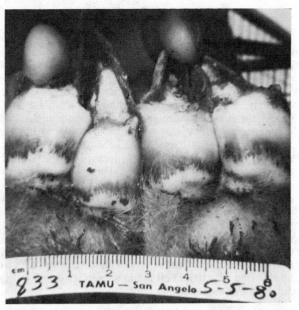

Figure 3. BTV infected sheep with inflamed coronary bands.

appear on lips and dental pads. Occasionally severe ulceration of the dental pad is seen. Anorexia and loss of condition occur often. Coronitis first manifested as a lameness is frequently seen. This lesion may appear about day 10 or 12 post-inoculation when the sensitive lamina of the hoof become inflamed (Fig. 3). The high fever producing tender or weak fleece may result in reduction of wool value.

Abortion and congenital deformities such as hydranencephaly may occur in sheep naturally infected with BTV. Viremia persisting up to two months has been found in blood and tissues of newborn lambs from ewes experimentally infected in mid gestation.

Newborn lambs have an effective immunity that may last up to six months. Spring lambs may lose this immunity when the incidence of BT is at its peak, resulting in serious economic loss to the producer.

DIAGNOSIS

A presumptive diagnosis of BT infection of sheep can be made on the basis of clinical disease. BT resembles but must be differentiated from contagious ecthyma (soremouth), mycotic stomatitis, photosensitization, infestation with nose bots, and the exotic diseases of foot-and-mouth disease and sheep pox. A confirmed diagnosis requires isolation and identification of the BTV or, alternatively, demonstration of a rise in specific antibody titer.

The BTV can be isolated from infected blood by inoculation of susceptible sheep, embryonating chicken eggs, or cell culture, preferably using blood taken during the acute phase (febrile period) of the disease. Blood should be collected with an anticoagulant and shipped to the diagnostic laboratory at refrigerator temperature or in wet ice. The modified direct complement fixation (MDCF) test and the agar gel immunodiffusion (AGID) test are group-specific tests. The neutralization test is used for serotype specificity, with the plaque neutralization test being the most sensitive.

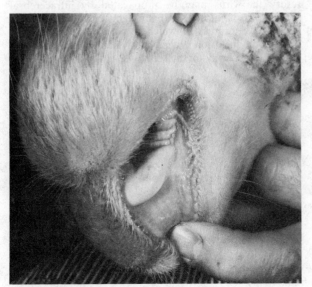

Figure 2. Shallow ulcer on the lip of a BTV infected sheep.

TREATMENT AND PREVENTION

Feed, water, and shade should be provided and sheep left alone. Drenching, administration of antibiotics, and driving of the sheep may produce edema of the lungs, resulting in increased deaths.

Good herd management may help control the spread of disease. Sheep should be sprayed with insecticide and, if possible, infected sheep should be housed at night.

Immunity to BTV can be artificially induced by the administration of inactivated or live vaccines. At present a modified live virus vaccine is licensed in the United States to control BT in sheep. The vaccine contains serotype 10, only one of the five serotypes known to be active in the U.S. An inactivated vaccine for sheep, developed by USDA-SEA, is being studied at the University of California at Davis. In addition, a polyvalent (four serotypes), live, attenuated BTV vaccine has been developed at Texas A&M University and used in Texas ruminants with excellent results. This vaccine appears to be safe and effective in all ruminant species tested but is not available commercially at this time.

Supplemental Reading

Barber, T. C.: Temporal appearance, geographic distribution and species of origin of bluetongue virus serotypes in the United States. AJVR 40:1654–1656, 1979.

Bowne, J. G.: Bluetongue disease. Adv. Vet. Sci. Comp. Med. 15:1–46, 1971.

Bruner, D. W., and Gillespie, J. H.: Hagan's Infectious Diseases of Domestic Animals. Cornell Univ. Press, Ithaca, 1973, 653–660.

Ovine Rotavirus

CHARLES A. MEBUS, D.V.M., Ph.D.

Ovine rotavirus belongs to the genus *Rotavirus* in the family Reoviridae. There is only one known serotype. Resistance of ovine rotavirus is similar to that of calf rotavirus. A two-hour exposure of infected intestinal contents to Lysol (5 per cent) or Formol-Saline inactivated the virus; a ten-second exposure had little effect.

EPIZOOTIOLOGY

The epizootiology of ovine rotavirus is similar to that of bovine rotavirus.

CLINICAL SIGNS AND LESIONS

Rotavirus diarrhea occurs in newborn lambs to three-week-old animals. The disease is more severe in few-day-old animals. The incubation period in experimental animals varies from 11 to 20 hours. The animals become depressed, anorectic, have abdominal discomfort, and develop diarrhea. Diarrhea continues for three to four days. Mortality will depend on secondary infection. Lesions are similar to those described for calf rotavirus infection.

DIAGNOSIS

The same procedures given for the diagnosis of calf rotavirus can be used for the diagnosis of ovine rotavirus.

PREVENTION

Rotavirus can be introduced into a flock by the addition of infected lambs or adult animals and by contaminated clothing and equipment. Therefore, management practices to minimize exposure are recommended.

Vaccine administered to the ewe during gestation has been shown to decrease the incidence of diarrhea.

Supplemental Reading

Snodgrass, D. R., Anguss, K. W., and Gray, E. W.: Rotavirus infection in lambs: pathogenesis and pathology. Arch. Virol. 55:263–274, 1977.

Snodgrass, D. R., and Wells, R. P.: The immunoprophylaxis of rotavirus infections in lambs. Vet. Rec. 102:146–148, 1978.

Nairobi Sheep Disease

HUGH W. REID, B.V.M.&S., D.T.V.M., Ph.D., M.R.C.V.S.

Nairobi sheep disease (NSD) is an arthropod-transmitted virus infection of sheep and goats characterized by a marked febrile response followed by profuse watery diarrhea that frequently becomes hemorrhagic. The course of disease may be peracute, acute, mild, or inapparent, with a case mortality frequently over 80 per cent.

The virus of NSD belongs to the *Nairovirus* genus within the family of arthropod-transmitted viruses known as the Bunyaviridae. Nairoviruses have distinct structural and antigenic characteristics and can be subdivided into six serogroups. The serogroup to which NSD virus belongs also contains Dugbe and Ganjam viruses isolated from ticks in Nigeria and India, respectively. The virus measures 90 to 100 nm in diameter and contains RNA, and all isolates appear to be antigenically identical. In the laboratory the virus may be propagated by intracerebral inoculation of mice or in baby hamster kidney cell line (BHK-21) cultures, in which it produces characteristic perinuclear inclusion bodies and forms plaques under an overlay of carboxy-methylcellulose.

EPIZOOTIOLOGY

NSD was first described in 1910 as a fatal gastroenteritis of trade sheep in Kenya. The subsequent studies of Montgomery in 1917 established that the disease was caused by a virus transmitted by *Rhipicephalus appendiculatus* ticks that had previously engorged on sheep reacting to infection. Thus NSD virus became the first identified tick-borne virus.

Following the recognition of NSD in the area around Nairobi, its distribution within Kenya was found to correspond generally to that of *R. appendiculatus*. The disease has subsequently been identified in Uganda, Northern Somalia, and probably Zaire and Ruanda. There is serologic evidence that it is present in Botswana, Ethiopia, Tanzania, and South Africa.

Natural transmission between sheep occurs only by tick bite. Both transtadial and transovarial transmission have been demonstrated in the tick vector.

Experimentally, *R. appendiculatus* is an efficient vector of the virus, and the distribution of the disease in Kenya corresponds to that of this tick. However, other ticks can transmit the virus, which has been isolated on a number of occasions from field collections of *Amblyomma variegatum*, suggesting that the epidemiology of NSD may be complex. Furthermore, in Somalia it is evident that *R. pulchellus* effectively transmits virus and appears to be the main vector in this region. Thus the suggestion by earlier workers that *R. appendiculatus* is the sole vector of NSD can no longer be accepted.

Naturally occurring infection of the native fauna of Africa has not been identified, and domestic animals other than sheep and goats are refractory to infection. Antibody detected in wild ruminants is probably due to infection with serologically related viruses. Thus it has been concluded that NSD is maintained in a sheep-tick-sheep cycle, and as Ganjam and NSD viruses appear to be identical, it is currently suggested that NSD may be a strain of Ganjam introduced into Africa from India.

CLINICAL SIGNS

All breeds of sheep and goats are susceptible. The mortality rate of African sheep tends to be high, even up to 80 per cent, whereas that of European breeds is seldom more than 50 per cent. Goats appear to be less susceptible, with a mortality rate of 10 per cent, but losses in the field have been reported to reach 88 per cent.

Following exposure to infected ticks, the incubation period is four to six days. Pyrexia of sudden onset is the first sign, with temperature rising rapidly to 40 to 42°C. Affected animals are dull and anorexic, and there may be a mucous nasal discharge. Shortly thereafter, watery green feces are voided and may become hemorrhagic. Distress and constant straining are evident, and the nasal discharge often becomes blood-tinged. The external genitalia of ewes swell, and pregnant animals frequently abort. Death may follow within 24 hours of the onset of signs but can be delayed for as long as six days. It is generally considered that the prognosis is poor if diarrhea develops.

At postmortem examination the hindquarters are usually soiled with feces and the nostrils caked with blood-tinged nasal discharge. The principal lesions are seen in the gastrointestinal tract, extending from the abomasum to the rectum. The mucosa of the abomasum and small intestine is edematous and hyperemic and may be hemorrhagic, particularly in the region of the pylorus and ileocecal valve. The most severe lesions are found in the large intestine, extending from the cecum sometimes as far as the rectum. The lumen may be filled with blood, and longitudinal hemorrhages extend along the tops of the folds that are edematous. Serosal hemorrhages may also be present.

In addition, the trachea is frequently hyperemic and may contain blood-tinged froth, whereas in a proportion of cases the lungs have lesions associated with secondary pasteurella pneumonia. Frequently ecchymoses are present on the endocardium and petechial hemorrhages on the epicardium. The genital tract, particularly of pregnant ewes, is edematous and hyperemic, and the mucous membranes are catarrhal. Lymph nodes are enlarged and moist, and the malpighian corpuscles of the spleen are prominent.

The only histologic changes that are consistently present and considered to be of diagnostic value are a severe glomerulotubular nephritis associated with hyaline and epithelial casts and a generalized vascular congestion of the kidney that is most marked around the glomeruli.

DIAGNOSIS

The clinical and postmortem picture cannot be relied on to provide a specific diagnosis, and confirmation depends on laboratory tests. From dead animals the isolation of virus from plasma, spleen, and mesenteric lymph node homogenates by intracerebral inoculation of suckling mice should be attempted. Tissue culture is less sensitive for primary isolation of virus, as generally isolates must be serially passaged two to five times before cytopathic effects can be detected. In recovered animals the detection of serum antibody will indicate previous infection with NSD. Animals that recover are immune for life, and though neutralizing antibody is not readily detected, high titers of antibody may be detected by fluorescent or indirect hemagglutination tests and are maintained for at least 15 months. Among the conditions that must be considered in the differential diagnosis are Rift Valley Fever, rinderpest, peste des petits ruminants, salmonellosis, pasteurellosis, babesiosis, coccidiosis, helminthiasis, heartwater, and poisoning.

PREVENTION

Virus serially passaged by intracerebral inoculation of mice or in tissue culture loses pathogenicity for sheep and has been used as attenuated live virus vaccines. However, the degree of attenuation is accompanied by a loss of immunogenicity. Thus, owing to the variability in susceptibility of different breeds of sheep, none of these vaccines has proved generally acceptable. An inactivated vaccine prepared from virus propagated in baby hamster kidney cells and then formalinized and precipitated with methanol produced a high level of resistance to laboratory challenge but has not yet been assessed in the field.

Supplemental Reading

Clerx, J. P. M., Casals, J., and Bishop, D. H. L.: Structural characteristics of Nairoviruses (genus *Nairovirus*, Bunyaviridae). J. Gen. Virol. 55:165–178, 1981.

Daubney, R., and Hudson, J. R.: Nairobi sheep disease. Parasitology 23:507–524, 1931.

Davies, F. G.: Nairobi sheep disease in Kenya. The isolation of virus from sheep and goats, ticks and possible maintenance hosts. J. Hyg. 81:259–265, 1978.

Rift Valley Fever in Sheep and Goats

R. J. YEDLOUTSCHNIG, D.V.M.
and J. S. WALKER, D.V.M., M.S.

Rift Valley fever (RVF) is caused by a pantropic arthropod-borne RNA virus of the family Bunyaviridae genus *Phlebovirus*. The virus is most stable within a pH range of 7 to 8 and is rapidly inactivated below pH 6.2. Two per cent acetic or citric acid or other chemicals with a very low pH are effective chemical inactivants of RVF virus (RVFV).

EPIZOOTIOLOGY

The disease naturally infects cattle, sheep, goats, and humans. Lambs and baby hamsters and mice are the most susceptible experimental animals. Outbreaks of RVF have usually been associated with years of high rainfall and high population densities of mosquitoes; RVFV has been isolated from *Aedes, Culex, Mansonia, Eretmopodites,* and *Anopheles* genera of mosquitoes.

More information is available in the article on RVF in cattle.

CLINICAL SIGNS

Newborn lambs and kids are highly susceptible to infection with RVFV, with mortality rates of 90 to 100 per cent. The incubation period in young lambs is about 12 hours, with a sudden temperature rise to 40.5 to 42.2°C followed by collapse and death within 36 hours. This acute form of the disease is less common in older sheep and goats, and mortality approximates 20 to 30 per cent.

Clinical signs in adults are not consistent but may include a rapid rise in temperature, vomiting, mucopurulent nasal discharge, unsteady gait, and, frequently, abortion. The disease in goats is less severe, although abortions are reported. The primary lesion produced by RVFV is a focal hepatic necrosis of varying degrees. Hepatic lesions in adult sheep are not as severe as those found in lambs, but multiple necrotic areas may be present. In some animals only small microscopic necrotic lesions develop.

DIAGNOSIS

The same diagnostic procedures used for RVF in cattle can be used in sheep and goats.

TREATMENT

No specific treatments are currently available.

PREVENTION AND CONTROL

Live attenuated and formalin-inactivated RVF vaccines have been developed for veterinary use in South Africa and Egypt. Two doses of the killed vaccine are recommended for use in nonenzootic zones. The Smithburn live attenuated vaccine is recommended in enzootic areas; this vaccine is associated with abortion in a small percentage of recipients and has been reported to cause arthrogryposis and hydroencephaly in ewes.

One means of control is to suppress mosquito vectors or at least to protect the animals from the vectors.

Supplemental Reading

Meegan, J. M., and Shope, R. E.: Emerging concepts on Rift Valley fever. *In* Pollard, M. (ed.): Perspectives in Virology, X1. Alan R. Liss, New York, 1981, 267–287.

Peters, C. J., and Meegan, J. M.: Rift Valley fever. *In* Steele, J. N. (ed.): Handbook Series in Zoonoses, Section B, Viral Zoonoses, Vol. 1. Boca Raton, CRC Press, 1981, 403–420.

Weiss, K. E.: Rift Valley fever—a review. Bull. Epizoot. Dis. Afr. 5:431–458, 1957.

Akabane Disease in Sheep and Goats

A. J. DELLA-PORTA, B.Sc., Ph.D.

Akabane disease is a congenital disease of cattle, sheep, and goats characterized by hydranencephaly (HE), arthrogryposis (AG), micrencephaly, and porencephaly. It usually occurs as localized epizootics and less frequently as sporadic cases. This disease is caused by Akabane virus, an insect-transmitted virus (arbovirus) belonging to the family Bunyaviridae, that occurs as an inapparent infection of nonimmune pregnant animals during the first trimester of pregnancy. The disease has been seen in lambs in Australia, Israel, and Turkey and in goats in Israel. Akabane virus is probably present throughout much of Africa and Asia.

CLINICAL SIGNS

Infection in the pregnant animal is inapparent. There may be an increase observed in the number of abortions or an apparent decrease in the number of ewes and goats reaching parturition. At birth, many of the lambs and kids may be suffering from hydranencephaly, micrencephaly, arthrogryposis, and other skeletal and nervous system impairments. These syndromes can overlap in sequence, and animals can be seen exhibiting more than one of these signs.

The central nervous lesions are similar to those seen in calves (see Akabane Disease in Cattle).

DIAGNOSIS

As Akabane virus has not been isolated from congenitally affected offspring born at term, proof of infection must be based on serologic and pathologic evidence. Serologic evidence is based on the presence of virus-neutralizing antibodies against Akabane virus in the precolostrum serum sample from the affected offspring.

Supplemental Reading

Kurogi, H., Inaba, Y., Takahashi, E., Sato, K., Goto, Y., and Omori, T.: Experimental infection of pregnant goats with Akabane virus. Natl. Inst. An. Hlth. Q. *17*:1–9, 1977.

Parsonson, I. M., Della-Porta, A. J., O'Halloran, M. L., Snowdon, W. A., Fahey, K. J., and Standfast, H. A.: Akabane virus infection in the pregnant ewe. 1. Growth of virus in the foetus and the development of the foetal immune response. Vet. Microbiol. 6:197–207, 1981.

Porterfield, J. S., and Della-Porta, A. J.: Bunyaviridae: Infections and diagnosis. In Kurstak, E., and Kurstak, C. (eds.): Comparative Diagnosis of Viral Diseases, Vol. 4, Part B. New York, Academic Press, 1981, 479–508.

Rabies in Sheep and Goats

GEORGE M. BAER, D.V.M.

Rabies is rare in sheep and goats. United States surveillance summaries from 1971 to 1981 indicate that a minimum of 3 cases and a maximum of 30 cases were reported annually, most occurring in states with many reported cases of wildlife rabies, such as Maine (fox rabies) and Texas, Iowa, and Oklahoma (skunk rabies). In the current European fox epizootic, the number of sheep reported rabid is slightly higher, 0.7 per cent of the total of 30,832 cases reported between 1954 and 1966. The seasonal peak usually comes in the spring, when most cases occur in foxes. Sheep and goats are usually bitten by rabid animals on the face, lips, and nose. The clinical signs include pruritus, sexual excitement, paresthesia, pica, excitation, aggressiveness, depression, and terminal paralysis. The incubation periods in one outbreak varied from 15 to 65 days. The attack rate may be high, and multiple deaths in affected herds are common. In the above-mentioned outbreak, 17 of the 22 animals bitten died of rabies. For a more complete description, refer to the overview by Wachendorfer. Diagnosis is made by the fluorescent antibody staining of brain impressions from sheep that have died. There are no recorded human rabies cases due to exposures to rabid sheep. There is only one vaccine currently licensed for use in sheep in the United States, which is an inactivated tissue culture vaccine.

Supplemental Reading

Feldkamp, R.: Atypical rabies in a flock of ewes. Vet. Med./Small Anim. Clin. 72:1496, 1977.

Wachendorfer, G.: Zur Epidemiologie und Klinik der Tollwut des Schafes. Sonderdruck aus Veterinär-Medizinische Nachrichten 1966. Heft 4:275–294, 1966.

Maedi-Visna (Progressive Pneumonia, Zwoegerziekte)

RANDALL C. CUTLIP, D.V.M., Ph.D.

Maedi-visna, meaning "dyspnea" and "wasting," respectively, are Icelandic terms for a chronic progressive viral disease of adult sheep known also as progressive pneumonia in the United States and zwoegerziekte in Holland. In Iceland the disease was initially described as two separate entities, pneumonitis (maedi) and encephalitis (visna).

ETIOLOGY

Maedi-visna is caused by an exogenous retrovirus that is closely related to the virus of caprine arthritis-encephalitis. Structurally, the virus contains a dense 40-nm core surrounded by a single envelope with 8-nm spikes. The core is formed in the peripheral cytoplasm of the infected cell and is encased in host cell membrane by a budding process. The mature virus is 80 to 120 nm in diameter. Major detectable antigenic components are polypeptides of the core and glycoproteins of the envelope. The core proteins are stable, but the glycoproteins, important in serum neutralization, are subject to antigenic drift. Thus, there are multiple minor variants when tested by serum neutralization. The virus is readily inactivated by heat, drying, and disinfectants but is stable at refrigeration temperature.

EPIZOOTIOLOGY

Infection with maedi-visna virus is unconventional in that a carrier state, in the presence of circulating homologous antibodies, is the rule rather than the exception. The RNA virus is carried as DNA copies (provirus) that are integrated into the chromosomal nucleic acid of infected cells. The provirus may be carried for the life of the sheep without clinical affect or it may induce disease. It is not known why some sheep are clinically affected and others are not. Disease is believed to be immune-mediated.

In most sheep-raising areas of the world, infection is common but clinical disease is uncommon. Australia and New Zealand are believed to be free of the virus. Rarely is there more than a 5 per cent annual loss in a flock, but infection may reach 100 per cent. Some breeds (Icelandic, Texel, Border Leicester, Finnish) appear to be more susceptible to clinical disease. Goats are the only species other than sheep known to be susceptible to infection. Transmission of virus can occur at any time by contact, after birth through the milk and, rarely, before birth. The lactogenic route is believed to be the most common.

CLINICAL SIGNS

The cardinal feature of maedi-visna is a continuous weight loss until death several weeks to months later. Respiration becomes progressively more labored. Rarely, there is a CNS disturbance characterized by listlessness and advancing hindquarter paralysis. Severe lameness because of chronic arthritis, especially of the carpal and tarsal joints, is occasionally seen. The incubation period is more than one year, and death is inevitable once signs appear. Affected sheep are afebrile and continue to eat. Signs may be exacerbated during times of stress such as lambing, nursing, or inclement weather.

At necropsy, the lungs fail to deflate fully and weigh two to three times normal weight. They are diffusely involved, grayish-pink with gray patches, of a firm spongy consistency, and dry. The anteroventral areas are frequently dark red and consolidated because of secondary bacterial infection. Thoracic lymph nodes are enlarged. Affected joints have focal necrosis of the articular cartilage and subchondral bone and fibroplasia of the synovium and capsule.

The characteristic histologic feature of maedi-visna is the presence of multiple lymphoid nodules in the interstitium of the lungs. Alveolar septa are thickened by an accumulation of mononuclear cells and, in many cases, by excessive fibromuscular tissue. Epithelial hyperplasia is usually minimal but may become extensive with secondary infections, resulting in an adenomatous appearance that has been confused with pulmonary adenomatosis (jaagsiekte). Neural lesions vary from a simple cuffing of blood vessels with lymphocytes to necrosis of the ependyma and the subependymal neuropile. Articular lesions are those of a chronic nonsuppurative inflammation.

DIAGNOSIS

Infection can be diagnosed by serologic testing or by isolating the virus from buffy coats. Diagnosis of disease is dependent upon finding typical signs and lesions.

TREATMENT

No treatment is effective.

PREVENTION AND CONTROL

The only known method of preventing infection is to avoid exposure to the virus. Once a flock is infected, the disease can be controlled by removing serologically positive animals from the flock or by isolating lambs from the flock at birth. Maedi-visna was eradicated from Iceland by slaughtering all sheep exposed to sheep with the clinical disease.

Supplemental Reading

Dawson, M.: Maedi/visna: A review. Vet. Rec. 106:212–216, 1980.
DeBoer, G. F., and Houwers, D. J.: Epizootiology of maedi/visna in sheep. In Tyrrell, D. A. J. (ed.): Aspects of Slow and Persistent Virus Infections. Martinus Nijhoff, Amsterdam, 1980, 192–220.

Caprine Arthritis-Encephalitis

D. SCOTT ADAMS, D.V.M., Ph.D.

Caprine arthritis-encephalitis virus (CAEV) is a non-oncogenic retrovirus of the subfamily Lentiviridae. It is antigenically related to progressive pneumonia virus and maedi/visna virus of sheep but not identical as determined by nucleic acid hybridization.

The virus has a lipid envelope and is inactivated by organic solvents such as ether and alcohol. It is also inactivated by heat at 56°C for one hour. No other stability trials have been done, but if CAEV stability is consistent with other related retroviruses, drying, UV light, and a wide range of disinfectants should inactivate it as well.

EPIZOOTIOLOGY

All breeds of goats appear to be susceptible to infection by CAEV and sheep have also been experimentally infected. Serologic surveys using an agar gel immunodiffusion (AGID) technique (which does not distinguish CAEV infection from infection by maedi/visna and progressive pneumonia viruses) indicate that infection is most common among the dairy goat breeds, particularly in Europe, the United States, and Australia. Indigenous goats and goats raised under pastoral conditions usually have a low level of infection.

In countries, such as the United States, where the prevalence of seropositive goats is high, disease expression is estimated to be from 0 to 25 per cent in any given herd. The factors that control disease expression are unknown, but virus strains, host, and environmental factors may play important roles.

The virus is most commonly and efficiently transmitted through milk and colostrum to neonatal kids. Intrauterine transmission may occur but does not appear to be a major mode of transmission. The virus can be transmitted horizontally but requires prolonged contact of several months. Artificial or natural breeding of infected bucks to uninfected does seems particularly unlikely to result in transmission. However, contact between infected and uninfected does that are lactating should be avoided. The virus appears to persist primarily in the host and not in the environment for any length of time. Seropositive goats should be considered infected for life.

DIAGNOSIS

The diagnosis of the arthritic form is based on a history of chronic arthritis of adult goats, especially involving the carpi and other peripheral joints, that is unresponsive to antibiotic therapy. Bursitis, unthriftiness, and failure to isolate bacteria from affected joints are additional findings. Analysis of synovial fluid with Wright's stain reveals a predominance of mononuclear cells except in very acute cases. The mineralization of soft tissues around joints, bursae, and tendon sheaths may be demonstrated by radiography or at postmortem. The finding of serum antibody against the virus is helpful to the diagnosis but is not pathognomonic. Chronic proliferative synovitis with infiltration by mononuclear cells and fibrin, necrosis, and mineralization are typical histologic findings.

The encephalitic form, leukoencephalomyelitis, usually affects kid goats two to four months of age with an afebrile, ascending paralysis, which may or may not proceed to seizures or death. Adult goats may develop encephalitis with variable signs depending on the location and extent of the lesions. Diagnosis is best determined by postmortem histologic examination of the brain and spinal cord.

TREATMENT

Treatment of the arthritis is only palliative. Affected goats may be made more comfortable with phenylbutazone at a dose of 5 to 10 mg/kg orally. No treatment of the encephalitic form is recommended.

PREVENTION AND CONTROL

Kids must be separated from infected does immediately at birth to prevent suckling, fed colostrum that has been heated to 56°C for one hour or colostrum from a known CAEV-free doe, fed pasteurized goat milk, cow milk, or milk replacer until weaning, and then tested for evidence of infection at six months of age and at six-month intervals thereafter. When no seropositive goats are found in two successive tests the group may be considered CAEV-free.

Supplemental Reading

Adams, D. S.: The meaning of the agar gel immunodiffusion test (AGID) for antibody against caprine arthritis encephalitis virus (CAEV). Dairy Goat J. *60*:633–635, 1982.

Adams, D. S., Klevjer-Anderson, P., Carlson, J. L., McGuire, T. C., and Gorham, J. R.: Transmission and control of caprine arthritis-encephalitis virus. Am. J. Vet. Res. *44*:1670–1675, 1983.

Crawford, T. B., and Adams, D. S.: Caprine arthritis-encephalitis: Clinical features and presence of antibody in selected goat populations. J. Am. Vet. Med. Assoc. *178*:713–719, 1981.

Ovine Astroviruses

JANICE C. BRIDGER, B.Sc., Ph.D.

By negative-stain electron microscopy, the 30-nm particles appear circular in outline with a five- or six-pointed stellate configuration on the surface. Although morphologically indistinguishable from astroviruses of other species, ovine astroviruses do not cross-react by immunofluorescence with convalescent antisera. Particles contain single-stranded RNA. To date, only one strain has been studied.

EPIZOOTIOLOGY

No information is available on the significance of astroviruses in ovine enteritis or on the prevalence of infection. The virus is recognized only in the United Kingdom, where it was identified in an outbreak of diarrhea in lambs four to six weeks old. Experimental infection can be produced by oral inoculation of bacteria-free fecal filtrates in gnotobiotic lambs one to three days old.

CLINICAL SIGNS

The single strain studied produced a mild diarrhea in gnotobiotic lambs one to three days old. Histologic damage was confined to the middle and posterior small intestine where villus height:crypt depth ratios were reduced and epithelial cells on the distal parts of villi immunofluoresced. Crystalline arrays of virus particles were seen in the cytoplasm of infected cells.

DIAGNOSIS

Electron microscopy, particularly with ammonium molybdate as the negative stain, is used to identify astroviruses in feces; a simple preparative procedure without centrifugation is adequate to demonstrate particles. Alternatively, immunofluorescent staining of cryostat sections of small intestine may be used but the highest rate of cell infection was found to be during the incubation period. Unlike human and bovine astroviruses, detection by cell culture inoculation is not possible, as ovine astro- viruses have not been shown to infect cell cultures, even on primary passage.

TREATMENT, PREVENTION, AND CONTROL

No specific therapeutic studies have been conducted but the pathogenesis suggests that oral rehydration would be beneficial. No vaccines are available. Passive protection by maternal antibody may be possible, but natural levels in the ovine population are unknown.

Supplemental Reading

Snodgrass, D. R.: Astroviruses in diarrhea of young animals and children. *In* Kurstak, E. and Kurstak, C. (eds.): Comparative Diagnosis of Viral Disease IVB. Academic Press, New York, 1981.

Scrapie

HOWARD W. WHITFORD, D.V.M., Ph.D.

The agent that causes scrapie, believed to be a virus, has some very extraordinary properties. The virus has never been visualized using the electron microscope, but filtration studies indicate that it is 50 to 60 nm in diameter. The virus is extremely resistant to heat and chemical disinfectants. Infected brain tissue that has been heated at 100°C for eight hours is capable of inducing disease when injected into susceptible sheep. Likewise, infected mouse brain stored in 10 per cent formalin for up to four months remains infective for goats and mice. It has been suggested that the scrapie agent may belong to the prion group of pathogens. (In its broadest sense, a prion is a subviral particle, consisting of a strand of nucleic acid, without an outer protein coat.)

The scrapie agent produces no detectable humoral or cellular antibody. The only method of demonstrating the presence of the scrapie agent is by inoculating tissue from an infected animal into a susceptible host, mice being the most commonly used laboratory animals.

EPIZOOTIOLOGY

The natural host for scrapie is believed to be sheep. Mink encephalopathy and Kuru in man appear to be caused by closely related agents. Scrapie has been experimentally reproduced in goats, mink, laboratory primates, and a variety of laboratory rodents.

Geographically, scrapie is widespread. The disease occurs in sheep in Great Britain, Belgium, France, Germany, Spain, India, Iceland, Canada, and the United States. The disease was also recognized in South Africa, Australia, and New Zealand following importation of infected sheep from Great Britain. Prompt quarantine and slaughter resulted in the eradication of the disease in these countries.

The incidence of the disease in sheep in the United States over the past ten years shows an apparent increase. Whether this is due to better reporting rather than an actual increase of diseased animals is questionable. The following summarizes the number of outbreaks for the past decade: 1974—2; 1975—2; 1976—6; 1977—3; 1978—1; 1979—4; 1980—11; 1981—11; 1982—18; 1983—15.

The 15 outbreaks in FY 1983 (October 1982 to September 1983) represented flocks located in ten states as follows: Illinois—1; Indiana—2; Louisiana—1; Massachusetts—1; Michigan—1; New Jersey—1; Oklahoma—3; Texas—1, Virginia—2; Wisconsin—2.

The most commonly affected breeds of sheep are Suffolk, Cheviots, and Swaledale, although experimentally no breed of sheep or goats has been found to be resistant.

Transmission of the disease can occur both vertically and horizontally. There is no evidence that lambs are infected *in utero,* although work is in progress to confirm that embryos harvested from infected sheep do not carry the agent when implanted in a susceptible recipient. The scrapie virus has not been recovered from milk of lactating ewes, and it is believed that lambs are infected at an early age via infected nasal secretions from the dam. Horizontal transmission probably occurs through fecal shedding of the agent since significant titers have been demonstrated in the intestines. Resistance to the virus increases with age.

The pathogenesis of scrapie has been laboriously worked out by Hadlow and Eklund. The virus in experimentally infected animals is initially in the lymphoreticular system, namely the retropharyngeal lymph nodes and spleen. Next the virus is detected in the intestine, where it replicates slowly for months or years. Although viremia has never been demonstrated, the virus is probably carried to the CNS by the blood. The virus reaches the brain stem most likely via the cranial nerves and replicates in those parts of the brain that result in the clinical signs (incoordination, pruritus, and so on). The virus is not cleared from the extraneural tissue and continues to be shed throughout the course of the disease.

CLINICAL SIGNS

In natural outbreaks of scrapie, clinical signs may occur in sheep between the ages of 18 months and 6 years, most commonly in animals 30 to 60 months of age. Neurologic manifestations are the only antemortem signs noted. These develop very slowly and insidiously. Initially the animals appear apprehensive. They then become excitable and overreact to routine stimuli. As the disease progresses, tremors of the head and neck with the head held high may be noted. Muscle tremors of the flanks and thighs may also develop. Pruritus, usually beginning at the tailhead and progressing anteriorly over the flanks and ribs, develops with resultant scratching and loss of wool (Fig. 1). Serpentine tongue movements accompany the scratching. Licking and wool biting affected areas are common. Incoordination that becomes progressively pronounced develops until the animal becomes recumbent and invariably dies. The clinical disease may occur over a period as short as a few weeks or as long as a year, but most cases last between six weeks and six months. During the clinical course, the animal remains alert with a good appetite but weight loss will occur.

Post-mortem examination of animals dying of scrapie shows no gross abnormalities with the exception of localized skin trauma due to scratching. Microscopically, the lesions are confined to the CNS where degenerative changes are seen. These changes are confined to the cerebellar cortex, medulla oblongata, pons, mid brain, diencephalon, and corpus striatum and consist of pyknotic and shrunken neurons, cytoplasmic vacuoles, and astrocytosis. Few, if any, changes are noted in the spinal cord or cerebral cortex.

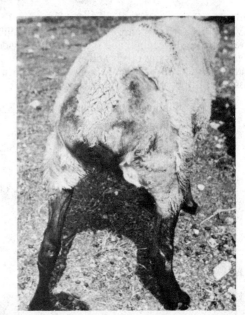

Figure 1. Scrapie-infected sheep showing wool loss due to pruritus and scratching. (Photograph courtesy of Dr. Wilbur Clark, Scrapie Field Trial, Mission, Texas.)

DIAGNOSIS

At the present time, scrapie in a live animal cannot be definitively diagnosed using current laboratory procedures. This is because the infectious agent has never been isolated, purified, or propagated outside the animal host. Without an antigen, there is no serologic test and humoral antibody response cannot be detected. An added frustration is that attempts to demonstrate a viremia have been unsuccessful.

A tentative diagnosis is based on history of exposure, long incubation period, age of the animal, and clinical signs (some animals may not have pruritus) progressing to death. Histopathologic lesions in the brain and transmission of the disease to mice by inoculation with infected tissue confirms the diagnosis.

Differential diagnosis includes encephalopathies due to other infectious agents (such as *Listeria,* louping ill, visna, maedi, caprine arthritis-encephalitis), polioencephalomalacia, and pruritic dermatitis caused by bacteria or fungi. The age of the animal and response to specific therapy should rule out other disease conditions.

Scrapie is a reportable disease, and the appropriate state and federal animal health officials should be contacted if scrapie is suspected.

TREATMENT

No treatment has been found to be effective and none should be attempted.

PREVENTION AND CONTROL

The historical approach to prevention and control of scrapie has been to slaughter herds that have experienced the disease, tracing back to herds of origin and destroying them also. This method proved successful in eradicating

Table 1. *Animals Requiring Slaughter in Scrapie Eradication Program*

1. Infected female
   a. 1st generation progeny (male and female)
   b. All succeeding female generations
   c. Dam of infected female
   d. Siblings of infected female
   e. Maternal grand dam of infected female
2. Infected male
   a. 1st generation progeny (male and female)
   b. Dam of infected male
   c. Siblings of infected male
   d. Maternal grand dam of infected male

Note: All other animals in a flock having scrapie-infected sheep are considered to be exposed and must be permanently identified and quarantined for a period of 42 months following the most recent exposure. Also considered to be exposed are all animals having been present in the flock with the infected animals even though these animals may not have been present at the time the disease was diagnosed.

the disease in New Zealand and Australia, probably owing more to the early recognition and prompt action than the method itself.

In the U.S. and Canada, eradication attempts have failed and the number of cases in the U.S. appears to be on the increase. Because of the danger of eliminating certain valuable blood lines of sheep in the U.S. and Canada, plus the expense of indemnity payments, a new approach to the control of the disease was adopted in April of 1983.

Briefly, the revised Scrapie Eradication Program calls for the provisions listed in Table 1 when an infected animal is discovered. For further information concerning the scrapie eradication program in the U.S., refer to Veterinary Services Memorandum No. 557.1 dated April 8, 1983, which is available from the Area Veterinarian in Charge, Animal and Plant Health Inspection Service, USDA.

Supplemental Reading

Eklund, C. M., and Hadlow, W. J.: The slow virus diseases. *In* Steele, J. H. (ed.): CRC Handbook Series in Zoonoses. CRC Press, Boca Raton, Fla., 1981.

Gadjusek, D. C., Gibbs, C. J., Jr., and Alpers, M.: Slow, Latent, and Temperate Virus Infections. U.S. Dept. Health, Education and Welfare, Public Health Service, National Institutes of Health, National Institute of Neurological Diseases and Blindness, 1965.

Hadlow, W. J., and Eklund, C. M.: Scrapie—A Virus-Induced Chronic Encephalopathy of Sheep. Infections of the Nervous System. Research Publication of The Association for Research in Nervous and Mental Disease, Vol. XLIV, 1968.

Jensen, F.: Diseases of Sheep. Lea & Febiger, Philadelphia, 1982.

Pulmonary Adenomatosis (Jaagsiekte)

RANDALL C. CUTLIP, D.V.M., Ph.D.

Pulmonary adenomatosis, or jaagsiekte, an Afrikaans term meaning "driving sickness," is an infectious adenocarcinoma of the lungs of sheep that metastasizes occasionally to regional lymph nodes and rarely to other organs.

ETIOLOGY

A causal agent has not been isolated; however, a retrovirus, believed to be the cause, has been seen with the electron microscope in the lungs of affected sheep. A herpesvirus associated with the disease has been discredited as the primary agent but may be involved in a secondary role.

EPIZOOTIOLOGY

Pulmonary adenomatosis was first described in South Africa in 1891. Since then, the disease has been found in many countries of the world. There are no known differences in susceptibility of breeds of sheep, and sheep appear to be the natural host of the disease. It has also been reported in goats. The disease can be transmitted experimentally by intratracheal administration of lung homogenates or pulmonary lavage fluids. Natural transmission is believed to be by direct contact and by contact with food or water contaminated by fluid from the respiratory tract of affected sheep. Annual death rates in a flock are usually less than 2 per cent but death rates as high as 50 per cent have been reported.

CLINICAL SIGNS AND LESIONS

The disease is characterized clinically by a long and variable incubation period of two months to two years, an insidious onset, and a slow progression until death results after several months. The chief signs are progressive dyspnea and loss of weight. Late in the disease, excess fluid produced in the lungs by neoplastic cells can be heard as moist rales and frequently runs from the nostrils when the rear of the affected sheep is elevated. In uncomplicated cases, temperature and appetite are normal and coughing is rare. Death from bacterial pneumonia is a common sequel to this neoplasm.

Macroscopic lesions are unevenly distributed in the lungs, with most in the ventral parts. They are usually bilateral and vary within the same lung from small discrete areas of less than 1 cm diameter to large confluent areas several centimeters in diameter. Affected areas of the lungs are reddish-gray to bluish-gray in color, firm in consistency, and wet on cut surface. Microscopically, the lesion is a papillary adenocarcinoma with a variable content of fibrous and myxomatous stroma. The neoplastic epithelial cells arise from type II alveolar epithelial cells and nonciliated bronchiolar epithelial cells. Metastatic lesions are usually small and mimic the primary lesion in microscopic appearance.

DIAGNOSIS

Pulmonary adenomatosis can be diagnosed only by microscopic examination of the lesion.

TREATMENT

No treatment is effective against the neoplasm, but life may be prolonged by treating with antibiotics to prevent secondary pneumonia.

PREVENTION AND CONTROL

The lack of a simple diagnostic test limits an effective control. The disease was eradicated from Iceland by slaughtering all affected sheep and their contacts. Based on epidemiologic data, removing affected sheep from a flock and rearing lambs in isolation would be useful control measures.

Supplemental Reading

Perk, K.: Slow virus infections of ovine lung. Adv. Vet. Sci. Comp. Med. *26*:267–287, 1982.
Sharp, J. M. : Slow virus infections of the respiratory tract of sheep. Vet. Rec. *108*:391–393, 1981.

Chlamydia-Induced Diseases of Sheep and Goats

J. STORZ, D.V.M., Ph.D.

Chlamydial agents were proved to cause abortions and genital disorders, pneumonia, and intestinal infections in sheep and goats as well as polyarthritis and keratoconjunctivitis in sheep.[1]

PROPERTIES OF CHLAMYDIAE OF OVINE ORIGIN

As obligate intracellular infectious agents that comprise antigenically related and culturally, tinctorially, and morphologically similar microorganisms, ovine chlamydiae can be propagated in the cells of yolk sacs of developing chicken embryos or in cultured cells, preferably mouse L cells, where they multiply in the cytoplasm and cause cell lysis toward the end of the development cycle. Chlamydiae of sheep have specific antigens that separate them into the immunotypes 1 and 2. Strains isolated from abortions, pneumonia, and intestinal infections fall into immunotype 1, whereas those isolated from keratoconjunctivitis and polyarthritis with the associated intestinal phase of infections comprise immunotype 2. Infectivity for cells of all these strains is enhanced by centrifugation. Pretreatment of cultured cells with diethylamino-ethyl-dextran (DEAE-D) enhances adsorption of immunotype 2 but not immunotype 1 strains. Specific antigenic and cultural properties of chlamydiae isolated from diseases of goats have not been studied.[2]

EPIZOOTIOLOGY

These infections have a worldwide distribution. The infectious chain is maintained directly in the sheep and goat population, and an important role is played by the intestinal infections, which persist over long periods with continued shedding. Entrance into new hosts may occur through oral, oropharyngeal, conjunctival, and respiratory infections. Chlamydiae were also isolated from the semen of rams.[1]

CLINICAL SIGNS

The intestinal chlamydial infection is clinically inapparent. Lambs respond with a fever two to six days after respiratory infection, when they are also depressed, anorectic, and have signs of respiratory distress with a dry cough.[3]

Chlamydial infection of pregnant ewes and goats may result in abortion, stillbirth, or the delivery of weak offspring. Abortions occur in the last month of gestation, but they were seen as early as the 100th day of gestation. The incidence of abortion may reach 30 per cent in flocks exposed for the first time. More commonly, 1 to 5 per cent of the pregnant animals in enzootically infected herds abort, and losses occur year after year. Dams of all ages may abort, but higher rates may be observed among the young ones. Rams with genital chlamydial infections have epididymitis, and their semen is of poor quality and contains large numbers of leukocytes.[2, 4]

Chlamydia-induced polyarthritis was observed among lambs out on ranges as well as in lambs from farm flocks and feedlots. Lambs that weighed 55 to 105 pounds appeared to be affected more often, and morbidity ranged from 2 to 75 per cent. Rectal temperatures of affected lambs were 39 to 42°C. The lambs had varying degrees of stiffness, lameness, and anorexia. Affected lambs were gaunt, depressed, and reluctant to move or stand or bear weight on their limbs. The highest incidence of disease among sheep on ranges was observed in July through September, whereas in feedlot lambs the disease was most prevalent in October through December.[1, 5]

The severity of chlamydial keratoconjunctivitis of sheep was variable. Early signs consisted of chemosis and dilation of conjunctival vessels at the lid margins. Diffuse reddening developed later in the lower fornices, where fine filaments of mucus were present. The development of lymphoid follicles signaled intermediate stages of conjunctival involvement. The bulbar surface of the third eyelid developed numerous follicles, which may form 2- to 4-mm high folds on the upper and lower fornix. Conjunctival hyperemia, edema, and follicle development caused swelling of the periorbital tissues. Lacrimal drainage was compromised, epiphora was common, and abundant seropurulent eye discharge was observed to seal the eyelids with a crust.[4]

LESIONS

Consolidation of the anterior lobes and of the lungs in the hilus region is observed in naturally occurring chlamydial pneumonia of sheep and goats. Sharply defined areas of consolidation have a dull, gray-pink color. The lungs are heavy and fail to collapse. Slightly opaque mucus appears in open bronchioli. The regional lymph nodes are enlarged.[3]

The prominent pathologic change in chlamydial abortions of ewes is placentitis. Various numbers of cotyledons are necrotic, and the periplacentome of affected cotyledons is thickened and has an opaque yellow-pink color. The placenta may be covered with a layer of flaky, clay-colored exudate. The margins of placental lesions consist of zones of hyperemia and hemorrhage.[1, 2]

Changes in the aborted fetuses depend on the stage of

gestation and the duration of infection. Lambs that are aborted near term usually have a rather clean appearance. Petechiae can be detected in the subcutis of many aborted lambs. The livers may be congested and slightly swollen. Pinpoint, whitish foci are seen on the visceral and cut surfaces of livers from some lambs.[1]

The most prominent lesions of lambs with chlamydial polyarthritis are associated with the joints and periarticular tissues. The synovial fluid is increased, has a turbid appearance, and may contain fibrin plaques. Affected tendons and tendon sheaths contain edema fluid and are swollen.[1, 5]

DIAGNOSIS

Clinical signs and the history of the disease episode may suggest chlamydial infection as a cause of keratoconjunctivitis, polyarthritis, or abortions. Laboratory diagnosis is the only reliable way to detect these infections. They can be identified through exfoliative cytologic methods applied to placental specimens or scrapings from the conjunctiva, trachea, or synovial membranes. Cytoplasmic chlamydial inclusions are demonstrable in conjunctival. synovial, or tracheal cells following staining with the Giemsa method. Chlamydial elementary bodies are present in placental impression smears. The Giemsa stain is best for revealing elementary bodies in these preparations. Immunofluorescent methods applied to the exfoliative cytologic preparations enhance both sensitivity and specificity.[1, 4]

Isolation of Chlamydiae from clinical specimens is the second diagnostic approach. Most strains multiply in the yolk sac cells of developing chicken embryos. Isolation in cultured cells employing infectivity enhancing methods is more sensitive and far less time consuming.[1]

Chlamydial antibodies to genus-specific antigens can be detected in the complement fixation or the enzyme-linked immunosorbent tests or by double immunodiffusion.

TREATMENT

Chlamydial multiplication is inhibited by tetracyclines or chlortetracyclines and by erythromycin. Liquamycin* (20 mg/kg) is also used. Polyarthritis strains have a fair degree of susceptibility to penicillin.[1]

PREVENTION AND CONTROL

An adjuvanted, killed chlamydial vaccine prepared with yolk sacs of infected chicken embryos is available in England to prevent chlamydial abortions and is also marketed in the United States. Recent evaluations, however, revealed that its efficacy is much less than previously claimed.[1] The live chlamydial vaccine against feline pneumonitis was also suggested for use to prevent chlamydial abortions in ewes and goats. This chlamydial strain differs so much from ovine chlamydial agents that its use in animals other than cats is presently not justified. Vaccination attempts to prevent other clinical manifestations

*Available from Pfizer and Co., New York, NY 10017

of chlamydial infections in sheep and goats have not been reported.

References

1. Storz, J.: Chlamydia and Chlamydia-Induced Diseases. Charles C. Thomas, Springfield, Ill, 1971.
2. McCauley, E. H., and Tieken, E. L.: Psittacosis-lymphogranuloma venereum agent isolated during an abortion epizootic in goats. J. Am. Vet. Med. Assoc. 152:1758–1765, 1968.
3. Dungworth, D. L., and Cordy, D. R.: The pathogenesis of ovine pneumonia. I. Isolation of a virus of the PL group. J. Comp. Pathol. Ther. 72:9–76, 1962.
4. Storz, J., Pierson, R. E., Marriott, M. E., and Chow, T. L.: Isolation of psittacosis agents from follicular conjunctivitis of sheep. Proc. Soc. Exp. Biol. Med. 125:857–860, 1967.
5. Mendlowski, B., and Segre, D.: Polyarthritis in sheep. I. Description of the disease and experimental transmission. Am. J. Vet. Res. 21:68–73, 1960.

Ovine and Caprine Mycoplasmosis

CHARLES W. LIVINGSTON, JR., D.V.M., Ph.D.

Worldwide, mycoplasmas are a threat to sheep and goat populations and are capable of producing major economic losses under certain conditions. The most pathogenic mycoplasmas *Mycoplasma agalactiae, M. mycoides* subsp. *mycoides,* and *M. mycoides* subsp. *capri* have been isolated only rarely in the United States and, if still present, appear to be limited only to certain isolated flocks. The remainder of the named species of ovine and caprine mycoplasma, ureaplasma, and acholeplasma are present in sheep and goat flocks in the United States. In fact, it is extremely difficult to identify a Texas flock of sheep or goats that is free of mycoplasmal or ureaplasmal infections. Fortunately, the infection produced by the species present in the United States is much less severe than that in the exotic species.

ETIOLOGY

The most prevalent species isolated from Texas sheep and goat flocks are *M. ovipneumoniae* from the respiratory tract, *M. conjunctivae* from lacrimal secretions, and *M.* sp. 2D and *Ureaplasma* spp. from the genitourinary tract. All appear to be susceptible to oxytetracycline, chlortetracycline, and tylosin, but attempts to eliminate mycoplasmas or ureaplasmas from infected flocks by antibiotic treatment appear to be futile. Since the mycoplasma group does not have a cell wall, viability outside the host is limited. Infection usually occurs by contact of infected aerosols or fluids.

EPIZOOTIOLOGY

Atypical or "summer" pneumonia is associated with *M. ovipneumoniae* and usually occurs in lambs placed in dusty feedlots. In severe outbreaks, 90 per cent of the lambs in pens can become infected, resulting in a 10 per cent condemnation rate at the abattoir. Young Angora goats also may experience this type of pneumonia as a result of stress and exposure after shearing. On culturing pneumonic lesions obtained from the abattoir, *M. ovipneumoniae* is usually isolated from 98 to 99 per cent of the specimens collected, and the *Pasteurella hemolytica* isolation rate from the same specimen is usually from 65 to 70 per cent.

Infectious keratoconjunctivitis (IKC) can be produced by experimental inoculation of *M. conjunctivae* into the eyes of susceptible lambs and kids. This disease condition usually appears after eyes are exposed to adverse environmental conditions, e.g., bright sunlight, dust, pollen, wind. Transporting sheep and particularly Angora goats in open trucks or trailers and on arrival placing them in dusty pens may result in a display of a mucopurulent lacrimal discharge in 70 to 90 per cent of the animals, with conjunctivitis progressing to corneal opacity (blindness) in 5 to 20 per cent. In a few normal-appearing eyes, *M. conjunctivae* may remain dormant for several months and then become active after the eyes are stressed. Close contact with other sheep in the flock will then permit the dissemination of the mycoplasma.

Ureaplasma sp. is the most common inhabitant of the genitourinary tract of sheep and goats, with up to 99 per cent of the flocks and from 5 to 95 per cent of the animals being infected. In man, certain serotypes of *Ureaplasma urealyticum* are recognized as a cause of nongonococcal urethritis and *U. diversum* is associated with pneumonia in cattle. *Ureaplasma* sp. is associated with infertility and reproductive failure in sheep, but a causal relationship is not certain.

CLINICAL SIGNS AND LESIONS

In pens containing lambs with atypical pneumonia, one will observe that many lambs will have a dry, "hacking" cough. The lambs may not appear to be noticeably sick, but the weight gain performance is significantly reduced. An increase in incidence of rectal prolapse may result from persistent coughing. In natural infections, the ventral portion of the apical, cardiac, and intermediate lobes of the lung may be pneumonic. Experimental infection of lambs with *M. ovipneumoniae* alone usually does not produce as severe pneumonic lesions as does the dual inoculation of *M. ovipneumoniae* and *P. hemolyticum*. Experimental infection of *M. ovipneumoniae* in gnotobiotes usually results in very mild pneumonic lesions and systematic lesions, particularly of the synovial tissues.

Although chlamydial and viral agents are isolated from eyes with conjunctivitis, clinical signs of IKC can be produced by experimental inoculation of *M. conjunctivae*. Usually *M. conjunctivae* appears in the greatest numbers, oftentimes in almost pure culture, in the first or mucopurulent lacrimal stage of IKC. Mild to severe conjunctivitis may follow the first stage. Then small blood vessels develop and invade the cornea from the periphery toward the center of the cornea. A white, opaque pannus may develop on the cornea, producing temporary blindness in the affected eye. Occasionally, ulcers may form on the cornea and, if severe, may cause a rupture resulting in permanent blindness. Usually the lesions in the eyes do not develop at the same rate, and vision, although impaired, does not prevent the affected animal from locating food and water. In those animals that become totally blind, food and water must be made easily available until sight is regained, usually within three weeks. Development of immunity is incomplete and of short duration; reinfection with signs of disease can recur within 70 days. Usually the signs are not as severe as first-time infections.

The pathogenicity of *Ureaplasma* sp. for sheep and goats has not been definitely established. Ureaplasmas have an affinity for attaching to cell surfaces and possess a urease capable of producing large quantities of ammonia. The pathogenic effects, if existent, may be attributed to these properties. In certain sheep flocks, the presence of a new mycoplasma, *M. sp 2D*, in the reproductive tract may have some involvement with ureaplasma in reproductive problems.

DIAGNOSIS

The diagnosis depends upon the isolation and identification of the mycoplasma involved.

TREATMENT

At the present time, the most practical means of treatment for mycoplasmal infections under range or feedlot conditions is to provide proper housing and feeding procedures. Lambs can be maintained until they are slaughtered and Angora kids until the course of the disease outbreak is complete. Antibiotics, such as tetracycline, oxytetracycline, and tylosin, may be beneficial in preventing death and shortening the course of the disease in the case of pneumonia, especially in Angora goats. In attempting to treat feedlot lambs with antibiotics, the benefits received may not exceed the cost of treatment.

In outbreaks of IKC, topical application of antibiotics in the eyes is not recommended on a flock basis. Individual animals may show improvement with treatment, but signs of infection will tend to persist longer in the treated flock than in the untreated flock. Usually, if shade, water, and food are provided and dusty conditions reduced, the course of untreated IKC in the flock will average 30 to 45 days with less than 0.5 per cent death loss.

Additional information concerning the deleterious effects of *Ureaplasma* sp. must be obtained before valid recommendations can be offered. Since almost all of the flocks in this area of Texas harbor *Ureaplasma* sp., one should recognize the infection as being present without undue concern until research results show otherwise.

Supplemental Reading

Cottew, G. S.: Caprine-ovine mycoplasmas. *In* Tully, J. G., and Whitcomb, R. F. (eds.): The Mycoplasmas, Vol. 2. Academic Press, New York, 1979, 103–132.

Porcine Pseudorabies (Aujeszky's Disease)

ROBERT A. CRANDELL, B.S., D.V.M., M.P.H.

Pseudorabies is an infectious, naturally occurring virus disease affecting many animal species. The disease is known as Aujeszky's disease, mad itch, and infectious bulbar paralysis. In cattle, sheep, dogs, and cats the disease is characterized by a severe local pruritus with a high mortality. The clinical disease in pigs varies with the age of the animal. There has been a marked increase in the incidence in the United States, Mexico, and some western European countries in recent years.

ETIOLOGY

Pseudorabies (PR) is caused by a herpesvirus, a large DNA virus measuring 150 to 180 nm in diameter. All PR viruses studied belong to one serotype. Although the virus strains are indistinguishable serologically, there are variations in virulence and biologic characteristics among strains. Like other herpesviruses, PR virus has the ability to persist in the host as a latent infection. The virus is relatively stable, and the survival time outside of the animal's body is dependent on the environmental conditions. The virus is readily inactivated with chloroform, ether, 1 per cent sodium hydroxide, and 5 per cent phenol. The virus replicates with cytopathic changes in a wide variety of cell cultures derived from different animal species. The rabbit is the most sensitive of the laboratory animals to infection.

EPIZOOTIOLOGY

Pseudorabies-infected swine are believed to be the primary source of infection for other animals and the host reservoir for the perpetuation of the virus in nature. The communicability of the virus from swine to other species, and particularly to other swine, is the most important single factor known in the transmission of PR virus. Infected swine transmit the virus through the nasal secretions, saliva, milk, and placenta and by boars during service.

Survivors of an outbreak develop a long-lasting antibody. The virus persists in recovered animals as a latent infection. These animals become carriers and, under certain stresses, the virus is re-activated and serves as a source of infection to susceptible animals.

The reservoirs of the virus and the nature of spread from farm to farm are not understood. Although the virus has been isolated from a number of wildlife species, their importance as a reservoir and role in the spread of the virus are not conclusive. Badgers, raccoons, skunks, rats, foxes, coyotes, and opossums have been found to be naturally infected. The source of infection is believed to be from feeding upon infected swine carcasses.

Dogs and cats are highly susceptible to infection by the oral route. It is common to have a sudden illness and death in these animals on swine farms before the disease is recognized in the swine.

CLINICAL SIGNS

Porcine PR occurs as both a clinical and subclinical infection; however, the morbidity and mortality are highest in the newborn pig. In the older pig the disease generally occurs as a milder clinical disease or an inapparent infection.

The illness in the very young and weaning-age pig has a sudden onset and progresses rapidly, resulting in high death losses. Newborn pigs from infected sows die as early as one day of age, with the average age of death being about one week; however, deaths may extend over a period of one month after farrowing. Temperature may exceed 40.5°C. Depression, tremors, incoordination, and convulsions are observed before death. Respiratory signs are the most predominant clinical feature with some strains of virus. Diarrhea and vomition may be present but are not constant features of the disease.

Disorientation is common, and if the pigs are not confined they will wander off and die. Pigs have been observed to rub their heads against walls and run into objects with their snouts to the ground. Death losses in litters of very young pigs may approach 100 per cent, whereas death losses may reach 40 to 60 per cent in three-to four-week-old pigs.

Outbreaks in feeder operations have occurred as late as one month after the addition of new animals. In the three- to five-month-old pig, the clinical signs may persist as long as seven or eight days after onset. The death losses are less than in the younger pigs. Temperatures may reach 41.5°C, and the animals usually stop eating and may vomit. Head and body tremors, circling, and paddling movements of varying degrees are characteristic. Some infected pigs weighing 45 to 68 kg have been described as having a "wobbly motion." Death is preceded by convulsions and prostration.

A respiratory form of the disease has also been observed in sows and gilts. The animals have fever, may cough or sneeze, and go off feed. Abortions may occur during the early or late stages of gestation. In the later stages of pregnancy, the fetus may be retained and become mummified. Some sows will absorb the fetuses, whereas others will farrow stillborn pigs. Many sows will have a fever, go off feed, and may vomit for several days at the time of farrowing or immediately thereafter. Occasionally a sow or gilt will die. A few animals may rub their noses or heads; however, the "mad itch" syndrome seen in other species is generally absent in swine. Some herds experience breeding problems with sows and gilts following an outbreak.

DIAGNOSIS

A clinical diagnosis of PR should always be confirmed by laboratory methods because the clinical signs mimic other diseases, and PR may also occur concurrently with another condition.

PR is confirmed by the isolation and identification of the virus and by the fluorescent antibody test (FAT). The recommended specimens for virus isolation from suspect pigs are the tonsils and portions of the olfactory lobes, pons, and medulla. The tonsil is the choice tissue for FAT. Although the virus may be present in other tissues, such as the lung, liver, and spleen, these tissues are not routinely examined. It is important that tissue from more than one animal from a suspect herd be submitted to the laboratory because the virus is not recovered from all animals and not all tonsils are positive by the FAT.

Some of the swine diseases from which PR must be differentiated are enterovirus infections, water deprivation (salt poisoning), and hog cholera. Rabies is of special concern with cattle and in peculiar acting wild animals.

Serologic methods are useful in surveys and monitoring

herds but are not recommended for the identification of an outbreak. Demonstrable antibodies are not present in the serum of animals during the acute stage of illness.

TREATMENT

There is no treatment that will reverse the course of illness after clinical signs appear. Although the administration of hyperimmune serum to baby pigs is effective in reducing death losses during an outbreak, there is no commercial source for the serum.

PUBLIC HEALTH CONSIDERATIONS

There are no known public health concerns associated with PRV infections in animals.

CONTROL

In Europe, where Aujeszky's disease has been a serious problem for many years, various approaches have been taken to control the disease. Inactivated and live attenuated vaccines and immune serum have been used in an effort to immunize pigs and reduce losses. The success of these programs has varied among the different countries. Pig losses were reduced in Hungary by vaccination with attenuated vaccine, but the disease was not eliminated. The vaccine did not prevent the pigs from becoming virus carriers. The present approach in Hungary is to attempt eradication by establishing disease-free breeding stock. Some countries (e.g., Switzerland), do not allow vaccination.

In the United States the present program is based on control rather than eradication. Modified live virus and inactivated PR vaccines are licensed and marketed in the United States. The vaccines are being used primarily to reduce death losses in infected herds and to prevent the development of disease in high-risk herds located in endemic areas. Some infected herds are being depopulated or are subjected to a test and removal program for eliminating the infection on an individual herd basis.

Serologic testing and restricting the movement of positive animals are important features of a control program. It is recommended that animals have a negative test before entering exhibitions and herds as replacement breeding stock. Replacement gilts and boars should be tested within 30 days of movement, held in isolation for 30 days, and retested negative before adding to the new herd.

Early recognition of the disease is important in controlling the spread of the virus. When PR is suspected in a herd, the sick animals should be isolated until a laboratory diagnosis can be made. When PR is confirmed, the herd should be quarantined and traffic to and from the premise should be controlled. All dead animals should be buried or burned. Dogs and cats should not be allowed to co-mingle with swine or eat dead pigs. Although difficult, every effort should be made to control wildlife.

Supplemental Reading

Gustafson, D. P.: Pseudorabies. *In* Dunne, H. W., and Leman, A. D. (eds.): Diseases of Swine, 4th ed. Ames, Ia., Iowa State University Press, 1975, 391.

Hill, H. T., Crandell, R. A., Kanitz, C. L., et al.: Recommended minimum standards for diagnostic tests employed in the diagnosis of pseudorabies (Aujeszky's disease). Proc. Am. Assoc. Vet. Lab. Diagn. 20th Ann. Meeting, 1977, 375.
Mock, R. E., Crandell, R. A., and Mesfin, G. M.: Induced latency in pseudorabies vaccinated pigs. Can. J. Comp. Med. 45:56–59, 1981.

Porcine Cytomegalovirus (Inclusion Body Rhinitis)

ROBERT ASSAF, AGR., M.SC.V.

Porcine cytomegalovirus (PCMV) is associated with pig inclusion body rhinitis and death in very young piglets and fetuses.

ETIOLOGY

PCMV is a DNA virus belonging to the herpesvirus family and is sensitive to ether and chloroform. Only one serotype has been reported. The virus grows in lung macrophages, porcine fallopian tube cell line, and primary pig testis cells.

EPIZOOTIOLOGY

PCMV is host-specific and probably occurs worldwide. The disease is most commonly propagated via the nasal route. Infected boars may also transmit the disease. The economic importance of the disease is not well known.

CLINICAL SIGNS AND LESIONS

Natural outbreaks include symptoms of shivering, sneezing, respiratory distress, and death in piglets. Usually, pigs older than three weeks are asymptomatic. Early post-natal or congenital infection also occurs and is associated with mummification, stillbirths, neonatal death, and runt pigs.

In piglets the infection produces widespread petechiae and edema involving most commonly the thoracic cavity and subcutaneous tissues. In older animals no macroscopic lesions are found. Basophilic intranuclear inclusion bodies and cytomegaly are seen in numerous cells.

DIAGNOSIS

Serologic diagnosis is based on the indirect immunofluorescence test (IIF) or enzyme-linked immunosorbent assay (ELISA). Virus may be isolated from nasal mucosa, lung, and kidney. Viral antigen can be detected by the IIF test on frozen sections of infected tissue.

TREATMENT AND PREVENTION

There is no specific treatment for PCMV infection. Good management and abstention of introducing new stock during the mating period and the first month of pregnancy should be practiced.

Supplemental Reading

Assaf, R., Bouilland, A. M. P., and Di Franco, E.: Enzyme-linked immunosorbent assay for the detection of antibodies to porcine cytomegalovirus. Can. J. Comp. Med. 46:183–185, 1982.

Edington, N.: Porcine cytomegalovirus infection. In Disease of Swine, 5th ed. Ames, Ia., Iowa State University Press, 1981, 271–277.

Swine Pox

DEOKI N. TRIPATHY, B.V.Sc.&A.H., Ph.D.

Swine pox is caused by swine poxvirus, which belongs to the genus *Suipoxvirus* of the Poxviridae family. This virus is highly host-specific, and the disease is characterized by the development of cutaneous lesions in susceptible young pigs.

EPIZOOTIOLOGY

Swine pox is worldwide in distribution and primariiy affects the susceptible population of young pigs. Once introduced in a large herd, the disease is maintained for a long time owing to constant availability of susceptible young pigs as replacement stock and the resistance of the virus to environmental conditions. The virus can survive in the dried crusts for at least one year.

Swine pox is transmitted by direct contact associated with skin injury. Under natural conditions, the louse *Hematopinus suis* acts as a mechanical vector of the virus and may carry the virus for weeks or months. The lice puncture the skin and provide injury necessary to permit entry of the virus. The severity of the disease is influenced by louse infestation and the degree of injury. Injuries from mechanical irritations or other blood-sucking external parasites can bring results similar to those seen with lice injuries. Skin lesion of poxvirus infection in a newborn piglet suggesting transplacental infection have been reported.

CLINICAL SIGNS AND LESIONS

The incubation period varies from 4 to 6 days and sometimes 12 to 14 days. The onset may be marked by a mild transient fever and inappetence. The initial skin lesions are small, round, erythematous spots that increase in size and thickness to form reddish papules of about 2 mm in diameter. These papules enlarge to 2 to 5 mm in diameter and become vesicles and then form umbilicated pustules. The vesicular stage is of short duration and is often missed. With rapid drying of the exudate, scabs are formed with depressed centers. Desquamation of the scabs or crusts leaves a small, white, discolored spot. The course of the disease is one and one half to three and one half

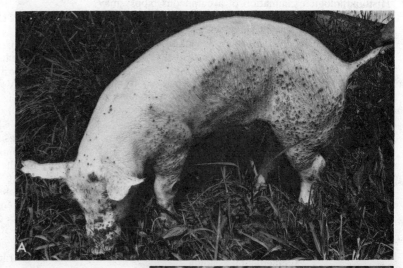

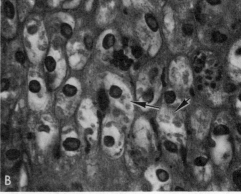

Figure 1. Swinepox.

A. Cutaneous lesions in a pig 14 days after intravenous inoculations with swine poxvirus. (Miller, R. B., and Olson, L. D.: Experimental induction of cutaneous streptococcal abscesses in swine as a sequela to swinepox. Am. J. Vet. Res. 41:341–347, 1980). (Courtesy of American Veterinary Medical Association.)

B. Microscopic epidermal changes characterized by hydropic degeneration, cytoplasmic inclusions (arrows), and nuclear vacuolations. H&E 450×. (Courtesy of Dr. Crandell.)

weeks. The lesions occur primarily on the abdomen and inner aspects of the thighs but may occur on other areas (Fig. 1A). Udder and teat lesions may occur in some sows that nurse infected piglets. In such cases, loss of piglets may occur because of low milk consumption resulting from painfully infected teats. Regional lymphadenopathy has been observed.

DIAGNOSIS

Swine pox may be suspected when characteristic cutaneous pox lesions are observed. Swine are susceptible to vaccinia virus *(Orthopoxvirus* genus of the Poxviridae family), which has a wide host range and causes similar lesions. However, because of discontinuation of human vaccination, chances of animal infection by vaccinia virus in the future are unlikely. Swine pox should be clinically differentiated from other cutaneous infections (e.g., vesicular exanthema, vesicular stomatitis, foot-and-mouth disease, erysipelas), parasitic skin diseases, and allergic skin conditions.

Virions of typical poxvirus morphology can be detected under the electron microscope in negatively stained preparations or in ultra-thin sections of cutaneous lesions. Swine poxvirus has a restricted host range, as it affects swine only, can be isolated in cell cultures of swine origin only, and does not grow in embryonated eggs or other laboratory animals.

Swine poxvirus has an affinity for epidermal cells. Histopathologic examination of a cutaneous biopsy may be helpful in diagnosis. Swine poxvirus causes hydropic degeneration and hyperplasia of epidermal cells. Infected cells contain eosinophilic cytoplasmic inclusion bodies and nuclear vacuolation that is characteristic of swine poxvirus infection (Fig. 1B).

Pigs recovered from swine pox are refractory to challenge with swine poxvirus, indicating development of active immunity.

TREATMENT

There is no specific therapy for swine pox. If the disease is associated with lice infestation, primary attempts should be aimed at eliminating the lice. Insecticides are applied by dipping or spraying the animals or dusting the bedding. Only those insecticides that are approved for use on swine to control lice should be used.

Supplemental Reading

Kasza, L.: Swinepox. *In* Leman, A. D., Glock, R. D., Mengeling, W. L., Penny, R. H. C., Scholl, E., and Straw, B. (eds.): Diseases of Swine, 5th ed. Ames, Ia., Iowa State University Press, 1981, 254–260.
Neufeld, J. L.: Spontaneous pustular dermatitis in a newborn piglet associated with a poxvirus. Can. Vet. J. 22:156–158, 1981.
Tripathy, D. N., Hanson, L. E., and Crandell, R. A.: Poxviruses of veterinary importance: Diagnosis of infections. *In* Kurstak, E., and Kurstak, C. (eds.): Comparative Diagnosis of Viral Diseases, Vol. III. Academic Press, New York, 1981, 267–346.

Porcine Adenoviruses*

DONALD MATTSON, D.V.M., Ph.D.

Porcine adenoviruses (PAVs) possess certain physiochemical properties in common with other members of the Adenoviridae family. There are currently five officially recognized types of PAV. Additional isolations have been reported and have been shown to vary antigenically from the recognized prototypes.

There have been no reports concerning the resistance of PAV to disinfectants. One isolate has been shown to withstand inactivation for ten days or more at 25°C.

EPIZOOTIOLOGY

Porcine adenoviruses are widely distributed and appear to be present in most countries. There may be some regional predominance of individual types. Few serologic survey studies have been undertaken, and an accurate figure concerning incidence of infection cannot be given. One study showed that the main period of infectivity was immediately after weaning. PAVs replicate extensively in the nasal cavity, tonsils, and alimentary tract. The method of viral transmission is probably by direct contact. Chronic infection takes place in the intestinal tract and kidney. The role of virus shedding in the urine and transmission of infection has not been investigated.

CLINICAL SIGNS AND LESIONS

Infection is usually not associated with disease, and most investigators consider PAV to be of little pathogenic significance with the possible exception of PAV type 4.

Some PAVs have been recovered from neonatal pigs with diarrhea. Experimental infectivity studies with gnotobiotic pigs have usually failed to reproduce the disease. In one study where enteritis was reproduced, the severity of disease was mild.

Some strains of PAV have been shown to have an affinity for the respiratory tract. In disease transmission studies, there was no clinical evidence of disease and minimal lesions were observed in the lungs. A synergistic effect between PAV type 4 and *Mycoplasma hyopneumoniae* has been proposed.

PAV type 4 was originally isolated from a ten-week-old pig with encephalitis. Several investigators have attempted to transmit the disease in gnotobiotic colostrum-deprived pigs. The virus was shown to replicate extensively in the intestinal tract during the first week of infection, but neurologic signs did not develop. Histopathologic changes consistent with meningoencephalitis were produced two to three weeks after infection; a complex pathogenesis for CNS infection was proposed.

*Oregon Agricultural Experiment Station Technical Paper No. 7019.

DIAGNOSIS

For viral isolation, samples should be taken from tissue or organs with pathologic changes. In the early stages of the disease, viral-infected cells can be detected by the fluorescent antibody technique.

Paired serum samples should be submitted for serologic diagnosis. An agar gel precipitation test has been used to test antibody titer increase to the group-specific antigen. For type-specific testing, the serum-viral neutralization test must be used. Most diagnostic laboratories do not provide serologic testing for PAV.

TREATMENT

There is no specific treatment for adenoviral infection.

PREVENTION AND CONTROL

There are no vaccines available for prevention of PAV infection.

Supplemental Reading

Coussement, W., Ducatelle, R., Charlier, G., and Hoorens, J.: Adeno-virus enteritis in pigs. Am. J. Vet. Res. *42*:1905–1911, 1981.
McFerran, J. B.: Adenoviruses of vertebrate animals. *In* Kurstak, E., and Kurstak, C. (eds.): Comparative Diagnosis of Viral Diseases. III. Vertebrate Animal and Related Viruses. Part A: DNA Viruses. Academic Press, New York, 1981, 125–128.

Porcine Parvovirus-Induced Reproductive Failure

WILLIAM L. MENGELING, D.V.M., Ph.D.

Porcine parvovirus (PPV)-induced reproductive failure is characterized by prenatal infection and death, usually without accompanying maternal clinical signs. Dams are most often exposed oronasally, and embryos and fetuses are subsequently infected transplacentally. A venereal route of exposure is also possible because PPV has been isolated from boar semen. The virus is distributed among swine throughout the world, and all strains that have been compared are antigenically similar or identical. In the United States, PPV is ubiquitous and the disease is common.

Reproductive failure is the probable consequence of exposure of nonimmune females to PPV any time during the first half (eight weeks) of gestation. Later exposure is often innocuous for fetuses because they may not be infected transplacentally for two or more weeks; by ten weeks of gestational age, fetuses are usually immunocompetent and relatively resistant. However, the effect of late fetal infection on neonatal survival has not been determined.

When an entire litter is infected at about the same time, the effects on both dam and litter can be considered according to the stage of gestation as follows. (1) Embryo (≤30 days): Embryos die and are resorbed and the dam returns to estrus. Subsequent copulation and conception are followed by an uneventful pregnancy. However, on the basis of observations of naturally occurring cases, older embryos may not always be completely resorbed. The result is that females return to estrus and accept the boar but do not conceive. The latter possibility is speculative and has not been confirmed experimentally. (2) Early fetus (~30 to ~70 days): Fetuses die and become relatively dehydrated (mummified). The dam does not return to estrus, and farrowing is often delayed. Many affected dams are marketed when they fail to farrow at the expected time, and they appear nonpregnant as a result of resorption of fetal and associated extrafetal fluids. (3) Late fetus (~70 days to term): Most infected fetuses survive *in utero* and produce antibody to PPV. Nevertheless, the virus persists, and it can be disseminated at farrowing in extrafetal fluids and by neonates.

When only part of a litter is infected transplacentally, then some or all littermates can be infected by intrauterine spread of virus. Because intrauterine spread is often relatively slow, particularly when fetuses are able to produce antibody, a litter may become infected progressively over almost the entire gestation. Therefore, all of the effects on embryos and fetuses that were described in the preceding paragraph can be represented in a single litter. Additionally, one or more pigs of a litter may be stillborn when dead littermates cause a prolonged gestation or farrowing interval or both. Note, however, that in such cases one would expect to find mummified fetuses as well as stillborn pigs.

CLINICAL SIGNS AND LESIONS

Maternal infection is usually subclinical. A mild, transient fever and leukopenia have been shown under experimental conditions. The possibility of PPV-induced reproductive failure can be considered when an unusually large number of bred females return to estrus, fail to farrow despite being anestrus, farrow small litters, or farrow a large proportion of mummified fetuses. When maternal exposure is near mid gestation, the abdominal girth of pregnant females will often decrease noticeably as fetuses die and associated fluids are resorbed. There is no evidence that abortion is a significant feature of the naturally occurring disease. The virus has not been associated unequivocally with any other disease syndrome, and boars seem clinically unaffected.

Most fetuses that die as a direct result of PPV infection are in an advanced stage of autolysis and mummification when they are farrowed. Consequently, a thorough necropsy examination is limited to the relatively few infected fetuses that die near term or are stillborn. Macroscopic lesions have not been reported for such fetuses, but microscopic lesions of meningoencephalitis have been suggested as pathognomonic for PPV infection. These lesions consist of perivascular cuffing with proliferating adventitial cells, histiocytes, and plasma cells in the leptomeninges and parenchymatous tissue of the brain, excluding the cerebellum.

DIAGNOSIS

A tentative diagnosis of PPV-induced reproductive failure is based on a high incidence of embryonic or fetal death or both, an absence of concurrent or previous maternal illness, and an absence or low incidence of abortion. Although numerous other agents have been associated with the same or a similar syndrome, recent studies suggest that PPV is the most common infectious cause.

For a confirmed diagnosis, tissue from affected fetuses must be submitted to a laboratory where it can be tested for viral antigen, viral hemagglutinin, and infectious virus. The tissue of choice is lung collected from mummified fetuses. Tissues from live and stillborn pigs are much less suitable because they are more likely to be either noninfected or contain antibody that would interfere with testing. Several whole mummified fetuses or their lungs should be sent refrigerated or frozen to the laboratory. The fastest and most definitive diagnostic method is the examination of cryostat-microtome sections of tissue by immunofluorescence microscopy. Viral antigen is extremely stable and remains reactive for months after fetal death. The usual finding is masses of viral antigen throughout the tissue. Tissue also can be triturated and tested for viral hemagglutinin or infectious virus or both. Infectivity is less stable than either antigenicity or hemagglutinating activity, however, and isolation of virus from mummified tissues is sometimes unsuccessful.

Results of testing maternal serums for hemagglutination inhibiting (HI) antibody are significant when serums collected at about the time of farrowing are free of antibody—and thus preclude the involvement of PPV—and when two or more serums collected at different times during gestation reveal seroconversion. When infection is early in gestation and embryos are resorbed, maternal seroconversion is the only means by which a probable diagnosis can be made. Because PPV is ubiquitous, the presence of antibody in maternal serum collected only at about the time of farrowing is of no diagnostic significance.

Serums collected from neonates before they ingest colostrum also can be tested for HI antibody, and often titers are as high as those of adults. Although the presence of antibody in serum of neonates of small litters or of litters with dead and mummified fetuses is reasonable evidence for a causal role for PPV, it obviously is less definitive than demonstrating viral antigen in tissue of dead fetuses.

TREATMENT

There is no treatment.

PREVENTION

Porcine parvovirus-induced reproductive failure can be prevented by vaccination or by exposing females to virulent virus several weeks before breeding to establish immunity. Boars also should be immune to minimize the chance of their disseminating the virus by various routes, including semen. Exposure to virulent virus can sometimes be accomplished by commingling gilts and boars with other swine that may be shedding PPV, e.g., older breeding stock, or by placing them in potentially contaminated quarters. However, neither procedure is dependable or selective. Vaccines are available commercially. To be effective, vaccines should be administered only after passively acquired (colostral) antibody has disappeared.

Supplemental Reading

Cartwright, S. F., and Huck, R. A.: Viruses isolated in association with herd infertility, abortions and stillbirths in pigs. Vet. Rec. 81:196–197, 1967.

Joo, H. S., Donaldson-Wood, C. R., and Johnson, R. H.: Observations on the pathogenesis of porcine parvovirus infection. Arch. Virol. 51:123–129, 1976.

Mengeling, W. L., Cutlip, R. C., Wilson, R. A., Parks, J. B., and Marshall, R. F.: Fetal mummification associated with porcine parvovirus infection. J. Am. Vet. Med. Assoc. 166:993–995, 1975.

Mengeling, W. L.: Prevalence of porcine parvovirus-induced reproductive failure: An abattoir study. J. Am. Vet. Med. Assoc. 172:1291–1294, 1978.

Mengeling, W. L., Paul, P. S., and Brown, T. T.: Transplacental infection and embryonic death following maternal exposure to porcine parvovirus near the time of conception. Arch. Virol. 65:55–62, 1980.

Iridovirus (African Swine Fever)

H. A. McDANIEL, D.V.M., Ph.D.

African swine fever (ASF) is a highly contagious viral disease that affects only swine. Acute, subacute, and chronic forms occur in domestic swine, and an inapparent form occurs in wild swine. There are notable differences between the disease produced by many strains of ASF virus. Mortality varies from nearly 100 per cent with the most virulent strains to less than 20 per cent with the least virulent strains. The form of ASF that produces approximately 50 per cent mortality will be used here as the reference form (since this form appeared to be the most prevalent during 1983 when this article was prepared).

ETIOLOGY

ASF is caused by a relatively large DNA virus that is highly resistant to inactivation by environmental factors and many disinfectants. This virus may remain viable in soil or in blood, bone marrow, or pork at room temperature for several months.

There are four types and numerous strains of ASF virus. Antibodies to ASF virus are usually present in high titers in recovered pigs, but they do not neutralize the virus.

Two commercially available disinfectants have been found to be effective against ASF virus. These are a 1 per cent solution of One-Stroke-Environ* and Vanodyne-FAM†. Both products are also sold under other trade names.

EPIZOOTIOLOGY

The first reports of ASF were from East Africa in 1909. Outbreaks have been reported in Spain, Portugal, France, and Italy. In France and Italy all infected and exposed swine were quickly slaughtered, and the disease was eradicated.

---

*Available from Vestal Laboratories, St. Louis, MO 63166
†Available from Vanodyne International Ltd., Eccles, Manchester, England, and Pfizer International, New York, NY 10017

In 1971, ASF first occurred in the Western Hemisphere in Cuba. Within a few months over 400,000 swine died or were slaughtered as infected or exposed, and no more cases occurred in Cuba. In 1978, ASF was found in four new, widely separated areas: Sardinia, Malta, the Dominican Republic, and Brazil. During the fall and winter of 1977, a marked increase in the incidence of ASF occurred in Spain and Portugal and may have been the source of the virus disclosed in new areas in 1978. From the Dominican Republic, it spread to Haiti and then to Cuba. There is no reason to believe the ASF virus found in Cuba in 1980 was due to the 1971 outbreak.

Elimination of all infected and exposed swine appears to have eradicated ASF virus from Malta, the Dominican Republic, Haiti, and Cuba.

In Sardinia all pigs associated with sick pigs were depopulated, but pigs with AFS antibodies are occasionally still found. An outbreak on mainland Italy in early 1983 was attributed to pork from Sardinia. Clinical illness and deaths were reported during this outbreak. All infected and exposed pigs were quickly killed and the outbreak was stopped. There is still much to be learned before we can explain the cyclic nature of ASF in enzootic areas and the factors that cause ASF to go from inapparent to a highly lethal disease.

Transmission is by direct or indirect contact. Soft ticks, *Ornithodoros moubata* and *O. erraticus,* serve as biologic reservoirs and vectors of ASF virus in Africa and the Iberian Peninsula.

O. puertoricensis and *O. turicata,* found in several Caribbean Islands and Florida, respectively, have experimentally transmitted ASF virus under laboratory conditions, but ticks collected in the Dominican Republic and Haiti did not contain ASF virus. Large areas where ASF-infected pigs were found earlier have more recently been repopulated with pigs that remained free of ASF.

CLINICAL SIGNS AND LESIONS

The first sign of ASF is often depression and fever, but one or two pigs may be found dead without apparent prior illness. In totally white pigs the most obvious change is red to reddish-blue hyperemia and congestion of the skin over the snout, ears, and fetlocks, under the belly, and up the sides and over the hindquarters. However, this discoloration is not apparent in swine with pigmented skin. The skin of yellow, almost white, or white-spotted swine remains normal in color. As soon as illness becomes apparent, AFS-infected pigs will usually have a body temperature of 41 to 42°C. Fever is an important differential diagnostic criteria and will indicate that the illness is not due to intoxication. Pigs with ASF do not usually huddle together as tightly as do those with hog cholera (Fig. 1).

Pregnant animals usually abort during the initial illness regardless of the stage of pregnancy, and these animals almost always die within a few days. Ecchymotic hemorrhagic spots from 1 to 3 cm in diameter may be seen on the fetal membranes or skin of aborted fetuses.

Infected swine usually continue to eat and drink until near death. They are more alert than might be expected with such a high body temperature. Incoordination, trembling, convulsions, and muscular twitching are unusual and, when present, are not as marked as those in hog cholera. However, coughing and dyspnea are more marked than in uncomplicated hog cholera. Diarrhea is seldom seen in uncomplicated ASF.

Ascites may be the first abnormality seen when the carcass is opened. Excessive straw-colored or blood-tinged fluid may be found in the pleural and peritoneal cavities and pericardial sac. If ascites has been present long enough for fibrin to form and fluids to be re-absorbed, fibrin tags may be present on any organ or tissue surface similar to the fibrin deposits seen in mycoplasmal and certain bacterial infections.

The vascular system is severely damaged, and edema and hemorrhage may be found in any tissue. Hemorrhage is more often seen in visceral organs, especially lymph nodes, lungs, heart, kidneys, on the serosal surface of intestines and diaphragm, and on the serosal or mucosal surface of the stomach. Some petechial-sized hemorrhages will usually be found, but many of the hemorrhagic foci are ecchymotic.

The spleen may be normal, but in about 50 per cent of the animals affected it will be swollen to two to three times normal, very friable with the splenic pulp having the consistency of currant jelly, or occasionally normal size with infarcts indistinguishable from those seen in hog cholera.

The liver is usually swollen, congested, and dark red or clay colored. The surface may have a fine granular or

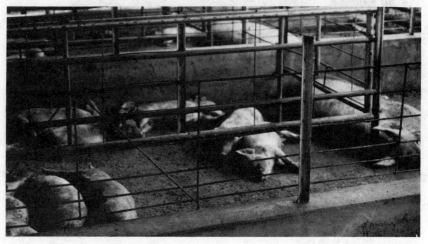

Figure 1. Swine infected with African swine fever (ASF) in Dominican Republic. Note that they do not pile together as in hog cholera.

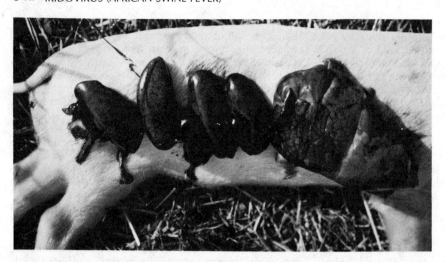

Figure 2. Kidneys and lungs from swine dying from ASF. Note the petechial and ecchymotic hemorrhage on the surface of the kidneys and the clotted blood adhering to the reflected renal capsules. In the lung, marked interlobular edema and hemorrhage are present in the dorsal anterior part of the lung, and pale blotchy areas can be seen on the surface of the diaphragmatic lobe.

slightly rough appearance due to parenchymatous tissue swelling more than interlobular connective tissue. Occasionally well-demarcated focal blotchy areas will be seen on the surface and extending into the parenchyma. They may be lighter or darker than the surrounding liver tissues.

The gall bladder is often edematous and may be over 0.5 cm thick and opaque. The blood vessels are distended with blood. The bile often contains sufficient blood to cause clotting of the blood-bile mixture, and fibrin from the clot may adhere to the wall of the gall bladder.

Lymph nodes throughout the body are usually edematous and hemorrhagic. The hemorrhage may be subcapsular, as in hog cholera, or diffuse. When lymph node hemorrhage is diffuse and extensive, the nodes have the appearance of a shiny blood clot and are two to four times larger than normal. The gastrohepatic and renal nodes are the ones most frequently and severely affected. Usually lymph nodes in the pleural and peritoneal cavities are more affected than the body nodes, but those in the neck and head region may also be severely affected.

In a small percentage of infected pigs, the mucosa of the stomach, especially the fundic portion, will appear bright blood red. Close examination will reveal that the mucosa is coated with a mixture of mucus and blood. Free blood in the stomach or intestine is rarely seen.

Peyer's patches throughout the small intestines may be edematous and occasionally necrotic. The intestinal contents are usually normal, but when bloody dysentery occurs, the colon will usually contain large amounts of blood.

Tonsillar abscesses and button ulcers near the cecal orifice are usually absent. Petechiae on the epiglottis and the mucosa of the urinary bladder are not seen as frequently as in hog cholera.

Kidney involvement may be extremely variable, even within the same infected herd. In approximately 10 per cent of the pigs dying of ASF, the kidney will appear normal, and in about 20 per cent the kidney will be extensively hemorrhagic (Fig. 2). In these pigs the kidneys appear to be contained in a transparent sac filled with blood. Apparently, when hemorrhage is extensive within the kidney, blood seeps through the renal capsule, forming a clot about 6.7 mm thick around the kidney. In these cases, free blood will usually be found in the pelvis and

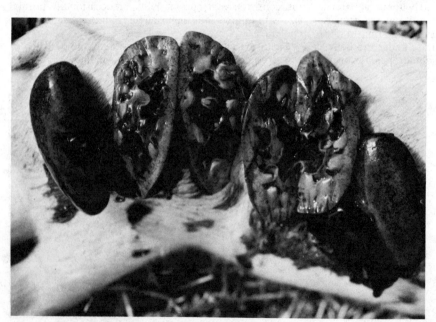

Figure 3. These are the same kidneys illustrated in Figure 2. Two have been opened to illustrate hemorrhage on the cut surface and clotted blood in the pelvis.

the cortex will be severely congested and hemorrhagic (Fig. 3). In other cases, only a few petechiae will be seen on the surface as typically seen in hog cholera.

The lungs are usually severely affected. Petechiae and ecchymotic hemorrhage may be seen on the surface and throughout the lungs. Pulmonary edema may be especially prominent in the interlobular connective tissue of the anterior dorsal quarter of the lung. Edematous fluids may contain sufficient blood to have the appearance of blood.

PREVENTION AND TREATMENT

There is no effective therapy. A satisfactory vaccine has not been developed, and there is little hope of one in the near future, since ASF antibodies do not neutralize the virus. Many seemingly recovered swine remain carriers of ASF virus for prolonged periods, probably as long as they live. They may be normal or appear unthrifty and frequently develop pneumonia, joint lesions, nephritis, and skin lesions.

CONTROL

Destruction of all infected and exposed swine, together with sound sanitary practices, has been effective in eradicating ASF from France, mainland Italy, Cuba, and parts of Africa. Most recently these measures were applied in Malta, the Dominican Republic, Haiti, and again in Cuba, and these areas appear to be free of ASF.

Preventing direct or indirect exposure to infected swine, especially swine in the incubation period of ASF, is effective in reducing spread. Veterinarians, feedmen, and other service personnel on infected premises must be extremely careful to avoid transmitting ASF.

When ASF enters a new area, it is often erroneously diagnosed as hog cholera, and large numbers of swine are quickly vaccinated against hog cholera. The vaccine is not only completely ineffective in prevention of ASF, but epidemiologic data indicate much ASF is spread in the process.

Spread via uncooked pork scraps from infected swine in garbage fed to swine is apparently the most frequent means of spread to distant locations, i.e., introduction into other countries or areas. Garbage from international carriers, airlines, and ships is especially hazardous.

Government officials responsible for animal health should be immediately notified when ASF is suspected so that appropriate measures can be taken to confirm the diagnosis and, if positive, to institute quarantines and take other appropriate actions to stop the spread and eliminate infected and exposed swine and reservoirs of the virus.

Supplemental Reading

Eradication of Hog Cholera and African Swine Fever. FAO Animal Production and Health Paper, AGA-716, 1976.

Mare, C. J.: African swine fever. In Foreign Animal Diseases: Their Prevention, Diagnosis and Control. Committee on Foreign Animal Diseases of the United States Animal Health Association, Richmond, Va., 1975, 43–54.

McDaniel, H. A.: African swine fever. In Diseases of Swine, 5th ed. Iowa State University Press, Ames, Ia., 1981, 237–245.

Mebus, C. A., and Dardiri, A. H.: Additional characterization of disease caused by African swine fever viruses isolated from Brazil and the Dominican Republic. Proceedings 83rd Annual Meeting of USAHA, 1979, 227–239.

Wesley, R. D., and Tuthill, A. E.: Genome relatedness among African swine fever virus field isolates by restriction endonuclease analysis. Unpublished report, USDA, ARS, Plum Island Animal Disease Center, Greenport, N.Y.

Wesley, R. D., and Pan, I. C.: African swine fever virus DNA: Restriction endonuclease cleavage patterns of wild-type Vero cell-adapted and plaque purified virus. J. Gen. Virol., 63:383–391, 1982.

Calicivirus (Vesicular Exanthema of Swine Virus)

ALVIN W. SMITH, D.V.M., Ph.D.

Vesicular exanthema of swine virus (VESV) belongs to the family Caliciviridae, of which VESV-A$_{48}$ (isolated in California from pigs with vesicular exanthema in 1948) is the prototype species. Caliciviruses are single-stranded RNA viruses about 34 to 36 nanometers in diameter. They are lipid solvent–resistant but are unstable at pH 3 and at 50°C. Divalent cations (Mg^{++}) further degrade them in the presence of heat. They can survive for long periods at 4°C and will survive for 14 days in 15°C sea water. Although they are de-activated by a variety of antiseptics, 2 per cent lye has been the disinfectant of choice.

There were 13 known serotypes of VESV isolated from swine between 1934 and 1956. Since that time there have been 13 more serotypes of caliciviruses indistinguishable from VESV isolated from marine mammals and marine fish. Six of these that have been tested do infect swine, and some are more virulent for swine than many of the original 13 VESV types. Other caliciviruses have been isolated from mink, dogs, reptiles, chimpanzees, and calves. Of these, only the calf isolate has been tested in swine, and it does produce clinical vesicular lesions in experimentally inoculated swine. There are now a total of 32 known serotypes of calicivirus worldwide, including the single serotype infecting cats. Of these, only the feline type is known not to infect swine.

EPIZOOTIOLOGY

Vesicular exanthema was said to be a new disease of pigs after its first documented appearance in 1932 in Orange County, California. That outbreak was treated as foot-and-mouth disease and eradicated; however, the disease re-appeared on an annual basis through 1936. Each outbreak was controlled and no more occurrences were reported between 1936 and 1939. From 1939 until it was eradicated in the mid 1950's the disease was endemic in California. In 1952, VES escaped California and spread throughout all the major swine-producing areas of the United States. The last outbreak occurred in 1956. The disease was declared eradicated and was classed as a foreign animal disease in 1959. Vesicular exanthema has never been reported outside the continental United States except for single occurrences in Hawaii and Iceland, which were each traceable to shipments of U.S. pork.

Prior to 1972, swine were the only known naturally occurring hosts for VESV. Now the more recent calicivirus isolates of marine origin can in some cases be shown to be antigenically closer to the VES viruses than some of the VES virus serotypes are to each other. This finding, plus the reports that caliciviruses from seals and fish will infect swine and the discovery that many unrelated species of feral mammals along the coastal zones have type-specific antibodies to both the recent isolates of marine origin and the original virus types isolated from swine, leaves little doubt that these agents have broad host spectrums. In one series of studies, one calicivirus serotype was shown to infect fish, seals, swine and monkeys.

The original outbreaks of disease were associated with feeding raw garbage, and it is now widely accepted that the virus-contaminated components in the garbage were marine products. Both marine mammals and fish are proven reservoirs for a calicivirus that causes typical vesicular lesions in experimentally exposed swine. In addition, the infection will spread horizontally and cause vesicular lesions in pen contact swine.

Although VESV has been reported only in the United States, marine mammals carrying caliciviruses infectious for swine are known to migrate along the Mexican, United States, Canadian, Alaskan, and Russian coasts. Northern fur seals harvested in Russia have type-specific antibodies for certain of these viruses. There has been no report of these agents in marine species outside the Pacific Basin and the Bering and Chukchi Seas.

CLINICAL SIGNS AND LESIONS

Vesicular exanthema of swine is indistinguishable clinically from foot-and-mouth disease (FMD), vesicular stomatitis (VS), and swine vesicular disease (SVD). Vesicular lesions will be seen around the coronary bands of the feet and on the snout and oral tissues. Swine will show lameness with reluctance to move and will not maintain a full level of food intake. In addition to these manifestations that occur as a result of the vesicular lesions, agalactia, abortion, myocarditis, and mild encephalitis have been reported. Consequently, runting and unthriftiness are common sequelae, even though the epidermal lesions usually heal rather quickly. Morbidity is variable but can approach 100 per cent; however, mortality is low. In the past, VES virus has been most often introduced into swine herds by feeding raw contaminated garbage, but infected pigs shedding virus in their body excretions can spread the disease.

DIAGNOSIS

Diagnosis is on the basis of virus isolation and serologic testing. Epithelial coverings of lesions and vesicular fluid frozen or placed in buffered glycerol are the laboratory samples of choice. Acute and convalescent serums are useful. Virus isolation can be accomplished in vero cells or pig kidney cells. Direct electron microscopic examination could be rapid and useful in differentiating this virus from those causing FMD, VS, and SVD. Serum neutralization tests are necessary to identify VESV serotypes; however, complement fixation has been used for group testing and monoclonal antibody techniques are now being developed for screening tests.

TREATMENT

Treatment should be directed toward the relief of signs and prevention of secondary infection. There are no specific chemotherapeutic agents for calicivirus infections. Should secondary infections become severe, administration of parenteral antibiotics could be indicated.

PREVENTION AND CONTROL

Vesicular exanthema of swine is classed as a foreign animal disease. Prompt reporting of all vesicular disease outbreaks is essential. Should VES be diagnosed, eradication procedures, which include slaughter, quarantine of premises, and restricted animal movements, are mandated. Recent findings confirm that these viruses are not host-specific and they may infect a variety of species. Additional strong evidence suggests that man may also become infected, and this should call for strong safeguards to minimize human exposure to infected materials and animals. These newly emerging concepts on the biology of caliciviruses suggests that their character is rapidly changing. As more new host species emerge and additional overviews of transmission develop, the probabilities increase that this virus could once again be introduced into domestic swine populations.

Supplemental Reading

Bankowski, R. A.: Vesicular exanthema. Adv. Vet. Sci. *10*:23–64, 1965.
Smith, A. W., and Akers, T. G.: Vesicular exanthema of swine. J. Am. Vet. Med. Assoc. *169*:700–703, 1976.
Smith, A. W.: Focus on Caliciviral Disease. Foreign Animal Disease Report, USDA-APHIS, 11–3:8–16, 1973.

Enteroviral Encephalomyelitis of Pigs (Teschen Disease)

TALMAGE T. BROWN, JR., D.V.M., Ph.D.

Porcine enteroviruses are ubiquitous in swine populations all over the world. Infections are usually inapparent but certain strains may cause clinical disorders including encephalomyelitis, diarrhea, pneumonia, myocarditis, and reproductive failure. Porcine enteroviruses have been classified into 11 serogroups with most of the neurogenic strains belonging to serogroups 1, 2, or 3. The small, RNA-containing enteroviruses are nonenveloped and, therefore, are resistant to many chemicals. In one test of disinfectants, only sodium hypochlorite and 70 per cent alcohol effectively inactivated enterovirus. Enteroviruses are capable of surviving in the environment for many months. The resistance of enteroviruses to environmental factors and chemicals makes it difficult to eliminate them from contaminated premises. This factor is probably the main reason enteroviral infections are so widespread in swine populations. Transmission can occur directly by the fecal-oral route and indirectly by housing susceptible pigs on contaminated premises or by feeding uncooked contaminated pork products.

EPIZOOTIOLOGY

The classical form of enteroviral encephalomyelitis (Teschen disease) was originally described in 1929 as a severe, devastating nervous disease in the Teschen district of Czechoslovakia. During World War II, Teschen disease spread into other eastern and central European countries and later was also reported in Madagascar. In recent years, the incidence of Teschen disease has diminished markedly. Enteroviral encephalomyelitis (EE) as seen currently is usually a mild disease characterized by some degree of ataxia and posterior paresis with low morbidity and mortality. These milder forms of EE have been given different names including Talfan disease, poliomyelitis suum, benign epizootic paresis, and polioencephalomyelitis. They have been described as occurring in various parts of Europe, North America, South America, and Australia. Currently, the worldwide incidence of EE is difficult to determine, as the reportable, severe form (Teschen disease) is seldom diagnosed and the diagnoses of the milder forms are usually not reported. The limited evidence available suggests a low incidence of EE in Europe and North America.

When EE does occur, morbidity is usually not over 50 per cent and then only when infection occurs for the first time in a population containing a high proportion of young pigs. After viral introduction, swine of all ages may become infected and show signs of disease, but once infection is established clinical disease is usually limited to pigs less than 12 weeks old. Among these, the disease is most severe in pigs less than two weeks old when exposed. Usually, not all litters in a given herd are affected, and among those that are, often less than 50 per cent of the pigs show clinical signs of disease.

Infection by the less virulent neurogenic strains of enteroviruses results in a low mortality rate. As the virulence of the infecting strains increases, the rate of mortality increases to a point where the introduction of a highly virulent strain into a susceptible population may result in death losses approaching 100 per cent of the infected pigs.

CLINICAL SIGNS AND LESIONS

The most typical form of EE currently seen is some degree of rear limb ataxia and weakness in pigs over 2 weeks and less than 12 weeks of age. These signs appear 14 to 21 days after exposure to enterovirus, often simultaneously in a number of pigs in the same litter or in different litters. During the early stages of the disease, affected pigs may also huddle or respond to noise, touch, or sudden movement by the development of generalized muscle tremors, tonic-clonic spasms of rear leg muscles, or convulsive seizures. Paresis may worsen for two to three days, extending from the rear to the front legs, and then gradually improve with recovery in a week or two. Occasionally, recovery may take three or more weeks or may be incomplete in that some neurologic deficiency may remain. The latter is more common in mature animals. If disease results from infection by one of the virulent neurogenic strains, paresis may be followed by paralysis, recumbency, and death, usually by the third or fourth day and nearly always within two weeks. Anorexia and lethargy have been reported in some outbreaks, whereas in others the pigs remained bright and alert and had good appetites. Early, there may be fever (40 to 41° C), but often the temperature remains normal. Vomiting and diarrhea are not usual features of the disease.

Gross findings at necropsy are nonspecific. Significant microscopic lesions are limited to the central nervous system where typically one sees a nonsuppurative inflammation involving the gray matter almost exclusively or at least to a greater degree than the white matter. Accompanying the inflammatory changes is neuronal necrosis seen mainly in dorsal root ganglia, ventral horns in the spinal cord, and multiple brain stem nuclei.

DIAGNOSIS

Signs of a locomotor disturbance suggesting spinal cord injury are characteristic of EE, but signs of cerebral dysfunction, such as blindness, aimless walking, and convulsions, are not typical. Enteroviral encephalomyelitis must be differentiated from a variety of neurologic disorders affecting swine, including pseudorabies, hog cholera, African swine fever, rabies, edema disease, and salt poisoning. The clinical signs of these disorders overlap; therefore, diagnosis should be based on a complete history, observation of the full spectrum of symptoms, postmortem examination of affected animals, and, if necessary, isolation and identification of the causative agent. For isolation and identification, fresh or frozen nervous tissue should be submitted to an appropriate laboratory for virus isolation. Paired serum samples taken at least 14 days apart may be of value in retrospectively establishing the cause of the disease.

TREATMENT

There is no treatment for EE, but supportive therapy to prevent secondary infections may be considered if the value of the animal warrants it.

In small to moderate-sized herds (50 to 150 animals), cases of EE may continue to appear for several months; then they disappear unless susceptible animals are brought into the herd. In large herds of 400 to 500 or more animals, disease may persist, and a few clinical cases may appear each year.

PREVENTION

Both inactivated and attenuated live virus vaccines exist, but their use has been restricted to parts of Europe and Madagascar where vaccination is economically necessary. If a virulent strain of virus is introduced into a herd, affected animals should be isolated from unaffected animals, especially those 12 weeks old or younger, and, if feasible, eliminated from the herd. In an endemic area, new breeding stock should be brought into the herd soon enough before breeding to give ample opportunity for exposure and infection with indigenous agents, thereby enhancing the chances of colostral antibody protection of the offspring.

Supplemental Reading

Jones, T. C.: Encephalomyelitides. *In* Dunne, H. W., and Leman, A. D. (eds.): Diseases of Swine. Iowa State University Press, Ames, Ia., 1975, 369–384.
Kaplan, M. M., and Meranze, D. R.: Porcine virus encephalomyelitis and its possible biological relationship to human poliomyelitis. Vet. Med. 43:330–341, 1948.
Mills, J. H. L., and Nielsen, S. W.: Porcine polioencephalomyelitides. Adv. Vet. Sci. 12:33–104, 1968.

Swine Vesicular Disease

ALVIN W. SMITH, D.V.M., Ph.D.

Swine vesicular disease (SVD) is classed as a foreign animal disease, and the causal agent is one of the picornaviruses (small RNA viruses) grouped as an enterovirus. It has icosahedral symmetry and appears generally round with a diameter of 28 nanometers. SVDV is serologically and biologically closely related to the human enterovirus coxsackie B-5 but not other porcine enteroviruses. However, there are strain differences between isolates of SVD virus. It is stable for many months in the environment and has been isolated from earthworms collected above the infected carcasses of buried pigs. Restocking of premises after depopulation has been difficult because of viral persistence in the environment. Hams taken from infected pigs and processed in the Parma tradition have been shown to consistently harbor viable virus for six months but not one year after slaughter. Salami and pepperoni containing dried contaminated pork retained residual infective virus for at least 200 days. The virus is acid resistant and heat stabilized in the presence of divalent cations ($50°$ C and 1 M Mg^{++}).

EPIZOOTIOLOGY

Swine and man are the only known hosts to be naturally infected. Newborn mice are susceptible by intracerebral and intraperitoneal inoculations but become refractory to infection by seven days of age. SVD is a new disease of pigs that was first recognized in 1966 in Lombardy, Italy, and initially was indistinguishable from foot-and-mouth disease. In 1971, the disease was diagnosed in Hong Kong, then the following year in Staffordshire, England. By 1974, SVD had been discovered in France, Poland, Austria, Germany, Switzerland, Japan, and Taiwan. Indirect evidence suggests that the People's Republic of China has also experienced occurrences of SVD. At this time it should be considered endemic in Asia and Europe. Efforts in England to eradicate the disease are continuing but have been unsuccessful.

The international spread of SVD virus has occurred primarily by the trans-shipment of exposed pigs and infected pork products. Once SVD becomes established, direct contact with infected swine, contaminated garbage, swine-holding facilities, or swine-handling equipment appears to be the major source of continuing exposure. There are no known reservoirs in nature other than swine. Although humans are susceptible to SVDV infection and this agent may have arisen as a variant of a human Coxsackie virus, there is no evidence of a human reservoir for SVD.

CLINICAL SIGNS AND LESIONS

The incubation period for SVD is two to six days, and seroconversion can be shown by day 4. Clinically the disease is indistinguishable from foot-and-mouth disease (FMD), vesicular stomatitis (VS), and vesicular exanthema of swine (VESV). Lameness of sudden onset is usually the first sign and is more obvious in larger and heavier animals. Temperatures may be elevated 2 to $4°$ C, and there is a reluctance to eat. Vesicles appear on the coronary band, dew claws, interdigital space, and heel of the foot. In natural infections, the snout, tongue, and lips are more frequently involved and fluid-filled vesicles, tags of epidermis, or erosions will be seen. Lesions other than vesicles on epithelial surfaces have not been described grossly. Recovery is usually rapid, and, barring secondary involvement, swine will usually return to normal within three weeks. Morbidity is high and mortality is low, except in newborn pigs, where mortality is also high.

DIAGNOSIS

Although the condition cannot be clinically differentiated from FMD, VESV, or VS, the presence of lesions in contact cattle would tend to eliminate SVD, and the absence of lesions in exposed cattle would suggest SVD. Laboratory diagnosis is essential, and both lesion material and serum should be submitted. The epithelial coverings of the vesicles and vesicular fluid are samples of choice. These should be placed in buffered glycerol or frozen for shipment. Virus isolation, complement fixation, and virus neutralization are the tests of choice. Direct electron microscopic examination may easily differentiate this virus from the bullet-shaped virus of VS or the typical caliciviruses of VES but not the enterovirus of FMD. Immunoelectron microscopy should rapidly differentiate SVD and FMDV if adequate quantities of antigen are available from processed laboratory specimens.

TREATMENT

Specific therapy is not available; however, the disease is self-limiting and recovery is usually complete within three weeks, except for newborn pigs. Symptomatic treatment and good sanitation to reduce secondary infections are useful. If secondary infection does occur, parenteral antimicrobials may be useful.

PREVENTION AND CONTROL

This is a foreign animal disease that has not been reported in the United States. All outbreaks of vesicular disease should be reported immediately to a regulatory veterinarian. If a diagnosed outbreak of SVD does occur, eradication measures would be instituted and would include slaughter of infected animals, quarantine of infected premises, and restriction of swine movements. Because of the resistance of this agent to environmental effects and to many of the accepted food-processing procedures, the threat of this disease being introduced into the United States is very real.

Supplemental Reading

Callis, J. J., Dardiri, A. H., Ferris, D. H., et al.: Illustrated Manual for the Recognition and Diagnosis of Certain Animal Diseases. Mexico-United States Commission for the Prevention of Foot and Mouth Disease. Plum Island Animal Disease Center, 1982, 19–21.

Graves, J. H., and McKercher, P. D.: Swine vesicular disease. Proc. 77th Ann. Mtg. U.S. Animal Health Assoc. 1973, 155–159.

SMEDI and Other Porcine Enteroviruses

WILLIAM L. MENGELING, D.V.M., Ph.D.

The acronym SMEDI was introduced into the veterinary literature in 1965 to designate porcine enteroviruses (SMEDI viruses) that caused a syndrome of reproductive failure of swine characterized by stillbirth, mummification, embryonic death, and infertility (SMEDI syndrome). Subsequent reports that several other viruses cause the same, or a similar, syndrome have resulted in the ambiguous usage and interpretation of SMEDI when used as an adjective to describe viruses associated with reproductive failure. Although some veterinary scientists and practitioners still adhere to the original definition of a SMEDI virus, perhaps the more common usage of the term is for any virus that causes embryonic or fetal death, or both, in the absence of maternal clinical signs and without ensuing abortion. Viruses in addition to porcine enteroviruses that have been reported to meet the aforementioned criteria are porcine parvovirus, reovirus, adenovirus, Japanese B encephalitis virus, and porcine cytomegalovirus. All but Japanese B encephalitis virus are present and common among swine in the United States; however, there is substantial evidence to indicate that porcine parvovirus is the cause of most such cases.

Porcine enteroviruses also have been reported to be associated with other clinical diseases, namely, enteritis, pneumonitis, pericarditis, myocarditis, and polioencephalomyelitis. With the exception of polioencephalomyelitis, however, their role in these conditions is unclear. The most severe form of polioencephalomyelitis caused by porcine enterovirus, i.e., Teschen disease, is discussed elsewhere.

Supplemental Reading

Huang, J., Gentry, R. F., and Zarkower, A.: Experimental infection of pregnant sows with porcine enteroviruses. Am. J. Vet. Res., *41*:469–473, 1980.

Encephalomyocarditis Virus

JOSEPH H. GAINER, D.V.M.

The encephalomyocarditis virus (EMCV) is a small picornavirus that survives well outside the host. It is inactivated by hypochlorites and iodinated compounds.

EPIZOOTIOLOGY

EMCV has been isolated worldwide since 1940 from several species: human, pig, rat, baboon, chimpanzee, and African elephant; the lion may be susceptible. The pig is the domestic animal most often infected, most infections in the U.S. occurring in Florida. Mortality in swine herds, although usually low, has been 100 per cent. The rat perhaps serves as a reservoir of the virus, contaminating the food and drinking water with infected feces. Immunotoxic chemicals may aggravate the infection in pigs. No field cases, to my knowledge, have been reported in pigs in the U.S. since 1975; but EMCV infections still occur in the north coastal region of New South Wales, where the swine industry is of the highly intensive variety.

CLINICAL SIGNS AND LESIONS

Sudden death, suggesting myocardial failure, in young, two- to four-month-old pigs, subhuman primates, and elephants, is the principal sign. Pathognomonic lesions are small (1 to 2 × 5 to 10 mm), grayish-white foci in the right myocardium consisting microscopically of calcium with lymphocytic, monocytic infiltration. The heart contains high levels of virus.

DIAGNOSIS

EMCV is diagnosed by virus isolation with specific antiserum. Sudden death of animals with characteristic heart lesions is strongly presumptive.

TREATMENT

At the present time there is no treatment available.

PREVENTION AND CONTROL

Rat control prevents spread. Outbreaks usually run a short course with immunity in surviving animals. No commercial vaccines have been developed.

Supplemental Reading

Acland, H. M., and Littlejohns, I. R.: Encephalomyocarditis virus infection of pigs, 1. An outbreak in New South Wales. Austr. Vet. J. *51*:409–415, 1975.
Gainer, J. H.: Effects of viruses on the heart. *In* Bourne, G. H. (ed.): Hearts and Heart-like Organs, Vol. 3. Pathology and Surgery of the Heart. Academic Press, New York, 1980, 189–237.
Littlejohns, I. R., and Acland, H. M.: Encephalomyocarditis virus infection in pigs, 2. Experimental disease. Aust. Vet. J. *51*:416–422, 1975.

Foot-and-Mouth Disease in Pigs

JERRY CALLIS, D.V.M., M.S., D.Sc.

Foot-and-mouth disease (FMD) is caused by a picornavirus. There are seven distinct serotypes and many subtypes within each owing to the antigenic lability of the virus. A shift in the pH to 6 and below or to 9 and above creates a less favorable environment for infectivity. Two per cent caustic soda, 4 per cent soda ash, and 2 per cent acetic acid are good disinfectants.

EPIZOOTIOLOGY

FMD virus infects all species of animals, domestic and wild, that have cloven hoofs. Other naturally infected

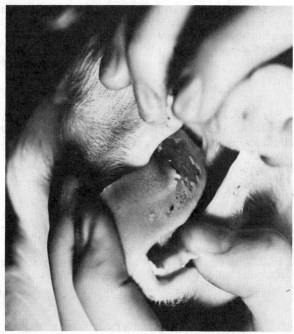

Figure 1. Erosion of epithelium on the tongue of a piglet infected with FMDV.

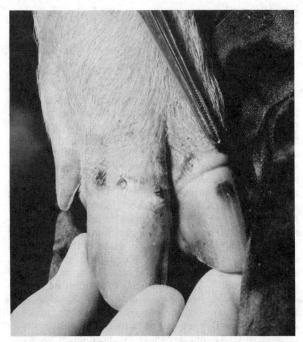

Figure 2. Unruptured vesicle on coronary band of pig.

species include armadillos, hedgehogs, rats, nutria, grizzly bears, and elephants. Dogs, cats, rabbits, guinea pigs, chickens, mice, and chinchilla may be experimentally infected. Swine, in contrast to cattle, sheep, and goats, have not been shown to become carriers following infection and recovery.

CLINICAL SIGNS AND LESIONS

The clinical signs of FMD infection in swine are vesicles or erosions on the snout, lips, and tongue; on the coronary band; and between the claws on the feet. Infected animals have an elevated temperature and are reluctant to stand or move because of pain caused by blisters on their feet (Figs. 1 and 2).

DIAGNOSIS

Blisters or vesicles in the mouth or snout or on the feet and an elevated temperature are characteristic of FMD in swine; however, these same lesions occur in three other vesicular infections in swine including vesicular stomatitis, vesicular exanthema of swine, and swine vesicular disease. For this reason a laboratory diagnosis is essential. Diagnosis can be made by isolation of the virus and identification by complement fixation, virus neutralization, agar-gel precipitin tests, and enzyme-linked immunosorbent assay.

TREATMENT

There is no specific cure for the disease. Palliative treatment may make the animals more comfortable.

PREVENTION AND CONTROL

The best way to prevent infection is to avoid contact with infected or recovered animals and their products. In the FMD-free countries the disease is eradicated by slaughter of the infected animals, destruction of the carcass, and disinfection of the premises. Vaccines have been available since the 1930's but are generally more effective for cattle than swine. In recent years vaccines have been used with more success in swine. In control programs it is also essential to control movement of infected animals and products so as to prevent aerosols of the viruses and transmission by air.

Supplemental Reading

Bachrach, H. L.: Foot-and-mouth disease. Ann. Rev. Microbiol. *22*:201, 1968.
Callis, J. J., and McKercher, P. D.: Foot-and-mouth disease. *In* Leman, A. D., et al. (eds.): Diseases of Swine, 5th ed. Iowa State University Press, Ames, Ia., 1981, 278–287.
Cottral, G. E.: Diagnosis of bovine vesicular disease. J. Am. Vet. Med. Assoc. *161*:1293, 1972.

Hog Cholera

EDWARD A. CARBREY, V.M.D., M.S.

Hog cholera (HC) is a highly contagious disease of swine caused by a small (40 to 50 nm) enveloped RNA-containing virus with cubic capsid symmetry that replicates in the cytoplasm of the cell. There is only one serotype but different strains will vary considerably in their virulence and pathogenicity. HC virus (HCV) is inactivated by heat (60 minutes at 56°C), lipolytic chemicals (detergents), or the common disinfectants including hypochlorite, cresol, sodium orthophenylphenate, and 2 per cent sodium hydroxide. Its survival in blood, feces, or saliva is dependent on the environment. HCV has been recovered from processed hams and bacon after 85 days. Natural freeze-drying in temperate zones during winter will permit long survival. Synonyms are classical swine fever, Virus-schweinepest, and peste du porc.

EPIZOOTIOLOGY

Hog cholera is found world wide except in countries in which it has been eradicated, e.g., Canada, Great Britain, and the United States. Although other animal species may be infected experimentally, the pig is the only natural host and reservoir. The virus is transmitted by lacrimal and nasal discharges, saliva, urine, feces, and tissues of infected pigs. Sources of infection include pig movement, garbage feeding, live virus vaccines, in utero infection in pregnant sows, insect transmission by mechanical means (winged needle), and persistent or immune tolerant infections (runt pigs). Infection of pregnant sows has resulted in the virus persisting in fetuses in utero for 109 days. Continuous farrowing may ensure persistence of virus of low virulence with continuing infection and losses in baby pigs.

CLINICAL SIGNS AND LESIONS

Pigs affected with acute HC look and act sick; the course of the disease is downhill and remissions are rare. Initially, only a few pigs are affected. They appear drowsy and stand with arched backs, drooping heads, and straight tails. The sick pigs appear to be cold. Anorexia shortly becomes complete, although pigs will continue to drink water. Fever is concurrent with temperatures as high as 42.2°C (most in the range of 41.1°C). There is marked lacrimal discharge with conjunctivitis so severe that the eyes may be pasted shut. Pigs huddle in the bedding and pile up on each other. Constipation develops during the fever and is followed by severe diarrhea. Eventually the pigs become gaunt and have a weak, staggering gait. Purple discoloration of the skin and convulsions may be observed just before death. In chronic HC clinical signs are less severe, pigs survive longer, and remissions occur. Pigs will resume eating but do not finish their ration so that weight is not gained and some pigs become runts. If secondary bacterial invaders become involved, other clinical signs may be observed.

Inapparent or unnoticed HC is caused by low-virulence strains that fail to produce clinical signs when inoculated experimentally into eight-week-old, SPF pigs. In affected herds the only clinical signs observed are baby pig deaths, stillbirths, abortions, and mummified fetuses. The administration of modified live virus vaccine to pregnant sows may cause this syndrome. Newborn pigs may show tremors or trembling (shakers) related to cerebellar hypoplasia and hypomyelinogenesis.

The pathogenesis and lesions of HCV are due to its affinity for epithelium and the reticuloendothelial system. Primary invasion is through the oronasal epithelium, and severe impairment of metabolism is caused by damage to the vascular endothelium. Entry of the virus is by ingestion or inhalation, with the tonsil as the primary site of viral replication. Secondary spread to the spleen occurs by viremia, with infected WBC detected as early as 16 hours after oral exposure. The parenchymatous organs are invaded after three to four days. Edema and swelling of the infected vascular endothelium result in thrombosis, infarction, and hemorrhage. Common lesions are infarcts of the spleen, button ulcers in the large intestine, and petechial hemorrhages in the lungs, epiglottis, bladder, and kidney. Other frequent lesions are edema and peripheral hemorrhage of the lymph nodes and hemorrhage and necrosis of the tonsil. In chronic HC, lesions are less severe and bronchopneumonia may be found.

DIAGNOSIS

The diagnosis may be confirmed by laboratory examinations to detect viral antigen, isolate the virus, and detect HC antibody titers in serums from convalescent pigs. Tonsil, spleen, and mandibular lymph nodes should be submitted. Thin sections of tonsil can be cut in a cryostat, and virus-infected cells in the tonsillar crypts may be detected by immunofluorescence. Splenic suspension may be inoculated into pig kidney cell cultures. After overnight incubation of the cultures, infected cells can be detected by immunofluorescence. Inapparent HC can be confirmed in nonvaccinated pigs by detecting HC antibody with the neutralization test.

PREVENTION AND CONTROL

There is no effective treatment for HC. Upon confirmation of the diagnosis, it may be possible to save some of the pigs by promptly vaccinating the herd with a potent modified live virus (MLV) vaccine and liberal doses of HC antiserum. If pregnant sows are present they should also be vaccinated, but surviving sows should be sent to slaughter before they farrow.

In a country where HC is enzootic, a regular vaccination program is the safest method of preventing the disease. Young pigs should be routinely vaccinated with MLV vaccine after weaning (eight to ten weeks of age), and the breeding herd should be vaccinated at least once a year. Sows should be vaccinated only when open, and baby pigs and pregnant sows should be isolated from vaccinated pigs for at least 30 days. HC antiserum should be administered with the vaccine in accordance with the recommendations of the producer. The virulence of the vaccine virus and the health status of the pigs should be considered in determining the appropriate dosage of antiserum.

Clinical HC can be controlled with an adequate vaccination program. However, ultimate HC control in a country or state must involve eradication of the virus. This requires the cooperation of the government, veterinary profession, and swine industry. An initial phase of intensive vaccination, followed by detection and quarantine of infected herds and finally slaughter and disposal of infected pigs, has successfully eradicated HC.

Supplemental Reading

Hog cholera and its eradication. Animal and Plant Health Inspection Service, U.S. Dept. Agric., 91–55:1, Sept., 1981.

Stewart, W. C.: Hog cholera. In Leman, A. D., et al. (eds.): Diseases of Swine, 5th ed. Iowa State University Press, Ames, Ia., 1981, 224–236.

Van Oirschot, J. T., and Terpstra, C. A.: Congenital persistent swine fever infection. I. Clinical and virologic observations. Vet. Microbiol., 2:121–132, 1977.

Flavivirus (Japanese Encephalitis)

EDWARD A. CARBREY, V.M.D., M.S.

Japanese encephalitis (JE) is caused by a small (40 to 50 nm) single-stranded RNA virus, genus *Flavivirus*, family Togaviridae.

EPIZOOTIOLOGY

The virus is mosquito-borne and infects humans, animals, and birds. Swine develop high concentrations of virus in their blood and serve as amplifying hosts. JE virus (JEV) is inactivated by heat (30 minutes at 56°C), lipid solvents, and sodium hypochlorite. JE is enzootic in Southeast Asia including USSR, China, Philippines, Indonesia, and India. Synonyms are Japanese B encephalitis, Russian autumnal encephalitis, and summer encephalitis.

CLINICAL SIGNS AND LESIONS

The clinical signs in humans are fever, headache, prostration, stiff neck, and encephalitis. Horses may develop encephalitis, whereas cattle, sheep, and goats have inapparent infections. When pregnant sows are infected, severe economic losses occur. JEV spreads to the fetuses, causing stillbirths, mummified fetuses, and weak pigs in approximately half of the infected sows. Some of the weak piglets have nervous signs and edema, whereas hydrocephalus is observed in stillborn pigs. JEV infection of boars causes infertility. The infected boars have edematous, congested testicles and hardening of the epididymis. Reduced sexual drive is observed, and JEV may be isolated from the semen. Otherwise, clinical signs are not observed except in very young pigs.

DIAGNOSIS

JEV may be isolated from the tissues of stillborn pigs in suckling mice, chick embryos, or cell cultures. A serologic diagnosis may be made by detecting a rise in antibody titer with a neutralization or hemagglutination-inhibition test performed on paired (acute and convalescent) serums.

PREVENTION AND CONTROL

Both attenuated live virus and inactivated vaccines are used to prevent baby pig losses. Young gilts and boars should be vaccinated before breeding. When using inactivated vaccines at least two doses should be given at an interval of two to three weeks. In temperate climates the vaccination should be done before the mosquito season.

Supplemental Reading

Huang, C. H.: Studies of Japanese encephalitis in China. Adv. Virus Res. 27:71–101, 1982.
Joo, H. S.: Japanese B encephalitis infection. *In* Leman, A. D., et al. (eds.): Diseases of Swine, 5th ed. Iowa State University Press, Ames, Ia., 1981, 347–351.
Lim, T. W., and Beran, G. W.: Japanese encephalitis. *In* Handbook Series in Zoonoses, Section B: Viral Zoonoses. CRC Press, Inc., Boca Raton, Fl., Vol. 1 1981, 449–456.

Porcine Reoviruses

SASHI B. MOHANTY, B.V.Sc.&A.H., Ph.D.

Reovirus types 1 and 3, isolated from apparently normal pigs and pigs with clinical disease, are serologically identical to human reoviruses. Antibodies to these agents are highly prevalent in swine populations. Porcine reoviruses grow and produce cytopathic effects (CPE) in cell cultures of porcine origin and a variety of other mammalian cells. They may produce initial CPE in HEP-2 and PK-15 cell lines, but they cannot be maintained by serial passages in these cells. Reovirus type 1 was isolated from healthy pigs, from pigs with respiratory illness, and from aborted fetuses. Type 3 was isolated from pigs with dyspnea.

CLINICAL SIGNS AND LESIONS

The pathogenic role of porcine reoviruses is not fully understood. Pigs experimentally infected with reovirus type 1 of human origin and with types 1 and 3 of porcine origin had only a mild, transient febrile reaction. Older pigs, however, had no reaction to type 3 reovirus. Experimental infection of sows between 40 and 80 days of gestation resulted in stillbirths, mummified fetuses, and small weak pigs.

No gross lesions have been described. Histologic changes confined to the lungs are mild and focal. Lobular alveolar emphysema, peribronchiolar lymphocytic infiltration, and thickened alveolar walls are seen in type 3 reoviral infection.

DIAGNOSIS, PREVENTION, AND CONTROL

Virus isolation and seroconversion are adequate for a diagnosis. Histopathologic changes may also be helpful. There is no vaccine.

Supplemental Reading

McAdaragh, J. P., and Robl, M. G.: Experimental reovirus infection of pregnant sows. Proc. 4th Int. Congr. Pig Vet. Soc. Iowa State Univ., 1976, pp. DDI.
McFerran, J. B.: Reovirus infection. *In* Leman, A. D., et al. (eds.): Diseases of Swine, 5th ed. Iowa State University Press, Ames, Ia., 1981, 330–334.

Porcine Rotavirus

EDWARD H. BOHL, D.V.M., Ph.D.

Rotavirus is a name given to a group of viruses that have similar characteristics and are generally capable of causing diarrhea in the young. At least two serotypes of porcine rotaviruses occur. Rotaviruses are very resistant to environmental conditions and chemicals.

EPIZOOTIOLOGY

Rotaviral infections of swine are very common and widespread. Undoubtedly, all herds have a persistent or enzootic infection. Most pigs probably become infected between two and one half weeks of age and one week after weaning, depending on the degree of passive immunity and viral exposure.

CLINICAL SIGNS AND LESIONS

Most pigs have a subclinical infection or only a transient diarrhea at one to five weeks of age, whereas a few have a more severe diarrhea with dehydration. Concurrent infections, decreased passive immunity, and stress (especially chilling) contribute to the severity of the infection.

DIAGNOSIS

At times, clinical signs can resemble those caused by TGE virus, pathogenic *Escherichia coli,* or coccidia. Laboratory diagnosis usually consists of the demonstration of the virus in stool samples by electronmicroscopy or of infected enterocytes by fluorescent antibody staining of jejunal mucosal smears.

TREATMENT

Keeping pigs warm and dry will help reduce severity of disease.

PREVENTION AND CONTROL

Sanitation measures to reduce the level of viral exposure, provision of optimal environmental conditions of pigs, and, possibly, vaccination may be helpful. A licensed vaccine for vaccinating pregnant swine and/or suckling pigs is available.

Supplemental Reading

Bohl, E. H., Jr.: Rotaviral diarrhea in pigs: a brief review. A.V.M.A. *174*:613–615, 1979.
Woode, G. N., and Bohl, E. H., Jr.: Rotavirus. *In* Leman, A. D., et al. (eds.): Diseases of Swine, 5th ed. Iowa State University Press, Ames, Ia., 310–322, 1981.

Transmissible Gastro-Enteritis Virus

EDWARD H. BOHL, D.V.M., Ph.D.

Transmissible gastro-enteritis (TGE) is one of the most serious and feared diseases of newborn pigs since mortality can approach 100 per cent and since vaccination and treatment are of limited value. This disease is caused by an enteric porcine coronavirus. Only 1 serotype is known, but transmissible gastro-enteritis virus (TGEV) is antigenically related to coronaviruses of dogs and cats (feline infectious peritonitis virus). TGEV causes an intestinal infection of swine of all ages, with diarrhea as one of the prominent clinical signs. The virus is rather sensitive to temperature (above $32°$ C), sunlight, and a variety of chemicals or disinfectants.

EPIZOOTIOLOGY

TGE is usually a seasonal, cold weather disease occurring most frequently from November to April. The common modes of transmission from herd to herd appear to be (1) starlings that tend to flock and feed around swine; (2) footwear, clothing, and vehicles contaminated with feces from recently infected pigs, as occurs during transport of swine or feed to or from farms; and (3) newly introduced infected animals, especially feeder pigs. Fecal shedding of virus usually lasts for less than two weeks. However, TGEV has been recovered from internal tissues of the respiratory and intestinal tracts for 104 days after infection, but it is not known if these persistently infected animals can actually shed viable virus from their bodies for longer than about two weeks.

Two distinct forms of the disease occur in herds: epizootic and enzootic TGE. Epizootic TGE occurs after the entrance of the infection into a herd where most, if not all, of the animals are susceptible (nonimmune). It is characterized by a rapid spread through the herd. Most swine of all ages will show some evidence of inappetence, lethargy, or diarrhea, and a few will vomit. Disease in young pigs is severe, with high mortality in those less than one to two weeks old. The disease in a herd runs its course in two to four weeks unless there is a continual source of susceptible animals.

Enzootic TGE is increasingly observed and refers to a persistence of infection in a herd. It is usually associated with a continuous farrowing program or frequent entrance of susceptible animals, whereby infection can be perpetuated. Sows in these herds have been previously infected and are immune. They provide a variable degree of passive immunity to suckling pigs for one to four weeks or until weaning. Diarrhea usually occurs in pigs from about one week of age to two weeks after weaning and results when the level of viral exposure overcomes the level of passive immunity. In some herds the "break" occurs, primarily after weaning, owing to the abrupt cessation of lactogenic immunity (ingestion of immune milk) and severe viral exposure. Feeder pig operations provide an ideal environment for the occurrence of enzootic TGE because of the frequent entrance of susceptible pigs and may account for the summer residence of infection, which then can serve as a focus for establishing epizootics during the winter. As revealed by serologic surveys, infection is rather common and widespread since about 50 per cent of the herds were positive in some studies.

CLINICAL SIGNS AND LESIONS

TGEV infects the villous enterocytes of the small intestines. These infected cells are shed from the villi, resulting in villous atrophy, an impairment in digestion, an accumulation of fluids in the intestines, and diarrhea. The severity of diarrhea and dehydration is greatest in newborn pigs, resulting in about 100 per cent mortality, but decreases so that few deaths usually occur in pigs older than four to five weeks of age unless there are complications or undue stress. Subclinical infections may occur in some feeder pigs or older animals, but some lactating animals become very sick. Refer to the section on epizootiology for disease pattern seen with epizootic or enzootic TGE.

DIAGNOSIS

Epizootic TGE in the U.S. and Canada can usually be accurately diagnosed from the herd history and clinical signs, especialy if piglets are involved. Porcine epidemic diarrhea, also caused by a coronavirus, occurs in Europe and can resemble TGE, but the infection has not been detected in the U.S. or Canada. Enzootic TGE is usually more difficult to diagnose and must be differentiated from other diseases with similar clinical signs, such as colibacillosis, coccidiosis, and rotaviral diarrhea. Examination of the mucosal surface of the small intestine will reveal villous atrophy, but this lesion is also seen in coccidiosis and rotaviral diarrhea. For the laboratory diagnosis of TGE in piglets, the fluorescent antibody staining test conducted on mucosal scrapings of the small intestines is recommended. For best results, specimens should be collected from animals euthanized as soon as possible after onset of diarrhea. Serologic tests are useful, especially if acute and convalescent serum samples are available.

TREATMENT

There is no specific treatment. Death losses can be reduced if pigs are kept warm (above 32° C) and dry and if they have access to electrolyte-glucose solution, water, or milk replacer. However, most sick pigs under three days of age will die regardless of treatment. If secondary bacterial infection, such as colibacillosis, is involved, antibacterial therapy may be helpful but this is questionable.

PREVENTION AND CONTROL

Precautions should be taken, especially in winter, to prevent entry of infection onto farms as discussed under epizootiology. Sows that have been previously infected at least two and one half weeks before farrowing will provide rather effective passive immunity to their suckling pigs, at least for the critical period of the first one to three weeks. This procedure can be duplicated by "planned" infection of pregnant swine with known virulent TGEV, but there are disadvantages.

There are several licensed vaccines available for use on pregnant swine that provide passive immunity to suckling pigs. These vaccines are composed of live attenuated TGEV and are administered orally, intramuscularly, or intramammarily on two to three occasions during the last six weeks of pregnancy. Most data indicate that these vaccines, when administered to serologically negative animals, are of limited effectiveness; that is, mortality is usually reduced but morbidity is not. However, these vaccines can be used to boost the existing immunity in previously infected swine, especially in enzootically infected herds. Their use may be more cost effective in this respect than when used to vaccinate serologically negative animals.

When epizootic TGE occurs, it may be advisable to purposefully expose all animals in the herd to TGE so that the infection can run its course as rapidly as possible and, thus, prevent enzootic TGE. Exceptions to this recommendation might be pregnant swine in the last two weeks of pregnancy, and their isolation from exposed animals during farrowing might be considered.

Supplemental Reading

Bohl, E. H.: Transmissible gastroenteritis. In Leman, A. D., et al. (eds.): Diseases of Swine, 5th ed. Iowa State University Press, Ames, Ia., 1981, 195–208.

Haelterman, E. O.: Viral diarrhea of swine: some suggestions for research. Proc. U.S. Anim. Health Assoc. 85:462–467, 1981.

Morin, M., et al.: Neonatal diarrhea of pigs in Quebec: infectious causes of significant outbreaks. Can. J. Comp. Med. 47:11–17, 1983.

Encephalitis-Vomiting and Wasting Disease Complex of Swine

WILLIAM L. MENGELING, D.V.M., Ph.D.

The term "encephalitis-vomiting and wasting disease complex" is used to encompass the variety of clinical manifestations of infection of swine with a neurotropic porcine coronavirus. The virus is named hemagglutinating encephalomyelitis virus (HEV) in reference to its ability to agglutinate erythrocytes of several species of animals and its neuropathogenicity.

There are two primary clinical forms of the disease complex. One form is peracute to acute. It is characterized clinically by nervous signs and histopathologically by lesions of nonsuppurative encephalomyelitis. This form does not have a specific name, but it is probably the same form as a condition first reported in Canada in 1959 and referred to as Ontario encephalomyelitis. The second primary form of the disease complex is subacute to chronic. It is characterized clinically by vomition and progressive emaciation and is called vomiting and wasting disease (VWD). Lesions of mild nonsuppurative encephalomyelitis have been found in pigs killed early in the course of VWD. Some European scientists have referred to isolates from pigs affected with VWD as VWD virus, but there is no evidence that such isolates differ from HEV either structurally or antigenically.

EPIZOOTIOLOGY

Infection with HEV is common, particularly in areas of concentrated swine production. Conversely, clinical disease is rare and confined almost exclusively to pigs within their first few weeks of life. Although epizootiology and pathogenesis have not been completely defined, the following events seem most probable on the basis of information currently available. Virus is disseminated through aerosols and by direct contact of infected and noninfected pigs. In most pigs, infection is subclinical and limited mainly to the initial sites of viral replication in the upper respiratory tract and tonsil. Occasionally, virus invades the central nervous system (CNS) by extension through peripheral nerves to cause disease. The extent of CNS damage apparently determines the type and severity of clinical signs. In at least some cases, HEV also can infect neurons of the digestive tract.

CLINICAL SIGNS AND LESIONS

Under experimental conditions, clinical signs appear four to eight days after oronasal exposure. A somewhat shorter incubation for some naturally occurring cases is suggested by case histories. Although signs are variable, they can be grouped according to the two main forms of clinical illness. Signs of the peracute to acute form are hyperesthesia, muscle tremors, incoordination, collapse, nystagmus, and paddling movements. Many affected pigs also vomit. Some pigs die within 24 hours after the initial appearance of signs. Signs of the subacute to chronic form are vomition and either progressive emaciation or failure to gain weight at a normal rate. Inappetence and listlessness are common to both forms, and occasionally these are the only signs that are observed. In such cases, pigs may recover completely. Sometimes there are marked differences in the susceptibility of pigs even within the same litter. Although morbidity and mortality are variable, they may reach 100 per cent of the baby pigs in some herds.

There are no consistent macroscopic lesions of pigs infected with HEV. In pigs affected with VWD, the gastrointestinal tract is usually relatively empty because of inappetence and vomition. The sparse stomach contents may be bile-stained. Areas of pulmonary consolidation have been observed in experimentally infected pigs.

Microscopic lesions of nonsuppurative encephalomyelitis are often extensive in pigs with nervous signs, and viral infection of neurons has been demonstrated by immunofluorescence microscopy. Lesions consist of perivascular cuffing with mononuclear cells, glial nodules, and neuronophagia. Most are in the gray matter of the brain stem and anterior spinal cord. Similar but less extensive lesions are found in pigs killed early in the course of VWD. This observation, plus the fact that HEV is seldom isolated from the gastrointestinal tract, has led to the hypothesis that VWD is due to limited but irreparable neuronal damage. Microscopic inflammatory lesions of the respiratory tract have been observed with both forms of the disease. The association of HEV with such lesions has been confirmed by virus isolation and immunofluorescence microscopy.

DIAGNOSIS

A tentative diagnosis of the encephalitis-vomiting and wasting disease complex is based on the occurrence of characteristic clinical signs mainly or entirely among pigs within the first few weeks of their life. Although pseudorabies virus and porcine enteroviruses can cause similar nervous signs and vomition, they more often affect older pigs as well. Transmissible gastro-enteritis virus also causes baby pigs to vomit, but the absence of nervous signs and the presence of diarrhea with transmissible gastro-enteritis are distinguishing features.

A definitive diagnosis depends on isolation of HEV from nervous tissue or demonstration of HEV-infected neurons by immunofluorescence microscopy. Because HEV is ubiquitous among swine, neither the detection of antibody nor the isolation of the virus from nonnervous tissue can be considered probable diagnostic evidence. The tissue of choice for diagnostic purposes is brain stem collected from a pig that has had clinical signs for no more than 48 hours and preferably less than 24 hours. The brain stem is cut symmetrically in halves, and one half is fixed in 10 per cent formalin for histologic examination. The other half is further divided into two parts. One part is used for attempted virus isolation, and the other is cut into thin sections with a cryostat-microtome for examination by direct immunofluorescence microscopy. Several studies have confirmed that virus isolation is usually unsuccessful after one or two days of clinical signs. One possible contributing factor is that because of the relatively long incubation period (perhaps reflecting the time required for the virus to reach the CNS), humoral antibody is present at or soon after the appearance of clinical signs.

TREATMENT

Treatment to reduce dehydration and electrolyte imbalance in cases of persistent vomition and to control secondary pathogens with antibiotics depends on the value of the affected pigs.

PREVENTION

Clinical disease is usually self-limiting. Most or all litters born over a period of one to two weeks may be affected, but eventually, through exposure of dams before farrowing, neonates are protected by colostral antibody. Passively acquired immunity may explain, in part, why the disease is so rare despite the probability that many pigs are initially exposed to HEV during the first few weeks of their life. Although the development of a vaccine is technically feasible, the sporadic nature of the disease makes vaccination economically unlikely.

Supplemental Reading

Andries, K., and Pensaert, M. B.: Virus isolation and immunofluorescence in different organs of pigs infected with hemagglutinating encephalomyelitis virus. Am. J. Vet. Res. 41:215–218, 1980.
Greig, A. S.: Hemagglutinating encephalomyelitis. In Leman, A. D., et al. (eds.): Diseases of Swine, 5th ed. Iowa State University Press, Ames, Ia., 1981, 246–253.
Mengeling, W. L., and Cutlip, R. C.: Pathogenicity of field isolates of hemagglutinating encephalomyelitis virus for neonatal pigs. J. Am. Vet. Med. Assoc. 168:236–239, 1976.

Swine Influenza

B. C. EASTERDAY, D.V.M., Ph.D.

Swine influenza (SI), also known as swine flu, hog flu, and pig flu, is a specific, acute, infectious, respiratory disease of swine caused by a type A influenza virus. The disease is characterized by sudden onset, coughing, dyspnea, fever, prostration, and rapid recovery. The mortality rate is low except in very young piglets and cases complicated by other infections or conditions.

ETIOLOGY

The cause of SI is a type A influenza virus. It is one of many such viruses of diverse antigenic characteristics found in humans, horses, and many domestic and wild avian species. The influenza viruses belong to the family Orthomyxoviridae. They have enveloped virions 80 to 120 nm in diameter that may be spherical, elongated, or pleomorphic. The structural proteins on the surface of the virion, hemagglutinin (H) and neuraminidase (N), are the significant surface antigens. Antibodies to the hemagglutinin are protective against viruses containing the same hemagglutinin. Antibodies are also formed against the neuraminidase antigen, but they are less important in providing protection from infection.

Swine influenza virus (SIV) has been remarkably stable in its antigenic characteristics over 60 years. However, there has been definite antigenic drifting, and the contemporary strains are clearly distinguishable from the older ones. Co-existing subpopulations with antigenically and biologically distinguishable hemagglutinins may be found in SIVs isolated from swine and humans. Influenza viruses with swine characteristics, but clearly distinguishable antigenically from classical swine strains, have been recovered from avian species.

It is clear that swine have become infected with at least four distinct type A influenza viruses. These include the "classical" SIV, with the antigenic characteristics H1N1 (formerly Hsw1N1), the Hong Kong influenza virus H3N2 and its antigenic variants, the "Russian" influenza virus, an H1N1 virus, and more recently, an H1N1 virus with some of the classic SIV antigenic characteristics but generally considered to be of avian origin.

EPIZOOTIOLOGY

The first appearance of SI in a swine population is generally associated with the movement of animals, e.g., the introduction of breeding stock, introduction of feeder pigs, or return of show stock to the farm. Once the infection has appeared in a swine-breeding operation or any environment where there is no complete depopulation, it is likely to be maintained in the herd with at least annual episodes of acute disease. It is generally reported that outbreaks are explosive, with all of the pigs in the herd becoming ill at the same time. However, owners who observe their herds closely are often aware of one or a few pigs with signs of the disease two to five days before the whole herd is involved. Although the precise method of transmission is not known, it is presumed to be direct pig-to-pig transmission by the nasopharyngeal route. Nasal secretions are laden with virus during the acute febrile stages of infection, providing an abundant source of infectious materials for susceptible animals.

It is quite clear that although outbreaks of SI are generally seasonal, especially in the north central United States, the infection and disease are present throughout the year.

It has been clear since 1976 that SIV may be transmitted from pigs to humans and may cause acute respiratory disease. The documented cases of transmission of SIV resulting in acute respiratory disease in humans in contact with swine have been in young men under 30 years of age. In the United States there is a plentiful source of virus in the pig populations, and there are thousands of contacts between humans beings and pigs every day. Such exposure constitutes an occupational hazard and a potential public health problem of undetermined magnitude and significance.

CLINICAL SIGNS AND LESIONS

Classical SI, as it occurs in nature, is a herd disease. It is most frequently described as a disease of autumn, winter, and early spring. There is a sudden onset of signs, most of which are referable to the respiratory tract. Coughing, inactivity, and inappetence are generally the first signs noticed. This proceeds to labored and jerky breathing and prolonged paroxysmal coughing. Great prostration and complete anorexia along with conjunctivitis, nasal discharge, and loss of weight are common. Body temperature is commonly elevated to 42.2°C (106°F) or greater. This state of severe illness remains practically unchanged for five to seven days, after which there is remarkably fast recovery. The morbidity rate will approach 100 per cent. The mortality rate in uncomplicated cases is usually less than 1 per cent. Most death losses are in suckling pigs.

The lesions observed in acute swine influenza are those of a viral pneumonia. The mucosa of the pharynx, larynx, trachea, and large bronchi is hyperemic and covered with mucus. The small bronchi and bronchioles are completely filled with exudate. There is a sharp line of demarcation between normal and pneumonic lung. Cervical and mediastinal lymph nodes are enlarged and edematous and may be congested.

In fatal cases with the more severe lesions, there is more fibrin in the bronchial exudate and accumulation of fibrin on the pleural surfaces of the lung and thoracic wall. In natural fatal cases there may be a lobular pneumonia involving about 60 per cent of all lobes. The involved areas were plum-colored and slightly firm.

DIAGNOSIS

SI may be suspected when there is an outbreak of acute respiratory disease involving most or all of the pigs in a herd. Although signs of the classical disease may be present, a clinical diagnosis is presumptive. There are conditions that are clinically identical to classical SI that are not caused by the SIV. Furthermore, the SIV has been recovered from cases of poorly defined respiratory disease that have no similarity to the classical disease. SI must be differentiated from enzootic pneumonia of pigs and other acute and chronic respiratory diseases.

A definitive diagnosis of SI can be made only by the isolation and identification of SIV or by demonstration of specific antibodies. The most common method for isolation of virus is by intra-amniotic or intra-allantoic inoculation of embryonated (10 to 12 days) chicken eggs. Nasal mucus is obtained by swabbing and is then suspended in a suitable transport medium such as glycerol-saline and injected into the embryonated eggs. Pharyngeal mucus may be obtained by swabbing in very small pigs, in which it is difficult to swab the nasal passages. Virus is more likely to be found in nasal secretion during the febrile period than after the fever has subsided.

Serologic diagnosis of SI requires the testing of paired serum samples, one obtained during the acute phase of the disease and the other three to four weeks after the first sample, to demonstrate an increase in amount of antibody. The hemagglutination-inhibition (HI) test is most commonly employed for serologic diagnosis of SI.

Positive diagnosis of the disease by serologic and virologic means among suckling or weanling pigs from dams with antibody to the virus may be complicated. Maternal antibody persists two to four months, depending on the initial level. It has been shown that weanling pigs with maternal antibody may be infected and may shed virus.

TREATMENT

There is no specific therapy for SI. Careful nursing is important, with the provision of a comfortable, draft-free shelter. Clean, dry, dust-free bedding should be provided. Pigs should not be moved or transported during the acute stages of the disease so as to avoid additional stress to the respiratory system.

Expectorants are commonly used as a herd treatment and are administered in the drinking water. Antimicrobial agents have been used on a herd basis to control concurrent or secondary bacterial infections.

PREVENTION

There are no licensed vaccines available in the United States for the prevention of SI.*

*Author's note: As of late 1983, acute respiratory disease of swine in Europe has been attributed to infection with H3N2 influenza virus.

Supplemental Reading

Easterday, B. C.: Swine influenza. In Leman, A. D., et al. (eds.): Diseases of Swine, 5th ed. Iowa State University Press, Ames, Ia., 1981, 184.
Gillespie, J. H., and Timoney, J. F.: Swine influenza. In Gillespie, J. H., and Timoney, J. F. (eds.): Hagan and Bruner's Infectious Diseases of Domestic Animals, 7th ed. Cornell University Press, Ithaca, N.Y., 1981, 711.
Kaplan, M. M., and Webster, R. G.: The epidemiology of influenza. Sci. Am. 237:88–105, 1977.

Vesicular Stomatitis Virus in Swine

ALVIN W. SMITH, D.V.M., Ph.D.

The etiologic agent, a Rhabdoviridae of the genus Vesiculovirus, has been discussed in detail in Vesicular Stomatitis Virus in Cattle. Also included in that article is additional information on epizootiology, clinical signs and lesions, diagnosis, treatment, prevention, and control.

There are some differences, however, between the virus in cattle and that in swine. During the periodic epizootics that occur, pigs have not been involved to the same extent as cattle and horses. Swine that ingest the virus will develop antibodies but not clinical disease, and garbage feeding has not been a means of transmission nor a

concern in the control of the disease in pigs. Intravenous injections of virus will cause foot and snout lesions. Fighting and abrading mucous membranes may be other primary means of spread in pigs. Pigs that contract the disease through natural exposure are seen to have foot lesions more often than snout lesions, and lameness may be the only sign noted on initial examination.

The diagnosis of vesicular stomatitis in swine is more complicated than it is in cattle because the disease must be differentiated from swine vesicular disease (an enterovirus) and vesicular exanthema of swine (a calicivirus) in addition to foot-and-mouth disease. All four of these virus diseases of swine occur with mouth and foot lesions that are clinically identical. Virus isolation or visualization and serologic examinations are essential for rapid and definitive diagnosis of this disease in pigs.

Rabies in Pigs

GEORGE M. BAER, D.V.M.

In the United States less than a dozen pigs are reported rabid each year. These are found in the midwestern states that have appreciable numbers of rabid skunks and in the northeastern states that have large numbers of rabid foxes. Rabid pigs show hyperexcitability, sexual excitement, and aggressiveness. In one outbreak pigs showed "a peculiar twitching and preoccupation with the nose similar to that observed in swine with rings recently placed in their noses" (one would suspect that the pigs were bitten on the nose). This was followed by prostration, rapid chewing movements, excessive salivation, and generalized clonic muscular spasms that gradually changed to fine tremors. The reported incubation period varies greatly, with an average of 70 days in one group of pigs.

Pigs appear to be quite resistant to the disease, and there have been reports of animals getting sick and then recovering fully. Little is known about the salivary excretion of the virus, but the salivary glands in rabid pigs are often infective.

Diagnosis is made by routine fluorescent antibody staining of brain impressions. No rabies vaccines are currently licensed for pigs in the United States.

Supplemental Reading

Dunne, H. W.: In Diseases of Swine. Iowa State University Press, Ames, Ia., 1975, 411–421.
Merriman, G. M.: Rabies in Tennessee swine. J. Am. Vet. Med. Assoc. 148:809–811, 1966.
Morehouse, L. G., Kintner, L. D., and Nelson, S. L.: Rabies in swine. J. Am. Vet. Med. Assoc. 153:57–64, 1968.

Chlamydial Infections of Swine

J. STORZ, D.V.M., Ph.D.

These obligate intracellular infectious agents comprise antigenically related and culturally, morphologically, and tinctorially similar microorganisms. The few porcine chlamydial strains studied were isolated from fecal samples, joint fluid, lungs, placentas, and conjunctival scrapings.[1]

They required numerous subpassages for adaptation to the yolk sac cells of developing chicken embryos. Porcine isolates were highly pathogenic after adaptation, but they produced relatively few elementary bodies in chicken embryos. Behavior in cell cultures separated them as biotypes 4 and 5 from ovine, bovine, feline, and avian chlamydial strains.[2]

EPIZOOTIOLOGY

Chlamydial infections of swine were detected in Canada, France, Austria, and Eastern European countries. Infected swine were found to shed them in respiratory and conjunctival exudates and in the feces. Transmission may occur through aerosols or by the oral-fecal route. Chlamydial elementary bodies are relatively stable in body fluids. Quaternary ammonium compounds inactivate their infectivity within five minutes.[1, 3, 4]

CLINICAL SIGNS

Chlamydiae were cultured from conjunctival scrapings of piglets with conjunctivitis, from feces of apparently normal pigs, from joint fluids of slaughter pigs with arthritic joint lesions, from lungs of piglets with pneumonia, and from placentas of sows that aborted.[1, 4] Experimental inoculation successfully induced conjunctivitis and complicating eye lesions, pneumonia, and intestinal infections.[2] Specific clinical signs differentiating Chlamydia-induced clinical signs from similar disease conditions associated with other infectious agents were not reported.

DIAGNOSIS

This infection of swine can be detected through exfoliative cytologic examination of conjunctival scrapings, joint fluids, or placental impression smears following Giemsa or Gimenez staining.[5] Fluorescent antibody methods should be applied to the exfoliative cytologic diagnostic approach, because they bring immunologic specificity and sensitivity to this technique. Attempts should also be made to isolate chlamydiae from specimens of affected animals. This is done most effectively with cell culture methods under conditions enhancing adsorption to host cells through centrifugal force or the use of diethylaminoethyl-dextran (DEAE-D).[2] Another method involves inoculating seven-day-old chicken embryos by the yolk sac route, a method that is more laborious and time-consuming. Antibodies against chlamydial agents were found at a relatively high rate in swine herds of Britain. The complement fixation test was used in these studies.[4, 5] Few laboratories provide modern diagnostic tests to detect these infections in swine.

TREATMENT

Chlamydial multiplication is arrested or inhibited by tetracyclines, chlortetracycline, oxytetracycline (Liquamycin* 20 mg/kg), and erythromycin.

_____
*Available from Pfizer and Co., New York, NY 10017

PREVENTION AND CONTROL

Approaches to prevent these infections in swine have not been explored.

References

1. Koelbl, O., Burtscher, H., and Hebenstreit, J.: Polyarthritis bei Schlachtschweinen. Microbiologische, histologische, und fleisch hygiensche Untersuchungen und Aspekte. Wien Tierarztl. Monatsschr. 57:355–361, 1970.
2. Spears, P., and Storz, J.: Biotyping of Chlamydia psittaci based on inclusion morphology and response to DEAE-dextran and cycloheximide. Infect. Immun. 24:224–232, 1979.
3. Pavlov, P., Milanov, M., and Tschilev, D.: Recherches sur la rickettsiose kerato-conjunctivale du porc en Bulgaria. Ann. Inst. Pasteur. 105:450–454, 1963.
4. Tolybekow, A. S., Wischnjakowa, L. A., and Dobin, M. A.: Die aetiologische Bedeutung eines Erregers aus der Bedsoniengruppe fur die enzootische Pneumonie der Schweine. Monatshft. Veterinarmed. 28:339–344, 1973.
5. Storz, J.: Chlamydia and Chlamydia-Induced Diseases. Springfield, Illinois, Charles C Thomas, 1971.

Swine Mycoplasmosis

C. H. ARMSTRONG, D.V.M., Ph.D.

PNEUMONIA CAUSED BY
Mycoplasma hyopneumonia

Mycoplasmal pneumonia of swine (MPS; also called enzootic pneumonia of pigs [EPP]) is a chronic disease that occurs in all of the major swine-producing regions of the world. Essentially all conventional (non-SPF) herds are affected. Annual losses in the U.S. have been estimated to be $200 million.

The causative agent of MPS is Mycoplasma (M.) hyopneumoniae (suipneumoniae). The only known host of M. hyopneumoniae is the pig. Transmission is from infected pig to susceptible pig via infective aerosols. Swine of all ages are susceptible to MPS; however, in affected herds young pigs are often resistant to infection as a result of maternal antibodies. These pigs become infected at two to four months of age when they are commingled with older swine in the growing and finishing units.

The development and progression of lesions follow the distribution of the causative agent; i.e., lesions generally begin at the ventral aspects of the lobes and progress dorsally. The typical lesion is purple in color and lobular in distribution and is most apt to be seen in the apical and cardiac lobes. During the active phase of infection, lobules are slightly swollen and have a lymphoid texture when cut. The airways of such lungs contain a sticky white exudate that is laden with M. hyopneumoniae organisms. Later, the lobules are contracted slightly and the airways contain little or no exudate.

MPS is characterized by high morbidity and zero mortality. Clinical signs include a chronic, dry, nonproductive cough; rough hair coat; retarded growth rate; and inefficient utilization of feed. The severity of these signs is influenced directly by the quality of the environment and by concurrent diseases such as bacterial pneumonias, atrophic rhinitis, and ascarid migration.

Most laboratories diagnose MPS entirely on the basis of gross and microscopic lesions. The lesions associated with MPS are characteristic but not pathognomonic. Consequently the use of lesions as the sole criterion of MPS can result in false-positive diagnoses. It also should be emphasized that the absence of gross lesions does not prove freedom from infection. A definitive diagnosis requires that *M. hyopneumoniae* be visualized in immunofluorescence (IF)-stained lung sections or that it be recovered culturally. The preferred specimen is a lung in the active stage of infection. The IF test should be performed first because it is rapid and relatively inexpensive. The IF test is specific and positive results are reliable; however, negative results do not prove absence of infection. Therefore, IF negative lungs should be examined culturally. Unfortunately, few diagnostic laboratories are capable of isolating and identifying *M. hyopneumoniae* owing to its fastidious nature. The complement fixation test, indirect hemagglutination test, and the enzyme-linked immunosorbent assay have been used to diagnose MPS ante mortem. These tests are useful when applied on a herd basis but lack the sensitivity and the specificity to reliably identify infected swine on an individual basis.

Control of MPS is best accomplished by providing good ventilation and optimal temperature, avoiding overcrowding, and controlling associated diseases such as bacterial pneumonias, atrophic rhinitis, and ascariasis. Tetracycline, lincomycin, tylosin, and tiamulin (not available in the U.S.), used according to the manufacturer's directions, reduce the incidence and severity of lesions and improve growth rate and feed utilization efficiency. They do not eliminate an existing *M. hyopneumoniae* infection.

POLYSEROSITIS AND ARTHRITIS CAUSED BY *Mycoplasma hyorhinis*

Mycoplasma hyorhinis is a common inhabitant of the nasal cavity of pigs in all parts of the world. Piglets acquire the infection early in life via aerosols from older pigs and infected littermates. *M. hyorhinis* remains localized in the nasal cavity in most pigs and causes no perceptible illness. Some sort of stress appears to be a prerequisite to clinical disease; i.e., stress leads to septicemia with a resulting localization of the organism in joints and on serosal membranes.

The disease occurs most commonly in pigs three to ten weeks of age and occasionally in young adult swine. First evidence of illness appears three to ten days following stress. Clinical signs include fever, restlessness, dull hair coat, reluctance to move, abdominal tenderness, labored breathing, swollen joints, and lameness. Acute-phase lesions consist of serofibrinous pleuritis, pericarditis, peritonitis, synovitis, and arthritis. There is regression of the signs associated with polyserositis in 10 to 14 days. The most severe signs of arthritis are seen after the acute phase of illness has passed. Arthritis generally persists for two to three months, and some swine may be lame for as long as six months.

Diagnosis depends on isolating *M. hyorhinis* from affected tissues. *M. hyorhinis* grows well on a variety of mycoplasmal media and is relatively easy to isolate and identify. Swine in the acute phase of the disease are preferred diagnostic specimens, especially for the polyserositis phase of infection. However, the organism can be recovered from joints for several weeks after the acute phase of the disease. Diseases that must be differentiated include Glassers disease (a polyserositis caused by *Hemophilus* species) and erysipelas arthritis.

M. hyorhinis is susceptible *in vitro* to a variety of antibiotics, but the use of such compounds clinically is disappointing. The best way to control the disease is to reduce stress, i.e., to control respiratory and intestinal infections and to provide a good environment.

ARTHRITIS CAUSED BY *Mycoplasma hyosynoviae*

A high percentage of sows in the U.S. harbor *M. hyosynoviae* in their nasopharynx. Pigs acquire the infection from adult carriers or from infected penmates via nasopharyngeal secretions. Most pigs are at least six to eight weeks of age before they become infected. Intranasal exposure is followed in two to four days by septicemia. The septicemia persists for eight to ten days and may lead to joint infection. The factors leading to joint disease have not been defined. Age may be important. It has been suggested that exposure prior to ten weeks of age results in inapparent disease and resistance to arthritis later in life. Arthritis reportedly is more severe in certain genetic strains of heavily muscled swine with straight legs. It also has been suggested that swine with osteochondrosis may experience more severe arthritis when infected with *M. hyosynoviae*.

M. hyosynoviae induces a nonsuppurative polyarthritis with little or no fever. There is no polyserositis. The disease is most common in swine 10 to 20 weeks of age. It is characterized by an acute lameness of sudden onset that persists three to ten days. The acute phase usually is followed by gradual recovery. Synovial fluid is increased in volume and at first is serosanguinous and later yellowish-brown.

A definitive diagnosis depends upon isolation of the causative agent. *M. hyosynoviae* is readily recovered from affected joints during the acute phase of illness but disappears rapidly thereafter. Synovial fluids should be collected from several untreated swine and examined by a microbiologist familiar with the mycoplasmas.

Swine in the acute phase of the disease respond well to intramuscular tylosin (5 mg/kg) or lincomycin (5 mg/kg) in combination with corticosteroids. Prevention includes use of breeding stock with good leg conformation and avoidance of stress during the period of greatest susceptibility. Early weaning and subsequent rearing in the absence of carrier swine also may be effective.

Supplemental Reading

Ross, R. F.: Mycoplasmal diseases. *In* Leman, A. D., et al. (eds.): Diseases of Swine, 5th ed. Iowa State University Press, Ames, Ia., 1981, 535–549.

Whittlestone, P.: Porcine mycoplasmas. *In* Tully, J. G., and Whitcomb, R. F. (eds.): The Mycoplasmas, Vol. II. Academic Press, New York, 1979, 133–176.

BACTERIAL AND FUNGAL DISEASES

JOHN N. BERG, D.V.M., Ph.D.
Consulting Editor

Streptococcal Diseases

JIMMY L. HOWARD, D.V.M., M.S.

Streptococcal infections affecting food animal species are numerous and varied in their clinical manifestations. *Streptococcus agalactia, S. dysglactiae, S. uberis, S. zooepidemicus, S. pneumoniae,* and rarely *S. pyogenes* are the causative agents in mastitis and are discussed in the article on mastitis. Other streptococcal related diseases include acute infectious septicemia of calves, sheep, and swine; pharyngitis and pneumonia of calves; meningoencephalitis and otitis media of calves and pigs; infectious dermatitis of piglets; cervical or "jowl" abscess of pigs; and omphalophlebitis of neonates. Acute streptococcal septicemia may occur in adult animals, particularly sows. Also, genital tract infections and abortions may occur in sows.

ETIOLOGY

The etiologic agents are gram-positive spherical organisms belonging to the genus *Streptococcus.* The organisms are classified as hemolytic or nonhemolytic. The hemolytic group is further classified by Lancefield's serologic method, which is based on the precipitation test. The original classification designated 5 types of streptococci, grouped as A, B, C, D, and E. The organisms are currently differentiated serologically into Lancefield groups A to T on the basis of the carbohydrate constituents of the cell walls. Not all strains now placed in the Lancefield groups are hemolytic. Most of the Lancefield groups have been isolated from food animals. Members of group C, the "animal pyogenes" type, are the most common causes of streptococcal diseases. *S. pyogenes* occasionally infects the udder of cattle, causing acute mastitis. *S. pyogenes* normally gains access to the mammary system by human exposure and can cause widespread outbreaks of scarlet fever or septic sore throat in humans.

EPIZOOTIOLOGY

Streptococcal infections are found worldwide. The organisms are prevalent in nature and infect both humans and animals.

The organism may be airborne and gains entry through any natural orifice, such as those of the respiratory, digestive, and urogenital systems. It can also gain entry through contaminated wounds. Streptococci are easily transported through the blood vascular system, resulting in a bacteremia. Almost all streptococci produce a toxin and septicemia results.

CLINICAL SIGNS AND PATHOGENESIS

Streptococcal Mastitis

Streptococci are probably the most common organism associated with inflammation of the mammary gland. *S. agalactiae* is an obligate pathogen of the mammary gland, and the mastitis produced is specific contagious disease. Mastitis is described more fully in another article.

Acute Septicemia

Acute septicemia has a sudden onset with possible death within 12 to 48 hr. There is high fever (40 to 42°C), anorexia, dyspnea, weakness, prostration, coma, and death. Frequently there is dysentery and hematuria. Occasionally, abscesses may be found and may be the seat of infection. Abscesses in critical organs usually result in death. Subserous or submucosal petechial or ecchymotic hemorrhages are seen at necropsy. Localization of infection in joints, heart valves, meninges, and eyes is common.

Pharyngitis and Pneumonia in Calves

Pharyngitis and pneumonia have a sudden onset of fever (40 to 42°C), anorexia, muscular soreness, and respiratory distress. The condition usually begins as a slight cough and develops into respiratory dyspnea. There are moist rales early in the course of the disease. Slight conjunctivitis with serous nasal and eye discharge is found. Ruptured lung abscesses usually result in death of the animal. Postmortem lesions are those of pneumonia.

Meningoencephalitis and Otitis Media in Calves and Pigs

The earliest signs of meningoencephalitis and otitis media are muscle soreness and stiffness accompanied by a high fever (41 to 42°C). The head is held up and forward or, in the case of otitis media, it is held to one side. The animal usually shows circling, ataxia, weakness, and paralysis. Opisthotonus, nystagmus, strabismus, and blindness may occur. The animal may show signs of convulsion or coma or both. The course of the disease is usually quite short, and death occurs within 12 hr of the first signs.

Infectious Dermatitis of Piglets

Contagious pyoderma is characterized by the formation of pustules primarily on the face and neck of young pigs. The lesions spread from wounds and abrasions caused by the needle teeth of other pigs. These pustules occasionally coalesce to form large, infected areas with scab formation. This condition is often confused with exudative epidermitis. Epidermitis is usually more generalized, and the skin develops an oily texture.

Cervical or Jowl Abscesses

Jowl abscesses are not infrequent in the cervical nodes of swine and are frequently observed at slaughter. Often the head or the entire carcass is condemned at slaughter because of these abscesses. Clinically, there is an enlargement of the lymph nodes of the head and neck. Pressure on the pharyngeal area causing respiratory distress may be evident.

Septic Joint Disease in Neonates

Septic joint disease in neonates is an acute infectious disease caused by various species of organisms, including *Steptococcus*. It is characterized by septicemia with or without localized infection. There is often a purulent focus of infection in the umbilicus, joints, tendon sheaths, kidney, liver, lungs, or other parts of the body. The early symptoms are usually those of acute septicemia, with later abscess formation, resulting in chronic infection. Weak animals seem to be more susceptible to the acute form and often succumb to the disease. Healthy animals are more prone to the chronic form, which often lingers and cripples or stunts the animal.

Meningitis, ophthalmitis, omphalophlebitis, and polyarthritis are the most common signs. Ophthalmitis usually only occurs in calves very soon after birth. Omphalophlebitis is first observed as a painful swelling of the navel. A purulent discharge and a patent urachus may occur. Polyarthritis is manifested by an apparent lameness with swelling and tenderness of the joints. The hock, stifle, and knee joints are most commonly affected. Clinically, the animal will show stiffness, anorexia, depression, and a fever of approximately 40°C.

Necropsy findings are often those of septicemia. In more chonic forms, there are suppurative lesions of the umbilicus and one or more joints. There may be multiple abscesses in the liver, kidney, spleen, and lungs. Valvular endocarditis may be present in pigs and lambs but only rarely in calves. In pigs dying of endocarditis, there is usually a large vegetative lesion on heart valves.

DIAGNOSIS

Streptococcal infections are usually diagnosed tentatively by clinical signs and associated circumstances. Laboratory test results will indicate various degrees of an inflammatory reaction. To make a definitive diagnosis, the organism must be isolated and identified. The organism is isolated from the blood, milk, or abscess in cases of septicemia, mastitis, or omphalophlebitis respectively.

In cases of meningoencephalitis or pneumonia, the organism is often isolated at necropsy. The response to treatment can be an aid to diagnosis.

TREATMENT

Penicillin is still the treatment of choice in most cases of streptococcal infection. The dosage should be high (20,000 to 30,000 units per kg body weight) and given daily for a period of 3 to 5 days. Procaine penicillin G given intramuscularly is the most effective form and route. Sulfonamides, such as sulfanilamide, sulfamerazine, or sulfadimethoxine, at the rate of 1 gm per 7 kg body weight are effective. A combination of penicillin and a sulfonamide have proved very effective in most streptococcal infections. In cases of septicemia or meningoencephalitis, crystalline penicillin can be given intravenously. It is not advisable to give large doses of potassium penicillin intravenously because of the adverse effects of the potassium ion. Where suppuration is already present, parenteral administration of enzymes may be beneficial. In some cases corticosteroids are given in combination with large doses of antibiotics.

Other antibiotics found very effective against most streptococci include lincomycin, ampicillin, bacitracin, chlortetracycline, oxytetracycline, erythromycin, and cephalothin.

Specific antitoxin sera have proved effective against streptococci that produce soluble toxins if given in the very early stages of infection. Whole blood at the rate of 5 to 10 ml/kg body weight may be given by intraperitoneal, intravenous, or subcutaneous routes. The intravenous route is the one of choice in my opinion. The dam's blood may be used in neonates, but other sources may be adequate.

Supportive therapy, including fluid administration and antipyretics, may be essential in treating critical cases. Economics will also be an important consideration, determining the extent of supportive therapy. Any obvious external abscesses should be opened and drained. Suppurative wounds should be cleaned, disinfected, and treated with topical antimicrobials.

PREVENTION

Preventive measures should include good sanitation practices. Environmental factors, such as cleanliness, proper ventilation, heat, and light, are essential in the control of streptococcal infection. Disinfection of maternity quarters and pasture rotation are recommended. Washing sows before farrowing, cutting of needle teeth in baby pigs, dipping the navel cord of the newborn in tincture of iodine, providing clean bedding, and insisting on clean handlers are sound management practices. Provide an adequate supply of colostrum either naturally or artificially. The need of the neonate for adequate colostrum within the first 12 hr is extremely important.

Chlortetracycline fed at the rate of 50 gm/ton of feed is an effective preventive for cervical abscess control in swine.

Recovery from a streptococcal infection does not generally confer any lasting immunity. Most bacterins or attentuated cultures have not been very effective as immunizing agents. Some bacterins, such as polyvalent aluminium hydroxide absorbed bacterins or alum precipitated bacterins, have produced temporary immunity and may be given in severe outbreaks of disease. Heat-killed and live cultures of *S. agalactiae* have been used in both treatment and prevention of bovine streptococcal mastitis with conflicting results. Streptococcal bacterins given to pregnant sows may help control abscesses (lymphadenitis) in piglets.

Staphylococcal Diseases

JIMMY L. HOWARD, D.V.M., M.S.

Staphylococcal infections are not uncommon in food animals and are usually classified as nonspecific suppurative disease processes. The most frequent pus-forming organism of humans belongs to the staphylococcal group, but that is not true of food animals. However, there is ample evidence that transmission between humans and animals occurs. Granulomatous staphylococcal mastitis, exudative epidermitis of pigs, and enzootic staphylococcosis of lambs are specific disease entities.

ETIOLOGY

The disease-causing agents are gram-positive coccoid bacterial organisms that occur in packets and belong to the genus *Staphylococcus*. The most frequent pathogenic species in animals are *S. aureus, S. albus,* and *S. hyos (S. hyicus)*. The pathogenic staphylococci produce one or more toxins. *S. aureus* produces a hemotoxin, a leukocidin, and a necrotizing toxin.

EPIZOOTIOLOGY

Staphylococcal infections are found worldwide. The organisms are widespread in nature and are often obligate pathogens.

The organism may be airborne and gains entrance through natural body openings. It may also be transmitted by biting arthropods or insects, such as the ticks causing pyemia (enzootic staphylococcosis) of lambs. The most common method of transmission is by wound contamination or by unsanitary environment conditions.

CLINICAL SIGNS AND PATHOGENESIS

Staphylococcal Mastitis

Staphylococcal mastitis appears to be a more prevalent form of mastitis now than in the past. The primary reason for this apparent increase is that effective antibiotic therapy has reduced streptococcal infections, and the antibiotic-resistant strains of *Staphylococcus* spp. have remained. Occasionally, staphylococci cause chronic granulomatous mastitis, *botyromycosis*. This has been mistakenly called "actinomycotic mastitis." Generalized staphylococcal mastitis is a fulminating septicemia with all the associated symptoms, while staphylococcal granulomatous mastitis usually affects 1 or 2 quarters of the udder but the general health of the animal is not affected. Further discussion of mastitis will be presented in that article.

Exudative Epidermitis of Pigs

Exudative epidermitis is caused by *S. hyos (S. hyicus)*, which enters through the umbilicus, feet abrasions, or lacerations. The entire body is usually covered with a greasy exudate, and in less acute cases the skin becomes thickened and more wrinkled. This condition is elucidated in the articles on dermatologic diseases.

Enzootic Staphylococcosis of Lambs

This disease, referred to as tick pyemia of lambs, is a staphylococcal infection caused by *S. aureus* and transmitted by the bites of ticks. The disease is manifested by septicemia and subsequent localization in many organs. It usually occurs in early summer in very young lambs. The symptoms are those of fulminating septicemia, arthritis, or meningitis. The organisms frequently localize in various organs, such as skin, muscles, tendon sheaths, joints, or viscera, and cause suppurative lesions. This condition seems to be limited to the lambs of Great Britain.

General Suppurative Disease

The most common form of staphylococcal infection is septicemia with or without abscess formation. It often starts as a localized wound infection or mammary infection that results in very acute septicemia, and the animal has signs of marked toxemia. There are high fever (40 to 42°C), anorexia, listlessness, weakness, prostration, coma, and death within a few days.

DIAGNOSIS

Staphylococcal infections are often diagnosed by the clinical signs and by the failure of the animal to respond to routine treatment. Clinical and laboratory findings are those of septicemic or bacterial toxemia and are not pathognomonic. A definitive diagnosis is made by isolation and identification of the organism. Staphylococci are frequently associated with other organisms in general disease processes, such as pneumonia, mastitis, dermatitis, and so on.

TREATMENT AND PREVENTION

Treatment and prevention of staphylococcal diseases are found in the article on streptococcal diseases. *Staphylococcus aureus*, however, is usually resistant to penicillin G, and a penicillinase-resistant semisynthetic penicillin, such as ampicillin or nafcillin, must be used. Other effective drugs are cephalosporin, erythromycin, vancomycin, and sulfonamides.

Bacterins and toxoids have been beneficial in preventing or decreasing the incidence of staphylococcal infections.

Swine Erysipelas

RICHARD L. WOOD, D.V.M., Ph.D.

Swine erysipelas is an infectious disease manifested by acute or subacute septicemia and chronic proliferative lesions. It is caused by *Erysipelothrix rhusiopathiae,* a gram-positive bacillus with a tendency to form elongated filaments. The organism is facultatively aerobic, weakly hemolytic, and forms tiny (0.5 to 1.0 mm) transparent colonies on solid medium. The disease it causes occurs in swine-producing areas throughout the world. Available information suggests that the prevalence of swine erysipelas in the United States has decreased since the 1950s, but the disease is still considered to be of economic importance.

Swine erysipelas appears in acute, subacute, and chronic forms. Acute erysipelas is characterized by septicemia of varying severity, usually occurring within 24 hr after exposure. Early changes involve damage to endothelium of microscopic blood vessels throughout the body, with hyaline thrombosis and deposition of fibrin in perivascular tissues. The process leads eventually to connective tissue proliferation in predisposed sites, such as synovial tissues. Subacute erysipelas is milder, with transient septicemia and local perivascular damage. Chronic erysipelas is characterized by proliferative lesions, primarily of the joints, and to a lesser extent, of the heart valves.

CLINICAL SIGNS AND PATHOGENESIS

Acute erysipelas is characterized by its sudden appearance, sometimes with sudden death of one or more pigs. Others may be noticeably sick, with temperatures of 41°C (105°F) or higher. Affected animals are depressed but irritable when disturbed. If able to get up, they move with a stiff, painful gait. Varying degrees of inappetence and firm, dry stools are usually observed. Rhomboid urticarial lesions may appear, commonly 3 days postexposure. When lesions are general, they indicate septicemia, and their intensity is related to the severity of the disease. In subacute erysipelas, clinical signs are mild. Urticarial lesions, if any, are mild, transient, and easily overlooked. Chronic erysipelas is generally characterized by signs of arthritis. Sudden death from cardiac insufficiency is infrequent. In arthritis, joints show various degrees of stiffness and enlargement, resulting in interference with function ranging from a slight limp to complete loss of use of the limb.

In uncomplicated acute erysipelas, leukopenia accompanied by a relative degree of lymphocytosis occurs during the first 3 to 5 days. Leukocytosis may be seen in some cases after several days or in cases of mixed infections. Hemoglobin and hematocrit values decrease, and sedimentation rates increase.

The characteristic rhomboid urticarial lesions of acute erysipelas are pathognomonic. Other lesions may be suggestive but are not specific, e.g., diffuse cutaneous hemostasis, congestion of internal organs, hemorrhage of gastric serosa, enlarged spleen, subcapsular hemorrhage of peripheral lymph nodes, and early proliferative synovitis. In chronic erysipelas, the predominant lesion is proliferative, nonsuppurative arthritis. Vegetative endocarditis is an occasional sign.

DIAGNOSIS

Erysipelas is most readily diagnosed by clinical and bacteriologic examinations. A presumptive diagnosis may be based on a combination of characteristic signs, e.g., a history of a few cases of sudden deaths and several other cases of fever and apparent stiffness, irritability and reluctance to move but unexpected vitality when aroused, clear and alert eyes, and characteristic rhomboid skin lesions. Hemoculture is useful in the acute form, but blood samples should be taken from more than 1 animal. At necropsy, cultures should be made from internal organs and joints. Care should be taken to avoid accidental skin infection, as the erysipelas organism is pathogenic for humans. Serologic examination by agglutination test has limited practical value; it is used primarily for detection of chronic infection. Mortality from erysipelas is usually not high, and the acute form responds well to treatment. However, chronic disease is a common sequela, regardless of the outcome of an acute or subacute outbreak.

TREATMENT

Treatment of acute erysipelas is aimed at elimination of the infection with antibiotics, sometimes in combination with hyperimmune serum (Table 1). Penicillin, to which the causative organism is highly sensitive, is generally considered the antibiotic of choice. Regimens usually involve giving penicillin with or without other antibiotics or antisera. Some practitioners favor a long-acting combination of benzathine penicillin G and procaine penicillin G administered to visibly sick animals in a single dose. Procaine penicillin G alone is sometimes given in less severe cases. Tetracycline, lincomycin, and tylosin are also used for treatment.

While visibly sick pigs are treated individually, the entire herd may be given tetracycline in the drinking water until 5 days after all signs of disease are gone. Antiserum may be used for herd treatment but is more commonly used for treatment of suckling pigs. There is no practical treatment for chronic erysipelas, but antibiotics may be helpful in early stages.

Table 1. *Common Drug Dosages of Swine*

Drug	Dose
Benzathine penicillin G and procaine penicillin G combination	5000 to 10,000 units/lb IM (single dose). *Caution:* Extra-label use. A legitimate veterinarian-client-patient relationship must exist. An appropriate, extended time period must elapse before treated animals can be used for human food.
Procaine penicillin G	3000 units/lb IM daily for not more than 4 days. Withdrawal period of 5 days.
Chlortetracycline	10 mg/lb daily in drinking water. Withdrawal period of 5 days.
Tetracycline	Dosage according to label directions. Withdrawal period of 5 days.
Oxytetracycline	Dosage according to label directions. Given in drinking water. Withdrawal period of 5 days.
Lincomycin	5 mg/lb IM daily for 3 to 7 days. Withdrawal period of 6 days.
Tylosin	100 to 200 mg/100 lb daily. Withdrawal period of 4 days.
Erysipelothrix rhusiopathiae antiserum, equine origin	Up to 50 lb, 5 to 10 ml; 50 to 75 lb, 10 to 20 ml; 75 to 100 lb, 15 to 30 ml; and 100 lb or more, 20 to 40 ml, injected into axillary space.

PREVENTION

Prevention of erysipelas is best accomplished by proper herd health management, including immunization. Replacement animals should be obtained from clean sources and should be isolated for 30 days. Chronically affected carriers should be eliminated. Sound husbandry relative to nutrition, housing, and sanitation should be practiced. Attenuated live and killed vaccines are available. A regular immunization program for both breeding and marketing animals is recommended.

Supplemental Reading

Wood, R. L.: Erysipelas. In Leman, A. D., Glock, R. D., Mengeling, W. L., et al. (eds.): Diseases of Swine, 5th ed. Ames, Iowa, Iowa State University Press, 457–470, 1981.
Wood, R. L.: Swine erysipelas—A review of prevalence and research. J. Am. Vet. Med. Assoc. 184:944–949, 1984.

Listeriosis
Circling Disease, Silage Sickness

STANLEY M. DENNIS, B.V.Sc., Ph.D., F.R.C.V.S., F.R.C.Path.

Listeriosis is an infectious disease caused by *Listeria monocytogenes*. In ruminants it is characterized by encephalitis or abortion in adults and by septicemia in fetuses and neonates. In monogastric animals, it is usually characterized by septicemia with focal hepatic necrosis. In ruminants, especially sheep, listeriosis has been called circling disease and in Iceland, silage sickness.

Listeriosis is worldwide in distribution and affects a wide variety of mammalian and avian species, including humans. It is more prevalent in temperate and cold climates.

ETIOLOGY

Four species of *Listeria* are now recognized: *L. monocytogenes*, *L. grayi*, *L. murrayi*, and *L. denitrificans*. *L. monocytogenes* is the most important species producing listeriosis in animals.

Listeria are small, motile, pleomorphic gram-positive nonsporing coccobacilli. *L. monocytogenes* is divided into at least 6 serovars with a number of subtypes. Serovars 1/2a and 4b account for 97 per cent of the isolates from animal and human diseases. Serovar 5 is a cause of sporadic or enzootic abortion in sheep and possibly in cattle. Serovars 2, 3, 4 (other than 4b), and 5 are rarely reported in the United States.

Primary isolation of *Listeria* is best accomplished under microaerophilic conditions. *Listeria* grows under a wide temperature range (4 to 44°C), with the optimum temperature between 30 and 37°C. Their ability to grow at 4°C is important diagnostically and is the basis for the "cold enrichment" method for primary isolation of *Listeria* from suspected cases of listeric encephalitis. Brain suspensions are held at 4°C and cultured weekly. This procedure is not necessary for fetal or placental tissues, as *L. monocytogenes* is present in large numbers.

EPIZOOTIOLOGY

The natural habitat of *Listeria* appears to be soil and the mammalian intestinal tract. Vegetation and silage become contaminated with soil or feces or both. Grazing animals, domestic and feral, ingest *Listeria* and further contaminate soil and vegetation, thereby establishing an ecologic listeric cycle, like *Salmonella*. Animal-to-animal transmission by fecal-to-oral route occurs (Fig. 1). Animal-to-human transmission may occur directly or indirectly via milk, meat, eggs, vegetables, and so forth. Listeriosis is more of a geonosis or saprozoonosis than a zoonosis.

L. monocytogenes has been isolated from the feces of apparently healthy animals (birds) and humans in several countries. Present evidence indicates that the majority of listeric infections are too mild to be recognized clinically or are latent.

Sporadic cases of listeric encephalitis are common and over a period of months, 5 per cent of a cattle herd or 10 per cent of a sheep flock may become infected. Listeriosis is primarily a winter-spring disease. Confined sheep and cattle, especially those fed silage, have a higher incidence than range animals. Listeriosis affects all breeds, sexes, and ages of animals.

Recovery of *Listeria* from milk of mastitic and apparently normal cows emphasizes the potential danger of milk-borne listeriosis in animal and human populations. Excretion of *Listeria* in milk is usually intermittent but may persist for periods exceeding a single lactation. *Listeria* has also been isolated from the milk of sheep, goats, and women.

The distal intestinal tract is regarded as a reservoir from which *Listeria* is able to invade tissues when the body's defense mechanisms are impaired. *L. monocytogenes* is so widespread that some consider it to be more of an epiphyte than an intracellular pathogen. The most important single cause of both clinical and nonclinical listeric infections is gross environmental contamination. *Listeria* are able to survive exposure at a wide range of ambient temperature and relative humidity, and can multiply in soil at 18 to 20°C. As a result, they are present on many types of grass, hay, and other crops. In a cool damp environment, *Listeria* can survive in organic matter for years. Their survival is good in grass, soil, and silage of near neutral pH but is poor in acid soil and good quality silage.

It is suggested that *Listeria* organisms are saprophytes living in a plant-soil environment and can be contracted by animals and humans practically anywhere. Outbreaks of listeriosis in sheep and cattle have been attributed to silage. Poor quality or poorly cured silage (pH 5.6 or greater) provides a favorable growth substrate for *Listeria* present on grass or crops. Pit silage appears to be involved more than tower-type silage, possibly by greater soil and fecal matter being introduced by tractors during filling and packing. Frequency of listeriosis tends to increase as the lower and damper layers of silage are consumed, shortly before animals are turned out to graze in spring. It is postulated that listeric-contaminated silage results in a large number of latent infections, often approaching 100 per cent of the herd or flock, but clinical listeriosis develops in only a few animals.

L. monocytogenes has high infectivity but low pathogenicity, and clinical listeric infection is usually not manifested unless the host's resistance is reduced by various stress factors, intercurrent diseases, or pregnancy. Although stress is important, certain intercurrent infections in cattle may facilitate entry of *Listeria* by damaging mucosal surfaces. Normal intestinal carriers from infected herds or flocks disseminate listeric infection to clean herds or flocks upon their introduction.

PATHOGENESIS

The initial route of exposure is probably ingestion of *Listeria*-contaminated soil, vegetation, or silage. The prevalence of encephalitis or septicemia in a group of animals during an outbreak of listeriosis under different environmental conditions suggests *Listeria* gains entry by several routes: encephalitis following minute wounds in buccal mucosa, inhalation, or conjunctival contamination and septicemia and latent infection by ingestion and inhalation. *L. monocytogenes* has a predilection to localize in the intestinal wall, placenta, and medulla oblongata.

Listeric encephalitis is essentially a local infection of the brain stem, resulting from *L. monocytogenes* ascending via cranial nerves. Susceptible animals are exposed to *L. monocytogenes* in contaminated feed, especially silage. Grass and grain awns can result in abrasions and small puncture wounds in the buccal mucosa, lips, muzzle, and nostrils. *Listeria* penetrates these tissues innervated by cranial nerves, especially the trigeminal, and centripetally migrates along one or more branches to the medulla oblongata and pons. The lesions are confined to the brain, and the clinical signs vary according to the functions of the damaged neurons. The selective localization of *L. monocytogenes* in the brain stem is often unilateral and accounts for the signs of facial paralysis and circling.

Septicemic or visceral listeriosis affects organs other than brain, and the principal manifestations are visceral lesions, especially hepatitis and placentitis with abortion. *Listeria* invading the body via the alimentary tract tend to localize in the intestinal wall, especially in Peyer's patches, and result in inapparent listeric infection and prolonged fecal excretion. In some cases, bacteremia with localization in various organs or even a fatal septicemia may develop. *Listeria* may also be excreted to the external environment in feces, milk, tears, nasal secretion, urine, and uterine discharge and perpetuate the listeric infection cycle.

The uterus of all pregnant domestic animals is highly susceptible to listeric infection, which results in placentitis, fetal death, abortion, stillbirths, neonatal deaths, and possibly viable carriers. The primary site of genital listeriosis is the placenta, which offers little or no resistance to invasion by *L. monocytogenes*. Fetal infection is secondary to placental damage and dysfunction. The uterus is extensively involved only when fetal and placental tissues are retained, and fatal listeric septicemia may follow but not when the infected uterine contents are aborted quickly and completely. Although listeric metritis is constant, it has little or no lasting effect on reproductive function, but *Listeria* may be shed for a month or more. Sporadic abortions, resulting from some stress in pregnancy and development of listeric congenital infection in individual animals, is more likely than abortions caused by a herd or flock pathogen spreading horizontally.

CLINICAL SIGNS

Listeric infection is generally associated with characteristic clinical signs: encephalitis in adult ruminants, septicemia in swine and neonatal ruminants, and abortion and

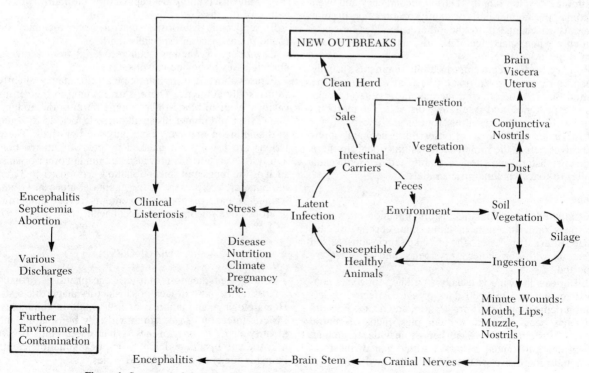

Figure 1. Summary of the animal-environment cycle of listeric infection in domestic animals.

perinatal mortality in all species, especially ruminants. Infection is more common in ruminants fed silage.

Ruminants

Encephalitis is the most frequently recognized form of listeric infection and is of economic importance. It affects sheep, cattle, goats, and occasionally pigs and generally occurs in winter and early spring. Although both sexes and all ages are affected, it is more common during the first 3 years of life. Morbidity is low, but mortality is high.

Listeric encephalitis in sheep and goats is acute, with death occurring as early as 4 to 48 hr after onset of signs, and recovery is rare. In cattle, the disease is more chronic, with most surviving 4 to 14 days. Spontaneous recovery is frequent, but long-lasting brain damage is also frequent.

Clinical signs of listeric encephalitis in ruminants are similar and differ only in severity. The incubation period is unknown, probably 2 to 3 weeks. Affected animals become depressed, disoriented, febrile, and indifferent to their surroundings, and usually separate themselves from the rest of the flock or herd. In the early stages, affected animals tend to crowd into corners and lean or push their heads against stationary objects, such as mangers and fences, as if unable to stand. Facial paralysis with drooping ear, dilated nostril, and lowered eyelid on the affected side often develops—this is more common in cattle than in sheep. Torticollis may develop. Often, intermittent twitching and paralysis of facial and throat muscles and the tongue, which usually protrudes, interfere with swallowing, resulting in profuse salivation. Marked nasal discharge and anorexia are common. Strabismus and conjunctivitis are common, and the animal may seem blind. If it walks, it stumbles and moves in circles, always in the same direction. Paralysis of limbs is progressive. In the terminal stages, the animal falls and is unable to rise without assistance. Prostration followed by coma and death may develop rapidly. During recumbency and even in coma, the animal lies constantly on one side despite attempts to change it to the other side. Deaths cease suddenly when silage feeding ends, and the sheep are turned out to pasture.

Primary listeric septicemia in adult ruminants, usually sheep, is reported in Europe but is relatively rare in the United States. The affected animals have general weakness, inappetence, and respiratory distress. The mortality is not as high as that resulting from listeric encephalitis.

Listeric encephalitis is not observed in neonatal lambs and calves before the rumen becomes functional. In these neonates, listeric infection is manifested by septicemia similar to that in monogastric animals.

Swine

Compared with ruminants, listeric infection in swine is relatively rare. It results in septicemia, encephalitis, localized internal abscesses, and pox-like skin lesions. Mixed infections with hog cholera, erysipelas, and influenza are reported.

Listeriosis in swine is usually sporadic septicemia confined to pigs less than 30 days of age. Affected piglets exhibit depression, fever, prostration, and death. Encephalitis has been reported in older pigs. Signs of central nervous system (CNS) disturbances include trembling, incoordination, caudal paralysis, stilted gait of the forelegs, and progressive weakness, followed by death.

Listeriosis in swine, either septicemic or encephalitic, usually runs a rapid and fatal course of 3 to 4 days. The majority of swine listeric infections, however, apparently do not manifest clinical signs.

Pregnant Animals

Regardless of animal species, stage of gestation, or route of infection, the uterine contents quickly become infected with *L. monocytogenes*. Most listeric abortions occur in the last trimester but may occur at any stage of gestation. Near term, the fetus may be stillborn, born alive and die in a few hours or days, or survive. No premonitory signs of abortion are observed, and most dams exhibit little or no signs of general infection and recover spontaneously. The abortion rate in sheep is reported to range from 1 to 20 per cent, with the average being about 10 per cent. Abortion in sheep occurs within 3 to 11 days after exposure, depending upon the route of infection.

NECROPSY FINDINGS

There are no gross lesions in animals dying from listeric encephalitis apart from some congestion of meningeal vessels and greater cerebrospinal fluid. Microscopic lesions are confined primarily to the pons, medulla, and anterior spinal cord. Marked perivascular cuffing of mononuclear cells and varying degrees of focal necrosis develop. In sheep and goats, neutrophils predominate in the necrotic foci, resulting in microabscesses. There are edema, hemorrhage, neuron degeneration, neuronophagia, congestion, and some thrombi. In cattle, the perivascular cuffs are smaller, and the focal lesions are usually limited to edema and small accumulations of microglial cells and lymphocytes. Rarely are lesions as extensive as those in sheep, an observation in keeping with the more chronic nature of the disease.

In septicemic listeriosis, small necrotic foci may be found in any viscera, especially the liver.

L. monocytogenes has been recovered from acute or chronic cases of bovine mastitis.

Fetuses aborting from listeric placentitis may be slightly to markedly autolytic. There is excess fluid in the serous cavities, clear to blood-tinged; some fibrin in the abdominal cavity; and numerous small necrotic foci, up to 2 mm in diameter, in the liver, especially the right half. These lesions are usually not masked by gross or microscopic autolysis. Necrotic foci may also be found in other organs, such as the lungs and spleen. Shallow erosions, 1 to 3 mm in diameter, are present in the abomasal mucosa. Gram-stained smears of abomasal contents reveal numerous gram-positive, pleomorphic coccobacilli.

DIAGNOSIS

Antemortem diagnosis of listeric encephalitis is virtually impossible because of lack of satisfactory diagnostic tests. Hematologic examination is of little value in ruminants. Listeric infection can be confirmed only by isolating and identifying *L. monocytogenes*. When encephalitis occurs in cattle and results in death, prompt examination should be made for both listeriosis and rabies.

Table 1. *Differential Diagnosis of Listeric Encephalitis*

Sheep	Cattle	Swine
Rabies	Rabies	Rabies
Polioencephalomalacia	Lead poisoning	Pseudorabies
Pregnancy toxemia	Ketosis	Hog cholera
Brain abscess	Acute gastroenteritis	Erysipelas
Gid	Aujesky's disease	Intoxication
	Viral encephalitis	Influenza
		Nutritional disturbance

Listeric encephalitis is diagnosed by typical abnormal CNS signs of circling, lateral inclination of the head, and facial paralysis. These signs, especially in sheep and cattle fed silage, suggest listeriosis.

Listeric encephalitis must be differentiated from other diseases listed in Table 1.

Listeric abortion must be differentiated from other causes of abortion, such as brucellosis, vibriosis, salmonellosis, infectious bovine rhinotracheitis, enzootic ovine abortion, leptospirosis, and parvovirus, depending upon species.

Laboratory diagnosis of listeriosis is based on isolating and identifying *L. monocytogenes*. Difficulties are often encountered in isolating *Listeria* from fresh tissues, especially brain. Directly stained smears, particularly of fetal or placental tissues, may reveal large numbers of pleomorphic, gram-positive, small rods suggestive of listeriosis. Fluorescent antibody techniques are effective for rapid diagnosis and identification of *L. monocytogenes* in smears from dead or aborted animals and from their milk and meat.

Serologic tests, such as agglutination and complement fixation, are not used routinely for diagnosing listeriosis, as they are unreliable. Enzyme-linked immunosorbent assay (ELISA) could be effective for detecting carrier cattle.

Inoculation of rabbits, guinea pigs, and mice may be used for confirming listeric isolates. Mice inoculated with bovine brain from victims suspected of having rabies that die within 48 to 72 hr should not be discarded without being cultured for *Listeria*. Intracerebral inoculation of listeric-infected material causes mice to die in 2 to 3 days, and *Listeria* can be cultured from their brains.

TREATMENT

Listeria is sensitive to ampicillin, chloramphenicol, erythromycin, gentamicin, penicillin, neomycin, and tetracycline. They rapidly become resistant to streptomycin and are resistant to polymyxin B. Ampicillin is reported to be most effective both *in vitro* and *in vivo*. Penicillin in high doses is the most economic antibiotic therapy for use in food animals.

Early treatment is essential, as animals with severe clinical signs of CNS involvement do not respond. Prognosis depends upon the duration of listeriosis prior to diagnosis, commencement of treatment, and mobility of the patient. If the animal is recumbent, treatment is of little use. Penicillin G intramuscularly (44,000 units/kg or 15 to 20 million units twice daily) for 7 to 14 days in cattle is reported to be effective. Dehydration, acid-base imbal-

ance, and electrolyte disturbance must also be corrected. Supportive therapy, such as transfer of ruminal contents, analgesics, and nursing, may be required.

Affected adult sheep seldom repond to treatment. Chloramphenicol and a combination of penicillin (300,000 units) and streptomycin (0.25 gm) have been successful in lambs with septicemic listeriosis. Penicillin G (1 to 2 million units) and gentamicin (1 mg/kg) intramuscularly, singly or in combination, have been effective in goats. Penicillin has been reported to be successful in swine.

IMMUNITY

Knowledge regarding immunization against listeriosis is scanty. Its sporadic occurrence and low morbidity have not stimulated wide study. Research has found that resistance to *L. monocytogenes* is primarily dependent on cell-mediated immunity.

Formol and heat-killed vaccines have given little protection. Viable, nonpathogenic, rough colonies of *L. monocytogenes* have been reported to give protection against challenge with virulent, smooth colonies. Living vaccines have been protective in sheep, but for public health reasons their use is not recommended.

Conclusions drawn from reports of various listeric vaccines used in feedlots with heavy sheep losses are that living or dead vaccines have no appreciable effect on the course of an outbreak or in preventing listeriosis in sheep in infected facilities.

CONTROL

Institution of control measures for infectious diseases and good hygiene are the only measures available at present. When listeriosis has broken out, affected animals should be isolated and disposed of as quickly as possible by a rendering plant, preferably by burning or by burying deeply under quicklime. Buildings housing affected animals or animals in contact with them should be thoroughly cleaned and disinfected, and all bedding and feed burned.

Reduce silage feeding and avoid feeding any spoiled silage. In affected feedlots, constant feeding of low-level doses of tetracyclines should be considered.

Animals with nonfatal listeric infections or those recovering following antibiotic therapy may be carriers for long periods and should therefore be eliminated as quickly as possible. Some lactating cows with listeric encephalitis may excrete *Listeria* via milk for long periods; such cows are a public health hazard.

Supplemental Reading

Blenden, D. C.: Listeriosis. *In* Dunne, H. W., and Leman, A. D. (eds.): Diseases of Swine, 4th ed. Ames, Iowa, Iowa State University Press, 461, 1975.

Gray, M. L., and Killinger, A. H.: *Listeria monocytogenes* and listeric infections. Bacteriol. Rev. *30*:309, 1966.

Ladds, P. W., Dennis, S. M., and Njoku, C. O.: Pathology of listeric infection in domestic animals. Vet. Bull. *44*:67, 1974.

Rebhun, W. C., and deLahunta, A.: Diagnosis and treatment of bovine listeriosis. J. Am. Vet. Med. Assoc. *180*:395, 1982.

Seeliger, H. P. R.: Listeriosis. New York, Hafner Publishing Co., 1961.

Woodbine, M. (ed.): Proceedings Sixth Symposium on Listeriosis, Nottingham, Leicester University Press, 1976.

Anthrax

ARNOLD F. KAUFMANN, D.V.M., M.S.

Anthrax is an acute infectious disease of food animals caused by *Bacillus anthracis*. The disease has a worldwide distribution and can affect a wide range of mammalian species, including humans.

B. anthracis is a member of the normal bacterial flora of numerous soil types sharing a pH higher than 6. Although naturally contaminated soil is the primary reservoir of infection, outbreaks have been traced to a variety of other sources, such as animal-origin feed and fertilizer, river water contaminated by wastes from animal-product processing, and even crops raised on contaminated soil.

Within the United States, anthrax tends to be restricted to certain regions, such as the lower Mississippi River Valley. Outbreaks, however, have occurred in virtually every state. Even in recognized areas of endemic disease, anthrax occurs very irregularly. Many years may elapse between sporadic cases and epizootics in a high-risk area. Multiple small sporadic outbreaks are reported each year in the United States, but epizootics are uncommon.

Outbreaks in grazing animals occur primarily in warm seasons of the year when the minimum daily temperature is above 16°C, but documented cases have occurred even in mid-winter in northern states. Epizootics tend to follow periods of marked climatic or ecologic change, such as heavy rainfall, flooding, or drought.

In food animals, infection usually results from ingestion of contaminated feed. Anthax is not communicable directly between animals except in instances such as swine feeding on carcasses. Transmission by biting flies can take place, but recent studies indicate that biting insects have an insignificant, if any, role in anthrax epizootics.

The attack rate in an outbreak is variable, but the case to fatality ratio is high, usually exceeding 90 per cent. Compared with cattle, sheep and goats are highly susceptible to experimental infection, whereas swine are much more resistant. Under field conditions, however, the attack rate by species on the same pasture does not necessarily correlate with relative species susceptibility, presumably because of differences in grazing patterns. Relative risk also varies with age (lambs and calves are seldom affected) and with sex (bulls are much more susceptible to infection than cows).

CLINICAL SIGNS

The incubation period of natural anthrax is typically 3 to 7 days, but it may range from 1 to 14 days or more. The clinical course is from peracute to chronic. Sudden death in animals that appeared normal a few hours earlier is common.

In ruminant livestock, the acute illness is characterized by abrupt onset of fever (temperature may rise to 42°C), variably followed by anorexia, ruminal stasis, signs of abdominal pain, hematuria, and blood-tinged diarrhea. Pregnant animals may abort, and milk production in lactating animals often abruptly declines, with milk being abnormal or blood being tinged. Subcutaneous edematous swellings may be present, particularly on the ventral aspect of the neck. Death usually occurs within 1 to 3 days after onset, with severe depression, respiratory distress, muscular tremors, and convulsions being common terminal events. Occasionally, animals survive the infection without treatment, but this is uncommon. Chronic infection rarely is found in cattle. When it is, however, it is characterized by localized edematous swelling, which can be quite extensive and most common on the ventral neck, thorax, and shoulders.

In swine, the disease is similar to that in ruminants except edematous swelling of the head and neck is much more common. The swelling may be so extensive as to interfere with breathing and swallowing. Chronic infection localized in the tonsils and cervical lymph nodes is common.

NECROPSY FINDINGS

The carcasses of animals that died of anthrax tend to putrify rapidly and develop incomplete rigor mortis. Blood may exude from the nose, mouth, and anus. The blood is dark, clots poorly, and flows freely from cut surfaces.

The lesions of anthrax result from widespread damage to the reticuloendothelial system and vasculature. In ruminants, the spleen is almost always greatly enlarged, dark, and soft. The necrotic and engorged red pulp will readily exude from incisions in the splenic capsule.

The lymph nodes, particularly in the region of the initial infection site, will be hemorrhagic and edematous. Hemorrhages of various sizes are common on the serosal surfaces of the abdomen and thorax, as well as the epicardium and endocardium. A localized to diffuse gelatinous edema is commonly present under the serosa of various organs, between skeletal muscle groups, and in the subcutis. A small amount of serous to blood-tinged fluid is usually present in the body cavities. Hemorrhages frequently occur along the gastrointestinal tract mucosa. Ulcers, particularly over Peyer's patches, may also be noted.

In swine, the lesions tend to be restricted to the tonsils, cervical lymph nodes, and surrounding tissues. The lymphatic tissues of the head and neck will be enlarged and appear a mottled salmon to a brick-red color on cut surface. Diphtheritic membranes or ulcers may develop over the pharyngeal surface of the tonsils. A thick layer of gelatinous edema generally surrounds the involved lymphatic tissues.

DIAGNOSIS

Anthrax may be confused with a wide range of diseases causing sudden death. Definitive diagnosis through isolation of *B. anthracis* from affected tissues, however, is generally not difficult.

If anthrax is suspected, complete necropsy of affected animals should be avoided to reduce environmental contamination and health risks to personnel. A small amount of blood collected aseptically from a superficial vessel such as the jugular vein is the preferred diagnostic specimen. For shipment to the laboratory, the blood can be left in the syringe, which in turn should be enclosed in a leakproof container. The blood can also be submitted to the laboratory as a dried specimen on a sterile swab or small piece of sterile cotton umbilical tape, or, if neces-

Table 1. Anthrax Vaccines

Name	Supplier	Dose	Vial Sizes
Anthrax Spore Vaccine	Colorado Serum Company Denver, Colorado 80216	1 ml for cattle, goats, sheep, swine	10 ml, 25 ml, 50 ml
Anvax	Jensen-Salsbery Laboratories Kansas City, Missouri 64141	2 ml for cattle, goats, sheep, swine	20 ml, 100 ml
Thraxol-2	Bayvet Division Cutter Laboratories Shawnee Mission, Kansas 66201	2 ml for cattle 1 ml for sheep, swine	20 ml, 100 ml

sary, as thin smears on microscopic slides. An ear from the carcass is not a desirable diagnostic specimen. In swine with localized disease, a small piece of affected lymphatic tissue that has been collected aseptically should be submitted. Tissue specimens other than dried blood should be shipped refrigerated or frozen.

Examination of blood smears from recently dead animals is used for field diagnosis but may be misleading. On Wright- or Giemsa-stained blood smears, *B. anthracis* will appear as single to short-chained bacilli with blunted ends. The presence of a capsule about the bacilli is the important distinguishing feature of the anthrax organism in such preparations. Fluorescent-antibody procedures are also used in the diagnosis of anthrax.

TREATMENT

The anthrax bacillus is highly susceptible to a number of antimicrobial agents. Under field conditions, penicillin and oxytetracycline have been reported most consistently as being therapeutically effective. The common recommended daily dose of penicillin for swine, sheep, and goats is 22,000 units/kg; the daily dose for cattle is 5 to 10 million units. Therapy should be continued for at least 5 days, and the daily dose should be administered in 2 equal parts at 12-hr intervals for the first 2 days. In severely ill animals, the initial dose should be administered intravenously.

The daily oxytetracycline dose, administered intravenously or intramuscularly, is 4.4 mg/kg for all species. The daily dose should be divided in 2 equal parts for the initial period of therapy, as with penicillin.

Antibiotics should not be administered to healthy animals recently vaccinated against anthrax. The only anthrax vaccines in common use are live spore products, which must germinate and grow in the vaccinated animal's body to provide protection. Experimental evidence indicates that concurrent administration of antibiotics and anthrax vaccine negates the protective effect of the vaccine.

Hyperimmune anthrax serum has been recommended for use in conjunction with antibiotic therapy. Such serum, however, is not available in the United States.

PREVENTION

Annual vaccination of livestock in areas of endemic anthrax is recommended. The nonencapsulated Sterne-strain vaccine is almost universally used for this purpose.

Vaccination should be done 2 to 4 weeks prior to the season outbreaks are expected. Animals should not be vaccinated within 60 days of anticipated slaughter. Antibiotics should not be administered within 7 days of vaccination.

The Sterne-strain anthrax vaccine (Anthrax Spore Vaccine, Anvax, and Thraxol-2; see Table 1) is administered subcutaneously. The dose recommended by the manufacturers varies from 1 to 2 ml. A second dose administered 2 to 4 weeks after the first dose is commonly recommended. Field evidence indicates that equal protection is given by either 1 or 2 doses. Immunity develops about 7 days after vaccination. Localized subcutaneous edema commonly develops within 24 hr at the injection site and lasts several days. This edema is rarely severe.

All outbreaks should be reported to local regulatory and public health officials. Quarantine should be placed on affected premises to prevent infected animals from being marketed. All susceptible livestock on affected and surrounding premises should be vaccinated. Prior to vaccination of dairy cattle at the time of an outbreak, the procedures required by state health authorities should be determined. Carcasses of animals that die of anthrax should be either burned completely or buried deeply (2 m of soil) to reduce environmental contamination. Covering the carcasses with a layer of quicklime (calcium oxide) at burial is often recommended; the benefit of this procedure is unknown. Bedding and other contaminated material should also be burned or buried.

Supplemental Reading

Kaufmann, A. F., Fox, M. D., and Kolb, R. C.: Anthrax in Louisiana, 1971: An evaluation of the Sterne strain anthrax vaccine. J. Am. Vet. Med. Assoc. *163*:442–445, 1973.
Lincoln, R. E., Walker, J. S., Klein, F., and Haines, B. W.: Anthrax. Adv. Vet. Sci. *9*:327–368, 1964.
Van Ness, G. B.: Ecology of anthrax. Science *172*:1303–1307, 1971.

Clostridial Bacteria and Clostridial Myositis

BENNIE G. ERWIN, D.V.M., M.S.

The control of clostridial diseases is important to the economic success of livestock owners. Clostridial diseases are infectious but not contagious. That is to say, these diseases seldom, if ever, are transmitted directly from animal to animal. Regardless of management conditions, animals are continuously exposed to clostridial organisms, which are normal inhabitants of soil and are part of the normal indigenous bacterial flora of the digestive tract of healthy animals. Clostridial diseases are, therefore, a constant threat wherever livestock are present.

Bacteria of the genus *Clostridium* have the ability to multiply only in the absence of oxygen (anaerobic environment). They survive in the soil and in the environment in the form of highly resistant spores, where they may remain infectious for many years. They are highly resistant to environmental changes and to disinfectants.

Only a few of the many clostridial species in the environment are pathogenic to livestock. The most significant are *Clostridium chauvoei (C. welchii), C. septicum, C. novyi* Type B, *C. haemolyticum (C. novyi,* Type D), *C. sordellii, C. perfringens* Types B, C, and D, and *C. tetani*. Clostridia may enter the animal's body as spores or vegetative cells through contaminated food, through inhalation, or through entrance to contaminated wounds. Circulating spores of some clostridial species may become temporarily sequestered in organs and tissues. Since spores are unable to germinate in normal tissue, they do not become involved in the development of disease until there is some type of predisposing insult to the organ or tissue in the vicinity of the bacterial spore. These insults provide the favorable environment that will support germination and continuous bacterial growth. Once a suitable anaerobic environment develops, the spore germinates into a vegetative, toxin-producing bacterial cell. A variety of potent toxins are released by multiplying clostridia. Each toxin affects its host in a rather specific manner. The actual types of toxins produced vary by clostridial species. Of greatest importance are the toxins that destroy tissue cells (necrotizing) and red blood cells (hemolyzing), and those that interrupt nerve impulses (neurotoxins). Some toxins produce their primary effect at the original site of infection. Others are disseminated by the blood stream, where they impair neurologic function or destroy tissues and organs at distant sites. The resulting clostridial diseases will be characteristic of the most proliferative clostridial species present at the site of insult. Although mixed clostridial infections can occur, in most instances 1 or possibly 2 species will predominate.

The reasons for the occurrence of a specific clostridial species in certain infection sites, such as muscle tissue, liver, and small intestine, are unclear. It may be that the specific disease-triggering mechanisms most often take place in these 3 sites and, subsequent to this, the tissues provide specific nutrients to support the growth and production of exotoxins. In most cases, these toxins cause severe necrosis that provides a suitable expanding environment for further clostridial growth. For whatever reason, it is well known that the muscle tissue is the principal infection site for *C. chauvoei, C. septicum, C. sordellii,* and *C. novyi* Type B; the liver for *C. novyi* Type B and *C. haemolyticum;* and the gastrointestinal tract for *C. perfringens* Types B, C, and D.

BLACKLEG, MALIGNANT EDEMA, AND SORDELLII OR SORD

Clostridial myositis in animals is analogous to gas gangrene in humans. Muscle tissue (primarily skeletal) is the principal site of infection for *C. chauvoei* (blackleg), *C. septicum* (malignant edema), *C. sordellii* (sordelli or sord), and occasionally *C. novyi* Type B. These pathogens may act alone or in combination with each other. On rare occasions, *C. carnis* and *C. perfringens* Type A are involved in cases of clostridial myositis. Similarities in the pathogenesis of diseases produced by these organisms provide the rationale for discussing blackleg, malignant edema, sordellii, and related diseases under the general heading Clostridial Myositis.

OCCURRENCE

Clostridial myositis occurs primarily in cattle, sheep, goats, and wildlife ruminants, and sometimes in swine and horses. Blackleg is a term primarily used to describe gangrenous myositis. Malignant edema is more likely to refer to a wound infection (myocellulitis) in which *C. septicum, C. novyi* Type B, and to a lesser extent, *C. sordellii* and *C. chauvoei* are involved. Conditions that cause muscle damage predispose cattle to clostridial myositis. These are bruises caused by butting and riding (i.e., estrus in cows and buller steers), scratches, and wounds. Under managed husbandry, conditions that may result in muscle damage are bruises from close confinement, feed bunks, shipping, and restraint in squeeze chutes, alleys, and so forth. Using a stockprod on animals or transporting them over long distances (causing muscle strain) may also trigger clostridial myositis. In the United States, sheep are quite susceptible to *C. septicum* myositis. An intestinal form of *C. septicum* gas gangrene, known as "Braxy," is found in sheep of northern European, but is uncommon in sheep of the United States. Like malignant edema, blackleg in sheep is almost always associated with wounds, such as those after shearing, docking, and unsanitary surgical procedures. At times, there are cases of clostridial myositis deaths following vaccination with contaminated needles or following the injection of products that cause tissue necrosis. A gangrenous myositis or cellulitis or both due to *C. novyi* Type B and *C. carnis* sometimes is seen in cattle and swine. *C. perfringens* Type A is a well known cause of gas gangrene in humans and may cause disease in animals at times.

These diseases affect animals without regard to age, sex, or breed. The highest incidence often occurs in animals over 3 months of age that are doing well. In the case of *C. chauvoei,* cattle apparently develop a natural resistance after 2 years of age. Such is not the case for the other clostridial diseases. Clostridial wound infections are not species specific, and it is usually impossible to differentiate the specific clostridial organism clinically or postmortem.

CLINICAL SIGNS

Clostridial myositis often escapes clinical detection, and animals are found dead. The incubation period for clostridial myositis ranges from 2 to 5 days, and the mortality rate approaches 100 per cent. In the case of blackleg, initial signs are lameness, depression, anorexia, rumen stasis, and high fever ($\geq 40°C$ or 104°F). The animal is reluctant to move. Upon close examination, a swelling of the thigh, rump, loin, shoulder, brisket, or neck can be felt. These swellings are a result of subcutaneous emphysema that crepitates when palpated. The swellings are warm initially but as the disease progresses they become cold and insensitive. The skin over these areas feels dry and is discolored. As the disease progresses, tremors, dyspnea, prostration, coma, and death from systemic toxemia are observed 12 to 24 hr after clinical signs begin.

Blackleg in sheep is less common than in cattle and is characterized by a less extensive local emphysematous-gangrenous myositis. Rams that are aggressive fighters are more susceptible to *C. chauvoei* infections.

All ages and species of animals are susceptible to *C. septicum* infections. Initially, there are high fever (often ≥ 106°F), depression, and anorexia. A rapidly spreading edema and sometimes emphysema develop around the wound. The edematous fluid is blood tinged and begins to gravitate to lower portions of the body. Animals with post-parturient genital malignant edema develop a severe depression with edema of the vulva, vagina, and uterus. The swelling may also involve the inside of the thighs and the udder. Serosanguinous fluid oozes from the vulva and often has a rancid odor. Cows or ewes with this type of infection usually die within a few hours. Phlegmon, as a result of castration, docking, or dehorning wounds, is often the result of *C. septicum* or *C. novyi* Type B contamination or both. In the case of *C. novyi* Type B, emphysema is less pronounced.

PATHOGENESIS

Autolysis and swelling of tissue begin shortly after death in animals that died from clostridial myositis. Blood-stained froth often flows from the nose and anus. The conjunctivae are severely congested.

The lesions of *C. chauvoei* are most commonly found in the large muscles of the shoulder and the hind limbs. However, lesions may be found in any striated muscle tissue, and on rare occasions the myocardium, the diaphragm, and the base of the tongue may be the primary sites of the infection. Swellings that crepitate upon palpation are more characteristic of *C. chauvoei* than of *C. septicum*. Upon excision, the subcutaneous tissue and fascia adjacent to the lesions are engorged with blood-stained fluid permeated with gas bubbles. In disease due to *C. chauvoei,* the affected muscles appear dark red and moist toward the periphery, but the center is lighter colored, drier, and porous as gas bubbles separate bundles of fibers. When squeezed, the tissue feels spongy and red fluid oozes out. The odor of the necrotic tissue is similar to that of rancid butter. In fresh carcasses, there is a definite demarcation between abnormal and normal tissues.

There are other changes in the carcass, although they are not consistent in degree and distribution. There is often severe parenchymatous tissue degeneration caused by systemically distributed toxins. It is not uncommon to find fibrinohemorrhagic pleuritis with extensive hemorrhage along the ventral borders of the lungs. The lungs may also be congested with some interstitial edema and hemorrhage. The myocardium is often pale and friable, and the endocardium of the right heart is hemorrhagic. The spleen may be normal or enlarged with a mushy type of pulp. The liver is usually pale and friable, and if autolyzed, is enlarged and very porous.

In sheep, the lesions resemble those of cattle except that crepitation is usually not as pronounced, and affected muscles are not as dry. A serosanguinous transudate is more abundant in lesions containing *C. septicum.*

Although *C. novyi* Type B is the well known cause of infectious necrotic hepatitis (black disease) in cattle and sheep, it is not unusual to find this organism as the cause of clostridial myositis. It has been identified in cases of "swell head" ("big head") in sheep and in cases of "black neck" in cattle. Clinical signs and necropsy findings are similar to those of *C. chauvoei* and *C. septicum.* This organism produces a serosanguineous, foul smelling myocellulitis. Internal organ changes are usually characterized by more edema than those with blackleg or malignant edema.

C. sordellii is an often overlooked, extremely pathogenic organism that produces a highly lethal protoplasmic exotoxin. It also produces lecithinase and hemolysin. In cattle and sheep, the clinical signs and gross pathology are consistent with those of clostridial myositis. However, the *C. sordellii* toxin is more toxic and deadly than the other clostridial myositis toxins. Infection due to *C. sordellii* is always fatal. *C. sordellii* has been isolated and incriminated in cases referred to as black neck syndrome, a malady that seems to be prevalent in feedlot cattle that bruise their necks and briskets in crowded feed bunk conditions. Although not proved, cases of "enterotoxemia," presumably caused by *C. sordellii*, have been reported. Horses are susceptible to *C. sordellii*, and the disease is characterized by massive local tissue reaction, high fever, severe toxemia, and death.

Clinical signs of *C. sordellii* in cattle are obscure because there is no notable rise in body temperature. Anorexia, tissue swellings, lameness, and toxicosis usually develop, but these signs are not observed until the patient is terminally ill. Most animals do not develop tissue emphysema because death is sudden. Rapid respiration is observed during the terminal phase, and death occurs with no agonal struggling. In the terminal stage, there may be hemolysis of red blood cells, but hemoglobinuria is seldom, if ever, observed. Death takes place within 24 to 48 hr after vegetative cells begin to produce toxins.

Gross necropsy findings of animals that died of *C. sordellii* infection include (1) massive subendocardial hemorrhages in the left ventricle but not the right ventricle, (2) submucosal congestion and sometimes hemorrhage throughout the trachea and bronchi, (3) an enlarged hemorrhagic thymus, (4) perirenal edema that extends into the pelvic inlet, (5) hemorrhage of the calyces of the kidney without blood or hemoglobin in the urine, (6) congestion of the parietal surface of the abomasum, reticulum, part of the rumen, and omentum, (7) hemorrhagic edema with little emphysema involving the tissue and lymph nodes adjacent to the lesions, (8) reddened serosal surface of the abdominal wall and contiguous musculature, (9) soft and friable spleen, and (10) edematous lungs at times with serosanguinous fluid in the thoracic and abdominal cavities.

DIAGNOSIS

The specific diagnosis of clostridial myositis in the field and in the laboratory is difficult because the various organisms produce similar clinical signs and pathology. Field diagnosis based on clinical signs is seldom possible because of the peracute nature of the diseases. Diagnosis is usually based on postmortem findings and laboratory studies. Unless the carcasses are fresh, differential diagnosis of the specific clostridial species involved is difficult or impossible because postmortem decomposition is particularly rapid when clostridial organisms are involved. In addition, clostridial toxins are rapidly destroyed during autolysis.

An accurate history, a systematic postmortem examination, a clear and concise description of the pathologic lesions, and the selection of appropriate samples that are carefully taken, properly preserved, packed, and quickly shipped to the laboratory are of great value for accurate diagnosis. It is important to establish the specific cause of death so that suitable prophylaxis can be initiated to protect the remainder of the herd.

Two to three impression smears on clean, glass microscopic slides should be made from the lesions. It is essential to get tissue smears and not just fluid on the slides. Such smears should be collected at the periphery of the lesion, air-dried, and properly labeled. Tissue specimens should also be collected, placed in a leak-proof container, and labeled. Blood and body fluids, which may be helpful to the laboratory, can also be collected in sterile containers. It is important to prevent multiplication of contaminating bacteria during shipment; therefore, the samples should be kept cold (use cold packs or crushed ice). Dry ice can be used if the samples are to be in transit more than 48 hrs.

Differentiation of various pathogenic and related species of *Clostridium* is based on fluorescent antibody (FA) staining, cultural characteristics, spore shape and position, and, if appropriate, serologic specificity of the toxin or somatic antigens. Specific FA reagents are available for identification of *C. chauvoei, C. septicum, C. sordelli,* and *C. novyi* Type B. It is well to remember that laboratory personnel do not diagnose; they identify and classify organisms from the samples provided.

PREVENTION

The need for immunization against all clostridial diseases is of critical importance because (1) clostridial spores are ubiquitous and reside within the animal's body, (2) the presence of spores within the animal does not stimulate a naturally acquired immunity to the vegetative forms of the organism or to the toxins they release, and (3) activated clostridia produce death before a protective response can be mounted.

Bacterin toxoids and toxoids are available for immunization against common clostridial diseases. Two doses are required for greater assurance of protection against all clostridial agents except possibly *C. chauvoei*. Multivalent bacterin toxoids are available that contain antigens against 2 or more clostridial species, including *C. chauvoei, C. septicum, C. novyi, C. sordellii,* and *C. perfrigens*. Animals can be vaccinated at any age; however, those less than 3 to 4 months old should be revaccinated at weaning. The duration of immunity is not long-lived, and booster vaccinations every 6 to 8 months greatly reduce the risk of death to these highly fatal diseases.

Carcasses should be removed by the rendering works, buried, or burned to minimize soil contamination with clostridial spores.

TREATMENT

Clinically ill animals, if observed, should be separated from healthy animals and treated with antibiotics, such as penicillin and tetracyclines. When appropriate, supportive therapy, such as fluids and vitamins, should be administered. Treatment should be repeated daily until the body temperature remains normal for 48 hr. Unvaccinated healthy animals should be vaccinated as soon as possible, and the owner should be advised that there may still be some loss for 10 days to 2 weeks, which is the approximate time to produce immunity after vaccination.

Supplemental Reading

Amstatz, H. E.: Bovine Medicine and Surgery and Herd Health Management, 2nd ed. Santa Barbara, American Veterinary Publications, Inc., 1980.

Blood, D. C., Radostits, O. M., and Henderson, J. A.: Veterinary Medicine, 6th ed. London, Bailliere Tindall, 1983.

Jubb, K. V. F., and Kennedy, P. C.: Pathology of Domestic Animals, 2nd ed. New York, Academic Press, 1970.

Mims, C. A.: The Pathogenesis of Infectious Diseases, 2nd ed. New York, Academic Press, 1982.

Williams, B. M.: *Clostridium myositis* in cattle: bacteriology and gross pathology. Vet. Rec., *100*:89–91, 1977.

Clostridial Hepatitis Black Disease and Bacillary Hemoglobinuria

BENNIE G. ERWIN, D.V.M., M.S.

Two highly fatal clostridial diseases for which the liver is the principal site of infection are black disease and bacillary hemoglobinuria. Black disease (infectious necrotic hepatitis) is caused by *Clostridium novyi* Type B, while bacillary hemoglobinuria (redwater disease, icterohemoglobinuria) is caused by *C. haemolyticum (C. novyi* Type D). Similarities in the bacteriologic properties and the pathogenic characteristics of these pathogens make it practical to discuss black disease and bacillary hemoglobinuria as a disease complex.

OCCURRENCE

Black disease occurs primarily in cattle, sheep, and wildlife ruminants. It is less common in swine and is only rarely observed in other species. Bacillary hemoglobinuria usually affects cattle, but may affect sheep and wildlife ruminants. Both diseases occur in animals of all ages, breeds, and sexes, although the highest incidence is in animals more than 4 months old. In the case of bacillary hemoglobinuria, adult cattle seem to be the most susceptible. The potential for disease is always present, irrespective of geographic location or season, since the causative bacteria are members of the normal flora of soil and the digestive tract and are shed in the feces of healthy animals. There is probably no area within the United States or the Western Hemisphere that is exempt from these 2 clostridial diseases. However, these diseases are more likely in cattle and sheep consuming forage in poorly drained or irrigated areas that are infested with snails, the intermediate host for liver flukes.

Spores of *C. novyi* and *C. haemolyticum* survive for long periods in contaminated soil or in bones of carcasses of previously diseased animals. These diseases are probably carried from one area to another by being shed in feces or urine of cattle and sheep with inapparent infections. Spores can also be transported by water, by migration of carrion-eating predators, and by vehicles used to transport livestock or feed.

Sudden outbreaks of disease and heavy losses can take place when infected cattle are moved to uninfected areas. When apparently healthy, nonvaccinated cattle from an infected area are moved and mixed with uninfected indigenous cattle, disease can develop in both the indigenous and nonvaccinated cattle. These types of outbreaks are probably due to organisms being shed in feces and urine of the transported cattle that were under stress either during or after shipment.

PATHOGENESIS

The disease is spread by ingestion of spores in contaminated food and water. Spores are moved from the gastrointestinal tract to body tissues and organs. Both bacteria have been isolated from the livers of healthy cattle and sheep. Prerequisites for development of disease are a susceptible host, the presence of spores, and an initial inflammation or necrosis in the liver that results in the formation of a hypoxic milieu favorable for spore germination and growth of toxin-producing vegetative cells. Vegetative cells release toxins that cause further necrosis of surrounding hepatic tissue, thus allowing extension of the infection. Some of the more common causes of the initial hepatic insult are (1) parasite migration, such as that of common liver fluke, *Fasciola hepatica,* (2) telangiectasis (sawdust liver), (3) liver abscesses, (4) chemicals, (5) fatty changes, (6) traumatic injury, (7) plant toxins, and (8) bacterial hepatitis.

Bacillary hemoglobinuria can be induced by intentionally damaging the liver (i.e., taking a liver biopsy from cattle raised in an area where the disease was endemic), thus supporting the belief that disease results from activation of *C. haemolyticum* spores present in the liver.

The principal exotoxins produced by strains of *C. novyi* Type B are the highly necrotizing lethal alpha toxin and a necrotizing and hemolytic beta toxin not usually formed in lethal amounts. *C. haemolyticum,* however, produces large amounts of a highly lethal beta toxin (phospholipase C). Although the alpha toxin of *C. novyi* Type B sometimes causes gas gangrene, its primary pathologic effect is damage to the capillary endothelium, resulting in extensive infiltration of fluid into connective tissue, i.e., edema. Accumulation of gas is seldom marked unless the infection is well advanced. In contrast, the lecithinolytic beta toxin of *C. haemolyticum* is responsible for the marked intravascular hemolysis of red blood cells. FA conjugates prepared from *C. novyi* Type B antisera cross-react with *C. haemolyticum;* however, there is no known cross-immunity between them.

A reproducible *C. haemolyticum* intrahepatic challenge procedure for cattle has been described by Erwin. Briefly, this open-surgery technique for intrahepatic inoculations of spores, suspected in 40 per cent calcium chloride as the hepatic debilitant, simulates concurrent hepatic necrosis and viable spores presence, a condition that apparently exists in the induction of bacillary hemoglobinuria and black disease in cattle and sheep under natural conditions. This same method has been used effectively to experimentally induce black disease in cattle.

CLINICAL SIGNS

Deaths from acute to peracute forms of black disease usually occur without clinical signs. The duration of illness ranges between 60 and 120 hr, and the mortality is high (> 90 per cent). The clinical signs in cattle and sheep are similar when they are present. Illness is initially characterized by central nervous system (CNS) depression. Body temperature may or may not be elevated. Appetite is poor, rumination is slow or nonexistent, respiration is rapid, and affected animals tend to remain segregated from the rest of the herd and are reluctant to move. When forced to move, they are inclined to lag behind, or they may temporarily appear to act normal. As the disease progresses, anorexia and depression are worse. Severely depressed animals may stand over water and periodically drink small amounts. The consistency of the feces may be normal or watery, but seldom, if ever, bloody. Animals in advanced stages of disease often appear heavily tranquilized and display varying degrees of hyperpnea or dyspnea or both, which in many cases is accompanied by an expiratory grunt. Death is apparently due to respiratory failure and toxemia. It usually occurs without struggling, even when respiration is severely distressed. The course of the disease in those animals showing overt clinical signs is seldom more than a few hours. With black disease, the red blood cell counts (RBC), white blood cell counts (WBC), packed cell volume (PCV), and hemoglobin (Hb) levels are usually elevated. Elevated PCV and Hb values correspond with the degree of dehydration as the disease progresses.

The duration of illness in cattle with bacillary hemoglobinuria is usually quite short (18 to 36 hr). Mortality is high ($\geq$ 95 per cent), and animals with peracute infections usually die before clinical signs are observed. When clinical signs are observed, onset is sudden. There is early evidence of CNS depression and anorexia. Affected animals often stand apart from others with head extended and back arched, and grunting is often evident when animals are forced to walk. Rumination, lactation, and sometimes defecation cease. Early body temperatures are usually elevated 40 to 41°C (104 to 106°F) but decline to normal or subnormal before death. Initially, breathing is rapid and shallow, becoming more distressed as the disease ensues. Small amounts of bright red blood may be observed in the external nares, and as breathing becomes severely impaired, blood tinged froth may ooze from the nostrils and mouth.

In animals that survive 24 hr or more, one of the most characteristic signs of bacillary hemoglobinuria is the passing of port wine–colored urine (hemoglobinuria). At this time, the urine is strongly positive for albumin but is usually negative for ketones and sugar. By the time hemoglobinuria is observed, 30 to 50 per cent of the circulating red blood cells have been hemolyzed. RBC, Hb, and PCV levels may drop to less than 4 million/mm³, 4 gm/100 ml, and 20 per cent, respectively. The clinical signs that accompany these low hematologic values are anemia and icterus, the intensity of which increases as the number of red blood cells decreases. Jugular vein pulsations are often present in anemic animals, the blood is thin (watery) and coagulates slowly. Extravasation of plasma into tissue spaces, especially the subcutaneous tissue in ventral areas of the body, is sometimes observed in advanced cases. Not uncommonly, the feces become soft, bile-stained, and bloody. Death is apparently due to hypoxemia and respiratory failure.

NECROPSY FINDINGS

Lesions in cattle and sheep that die of black disease are not well defined because postmortem decomposition is rapid. In fresh carcasses, there may be varying degrees of subcutaneous edema, especially in the sternal area. The subcutaneous tissues may have a dark appearance due to seepage of blood from the damaged capillaries. This finding, which is more pronounced in sheep than in cattle, has given rise to the name black disease. A straw-colored gelatinous exudate may be observed along fascial planes in the muscles covering the abdomen, thorax, and neck.

The peritracheal tissue, from the pharynx to the thoracic inlet, is usually congested but not necessarily hemorrhagic in animals dead less than 2 hr. In animals that have been dead more than 2 hr, these same tissues often appear to contain extensive hemorrhage owing to postmortem changes. The accumulation of black, bloody fluid has given rise to the name "black neck." This finding is usually due to imbibition of blood from damaged capillaries into the tissues of the neck that are undergoing early postmortem autolysis. These areas of blood imbibition may occur in other body parts, such as the flanks and thighs. Other bacteria, such as *C. sordelli, C. chauvoei, C. septicum, C. carnis, C. perfringens* as well as *C. Novyi* and a variety of other nonpathogenc anaerobes, are often isolated either singly or in combination from carcasses that appear to have died of "black neck." It is well to remember that black neck, irrespective of its cause, is of diagnostic value only when it is accompanied by microscopic evidence of tissue damage (necrosis), vascular thrombi, hemolyzed erythrocytes, some leukocyte infiltration, and a positive identification of the actual etiologic agent in the affected tissue. However, in fresh carcasses it is not uncommon to find congestion and hemorrhage in the thymus gland and prescapsular and peripharyngeal lymph nodes. There is also little or no evidence of gas in body tissues by *C. novyi* Type B unless putrefaction is advanced.

In the abdominal cavity, the parietal peritoneum and omentum are usually severely congested. The perirenal fat is congested and often edematous. The kidneys are usually normal in appearance, and only rarely does the urine contain hemoglobin or blood. The peritoneal, pleural, and pericardial cavities contain serosanguineous fluid. Subendocardial hemorrhages in the left ventricle are common. The endocardium of the right ventricle is often congested and stained with hemoglobin but is not

hemorrhagic. The spleen may be enlarged and contain subcapsular hemorrhage. The adrenal glands are enlarged, congested, and hemorrhagic, and lack consistency. Small areas of congestion, petechiae, and suffusive hemorrhages may be present in the serosa of the intestinal tract.

The liver is usually enlarged, dark brown to mahogany, with small areas (1 to 8 cm in diameter) of necrosis on the capsular surface. The liver should be sliced carefully in several directions to find these focal areas of necrosis, which are gray, yellow, or occasionally dark red. Areas of necrosis that are slightly larger, conical in shape, light in color, and surrounded by a zone of hyperemia are sometimes seen. These necrotic areas are similar to the large and usually single anemic liver infarct described in animals that have died of bacillary hemoglobinuria. There is sometimes evidence of fluke infestation in the form of migration tracts or parasites or both in the bile ducts.

The principal lesions associated with bacillary hemoglobinuria are liver necrosis and hemoglobinuria. However, about 30 per cent of the cattle that die of peracute disease have poorly defined liver lesions and no hemoglobin in their urine; consequently, these cases are indistinguishable from those of peracute or acute black disease. Cattle that survive long enough to develop anemia are relatively easy to diagnose at necropsy. The most common and characteristic necropsy lesion is an anemic infarct in the liver, which is considered to be pathognomonic. It is uncommon to find more than 1 infarct, and it may be found in any part of the liver, ranging from 5 to 30 cm in diameter. The infarct is pale, conical in shape on cut surface, and surrounded by a reddish zone of congestion. It is composed of necrotic tissue, the core of which may be liquified, with thrombi in large vessels at its apex. The gallbladder is usually filled with dark-colored granular appearing bile, and there is generalized icterus. Adult flukes may be found in bile ducts. The spleen is usually enlarged and often shows subcapsular hemorrhages. The kidneys may or may not have petechiae. The urinary bladder contains dark-red urine. In pregnant females, the uterus has serosal hemorrhages, and the amniotic fluid is red. Most of the lymph nodes in the abdominal cavity are either severely congested or hemorrhagic. The parietal and visceral peritoneums usually are observed to have petechial, ecchymotic, or suffusive types of hemorrhages. Serosanguineous fluid is present in the peritoneal, pleural, and pericardial cavities. Changes in the gastrointestinal tract range from mild inflammation of the mucosal lining to hemorrhage into the lumen of the large and sometimes small intestine.

In the thoracic cavity, the trachea and bronchi are frequently filled with a blood-tinged frothy exudate. Various degrees of hyperemia, hemorrhage, interstitial edema, and emphysema are observed in pulmonary tissue, especially in the dorsal parts of the lung. The cardiac musculature is congested, and the left ventricle generally is found with subendocardial hemorrhages.

DIAGNOSIS

A diagnosis of black disease or bacillary hemoglobinuria can be made in animals that have clinical signs or postmortem lesions or both that are typical of the disease. However, peracute infections may be difficult to diagnose because of similarities in gross pathology. In deaths from peracute infections, the veterinarian must rely on the aid of diagnostic laboratory test results in an attempt to make a final diagnosis. Appropriate specimens from a recently dead animal should be collected, including tissues showing pathologic lesions, blood, and exudates from the peritoneal, thoracic, or pericardial cavities. These should be submitted with a detailed history and a concise description of necropsy findings to the laboratory personnel. Also, air-dried blood smears, impression smears from the periphery of liver lesions, and a smear from the cut surface of the spleen are of value for aiding in diagnoses of these diseases. If samples cannot be delivered directly, they should be shipped cold or frozen.

Laboratory-assisted diagnosis depends upon isolation and identification of the actual causative organism. FA tests are useful for identification of *C. novyi;* however, the demonstration of *C. novyi* by FA techniques must be interpreted with caution, since many animals carry these organisms as part of their normal flora, and after death they multiply appreciably and can be demonstrated by FA with ease. FA conjugates prepared from *C. novyi* Type B will cross-react with *C. haemolyticum* (*C. novyi* Type D). Thus, a positive FA test does not differentiate *C. novyi* Type B from *C. haemolyticum.* Unless extensive biochemical and toxin identification tests are carried out, *C. novyi* Type B and *C. haemolyticum* are indistinguishable. FA tests are quite useful in differentiating clostridial diseases with signs and pathology that are similar to those of black disease and bacillary hemoglobinuria.

PREVENTION

Black disease and bacillary hemoglobinuria can be prevented by vaccination. Commercial bacterins are available against *C. novyi* Type B and *C. haemolyticum (C. novyi* Type D). For primary immunization, 2 doses 3 to 4 weeks apart are required. Duration of immunity against these diseases is not well established. Based on field information, both naturally acquired immunity and vaccination acquired immunity are apparently short lived (4 to 6 months). Animals can be vaccinated at any age; however, those less than 3 to 4 months old should be revaccinated at weaning. Because of the relatively short duration of immunity, animals should be revaccinated every 5 to 6 months. Unvaccinated cattle should not be mixed with cattle from an endemic area and should not be transported to endemic areas.

TREATMENT

If treatment is attempted, affected animals should be given penicillin or tetracycline to control the infection and fluids either intravenously or intraruminally to combat dehydration. Cattle with bacillary hemoglobinuria may be given blood transfusions, which should be given slowly and repeatedly if necessary. Affected animals should be handled carefully to avoid excitement. Other supportive therapy includes the parenteral administration of vitamins, especially those containing liver extracts, and possibly iron.

Supplemental Reading

Erwin, B. G.: Experimental induction of bacillary hemoglobinuria in cattle. Am. J. Vet. Res. 38:1625–1627, 1977.
Macheak, M. E.: Clostridial diseases of cattle. Vet. Med. Small Anim. Clin. 73:195–200, 1978.
Nillo, L., Dorward, W. J., and Avery, R. L.: The role of *Clostridium novyi* in bovine disease in Alberta. Can. Vet. J. 10:159–169, 1969.
Smith, L. D. S., and Jasmin, A. M.: The recovery of *Clostridium haemolyticum* from the livers and kidneys of apparently normal cattle. J. Am. Vet. Med. Assoc. 129:68–71, 1956.
Williams, B. M.: *Clostridium oedematiens* infections (black disease and bacillary hemoglobinuria) of cattle in mid-Wales. Vet. Rec. 76:591–596, 1964.

Enterotoxemia
(Clostridium perfringens)

DEAN H. SMITH, D.V.M., M.S.

Clostridium perfringens is the causative organism of a number of animal diseases, usually lumped together as enterotoxemia, although a variety of signs and lesions may occur. Enterotoxemia is an acute, infectious, noncontagious disease that apparently originates in the gut and often affects apparently healthy animals on full feed. It is caused by several toxigenic types of the anaerobic spore-forming bacterium *C. perfringens,* which has worldwide distribution. The disease affects many species of animals and is economically important in cattle, sheep, goats, and swine.

Five types of *C. perfringens* are known to infect food animals. These are designated as Types A, B, C, D, or E, depending upon specific toxin production. Types C and D are of major concern in the United States, while Types A and E are of limited concern. Type B is not known to be a problem in the United States. All types have certain common characteristics. The bacteria are often found in small numbers in the intestinal tracts of healthy individuals. They cause problems only when conditions permit a dramatic increase in their population and the intestinal environment becomes favorable for toxin production. Infections tend to recur on the same premises, a trait common to all related groups of anaerobic spore-forming pathogens.

Clinically the *C. perfringens* types differ in the signs and lesions they cause and are described separately. The elements of diagnosis, treatment, and prevention, however, will be presented together because of their similarity for all types.

TYPE A ENTEROTOXEMIA

The occurrence of Type A enterotoxemia is sporadic. It usually occurs in the spring in lambs and calves less than 3 months of age. Faster gaining animals are most often infected, and the disease is more severe in lambs than in calves. Morbidity varies widely, sometimes reaching 30 per cent or more, while mortality approaches 100 per cent. Alpha toxin is produced in abundance and results in massive intravenous hemolysis and destruction of capillary walls principally in the thoracic and abdominal cavities. Clinically different Type A infections also appear in piglets and chicks.

Clinical Signs

Clinically, Type A enterotoxemia in lambs is characterized by severe anemia followed by icterus and a rapid course from onset to termination. Icteric discoloration is visible on all exposed mucous membranes and is responsible for the term "yellow lamb disease." The initial sign, colic, is followed by an interruption of gastric activity. Erythrocyte count and packed cell volume drop precipitously, and the blood serum is icteric or blood tinged. Marked hemoglobinuria appears near the termination of the clinical disease, and mortality can reach 100 per cent. In cattle, the signs, lesions, and mortality are much less severe. In piglets, Type A infection has a low morbidity, low mortality, slowly developing arthritis, and keratosis that are associated with a high protein diet.

Findings

In lambs, changes observed at necropsy are thin watery blood, generalized icterus, and severe hemoglobinuria. The kidneys are dark brown in color and soft in consistency. Excess amber or blood tinged fluid is often present in the body cavities. The kidneys, liver, and spleen are congested, and there may be multiple suffusion type hemorrhages on these organs as well as on the heart. In cattle the lesions are less severe, and both morbidity and mortality are lower than in lambs. In swine, an arthritic-keratotic disease persists over a period of weeks to months with the ultimate development of joint deformities.

TYPE B ENTEROTOXEMIA

"Lamb dysentery" is a highly fatal disease of lambs caused by C. perfringens Type B. Also affected are calves and foals less than 3 weeks of age. It has been reported from England, Europe, South Africa, and the Near East, but has not been reported from the United States, Australia, or New Zealand.

Since C. perfringens Type B produces all 3 major lethal toxins, the clinical signs and lesions of Type B enterotoxemia can resemble other C. perfringens infections, and accurate determination can be made only by isolating and identifying the causative organism.

Clinical Signs

Death may supersede the development of any clinical signs. Animals that develop clinical signs stop nursing and are listless and recumbent. A fetid diarrhea is produced that may become blood tinged shortly before death. Death is usually in a few hours, but some individuals survive for several days. Mortality approaches 100 per cent.

Necropsy Findings

There is severe inflammation of the intestine. Ulcerated and necrotic areas are found in the walls of the small and large intestines. These areas are typically surrounded by hemorrhagic zones that form composite lesions typical of this disease. The colon mucosa is often highly inflamed. Mediastinal lymph nodes are enlarged and edematous, and the liver is enlarged and friable.

TYPE C ENTEROTOXEMIA

C. perfringens Type C causes an acute hemorrhagic enteritis with high mortality in calves, lambs, and piglets less than 2 weeks old. The disease also affects chickens and kids. The young animals are almost always offspring of high-producing mothers. Older cattle and sheep on full feed are also infected. The disease in sheep is termed "struck" and was first described in England. Type C infections have since been found in sheep and other species throughout the world.

Very young animals seem to become infected at or shortly after birth. Those few diseased individuals that survive do not gain normally and may eventually die. The disease in the very young is not well unerstood but may result from the ingestion of a large quantity of milk, which provides a favorable environment for rapid multiplication of C. perfringens Type C.

Clinical Signs

Death often occurs before any clinical signs of disease. Before death, animals show evidence of abdominal pain and depression. They become listless, and the young stop nursing. Animals that survive for a time may have bloody diarrhea and central nervous system (CNS) involvement.

Necropsy Findings

Both alpha and beta toxins are produced by Type C. Clinical and postmortem changes are dependent upon the amount of each toxin produced and the length of illness. Should alpha toxin predominate, extensive hemorrhage will occur in the small intestine and mesenteric lymph nodes, and the jejunum and ileum will consistently show extensive hemorrhage and blood stained intestinal contents throughout the lower intestine and colon. If beta toxin is present in pathogenic amount, there will be necrosis of the intestine and peritonitis. This lesion is often seen in piglets. Petechiae will be found on the heart, spleen, thymus, and serosal surfaces. There may also be edema and neuronal degeneration in the brain.

TYPE D ENTEROTOXEMIA

"Overeating disease" caused by C. perfringens Type D is of considerable economic importance in feedlot cattle, although cattle are less often affected than goats or sheep. Type D enterotoxemia is a common disease of unvaccinated feeder lambs and older animals on full grain rations. Single lambs less than 12 weeks of age nursing high-producing ewes are most often involved, but twins are seldom involved, since they are not receiving the same high nutritional diet.

In feeder animals as the ratio of concentrate to roughage becomes high, the pH of rumen content becomes low. Fermented grain passes into the small intestine, and the clostridial pathogens multiply with subsequent toxin production. Type D C. perfringens produces alpha hemolytic toxin and the predominating epsilon toxin that, when trypsinized in the small intestine, causes necrosis. Epsilon toxin increases vascular permeability, resulting in hemorrhage and edema in the tissues. The epsilon toxin acts as an initial stimulant to the CNS but ultimately produces soft foci and liquefaction necrosis in the brain tissue. The lesions apparently arise from vascular permeability and edema.

Clinical Signs

The clinical signs of this disease are similar in all species of animals. In a majority of cases, animals previously thought to be healthy are found dead. Affected animals consistently have a history of full feed diets or of nursing high-producing dams. Feeder lambs have been observed to drop to the ground, convulse, and die within minutes. Those that survive for a time usually lie on their sternum with the head held back and to one side. Animals that remain on their feet may circle. There is usually a mild temperature rise of 2 or 3 degrees accompanied by drooling. Diarrhea may or may not be present. Some animals with protracted diarrhea recover after about 1 week. Posterior paralysis may occur, followed by coma and death in 8 to 12 hr. Sudden external stimuli may provoke convulsions and opisthotonos.

Necropsy Findings

Observable lesions depend upon the length of the illness. Individuals that die suddenly usually have a rumen and abomasum filled with concentrated feed. Petechial and ecchymotic hemorrhages occur on the serosal surface of the rumen, abomasum, and duodenum and may appear on the diaphragm and abdominal muscles. There is excess pericardial fluid, and hemorrhages may occur on the epicardium and the endocardium. These hemorrhages are often more severe in the left ventricle. The abdominal and duodenal mucosae are inflamed. There is excess fluid in some portions of the small intestine, particularly in the ileum. Intestinal lymph nodes are swollen and reddened. Animals that survive for a time accumulate fluid in the lungs and develop focal necrosis and edema of the brain.

Tissues of animals that die from overeating disease tend to decompose rapidly. This is especially noticeable in the kidneys of sheep, a change that accounts for the name "pulpy kidney disease" that has been applied to this condition.

TYPE E ENTEROTOXEMIA

Type E enterotoxemia is a rare disease of calves that has been reported from the Barkly Tablelands in Northern Territory of Australia. The disease has symptoms similar to Type C enterotoxemia, and postmortem examination reveals hemorrhagic enteritis and separation of the intestinal mucosa from the submucosa.

Quite probably, Type E enterotoxemia involves both alpha and iota toxins. Alpha toxin produces hemorrhages, and iota toxin is a necrotoxin that can be activated from its prototoxin form by proteolytic enzymes in the gut. Type E strains of *C. perfringens* were isolated from kidneys but not from the gut of animals that died of the disease.

DIAGNOSIS OF ENTEROTOXEMIA

Sudden and unexplained death of apparently healthy young calves, lambs, pigs, or of older animals on full feed is sufficient reason to suspect enterotoxemia. Examination of stained smears of intestinal content selected from several locations along the intestine will often aid the diagnostician. Replacement of normal intestinal bacteria flora by large numbers of gram-positive rods, occurring singly or in short chains, is presumptive evidence of enterotoxemia. Hypoglycemia and glycosuria are inconsistent changes but are an aid to diagnosis when present. Laboratory assistance is essential to determine the *C.*

perfringens type that is involved. This can be done either by isolation and identification of the organisms or by identifying the toxin present in the small intestine. Intestinal contents (fluid) should be removed shortly after death and placed in a container and refrigerated. The toxin is fragile and will disappear within a few hours unless this is done. One drop of chloroform added to approximately 10 ml of sample will aid in stabilizing the toxin. Toxin shipped to the laboratory should be kept cold. Specific typing antisera are available for laboratory animal protection tests or for intradermal toxin neutralization procedures.

Acute bloat, thromboembolic meningoencephalitis (TEME), polioencephalomalacia (PEM), and acute poisoning can appear quite similar to enterotoxemia. Animals dying from bloat usually have a distended rumen containing frothy material, and there will be engorgement of the superficial blood vessels, especially in the anterior parts of the body. Animals with TEME and PEM usually live longer and at necropsy have gross and microscopic changes. The availability of toxic material and chemical analysis will help determine poisoning cases. The cardiac form of white muscle disease can be confused with enterotoxemia but can be differentiated by gross lesions at necropsy.

Type A enterotoxemia may resemble subacute or chronic copper poisoning. It can also be confused with leptospirosis and bacillary hemoglobinuria. Liver levels below 150 ppm on a wet-weight basis will eliminate copper poisoning as a diagnosis. Serologic tests on several animals in the herd and histopathologic changes will differentiate leptospirosis. Bacillary hemoglobinuria can be eliminated as a cause if a typical liver infarct is not present.

TREATMENT AND PREVENTION OF ENTEROTOXEMIA

Animals with clinical cases of enterotoxemia respond poorly to treatment. Once sufficient toxin is produced, the course of the disease is usually irreversible. Antitoxin can be given intravenously, and antibiotics can also be given.

Losses in feed lots can best be controlled by reducing the concentrate in the ration and by increasing the roughage. Economic factors sometimes make this course of action unacceptable. Immunization of all animals with Type C and D toxoids before they enter the feed lot is effective. Two injections administered 2 weeks apart will normally protect individuals through the feeding period.

Protection of newborn animals can be provided by vaccinating the dam 2 to 3 months prior to parturition and again 3 to 5 weeks later with Type B, C, and D toxoids. Annual booster injections administered thereafter previous to parturition will maintain protection to offspring through the colostral milk. Passive immunity can be provided offspring of nonimmunized dams by parenteral injection of hyperimmune serum at birth. This protection lasts for about 3 weeks, a critical period for many outbreaks, especially those caused by *C. perfringens* Type B. Active immunity can then be produced by the administration of toxoid.

Type A *C. perfringens* is a poor antigen, and effective biologics are not available. Outbreaks must be controlled by changes in management practices.

Supplemental Reading

Jensen, R., and Mackey, D. R.: Diseases of Feedlot Cattle, 3rd ed. Lea & Febiger, Philadelphia, 1979.

Martin, W. B.: Diseases of Sheep. Boston, Blackwell Scientific Publications, 1983.

Niilo, L., Harries, W. N., and Jones, G. A.: *Clostridium perfringens* Type C in neonatal calves in Alberta. Can. Vet. J. *15*:224–226, 1974.

Smith, L. D. S.: The Pathogenic Anaerobic Bacteria, 2nd ed. Springfield, Illinois, Charles C Thomas, 1975.

Salmonellosis

CLAIR M. HIBBS, D.V.M., Ph.D.
and GEORGE A. KENNEDY, D.V.M., Ph.D

Salmonellosis is a ubiquitous disease affecting nearly all species of vertebrates. It is caused by a large number (more than 1500) of serotypes of *Salmonella* spp., which are gram-negative, pleomorphic, motile, aerobic and facultative anaerobic rods that produce potent tissue-damaging toxins. Clinically, the disease may be systemic or enteric and may be acute or chronic. The disease tends to occur in the very young, the debilitated, or the very old, although any animal may be affected.

Carriers that do not appear ill are common in all species, which makes salmonellosis difficult to control. Carrier animals that are hauled or stressed shed organisms more readily. Concentrated animal populations and poor sanitation also enhance the maintenance of this organism in the environment. Salmonellae may survive in soil or stagnant water for several months. The organisms survive freezing but are readily inactivated by heat and sunlight.

Mortality and morbidity may be quite high, depending on type of husbandry techniques, weather, other environmental circumstances, and concomitant diseases. There seems to have been an increase in the number of cases of salmonellosis in recent years. This can probably be attributed to more concentrated husbandry and better diagnostic capabilities. Contaminated water, feed, pasture, and carrier animals are all possible sources of the organism. Liquid slurries from manure pits are excellent sources for contamination of pastures and other fields.

Transmission is usually by ingestion of live organisms. The organisms are facultative, intracellular organisms that can invade cells and localize in lymphoid tissue and in macrophages of the reticuloendothelial (RE) system. As salmonellae die or are killed, endotoxin is released, often resulting in endotoxic shock. Other disease producing agents are frequently associated with salmonella infection. In fact, salmonellae are frequently opportunistic pathogens secondary to primary disease.

Some *Salmonella* spp. are nonhost-adapted, while others are quite specifically host-adapted. *S. typhimurium*, the most commonly isolated serotype from all animals, is an example of a nonhost-adapted serotype. *S. choleraesuis* and *S. typhisuis* are common disease pathogens of swine only, whereas *S. dublin* is a rare disease pathogen of ruminants.

CLINICAL SIGNS

Pigs

Salmonellosis can occur in all ages of pigs but is most likely to occur in weanling or feeder pigs. The clinical signs may vary from peracute septicemia to chronic enterocolitis. It is not a common problem in nursing pigs but occasionally is a cause of diarrhea, septicemia, and even abnormal central nervous system (CNS) signs. In piglets, depression and rapid death are the main features, but enteritis, particularly necrotic enteritis, may be a feature. Laboratory identification methods are necessary to differentiate *Salmonella* spp. from *Escherichia coli*, intestinal viruses, coccidia, streptococci that cause septicemia, or *Clostridium perfringens* Type C.

Septicemic salmonellosis is generally due to *S. choleraesuis*. It occurs mainly in weanling or young feeder pigs and frequently follows some form of stress. Fever, depression, prostration, and sudden death are characteristic of the acute septicemic form. Pigs may huddle together, as if cold. Reddish or purplish skin blotches that blanch on pressure are a common but nonspecific sign of septicemia. Abnormal central nervous system (CNS) signs owing to meningitis or encephalitis or both may occur in a variable number of pigs. Diarrhea is usually not a prominent feature of septicemic salmonellosis. Mortality is high, but morbidity tends to be lower than with the enteric forms.

Acute enteric salmonellosis is characterized by watery to mucohemorrhagic, fetid diarrhea along with fever, weakness, and anorexia. Shreds of fibrin, sloughing mucosa, and some fresh blood are often present in the feces. Morbidity and mortality may be high. Many survivors of the enteric form will be unthrifty and may remain carriers. Rectal stricture syndrome may also be a sequel to enteric salmonellosis. *S. typhimurium* is the most common cause of enteric salmonellosis in swine and probably the sole cause of rectal stricture syndrome.

The chronic enteric form is not uncommon and may or may not follow an outbreak of the acute enteric form. It is characterized by persistent watery, yellowish diarrhea, unthriftiness, and intermittent fever. Growth of recovered pigs may remain permanently stunted.

Differential diagnosis of septicemic salmonellosis should include hog cholera, erysipelas, streptococcal septicemia, edema, and pseudorabies. For the enteric form, swine dysentery, necroproliferative ileitis (campylobacteriosis), and whipworms need to be diagnostically differentiated. Mixed infections are common.

Cattle

Samonellosis affects both dairy and beef cattle. It is more difficult to strictly categorize the disease in cattle as systemic or enteric, since in any given case one form may merge into the other, particularly in calves. Prevalence of the various serotypes changes with different geographic localities, but *S. typhimurium* tends to be common worldwide. *S. newport* and *S. dublin* are also important in cattle but tend to have more patchy distribution. *S. dublin* seems to be spreading in the United States, and recovered cattle have a greater tendency to remain as chronic carriers of *S. dublin* than other serotypes.

Acute salmonellosis is more common in dairy than beef calves. It usually does not occur in calves less than 2 weeks old. However, it has been reported in beef calves on pasture and in calves less than 1 week old. A common history includes a moderately high incidence of intractable diarrhea with some deaths, and calves continue to develop the disease over an extended period. The initial fever may or may not have subsided by the time the calf is examined. The temperature commonly drops upon initiation of diarrhea. Extreme weakness is often a prominent sign. The most characteristic feature is brownish, watery diarrhea with shreds and flakes of fibrin and sloughing mucosa, and streaks of fresh blood. Meningitis, polyarthritis, and pneumonia may occur in septicemic cases. In the enteric form, most calves will be terminally septicemic, and those that survive may remain unthrifty.

Sources of infection may be carrier animals or newly purchased calves, contaminated feed, water, or bedding. Hauling, lack of colostrum, and cold or wet weather are often predisposing factors.

Signs in adult cattle are acute illness with depression, fever, cessation of milk flow, and severe diarrhea. The stress of parturition can be a precipitating factor. The diarrheic feces tend to be fetid and watery, and contain mucus, fibrinous casts, and sometimes considerable quantities of fresh blood. Persistent diarrhea and unthriftiness characterize the more chronic syndrome. Pregnant animals may abort. Abortion is more commonly associated with *S. dublin* than with other serotypes. The disease may become enzootic on some premises, particularly dairies.

Salmonellosis in the feed lot may occur at any time during the fattening period. It generally appears soon after cattle arrive in the feedlot, owing to the stresses encountered in shipping. It has been noted that feeding green chopped alfalfa and green chopped corn may enhance the disease. A sudden onset of semifluid to mucohemorrhagic diarrhea accompanied by depression, fever, and weakness is characteristic. The character of the diarrhea may mimic bovine viral diarrhea (BVD) or coccidiosis.

Differential diagnosis includes colibacillosis and viral diarrhea in calves; and pasteurellosis, BVD, Johne's disease, coccidiosis, parasites, and certain poisonings in older calves and adults.

Blood studies may reveal leukopenia early in the course of the disease, but there are no consistent clinicopathologic findings.

Sheep and Goats

Salmonellosis is most frequent and is economically most important in feeder lambs. It is found in ewe and lamb flocks as the septicemic or enteric form and may cause abortions. The aborting ewe is usually sick at the time. Feeder lambs generally are affected soon after arrival at the lot. There is watery diarrhea that often contains mucus and streaks of blood. Fever and depression are less specific features. Twenty-five per cent or more of the lambs may be affected, and mortality may be high. Salmonellosis must be differentiated from coccidiosis. Coccidiosis is more common, tends to appear 1 to 3 weeks after arrival, and commonly causes more blood in the feces.

Blood in feces of salmonella affected goats may or may not be a prominent feature of the diarrhea. It has been reported in neonatal kids, older nursing kids, and adults. Coccidiosis, parasitism, and enterotoxemia must be included in the differential diagnosis.

NECROPSY FINDINGS

No gross lesions can be considered pathognomonic, but some may be highly suggestive. Ingestion of the organism is followed by invasion of the intestinal epithelial cells and a subsequent localization in the RE cells of the lymphoid follicles of the digestive tract. The high concentration of lymphoid tissue in the ileum, cecum, and colon predisposes these areas to severe lesions. Cellular invasion, elaboration of an *E. coli*–like enterotoxin, and a cytotoxin are speculated to be involved in the pathogenesis of the lesions. Depending on various factors, such as serotype and host resistance, the organisms may remain localized in the intestinal mucosa and mesenteric lymph nodes or gain entrance to the blood and become disseminated. Invasion of epithelial and RE cells is followed by multiplication of the organisms and an acute inflammatory reaction with vascular damage, thrombosis, hemorrhage, and necrosis. Pneumonia frequently appears after systemic invasion; thus in systemic salmonellosis the lungs are often a tissue of choice for culturing salmonellae. The stomachs of monogastric animals generally have reddened mucosae, while the abomasums of ruminants may or may not have reddened mucosae. Miliary foci of necrosis and inflammation are rarely observed grossly in the liver but are frequently observed histologically. Occasionally, there is edema of the gallbladder wall.

Splenic enlargement is a common finding in swine and may occur in ruminants but not as consistently. There is usually generalized lymphadenopathy in systemic cases, and in enteric cases the mesenteric lymph nodes are consistently enlarged and frequently hemorrhagic. In pigs, petechial hemorrhages may be present on the cortical surface of the kidneys ("turkey egg kidney") and on the mucosal surface of the urinary bladder. Serosal hemorrhages may be found on any of the visceral organs.

Intestinal changes are generally confined to the ileum, cecum, and colon. This can be an important point of differentiation, as swine dysentery owing to *Treponema* is always confined to the cecum and colon. The mucosal surface may vary from red to grayish yellow. The latter is associated with the more chronic form of the disease. Pseudomembranes, ulceration, serosanguineous material, and whitish flecks of fibrin and sloughing mucosa, sometimes forming casts of the intestinal lumen, are observed within the intestines. The intestinal wall may become thickened and rigid, especially in pigs, giving rise to the term "garden hose gut." In these cases, necroproliferative ileitis caused by *Campylobacter sputorum* is the main cause. Septic polyarthritis is a less frequently observed lesion.

Lung, tied-off sections of affected intestine, and mesenteric lymph nodes have been the most productive tissues for recovery of salmonellae. These organs are followed, in frequency of successful isolations, by liver, spleen, and kidney. Thinly sliced pieces of tissue should also be submitted in 10-per cent buffered formalin for histologic examination. Histologic lesions are suggestive but not specific for salmonellosis. On the other hand, simply isolating a salmonella from tissues is not proof of its involvement in the animal's illness.

PREVENTION

Salmonellae are widespread in the environment, and clinically normal carriers do occur; thus prevention is not always easy. Prevention of the disease involves considerable labor and dedication on the part of both owner and veterinarian. Common medical sense should prevail. Closed herd operations are best when possible. Quarantine of replacement stock for 2 to 4 weeks is helpful but is not 100 per cent effective owing to carrier animals. Many cases occur as a result of exposure of susceptible animals to carriers; therefore purchase of replacement stock from herds with no history of salmonellosis is helpful.

It is advisable to purchase feed stuffs from reputable manufacturers and dealers. Dried milk, meat scraps, bone meal, and other animal or fish products are potential sources of salmonellae unless properly processed. Forages and grains are not generally a source of salmonellae, but contaminated haylage has been a source.

Effluent from human sewage is an excellent origin of salmonellae. Some rural homes have effluent discharging directly into lots or fields. Two severe cases of salmonellosis in beef calves, investigated by one of us, involved household effluents running into the calving areas.

Vaccination as a preventive may have value in some situations. Commercial *S. typhimurium* and *S. dublin* bacterins are available. Autogenous bacterins have been used with limited success. Live vaccines have reportedly good success in the United Kingdom, and research using metabolically altered strains is promising.

Livestock owners with infected animals should use precautions when disposing of infected carcasses, so as to prevent contamination of barns, pens, and equipment. Several years ago, one of us performed a bacteriologic survey of a horse slaughter plant. Salmonellae were isolated from the holding pens, sewer drain, shackle hooks used to transport carcasses, doorway to the cooler, boning knives, and other areas and objects. This demonstrates the importance of careful prevention of contamination. There are numerous reports of different ways of spreading salmonellae by contaminated equipment. Cleaning and disinfection will help to prevent spread of the organism. The common phenolic-, chlorine-, and iodine-based disinfectants are all effective.

TREATMENT

Basically, therapy of animals with clinical salmonellosis involves the use of antibiotics, supportive measures, good nursing care, good hygiene, and if possible, separation of the sick from the healthy.

The role of antibiotics is controversial, as they apparently do not eliminate the carrier state and may contribute to the development of antibiotic-resistant strains. Furthermore, the results are often disappointing, particularly if not instituted early in the course of the disease. Experimental studies in swine suggest that continuous inclusion of an antibiotic in the feed to which the resident salmonellae are susceptible should reduce the prevalence and severity of the disease, although it may not affect the infection rate and may be of little benefit if initiated once clinical signs have appeared.

In clinically ill animals, the usual approach is to administer antibiotics orally and, when feasible, parenterally. When dealing with the septicemic form and treating the animal with oral antibiotics, a drug that is absorbed and reaches effective blood levels should be used. The choice of antibiotics should be based on sensitivity tests and approval for use in food animals. When sensitivity results are not available, the choice should be one of the drugs usually effective against salmonellae. This may vary in different geographic locations. In our laboratory, antibacterial drugs to which currently there are the fewest resistant strains of salmonellae are ampicillin, gentamicin, trimethoprim-sulfadiazine, and nitrofuran. Strains resistant to neomycin, tetracycline, and sulfa are becoming more common. Carbadox, a synthetic antibacterial compound, has been shown to diminish the extent and severity of enteric lesions induced by salmonellae but has the disadvantage of a 70-day withdrawal period and is not absorbed from the intestine. In our laboratory, we have been finding greater numbers of strains showing in vitro resistance to carbadox.

In most herds, individual parenteral treatment is difficult to administer, and medication via the water source is most practical. Medicated water is better than medicated feed, as ill animals will generally continue to drink but will reduce feed intake greatly.

When conditions permit, individual treatment may be practical, and parenteral antibiotics and fluids to combat dehydration are indicated. Management manipulations that reduce stress and fecal-oral contamination will be helpful. Strict sanitation to lower exposure is frequently the most beneficial treatment and preventive measure. Switching to an easily digestible, higher roughage ration is sometimes of benefit. Culling chronically unthrifty animals is a useful management procedure, as these animals often remain sources of environmental contamination.

PUBLIC HEALTH CONSIDERATIONS

Salmonellosis is reported to be the most important animal-borne bacterial infection of humans. Most serotypes are infective for humans; even such animal-adapted strains as *S. choleraesuis* and *S. dublin* can be serious pathogens for humans. The disease usually takes the form of gastroenteritis, but systemic disease with fatalities have occured. Human salmonellosis may be contracted by direct or indirect contact with actively or latently infected animals, their excreta, or their food products. Human to human transmission is also important.

The stress of being shipped to slaughter often increases fecal shedding in latent carriers. This and constant recontamination of holding pens at slaughter facilities can result in widespread contamination of carcasses and food products. More often, food products become contaminated by breakdown in hygienic precautions at the time of processing, display, preparation, or storage.

Poultry and poultry products are considered the most frequent animal source of human infection but other meats, particularly pork, are also frequently incriminated. Even some smoked and cooked meat products may harbor salmonellae. Milk is less frequently a problem, as pasteurization destroys the organism.

Although cases of clinical salmonellosis have not been found to be more prevalent in livestock owners or their families than in other families, the potential danger needs to be recognized by attending veterinarians when dealing with suspected or confirmed cases of salmonellosis. Cases of serious salmonellosis in veterinarians are documented.

Supplemental Reading

Bulgin, M. S.: *Salmonella dublin*: What veterinarians should know. J. Am. Vet. Assoc. *182*:116–118, 1983.

Bulgin, M. S., and Anderson, B. C.: Salmonellosis in goats. J. Am. Vet. Med. Assoc. *178*:720–723, 1981.

Galton, M. M., Smith, W. V., McElrath, H. B., and Hardy, A. V.: Salmonella in swine, cattle, and the environment of abattoirs. J. Infect. Dis. *95*:236–245, 1954.

Hibbs, C. M., and Foltz, V. D.: Bovine salmonellosis associated with contaminated creek water and human infection. Vet. Med. Small Anim. Clin. 59:1153–1155, 1964.

Lindberg, A. A., and Roberston, J. A.: S. typhimurium infection in calves: cell-mediated and humoral immune reactions before and after challenge with live virulent bacteria in calves given live or inactivated vaccines. Infect. Immun. 41:742–750, 1983.

Mair, N. S., and Ross, A. I.: Survival of Salmonella typhimurium in the soil. Mon. Bull. Minist. Health 19:39–41, 1960.

Morehouse, L. G.: Salmonellosis in swine and its control. J. Am. Vet. Med. Assoc. 160:593–602, 1972.

Smith, B. P., Habasha, F. G., Reina-Guerra, M., and Hardy, A. J.: Immunization of calves against salmonellosis. Am. J. Vet. Res. 41:1947–1951, 1980.

Wilcock, B. P., Armstrong, C. H., and Olander, H. J.: The significance of serotype in the clinical and pathological features of naturally occurring porcine salmonellosis. Can. J. Comp. Med. 40:80–88, 1976.

Wilcock, B., and Olander, H. J.: Influence of oral antibiotic feeding on the duration and severity of clinical disease, growth performance, and pattern of shedding in swine inoculated with Salmonella typhimurium. J. Am. Vet. Med. Assoc. 172:472–477, 1978.

Wray, C., and Sojka, W. J.: Reviews of the progress of dairy science; bovine salmonellosis. J. Dairy Res. 44:383–425, 1977.

Swine Dysentery

ROBERT D. GLOCK, D.V.M., Ph.D.

Swine dysentery (bloody scours) is a common diarrheal disease in swine-rearing areas throughout the world. It is feared by swine producers because it is easily transmitted and tends to cause long-term economic losses. Exact incidence is not known because of a current lack of reliable methods for determining whether there may be carrier animals in a particular herd. However, some estimates place the infection rate at up to 40 per cent of the swine herds in the United States.

The term swine dysentery refers to a specific disease. The primary causative agent and the key to transmission of the disease is an anaerobic spirochete, Treponema hyodysenteriae. Other gram-negative, anaerobic bacteria, which are normally present in swine intestines, may play a synergistic role in the pathogenesis.

Mechanisms of pathogenesis in swine dysentery have not been clearly defined, but T. hyodysenteriae are located deep in crypts and often invade in or through the epithelial layer of the large intestine. Systemic invasion is not characteristic, and the effects on the host are usually the result of the severe dysentery resulting from enteritis diffusely affecting the large intestine.

CLINICAL SIGNS

All ages of swine are susceptible to swine dysentery, but pigs in the postweaning and early fattening periods are most frequently affected. The disease is seen only occasionally in suckling pigs. Deaths of unknown peracute pathogenesis are infrequently encountered. These pigs usually have typical enteric lesions but may die prior to the onset of diarrhea. Clinical signs in most pigs begin as mucoid diarrhea that often progresses to dysentery with excess blood, mucus, and fibrin in the feces. Initially, flecks of blood may be found scattered in the mucoid feces. If the disease progresses, the blood may be thoroughly mixed in watery feces. Abdominal pain and dehydration cause a very gaunt, arched-back appearance.

The diarrhea and anorexia result in depletion of serum electrolytes, metabolic acidosis, and some deaths. However, the majority of economic losses are the result of reduced performance, cost of continuous medication, and loss of breeding stock markets.

DIAGNOSIS

It is important to recognize that there are many causes of diarrhea or dysentery. A diagnosis of swine dysentery should include an appropriate history such as the recent movement of swine into a clean herd. Previously infected pigs may have no clinical signs until after the stress of movement, environmental change, or altered feeding routine. The incubation period of swine dysentery may range from 2 to 3 days to a number of months, depending on the amount of exposure and the condition of the host pig. Some swine apparently carry the disease without showing any clinical signs. However, clinical signs often appear within 1 to 2 weeks after exposure.

Clinical signs of dysentery with blood in the feces may be caused by other diseases, such as salmonellosis, trichuriasis, and necroproliferative enteritis (intestinal adenomatosis). Gastric ulcers can also cause blood-stained feces, although the feces are usually darker in color and more firm than those of swine dysentery.

Necropsy of an acutely affected pig may be essential. Specific lesions of swine dysentery are limited to the large intestine, which is usually hyperemic and often edematous. The mucosa is diffusely inflamed, swollen, and covered by variable combinations of mucus, fibrin, blood, and some cellular debris, depending on the stage of development of the disease. The lesions of salmonellosis differ because they may be found in other parts of the intestine or in other organs. The best differential diagnostic procedure for trichuriasis is to inspect the cecal and colonic mucosa for the parasites. Necroproliferative enteritis is differentiated by type of lesions and the location of the lesions in the small intestine.

Laboratory aids to the diagnosis of swine dysentery may include visual examination of mucosal scrapings (or dysenteric feces) by darkfield or phase microscopy to identify numerous large, motile spirochetes with tapered ends. These can also be identified by smears stained with crystal violet or Victoria blue 4-R, and they can also be visualized on histologic sections of the large intestine by using silver stains. The intestine has characteristic diffuse lesions of edema, crypt dilation, superficial erosion, and mucosal hyperemia. The reliability of these presumptive diagnostic aids is jeopardized by the fact that nonpathogenic spirochetes, T. innocens, may rarely be found in large numbers in pigs without swine dysentery.

Definitive diagnosis of swine dysentery is based on isolation and identification of T. hyodysenteriae from colonic mucosal or rectal swabs. Trypticase soy agar with 5-per cent bovine blood and 400 µg/ml of spectinomycin may be streaked, incubated anaerobically at 42°C, and examined for the presence of typical complete hemolysis. Specimens submitted for culture should be kept cool and moist but not frozen. It is important to also culture for Salmonella spp. Combinations of infections with swine dysentery, salmonellosis, and trichuriasis are not uncommon, so the mere presence of one organism does not exclude the presence of others.

Table 1. *Some Drugs Commonly Used for Treatment of Swine Dysentery**

Compound	Dose	Duration (days)	Control or Preventive Level	Withdrawal Time (days)
Bacitracin	1 gm/gal water	14	250 gm/ton feed	0
Carbadox	50 gm/ton feed	Continuous	50 gm/ton feed	70
Dimetridazole†	0.025% in water	5	100 gm/ton feed	ND‡
Furazolidone	300 gm/ton feed	14	100 gm/ton feed	0
Gentamicin†	50 mg/gal	3–5	ND	ND
Ipronidazole†	0.005% in water	7	50 gm/ton feed	ND
Lincomycin	0.025% in water	10	ND	6
	100 gm/ton feed	21	40 gm/ton feed	6
Neomycin	300 gm/ton feed	3–5	ND	20
Ronidazole†	0.006% in water	3–5	60 gm/ton feed	ND
Sodium arsanilate	4.5 grains/gal water	5–7	ND	5
	90 gm/ton feed	5–7	90 gm/ton feed	5
Tiamulin	0.006% in water	5	25 gm/ton feed	ND
Tylosin	0.25 gm/gal water	3–10	100 gm/tn feed	0 (feed), 2 (water)
	1.0–4.0 mg/lb (injectable)	1–3	ND	4
Virginiamycin	100 gm/ton feed	14	25 gm/ton feed§	0

*Modified from Harris, D. L., and Glock, R. D.: Swine dysentery. *In* Dunne, H. W., and Leman, A. D. (eds.): Diseases of Swine. Ames, Iowa, Iowa State University Press, 441, 1981.
†These compounds were not approved for administration to swine in the United States at the time this table was compiled.
‡Not determined.
§Up to 120 lb of body weight.

Detection of individual carrier animals is very difficult, but rectal swab cultures and serologic tests on specimens from numerous animals have some promise as methods of determining carrier animals in the herd.

CONTROL

After establishing a diagnosis of swine dysentery, medication in the feed or water is recommended. In a very acute outbreak, medication of water is preferred because of reduced feed consumption by sick pigs. Parenteral treatment with drugs, such as tylosin or lincomycin, is also useful in some cases. Initial medication can then be followed by the use of therapeutic or control levels of medications available as feed additives. The disease is likely to persist in infected premises, so it is frequently necessary to medicate continuously or, at least, repeatedly. Table 1 lists some drugs commonly used for treatment of swine dysentery.

It is imperative that pig comfort and sanitation be given primary attention in any control program. There is a direct correlation between levels of contamination and severity of the disease.

PREVENTION

The most important consideration in prevention of swine dysentery is to maintain a closed herd. Any new stock should be purchased from a reliable supplier who can provide a history free of swine dysentery. Any new arrivals should be isolated and observed for several weeks before entry into the main herd. If diarrhea should occur, cultures should be analyzed to determine if *T. hyodysenteriae* is present. It is also imperative that animals be transported in a truck that has been thoroughly cleaned.

T. hyodysenteriae can survive for at least a few days in moist, cool feces, so infection can also be easily transmitted by fomites, such as truck tires and boots. The organisms can survive passage through the digestive tracts of dogs. This has not been proved to be a common method of transmission, but it is a potential hazard. Mice have been shown to be long-term carriers of infection.

It may be wise to use preventive levels of medications (Table 1) in situations where animals of unknown origin are combined with the herd, or where previously contaminated facilities are used. Survival times of *T. hyodysenteriae* range from a few hours or less on clean, dry surfaces to a number of weeks in cool, moist feces. Survival time in anaerobically stored wastes may be quite long.

Supplemental Reading

Harris, D. L., and Glock, R. D.: Swine dysentery. *In* Dunne, H. W., and Leman, A. D. (eds.): Diseases of Swine. Ames, Iowa, Iowa State University Press, 541–553, 1975.
Kinyon, J. M., Harris, D. L., and Glock, R. D.: Enteropathogenicity of various isolates of *Treponema hyodysenteriae*. Infect. Immunol. *15*:638–646, 1977.
Kinyon, J. M., and Harris, D. L.: *Treponema innocens*, a new species of intestinal bacteria, and emended description of the type strain of *Treponema hyodysenteriae*. Internat. J. Systemic Bact. *29*:102–109, 1979.
Songer, J. G., Kinyon, J. M., and Harris, D. L.: Selective medium for isolation of *Treponema hyodysenteriae*. J. Clin. Microbial. *4*:57–60, 1976.

Swine Proliferative Enteritis

(Necroproliferative Enteritis, Intestinal Adenomatosis, Hemorrhagic and Bloody Bowel Syndrome, Terminal and Regional Ileitis, and Necrotic Enteritis)

HAROLD J. KURTZ, M.S., D.V.M., Ph.D.

Swine proliferative enteritis is a disease of pigs that has been recognized in the swine producing areas of the United States as a serious entity for at least a decade. This infectious intestinal disease appears to be rising in incidence in the heavily concentrated swine producing areas of the United States. The disease is present in other parts of the world, and the first extensive research and subsequent publication of data about this syndrome were in Scotland. The disease has also been investigated in Sweden, Australia, Denmark, Taiwan, and other countries. Enteric swine disease has been given a number of eponyms, but it is generally agreed to be a disease with a variety of pathologic syndromes. It has numerous clinical signs and this fact has led to the various names that appear in the medical literature.

Swine proliferative enteritis is characterized as a non-septicemic disease with pathologic lesions confined to the lower half of the small intestine and, occasionally the cecum and spiral colon. Although the mesenteric lymph nodes and the mesentery are edematous, this observation is not pathognomonic for the syndrome. Enteric disease usually exhibits an incidence of between 1 and 10 per cent of the affected herd, although it is reasonable to suggest that there is probably 100 per cent morbidity with all animals in the herd infected as carriers of the organism. The pathogenesis of the disease is related to secondary stress factors that allow the organism to invade the intestinal mucosa and produce characteristic lesions. These stressful situations are transportation, breeding, nutritional changes, environmental changes, and other secondary intestinal pathogens.

The disease affects weaned pigs of all ages, including sows and boars. Minnesota investigators have discovered that the majority of adult pigs carry antibodies against the *Campylobacter* organisms, and the antibodies decay to undetectable levels in the nursing pig when it reaches approximately 4 weeks of age. This may explain why the disease rarely, if ever, occurs in young nursing pigs but occurs in feeder pigs. The cause of porcine proliferative enteritis is generally accepted to be *Campylobacter (Vibrio) sputorum* subsp. *mucosalis.* Recently another organism (*C. hyointestinalis*) has been associated with the disease. There are other distinct species in the intestinal microflora of the pig (*C. jejuni* and *C. coli*). *C. coli* is thought to be nonpathogenic. All of the 4 species can be separated by cultural and biochemical characteristics. A University of Minnesota research group used the direct fluorescent antibody technique and showed that the infected intestinal epithelial cells contain both *C. sputorum* subsp. *mucosalis* and *C. hyointestinalis.*

Attempts to consistently reproduce the disease under experimental conditions have been disappointing. Perhaps this is due to the inability to define the factors that potentiate the predisposition of the disease in the pig experimentally. It is possible that these pigs may have specific antibodies that prevent the organism from gaining entry into the intestinal epithelial cell.

CLINICAL SIGNS

The clinical forms of this disease fall into 3 main categories. The peracute form is characterized by massive hemorrhagic diapedesis into the terminal portion of the small intestine. Whole blood migrates from the lower small intestine into the large bowel and, if the pig survives for a sufficient time, whole blood will be passed with the stool. The pigs with this form of the disease usually have a high mortality rate, and death occurs with relative suddenness. The causes of death in cases of the hemorrhagic form are anemia and hemorrhagic shock. This form of the diseae is seen most frequently in adult animals, and stress factors may be estrus or pregnancy. Boars that are breeding sows may hemorrhage profusely, and pregnant sows may abort owing to severe anemia resulting from intestinal hemorrhage. Occasionally, this type of clinical form is seen in feeder pigs approaching market weight.

The second clinical form is that of mucohemorrhagic diarrhea. This form of the disease is common in feeder pigs, and fresh blood in the stool is not a consistent finding. Usually 10 per cent of the herd may be showing signs of diarrhea, although the incidence may be as high as 80 to 100 per cent. These animals show contraction of the abdominal and lumbar areas with a rough hair coat. Feed efficiency is decreased, and some anorexia is observed. Pigs may die during this phase of the disease, but usually death is delayed until the chronic phase has passed. The chronic phase of the disease is characterized by a fibrinonecrotic enteritis with numerous diphtheritic casts present in the lumen of the lower intestinal tract. Animals with the disease have a chronic watery diarrhea, which is usually very odoriferous. The animals in the chronic phase of the disease are very thin and usually die from malabsorption syndrome. The clinical pathogenesis of the affected animals may include anemia, neutrophilia, or hypoproteinemia, depending upon the stage of the disease. Animals with the disease are not generally pyrexic unless there are secondary infections.

NECROPSY FINDINGS

Pigs dying as the result of a hemorrhagic episode of swine proliferative enteritis usually have large colons full of clotted blood. The gross appearance of the animal with a pale carcass indicates severe anemia. The serosal surface of the lower small intestine may show thickening with a reticulated edematous surface. When the intestinal lumen is opened, there may or may not be gross evidence of a thickened mucosa. If one examines the ileum microscopically, there is always a proliferation of the epithelial cells in the ileal mucosa. Occasionally animals dying from hemorrhage will have a dilated small intestine which has no gross evidence of thickening. The usual lesion in the feeder pig is a thickened lower small intestinal wall. When the intestine is incised and the mucosa examined, one may see a polypoid-like proliferation of the mucosal surface. The changes are characterized histologically as severe proliferation of the intestinal mucosal cells, especially those cells lining the intestinal crypts; hence the term "intestinal adenomatosis" (these lesions will occasionally mimic the lesions of intestinal adenoma).

The chronic phase of the disease is characterized grossly as a fibrinonecrotic, ulcerative, terminal ileitis. The lower portion of the small intestine is usually dilated and filled with a diphtheritic cast, and the colon is filled with a watery type of fluid that contains remnants of necrotic intestinal mucosa. The terminal portion of the small intestinal wall may be very thin due to the necrosis of the mucosa, and histologically, the only remnants of mucosa remaining are the deeper crypts beneath the ulcerated surface. The animals are very thin and are sometimes referred to as having "necro-gut."

DIAGNOSIS

The diagnosis of swine proliferative enteritis is based upon the postmortem lesions. The important differential diagnoses that one must consider include the following: gastric ulceration, swine dysentery, trichuriasis, salmonellosis, volvulus, and acute hemorrhagic enteropathy of unknown causes. The definitive diagnosis is based on pathologic findings. The affected portion of the terminal small intestine has characteristic proliferation of the mucosal epithelial cells, but one must use the Warthin-Starry silver stain in order to visualize the *Campylobacter* organisms intracellularly. These organisms are present in the epithelial cells of the thickened and corrugated mucosal glands. They are usually numerous in the cytoplasm of the intestinal epithelial cell. Specific fluorescent antibody studies can be used to identify the organism either as *C. sputorum* subsp. *mucosalis* or as *C. hyointestinalis*. A competent microbiologist can isolate either of these organisms from the scrapings of the mucosal surface, but special techniques must be employed to grow and identify these microaerophilic organisms. Frozen or fresh ligated segments of ileum may be submitted to the laboratory staff for culture. Submission of sections in formalin for histopathologic examination is essential.

Serologic studies indicate that infected animals may have low antibody titers to the organism, but diagnoses based on serologic findings are tenuous.

TREATMENT

Evaluation of the therapeutics for controlling this disease is hampered by inconsistent experimental reproduction. Numerous antimicrobial agents have been evaluated *in vitro* for their effectiveness against field isolates of *C. coli*, *C. sputorum* subsp. *mucosalis*, and *C. hyointestinalis*, using agar dilution techniques. The following agents were most efficacious *in vitro*: carbadox, furazolidone, ampicillin, nitrofurantoin, gentamicin, and dimetridazole. Some of the least useful drugs in this trial were the sulfa drugs, novobiocin, vancomycin, cycloheximide, bacitracin, arsanilic acid, imidazole, and polymyxin E. Many antimicrobic agents, such as tetracycline and erythromycin, had intermediate levels of activity against these 3 species of *Campylobacter*. Although tylosin and spectinomycin had previously been suggested as drugs of choice for this disease, laboratory studies indicate that it has a low *in vitro* activity against the *Campylobacter* species tested. Neomycin and chloramphenicol are efficacious, but the results with lincomycin were disappointing in our laboratory trials. One must realize that some drugs perform differently under field conditions than under laboratory conditions.

CONTROL

Swine operations that have endemic chronic proliferative enteritis may benefit from periodic high level antibiotic supplementation in the feed for periods of 2 or 4 days duration. Minimizing recognizable stress factors may be beneficial in reducing the number of clinical cases of proliferative enteritis. However, genetic predisposition cannot be completely ignored, since to date no controlled scientific studies have investigated this aspect of the disease.

Supplemental Reading

Chang, K., Kurtz, H. J., Ward, G. E., and Gebhart, C. J.: Immunofluorescence demonstration of *Campylobacter hyointestinalis* and *Campylobacter sputorum* spp. *mucosalis* in swine intestines with lesions of proliferative enteritis. Am. J. Vet. Res. *45*:703–710, 1984.

Ensbo, P.: Terminal or regional ileitis in swine. Nord. Vet. Med. *3*:1–28, 1951.

Gebhart, C. J., Ward, G. E., Chang, K., and Kurtz, H. J.: *Campylobacter hyointestinalis* (new species) isolated from swine with lesions of proliferative ileitis. Am. J. Vet. Res. *44*:361–367, 1983.

Johnsson, L., and Martinsson, K.: Regional ileitis pigs—morphological and pathogenic aspects. Acta. Vet. Scand. *17*:223–232, 1976.

Lawson, G. H. K., and Rowland, A. C.: Intestinal adenomatosis in the pig; a bacteriological study. Res. Vet. Sci. *178*:331–336, 1974.

Love, D. N., and Love, R. J.: Pathology of proliferative hemorrhagic enteropathy in pigs. Vet. Pathol. *16*:41–48, 1979.

Pasteurellosis

C. A. HJERPE, D.V.M.

The term pasteurellosis refers to pneumonic and septicemic diseases of cattle, sheep, goats, and swine from which *Pasteurella multocida* or *P. haemolytica* or both are isolated.

ETIOLOGY

Pneumonic pasteurellosis of cattle is discussed in The Bovine Respiratory Disease Complex (Section 10). *P. multocida* Types A and *P. haemolytica* Type A1 are considered to be the usual causative organisms of the severe clinical signs and pneumonic lesions. Septicemic pasteurellosis of cattle occurs rarely except in southern Asia, where *P. multocida* Type B is the causative agent. Pasteurellosis of swine is nearly always of the pneumonic form and is caused by *P. multocida* Types A and D. Pasteurellosis of sheep is most common as the pneumonic form, but septicemia is not unusual. *P. haemolytica* is usually the causative agent. Pneumonic pasteurellosis is most frequently observed in lambs, but sheep of all ages are susceptible. Septicemic pasteurellosis is found only in lambs. Pasteurellosis of goats is probably similar to that of sheep, although little information has been reported about it.

The origin of pneumonic pasteurellosis in sheep, goats, and swine is probably very similar to that of cattle. *P. haemolytica* and *P. multocida* are common saprophytes in the nasal passages and oropharynx of normal sheep and swine, respectively. Clinical disease does not usually develop except in animals subjected to stresses, such as weaning, transportation, exposure to inclement weather, chilling, overheating, exposure to drafts, confinement in poorly ventilated barns, overcrowding, ration changes, shearing, deworming, malnutrition, and severe parasitism. Presumably, as in cattle, the efficiency of pulmonary clearance by the mucociliary apparatus and the pulmonary alveolar macrophages is impaired by exposure to stress. As a result, *Pasteurella* bacteria, which are inhaled in droplet nuclei from the nasal and oropharyngeal mucosae of carrier animals, are able to colonize the lower respiratory tract and initiate inflammatory disease. No respiratory viruses have been implicated as primary pathogens in sheep and swine as they have been in cattle.

Pneumonic pasteurellosis of swine is almost invariably associated with enzootic pneumonia caused by *Mycoplasma hyopneumoniae*. It is believed that the swine lung predisposes them to pneumonic pasteurellosis by the lesions of enzootic pneumonia. In the absence of super-infection with *P. multocida* or other bacteria, enzootic pneumonia of swine is a mild or subclinical disease. Pneumonic pasteurellosis also occurs as a complication of hog cholera.

Similarly, sheep affected with chronic, subclinical enzootic pneumonia caused by *Chlamydia* spp. have a greater suceptibility to pneumonic pasteurellosis. Septicemic pasteurellosis of lambs occurs under the conditions of stress that can also precipitate pneumonia. It is not known why some outbreaks take the septicemic form and why others take the pneumonic form.

Transmission of pasteurellosis is by direct contact, by inhalation of aerosols induced by coughing, and by consumption of feed or water that is contaminated by nasal discharge or drool from infected animals. Nursing lambs have also been infected from ewes with mastitis caused by *P. haemolytica*.

CLINICAL SIGNS

Pneumonic pasteurellosis of sheep and swine is characterized by depression, inappetance, fever, cough, nasal discharge, and dyspnea. Morbidity and mortality rates of 40 per cent and 5 per cent, respectively, are not unusual. Auscultation of the lung fields may help detect increased vesicular breath sounds, bronchial tones, rales, and exaggerated expiratory sounds.

In septicemic pasteurellosis of lambs, sudden death in animals not noted to be sick is the usual manifestation. In septicemic pasteurellosis of cattle, the course is usually about 24 hr. High fever, severe depression, salivation, mucosal petechiae, and subcutaneous swellings have been described.

PATHOLOGY

Pneumonic lesions in sheep, goats, and swine are similar to those described in cattle with the bovine respiratory disease complex (see Section 10).

In septicemic pasteurellosis of cattle there is generalized petechiae, and pulmonary edema and gastroenteritis may be present.

In septicemic pasteurellosis of lambs, there are widespread hemorrhages, ulcerative and hemorrhagic gastroenteritis may be present, and the lungs are congested and edematous. Small (0.2 to 1.0 mm) pale foci of infection are visible on the serosal and cut surfaces of liver and lungs. Diagnosis is based upon the occurrence of sudden deaths in lambs under stress and upon the isolation of *P. haemolytica* from the liver and spleen of animals with lesions of septicemia.

TREATMENT

Treatment of pasteurellosis is discussed in The Bovine Respiratory Disease Complex (Section 10). Oxytetracycline, procaine penicillin G, and sodium sulfamethazine are approved by the FDA for parenteral administration in swine. Sodium sulfamethazine is usually administered by intraperitoneal injection. Tetracycline, chlortetracycline, ampicillin trihydrate, sodium sulfachlorpyridazine,

and sodium sulfathiazole are approved for oral administration in swine. Rational dosage recommendations are lacking for oral administration of ampicillin and tetracycline in swine.

Procaine penicillin G and sodium sulfamethazine are approved for parenteral adminstration in sheep and goats, and sulfamethazine is approved for oral adminstration.

CONTROL

Control of pasteurellosis in swine is based upon eradication of enzootic pneumonia from the herd, usually by depopulation and restocking with specific pathogen-free swine. Pasteurella bacterins in swine are ineffective.

Control of pasteurellosis in sheep is based upon eliminating or reducing stresses and upon administering mass medication with appropriate antimicrobics in full therapeutic dosages during outbreaks. Pasteurella bacterins do not prevent pneumonia, but mortality may be reduced by vaccinating at 3 weeks and again at 5 weeks of age.

An effective bacterin is available for prevention of septicemic pasteurellosis in cattle.

Supplemental Reading

Blood, D. C., and Henderson, J. A.: Veterinary Medicine, 4th ed. Baltimore, Williams & Wilkins, 363–371, 1974.

Carter, G. C.: Pasteurellosis. *In* Dunne, H. W., and Leman, A. D. (eds.). Diseases of Swine, 4th ed. Ames, Iowa, Iowa State University Press, 621–629, 1975.

Jensen, R.: Diseases of Sheep. Philadelphia, Lea and Febiger, 171–178, 1974.

The *Haemophilus somnus* Complex

PETER B. LITTLE, D.V.M., Ph.D.

Haemophilus somnus was first recognized as the cause of a fatal septicemic disease of feed lot cattle with severe neurologic complications (thromboembolic meningoencephalitis (TME), sleeper syndrome). The organism is now known to be involved in bovine pneumonia, arthritis, endometritis, abortion, and more recently in conjunctivitis.

ETIOLOGY

H. somnus is a gram-negative nonspore-forming coccobacillary organism that requires 10-per cent carbon dioxide in air for optimal growth. It does not need an X or V factor for growth, a requirement for placement in the genus *Haemophilus*; therefore, the bacterium will likely be placed in a different genus in the future. The bacterium can be isolated on brain-heart infusion agar supplemented with 10 per cent bovine blood and 0.5 per cent yeast extract. Growth occurs as 1 to 2 mm regularly convex, slightly yellow, glistening colonies in 2 or 3 days. Thiamine monophosphate, cysteine hydrochloride, and soluble starch potentiate growth of *H. somnus*.

OCCURRENCE

Infectious TME was first recognized in Colorado in 1956, and *H. somnus* was connected with it in California in 1960. Over the last 2 decades, the disease has moved in northerly and westerly directions across the continent probably in association with feeder cattle movement. There appears to be little doubt that similar, or even identical, organisms were isolated from bovine disease as early as 1927 in the United States and 1950 in Canada. *H. somnus* syndromes have been reported from the United States, Canada, Switzerland, Belgium, Italy, Germany, Australia, Poland, Japan, Romania, and Russia. It is likely that there are few countries that import cattle in which it does not exist. A sheep pathogen related to *H. somnus* called *Histophilus ovis* has been identified in New Zealand, Australia, and Canada by Humphrey and Stephens. *H. ovis* experimentally produces lesions of TME in cattle.

INCIDENCE

The total incidence of TME in its various forms is not known. However, when TME occurs in a feed lot, from 0.1 to 1 per cent of the cattle are affected with the acute and often fatal disease. In a 2-year-long Canadian study, only 11 per cent of feed lots had the disease in both years, and the average overall population mortality rate for 3 years was 0.1 per cent. Serologic studies suggest that 20 to 50 per cent of cattle are seropositive to *Haemophilus somnus*, although cross-reactivity induced by *H. agni*, *Actinobacillus lignieresii*, *Listeria monocytogenes*, *Campylobacter fetus*, and other bacteria may account for some positive test results. As many as 20 per cent of cases of pneumonia in calves are associated with *H. somnus* as pure or mixed infections. There is a 70 per cent genital carrier rate in affected bulls, which is considerably lower in cows. The organism is seldom isolated from the upper respiratory tract of healthy cattle.

PATHOGENESIS

Experimental work has clarified some aspects of the pathogenesis of *H. somnus* septicemic disease. The mode of entry is unresolved, although the nasopharyngeal and pulmonary routes are the most likely. Intratracheal instillation or intravenous administration of *H. somnus* is capable of reproducing the pulmonary and acute septicemic disease and TME lesions. Serum antibody levels give no indication of an animal's vulnerability to infection, suggesting that a complex host-bacterial relationship exists, which produces the fatal effects. This probably includes cell mediated factors such as neutrophil killing and perhaps the rapidity of the neutrophil response. The organism has a cell-associated cytotoxic effect that separates endothelial cells and activates clotting. This appears to be responsible for the widespread thrombotic phenomena in the organs of affected animals. Little is known of the pathogenesis of the pulmonary lesions; however, the response is typical of other acute bacterial pneumonic processes. In abortion, thrombotic phenomena in the fetus and necrosis of the placenta lead to death of the fetus.

CLINICAL SIGNS

TME is found in cattle 4 months to 3 years of age but most frequently in 7- to 9-month-old feed lot calves. The onset of disease in a group of calves usually is within 4 weeks of commencement of the feeder period, sometimes in association with respiratory disease. Animals affected with TME are found dead or are separated from the group. They are depressed and walk reluctantly, often with a stiff knuckling gait. Fever of 41°C (106°F), muscle tremor, weakness, and recumbency rapidly supervene in untreated cases. The severe septicemic shock often obscures neurologic signs, but ataxia, stiff neck, blindness, nystagmus, and circling are reported. Premortal coma accounts for the sleeper syndrome. At this stage, the temperature is subnormal, and the respiration has an interrupted expiratory phase. Pathognomonic multifocal hemorrhagic retinal infarcts are observed in 20 per cent of cases. Cerebrospinal fluid (CSF) of a comatose animal is cloudy. Smear or culture results help confirm the presence of the coccobacillus.

In calves, the signs of brochopneumonic respiratory syndrome due to *H. somnus* are poor condition, fever, and hacking cough. Bilateral consolidation of the anteroventral lung lobes occurs, and moist rales may be auscultated. An acute respiratory form has a shorter course with fever, rapid weight loss, dyspnea, and extensive consolidation of the lungs. Pleuritic rubs may be auscultated.

Arthritis, an uncommon chronic form of the disease, is seen in animals that have averted the fatal septicemic form. It is characterized by swollen joints and tendon sheaths. The joint fluid is serosanguineous with fibrin flecks; purulent exudate is not seen. Infected cattle are in poor condition.

The endometritis syndrome (described principally in Australia and Europe) is characterized by a purulent vaginal discharge and, frequently, by red granular vaginitis and cervicitis after breeding. The period between calving and conception may be significantly prolonged. *Ureaplasma* and *H. somnus* may coexist. Abortion with retained placenta occurs at 7 to 9 months of gestation but is rare. Diagnosis is confirmed by microscopic demonstration of fetal and placental lesions and by bacterial culture.

PATHOLOGY AND NECROPSY FINDINGS

Septicemic *H. somnus* produces lesions in many organs but particularly in the nervous system. Lesions are found in the brain, eye, spinal cord, skeletal muscles, urinary bladder, heart, kidney, joints, tendon sheaths, lungs, and retropharyngeal lymph nodes. In genital carriers the organism may be isolated from the prepuce and from the region of Bartholin's glands in the vagina.

The hematologic pattern of septicemic *H. somnus* is that of endotoxic shock with pronounced neutropenia and the presence of fibrin split products. Neutrophilic pleocytosis is present in the CSF with counts as high as 500/cmm. Pandy's test for CSF globulin is positive, and the creatine phosphokinase levels in the CSF may be elevated.

Petechial and ecchymotic hemorrhages are found in the subcutaneous tissues, fascial planes, and muscle of cattle with TME. Endocardial and epicardial ecchymotic hemmorhages may be severe. Joints and tendon sheaths

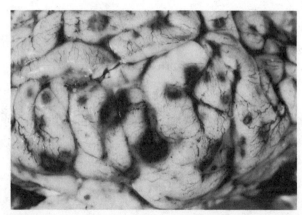

Figure 1. Feedlot steer with multiple focal septal infarcts in the parietal cortex caused by *H. somnus* (TME).

frequently contain excess fluid and fibrin strands. This is often very noticeable in the atlanto-occipital joint, when the head is removed. The retropharyngeal lymph nodes are enlarged and red. Focal 0.5 to 2 cm hemorrhagic lesions are often found in the larynx, heart, retina, intestines, kidneys, and mucosal surface of the bladder. Pathognomonic lesions are seen in the brain in 75 to 80 per cent of cases. Grossly, these lesions are multifocal hemorrhagic infarcts, generally 2 mm to 2 cm in diameter, bright red, and found over the cortex as well as on cut section (Fig. 1). Focal red lesions of the spinal cord are best observed on cut surface. A slight to moderate cloudiness of the meninges and CSF indicates the prominent acute meningitis that is always present.

The acute fibrinous pneumonic and pleuritic lesions of *H. somnus* infection in feed lot cattle are comparable to the more common *Pasteurella haemolytica* lesions. Microscopically, fibrinous pneumonia and necrotic bronchiolitis are evident. In younger calves, the respiratory lesions of *H. somnus* are those of chronic, suppurative bronchopneumonia. There are anteroventral consolidation, prominent pus-filled bronchioles, and frequently gray necrotic foci (2 to 4 mm). Tissue from the junction between normal and affected lung gives the best yield of the organism in culture.

Aborted fetuses may have gross petechial hemorrhages in tissues with focal necrotic placentitis. Microscopic and bacteriologic analyses of placenta and fetus are usually necessary for diagnosis, however. Little is known about the uterine lesions in the endometrial form of the disease.

DIAGNOSIS

H. somnus septicemia should be suspected in feed lot cattle when sudden death occurs, or when they are afflicted with pyrexia, depression, and stiffness. Ophthalmoscopic examination can help confirm the diagnosis in 20 per cent of live animals with retinal infarcts. The presence of acute meningitis can be confirmed with a cisternal CSF tap. Multifocal hemorrhagic infarcts in the brain at necropsy are characteristic. Culture on brain-heart infusion agar with 5-per cent bovine blood and 0.5-per cent yeast extract (Difco) in 10 per cent carbon dioxide will assist the veterinarian in confirming the diagnosis.

TME is frequently confused with other feed lot cattle diseases involving the CNS. Cattle with polioencephalomalacia (PE) separate from the group in a manner similar to those with TME, but fever is usually absent. In PE there are consistent neurologic signs of bilateral blindness and preserved pupillary light reflexes, with moderate to severe opisthotonos, hyperesthesia, and clonic convulsions in later stages. A CSF analysis may show some macrophages, but the suppurative meningitic exudate typical of TME is not found. Listeriosis is characterized by fever and depression, but in most cases the cranial nerve signs indicative of focal medullary lesions will assist in separating the diagnosis of listeriosis from TME. In listeriosis, the CSF analysis indicates mild to moderate lymphocytic meningitis.

TME cases that are treated early and that have predominantly spinal infarctive lesions are a special problem in regard to differential diagnosis of rabies, spinal abscess, and vertebral fractures associated with calcium and phosphorus dietary imbalances. The history of acute febrile disease that rapidly resolved with antibiotic treatment, leaving residual paralysis without progressively abnormal neurologic signs, separates TME spinal disease from rabies, vertebral fracture, and abscesses. Treated animals are bright and alert, and eat well. They become star boarders until the owner recognizes the futility of continuous special care.

Respiratory disease caused by *H. somnus* must be differentiated from respiratory disease caused by *Pasteurella haemolytica*, *P. multocida*, *Corynebacterium pyogenes*, and *Mycoplasma* sp. Necropsy with microbiologic confirmation is usually necessary for diagnosis, although *H. somnus* can often be isolated from the noses of animals with *H. somnus* pneumonia, using swabs.

H. somnus should be suspected as a cause of infertility in beef and dairy cows if the disease is associated with post-breeding endometritis, vaginitis, and purulent discharge. The disease must be differentiated from trichomoniasis, *Ureaplasma* infection, vibriosis, and infectious pustular vulvovaginitis. Microbiologic studies of the vaginal exudate are required to accurately identify each of these conditions. Special cultural procedures may be required, since *H. somnus* is often overgrown with aerobic bacteria, such as *Proteus*, *Corynebacterium*, and *Streptococcus* in these cases.

A clinical diagnosis on the basis of symptoms and lesions is not usually possible in cases of abortion, conjunctivitis, and mastitis caused by *H. somnus*. Cultural confirmation is required in order to make a diagnosis.

Resistance to *H. somnus* infection does not correlate with serum antibody levels. Therefore, the use of antibody determination as a means of identifying infected groups is also of no purpose, since virtually all cattle carry antibody levels from exposure either to *H. somnus* or to bacteria that cross-react in the *H. somnus* test.

PROGNOSIS

Early treatment of TME while the animal is still ambulatory generally results in dramatic recovery, since the organism is highly sensitive to most systemic antibiotics. Recumbent animals having advanced septicemia and the attendant brain and spinal cord infarcts are poor candidates for treatment and should be destroyed. Recumbent animals with only spinal cord lesions may recover in 4 to

6 weeks with good nursing care if this is economically justified.

PREVENTION AND THERAPY

H. somnus will survive for long periods on fomites contaminated with infected exudate and blood; therefore, pressure spraying of watering areas, feedbunks, and yards with a period of drying and sunlight will reduce bacterial contamination when yards are quickly restocked. More important is the recognition that many cattle are carriers of genital infections. Intermingling of cattle groups heightens the opportunity for cross-infection of susceptible cattle. Overcrowding of cattle similarly increases the chances of infection of susceptible cattle from the respiratory droplets and urinary or genital secretions of infected cattle.

Several bacterins are currently available for use against *H. somnus*. All require 2 doses, and many contain antigens to other common bacterial diseases. The economic value of vaccination to prevent TME has been questioned because of the sporadic nature of the disease. Under good management conditions and reliable surveillance, early antibiotic therapy is probably the most economical. However, if cattle surveillance is less than optimal, vaccination may be indicated to prevent TME. The efficacy of vaccination to prevent respiratory and other forms of the disease has not been demonstrated.

Antibiotics

Acute cases of TME should be treated with intravenous oxytetracycline (10 mg/kg). Chloramphenicol is also effective but is not approved for food animal use in the United States.

Neomycin, sulfonamide, lincomycin, and spectinomycin are often ineffective.

Supplemental Readings

Davidson, J. N., Carpenter, T. E., and Hjerpe, C. A.: An example of an economic decision analysis approach to the problem of thromboembolic meningoencephalitis (TME) in feedlot cattle. Cornell Vet. *71*:383–390, 1981.

Humphrey, J. D., and Stephens, L. R.: *Haemophilus somnus:* A review. Vet. Bull. *53*:987–1004, 1983.

Little, P. B., and Sorensen, D. K.: Bovine polioencephalomalacia, infectious embolic meningoencephalitis, and acute lead poisoning in feedlot cattle. J. Am. Vet. Med. Assoc. *155*:1892–1903, 1969.

Stephens, L. R., Humphrey, J. D., Little, P. B., and Barnum, D. A.: Morphological, biochemical, antigenic and cytochemical relationships among *Haemophilus somnus, Haemophilus agni, Haemophilus haemoglobinophilus, Histophilus ovis* and *Actinobacillus seminis.* J. Clin. Micro. *17*:728–737, 1983.

Stephens, L. R., Little, P. B., et al.: Vaccination of cattle against experimentally induced thromboembolic meningoencephalitis with a *Haemophilus somnus* bacterin. Am. J. Vet. Res. *43*:1339–1342, 1982.

Haemophilus pleuropneumoniae

ROY A. SCHULTZ, D.V.M., M.S.

Haemophilus pleuropneumoniae (HPP) causes a disease of swine characterized by pneumonia and pleuritis. It can manifest itself as an acute form, causing sudden deaths in growing and finishing hogs. The more chronic form causes lung abscesses and adhesions of the lungs to the thoracic cavity, resulting in slow growing and unthrifty hogs.

ETIOLOGY

H. pleuropneumoniae is a gram-negative coccobacillary rod. It requires the V factor (NAD) for growth and is hemolytic. The production of urease and the fermentation of mannitol, xylose, and deoxyribose differentiate *H. pleuropneumoniae* from other V factor–dependent *Haemophilus* species of porcine and human origin.

PATHOGENESIS

The disease is most often found in pigs during the growing and finishing periods but is not limited to those periods. The incubation period can be as short as 6 to 8 hr. An outbreak often follows a stressful event, such as moving, mixing, and sudden weather changes. The organisms are spread by aerosol droplets, and 100 per cent of a group can be infected, with death rates of 7 to 30 per cent or more being common if immediate and effective treatment is not initiated. As few as 10,000 organisms can kill a 100-lb pig in 8 to 12 hr, and as few as 100 organisms can cause a lung abscess. Researchers in Switzerland have incriminated the boar and breeding stock as the predominant transmitters of the disease between susceptible herds. They have found no evidence of transmission by birds, rodents, cats, or stockworkers, or through air, other than short distances. The severity of the disease will depend on the environment and climate as well as promptness and effectiveness of treatment. A certain percentage of recovered animals will have small abscesses in their lungs or tonsils or both, which serve as reservoirs of infection to susceptible individuals added to the group. There are 9 known serotypes in the world, 5 of which have been identified in the United States. Serotype 5 is the most prevalent followed by serotypes 1 and 7. Serotypes 3 and 4 account for a small percentage of the isolates.

CLINICAL SIGNS

The clinical signs of the disease vary, but the first sign of acute HPP infection is quite often 1 or several dead pigs. Other pigs may show mild to severe coughing, a rough hair coat, lack of appetite, elevated temperature (40 to 42°C), and a stilted gait. As the disease progresses, thumping and severe respiratory distress with cyanosis or purpling of the ears, nose, and abdomen may occur.

DIAGNOSIS

A preliminary diagnosis of HPP may be made by history, typical gross lesions, age, respiratory distress, and sudden death. A definitive diagnosis may require the results of a culture of the organism from a typical lesion. Culture on sheep blood agar cross streaked with nonhemolytic *Staphylococcus* reveals satellite hemolytic colonies. Culturing should be done as soon after death as possible. If this is not possible, the lung should be stored in a glycerol and water solution for transport to a diagnostic laboratory.

There is often a bloody, foamy discharge from the noses and mouths of pigs that die of the acute form. Postmortem examination of affected swine shows massive pulmonary hemorrhage. Circumscribed necrotic and hemorrhagic areas are common, especially in the diaphragmatic lobe of the lung. Fibrin on the pleural surfaces is frequently present, and adherence of the lungs to the thoracic wall is common.

TREATMENT

The disease-causing organisms are located deep in lung abscesses that have poor blood supplies. Drug concentrations at these sites are usually low unless high drug concentrations are used. Oral antibiotics often do not adequately control the disease because drug concentrations at the site of infection are not sufficiently high to kill the organism. Ideally, treatment should be with an antibiotic to which the organism has been found to be sensitive. In an outbreak of the acute form, time does not permit sensitivity testing, so the entire group of animals in the same air space should be injected with a high dose of long-acting penicillin (60,000 units/kg) or long-acting oxytetracycline (18 mg/kg). In a recent study of 50 field isolates of HPP, 16 per cent were resistant to penicillin, and 18 per cent were resistant to tetracycline. Over 50 per cent were resistant to sulfa. Sensitivity testing requires about 24 to 48 hr to complete, and an antibiotic that is most effective can be chosen for any follow-up therapy. In the United States, injections of spectinomycin or gentamicin, or the addition of tiamulin to the water (180 ppm) has been beneficial in those cases resistant to penicillin or tetracycline. Chloramphenicol has been effective and can be used in those countries where it is legal for use in food animal production.

Injection of the pigs with the antibiotic of choice is usually followed by adding a high dose of an appropriate antimicrobial, such as tetracycline or sulfathiazole, to the feed or water, in spite of the fact that this does not control the initial outbreak. The rationale of this therapy is to reduce the level of other respiratory pathogens and to reduce the level of *H. pleuropneumoniae* in tissues the drugs can reach.

Along with antibiotic therapy, good management procedures may help minimize the number of deaths. Decreasing the number of pigs per pen, increasing pig comfort, improving ventilation, reducing dust level, and maintaining a constant temperature all may help minimize the effects of the outbreak. Some producers have fogged the air with 2-per cent chlorine dioxide to minimize the number of airborne organisms. Prompt action during diagnosis and treatment is necessary to keep losses down.

CONTROL

Control methods will vary for different operations. Finishing operations that buy pigs from many sources, and those with a closed herd, "farrow to finish" operation may have different approaches. In general, anything to reduce the stress will help to reduce the incidence as well as the chances for an explosive outbreak. Good management procedures, such as all-in, all-out movement, not mixing older hogs with younger hogs, proper stocking densities, and maximum pig comfort with optimum ven-

tilation all help to check the disease. Vaccination with bacterins (twice at 2 and 4 weeks before exposure) has aided in controlling losses and reducing lung lesions in many operations. Autogenous bacterins made with young cultures and with proper adjuvants have helped tremendously in many farrow to finish operations. Only 3 approved vaccines are presently available in the United States, but 2 or 3 more are in the final stages of approval. A massive exposure, however, can override any vaccination program.

The use of the complement fixation test is available to detect antibodies in sera in order to identify individuals and herds with chronic infections. In farrow to finish operations, testing of 10 breeding animals will give owners a 95 per cent probability of finding evidence of antibodies. If they are present, it can be assumed that sooner or later there will be problems in the finishing area if conditions are right. If antibodies are not present, owners should test any new breeding stock to prevent the entrance of HPP into the herd. Care must also be exercised when introducing "clean" boars or other breeding stock into an infected herd. The exposure of a susceptible animal to HPP may precipitate the disease.

Supplementary Reading

Nicolet, J., and Scholl, E. D. O.: *In* Leman, A. D., Glock, R. D., Mongeling, W. L., et al. (eds.): Diseases of Swine, 5th ed. Ames, Iowa, Iowa State University Press, 368–375, 1981.
Nielsen, R.: *Haemophilus parahaemolyticus* serotypes pathogenicity and cross immunity. Nord. Vet. Med. *31*:407–413, 1979.
Schultz, R., Ross, R., Gunnarsson, A., and Nielsen, R.: Serotyping of 50 different isolates of *Haemophilus pleuropneumoniae* from swine pneumonia in Iowa and surrounding states. Vet. Med. Small Anim. Clin. 78:9, 1451–1453, 1983.

Swine Rhinitis

JAMES D. McKEAN, D.V.M., M.S.

Rhinitis is an inflammation of the nasal mucosa resulting from either an infectious or an environmental insult. Normally, the nasal turbinates function to filter large dust particles and infectious agents and to warm and moisten inspired air. Failure to function properly exposes the lower respiratory tract to a greater number of pathogens and dust particles and may increase the possibility of pneumonia. Three major types of swine rhinitis can be clinically defined by differences in morphologic and clinical appearance: necrotic rhinitis, infectious atrophic rhinitis, and inclusion-body rhinitis.

NECROTIC RHINITIS (BULLNOSE)

Necrotic rhinitis is an uncommon disease in swine caused by *Fusiformis (Sphaerophorus) necrophorus*. Animals of all ages may be affected, but infection generally begins in animals less than 2 months old. Invasion by the organism is assisted by breaks in the skin or the buccal mucosa, such as wounds from fighting, traumatic wounds from improper canine tooth clipping, and wounds from the lodging of penetrating objects between teeth. Bacterial invasion is more common in dirty or highly contaminated environments. Sporadic incidences have declined with better sanitation and cleaner facilities necessary to modern pork production.

Clinical Signs

Signs of infection are facial swelling and abscesses at the affected site. Lesions are generally unilateral. As abscesses enlarge, rarefaction and necrosis of underlying bone may occur. Large abscesses may interfere with normal respiration and mastication. Reduced feed consumption causes poor growth and, occasionally, toxemia may result in death.

Treatment

Treatment of necrotic rhinitis is generally ineffective because of the large amounts of pus and the difficulty of achieving therapeutic drug levels at the site of organism multiplication. Use of locally applied antibiotics and sulfa drugs may have an ameliorative effect. Prevention is by removal of objects causing abrasions, by use of proper techniques for clipping needle teeth, and by cleaning and disinfecting of infected premises.

ATROPHIC RHINITIS

In contrast to necrotic rhinitis, atrophic rhinitis (AR) is a highly contagious, infectious disease localized on the nasal mucosa. AR is a "lesion" disease generally resulting from chronic inflammation of the nasal mucous membranes. Although this chronic irritation can be caused experimentally by a variety of agents, *Bordella bronchiseptica* is a major cause of AR in swine of the midwestern United States. Other organisms, including *Pasteurella, Haemophilus,* and cytomegalovirus (inclusion-body rhinitis), have been implicated as initiating or contributing to AR lesion development.

Epidemiology

B. bronchiseptica is an ubiquitous organism in mammalian populations. Isolations have been made from swine, humans, dogs, cats, rats, and other animals commonly found on swine farms. Nonswine isolates may infect swine, but some require several swine passages to develop significant AR pathogenicity. Swine are the major carriers of turbinate atrophy–causing *B. bronchiseptica*. Sow-to-litter and pig-to-pig aerosol transmissions are the most common methods of transmission. Swine can be infected at any age, but severe lesion development with *B. bronchiseptica* requires infection at an early age (usually less than 3 to 6 weeks). *Pasteurella* isolations are less common than *B. bronchiseptica* isolations, but transmission is by the same mechanism. *Pasteurella* infections may extend the time for severe lesion development to 10 to 12 weeks.

Intensification of existing *B. bronchiseptica* infections or initiation of nasal mucosal damage by *B. bronchiseptica* along with greater growth of other organisms causes more severe turbinate damage than with a single infection. Acting synergistically, *Pasteurella multocida* Type A and *Haemophilus parasuis* may cause mild rhinitis in the absence of *B. bronchiseptica*.[1] Type D strains of *Pasteurella* have been found to produce severe turbinate damage. The identification of a specific heat-labile toxin capable of producing turbinate atrophy when injected intramuscularly has increased interest in the study of Type D *Pasteurella* strains. Generally, these *Pasteurella* strains require assistance in establishing nasal or pulmonary in-

fections. This may be the role of *B. bronchiseptica* in some severely affected herds. Other factors that may contribute to greater severity, irrespective of initiating cause, are concurrent diarrhea or pneumonia, drafts, dampness, and chilling conditions, overcrowding, keeping variously aged pigs together, and high ammonia and dust concentrations. Further work is needed to clarify these interactions in field situations.

Clinical Signs

Clinical signs of AR infection are nonspecific. Sneezing and sniffling, mucopurulent nasal discharge with occasional flecks of blood or, in severe cases, nasal bleeding, tear strains under the eyes due to increased lacrimal spillage, and retarded growth are signs of AR. Clinical signs are seen in young swine, sometimes as young as 1 week of age. Although pathognomonic when present, nasal distortion does not frequently occur in affected pigs. Severe turbinate atrophy results in abnormal facial bone growth. If unilateral, the nose grows more slowly on the affected side, causing deviation to that side; if bilateral, the snout is shorter. The lower jaw and skin covering the snout grow at normal rates, causing an abnormally short snout (brachygnathia superior) and excessively wrinkled skin over the snout. Within an infected herd the entire continuum from mild to severe turbinate atrophy may be observed. With severe infections, growth rate and feed efficiency retardation of up to 10 per cent were reported.[2] Clinical observations indicate severe infections may reduce performance by up to 30 per cent. Lesion development and performance are not directly linked. Severely affected animals may grow as rapidly as unaffected herd mates. A higher incidence and severity of pneumonia lesions may explain some of the lowered performances in severely affected swine. The mechanism for increased pneumonic lesions is not well understood but may result from the greater pulmonary insult caused by reduced filtration of bacteria and dust. Alternately, AR lesions and poor performance may be secondary to the release of AR-associated toxins by Type D *Pasteurella* localized in pneumonic lesions.

Diagnosis

Diagnosis of atrophic rhinitis is by observation of typical clinical signs and by postmortem turbinate atrophy. Generally, the ventral turbinates are the first affected, followed by the dorsal and ethmoid turbinates. In severe cases, only remnants of turbinates may be found. It is only by observation of the morphologic condition of the nasal turbinates that this disease can be definitely diagnosed. At necropsy of all pigs over 15 kg, the snout should be cut to the second premolar tooth level and observed for typical lesions. Radiographic techniques have been attempted for lesion detection in live animals, but difficulties in uniform positioning and radiographic interpretation make this procedure impractical for field application.

Treatment

Treatment of AR-affected swine is generally unrewarding because of the irreversibility of most lesions. Feeding of tetracycline, tylosin, or sulfonamides or combinations of all 3 at 100 gm/ton each in starter and grower rations may help suppress other respiratory diseases and improve feed efficiency and growth rates in the presence of AR.

Control should be directed at (1) reducing carrier

animal numbers, (2) minimizing transmission to susceptible swine, and (3) rapid removing of pathogenic organisms from the respiratory tract of infected swine. All 3 can be done with a combination of management, vaccination, and medication programs. Sulfamethazine, sulfathiazole, and potentiated sulfas are the most commonly used antibacterial drugs in AR suppression. They must be fed for 1 to 3 weeks for maximal effect. Treatment of sows prior to farrowing and of pigs eating creep and grower rations can reduce AR lesions significantly. Levels of 100 to 150 gm/ton sulfamethazine or sulfathiazole in creepfeed, 800 mg trimethoprim and 4 gm sulfadiazine for each sow daily for 10 days, or sulfathiazole at 0.13 to 26 gm/L of drinking water for 7 to 10 days have proved successful.

Treatment programs based on multiple injections of antibacterial compounds in suckling pigs have reduced lesion development. Oxytetracycline (OTC), potentiated sulfas (Tiamulin), tylosin, and lincomycin have all been used. A sustained-release tetracycline (LA-200) injected on days 1, 7, 14, and 21 of life—0.5 ml for the first 2 injections and 1 ml for the next 2—resulted in reduced AR and pneumonia scores and improved growth performance. A 5-per cent OTC soluble powder sprayed in each nostril once or twice a week for 2 to 3 weeks has produced good results. Therapeutic levels of tylosin, lincomycin, or potentiated sulfa have been injected at days 1, 6, 10, and 14 or days 3, 6, and 12 with reported success. Before beginning an intensive treatment program, antibiograms for *B. bronchiseptica* and *Pasteurella* strains in the herd should be evaluated. Many of these strains are sulfa and tetracycline resistant. This resistance emphasizes the need for concurrent immunologic and environmental control.

Prevention and Control

Vaccination of suckling pigs with *Bordetella* bacterin has been a successful addition to some AR control programs. For maximum effect, the initial vaccination should be during the first week of life, followed by a second immunization at the second or fourth week of life. The immunity produced decreases the number and the longevity of *B. bronchiseptica* on the nasal mucosa. This helps diminish the severity of AR lesion development. Vaccination of sows before farrowing lessens the number of carrier animals and provides additional colostral immunity to the litter. Both activities decrease the exposure of pigs nursing immune sows. Some herds respond better to vaccination with *B. bronchiseptica* and *Pasteurella* bacterin together than with a *B. bronchiseptica* or *Pasteurella* bacterin alone. Experimental work with mixed infections of *B. bronchiseptica* and toxin-producing *Pasteurella* strains have shown partial protection from either *B. bronchiseptica* or *Pasteurella* vaccines, but more complete protection from a vaccine containing both.

Environmental control includes an all-in, all-out farrowing house and a clean and disinfected nursery to reduce spread of infection of younger susceptible swine. *Bordetella* and *Pasteurella* are very susceptible to all common disinfectants and to drying. However, under favorable conditions, survival of *Bordetella* and *Pasteurella* for several weeks in vacated swine facilities is possible. Since concurrent infections or stress conditions can increase AR severity, provision of warm, dry, draft-free facilities and prompt treatment of other diseases in young swine will help reduce AR.

Introduction of AR-infected breeding stock is a major method of interherd spread. Accredited, specific pathogen-free herds with recent slaughter inspections showing no disease are good sources of AR-free breeding animals. Nasal swabs and bacteriologic cultures for *B. bronchiseptica* and *Pasteurella* with negative results prior to herd entry may assist in reducing potential for AR carrier introduction. For maximal protection, new animals should have negative results on 3 consecutive nasal swabs collected at weekly intervals.

The highest percentage of pathogen-positive swine (approaching 100 per cent) in an infected herd is at 8 to 10 weeks of age, with a gradual reduction to 10 to 15 per cent by 1 year of age and further reductions thereafter.[3] Maintaining an older sow herd may reduce the spread of infection of the offspring. This pressure along with medical, environmental, and immunologic measures generally will control AR. When these methods fail or when production losses eliminate the profitability of the operation, total depopulation should be considered.

References

1. Ross, R., and Gois, M.: Personal communications. 1978.
2. Hasebe, H.: Occurrence and epizootiological surveys of infectious atrophic rhinitis in swine. Nip. Vet. Zoo. Tech. Col. Bull. *19*:92, 1971.
3. Switzer, W. P., and Farrington, D. O.: Diseases of Swine, 5th ed. Ames, Iowa, Iowa State University Press, 497–507, 1981.

Brucellosis

PAUL NICOLETTI, D.V.M., M.S.

Brucellosis in food-producing animals is caused by 4 of the 6 members of the genus *Brucella*. Infections in cattle are caused primarily by *B. abortus*, in swine by *B. suis*, in goats by *B. melitensis*, and in sheep by *B. ovis* and *B. melitensis*. Cross-species infections are uncommon and clinical symptoms are rare.

HISTORY

In 1886, a micrococcus was isolated from the spleen of human patients, and the disease it caused was called undulant fever in 1897. In 1904, a young British physician, Bruce, was commissioned to determine the cause of the human malady on the Isle of Malta. In the meantime, a Danish veterinarian, Bang, had isolated a microorganism from an aborting heifer that was later to be called *B. abortus*. Traum in California, in 1914, isolated *B. suis* from a sow. In 1953, Buddle and Boyes in Australia and New Zealand identified *B. ovis* as a cause of epididymitis in sheep.

Brucellosis is the term now used for infections by any member of the genus *Brucella*. In humans, it is occasionally referred to as undulant fever or Malta fever and in cattle as Bang's disease. All species infect humans except *B. ovis* and *B. neotomae*. There are no residual *B. melitensis* infections in the United States. Sporadic cases occur in goats and humans when introduced from and contracted in other countries, respectively.

The incidence of cattle brucellosis in the United States had been reduced from 5 per cent in 1957 to approximately 0.4 per cent in 1983, according the United States Department of Agriculture (USDA) statistics. The actual losses due to the disease are difficult to estimate but are given

Table 1. *Some General Characteristics of Four Species of*
Brucella*

Species	Number of Biotypes	Growth Requirements			
		CO_2	H_2S	Basic Fuchsin	Thionin
B. melitensis	3	−	−	+	+
B. abortus	9	+	+	+	−
B. suis	4	−	+	−	+
B. ovis	1	+	−	+	+

*Variations occur among some biotypes.

as approximately $35 million annually from abortions, decreased milk yield (especially owing to early calving), temporary or occasionally permanent sterility, and sale and replacement of diseased cattle. Estimates of losses are not available for human, swine, or sheep infections. The incidence of swine brucellosis has declined to approximately 0.04 per cent among marketed swine. Approximately one half of the states of the United States are validated brucellosis-free.

ETIOLOGY

Brucellae are gram-negative coccobacilli that are nonmotile and noncapsulated. They are aerobic, but some species require CO_2 for cultivation. The colonies appear in approximately 4 to 5 days and are round and convex, displaying a somewhat characteristic bluish color when examined with light transmitted at a 45-degree angle.

Differentiation of species and biotypes in the genus *Brucella* is based upon various growth requirements, dye sensitivities, metabolic substrates, serologic reactions, and bacteriophage susceptibility (Table 1).

CLINICAL SIGNS

Cattle

After ingestion of the coccobacilli there is temporary septicemia with phagocytosis by neutrophils and fixed macrophages of local lymph nodes. The predilection sites are the endometrium and fetal placenta in the pregnant cow and the supramammary lymph nodes and udder. Uterine infection is probably related to the presence of a natural compound erythritol, which stimulates the growth of *B. abortus*. The severity of uterine infection varies, but the numbers of organisms are greatest at the time of abortion or parturition. Genital infection usually disappears within 30 days after calving but may recur at subsequent pregnancies. Inflammation of the allantochorion may interfere with circulation to the fetus and cause subsequent death and expulsion. Abortions frequently occur after the fifth month of pregnancy, and a retained placenta may follow. Not all infections result in abortion, and few cattle abort more than once. A small percentage of cattle spontaneously recover. A high percentage of cattle have permanent udder infection with shedding of organisms in the milk.

In the bull, *B. abortus* may produce orchitis with abscesses, epididymitis (Fig. 1), and inflammation of accessory reproductive organs. Orchitis is usually unilateral and results in reduced libido and impaired fertility. Brucellae may be discharged in the semen.

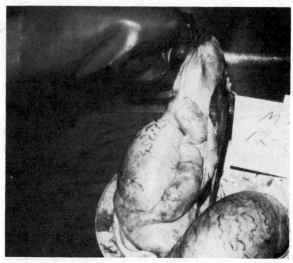

Figure 1. Epididymitis in a bull with *Brucella abortus* infection.

Swine

Clinical evidence of *B. suis* infections varies and is influenced by many factors. The typical syndrome is that of abortion or birth of stillborn or weak pigs, infertility, orchitis (Fig. 2), and sometimes posterior paralysis or lameness due to spondylitis. Genital infection is more permanent in boars than in sows. The semen usually contains large numbers of organisms and infects sows during breeding.

Sheep and Goats

B. melitensis infections are formed in both sheep and goats and produce abortions in late pregnancy (Fig. 3). The abortion rate varies considerably. Infected ewes and

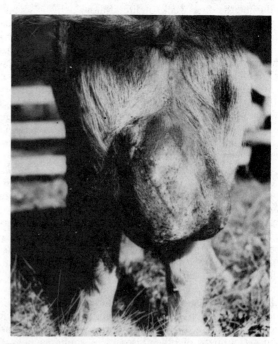

Figure 2. Unilateral orchitis from *B. suis*. (Courtesy of Dr. B. Deyoe.)

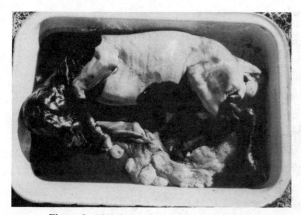

Figure 3. Abortion in sheep with brucellosis.

goats excrete organisms in the milk and in vaginal discharges.

B. ovis infections in sheep are usually demonstrated by epididymitis and orchitis. There may be abortions even though the ewe appears to be more resistant than the ram, and the disease may not persist. Gross lesions of scrotal edema, fibrosis, and adhesions are observed. There may be aspermia and abnormalities in motility or morphology of spermatozoa. Transmission is from ram to ram during preputial or rectal contact and from ram to ewe during mating.

DIAGNOSIS

A correct diagnosis depends upon herd or flock history along with information concerning the individual. Serologic, bacteriologic, or pathologic examinations may be necessary.

Antibodies to *Brucella* are found in a number of fluids, but most tests are performed on serum or milk. Herd surveillance methods include milk-ring and blood tests on marketed cattle. The milk-ring test is much more efficient, as it surveys nearly all of the population at one time. Identification of infected herds is through blood tests for marketed cattle. This method depends upon the sale of an animal with positive results and may be slow to identify infected herds.

SEROLOGY

Positive results from serologic tests indicate present or past exposure to an antigenic stimulus and cannot always be equated with infection. They also do not measure immunity.

The only international standard for the diagnosis of brucellosis in individual cattle is the tube agglutination test (Fig. 4), which measures in international units. The test methods and the interpretation of results vary in both veterinary and human medicine and from country to country. In the United States, tests on cattle are considered positive if the serum reacts in the 1:100 or greater dilution and is from a nonvaccinate and in the 1:200 dilution and from a vaccinate. Test results from cattle with lower titers are classified as suspect or negative, depending upon vaccination status. The tube agglutination test is influenced by many factors, and there are many false-positive and false-negative results. Causes of false results are early or chronic infections, vaccination, and heterospecific antigens. The difficulties in performing the test and in interpreting results have led to development and use of several other procedures.

Plate Agglutination Test. This rapid test is comparable to the tube agglutination test in sensitivity and is subject to most of the same factors that influence the results.

Card Test or Rose Bengal Test. This test (Fig. 5) is performed with card, tile, or machine. It is simple and can be done at the farm, ranch, market facility, or laboratory. The test is a good screening procedure (there are few false-negative results) and should generally be supported by other tests (there may be many false-positive results, especially in vaccinated populations) and information on herd and individual history.

Rivanol Precipitation Test. This procedure depends upon the precipitation of high molecular weight agglutinins and examination of the supernatant with a special antigen. It is less sensitive than the standard agglutination

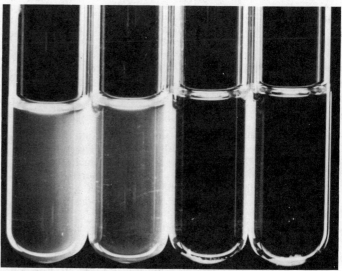

Figure 4. Tube agglutination test with negative (left) and positive (right) results.

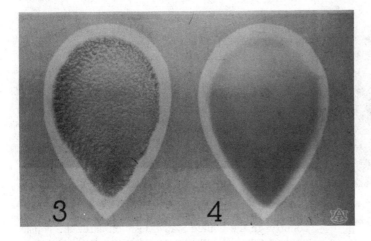

Figure 5. Card test showing agglutination (left).

or card test and is more simple than the complement fixation test.

Complement Fixation Test. Many studies have shown the superiority of this test in specificity and sensitivity, especially for chronically infected cattle and vaccinated cattle.

Other test methods that have been used are ELISA, serum buffered acid antigen, heat inactivation, mercaptoethanol, Coombs' antiglobulin, hemagglutination, milk-ring and whey tests, vaginal mucous and semen plasma agglutination, and fluorescent antibody examination of tissues or excretions.

Regardless of the test used, the results should be properly evaluated. Emphasis should be placed upon kinds of antibodies (qualitative) instead of numbers of antibodies (quantitative).

BACTERIOLOGY

The milk and other udder secretions are good sources of organisms. The supramammary lymph nodes are the preferential site at necropsy, but other lymph nodes are also useful. Abomasal fluids should be cultured from the fetus.

Swine

There is agreement that individual animal test results are less accurate in swine than in cattle. There may be false-negative or false-positive results. A herd test result profile is best. The card test is very useful, and supplemental procedures can be used. Sites for cultures should include the lymph nodes, especially those in the cervical region, and the seminal vesicles.

Sheep and Goats

There is no international standard for test or interpretation of results for *B. melitensis* infections. The tube agglutination test is generally used, but complement fixation and dermal hypersensitivity tests are preferred by many workers. Bacteriologic examinations are of vaginal discharges, milk, spleen, lymph nodes, placentae, and aborted fetuses.

The diagnosis of *B. ovis* infection requires a clinical examination, semen evaluation, and interpretation of results of the complement fixation tests on blood sera and cultures if indicated. A gel diffusion test has also given good results.

EPIDEMIOLOGY

Cattle

The infected cow is the source of most infections through discharges and products associated with parturition (Fig. 6). She is generally not infectious to other cattle by 2 to 4 weeks after parturition. Hygienic measures are important but may not be effective to control the disease due to seronegatively infected cattle that abort or calve normally. The variable incubation period of a few weeks to several months is related to the gestation period and severity of exposure.

Brucellae are intracellular parasites and, in this environment, are not antigenic and are protected from host defenses and chemotherapy.

Calves born to infected cows and those ingesting contaminated milk are temporarily infected. The permanency of this infection has been disputed. However, it is now certain that latent infections occur, but the frequency and contributing factors are unknown. An additional problem is that the heifer becomes seronegative during most of prepuberty and prior to calving. There have been many reports of latent infections that have resulted in new herd infections, or reinfections of herds considered free of brucellosis.

Under natural conditions, the bull appears to play a minor, if any, role in the transmission of brucellosis. However, contaminated semen used in artificial insemination may result in infections.

Brucellosis in wildlife species has not proved to be a problem in transmission to domesticated livestock except under special circumstances. The disease has persisted in certain bison populations in the United States and in caribou and reindeer populations in the Arctic.

Brucella organisms may survive within protected environments for several weeks, but sunlight kills them within a few hours. The virulence of strains varies, but no satisfactory *in vitro* method for its measurement has been developed.

TREATMENT

No satisfactory treatment for brucellosis in domestic animals has been discovered. Spontaneous recoveries occur among all species, and the percentages vary.

There has been success in treating *B. ovis* infections

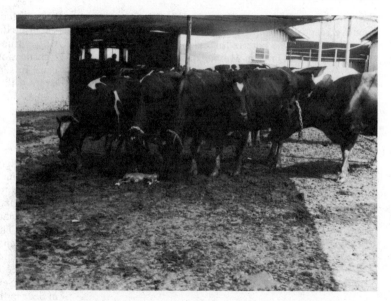

Figure 6. Ingestion is the most common source of *Brucella* infection, such as an aborted fetus.

with chlortetracycline and streptomycin, but the costs were high.

PUBLIC HEALTH CONSIDERATIONS

Brucellosis is a true zoonosis, and control in humans is directly related to its prevalence among other animals. Occupationally related infections predominate, with slaughterhouse workers the highest risk group.

B. melitensis is considered the most virulent species for humans, followed by *B. suis* and *B. abortus* in that order.

Direct contact with contaminated fluids and tissues is the chief source of infection. Outbreaks in slaughterhouses have been reported due to inhalation of *B. suis*. Accidental inoculation of strain 19 among veterinarians and laboratory workers is not uncommon. Ingestion of contaminated and unpasteurized dairy products is a very serious public health problem where *B. melitensis* is prevalent.

The symptoms in humans vary in severity from acute to chronic, and many infections are undiagnosed. The classic symptoms are headache, undulating fever, joint pains, chills, and weakness. Relapses after apparently successful treatment are not uncommon. The serum agglutination test is most often used to aid in the diagnosis, but methods of performing the test and interpretations of results may vary. The card test is very useful for acute infections. Intradermic tests should be avoided.

Acute infections respond well to oral tetracycline and intramuscular streptomycin. An early diagnosis combined with proper and prolonged treatment is important.

CONTROL

The control of brucellosis is both a herd owner's and a regulatory agent's responsibility. The major phases are identification and slaughter of diseased livestock, vaccination, herd management, and livestock movement control.

Strain 19 is the only approved vaccine in the United States for *B. abortus* infections. Other vaccines such as 45/20 and H38 have been studied by many investigators, often with conflicting findings. An attenuated strain of *B.*

melitensis, Rev 1, is used in other countries and is very effective. A commercial adjuvant vaccine is available to prevent *B. ovis* infections.

Currently, strain 19 is recommended for vaccination of calves at 2 to 6 months of age in dairy breeds and at 2 to 10 months of age in beef breeds. It can also be used for adult cattle in a lowered dose and under restricted conditions. High rates of vaccination in herds are important to reduction of herd infection rates.

The immunity produced by *Brucella* vaccines is cell mediated and related to dose and virulence of the challenge strain. The effectiveness of vaccination is best when a high percentage of the herd is immunized so that exposure potential is minimized. Individual effectiveness is often quoted to be about 65 to 70 per cent, but herd effectiveness is much greater. Vaccinated animals are much more likely to resist the disease or to have less severe cases, so that fewer organisms are excreted.

The herd size is very important in brucellosis control, especially if there is close confinement. Introduction of replacement animals raises the risk of herd infection. The status of the herd of origin is very important. Negative test results on purchased animals are not a satisfactory means of preventing introduction of cattle that are incubating the disease.

A cooperative program for control and eradication of bovine brucellosis began in 1934 largely as a drought relief effort. It received special emphasis in the early 1950s, and the current budget of public funds in the United States is about $85 million annually. The Uniform Methods and Rules are administered by the USDA. Strain 19 vaccination has been an integral part of the program with peak usage in 1983 when over 8 million calves were vaccinated. The program emphasizes surveillance of dairy and beef herds with test and slaughter of reactors until at least 120 days elapse without additional reactors. The effectiveness varies considerably with surveillance method, herd size, vaccination levels, and owner cooperation.

Swine

Purchase of swine from *Brucella*-free herds or rearing replacements is the best prevention. If brucellosis exists it is best to depopulate the herd. A second proposal is to retain young pigs and test them prior to breeding and farrowing. A third but inferior approach is to test and remove reactors until the last 2 herd tests reveal no more infected swine. The criteria for validating herds and areas are given in the Uniform Methods and Rules.

Sheep and Goats

Where *B. melitensis* exists, consideration is given to slaughter of the entire flock or herd. Use of Rev 1 vaccine with or without identification and slaughter of infected animals is another form of control.

The control of *B. ovis* is accomplished by maintaining young rams separate from mature rams. In addition, mature sheep are examined, and those with clinical and serologic evidence of infection are slaughtered. Vaccination of young rams is also recommended.

Supplemental Reading

Alton, G. G., Jones, L. M., and Pietz, D. E.: Laboratory Techniques in Brucellosis. World Health Organization Monograph Series no. 55, 2nd ed., 1975.

Crawford, R. P., and Hidalgo, R. J. (eds.): Bovine Brucellosis: An International Symposium. Texas, Texas A and M University Press, 1977.

Deyoe, B. L., and Manthei, C. A.: Brucellosis: *In* Disease of Swine, 4th ed. Iowa, Iowa State University Press, 492–515, 1975.

Jensen, R.: Diseases of Sheep. Philadelphia, Lea and Febiger, 51–57, 1974.

Nicoletti, P.: The Epidemiology of Bovine Brucellosis. *In* Advances in Veterinary Science and Comparative Medicine, vol. 24. New York, Academic Press, Inc., 1980.

Wilesmith, J. W.: The persistence of *Brucella abortus* in calves: a retrospective study of heavily infected herds. Vet. Rec. *103*:149–153, 1978.

Leptospirosis

LYLE E. HANSON, D.V.M., Ph.D.

Leptospirosis is an important infectious disease that affects all domestic animals as well as humans and wild animals. The disease is responsible for significant economic losses to the livestock industry, primarily due to abortion, reduction of milk and weight gain, and secondarily due to death. Human infections, which may vary from mild to serious, result from contact with pathogens in the urine of domestic or wild animals.

Incidence of leptospirosis in domestic animals is highest in cattle and lowest in sheep and goats. In a serologic survey involving reports from diagnostic laboratories in the United States in 1974, the combined serovar (serotype) reactor rate was more than 15 per cent in cattle and 3 per cent in swine.

The primary hosts vary with leptospiral serovars (serotypes), and usually only 1 to 2 host species are the principal carriers. *Pomona* serovar commonly affecting cattle and swine and occasionally wildlife often causes a severe disease. *Hardjo* is the predominant leptospiral serovar involving cattle, which are the reservoir hosts. Isolations of *hardjo* have been made from sheep, horses, and humans. *Grippotyphosa*, which has its reservoir in wildlife (especially small carnivores), sometimes is responsible for serious herd infections in both cattle and swine. *Icterohaemorrhagiae*, a serovar with its major reservoir in rats, and *canicola*, a serovar primarily affecting dogs, both can cause infections in cattle and swine.

Leptospires are usually shed in the urine and are transmitted to other hosts that have direct contact with the urine droplets or whose abraded skin comes in contact with urine-contaminated surface waters. Occasionally, transmission also occurs during coitus by contaminated urine or semen. Food chain transmission may be found in swine if they are allowed to consume leptospiral-infected rodent carcasses.

ETIOLOGY

Although over 100 leptospiral serovars have been isolated from animals, only 7 serovars have been isolated from livestock in the United States. The serovars *canicola*, *grippotyphosa*, *icterohaemorrhagiae*, and *pomona* have been isolated from both swine and cattle as well as wildlife. Three closely related serovars, *hardjo*, *balcanica*, and *szwajizak*, have been isolated only from cattle and humans in the United States. *Hardjo* has been isolated from sheep in New Zealand and from horse fetuses in Ireland. Serologic evidence indicates infections may occur in deer in the United States. Serologic studies also suggest that *autumnalis*, *bratislava*, *ballum*, and *tarassovi* serovars may cause cattle and swine infections in the United States.

Leptospires are filamentous organisms tightly coiled around an axial filament, ranging from 0.1 to 0.3 μm in width to 6 to 20 μm in length. A hook is generally present at one or both ends. The motility of the organisms is accomplished by rapid rotation along the long axis. Dark-field microscopy is generally used for visualization, as it provides an opportunity to observe both the morphologic condition and the characteristic motility. Leptospiral organisms can be stained either with Giemsa stain or with silver impregnation but not with aniline dyes.

PATHOGENESIS

Pathogenic leptospires actively penetrate exposed mucous membranes and abraded skin. The invading leptospires first multiply in the liver tissue, causing cellular necrosis and separation of liver cord cells. Leptospiremia following primary multiplication of the organisms in the liver usually results in the development of secondary sites of multiplication in the kidneys, lungs, reproductive organs, and brain.

Generally, the first antibodies (agglutinins) are detectable in the serum with a microscopic agglutination test 5 to 10 days after infection. Following the appearance of antibodies in the serum, leptospires can be isolated only intermittently from the blood. Agglutinins are elevated in concentration from 1 to 3 weeks following the initial signs of infection and persist from a few weeks to many months, and in some cattle and horses may remain active for many years.

Acute leptospiral infections generally involve the kidney, brain, and uterus and may become chronic. Leptospires have been isolated from kidneys and urine of both cattle and swine for as long as 1 year after the acute stage of the disease. Uterine penetration can occur during the immediate infection in pregnant animals of all susceptible species, resulting in infections of the fetuses. This may cause deaths, abortions, stillbirths, or persistent infections in newborns for several weeks. Both bovine and porcine fetuses have a limited capacity to produce agglutinating antibodies that may be detected in the blood of stillborn or newborn calves and pigs.

Chronic leptospiral infections have been demonstrated in the kidney, uterus, mammary gland, and brain. Persistent tissue infections can cause extensive destruction of glomeruli and tubules; interstitial and glomerular infiltrations in kidneys; and lymphocytes, plasma cells, and fibroblast infiltrations in other organs.

CLINICAL SIGNS

Acute leptospirosis is evident initially by an elevation of temperature that may persist from only a few hours to several days. Recurrent hyperemia is observed in some animals. Other signs associated with more severe infections are hemoglobinuria, anemia (cattle), jaundice, muscular weakness, pulmonary congestion, encephalitis, and death. Production of yellow-clotted milk followed by agalactia without notable inflammation is a frequent sign in cows. This condition has been commonly identified as "cold" mastitis. Agalactia usually lasts for 5 to 10 days, but reduced milk production may last throughout the entire lactation period. *Hardjo* has been isolated from mammary tissues of goats 3 weeks after inoculation, indicating this route may be involved in field infections.

In bulls, orchitis with reduced spermatogenesis occurs inconsistently. Semen produced during the acute stage of infection may contain leptospires for a short period. Though the transmission during coitus has been verified, it has not been determined whether the leptospires originate from semen or urine.

Abortions occur a few days to several weeks following initial infection of the fetuses. In swine, abortion usually is within a few days of the fetal infection, and live leptospires are frequently detected in the tissue of the fetus. However, dead cattle and sheep fetuses are retained for a longer period in the uterus, and the autolytic changes that result kill the leptospires before the fetus is expelled.

DIAGNOSIS

A correlation of clinical signs with serologic test results provides the most effective diagnostic aid. Titers of 1:100 or greater with either the microscope agglutination (MA) or microtiter technique are considered significant reactions. If serum is collected early in the acute stage of the disease, when serologic tests are usually negative, a sample should be tested 1 to 2 weeks later when an adequate antibody response would be measurable. A single positive serologic test result cannot reliably indicate the course of the disease, as it does not identify the stage. MA titers in some animals disappear before shedding from the kidney ceases. Some animals develop MA titers of 1:100 or greater for 2 to 3 months following vaccination, but these titers fall below diagnostically relevant levels by 4 to 5 months.

Isolation of leptospires from domestic animals is most successful during or immediately after the acute stage of the disease. Isolations are often made from swine fetuses but usually not from cattle or sheep fetuses, as autolysis usually is more extensive. Isolates can be taken from the blood during the short leptospiremic period or for longer periods from the urine. Isolation can be obtained either in special media or in laboratory animals, such as weanling hamsters, if proper specimens are used.

TREATMENT

Antibiotic therapy has been effective in reducing leptospiremia and the severity of clinical signs if administered during the acute stage. A single dose of 25 mg/kg of dihydrostreptomycin has been recommended as an effective procedure. However, several daily administrations of the same dose are more reliable. If renal failure occurs in a case of severe infection and the value of the animal warrants extensive measures, supportive therapy may include the administration of electrolytes and peritoneal dialysis. Antibiotics, such as dihydrostreptomycin or tetracycline, should be incorporated into the dialyzing fluid.

A leptospiral bacterin can be administered concurrently with an antibiotic to reduce dissemination of the infection within the herd if it is initiated early in the course of the epidemic. The bacterin must be an homologous serotype and will be effective only if the animal received it prior to exposure.

PREVENTION

Strict adherence to disease preventive management procedures will significantly reduce the dissemination of leptospiral infections. Domestic animals should be fenced in away from ponds, marshes, and streams that may be contaminated by leptospires. All new animals should be tested before being added to the herd. Annual testing of 10 per cent of the herd provides a continuous evaluation of herd status.

Administration of tetracycline for 10 to 14 days at 200 to 400 gm/ton of feed is an effective prophylactic procedure. However, the antibiotic would have to be fed on a continuous basis to prevent infection.

Administration of leptospiral bacterins can result in the development of protection against the homologous serovars for 6 months to 1 year. Although agglutinins may be detectable following vaccination for 2 to 3 months, neutralizing antibodies persist for longer periods. As cross-protection among serovars is minimal, the homologous serovar must be contained in the bacterin to provide adequate clinical protection. Revaccination of cattle in open herds should be conducted every 6 months and in closed herds every 12 months. Swine should be vaccinated twice at about 2-week intervals initially and again at 6-month intervals if the breeding animals are retained for several years. Currently, polyvalent bacterins containing *grippotyphosa, hardjo, pomona, canicola,* and *icterohaemorrhagiae* serovars are the most extensively used.

Persistent serologic reactions with low titer results are a serious problem for bull stud and for purebred cattle owners. Although isolations, except for *hardjo*, have not been made from cattle for longer than 15 months following an initial infection, titers may persist many years. Treatment with dihydrostreptomycin and vaccination is recommended for prophylactic purposes, but neither treatment significantly alters the subsequent serologic responses.

Supplemental Reading

Hanson, L. E., and Tripathy, D. N.: Leptospirosis. *In* Lehman, A. D., Glock, R. D., Mengeling, W. L., et al. (eds.): Diseases of Swine, 5th ed. Ames Iowa, Iowa State University Press, 1981.

South, P. J., and Stoenner, H. G.: The control of outbreaks of leptospirosis in beef cattle by simultaneous vaccination and treatment with dihydrostreptomycin. Proc. U.S. Anim. Health Assoc. 78:126, 1974.

Stalheim, O. H. V.: Chemotherapy of renal leptospirosis in cattle. Am. J. Vet. Res. 30:1317, 1969.

Vibriosis

(Bovine Genital Vibriosis and Ovine Vibrionic Abortion)

ALVIN B. HOERLEIN, D.V.M., Ph.D.

BOVINE GENITAL VIBRIOSIS

Bovine genital vibriosis is a venereal disease of cattle caused by *Vibrio fetus* var. *venerealis*,* which is transmitted from infected to noninfected animals during copulation and is characterized by temporary infertility of the female. The disease is widespread and is an important cause of infertility in cattle.

Clinical Signs

The chief clinical sign of infection is return to estrus by a bred cow. Exudate is not noted because the embryo is killed at an early stage. Abortions are infrequent. In some cows with the disease, pregnancy may result after 2 or 3 breedings and if the cows are left with the bulls, most will be pregnant within 9 months after initial exposure. The variable recovery times of individuals in the herd result in a prolonged calving season. Pregnancy examinations after the breeding season will reveal a large variation in ages of the fetuses. Depending on factors associated with carrier rates, susceptible animals, immune status, and management procedures, pregnancy rates may vary from 30 to 85 per cent in seasonally bred herds.

Pathogenesis

A thorough understanding of the pathogenesis of the disease in the individual animal and its transmission through the herd is invaluable in helping to make a diagnosis. The infected bull deposits semen and vibrios in the area of the cervix during breeding. The ovum is fertilized after initial exposure. The bacteria multiply and by 7 to 14 days will invade the oviducts. The fertilized ovum is destroyed by the bacteria so early that most susceptible heifers return to estrus at the normal interval. In subsequent breedings fertilization may not occur, since it has been shown that the vibrios adversely affect the cilia of the epithelial cells of the oviducts. Large numbers of bacteria will usually be found in cervicovaginal mucus from 3 weeks to 3 months after exposure. Eventually most of the infected cattle will conceive if bred repeatedly and will give birth to normal calves. Some cows remain carriers of the disease after normal parturition, and there is a measure of convalescent immunity. When bred again,

they become infected as evidenced by the temporary presence of *V. fetus* in cervical mucus, but fertility is normal. Infected cows bred to noninfected bulls for 2 or 3 years before being bred by an infected bull are still susceptible to reinfection. An annual "booster" infection appears essential for continued immunity.

Bulls contract the infection from infected females during breeding. The vibrios grow in the epithelial crypts of the penis and prepuce. Bulls may be transiently or chronically infected. Permanent infections are more common in older bulls. Bulls do not develop convalescent immunity from infection, since they can be reinfected after successful treatment. In beef cattle herds, where bulls do not get very old, it appears that carrier cows perpetuate the infection from year to year. The superficial nature of the infection in bulls precludes signs of disease, but in recently infected herds the burden of repeated breeding may result in temporary infertility.

Diagnosis

A tentative diagnosis of vibriosis can be made by thorough study of the herd history and by application of the knowledge of the pathogenesis of the disease.[1] The classic disease syndrome is characterized by repeated breeding and delayed conception, and a 20 to 30 per cent pregnancy rate after 60 days of breeding is not often seen, since it requires that all of the bulls be infected from the start of breeding and that all of the cows be susceptible to infection. Normal pregnancy rate is 90 per cent.

In most herds there are a small number of infected cattle during the first year of the disease, with greater numbers of infected cattle in the subsequent years. In many herds that have been infected for years, annual pregnancy rates may be from 70 to 80 per cent. A "strung out" calving season is an excellent indication of vibriosis. While all cattle are susceptible to infection, the usual herd will have a mixed population in relation to vibriosis at the beginning of each breeding season. A few of the cattle infected the previous year will still be carriers. Cows previously infected will have varying degrees of convalescent immunity. Some animals will be susceptible. Most of the bulls in seasonally bred beef herds will eliminate the organisms during the nonbreeding season. Thus, variable patterns of infertility can be expected from herd to herd.

In Western beef cattle herds, the highest pregnancy rates are often found in the heifers when they are bred separately to young bulls not previously exposed to infection. The lowest pregnancy rates often occur in young cows being bred for their second calf in the cow herd with old bulls.

In dairy herds, where artificial insemination is used exclusively, vibriosis seldom spreads. However, in many dairy herds bulls are used to breed the heifers and to breed those cows that have not become pregnant after several inseminations. If infection is present, the pregnancy rates in the replacement heifers may be very low.

A tentative diagnosis of vibriosis is most easily confirmed by bacteriologic examination of a freshly aborted fetus. Under most husbandry conditions, the small number of aborted fetuses either are not found while fresh enough for examination or are destroyed by predators.

The most practicable method of diagnosing vibriosis is through bacteriologic examination of cervicovaginal mucus. The techniques are not difficult to implement and have been well tested and described in detail.[2] Success

---

*Classified in Bergey's Manual of Systematic Bacteriology (Vol. 1, 1984) as *Campylobacter fetus* subsp. *venerealis*.

will be enhanced by selection of those animals for sampling that are most likely to yield positive results in cultures. Almost all susceptible, nonpregnant cows will be positive from 3 weeks to 3 months after initial exposure, and 5 to 10 mucus samples are adequate. Six months after initial exposure, only 20 per cent of the nonpregnant cows are still positive, so 20 or more cows need to be sampled for reliable results for diagnosis. Heifers or young cows bred for the first time by the old herd bulls are preferred, since the older cows may have convalescent immunity. Sampling of pregnant or postpartum cows is rarely successful. Mucus samples may be cultured in the laboratory within 6 hr after collection, but for long transport (up to 3 or 4 days) plastic pipettes containing samples should be frozen immediately on dry ice. Australian researchers have developed a complex transport medium for *V. fetus* specimens that has now been tested in the United States, which holds promise for transportation of specimens.[3] A single positive culture of *V. fetus* indicates herd infection. Immunologic test methods are so unreliable that few laboratories do them.

The *V. fetus* carrier state in the bull can be determined by bacteriologic culture and by identification of the organisms in semen, artificial vaginal washings, and preputial smegma. Smegma is preferred. Some laboratory staffs are capable of competent bacteriologic examination, but the methods are difficult and require considerable experience.

Diagnosis of infection in bulls is most easily accomplished by breeding virgin test heifers. Cervicovaginal mucus is examined bacteriologically in 3 weeks. Stud bulls used for artificial insemination can be tested by collection of smegma for introduction into virgin test heifers.

Control and Prevention

Exclusive use of artificial insemination with properly treated semen from noninfected bulls is an efficient method of controlling vibriosis. While useful in most dairy herds, it is useful in few beef cattle herds, owing to unsatisfactory pregnancy rates. The use of "clean-up" bulls after artificial insemination negates its value.

When exclusive artificial insemination is impracticable, the best method of disease control is vaccination of all female cattle. Oil adjuvant bacterins with heavy concentrations of highly immunogenic strains of *V. fetus* give adequate protection against the infertility caused by Vibriosis. For best results, a single injection of the vaccine should be given 60 to 90 days before breeding. Since both convalescent and vaccinal immunity wane with the passage of time, annual revaccination is required to maintain maximal reproductive rates. Revaccination of beef cows at weaning has been shown to be effective. In the absence of other reproductive problems, properly vaccinated Vibrioinfected herds should have pregnancy rates greater than 90 per cent.

Vaccination of bulls has not usually been recommended, but recent research in Australia and Belgium suggests that the carrier state of bulls may be modified by vaccination. The vaccines must have especially high antigen content. Recent controlled experiments in Colorado demonstrated that vaccination of infected bulls had value in elimination of the bacteria from most of the bulls. An exclusive bull vaccination program should be approached with caution until additional research demonstrates its value.

Treatment

Dihydrostreptomycin injected subcutaneously at 22 mg/kg, and 5 gm of a 50-per cent solution applied locally to the penis and prepuce will eliminate the infection from bulls. The bulls thus cured are still susceptible to reinfection. While antibiotics are not of value in treatment of the infection in the female, vaccination will hasten recovery.

OVINE VIBRIONIC ABORTION

Ovine vibrionic abortion is an acute contagious disease of sheep caused by *Vibrio fetus* var. *intestinalis** and is characterized by late abortion or birth of dead or weak lambs. The disease is found in all parts of the world but is a serious threat only in flocks having partial or complete confinement.

Clinical Signs

The clinical signs of vibriosis consist of abortions in the last trimester of pregnancy, especially in the last month. Some lambs are dead, while others are weak and may live for several days.

Pathogenesis

The organisms are carried in the gallbladder of some previously infected sheep and are spread through fecal contamination of feed and water. After ingestion of the organisms, the ewe has bacteremia for 1 to 2 weeks, during which time, if she is in the later part of gestation, the placenta and eventually the fetus may become infected.[4] Abortion by one or a small number of ewes is often followed by a "storm" of abortions in the flock. This results from massive exposure of pregnant ewes nosing an aborted fetus and placenta. There is no spread of the venereal disease. The abortion rate may be as high as 70 per cent, but usually it is 20 to 30 per cent. Five per cent of the aborting ewes may die of other complications. There is convalescent immunity, since those ewes that abort will produce normal lambs the next season. They appear to be immune for 2 or 3 years.

Diagnosis

The diagnosis of ovine vibriosis is made by bacteriologic examination of the stomach contents of an aborted fetus. A direct stain for bacteria in the stomach contents or affected cotyledons may be adequate. Dead or weak full term lambs may have typical liver lesions that are depressed, light-colored areas (2 to 3 cm in diameter) on the surface.

Control and Prevention

Bacterins that stimulate effective immunity are available, but they must be given before exposure to infection. If a diagnosis can be made early enough in an epizootic, vaccination will probably protect those ewes not yet exposed. After an outbreak of infection, vaccination of all ewes and subsequent additional ewes to the flock will prevent the disease.

---

*Classified in Bergey's Manual of Systematic Bacteriology (Vol. 1, 1984) as *Campylobacter fetus* subsp. *fetus*.

References

1. Carroll, E. J., and Hoerlein, A. B.: Diagnosis and control of bovine genital vibriosis. J. Am. Vet. Med. Assoc. *161*:1359, 1972.
2. Hoerlein, A. B.: Vibriosis. *In* Amstutz, H. E. (ed.): Bovine Medicine and Surgery, 2nd ed. Santa Barbara, California, American Veterinary Publications, 298–312, 1980.
3. Winter, A. J., and Caveney, N. T.: Evaluation of a transport medium for *Campylobacter (Vibrio) fetus*. J. Am. Vet. Med. Assoc. *173*:472, 1978.
4. Jensen, R.: Diseases of Sheep. Philadelphia, Lea and Febiger, 60, 1974.

Tuberculosis

L. D. KONYHA, D.V.M., M.S.

Tuberculosis is an infectious disease caused by certain pathogenic acid-fast organisms of the genus *Mycobacterium* and is usually characterized by the formation of nodular granulomas known as tubercles. Although commonly a chronic, debilitating disease, tuberculosis can occasionally assume a rapidly progressive course.

ETIOLOGY

Three types of tubercle bacilli are recognized in warm-blooded animals: human, bovine, and fowl. Their causative organisms are classified in *Bergey's Manual of Determinative Bacteriology* (8th ed.) as *Mycobacterium tuberculosis*, *M. bovis*, and *M. avium*, respectively. Since tubercle bacilli do not multiply except in infected animals, their principal reservoirs in nature are the three groups of animals mentioned earlier. Though certain morphologic and cultural differences are described, these can vary considerably and cannot be depended upon for accurate identification. Many biochemical tests have been devised that are extremely useful in classifying mycobacteria. The most common are niacin, catalase, arylsulfatase, and growth inhibition tests. The mycobacterial tube agglutination test described by Schaefer has provided a useful procedure for the classification of *M. avium* organisms. Cattle are susceptible to human tuberculosis, but lesions of this infection are seldom reported. Although there are cases on record of generalized bovine tuberculosis caused by the avian strain, they are unusual. If the avian infection becomes established in bovines, gross lesions generally are limited to the mesenteric lymph nodes. During a 10-year period (July 1, 1972 to June 30, 1982), *M. bovis* accounted for 71 per cent of the total isolations of Mycobacteria from bovine tuberculous specimens submitted to the National Veterinary Services Laboratory for culturing.

EPIDEMIOLOGY

Bovine tuberculosis is known to exist in all parts of the world. Of the 164 countries reporting in the 1982 Animal Health Yearbook, 26 indicated bovine tuberculosis to be an exceptional occurrence, 54 indicated a low sporadic incidence, 26 indicated a moderate incidence, and 3 indicated a high incidence. Even though tuberculosis in cattle in the United States has been reduced to an exceptional occurrence, there were still 14 *M. bovis* infected herds in fiscal year 1983, and reports of epizootics of the disease continue.

PATHOGENESIS

The disease commences with the formation of the primary focus, which is in the lungs in about 90 per cent of the cases. Lymphatic drainage from the primary focus leads to the formation of a caseous lesion in the corresponding lymph node, and this lesion, together with the primary focus, is known as the primary complex.

Whenever the organisms localize, their activity stimulates the formation of tumor-like masses called tubercles. Any tissue can be affected, but lesions are most frequent in lymph nodes (bronchial, mediastinal, portal, and cervical), lungs, liver, spleen, and surfaces of the body cavities. The bacilli spread throughout tissues by extension onto surfaces in contact with a lesion, or they may be transported in body cavity fluids and disseminated in the vascular system subsequent to vessel erosion at a lesion site.

DISSEMINATION

The tuberculous cow is the greatest source of danger to healthy cattle, and an infected animal not promptly removed from the herd is a source of potential reinfection. Active lesions can contain myriads of bacilli, and when they communicate with natural body openings, the bacilli can be widely disseminated. In diseased cattle, this is most frequently by way of the respiratory tract. Bronchial exudates, which are teeming with organisms, may be expelled into the manger or watering trough by coughing, or exudates may be swallowed and expelled in the feces. Animals that ingest contaminated feed or water may contract the disease. Inhalation of contaminated aerosols is an important way in which the disease is disseminated in closed barns with poor ventilation. Contaminated dust, droplets, or dried secretions can enter the respiratory tract to cause infection in susceptible animals.

Viable organisms can also be eliminated in the milk, even though there are no lesions in the udder. Calves sometimes are infected during the first few hours or days of life when nursing an infected dam. Many calves in the past were infected by ingestion of unpasteurized skimmed milk from diseased cows. Calves may infrequently be infected as a result of intrauterine exposure.

CLINICAL SIGNS

Clinical signs of tuberculosis in cattle in the United States are seldom encountered today because intradermal tuberculin test results facilitate presumptive diagnosis and elimination of infected animals before signs appear. Prior to the national bovine tuberculosis eradication program, however, the signs associated with this disease were common.

The evidence of tuberculosis exhibited by any animal depends upon the extent and location of lesions. In many instances, characteristic signs are lacking even in advanced stages of the disease when many organs are involved.

Lung involvement may be manifested by a cough that can be induced by changes in temperature or by manual pressure on the trachea. Dyspnea and other signs of low-grade pneumonia are also evidence of lung involvement. In advanced cases, lymph nodes are frequently greatly enlarged and may obstruct air passages, the alimentary tract, or blood vessels. Lymph nodes of the head and neck may become visibly affected and sometimes rupture and drain to the outside. Involvement of the digestive tract is characterized by intermittent diarrhea and by constipation in some cases. Extreme emaciation and acute respiratory distress may occur during the terminal stages. Lesions involving the female genitalia are possible. Primary uterine infection may be found following service by an infected bull or even following artificial insemination by contaminated semen. The male genitalia are seldom involved; however, when penile lesions are present, they appear to be limited to the submucosa of the glans, sheath, and adjacent lymphatics.

NECROPSY FINDINGS

On necropsy, tuberculous granulomas usually have a yellowish appearance and are caseous, caseocalcareous, or calcified in consistency. The appearance may sometimes be purulent. The caseous center is usually dry and firm and covered by a fibrous connective capsule of varying thickness. In recent years, calcification has been seen less commonly. The lesions may be so small as to be missed by the unaided eye or so large as to involve the greater part of an organ. Bronchopneumonia may be observed grossly in instances of lung lesions, and there may be little evidence of fluid accumulations microscopically. Lesions may be situated in any one of the lung lobes, causing productive bronchopneumonia that, in turn, gives rise to lesions in the bronchotracheal tree and regional lymph nodes.

When tubercle bacilli enter the body they usually are phagocytized by neutrophils almost immediately. The neutrophils are destroyed by multiplying mycobacteria, and as dead cells they stimulate the accumulation of epithelioid cells that engulf the neutrophils and mycobacteria. The bacilli are not destroyed, but multiply within the epithelioid cells and apparently produce a toxic substance that destroys adjoining cells. This causes an area of caseous necrosis and the beginning of a tubercle. More epithelioid cells encircle the necrotic area, while in the center of the tubercle the cellular nuclei disappear and structural detail is lost.

A number of epithelioid cells coalesce, forming multi-nucleated giant cells (Langhans' cells). These cells are characteristic but not pathognomonic of tubercles. They are also found in granulomatous lesions of other chronic inflammatory diseases. Acid-fast bacilli may be demonstrated throughout a lesion in epithelioid cells, in giant cells, and in necrotic debris. Granulation tissue forms and is usually surrounded by a zone of lymphocytes and fibroblasts, frequently near a blood vessel.

DIAGNOSIS

Clinical evidence of tuberculosis is usually lacking; therefore, its diagnosis in individual animals and an erad-

ication program were not possible prior to the development of tuberculin by Koch in 1890. Tuberculin, a concentrated sterile culture filtrate of tubercle bacilli grown on glycerinated beef broth, and more recently on synthetic media, provides a means of detecting a diseased animal. Animals affected with tuberculosis are allergic to the proteins contained in the tuberculin and give characteristically delayed hypersensitivity reactions when exposed to them. If tuberculin is deposited in the deep layers of the skin (intradermally), a local reaction characterized by swelling and inflammation is induced in infected animals. In the United States, the caudal fold is the preferred injection site for the intradermal tuberculin test. The injection sites are examined by observation and palpation 72 hr postinjection.

Nearly all countries of the world are now using a strain of *M. bovis* for the preparation of this mammalian tuberculin. Heat-concentrated synthetic media tuberculin (OT) is still used in some countries, but a majority (including the United States) are now using purified protein derivative (PPD) tuberculin at a protein concentration of 1 mg/ml (3 mg/ml in Australia). PPD are preferable because they are easier to standardize, are more stable, and are more specific.

Although remarkably effective, the intradermal test has certain limitations, as do all diagnostic tests. No antigen (tuberculin) is entirely specific, and significant intradermal responses are induced not only by infection with the homologous organism *(M. bovis)* but also to varying degrees by several heterologous organisms, primarily other mycobacteria. All animals with a positive response in herds that are not known to be infected with *M. bovis* and animals with a positive response in areas of the world where bovine tuberculosis has been nearly eradicated (such as the United States) should be retested by the comparative-cervical (c-c) test. In the United States, only veterinarians specifically approved by state or federal regulatory agencies are permitted to conduct the c-c test using PPD tuberculins of equal biologic potency, as determined in sensitized guinea pigs. The c-c test is contraindicated in cattle in known *M. bovis* infected herds.

TREATMENT

Until the discovery of the antituberculosis drug isoniazid or isonicotinic acid hydrazide (INH), there was no practical therapeutic agent available for bovine tuberculosis. Reports from South Africa indicate that it is economically feasible to treat cattle with isoniazid. See Table 1 for the treatment protocol in South Africa.

Isoniazid therapy may have potential value in countries where the incidence of bovine tuberculosis is high and

Table 1. *INH Treatment for Bovine Tuberculosis*

Choice of Herds for Treatment
Large herds ($\geq$ 200), high producers, and herds with infection rates over 30 per cent.
Positively reacting herds of valuable stud animals or special blood lines.

Dosages
Infected cattle and cattle with suspicious reactions: 20 mg/kg daily (maximum 12 gm/day for bulls and 10 gm/day for cows) for 2 months. Same dose 3 times weekly for another 5 months.
Cattle with negative reactions: 10 mg/kg daily (maximum 4.5 gm/day for adults, and 2.2 gm/day for calves) for 2 months.

"test and slaughter" methods are not yet feasible. The disadvantages of using INH are so great (up to 25 per cent refractory cases, emergence of drug-resistant strains, elimination of INH in the milk, and the danger of relapse when the drug is withdrawn) that the treatment of bovine tuberculosis is not permitted in the United States.

PREVENTION AND CONTROL

Eradication of bovine tuberculosis is a major objective that has nearly been achieved in many countries of Europe, North America (including the United States), Japan, New Zealand, and Australia. The basis of these eradication programs has been the systemic application of the tuberculin test and the slaughter of reactors.

The best preventive measure against introduction of bovine tuberculosis is a negative tuberculin test result in the animal before change of ownership, whether change is international, interstate, or local in nature. A complete epidemiologic investigation, with testing where indicated, should be conducted on every animal found to have lesions of tuberculosis on routine postmortem examination.

Since 1890 various types of vaccines have been advocated for cattle, but none have produced effective immunity to bovine tuberculosis. Recent investigations in Malawi confirm that while BCG vaccine (the most successful immunizing agent in humans) reduces the severity of the initial disease in cattle, it does not completely prevent infection. Besides affording no practical protection to cattle, vaccination induces hypersensitivity to tuberculin and, thus, interferes with diagnostic test results. Countries that have attempted to use vaccination as the basis of a control program ultimately abandon the procedure in favor of the "test and slaughter" method.

Supplemental Reading

Animal Health Yearbook, FAO, WHO, OIE, 1977.
Francis, J.: Tuberculosis in Animals and Man. London, Cassel and Co., Ltd., 1958.
Konyha, L. D., and Chaloux, P. A.: Bacterial diseases. In Amstutz, H. E. (ed.): Tuberculosis, Bovine Medicine and Surgery, 3rd ed. Santa Barbara, California, American Veterinary Publications, 1980.
Rich, A. R.: The Pathogenesis of Tuberculosis, 2nd ed. Springfield, Illinois, Charles C Thomas, 3–118, 1950.
Schaefer, W. B.: Serologic identification and classification of the atypical mycobacteria by agglutination. Am. Rev. Resp. Dis. 96:115, 1965.
Smith, H. A., Jones, T. C., and Hunt, R. D.: Veterinary Pathology, 5th ed. Philadelphia, Lea and Febiger, 1983.

Swine Tuberculosis

J. GLENN SONGER, Ph.D.

Tuberculosis as it occurs in pigs today bears little resemblance to tuberculosis in cattle or in humans. The disease in pigs has no apparent effect on the health of the animal, and no evidence exists that it can be transmitted from pigs to humans, either by direct contact or by eating pork products. It is found in about 0.4 per cent of all pigs slaughtered under United States federal government inspection, costing the pork industry an estimated $2.5 to 3 million annually. Since the disease in pigs is different in so many ways from the disease in cattle and in humans, some workers have suggested that it be called swine mycobacteriosis rather than tuberculosis.

ETIOLOGY

In the early part of this century, when both human and bovine tuberculosis were more prevalent, bacteria found in swine with tuberculosis were often shown to be either bovine (Mycobacterium bovis) or human (M. tuberculosis) type. As early as 1925, however, M. avium began to appear more frequently in swine with tuberculosis, and this trend has continued. Today, isolation from swine of mycobacteria other than M. avium is uncommon. A few workers have, in recent years, reported the extensive involvement of bovine tubercle bacilli in tuberculosis of swine, usually in animals from countries other than the United States or in animals fed improperly cooked wastes from cattle slaughtering plants.

PATHOGENESIS

Pigs are usually infected by ingestion of feed contaminated with the bacteria. When swallowed, M. avium penetrates the wall of the gastrointestinal tract and is carried to regional lymph nodes, usually cervical or mesenteric nodes. Lesions develop in these nodes, but progressive disease is rare. For this reason, the health and condition of the pig remain unaffected in the majority of cases. It is usually impossible, therefore, to diagnose tuberculosis in pigs based on clinical signs.

Lesions in the lymph nodes are found, however, when pigs are slaughtered. Prior to 1972, tissues with these lesions were trimmed and discarded. In 1972, a regulation was adopted that called for cooking at 170°F for 30 minutes all of the carcasses found to have at least 2 isolated lesions of tuberculosis; these carcasses are designated "passed for cooking" or PFC. Carcasses processed in this manner lose most of their economic worth, and the additional labor required at slaughter increases the cost. In addition, many processing plants have no facilities for cooking carcasses and they must, therefore, be condemned.

EPIDEMIOLOGY

Incidence of the disease is determined from findings of meat inspectors at slaughter. On this basis, the prevalence of lesions is about 0.4 per cent of all hogs slaughtered each year under federal government inspection. The infection rate may be higher since mycobacteria can be in lymph nodes in the absence of gross lesions, and some lesions are not detected by inspectors. Lesions induced by Corynebacterium equi may be mistaken for tuberculous lesions, thus yielding false-positive findings.

Poultry with tuberculosis are still occasionally found to be the source of infection for swine but to a much lesser extent than previously. Pig-to-pig transmission of tuberculosis has been reported and is probably due to the presence of infected sites in the intestinal wall that allow shedding of mycobacteria in the feces. Infections of the lungs, mammary glands, and uterus also occur and may be a means of transmission or of introduction of the disease into a herd. Garbage feeding, although relatively rare, is another possible means for the spread of swine tuberculosis.

In recent years, work has shown that sawdust or woodshavings used for bedding may be a source of the infection for swine. *M. avium* can often be found in samples of sawdust and woodshavings, where it survives for long periods and may even multiply under proper conditions of moisture and temperature. This may explain the seasonal occurrence of tuberculosis in some herds.

Soil is another possible reservoir. *M. avium* may survive for more than 4 years in soil and litter contaminated by chickens with tuberculosis.

LESIONS

Lesions of *M. avium* infection are usually confined to the lymph nodes associated with the digestive tract. Grossly, lesions are white to yellow, raised, and usually ranging in size from barely visible to 10 mm in diameter. Active lesions are rarely calcified, but older lesions (of several months) may be calcified, as suggested by their gritty texture on cutting. Caseous, rather than purulent, exudate is usually seen, as is diffuse fibrosis and proliferation of epithelioid and giant cells. Calcification often is found in older lesions, and necrosis is limited. Gross and microscopic lesions in pigs due to *M. avium* infection cannot be reliably distinguished from those caused by *M. bovis* or *M. tuberculosis* without bacteriologic examination.

DIAGNOSIS

Diagnosis of *M. avium* infection should be accomplished by detection of typical gross and microscopic lesions and isolation and identification of *M. avium*. The tuberculin skin test, using 0.1 ml tuberculin or PPD intradermally in the dorsal surface of the ear, may be helpful as a herd test, but displays high false-positive and false-negative rates. Other diagnostic tests are not in common use.

THERAPY

No vaccine is available at present. No antimicrobial agents have been shown to be effective in preventing or treating the infection.

PREVENTION AND CONTROL

It is important not to mix swine and poultry production on the same farm. Feeding uncooked garbage or other material that might contain viable tubercle bacilli to pigs must be avoided. The purchase of breeding stock from tuberculosis-free herds should be practiced.

Infected herds may be depopulated and then repopulated with stock from tuberculosis-free herds. Little is known about effective procedures for decontamination of infected soil; concrete lots should be used whenever possible. Concrete surfaces and equipment such as farrowing crates and feeders must be disinfected with a phenol-based disinfectant (e.g., Amphyl) or a 2 to 3 per cent cresylic acid solution. Quaternary-ammonium disinfectants are not effective against mycobacteria.

Lesions caused by *M. avium* usually regress and disappear with age. Therefore, gilts can be kept, thus adding to the herd size or to the breeding animals. When these animals are sold at the end of their usefulness as breeding animals, the lesions may have disappeared.

If the source of the infection can be found and eliminated (e.g., infected bedding), the producer may be able to wait for the approximate 6-month period until all exposed pigs have been slaughtered.

Swine tuberculosis is obviously a disease that is better prevented than controlled. Efforts should be made to avoid all contact between hogs and birds. Hogs should not be housed in old poultry buildings unless they are constructed in such a way as to allow thorough cleaning and disinfection.

If at all possible, the use of woodshavings for bedding (especially in farrowing buildings) should be eliminated. Some producers have used woodshavings as bedding and experienced no problems, while others have been forced out of business due to tuberculosis in their animals. If woodshavings must be used, they should be kept dry, both at the sawmill and on the farm. Wild birds should also be kept away from storage areas.

Supplemental Reading

Songer, J. Glenn.: Environmental sources of *Mycobacterium avium* for infection of animals and man. Proc. Ann. Meeting United States Animal Health Assoc. *84*:528–535,1980.
Thoen, C. O., and Karlson, A. G.: Tuberculosis. *In* Leman, A. D., et al. (eds.). Diseases of Swine. Ames, Iowa, Iowa State University Press, 508–516, 1981.

Johne's Disease
(Paratuberculosis)

AUBREY B. LARSEN, D.V.M., M.S.

Johne's disease, paratuberculosis, is a chronic infectious disease of ruminants and has been diagnosed in almost every state in the United States.

ETIOLOGY

Johne's disease is caused by *Mycobacterium paratuberculosis*, a small, acid-fast bacillus about 1 to 2 μ in length and 0.5 μ in diameter. These organisms inhabit primarily the intestinal mucosa of the ileocecal valve region and the neighboring mesenteric lymph nodes. They may be found from the upper portion of the small intestines to the rectum, however. *M. paratuberculosis* is seen in typical clumps and can be seen singly or in clumps in smears of infected intestinal mucosa with an acid-fast stain. The organisms may be extracellular or intracellular, as observed from tissue sections. They may be found occasionally upon microscopic examination of stained sections, when they cannot be found in stained smears.

Guinea pigs, hamsters, mice, rats, and rabbits are not susceptible to natural infections with *M. paratuberculosis*.

CLINICAL SIGNS

Johne's disease affects adults, and usually only 1 or 2 cattle in the herd will have clinical signs of the disease at any one time. Chronic diarrhea accompanied by a gradual loss of weight is considered typical of the clinical disease.

However, in some cases, a gradual weight loss may precede diarrhea by several months, and in sheep and goats there may be a gradual weight loss and eventually death without diarrhea. Affected animals have an unthrifty appearance, rough coat, dry skin, and reduced milk production. The temperature may or may not be elevated.

DIAGNOSIS

Johne's disease may be confused with malnutrition, chronic traumatic gastritis, abscesses of liver, coccidiosis, winter dysentery, pyelonephritis, and helminth parasitism. A thorough examination by the clinician will help rule out most of these conditions.

Most heavily infected cattle react to the intravenous johnin test. This test is more reliable than either the intradermic johnin test or the serologic tests for assistance in diagnosing the disease in clinically ill animals. The intravenous johnin test should be conducted only on days when the environmental temperature is less than 30.6°C. The test is conducted as follows: a preinjection rectal temperature is obtained, 2 to 4 ml of johnin is administered, and temperature is recorded at 4½, 6, and 7½ hr postinjection. A rectal temperature rise of 0.83°C or more over the preinjection temperature is considered a positive result, provided the highest temperature recorded is at least 39.6°C. Some infected cattle will develop temperatures of 41.7°C during the test. If the preinjection temperature is 39.4°C or more, the animal cannot be tested.

In addition to the intravenous johnin test, a diagnosis can be confirmed by demonstrating typical acid-fast bacilli in stained smears prepared from intestinal mucosa or from feces. Failure to find the bacillus in smears prepared from material obtained from the living animal does not negate the diagnosis of paratuberculosis, especially if the intravenous johnin test was positive. The animal should be examined postmortem to confirm the accuracy of the diagnosis. If a postmortem examination is made of an animal suspected of having had Johne's disease, the practitioner should not depend on the presence of macroscopic lesions to confirm the cause of death. Some infected cattle do not have gross changes in the intestine or other tissues. To confirm the cause of death, select a specimen that includes the terminal 6 in. of ileum, ileocecal valve, and an adjacent mesenteric lymph node. A piece of intestine about 2 cm square and one half of the mesenteric lymph node should be placed in a 10-per cent formalin solution and sent to the laboratory for histologic examination. The remainder of the specimen should be frozen and sent to the laboratory for culturing. The identfication of *M. paratuberculosis* requires special procedures and equipment available only in the laboratory.

TREATMENT

Treatment of Johne's disease is not recommended because clinical signs are observed only in the terminal stage of the disease. Drugs useful in the treatment of other mycobacterial infections have been used, and none have been satisfactory.

PREVENTION

Johne's disease is usually introduced into clean herds through the purchase of diseased cattle. Therefore, herd owners should be advised to raise their own replacements and to avoid purchasing or leasing cattle. Improved blood lines can be obtained by artificial insemination.

When herd additions are necessary, they should not be purchased from any herd with a history of Johne's disease.

CONTROL AND ERADICATION

The disease is self-limiting in some cattle, and other cattle may recover completely. The numbers of infected cattle that appear healthy usually exceed those that actually develop signs of disease. The intradermal johnin skin test has been disappointing as a control measure. All cattle that show clinical signs of disease should be removed from the herd at once and slaughtered. Feces of all remaining cattle 2 years of age or older should be cultured annually for the presence of *M. paratuberculosis*, and those with positive results should also be removed from the herd and sold for slaughter.

Calves are very susceptible and become infected by ingesting feces of diseased animals. However, they do develop some natural resistance as they mature, and it has been found that raising young animals separately from adults greatly reduces losses in infected herds. Manure from the adults should not be spread on pastures. Fecal contamination of all feed and water should be avoided. The herd should be maintained on an adequate ration containing all the requirements for good growth and production. There is evidence that a poor ration increases the incidence of the disease, although definite proof is lacking. Keeping the premises clean and sanitary also reduces losses from the disease. Cresylic acid disinfectant and sodium orthophenylphenate (used in the same dilutions recommended for disinfecting premises contaminated with *M. bovis*) are suitable for use on premises contaminated with *M. paratuberculosis*.

IMMUNIZATION

It has been found that good management, separation of calves from adults, and good sanitary practices reduce losses from Johne's disease but in many instances will not eradicate it from the herd. Therefore, vaccination has been investigated as an additional means of control. In experimental field studies, it has been found that there is a substantial reduction in clinical Johne's disease in herds in which a vaccine is used.

In Great Britain and European countries, live bacterial vaccines are used. However, in the United States only killed bacterial vaccines have been used. Calves are vaccinated before they reach 30 days of age. A fibrocaseous nodule develops at the vaccination site and may remain for the life of the animal.

Advantages of killed vaccines are (1) the bacillus cannot mutate and become virulent, (2) they are less likely to change during storage than live products, and (3) persistent infections with vaccine strains do not occur.

It has been assumed that cattle vaccinated against paratuberculosis would become hypersensitive to tuberculin and would therefore interfere with tuberculosis eradication programs. Experiments have shown, however, that cattle that were vaccinated against paratuberculosis that later became infected with bovine tuberculosis could be identified with appropriate tests.

In 1982 a vaccine offering protection against Johne's disease was licensed in the United States. Before a state can receive approval for use of the vaccine, federal government authorities require the State Regulatory Agency to present an acceptable Johne's disease control program for the state.

An effective vaccine, when used in conjunction with other control measures, should make it possible to eliminate the disease from affected herds in most instances.

JOHNE'S DISEASE IN OTHER DOMESTIC ANIMALS

Johne's disease is often diagnosed in goats and sometimes in sheep in the United States. Diarrhea is not as severe in these species. Diseased sheep may lose part of their wool. Affected animals lose weight, and the clinical signs are often confused with those of parasitism. The diagnosis is confirmed by demonstrating the bacillus in intestinal mucosa or in feces, or by culturing the bacillus.

Johne's disease in sheep and goats is difficult to control since it is usually not practical to separate the young from their dams. The disease may be eliminated by disposing of the entire flock, thoroughly cleaning and disinfecting the premises, and keeping the premises free from livestock for at least 1 year. Vaccination of lambs has also been an effective control method.

Supplemental Reading

Larsen, A. B., and Kopecky, K. E.: Studies on the intravenous administration of johnin to diagnose Johne's disease. Am. J. Vet. Res. 26:673–675, 1965.
Larsen, A. B., Moyle, A. I., and Himes, E. M.: Experimental vaccination of cattle against paratuberculosis (Johne's disease) with killed bacterial vaccines: a controlled field study. Am. J. Vet. Res. 39:65–69, 1978.
Larsen, A. B., Vardaman, T. H., and Merkal, R. S.: An extended study of a herd of cattle naturally infected with Johne's disease. I. The significance of the intradermal johnin test. Am. J. Vet. Res. 24:91–93, 1963.

Corynebacterial Infections

JESS L. AYERS, D.V.M., Ph.D.

Members of the genus *Corynebacterium* are common causes of infection in cattle, sheep, and swine. The bacteria in this genera are gram-positive, nonmotile, nonsporeforming, pleomorphic short rods. If there is a unifying characteristic of infection by members of the genus *Corynebacterium*, it is the production of purulent exudates. The exudates are dirty-white to yellow, sometimes with a green tinge, and are of varying consistency. Good management practices may be the most important means of control of corynebacterial infections, since traditional manipulation of the immune system by natural or artificial methods does not appear to adequately stimulate acquired resistance.

CATTLE

The specific diseases occurring in cattle are ulcerative lymphangitis and caseous lymphadenitis caused by *C. pseudotuberculosis* and contagious bovine pyelonephritis caused by *C. renale*. However, infection by *C. pyogenes* is far more frequent and economically serious than any of the first 3 conditions.

Both *C. pyogenes* and *C. renale* are sometimes isolated from uterovaginal scretions and from milk of cows with metritis. *C. pyogenes* infection has been associated with embryonic and fetal deaths and is a minor cause of footrot in cattle. The organism has been isolated from suppurative processes of the central nervous system and from embolic suppurative nephritis in cattle. Chronic suppurative arthritis in cattle is often associated with *C. pyogenes* infection. There have been occasional reports of bone lesions in the radius, metacarpus, and metatarsus where focal destructive lesions and sequestrations occur. Abscesses and vertebral body necrosis caused by *C. pyogenes* and *Fusobacterium necrophorum* result in paralysis in a small percentage of cattle.

Various predisposing factors aid in the establishment of *C. pyogenes* infection. For example, its ability to produce disease is apparently greatly enhanced by trauma, such as bruising of muscle. Abscesses in the lungs due to *C. pyogenes* are common sequelae of bronchopneumonia of calves and feedlot cattle and are considered secondary to the primary pneumonia caused by other agents such as *Pasteurella* spp.

Abscesses that are readily accessible respond to surgical drainage and systemic penicillin. It is important to maintain drainage while interior healing of the abscess takes place. However, internal abscesses create diagnostic and therapeutic problems for which there are no apparent answers.

Corynebacterial mastitis in cattle is currently provoking a great deal of interest. *C. bovis* is a common skin and teat canal inhabitant that rarely causes mastitis. Mastitis caused by *C. pyogenes,* however, is a very severe disease of the udder that usually terminates the productivity and often the life of the animal. In the United States, it is not common, and it is found only sporadically within a herd, usually accounting for only 1 to 2 per cent of the acute cases of mastitis. Onset is sudden, with the gland undergoing extensive necrosis and abscesses. The development of fistulous tracts is a unique characteristic of *C. pyogenes* mastitis. Metastasis to other organs will often lead to chronic debilitation.

In the United States, the disease occurs at any time of the year and usually occurs in lactating cattle. Quite a different epizootiology seems to exist in England and western Europe where acute *C. pyogenes* mastitis is commonly known as "summer mastitis" and accounts for about 10 per cent of the cases of acute mastitis. The name originated because of the higher incidence of the disease in the summer than in the other seasons of the year. There is a direct relationship between the rate of infection and the amount of rainfall. There is evidence that the bacteria may be transmitted by insects. The number of cases is higher in animals using pastures near forests where insect populations are greatest. Studies have shown that insecticide treatment of pastures reduces infection. Summer mastitis is more common in dry cows and in nonlactating heifers, occurring very commonly in heifers less than 10 months of age.

Treatment of acute causes of *C. pyogenes* mastitis probably has little value in restoring productive usefulness to the affected cow. The animal may be salvaged for slaughter by abscess drainage via teat amputation coupled with daily subcutaneous penicillin at 44,000 units/kg for 7 to 10 days.

The predominance of the disease in dry cows in Europe facilitates their treatment. Procaine benzylpenicillin (300,000 units) administered into the gland has given reasonable protection against summer mastitis. A polyvalent vaccine *(Escherichia coli, C. pyogenes, C. renale, Streptococcus agalactiae, S. uberis, S. zooepidermicus,* and *Staphylococcus aureus)* has been reported to be capable of protecting the udder from infection during lactation.

GOATS AND SHEEP

Goats and sheep are discussed here because the current state of knowledge does not differentiate between the nonspecific cornyebacterial infections of these 2 species. Further, *C. pyogenes* produces abscesses and mastitis in goats and sheep that seem to have pathogeneses and treatments similar to those in cattle.

Epididymitis and orchitis have been produced by *C. pseudotuberculosis* in rams. The cellulitis of *Brucella ovis* infection, the usual cause of ram epididymitis, may predispose the ram to testicular and scrotal abscesses containing *C. pseudotuberculosis.* Treatment of these abscesses should not spread the organism to other animals. This treatment, including surgical drainage and packing the abscess with gauze, would likely be in order for only valuable rams because of the difficulty and expense of confinement.

C. pyogenes or *C. pseudotuberculosis* arthritis may be a sequel to umbilical infection in lambs and kids; it may also follow dipping of lambs in which the fluid becomes contaminated with either of these 2 organisms. If detected early, high doses of penicillin may be of value in purebred animals or in animals being raised as a project by young owners. The prognosis is guarded, however, and the greatest effort should be made to prevent navel infections by lambing or kidding on clean pasture or by disinfecting the navel with an iodine preparation when the young are delivered in confinement.

Bronchopneumonia in sheep is most commonly associated with *Pasteurella* spp. and *C. pyogenes;* however, *C. equi* has occasionally been isolated in pure culture from pneumonic lung tissue. Since more than 1 organism is often involved, treatment is nonspecific. Oxytetracycline and sulfonamide are helpful, especially if administered early in the case. As with all species of food-producing animals, young kids and lambs exposed to daily temperature fluctuations of 15° to 30°C are very susceptible to pneumonia. During spring and fall when these tempera-ture fluctuations occur, managers should be particularly watchful in order to detect illness early.

In cases of mastitis, uncommonly caused by *C. pyogenes* and *C. pseudotuberculosis,* the prognosis and treatment will be similar to that for cattle. The economic advantage of treatment in order to salvage the animals for slaughter is not as great as with cattle and in most cases does not merit the greater risk of infection to other animals in contact with one that is shedding the organism.

A form of necrotic laryngitis caused by *C. pyogenes* has resulted in abscesses of the arytenoid cartilage of rams. Death is certain in the untreated animal, but oral sulfamethazine at 140 mg/kg daily as needed has been a somewhat successful treatment.

Corynebacterial infections are found sporadically in other conditions. *C. pyogenes* and *Fusobacterium necrophorum* are the causes of foot abscesses in sheep. Reduced ewe fertility and general debilitation have been associated with pathologic changes in the reproductive tract and pelvic lymph nodes from which *C. pseudotuberculosis* has been isolated. *C. pseudotuberculosis* has also been isolated in pure culture from brain abscesses. *C. pyogenes* is associated with vegetative endocarditis.

SWINE

C. pyogenes is found in many suppurative lesions of the pig. It is common in suppurative pneumonia, seemingly as the primary agent, but it is also seen with primary pasteurellosis. Suppurative arthritis due to *C. pyogenes* infection often appears after farrowing, suggesting that the uterus may be the primary route of entry. Stiffness, lameness, cachexia, pneumonia, and paralysis may result.

C. pyogenes has also been observed as a cause of vertebral osteomyelitis in the pig. It is occasionally a secondary invader in atrophic rhinitis and porcine enzootic pneumonia *(Mycoplasma hyopneumoniae* infection). *C. pyogenes* is among the less frequent primary agents in porcine agalactia syndrome and septicemic abortion.

C. equi has been isolated from granulomatous lesions in the lymph nodes of the neck and head regions of swine. The presence of this bacterium in these tissues has introduced the question and the subsequent controversy as to whether it might be responsible for the tuberculosis-like lesions sometimes found in these nodules.

C. suis has been implicated as a cause of cystitis and pyelonephritis in breeding swine. The diseases are apparently transmitted venereally. Affected animals develop mild to severe pyelonephritis characterized by fever, blood in the urine, excessive thirst, and abdominal pain. Animals with the diseases can be treated with penicillin or ampicillin.

Supplemental Reading

Blood, D. C., Radostits, O. M., and Henderson, J. A.: Veterinary Medicine, 6th ed. Philadelphia, Lea and Febiger, 1983.
Leman, A. D., Glock, R. D., and Mengeling, W. L., et al.: Diseases of Swine, 5th ed. Ames, Iowa, Iowa State University Press, 1981.
Jensen, R.: Diseases of Sheep, 2nd ed. Philadelphia, Lea and Febiger, 1972.
Jensen, R., and Mackey, D. R.: Diseases of Feedlot Cattle, 3rd ed. Philadelphia, Lea and Febiger, 1979.

Caseous Lymphadenitis

JESS L. AYERS, D.V.M., Ph.D.

Caseous lymphadenitis is a common disease of sheep and goats and a rare disease of cattle. In sheep, caseous lymphadenitis can produce a serious economic problem as a result of carcass condemnation at slaughter plants. It is viewed by both veterinarians and goat producers as the most common caprine disease in the United States. The disease is usually characterized by abscesses of 1 or more superficial lymph nodes. The exudate of the mature abscess is thick, putty-like, and white, yellow, or tan. In sheep, the exudate may be extremely dry and formed in layers that have been referred to as "concentric lamination" and compared to the layers of an onion. This phenomenon is not commonly observed in goat abscesses. The etiologic agent is generally *Corynebacterium pseudotuberculosis*, although other organisms may occasionally produce similar abscesses.

In sheep, the most commonly involved lymph nodes are the precrural and precapsular, whereas in goats the most commonly involved lymph nodes are the parotid followed by the precapsular.

Mode of transmission is not known; however, one means is probably mechanical transmission from sheep to sheep by contaminated shears. Until recently, it was thought that a skin wound or some other mode of traumatic inoculation was necessary for entrance of the organism into the body. In the dairy goat, however, infection cannot be associated with shearing. While goats are wholebody clipped as part of grooming for conformation contests, this procedure usually does not produce skin wounds, and the postclipping incidence of caseous lymphadenitis is apparently no greater than at any other time. It has been reported that the organism can penetrate directly into intact skin. My preliminary work indicates that a suspension of the organisms applied with a toothbrush can pass through skin in which the only treatment has been close clipping of the hair minutes before. Contiguous lymph nodes contain the organism as early as 3 days after application.

In goats, transmission does appear to be directly from animal to animal or from fomites. Producers insist that the incidence is much greater after animals are assembled at fairs or other similar events. There is also evidence that the organism can enter the body by ingestion.

It appears that some animals in an infected herd or flock never develop caseous lymphadenitis, others become infected only once, while still others are continually plagued. A very small percentage develop internal abscesses primarily of the mediastinal and bronchial lymph nodes and lung parenchyma. These internal abscesses, which are found at necropsy or slaughter, are usually observed in animals that have been undergoing progressive debilitation. Internal abscesses are also occasionally found in apparently healthy sheep.

DIAGNOSIS

Clinical diagnosis of caseous lymphadenitis in the goat is seldom problematical. The presence of enlarged superficial lymph nodes is the first indication. The palpable consistency of the nodes varies with stage of development of the lesion; they are firm and unyielding initially and semisoft and doughy later. An inaccurate diagnosis may be made if there is an encapsulated abscess in an area not known to contain a lymph node or if there is an abscess of distinctly liquid consistency.

Enlarged superficial lymph nodes of sheep may be hidden by the wool and are detected by palpation. Further, the incidence of nonvisible or nonpalpable abscesses is apparently higher in sheep than in goats. Detection of an inapparent carrier, if necessary, would require use of serologic test results.

A diagnosis is confirmed by isolation and identification of *C. pseudotuberculosis* using laboratory test results. Colonies appear on blood agar after 36 to 96 hr incubation at 37°C. They are small (2 to 3 mm in diameter), white or yellow, and may have a 1-mm zone of clear hemolysis. Colonies are very dry and crumbly, with a wrinkled surface, and are easily pushed intact with an inoculating loop across the medium. The organisms are gram-positive, extremely short rods that are very easily mistaken for cocci. In contrast to *C. pyogenes*, *C. pseudotuberculosis* is catalase-positive. Culturing, gram-staining, and catalase testing are simply done in a small clinical laboratory, and the results are usually sufficient for confirmation of the correct diagnosis. Absolute confirmation can be made by demonstrating that the organism is nonmotile, hydrolyzes urea, and ferments dextrose but not lactose.

It is tempting, in a busy practice, to neglect isolation and identification of the organism. As a practical compromise, it is suggested that culturing be conducted (1) when the disease first appears in a flock or herd, (2) when any abscess that varies from the typical characteristics of *C. pseudotuberculosis* lesions appears, and (3) when a small percentage of typical abscesses appear after the initial diagnosis is made.

Clinical differential diagnosis is seldom a problem except when caseous lymphadenitis is considered as the cause of chronic debilitation. In such a case, it is difficult to distinguish it clinically from Johne's disease in goats or other nonspecific debilitating diseases. Necropsy examination is usually needed to distinguish these conditions. Antemortem differentiation of the organism can be done by acid-fast staining of fecal smears or by culturing feces for the presence of *Mycobacterium paratuberculosis*. Bacteriologic isolation of the latter organism requires special techniques, however.

TREATMENT AND PREVENTION

Caseous lymphadenitis is absolutely refractory to chemotherapy, presumably because of the abscess' very thick capsule. Because of this, antibiotic sensitivity tests on the isolated organism should not be expected to supply useful treatment information. Whether or not there is an early stage in the disease when the unprotected organism is susceptible to antibiotic therapy is apparently not known.

The primary treatment is incision and drainage of the abscess. The abscess should be mature, as determined by the soft doughy consistency; however, some abscesses are so tightly filled that they feel rather hard. The area dorsal and ventral to the lesion should be clipped, and the incision site should be cleaned and disinfected. When possible, the incision is made about 2 cm long at the most ventral portion of the superficial enlargement. An elliptical strip of skin 1 cm wide should be excised in order to create an opening to allow continuous drainage. The exudate is removed from the abscess and collected carefully for complete disposal. Equal portions of 0.2-per cent nitrofurazone solution and 3-per cent hydrogen peroxide are mixed and about 50 to 100 ml are used to flush the abscess. Rolled gauze (5 to 8 cm wide), which had been presoaked and stored in a vial containing either 0.5-per cent povidone-iodine solution or 0.2-per cent nitrofurazone solution, is used to pack the abscess cavity. The owner is instructed to remove one third of the gauze each day. The initial incision is kept to 2 cm or less so that the gauze will not easily fall from the cavity. If the abscess is not packed, the incision should be made as long as possible. Great care must be taken to avoid major vessels when excising posterior to the mandible or ventral to the ear, and the incision length may well be limited by these vessels. It must be emphasized when instructing owners to keep the wound open by soaking it with warm soapy water and debriding it daily. They must ensure that the abscess heals from the inside.

Prevention of the spread of the organism by culling all infected animals is by far the most efficient way to control the disease. However, there are other factors, primarily economic, that owners consider when they are advised to slaughter infected animals. Some breeders may knowingly purchase infected animals when improving their bloodlines.

Isolation should be used as an alternate method of control when owners will not slaughter infected animals. Although not all the conditions under which an infected animal transmits the organism are known, certainly it is shed from an open abscess. The organism is excreted from the wound until it is completely healed. Therefore, animals that have mature abscesses or that have been treated should be isolated until their wounds have completely healed.

In commercial sheep flocks, a fairly good degree of control can be maintained if lymph nodes are routinely palpated and animals with enlarged lymph nodes slaughtered. The incidence of caseous lymphadenitis in sheep is much higher in older animals; thus the sheep owner finds it easier to control by culling than does the goat owner, whose animals do not have this age discrimination.

Two further recommendations that might lessen the spread of infection are (1) feeders designed so that animals are not required to insert their heads (the very popular keyhole feeders are easily contaminated with the organism) and (2) implementation and support of strict enforcement rules by veterinarians to prevent animals with abscesses from being unloaded at fairs and shows.

Resistance to *C. pseudotuberculosis* is not well understood. Some clinicians have used autogenous bacterins and quite often have reported positive results. Those who use autogenous bacterins usually also make management improvements. The latter may be the basis for their success in controlling the disease. Resistance to infection, if it occurs, is likely to be of the cellular type. Perhaps a greater understanding of cell-mediated immunity will break down the barriers to research progress on this aspect of the disease and give immunization some potential in caseous lymphadenitis control. As with many diseases of food-producing animals, however, good management is probably the most important factor contributing to successful control.

Supplemental Reading

Ayers, J. L.: Caseous lymphadenitis in goats and sheep: a review of diagnosis, pathogenesis and immunity. J. Am. Vet. Med. Assoc. *171*:1251–1254, 1977.

Ulcerative Lymphangitis of Cattle

JESS L. AYERS, D.V.M., Ph.D.
and ALYN McCLURE, D.V.M.

Ulcerative lymphangitis is an extremely rare disease, especially in cattle. The etiologic agent is *Corynebacterium pseudotuberculosis*, which is reputed to gain entrance through wounds of the feet and fetlocks. The initial sign is nodular swelling of these lower areas of the leg, and minimal lameness is a variable finding. Inflammatory swelling of the lymphatic vessels and lymph nodes produces nodules and cords in the subcutis. The nodules are abscesses that can grow to 5 cm in diameter. If not excised they will rupture, leaving a necrotic base that extends beneath the surrounding skin edges. The exudate is predominantly yellow or white and seropurulent but may be darkened with blood. It contains detritus that is produced from the necrotizing process.

DIAGNOSIS

Diagnosis is made on the presence of rather distinct clinical signs and bacteriologic isolation of *C. pseudotuberculosis*.

TREATMENT

Sodium iodide (20 per cent) is given intravenously once at the rate of 16.5 ml/50 kg. Additionally, penicillin at 44,000 units/kg once daily and streptomycin at 22 mg/kg twice daily is administered subcutaneously for 10 days. The abscesses are excised, drained, and dressed vigorously with 7-per cent tincture of iodine.

Actinobacillosis

JIMMY L. HOWARD, D.V.M., M.S.

Actinobacillosis, also known as "woody tongue" or "big head," is a chronic infectious disease of cattle and, secondarily, of swine and sheep. It is characterized by thick-walled abscesses of the soft tissues of the head. In cattle, lesions are confined primarily to the tongue and cervical lymph nodes with only occasional involvement of the pharyngeal lymph nodes and esophageal groove. In sheep, the lesions primarily involve soft tissues of the head, neck, and nasal cavities but not the tongue. The organism can occasionally be isolated from udder abscesses in swine.

ETIOLOGY

The etiologic agent is *Actinobacillus lignieresii,* an aerobic, gram-negative coccobacillus. The organism appears singly or in short chains in abscesses and forms "sulfur granules" in tissues. The bacteria are highly sensitive to normal environments and live only for approximately 5 days outside the animal host. *A. seminis* has been found to cause acute purulent epididymitis of rams in Australia and South Africa.

EPIZOOTIOLOGY

The disease is found worldwide. It is very common in western and southwestern United States. Transmission and pathogenesis are not well defined. *A. lignieresii* is widespread in soil and manure and has been isolated from saliva and the alimentary tract of healthy cattle. It appears to be an obligate parasite of the upper respiratory and alimentary tract mucosae. The organism cannot normally invade healthy skin and therefore needs some type of trauma to allow entry. Sharp awns, stickers, and food particles cause oral wounds that assist in the organisms' invasion of the tissues.

Susceptible hosts are primarily cattle and, secondarily, sheep and swine. Humans are rarely infected. Over 90 per cent of cattle infections involve the cervical lymph nodes, and less than 5 per cent involve the tongue. *A. seminis* may be excreted in the semen of apparently healthy rams.

CLINICAL SIGNS AND PATHOGENESIS

Infectious granuloma produces chronic inflammation. There are circumscribed, small, diffuse, or multiple swellings in the subcutis or lymph glands of the submaxillary, parotid, and retropharyngeal areas of the head and neck. These swellings gradually enlarge to form thick-walled abscesses that are not hot or painful. They persist for several weeks or months and usually rupture and discharge a viscid, odorless, white or slightly greenish pus. Sinus tracts often occur to the outside. Occasionally, there is hematogenous dissemination of infection, and the lung and liver are the internal organs most often affected. When generalized dissemination occurs the condition is usually progressive and fatal.

Clinical signs are multiple abscesses, particularly of the head and neck. The animal may show signs of dysphagia when there are abscesses of the soft palate or retropharyngeal areas. Respiratory dyspnea and even sonorous rales may be observed when there is impingement on the trachea or lungs.

Lingual actinobacillosis (woody tongue) has a sudden onset with excessive salivation and difficult mastication. The tongue is enlarged and firm. In chronic cases, the tongue will protrude from the mouth and may be immobile. Epididymitis of rams caused by *A. seminis* shows a mixed purulent and nonpurulent inflammation of the epididymis, cystic hyperplasia of the ductus epididymis, interstitial fibrosis, and spermatic granulomas. The clinical signs and lesions are similar to those of the epididymitis caused by *Brucella ovis.*

DIAGNOSIS

Clinical diagnosis is usually made from clinical signs and physical examination. Differential diagnosis includes actinomycosis, tuberculosis, pyogenic bacterial abscesses, and neoplasms.

Actinomycosis usually involves bone, and the lesion is hard and fibrous. The sulfur granules can be felt in the exudate as a sand-like material. A tuberculin test may be used to help diagnose tuberculosis. Pyogenic bacterial abscesses are often hot and painful. They commonly have a less viscous pus with a pungent odor. Neoplasms are confined to a single large area with no pus. A large 10- to 12-gauge needle may be used to aspirate a sample of pus.

Laboratory diagnostic assistance involves microscopic examination and culture evaluation.

TREATMENT

Instructions for treatment of actinobacillosis are found in the article on actinomycosis.

Actinomycosis

JIMMY L. HOWARD, D.V.M., M.S.

Actinomycosis, also known as "lumpy jaw," is a subacute or chronic infectious disease of animals and humans characterized by a suppurative granulomatous tissue reaction. The disease is most common in cattle and is primarily manifested by rarefying osteomyelitis of the bones of the skull, particularly the mandible and maxilla. Rarely, there is visceral actinomycosis in swine, but more commonly there are granulomatous lesions of the skin under the udder. In severe cases of actinomycosis, there may be extensive soft tissue involvement, particularly of the muscles and fascia of the head and neck.

ETIOLOGY

The etiologic agent is *Actinomyces bovis,* a gram-positive, nonspore-forming, noncapsulating, nonacid-fast, filamentous anaerobe. The organism forms clumps called "sulfur granules" or "rosettes" that may appear as sand-like granular material when examined macroscopically. Microscopically, it often appears as a "ray fungus," hence the name *Actinomyces.* *A. bovis* is a normal inhabitant of the mucous membranes of the oral cavity, upper respiratory tract, and digestive tracts of animals and humans.

EPIZOOTIOLOGY

Geographically, the disease is found worldwide in areas primarily devoted to grazing cattle. In the United States, it occurs more commonly in the western and midwestern states. The transmission and pathogenesis are not clearly understood, but the organism is a common inhabitant of the bovine mouth, and infection is introduced through the buccal mucosa by sharp objects, such as thorns, grass awns, or other foreign material. Infection may enter through dental alveoli when deciduous teeth are shed and permanent teeth erupt. This may account for the disease being more prevalent in young cattle 2 to 5 years of age.

A. bovis enters the soft tissues of the head by way of sharp objects or erupting teeth, and the tissue necrosis that follows results in the anaerobic conditions necessary for the growth of the organism.

Susceptible hosts are primarily cattle, secondarily swine, and rarely sheep. The disease is infrequent in humans.

CLINICAL SIGNS AND PATHOGENESIS

The organism causes a low grade inflammatory reaction. There is proliferation of connective tissue and leucocytic infiltration that results in a walled, tumor-like mass. This granulomatous lesion invades the bones of the skull, particularly the mandible or maxilla, often at the level of the third or fourth molar. This circumscribed, immovable bony swelling may reach considerable size (10 to 14 cm in diameter) and interferes with mastication. Some lesions develop rapidly within a few weeks, while others develop within months. The swellings may be diffuse or discrete, and are hard, immovable, and usually painful in early stages. The lesions contain intercommunicating pockets of pus that often rupture to the outside, forming a fistulous tract. The pus formed in these lesions does not have a disagreeable odor, an important consideration in differential diagnosis. The amount of purulent discharge is small and is a thick, honey-like fluid containing minute, hard, yellow-white granules (sulfur granules) with a sand-like consistency.

Occasionally, the swellings will involve the soft tissues of the head and neck. This may result in dysphagia or dyspnea. The most common and severe form of soft tissue involvement is invasion of the esophageal groove and reticulum, which impairs digestion. There are confirmed cases of bovine orchitis caused by A. bovis.

The course of the disease is nearly always chronic and is accompanied by anorexia and progressive emaciation.

The most common form of the disease in pigs is a tumor-like granulomatous lesion of the mammae. The infection probably is introduced from wounds caused by the teeth of baby pigs. Occasionally, visceral actinomycosis results in a wasting disease.

The pathologic findings in cattle are rarefying ostitis and osteoporosis with interspersed granulomatous tissue and pockets of whey-like pus with small, gritty sulfur granules. These granules are about the size of a pin's head and contain microscopic gram-positive mycelium and short rods surrounded by a zone of gram-negative, club-shaped bodies. Granulomatous lesions containing pockets of pus may be found in the soft tissues of the head, the esophageal groove, the lower esophagus, and the wall of the reticulum. Involvement of the lymph nodes does not occur.

DIAGNOSIS

Clinical diagnosis is usually made from signs and physical examination. Differential diagnosis includes actino-bacillosis, pyogenic bacterial abscesses, neoplasms, and rarely coccidioidomycosis. Actinobacillosis does not involve bone and is a fluctuating mass. Pyogenic bacterial abscesses are movable masses with a very offensive odor to the pus and no granule formation. Neoplasms are nonpyogenic.

Diagnosis is assisted by laboratory demonstration of sulfur granules, gram-positive rods, and ray fungus on microscopic examination.

TREATMENT

Actinomycosis and Actinobacillosis

Treatment for both actinomycosis and actinobacillosis will be discussed here.

Most treatments for actinomycosis are unsatisfactory. However, early treatment of actinobacillosis is very effective. Sulfanilamide, sulfapyridine, and sulfathiazole at the rate of 1 gm/kg for 5 to 6 days have given some apparent benefit. This is the recommended treatment in human cases of actinomycosis.

Penicillin is of some value in the treatment of actinomycosis. Streptomycin given intramuscularly at the rate of 15 to 20 mg/kg for 5 to 7 days has been effective in both conditions. These drugs seem to work best when injected into the lesion and when given in combination with iodides or local surgical treatment. Isoniazid at the rate of 6 to 10 mg/kg daily, given orally or intramuscularly for a period of 2 to 3 weeks, has given favorable results if in combination with iodide therapy. The organisms are sensitive to tetracycline. However, it is difficult to obtain satisfactory blood levels of the antibiotic to penetrate the thick-walled abscesses or bony matrix.

Proteolytic enzymes such as chymotrypsin (Kymar)* given intramuscularly at the rate of 25,000 units daily for 5 to 6 days have proved beneficial in some cases.

Iodides are still the treatment of choice for both actinomycosis and actinobacillosis. Iodides have little bactericidal effect on the organisms and apparently exert a beneficial effect by reducing the granulomatous tissue reaction.

Both oral and intravenous iodides may be used. Sodium iodide at the rate of 1.0 gm 15 kg can be given intravenously as a 10- or 20-per cent solution to both cattle and sheep. One or 2 additional treatments at 10 to 14 day intervals are recommended. The standard treatment for sheep is a subcutaneous injection of 20 ml of a 10-per cent sodium iodide solution repeated at weekly intervals for 4 to 5 weeks. Potassium iodide at the rate of 6 to 10 gm/day for 7 to 10 days can be given orally as a drench or placed on the feed for cattle. Potassium iodide is unpalatable, and cattle are reluctant to eat it. Organic iodide salts such as ethylenediamine dihydriodide (Hi-Amine)† are palatable and can be given in the feed. The recommended dosage of Hi-Amine for cattle is 15 to 30 gm/head/day for 2 to 3 weeks and 7.5 to 15 gm/head/day for sheep. As an aid in the prevention of lumpy jaw in cattle and sheep, 450 gm of Hi-Amine mixed with 25 kg of feeding salt, should be self-fed continuously, as the sole source of salt.

Treatment with iodides may be continued until signs of iodism appear. Lacrimation, anorexia, and dry, scaly

---

*Available from Pitman-Moore, Inc., Washington Crossing, NJ 08560.
†Available from Burns-Biotec Laboratories, Omaha, NE 68127.

haircoat (dandruff) are signs of iodism and indicate the maximum iodide dose has been reached.

In cases of pregnant females and breeding males, there is a possibility that the heavy dosage could cause abortion, premature births, or temporary sterility. This is apparently very rare, however.

When bony lesions are extensive, the most that can be expected with any treatment for actinomycosis is an arrest of its development.

Surgical treatment consists of extensive incision of the lesions, providing drainage and packing the wound with gauze soaked in tincture of iodine.

Radiation treatment has been attempted with little permanent benefit. X-ray therapy has proved to be of value in arresting the growth of the lesion but is only of temporary value and should be used only on extremely valuable animals.

CONTROL

The primary control measure is to isolate or dispose of affected animals. Animals being treated should be isolated from the remainder of the flock or herd. Sanitation to prevent contamination of feeding facilities is important. In cases where several animals in 1 herd are involved, the extended use of organic iodides in the feed may be beneficial.

Nocardiosis

ERNST L. BIBERSTEIN, D.V.M., Ph.D.

Nocardiosis is a pyogranulomatous infection of humans and animals caused by a group of soil bacteria belonging to the genus *Nocardia*. *N. asteroides* is by far the most frequent species involved. *N. brasiliensis* and *N. caviae* have been implicated occasionally. The 3 species are morphologically indistinguishable and cause the same types of diseases. They can be differentiated by cultural and biochemical tests.

A tropical chronic skin disease of cattle, bovine farcy, or tropical actinomycosis, is caused by *N. farcinica,* which shares morphologic and staining characteristics as well as some antigens with *N. asteroides.* (Bovine farcy is not considered "nocardiosis" as it is used in this discussion.) Because the diseases have resemblances of pathologic, clinical, and epidemiologic features, nocardiosis is commonly lumped with mycosis in the literature. It is important, therefore, to stress the bacterial nature of nocardiosis, including the susceptibility of *Nocardia* to certain antibacterial drugs, and the insusceptibility to common antifungal agents.

EPIDEMIOLOGY

Nocardia spp. are soil organisms that find their way into animals most commonly by inhalation, wound infection, ingestion, and unsanitary and misguided surgical manipulations of the bovine udder as well as inadequate milking hygiene. Except for the milking herd, nocardiosis is not transmissible from infected individuals to noninfected individuals. In many circumstances of nocardiosis, an underlying immunologic inadequacy is present. The organism has remarkable powers of survival, and some strains are capable of withstanding pasteurization.

Distribution and Pathogenesis

There are no geographic restrictions for nocardiosis, and it has been described in all the major food-producing mammals. The most important form, in frequency and economic impact, is bovine nocardial mastitis, which often assumes epidemic proportions. In other species, such as swine, sheep, and goats, only sporadic cases of pneumonia, abortion, lymphadenitis, and mastitis have been observed. Sporadic pneumonia and abortion and other extramammary infections also occur in cattle. In all instances, nocardiosis tends to be a local to regional infection, i.e., there is little tendency for systemic dissemination. In view of the rarity, unpredictability, and frequent intractability of this type of nocardiosis, the remainder of the discussion will be concentrated on bovine mastitis.

CLINICAL SIGNS AND PATHOLOGY

Nocardial mastitis is an ascending infection that is often introduced by intramammary infusions, contaminated teat cups, wash rags, or milker's hands. Clinical onset may be sudden, with reduced milk yield and fairly high fever (42°C). The affected quarter is painful and swollen. Enlarged lymph nodes, especially the supramammary nodes, are common. Mammary secretions are watery at first, then become serum-like with flakes. They may become mucopurulent and finally become creamy thick. There is usually no odor or evidence of blood in the secretion. Among systemic signs, leukopenia with a pronounced left shift may be found and urinary abnormalities with proteinuria and cellular admixtures may also be found. The pathologic events in the udder begin with an exudative necrotic reaction in the acute stage. This is followed by extensive abscess formations, sometimes with percutaneous rupture and establishment of a permanent sinus tract. Granuloma formation and fibrosis characterize the subsequent chronic course.

Some cases are chronic from the onset, mimicking mastitis due to other more common agents. The eventual fibrosis and atrophy is typical of these agents as well. Animals acutely affected may die during the febrile stage. Death due to rupture of the udder may also occur.

DIAGNOSIS

Nocardia appears on direct, Gram's stain smears as gram-positive, branching beaded filaments that are indistinguishable from *Actinomyces* spp. When such structures are seen, another smear should be stained by an acid-fast procedure (preferably Kinyoun's acid-fast procedure). *Nocardia* will be typically acid-fast.

Culture on blood agar, after several days of incubation at either room temperature or 37°C, will yield colonies with a dull waxy to velvety surface and pigmentation that may vary from chalky white to ivory yellow to coral pink. The crumbly, dry consistency combined with a Gram's stain should provide adequate hints as to the likely identity of the isolate. Any culture of this type should be sent to a medical or veterinary microbiology laboratory for confirmation of identification. Since the organism has some capability of infecting humans by the respiratory route, manipulations of the culture are best done under a properly vented hood.

Dermal hypersensitivity and circulating antibody tests (complement fixation) have been described for *Nocardia* but are not generally available for diagnostic use.

TREATMENT

The response to treatment of nocardial mastitis is almost uniformly unsatisfactory. Although numerous antimicrobials, particularly sulfa drugs, show *in vitro* activity, they have been of little benefit in curing mastitis in the sense of restoring glands to acceptable productivity. Clinical improvement and bacteriologic cures have been obtained on a 4- to 5-day regimen of 2 daily intramammary infusions of 500 mg novobiocin in 25 ml of vehicle containing 0.2-per cent nitrofurazone. The consistent failure of antimicrobial therapy may be due to the advanced nature of the lesion by the time treatment is instituted.

In other forms of nocardiosis, trimethoprim-sulfonamide combinations are the current drugs of choice.

CONTROL AND PREVENTION

The best control of nocardial mastitis consists of the culling of affected cows and the adhering to of sound sanitary practices. Disinfection can be accomplished with 5 minutes exposure to chlorine (100 ppm) or Roccal (200 ppm). Unlike all other forms of nocardiosis, nocardial mastitis is an indirectly contagious disease transmitted by infected mammary secretions on milking equipment, bedding, and other fomites. It will be eliminated only when the chain of transmission is broken.

Supplemental Reading

Ainsworth, G. C., and Austwick, P. K. C.: Fungal Disease of Animals, 2nd ed. England, Commonwealth Agricultural Bureaux, Farnham Royal, 1973.

Anderson, K. L., and Wilcke, J. R.: Potentiated sulfonamides in the treatment of bovine pulmonary nocardiosis. J. Vet. Pharm. Ther. 3:217–220, 1980.

Jungerman, P. F., and Schwartzman, R. M.: Veterinary Medical Mycology, Philadelphia, Lea and Febiger, 1973.

Pier, A. C., Gray, D. M., and Fossatti, M. S.: *Nocardia asteroides*, a newly recognized pathogen of the mastitis complex. Am. J. Vet. Res. 19:319–331, 1958.

Dermatophilosis

JOHN N. BERG, D.V.M., Ph.D.

Dermatophilosis is a chronic cutaneous disease caused by the actinomycete *Dermatophilus congolensis*. The disease is characterized as an ulcerative, exudative dermatitis. Infection occurs in a wide variety of animal species and humans but most commonly occurs in cattle, horses, goats, and sheep. In sheep, the disease is known as mycotic dermatitis or lumpy wool disease when the body but not the limbs are involved, and proliferative dermatitis or strawberry-foot rot when the lower limbs are involved. In other species it has been called cutaneous streptotri-cosis. Dermatophilosis has been reported world wide. It usually appears during periods of high rainfall. It is very common in many tropical and semitropical countries. The disease was first recognized in the United States in 1961 and has since been reported in at least 14 states. Dermatophilosis is a zoonotic disease, i.e., infecting humans that have handled infected animals.

ETIOLOGY AND PATHOGENESIS

D. congolensis, an actinomycete, is a gram-positive branching rod whose hyphal elements show various stages of segmentation due to the septa of the hyphae. The septa form motile zoospores in water. The bacterium can be cultivated aerobically on enriched blood agar where it forms hemolytic pigmented colonies that adhere to the agar.

Animals of all ages and both sexes are susceptible to infection. The disease is commonly associated with moist climatic conditions. Continuous wetting of the skin may cause softening and swelling of the epidermal layers that allow *D. congolensis* to more readily invade and grow in the epidermis. However, invasion is probably through breaks in the skin due to mechanical injury. Injuries to the skin during shearing of sheep often precipitate infection in endemic areas.

Transmission of *D. congolensis* is through direct contact with infected animals. Ticks and biting flies may also spread the infection.

CLINICAL SIGNS

Dermatophilosis in cattle occurs as an exudative dermatitis with subsequent formation of scabs and crusts with matted hair at their bases. The crusts may become thickened and horny and project from the skin. The crusts will separate from the underlying skin during the healing process, leaving areas of alopecia. Lesions vary in size from less than 1 cm to confluent lesions that cover large areas of the body surface. The lesions are most common over the back, sides, shoulders, neck, and head, although other areas may be involved. In calves, the lesions often start at the muzzle and spread over the head and neck. Animals with mild lesions may suffer little discomfort, but animals with severe lesions may suffer depression and anorexia with subsequent debility and death. Often, only 1 or 2 animals in a group are affected, although a higher incidence may be noted.

Dermatophilosis in sheep has been reported as 2 clinical entities: mycotic dermatitis and proliferative dermatitis. Neither is common in the United States, but the presence of the mycotic dermatitis type has been confirmed. Ovine dermatophilosis is often mild, with only a slight loss of wool or localized infections on the ears and nose. However, severely infected animals may have extensive regions of crusting that may be palpated under the wool. The crusts may remain attached to the wool fibers or become detached, exposing a pink moist skin surface.

Dermatophilus infection of the lower limbs in sheep is called proliferative dermatitis or strawberry-foot rot. The condition has not been reported in the United States. The syndrome is characterized as an inflammatory scabbing with swelling on the legs between the coronet and the back. Removal of the scabbing reveals a fleshy mass with many fine bleeding points that resembles a strawberry. Severely affected animals may become lame.

DIAGNOSIS

The clinical lesions of dermatophilosis are suggestive of the disease, especially if associated with conditions of excessive dampness. Diagnosis is easily confirmed by direct microscopic examination of stained smears. Recently formed exudates or crusts should be macerated into a few drops of sterile water and spread on a glass slide and allowed to dry. The slide should be stained with Giemsa stain (Wright's stain or methylene blue will also work) and examined under oil-immersion magnification. Typical branched filaments dividing both transversely and longitudinally into thick parallel rows of coccoid cells helps confirm *D. congolensis*. The bacterium may be cultured on enriched media such as blood agar, but care must be taken in selection of material to be cultured since the lesions are often contaminated with other microorganisms.

THERAPY

Spontaneous healing often occurs in mild cases, especially if the animal is placed in dry surroundings. In more severe or chronic cases, the animal should be kept in a dry environment. Although topical therapy has been unrewarding, gentle bathing with warm water and soap or an iodine shampoo will help remove crusts and exudate. In infected herds, spontaneous recovery usually occurs with the advent of dry weather.

In severely affected animals, large doses of antibiotics have been effective. Penicillin and streptomycin as a single dose (70,000 units/kg and 70 mg/kg, respectively) or in 5 daily doses (5000 units/kg and 5 mg/kg, respectively) may be used. Tetracycline given for 5 days (5 mg/kg/day) or a single injection of long-acting oxytetracycline (20 mg/kg) has also been used.

Topical treatments have been applied, such as dips and sprays of 0.2- to 0.5-per cent zinc sulfate and 0.2-per cent copper sulfate (affects dyeing qualities of wool) or alum (potassium aluminum sulfate) as a 1-per cent dip of 57-per cent dust. The zinc sulfate spray applied immediately after shearing may prevent infection from shearing injuries.

PREVENTION

Control of the disease is primarily aimed at minimizing predisposing factors and contact with infected animals. Animals should be kept in a good nutritional state. Avoid procedures that cause injury to the skin such as shearing during damp weather. In infected herds, dipping of sheep should be delayed for 10 days after shearing to avoid spread of infection through the dipping vats into shearing wounds. If possible, isolate infected animals from other animals in the herd. Currently, no vaccine is available.

Supplemental Reading

Harris, S. T.: Proliferative dermatitis of the legs ("strawberry foot rot") in sheep. J. Comp. Pathol. 58:314–328, 1948.

Kaplan, W.: Dermatophilosis—A recently recognized disease in the United States. Southwest. Vet. 20:14–19, 1966.
Lloyd, D. H., and Sellers, K. C. (eds.): Dermatophilus Infection in Animals and Man. New York, Academic Press, 1976.
Roberts, D. S.: Dermatophilus infection. Vet. Bull. 37:513–521, 1967.

Systemic Mycoses

ERNST L. BIBERSTEIN, D.V.M., Ph.D.

This discussion of systemic mycoses considers those fungal infections of food-producing mammals that affect any organ except the superficial layers of the skin. While some of the infections, such as bovine mastitis and those causing abortion, may not be systemic diseases in the literal sense, they represent conditions from which systemic dissemination or localized signs of an otherwise inapparent generalized infection may develop.

The systemic or deep mycoses do not occupy a place of prominence among the various diseases of livestock. The agents that cause systemic mycoses are, without exception, components of the natural microbial flora of the external or internal environment. Those inhabiting the external environment, which constitute the large majority of the organisms to be considered, are of low virulence to the normal animal. Animals are constantly exposed to such organisms via the respiratory or intestinal route without any observable adverse effects. Their assumption of a pathogenic role depends on 1 or more of 3 possible developments that change this environmental equilibrium.

1. A derangement in the physiology of the animal, e.g., hormonal changes caused by advanced pregnancy and certain pituitary tumors or changes caused by medication, particularly antimicrobial drugs that encourage fungal colonization and proliferation by eliminating bacterial competition or by other direct stimulatory effects.

2. An abnormal increase in the abundance of the fungi in the immediate environment, such as moldy feed and bedding.

3. The introduction of fungal cells by routes other than the respiratory or alimentary tract. The most important example of this is the infection of the mammary gland, usually directly or indirectly by human interference. Wounds and uterine infections are other possibilities.

In many systemic infections, an underlying change that causes stress and alters host resistance can be shown. These circumstances would place such infections among the "opportunistic diseases," a much abused and overused term that should be applied only to infections the clinical manifestations of which are predicated on breakdown of normal host defenses.

Under these conditions, it is not surprising that the bulk of systemic mycoses are sporadic, most often in individual animals or in groups of animals subjected to comparable stress and exposure. One consequence of this sporadic and unpredictable occurrence is a lessened likelihood of a clinical diagnosis, especially in early stages of the infection. Confirmation of these diseases involves pathologic (including histopathologic) and cultural confirmations.

To describe the therapy of deep mycoses of food animals as being in its infancy would be an extravagant overstatement. Infections in food animal populations either are subclinical or are not diagnosed until the disease has progressed past a point where therapy is of any possible benefit. Rationally based treatment is rarely attempted, and, if attempted, is rarely successful. Moreover, the antimycotic drugs now available have had only limited application in food animals. The proven means of dealing with systemic mycoses in food-producing mammals are largely confined to reasonable preventive measures to be instituted when the cause of condition has been established by diagnostic laboratory tests.

ETIOLOGY

The most important and economically significant mycotic syndromes recognized in food animals, primarily bovine abortion and mastitis, can be caused by a variety of fungal agents, and a brief characterization follows.

With the exception of some of the *Candida* spp. (especially *Candida albicans*) and, possibly, *Rhinosporidium seeberi*, all the fungi involved are saprophytes; i.e., they live upon dead or decaying organic matter, which is their normal and preferred habitat, and are not associated with the animal in their normal habitat.

Aspergillus

Aspergillus spp. are very common molds found in virtually every habitat in all parts of the world. They grow as branching filaments (hyphae) with frequent subdivisions (septa). When propagating on a surface under abundant air supply, as in the respiratory tract (or on an agar plate), they also develop pigmented fruiting bodies (broom-like structures) at their free ends in whose bristles chains of spores (conidia) form. The color and structure of the fruiting bodies are characteristic for each species. The most common species that affects animals is *A. fumigatus*. Septated hyphae can be demonstrated in unstained wet mounts, gram-stained fixed smears, and stained sections of pathologic material. For practical purposes, their presence in lesions justifies a provisional diagnosis of aspergillosis, for while *Aspergillus* is not the only potentially pathogenic mold producing septated hyphae in tissue, it is by far the most common.

Zygomycetes or Phycomycetes

The Zygomycetes or Phycomycetes, also sometimes called the mucoraceous fungi, are as abundant and cosmopolitan as *Aspergillus*. They differ most obviously from the latter in possessing few or no subdivisions in their usually broader hyphae, the only structures found in tissue. The fruiting bodies, which develop in culture, are spherical or oblong vesicles (sporangia), in which spores are formed. The shape of the sporangia, their support stalks (sporangiophores), and their relation to other hyphal features are important in determining genus and species. The genera important in animal diseases are *Mucor, Rhizopus, Absidia,* and *Mortierella.* A zygomycotic infection is suggested by the presence of broad, readily collapsing and twisting, nonseptate hyphae, in smears or sections. A more precise diagnosis requires interpretation of culture results.

Histoplasma

Histoplasma capsulatum is a saprophytic fungus of more restricted geographic distribution than *Aspergillus* and the Zygomycetes. It is most concentrated in the eastern central United States, but endemic foci are known in many parts of the world. *H. capsulatum* is 1 of several of the so-called dimorphic fungi, i.e., fungi occurring as mycelial forms (molds) in their saprophytic phase and as nonmycelial forms in their tissue phase. In the case of *H. capsulatum,* the tissue phase is the yeast form. The yeasts, occasionally budding, can be demonstrated in stained smears or sections within phagocytic cells of infected host animals, usually macrophages in fluids or tissue. In culture, especially at room temperature, these yeasts grow into the mold phase again, producing characteristic thick-walled spores called "tuberculate" because of their studded exterior. At 37°C on rich media, they may grow as yeasts. *H. capsulatum* will certainly grow as yeasts in experimental animals (e.g., mice) when culture of yeast phase, mold phase, or lesion material is injected intraperitoneally. Demonstration of the 2 phases is required for definitive identification.

Coccidioides

Coccidioides immitis, the agent of coccidioidomycosis, is another dimorphic fungus. It is confined to certain parts of the Western Hemisphere, where soil and climate favor its growth, and all authentic instances of diseases in humans and animals are traceable to these areas. In the United States, they are in parts of California, Arizona, New Mexico, and Texas. The saprophytic phase of *C. immitis* is mycelial, which is also the form in which the fungus grows on agar plates at either room temperature or 37°C. The spores produced in this phase are arthrospores (or arthroconidia), i.e., specialized thick-walled, cask-shaped hyphal cells that alternate with empty cells so that the arthrospore-bearing hypha appears as a broken line ("barber pole" effect). In the parasitic phase, following inhalation or, rarely, traumatic introduction, the arthrospore is transformed into a spherical structure (spherule, sporangium) in which nonbudding endospores develop. These, upon liberation from the mature spherule, may be disseminated to other areas and tissues of the host where another cycle of sporangium and endospore formation can be initiated. Culturing the sporangial phase on the usual agar media results in reversion to the filamentous mold form. The spherules can be demonstrated in wet mounts of bronchial washes or exudate and in stained sections of tissue.

Paracoccidioides

Paracoccidioides brasiliensis is the dimorphic fungus responsible for so-called South American blastomycosis, an often progressive systemic disease of humans. The tissue form consists of multiply budding yeasts, which can also be cultured on rich media at body temperature. The mycelial phase, which grows at room temperature on plain media—and presumably in nature in the endemic areas of Lation America—lacks distinctive diagnostic structures. No natural infections in animals have been reported, and experimental infections in cattle have produced only localized granulomatous lesions. There is an abundance of reactors to the specific skin test, however, among cattle, sheep, and horses of endemic areas, suggesting exposure of, and at least subclinical infections in, these hosts.

Cryptococcus

Cryptococcus neoformans differs from the previously mentioned fungi because it is encountered only in the yeast form. Strains exibiting hyphal formation have been described but are more of taxonomic interest than of practical diagnostic importance. The organism ordinarily leads a saprophytic existence in the soil, its growth being enhanced by bird, especially pigeon, feces. Morphologically, *C. neoformans* is a spherical cell that reproduces by budding. The most striking feature is the presence of a mucoid capsule of varying thickness that can be demonstrated in wet mounts of exudates in India ink or by special stains in tissue sections (mucicarmine). The finding of budding yeast cells surrounded by large halos in pathologic fluids is pathognomonic of cryptococcosis.

Candida

Candida spp. (formerly *Monilia*) also occupy an exceptional place among the fungi under consideration. Although they have been encountered in a variety of habitats including the soil and vegetation, they are generally much more closely associated with animals than the agents discussed previously. *C. albicans,* the one most prevalent in infections of humans and animals, is in fact a parasite normally present on the mucous membranes, especially of the alimentary tract. Infections are most commonly endogenous, i.e., produced by the strain carried commensally by the affected host.

Candida spp. are basically yeasts that propagate by budding. The predominant cell shape is oval, and buds may be single or multiple. Under altered nutritional and atmospheric conditions, *Candida* spp. form mycelium by spore germination or pseudomycelium by cellular elongation and filament formation, which provides a morphologic basis for separating *Candida* spp. from *Cryptococcus* spp. This is also characteristic of *Candida* in its invasive phase, i.e., when actively growing in tissue rather than on mucus-containing membranes.

Candida in its yeast, mycelial, and pseudomycelial forms is readily demonstrable in fixed Gram's stain smears of infected material in tissue sections stained specifically for fungi.

Rhinosporidium seeberi

Rhinosporidium seeberi has been reported from all continents. Most cases of infection are in tropical or subtropical climates. The pathogen has never been convincingly cultured on artificial media. In the parasitic state, it forms large vesicles, up to several hundred μm in diameter, in which endospores are generated. Their large size and anatomic predilection for the nasal mucosa differentiates them from the spherules (sporangia) of *C. immitis.* The natural reservoir of the agent is unknown. It is not likely to be the infected individual since transmission among members of susceptible species has not been demonstrated, and attempts at experimental infection have been unsuccessful. The firmest evidence that this is in fact a fungus rests on cytochemical reactions.

Prototheca

Prototheca spp. are actually not fungi but algae devoid of chlorophyll. They resemble yeasts superficially in being basically unicellular nucleated organisms enclosed by rigid cell walls. Their mode of reproduction is reminiscent of that of *Coccidioides* in that they undergo endosporulation, forming a sporangium from which, through internal cleavage, a new crop of organisms is produced and eventually liberated. Sporangia are readily demonstrated in unstained exudates and in culture suspensions as spherical to oval bodies, about 20 μm in diameter, containing a variable number of endospores. Alternatively, they may be stained with a type of Romanovsky stain (Wright-Leishman) or fungal stain (Gridley's, Gomori's methenamine silver, periodic acid–Schiff). They grow readily on common isolation media like blood, infusion, or tryptose agars in 48 hr at room or incubator-range temperature. The colonies also resemble those of yeasts, being white to off-white in color and creamy in consistency. Microscopic examination will reveal the characteristic pattern of spherical to oval cells at varying stages of endosporulation.

The etiologic agents are generally noncontagious in these systemic fungal infections. The vast majority of cases are a result of exposure to a common reservoir (given the physiologic or immunologic inadequacies that may be prerequisite to clinical infection). In the instance of many *Candida* infections, instead of the common extraneous source, part of the normal flora constitutes the reservoir of infection. Regardless, the infected animal poses no added threat to other animals in close contact. An exception to this rule may be the case of bovine mastitis, as will be noted.

All the agents mentioned are potentially pathogenic to humans under much the same condition as animals. The noncontagious nature of the diseases makes transmission from infected animals to humans a rather minor concern. The exclusion of infected animal products, particularly milk and its derivatives, from human consumption would be prompted by consideration of esthetics almost as much as of public health.

GENITAL INFECTIONS AND ABORTIONS

Incidence

The most prominent mycotic problem in food animal medicine concerns bovine genital infections, particularly abortions. While less than 40 per cent of all abortions in cattle can be associated with an infectious agent, fungal agents are blamed for about 2 to 30 per cent of this total. The rate varies from year to year and from place to place. In several surveys during the last decade, fungal agents ranked in first or second place among the microbial causes of abortion, competing in the United States with viral abortion due to IBR virus and in Europe with various bacteria, including *Brucella abortus* and streptococci.

Etiology

A wide variety of fungal species have been implicated. Current compilations bring the total to about 40. *Aspergillus fumigatus* accounts for about two thirds or more of all mycotic abortions. It is followed in frequency by the zygomycotic fungi (*Mucor, Rhizopus, Mortierella,* and *Absidia*). A low percentage of abortions are due to yeast-like fungi, especially *Candida* spp. Among the very sporadic causes recorded in recent years, the molds *Pseudallescheria (Petriellidium) boydii* and *Penicillium* spp. may be mentioned, as well as the yeasts *Torulopsis glabrata* and *Saccharomyces fragilis.*

Epidemiology

As is apparent from the identity of the leading agents implicated in mycotic abortions, the source of infection in most cases is external. Fungal spores are present in varying amounts in the feed and air, and evidence points accordingly to the alimentary and respiratory tracts as the important portals of infection. Genital infections also develop endogenously, i.e., from commensal flora of the vagina or from contaminated semen. Breeding problems due to this type of infection appear to involve yeasts more often than molds and appear to be manifested not so much in abortions as in failures to conceive. Semen used for artificial insemination has repeatedly been shown to contain yeasts. In some instances, such contamination has been related to breeding problems, metritis, and even early abortion. Although various fungi of preputial origin have been demonstrated in semen, an important source of the fungi is semen extenders and other additives.

Epidemic seminovesiculitis and epididymitis of a Hungarian bull stud due to infection with *Candida guillermondii* has been reported. Apart from local tissue lesions and deterioration in semen quality, there was hematogenous spread to the abdominal viscera and, as a further sequela, porphyria resulting in additional damage to sperm viability as well as to red blood cell survival. The disease could be reproduced by feeding the agent, and the natural outbreak was blamed on the abundance of *C. guillermondii* in bedding and feed, its severity possibly aggravated by the use of tetracycline early in the outbreak before its etiology was established.

Mycotic abortions may occur at almost any time of gestation beginning in the third month, but they are most common in later pregnancy, i.e., in the sixth month or later. The seasonal incidence shows a decisive preponderance during winter. The circumstances probably responsible for this are (1) confinement in stables with its greater likelihood of prolonged respiratory exposure to suspended spores in high concentration, (2) the use of harvested feeds in which there has been fungal growth, and, in many parts of the world, (3) the prevalence of animals in the advanced stages of pregnancy.

The higher incidence of fungus-induced abortions, which has been reported from various countries and continents in recent times, has been credited to the following:

1. The greater concentration of animals, subjecting them not only to more individual stress but to identical environments where factors produce their effects on large numbers of animals simultaneously.

2. The indiscriminate use of antibacterial drugs in feed and otherwise upsetting the microbial balance in favor of fungal proliferation, or possibly even stimulating fungal proliferation directly.

3. The widespread use in cattle operations of steroids with their immunodepressant action as well as their more subtle biochemical effects believed to favor fungal growth.

4. The increasingly artificial conditions of cattle husbandry involving greater use of harvested and stored feeds (hay, silage) in which fungal growth is high, as opposed to use of pasture in which fungal concentration is low.

Moisture and pH of hay and of silage have been related to mold infestation. *Absidia* and *Aspergillus fumigatus* abounded at 30 to 40 per cent water content of hay. Rotting hay contained both these agents as well as *Mortierella wolfii*. Moldy (pH 7.2) and rotten (pH 8.0) silage harbored *Absidia ramosa* and *M. wolfii*.

While the outcome of exposure to possible agents of mycotic abortion depends to a considerable extent on host factors, quantitative aspects appear to be of great importance, as abortions in cattle have frequently been related to the use of obviously moldy feed.

Pathogenesis

The bulk of pathologic and experimental evidence points to the conclusion that most bovine mycotic abortions are the result of generalized infections via the respiratory and alimentary routes. Manifestations in these systems, e.g., granulomas in the lung and ulcers in the stomach, may be subclinical but lead to blood-borne dissemination. Localization in the placenta results in placentitis, necrosis, and hemorrhage, with eventual separation of the chorion from the maternal placental tissue by an exudate in which fungal structures, usually hyphae, abound. Penetration of tissue and blood vessels is thought to be aided, at least in the case of certain fungi, by necrotizing enzymes. Attempts to account for the placental localization of fungi have revealed substances in tissue extracts of cattle that stimulate germination of fungal spores and growth of fungi. While these activities were demonstrated in extracts of a variety of tissues, they were highest in those of placental origin. The chemical nature of such substances has not been adequately defined, nor is it necessarily the total explanation of the abortion process. Immunologic factors have been suspected to play a part, including perhaps a rejection of the fetus by the dam analogous to a "graft vs. host reaction." This might be initiated by the breakdown, as a result of placental necrosis, of the division between fetal antigens and maternal circulation. The observation that experimental infection of pregnant ewes evoked an antibody response directed against placental constituents may be relevant in this context.

Clinical Signs and Pathology

Clinically, there are generally few distinguishing features that would differentiate mycotic from other abortions at the same stage of pregnancy. In the majority of cases, no general illness is present in the aborting cow, although fatal, fulminating pneumonia following *M. wolfii* infection has been reported in New Zealand, which were followed within 1 to 5 days by fulminating and ultimately fatal pneumonia in the majority of affected animals. Such systemic complications by *M. wolfii* abortions have not been common in Europe and the United States.

The aborted fetuses may be grossly normal. A variable percentage (2 to 25 per cent) have ringworm-like skin lesions in which fungal elements can be demonstrated. They are concentrated in the head and neck region. Such lesions are observed with *Aspergillus*- and zygomycete-induced abortions. Internal lesions of the fetus may include general lymphadenitis, dehydration, and emaciation. Mycotic colonization of lungs, liver, spleen, and brain may occur. Grossly recognizable mold colonies may be floating in the abomasal or amniotic fluid.

The most significant lesions of mycotic abortion are those of necrotizing, hemorrhagic placentitis, manifested grossly by brownish discoloration and swollen necrotic placentomas with thickened edges, distorting the structure into a cup-like shape. There is much adventitious placentation and thickening of intercotyledonary areas. The cotyledons adhere firmly to the maternal caruncles, so that retention of the placenta is very common. Attempts to detach the placenta often result in removal of the caruncles as well.

Microscopically, the basic lesion is one of vasculitis, with apparent hyphal invasion of the vessel walls, especially when zygomycotic agents are involved. Thrombosis, hemorrhage, necrosis, and inflammation with neutrophilic components predominating follow, beginning at the placentomal base and extending to the zone of arcade. Microscopic fetal lesions include bronchopneumonia and, where skin lesions are present, necrotizing epidermitis.

Extragenital lesions in the cows consist of pyogranulomatous nodules in various internal organs, particularly lung and kidneys. In cases of fatal pneumonia described as abortion sequela due to *M. wolfii*, a fibrinohemorrhagic process is evident.

Diagnosis

The diagnosis of mycotic abortion rests on the demonstration of fungi in association with significant lesions. It is important to realize that the mere demonstration or, even less conclusively, culture of fungi from specimens obtained after abortions or from genital tracts does not constitute adequate evidence of a causative role played by fungi in the abortion. The ubiquity of fungi in the bovine environment and the almost invariable contamination of placenta and fetus prior to examination render the presence of fungi in such material very likely. Fungi must be demonstrated as integral parts of the histopathology before their etiologic significance can be fully established.

For pathologic examination, placental tissues, especially cotyledons, should be submitted. If the entire fetus cannot be promptly forwarded to a laboratory, skin lesions, lymph nodes, lung, and stomach with its contents securely tied off should be forwarded. Duplicate tissue samples can be placed into 10-per cent formalin. The stomach contents may be preserved for microscopic examination by addition of 1 part formalin to 9 parts fluid (final concentration of formaldehyde, 2 to 5 per cent).

For diagnostic mycologic identification, prompt forwarding of specimens for culturing is essential. Fungi do not tolerate putrefactive tissue changes well nor do they benefit from freezing. Reportedly, *Aspergillus* spp. survive postmortem autolysis better than do zygomycetes, a circumstance possibly distorting some of the data given earlier on the frequency of various fungi in abortion.

Treatment and Control

The varied etiology and sporadic and usually low incidence of mycotic abortion would make specific control measures difficult to develop and their adoption doubtful. To date, none are available. A reasonable preventive step, however, is the elimination of moldy feeds, as there appears to be a fairly firm correlation between conditions favoring mold growth and the occurrence of mycotic abortions. Most cows that survive an episode of fungal abortion return to breed normally, without special treatment.

MYCOTIC ABORTIONS IN NONBOVINE SPECIES

Abortions in food animals other than cattle due to fungal agents are quite rare. Isolated abortions caused by *A. fumigatus* have been reported in sheep and swine. *Gliomastix* spp., *P. (Petriellidium) boydii*, and *Exophiala jeanselmii* have also been identified in swine placentitis and fetal pneumonia.

MYCOTIC MASTITIS

Incidence

The reported incidence of mycotic mastitis ranges from about 1 to 10 per cent of total mastitis of infectious origin. These figures may have little relevance to individual herds, where outbreaks, usually triggered by some management factor, may involve the majority of milking cows.

As is the case with bacterial mastitis, a large variety of fungal agents have been implicated. The most frequent appear to be the yeast-like fungi, particularly *Candida* spp. and *Cryptococcus* spp. Other genera are *Hansenula, Pichia, Rhodotorula, Torulopsis, Trichosporon,* and *Saccharomyces.* Mold mastitis is less frequently encountered, but there have been incriminations of *Aspergillus fumigatus* in a greater number of instances in recent years, particularly in Europe. *Pseudallescheria (Petriellidium) boydii* has been implicated on occasion, and there is growing awareness of the possibility of the alga *Prototheca* sp. (usually *P. zopfii*) causing mastitis.

Epidemiology

Like all cases of mastitis, mycotic mastitis is decisively influenced by management factors. Two aspects of dairy routine are particularly pertinent, milking hygiene and the use of antimicrobial drugs, especially by intramammary infusion. Inadequate milking hygiene may permit the passage of mastitis-producing agents from one mammary gland to another, converting a basically fortuitous, sporadic infection into a transmissible disease of potentially epidemic proportions. Mycotic mastitis as a herd problem is related to machine milking and other practices involving rapid successive contact of udders with persons or equipment capable of acting as vehicles of transmission.

The use of antibacterial drugs can play a part in the production of mastitis in 2 possible ways. First, it can provide the mechanical means of introducing fungal spores into the gland, since these are abundant in the environment, including the skin of the udder. Yeasts have also been found in freshly opened antibiotic preparations. Secondly, some antimicrobials are suspected of stimulating fungal growth and depressing certain host defense factors. Tetracycline has been described as having both these effects with regard to *Candida albicans*. Experimental attempts at demonstrating the stimulatory effects of antibiotics on fungal mastitis have had equivocal results, but circumstances surrounding mycotic mastitis outbreaks frequently include preceding or ongoing antibacterial intramammary therapy.

Clinical Signs, Pathogenesis, and Pathology

Fungal mastitis has no consistent peculiarities to differentiate it from bacterial mastitis. Reduced milk flow, swelling, and greater firmness of the affected gland are observed along with varying abnormalities in the appearance of the milk and positive results of the California Mastitis Test. Fevers with "spiking" temperatures may occur but have not been correlated with demonstrable fungemia. The duration and course of the disease are highly variable, depending on the infecting agent and on the size of the infecting dose. The most severe fungal mastitis is caused by *Cryptococcus neoformans,* which can extend over weeks and months, lead to complete suppression of milk flow, and leave glands with diminished or lost milk-secreting ability. By contrast, infection with other yeasts (*Candida* spp., *Trichosporon* spp.) takes a more benign and frequently self-limiting course. Whenever herds undergoing outbreaks of fungal mastitis have been investigated, a large proportion of infected but clinically normal animals were identified, even when *C. neoformans* was present.

Pathologically, yeasts evoke pyogranulomatous reactions. The acute phase is characterized by neutrophilic and eosinophilic exudates. Histiocytic infiltration and granuloma formation follow. Grossly, edema predominates early, with granulomatous foci and fibrotic changes occurring in advanced lesions.

In *A. fumigatus* mastitis, a chronic progressive course is usually observed with suppurative lesions predominating at necropsy. Prototothecal mastitis, although varying from acute to chronic to inapparent, also appears to follow a progressive, irreversible course ending eventually in the destruction of the infected gland.

Diagnosis

In the absence of specific clinical criteria, the demonstration of the causative agent by direct microscopic findings and culture is a firm requirement for establishing a diagnosis of fungal mastitis. The manner of collection, promptness of handling, and method of processing are of critical importance in determining results. The presence of fungi (e.g., *Candida* spp.) in the bovine's environment, on the skin, and even in the teat canal and sinus would render the isolation of small numbers of the organisms of doubtful significance. Similarly, the finding of fungal growth from milk that has been incubated prior to being cultured may mean very little. However, finding yeast cells in fresh milk by direct microscopic examinations of fixed stained smears indicates the presence of considerable numbers ($\geq 10^4$ to 10^5 cells/ml) and points to infection. *Candida* cells are readily stained by Gram's stain and appear as predominantly purple, often budding ovoids. Cryptococcal cells do not show any consistent staining patterns with Gram's stain and are apt to be overlooked unless the observer is specifically looking for *Cryptococcus*. In the latter case, the preferred method is to mix a drop of milk with a drop of high grade India ink on a slide and cover the preparation with a coverslip. The spherical yeast cells, sometimes with 1 bud, rarely with more, will appear under high dry magnification (400X) in the black background surrounded by bright unstained spherical capsules, the width of which may approach the diameter of the yeast cells themselves.

Both *Candida* and *Cryptococcus* will grow on most common culture media, including blood and Sabouraud's agar at either room temperature or 37°C. Media containing cycloheximides (e.g., cycloheximide-chloramphenicol agar and Dermatophyte test medium) should be avoided since they are inhibitory to *Cryptococcus neoformans* and some species of *Candida*. Several days should be allowed for colonial growth to develop. The specific identification of the yeast is based on morphologic and physiologic tests. Several simple 1-step commercially available systems (e.g., API-C20, Analytab*) of yeast identification exist for clinically prominent species. Hyphal fragments can be demonstrated in centrifuged mammary secretions by wet

mounts in 15-per cent potassium hydroxide. *A. fumigatus* grows well on blood agar and most other common media and is identified on the basis of fruiting structure morphology. Demonstration and culture of *Prototheca* spp. have been described earlier.

Treatment and Control

There is at present no established treatment for fungal mastitis. In fact, no intramammary antimycotic drug has been approved to date for use in the United States. Mycostatin has been given for both cryptococcal and candidal infections. In the former, it had little advantage over nonspecific measures. In the latter, its effects were difficult to assess since many infections of this type subside spontaneously. Recommendations followed in Europe include intramammary nystatin ointment at the rate of 3 gm on 3 successive days, or nystatin solution at the rate of 250,000 units in 2.5 ml on at least 2 successive days but to no more than 2 quarters at one time due to the toxic local and systemic effects that the aqueous solution may elicit. Clotrimazole is also suggested and can be used as ointment or as aqueous solution at the rate of 100 to 200 mg/quarter in 10 to 20 ml, 2 to 4 times at 24-hr intervals. Another drug that has been suggested for treatment of *Candida* mastitis is intramammary natamycin (Pimaricin) given as 2.5- or 5-per cent solution in 20 or 10 ml, respectively, on 3 successive days.

In vitro test results showed yeasts isolated from bovine mastitis most susceptible to clotrimazole. Results varied with regard to other antimycotics, including miconazole, nystatin, and 5-fluorocytosine. One study rated ketoconazole next best to clotrimazole.

There are no recommendations, based on adequate field or experimental studies, concerning the treatment of mastitis due to molds.

OTHER MYCOSES

Aspergillosis

Sporadic clinical aspergillosis in cattle, sheep, and swine as either isolated cases or limited outbreaks have been reported from all parts of the world. They involve primarily young animals or debilitated animals. Either the respiratory or alimentary tract is affected and constitutes the likely portal of infection. General cases with lesions in kidney, liver, and lungs are also sometimes observed. The involvement of *Aspergillus* spp. in bovine hypersensitivity pneumonitis, resembling farmer's lung, is not firmly established. Multiple infections with *Aspergillus* combined with *Candida* spp. or Zygomycetes have been repeatedly observed.

Massive exposure to moldy feed and bedding, dietary acidosis, and extended administration of antimicrobial drugs have been found associated with outbreaks. Subclinical infections have been shown to be widespread in cattle, with both pulmonary and intestinal localizations reported. Several instances of fatal infections in newborn animals, especially lambs, point to the likelihood of prenatal exposure.

Acute cases exhibit hemorrhagic, necrotic lesions associated with vasculitis and thrombosis. More chronic cases are characterized by granuloma formation and fibrosis. Eosinophils may be prominent in association with the lesions and in the circulating blood. The agent will appear

---

*Available from Analytab Products, 200 Express St., Plainview, New York, 11380.

as septate filaments, 2 to 3 μm in caliber, fairly regular in outline, and generally branching at acute angles. In progressive pulmonary aspergillosis, cavitation may occur, with the fungus growing freely in the lumen of the cavities, producing cottony, aerial mycelia, complete with pigmented fruiting bodies. A frequent feature of chronic and subclinical aspergillosis is the presence of "asteroid" bodies, i.e., hyphal nests surrounded by radiating acidophilic projections. These have been identified as host immunoglobulins and have been observed in a number of other fungal infections (coccidioidomycosis, sporotrichosis).

Reports from Europe mention nystatin as useful treatment for intestinal infections of pigs.

Zygomycoses (Phycomycoses)

Systemic infection with Zygomycetes is primarily in cattle but also in swine. Reports of infections in sheep are extremely rare. The genera involved are mainly *Mucor, Absidia,* and *Rhizopus*. Many cases are based on histopathologic findings only, so that no genus, let alone species, identification is possible. A noteworthy incidence of *Mortierella* infections has been reported only from New Zealand, although there are sporadic incidences elsewhere.

The epidemiology of these infections, like that of aspergillosis, often appears related to stressful experiences like parturition, inappropriate diet, and concurrent infection due to other fungi, bacteria, or viruses. A case developing after experimental irradiation also fits this pattern. Unusually concentrated exposure to the agents is also thought to play a part. Gastrointestinal tract involvement predominates, especially in pigs. Several cases of neonatal encephalitis have been observed in cattle.

Reports of zygomycotic infections, especially in young animals, describe acute signs and lesions more often than is the case with aspergillosis. Gastrointestinal tract disturbances are frequently the first sign, including anorexia and mucosanguineous diarrhea. Ruminal atony, bloat, and colic have been observed in affected cattle. Other forms affect mainly the lymph nodes of the intestinal tract or thorax.

The gross lesions in the gastrointestinal tract are ulcerations of stomach and intestine. Any part of the stomach can be involved. In ruminants, the rumen and abomasum are the usual sites. Depending on the acuteness of the condition, hemorrhagic, necrotic, suppurative, and nodular, granulomatous features will predominate in that order. In the lymphadenitic form, the only lesions may be granulomas in the nodes that range from a few millimeters in diameter to those that have replaced all recognizable lymph node tissue. Microscopically, the basic lesion is vasculitis, affecting either arteries or veins and initiated by hyphal invasion of the vessel wall. Thrombosis and vascular disintegration follow, causing hemorrhage, necrosis, and suppuration that are grossly observable. Hyphae will be apparent and distinguishable from those of *Aspergillus* spp. by their larger size (up to 7 μm), their irregular outline, their relative lack of septa, and their greater tendency to branch to right angles.

No successful treatment has been established.

Candidiasis

Most *Candida* infections have been encountered in cattle and swine. The localization, other than in bovine mastitis, has been predominantly in the alimentary tract from the mouth to the intestine. Septicemic and pneumonic infections are sometimes seen.

The source of the causative agents may be the mucous membranes of the animals themselves containing *C. albicans,* as well as the skin and external environment containing other *Candida* spp. The prolonged use of broad-spectrum antibacterial drugs is frequently a factor in initiating clinical candidiasis. The disruption of the normal microbial balance in the digestive tract is thought to produce the overgrowth and pathogenesis by the yeasts. A more direct role of tetracycline in stimulating growth of *Candida* has also been suspected. In some cases, massive prolonged exposure to contaminated feed has been implicated in the absence of, or in addition to, antibiotics.

The common clinical form of candidiasis is thrush and enteritis in calves and young pigs. Thrush is an ulcerative pseudomembranous inflammation of the mucous membranes of the mouth, esophagus, and stomach (rumen). The process in the intestine is similar but not usually referred to as thrush. Clinical signs will reflect the location of the process: inappetence, excessive salivation, and vomiting occur in oral and upper digestive tract infections. Intestinal infections are also characterized by diarrhea.

Lesions are those of ulcerative inflammation with varying amounts of overlying fibrinous exudate. As long as the process is relatively superficial, the yeast forms of *Candida* predominate. With invasion of deeper tissue, pseudomycelial and mycelial structures replace the yeasts.

Confirmation of candidiasis requires demonstration of *Candida* spp. in significant numbers in association with compatible lesions. The recovery of *Candida* from oral or rectal swabs and even from tracheobronchial washes does not establish the diagnosis. Overgrowth without significant pathogenic activity is a distinct possibility with these fungi. Finding a preponderance of filamentous forms would be much more suggestive of a disease. Microbiologic observations must be evaluated in the light of pathologic and clinical evidence.

The agents of candidiasis are readily cultured on common media over a wide range of temperatures (see Mycotic Mastitis). There are few reports of successful treatment of clinical candidiasis, especially from this country. Experience in Europe showed favorable results with oral nystatin and amphotericin-B in isolated instances. Since most cases of candidiasis are related to some inadequacy in host defenses or to mismanagement or to unusually heavy exposure, control measures should be directed at removing these underlying causes.

Histoplasmosis

Instances of clinical histoplasmosis in livestock are extremely rare. Existing reports concern cattle and pigs. Respiratory lesions were present in all 6 cases but 1, where the lesions were in the liver. All evidence points to the absence of histoplasmosis as a problem in food animals.

Coccidioidomycosis

Among food-producing mammals, only cattle are infected with *Coccidioides immitis* to any significant extent. The infection is quite common in endemic areas but invariably subclinical and evident only at postmortem examination, when thoracic lymphadenitis and small lung lesions may be noted. Coccidioidomycosis in sheep has been reported. The infection is of no economic importance in livestock, since even the bovine cases are not extensive enough to cause carcass condemnation.

Mycotic Nasal Infections

A variety of fungi have been implicated in nasal infections. Among food-producing animals only cattle have been involved. The lesions are nasal granulomas and polyps, which lead to respiratory distress of varying severity. Best known among the polyp-forming infections is rhinosporidiosis, a disease mostly seen in tropical and subtropical climates but occasionally seen in the United States. Polyps, pedunculated or not, form in 1 nostril. They are soft and pink and bleed readily. The whitish specks they contain are the spherules (sporangia) previously mentioned. Little is known about the life cycle of the agent. A free-living form is suspected by some workers, since direct transmission does not take place. Treatment is through surgical excision. A report from Argentina refers to cures in 9 cases following treatment with calcium, isoniazid (isonicotinic acid hydrazide), and 60-per cent sodium iodide.

Bovine granulomas with and without polyp formations have been found associated with infections by pigmented saprophytic fungi (phaeohyphomycosis). Some of these infections were accompanied by fairly widespread involvement of skin and lymph nodes. The agents included among other black (dematiaceous) fungi mainly *Drechslera (Helminthosporium) rostrata* and *D. (H.) spicifera*. The lesions have been described as mycetomas and allergy is assumed by many workers to be involved. No medical treatment is known.

DEEP MYCOSES

Diagnosis

In addition to discussion of diagnoses of the various infections, the following observations apply to diagnoses of deep fungal infections in general:

1. As a rule, no distinctive lesions, signs, or symptoms differentiate fungal infections from other infections of the same organ system. Exceptions are certain bovine abortions in which fetal skin lesions are observed in a minority of cases. Another exception is aspergillosis in an aerated space, e.g., respiratory passages or pulmonary cavitations. In all other cases, the correct diagnosis depends on the demonstration of the fungus in association with the disease.

2. The isolation of fungi, especially in small numbers, does not of itself establish the presence of mycotic disease. The agent must be related histopathologically to the lesions from which it was recovered. Most fungi are detectable in tissue stained routinely with hematoxylin-eosin, but some are not, especially in their most typical form. Special fungal stains (periodic acid–Schiff, Gridley's, Gomori's methenamine silver) are often useful.

3. Direct demonstration of fungal structures in wet mounts or stained smears is somewhat more convincing than isolation because of the large number of such structures that would have to be present in order to be detectable by direct microscopic examination (10^4 to 10^5/ml). It would still not be conclusive evidence but could reflect fungal overgrowth in the absence of pathogenic activity. The finding of branching hyphae or budding

yeasts would mean more than the mere presence of spores, and the finding of the tissue phase or dimorphic fungi would be acceptable evidence of infection.

4. Culture of fungi responsible for deep mycoses does not require special media. All the fungi referred to in this article (except *Rhinosporidium*) grow well on blood agar under atmospheric conditions and over a wide range of temperatures. Long incubation periods (up to 10 days) may have to be allowed, a circumstance increasing the likelihood of bacterial overgrowth. Commercially available selective fungal media are commonly designed for dermatophyte culture and contain inhibitors that would suppress growth of many of the agents potentially involved in deep mycoses.

5. Most of the agents of deep mycoses are provisionally identifiable as to their major group from their appearance on direct microscopic examination and from their primary growth on isolation media. The salient features of these groups have been described previously. Specific identification requires appropriate laboratory facilities and laboratory staff expertise. It is important to realize that spores of many fungi, especially molds, are readily dispersed from cultures, constituting a potential health hazard to humans. Cultures should therefore be handled with caution, optimally under properly ventilated safety hoods by trained, experienced personnel.

5. Pathologic materials for laboratory-assisted diagnosis should be handled much like other samples intended for microbiologic processing, except that they should not be frozen. Place tissue intended for histopathologic examination in 10-per cent buffered formalin. For details on identification and laboratory techniques, consult a medical mycology reference.

ANTIFUNGAL DRUGS

As has been stated, medical treatment of deep mycosis in food animals is a virtually unexplored field, in part because antifungal drugs suitable for such treatment are relatively new and have not been adequately tested in food-producing mammals. It is to be expected that this situation will change and that drugs presently in use on humans and companion animals will also be utilized to some extent on meat and dairy stock. A brief characterization of the types of drugs used on fungal infections is therefore appropriate. Present antifungal drugs fall into 3 chemical categories.

1. The polyenes are represented by nystatin (Mycostatin*) and amphotericin-B (Fungizone*). They are characterized by limited solubility in water and poor absorbability from the gastrointestinal tract. They are also quite toxic. As a result, nystatin is useful only for topical application or intestinal infection. Amphotericin-B, which is at present the mainstay of antifungal therapy in humans, is given by intravenous injection. Systemic amphotericin-B has not been used in food animals.

2. A more recently introduced antimycotic is 5-fluorocytosine (flucytosine, e.g., Ancobon†), which is readily absorbed from the gastrointestinal tract and is generally well tolerated. Its usefulness so far has been confined largely to the treatment of infections due to yeast-like

---

*Available from E.R. Squibb & Sons, Princeton, NJ 08540.
†Available from Hoffmann-La Roche, Inc., Nutley, NJ 07110.

fungi, particularly candidiasis and cryptococcosis. A further limitation to the use of 5-fluorocytosine is the existence of resistant strains of these yeasts in nature and the common emergence of resistance in the course of treatment. Susceptibility tests are advisable for establishing the appropriateness of this drug in each instance its use is considered.

3. The most recent additions to the antimycotic armamentarium are the various imidazole derivatives, e.g., miconazole (Monistat*), clotrimazole (Lotrimin†), and ketoconazole (Nizoral*). Some of these drugs, e.g., miconazole, can be used both topically and systemically, while others are dependable for topical use only, e.g., clotrimazole, which is inactivated by a liver enzyme induced by the drug itself. The imidazole derivatives have a rather broad spectrum of activity and affect both yeasts and mycelial fungi. They are effective when administered orally. Resistance has so far not been a major problem. The drugs even have some antibacterial activity and inhibit dermatophytes as well. Their toxicity is much less than

that of amphotericin-B. In humans, toxicity is manifested by nausea, vomiting, depression, and mental disturbances. Ketoconazole has been used in the treatment of systemic mycosis of companion animals with encouraging results.

Supplemental Reading

Ainsworth, G. C., and Austwick, P. K. C.: Fungal Diseases of Animals, 2nd ed. England, Commonwealth Agricultural Bureaux, Farnham Royal, 1973.

Jungerman, P. F., and Schwartzman, R. M.: Veterinary Medical Mycology. Philadelphia, Lea and Febiger, 1973.

McDonald, J. S., Richard, J. L., Anderson, A. J., and Fichter, R. E.: In vitro antimycotic sensitivity of yeasts isolated from infected bovine mammary glands. Am. J. Vet. Res. 41:1987–1990, 1980.

Pepin, G. A.: Bovine mycotic abortion. Vet. Annual 23:79–90, 1983.

Rippon, J. W.: Medical Mycology, 2nd ed. Philadelphia, W.B. Saunders Company, 1982.

Weigt, V., and Ahlers, D.: Zur Atiologie, Symptomatologie und Therapie der Hefemastitis bein Rind. Deutsche Tieraerztl. Wochenschr. 89:234–238, 1982.

*Available from Janssen Pharmaceutical, Inc., New Brunswick, NJ 08903.

†Available from Schering Corporation, Kenilworth, NJ 07033.

Refer to the first volume of *Current Veterinary Therapy: Food Animal Practice* for the following: Schoneweis, D. A., and Henry, S. C.: Colibacillosis in Swine. Section 8, Bacterial and Fungal Disease.

PROTOZOAL AND RICKETTSIAL DISEASES

JIMMY L. HOWARD, D.V.M., M.S.
Consulting Editor

Babesioses

(Piroplasmosis, Redwater Disease, Texas Cattle Fever)

THOMAS M. CRAIG, D.V.M., Ph.D.

Babesiosis is a tick-transmitted disease caused by various *Babesia* spp. The disease is found in cattle, sheep, goats, and swine throughout much of the world. In the Western Hemisphere babesiosis is a disease of cattle caused by either *B. bovis* or *B. bigemina,* where the vectors are extant from Mexico to Argentina. The disease is characterized by anemia, icterus, fever, hemoglobinuria, and, occasionally, abnormal central nervous system signs and death.

EPIZOOTIOLOGY

Although not necessarily a tropical disease, bovine babesiasis in the Western Hemisphere is limited to lowland tropical and subtropical regions. Much of the southern United States was an endemic region for bovine *Babesia,* but the vectors and disease were eradicated.

In endemic regions the effects of *Babesia* on cattle are largely unrecognized, as the infection is acquired at a young age. Calves are resistant to the effects of the organism both from a standpoint of immunity derived from their mothers and from a standpoint of resistance waning with age. Calves become carriers of the organism without clinical signs of disease and as long as they remain infected, they are resistant. This state of resistance to disease while remaining a carrier is called premunition. Constant reinfection occurs in endemic areas, and cattle go through life infected by the organisms without signs of disease. If for some reason reinfection fails to occur, the cattle may lose the infection and within a few months become susceptible to the disease. The disease is seen in areas where susceptible cattle are transported into endemic regions, or where because of weather conditions or tick control programs the vector population falls below the threshold necessary to maintain infection in the herd. The prevalence of infection in endemic areas approaches 100 per cent, but the incidence of disease is extremely low. Conversely, in epidemic regions or in transported cattle, the prevalence of disease may be extremely high at times. In untreated cases, the mortality rate may be as high as 50 to 90 per cent.

ETIOLOGY

The taxonomy of *Babesia* has been the subject of much controversy, partially arising from the confusion in the scientific literature concerning its life cycle. At this time, *Babesia* organisms are considered to be members of the Phylum Apicomplexa, Class Piroplasmasida, Family Babesiidae. Species of *Babesia* are host specific. The 2 species in the Western Hemisphere are *B. bovis* and *B. bigemina.* The species are differentiated by their morphology and by the clinical diseases they cause. *B. bovis* is the smaller of the two, and the piroplasms are approximately 2.4×1 μm, whereas the intraerythrocytic piroplasms of *B. bigemina* are 4.5×2.5 μm.

Transmission of the organism can be accomplished by the transfusion of blood from a carrier animal or by *Boophilus* ticks. Transmission by the tick is transovarian. The female tick becomes infected by the ingestion of piroplasms during engorgement. It then drops off the host and the organism reproduces within the tick's tissues with some of the organisms being incorporated within developing tick embryos. Larval ticks transmit *B. bovis* but do not transmit *B. bigemina* until the larvae have molted into the nymph or adult.

Within the cow, the erythrocyte is the only known host cell. The organism divides, forming 2 daughter cells, and then leaves its host cell, destroying it. Each daughter cell repeats the process of division in other erythrocytes.

CLINICAL SIGNS AND LESIONS

Reproduction of piroplasms by binary fission and invasion of erythrocytes occurs within the circulatory system. The incubation period is usually 2 to 3 weeks from the time of tick infestation, then destruction of erythrocytes results in anemia, hemoglobinemia, and hemoglobinuria. Clinical signs are fever (40 to 41.5°C), depression, dehydration, icterus, anorexia, elevated heart and respiratory rates, and abortion. Cerebral babesiasis, characterized by convulsions, opisthotonus, and coma, is observed in cattle infected with *B. bovis.* The abnormal cerebral signs are due to brain anoxia, resulting from severe anemia or clogging of capillaries by infected erythrocytes or both. Death is due to a shock-like syndrome associated with the release of vasoactive substances, accumulation of toxic substances, and anemic anoxia. Postmortem findings include icterus, enlarged soft spleen, enlarged yellow-brown liver, swollen dark-colored kidneys, and dark red urine in the bladder. The blood is watery, the lymph nodes are edematous, and there may be hemorrhages of the subserosa of the abomasum and small intestine. There may be pericardial and endocardial hemorrhages, and the pericardial sac may contain serosanguineous fluid. The lungs may be edematous, especially in acute cases. Most of the deaths are within 5 to 7 days of the onset of clinical signs, but this period varies with the susceptibility of the cattle, virulence of the organism, and environmental factors.

Cattle that survive the acute phase may completely recover with time, but those infected with *B. bigemina* will often experience 2 or 3 episodes of recrudescence, following initial onset. Some will become poor doers, or they will die because of secondary infections. The survivors become chronic carriers and are resistant to reinfection.

DIAGNOSIS

Clinical signs, history, and geographic region may be sufficient data for a presumptive diagnosis. However, confirmation of this diagnosis can only be made by observing the organisms. Either thick or thin blood films will reveal *B. bigemina*. *B. bovis* is often an elusive parasite because of its predilection for capillary beds. The chances for detecting *B. bovis* are increased by examining capillary blood from the end of the tail or by searching for the organism in capillaries, such as that obtained in cerebral or renal impression smears when the organisms cannot be found in blood smears.

In recent years, serologic tests for *Babesia* infections have been widely used to identify carrier cattle. The complement fixation and indirect fluorescent antibody tests are the most widely utilized, but other methods such as the ELSIA show promise. Confirmation of infection in a chronic carrier can be made by the inoculation of blood containing piroplasms into a splenectomized calf.

TREATMENT

Supportive treatment of acute babesiosis is quite important. However, the clinician may decide that animals with intractable cases, especially during hot weather, may benefit from benign neglect, as the excitement of handling may precipitate an anoxic crisis. Fluids and blood replacement are important to supportive therapy. A number of drugs that have specific effects against *Babesia* infections have been developed over the years, and a few of them will be discussed.

Trypan Blue

Trypan blue was the first really effective drug against *B. bigemina,* and it is given to cattle as a 1-per cent intravenous solution. It will not completely eradicate the infection but will lower parasitemia sufficiently that the animal's immunologic defenses will take over. Trypan blue gives a bluish tinge to cattle, which is especially noticeable in the sclera. The drug also causes extensive sloughing of tissues if administered perivascularly.

Babesiacides

Four compounds with babesiacidal activity are Diminazene (4,4′-diamidinodiazoaminobenzene diaceturate, Berenil,* or Ganasag†) at 2 to 5 mg/kg; Phenamidine (4,4′-diamidinodiphenyl ether, Lomidine‡) at 8 to 13 mg/kg; Amicarbalide (3,3′-diamidinocarbanilide, Diampron‡) at 5 to 10 mg/kg; and Imidocarb§ (3,3′-bis(2-imidazolin-2-yl carbanilide, Imizol§) at 0.5 to 2.5 mg/kg.

Imidocarb has both therapeutic and prophylactic activities. The drug has been withdrawn from the market in some countries because of its persistence in the tissues of treated animals. It is administered either subcutaneously or intramuscularly.

If the organisms are rapidly killed with the use of a chemotherapeutic agent, anemia may be temporarily exacerbated. In general, clinical cure rather than radical cure (sterilization) is desired, and as babesiacides are generally toxic, the lowest possible effective dose is desirable. Treated cattle then become chronic carriers but are resistant to further episodes of the disease.

PREVENTION

Eradication of tick vectors was the method of control in the United States. *Boophilus* are ticks that spend their entire feeding period on a single host rather than dropping off the host to molt and then feed on another host. They normally feed only on cattle for approximately 21 days, therefore, if the cattle are dipped regularly and no cattle are overlooked, eradication should be accomplished. Eradication schemes have been attempted elsewhere, such as in parts of Australia and Mexico, but have met with little success in these countries for several reasons. Probably the most important is the development of resistance by ticks to acaricides. Another reason for failure is the ability of some of the ticks to use alternate hosts such as white-tailed deer (which are not dipped) and the failure of the programs to require 100 per cent support by livestock owners. If only a few animals are not dipped, it is enough to allow the survival of ticks.

In addition to eradicating the ticks by use of acaricides, practices such as controlled burning and cultivating or resting pastures for prolonged periods will aid in keeping tick numbers low. In endemic areas, it is not desirable to get rid of all the ticks, but it is desirable to keep the tick numbers below the threshold value where "tick worry" becomes economically important.

If calves are exposed to infected ticks early in life, there will be no disease, and the calves will become naturally immunized by the bite of the infected tick. If, however, exposure to ticks is not a certainty, artificial infection may be needed at an early age. Inoculating blood from a carrier will cause infection, and if the recipient is young enough, it will not produce signs of disease. The same thing can be done to older cattle if care is taken to

---

*Manufactured by Hoechst-Roussel Pharmaceuticals Inc., Somerville, NJ 08876

†Manufactured by E.R. Squibb & Sons Inc., Princeton, NJ 08540

‡Manufactured by May & Baker Ltd., Dageham, United Kingdom

§Manufactured by Wellcome Animal Health, Kansas City, MO 64116

monitor the infection and treat it with a nonsterilizing dose of a babesiacide. Older cattle can also be protected by administering a defined dose of attenuated organisms that will cause infection but not disease. This method of protection is widely used in Australia, Republic of South Africa, and other areas where babesiosis is a threat.

Methods of attenuating the organisms vary from that of selection of a field isolate that causes mild clinical signs in susceptible cattle to the rapid passage of *B. bovis* in splenectomized calves. Irradiation of blood containing virulent organisms will cause attenuation of some species of *Babesia*.

Imidocarb has been used prophylactically in cattle introduced into endemic areas. As the effect of the drug wanes with time, a few of the organisms are able to establish an infection, but there is enough residual activity that the cattle are protected from disease. A state of premunition then follows. Attempts to produce vaccine with killed organisms have been unsuccessful, as only a very short duration of protection has been demonstrated. In the absence of reinfection, the inoculation of viable organisms may only protect for a few months, so in herds with a high risk potential reinoculating viable organisms must be repeated frequently.

Supplemental Reading

Joyner, L. P., and Donnelly, J.: The epidemiology of babesial infections. Adv. Parasitol. *17*:115–140, 1979.

Kuttler, K. L., and Todorovic, R. A.: Babesiasis. Foreign Animal Diseases, U.S.A.H.A. 297–307, 1975.

Kuttler, K. L.: Chemotherapy of babesiasis: a review in Babesiasis. Ristic, M. and Kreier, J. P. (eds.). New York, Academic Press, 65–85, 1981.

Mahoney, D. F.: *Babesia* of domestic animals. *In* Kreier, J. P. (ed.). Parasitic Protozoa, vol. 4. New York, Academic Press, 1–51, 1977.

Zwart, D.: Babesiasis: nonspecific resistance, immunological factors and pathogenesis. Adv. Parasitol. *17*:49–113, 1979.

Bovine Anaplasmosis

E. J. RICHEY, D.V.M.

Anaplasmosis is an infectious, noncontagious, transmissible disease of cattle caused by the intraerythrocytic parasite *Anaplasma marginale*.

EPIZOOTIOLOGY

In the United States, anaplasmosis is enzootic in the southern Atlantic states, the Gulf Coast states, the lower plains and western states but is sporadic in the northern states. All ages of cattle may become infected with anaplasmosis. The severity of illness and the percentage of deaths increases with age. Calves less than 6 months old seldom exhibit clinical signs of anaplasmosis. Cattle, ages 6 months to 3 years, become more ill, and more deaths occur with age. After 3 years of age, a 30 to 50 per cent mortality rate is reported in cattle exhibiting clinical anaplasmosis.

CLINICAL SIGNS AND LESIONS

The gross clinical signs of bovine anaplasmosis are predominantly related to acute anemia. A febrile response is noted, coinciding with the beginning of detectable parasitemia in the blood. The fever usually persists through the period of increasing parasitemia and may reach 41°C (106°F); however, subnormal temperatures are noted prior to death.

Acute anemia results in pallor of the mucosa, muscular weakness, depression, dehydration, anorexia, elevated heart rate, and, upon exertion, respiratory distress. The animal may be belligerent if inadequate tissue oxygenation has affected the brain. Examination of the blood shows it to be grossly thin and watery. Since the disease is characteristically hemolytic, i.e., the parasitized erythrocytes are destroyed in the reticuloendothelial system without release of free hemoglobin, hemoglobinuria is not observed.

Anaplasmosis can be divided into 4 stages: incubation, developmental, convalescent, and carrier. The *incubation stage* is that time from introduction of *Anaplasma* into a susceptible animal until the time 1 per cent of the red blood cells are infected. The length of this stage appears to vary directly with the number of organisms introduced into the animal. Under natural conditions, the time may be from 3 to 8 weeks, although shorter and longer times have been recorded. No clinical signs are evident during this stage. The end of the period coincides with the first rise in body temperature.

The *developmental stage* is that time when characteristic anemia is developing. It begins with 1 per cent infected red blood cells and ends with reticulocytes appearing in the peripheral circulation. The length of this stage varies from 4 to 9 days. During this period, most of the signs characteristic of anaplasmosis appear. The infected animal usually shows the first clinical signs about midway through the stage or about the third or fourth day. This is the time when owners who observe their cattle carefully each day will notice cattle are ill.

The *convalescent stage* extends from the appearance of reticulocytes to the return of normal for the various blood values. The length of this stage varies greatly and may extend from a few weeks to a few months.

The *carrier stage* is usually thought of as that time extending from the disappearance of discernible anaplasmic bodies sometime during the convalescent stage to the end of the animal's life. Clinically recovered animals remain carriers with nondetectable parasitemia and thus act as reservoirs of the disease.

The differentiation between developmental and convalescent stages is through evidence of greater erythropoiesis on stained blood smears. The signs of increased erythropoiesis in the peripheral blood, which identifies the convalescent stage, are reticulocytes, polychromatophils, basophilic stippled cells, normoblasts, high hemoglobin levels, and high total white blood cell counts.

Lesions at necropsy are typical of severe anemia with pallor of the tissues, thin watery blood and occasionally icterus. Since erythrocyte destruction took place, in the reticuloendothelial system, the spleen is greatly enlarged, with reddish brown pulp and enlarged splenic follicles; the liver is enlarged, with rounded edges; and the gallbladder is distended with dark bile.

DIAGNOSIS

Diagnosis of anaplasmosis can be based upon clinical signs, necropsy lesions, and the demonstration of *A.*

Table 1. *Stage of Anaplasmosis in Respect to Parasitemia, Positive Serologic Reactions, and Clinical Signs*

Stage of Disease	A. marginale on Blood Smear	Reaction to Serologic Test	Clinical Signs
Unexpected	No	Negative	None
Incubation	No	Negative	None
Developmental	Yes	Positive	Present
Convalescent	Yes*	Positive	Present
Carrier	No	Positive	None

*Immature RBCs also present.

marginale on stained blood smears. Use of serologic tests is of little value during an acute outbreak or during the anaplasmosis season, since animals in the incubation stage would test negatively. Positive diagnosis of acute cases (developmental or convalescent stages) can more easily and readily be made using stained blood smears. Carrier animals would react positively to the serologic test but would not exhibit detectable parasitemia on stained blood smears. A brief summary of the presence of parasitemia, serologic reactions, and clinical signs in relationship to the stage of disease are in Table 1.

The rapid card agglutination and complement fixation tests are the most common serologic tests used for the detection of anaplasma. Infected animals begin to exhibit positive reactions at about the same time that anaplasma bodies can first be seen in the red blood cells. The test reaction is, therefore, negative during the incubation period and positive during the developmental, convalescent, and carrier stages.

On a thin blood smear, stained with Giemsa or Wright's stain, *A. marginale* bodies appear as spherical granules 0.2 to 0.5 microns in diameter located near the periphery of the red blood cell. The anaplasma bodies would be detected during the developmental and convalescent stages.

Anaplasmosis outbreaks are related to the lack of a control program, to the per cent of herd that are anaplasmosis carriers, and to the amount of vector transmission.

NO CONTROLS + CARRIERS + VECTORS = OUTBREAKS

Either an increase in per cent of carriers or in amount of vector transmission can influence the severity of an outbreak. With this in mind, reducing vector transmission, instituting control programs to prevent outbreaks, eliminating the carrier state, and handling an outbreak of anaplasmosis need consideration.

TREATMENT AND CONTROL

Reducing Vector Transmission

Anaplasmosis is spread by a transfer of blood from an infected animal to a susceptible animal. Transmission is primarily a mechanical Fraufer of infected bovine blood; i.e., it is transmitted by biting insects or by instruments used by humans. There are also certain biologic vectors, such as *Dermacentor occidentalis* and *D. andersoni* ticks, which are capable of harboring the *Anaplasma* parasite through several life stages. Biting insects, such as the horsefly, stable fly, and mosquito, have been either proved

to be or incriminated to be mechanical vectors of anaplasmosis. These natural mechanical and biologic vectors are usually quite seasonal, and most outbreaks of anaplasmosis coincide with or immediately follow the vector season.

Control of biting insects quite often can be frustrating and generally can not be considered a practical, reliable method of totally preventing transmission of anaplasmosis. Application of insecticides that reduce the biting insect population will substantially reduce the number of clinical anaplasmosis cases occurring in a herd, however. Periodic spraying and dipping as well as use of dust bags and back rubbers, are common methods of insecticide application.

Contaminated surgical instruments, dehorners, and hypodermic needles are known mechanical vectors used by humans. This type of mechanical transmission takes place only when the disease organism is exchanged immediately—within minutes. A quick rinse of the contaminated instrument in clean water or disinfectant immediately after use will usually prevent transmission. When this type of transmission occurs, a large number of cattle in the herd show signs of anaplasmosis at nearly the same time, without a few cases having appeared earlier.

Programs for Control of Anaplasmosis

Test the Herd and Separate Carriers from Noncarriers. This program necessitates the collection of blood samples from and subsequent identification of each animal. It also requires that 2 separate herds be maintained during the vector season or that one group (carriers or noncarriers) be disposed of. There are no susceptible animals in a 100 per cent carrier herd. New additions must be protected, however, and there are regulations governing interstate movement of carrier animals.

Test the Herd and Eliminate the Carriers with Tetracycline Therapy.[1] (See Clearing the Carrier Stage.)

Anaplasmosis Vaccination (Anaplaz*) Control Program.[2] For an effective vaccination program, the herd owner should follow these recommendations:

1. The *initial vaccination* (first year) consists of 2 doses given 4 weeks apart, scheduled so that the second dose is given at least 2 weeks before the vector season.

2. A booster should be administered 2 weeks or more before the next vector season. After the first booster, additional boosters should be administered at least every other year to provide adequate protection. A vaccinated animal is still capable of becoming infected with *A. marginale* and subsequently can become a carrier. The vaccine does not prevent infection but aids in prevention of clinical symptoms.

Continuous Oxytetracycline Medication During the Vector Season. An injection of oxytetracycline is administered every 21 to 28 days,[3] beginning with the start of the vector season and extending 1 to 2 months after the vector season ends. The recommended dose is 6.6 to 11 mg/kg when using 50 to 100 mg/ml oxytetracycline or 20 mg/kg when using LA–200.†[4]

Continuous Chlortetracycline Medication During the Vector Season. For control of anaplasmosis, chlortetracycline may be administered by the following methods:

1. Medicated feed (1.1 mg/kg daily).

2. Medicated salt-mineral mixes offered free-choice, prepared to approximate daily consumption of 1.1 mg/kg.

3. Medicated feed blocks.[5]

*Available from Fort Dodge Laboratories, Fort Dodge, IA 50501
†Available from Pfizer Inc., New York, NY 10017

Consumption data should be available from the manufacturers.

Continuous Chlortetracycline Medication During the Entire Year. Chlortectracycline can be administered continously throughout the year in feed or salt-mineral mixes.

Oral daily doses of 0.22 to 0.55 mg/kg of chlortetracycline administered daily will prevent clinical anaplasmosis but will allow carrier infections to develop.[6] If medication, using this dosage of chlortetracycline is withdrawn shortly after a field challenge, expect clinical anaplasmosis to appear after a prolonged incubation stage.

It is essential that cattle receive an adequate amount of chlortetracycline. When using salt-mineral mixes or feed blocks as the vehicles for medication, place the mix or blocks near water holes, provide sufficient protection from the sun and rain, and replenish at frequent intervals. Cattle often prefer natural salt licks or salt licks associated with oil wells to salt-mineral mixes. It is advisable to routinely check to ensure that the cattle are consuming the medicated mix.

Bulls apparently do not consume adequate chlortetracycline and require additional protection, such as vaccination.

Eliminating the Carrier Stage

Anaplasmosis carrier cattle may be cured of the infection by treatment with certain tetracycline antibiotics. Carrier stage elimination programs must include postmedication serologic testing. The complement fixation test results can remain positive for months after treatment, but the reactor's blood may not be infective. When testing 6 months after treatment ceases, all cases with positive results should be considered as "treatment failures." Failures should be retreated or separated from the rest of the herd. Animals that have been cleared of the carrier state are susceptible to reinfection but exhibit resistance to clinical anaplasmosis for as long as 30 months.[7]

Oxytetracycline (50 to 100 mg/ml): 5-Day Treatment.[8] Administer 22 mg/kg daily for 5 days: intramuscularly, not over 10 ml per injection site and intravenously dilute with physiologic saline.

Oxytetracycline (50 to 100 mg/ml): 10-Day Treatment.[9] Administer 11 mg/kg daily for 10 days: intramuscularly, not over 10 ml per injection site and intravenously dilute with physiologic saline.

Oxytetracycline (LA–200): 4 Treatments at 3-Day Intervals.[10] Each animal receives 4 treatments of LA–200 at 3-day intervals at a dose of 20 mg/kg. The total dose should be divided between 2 injection sites and given by deep intramuscular injection.

Chlortetracycline (11 mg/kg): 60-Day Treatment.[11] It is recommended that chlortetracycline be fed at 11 mg/kg daily for 60 days. At this level, chlortetracycline will eliminate the carrier stage. Oral administration permits treatment on a herd basis and the use of economical antibiotic premixes. This oral dose may cause diarrhea, anorexia, and weight loss during the first week, but the cattle return to normal rapidly after that time. The medicated feed should nevertheless be offered during this time.

Chlortetracycline (1.1 mg/kg): 120-Day Treatment.[12] Chlortetracycline fed at the rate of 1.1 mg/kg/day for 120 days eliminates the carrier state of anaplasmosis. This low dosage fed for 120 days makes clearing of the carrier state very simple while feeding range cattle in winter.

Note: Programs for the elimination of the carrier state should be conducted after the vector season has ended.

The effect of a continuous field challenge exposure while attempting carrier state elimination has not been fully investigated.

Handling an Anaplasmosis Outbreak

Regardless of the availability of adequate control programs, many producers either choose not to use a program or have no reason to do so. In either event, it is necessary to describe the methods available to veterinarians and producers for controlling anaplasmosis outbreaks in herds. The proper handling of an outbreak should include the treatment of clinically ill animals *and* the adequate protection of the remainder of the animals. The clinically ill animal may only be the first of many that will become ill from or exposed to anaplasmosis.

When considering the treatment of clinical anaplasmosis, it must be realized that the important stages are the developmental and convalescent stages. Normally, it is during 1 of these 2 stages that the veterinarian is called to examine the sick animal. Clinical signs are first evident about midway through the developmental stage. Animals treated with parenteral oxytetracycline at this time have better than average chances for recovery. Any delay in treatment during the developmental stage decreases the animal's chances for recovery. A single parenteral injection of oxytetracycline, administered while the percentage of infected cells is less than 15 per cent, can be very effective in reducing the severity of the disease. Oxytetracycline will stop the increase in infected red blood cells, and since it is mainly the infected red blood cells that are destroyed to produce the anemia, the red blood cell count should not drop below the critical level. When infected cells are more than 15 per cent, oxytetracycline effectiveness is reduced. Recovery then is due to the natural ability of the bone marrow to produce red blood cells in sufficient numbers to compensate for the loss of the infected cells.

Frequently, towards the end of the developmental stage and the beginning of the convalescent stage, the best treatment is no treatment. At all times, *Anaplasma* infected cattle should be handled gently and without excitement, especially at this time when anemia is most severe. There are reasons for not treating at this time. First, the animal may suddenly die from anoxia if forced to move or if excited. Second, treatment given at this time does little or nothing to change the outcome of the disease. Tetracycline is of little value since it acts only to reduce the number of infected red blood cells, and the number is already being rapidly reduced by the reticuloendothelial system. Hematinic drugs do not have enough time to stimulate erythropoiesis, and a blood transfusion in sufficient amount to be beneficial may overload the heart that is weakened by anoxia.

In addition to treating the clinically ill animals, the remainder of the animals must be adequately protected. Since no clinical symptoms are being exhibited by the animals in the remainder of the herd, it is assumed that they are *unexposed,* in the *incubation stage,* or in the *convalescent stage* (see Table 1). The unexposed animals and the animals in the incubation stage must be provided with temporary protection until prolonged protection can be established.

Drug Therapy

Temporary protection is accomplished by administering parenteral injections of oxytetracycline. Parenteral injections of oxytetracycline prior to exposure have no effect on a later infection, but animals injected with a single parenteral dose of oxytetracycline during the incubation stage exhibit a prolonged incubation stage for 2 to 3 weeks. A single dose of oxytetracycline administered to animals early in the developmental stage will suppress clinical disease for 3 to 4 weeks. In both cases, clinical anaplasmosis is delayed for approximately 28 days.

Prolonged protection can be accomplished in several ways: treating with oxytetracycline, vaccinating, or feeding with chlortetracycline.

Oxytetracycline treatments repeated at 28-day intervals will continue to suppress the clinical disease but will not prevent immunological response to the presence of the *Anaplasma* organism. In time, the exposed animals would become immunologically protected and would exhibit positive results in response to the serologic tests for anaplasmosis.

Prolonged protection can also be accomplished by *vaccinating* the animals with the required 2 doses of inactivated anaplasmosis vaccine (Anaplaz). The 2 doses of vaccine must be administered at least 4 weeks apart. Protection is afforded the animals 2 weeks after the second dose of vaccine is given. Thus temporary protection against clinical anaplasmosis, i.e., injectable oxytetracycline, must be provided for 6 weeks after the first dose of Anaplaz is administered.

Chlortetracycline administered orally at the rate of 1.1 mg/kg/day will prevent infection, suppress clinical disease, and eliminate the carrier state, depending upon the duration of the treatment and the stage of the disease when treatment began. Chlortetracycline administered at this rate for 60 days will prevent infection in subsequently exposed animals and suppress clinical disease in those animals in the incubation stage and early developmental stage. It may require days and sometimes at least a week to obtain the medicated feed or mineral mix. In addition, it must be ensured that the animals are consuming adequate amounts of the medicated feed or mineral to obtain sufficient chlortetracycline. Again, temporary protection must be provided during this period of delay.

Treatment

By the time the producer usually sees an animal with clinical anaplasmosis, it is almost over the acute infection and is suffering from anemia. Any excitement or exertion could cause the animal to collapse, resulting in death. Confirmation of anaplasmosis and subsequent treatment of the affected animals should be begun by the veterinarian.

If treatment is initiated, it is recommended that a single dosage of Liquamycin LA–200 (200 mg/ml) at the rate of 20 mg/kg[13] be administered rather than the daily treatments with a lower concentration of oxytetracycline (50 to 100 mg/ml). If Liquamycin LA–200 is not available, use a lower concentration of oxytetracycline (11 mg/kg).

Regardless of the concentration, administer no more than 10 ml of oxytetracycline intramuscularly per injection site.

The blood of an animal with clinical anaplasmosis is at least 20 times more infective than the blood of a healthy carrier. Move the healthy animals away from the sick animals (exertion could kill the sick animals) and provide adequate protection for the healthy animals (carriers and exposed animals).

Temporary and Prolonged Protection

In addition to treating the sick animals, one of the following methods should be followed to provide protection for the remainder of the herd:

Use Injectable Oxytetracycline.[3] At the first indication of anaplasmosis, gather all susceptible animals and administer oxytetracycline at the rate of 6.6 to 11 mg/kg for temporary protection. For prolonged protection, this treatment must be repeated at 21- to 28-day intervals throughout the vector season. After withdrawal of the medication, close observation should be continued for symptoms of anaplasmosis.

Use Anaplaz Vaccine and Oxytetracycline.[14] At the first indication of anaplasmosis, gather all susceptible animals

Table 2. *Tetracycline Treatment Regimens for Anaplasmosis Control, Carrier Stage Elimination, and Outbreaks*

Drug*	Route	Dose (mg/kg)	Frequency
Anaplasmosis Control			
Chlortetracycline	Oral	0.22 to 0.55	Daily free choice in salt-mineral mix all year
Chlortetracycline	Oral	1.1	Daily in feed or salt-mineral mix for duration of vector season
Oxytetracycline (50 to 100 mg/ml)	IV or IM	6.6 to 11	One injection every 28 days during the vector season
Oxytetracycline (LA–200)	IM	20	One injection every 28 days during the vector season
Carrier State Elimination			
Chlortetracycline	Oral	1.1	Daily in feed for 120 days
Chlortetracycline	Oral	11	Daily in feed for 60 days
Oxytetracycline (50 to 100 mg/ml)	IV or IM	11	Once daily for 10 days
Oxytetracycline (50 to 100 mg/ml)	IV or IM	22	Once daily for 5 days
Oxytetracycline (LA–200)	IM	20	4 treatments at 3-day intervals
Outbreaks			
Treatment of Sick			
Oxytetracycline (50 to 100 ml)	IM	11	May require > 1 treatment
Oxytetracycline (LA–200)	IM	20	One treatment
Temporary Protection			
Oxytetracycline (50 to 100 mg/ml)	IM	6.6 to 11	One treatment
Oxytetracycline (LA–200)	IM	20	One treatment
Prolonged Protection			
Oxytetracycline (50 to 100 mg/ml)	IM	6.6 to 11	One injection every 28 days during the vector season
Oxytetracycline (LA–200)	IM	20	One injection every 28 days during the vector season
Chlortetracycline	Oral	1.1	Daily in salt-mineral mix or block for 60 days

*Anaplaz vaccine can be used to elicit prolonged protection. For temporary protection, oxytetracycline should also be injected when each dose of vaccine is administered.

and administer oxytetracycline at the rate of 6.6 to 11 mg/kg for temporary protection. For prolonged protection, give each animal the first dose of Anaplaz vaccine. Twenty eight days later, give the second dose of Anaplaz vaccine and another dose of oxytetracycline.

If anaplasmosis occurs because an Anaplaz booster injection was skipped, administer oxytetracycline at the rate of 6.6 to 11 mg/kg and an Anaplaz vaccination to all susceptible animals. The previously nonvaccinated animals should receive a second dose of both Anaplaz and oxytetracycline in 28 days.

Use of Injectable Oxytetracycline and Oral Chlortetracycline.[15] At the first indication of anaplasmosis, gather all susceptible animals and administer oxytetracycline at the rate of 6.6 to 11 mg/kg for temporary protection. For prolonged protection, immediately offer chlortetracycline free-choice in a medicated salt-mineral mix or feed block, (1.1 mg/kg). Chlortetracycline-mediated mixes or blocks should be offered for at least 60 days. Adequate consumption of the medicated mixes or feed blocks should be ensured.

Tetracycline treatment regimens for anaplasmosis control, carrier stage elimination, and outbreaks are illustrated in Table 2.

References

1. Brock, W. E., Pearson, C. C., and Kliewer, I. O.: Anaplasmosis Control by Test and Subsequent Treatment with Chlortetracycline. Proceedings Sixty-second Annual Meeting United States Livestock Association, San Antonio, 66–70, 1958.
2. Brock, W. E., Kliewer, I. O., and Pearson, C. C.: A vaccine for anaplasmosis. J. Am. Vet. Med. Assoc. 147:948–951, 1965.
3. Miller, J. G.: Protective Measures Against Anaplasmosis in Jamaica for Imported Animals. Proceedings Fourth National Anaplasmosis Conference, 49–50, 1962.
4. Lincoln, S. D., and Magonigle, R. A.: The Prophylatic Efficacy of Long-Acting Oxytetracycline (Terramycin LA–200) in Experimental Bovine Anaplasmosis. Proceedings Seventh National Anaplasmosis Conference, Mississippi State University, Mississippi, 589–599, 1981.
5. Richey, E. J., and Kliewer, I. O.: Efficacy of Chlortetracycline Against Bovine Anaplasmosis When Administered Free Choice to Cattle in a Medicated Feed Block and Salt-Mineral Mix. Proceedings Seventh National Anaplasmosis Conference, Mississippi State University, Mississippi, 635–647, 1981.
6. Pearson, C. C.: Preventive Therapy of Anaplasmosis by Feeding Chlortetracycline. Proceedings Third National Anaplasmosis Conference, Manhattan, Kansas, 64–66, 1957.
7. Renshaw, H. W., Magonigle, R. A., Eckbald, W. P., et al: Immunity to Bovine Anaplasmosis After Elimination of the Carrier Status with Oxytetracycline Hydrochloride. Proceedings Annual Meeting United States Animal Health Association, 79–88, 1976.
8. Pearson, C. C., Brock, W. E., and Kliewer, I. O.: A study of tetracycline dosage in cattle which are anaplasmosis carriers. J. Am. Vet. Med. Assoc. 130:290–292, 1957.
9. Magonigle, R. A., Renshaw, H. W., Vaugh, H. W., et al: Effect of five daily intravenous treatments with oxytetracycline hydrochloride on the carrier status of bovine anaplasmosis. J. Am. Vet. Med. Assoc. 167:1080–1083, 1975.
10. Magonigle, R. A., and Newby, T. J.: Elimination of naturally acquired chronic anaplasma marginale infection with a long acting oxytetracycline. Am. J. Vet. Res. 43:2170–2172, 1982.
11. Franklin, T. E., Huff, J. W., and Grumbles, L. C.: Chlortetracycline for elimination of anaplasmosis in carrier cattle. J. Am. Vet. Med. Assoc. 147:353–356, 1965.
12. Richey, E. J., Brock, W. E., Kliewer, I. O., and Jones, E. W.: Low levels of chlortetracycline for anaplasmosis. Am. J. Vet. Res. 38:171–172, 1977.
13. Magonigle, R. A., Simpson, J. E., and Frank, W. F.: Efficacy of a new oxytetracycline formulation against clinical anaplasmosis. Am. J. Vet. Res. 39:1407–1410, 1978.
14. Bedell, D. M., and Slater, M.: The use of a combination of the therapeutic and immunological regimen in an anaplasmosis epizootic. Biochem. Rev. 33:15–18, 1971.
15. Richey, E. J., and Kliewer, I. O.: Controlling An Acute Outbreak of Bovine Anaplasmosis with Oxytetracycline and Chlortetracycline. Proceedings Seventh National Anaplasmosis Conference, Mississippi State University, Mississippi, 615–627, 1981.

Porcine Eperythrozoonosis

A. R. SMITH, D.V.M., Ph.D.

Eperythrozoonosis is a disease of swine that results from infection with the rickettsial organism *Eperythrozoon suis*. Prior to the development of the indirect hemagglutination (IHA) test for diagnosis of eperythrozoonosis, *E. suis* was principally considered a pathogen of feeder pigs in which acute icteroanemia with apparently low morbidity and high mortality was observed. A correlation between titers for eperythrozoonosis was observed in swine and the following clinical disease syndromes:

1. Newborn to postweaning pigs with anemia, weakness, and increased susceptibility to infection.
2. Stressed feeder pigs with the classic symptoms of icteroanemia accompanied by splenomegaly.
3. Market weight hogs with "delayed-marketing syndrome" (animals required longer time to reach market weight).
4. Sows with delayed estrus, embryonic death, and multiple estrus.

Clinical diagnosis of eperythrozoonosis is difficult, since a variety of other infectious diseases and management conditions can cause the same symptoms.

ETIOLOGY

The etiologic agent of porcine eperythrozoonosis, *E. suis*, is an obligate, intracellular parasite of porcine erythrocytes. The majority of organisms are coccoid, with an average diameter of 0.8 to 1.0 μ. Organisms may be seen in blood films prepared from infected, febrile pigs stained with any of the Romanovsky's stains. Blood films should be stained with either Wright-Giemsa or Diff-Quik Stain* (has a staining time of only 30 seconds). Parasites may vary from an occasional organism to approximately 5 organisms per erythrocyte. Organisms are also frequently observed free in the plasma.

EPIDEMIOLOGY

The vertebrate host for *E. suis* is apparently restricted to *Sus scrofa*. Early observers of eperythrozoonosis noted that the majority of clinical cases occurred in the summer, suggesting arthropod vectors.

Presence of the hog louse *Haematopinus suis* has been implicated in transmission. Mosquitoes may also be able to transmit infection. Researchers at Purdue University are attempting to show experimental transmission by lice and biting flies.

---

*Available from Harleco, Gibbstown, NJ 08027.

The seasonal nature of the disease appears to have been minimized with the rearing of swine in confinement. Ample opportunities for mechanical transmission through needles and surgical instruments exist in many units. Research at the University of Illinois has shown transmission in utero and transmission by giving infected blood orally.

CLINICAL SIGNS

Field Infections

Pigs less than 5 days old are the most likely group within a herd to have clinical signs. Dr. Steve Henry, a practitioner at Abilene, Kansas, reported observing skin pallor and mild icterus when examining affected pigs in good light. When light was transmitted through the pinna of the ear, subtle color differences were quite obvious. For white breeds, this visual examination procedure was preferred, but examination of sclera and mucous membranes sufficed for colored breeds. Observation of the network of small vessels in the pinna and their refilling, following manual blanching, gave a good estimation of anemia in normally hydrated pigs. In the most severely affected pigs, vessels could not be seen in the pinna, and icterus was prominent. Mild icterus was evident in most infected pigs but varied in intensity within a litter. When a group of pigs was examined, this variability gave the impression of some pigs being affected and others being normal; however, this was not always the case, as few were normal on careful individual examination. After pigs with uncomplicated infections are approximately 1 week old, icterus usually disappears and the vascular network in the pinna is seen, giving the ear a more normal, pink color. These recovering pigs then show effects of the infection by a wide variation in size and vigor. Resolution seemed to occur at different rates within a litter and among affected litters. By weaning time, an uneven group of pigs is often the principal remaining clinical sign, although icterus and anemia are seen occasionally in severely affected herds at weaning.

In pigs with concurrent bacterial or parasitic disease, early anemia is not resolved; in fact, chronic, nonresponsive anemia with skin pallor and general unthriftiness develops. Chronic bacterial pneumonia and enteritis usually observed in a number of pigs in affected herds. Control of concurrent infections is more difficult than expected.

Feeder Pigs

In herds of feeder pigs with eperythrozoonosis (clinical or subclinical), classic icteroanemia is not observed. However, it was observed in feedlots where sets of pigs of different origins were grouped.

Sows

Signs of infection is sows fall into 2 categories—acute and chronic. Acutely affected sows typically are anorectic for 1 to 3 days, have a temperature ranging from 40.0 to 41.7° C, and occasionally develop mammary and vulvar edema. Acute episodes are usually limited to sows under stress, most commonly immediately postpartum in the first 2 to 4 days after being moved into the farrowing house or when regrouped for breeding. Fever often lasts into the farrowing and early postfarrowing periods, which complicates diagnosis. Predictably, the most severely affected pigs are from anoretic and febrile dams. In such dams, milk flow is depressed, and maternal behavior is subnormal or lacking. Recovery without treatment often occurs by the third day postfarrowing, with milk flow and maternal behavior returning, thus differentiating an *E. suis* infection from other bacterial infections. Immunity apparently does not persist for long periods, inasmuch as some individuals develop the same signs on subsequent farrowings. Acute infections in sows at weaning and at regrouping are often noticed by the producer as transient anorexia and lethargy, but little attention is generally given to these signs because sows are often uncomfortable for a few days after their pigs are weaned. When examined, the sows are febrile (40.0 to 41.7° C). Acute infections at weaning resulted in a marked decline in first-breeding conception rate, but sows generally conceived readily on second estrus, as compared with the gradual decline in conception rate noticed with chronic infections. Acute infections in sows typically resolve to clinical recovery without treatment, yet their poor reproductive efficiency, inadequate milk production, and lowered performance of their pigs represent economic losses.

Sows with chronic infection have much the same clinical appearance as other pigs with chronic infections; that is, a portion of the herd becomes debilitated, pale, and icteric. Many of these sows will not conceive on multiple matings and some do not show estrus, causing a slow decline in conception rates. Concurrent infectious disease, especially sarcoptic mange, along with poor environmental and nutritional conditions contribute to the development of debility and anemia. Death from secondary infection is common, and affected sows do not gain weight even when segregated and placed on ad lib feeding.

Laboratory Infections

Splenectomized pigs ranging from 10 to 17 weeks old have been injected with eperythrozoon-infected blood. One ml of blood containing detectable organisms produced a febrile response 7 to 8 days postinjection. Pigs became anorectic, temperatures were in the 41.1 to 41.7° C range, eperythrozoon organisms were numerous in the erythrocytes, and the animals became hypoglycemic. If animals were left untreated, the fever persisted until death. Some extremely hypoglycemic (<10 mg/100 ml blood glucose) pigs went into convulsions, quickly followed by coma and death. If animals survive the initial hypoglycemic crisis, the glucose levels return to nearly normal within 24 hours. Anemia develops gradually, often requiring 1 week to become clinically obvious. At this time, respiration rate was increased, and sometimes icterus was visible. The blood appears thin, pale, and watery. The erythrocyte sedimentation rate is higher and the platelet count is lower. Affected pigs are often listless, depressed, and constipated. Hemoglobinuria is not observed. Weight loss during the 24-hr period preceding death often exceeds 10 per cent of body weight.

The following lesions have been noted on postmortem examination of anemic pigs: icterus; thin, watery blood; fluid in the pericardial sac and thoracic cavity; yellow liver; dark, bile-stained intestinal contents; enlarged kidneys; and depressed bone marrow.

DIAGNOSIS

Preliminary diagnosis can be made by consideration of history and clinical symptoms with confirmation by finding of the organisms in a stained blood film or positive IHA test results. Organisms can be identified most easily in acutely infected febrile animals, especially pigs younger than 5 days. Organisms are difficult to detect in recovered carrier (latently) infected pigs. Carrier animals develop clinical eperythrozoonosis following splenectomy. Normal, splenectomized pigs develop clinical disease when injected with fresh blood containing anticoagulants obtained from sows with IHA titers. Pigs younger than 12 weeks of age (even carriers) do not react to the IHA test. Infected boars react with low titers in the IHA test.

Experimentally infected pigs develop IHA titers of 40 or greater. Titers are detected after the febrile and parasitemic period. The titer of 40 appears to be significant. In an infected herd, 10 per cent or more of the samples should have titers of 80 or more.

TREATMENT

The United States Food and Drug Administration has not approved any product for the treatment of eperythrozoonosis in swine. However, arsenical compounds (arsanilic acid, sodium arsanilate, and 3-nitro) and tetracyclines are used. Experimentally infected, splenectomized swine have not been cleared of the carrier state through the use of tetracycline. Injection of oxytetracycline has been quite effective in reducing clinical signs (anemia and icterus in pigs and debility in sows). Oxytetracycline has been administered[3] to sows at the rate of 11 mg/kg as a prefarrowing injection in an attempt to limit the expected recrudescence of parasitemia during stress of farrowing. Pigs have been given oxytetracycline when 1 day old in an attempt to kill organisms of transplacentally infected pigs. Retreatment of pigs appears necessary in affected herds, because cessation of such treatment results in greater anemia and mortality in young pigs. Many veterinarians give 2 injections of iron dextran at weekly intervals in infected herds to replace the iron eliminated through erythrocyte destruction. Tetracycline at the nursing ration of 200 gm/ton may also be helpful.

Various treatment regimens are being used to control eperythrozoonosis in swine. More research is needed to formulate totally effective control methods.

Some of the regimens using arsanilic acid therapy are listed next.

1. Arsanilic acid is incorporated in the gestation ration and fed to gestating females from day 21 to 105 at 90 gm/ton (each animal would receive approximately 150 mg of arsanilic acid daily). With this regimen, arsanilic acid is not incorporated in the lactation ration.

2. Arsanilic acid is incorporated for use only in the farrowing house ration. With this plan, arsanilic acid is fed for 1 week prefarrowing at 180 gm/ton (500 mg arsanilic acid/sow/day). The level of arsanilic acid is then decreased to 90 gm/ton and fed until the pigs are weaned.

3. When clinical eperythrozoonosis develops, the whole herd (with the exception of animals in the farrowing house) can be placed on 180 gm/ton for 1 week. Later, reduce the dose to 90 gm/ton for 1 month. Some operations incoporate arsanilic acid in the ration for 1 month and then alternate with an arsanilic acid free–ration for 1 month.

4. In the chronically affected herd, the producer should feed replacement gilts arsanilic acid at 90 gm/ton from time of selection as breeding animals until bred.

There can be problems of cumulative arsenic toxicosis if many sows are penned together and a level of arsanilic acid of 180 gm/ton is fed for extended periods. Toxicosis is most often observed in blind sows. The 3-nitro arsenicals should be used at 50 per cent of those levels for arsanilic acid.

The Feed Additive Compendium does not list any feed additives specifically for treatment of eperythrozoonosis. Therefore, feed mills are unable to add arsanilic acid or tetracycline. Veterinarians recommending on-farm mixing of these drugs for eperythrozoonosis assume legal responsibility for any problems. Approved feed assay guides for arsanilic acid in treatment of swine dysentery and for tetracycline in treatment of leptospirosis may be helpful. A withdrawal period of 5 days is required for the arsenicals.

CONTROL

A number of herds with eperythrozoonosis have moderate to severe sarcoptic mange and lice infestation. Field experience conclusively shows that eperythrozoonosis cannot be controlled by drug therapy in the presence of vectors. Inherent in any control program is the necessity for procedures that limit transmission of the organism and that minimize other diseases, including parasitism. Transmission with blood-contaminated syringes, needles, and surgical instruments can be controlled in sows by changing needles between injections and blood samplings, and in pigs by changing needles between litters. In addition, surgical instruments should be dipped in disinfectant solution between each animal. A major effort has to be directed to also control sarcoptic mange, pediculosis, and helminth infections.

References

1. Baker, H. J., Cassell, G. H., and Lindsay, J. R.: Research complications due to *Haemobartonella* and *Eperythrozoon* infections in experimental animals. Am. J. Path. *64*:624–650, 1971.
2. Berrier, H. H., and Gouge, R. E.: Eperythrozoonosis transmitted *in utero* from carrier sows to their pigs. J. Am. Vet. Med. Assn. *124*:98–100, 1954.
3. Henry, S. C.: Clinical observations on Eperythrozoonosis. J. Am. Vet. Med. Assn. *174*:601–603, 1979.
4. Splitter, E. J., and Williamson, R. L.: Eperythrozoonosis in swine. J. Am. Vet. Med. Assn. *116*:360–364, 1950.
5. Williams, R.: Purdue University, West Lafayette, Indiana, personal communication.

Theileriosis

NORMAN D. LEVINE, Ph.D.

Theileriosis is caused by protozoan parasites of the genus *Theileria* (synonyms, *Gonderia, Cytauxzoon, Haematoxenus*). Several species are involved: *T. parva* is the cause of East Coast fever of cattle in Africa; *T. lawrencei* is the cause of corridor disease of buffalo and cattle in South Africa; *T. annulata* is the cause of tropical theilerosis of cattle in the Middle East, other parts of Asia, and the Mediterranean basin. *T. mutans* is nonpathogenic or produces benign theileriosis of cattle in Africa, and *T. orientalis* does the same in Eurasia, North Africa, and Australia. A single case of *T. mutans* infection has been reported in Kansas in the United States. *T. lestoquardi* and *T. ovis* are the agents of theileriosis in goats and sheep in Africa, Asia, the southern areas of the USSR, and parts of Europe. *T. felis* is the infective organism of theileriosis in cats in the United States. All are transmitted by ticks. *Theileria* spp. do not invade tick eggs like *Babesia* spp. but pass from one stage to the next. The most important vector of *T. parva* is *Rhipicephalus appendiculatus;* of *T. annulata, Hyalomma;* of *T. mutans, Amblyomma;* of *T. ovis, R. bursa;* those of *T. lestoquardi* and *T. felis* are unknown.

LIFE CYCLE

When a parasite-infected tick bites a susceptible animal, the parasites first go to the lymph nodes and spleen, where they invade the lymphocytes. Here they multiply, producing "Koch's blue bodies," which are meronts (cysts, pseudocysts, or terminal colonies) that produce merozoites within them. Early in the infection a relatively few, large merozoites (macromerozoites) are produced by each meront; later, each meront produces a larger number of smaller ones (micromerozoites). The micromerozoites enter the blood as piroplasms, and these then invade the red blood cells. The forms in the erythrocytes are rod-shaped (about 1.5 to 2.0 × 0.5 to 1.0 μm), round (0.5 to 1.5 μm in diameter), oval (about 2.0 × 0.6 μm), comma-shaped, or even granule-like. The sexual stage of the life cycle takes place in the ticks.

T. parva is the most pathogenic of the bovine species, killing up to 90 to 100 per cent of affected animals. *T. annulata* kills perhaps about 50 per cent, and *T. mutans* and *T. orientalis* are seldom more than slightly, if at all, pathogenic. *T. lestoquardi* is highly pathogenic for adult sheep and goats, while *T. ovis* is nonpathogenic or almost so. *T. felis* causes a serious disease in cats (especially pregnant ones).

CLINICAL SIGNS AND LESIONS

Theileriosis is a febrile disease. The incubation period averages about 2 weeks. Fever is followed by cessation of rumination, a serous nasal discharge, lacrimation, swelling of the superficial lymph nodes and sometimes of the eyelids, ears, and jowl region, rapid heartbeat, general weakness, decreased milk production, diarrhea (frequently with blood and mucus in the feces), emaciation, coughing, and sometimes icterus. Oliogocythemic anemia is present, but there is no hematuria in uncomplicated cases. Adult animals are more susceptible than young animals.

The lymph nodes are markedly swollen and hyperemic. The spleen and liver are enlarged, the liver is friable, brownish yellow to lemon yellow, with parenchymatous degeneration. The kidneys are either congested or pale brown, with a varying number of hemorrhagic "infarcts" or grayish-white lymphomatomata. There are characteristic ulcers with a central necrotic area surrounded by hemorrage in the abomasum and intestines.

DIAGNOSIS

Meronts in Giemsa-stained aspirates of the lymph nodes or parasites in Giemsa-stained erythrocytes in blood smears are pathognomonic.

TREATMENT

No drug is effective once signs of disease have appeared. Chlortetracycline and oxytetracycline may prevent clinical disease if given repeatedly during the incubation period.

PREVENTION

Prevention depends upon tick control and quarantine. Ticks can be eliminated by repeated dipping, even though arsenic-resistant strains of ticks have appeared.

Quarantine measures will prevent the spread of theileriosis. In isolated outbreaks, the whole herd may be slaughtered, and the farm kept free of infected animals for 18 months before restocking.

Supplemental Reading

Levine, N. D.: Protozoan Parasites of Domestic Animals and of Man, 2nd ed. Minneapolis, Minnesota, Burgess Publishing Co., 336–346, 1973.

Toxoplasmosis

NORMAN D. LEVINE, Ph.D.

Toxoplasmosis is caused by the euryxenous coccidial protozoon, *Toxoplasma gondii*. There are a few other species, but little is known about them. *Hammondia* is a synonym of *Toxoplasma*. The complete life cycle requires 2 hosts, and transmission can occur from one intermediate host to another. Oocysts produced sexually are found in the feces of cats and other felids; they are the definitive hosts. Meronts (often called cysts, pseudocysts or terminal colonies) containing merozoites occur in about 200 species of mammals and birds, including humans and all the domestic animals; they are the intermediate hosts. Transmission can be by means of oocysts from felids to various animals or by means of merozoites from one intermediate host to another.

Toxoplasma is found within many types of cells, such as neurons, microglia, endoplasmic reticulum, hepatocytes, lung, glandular epithelium, cardiac muscle, skeletal muscle, fetal membranes, and leukocytes. In early infections of an intermediate host, the meronts in the tissues are in the form of groups containing relatively nonresistant merozoites known as tachyzoites. Later, the meronts are found primarily in the brain; they are often called cysts and contain relatively resistant merozoites known as bradyzoites. In the cat, there is a generation of meronts in the intestinal epithelial cells. These produce male and female gamonts, which, after fertilization, produce resistant oocysts that pass out in the feces. Newly passed oocysts are 11 to 14 × 9 to 11 μm. They are not infective, but must first form sporozoites within them, a process that takes 2 to 3 days at 24° C. Every sporulated, infective oocyst contains 4 sporocysts, each containing 2 sporozoites.

Infections in mature animals are usually inapparent, but the clinical signs may vary from none to those of an acutely fatal disease. Death of newborns or abortions may occur if mothers are infected while pregnant. Perinatal mortality is especially characteristic in sheep.

CLINICAL SIGNS AND LESIONS

These may vary from no disease to an acute, fatal disease. Signs are highly variable. In newborn animals there may be encephalitis, rash, jaundice, and hepatomegaly, sometimes associated with chorioretinitis, hydrocephalus, and microcephaly. Abortion or early death may occur. In adult animals there may be fever, cough, anorexia, weakness, or depression. The disease may be characterized by lymphadenopathy, exanthema, pneumonitis, encephalitis, and chronic chorioretinitis. There may be other signs.

T. gondii may cause cellular or interstitial necrosis in any part of the brain or spinal cord. Periventricular vasculitis and necrosis are often present. There may be small, sharply delimited areas of coagulation necrosis in any part of the liver lobules. Small, gray, tumor-like nodules may be scattered through one or all lobes of the lungs; they fill the alveoli with large mononuclear cells and leukocytes. The lymph nodes may be markedly enlarged and contain extensive areas of coagulation necrosis. Ulcers may be seen in the intestine. Ocular infections are rare except in cats and humans. The disease is often associated with the distemper of dogs.

DIAGNOSIS

Because the signs and lesions are so varied and mimic those of many other diseases, a definitive diagnosis cannot be made. It depends upon recognition or isolation of the causative organism. The most certain method is isolation of the parasite itself. Experimental animals should be inoculated, preferably intraperitoneally. Mice, hamsters, and guinea pigs are especially sensitive; the administration of cortisone for 3 to 5 days before inoculation may or may not increase the chance of isolating the organism.

The organisms may be recognized in tissue sections, but they may also not be recognized.

Serologic tests are commonly useful in surveys, but they are not useful in diagnosis because such high proportions of adult animals produce positive results. It has been estimated, for example, that about 30 per cent of humans in the United States are serologically positive. Newly infected animals may have negative test results but die. A rise in titer between 2 tests a few weeks apart indicates active infection.

The dye test and the indirect hemagglutination test are perhaps the most satisfactory.

TREATMENT

No satisfactory treatment is known for toxoplasmosis. Best results have been obtained by the use of pyrimethamine and sulfonamides simultaneously; the 2 drugs act synergistically.

Although treatment is not usually employed in food animals, 66 mg/kg sulfathiazole orally every 4 hr plus 0.44 mg/kg pyrimethamine daily for about 5 weeks might be helpful.

PREVENTION

Toxoplasmosis can be acquired by ingestion of sporulated oocysts in cat feces or of bradyzoites in mice, rats, other animals, or raw meat. Infection can also be induced by parenteral inoculation. Human infections have resulted from contaminated needle scratches.

The practice of keeping cats in the barn to control mice provides perhaps the most important source of infection for food animals. The oocysts are resistant to acids, alkalies, and common detergents, but they are not resistant to ammonia, drying, and a temperature of 55° C.

Toxoplasmosis can be prevented in food animals by keeping them separated from cats and by not allowing them to eat the meat or the carcasses of other animals. The latter applies particularly to swine. The placentas of infected sheep should be considered a particularly good source of infection.

Since toxoplasmosis is a zoonosis and can affect humans, adequate precaution should be taken by veterinarians to avoid infection. Protective clothing and gloves should be worn while carrying out necropsies on potentially infected animals.

Supplemental Reading*

Dubey, J. P.: *Toxoplasma, Hammondia, Besnoitia, Sarcocystis,* and other tissue cyst-forming coccidia of man and animals. *In* Kreier, J. P. (ed.), Parasitic Protozoa. New York, Academic Press, 101–237, 1977.
Jira, J., and Kozojed, V.: Toxoplasmose—1908–1967. Stuttgart, Germany, G. Fischer, 1970.
Levine, N. D.: Taxonomy of *Toxoplasma.* J. Protozool. *24*:36–41, 1971.
Levine, N. D.: Protozoan Parasites of Domestic Animals and of Man, 2nd ed. Minneapolis, Minnesota, Burgess Publishing Co., 294–307, 1973.

*Over 9000 papers have been published on *Toxoplasma* (see Jira and Kozojed, 1970). The references cite most of them and give sufficient information for our purposes.

Sarcocystosis

NORMAN D. LEVINE, Ph.D.

Sarcocystosis is caused by a coccidial protozoan, *Sarcocystis,* which has a predator-prey life cycle. In prey animals, the first 2 meront generations occur in the endothelium of the blood vessels. It is these stages that cause disease. Sarcocysts (last generation meronts), often visible to the naked eye and containing thousands of merozoites, are found in the muscles. Microscopic sporocysts and a few oocysts are found in the feces of predator animals. This particular life cycle was not recognized until

Supplemental Reading

 Toxoplasma, Hammondia, Besnoitia, Sarcocystis, and other
 forming coccidia of man and animals. *In* Kreier, J. P. (ed.).
 rotozoa. New York, Academic Press, 101–237, 1977.
)., and Tadros, W.: Named species and hosts of *Sarcocystis*
 Apicomplexa: Sarcocystidae). System. Parasitol. 2:41–59,

tosporidiosis

J. PANCIERA, D.V.M., M.S., Ph.D.

ers of the genus *Cryptosporidium* are coccidia of
ily Cryptosporidiidae, suborder Eimeriorina.
poridial infections have been reported in many
hosts including cattle, swine, sheep, and goats.
has been assumed that there are several species
tosporidium, each host specific, recent research
s that the species infecting calves can be experi-
y transmitted to swine, sheep, goats, rats, mice,
pigs, dogs, and cats. Cryptosporidial infections of
s have been experimentally transmitted to calves,
ats, dogs, goats, and swine. Natural transmission
ntly is by ingestion of infected fecal material.
gh many details of the life cycle of cryptosporidia
t known, asexual and sexual phases of reproduction
r to other coccidia are found in the intestinal tract.
arasites exist both free in the intestinal lumen and
ed to the lumenal surface of intestinal epithelial
At points of parasitic attachment, intestinal micro-
re absent or altered, thereby reducing the surface
of intestine available for absorption of nutrients.

CLINICAL SIGNS AND LESIONS

Cryptosporidial infections of cattle have been recognized more and more frequently in recent years, usually but not always in animals afflicted with acute or chronic diarrhea. Most cases thus far reported have been in calves less than 3 weeks old. The character of diarrheic feces is similar to that of many other enteric diseases and may be accompanied by anorexia, dehydration, weight loss, debility, and sometimes death. Organisms are usually shed in the feces of calves within 5 days after infection and continue to be shed for about 10 days. Diarrhea usually develops within 3 to 5 days after experimental infection and persists for several days after fecal shedding ceases. While it cannot be unequivocally stated that *Cryptosporidium* is a primary and important cause of diarrhea in calves and other species, field and laboratory observations strongly indicate a significant role in calf diarrhea. Several reports indicate individual cases of disease; other reports indicate significant morbidity from natural infections.

Gross necropsy lesions range from mild to moderate enteritis, the most severe characterized by adherent mucofibrinous exudate in the lower small intestinal and colonic mucosae. Histologically, there are organisms adhering to the villous epithelium, and there is villous atrophy and mononuclear cell infiltration of the lamina propria. Parasites are most frequently present and most numerous in the ileum but are present in the jejunum and colon as well. Fecal cryptosporidial forms are demonstrable by Giemsa-stained fecal smears and scrapings of ileal mucosa and by fecal flotation techniques.

pigs depends upon recognition of sarcocysts in the muscles. The first 2 generations of meronts in the endothelial cells of the small blood vessels are too small to see without magnification. The sarcocysts of the species that mature in cats are whitish or pale-yellowish tubular or ellipsoidal bodies that may be several millimeters long. They are easily visible without magnification. The sarcocysts of the species that mature in dogs are ordinarily microscopic. This can be readily identified in stained sections, and are packed with bradyzoites whose nuclei stain dark blue with hematoxylin. Since the muscle fibers stain pink, it is easy to see them.

TREATMENT

There is no satisfactory treatment for sarcocystosis, but supportive measures may be helpful.

PREVENTION

Infection of food animals with *Sarcocystis* can be avoided by preventing contact with the feces of dogs, cats, and other predatory animals, so that the food animals do not ingest the sporocysts when feeding and grazing. Human feces should be disposed of so that they are inaccessible to food animals.

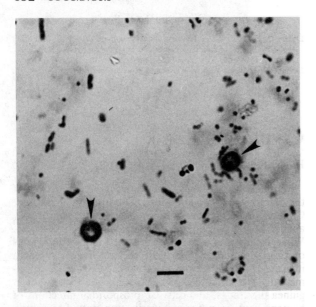

Figure 1. Cryptosporidia in fecal smear–Giemsa stain. (Courtesy of Dr. H. Moon.) Bar equals 5 μm.

DIAGNOSIS

Giemsa-stained cysts are round, 4 to 5 μm in diameter, and have blue-stained cytoplasm containing 2 to 5 dense red granules (Fig. 1). Organisms are present in histologic sections of intestine provided it is fixed immediately after death. Postmortem autolysis severely diminishes the chance of their demonstration.

TREATMENT AND PREVENTION

An effective treatment protocol has not been documented. The use of coccidiostats has been suggested as a preventive measure. The usually mild and transient nature of the enteric lesion suggests that conservative, supportive therapy may be effective.

Supplemental Reading

Anderson, B. C.: Patterns of shedding of cryptosporidial oocysts in calves. J. Am. Vet. Med. Assoc. *178*:982, 1981.
Anderson, B. C.: Cryptosporidiosis: a review. J. Am. Vet. Med. Assoc. *180*:1455, 1982.
Pohlenz, J., Moon, H. W., et al.: Cryptosporidial infection as a probable factor in neonatal diarrhea of calves. J. Am. Vet. Med. Assoc. *172*:452, 1978.

Coccidiosis

KENNETH S. TODD, JR., Ph.D.,
JOSEPH A. DIPIETRO, D.V.M., M.S.,
and WALTER M. GUTERBOCK, D.V.M., M.S.

Coccidiosis in food-producing animals is caused by intracellular protozoan parasites of the genera *Isospora* and *Eimeria*. In addition, *Cryptosporidium muris* has been described from cattle, sheep, goats, and pigs, as well as other mammals. Coccidia usually inhabit the intestinal tract. Coccidia of the genera *Eimeria* and *Isospora* are highly host and organ specific. Many species parasitize only specific parts of the intestine. Some species are found in a particular site within infected cells. Transmission of the genera *Eimeria* and *Isospora* between host species is not possible. Sheep and goats, however, may share some of the same species of coccidia. *C. muris* is not as host specific, and evidence indicates the same species is present in all mammals.[13]

EPIZOOTIOLOGY

The species of coccidia found in cattle, sheep, goats, and pigs are listed in Table 1. The species tabulated are those considered to be valid.[12, 13, 18] Taxonomists do not agree on the number of species found in each host, and mixed infections are common.

Coccidia Life Cycle

The life cycle of coccidia is complex and includes both asexual and sexual cycles within the host. Some development also takes place outside the host. A generalized life cycle is illustrated in Figure 1.

Oocysts of *Eimeria* spp. or *Isospora* spp. passed in the feces contain a single cell. *C. muris* oocysts are sporulated when passed and contain sporozoites. In the presence of oxygen and moisture and at the proper temperature, they sporulate to the infective state. Sporulated oocysts may be recognized by the presence of 2 or 4 sporocyts (depending upon the genus) within the oocyst wall. After a sporulated oocyst is ingested by a suitable host, sporozoites are liberated into the lumen of the intestine. The sporozoites penetrate intestinal cells and form spheres called trophozoites. These divide (merogony or schizogony) to form meronts or schizonts. Each schizont (meront) contains many merozoites. Mature merozoites are released from the schizonts into the gut lumen, as the host cell is ruptured and destroyed.

After they are released from the schizont, the merozoites penetrate other intestinal cells. They may form new generations of schizonts or gametes. There are 1 to 3

Table 1. *Species of* Eimeria, Isospora, *and* Cryptosporidium *Present in Cattle, Goats, Sheep, and Swine*

Host	Coccidium	Host	Coccidium
Ox	E. alabamensis	Sheep	E. weybridgensis
	E. auburnensis	*Continued*	C. muris
	E. bovis	Goat	E. arloingi
	E. brasiliensis		E. christenseni
	E. bukidnonensis		E. crandallis
	E. canadensis		E. faurei
	E. ellipsoidalis		E. gilruthi
	E. illinoisensis		E. granulosa
	E. kosti		E. hawkinsi
	E. pellita		E. intricata
	E. subspherica		E. ninakohlyakimovae
	E. wyomingensis		E. pallida
	E. zuernii		E. parva
	I. aksaica		E. punctata
	C. muris		C. muris
Zebu	E. bombayensis	Swine	E. cerdouis
	E. mundiragi		E. debliecki
Sheep	E. ahsata		E. guevarai
	E. crandallis		E. neodebliecki
	E. faurei		E. perminuta
	E. gilruthi		E. polita
	E. gonzalezi		E. porci
	E. granulosa		E. romaniae
	E. hawkinsi		E. scabra
	E. intricata		E. scrofae
	E. marsica		E. spinosa
	E. ovinoidalis		I. almaataensis
	E. ovina		I. neyrai
	E. pallida		I. suis
	E. parva		C. muris
	E. punctata		

generations of schizonts preceding gametogony; the number depends on the species. All species eventually form gametes.

The sexual stages are macrogametes or microgametocytes. Macrogametes contain only 1 nucleus. Microgametocytes are less numerous and contain many highly motile, thread-like, flagellated microgametes, which correspond to spermatozoa of higher animals. Eventually, the host cell containing the microgametocyte ruptures, and microgametes are released into the intestinal lumen. These penetrate the intestinal cells containing the macrogametes and fertilize them.

After fertilization, the zygotes form walls and become oocysts. The host cells rupture after the oocysts mature, each cell releasing its oocyst into the lumen of the gut. The oocysts then pass out in the feces unsporulated. Sporulation takes place and has already been described.

The life cycle of *Cryptosporidium muris* is similar, but the parasites are located in the brush border of epithelial cells of the intestine. Some workers have reported sporocysts are not found in oocysts, but other workers have described them.

The host's cells are destroyed by schizogony, gametogony, and the release of oocysts. Since each schizont contains hundreds or thousands of merozoites, and since there may be several generations of schizonts, each oocyst ingested has the potential of destroying thousands or millions of intestinal cells. The location of the sexual and asexual stages, the number of asexual stages, and the number of merozoites released by the schizonts vary with

the species of coccidium, as does the time required to complete the life cycle. For each species of coccidium, the number of asexual stages, the number of merozoites, and the prepatent period are relatively constant. Thus, each species has the intrinsic ability to destroy a certain number of host cells.

Each oocyst ingested can theoretically cause the destruction of a limited number of host cells, assuming all merozoites survive. Once the gametes are formed, the organism is unable to multiply further. If exposure to oocysts is stopped, the infection will run its course but no more proliferation of coccidia can occur. This is in contrast to viruses or bacteria, which can multiply freely. The severity of coccidiosis may depend on the number of oocysts ingested. Since the turnover of intestinal epithelial cells is rapid (1 to 2 days) even in healthy animals, coccidia must destroy large numbers of cells in a short time to cause disease. Poor sanitation and crowded conditions enhance the number of oocysts available to each animal, and therefore predispose the animals to outbreaks of clinical coccidiosis.

Coccidia harm their hosts by destruction of host cells and tissues. This may be followed by secondary bacterial invasion. The loss of intestinal epithelium may lead to blood and electrolyte losses and malabsorption.

Coccidiosis is frequently a disease of young, nonimmune animals. Animals that survive an outbreak of coccidiosis are usually immune. When reinoculated, they may pass small numbers of oocysts but generally will not get sick unless the inoculum is very large.

CLINICAL SIGNS AND LESIONS

As with other parasitic diseases, clinical signs vary and may be vague. Sloughed intestinal tissue and frank blood may be present in the feces. Rough hair coat, poor weight gain, weight loss, weakness, emaciation, and death may result. Central nervous system disorders have been reported in cattle with coccidiosis. In most cases, animals were infected with *Eimeria zuernii*. *C. muris* may cause mild to severe diarrhea.

Congestion, erosion, and hemorrhage may be found in the intestinal mucosa. The intestinal contents may be watery and contain sloughed intestinal mucosa and blood. Endogenous stages may be observed by histologic examination of smears or sections. The feces and intestinal mucosae of dead animals should be examined for oocysts.

DIAGNOSIS

A diagnosis of coccidiosis cannot be made unless clinical signs are present. Many species of coccidia are nonpathogenic, and even pathogenic species may cause no problems in small numbers or in immune animals. For example, almost all of the fecal samples from healthy sheep and goats examined in our laboratory contain coccidian oocysts.

The classic coccidiosis patient is young and passes large numbers of oocysts in the feces. In peracute cases, however, the animal may die before oocysts are passed. Adult animals that remain in their herd of origin are usually

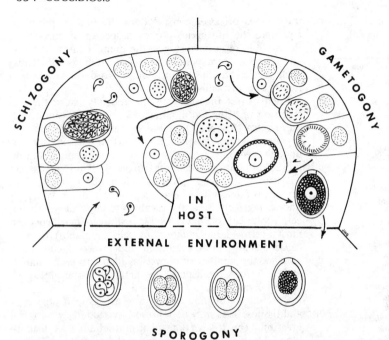

Figure 1. Diagram of a typical coccidian life cycle. (Adapted from Todd, 1975.)

immune to the local coccidia. The introduction of new animals can lead to outbreaks in the new animals, or if the new animals are passing oocysts of an unfamiliar species, in the animals of recipient herd. The moving of animals to pens that are heavily contaminated with oocysts can also precipitate an outbreak. Immunity to coccidia usually can be achieved with a large inoculum, but immunity to one species does not confer immunity to other species.

The number of oocysts passed in each gram of feces gives some indication of the severity of an infection, since each oocyst represents a destroyed intestinal epithelial cell. This is in marked contrast to helminth infections, where egg counts tell the clinician relatively little about the number of worms present. A diagnosis should not be based on the presence or absence of a certain number of oocysts. The presence of many oocysts of the same size and shape in a fecal specimen from an animal with clinical signs consistent with the disease, however, is sufficient basis for diagnosis.

Routine fecal flotation techniques can be used to examine the feces for coccidia. Any of the usual salt or sugar solutions will work. Routine examinations of feces from healthy animals will familiarize clinicians with the normal level of oocysts for animals in their area. This practice will alert them when they see more than the usual number of coccidia.

In the past, *Cryptosporidium muris* infection was usually confirmed only by histologic examination of the intestine. Methods to detect oocysts by fecal flotation[2, 10] and Giemsa-stained feces[19] have since been described. In cattle, coccidiosis is found mostly in feedlot stock. Outbreaks often are in winter in calves under the stresses of weaning, crowding, malnutrition, and poor weather. *E. zuernii* and *E. bovis* are often involved in outbreaks of clinical coccidiosis. The oocysts of *E. zuernii* are 12 to 29 × 10 to 21 μm, and those of *E. bovis* are 23 to 34 × 17 to 23 μm. Both contain 4 sporocysts.

In the United States, sheep coccidiosis is usually a disease of feedlot lambs. Individual sheep may develop coccidiosis when they are introduced into a new flock. In the United Kingdom, ovine coccidiosis is most frequent in unweaned lambs that are intensively grazed.[8] Several species of coccidia may be involved, but *E. ahsata* and *E. ovinodalis* are evidently the most pathogenic.

Coccidiosis of goats is generally a disease of young kids and may cause sudden, otherwise unexplained deaths. Several species of coccidia may be involved.

Clinical coccidiosis in swine occurs almost exclusively in young piglets infected with *Isospora suis*. The oocysts of this species are ovoid, 17 to 24 × 17 to 21 μm, and contain 2 sporocysts after sporulation. Diagnosis is usually confirmed by histopathologic examination of intestinal sections, since piglets often die before passing oocysts. The feces are yellow to brown, fluid, and frothy.

TREATMENT

The following compounds are approved for treatment or prophylaxis of bovine coccidiosis in the United States: amprolium, sulfaquinoxaline, and decoquinate. Decoquinate (Deccox*) is available as a feed additive to be used in ruminating calves and cattle at a rate of 22.7 mg/100 lb of body weight. It should be added to the feed for at least 28 days during coccidiosis exposure or during periods when coccidiosis is likely to be a hazard.

Sulfaquinoxaline (S.Q.†) is given at a dosage of 5 oz/50 gal of water for 3 to 5 days to prevent outbreaks of coccidiosis in cattle.

Amprolium (Corid†, Amprovine†) is given at a dosage of 10 mg/kg for 5 days for treatment of coccidiosis and at a rate of 5 mg/kg for 21 days for prevention.

Nitrofurazone has been found to be effective in treating coccidiosis of sheep and goats. Tarlatzis and coworkers

*Available from Rhodia Inc., Ashland, OH 44805
†Available from Merck, Sharp, & Dohme, Rahway, NJ 07065

successfully used crystalline nitrofurazone at 7 to 10 mg/kg in young lambs and goats naturally infected with *Eimeria faurei*.[24] Better results were obtained with higher doses. They used 50 mg tablets of nitrofurazone to treat 5-kg kids infected with *E. faurei*.[25] In treated animals, cessation of diarrhea, re-establishment of appetite, and improvement of general condition were observed. Trials with 2 tablets per animal gave better results than trials with 1 tablet per animal.

Amprolium has been used to treat lambs experimentally infected with coccidia. Hammond and coworkers used 25 mg/lb for 14 to 19 days in lambs inoculated with *E. ninakohlyakimovae*.[9] No clinical signs of coccidiosis were noted in treated lambs, while control lambs had severe coccidiosis. Baker and coworkers fed amprolium at 50 mg/kg for 20 days to lambs in a feedlot where coccidiosis had been a problem.[3] Treated lambs had lower oocyst outputs than untreated lambs. There was no significant difference in weight gain or feed conversion between the treated and untreated groups.

Fitzgerald and Mansfield found that when monensin was given at 10 to 20 ppm in the feed, lambs naturally infected with coccidia and experimentally infected with *E. ninakohlyakimovae* gained more weight and had better feed conversion than naturally or experimentally infected lambs not given monensin. A report by Leek and colleagues stated that when monensin was fed to lambs experimentally infected with *E. ninakohlyakimovae*, there was some decline in fecal oocyst output compared with untreated controls, but the treated lambs had a reduced feed intake and weight gain.[11] Monensin was used at 17 and 33 mg/kg in the feed for 24 days in lambs experimentally inoculated with *Eimeria* spp. by Foreyt and workers.[7] The compound was effective in eliminating oocyst output and caused treated lambs to gain more weight than control lambs.

Lasalocid has been reported to be effective against ovine coccidiosis. It was used in feed at a dosage of 100 mg/kg for 100 days in experimentally inoculated lambs, and it was effective in eliminating oocyst output. Treated lambs gained more weight than control lambs.[7]

Sulfonamides have been used for therapy of ovine and caprine coccidiosis with variable results.

In a review by Gregory and colleagues, the most effective compounds to prevent ovine coccidiosis were lasalocid, monensin, and amprolium.[8] Monensin was of little value as a curative medication. Sulfonamides gave the best results for treatment.

Various compounds have been used experimentally to treat porcine coccidiosis. Sulfaguanidine mixed in feed at a rate of 1 gm/10 lbs was fed for 7 to 10 or more days for prophylaxis of *E. debliecki* and *E. scabra* infections.[1] The compound suppressed oocyst output. It was reported that 0.44 gm nitrofurazone was effective in treating coccidiosis caused by *E. debliecki* in 2 pigs when administered in the feed for 7 days.[5]

The use of amprolium was recommended at 25 to 65 mg/kg once or twice daily for 3 to 4 days to treat coccidiosis in swine.[18] In pigs experimentally infected with coccidian oocysts, it was reported that chlortetracycline plus sulfamethazine and penicillin, buquinolate, and lincomycin suppressed oocyst production.

Roberts and coworkers have described control methods for *Isospora suis*.[20] In one herd, piglets were given amprolium orally at 25 mg/kg for the first 3 or 4 days of life. This was effective in controlling diarrhea. They also used amprolium successfully for sows, which was reported to be effective in preventing coccidiosis in unweaned piglets, but the dosage used is not clear.

The following steps to control coccidiosis were recommended in a report by Lindsay and colleagues:[14]

1. Fecal examination for *I. suis* in piglets from litters that are 7 to 10 days old.

2. Routine laboratory examinations for *I. suis* and other possible enteropathogens associated with neonatal scours complex.

3. Disinfection of farrowing crates using ammonia solutions or commercial bleach (50-per cent) solutions. Steam cleaning if available.

4. Limited access to crates by workers, especially after scours, to prevent crate to crate contamination of oocysts.

5. Feeding of coccidiostats to sows beginning 2 weeks before farrowing and continuing throughout lactation.

6. Administration of coccidiostats to newborn piglets as soon as possible and until weaning (minimum 2 weeks). This can be achieved by individual dosing or by adding to the water, crop feed, or oral iron mixture.

Treating sows with 0.5 oz amprolium for 5 to 7 days prior to farrowing helped prevent coccidiosis in 8-day-old pigs, but the response was not complete.[4] Best results in preventing neonatal coccidiosis were obtained by adding 8 oz of amprolium per 100 gal of water for 3 weeks.

When amprolium or decoquinate was mixed in the sow ration, at 1 kg/ton for 3 weeks prior to and 3 weeks after farrowing, there was a reduction or cessation of neonatal diarrhea. The program was considered to be moderately successful.[23]

The treatment with amprolium of sows 2 weeks prior to and 2 weeks after farrowing gave variable results from herd to herd.[21] Researchers were of the opinion that when amprolium was given to 2- or 3-day-old pigs for 5 days, poor results were obtained. The best means of control was considered to be strict sanitation in the farrowing house.

Treatment of cryptosporidiosis has not generally been successful. In a review, it was reported that more than 40 compounds, including coccidiostats, other antiprotozoal agents, broad-spectrum antibiotics, and anthelmintics, evaluated against *Cryptosporidium*, none were effective.[26] Lasalocid was used to treat cryptosporidiosis in calves, but the effective dose was toxic.[16]

PUBLIC HEALTH CONSIDERATIONS

The genera *Eimeria* and *Isospora* in food-producing animals are host specific and cannot be transmitted to humans. *Cryptosporidium muris*, however, can be transmitted to humans.

Sarcocystis and *Toxoplasma* are coccidia but do not have intestinal stages in food-producing animals. These animals are intermediate hosts for certain species that may be transmitted to humans in undercooked meat. *Sarcocystis* spp. and *Toxoplasma* spp. are discussed separately elsewhere in this section.

References

1. Alicata, J. E., and Willett, E. L.: Observations on the prophylactic and curative value of sulfaguanidine in swine coccidiosis. Am. J. Vet. Res. 7:94–100, 1946.

2. Anderson, B. C.: Patterns of shedding of cryptosporidiae oocysts in Idaho calves. J. Am. Vet. Med. Assoc. *178*:982–984, 1981.
3. Baker, N. F., Walters, G. T., and Fisk, R. A.: Amprolium for control of coccidiosis in feedlot lambs. Am. J. Vet. Res. *33*:83–86, 1972.
4. Clark, L. K.: Coccidiosis in baby pigs. Mod. Vet. Pract. *61*:605–606, 1980.
5. Deom, J., and Mortelmans, J.: Essai therapeutique de la coccidiose du porc par la nitrofurazone. Ann. Med. Vet. *98*:82–86, 1954.
6. Fitzgerald, P. R., and Mansfield, M. E.: Ovine coccidiosis: effect of the antibiotic monensin against *Eimeria ninakohlyakimovae* and other naturally occurring coccidia of sheep. Am. J. Vet. Res. *39*:7–10, 1978.
7. Foreyt, W. J., Gates, N. L., and Wescott, R. B.: Effects of lasalocid and monensin against experimentally induced coccidiosis in confinement-reared lambs from weaning to market weight. Am. J. Vet. Res. *40*:97–100, 1979.
8. Gregory, M. W., Joyner, L. P., Catchpole, J., and Norton, C. C.: Ovine coccidiosis in England and Wales 1978–1979. Vet. Rec. *106*:461–462, 1980.
9. Hammond, D. M., Kuta, J. E., and Miner, M. L.: Amprolium for control of experimental coccidiosis in lambs. Cornell Vet. *57*:611–623, 1967.
10. Iseki, M.: *Cryptosporidium felis* sp. n. (Protozoa: Eimeriorina) from the domestic cat. Jpn. J. Parasitol. *28*:285–307, 1979.
11. Leek, R. G., Fayer, R., and McLoughlin, D. K.: Effect of monensin on experimental infections of *Eimeria ninakohlyakimovae* in lambs. Am. J. Vet. Res. *37*:339–341, 1976.
12. Levine, N. D.: Textbook of Veterinary Parasitology. Minneapolis, Minnesota, Burgess Publishing Co., 1977.
13. Levine, N. D.: Taxonomy and review of the coccidian genus *Cryptosporidium* (Protozoa, Apicomplexa). J. Protozool. *31*:94–98, 1984.
14. Lindsay, D. S., Current, W. L., Ernst, J. V., and Stuart, B. P.: Diagnosis of neonatal porcine coccidiosis caused by *Isospora suis*, Vet. Med./Small Anim. Clin. *78*:89–94, 1983.
15. Long, P. L.: Pathology and pathogenicity of coccidial infections. *In* Hammond, D. M., and Long, P. L. (eds.). The Coccidia: *Eimeria, Isospora, Toxoplasma,* and Related Genera. Baltimore, University Park Press, 1973.
16. Moon, H. W., Woode, G. N. and Ahrens, F. A.: Attempted chemoprophylaxis of cryptosporidiosis in calves. Vet. Rec. *110*:181, 1982.
17. Onawunmi, O. A., and Todd, A. C.: Suppression and control of experimentally induced porcine coccidiosis with chlortetracycline combination buquinolate and lincomycin hydrochloride. Am. J. Vet. Res. *37*:657–660, 1976.
18. Pellerdy, L. P.: Coccidia and Coccidiosis, 2nd ed. Berlin, Paul Parey, 1974.
19. Pohleny, J., Moon, H. W., Cheville, N. F., and Bemrich, W. J.: Cryptosporidiosis as a probable factor in neonatal diarrhea of calves. J. Am. Vet. Assoc. *172*:452–457, 1978.
20. Roberts, L., and Walker, E. J.: Field study of coccidial and rotaviral diarrhea in unweaned pigs. Vet. Rec. *110*:11–13, 1982.
21. Robinson, Y., and Norin, M.: Porcine neonatal coccidiosis in Quebec. Can. Vet. J. *23*:212–216, 1982.
22. Ryley, J. F.: Why and how are coccidia harmful to their host. Symp. Brit. Soc. Parasit. *13*:43–58, 1975.
23. Sanford, S. E. and Josephson, G. K. A.: Porcine neonatal coccidiosis. Can. Vet. J. *22*:282–285, 1981.
24. Tarlatzis, C., Panetsos, A., and Dragonas, P.: Further experiences with furacin in treatment of ovine and caprine coccidiosis. *131*:474, 1957.
25. Tarlatzis, C., Panetsos, A., and Dragonas, P.: Furacin in the treatment of ovine and caprine coccidiosis. J. Am. Vet. Med. Assoc. *126*:391–392, 1955.
26. Tzipori, S.: Cryptosporidiosis in animals and humans. Microbiol. Rev. *47*:84–96, 1983.

Balantidiasis

KENNETH S. TODD, JR., Ph.D.,
JOSEPH A. DIPIETRO, D.V.M., M.S.,
and WALTER M. GUTERBOCK, D.V.M., M.S.

Balantidiasis is caused by the ciliated protozoan *Balantidium coli*. The organism has been found in the cecum and colon of the pig, humans, some other primates, but rarely in other hosts, such as horses and cattle. Lubinsky considered a similar protozoan reported in cattle to be *Buxtonella sulcata*.[7] *Balantidium coli* is most common in swine, and various surveys show its incidence to be 17 to 100 per cent. Reproduction is by transverse binary fission. Cysts may be formed, and these can survive outside the host. Trophozoites of *B. coli* are 30 to 150 μm × 25 to 120 μm, and cysts are 40 to 60 μm in diameter.[6] Dimensions of the trophozoites vary greatly, depending on the amount of starch they have ingested.[5] Transmission takes place by the ingestion of trophozoites or cysts.

EPIZOOTIOLOGY

B. coli is usually not considered to be a pathogen except in humans. In pigs, the protozoan generally is found in the lumen of the intestine but may invade the intestinal wall. Whether it can invade the intact intestinal wall or is a secondary invader of a lesion is not known. It does produce hyaluronidase.

B. coli was considered to be an important cause of hemorrhagic enteritis in swine in Zaire.[12] Large numbers of *B. coli* were found in 21 of 42 pigs with hemorrhagic enteritis from farms all over France.[11] Few, if any, *B. coli* were found in healthy pigs. Lesions caused by larval and adult *Trichuris* and larval *Œsophagostomum* may have favored invasion of the mucosa by *B. coli*. In one study, *B. coli* was considered a factor in the etiology of hemorrhagic gastroenteritis of swine, but no attempts to reproduce the disease were made.[12] *B. coli* was very numerous and regularly found in the depths of the mucosal crypts of the intestines of pigs with hemorrhagic enteritis in France.[9]

CLINICAL SIGNS AND LESIONS

Weight loss, emaciation, diarrhea, anemia, and death have been reported in pigs that were presumed to have balantidiasis. Clinical signs commonly appear after or during outbreaks of colibacillosis and at weaning.

Enteritis and numerous yellow nodules appear throughout the intestines of infected pigs. Histologic examination of the lesions reveals a diffuse inflammatory reaction, necrosis of the villi, mucosal ulceration, and numerous *B. coli* at their edges. Nodules containing *B. coli* and necrotic caseous centers, surrounded by granular tissue, are also present in the submucosa and muscularis. Ulcerations were reported in the large intestine of swine from herds in which *B. coli* may have been responsible for a mortality rate of 40 to 80 per cent.[4]

DIAGNOSIS

Trophozoites and cysts may be found by fecal flotation using standard techniques. *B. coli* is easy to recognize in stained fecal smears or histologic sections because of its large size and the darkly staining, often bean- or U-shaped macronucleus. Antemortem histologic examination revealed 50 per cent more animals with *B. coli* than did antemortem fecal examination.[3]

TREATMENT

Fatal balantidiasis has been reported in swine in Zaire in which the mortality rate was 30 to 40 per cent in pigs between 2 and 6 months of age.[10] Terramycin* was mixed with feed given to 20 pigs 3 months of age at a rate of 15 mg/kg twice daily for 5 days. After 3 days of treatment, diarrhea had stopped in 50 per cent of the pigs and by the fourth day, it had stopped in all 20 pigs. *B. coli* was not present in the feces of 14 of the 20 treated pigs, and the 6 pigs still passing the organism had lower numbers than prior to treatment. In an untreated group, 4 of 15 pigs died by the 5th day, the rest continued to lose condition, and the numbers of *B. coli* in feces increased. Tetracycline is the drug of choice for human balantidiasis.

A single dose of furazolidone at the rate of 45 mg/kg each day for 3 days has been reported to be effective treatment.

Metronidazole, when given at a dose of 0.25 gm twice daily for 3 days, is therapeutic.

Acetarsol at 1 mg/20 to 30 kg was found to be successful when antibiotics were also given. Also, dimetridazole at 50 mg/kg is helpful with or without antibiotics.

Treatment of porcine balantidiasis was reported using niridazole (Ambilhar†) at 20 to 40 mg/kg daily for 4 days and furazolidone at 45 mg/kg daily for 4 days.[13] Both compounds were 93 per cent effective in eliminating *B. coli* from the feces. Chloroquine at 5 mg/kg daily for 6 days was only 30 per cent effective.

Furazolidone was administered orally at 10 mg/kg twice daily for 6 days, and the treatment was considered to be effective.[8]

Diet may contribute to the overgrowth of *B. coli,* and diet modification may have a place in the treatment of porcine balantidiasis. Dietary starch is thought to be the main source of nourishment for *B. coli* in the intestinal lumen. In culture, rice starch is the main substrate for the organism.[5] Three human patients with *B. coli* enteritis were successfully treated with a diet of milk and the initial use of bismuth subnitrate to control tenesmus and diarrhea.[2] These patients felt prompt relief of pain and diarrhea, and the parasites disappeared from the feces. At that time, no drugs were known to be effective against *B. coli* although many had been tested.

PREVENTION

The protozoan is transmitted in the feces. Cysts are infective when passed. Sanitation, cleanliness, and good management are therefore the primary preventive measures.

PUBLIC HEALTH CONSIDERATIONS

Transmission from swine to humans is possible, and more than 50 per cent of humans with *B. coli* infections have a history of contact with pigs.[1]

---

*Available from Pfizer, Inc., New York, NY 10017

†Available from CIBA Pharmaceutical Co., Summit, NJ 07901

References

1. Aréan, V. M., and Echevarria, R.: Balantidiasis. *In* Marcial-Rojas, R. A. (ed.). Pathology of Protozoal and Helminthic Diseases. Baltimore, Williams & Wilkins, 1971.
2. Greene, J. L., and Scully, F. J.: Diet in the treatment of *Balantidium coli* infection. J. Am. Med. Assn. *81*:291–292, 1923.
3. Indermühle, N. A.: Endoparasitenbefall beim Schwein. Schweiz. Arch. Tierheilkd. *120*:513–525, 1978.
4. Karpenko, I. G.: Control of *Balantidium* infection in pigs (using metronidazole). Veterinariia. *3*:69–71, 1970.
5. Levine, N. D.: The effect of food intake upon the dimensions of *Balantidium* from swine in culture. Am. J. Hyg. *32*:81–87, 1940.
6. Levine, N. D.: Protozoan Parasites of Domestic Animals and of Man, 2nd ed. Minneapolis, Minnesota, Burgess Publishing Co., 369–370, 1973.
7. Lubinsky, G.: *Buxtonella sulcata* (Ciliata: Holotricha), a parasite of *Bos indicus* and *Bubalus bubalus* in the Western Punjab. Can. J. Zool. *35*:545–548, 1957.
8. Manichan, R., Gopalahrishan, C. A., Chellappa, D. J., and Moohlnapan, M.: Acute balantidial dysentery in pigs. Cherion. *9*:345–347, 1980.
9. Marchand, M.: L'enterite hémorragique du porc dans le Pas-de-Calais. Bull. Soc. Vet. Pract. *55*:183–188, 1971.
10. Mwamba, T., and Pandey, V. S.: Effect of terramycin in balantidiosis of pigs. Ann. Rech. Vet. *8*:167–169, 1977.
11. Vaissaire, J., Renault, L., Maire, C., et al.: Contribution a l'étude de l'entérite hémorragique du porc. Rec Med. Vet. *145*:433, 1970.
12. Verhulst, A., and Cornet, R.: La balantidiose du porc en République du Zäire et son traitement par le niridazole (Ambilhar). Rev. Elev. Med. Vet. Pays Trop. *28*:301–304, 1975.
13. Verhulst, A., and Shukla, R. R.: Etude comparée de l'efficacité du niridazole, de la furazolidone et de la chloroquine dans le traitement de la balantidiose porcine. Proc. Twentieth World Vet. Cong., Thessaloniki. *3*:2237–2239, 1976.
14. Walzer, P. D., and G. R., Healy, Balantidiasis. *In* Steele, J. H. (ed.). Handbook Series in Zoonoses. Section C. Parasitic Zoonoses, vol. 1. Boca Raton, Florida, CRC Press, 1982.
15. Zaman, V.: *Balantidium coli. In* Kreier, J. P. (ed.): Parasitic Protozoa. New York, Academic Press, 1978.

Amoebiasis

KENNETH S. TODD, JR., Ph.D.,
WALTER M. GUTERBOCK, D.V.M., M.S.,
and JOSEPH A. DIPIETRO, D.V.M., M.S.

Amoebiasis or amoebic dysentery is caused by the protozoan *Entamoeba histolytica,* which has been reported from many species of animals including dogs, pigs, and possibly cattle. It is primarily a pathogen of humans, infecting the large intestine and occasionally other organs, such as the liver. The parasite has a worldwide distribution.

Two forms of the parasite are known, trophozoites and cysts. The trophozoites of the large pathogenic race are 20 to 30 μm in diameter, while those of the small nonpathogenic race are 12 to 15 μm in diameter. Reproduction of the trophozoites is by binary fission. Cysts of both the large and small races are 10 to 20 μm in diameter, and the cysts contain 4 nuclei.

EPIZOOTIOLOGY

E. histolytica is a pathogen in humans. Nothing is known about its pathogenicity in food-producing animals. Researchers were unable to establish *E. histolytica* infections by repeated direct injections of known virulent organisms from an active case of human amoebiasis into the intestine and liver of conventionally raised 3-month-old pigs.[3] Transmission also failed when the pigs were put on a high carbohydrate diet. The inoculum used was virulent for kittens, however.

Some species of amoebae have been reported from food-producing animals. These include *Vahlkampfia* sp., *E. coli, E. wenyoni, E. bovis, E. ovis, E. dilimani, E. suis, E. caprae, Endolimax nana,* and *Iodamoeba buetsch-*

lii. Entamoeba polecki was first described in swine but has also been described in humans, cattle, goats, sheep, and other mammals. The pathogenicity of the listed species in food-producing animals is unknown.

CLINICAL SIGNS AND LESIONS

There are no known clinical signs and lesions of *E. histolytica*–induced amoebiasis in food-producing animals.

DIAGNOSIS

Living amoebae may be found in fresh fecal smears that have been diluted with 0.9 per cent saline. Amoebae are difficult to identify, especially if the aperture on the condenser of the microscope is open too wide and the light is too bright. Staining the smears with Lugol's solution makes identification easier, allowing the nuclei to be studied. Confirmation of the presence of amoebae requires practice, and samples should be sent to a diagnostic laboratory for this reason. If fecal smears are submitted, they should be fixed in Schaudinn's fluid. Bulk feces may be sent if preserved by the MIF (merthiolate–iodine–formalin) technique. Samples should be taken directly from a living animal and fixed immediately.

TREATMENT

Because amoebae are usually considered to be non-pathogenic in food-producing animals, treatment is non-existent.

PUBLIC HEALTH CONSIDERATIONS

Transmission of *E. histolytica* from animals to humans has not been reported. *E. histolytica* can be a serious pathogen in humans and is transmitted from person to person in the feces.

References

1. Albach, R. A., and Boodin, T.: Amoebae. *In* Krier, J. P. (ed.). Parasitic Protozoa, vol. 2. New York, Academic Press, 1978.
2. Frye, W. W., and Meleney, H. E.: Investigations of *Entamoeba histolytica* and other intestinal protozoa in Tennessee. IV. A study of flies, rats, mice, and some domestic animals as possible carriers of the intestinal protozoa of man in a rural community. Am. J. Hyg. *16*:729–749, 1932.
3. Frye, W. W., and Meleney, H. E.: Studies of *Entamoeba histolytica* and other intestinal protozoa in Tennessee. VIII. Observations on the intestinal protozoa in young pigs and attempts to produce infection with a human strain of *E. histolytica*. Am. J. Hyg. *20*:404–415, 1934.
4. Levine, N. D.: Protozoan Parasites of Domestic Animals and of Man. Minneapolis, Minnesota, Burgess Publishing Co., 1973.
5. Lushbaugh, W. B., and Pittman, F. E.: Amebiasis. *In* Steele, J. H. (ed.). Handbook Series in Zoonoses. Section C: Parasitic Zoonosis, vol. 1. Boca Raton, Florida, CRC Press, 1982.
6. Noble, G. A., and Noble, E. R.: Entamoebae in farm mammals. J. Parasitol. *38*:571–595, 1952.
7. Pérez-Tamayo, R., and Brandt, H.: Amoebiasis. *In* Marcial-Rojas, R. A. (ed.). Pathology of Protozoal and Helminthic Diseases. Baltimore, Williams & Wilkins, 1971.
8. Walkiers, J.: Un cas d'amibiase intestinale chez un bovidé. Ann. Soc. Belge Med. Trop. *31*:379–380, 1930.

Trichomoniasis in Cattle

BRUCE ABBITT, D.V.M., M.S.

Bovine trichomoniasis is a venereal disease of worldwide distribution caused by the protozoan, *Trichomonas foetus* (Fig. 1). The disease is characterized primarily by abortion (the majority during the first 5 months of gestation) and by postbreeding pyometra. The only proven method of natural transmission is coitus, although fomites (artificial insemination [AI] pipettes, artificial vaginas, and so forth) have helped spread the disease. Transfer of the disease by frozen semen collected from infected bulls is theoretically possible but highly unlikely. Incidence of trichomoniasis is often high in areas characterized by agricultural practices such as use of older bulls for natural service and large, often comingling herds, and is often low in areas characterized by agricultural practice such as use of young bulls and artificial insemination and small, separated herds.

The number of cases in the United States is difficult to ascertain because of the nonreportable status of the disease. Limited information on trichomoniasis prevalence in 2 small geographic areas was obtained in 2 surveys in the 1970's. Approximately 8 per cent of the bulls passing through a "sale ring" in an Oklahoma[1] and a Florida abattoir[2] were found to be infected.

CLINICAL SIGNS AND LESIONS

The protozoan localizes in the secretions of the vagina, uterus, and oviduct, and initially does not interfere with

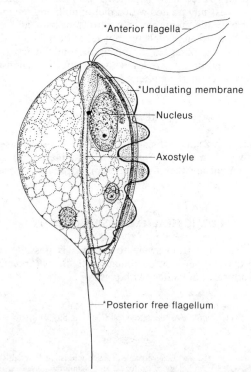

*Anterior flagella

*Undulating membrane

Nucleus

Axostyle

*Posterior free flagellum

Figure 1. *Trichomonas foetus.* Approximate size 10 to 25 μ in length by 5 to 10 μ in width. (Structures with asterisks can be seen without staining.)

conception.[3] A mucopurulent discharge associated with vaginitis or endometritis, or both, is present in some but not in all cases. The discharge is often of small quantity and therefore seldom observed. Embryonic wastage is attributed to the inflammatory changes in the uterus and fetal membranes that could be initially detected by approximately 50 days of gestation in heifers bred by an infected bull.[3] This finding agrees well with the average stage of gestation (3 months, with a range of 1 to 9 months) at the time of abortion in a study of 840 naturally occurring trichomonad-induced abortions.[4] In another study spanning 3 years, cows continuously joined by trichomonad-infected bulls were compared to cows continuously joined by noninfected bulls.[5] Primary initial infection in this study resulted in an average delay in calving of approximately 3 months. Subsequent susceptibility to reinfection and severity of reinfection (delay in calving) was shown to depend on the infection-free interval preceding re-exposure. Thus, cows free of infection for 1 month and then re-exposed did not become reinfected. Re-exposure after a 10.3-month interval resulted in a 72 per cent incidence of reinfection, and re-exposure after a 19.7-month interval resulted in a 100 per cent reinfection rate. Cows reinfected after less than a 15-month interval free of infection experienced a 20- to 26-day delay in calving; those reinfected after a 19.7-month interval free of infection experienced a delay in calving similar to a primary infection (3 months). The cow can sometimes carry the infection through a normal gestation.[6, 7] Although this is rarely reported, it raises the possibility of "carrier" cows. Palpable postcoital pyometra and abortion after the fifth month of gestation are sporadic and seemingly occur more frequently in chronically infected herds.

Trichomoniasis is asymptomatic in the male. The protozoan localizes in the secretions and epithelium lining of the penis, prepuce, and anterior portion of the urethra.[8] Empirical evidence and attempts to infect bulls at various ages have shown that bulls less than 4 years of age are seldom naturally infected.[1, 9] and are difficult to infect experimentally.[10, 11] This may not be true for all breeds, however. My experience indicates that young Brangus and Santa Gertrudis bulls may not recover spontaneously from infection. Others have noted apparent chronic infection in young Texas Longhorns.[12]

Since abortions during the first 3 to 4 months of gestation often go unnoticed, trichomoniasis is manifested primarily on a herd basis by infertility, the severity of which depends on the extent of exposure.

DIAGNOSIS

A tentative diagnosis is often based on clinical signs after eliminating other common causes of herd infertility. Chief among the latter are inadequate nutrition, vibriosis, and bull infertility. Definitive diagnosis depends on demonstrating the presence of T. foetus. The protozoan often is found in great numbers in the fetal fluids associated with trichomonad-induced abortion (amniotic, abomasal, pharyngeal) and exudates associated with pyometra. Microscopic examination of these fluids often yields conclusive proof of infection.* Unfortunately, these fluids are not always available for examination. Since the bull is usually the source of continued infection in a herd and is

also a sentinel for introduction of infection, microscopic evaluation of preputial smegma following centrifugation or culture is the most common method employed to confirm diagnosis. Samples of smegma can be collected by several methods.

Douche. The sheath is infused with approximately 200 ml of physiological saline solution (PSS). The preputial opening is occluded, and the trapped fluid is massaged and recollected. The fluid is than centrifuged (2000 rpm for 10 minutes), and the sediment is examined microscopically.*

Swab. A cotton swab is used to obtain a sample of smegma from the fornix of the bull's prepuce. The swab is rinsed in 5 to 10 ml of PSS, centrifuged (2000 rpm for 10 minutes), and the sediment is examined microscopically.*

Pipette. An AI pipette is introduced into the fornix of the bull's prepuce, and smegma is collected by a combination of scraping and aspirating via an attached rubber bulb or syringe. The use of an experimentally designed instrument to scrape the epithelium resulted in a significant increase in the percentage of samples with positive findings from infected bulls and thus suggests that the scraping should be fairly vigrous.[13] The epithelial cells and the smegma that are collected are mixed with 5 to 10 ml of PSS, centrifuged at 2000 rpm for 10 minutes, and the sediment is examined microscopically.*

The douche method is reportedly the most efficient of these 3 techniques.[14] However, in bulls known to be infected, the pipette method used in conjunction with culture medium has been shown to be at least 97 per cent accurate under ideal conditions, which is superior to the other methods.[15] The directions for preparation of a commonly used medium, Diamond's medium, are given in Table 1.[16] Smegma obtained by scraping the bull's prepuce is layered on approximately 10 ml of the Diamond's medium. The anaerobic, motile trichomonads swim to the bottom and multiply, leaving competitive bacteria to multiply in the upper layers. If the smegma is accidentally mixed with the culture medium, a subsample can be taken from the first tube and layered on a fresh column of medium. If necessary, the inoculated medium can be refrigerated for 24 hr prior to incubation. The smegma can be mixed with United States Pharmacopeia† lactated Ringer's solution and stored refrigerated for up to 48 hr prior to inoculation in culture medium.[12] The culture medium is incubated at 37° C; fluid is taken from the bottom of the tube by pipette and examined microscopically (as described previously) at 24 hr and, if necessary, 48 hr. Bacterial overgrowth, indicated by cloudiness of the normally clear medium, begins at the top of the column and usually approaches the bottom by approximately 48 hr. Samples should be examined before the cloudiness reaches the bottom of the test tube. Sam-

---

*In each case, a drop of the sediment, fluid, or culture medium is examined at 100 × magnification for the trichomonads, which move in an irregular, jerky manner associated with continual rolling. Reducing the light to a low level by closing the condenser diaphragm will aid in visualizing the semitransparent trichomonads. In preparations of sediment, movement of tissue debris in association with individual trichomonads is all that is generally observable under low power. Confirmation in each case is by examination (using a coverslip) at 400 × magnification, at which time the undulating membrane and flagellae can be seen coming in and out of view as the organism moves and rolls (see Fig. 1).

†United States Pharmacopeia lactated Ringer's is required as other formulations often contain preservatives that will kill the trichomonads.

Table 1. *Preparation of Diamond's Medium (100 ml)*

Ingredient	Gm
Trypticase peptone	2.0
Yeast extract	1.0
Maltose	0.5
L-cystine hydrochloride	0.1
L-ascorbic acid	0.02
Distilled water to make 90 ml	—
K_2HPO_4*	0.08
KH_2PO_4*	0.08

1. Mix all ingredients. Adjust pH to 7.2 to 7.4 with NaOH or HCl if necessary.

2. Add 0.05 gm of agar and autoclave for 10 minutes at 121° C.

3. Cool to 49° C and aseptically add 10 ml of inactivated (56° C for 30 minutes) bovine serum,* 100,000 units of penicillin G (1 ml of a stock solution prepared by adding 10 ml of sterile H_2O to 10^6 units of penicillin G), and 0.1 gm of streptomycin in sulfate (0.5 ml of stock solution prepared by adding 5 ml of sterile H_2O to 1 gm of streptomycin sulfate).

4. Aseptically dipense 10 ml per sterile 16 × 125 mm screw cap vial. Check for sterility by incubating 24 hr at 37° C.

*Original media as reported by L. S. Diamond did not contain K_2HPO_4 or KH_2PO_4, were adjusted to a pH of 6.8 to 7.0, and contained 10 ml/100 ml of inactivated sheep serum. All asterisks refer to slight modifications in media. The modifications are a result of experience in field and laboratory use of the media in conjunction with the identification of *Trichomonas foetus* for diagnostic purposes by Dr. C. P. Hibler of the Pathology Department, College of Veterinary Medicine and Biomedical Sciences, Colorado State University, Fort Collins, Colorado 80523.

ples with positive results will generally have large numbers of trichomonads present by 24 to 48 hr of incubation.

Cervicovaginal mucus (CVM) culture can be a valuable diagnostic aid. This method proved to be extremely accurate in a group of 20 experimentally infected heifers.[3] I have found that CVM samples cultured in Diamond's medium may also be valuable as an indicator of impending abortion. In one infected herd, approximately 50 per cent of the pregnant females with positive culture results (average 81 days gestation at the time of culture) subsequently aborted. These findings suggest that culturing of CVM samples may be a reliable method for confirming diagnosis. However, additional studies are required before this technique can be recommended as a standard procedure for identifying infected cows.

HERD CONTROL

The prognosis for the infected herd is generally good provided control measures are adequately implemented. Details involving the implementation of control measures for a specific herd will vary. Control measures should be based on both a knowledge of the epidemiology of the disease and the particular herd. Proven control methods can be grouped into 5 broad categories.

1. Depopulation. Obviously often effective, but also often impractical because of economic considerations.

2. Artificial Insemination. This is effective but often impractical because of managerial or economic factors, or both.

3. Quarantine. The herd can be separated into 2 groups, 1 containing exposed cows, the other unexposed cows. Heifers and purchased unexposed cows can be added to the unexposed group, while allowing natural attrition to eliminate cows in the exposed group. This method is

potentially effective but is generally not practical because of the difficulty in maintaing 100 per cent separation of 2 sexually active groups of cattle on the same premises.

4. Removal of Infected Bulls and Sexual Rest. Various modifications of this basic program have been reported as effective.[17, 18] Briefly, these methods require that exposed cows be sexually rested for at least 90 days postpartum. Allowing 2 normal estrous cycles has also been recommended prior to rebreeding. This measure often has limited appeal because of the economic factors associated with a 90-day delay of breeding and the difficulty involved, particularly verification of postpartum estrous cycles.

5. Selective Culling Combined with the Use of Young Bulls. Cows failing either to conceive or to calve before the next breeding season are culled, and breeding is limited to bulls with negative culture results for trichomoniasis that are less than 4 years of age. This procedure is repeated for several years, with the progress of the herd monitored by testing the bulls for trichomoniasis after each breeding season. This method is reportedly effective and has the added benefit of promoting management practices (culling of infertile cows and use of young bulls) that may increase herd productivity and genetic progress.[1] However, it may not be effective in certain breeds (see Clinical Signs and Lesions).

Surveillance for trichomoniasis in conjunction with all of the control programs should include periodic culture of the breeding bulls and astute observation of the cows for abnormal estrous cycles, abortions, and pyometra.

TREATMENT

Treatment of individual cows has not been thoroughly investigated, probably because of the temporary nature of the infection. The prognosis for treatment of the individual bull is excellent. Because of their ability to recovery spontaneously, it is often not necessary to treat bulls of less than 4 years of age.

Three 5-nitroimidazoles (dimetridazole,* ipronidazole† and metronidazole‡) are all effective as systemic treatment agents, but these drugs are not approved for use in the bovine species in the United States.

Dimetridazole

Dimetridazole (1,2-dimethyl-5-nitroimidazole), available as a powder in the United States, is effective orally at 50 mg/kg daily for 5 days.[19] The drug can be administered as a bolus, as a drench, or as a feed additive. Feed refusal or temporary inappetance is often observed in bulls following initial consumption of dimetridazole, and thus the use of dimetridazole as a feed additive should be cautioned because resistant strains of trichomonads may develop if subtherapeutic levels are administered.[20] Rumen stasis is frequently observed during or after treatment of bulls on high concentrate rations. This can usually be prevented by feeding a diet high in roughage for several days before and during treatment.

Dimetridazole is also effective when given intravenously

*Available from Salsbury Laboratories, Charles City, IA 50616
†Available from Hoffman-LaRoche, Inc., Nutley, NJ 07110
‡Available from G. D. Searle & Co., Chicago, IL 60680

in dosages ranging from 10 mg/kg daily for 5 days to 50 to 100 mg/kg in a single injection.[21] The drug is soluble only in relatively low pH solutions, such as 10 to 20 per cent sulfuric acid. The clinical response to injection of the volume of acidic solution (13 to 27 ml/100 kg) needed to supply the necessary dosage of dimetridazole varied among bulls. Some experienced respiratory difficulty, ataxia, recumbency for up to 15 minutes, and weakness for up to 2 days. Although these effects are transitory, they are manifestations of severe interruptions of homeostases. Forced oral treatment is preferable in most instances, as it assures adequate dosage without the risks involved with intravenous treatment.

Ipronidazole

Ipronidazole (1-methyl-2-isopropyl-5-nitroimidazole), available as a powder in the United States, is reported to be effective for herd or individual treatment when administered as a single intramuscular injection of 15 gm in cows or 30 gm in bulls.[22] Treatment in bulls was preceded by 3 days of a broad-spectrum antibiotic therapy to eliminate micrococci from the sheath that might metabolize or inactivate the drug. Researchers at Colorado State University (Drs. Les Ball and John Cheney, personal communication) found that pretreatment with a broad-spectrum antibiotic followed by a single intramuscular injection of 30 gm of ipronidazole effected a cure rate of approximately 50 per cent of the bulls treated. All treated bulls had negative culture results for the first few weeks post-treatment, but approximately 50 per cent had positive culture results by 4 to 6 weeks post-treatment. These same researchers were able to achieve a 100 per cent cure rate in a small group of bulls given 15 gm ipronidazole daily for 3 days (treatment was preceded by 3 days of broad-spectrum antibiotic administration). Ipronidazole, while being very similar to dimetridazole, has the distinct advantage of being highly soluble in aqueous solution. The aqueous solution obtained must be carefully handled, as it is easily inactivated by exposure to light, bases, or reducing agents.

Metronidazole

Metronidazole (1-β-hydroxyethyl-2-methyl-5-nitroimidazole) (availabe as a tablet and as a vaginal suppository in the United States) has been reported effective when given intravenously at dosages ranging from 75 mg/kg for 3 successive injections at 12-hr intervals to 10 mg/kg once daily for 2 days.[23]

Trichomonads that became resistant to dimetridazole because of subtherapeutic regimens were also resistant to metronidazole.[20] It is reasonable to assume that these trichomonads would also be resistant to ipronidazole, since all 3 of these drugs are similar.

PREVENTION

Trichomoniasis can be prevented by adequate screening, testing, and isolating procedures for all additions to an established herd. Prior to use, bulls, unless virgins, should be tested by using culture methods at least 3 times at weekly intervals. As testing procedures for individual cows are not well established, additions to established herds should, if possible, be limited to animals that are virgins or that originate from herds free from infection. All other female additions should be tested using culture techniques prior to entering the herds. Pregnant females should be isolated from bulls during gestation and, ideally, for 90 days after calving. Open cows should be bred by AI or "sacrifice" bulls and should remain separate from other bulls during gestation and, ideally, for 90 days after calving. Bulls exposed to these cows should be tested for trichomoniasis prior to further use in the herd.

Vaccination

An experimental vaccine produced in Australia has been shown to be efficacious both prophylactically and therapeutically in bulls less than 5.5 years of age but was not efficacious in bulls more than 5.5 years of age.[23] This vaccine could be used to extend the period of natural resistance in young bulls, an effect that would be of practical benefit in control programs based on use of young bulls, This vaccine, however, is not at this time commercially available.

References

1. Wilson, K. W., Gandy, E. T., and Goodwin, D.: The prevalence of trichomoniasis in Oklahoma beef bulls. Okla. Vet. 31:40, 1979.
2. Abbitt, B., and Meyerholz, G. W.: Trichomonas fetus infection of range bulls in South Florida. Vet. Med./Small Anim. Clin. 1339, 1979.
3. Parsonson, I. M., Clark, B. L., and Dufty, J. H.: Early pathogenesis and pathology of Trichomonas fetus infection in virgin heifers. J. Comp. Path. 86:59, 1976.
4. Hess, V. E., and Brunner, J.: Untersuchungen über verschiedene abortusursachen beim rind. Schweizer Archiv fur Tierheilkunde. 285, 1949.
5. Clark, B. L., Dufty, J. H., and Parsonson, I. M.: The effect of Tritrichomonas foetus infection on calving rates in beef cattle. Aust. Vet. J. 60:71, 1983.
6. Morgan, B. B.: Bovine Trichomoniasis. Minneapolis, Minnesota, Burgess Publishing Co., 1–150, 1964.
7. Morgan, B. B.: Studies on the trichomonad carrier-cow problem. J. Anim. Sci. 3:437, 1944.
8. Parsonson, I. M., Clark, B. L., and Dufty, J. H.: The pathogenesis of Tritrichomonas foetus infection in the bull. Aust. Vet. J. 50:421, 1974.
9. Ladds, P. W., Dennett, D. P., and Glazebrook, J. S.: A survey of the genitalia of bulls in Northern Australia. Aust. Vet. J. 49:335, 1973.
10. Clark, B. L., Personson, I. M., and Dufty, J. H.: Experimental infection of bulls with Tritrichomonas foetus. Aust. Vet. J. 50:189, 1974.
11. Clark, B. L., Parsonson, I. M., White, M. B., et al.: Control of trichomoniasis in a large herd of beef cattle. Aust. Vet. J. 50:424, 1974.
12. Kimsey, P. B., Darien, J., Kendrick, J. W., and Franti, C. E.: Bovine trichomoniasis: diagnosis and treatment. J. Am. Vet. Med. Assoc. 177:616, 1980.
13. Tedesco, L. F., Errico, F., and Del Baglivi, L. P.: Diagnosis of Tritrichomonas foetus infection in bulls using two sampling methods and a transport medium. Aust. Vet. J. 55:322, 1979.
14. Fitzgerald, P. R., Hammond, D. M., Miner, M. L., and Binns, W.: Relative efficacy of various methods of obtaining preputial samples for diagnosis of trichomoniasis in the bulls. Am. J. Vet. Res. 49:452, 1952.
15. Clark, B. L., White, M. B., and Banfield, J. C.: Diagnosis of Tritrichomonas foetus infection in bulls. Aust. Vet. J. 47:181, 1971.
16. Diamond, L. S.: The establishment of various trichomonads of animals and man in axenic cultures. J. Parasit. 43:488, 1957.
17. Bartlett, D. E.: Further observations on experimental treatments of Trichomonas foetus infection in bulls. Am. J. Vet. Res. 9:351, 1948.
18. Bartlett, D. E., and Dikmans, G.: Field studies on bovine venereal trichomoniasis effects on herds and efficacy of certain practices in control. Am. J. Vet. Res. 10:30, 1949.
19. McLoughlin, D. K.: Dimetridazole, a systemic treatment for bovine venereal trichomoniasis. I. Oral administration. J. Parasit. 51:835, 1965.
20. McLoughlin, D. K.: Drug tolerance by Tritrichomonas fetus. J. Parasit. 53:646, 1967.

21. McLoughlin, D. K.: Dimetridazole, a systemic treatment for bovine venereal trichomoniasis. II. Intravenous administration. J. Parasit. *54*:1038, 1968.
22. Retief, G. P.: Trichomoniasis treatment in cattle. South Afric. Vet. Clin. June, July:23, 1978.
23. Gasparini, G., Vaughi, M., and Tardani, A.: Treatment of bovine trichomoniasis with metronidazole (8823 R.P.). Vet. Rec. *75*:940, 1963.
24. Clark, B. L., Dufty, J. H., and Parsonson, I. M.: Immunization of bulls against trichomoniasis. Aust. Vet. J. *60*:178, 1983.

Trypanosomiasis

(Nagana, Samore, Tsetse-Fly Disease)

ALBERT A. ILEMOBADE, D.V.M., M.S., Ph.D.

Trypanosomiasis is a disease affecting cattle, camels, buffaloes, horses, pigs, sheep, goats, and dogs. Clinically, it is usually a chronic but sometimes acute condition characterized by intermittent fever, debilitation, loss of condition, and death if not treated.

DISTRIBUTION

Livestock in all continents except Australia are affected with trypanosomiasis. It is only in Africa, south of the Sahara, where tsetse flies (*Glossina* spp.) occur that trypanosomiasis assumes economic importance, causing stock mortality and depressed productive capability, which may be of meat, milk, reproduction, or traction.

The distribution of pathogenic trypanosomes coincides with that of their vectors, the tsetse flies, which are found between latitudes of 14 degrees north and 29 degrees south. Areas within this geographic zone are very arid and tsetse flies are not present, but camel trypanosomiasis caused by *Trypanosoma evansi* is present and transmitted mechanically by biting flies. *T. evansi* is also important as a cause of trypanosomiasis in cattle and buffaloes in India, USSR, and the Far East. A species of animal trypanosome that is pathogenic to livestock in Africa (*T. vivax*) occurs in cattle in South America where it is transmitted by biting flies.

ETIOLOGY

The most important pathogenic trypanosomes transmitted by tsetse flies are *Trypanosoma brucei, T. congolense, T. vivax,* and *T. simiae*. All species, apart from *T. simiae*, are pathogenic to cattle, sheep, and goats, although *T. brucei* is frequently less pathogenic.

T. simiae causes virulent disease in pigs. *T. evansi* is pathogenic to camels in Africa and to cattle and buffaloes in India and the Far East.

EPIZOOTIOLOGY

Nearly all species of tsetse flies harbor trypanosomes that are pathogenic to livestock. Animals become infected when they intrude upon the natural sylvatic cycle of trypanosomes involving wild game and tsetse flies. Once domestic stock are infected, the transmission continues back and forth between the 2 cycles. Tsetse flies become infected when they feed on an infected host. The ingested trypanosomes undergo a cycle of development in the flies, lasting between 1 and 5 weeks when trypanosomes that are infective to animals, called metacyclics (metatrypanosomes), are produced.

The severity of trypanosomiasis is related to fly density, fly vectorial capacity and trypanosome virulence. Although all domestic stock are susceptible to trypanosomiasis, susceptibility varies, depending on the breed, previous exposure, and stress factors. The N'Dama and Muturu cattle of West and Central Africa possess a degree of tolerance to trypanosomiasis, a characteristic commonly referred to as trypanotolerance.

PATHOGENESIS

The disease is initiated by the bite of an infected tsetse fly; the site of bite is sometimes marked by a reaction, frequently referred to as chancre. This is more marked in human trypanosomiasis than in animal trypanosomiasis. From the initial site of inoculation, the metacyclic trypanosomes are believed to multiply in the subcutaneous tissues of the skin; from there they invade the bloodstream either directly or indirectly via the lymphatic system. In the blood stream, the trypanosomes become transformed to the trypomastigote and divide equally by longitudinal binary fission. In general, the different species of trypanosomes occupy different sites in the body: *T. congolense* and *T. vivax* are normally confined to the blood, while *T. brucei* is found both in the blood and in the tissues. Consequently, *T. brucei* causes relatively more tissue damage than does either *T. congolense* or *T. vivax*.

The appearance of trypanosomes in the peripheral circulation is often heralded by an elevated body temperature, and the initial parasitemia and fever usually persist for several days before a trypanolytic crisis develops with parasites becoming scanty and temperature returning to normal. The first trypanolytic crisis is followed by further intermittent parasitemia and associated fever, leading to anemia that is related to the intensity and duration of parasitemia.

All 3 species of trypanosomes (*T. brucei, T. congolense,* and *T. vivax*) undergo antigenic variation and, therefore, in most animals, there is little or no protective immunity. Ineffective immune responses bring about some undesirable immunopathologic changes.

CLINICAL SIGNS AND LESIONS

Animals that are exposed to infection by tsetse flies develop patency after variable prepatent periods, depending on the strain and species of the infecting trypanosomes and on the number of trypanosomes introduced. In general, the prepatent period varies from 3 to 20 days or more. The disease may be peracute (as in *T. simiae* of pigs), acute, subacute, or chronic (*T. brucei, T. congolense,* and *T. vivax*). In peracute cases, clinical signs are hardly evident before death. Acute cases are characterized by dullness and slightly reduced feed intake that may not attract an observer's attention. Pulse and respiration rates are accelerated, and fever (39.5 to 41.2° C) is a regular finding. The visible mucous membranes are pale, and the superficial lymph nodes, especially the prescapulars and prefemorals, may become swollen and thus prominent. If an animal survives the acute phase, it passes into the subacute or chronic phase.

Most cases of trypanosomiasis are chronic and are characterized by wasting, intermittent fever, anemia, dull coat, shallow and rapid respiration, and marked jugular pulse. At this stage, animals may become recumbent, and pregnant cows may abort. If the disease is not treated it may cause death. In few cases, an untreated animal recovers. It would appear from field observations that treatment may not be beneficial unless given before irreversible changes set in, usually before the packed cell volume (PCV) falls below 17 to 20 per cent, depending on the age of the animal.

CLINICAL PATHOLOGY

The only constant finding is anemia characterized by elevated extravascular erythrocyte destruction and frequently the presence of the causative trypanosome.

NECROPSY FINDINGS

The lesions are not particularly remarkable and certainly not pathognomonic. In peracute and acute cases, as in *T. simiae* or *T. vivax* infections, there are diffuse hemorrhages in the serosal and mucosal membranes of the gastrointestinal tract and other visceral organs and areas of emphysema in the lungs. In chronic disease, the carcass is usually emaciated and anemic with enlarged lymph nodes. Serous atrophy of fat is usually observed in the adipose connective tissue around the heart, the kidney, and the mesentery.

DIAGNOSIS

The history of the affected animals, the geographic incidence of tsetse flies and trypanosomiasis, and the clinical signs of infection are suggestive. Definite diagnosis is, however, based on microscopic detection of the trypanosomes in stained blood smears. Wet blood smears

can be examined microscopically under a coverslip (thick or thin). The so-called standard trypanosome detection methods (STDM) include the following:

1. Wet, thick, and thin blood films.
2. Subinoculation of susceptible laboratory animals (mice).
3. Hematocrit centrifuge test (HCT) and darkground phase contrast buffy coat technique.

The methods used will be dictated by the species of trypanosomes involved. A combination of thick blood smear and HCT is considered the best for detection of *T. vivax*, whereas subinoculation of laboratory mice is the most sensitive method for detecting *T. brucei*.

Since trypanosomiasis is an occult disease, parasitemia may be low and sporadic, and may not be detected by any of the methods described. The absence of trypanosomes does not necessarily imply the absence of trypanosomiasis until persistent blood examination for many days has proved otherwise. This is the main reason why diagnosis is made on a herd basis. Serologic tests, for example, IHA, CFT, IFAT, ELISA, have been developed, but results still need to be correlated with a parasitologic finding.

Trypanosomiasis may be confused with other chronic wasting diseases, notably helminthiasis and malnutrition, but a differential diagnosis can be made on the basis of the demonstration and identification of the pathogenic trypanosomes and fecal examination. Babesiasis and anaplasmosis may also be confused with trypanosomiasis, but both can be differentiated on blood smear examination and other clinical features. Acute anthrax in pigs, which may be confused with *T. simiae* infection in pigs, is characterized by subcutaneous gelatinous edema of the throat region and exudation of tarry blood from the natural orifices of the cadaver.

TREATMENT

The drugs in current use for the treatment of tsetse-transmitted trypanosomal infections and indications for their use are given in Tables 1 and 2. Because of the seminomadic husbandry practiced by cattle owners in Africa, and the fact that trypanosomiasis is an occult disease, treatment is on a herd basis, each animal being treated with a single dose of trypanocide. Single-dose treatment is the order in trypanosomiasis.

Because drug resistance is found with distressing fre-

Table 1. *Drugs Used in the Treatment of Trypanosomiasis of Food Animals**

Drug	Proprietary Name	Solution	Dosage (mg/kg)	Route	Host	*Trypanosoma*
Diminazine aceturate	Berenil Ganaseg	7% cold water	3.5	SC or IM	Cattle, sheep, goats, pigs, camels	*T. vivax, T. congolense, T. brucei, T. evansi*
Homidium chloride or Homidium bromide	Novidium Ethidium	2% cold water	1.0	IM	Cattle, sheep, goats	*T. vivax, T. congolense*
Isometamidium	Samorin Trypamidium	1 or 2% cold water	0.25–0.75	IM	Cattle, sheep, goats	*T. vivax, T. congolense*
Quinapyramine dimethosulfate	Antrycide	10% cold water	5.0	SC	Cattle, sheep, goats, camels	*T. vivax, T. congolense, T. brucei, T. evansi,*
Suramin	Antrypol Naganol	10% cold water	10.0	IM	Camels	*T. brucei, T. evansi*

*See Appendix for suppliers.

Table 2. *Drugs Used for Prophylaxis in Animal Trypanosomiasis**

Drug	Proprietary Name	Solution	Dosage (mg/kg)	Route	Trypanosoma	Length of Protection (months)	Host
Isomatamidium	Samorin	1–2% cold water	0.75–1.0	IM	*T. vivax* *T. congolense* *T. brucei* *T. evansi*	2–4	Cattle, goats, sheep, camels
Pyrithidium bromide	Prothidium	2% boiling water	2.0	IM	*T. vivax* *T. congolense* *T. brucei* *T. evansi*	2–4	Cattle, sheep, goats, camels
Quinapyramine chloride plus dimethosulfate	Antrycide Prosalt	16.6% cold water	7.4	SC	*T. brucei* *T. evansi*		Cattle, sheep, goats, camels

*See Appendix for suppliers.

quency in trypanosomiasis, the need for great care in preparing solutions of trypanocides and for correct doses in the field cannot be overemphasized. The problem of drug resistance is particularly critical because no new drugs have been marketed for more than 20 years. In addition, the currently available trypanocides are related chemically and therefore liable to cross-resistance, and the trypanocides now available are too few. Recent efforts at screening drugs effective against trypanosomes have yielded few positive leads.

In many field cases, supportive treatment in the form of hematinics, fluids, and green feeds, is indicated and may make the difference between immediate or protracted recovery.

Several prophylactic drugs are also available (see Table 2) for the prevention of trypanosomiasis. In principle, trypanoprophylaxis is practiced in cattle under low trypanosomiasis risk, and where husbandry and management practices are good.

Cattle

The drugs to use in any given area may depend on the drug-resistant status of the circulating *Trypanosoma* species or the prevalent *Trypanosoma* species in the area. It is generally accepted that homidium compounds are to be preferred where *T. vivax* predominates, and diminazine aceturate where *T. congolense* predominates. Block treatment is usually given in herds where trypanosomiasis has been diagnosed, even if only a few cases were identified. Relapse infections must be treated with chemically unrelated drugs. Because several trypanocidal drugs sometimes cause severe local reactions, subcutaneous injections should be made preferably in the dewlap, and intramuscular injections should be made deep in the muscles of the midneck.

Sheep and Goats

The treatment of cattle is the same as the treatment of sheep and goats.

Pigs

Infections due to *T. brucei* and *T. congolense* can be treated in the same way as infections in cattle. There is as yet no effective drug against *T. simiae* infections probably because of the rapidity with which the disease causes death. Thus, reliance is better placed on prophylactic than curative therapy. For prophylaxis, quinapyramine dimethosulfate in 5 per cent cold water is given

subcutaneously at 40 mg/kg; or isometamidium is given at 12.5 to 35 mg/kg. A combination of subcutaneous quinapyramine dimethosulfate (7.5 mg/kg) and diminazine aceturate (5 mg/kg) has also been used.

Camels

Quinapyramine remains the drug of choice in camel trypanosomiasis caused by *T. evansi*, but suramin in a 10 per cent aqueous solution given at 7 to 10 mg/kg intravenously is also effective but more expensive. Furthermore, isolates of *T. evansi* resistant to suramin are becoming more common, while such isolates remain sensitive to quinapyramine. Although suramin has a narrow margin of safety and causes toxic reactions in the liver and kidneys of other animal species, camels seem to be unaffected.

CONTROL

The control of animal trypanosomiasis has been directed at both the organism and the vector, the tsetse fly. Only limited success has been achieved in eradicating tsetse flies because of their ecologic distribution and habits. Most control or eradication programs have been based on ground application of insecticides (DDT, dieldrin, endosulfan) by discriminate spraying or by aerial application using helicopters or fixed-wing planes. Because re-infestation has been one of the problems in large scale eradication programs, and because residual tsetse flies that survive insecticide application may, though undetectable, cause significant disease problems, biologic control using the sterile insect technique (SIT) has been introduced as a mop-up operation and possibly as a barrier.

Because some animals are able to tolerate a certain degree of trypanosomiasis risk, they are regarded as trypanotolerant. Such trypanotolerant animals are being used more frequently in areas where tsetse fly eradication is both economically and technically infeasible.

Vaccination against trypanosomiasis appears promising based on the facts that some animals are trypanotolerant and that some acquire protective immunity following exposure and treatment. This method of control has to overcome the problem of antigenic variation, however. In the final analysis, it is probably a measure of integrating chemotherapy, vector control, and effective immune response that will guarantee the control or eradication of animal trypanosomiasis.

Supplemental Reading

FAO-WHO: The African Trypanosomiases. Report of a Joint WHO Expert Committee and FAO Expert Consultation. Rome, 1979.

Ilemobade, A. A. (ed.): Proceedings of the First National Conference on Tsetse and Trypanosomiasis Research in Nigeria. Kaduna, Nigeria, 1981.

Losos, G., and Ikede, B. O.: Review of pathology of diseases in domestic and laboratory animals caused by *Trypanosoma congolense, T. vivax, T. brucei, T. rhodesiense* and *T. gambiense.* Vet. Pathol. Suppl. *9:*1–71, 1972.

Mulligan, H. W. (ed.): The African Trypanosomiases. London, George & Unwin Ltd., 1970.

Williamson, J.: Chemotherapy of African trypanosomiasis. Trop. Dis. Bull. *73:*531–542, 1976.

Tick-Borne Fever

ERVIN J. BAAS, D.V.M., Ph.D.

Tick-borne fever (TBF) is a mild to acute infectious, noncontagious disease of sheep, goats, and cattle, and is characterized by fever, anorexia, weight loss, abortion, and infertility. The disease is caused by *Rickettsia phagocytophilia (Cytoectes phagocytophilia, C. ovis* var. *decani, Ehrlichia ovis,* and *E. phagocytophilia).* TBF is widely distributed and of economic concern in endemic areas of the United Kingdom, some European countries, Africa, and India, wherever the raising of cattle, sheep, and goats is prevalent.

EPIZOOTIOLOGY

Natural transmission requires *Ixodes ricinus* ticks in Europe and *Rhipicephalus haemophysaloides* ticks in India. Female nymphs and adult ticks spread the organism during the sucking of blood. The organism does not pass transovarially in the female tick. In the blood of the mammalian host, the organism enters the cytoplasm of granulocytes and monocytes, replicates, and discharges substances that induce a febrile reaction.

In endemic areas, latent carriers are a source of infection to young animals that may have only inapparent or minor infections. Mortality may reach 10 per cent, and the survivors develop an immunity lasting up to 1 year. A higher incidence of severe disease is found in unexposed, older animals that are brought into endemic areas.

CLINICAL SIGNS AND LESIONS

The incubation period varies from 3 to 13 days. The host's temperature rises abruptly to 39 to 42°C, persists 2 to 12 days, and then falls to normal. Animals with mild disease develop listlessness, inappetence, and weight loss. There is a low mortality rate. Animals with more severe disease may have lameness, a drop in milk production, and 30 per cent may abort in late pregnancy. A 7-per cent mortality rate is observed in these animals. Breeding males may become infertile for up to 2 months because of impaired spermatogenesis. TBF may exacerbate other illnesses. Thus, more severe signs and higher mortality rates may be caused by secondary disorders.

The causative agent, which can persist in blood for several weeks after cessation of signs, forms cytoplasmic inclusions in up to 95 per cent of the granulocytes and monocytes. Inclusions appear as single pleomorphic 1 to 2 μm elementary particles or as 2 to 4 μm aggregates, taking different forms (as seen with light microscopy) that include small, tightly packed homogeneous masses, fragmented and ring forms dispersed by "vacuole fluids," and large inclusions with many particles called "morula." Inclusions stain gray, black, or blue with Romanowsky's, methylene blue, or Geimsa stain. Neutropenia, lymphocytopenia, thrombocytopenia, and anemia may develop.

An enlarged spleen is the primary lesion found during the postfebrile state of TBF. There may be secondary infections with pyogenic *Staphylococcus* and *Pasteurella* spp., causing lameness, pneumonia, or hemorrhagic enteritis.

Additional lesions must not be overlooked, as more dual infections have been recognized and reported in recent medical literature. Listeriosis with TBF can induce low serum iron and albumin levels, swollen livers and spleens, and miliary granulomas in the liver, spleen, adrenals, and kidneys. Lymphopenia induced by *R. phagocytophilia* is associated with a profound decline in circulating B-lymphocytes and a decline in humoral antibody responses during clinical episodes. Experimentally, vaccination with *Clostridium chauvoei* has produced significantly low titers in sheep infected with TBF.

DIAGNOSIS

A tentative diagnosis can be based on evidence of tick infestation and typical clinical signs, but confirmation depends upon the presence of inclusions. Serologically, complement fixation test results are reliable. Differential diagnosis should include other diseases characterized by abortions, such as louping ill, enzootic abortion, and vibriosis. TBF should be considered as a predisposing condition in other diseases. *Listeria* septicemia can be more severe with TBF, but meningoencephalitis hasn't been reported. When lambs were infected simultaneously with parainfluenza type 3 virus, TBF induced longer viral excretion and depressed antiviral antibody production. This supports the postulated role of TBF in outbreaks of sheep pneumonia, prevalent in sheep of Scotland.

IMMUNITY, TREATMENT, AND PREVENTION

A short, variable immunity develops, the duration of which may be influenced by the different degrees of virulence among the strains found in ruminant species.

Individual animals may be treated effectively with tetracycline (5 to 10 mg/kg intravenously or orally). Secondary diseases will require appropriate treatment.

Tick control is difficult because there are no acaricides available that have sufficient residual activity for use on pastures. Exposure of susceptible and, especially, pregnant animals to pastures heavily infested with ticks should be avoided. Exposure during low tick activity may help animals develop immunity without severe disease. This immunity can be sustained with continual exposure. Isolation of TBF from wild deer and goats indicates that they may serve as carriers and potential sources of infection for susceptible sheep and goats in areas where suitable vectors exist.

Supplemental Reading

Batungbacal, M. R., and Scott, G. R.: Tick-borne fever and concurrent parainfluenza-3 virus infections in sheep. J. Comp. Path. 92:415–428, 1982.

Greig, A., and MacLeod, N. S. M.: Tick-borne fever in association with mucosal disease and cobalt deficiency in calves. Vet. Record. 100:562–564, 1977.

Gronstol, H., and Overas, J.: Listeriosis in sheep: tick-borne fever used as a model to study predisposing factors. Acta Vet. Scand. 21:533–545, 1980.

Jensen, R.: Tick-borne Fever in Diseases of Sheep. Philadelphia, Lea & Febiger, 43–46, 1974.

Snodgrass, D. R., and Ramachandran, S.: A complement fixation test for tick-borne fever of sheep. Brit. Vet. J. 127:14, 1971.

Heartwater

(Cowdriosis, Blacklung, Daji Enguruti, Kabowa, Khadar, Magak)

ALBERT A. ILEMOBADE, D.V.M., M.S., Ph.D.

Heartwater is a tick-borne septicemic disease of ruminants caused by a rickettsial organism, *Cowdria ruminantium,* characterized by high fever, abnormal nervous system signs, and sudden death.

DISTRIBUTION

Heartwater is found in Africa, south of the Sahara, including Madagascar. The statement that the disease is confined to those areas where ticks belonging to the genus *Amblyomma* are found, is to some extent supported by the recent confirmation of its presence in the Caribbean islands, raising the specter of the disease's spreading to the American continent. A heartwater-like disease has been reported from Yugoslavia and Malaysia.

ETIOLOGY

C. ruminantium is an intracellular rickettsial organism growing singly in colonies or in clumps (Fig. 1) with a predilection for the vascular endothelium of the ruminant host. Recently, 2 strains of *C. ruminantium* isolated from field cases were reported to be infective to mice. Some other reports have indicated that ferrets are, to some degree, susceptible. Although attempts to grow the organism in chicken embryo or cell culture have not been successful, there is indication that the organism is able to survive for 2 weeks or more in primary goat kidney cell culture.

Morphologically, the organism is pleomorphic and consists of small coccus-shaped, spherical, ellipsoidal, and occasionally rod-shaped bodies ranging from 0.2 to 2.5 microns in diameter. The organism is gram-negative and stains blue with Romanovsky's preparation.

TRANSMISSION

Only 5 of the known 16 species of *Amblyomma* ticks that feed on mammals have been shown to transmit the disease in nature. These are *A. gemma, A. hebraeum, A. lepidum, A. pomposum,* and *A. variegatum.* Transmission is stage to stage but not transovarial. Recovered ruminants remain carriers for at least 60 days, and adult *A. variegatum* retain infectivity for over 15 months after infected nymphs have molted. Two species of American *Amblyomma* (*A. maculatum* and *A. cajannense*) have been shown experimentally to be capable of transmitting the disease.

PATHOGENESIS

There are still gaps in our knowledge of the pathogenesis of heartwater. When *C. ruminantium* is introduced into the ruminant host either by ticks or by needle, it is removed from circulation by free mononuclear phagocytes and by those lining blood and lymph sinuses. The organism is subsequently transported to the regional lymph nodes, which probably serve as the primary replication site. Rupture of lymph node endothelial cells leads to release of *C. ruminantium* into lymph sinuses, and from there organisms are then transported by the different lymph tissue into blood circulation, with subsequent parasitization of vascular endothelium of body organs. The cause of death is still undetermined.

CLINICAL SIGNS AND LESIONS

Generally, the incubation period in goats and sheep, irrespective of the mode of infection, varies between 14 and 17 days. In cattle, it is between 10 and 16 days but may be as long as 35 days. Depending on the susceptibility of individual animals and breeds and on the virulence of the infecting organism, different forms of heartwater have been recognized. These are peracute, acute, subacute, and mild or inapparent cases.

Peracute Cases

These are characterized by sudden death with the presence of clinical signs not longer than 36 hr. Affected

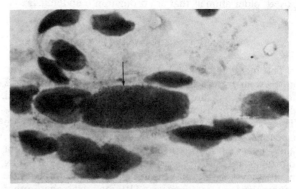

Figure 1. A large colony of *Cowdria ruminantium* (arrow) in the endothelial cell of brain capillary.

animals suddenly develop febrile reactions with a rectal temperature of 41°C or above within 6 to 12 hr. This is usually followed by prostration, collapse, and death after paroxysmal convulsions.

Acute Cases

Acute cases are the most common clinical forms in susceptible animals, with temperature elevation being the first sign. Temperatures of 41°C or higher are common and usually develop within 12 hr. Initially, feeding and rumination are normal, but later some sluggishness may be observed. This is frequently followed by reduced appetite, cessation of rumination, and difficult respiration, often of the abdominal type. Affected animals show progressively unsteady gait and commonly stand with legs apart. In an apparent attempt to steady themselves, they frequently lean against the wall for support. In fatal cases, animals assume lateral recumbency with legs stretched out and, subsequently, pedaling movements that may last 2 minutes at a time may be observed. Animals exhibit chewing movements, frothy mouth, continual licking of the lips, and opisthotonos. Nystagmus is commonly observed and becomes more intense with the progress of nervous convulsions. Abortion may occur, and diarrhea, which occurs more frequently in cattle than in sheep and goats, may be observed. The course of the disease runs between 2 and 6 days, and recovery, which is infrequent, is usually prolonged and protracted. In susceptible animals, morbidity and mortality may approach 100 per cent.

Subacute Cases

These cases are similar to the acute cases except that they are usually less intense. The course runs for up to 10 days when affected animals may suddenly collapse and die. Recovery seldom occurs and is usually prolonged.

Mild Cases

In this type, affected animals do not exhibit any clinical signs. The significance of the mild form is that it serves as a good source of infection for ticks and of perpetuation of infection in endemic areas.

CLINICAL PATHOLOGY

A common finding is eosinopenia. Lymphopenia and neutropenia have been observed in experimentally infected goats. The packed cell volume is usually normal, although a marked decline may be observed immediately prior to death. Notable disturbances of the acid-base balance have been reported.

NECROPSY FINDINGS

In general, the cadaver has no unusual pathological lesions. The lesions in peracute forms are limited to subepicardial and subendocardial hemorrhages. In other forms of the disease, typical lesions commonly include abrasions due to mechanical injury sustained during nervous convulsions, ascites, hydrothorax, and hydropericardium (hence, the name heartwater). The pericardial fluid is usually straw-colored and clots on exposure to air. In addition, pulmonary edema, congestion of lungs, subepi-cardial and subendocardial hemorrhages, hyperemia of the gastrointestinal tract, and edema of the lymph nodes (particularly those of the mesentery) are commonly observed. Histopathologic examination reveals very little, apart from leukostasis of the brain and perivascular infiltration of mononuclear cells.

DIAGNOSIS

Since there are no pathognomonic signs, antemortem confirmation of diagnosis is extremely difficult. Brain biopsy techniques have been successful under experimental conditions in goats but are not feasible under field conditions. Sudden deaths following nervous convulsions with pedaling movements, a history of heartwater in the area, and the presence of *Amblyomma* ticks are helpful towards arriving at a tentative diagnosis. Confirmation of diagnosis is based on the microscopic demonstration of *C. ruminantium* in Giemsa-stained squash smears of brain cortex. Preferably, smears should be made within 24 hr of death because the organism progressively loses stainability postmortem.

Differentiation of heartwater from anthrax, tetanus, strychnine poisoning, cerebral babesiosis, rabies, and hypomagnesemic tetany is necessary. The peracute and acute forms resemble anthrax, but the presence in natural orifices of dark tarry blood that fails to clot on exposure to air, and the presence of *Bacillus anthracis* in the blood differentiates this condition from heartwater. In tetanus, prolapse of the third eyelid, tetany of the masseter muscles, and normal temperature and pulse are commonly observed; such signs are not observed in heartwater. Strychnine poisoning is uncommon in farm animals and when it occurs, it usually results from overdosing, and the history is usually conclusive. In cerebral babesiosis, the abnormal nervous system signs are usually less severe, and there is commonly evidence of anemia and *Babesia bovis* in brain squash smears. Decreased sensation following the initial nervous system's reaction, weakness especially of the hindquarters, lack of gross abnormalities at postmortem examination, and the presence of Negri bodies help differentiate rabies from heartwater. Hypomagnesemic tetany can be identified by the brief period of tetany, by the progressive depression of consciousness, and by the favorable response to administration of calcium-magnesium preparations.

TREATMENT

Under field conditions, treatment is generally disappointing because of the difficulty of early diagnosis and poor response in the later stages of the disease. Tetracyclines are the drugs of choice, with 2 doses of 5 mg/kg intramuscularly at intervals of 24 hr at the early stages of the disease usually sufficing. Recent investigations have shown that a new, long-acting oxytetracycline (Terramycin/LA*) is equally effective when given as a single dose of 20 mg/kg intramuscularly. Once abnormal nervous system reactions are supervened, the prognosis is poor, although a recent investigation showed that Terramy-

---

*Available from Pfizer, Inc., New York, NY 10017.

cin/LA was effective in approximately 50 per cent of such cases, when the total dosage was divided into 2; 1 dose given intramuscularly and the other dose given intravenously.

CONTROL

Calves and lambs up to 4 weeks old and kids up to 6 weeks old possess natural resistance to the disease, and can, therefore, be vaccinated with virulent organisms in blood. More than 90 per cent of animals vaccinated in this way resist subsequent lethal challenge. Older animals can be immunized by the method of "infection and treatment," using blood or ground tick stabilate. Since the infective blood or tick stabilate must be given intravenously in order to produce the appropriate reaction, more convenient routes of inoculation have been ex-plored. Brain homogenates from infected animals have now been shown to be equally reliable when given subcutaneously. Strategic tick control is crucial as a complement to any method aimed at controlling the disease.

Supplemental Reading

Camus, E., and Barre, N.: La Cowdriose, revue générale des connaissances. Maisons-Alfort, France, Institut d'Élevage et de Médecine Vétérinaire des Pays Tropicaux, 147, 1983.

Haig, D. A.: Tick-borne rickettsioses in South Africa. Adv. Vet. Sci. 2:307–325, 1955.

Ilemobade, A. A., and Leeflang, P.: Epidemiology of heartwater in Nigeria. Rev. Elev. Med. Vet. Pays. Trop. 30:149–155, 1977.

Ilemobade, A. A., and Blotkamp, C.: Heartwater in Nigeria. II. The isolation of Cowdria ruminantium from live and dead animals and the importance of routes of inoculation. Trop. Anim. Health Prod. 10:39–44, 1978.

Uilenberg, G.: Heartwater disease. In Ristic, M. and McIntyre, I. (eds.). Diseases of Cattle in the Tropics. The Hague, Nijhoff Publishers, 345–360, 1981.

DISEASES OF THE RESPIRATORY SYSTEM

JEROME G. VESTWEBER, D.V.M., Ph.D.
Consulting Editor

Pathophysiology of the Bovine, Ovine, and Porcine Respiratory Tract*

JEROME G. VESTWEBER, D.V.M., Ph.D.

ANATOMY AND FUNCTION OF THE RESPIRATORY TRACT

The primary function of the respiratory system is the transport of oxygen from the external environment to body cells and of carbon dioxide from the cells to the external environment (Fig. 1). For effective respiration to take place, three inter-related mechanisms must function: (1) alveolar ventilation of the lung, (2) diffusion of gases to and from the alveoli–pulmonary capillary system, and (3) pulmonary blood flow. Respiratory disease includes any abnormality that causes disruption or failure of these mechanisms.

The pulmonary system includes structures necessary for external respiration (the upper and lower airways, thoracic wall and diaphragm, pleural space, gas exchange area, and supporting structures of the lung) as well as structures necessary for internal respiration (metabolizing cells and cardiovascular system). The respiratory tract is designed so that air can be conducted easily from the nose to the peripheral alveoli. For efficient gaseous exchange to take place, a large alveolar surface area is required. There are approximately 300×10^6 alveoli in animals the size of a sheep, providing a gaseous exchange area of approximately 80 m². The remaining portion of the respiratory tract is made up of tubing for conducting air from the nose to the alveoli. This tubing must remain patent so there is no obstruction to airflow.

The pulmonary system also serves the important functions of metabolic activity and lung defense. Metabolic functions include regulation of body temperature, acid/base balance, blood pressure regulation (enzymatic activation of angiotensin I to angiotensin II), and the production of histamines, prostaglandins E and F, serotonin, norepinephrine, and bradykinin.

The lungs are continuously exposed to air that contains dust, bacteria, fungi, viruses, and various noxious agents; defense against these potentially harmful materials is controlled by a complex of protective mechanisms. The structure and function of the respiratory tract is important in this defense mechanism because of the vulnerability of the system.

Nasal Cavity and Oropharynx

The nasal cavity, which has a large internal surface area because of the turbinates, functions in warming and

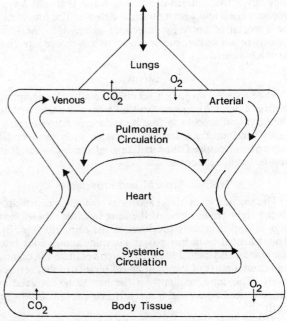

Figure 1. Total respiratory system includes the external respiratory section (upper airways, lungs, and chest wall) and internal respiratory section (metabolizing cells and cardiovascular systems).

*Kansas Agricultural Experimental Station, Contribution #84-252-B.

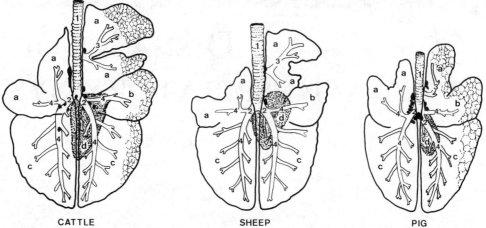

Figure 2. Trachea, bronchi and lungs of cattle, sheep and pig; dorsal aspect. a. Apical lobe; b. Middle lobe; c. Caudal lobe; d. Accessory lobe. 1. Trachea, 2. Principal bronchus, 3. Tracheal bronchus, 4. Bronchi.

humidifying incoming air. Additionally, it functions in aerodynamic filtration of particles larger than 10 microns by inertial impaction of these particles on the mucous membrane. Humidification of incoming air is important because it increases particle size and helps particles to settle out anteriorly in the respiratory tract. Impinged particles and secreted mucus are moved posteriorly by ciliary action to the oropharynx and swallowed. Drying of the mucous membrane is the most important cause of interference with ciliary action and, hence, the clearance mechanism. The temperature of the nasal cavity is lower than deeper parts of the body. This phenomenon is important when temperature-sensitive mutants of viruses are employed as vaccines.

The tonsils are located strategically at the site of greatest impaction in the nasopharynx and function as immunologically active antigen-processing tissue that aids laryngopharyngeal and gastrointestinal defense. The tonsils can be a portal of entry for infectious agents into the lymphatics or adjacent tissue or can act as a source of infection to other animals.

Larynx

The laryngeal opening is relatively small and is a limiting orifice. Forceful or rapid breathing may dry and irritate the laryngeal mucosa so that bacteria may become established and produce laryngeal lesions such as necrotic laryngitis of cattle. Other irritating inhalants can result in severe laryngeal edema.

Trachea, Bronchi, and Bronchioles

The trachea gives off an accessory asymmetric bronchus to the right cranial lobe of the lung in cattle, sheep, and pigs at approximately the level of the third rib (Fig. 2). This tracheal bronchus passes laterally and divides into the cranial and caudal bronchi, which ventilate the cranial and caudal parts of the right apical (cranial) lobe, respectively. This lobe frequently is the first to be involved in bronchopneumonia and frequently is atelectatic following birth.

The trachea bifurcates distal to the accessory bronchus into the right and left principal bronchi, which give off additional bronchi to different lobes of the lung (see Fig. 2). Further division occurs into secondary bronchi and

into one terminal bronchiole that serves a primary lobule of the lung. Bronchioles are defined as airways not having cartilage in their walls; they may collapse by pressure from surrounding pneumonic tissue, spasms of smooth muscle in walls, or during anaphylactic shock. The primary lobules are considered the basic respiratory portions of the lung.

Inhaled particulate matter that ranges in size from 2 to 10 microns is deposited from the larynx to the terminal bronchioles on airways lined by mucus-covered ciliated epithelium and is removed by the mucociliary transport system or by the cough mechanism. The ciliated airways transport this mucus-particulate matter to the oropharynx, to be swallowed there at a rate of approximately 15 mm per minute. Ciliated cells extend down to the terminal bronchioles, but their numbers are few in comparison with the major bronchi and trachea. Intercellular connections between ciliated cells allow coordination of movement, primarily upward toward the oropharynx. Destruction of the ciliated cells by infectious agents, high levels of gaseous irritants, or extremes in temperature or humidity may hinder flow rate.

Mucus has the physical properties of viscosity and elasticity. Infected mucus resulting from bronchitis is transported poorly because of increased viscosity and reduced elasticity. Mucus is made up of two layers: an outer gel layer derived primarily from goblet cells, and an inner sol layer contributed by submucosal glands. Mucus serves to prevent epithelial dehydration and has protective factors against infectious agents. Ninety per cent of the material deposited on the mucociliary blanket is cleared effectively within one hour. Factors such as dehydration, extremely cold inspired air, irritant gases such as ammonia, abnormal body electrolytes, anesthetics, general hypoxemia, or infectious agents such as viruses will impede mucociliary activity. If the presence of these factors allows pathogenic bacterial agents to colonize or remain in the upper respiratory tract for as long as three to four hours, infection probably will occur.

The cough reflex occurs in response to irritation of the respiratory tract, and the stimulus may arise anywhere between the pharynx and secondary branches of the bronchi. The most sensitive areas are in the region of the larynx and tracheal bifurcation. The smaller bronchioles are relatively insensitive. A cough may not result in expulsion of mucus from peripheral airways because of relatively low airflow rates, but compression of small airways resulting from high intrathoracic pressures can help produce a milking action that clears mucus to larger airways for subsequent removal. Difficulty in clearing secretions by this method is due mainly to increased viscosity and decreased elasticity of secretions.

Mechanical irritation of the larynx or trachea by inhalation of irritant gases, aerosols, and chemically inert dusts can produce bronchoconstriction. Reflex bronchoconstriction is a physiologic protective mechanism to prevent penetration of mechanical or chemical irritants further into the lungs.

Lungs

The right lung is divided into the apical (cranial), middle, diaphragmatic (caudal), and accessory lobes, whereas the left lung is divided into the apical (cranial) and diaphragmatic (caudal) lobes (see Fig. 2). The right lung has 55 to 60 per cent of the total lung volume. A lobule is the functional unit of the lungs and consists of a terminal bronchiole, poorly developed respiratory bronchiole, alveolar duct, alveolar sacs, and alveoli. In comparison with other domestic animals, cattle, sheep, and pigs have very extensive interlobular connective tissue or septa around these lobules that is continuous with a thick pleura covering the lung. This complete septum results in a lack of collateral ventilation between adjacent lobules.

In cattle, sheep, and pigs, the terminal bronchiole is the last airway into the lobule and the respiratory bronchiole is poorly developed. Respiratory bronchioles have alveoli developing from their walls, although this is not characteristic of terminal bronchioles. This creates difficulty in clearing plugs of mucus exudates from these distal terminal bronchioles because of the lack of collateral ventilation.

Interalveolar pores (pores of Kohn) occur infrequently between alveoli of the bovine. These pores communicate between alveoli and are important in the clearance mechanisms of the lung, especially if terminal bronchioles are plugged. Normally, air from unaffected alveoli will pass through the pores of Kohn and help force exudate out of the alveolus up to the mucociliary transport system. If an infected mucus plug is not cleared from the terminal bronchiole, it may become organized by fibrous connective tissue and completely occlude the bronchiole, resulting in collapse or emphysema of the affected lobule.

The three primary cells in the alveoli are the type I and II pneumocytes and the macrophages. Most of the alveolus is lined by the cytoplasm of type I pneumocytes and forms part of the blood-air barrier. At its thinnest, the barrier consists of type I pneumocyte cytoplasm, fused basement membranes, and vascular endothelial cell cytoplasm. These structures can be damaged easily, resulting in exudation of edema fluid, fibrinogen, and blood cells into the alveolus.

The type II pneumocyte is regarded as a precursor of the type I cell, and if there is lung damage, it rapidly proliferates to line the alveolus, producing what is called "epithelialization," "fetalization," or an "adenomatous" response. The type II pneumocyte also produces surfactant, a complex lipoprotein that forms a thin layer over the entire surface of the alveolus. Surfactant is responsible for maintaining low surface tension in the lung and preventing alveolar collapse. A lack of adequate levels of surfactant at birth can cause respiratory distress syndrome in the first day of life because the lungs will not remain inflated.

The alveolar macrophages are capable of killing bacteria by phagocytosis, engulfing debris in the alveoli, producing interferon, and, possibly, assisting in maintaining alveolar surfactant levels. Cattle appear to have fewer alveolar macrophages in the alveolar lumen than other mammals. Unlike peritoneal macrophages that function with lower pO_2 levels, alveolar macrophages function poorly in hypoventilated alveoli. Inflation of irritant materials will increase their numbers up to four times. The metabolic activity of macrophages has proved to require high levels of pO_2, the divalent cations (Ca^{++}, Mg^{++}), an energy source, proper pH, and isotonicity for optimum phagocytosis. Hypoxia, starvation, and acidosis will slow pulmonary clearance by alveolar macrophages.

Macrophage function also has been shown to diminish after infection with viruses. At least two bovine respiratory viruses infect alveolar macrophages. Parainfluenza-3 infects macrophages *in vivo* and *in vitro,* resulting in persistent infection. *In vitro* infection with infectious bovine rhinotracheitis virus results in reduced competence of the macrophages and subsequent cell death. Macrophage function also may be reduced under the influence of high endogenous concentrations of adrenal corticosteroid. Large concentrations of *Pasteurella haemolytica* in cattle (following viral- or steroid-induced impairment of macrophage function) may be able to further impair macrophage function and produce cytotoxicity toward macrophages.

Interferon is a product of the respiratory epithelium and alveolar macrophages and is present in respiratory secretions. To induce interferon synthesis, it is necessary for viruses, virus vaccines, or other synthetic polymers to penetrate respiratory cells. The affected cells release interferon, which enters unaffected cells to provide them with viral resistance by preventing viral replication. The principle of intranasal vaccination against infectious bovine rhinotracheitis and parainfluenza-3 is, in addition to local and systemic immunologic response, the production of interferon, which occurs within one to two days following administration. It also has been shown that intranasal vaccine strain infectious bovine rhinotracheitis virus will induce nasal secretion interferon, which will help protect against bovine rhinovirus and adenovirus.

Lysozymes produced by neutrophils, macrophages, alveolar macrophages, and glandular epithelial cells participate in bacteriolysis of gram-positive bacterial cell walls. These enzymes also participate in complement-antibody complex lysis of target cells. In addition, lactoferrin synthesized by glandular mucosal cells and polymorphonuclear leukocytes has potent bacteriostatic activity.

Bacteria, viruses, and fungi contain a wide variety of antigens to which the immune system can respond. The four classes of immunoglobulins defined at present are immunoglobulins (Ig) G, M, A, and E. There are two subclasses of IgG: IgG_1 and IgG_2. IgG_1 is the most important immunoglobulin transferred to the newborn animal in the colostrum.

IgM is a large immunoglobulin and remains within the intact blood vascular system. IgE is produced by plasma cells located within the respiratory and gastrointestinal mucous membranes. In some species, IgE is the immunoglobulin responsible for acute allergic reactions.

The respiratory tract produces local immunoglobulins,

such as IgA, that have virus-neutralizing properties and are a major component of local mucosal immunity. The antigenic stimulation for immunoglobulin production in pig lungs is reported to be initiated in lymphoid tissue along major bronchi and bronchioles called bronchus-associated lymphoid tissue (BALT). Immature B lymphocytes (thymus-independent) proliferate and differentiate in BALT and eventually migrate to areas of the respiratory epithelium. Respiratory immunoglobulins originating from other sources also may be present in the respiratory mucus. IgA and IgG from the systemic circulation may diffuse into the respiratory mucus.

PATHOLOGIC REACTIONS OF THE RESPIRATORY TRACT

Major components of any disease are the morphologic reactions involved in the affected tissue: the structural damage caused directly by the agent and the subsequent inflammatory response and repair process.

Mucous Membranes

The pathologic changes that occur with insult to the mucous membranes are similar for trauma, toxic chemical or bacterial exposure, or viral infection. The earliest changes are associated with destruction of ciliated or mucus-secretory cells which will be sloughed into the lumen. Often, in the early stages of infection viral-infected cells will be shed before they are dead, and these cells are good specimens for viral isolation or fluorescent antibody studies. Gradually, inflammation of the destroyed area develops with local intercellular edema, congestion, and leukocytic infiltration. Interferon production, secretion of IgA, and leakage of serum immunoglobulins occur with infectious agents.

The time needed for complete repair of epithelial surfaces depends on the species of animal, cause of injury, and the occurrence of secondary infection. Following mechanical injury, most of the epithelium is replaced by 14 days and is fully functional by 28 days. The repair rate following viral infection varies depending on the properties of the virus. Hyperplastic changes and the presence of viral inclusion bodies are seen with viral infections.

Nasal Cavity and Larynx

Inflammatory reactions in the nasal passages are common, especially when associated with upper respiratory tract viruses, such as infectious bovine rhinotracheitis of cattle. Observation of these mucous membranes will reveal an inflamed red color. A variety of organisms, such as *Pasteurella haemolytica, Pasteurella multocida,* and *Haemophilus somnus,* is able to colonize and reside in the nasal cavity. Organisms wait for the opportunity for the defense mechanism to be compromised, which allows their establishment in the lower respiratory tract.

Inflammation of the larynx reduces the luminal size dramatically, resulting in inspiratory dyspnea. Invasion of mucous membranes and supporting cartilage by micro-organisms can produce necrosis of these tissues and can result in more permanent problems such as intraluminal granulation tissue, necrotic cartilage, and hemiplegia.

Trachea, Bronchi, and Bronchioles

Mild tracheitis, which can only be detected microscopically, is not uncommon. Severe tracheitis is most usually due to viruses, such as infectious bovine rhinotracheitis, and also is associated with upper respiratory tract diseases, such as aspiration of infected debris from oral or pharyngeal lesions or accidental administration of liquids into the trachea.

Acute bronchitis frequently is associated with many viruses or bacteria. Chronic bronchitis may be recognized clinically by a persistent cough and excessive mucus secretion because of hypertrophy of mucus-secretory glands.

The bronchiolar epithelium is very sensitive to insult from chemical agents, viruses, and parasites. Necrosis, sloughing, regeneration, hyperplasia, and organization of mucus plugs are typical responses to injury in the bronchioles. The identification of viral inclusion bodies or the finding of lungworms is the only positive indication of cause. Bronchiolitis obliterans can result from severe local injury to the bronchiolar epithelium by bacterial, viral, parasitic, or chemical agents and is a feature of chronic bronchopneumonia. Areas of injury will have the basement membrane denuded; fibrinous exudate excretes into the lumen, followed by formation of fibroblasts that organize the exudate. Eventually the fibrinous cellular exudate is re-epithelialized, but the bronchiole will be partially or completely occluded. In experiments in which horses were given 3-methylindole to induce injury to the lungs, bronchiolitis obliterans could be found six days following administration. Severe mucus exudate accumulation or bronchiole obliteration within a specific bronchiole can result in several complications in the alveoli supplied: interference with airflow either in or out of the acini with resulting overinflation or collapse, reduced resistance to inhaled micro-organisms and resulting pneumonia, and release of inflammatory mediators and intracellular proteases that could be involved in the pathogenesis of emphysema.

Alveolar Atelectasis or Collapse

Atelectasis is described classically as an incomplete expansion of the lungs at birth, whereas the term "collapse" is reserved for previously inflated lungs. Although complete atelectasis of the lungs is found in the stillborn animal, partial atelectasis of the anterior ventral aspect of the lungs can be found in perinatal animals following the aspiration of fluid during birth. Areas of atelectasis potentially can predispose to the development of pneumonia at a later age. Atelectasis also is associated with hyaline membrane disease of human infants, the cause of which is believed to be a deficiency of saturated phospholipids of pulmonary surfactant. This disease is also seen in full-term neonatal pigs and cattle, but whether it is caused by a surfactant deficiency is not known.

Collapse of a lobule or lobules can be due to either bronchiolar obstruction or compression by surrounding pneumonic consolidation, abscesses, or extrapulmonary lesions such as hydrothorax, pneumothorax, or neoplasms. Collapse due to bronchiolar obstruction often is encountered in cattle, sheep, and pigs because of inadequate collateral ventilation.

Emphysema

Emphysema of the lung is characterized by an increase beyond normal in the size of the air spaces distal to the terminal bronchiole and destructive changes in the alveolar walls. This distinguishes emphysema from pulmonary overinflation, in which air spaces are enlarged but destructive changes are not present in the alveolar walls. Collateral ventilation through the pores of Kohn normally allows passage of air between adjacent normal alveoli of a lobule or between functioning alveoli of adjacent lobules. If the bronchiole supplying the alveoli is obstructed, the air within the alveoli is trapped and the volume increases with inspiration, but expiratory reduction does not occur. The walls of the alveoli become overdistended and thin, vascular supply is reduced, and walls rupture to produce cystic cavities. Emphysema is associated with chronic bronchopneumonia and is found outside areas of consolidation or atelectasis.

Interstitial emphysema is a necropsy finding of cattle and pigs owing to the entrance of air into the connective tissue of the interlobular septa. It is often a necropsy observation associated with agonal death following severe toxemia. Air may escape from the lungs and travel beneath the pleura into the mediastinum, then via the thoracic inlet to the subcutaneous tissues of the neck and back. The cause of interstitial emphysema is not fully known, but increased intrapulmonary pressure due to disease may cause rupture of terminal bronchioles and may result in passage of air to the interlobular septa.

Pulmonary Edema and Congestion

The barriers separating the vascular and alveolar spaces that are concerned with fluid balance are the capillary endothelium, basement membrane, alveolar epithelium, interstitial compartment, and pulmonary lymphatics. Movement of water into the alveolus or interstitium generally is associated with an alteration of structure and is caused by noxious agents, increased blood volume, or hydrostatic pressure. The equilibrium normally is maintained such that the alveolar surface is moist, but there is no large flux of water from the capillary bed into the alveolus. Pulmonary hypertension, heart failure, heart valve lesions, or mediastinal masses prevent the clearing of blood that comes from the lungs and may cause increased pulmonary venous pressure, with resulting congestion and edema of the lungs.

The permeability of the capillary-alveolar membranes also may be increased by infection (bacterial or viral pneumonia), endotoxins, inhaled noxious substances, uremia, allergic reactions, disseminated intravascular coagulation, and aspiration pneumonia.

Two stages of pulmonary edema are recognized. The first is interstitial edema, which is characterized by engorgement of the perivascular and peribronchial interstitial tissue. Pulmonary function usually is not affected at this stage. The second stage is alveolar edema; its development is not fully understood, but lymphatics may become overloaded, so that interstitial edema increases until fluid enters the alveoli.

The principal clinical signs of pulmonary edema are severe dyspnea, cyanosis, harsh vesicular sounds or moist rales (depending on amount of fluid present), and possible expectoration of foam or water from the trachea or nares.

Pneumonia

The conventional term "pneumonia" is reserved for the pathologic condition of inflammation of the lungs. Further division of pneumonia into exudative reaction of the alveolar space and cellular infiltration or proliferation of the alveolar wall or interstitial space will cover most of the pneumonias of cattle, sheep, and swine.

Bronchopneumonia or fibrinous pneumonia caused by pasteurellosis is the most common type of exudative reaction of the alveolar space. Exudation of fluid and infiltration of neutrophils into the air spaces are the major features of this disease.

Experimental production of *Pasteurella haemolytica* infection of the lungs in cattle produced the following sequence of lesions. Eighteen hours following intratracheal inoculation there were varying degrees of atelectasis, infiltration of neutrophils into alveolar spaces and bronchioles, and accumulation of macrophages and fibrin in alveoli. Exudate was prominent in and around the bronchioles. By three days, there was general distention of lymphatic vessels with fibrin and neutrophils; thrombosis of these vessels was common. A purulent exudate consisting of neutrophils and necrotic debris was present in bronchioles. Alveolar spaces contained large numbers of neutrophils, macrophages, occasional syncytial giant cells, and eosinophilic clots of fibrin. Small areas of coagulation necrosis were found in many calves. By seven days, lymphoid hyperplasia was extensive around bronchi and bronchioles; organizing obliterative bronchiolitis was observed. Small areas of necrosis were replaced by granulation tissue, and large areas of coagulation necrosis were still present. Fibrinous exudate in lymphatics and on the pleura was well organized.

As a general concept, it is well to think of any bronchopneumonic area of lung as passing through four successive stages. With treatment, the response may be abbreviated or aborted at any phase, and, frequently, the morphologic changes do not fit the classical descriptions. Furthermore, these divisions are arbitrary and all four stages represent a continuum of a single inflammatory reaction.

The first stage of active hyperemia (congestion) involves principally the development of extensive serous exudation and vascular distention. In this phase the alveolar septa are thickened by the engorged capillaries that contain aggregations of neutrophils, and the alveolar spaces are filled by a proteinaceous serous exudate. A few leukocytes may be present, chiefly neutrophils and macrophages. When the cause is an infectious agent, its development requires only a few hours.

In the second stage of early consolidation (so-called red hepatization), the affected area of lung is consolidated so that it has about the same degree of firmness as liver tissue. Although a considerable quantity of serous exudate may still remain in the alveoli, the consolidation (or hepatization) results from the filling of the alveoli with a cellular exudate usually mixed with fibrin. With the erythrocytes there are neutrophils, lymphocytes, and large mononuclear cells; the proportions depend upon the type and virulence of the causative agent.

In the third stage of late consolidation (gray hepatization), the lung tissue is still firm but less red than in the second stage. Microscopically, the hyperemia is not as apparent as in the second stage and the erythrocytes have disappeared from the alveolar contents, giving way to leukocytes and fibrin. The proportions of the different components of the exudate vary with the type and amount of the causative agent. If a pyogenic organism is the primary pathogen, the exudate consists largely of neutrophils and the lesion is described as a purulent pneumonia. Occasionally, depending on the causative agent, a predominantly fibrous pneumonia is seen.

The fourth phase, or the stage of resolution, occurs about a week after the onset of pneumonia. The causative agent has been eliminated or destroyed and the hyperemia has subsided. The cells and fibrin that fill the alveoli are liquified by proteolytic enzymes produced to a large extent by the leukocytes in the exudate. In a few days, the material that filled the alveoli is coughed up as a semisolid material and is drained away by the veins and lymphatics in a completely liquified state. The lining cells of the alveoli, most of which were destroyed during the inflammatory period, are regenerated within a few days, and the lung returns to morphologic and then to functional normality.

Pulmonary adenomatosis, chronic progressive pneumonia, and atypical interstitial pneumonia are examples of cellular infiltration or proliferation of the alveolar wall or interstitial space. Chronic progressive pneumonia and pulmonary adenomatosis are important diseases in sheep. In regard to the pathogenesis of chronic progressive pneumonia, it is thought that a virus stimulates reticular and lymphocyte cells to proliferate. This results in thickening of interalveolar septa from the presence of numerous histiocytes, new fibrocytes, and collagenous fibers. As the septa thicken, the squamous epithelial cells lining the alveoli morphologically transform into cuboidal cells. In addition, the peribronchiolar and perivascular lymphoid tissues undergo hyperplasia.

Pulmonary adenomatosis is characterized by adenomatous proliferation of the epithelial cells of the smallest bronchioles and alveoli after the prolonged, slow action of a virus of the epithelial cells.

Atypical interstitial pneumonia is also called acute bovine pulmonary emphysema and is an important disease in certain areas of the United States. The disease is characterized by pulmonary edema and emphysema with exudation into the alveoli of a protein-rich fluid, formation of hyaline membranes, epithelialization of the alveolar lining, and fibrous thickening of the alveolar septa. The current hypothesis of pathogenesis is that tryptophan, indoleacetic acid, or similar indolic compounds present in certain feeds or forages are converted to 3-methylindole by the action of rumen bacteria and are transported to the lungs, causing capillary endothelial and alveolar epithelial cell damage. The bovine respiratory syncytial virus has also been incriminated in this disease.

Supplemental Reading

Ardans, A. A.: Pulmonary structure, function and defense mechanisms. Proc. 8th Ann. A.A.B.P., 1975, 25–28.
Baskerville, A.: Mechanisms of infection in the respiratory tract. N. Z. Vet. J. 29:235–238, 1981.
Befus, A. D., and Bienenstock, J.: Immunology of the respiratory tract. Ill. Vet. Resp. Symp., 1978, 11–16.
Breeze, R.: Reactions to injury in the respiratory system. Ill. Vet. Resp. Symp., 1978, 204–228.
Breeze, R.: Structure and function in the respiratory system. Ill. Vet. Resp. Symp., 1978, 229–253.
Cummins, J. W., and Rosenquist, B. D.: Protection of calves against rhinovirus infection by nasal secretion interferon induced by infectious bovine rhinotracheitis virus. Am. J. Vet. Res. 41:161–165, 1980.
Cummins, J. W., and Rosenquist, B. D.: Temporary protection of calves against adenovirus infection by nasal secretion interferon induced by infectious bovine rhinotracheitis virus. Am. J. Vet. Res. 43:955–959, 1982.
Forman, A. J., Babuik, L. A., Baldwin, F., and Friend, S. C. E.: Effect of infectious bovine rhinotracheitis virus infection in calves on cell populations recovered by lung lavage. Am. J. Vet. Res. 43:1174–1179, 1982.
Frank, G. H.: Pasteurella haemolytica and respiratory disease in cattle. Proc. Ann. U.S. Animal Health Assoc., 83:153–160, 1979.
Friend, S. C., Thomson, R. G., and Wilkie, B. N.: Pulmonary lesions
Green, G. M., Jakab, G. J., Low, R. B., and Davis, G. S.: Defense mechanisms of the respiratory membrane. Am. Rev. Respir. Dis. 115:479–514, 1977.
Jubb, K. F., and Kennedy, P. C.: Pathology of Domestic Animals. Academic Press, New York, 154–281.
Markham, R. J., and Wilkie, B. N.: Interaction between Pasteurella haemolytica and bovine alveolar macrophages: Cytotoxic effect on macrophages and impaired phagocytosis. Am. J. Vet. Res. 41:18–22, 1980.
Osburn, B. I.: Immunologic concepts relating to the bovine respiratory system. Proc. 8th Ann. A.A.B.P., 1975, 30–32.
Veit, H. P., and Farrell, R. L.: The anatomy and physiology of the bovine respiratory system relating to pulmonary disease. Cornell Vet. 68:555–581, 1978.
Wilkie, B. N., and Markham, R. J. F.: Bronchoalveolar washing cells and immunoglobulins of clinically normal calves. Am. J. Vet. Res. 42:241–243, 1981.
induced by Pasteurella hemolytica in cattle. Can. J. Comp. Med. 41:219–223, 1977.

Upper Respiratory System

VAUGHN L. LARSON, D.V.M., Ph.D.

RHINITIS

Rhinosporidium spp. and Helminthosporium sp. fungi infect the nasal cavities of cattle, causing rhinitis. Allergic rhinitis is seen in pastured cattle and is called "summer snuffles." The inhalation of chemical fumes, smoke and exhaust fumes causes an irritant rhinitis. Calves raised in confinement over pits with inadequate ventilation often exhibit the signs of rhinitis.

Clinical Signs

Nasal discharge is the most prominent sign of rhinitis. This may be serous, mucoid, or suppurative, depending on the severity and chronicity of the disease. Usually serous discharge is seen early in the clinical course and this progresses to a mucoid discharge and then to a thick, suppurative exudate. Suppurative discharge is seen early in bacterial rhinitis but may not be seen in viral infections for several days or until secondary bacterial infection occurs. Nasal discharge may be blood-tinged in ulcerative rhinitis. Snorting and sneezing may be observed early in the course of rhinitis. Inspiratory dyspnea is usually only seen in severe infections or allergic reactions of the mucosa. Congestion of the mucous membranes is common, and erosions or ulcers are seen in some diseases.

Clinical Pathology

The laboratory findings and pathologic lesions of rhinitis in most cases depend on the causative disease and are discussed under those headings elsewhere in the text. The nasal cavity is a convenient site for obtaining specimens for bacterial and viral isolation of causative agents.

Treatment

Bacterial rhinitis is treated with parenterally administered antimicrobials. Since rhinitis usually is part of the respiratory disease complex, the reader is referred to that section for specific therapeutic recommendations. Allergic rhinitis can be relieved by irrigation of the nasal cavities with epinephrine solutions (1 ml 1:1000 epinephrine in

100 ml water) or parenteral corticosteroids (e.g., 0.02 mg/kg BW dexamethasone).

EPISTAXIS

Etiology

Bleeding from the nose can be due to either nasal cavity or pulmonary hemorrhage. Bleeding in the bronchial tree or hemoptysis is not always manifested as epistaxis unless it is extensive or unless the head is held low.

External trauma to the nasal and maxilla bones, dehorning and internal trauma from lodgement of objects in the nasal cavity, and passage of a nasogastric tube are common causes of nasal cavity hemorrhage. Usually slight hemorrhage is also observed in some cases of ulcerative rhinitis in cattle and atrophic rhinitis of swine. Nasal tumors and granulation tissue may ulcerate, causing slight recurrent epistaxis.

Severe pulmonary hemorrhage may be associated with erosion of pulmonary vessels by abscesses in chronic pneumonia. Also, severe hemorrhage may be seen following embolic showering of the lung in animals with vegetative endocarditis or thrombosis of the vena cava.

Epistaxis commonly is an early and prominent sign seen in diseases of blood coagulation. Disseminated intravascular coagulation may intervene in the course of many diseases, particularly those with endotoxemia such as Gram-negative bacterial infections of the uterus and mammary gland or in enteric diseases. Liver disease and the consumption of bracken fern or moldy sweet clover are causes of epistaxis due to coagulation deficiencies.

Clinical Signs

Epistaxis may vary from slight to profuse, may be unilateral or bilateral, and may be continuous or recurrent. Some recurrent cases may only present with evidence of previous bleeding such as nasal cavity clots or blood stains on the nostrils. Unilateral epistaxis is usually due to nasal cavity or paranasal sinus hemorrhage. Epistaxis due to pulmonary hemorrhage is usually bilateral, and in severe cases the blood may run in streams from both nostrils when the head is lowered. Coughing usually accompanies hemoptysis. Blood is swallowed, with resulting melena in chronic cases. Examination of the nasal cavity, pharynx, larynx, and trachea with a flexible fiberoptic endoscope usually is helpful in determining the source of hemorrhage.

Clinical signs in animals with epistaxis vary depending on the cause of hemorrhage. That due to trauma often is obvious. Bleeding associated with nasal cavity disease usually is accompanied by evidence of obstruction and inspiratory dyspnea. There is evidence of hemorrhage in other areas of the body in coagulopathies. Auscultation of the lungs and heart may reveal evidence of pneumonia or endocarditis if epistaxis is due to pulmonary hemorrhage.

Treatment

Epistaxis that is secondary to other diseases will resolve with successful treatment of the primary disease. Blood transfusions usually result in only transient improvement in severely anemic cases unless the primary cause of the hemorrhage is corrected. Traumatic epistaxis usually spontaneously resolves; however, bleeding time often can be reduced by repeated irrigation of the nasal cavity with epinephrine solutions (1 ml 1:1000 epinephrine in 100 ml water).

NASAL CAVITY OBSTRUCTION

Etiology

Partial obstruction of the nasal cavity commonly occurs in rhinitis because of inflammation of the mucosal lining and accumulation of exudates. Chronic obstructions are usually due to space-occupying lesions. Nasal polyps are common in cattle and sheep and rarely attain sufficient size to cause obstruction. Granulation tissue resulting from chronic infection or trauma or in reaction to foreign bodies occurs in the nasal passages. There are a few reports of nasal carcinomas and sarcomas in older food animals. Nasal adenocarcinoma of sheep and goats occurs endemically in some flocks and is thought to be due to a virus. Large obstructive growths can be caused by *Rhinosporidium* spp. and *Helminthosporium* sp. fungal infections.

Clinical Signs

Partial or unilateral obstruction may cause minimal signs in the nonstressed animal. Nasal discharge, inspiratory dyspnea, and stertor are usually exhibited variably depending on the degree of obstruction. Reduction or differences in airflow on expiration can be determined by placing the backs of the hands near the nostrils. Bilateral or complete occlusion of the passages causes significant distress, with the animal exhibiting mouth breathing.

The degree of obstruction and the location of the lesion can be determined by passing tubing of various sizes up the ventral meatus. Endoscopy may be used to visualize the lesion for biopsy and specific diagnosis.

Treatment

The prognosis of nasal obstruction is generally poor because of the limitations of treatment. Surgical removal of foreign bodies and polyps is possible in some cases.

SINUSITIS

Etiology

Frontal sinusitis is a common sequela of dehorning in cattle since the sinus is opened in this operation. Usually the problem spontaneously resolves. However, if the opening to the ethmoid meatus becomes occluded with exudates then the sinusitis becomes chronic. This becomes a significant problem if the dehorning incision closes prior to resolution of the sinus infection. The frontal sinuses as well as the maxillary and other paranasal sinuses can become infected as an extension of nasal cavity infections. The bones of the walls and septae can become infected by *Actinomyces bovis*. Sinus tumors of food animals rarely occur. *Oestrus ovis* larvae usually migrate to the maxillary and frontal sinuses, causing sinusitis in sheep.

Clinical Signs

A diagnosis of acute frontal sinusitis due to dehorning is usually obvious because of evidence of recent surgery.

Nasal discharge is prominent, as is the spillage of exudate from the surgical opening.

Animals with acute sinusitis due to ascending infection also exhibit nasal discharge. Percussion of the sinus regions elicits a dull sound.

In chronic sinusitis there may or may not be nasal discharge, depending on the patency of the openings to the nasal cavities. Some very chronic cases will persist for months or well beyond closure of the dehorning incision. The bones over the affected sinuses may become asymmetrically elevated. Dull percussion sounds are heard over the sinuses. The swelling of the sinus cavities can cause exophthalmus and strabismus. Pressure on the brain often causes neurologic signs such as opisthotonos and ataxia. The infection may extend to the meninges with the onset of acute meningitis. Radiographs usually reveal evidence of fluid accumulation and bone lysis.

Treatment

Acute sinusitis that persists following dehorning usually resolves following irrigation via the surgical incision with disinfectants (equal parts hydrogen peroxide [3 per cent] and povidone-iodine solution [10 per cent]). The treatment of chronic sinusitis must be more intensive and is less often successful. Animals showing evidence of extension of the disease should be treated with parenteral antibiotics (10 mg/kg oxytetracycline IV or IM SID). Successful treatment of chronic sinusitis requires opening of the sinuses for local treatment. The sinus should be opened at the dehorning site if the condition is a dehorning sequela or by a trephine opening over the most dependent area of the affected sinus, taking care not to damage vital structures. Long-term disinfectant irrigation is required in these cases.

PHARYNGITIS, LARYNGITIS, TRACHEITIS

Etiology

The upper air passages are usually involved along with the whole respiratory system in diseases grouped in the respiratory disease complex. Many of the etiologic agents colonize and replicate in the upper airways early in these diseases so that early clinical signs may be restricted to these anatomic sites. The following diseases are specific to the upper respiratory tract: infectious bovine rhinotracheitis and calf diphtheria in cattle, influenza in swine, and *Corynebacterium pyogenes* laryngitis of sheep.

Clinical Signs

A nonproductive cough is the most consistent clinical sign. The cough may be painful so that the animal may extend the head and mouth breathe between coughs. The lower trachea should be auscultated during coughing, since absence of rales indicates that the origin of the cough is due to upper respiratory irritation. Manual manipulation of the throat, cold air, and dust will induce coughing. Inspiratory dyspnea and stertorous breathing are seen with severe inflammation. Extreme irritation of the pharynx occasionally causes dysphagia. The regional soft tissues and lymph nodes are uncommonly involved.

The upper respiratory system of adult cattle can be thoroughly examined with a flexible endoscope. The larynx can usually be visualized via the mouth with the aid of a bright light and a cylindrical speculum.

Treatment

Infections of the upper respiratory system are treated with parenteral antibiotics at the same dosages as those recommended for the respiratory disease complex. The reader is referred to that section for specific therapeutic recommendations.

TRAUMATIC PHARYNGITIS

Etiology

Food animals are often treated by forced oral administration of medicants with minimal restraint by laymen with resulting damage to the pharynx. The injudicious administration of pills and magnets with a balling gun, liquids with a dose syringe, and fluids by esophageal feeders and the forceful passage of stiff stomach tubes cause the damage. Animals may cause similar trauma by inadvertently swallowing sharp objects. The problem with lacerations in this region is that ingesta impacts in the defects with resulting abscess or phlegmon.

Clinical Signs

The history of prior oral therapy is helpful in diagnosing this condition. Even in animals that were ill at the time of treatment there is usually a sudden deterioration in their condition. Anorexia is common, and many animals will not drink and become dehydrated. Inspiratory dyspnea is exhibited when severe inflammation of the pharynx develops. Usually there is some soft tissue swelling or fullness noted in the throat region. In severe cases, very large abscesses may form submucosally or in the regional lymph nodes. Occasionally, severe phlegmon will develop in the throat and extend to the intermandibular space or gravitate down the neck to the thoracic inlet.

In larger calves and cattle it is usually possible, via the mouth, to digitally palpate the damage in the pharyngeal mucosa. Endoscopy may be required for specific diagnosis in smaller food animals.

Treatment

In animals with extensive damage, therapy is usually unsuccessful and the best option is slaughter. Adult cattle with moderately superficial lesions can be managed by digitally removing ingesta from the defects twice a day and feeding a semi-fluid diet. This is done until granulation tissue fills the defect. Early in the disease a broad-spectrum antimicrobial therapy is indicated in those animals that are not to be slaughtered. Abscesses may point up later in the clinical course and can then be surgically drained.

OBSTRUCTION OF THE UPPER RESPIRATORY TRACT

Etiology

Partial and complete obstructions can occur in the pharynx, larynx, or trachea. Impediments to air movement through these structures can be due to a variety of causes. The pharynx can be impinged on by cellulitis of the throat or from abscesses or tumors in the retropharyngeal lymph nodes. In cattle and particularly calves, lymphosarcoma of these nodes often causes partial obstruction. Calf diphtheria and *Corynebacterium pyogenes* laryngitis of sheep can obstruct the larynx. Edema of the larynx may occur in allergic reactions in all species, as part of edema disease in swine, and as a reaction to irritation from trauma or the inhalation of smoke or chemical fumes. Perivascular cellulitis of the jugular veins can partially collapse the trachea. The tracheal diameter is also decreased when tracheal rings are fractured and in calves with congenital malformation of the rings.

Clinical Signs

Acute obstructions are manifested by severe dyspnea, anxiety, and cyanosis or even fatal asphyxia. Partial obstructions or those of a progressive nature are characterized by increasingly prominent thoracic movements during inspiration. Mouth breathing with extension of the head and loud stertor are prominent signs in advanced cases. Syncope or fatal asphyxia can result from agitation or forced exercise in these cases.

Treatment

Therapy is largely dependent on the cause and therefore varies from case to case. Regardless of cause, a tracheotomy will relieve the dyspnea and facilitate examination. The prompt administration of a corticosteroid and epinephrine is indicated in animals with laryngeal edema.

Supplemental Reading

Blood, D. C., Henderson, J. A., Radiostitis, O. M., et al.: Veterinary Medicine, 5th ed. Lea & Febiger, Philadelphia, 1979.
Jensen, R., and Swift, B. L.: Diseases of Sheep, 2nd ed. Lea & Febiger, Philadelphia, 1982.
Leman, A. D., et al.: Diseases of Swine, 5th ed. Iowa State University Press, Ames, Iowa, 1981.

Pneumonia

JEROME G. VESTWEBER, D.V.M., Ph.D.

Pneumonia occurs in all the food animal species (cattle, sheep, and swine) from a variety of causes, most of which are infectious. The most typical description of the disease when caused by a bacterial agent is a widespread exudative inflammatory reaction characterized by the formation of a fibrinosuppurative exudate that totally fills alveoli over a large area of the lung parenchyma. This inflammatory response follows the basic pattern of all inflammations and begins with serous exudation accompanied by active hyperemia. This is followed by a fibrinous exudation that creates the consolidation that is characteristic of pneumonia. Involvement of bronchi, bronchioles, and pleura also accompanies this disorder of the lung. The disease ranks high in economic importance to the food animal industry and is extremely costly for several reasons: immunity to some of the infectious agents is generally poor, vaccination has some limitations, and antibiotic therapy must be extensively applied to control the disease. Treatment may be life-saving, but loss in production by surviving animals may also result in economic liability.

ETIOLOGY

Respiratory disease in food animals is due to a complex of factors that often interact to produce disease. The management and environmental stresses placed on these animals are often the difference between the development of clinical diseases and the disease remaining subclinical.

Most of the viruses isolated will produce mild disease if not complicated by other factors, but they are capable of destroying the mucociliary transport system and depressing alveolar macrophage activity. The damaged respiratory tract offers a prime medium for secondary bacterial invaders. It is difficult to attribute primary responsibility of an infectious agent to specific pathologic changes, but in general viral agents are associated with upper respiratory tract disease and mild pathologic changes in lungs. The severe pathologic changes associated with pneumonia are primarily attributed to bacterial agents. Less frequently, mycotic agents and lungworms are involved in pneumonia or act in concert with viral and bacterial agents.

Cattle

Many infectious agents have been implicated as the cause of pneumonia and these include *Pasteurella multocida*, *Pasteurella haemolytica*, *Mycoplasma* spp., and parainfluenza-3 virus. Infectious bovine rhinotracheitis (IBR) virus and bovine virus diarrhea (BVD) virus may also be involved in pneumonia, but these two viruses usually produce separate, distinct clinical respiratory or digestive diseases, respectively. *Corynebacterium pyogenes* may be found as a secondary invader, especially if the pneumonia is chronic, and the organism usually produces abscessation of the lung. *Haemophilus somnus* is being found with increased frequency in pneumonia, but the role it plays in the respiratory tract is not as well defined as that in the central nervous system. The bovine respiratory syncytial virus and DN-599 virus have recently been isolated from respiratory disease of calves.

Parainfluenza-3 virus, adenovirus, rhinovirus, reovirus, enterovirus, herpesvirus, chlamydia agents, *Mycoplasma* spp., and *Pasteurella multocida* and *P. haemolytica* have all been isolated from cases of enzootic pneumonia of calves that characteristically occur during the animals' first six months of life when kept in enclosed crowded conditions where ventilation is inadequate and humidity high.

Atypical interstitial pneumonia has many synonyms such as acute pulmonary emphysema in nursing beef cows on recently occupied fall pasture, pulmonary adenomatosis in feedlot and pasture cattle, and the British names of "fog fever" in nursing cows on newly changed autumn pasture and "bovine farmer's lung disease" in cows in winter housing. Investigators have found that 3-methylindole, converted from tryptophan, and hypersensitivity to certain organisms, such as might occur with feeding moldy hay, are possible causal factors.

Swine

The most important cause of chronic pneumonia (enzootic pneumonia) in swine is *Mycoplasma hypopneumoniae*, whereas *Pasteurella multocida* is frequently involved in a secondary capacity in this disease.

Primary *Pasteurella multocida* infection is less frequent and will produce a fibrinous pneumonia. Often the migrating ascarid larvae have a predisposing capacity.

Young pigs can develop a severe pneumonia when exposed to swine influenza virus during the migration of swine Ascarid larvae through the lung. *Bordetella bronchiseptica* is capable of producing a chronic fibrosing bronchopneumonia in young pigs.

The reovirus, parovirus, pseudorabies virus, and enterovirus are all capable of producing an interstitial type of pneumonia in conjunction with other clinical involvement of the digestive, reproductive, or central nervous system.

Streptococcus spp. have been associated with pneumonia, and the lungworm *Metastrongylus elongatus* will produce a verminous pneumonia. Recently pleuropneumonia caused by *Haemophilus pleuropneumoniae* has been found in certain areas of the United States.

Sheep

The current knowledge of respiratory disease in sheep stems from pathologic descriptions of types of pneumonia rather than etiologic agents. Few viruses have been isolated.

Enzootic pneumonia (acute exudative) has been associated primarily with *Pasteurella multocida* and *P. haemolytica*. Stress factors will influence the severity of this pneumonia. This type of pneumonia is commonly preceded by infection with parainfluenza-3 virus or chlamydia agents.

Chronic progressive pneumonia (maedi) and pulmonary adenomatosis (jaagsiekte) are slowly progressive types of pulmonary disease thought to be caused by slow-acting viral agents. These viral agents cause a slow wasting type of respiratory disease in older sheep. Lungworm pneumonia also occurs in sheep.

PATHOGENESIS

There are two routes by which pathogenic organisms may enter the lungs: bronchogenic, which is the most frequent, and hematogenous. Around affected bronchioles, a pneumonic area forms and extends to the limits of the histologic lobule supplied by the bronchiole in question. Other lobules may also be affected, resulting in the affected portion of the lung being spotted with consolidated and relatively normal lobules in an irregular pattern. In the majority of penumonias that are bronchogenic in origin the anterior and ventral portions of the apical (cranial) and middle lobes of the lungs are first and most extensively affected. The disease may start and localize in the right lung because of the anterior asymmetrical bronchus coming off the trachea, but frequently both lungs are affected. It is not unusual for more than a third of the total of the two lungs to be consolidated, but frequently the process is much more limited.

Pneumonia of hematogenous origin may be lobular or lobar. The term "lobar" means that inflammation affects all lobules in a considerable area, even an entire lobe. Most pneumonias in food animals are lobular.

Although pneumonia is an inflammatory reaction taking place in the alveoli and their walls, the interlobular septa and other connective tissue structures are also distended with serous exudate. Bronchitis and bronchiolitis are often present in the pneumonic area. This is recognized by desquamation and disappearance of the epithelial lining cells, by an infiltration of lymphocytes and other leukocytes in the wall of the bronchus or bronchiole, and by

an accumulation of exudate in the lumen. The pleura over the pneumonic area may or may not share in the inflammatory process.

Some complications of pneumonia are the spread of the pneumonic process to new areas of lung tissue, and in the vicinity of the pneumonic changes there may be areas of lung collapse and overinflation or emphysema. Bronchiolar epithelium that has become ulcerated or plugged with necrotic inflammatory exudate can become organized with connective tissue from the ulcerated tissue resulting in a permanent bronchiole plug (bronchiolitis obliterans); this can further result in either collapse of lung tissue or emphysema. Overinflation or emphysema can also involve alveoli that expand beyond normal limits because of decreased space occupied by neighboring alveoli that are either collapsed or consolidated. The severity of collapse or emphysema is also in part proportional to the number of bronchioles that become partially or completely obliterated, thus allowing collateral ventilation of alveoli, trapping of air, and consequent rupture of alveolar walls. If fibrinous exudate remains for two weeks or longer in the alveoli, the same process occurs as when fibrin persists in a thrombus or in a fibrinous exudate elsewhere. The fibrin is organized by fibroblasts that grow into it from surrounding issues. Such an area is then converted permanently into fibrous connective tissue. This area of lung is now organized, and the original pulmonary parenchyma has been destroyed. With delayed resolution in a given area, other chronic changes may develop. The alveolar lining cells, normally flat and inconspicuous, may undergo hyperplasia and resemble cuboidal epithelium. The condition has also been called "fetalization" of the lining cells, since it resembles fetal lung. In pulmonary adenomatosis this change becomes extreme so that the area may resemble an adenoma.

CLINICAL SIGNS

Pneumonia will vary from the mildest syndrome, such as occurs with some cases of enzootic pneumonia of calves or pigs, to a rapidly fatal disease.

A bilateral mucopurulent nasal discharge may or may not be present depending upon the stage or duration of the disease. With acute pneumonia the nasal discharge is usually present, whereas if the disease is more chronic, the nasal discharge may be absent.

Coughing will be exhibited and will be moist and productive if the pneumonic process involves bronchi and bronchioles, and there is an accumulation of loose exudate within these respiratory passages. The cough will be more of a dry character if some of the following are present: the pneumonic process is in the early stages of hyperemia, there are chronic pathologic changes in the lung, or the pneumonia is more interstitial in character.

A fever is a good indicator of acute pneumonia and may range from 40 to 41°C. With response to treatment the fever will again decrease to the normal range, but lack of response suggests a viral pneumonia or lack of susceptibility of the causative organism. A fever that is slightly elevated (39 to 40°C) in an animal with some respiratory signs for a duration of five to seven days suggests incomplete resolution of the pneumonic process and permanent pathologic changes of the lungs.

Most animals will have an increased depth of respiration, whereas a few exhibit primarily shallow abdominal breathing. Most will have an inspiratory dyspnea, whereas fewer will have primarily an expiratory dyspnea.

If severe pain is present with pneumonia, it is usually indicative of a purulent pleuritis and will result in shallow respiratory movement and reluctance to move.

Extensive involvement of both lungs can result in open mouth breathing, extension of the head, dilation of the nostrils, abduction of the elbows, and the presence of thoracic inlet movement. Animals with chronic cases of pneumonia will be depressed, have gaunt appearance, exhibit inappetence, have fast, shallow, or labored respirations, expiratory grunt, some coughing, and usually a body temperature within the normal range.

AUSCULTATION OF THE LUNGS

When normal lung tissue is auscultated, vesicular sounds are heard. With abnormalities of the lungs, there will be harsh vesicular sounds in certain portions of the lung that remain functional. Bronchial sounds, which are normal over the trachea and the primary bronchi, are distinctly abnormal when they are heard over an extensive area of the lung field and usually indicate consolidation of the lungs. The absence of respiratory sounds is as important as the presence of abnormal sounds because no sounds imply that nonfunctional lung tissue is beneath the stethoscope unless the animal's breathing is very shallow.

Rales are always a sign of disease and are audible whenever movable exudate accumulates within the respiratory tract. Moist rales are often heard in early stages of pneumonia and they are heard throughout inspiration and expiration. They are heard as short, discontinuous crackling sounds produced by bubbles bursting in bronchial secretions. Moist rales indicate that transudate, mucus, pus, or blood is present in the bronchi, and if the rales are numerous there is considerable fluid present.

When pneumonia becomes more advanced or is resolved, the rales will become dry. The biggest difference between moist and dry rales is the consistency of fluid that produces the rales. Dry rales may vary from a shrill whistle to a deep hum and indicate inflammation of the mucous membranes of the bronchi or bronchioles and the presence of tenacious mucus partially occluding these respiratory passages.

Harsh vesicular sounds occur in showers in the terminal bronchi or bronchioles in the early and late stages of pneumonia. These sounds are a variety of moist rales, occur mostly on inspiration, and resemble hair rubbed between fingers close to the ear. They are produced by the passage of air into alveoli containing fluid and are suggestive of pulmonary edema or thin inflammatory fluid.

A pleural friction rub is pathognomonic for fibrinous pleuritis and sounds like squeaking leather. This sound is produced by roughening of the pleural surfaces and is usually best heard near the diaphragmatic portion of the lung, where the lung and pleura are making the greatest movement. Friction rubs are heard during both inspiration and expiration and are associated with a primary pleuritis, pneumonia, or secondary pleuritis. If frictional pleural sounds disappear, it may mean development of pleural adhesions so that the friction sounds no longer occur, or it may mean the secretion of fluid (exudate) so that the two pleural surfaces are separated and, therefore, again lubricated by fluid.

Emphysematous sounds are often heard as a squeak or whistle following the expiratory effort, or the sound simulates that produced by crushing a sheet of soft paper into a ball.

CLINICAL PATHOLOGY

A laboratory examination is indicated when the presented animal is representative of a herd problem or the economic value of the animal justifies in-depth investigation. Nasal or tracheal swabs may be utilized for either bacteriologic or viral isolation, but caution should be used in interpreting the bacterial findings from this method because it may not express the true pathogenic organisms responsible for the pneumonia. A transtracheal aspiration is more valuable in identifying the probable pathogenic bacteria and their spectrum of antibiotic sensitivity. A sterile disposable male canine catheter introduced through a 14-gauge needle placed between the tracheal rings anterior to the thoracic inlet will allow retrieval of organisms found deeper in the bronchi. Twenty-five ml of saline works well as a wash medium. Retrieval of 1 to 5 ml of the saline wash is all that is necessary for bacteriologic isolation.

Nasal scrapings of the mucosa cells with a chemical spatula can be placed on a clean, dry slide for viral fluorescent antibody studies. This method has the advantage over virus isolation of being a shorter laboratory test. Serologic testing of serum samples during the acute febrile and convalescent periods lends itself to viral identification. The disadvantage is the wait of two to four weeks to see if there is a fourfold increase in the titer.

Most white blood cell counts are within the upper normal range and will shift to the left with bacterial pneumonias, whereas a leukopenia and lymphopenia are more common with acute cases of viral pneumonia. The blood chemistry values for fibrinogen are usually elevated and are relative to the severity of the inflammatory process. With the availability of venous or arterial blood gases, a determination can be made of pulmonary function status. Radiographic examination will readily identify areas of abscessation, fibrosis, atelectasis, plugged bronchi and bronchioles, consolidation, and emphysema in calves, sheep, goats, and pigs, but size of cattle limits this procedure.

PATHOLOGY

Most of the pneumonias are bilateral, with the right apical lobe being affected first in bronchopneumonia because of the anterior bronchus supplying this lobe. Some animals die in the acute stages, and characteristic lesions are found. Extensive anteroventral portions of the cranial, middle, and caudal lobes are dark, red, gray, or red-black from infarction. The affected areas are hard and heavy, and the dark areas of consolidation are covered with varying amounts of fibrin on the pleural surface. Interlobular connective tissue is widened because of extensive edema, and lobulation is emphasized. Fibrin is also evident between lobules on the cut surface. Small, irregularly shaped pale areas of coagulation necrosis may develop in the parenchyma. Extensive lesions may be accompanied by emphysema of the remaining normal lung tissue.

Many animals not dying from acute disease develop debilitating chronic pneumonia. Pathologic findings include collapse due to obstruction of bronchioles. These affected areas are dark red and heavy but depressed below the surface of normal lung. The lung is variegated in color, consisting on cross sections of exaggerated lobular patterns with widened interlobular septa. There is progressive thickening of the alveolar septa and induration of the lung with some possibility of bronchiectasis. Organization of pleural exudate will result in permanent pleural adhesions. If the causative organisms are pyogenic, frank abscesses may occur. Lobular emphysema is common in chronic pneumonia and can be found between areas of pneumonia and collapse, whereas bullous areas are commonly found in more dorsal areas of the lung. Both alveolar and interstitial emphysema is prominent at the junction of the pneumonia and normal tissue.

The interstitial type of pneumonia usually involves both lungs and is characterized by uncollapsed, enlarged, and firm lungs. The caudal lobes are most commonly affected. The cut surface demonstrates pleural thickening and edema. Emphysema of interlobular, subpleural connective tissue and lymphatics is common.

Any bacterial or viral isolation taken from pathologic specimens should be accomplished in the early stages of pneumonia. If specimens are taken in the later stages, the primary pathogen may have disappeared and may be masked by changes induced by secondary agents.

DIAGNOSIS

A decision has to be made with an animal demonstrating respiratory insufficiency as to whether the problem is strictly confined to the respiratory system. Respiratory signs may be secondary to disease such as an infectious systemic disease, toxemia from a variety of causes, cardiac insufficiency, severe anemia, CNS disturbance, neoplasm of the thoracic cavity, poisoning, acid-base imbalance, diaphragmatic hernia, pleuritis, or obstructive upper respiratory disease. A thorough physical examination and basic clinical pathology parameters will help in making the decision whether this is primary respiratory disease.

The next decision to be made is whether the total respiratory system is involved or only part. To establish the area of the respiratory system involved, the character of respiration should be observed. Upper respiratory disease commonly produces an inspiratory dyspnea. Also, the sounds heard from the respiratory system are stenotic owing to narrowing of the air passageways. These sounds are whistling, roaring, or stenotic in character. The visual presence of hyperemia or swelling typical of inflammation or the presence of rales on auscultation of the trachea will clarify involvement of the upper respiratory system. Restrictive disease outside the lung caused by such diseases as pleuritis, hydrothorax, or diaphragmatic hernia commonly produces an expiratory type of dyspnea. Auscultation of the thorax will commonly produce no lung sounds in the ventral areas of the lung field. Thoracentesis will help make a diagnosis of these diseases.

Lastly, involvement of the lung itself with pneumonia or emphysema should be determined. Both diseases may be present concurrently. Emphysema commonly produces an expiratory dyspnea, whereas pneumonia demonstrates both inspiratory and expiratory dyspnea. The presence of a fever, the typical rales on auscultation, and the character of respiration will help establish pneumonia as a diagnosis. There is a need to determine if the pneumonia is primary or secondary to some other disease process, and if this is a herd problem the etiologic agent should be determined.

TREATMENT AND PREVENTION

Antibiotic selection is usually the initial consideration in the development of a therapeutic rationale for pneumonia cases. This is based upon the evidence that *Pasteurella* spp. are the principal causes of severe clinical signs, terminal lesions, and death loss to pneumonia regardless of the primary cause of respiratory disease. Other bacteria such as *Haemophilus* spp., *Corynebacterium* spp., and *Mycoplasma* spp. may also contribute in a primary or secondary capacity. Usually, *Pasteurella* spp. are sensitive to antibiotics and sulfonamides. However, the antibiotic sensitivity is variable, especially in cases treated only one or two days, owing to the development of resistance. Antibiotics should be administered for a minimum of three to four days (longer if response is not complete). Short duration and inadequate dosage therapy will result in clinical relapse and are conducive to the development of antibiotic resistance in respiratory bacteria.

Antibiotic drugs approved by the Food and Drug Administration (FDA) for parenteral use in food-producing animals are aqueous procaine penicillin G, benzathine penicillin G, ampicillin trihydrate, oxytetracycline hydrochloride, tetracycline hydrochloride, dihydrostreptomycin sulfate, erythromycin, amoxicillin, and tylosin. The recommended dosages, routes of administration, and withdrawal times before slaughter need to be closely observed to safeguard our milk and meat supplies.

The failure to get response to antibiotics may not always be explained by bacterial resistance but may be due to lack of early detection of the disease, advanced irreversible pathologic changes of the disease, and inadequate levels of previous therapy. Thus serious consideration of these factors should be made before using nonapproved drugs in the treatment of pneumonia.

Both parenteral and oral sulfonamides such as sulfathiazole, sulfamethazine, sulfamerazine, and sulfadimethoxine continue to be effective individual animal treatments as well as herd medication in the water supply in combination with electrolytes. Sulfonamides in combination with oxytetracycline administered parenterally continue to be a favorite treatment of many veterinarians. Most sulfonamides should be used at 200 mg/kg for the initial treatment and continued at 130 mg/kg for no more than a five-day period.

Slow-release sulfonamides have the advantage of requiring only one episode of cattle handling, but if the pneumonia is extensive they may not provide enough medication to resolve the infection.

Intratracheal administration of antibiotics can be an additive method of increasing antibiotic levels down in the bronchi and possibly lung parenchyma. Antibiotics and dosages (for a 230-kg animal) that have been used by this method are oxytetracycline (500 mg), and crystalline potassium penicillin (1 million units). Dissolve any of these in 10 to 30 ml of saline, and administer midtracheally with the head held in an upward position.

Individual patients may warrant the use of aerosol

therapy in which the goal is the deposition of aerosolized fluids on the mucosal surfaces of the airways. The therapeutic goals of these aerosols can be listed under three headings: (1) relief of bronchospasm, (2) decrease of mucosal edema, and (3) mobilization of released secretions. Mucolytic agents such as N-acetylcysteine (Mucomyst*) are available to break down mucus and purulent secretions. Antibiotics administered as aerosols should be limited to those with poor respiratory mucosal surface absorption (i.e., the aminoglycosides) and only when systemic administration has proved ineffective. Other groups of drugs that can be used for aerosol therapy include steroids and detergents.

Other forms of therapy for consideration in treating pneumonia are bronchodilators such as isoproterenol and theophylline. These are indicated if bronchospasm is present.

Controversy has existed over the use of corticosteroids in the treatment of pneumonia. Administration of corticosteroids early in the course of pneumonia will usually result in a clinical improvement (often a decrease in febrile response and an increase in appetite due to a euphroic effect), but these drugs at the common recommended dosages possibly increase the number of relapses and prolong the course of disease.

A highly effective method for preventing pneumonia has not been found. The bovine viral vaccines that contain infectious bovine rhinotracheitis virus, bovine diarrhea virus, and parainfluenza-3 virus (intranasal and intramuscular) are effective vaccines in cattle provided they are used at the correct time and before the animal becomes sick. They will also help prevent some of the predisposing effects that viral agents have on compromising the respiratory tract and allowing secondary bacterial infection.

Pasteurella vaccines are questionable immunizing agents, but benefit may be derived by frequent repeated injections at two- to three-week intervals. The help derived from Haemophilus vaccine in preventing respiratory disease has not been well determined.

The administration of hyperimmune serum derived from other animals previously inoculated with viral or bacterial antigens is considered to be of little value. Antibody levels produced are not at effective levels to justify the cost of their use.

Avoidance of "stress" factors is sometimes unpredictable from both management and environmental standpoints, but decreasing or eliminating as many possible adverse effects to the animal will help in preventing pneumonia. The timing of management events is very critical.

*Available from Mead Johnson Laboratories, Evansville, IN 47721.

Supplemental Reading

Breeze, R.: Reactions to injury in the respiratory system. Ill. Vet. Resp. Symp., 1978, 204–228.

Hjerpe, C. A.: Treatment of bacterial pneumonia in feedlot cattle. Proc. 8th Ann. A.A.B.P., 1975, 33–47.

Hjerpe, C. A., and Routen, T. A.: Practical and theoretical considerations concerning treatment of bacterial pneumonia in feedlot cattle with special reference to antimicrobic therapy. Proc. 9th Ann. A.A.B.P., 1976, 97–140.

Hore, D. E.: A review of respiratory agents associated with disease of sheep, cattle, and pigs in Australia and overseas. Aust. Vet. J. 52:502–509, 1976.

Jensen, R., Pierson, R., Braddy, P., Saari, D., Lauerman, L., England, J., Keyvanfar, H., Collier, J., Horton, D., McChesney, A., Benitez, A., and Christie, R.: Shipping fever pneumonia in yearling feedlot cattle. J. Am. Vet. Med. Assoc., 169:500–506, 1976.

Lillie, L. E.: The bovine respiratory disease complex. Can. Vet. J. 15:233–242, 1974.

Thomson, R. G.: Pathology and pathogenesis of the common diseases of the respiratory tract of cattle. Can. Vet. J. 15:249–251, 1974.

Vestweber, J., Guffy, M., Kelley, B., and Leipold, H.: Chronic bronchopneumonia in cattle. Bov. Pract. 12:55–62, 1977.

Acute Bovine Pulmonary Edema and Emphysema

ROGER BREEZE, B.V.M.S., Ph.D., M.R.C.V.S. and JAMES R. CARLSON, Ph.D.

Acute bovine pulmonary edema and emphysema (ABPE) is an acute respiratory distress syndrome that usually occurs in the fall in adult (over two years old) beef cattle moved from dry, sparse grazing to lush, green pastures. The disease has been known as fog fever in Europe for at least 200 years, the word "fog" having epidemiologic connotations in that the condition is often seen in cattle on "fog" pastures (that is, aftermath or foggage, the regrowth after a hay or silage cut). There is no association with atmospheric smog or fog. ABPE is consistently related to management practices resulting in sudden introduction of hungry adult cattle to lush grazing. In cow-calf operations in the western U.S.A., this typically occurs when the herd is brought from dry summer range onto irrigated or fertilized aftermath pasture. The species composition of the pasture does not appear to be important, provided it is lush. ABPE has been reported on a wide variety of grasses, alfalfa, rape, kale, and turnip tops. The disease is rare in dairy cattle probably because the necessary abrupt pasture movements are unusual in a well-managed milking herd. APBE appears to be more frequent in the Hereford breed and its crosses, apparently because this is the most prevalent type of animal in cow-calf operations. No breed appears to be unaffected under the right management conditions. The available evidence supports the view that ABPE is caused by ruminal production of 3-methylindole (3MI) from ingested L-tryptophan (TRP) in herbage.[1, 2] The 3MI is absorbed into the blood stream from the rumen and metabolized by a mixed function oxidase (MFO) system in the lung to produce pneumotoxicity (Fig. 1).

CLINICAL DISEASE

The terms "ABPE" and "fog fever" have been applied to a farrago of different respiratory conditions in which interstitial emphysema has been detected clinically or at necropsy (Figs. 2, 3, 4, and 5). In this context ABPE and fog fever refer only to the pasture-associated syndrome, which is defined in clinical, epidemiologic, and pathologic terms.[3] Almost all outbreaks of ABPE arise within two weeks of pasture change, and the condition is usually limited to fat, brood cows, usually of the Hereford type. The morbidity rate is variable but often approaches 50 percent; 30 per cent of severely affected animals die, usually within two days of the onset of clinical signs. In severe cases there is labored breathing with loud expira-

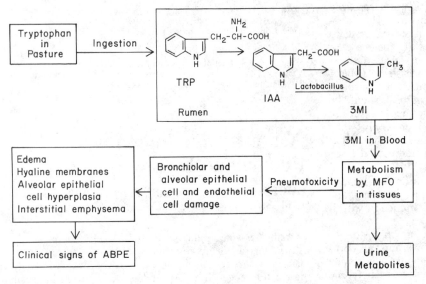

Figure 1. An outline of the pathogenesis of acute bovine pulmonary edema and emphysema (Key: TRP, tryptophan; IAA, indoleacetic acid; 3MI, 3-methylindole; MFO, mixed function oxidase).

tory grunt, frothing at the mouth, and mouth-breathing. On auscultation, inspiratory and expiratory sounds are usually surprisingly soft in view of the respiratory rate, and crackles (harsh or soft crackling sounds) are only occasionally detected. Severe cases improve dramatically after three days, and in these animals and in others that have not shown severe signs (and that may not be immediately apparent to the inexperienced observer) it is quite common to note only increased rate (50 to 80 per minute) and depth of breathing. Harsh respiratory sounds are common on auscultation, and crackles and rhonchi (whistling or musical adventitious sounds) may also be noted, particularly in caudal lung fields, in this later stage. Subcutaneous emphysema may be detected in a few of these convalescing animals. In addition to these signs of respiratory disease within an affected group, there is also a tendency for the demeanor of the group to change so that the animals become more tranquil. It should be particularly noted that coughing is not a dominant feature in affected individuals nor in the group as a whole.[4,5] In animals that die there are ecchymotic and petechial hemorrhages in the larynx, trachea, and bronchi, and the airways are filled with frothy edema fluid. Cranial lung lobes are deep red or purple, and the cut surface of the lobules has a smooth, glistening, glass-like appearance, the result of severe congestion, edema, and hyaline membranes. Interstitial emphysema with large gas bullae is apparent in all parts of the lung and occasionally may also extend along the back. Pulmonary edema is very noticeable, especially in the ventral segments of the lungs, and gelatinous yellow edema fluid can be found in the interlobular septa and perivascular connective tissue. Histolog-

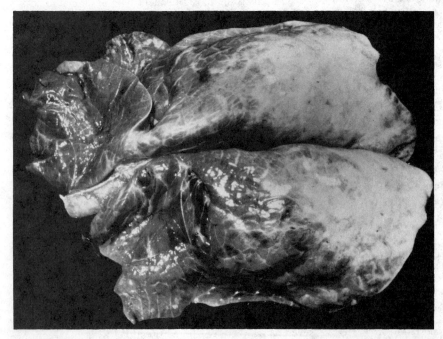

Figure 2. Fog fever: the cranial lobes are dark-red and congested. There is pleural edema and interstitial emphysema in the caudal lobes, which are distended by gas bullae. The lungs are from a fatal case.

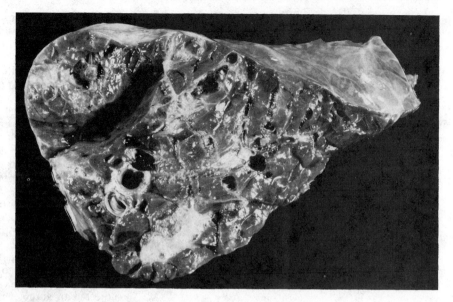

Figure 3. Fog fever: cross section of caudal lung lobe in Figure 2. Interstitial emphysema and gas bullae are evident. The lung lobes are dark-red and have a smooth, shiny cut surface indicative of the presence of congestion, edema, and hyaline membranes.

ically, alveoli and alveolar ducts are usually lined by eosinophilic hyaline membranes; edema fluid, a few eosinophils, neutrophils, alveolar macrophages, and multinucleated giant cells are found in the air spaces. In most animals there is some proliferation of alveolar epithelial cells. In animals that are slaughtererd after at least three to four days of illness, interstitial emphysema and pulmonary edema are usually minimal. However, all the lung tissue is fawn and rubbery as a result of severe, diffuse alveolar epithelial hyperplasia, in which the alveoli in all acini are lined by a single layer of cuboidal type 2 pneumonocytes containing frequent mitotic figures. Large mononuclear cells and a mixture of alveolar macrophages and type 2 pneumonocytes are found in the alveolar spaces, together with condensed hyaline deposits and multinucleated giant cells. Interalveolar septa are edematous, and many interstitial cells and eosinophils are apparent.[6] The pulmonary lesions are obligatory for diagnosis but are not pathognomonic. This is very important diagnostically. All cases of ABPE have some combination of the lesions mentioned previously, but all animals with some combination of these lesions do not have ABPE.

TREATMENT

Many different drugs, including corticosteroids, atropine, diethylcarbamazine, epinephrine, and diuretics, are alleged to be of value in the treatment of ABPE, but none have been properly tested. Our experience is that supportive therapy is only useful if it can be given with minimal stress to the animal involved and that recovery often occurs without drug treatment. Laboratory observation of cattle given TRP or 3MI confirms that many recover spontaneously over about ten days; relapses do not occur. Therapeutic trials using 3MI-induced pulmonary disease as a model have been limited thus far.[7] However, drugs acting as antagonists to postulated mediators of bovine anaphylaxis or hypersensitivity do not appear to alter the course of 3MI-induced ABPE significantly, even when given before 3MI dosage. This includes the following: acetylsalicylic acid (100 mg/kg B.W. orally every 12 hours); mepyramine (5 mg/kg B.W. intramuscularly every 12 hours); sodium meclofenamate (20 mg/kg B.W. intramuscularly daily); diethylcarbamazine citrate (1 ml 40 per cent w/v solution / 20 kg B.W. intramuscularly

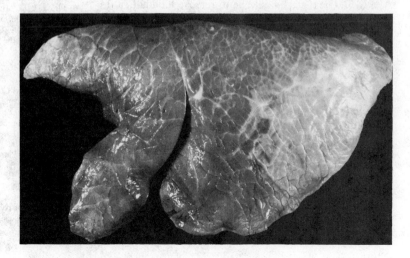

Figure 4. Fog fever: lungs of a slaughtered animal ill for four days. The lungs were fawn colored and very heavy.

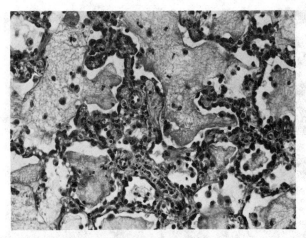

Figure 5. Histologic appearance of the lungs in fog fever. There are edema of the alveolar spaces and interalveolar septa and marked proliferation of cuboidal alveolar epithelial cells (type 2 pneumonocytes). (H & E, × 250)

every 12 hours); betamethasone (2 mg/kg intramuscularly every 12 hours).

In the absence of any proven effective therapy, our current recommendation for ABPE treatment, if this must be attempted, is furosemide (0.5 to 1.0 mg/kg B.W. intravenously or intramuscularly every 12 hours) with restriction of drinking water. Temporary hospital pens should be erected to avoid driving sick animals for long distances and to facilitate handling.

PREVENTION AND CONTROL

1. The first step in dealing with suspected ABPE is to consider the differential diagnosis and rule out other possibilities. Careful clinical or pathologic examination can distinguish a number of different disease entities frequently mistaken for ABPE.[5] Such conditions appear unlikely to cause differential diagnostic problems in typical epidemiologic situations in the western U.S.A. and elsewhere. In any event, the presence of interstitial emphysema should not be used as the sole diagnostic criterion.

2. Having established that the problem is indeed ABPE, the next step should be to remove all adult cattle and their calves from the pasture involved, taking great care to prevent unnecessary excitement or exertion in the process. In this respect, it is worth noting that cows and their calves should not be separated for any reason within the first three weeks of a move to lush pasture. The best preventive measure thereafter is to organize grazing management so as to avoid sudden introduction of hungry adult cattle to better pastures. This is often easier said than done but can be achieved by pregrazing lush pastures with less susceptible stock, such as sheep, horses, or immature cattle; by moving cattle on to new pasture before it becomes particularly lush; or by continuous strip-grazing. Some have recommended limiting intake of pasture by offering hay or concentrates daily or by restricting grazing time during the changeover period. Others suggest that cattle should be fed only grass that has been cut and

allowed to wilt during this time. All these measures may find a use under individual circumstances but are at best unreliable methods of preventing disease or limiting losses.

3. Pretreatment with piperonyl butoxide, an inhibitor of the MFO system, prevents 3MI-induced respiratory disease in goats and cattle. However, general understanding of the total animal effects of known MFO inhibitors is limited and at the present time it seems unlikely that dosing breeding stock on a regular basis with the large amounts of inhibitor necessary (0.5 ml/kg B.W. at 12-hour intervals) would prove to be a practical means of prophylaxis or would readily gain approval from regulatory agencies.

4. The most promising area for prevention of ABPE appears to be in the alteration of ruminal metabolism to inhibit or lower 3MI production. Oral doses of 200 mg monensin/head/day in gelatin capsules prevent TRP-induced ABPE in experimental cattle by reducing the conversion of TRP to 3MI in the rumen. The same treatment also reduces ruminal 3MI production in cattle subjected to abrupt change to lush pasture.[7] If current understanding of the pathogenesis of ABPE is correct, dosing with monensin for the first seven to ten days after introduction to lush pasture should prevent the disease. At present, use of monensin in brood cows is not approved by the Food and Drug Administration in the U.S.A. The best means of delivering the drug reliably under practical field conditions has yet to be determined. No beneficial effect of monensin is to be expected when the drug is given *after* clinical signs appear, since by this time 3MI-induced pneumotoxicity has been expressed.

References

1. Selman, I. E., Wiseman, A., Breeze, R. G., and Pirie, H. M.: Fog fever in cattle: various theories on its aetiology. Vet. Rec. 99:181–184, 1976.
2. Carlson, J. R., and Dickinson, E. O.: Tryptophan induced pulmonary edema and emphysema in ruminants. *In* Keeler, R. F., van Kampen, K. R., and James, L. F. (eds.): Effects of Poisonous Plants on Livestock. Academic Press, New York, 1978, 261, 272.
3. Breeze, R. G., Pirie, H. M., Selman, I. E., and Wiseman, A.: Acute respiratory distress in cattle. Vet. Rec. 97:226–229, 1975.
4. Selman, I. E., Wiseman, A., Pirie, H. M., and Breeze, R. G.: Fog fever in cattle: clinical and epidemiological features. Vet. Rec. 95:139–142, 1974.
5. Selman, I. E., Wiseman, A., Breeze, R. G., and Pirie, H. M.: Differential diagnosis of pulmonary disease in adult cattle in Britain. Bovine Pract. 12:63–74, 1977.
6. Pirie, H. M., Breeze, R. G., Selman, I. E., and, Wiseman, A.: Fog fever in cattle: pathology. Vet. Rec. 95:479–483, 1974.
7. Hammond, A. C., Carlson, J. R., Breeze, R. G., and Selman, I. E.: Progress in the prevention of acute bovine pulmonary emphysema. Bovine Pract. 14:9–14, 1979.

Supplemental Reading

Bray, T. J., and Carlson, J. R.: The role of mixed function oxidase in 3-methylindole induced acute pulmonary edema in goats. Am. J. Vet. Res. 40:268–272, 1979.
Breeze, R. G., Selman, I. E., Pirie, H. M., and Wiseman, A.: A reapprasial of atypical interstitial pneumonia in cattle. Bovine Pract. 13:75–81, 1978.
Breeze, P. G.: Parasitic bronchitis and pneumonia. Vet. Clin. North Am. 1:219–229, 1985.
Breeze, R. G.: Respiratory disease in adult cattle. Vet. Clin. North Am. 1:335–370, 1985.
Hammond, A. C., Carlson, J. R., and Breeze, R. G.: Monensin and the prevention of tryptophan-induced acute bovine pulmonary edema and emphysema. Science 201:153–155, 1978.

Vena Caval Thrombosis

ROGER BREEZE, B.V.M.S., Ph.D., M.R.C.V.S.

Hemoptysis, the coughing up of blood or blood-stained sputum, can be a dramatic clinical sign in cattle. A minor degree of hemoptysis may infrequently be observed in animals with right-sided infective endocarditis, but in the author's experience massive hemoptysis is virtually indicative of one disease: thrombosis of the caudal vena cava (CVCT, caval thrombosis).

THROMBOSIS OF THE CAUDAL VENA CAVA

History, Distribution, and Epidemiology

CVCT has been known in Europe for over 80 years and is now recognized as an increasing problem in the U.S.A.[1] CVCT is an important and common cause of cardiovascular disease in adult cattle, in the same ranks as infective endocarditis and traumatic pericarditis.[2, 3] In a survey of 1,998 yearling feedlot cattle, CVCT was the cause of death in 1.3 per cent. Of these, 40 per cent were affected in the first 45 days on the feedlot and a further 28 per cent during the next 45 days.[1] CVCT is associated with the rumenitis–hepatic abscess complex most prevalent in the fattening and finishing periods of feedlot management. In a Canadian survey, CVCT was present in 19.3 per cent of cattle with hepatic abscesses and was most frequent in one- to two-year-old cattle.[4]

Clinical Disease

CVCT may present in two forms. The most important and common is a respiratory syndrome that follows pulmonary arterial thromboembolism and the formation and rupture of pulmonary arterial aneurysms.[5] Much less frequently, cases are encountered in which the main presenting sign is gross abdominal distention due to hepatomegaly and massive ascites, but in such instances respiratory signs and pulmonary arterial lesions are also found.[6] CVCT is also reported as a cause of "sudden death" without prodromal signs. Death often occurs unexpectedly in CVCT, usually soon after an episode of severe intrapulmonary hemorrhage or hemoptysis, but this is usually preceded by other respiratory signs of at least several days' duration. It seems likely that in cases of "sudden death" these signs have passed unnoticed, the only exception being when sudden intravascular rupture of a hepatic abscess leads to rapidly fatal septicemia and septic shock.

In about half the cases there is a history of respiratory disease of only a few days' duration. These animals usually deteriorate rapidly once hemoptysis begins. Other cattle have a history of weight loss and coughing for weeks or months. Thoracic pain is often present and may be the reason for referral, but the respiratory signs are often such that the initial clinical diagnosis would appear to be chronic suppurative pneumonia—that is, until the onset of hemoptysis.

Increased rate of breathing (> 30 per minute at rest), increased depth of breathing, and coughing are present in every case. These signs are of little help in establishing a diagnosis, but three features are found sufficiently frequently to make this fairly straightforward, particularly when they occur together. These signs are (1) *anemia,* manifested as mucosal pallor, hemic murmur, and lowered packed cell volume (range 10 to 20 per cent; normal 28 to 35 per cent); (2) *hemoptysis;* and (3) *widespread rhonchi.* Other useful signs, which are common but not detectable in every case, are (4) *thoracic pain* at rest, while walking, or after coughing; (5) *hepatomegaly,* considered to be present if the liver projects into the right paralumbar fossa; (6) *melena;* and (7) *fever,* rectal temperature > 39°C. Finally, signs of congestive cardiac failure, including jugular distention and brisket edema, may be superimposed in a few animals developing chronic cor pulmonale following widespread pulmonary arterial thromboembolism.[5]

Pathogenesis
(Figs. 1 to 5)

A thrombus is always present in the hepatic or intrathoracic portion of the CVC between the liver and the right atrium. Almost all thrombi are the result of thrombophlebitis, where the wall of the CVC has been infiltrated by a perivascular hepatic or postdiaphragmatic abscess from which *Sphaerophorus* (Fusobacterium) *necrophorus, Corynebacterium pyogenes,* or *Staphylococcus* is often recovered. Most thrombi are large and often occlude the lumen of the CVC at or anterior to the openings of the hepatic veins. This gives rise to chronic venus congestion of the liver, hepatomegaly, and the development of a collateral venous circulation, which utilizes the hemiazygos, vertebral, and mammary veins to return blood to the heart. Gross abdominal enlargement due to ascites and massive hepatomegaly is uncommon and occurs only when the thrombus extends into and obstructs hepatic veins so that this collateral drainage is blocked.

Pulmonary arterial thromboembolism from the CVC thrombus is very widespread and has the following consequences: (1) there is extensive embolic occlusion of small arteries; (2) aneurysms form at sites of arterial obstruction; (3) sudden blockage of lobar or larger arteries can cause acute clinical crises or death; (4) arterial occlusion results in development of pulmonary arterial hypertension; and (5) pulmonary hypertension promotes and accelerates the formation of aneurysms and leads to cor pulmonale.[2, 3]

A peculiar feature of CVCT is the formation of multiple pulmonary arterial aneurysms at sites of thromboembolism or where the vessel wall has been weakened by arteritis, endarteritis, and thromboarteritis. Eventually, the wall of the aneurysmal sac becomes so attentuated that rupture occurs and blood is ejected into the adjacent pulmonary tissue,where it passes into the bronchial system (resulting in hemoptysis) or it forms large hematomata in the interstitium of the lung. Hemoptysis usually develops when an embolic abscess is located between the artery and bronchus in such a way that the bronchial and arterial walls are eroded simultaneously. Rupture of the aneurysm is immediately followed by hemoptysis, since the blood is ejected directly into the bronchial system. If only the arterial wall is eroded and the bronchus remains intact, blood ejected from ruptured aneurysms cannot gain access to the bronchial system and gathers in large, lamellated interstitial hematomata that may be 20 cm or more in diameter. Such intrapulmonary hemorrhage is the cause of anemia in the absence of hemoptysis. Thoracic pain may be the result of intrapulmonary hematomata, sup-

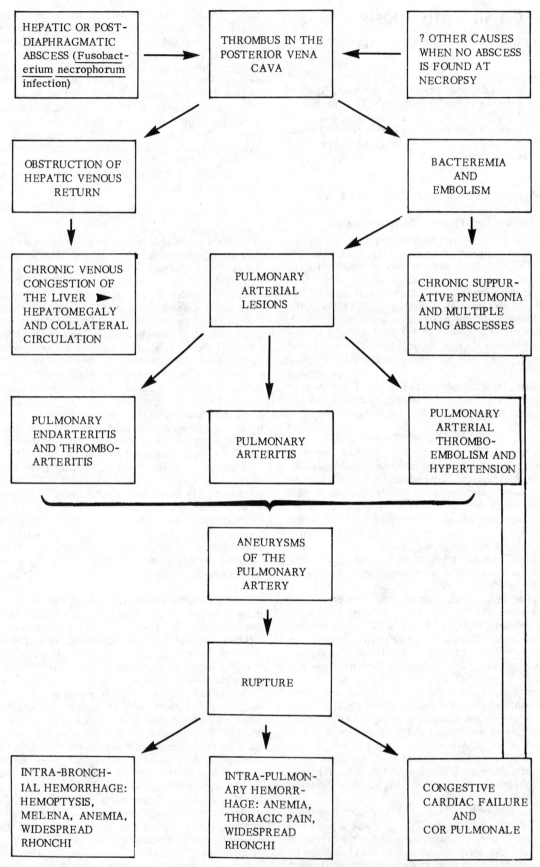

Figure 1. The pathogenesis of caudal vena caval thrombosis in cattle.

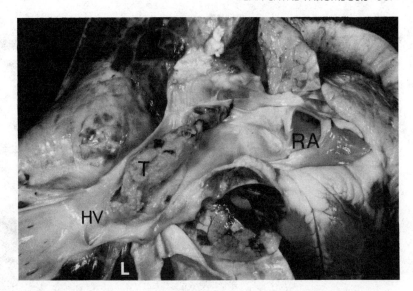

Figure 2. A rough-surfaced thrombus (T) almost occludes the lumen of the intrathoracic caudal vena cava. The liver (L), orifices of the hepatic veins (HV), and right atrium (RA) are marked.

purative pneumonia, and pleuritis, or dissecting aneurysms in which blood separates the tissue planes of the arterial media.

Diagnosis

Three features are of particular value in making a clinical diagnosis of CVCT: (1) anemia; (2) hemoptysis; and (3) widespread rhonchi. Thoracic pain, hepatomegaly, and melena, when present, are also useful. Hemoptysis should be distinguished from epistaxis, which might occur in infectious bovine rhinotracheitis, for example. Widespread rhonchi are detectable in many affected cattle, and the diagnostic possibilities when these sounds are scattered over a wide lung area are generally limited to CVCT, parasitic bronchitis, and fibrosing alveolitis.[7] When other findings are considered, there is little difficulty in differentiating CVCT from the latter two conditions.

Diagnosis of CVCT at necropsy presents no problem, providing the CVC is opened. This is best achieved by removing the larynx, trachea, lungs, heart, liver, and diaphragm together, then opening the vascular system; this procedure preserves the relationships of the organs and facilitates demonstration of the lesions. Hemoptysis may be wrongly attributed to the presence of primary lung abscesses if the CVC is not examined.

THROMBOSIS OF THE CRANIAL VENA CAVA

Thrombosis of the cranial vena cava is very uncommon but gives rise to venous obstruction, the development of a collateral venous circulation, embolic pneumonia, and pulmonary arterial aneurysms and thromboembolism.[8, 9]

Clinical Disease
(Fig. 6)

As in CVCT, presenting signs usually suggest chronic suppurative pneumonia. The frequency of hemoptysis has not been determined. Differential diagnosis is facilitated when additional signs are present, including: (1) edema of the head; (2) jugular distention in the absence of endocarditis or traumatic pericarditis; (3) widespread rhonchi; and (4) elevated venous pressure in the head and neck.

At necropsy, significant lesions include a septic thrombus in the cranial vena cava, pulmonary arterial thromboembolism, pulmonary arteritis, aneurysm formation, and embolic pneumonia. Massive edema of the head or severe jugular distension probably develops only when the collateral circulation is inadequate.

PULMONARY THROMBOEMBOLISM

Pulmonary thromboembolism and suppurative pneumonia may be consequences of infectious processes in various areas of the body including phlebitis of the jugular veins, endocarditis, hepatic abscess, mastitis, and metritis. Hemoptysis and aneurysm formation are not recorded in these situations. The reason for this is unclear. Pulmonary vascular hemodynamics may be unusual in vena caval thrombosis. Certainly the distribution of emboli to periarterial sites is unlike that of other diseases. It is possible that the emboli reach these unusual sites in VCT because they arrive in lymphatics or via the collateral circulation.

Treatment

Surgical removal of arterial aneurysms with ligation of the vena cava has successfully cured similar cases in man, but this is clearly impractical for all but the most valuable cattle.

Antibiotic treatment may remove or suppress the hepatic abscess and render emboli sterile in some cases, but in the majority significant penetration and resolution of the primary lesions would appear unlikely, even supposing these could be diagnosed. Once hemoptysis and anemia are noted, prompt slaughter and salvage are the only answer. Mortality rate at present is 100 per cent.

Prevention

On the assumption that CVCT is part of the rumenitis–hepatic abscess complex, measures taken to reduce the incidence of the latter problem in the feedlot might be expected to be beneficial.

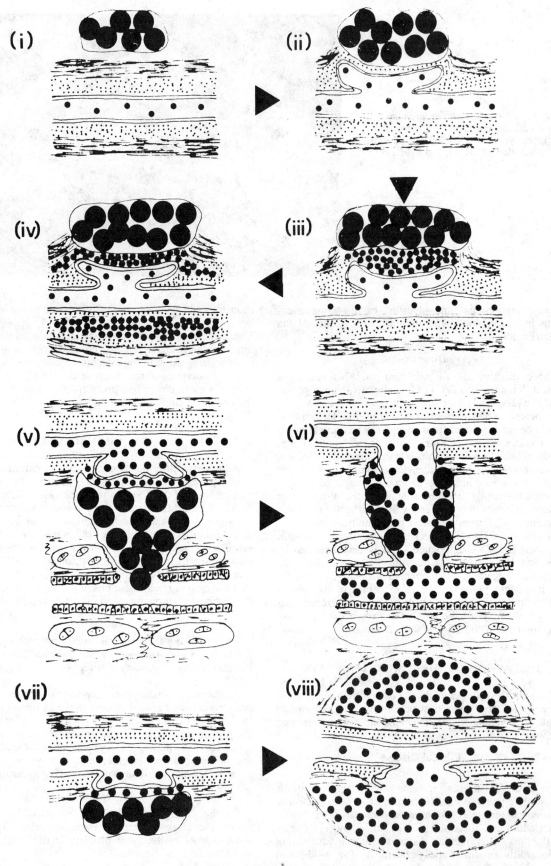

Figure 3. *See legend on opposite page.*

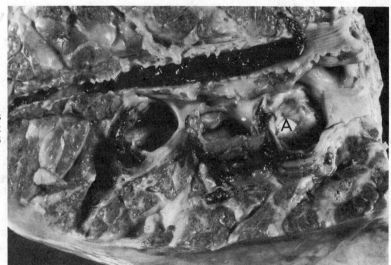

Figure 4. Three pulmonary arterial aneurysms (A) adjacent to a bronchus, which contains a cast of clotted blood. This corresponds to Figure 3 (iii).

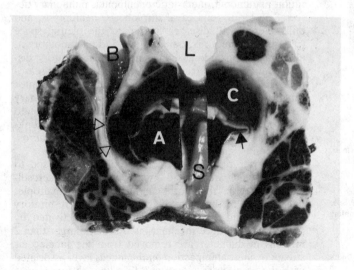

Figure 5. Cross section through a pulmonary arterial aneurysm comparable to Figure 3 (v). A lobar artery (L) gives off a segmental branch (S) in which there is an aneurysm (A) (solid arrows). Clotted blood (C) and pus surround the base of the aneurysm. The wall of the bronchus (B) is almost completely eroded (open arrows).

Figure 3. Diagrammatic representation of the pathogenesis of hemoptysis and hematomata resulting from pulmonary arteritis. (i) An embolic abscess is situated adjacent to the pulmonary artery. The endothelium, intima, media, and adventitia making up the arterial wall are indicated. (ii) Extension of the abscess results in erosion of the adventitia and media of an arc of the pulmonary artery and the formation of a saccular aneurysm at the site. (iii) Erosion of vasa vasorum in the wall of the pulmonary artery results in intramural and perivascular hemorrhage between the base of the aneurysm and the surrounding abscess. (iv) There is dissection of blood between the tissue planes of the media in the vicinity of the aneurysm and a dissecting aneurysm is formed. (v) A perivascular abscess erodes the wall of the bronchus to form a communication with the lumen. At the same time, it erodes an arc of the wall of the pulmonary artery to form a saccular aneurysm surrounded by clotted blood derived from eroded vasa vasorum. (vi) Rupture of the aneurysm in (v) results in hemoptysis and the contents of the abscess are flushed into the bronchus. (vii) A perivascular abscess that results in pulmonary arteritis and the formation of a pulmonary arterial aneurysm, but that does not erode the accompanying bronchus. (viii) Massive lamellated hematoma in the interstitium as a result of rupture of the lesion described in (vii) above. The blood cannot gain access to the bronchus (cf. vi).[3]

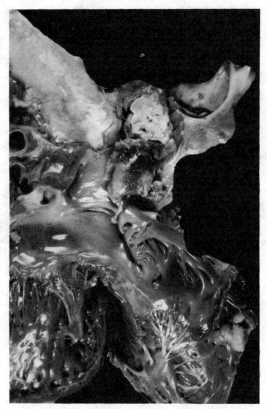

Figure 6. A septic thrombus occludes the cranial vena cava.

References

1. Jensen, R., Pierson, R. E., Braddy, P. M., Saari, D. A., Lauerman, L. H., England, J. J., Benitez, A., Horton, D. P., and McChesney, A. E.: Embolic pulmonary aneurysms in yearling feedlot cattle. J. Am. Vet. Med. Assoc. *169*:518–520, 1976.
2. Breeze, R. G., Pirie, H. M., Selman, I. E., and Wiseman, A.: Pulmonary arterial thromboembolism and pulmonary arterial mycotic aneurysms in cattle with vena caval thrombosis: a condition resembling the Hughes-Stovin syndrome. J. Path. *119*:229–237, 1976a.
3. Breeze, R. G., Pirie, H. M., Selman, I. E., and Wiseman, A.: Hemoptysis in cattle. Bovine Pract. *12*:64–72, 1976b.
4. Gudmundson, J., Radostits, O. M., and Doige, C. E.: Pulmonary thromboembolism in cattle due to thrombosis of the posterior vena cava associated with hepatic abscessation. Can. Vet. J. *19*:304–309, 1978.
5. Selman, I. E., Wiseman, A., Petrie, L., Pirie, H. M., and Breeze, R. G.: A respiratory syndrome in cattle resulting from thrombosis of the posterior vena cava. Vet. Rec. *94*:459–466, 1974.
6. Stöber, M., von: Pyogene Thrombosen der Vena cava caudalis beim Rind. Proc. IVth Int. Conf. Buiatrics (Zurich), 1–8, 1966.
7. Selman, I. E., Wiseman, A., Breeze, R. G., and Pirie, H. M.: Differential diagnosis of pulmonary disease in adult cattle in Britian. Bovine Pract. *13*:63–74, 1977.
8. Fisher, E. W., and Pirie, H. M.: Cardiovascular disease in domestic animals. Ann. N.Y. Acad. Sci. *127*:606–616, 1965.
9. Breeze, R. G., and Petrie, L.: Thrombosis of the cranial vena cava in a cow. Vet. Rec. *101*:130–131, 1977.

The Bovine Respiratory Disease Complex

C. A. HJERPE, D.V.M.

The etiology of the bovine respiratory disease complex is multifactorial and incompletely defined. It is believed that complex interactions between viruses, bacteria, and physical, psychological, physiologic, and environmental stress factors are involved. When primary, uncomplicated viral respiratory infections occur, the disease that results is, in most cases, subclinical or mild in nature. When severe clinical disease occurs, a bacterial bronchopneumonia and/or fibrinous pneumonia (B & FP) is nearly always present. The bacteria most frequently isolated from pneumonic bovine lungs are also commonly isolated from the oral, nasal, and oropharyngeal mucosae of normal cattle.

This definition of the bovine respiratory disease complex excludes all diseases that are limited to the upper respiratory tract (sinusitis, rhinitis, rhinosporidiosis/nasal granuloma, summer snuffles, epistaxis, pharyngitis, laryngitis, laryngeal edema, tracheitis, and tracheal edema), all sporadic diseases of the lower respiratory tract (aspiration pneumonia, metastatic pneumonia, pulmonary abscess, posterior vena caval thrombosis, hemoptysis, and milk allergy), all diseases limited to the pleural space (pleurisy, hydrothorax, hemothorax, and pneumothorax), all parasitic pneumonias, all congenital respiratory diseases, all neoplastic respiratory diseases, and all diseases included in the bovine interstitial pneumonia complex (atypical interstitial pneumonia, acute bovine pulmonary emphysema/3-methyl indole toxicosis, moldy sweet potato toxicosis, perilla mint toxicosis, paraquat toxicosis, stinkwood toxicosis, extrinsic allergic alveolitis, diffuse fibrosing alveolitis, and bacteremic interstitial pneumonia).

The lower respiratory tract is constantly exposed to bacteria, which are inhaled on dust particles and aerosolized from the nasal and oropharyngeal mucosae in droplet nuclei. Most of these particles impact on the respiratory membrane and are rapidly removed or inactivated by pulmonary clearance mechanisms. Particles larger than 2 microns in diameter are removed from the inhaled air stream by inertial impaction on the mucus layer associated with the respiratory membrane that lines the nasal passages, trachea, bronchi, and bronchioles. The nasal passages are particularly efficient in this regard. This mucus layer and the associated ciliated respiratory epithelial cells are collectively termed the "mucociliary apparatus." The mucus and associated inhaled bacteria and debris are propelled to the oropharynx by beating cilia, where they are disposed of by swallowing. Removal from the major bronchi and trachea is aided by the cough reflex.

Particles ranging in size from 0.5 to 2 microns in diameter may reach the alveoli and impact on the alveolar surface fluid film by sedimentation or Brownian movement. These particles are rapidly phagocytized and digested by pulmonary alveolar macrophages (PAM).

The lower respiratory tract of the healthy, unstressed bovine is highly resistant to bacterial invasion by the aerogenous route, even with massive experimental exposure by aerosol or by intratracheal or endobronchial inoculation. However, the efficiency of the mucociliary apparatus may be adversely affected by systemic dehydration, prolonged exposure to cold air, exposure to irritant gases, and infection with certain respiratory viruses. The efficiency of the PAM may be adversely affected by starvation, exposure to cold, systemic acidosis, hypoxia, and treatment with glucocorticoids (and inferentially by stress). In man, PAM function is also depressed by several respiratory viruses. Experimental infection with PI-3 virus in cattle reduces pulmonary clearance of *Pasteurella hemolytica* and, in combination with stress, favors development of a pasteurella pneumonia. It is not known whether depressed mucociliary clearance, depressed PAM clearance, or both are involved. Although *in vitro* PI-3 infections in calf trachea organ cultures cause severe destruction of ciliated respiratory epithelial cells, a similar effect is not usually observed *in vivo*.

To summarize, the term "bovine respiratory disease complex" refers to bacterial infections of the lower respiratory tract with organisms that are normal saprophytes in the upper respiratory tract and to which the normal lower tract is constantly exposed. Clinical disease results when mucociliary and/or PAM clearance is depressed by the combined effects of respiratory viruses and stress, permitting initiation of a bacterial bronchopneumonia and/or fibrinous pneumonia.

A large number of respiratory viruses have been isolated from cattle affected with clinical respiratory disease. These include IBR virus, African malignant catarrhal fever virus, bovine herpesvirus type 4, BVD virus, PI-3 virus, bovine adenovirus (eight types) bovine rhinovirus (two types), bovine respiratory syncytial virus (BRSV), reovirus (three types), bovine enterovirus (seven types), a calicivirus, and a coronavirus.

IBR virus, malignant catarrhal fever virus, bovine herpesvirus type 4, BVD virus, and BRSV are capable of causing severe primary disease. Experimental infections with PI-3 virus, IBR virus, and bovine herpesvirus type 4 have all been shown to reduce respiratory tract resistance to pasteurella bacteria.

Experimental infections with bovine adenovirus (types 1 to 6), reovirus (type 1), and bovine rhinovirus (types 1 and 2) produce only a mild primary respiratory disease syndrome. Experimental BRSV infections are generally mild, but severe primary disease results from simultaneous intranasal and intratracheal inoculations. Experimental infections with reovirus type 1 did not affect respiratory tract resistance to *P. multocida.*

Experimental infections with bovine adenovirus type 8, PI-3 virus, reovirus (types 2 and 3), and calicivirus produce subclinical primary respiratory disease. Respiratory disease has not been produced by experimental infections with bovine enterovirus (types 1 to 7). Experimental pulmonary infections with bovine adenovirus type 7 and coronavirus have not been reported.

Except for IBR virus and BRSV, information concerning the relative importance of these viruses in B & FP is lacking. Serologic evidence, implicating BRSV in as high as 60 per cent of field outbreaks of bovine respiratory disease, has been reported from the midwestern United States. Except for PI-3 and BVD, the effects of these viruses on pulmonary clearance mechanisms have not been studied. It has been found that BVD infection does not affect the clearance rate of inhaled *P. hemolytica* organisms.

Pasteurellae, especially *P. hemolytica* and *P. multocida,* are the bacteria most frequently isolated from pneumonic bovine lungs. Less frequently isolated bacteria include *Haemophilus somnus, Salmonella* spp., streptococci, *Staphylococcus aureus, E. coli,* and *Neisseria* spp. *Corynebacterium pyogenes* is frequently isolated with *Bacteroides melaninogenicus* from chronic lesions and pulmonary abscesses.

Stress factors that are thought to contribute to B & FP include exhaustion, starvation, and dehydration (often resulting from transportation); weaning, ration changes, castration, dehorning, overcrowding, chilling (from confinement in cold, damp quarters or from exposure to drafts or inclement weather), overheating (especially when alternated with chilling), confinement in poorly ventilated quarters, exposure to stagnant air or excessive humidity, and the social adjustments associated with commingling of cattle from different sources. The occurrence of nonrespiratory diseases, such as digestive upsets from improper feeding, is an additional stress factor. Irregular consumption of high energy rations and feeding of rations excessively high in energy prior to ruminal adaptation can result in overproduction of lactic acid in the rumen and systemic acidosis. This is an unusually serious occurrence in relation to B & FP, in view of the depressing effect of systemic acidosis on PAM function.

Mycoplasmas are frequently isolated from pneumonic bovine lungs, but their significance is unclear. Eleven species of mycoplasmas and acholeplasmas have been isolated from the bovine respiratory tract. *Mycoplasma mycoides* subsp. *mycoides* is the cause of contagious bovine pleuropneumonia. Of the remaining ten species, only three *(M. bovis, M. dispar, Ureaplasma* spp.) have been shown to be capable of causing pneumonic lesions, but clinical primary respiratory disease does not occur. Pulmonary mycoplasma infections with *M. bovis* do not affect the rate of pulmonary clearance of inhaled *P. hemolytica* organisms. Inclusion of *M. bovis* with *P. hemolytica* in intranasal inoculations has been reported to enhance the pathogenicity of *P. hemolytica* for calves, but the number of animals utilized was small.

Chlamydia spp. are occasionally isolated from pneumonic bovine lungs but are apparently not a part of the upper respiratory microflora of normal cattle. Chlamydias are obligate intracellular bacteria. Experimental intratracheal inoculation of *Chlamydia* spp. in cattle produces a subclinical exudative bronchopneumonia. Intratracheal inoculation with a *Chlamydia* spp. isolate from a case of sporadic bovine encephalomyelitis reduced the resistance of the bovine lung to challenge by *P. hemolytica.* The relative importance of chlamydia in B & FP is unknown.

The potential for an outbreak of B & FP exists in virtually any population of cattle subjected to stress, in view of the ubiquity of pasteurella bacteria and many of the bovine respiratory viruses. The probability that clinical disease may result is increased by mismanagement, which increases and compounds stresses, and by commingling cattle from different sources so as to introduce new respiratory viruses for which herd immunity is lacking.

Morbidity and mortality rates may rise to 100 per cent and to 30 per cent or higher, respectively, depending on the degree of mismanagement. Susceptibility to B & FP decreases with age, although outbreaks are occasionally encountered in cattle of all ages.

Transmission of respiratory viruses and bacteria occurs by direct contact, by inhalation of aerosols induced by coughing, and by ingestion of feed or water contaminated by nasal discharges and drool from infected animals.

CLINICAL SIGNS

Clinical disease does not usually occur until six to ten days after cattle are stressed or new animals are introduced to the herd. The first observable signs are slight depression and inappetence, manifested by gauntness. Affected animals often stand apart from the group with lowered head, drooping ears, and half-closed eyes, as if dozing. A human observer is often viewed out of the "corner" of one eye, as if discomfort results from turning the head and neck for direct, binocular viewing. In the early stages there is no dyspnea, although the respiratory rate may be elevated when there is high fever, especially when the ambient temperature is high. The muzzle may be dry and scabby in appearance. Nasal discharge may or may not be present, and it is often more indicative of the severity of the predisposing upper respiratory viral disease than of pneumonia. Coughing is never a prominent sign and is usually soft, moist, and occasional rather than paroxysmal. The rectal temperature may range from slightly above normal to 108°F. Diarrhea is occasionally present.

With extensive lung consolidation, there is marked depression, inappetence, and dyspnea with extended head and open mouth breathing. The rectal temperature may be elevated, normal, or subnormal. If the animal should respond to treatment at this stage, there is a marked tendency for relapse to occur within a few days to a few weeks after antimicrobial therapy is terminated. Those animals that do recover permanently may remain thin, grow slowly, and have a rough hair coat.

The distribution of the pneumonic lesion is anteroventral. Auscultation of the dorsal lung is usually normal. Rales, increased vesicular breath sounds, bronchial tones, and/or exaggerated expiratory sounds are evident upon auscultation of the anteroventral lung fields. When pleural effusion is present, there may be complete absence of respiratory sounds over the lung field below the fluid line.

PATHOLOGY

The lesions usually develop initially in the anteroventral lung. The disease is often subclinical until more than 10 to 15 per cent of the lungs are consolidated. From 60 to 80 per cent of the lungs are usually affected in fatal cases of uncomplicated B & FP. When other diseases such as IBR, BVD, salmonellosis, mycotic rumenitis, or traumatic pharyngitis occur primarily or secondarily, only 30 to 50 per cent of the lungs may be affected. Calves younger than four weeks of age are an exception, in that fatal infections, which involve only 10 to 20 per cent of the lung, are often encountered. Both lungs are usually involved, although the lesions are occasionally unilateral.

Healed, resolving, and inflamed areas of varying chronicity are often encountered in the same individual and can usually be correlated with a history of repeated relapses. Actively inflamed areas are swollen, firm, and engorged with blood. Inactive, resolving lesions are more nearly normal in size and are flaccid.

Pneumonic pasteurellosis usually takes the same course as a bronchopneumonia, and *P. multocida* is the bacterium most commonly isolated. Fibrinous pleuritis may or may not be present. In the less resistant host, or with more virulent bacteria (especially *P. haemolytica*), a more fulminating disease referred to as fibrinous (or lobar) pneumonia may occur. A fibrinous pleuritis is invariably present, often accompanied by pleural effusion. Individual lobules are often widely separated by edematous interlobular septa. Gross evidence of airway orientation is lacking.

It is possible to determine, within limits, the approximate duration of the clinical course by a careful gross postmortem examination of the sectioned pneumonic pulmonary lobules. This determination is of value in helping to fix responsibility when it is suspected that unhealthy cattle have been purchased or that disease detection has been faulty.

In fatal cases of bronchopneumonia, in which the clinical course is less than seven days, the cut surface of the lobules is reddish-brown in color. After a seven- to ten-day course, a few tiny white foci are visible against the reddish-brown cut lobular surface. These are focal accumulations of leukocytes within and around intralobular bronchioles. After a 10- to 14-day course, increased numbers of white foci, 1 to 2 mm in diameter, are visible against the reddish-brown congested lobular parenchyma. After a 14- to 21-day course, the white foci reach maximum numbers and size (2 mm) and are packed closely together. The lobules appear yellow to white in color, as little congestion is present. Thick ribbons of yellow exudate may be expressed from the cut ends of bronchioles when the lung is compressed. After a 21- to 30-day course, beginning resolution can be noted. The sectioned lobules are yellow to white or sometimes greenish in color, and the margins of the white foci are indistinct. A thin, purulent exudate may ooze from the cut surface. Inspissated exudate may be present within necrotic foci and within some of the larger airways. Beginning abscess formation may be noted, but the capsule is poorly developed. After a 30- to 60-day course, mature abscesses may be present. The lobules are smaller than normal. The cut ends of intralobular bronchioles are dilated and the bronchiolar walls are thickened and fibrotic. The interlobular septa are thickened by fibrosis in varying degrees. The area between bronchioles is congested and red in color. The visceral pleura may be thickened and fibrotic, and fibrous adhesions may be present between the lobes of the lung and between the pleura and the chest wall.

In fatal cases of fibrinous pneumonia, in which the clinical course is less than three days, the cut lobular surface is reddish-black in color. After a course of three to five days, there are red as well as reddish-black areas on the lobular surface. After a five- to seven-day course, the lobular surface is red to reddish-yellow in color. After a 7- to 14-day course the lobular surface is yellow in color. Patients that survive for longer than seven to ten days will usually recover. More chronic lesions than this may be noted in cattle that die from other causes. By 14 to 30 days after the onset of signs, resolution is occurring. The majority of affected lobules are necrotic. Beginning abscess formation may be noted within some lobules. In others, the necrotic lobule may separate from the septal wall, forming an inspissated central mass. By 30 to 60 days, mature abscesses may be present. The pleura is markedly thickened and fibrotic, and the lung is adhered to the chest wall.

Pure cases of fibrinous pneumonia are seldom encountered, as some areas of bronchopneumonia are nearly always present. Sometimes fibrinous pneumonia is superimposed on lobules previously affected with bronchopneumonia. Renal infarcts are a common secondary finding with either type of process.

With either kind of pneumonia, healing is usually complete by 60 to 90 days after the onset of clinical signs, except when there is extensive pulmonary abscessation. Affected areas heal by involution of alveolar tissue, resorption of exudates, and fibrosis. Normal respiratory function is not re-established in areas of lung in which severe bacterial infection has occurred.

TREATMENT

When effective antimicrobial therapy can be initiated on the first day that clinical signs are evident to an experienced observer and continued for 48 hours after fever, dyspnea, and toxemia have abated, and if appropriate shelter, nutrition, and nursing care are provided, mortality from acute, uncomplicated bacterial pneumonia in cattle will be negligible. Mortality is increased when disease detection is inadequate, resulting in delayed treatment, when ineffective antimicrobial drugs are utilized, when inappropriate dosages, routes of administration, or treatment intervals are selected, or when treatment is irregularly administered or prematurely terminated. Failure to promptly re-institute treatment when relapses occur is often a factor in excessive mortality. When disease detection is adequate and a satisfactory treatment program is maintained, most fatalities from B & FP can be explained in terms of antimicrobial-resistant pasteurella bacteria. Consequently, alternative antimicrobial therapy should be considered when a satisfactory clinical response is not evident by 48 hours after initiation of primary treatment. To minimize the risk of relapse, treatment with an effective antimicrobial drug should be continued for at least two days after the rectal temperature has returned to the normal range (less than 103°F) and signs of depression and dyspnea have abated. In severely affected cattle, it is wise to continue treatment for five to seven days after the rectal temperature has returned to the normal range.

Sick cattle should be kept dry and provided with shelter from cold winds or hot sun. Sick cattle penned together should be of similar size and should not be overcrowded. At least 12 linear inches and preferably 24 linear inches of feed bunk space and at least 40 square feet and preferably 100 square feet of pen space should be provided per animal.

Good quality longstem pasture grass or grain hay should be available at all times. Legume hays are not recommended for sick cattle, as their use is often associated with fatal bloat. In addition to hay, a starting ration should be fed free-choice to feedlot cattle. Clean, fresh water should be available at all times. Supplementary feeding is not required for cattle on good pasture.

When more than 50 to 60 per cent of an animal's lungs have become consolidated, response to treatment is nearly always unsatisfactory regardless of the treatment chosen or the antimicrobial sensitivity of the infecting organism. In those few cases that do respond, relapses are to be expected.

Relatively unsatisfactory response rates may be observed in calves shipped long distances to western feedlots, especially out of southeastern states. These cattle may be exhausted, if not debilitated, when they finally arrive in the feedlot and are often too tired and weak to eat for several days after arrival. If sick on arrival, or if they should become sick before recovering from the effects of shipping, response to treatment may be unsatisfactory.

B & FP in cattle is most frequently associated with *Pasteurella haemolytica, P. multocida,* and *Corynebacterium pyogenes. P. haemolytica* and *P. multocida* are usually sensitive to sulfonamides, penicillin G, ampicillin, amoxicillin, tetracyclines, chloramphenicol, spectinomycin, neomycin, kanamycin, gentamicin, polymyxin B, cephalothin, cephaloridine, and a combination of trimethoprim and a sulfonamide; they are usually resistant to dihydrostreptomycin and erythromycin; and they are always resistant to tylosin. *C. pyogenes* is always sensitive to penicillin G, ampicillin, amoxicillin, cephalothin, and cephaloridine; it is usually sensitive to chloramphenicol, spectinomycin, neomycin, kanamycin, and a combination of trimethoprim and a sulfonamide; it is frequently resistant to erythromycin and tylosin; it is usually resistant to oxytetracycline and dihydrostreptomycin; and it is always resistant to sulfonamides and polymyxin B.

Use of Sulfonamides in Treatment of B & FP

All sulfonamides are bacteriostatic through competitive inhibition of bacterial para-aminobenzoic acid utilization for the synthesis of folic acid. Since bacterial cross-resistance generally occurs between all sulfonamides, selection of a specific one for treatment of B & FP in cattle should be based only upon such considerations as (1) relative risk of toxicosis, (2) gastrointestinal absorption characteristics, (3) urinary excretion characteristics, (4) concentrations of free (active, unbound) drug achieved in blood serum, and (5) cost.

It is essential that continuously bacteriostatic blood concentrations be maintained during treatment with sulfonamides. A concentration of at least 8 to 15 mg per 100 ml of blood is desired, with 5 mg per 100 ml being the minimum effective concentration. When using sulfonamides such as sulfadimethoxine or sulfaethoxypyridazine, in which the ratio of active drug to protein-bound drug in blood is low, even higher concentrations are probably desirable. In general, the greater the blood concentration, the better the therapeutic response (toxicosis being the limiting factor). Recommendations concerning dosages, treatment intervals, and withdrawal periods are summarized in Table 1.

From 78 to 91 per cent of *P. haemolytica* and *P. multocida* isolates, recovered from nasal secretions of cattle with B & FP, are sensitive to sulfonamides. *C. pyogenes* is resistant to sulfonamides. In a series of acute feedlot B & FP cases summarized by the author, 81.9 per cent responded satisfactorily when treated with sulfamethazine USP boluses as recommended (see Table 1).

Sulfonamides are potentially toxic. Recommended dosages should not be exceeded. The treatment period should not exceed five to seven days. Water should be continu-

Table 1. *Recommendations Concerning Dosages, Treatment Intervals, and Withdrawal Periods for Some Sulfonamide Formulations Used in Treatment of Bronchopneumonia and Fibrinous Pneumonia in Cattle*

Sulfonamide	Dosage Priming	Dosage Maintenance	Treatment Interval	Withdrawal for Slaughter (days)	Withdrawal for Milk (days)
Sulfamethazine, USP	200 mg/kg	100–130 mg/kg	24 hr	10	4
Sulfamerazine	200 mg/kg	66 mg/kg	12 hr	10	—
Sulfapyridine	130 mg/kg	66 mg/kg	12 hr	10	—
Sulfathiazole	200 mg/kg	66 mg/kg	6–8 hr	10	—
Vetisulid[a]	33–50 mg/kg	33–50 mg/kg	12 hr	5[b]–7[c]	NA
Albon[d, e]	55 mg/kg	28 mg/kg	24 hr	5[b]–7[c]	2½
Albon-S.R.[d, e]	138 mg/kg	—	4 days	21	NA
S.E.Z.[f]	55 mg/kg	55 mg/kg	24 hr	16	NA
S.E.Z.C.-R[f]	220 mg/kg	—	3 days	16	NA
Sulfabrom[g, h]	200 mg/kg	—	48 hr	10	4
Spanbolet II[i]	1 bolus/68 kg	—	5 days	28	NA
Hava-Span[i, j]	1 bolus/90 kg	—	3½ days	16	NA
	1 bolus/45 kg	—	5 days	16	NA

[a]Sulfachlorpyridazine.
[b]After intravenous administration.
[c]After oral administration.
[d]Sulfadimethoxine.
[e]Blood levels reported by the manufacturer with the recommended dose are only marginally therapeutic.
[f]Sulfaethoxypyridazine.
[g]Sulfabromomethazine.
[h]Absorption from digestive tract not always reliable.
[i]Sustained-release sulfamethazine formulations.
[j]Therapeutic blood concentrations not obtained during the first 14 to 18 hours after administration.
NA = Not approved for use in lactating cattle.

ously available to treated animals. Acute toxicosis, characterized by weakness, ataxia, and collapse, may occur when sulfonamides are administered by rapid intravenous injection. The problem is avoided by proper technique. In reality, sulfonamide toxicity in cattle is a relatively rare occurrence. Most toxicosis problems have involved sulfathiazole or sulfapyridine, both of which are no longer commonly used.

A combination of trimethoprim and sulfadiazine is formulated in a fixed 1:5 ratio and has been used for treatment of B & FP in pre-ruminant calves on a prescription basis. Marked synergistic antimicrobial activity results from sequential blockage of two successive steps in microbial synthesis of folic acid. Twice daily oral administration in a dose of 48 mg per kg of body weight of combined drug has been recommended for use in pre-ruminant calves. This drug combination is ineffective in cattle with a functional rumen, owing to rapid removal and inactivation of trimethoprim by hepatic metabolism.

Use of Antibiotics in Treatment of B & FP in Cattle

"Approved" drugs have been approved by the Food and Drug Administration (FDA) of the United States Department of Health, Education, and Welfare for use in food-producing animals. Most, but not all, approved drugs are freely available to the livestock owner through over-the-counter sales but must be used according to label instructions with regard to dose, route of administration, maximum duration of treatment, and withdrawal period from treated animals before slaughter or marketing of milk. Procaine penicillin G in aqueous suspension, benzathine penicillin G, ampicillin trihydrate, amoxicillin trihydrate, oxytetracycline hydrochloride, tetracycline hydrochloride, dihydrostreptomycin sulfate, erythromycin, and tylosin are approved by the FDA for parenteral administration in cattle.

"Prescription legend" drugs are available to livestock owners only from a licensed veterinarian or by his prescription. Withdrawal recommendations have not been established for most prescription drugs. A veterinarian can legally use and prescribe these drugs for use in food-producing animals that are directly under his care or supervision. However, in so doing, the veterinarian assumes legal responsibility for any drug residues that are subsequently detected in meat or milk from treated animals. A veterinarian is also legally responsible when a residue is found in an animal treated with an FDA-approved drug if he has administered the drug without informing the owner or caretaker as to the proper withdrawal period or when he has used or recommended the drug in a dose or by a route of administration that is contrary to label recommendations.

The use of nonapproved drugs or the nonapproved use of approved drugs in treatment of livestock diseases should be undertaken by the veterinarian only when he has considered all other alternatives and is satisfied that (1) such use is truly in the best economic interest of his client, and (2) a suitably long drug withdrawal period can be enforced. In the case of aminoglycoside antibiotics (neomycin, kanamycin, gentamicin), no period of less than four months should be considered safe. Other prescription antibiotics should not be used unless a withdrawal period of at least two months can be ensured. Fortunately, most B & FP cases can be successfully managed with one or the other of three approved antimicrobial drugs: a sulfonamide (especially sulfamethazine), procaine penicillin G, or a tetracycline (especially oxytetracycline). Of the "prescription legend" antibiotics, only chloramphenicol, spectinomycin, and neomycin sulfate are sufficiently inexpensive to permit systemic use for treatment of B & FP in commercial cattle (Table 2).

Label recommendations concerning dosages, routes of administration, and treatment intervals have been determined empirically for nearly all existing FDA-approved antibiotics. In many instances, the label recommendation does not permit the most effective use with respect to the organisms most commonly associated with B & FP in cattle. Unfortunately, the veterinarian is in the position

Table 2. *Summary of Suggested Antibiotic Treatment Regimens for Bronchopneumonia and Fibrinous Pneumonia in Cattle*

Antibiotic	Proprietary Name	Manufacturer	Packaging	Mode of Action	Antibacterial Spectrum	Treatment Interval (hrs)	Dosage/ Treatment	Route of Administration	Withdrawal Period for Slaughter (days)
Oxytetracycline	Terramycin Injectable[a]	Pfizer	500-ml vial 50 mg/ml	Bacteriostatic	Broad-spectrum	24	11 mg/kg B.W.	SC	20[b]
	Liquamycin LA-200[a, c]	Pfizer	500-ml vial 200 mg/ml			48	20 mg/kg B.W.	IM	28[b]
Procaine penicillin G[a]	Crysticillin	Squibb	100-ml vial 300,000 units/ml	Bactericidal	Mainly gram-positive	24	66,000 u/kg B.W.	IM, SC	20[d]
Ampicillin[a]	Polyflex	Bristol	10-gm vial	Bactericidal	Broad-spectrum	12	22 mg/kg B.W.	SC	60[d]
Amoxicillin[c]	Amoxi-inject	Beecham	25-gm vial	Bactericidal	Broad-spectrum	12	11 mg/kg B.W.	IM, SC	25[b]
Erythromycin[a]	Gallimycin Injectable	Abbott	200-ml vial 200 mg/ml	Bacteriostatic	Mainly gram-positive	24	44 mg/kg B.W.	IM	30[d]
Tylosin[e]	Tylan 200	Elanco	250-ml vial 200 mg/ml	Bacteriostatic	Mainly gram-positive	24	44 mg/kg B.W.	IM	21[d]
Chloramphenicol[a]	P/M Chloramphenicol, Oral Solution	Pitman-Moore	200-ml vial 100 mg/ml	Bacteriostatic	Broad-spectrum	12	16.5 mg/kg B.W.	SC	60[d]
	Chloromycetin Na Succinate	Parke Davis	1-gm vial			24 / 12	44 mg/kg B.W. / 33 mg/kg B.W.	SC / SC, IM	
Spectinomycin[f]	Spectinomycin Injectable	Diamond	30-ml vial 100 mg/ml	Bacteriostatic	Broad-spectrum	8	33 mg/kg B.W.	SC	60[d]
Neomycin[a, g]	Biosol Liquid	Upjohn	1 pint 140 mg/ml	Bactericidal	Broad spectrum	8	88 mg/kg B.W.	IM, SC	120[d]

[a]Dosage, treatment interval, and route of administration adjusted so as to assure an antibiotic concentration in the serum that is equal to or greater than the minimum inhibitory concentration for sensitive P. haemolytica and P. multocida isolates for no less than 67 per cent of the period between treatments.

[b]Recommended by the FDA.

[c]Approved by the FDA for use in beef cattle as indicated in the table.

[d]Suggested by the author.

[e]Not recommended for treatment of Pasteurella infections.

[f]Dosage, treatment interval, and route of administration adjusted so as to assure an antibiotic concentration in the serum that is equal to or greater than the minimum inhibitory concentration for sensitive P. hemolytica and P. multocida isolates for no less than 50 per cent of the period between treatments.

[g]Approved only for oral and intramammary use.

of being forced to choose between a treatment regimen that is less than optimally effective in a substantial proportion of his cases and one that is effective in a greater number of cases but for which reliable drug withdrawal information is lacking. The author has summarized suggested dosage, administration route, and treatment interval regimens for oxytetracycline hydrochloride, procaine penicillin G in aqueous suspension, ampicillin trihydrate, amoxicillin trihydrate, erythromycin, tylosin, chloramphenicol, spectinomycin, and neomycin sulfate (see Table 2). The suggested regimens, in general, will maintain blood serum concentrations that are inhibitory for antibiotic-sensitive *P. haemolytica* and *P. multocida* isolates for at least two thirds of the time period between treatments.

Tetracyclines

From 63 to 97 per cent of *P. haemolytica* and *P. multocida* isolates recovered from nasal secretions of cattle with B & FP and approximately 20 per cent of *C. pyogenes* isolates are sensitive to tetracyclines. Chlortetracycline (CTC) and oxytetracycline (OTC) are both available in forms suitable for feed or water medication, but absorption from the digestive tract of cattle is limited. Doses of 88 mg per kg of body weight per day are required to achieve inhibitory (1 to 2 μgm/ml) serum concentrations. Adverse effects on ruminal microflora preclude the use of large doses of tetracyclines by the oral route for management of acute bacterial infections in cattle.

Of the three major tetracyclines, only oxytetracycline hydrochloride is suitable for intramuscular (IM) or subcutaneous (SC) injection. Consequently, it is the one most frequently utilized for systemic therapy. Subcutaneous administration, though not an FDA-approved procedure, is considered by the author to be the preferred method. Inhibitory serum OTC concentrations are obtained within one to four hours after subcutaneous injection. With some proprietary preparations, a substantial concentration advantage over intravenous and intramuscular administration is obtained during the last 8 to 16 hours of a 24-hour treatment interval. The frequency of post-injection abscessation is thought to be less with subcutaneous administration than with intramuscular administration. When abscessation does occur, less damage results to edible tissues. OTC is usually injected into the dorsal midcervical muscles or the cervical subcutaneous tissues. To minimize local tissue irritation, the calculated dose is administered in multiple injection sites, using a maximum volume of 10 ml per site. In a series of acute feedlot B & FP cases summarized by the author, 70.8 per cent responded satisfactorily when treated with OTC as suggested (see Table 2).

Penicillin G

From 63 to 78 per cent of *P. haemolytica* and *P. multocida* isolates recovered from nasal secretions of cattle with B & FP are sensitive to penicillin G. All *C. pyogenes* isolates are sensitive to penicillin G.

Because of rapid absorption from injection sites and rapid urinary excretion, multiple daily administration is required when treating with sodium or potassium penicillin G.

Serum concentrations of penicillin G are inhibitory for penicillin G–sensitive *P. haemolytica* and *P. multocida*

isolates (0.5 to 2 μgm/ml) for only four hours following administration of benzathine penicillin G (Bicillin Fortified* [benzathine penicillin G and procaine penicillin G in aqueous suspension]) in the FDA-approved regimen of 2 ml per 68 kg of body weight, injected subcutaneously. Even at five times the approved dose, serum penicillin G concentrations are inhibitory for only 12 hours following injection.

Procaine penicillin G, aqueous suspension, is the form of penicillin G best suited for treatment of B & FP in cattle. With the FDA-approved regimen of 6600 units per kg of body weight injected intramuscularly, serum penicillin G concentrations are inhibitory for penicillin G–sensitive *P. haemolytica* and *P. multocida* isolates for only two to four hours after administration. In a series of acute feedlot B & FP cases summarized by the author, 78.6 per cent responded satisfactorily when treated with procaine penicillin G as suggested (see Table 2).

Ampicillin Trihydrate and Amoxicillin Trihydrate

Sensitivity of *P. haemolytica* and *P. multocida* isolates to ampicillin and amoxicillin closely parallels sensitivity to penicillin G. Of 390 penicillin G–resistant isolates, 82.8 per cent were also resistant to ampicillin. As with penicillin G, all *C. pyogenes* isolates are sensitive to ampicillin and amoxicillin. The suggested treatment regimen (see Table 2) provides serum ampicillin concentrations that are continuously inhibitory for 96 per cent of ampicillin-sensitive *P. haemolytica* and *P. multocida* isolates.

Erythromycin

Erythromycin is marketed for use in cattle as Erythro-200.† With the FDA-approved treatment regimen of 4.4 mg per kg of body weight injected intramuscularly at 24-hour intervals, serum erythromycin concentrations are not inhibitory for *P. haemolytica* and *P. multocida* isolates. Approximately 29 per cent of *C. pyogenes* isolates are inhibited by similar erythromycin concentrations.

The author has utilized Erythro-200 for treatment in a large series of feedlot B & FP cases as suggested (see Table 2). Response rates ranging from 16 to 43 per cent were recorded. Severe local tissue reactions are associated with the use of Erythro-200 in this dosage. No more than 10 ml should be administered in any one injection site. Extreme care should be taken to avoid administering the drug into previously injected muscle masses. The first dose is divided equally between the gluteal and lateral hamstring muscles of the left rear limb. The second dose is similarly distributed in the opposite limb. The third and fourth doses are injected into the medial hamstring muscles of the left and right rear limbs, respectively. Treatment is usually limited to a maximum of four days. Relapsing cattle, previously treated with Erythro-200, are not retreated with it. Erythro-200 should be reserved for treatment of B & FP associated with bacteria that are sensitive to erythromycin and resistant to sulfonamides, penicillin G, and tetracyclines.

Peak serum erythromycin concentrations are achieved more rapidly and are significantly higher with intramuscular administration of Erythro-200 than with subcutaneous administration.

*Available from Wyeth Laboratories, Inc., Philadelphia, PA 19101.
†Available from Abbott Laboratories, North Chicago, IL 60064.

Tylosin

The author has successfully utilized tylosin as suggested (see Table 2) as an alternative to penicillin G therapy in refractory *C. pyogenes* infections. Sensitive *C. pyogenes* isolates are inhibited by substantially lower concentrations of tylosin than of penicillin G. In addition, tylosin, being a lipophilic antimicrobial, is better able to penetrate cellular membranes (such as the capsule of abscesses) than is penicillin G, which is an ionized antimicrobial.

Intramuscular administration is preferred to subcutaneous administration, since absorption from subcutaneous sites is significantly retarded.

Use of tylosin in the treatment of B & FP should be limited to penicillin G–refractory *C. pyogenes* infections and to infections with unusual organisms that are sensitive to tylosin and resistant to sulfonamides, penicillin G, and tetracyclines. In a series of acute feedlot B & FP cases treated with tylosin as suggested (see Table 2), 23 per cent responded favorably. Response rates of up to 37 per cent were obtained in chronic cases, which were more commonly associated with a *C. pyogenes* component.

Dihydrostreptomycin sulfate (DHS)

Approximately 72 per cent of *P. haemolytica* and *P. multocida* isolates and approximately 81 per cent of *C. pyogenes* isolates are *not* inhibited by the concentrations of DHS achieved in serum with the FDA-approved regimen of 11 mg per kg of body weight, injected intramuscularly. With this dosage, DHS must be administered at eight-hour intervals to maintain serum concentrations in the 8 to 18 μgm/ml range that is inhibitory for DHS-sensitive Pasteurellae. Consequently, DHS is not recommended for treatment of routine cases of bovine B & FP but should be reserved for those cases in which the infecting organism is sensitive to DHS but resistant to sulfonamides, penicillin G, tetracyclines, erythromycin, and tylosin. Serum concentrations of DHS are better sustained following intramuscular injection than following subcutaneous injection.

Chloramphenicol

Virtually all chloramphenicol-sensitive *P. haemolytica* and *P. multocida* isolates are inhibited by the serum concentrations resulting from the treatment regimens suggested (see Table 2). Approximately 56 per cent of *C. pyogenes* isolates are inhibited by these same regimens. In a series of acute B & FP cases summarized by the author, 82.6 per cent responded satisfactorily when treated with chloramphenicol as recommended (see Table 2). Because of (1) the comparative rarity of chloramphenicol-resistant pasteurella bacteria, (2) the persistence of inhibitory blood serum concentrations with once-daily subcutaneous administration, (3) safety, and (4) moderate cost, chloramphenicol is the "prescription legend" drug of choice for treatment of B & FP cases that have proven to be refractory to standard antimicrobial therapy. Unfortunately, it is now unlawful to administer chloramphenicol to food animals.

Spectinomycin

Approximately 79 per cent of *P. haemolytica* and *P. multocida* isolates from the lungs of fatal cases of feedlot B & FP (not treated with spectinomycin) are sensitive to spectinomycin. Approximately 69 per cent of *C. pyogenes* isolates are sensitive to spectinomycin. The suggested treatment regimen (see Table 2) provides serum spectinomycin concentrations that are inhibitory for most spectinomycin-sensitive *P. haemolytica* and *P. multocida* isolates during about 50 per cent of the time interval between treatments. When used as suggested (see Table 2) in clinical cases of B & FP, the efficacy of spectinomycin therapy is comparable to that reported with sulfamethazine, procaine penicillin G, and chloramphenicol.

Neomycin

With the suggested treatment regimen of 88 mg per kg of body weight (see Table 2), serum neomycin concentrations are inhibitory for virtually all *P. haemolytica* and *P. multocida* isolates and for approximately 74 per cent of *C. pyogenes* isolates. Neomycin sulfate should be used only as a treatment of last resort because of notoriously persistent tissue drug residues and because of the risk of nephrotoxicosis. Nephrotoxicosis has occurred in cattle treated twice daily with neomycin sulfate by intramuscular injection with dosages as low as 11 mg per kg of body weight and with a course of treatment as short as seven days. It is recommended, when possible, that the blood urea nitrogen (BUN) concentration be monitored during treatment to detect the possible onset of nephrotoxicosis. The renal lesion may be resolved if treatment is terminated promptly when BUN levels begin to rise. Irreversible auditory toxicosis may also result, particularly if therapy is prolonged.

Supportive Therapy

In the opinion of the author, supportive treatment (other than good husbandry as previously discussed) has little application in the treatment of uncomplicated B & FP in commercial cattle. Any benefits are usually only in the relief of symptoms and are unlikely to influence final mortality or culling rates. Use of corticosteroids in uncomplicated cases should be discouraged since efficacy of bacteriostatic antimicrobials may be reduced. In addition, corticosteroid therapy may cause remission of fever and toxemia, resulting in premature termination of antimicrobial therapy and leading to subsequent exacerbation of clinical signs.

PREVENTION AND CONTROL

Recommendations for control of B & FP must consider the geographic location of the individual production unit and the production system utilized. The objective of a preventative program is to minimize economic losses from B & FP by preventing IBR, BVD, PI-3, and perhaps BRSV infections through vaccination, by eliminating or decreasing stresses, and by avoiding management practices that favor a high incidence of B & FP.

Controlling B & FP in Feedlot Cattle

The B & FP problem can be reduced by utilization of "preconditioned" cattle. "Preconditioned" cattle have been weaned and fed a milled concentrate ration on the ranch of origin for a minimum period of 30 days prior to shipment to the feedlot. Processing is performed at least 14 days prior to shipment and should include necessary vaccinations, implantation with a growth stimulant, administration of a systemic organophosphate insecticide, and treatment with an anthelmintic, if required. B & FP losses are minimized by avoiding saleyard cattle and buying directly from ranchers. In a feedlot serviced by the author, the mortality rate was 1.5 per cent, the culling rate was 3.2 per cent, and the medicine cost was $5.09 per head in 1,070 yearling saleyard steers. Corresponding values were 1.0 per cent, 1.3 per cent, and $4.20 per head in 6,057 yearling ranch steers fed during the same two-year period. It was necessary to discount the saleyard cattle approximately $3.25 per head to compensate for increased health problems, especially B & FP.

If cattle have not previously been vaccinated for IBR and BVD, this should be done as soon as possible after arrival at the feedlot. IBR vaccination is absolutely essential. BVD vaccination is not as critical because most infections are subclinical. Additionally, cattle arriving in feedlots are usually protected by colostral BVD antibodies or are immune from natural exposure. Susceptible groups are occasionally encountered, however, and heavy losses can be expected when B & FP and BVD occur coincidentally. It is thought that the leukopenia and cellular and humoral immune system suppression resulting from BVD infection enhance the pathogenicity of pasteurella bacteria. The occurrence of post-vaccinal mucosal disease has been a deterrent to widespread acceptance of BVD vaccination. This problem is associated with the use of specific commercial modified live virus (MLV) vaccines, which should be avoided since they appear to be insufficiently attenuated. Two different groups of workers have reported adverse effects (increased morbidity rates from clinical BVD and respiratory disease) associated with the use of MLV BVD vaccines in stressed cattle. Nevertheless, the author prefers MLV IBR and BVD vaccines over inactivated vaccines when cattle cannot be immunized prior to arrival in the feedlot. Rapid achievement of immunity is paramount in an environment where instant exposure to virulent virus is virtually assured. Intramuscular MLV IBR vaccines are favored over intranasal MLV IBR vaccines because of cost advantages and negligible differences in efficacy.

Administration of either MLV or inactivated PI-3 vaccines to cattle after arrival in the feedlot should not be expected to provide cost-effective control of B & FP. Exposure to PI-3 virus may occur before effective immunity can develop. Additionally, a high proportion of cattle of feedlot age have significant serum antibody titers to PI-3 virus and may not benefit from immunization. Since PI-3 vaccination almost routinely fails to reduce the incidence of B & FP, it is likely that PI-3 is less important than other viruses in the etiology of B & FP. PI-3 vaccination may be desirable if it can be performed on the ranch of origin at least two weeks prior to transportation to the feedlot. MLV PI-3 vaccines, especially intranasal vaccines, are favored over inactivated virus vaccines, since nasal (secretory) antibody production is more important in resistance than humoral antibody production.

The importance and effectiveness of the new MLV BRSV vaccines for control of B & FP have yet to be determined under field conditions. The results of some limited field studies have shown promise, however.

Upon arrival at the feedlot, cattle should be re-fed on hay for several days before feeding concentrate rations to avoid overconsumption and lactic acidosis in hungry cat-

tle. Alternatively, cattle may be started on a milled ration containing 50 per cent roughage.

The incidence of B & FP is usually highest in groups of cattle that are least inclined to consume feedlot rations. Consequently, a major effort should be undertaken to encourage feed consumption in newly received cattle by offering a palatable ration kept fresh by frequent feeding of small quantities, by promptly removing stale feed, by preventing the accumulation of "fines" and by avoiding unnecessary ration changes. Receiving pens should be wide and shallow to keep the cattle in close proximity to the feedbunks. If cattle are reluctant to feed they can usually be coaxed to the feedbunks by frequent offerings of longstem baled hay placed on top of the milled feed. Premature utilization of very high energy rations before ruminal adaptation has occurred will aggravate the B & FP problem. Once feeding of a high energy ration has begun, it must be available free-choice at all times or lactic acidosis is likely to result.

It is especially important that cattle not be overcrowded during the first 30 days after arrival. A minimum of 40 square feet of pen space and 12 linear inches of feedbunk space per head should be provided. An allowance of approximately 100 square feet of pen space per head appears optimal in terms of stress reduction.

Except for initial processing, cattle should not be handled for 30 days after arrival to minimize stress and avoid disturbing their feeding patterns.

Cattle from different sources should not be commingled during the first 30 days after arrival to minimize cross-infection with respiratory viruses and to avoid stresses associated with establishing a new "pecking order."

Cattle of unequal size should not be penned together, since the smaller animals cannot effectively compete for feedbunk space.

The B & FP problem is aggravated when cattle are started in an excessively dusty or muddy environment. Corral dust is controlled in starting pens with sprinkler systems. After 30 days, the problem can be controlled by increasing the stocking rate, except where shade must be provided. Mud is harder to control. This is accomplished by hauling in dirt and building mounds for cattle to rest upon, by reducing stocking rates, and by frequent scraping of pens and removal of manure.

Mass medication may help to reduce the incidence of B & FP. Sulfonamides are administered in full therapeutic dosages for five to seven days in feed or water or individually in the form of sustained-release boluses (see Table 1). Antibiotics such as procaine penicillin G, aqueous suspension, or oxytetracycline hydrochloride are administered parenterally in full therapeutic dosages, usually for one to three days. Alternatively CTC or OTC may be administered in feed or water over a two- to four-week period utilizing a "prophylactic" dosage of 2.2 mg per kg of body weight per day. Mass medication of antimicrobials in full therapeutic dosages is very effective in preventing occurrence of clinical disease during the period that a therapeutic blood antimicrobial concentration is maintained and for a few days thereafter. It is more effective in highly stressed cattle, in which the occurrence of B & FP tends to be compressed into a relatively short seven- to ten-day period. Results are maximized when initiation of treatment is delayed until significant numbers of animals are beginning to show clinical signs of B & FP. The occurrence of B & FP may be spread out over a four- to six-week period in groups of cattle that have not been significantly stressed prior to arrival in the feedlot. In such groups, short periods of mass medication may have relatively insignificant effects on final morbidity rates. A 30-day "prophylactic"course of feed or water medication with CTC or OTC may be of greater value. Reductions of up to 50 per cent in the morbidity rate have been commonly reported. In the experience of the author, however, this method of control has been without merit under commercial feedlot conditions. Oral administration of CTC or OTC does not produce blood serum antibiotic concentrations that are inhibitory for pasteurella bacteria, so that sick cattle must be individually treated. Administration of a combination of procaine penicillin G and benzathine penicillin G to calves by subcutaneous injection in a single dose of 8800 units per kg of body weight within 24 hours after arrival at the feedlot has been said to reduce the occurrence of B & FP.

It should be appreciated that any mass medication scheme will suppress antimicrobial-sensitive bacteria and permit antimicrobial-resistant bacteria to increase their relative importance in the gastrointestinal and upper respiratory tract flora. An increased number of antimicrobial-resistant pasteurella pneumonia cases can be anticipated when mass medication is utilized, even though morbidity and mortality rates may be reduced by the practice. For this reason, mass medication is best reserved for use in highly stressed groups, in which a high percentage would be treated anyway. Newly received cattle should be isolated, especially from cattle that have received mass medication, until the period of highest susceptibility to B & FB has passed to minimize exposure to antimicrobial-resistant pasteurella bacteria.

Pasteurella bacterins and antisera prepared against pasteurella bacteria have been found valueless where controlled field studies have been conducted. However, preliminary results with modified live pasteurella vaccines appear promising. A modified live *P. haemolytica* vaccine has recently become commercially available. It can be predicted that (1) effective immunization against both *P. haemolytica* and *P. multocida* will be required for effective control of B & FP and that (2) the new modified live pasteurella vaccines will be most effective when they can be administered several weeks or more before cattle are introduced to the feedlot environment.

Commercial *Haemophilus somnus* bacterins are clearly effective for prevention of thromboembolic meningoencephalitis. However, the extent to which they may be effective in reducing the incidence of B & FP is, as yet, undetermined. Because of the difficulty with which *H. somnus* is isolated from tissues, the extent to which it is involved in the etiology of B & FP is, as yet, unknown. Various authors have reported its isolation from between 1.4 and 5 per cent of fatal cases of B & FP. In one large Canadian study, the mortality rate (from all causes) was not significantly influenced by administration of an *H. somnus* bacterin to calves upon arrival in feedlots. In three small Indian field trials, administration of an *H. somnus* bacterin to calves upon arrival in a feedlot did not influence the mortality rate or feedlot weight gains. In the initial trial, the morbidity rate from respiratory disease was significantly reduced from 30.8 to 19.8 per cent. In two subsequent trials, however, the morbidity

rate was not reduced by vaccination. It seems clear that vaccination of cattle with an inactivated product, subsequent to arrival at the feedlot, has limited potential for effective control of a disease like B & FP (in which significant morbidity often occurs within the first one to two weeks after arrival).

Since it is not currently possible to totally prevent B & FP, effective control is highly dependent on early disease detection and prompt, rational treatment of clinical cases. It is imperative that sufficient numbers of experienced pencheckers be provided.

Controlling B & FP in Beef Calves on Pasture

Pre-weaning vaccination against PI-3 virus infection has apparently prevented or reduced the post-weaning B & FP problem on individual ranches. Vaccination should be performed at least two to four weeks prior to weaning. Intranasal vaccine is preferred. Vaccination for IBR and BVD is also desirable where there is a post-weaning B & FP problem. Intranasal MLV or inactivated IBR vaccine is recommended if vaccinated calves are to be put back with pregnant cows to avoid the risk of vaccine virus IBR abortion. It remains to be determined how useful the new MLV BRSV vaccines and the new modified live *Pasteurella* vaccines may prove to be in this environment.

To minimize stress, calves should not be handled for two weeks before and after weaning. Weaning stress can be reduced by avoiding corral weaning; cows and calves are moved to a relatively small, well-fenced field with abundant forage. After seven to ten days, weaning is accomplished by removing one third of the cows each day over a three-day period. Two weeks after weaning, the calves can be moved to other pastures.

If corral weaning cannot be avoided, dusty or muddy conditions should be controlled. Preventive mass medication can be expected to reduce the incidence of B & FP with minimal risk of antimicrobial-resistant pasteurella pneumonia. By the time bacteria have developed resistance, the cattle are no longer under stress and are not highly susceptible to B & FP. Continuous medication of feed or water with tetracycline, CTC, or OTC in a dose of 2.2 mg per kg of body weight per day for two to four weeks after weaning is the method of choice.

Preventing B & FP in Dairy Calves

Calves should be vaccinated against PI-3 virus infection, preferably with intranasal MLV vaccine, approximately two to four weeks before they are weaned and placed in group pens. Vaccination for IBR, BVD, and perhaps BRSV is also recommended at this time.

Calves should be kept in individual crates for two weeks following weaning, after which time they can be placed in group pens, together with no more than 10 to 20 calves of similar age and size. Stressful procedures such as dehorning and castration should be done at least one month prior to weaning. Ideally, each group pen should be isolated from other group pens by at least 20 feet of open air space, so that a respiratory disease outbreak can be confined to an affected group of calves. Each group of calves should be raised together in isolation until they are four to six months of age, after which time their susceptibility to B & FP is dramatically reduced.

Corral dust or mud must be controlled. Calves should not be overcrowded. A minimum of 25 square feet of pen space and 12 linear inches of feedbunk space should be provided. This should be increased to 100 square feet of pen space per head should B & FP become a problem.

Whenever possible, housing of calves in enclosed buildings should be avoided. Adequate ventilation (in terms of the number of air changes per hour) of such structures is essential for satisfactory respiratory health and is seldom achieved. Any detectable odor of ammonia in a calf barn should be considered dangerous. Calves can tolerate very low temperatures if kept dry with adequate bedding and overhead cover and protected from drafts. Open sheds, enclosed on three sides and facing south, provide adequate shelter in severe climates with a minimum of ventilation problems. If calves must be housed, serious problems with B & FP can generally be avoided if the structure can be uniformly ventilated at a minimum rate of four air changes per hour, and draftiness, extreme temperatures, and temperature fluctuations prevented.

Calves that are debilitated by parasitism, malnutrition, or viral and/or bacterial gastrointestinal infections are highly susceptible to B & FP; therefore, these problems, if present, should be corrected.

Vaccination for brucellosis with strain 19 vaccine is a stress that often triggers outbreaks of B & FP in dairy calves. Strain 19 vaccine should not be simultaneously administered with any other live vaccine. Administration of strain 19 vaccine should be timed so as to avoid periods of high susceptibility to B & FP such as within two weeks of weaning, grouping, processing, vaccination with MLV vaccines, and so on.

Preventive mass medication should be avoided when other control measures are economically feasible; otherwise problems with antimicrobial-resistant *Pasteurella* pneumonia can be anticipated. Medication of feed or water with tetracycline, CTC, or OTC for the first 30 days after placement in group pens has not resulted in satisfactory control, in the experience of the author.

Early disease detection and prompt, rational treatment of clinical cases are necessary for satisfactory control. It is possible that the new modified live pasteurella vaccines may prove useful in the control of this problem.

FIBRINOUS PLEURITIS AND PLEUROPNEUMONIA

The term "fibrinous pleuritis and pleuropneumonia" (FPPP) has been proposed by the author for a unique and rather uncommon disease syndrome that deserves to be included under the umbrella of the bovine respiratory disease complex.

Etiology and Epidemiology

FPPP is an acute infection of the lung and/or pleura with *Haemophilus somnus,* often in conjunction with Pasteurella bacteria. It is thought that stress and concurrent respiratory viral infections are prerequisites, as in B & FP. Cattle are usually affected between the fourteenth and thirtieth day after arrival in the feedlot.

FPPP usually occurs sporadically and is usually of minor economic significance. A total of 11 fatal cases were diagnosed in a total of 96,092 head of cattle received by a single feedlot over a five-year period (a mortality of 0.01 per cent). Then, during the subsequent year, an outbreak of FPPP occurred and 40 fatal cases were diagnosed. Thirty three of these occurred in a population of 8,682 cattle received during a single month (a mortality rate of 0.38 per cent). Mortality rates in affected groups ranged from 0.18 to 2.03 per cent.

The precise morbidity rate of FPPP cannot be determined under commercial feedlot conditions. Because exacerbations of pleuritis and pneumonia and chronic unthriftiness would be anticipated in survivors and because only five such cases were recognized during an eight-year period of observation, it is believed that most affected cattle die. All ages, breeds, and sexes of feedlot cattle appear to be equally susceptible to FPPP.

FPPP is sometimes associated with the occurrence of *Haemophilus* thromboembolic meningoencephalitis (TEME). In the outbreak of FPPP observed by the author, six cases of TEME occurred within three days of the time that sister cattle, in the same lots (groups) as the cattle with TEME, were affected with fatal FPPP.

Clinical Signs

Onset is sudden and usually characterized by high fever, anorexia, marked depression, and expiratory dyspnea. The course was two days or less in 42 of 55 fatalities (76 per cent) in the author's series. Occasionally the course was as long as 57 days.

Pathology

When the chest is opened, one or both pleural spaces are found to be completely obliterated by massive accumulations of yellow fibrin and straw-colored fluid. A 5- to 8-cm thick sheet of fibrin is adhered to the pleura of the affected lung. In a few cases, only the pleura and pleural space are affected. Usually, however, a pleuropneumonia is also present. In these instances, the dependent parts of the affected lung are firm. Affected lobules are pinkish-tan and separated by enlarged, white interlobular septa. In some cases, lesions of acute or subacute B & FP accompany those of pleuropneumonia.

On histopathologic examination the interlobular septa are dilated with edema fluid and fibrin, are focally necrotic, and are separated from adjacent lung parenchyma by a zone of leukocytes. Airways are normal or mildly infiltrated with leukocytes. Alveoli are congested, flooded with edema fluid, atelectatic, or mildly infiltrated with leukocytes.

Treatment

The treatment regimens recommended for B & FP are also recommended for treatment of FPPP, although most cases are probably not amenable to treatment.

Control

As with TEME (and unlike B & FP), losses from FPPP are abruptly terminated when CTC or OTC is administered in the ration to affected groups in a dosage of 2.2 mg per kg of body weight per day for ten days. New cases are prevented from the third day of the medication period and more do not recur when treatment is terminated.

Commercial *H. somnus* bacterins would presumably afford protection if administered a sufficient period of time prior to exposure for immunity to develop. With usual and expected rates of occurrence, bacterins are not a cost-effective means of control.

Supplemental Reading

Hjerpe, C. A., and Routen, T. A.: Practical and theoretical considerations concerning treatment of bacterial pneumonia in feedlot cattle, with special reference to antimicrobic therapy. Proc. 9th Ann. Meeting A.A.B.P., 1976, 97–140.

Mohanty, S. B.: Bovine respiratory viruses. Adv. Vet. Sci. Comp. Med. 22:83–109, 1978.

Veit, H. P., and Farrell, R. L.: The anatomy and physiology of the bovine respiratory system relating to pulmonary disease. Cornell Vet. 68:555–581, 1978.

Chronic Respiratory Disease in the Pig

HARVEY D. HILLEY, D.V.M., Ph.D.,
BARBARA KOTT, D.V.M., M.S.,
and GARY D. DIAL, D.V.M., Ph.D.

The chronic respiratory disease complex has classically been divided into two general categories: atrophic rhinitis, in which lesions are confined to the upper respiratory tract, and chronic pneumonia, in which the lower respiratory tract is affected. Because the pathogenesis of atrophic rhinitis and of chronic pneumonia are similar, it is difficult to consider the lower respiratory tract without considering the upper. As discussed in this article, diseases of the upper and lower airways have a multifactorial etiology with a pathogenesis that is influenced by age of the host, pathogens involved, management practices, and environmental conditions. Although this article deals with chronic pneumonia, a discussion of atrophic rhinitis appears elsewhere in this volume.

IMPORTANCE OF CHRONIC PNEUMONIA

Chronic respiratory disease reduces growth performance, thereby decreasing profits in the growing and finishing phases of swine production. Although mortality due to chronic pneumonia is usually low, most economic losses are attributable to its high morbidity. The cost of chronic pneumonia to the American swine industry has recently been estimated to be approximately $250 million. Losses largely result from decreased productivity, reduced rates of gain, decreased feeding efficiency, marketing of light animals that never reach market weight, and condemnations at slaughter. Various surveys have found that between 25 per cent and 90 per cent of animals slaughtered have gross lesions of pneumonia, indicating that the morbidity of the disease is high in most swine operations. Although herds with chronic pneumonia have been suggested to have a reduction in average daily gain of between 0 and 10 per cent, experimental trials indicate that growth rates may be reduced as much as 25 per cent.

FACTORS INFLUENCING THE OCCURRENCE OF CHRONIC PNEUMONIA

Infectious Etiologies

Mycoplasmas, bacteria, viruses, and endoparasites can be associated with chronic pneumonia (Fig. 1). The progression of pneumonia is so dynamic that infectious agents present in early stages of disease may be absent or masked by other microbes that are isolated from the chronically infected animal. Thus, when evaluating the chronic pneumonia problem, identification of a single infectious agent is rare. Because various mycoplasmal, bacterial, viral, and endoparasitic agents complicate the disease, determining the true etiology of an outbreak of pneumonia is difficult.

Presently, most investigators consider *Mycoplasma hyopneumoniae* as the most common primary pathogen involved in chronic (enzootic) pneumonia of pigs. Secondary pathogens increase the course and severity of the Mycoplasma pneumonia. *Pasteurella multocida* type A is the most common opportunist but has not been found to be a primary cause of pneumonia. *Pasteurella multocida* type D (a toxin producer) is often associated with atrophic rhinitis but may also be capable of causing pneumonia. *Haemophilus pleuropneumoniae, Salmonella typhimurium* var. *copenhagen,* and *Salmonella cholerasuis* are well-recognized causes of acute epizootic pneumonia and also have been isolated from chronic cases of pneumonia. Other microbes that may be isolated from swine having chronic pneumonia include *Mycoplasma hyorhinis, Bordetella bronchiseptica, Haemophilus parasuis, Haemophilus* sp. (Taxon "minor group"), Streptococcus spp., and *Corynebacterium* spp. These organisms have been isolated from the respiratory tracts of young pigs and appear to be ubiquitous in older animals. Viral pathogens of the respiratory tracts of swine in the United States include inclusion body rhinitis (porcine cytomegalovirus), swine influenza virus, pseudorabies virus, and adenovirus. The importance of these viruses in the development of chronic pneumonia has not been investigated but is thought to be less than that of mycoplasmas and bacteria. Pulmonary migration of *Ascaris suum* larvae and *Metastrongylus* spp. in the presence of mycoplasmal, bacterial, or viral agents also has been shown to increase the severity of chronic pneumonia.

The most commonly observed lung lesion indicative of chronic pneumonia is consolidation of the ventral apical, cardiac, and intermediate lobes and anterior diaphragmatic lobes. Affected areas are purple to gray, often have a catarrhal exudate in the bronchioles, and have enlarged bronchial and mediastinal lymph nodes. If *H. pleuropneumoniae* is present, caseous nodules with thick capsules will be observed (primarily in the dorsal aspect of the diaphragmatic lobes) and there may be a fibrinous pleuritis. These caseous nodules should be differentiated from abscesses caused by *Corynebacterium pyogenes* and *Streptococcus* species. A fibrinous pleuritis may also be observed in pneumonias complicated by *P. multocida*. The pathogenesis of respiratory disease caused by mycoplasma, bacteria, viruses, and endoparasites has been covered in other articles. Nevertheless, their contribution to the chronic respiratory disease complex of swine should not be overlooked and must be considered in light of the host, management, and environmental influences on pneumonia.

Management

Various management practices have been shown to influence the incidence and severity of chronic pneumonia. Herds in which attention is paid to individual therapy of sick animals during post-weaning phases of production and in which an effort is made to keep facilities clean will have lower incidences of pneumonia. Minimizing the number of animals from different sources that are to be

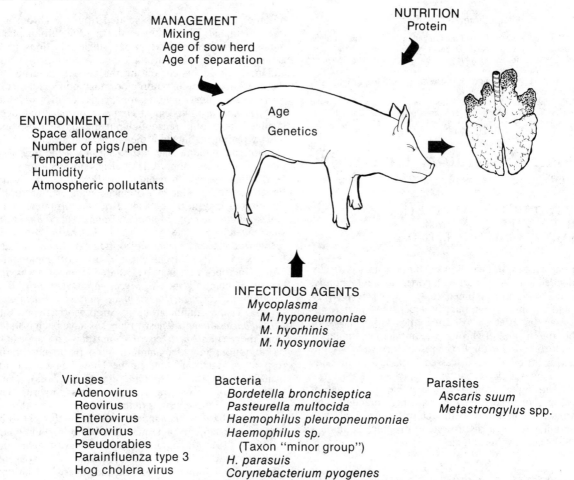

Figure 1. Factors affecting chronic pneumonia.

placed in the same facility has been shown to aid in the control of chronic pneumonia. Maintaining animals of similar age in groups that are kept intact and separate from groups of animals of other ages through the various stages of production results in a lower incidence of pneumonia than when young animals are continuously being added into a facility that also houses market-weight animals (continuous production). Development of an "all-in, all-out" system in which a group of animals is moved out before younger animals are moved into a section of a building prevents the horizontal transmission of infectious organisms from older, chronically infected animals to young, susceptible swine. The development of "all-in, all-out" animal flow also allows for cleaning between groups. It is not unusual to find operations with slow-growing swine in which there is a continuous flow of animals through facilities that are never cleaned.

Housing

The number of times an animal is moved during various phases of production influences the incidence of pneumonia. The incidence increases as animals are moved more frequently. One explanation for this observation is that since the dominance order of the pigs is relatively unstable, the movement of a group from one pen to another is sufficient to disrupt the social hierarchy. The resulting increased antagonistic interactions may alter an animal's resistance even when penmates have been kept together. In most operations, moving swine from one place of production to another is also accompanied by sorting and mixing, both of which further exacerbate the unstable social hierarchy.

Producers can also create increased instability of the social hierarchy and, consequently, increase the incidence of pneumonia by providing inadequate floor space. To minimize the impact that animal density has on pneumonia, several recommendations on the space allowances per pig have been made. These vary with age, floor type, and temperature. Common guidelines are 3 square feet per pig to 40 lb body weight, 4 square feet per pig to 100 lb body weight, 6 square feet per pig to 150 lb body weight, and 8 square feet per pig to 220 lb body weight. Floor space can be increased by 15 per cent during warm weather.

The number of animals in each group and the total number in a building are related to the incidence and severity of pneumonia. As the number of animals (n) in a facility is increased, the number of possible transmissions (N) between the animals increases exponentially ($N = n^2 - n$). Two different studies have documented that the incidence of pneumonia increases as the number of animals in a building increases. One study found that prevalence of pneumonia increased as capacity of buildings increased from less than 100, 100 to 200, 200 to 300, to more than 300 animals per building section. In another study, the severity of pneumonia was greater in farms that housed more than 500 animals per section as compared with farms that housed less than 500 animals per section. Although the ideal number of animals in a building needed to achieve the lowest incidence of pneumonia and the highest growth rates has not yet been elucidated, it appears that low numbers are most compatible with high performance.

Environment

Environmental factors have generally been considered to play a major role in the development of chronic pneumonia. Various parameters, such as temperature, humidity, aerosolized particulate matter, and various noxious gases, have been incriminated in the development of enzootic pneumonia. At present, there is very little information about the extent to which these environmental parameters influence the development of chronic pneumonia. It is currently thought by many that these parameters may indirectly affect the dose of a respiratory pathogen to which the animal is exposed and thereby directly affect the animal's defense mechanisms.

When an animal coughs or sneezes, microbes are expelled in aerosolized form. Large droplets (greater than 50 microns) will settle out rapidly, whereas smaller droplets (less than 20 microns) may evaporate to form droplet nuclei. These are capable of remaining suspended in the air for several hours. The aerodynamic size of these droplet nuclei is dependent upon the environmental temperature and humidity. A low temperature with low to moderate humidity (as occurs during the winter months) results in a higher number of small droplets remaining airborne for longer periods of time. The aerodynamic size of these particles also determines where they impact in the respiratory system. Particles around 10 microns in size usually impact in the nares, whereas particles of 5 microns or less in size have the ability to bypass the mucociliary apparatus and enter the terminal bronchioles and alveoli.

Temperature and moisture content not only influence the aerodynamic size of an infected droplet but also affect the survival of microbes in the environment. For most airborne microbes, the higher the temperature, the more quickly they die. Survivability at various humidities is dependent on the type of organism. Ultraviolet radiation in sunlight is also bactericidal and viricidal.

Dust particles that are found in swine confinement units are largely derived from the feed. Many of these particles (25 to 30 per cent) have an aerodynamic size (greater than 5 microns) that allows them to impact in the terminal bronchioles and alveoli. These small dust particles may act as vectors for gases and microbes to be carried to the lower respiratory tract. Dust may also exert a direct effect on the clearance mechanisms of the respiratory tracts of the pig. Practices such as adding liquid fat to diets, feeding a gruel, and cleaning facilities can be instituted to decrease the generation of aerosolized dust particles.

The type of waste disposal system that is being utilized within a facility has been shown to affect the severity of pneumonia. In the United States, it is a common practice to house swine on totally or partially slatted floors above anaerobic pits. This system is much more detrimental to the health of the animal than other systems. Hydrogen sulfide, ammonia, carbon dioxide, and methane are the major gases liberated from fermentation in anaerobic pits. The latter three are soluble in water. Ammonia is, in fact, so highly soluble in water that very little of what is inhaled ever reaches the lungs unless it is carried by a dust particle. However, even though ammonia only produces a slight change in the epithelium of the upper respiratory tract even at high concentrations, at relatively low ambient concentrations (50 to 75 ppm) it has been found to detrimentally influence the pulmonary clearance mechanisms of young pigs. Hydrogen sulfide (normally around 10 ppm in confinement buildings) may become an acute toxin if agitation of the pits causes release of high levels (> 400 ppm) into the air.

Buildings are ventilated to control microbial concentrations, temperature, humidity, dust content, and gases. Frequent subjective evaluation of the ventilation systems will in most cases reduce the incidence and severity of the pneumonia observed at slaughter. Finishing facilities in which the daily temperature fluctuations are minimized have a lower incidence of severely affected lungs at slaughter. Drafts, as expressed as an air velocity–temperature fluctuation index, are also related to the prevalence of severely affected lungs at slaughter. Draft-induced changes in air temperature predispose animals to pneumonia. Future studies that derive optimal ranges for effective environmental temperature and concentrations of moisture, gas, and dust will likely facilitate the control of chronic pneumonia.

Control

An effective control program is dependent upon maintaining a complete set of records so existing performance can be regularly evaluated. Goals should be established for the per cent mortality, rate of gain, number of animals culled at light market weights because of slow growth, and feed efficiency. With very little effort, producers can record the mortality rates of the nursery, growing, and finishing phases of production, the number of culled animals sold, rate of gain, and number of days from birth to market. However, it is usually more difficult to obtain the information needed for the calculation of feed efficiency. Since feed contributes to the major cost of production for raising weaned pigs, it is probably the best measure of the productivity of market swine. Feed efficiency can be monitored most accurately in facilities that feed groups of animals in batches or in ones that have specific pens in which weight hoppers are used to test representative pens of animals. Once objective assessments of productivity have been made, they can be related to subjective estimates of the severity and incidence of pneumonia. This can then be used to determine the impact of chronic pneumonia on the herd and to formulate control strategies.

There are several ways to assess the severity and incidence of pneumonia. On the farm, post-mortem evaluation of animals that have died will document the number of deaths due to pneumonia and provide some indication of the age at which pneumonia initially develops. It should be remembered that even though pneumonia is not as common a cause of death in suckling and nursery pigs as in growing/market swine, it has been observed in young swine. As discussed previously, examination of acutely affected animals is usually required if the pathogen of a respiratory problem is to be identified. Slaughterhouse investigation is another excellent clinical tool for estimating the degree to which decreased growth performance is attributable to pneumonia. One should remember that there may be a seasonal variation in the severity of pneumonia observed at slaughter; pneumonia may be more commonly observed in animals killed during March, April, May, and June, depending on facility type and location. Slaughterhouse investigations in conjunction with reviews of records not only establish the severity and cost of pneumonia but also determine if control measures are effective.

Vaccination and treatment are usually of minimal value in controlling chronic pneumonia. Products are commercially available for the control of *H. pleuropneumoniae, P. multocida,* and pseudorabies. Even though they may be beneficial in reducing mortality in acute outbreaks, they have questionable benefit in controlling chronic pneumonia. There are no vaccines available for any of the other infectious agents that have been shown to be involved in cases of chronic pneumonia.

Oral therapy of a groups of animals via the feed or water is often helpful in controlling an acute outbreak of pneumonia. Water medication is preferable, since sick animals are usually anorexic. Therapy ideally should be initiated after antibiotic sensitivity testing. Obviously, the effectiveness of the antimicrobial must be taken into account in light of its cost. Common water medications used in the treatment of swine pneumonias include various tetracyclines, sulfonamides, ampicillin, and lincomycin. Although presently cleared only for use in swine dysentery, tiamulin also has been found to be effective against *H. pleuropneumoniae* and *M. hyopneumoniae*. Injectable products include the tetracyclines, erythromycin, ampicillin, lincomycin, tylosin, penicillin, and streptomycin. Even though treatment of acute pneumonias is often rewarding, mass medication of swine having chronic pneumonia is of questionable benefit. When antimicrobials are used to combat pneumonia, efforts must be made to prevent reinfection after discontinuation of treatment. Individual therapy of the clinically ill animal is often possible with herds that have a low prevalence of pneumonia.

In addition to medical therapy, management can be altered in an attempt to control pneumonia. Hospital pens should be established and located outside the facility whenever possible. If internal parasites are a problem, an effective control program utilizing sanitation and anthelmintic treatment of sows and market swine should be initiated. In some herds, animal flow can be altered to allow for age separation. In others, the partitioning of facilities to handle individual groups may be economical. Such changes will allow for age separation, the close regulation of the environment needed for the specific age of animals, and the clean-up of the facility between groups. The number of sources of animals should be minimized and overcrowding avoided. The ventilation system should have the appropriate fan capacities, inlet sizes, and fan placement to provide adequate ventilation with even air distribution. If inexperienced, the practitioner should consult with an agricultural engineer who has expertise in the management of ventilation systems of hog confinement facilities. Although very seldom done, a regular maintenance schedule should be followed for thermostats, fans, curtain controllers, and inlets. Thermometers that monitor the high and low temperatures of the day can be used to monitor fluctuations and, thereby, optimize the pig's environment. In naturally ventilated facilities or in wide barns with poor air distribution, internal recirculation fans can be used to improve the air distribution. Space and ventilation requirements for various ages of animals can be found in the *Midwest Plan Services Structures and Facilities* (1980).

Since animal waste is the primary source of noxious gases that influence growth performance, special attention should be paid to regulating and monitoring waste disposal. If gasses are thought to contribute to a chronic pneumonia problem, waste-handling procedures may warrant modification. Facilities with anaerobic pits can be modified to a flush system. If this is not possible, a pit recharge system can be developed in which the manure in the pit is emptied every week and refilled with 8 to 12 inches of recycled lagoon water.

In summary, it cannot be overemphasized that improvement of management, facilities, and environment is the most cost-effective means of controlling chronic pneumonia.

Supplemental Reading

Backstrom, L., and Bremer, H.: The relationship between disease incidences of fatteners registered at slaughter and environmental factors in herd. Nord. Vet. Med. *30*:526, 1978.

Curtis, S. E.: Environmental Management in Animal Agriculture. Illinois Animal Environment Services, Mahomet, 1981, Ch. 20, 23, 24.

Hatch, T. F.: Distribution and deposition of inhaled particles in respiratory tract. Bacterial. Rev. *25*:237–240, 1961.

Lindqvist, J. O.: Animal health and environment in the production of fattening pigs. Acta Vet. Scand. *51*(Supp.):1–78, 1974.

Little, T. W. A.: Respiratory diseases in pigs: A study. Vet. Rec. *96*:540–544, 1975.

Midwest Plan Service: Swine Handbook: Housing and Equipment. Iowa State University Press, Ames, IA, 1972.

Ross, R. F.: Chronic pneumonia of swine with emphasis on mycoplasma pneumonia. Proc. Am. Assoc.: Swine Pract., 79–96, 1984.

Tielen, M. J. M.: Buildings, environmental conditions, and disease. Proc. 29th Ann. Meet. Eur. Assoc. Anim. Prod., 747, 1978.

Parasites of the Respiratory System

DWIGHT G. BENNETT, D.V.M., Ph.D.

Lungworms are common parasites of cattle, sheep, and swine. *Dictyocaulus viviparus* is the only lungworm of cattle. It is usually associated with areas of high moisture and moderate temperatures but is widely, though sporadically, distributed in North America.

Dictyocaulus filaria is the large lungworm of sheep. Its distribution is similar to that of the cattle lungworm. *Muellerius capillaris* is the hair lungworm of sheep and goats. It is found in the lungs of lambs at necropsy, and its presence is rarely diagnosed ante mortem. *Protostrongylus rufescens* is the red lungworm of sheep and goats. It is uncommon in North America.

There are three species of the genus *Metastrongylus* found in the lungs of swiine. *M. apri* is the most prevalent, being common in pigs all over North America. *M. salmi* and *M. pudendotectus* have a similar distribution but are less numerous.

LIFE CYCLES

Dictyocaulus viviparus and *D. filaria* have direct life cycles. The eggs are coughed up, and a few are coughed out of the mouth. However, most of the eggs are swallowed and hatch in the intestine, so first-stage larvae are ordinarily passed in the feces. The larvae on the ground develop to the infective stage in about four days. Drying, sunlight, and cold have been reported to be harmful to the larvae, but sufficient numbers survive the winter on pastures to establish infections the following spring. Cattle and sheep become infected by ingesting the third-stage larvae.

The remaining lumgworms have indirect life cycles involving earthworms *(Metastrongylus)* or snails and slugs *(Muellerius* and *Protostrongylus)* as intermediate hosts. The first-stage larvae or, in the case of *Metastrongylus*, eggs pass in the feces and develop no further until or unless they are eaten by the intermediate host. The definitive host becomes infected by eating the intermediate host.

In all cases the third-stage larvae penetrate the intestine of the definitive host and migrate via lymphatics to mesenteric lymph nodes and then via the circulatory system to the lungs. Prepatent periods vary from three to six weeks.

PATHOGENESIS AND CLINICAL EFFECTS

The pathogenesis and clinical effects of *Dictyocaulus* spp. and *Metastrongylus* spp. are similar. Larvae migrating through the alveoli and bronchioles to the bronchi are responsible for an inflammatory response that may result in the blockage of small bronchi and bronchioles with exudate. This lends to the collapse of alveoli. In heavy infections there is edema and an accumulation of gelatinous fluid in consolidated lobules. The bronchi contain frothy fluid and immature lungworms. The reaction to *Dictyocaulus viviparus* is generally more severe than the reaction to the other species.

Later in the infection there is blockage of the bronchi by adult worms and the exudation they provoke. The aspiration of eggs leads to an inflammatory reaction in the alveoli. Emphysema may result from blockage of the bronchioles. Secondary bacterial pneumonia may be a complication, and concurrent viral infections may be potentiated.

In mild infections (i.e., low numbers of parasites) there may be no clinical signs. As infections become more severe signs range from a mild cough with no loss of condition to mild weight loss, dyspnea, anorexia, rapid weight loss, and death.

Muellerius capillaris lives in the alveoli and lung parenchyma, each worm being surrounded by a nodule consisting of necrotic material, inflammatory cells, and connective tissue. *Protostrongylus rufescens* lives in the bronchioles where it irritates the mucosa and causes local areas of inflammation. The inflammatory exudate fills the alveoli distal to the parasitized bronchiole. Cellular infiltration and connective tissue proliferation result in the formation of small, yellowish-gray, conical foci in the lung parenchyma. Sheep and goats infected with *Protostrongylus* and *Muellerius* seldom show clinical signs, but the parasites may potentiate bacterial or viral pneumonia.

DIAGNOSIS

A history of repeated coughing, difficult breathing, and poor weight gains suggests infection with *Dictyocaulus viviparus, D. filaria,* or *Metastrongylus* spp. However, other respiratory diseases may have a similar history, so it is necessary to rely upon the demonstration of larvae *(Dictyocaulus)* or eggs *(Metastrongylus)* in the feces or immature worms and adults at necropsy to make a diagnosis of lungworm infection.

Diagnosis of Cattle Lungworms

The larvae of *D. viviparus* are the only nematode larvae found in fresh cattle feces uncontaminated with soil, so the demonstration of free larvae in such feces justifies a diagnosis of lungworm infection. The larvae may be found on fecal flotation, but the use of the Baermann technique is more efficient. In this technique a few grams of fresh feces are wrapped in gauze and placed in the top of a funnel, which is equipped with a piece of rubber tubing and a pinch clap at its tip. The funnel is filled with lukewarm water so that the feces are immersed. The larvae will swim out of the feces, through the gauze into the water, and gravity will carry them into the neck of the funnel. In two or three hours the water may be withdrawn from the neck of the funnel and examined for larvae with a microscope.

No larvae may be present in the feces when the disease is due to immature parasites in the bronchioles and alveoli. The worms may be easily recognized in the bronchi at necropsy.

Diagnosis of Sheep and Goat Lungworms

The diagnosis is complicated by the fact that the larvae of the three species must be differentiated when they are found in feces. The larvae are best recovered by the Baermann technique. *Dictyocaulus filaria* is found far more commonly than the other two species of lungworms, and its first-stage larvae are more than 0.5 mm long, whereas those of the other two species are approximately 0.3 mm long.

Diagnosis of Swine Lungworms

The eggs of *Metastrongylus* spp. have rough shells and contain fully developed first-stage larvae. They are easily recognized when seen on fecal flotation.

TREATMENT

Treatment for lungworms is justified whenever larvae or eggs are found in the feces or the parasites are found at necropsy in conjunction with clinical signs. Considering the prepatent periods, treatment might be indicated at six-week intervals to approach total control in the face of constant re-exposure. However, the development of immunity on the part of the hosts usually renders such frequent treatment unnecessary and uneconomical. Fortunately all of the anthelmintics recommended hereafter are also relatively effective against the major and more economically important gastrointestinal nematode parasites, so their use against these will also control lungworms.

In all species infected with lungworms there may be increased coughing immediately after treatment as the lungworms are killed. This coughing generally will not presist for more than a few hours.

Cattle Lungworms

L-tetramisole (Ripercol*, Levasol†, Levamisole†, Tramisole*) has been shown to be highly effective against mature and immature *Dictyocaulus viviparus*. It may be given in the feed or as a drench or bolus at doses of 2.5 to 5.0 mg/lb (5.5 to 11.0 mg/kg). It may also be given subcutaneously at a dosage of 1.5 to 3.6 mg/lb (3.3 to 8.0 mg/kg) in a 5 per cent solution. Toxicity is rarely seen in therapeutic doses. At two to three times the normal doses there may be excitement and trembling, salivation, licking of the lips, and shaking of the head. These signs are usually gone within 2 hours and nearly always within 24 hours. Toxic reactions are more likely, especially with the injectible form, if L-tetramisole is used at the same time as organophosphate insecticides.

Fenbendazole (Panacur‡) at a dosage of 5 mg/kg in an oral suspension or as a feed additive removed 99 to 100 per cent of adult cattle lungworms.

The following drugs are not yet available at this writing for use in cattle in North America. Cambendazole at doses of 9 to 11 mg/lb (20 to 40 mg/kg) is effective against mature cattle lungworms and somewhat less effective against immature cattle lungworms. Albendazole in a paste formulation at a dosage of 7.5 mg/kg is highly effective against mature cattle lungworms. Ivermectin (Ivome§) at 200 μgm/kg given by subcutaneous injection has approached 100 per cent efficacy.

Lungworms of Sheep and Goats

L-tetramisole given orally at 3.7 mg/lb (8 mg/kg) is effective against *Dictyocaulus filaria*. Albendazole and Ivermectin at dosages similar to those used for cattle are effective against *Dictyocaulus filaria,* but neither of these drugs is currently approved for use in sheep in North America.

Treatment is seldom, if ever, indicated for *Protostrongylus rufescens* or *Muellerius capillaris* infestation, although preliminary data indicate that Fenbendazole may be effective against *Protostrongylus* in bighorn sheep.

Lungworms of Swine

Levamisole at a dosage of 8 mg/kg in feed or water is highly effective against swine lungworms. Oxfendazole at 3 mg/kg in the feed eliminated all lungworms from pigs. Invermectin subcutaneously at 100 μgm/kg removed 99.9 per cent of *Metastrongylus* spp.

PREVENTION AND CONTROL

One method of preventing lungworm infection is to prevent animals from coming into contact with the infective larvae or the infected intermediate host. This often happens with no effort because many areas and individual farms are free of the parasites. Confinement rearing of swine frequently manages lungworms out of existence and certainly markedly reduces their prevalence. However, it

*Available from American Cyanamid Co., Princeton, NJ 08540
†Available from Pitman-Moore Co., Washington Crossing, NJ 08560
‡Available from Hoechst-Roussel Pharmaceutical, Inc., Somerville, NJ 08876
§Available from Merck and Company, Inc., Rahway, NJ 07065

must be remembered that the earthworm intermediate hosts may gain unexpected access via such things as drainage tiles.

When it is not possible to prevent all possible contact of the animals with the parasites, it is of value to take whatever measures are possible to ensure that the initial exposure is to a relatively small number of parasites. The smaller numbers at the exposure the more likely the young animal is to withstand the effects and develop immunity to further exposure without severe disease. Avoidance of overcrowding, overgrazing, and grazing of excessively moist areas will help prevent heavy exposures. Strategic anthelmintic treatment to reduce contamination of the premises with eggs and larvae is also helpful. Any measures to prevent pigs from ingesting earthworms (such as nose rings to discourage rooting) will reduce exposure.

Dictyocaulus viviparus is one of the very few parasites for which a highly effective vaccine has been developed. The vaccine consists of X-irradiated larvae and is given *per os* in two doses at a 28-day interval. The success of the vaccine is probably attributable to the lymphatic migration of the larvae. The irradiated larvae survive long enough to migrate into mesenteric lymph nodes and moult, thus stimulating immunity, but most of them die before reaching the lungs and causing disease. To maintain immunity vaccinated calves must be subjected to continued natural exposure. The fact that a few of the irradiated larvae reach sexual maturity in the lungs and produce eggs and larvae makes it inadvisable to use the vaccine in areas not known to be already contaminated with *Dictyocaulus* larvae.

NASAL BOT INFECTION

Oestrus ovis, the sheep nasal bot fly, is found wherever sheep are raised. The larvae are common in the nasal passages, turbinate bones, and paransal sinuses of sheep but much less common in goats.

Life Cycle

The adult flies appear during the warmer months of the year: only in summer in northern climates, spring through autumn in less severe climates, and year-round in warmer climates. An individual adult fly survives for less than 30 days. The flies rest during the cooler morning and evening hours and are active only during the middle of the day.

The female fly deposits first instar larvae (not eggs) one at a time around the nostrils of a sheep. The larvae migrate into the nasal passages. The larvae may remain in the first instar from two weeks to nine months. The second instar larvae pass into the sinuses and may remain there for a few weeks to several months. The third instar larvae crawl back out the nostrils and drop to the ground. The parasitic phase of the life cycle may be completed in as short a time as one month but may require more than a year. The parasites pupate in the ground for three to six weeks, or longer during cold seasons, before the adult fly emerges.

Pathogenesis and Clinical Effects

Adult females depositing their larvae annoy and frighten sheep, leading to head shaking and attempts to hide the nostrils against the ground or other sheep. The larvae irritate the mucosa by moving through the nasal passages and especially with their oral hooks and ventral spines. The irritation results in the secretion of a thick exudate, which may be tinged with blood. Some larvae may become entrapped in the sinuses and cause a sinusitis. Occasionally erosion of the bones of the skull and even damage to the brain may occur with resulting ataxia and hypermetria. As mature larvae migrate back down the nasal passages sheep may sneeze repeatedly in attempting to dislodge and expel them.

Diagnosis

Diagnosis may ordinarily be made only tentatively based on signs of nasal discharge, sneezing, and occasionally head shaking. Rarely expelled larvae may be found in feed troughs or waterers.

Treatment

Treatment has been difficult because the larvae are relatively inaccessible. Instillation of various insecticides and oils through the nostrils has been of very limited effectiveness.

Trichlorfon (Neguvon) used as a "pour on" onto the skin, not the wool, at 1.5 ml of an 8 per cent solution per 10 lb (4.5 kg) up to a total of 15 ml per sheep is effective as are other systemic organophosphates. Ivermectin at 200 μgm/kg given orally removed 100 per cent of first instar larvae. Neither the organophosphates nor ivermectin is approved for use in sheep in the United States.

Prevention and Control

Most attempts to prevent *Oestrus ovis* infestation have involved construction of feeders or salt dispensers that spray or rub pine tar or oil repellents on the nostril of sheep when they feed. However, the effectiveness of such repellents has not been encouraging.

Supplemental Reading

Benz, G. W., and Ernst, J. V.: Anthelmintic efficacy of ivermectin against immature gastrointestinal pulmonary nematodes of calves. Am. J. Vet. Res. 42:2097–2098, 1982.
Stewart, T. B., Marti, O. G., and Hale, O. M.: Efficacy of ivermectin against five genera of swine nematodes and the hog louse, *Haematopinus suis*. Am. J. Vet. Res. 42:1425–1426, 1981.
Wascott, R. B., and LeaMaster, B. R.: Efficacy of ivermectin against naturally acquired and experimentally induced nematode infections in sheep. Am. J. Vet. Res. 43:531–533, 1982.
Yazinski, T. A., Greenway, T., Presson, B. L., Pate, L. M., Featherstone, H., and William, M.: Antiparasitic efficacy of ivermectin in naturally parasitized sheep. Am. J. Vet. Res. 44:2186–2187, 1985.

Diagnostic Methods Applied to the Respiratory System*

JEROME G. VESTWEBER, D.V.M., Ph.D.

When clinical signs of dyspnea appear, it must be determined whether the problem is confined to the respiratory tract or the cardiovascular system or involves utilization of oxygen at the tissue level. Respiratory signs also may be exhibited secondary to systemic infectious diseases, toxemia, central nervous system disturbances, neoplasms of the thoracic cavity, poisoning, acid base

*Kansas Agricultural Experiment Station, Contribution #84–212–B.

imbalance, diaphragmatic hernias, and pleuritis. A thorough physical examination plus basic laboratory tests will aid in determining whether the clinical signs of dyspnea are due to primary respiratory disease.

The next decision to be made is what portion of the respiratory system is involved. This may be established by observing the character of respiratory effort. During a normal breathing pattern, the time duration ratio for inspiration to expiration is approximately 1:1 with a very short pause at the end of expiration. Difficulty in breathing, accompanied by a change from this normal breathing pattern, is called either inspiratory or expiratory dyspnea. Inspiratory dyspnea is characterized most frequently by breathing of a costal-thoracic type with a strong and long inspiration. This type of respiratory pattern is commonly associated with an upper respiratory disease and some forms of bronchopneumonia. If expiratory dyspnea, which is mainly an abdominal type of breathing pattern, occurs, one should be concerned that there is emphysema or other restrictive diseases of the lungs, such as pleuritis, hydrothorax, or diaphragmatic hernia. Dyspnea that is both inspiratory and expiratory is associated commonly with bronchopneumonia plus emphysema.

Audible sounds also are helpful in establishing the area of the respiratory tract that is involved. Normal breathing usually produces sounds that are not audible, whereas stenotic sounds are produced by constriction of the upper respiratory tract and are called stridor. These sounds often are associated with the breathing pattern. Snorting will occur with an obstructive type of lesion of the nasal mucosa such as mucosal swelling, collections of exudates and secretions, or a foreign body or neoplasm. The sound produced by pharyngeal stenosis is called snoring and is produced by constriction in the pharynx with vibration of the soft palate. This occurs with enlargement of retropharyngeal lymph nodes, abscesses of the pharyngeal wall, or generalized cellulitis in the surrounding pharyngeal area. Laryngeal stenosis produces roaring. This usually is caused by an inflammatory, edematous, or purulent necrotic process of the laryngeal mucosa. Stenosis of the trachea can produce stridor in the form of a loud purring sound that can be localized by compression or auscultation along the trachea. This may be caused by extreme swelling of the tracheal mucosa or collapse of tracheal rings. Groaning may accompany expiration when there is extensive emphysema or a painful lesion within the thoracic or abdominal cavity.

AUSCULTATION AND PERCUSSION OF THE LUNGS

Auscultation is one of the most useful diagnostic procedures, especially if pathologic changes of the lung are implied or suggested by the sounds that are heard with the stethoscope. A good quality stethoscope should be used in quiet surroundings. A routine should be established for auscultating the lung field, keeping in mind that there is a significant portion of the lung that cannot be evaluated readily beneath the front legs. Proceed in a definite horizontal pattern, progressing from cranial to caudal in the dorsal part of the lung field, and then repeat this routine more ventrally. Mental notes should be made about audible differences in the dorsal and ventral regions of the lung fields. The anatomic location of the major bronchi as they are distributed through the lung parenchyma should be kept in mind when interpreting lung sounds. The left lung field should be compared to the right lung field, because often one side is more significantly involved than the other. At each site one should listen for at least one or two breaths. To amplify any abnormal breathing sounds, deep respiratory efforts can be produced by placing a plastic bag loosely over the muzzle of the animal.

When normal lung tissue is auscultated, one of the following three sounds will be heard: bronchial, vesicular, or bronchovesicular. Most of the normal lung sounds heard are considered to be a mixture of bronchovesicular breathing. Normal bronchial sounds are sounds heard over the trachea and major branching of the bronchi. These sounds are distinctively abnormal when they are heard over an extensive area of the lung field and usually indicate consolidation of lung tissue. These sounds become louder than normal with stenosis of the upper respiratory tract due to laryngitis, tracheitis, or bronchitis. Vesicular sounds are normal sounds most commonly heard in the caudal dorsal aspect of the lung field and are generated by air passage through small airways.

If vesicular sounds become intensified, they may be called harsh vesicular sounds. Such sounds occur mostly on inspiration, resemble the sound of hair being rubbed between the fingers close to the ear, and are associated with early congestive stages of pneumonia or early pulmonary edema. Other discontinuous adventitious sounds are known as crackles. These sounds have been divided into coarse and fine crackles, a distinction previously reserved for moist and dry rales, respectively. Crackles are always a sign of disease and are heard as short discontinuous sounds produced by movable accumulating transudate, exudate, mucus, or blood present in the bronchi or bronchioles. Coarse crackles are often heard in the early stages of pneumonia when large quantities of inflammatory fluid are accumulating. When pneumonia becomes more advanced or is resolving, the crackles become fine. Fine crackles will range from a shrill whistle to a deep hum and still indicate inflammation of the mucous membranes of the bronchi or bronchioles. The amount of fluid is reduced, with tenacious mucus partially occluding respiratory passages.

Adventitious sounds of a continuous type are known as wheezes. These sounds are produced when a narrowed airway oscillates between being opened and nearly closed as air passes through it. Wheezes can be high-pitched (sibilant) or low-pitched (sonorous). Most wheezes occur during expiration, although upper respiratory obstruction can produce an inspiratory wheeze (stridor). Wheezes are heard most often with problems such as allergic bronchospasm, mucosal swelling, foreign bodies, tumors, and airway compression by enlarged lymph nodes.

A pleural friction rub sounds like squeaking leather and is suggestive of fibrinous pleuritis. The sound is produced by roughened pleural surfaces and is best heard near the diaphragmatic portion of the lungs. Friction rubs are heard during both inspiration and expiration and are associated with a primary pleuritis, pneumonia, or secondary pleuritis. Emphysematous sounds are heard most frequently as a squeak or a whistle following the expiratory effort and simulate the sound produced by crushing a sheet of soft paper into a ball or squeezing a balloon. These sounds

are heard most commonly over a bullous area of emphysema.

The absence of respiratory sounds is as important as the presence of abnormal sounds, because no sounds imply that nonfunctional lung tissue is beneath the stethoscope unless the animal is breathing very shallowly. Pleural effusion, pneumothorax, diaphragmatic hernia, or other space-occupying lesions of the thorax may be responsible for a silent lung.

Percussion is a useful diagnostic procedure when proficiency is obtained, and a systematic approach similar to auscultation needs to be established. The procedure is useful for making a diagnosis of excessive pleural fluid, pulmonary consolidation, or emphysema. The normal resonance will be replaced by dull solid sounds in cases of pleural fluid or pulmonary consolidation. There also will be a distinct line between dullness and normal resonance in cases of excessive pleural fluid accumulation. Emphysema produces a tympani-like resonance during percussion.

VIRAL ISOLATION AND FLUORESCENT ANTIBODY SPECIMENS FROM THE NASAL CAVITY

The mucous membranes of the nasal cavity are often the first tissues to be involved in a viral infection. In response to early infection, viral-infected, live, and dead mucociliary cells are sloughed into the lumen of the nasal cavity, and these cells are good specimens for viral isolation or fluorescent antibody studies. Specimens for viral isolation can be made of nasal secretions by brushing sterile cotton swabs against the walls of the nasal cavity and then placing the swabs in a viral transport medium* before sending them to a diagnostic laboratory. A specimen for the fluorescent antibody technique can be collected by introducing a chemical spatula approximately 8 to 10 cm into the nasal cavity and lightly scraping against the nasal septum to obtain virus-infected cells. The cells are then are transferred gently to clean microscopic slides and submitted for fluorescent antibody studies of the common viral agents involved in respiratory disease.

TRANSTRACHEAL ASPIRATION

A transtracheal aspiration is a valuable method for retrieving cells for cytology, isolating pathogenic bacteria, and identifying the spectrum of antibiotic sensitivity within the lower respiratory tract. One technique for this procedure involves first restraining the animal, preferably standing, with the head and neck extended dorsally. The midcervical tracheal area is clipped, surgically prepared, and infiltrated with local anesthetic. One hand then grasps the trachea, a small 1-cm incision is made in the skin, an Edwards 5½-in (14-cm) 9-gauge bleeding trocar is introduced between the tracheal rings, and a 90-cm polyethylene tube (PE 260) is passed through the trocar into the trachea. Once the polyethylene tubing is within the trachea, the trocar is removed to prevent any accidental

---

*Hank's Balanced Salt Solution, GIBCO Laboratories, Grand Island, NY 14072.

cutting of the tube. The tube is passed distally into the lung until slight resistance is felt. Then 30 ml of sterilized physiologic saline solution is injected via a 15-gauge needle that is placed in the end of the polyethylene tubing. Retrieval of 5 ml of saline wash is all that is necessary for bacterial isolation. Numerous other needle-catheter combinations are available for sample collection. An effective through-the-needle catheter combination consists of a 12-gauge 14-cm over-the-needle catheter* and a plastic 5 French canine urinary catheter.† In larger animals, a 10-gauge 14-cm over-the-needle catheter can be used with an 8 French urinary catheter. The 12-gauge catheter is positioned in the trachea, the inner needle stylet is removed, and the urinary catheter is passed through the 12-gauge plastic cannula. Flushing and aspiration are performed as previously described.

BRONCHOPULMONARY LAVAGE

Another method to study the cellular constituency of the lung involves a through-the-mouth approach. First a calf is restrained by using nose tongs to control the head. The tongue is grasped, extended, and pulled to the side of the mouth. A speculum is placed in the mouth to hold the jaws open, and a laryngoscope is used to help locate the larynx. A disposable guarded culture instrument‡ is inserted into the calf's trachea. The guarded tip of the culture instrument is then forced open with the swab. The swab is then removed, leaving the outer tube in the trachea as a cannula. For lavage, sterile 180-cm long polyethylene tubing§ (PE 320) with a 1-cm latex tubing tip is passed through the cannula into an airway of the lung until firm resistance is encountered. Approximately 60 ml of saline is infused, and between 25 and 40 ml of fluid will be retrieved.

Bronchial aspiration also can be taken during a bronchoscopy. This method offers an advantage in that the examination of the tracheobronchial tree can be carried out during the bronchoscopy in addition to obtaining a bronchial aspirate. The amount of saline infused varies with the size of the patient and preference of the operator.

THORACOCENTESIS

Large accumulations of fluid within the thoracic cavity are rare, but fluid can accumulate with a fibrinous type of bronchopneumonia or pleuritis. Following surgical skin preparation, aspiration with an 8-cm 16-gauge needle is best accomplished on the right side in the fifth or sixth intercostal space just dorsal or ventral to the humeroradial joint. Any excessive fluid can be removed if necessary, and fluid obtained can be cultured or examined cytologically to determine the characteristics of the cells found. Care needs to be taken not to allow entrance of air into the pleural cavity. If necessary, a drain tube can be inserted into the pleural cavity for the continued drainage of fluid and administration of medication.

*Medicut, Sherwood Medical Industries, St. Louis, MO 63103.
†Sovereign polypropylene catheter, Monoject Division of Sherwood Medical Industries, St. Louis, MO 63103.
‡Kalayjan Industries, Inc., Long Beach, CA 90803.
§Clay Adams, Division of Becton, Dickinson and Co., Parsippany, NJ 07054.

LUNG TISSUE BIOPSY

It is possible to obtain lung tissue biopsy specimens for histologic examination. The necessary equipment consists of a trephine with stylet (13 cm in length and 5 to 6 mm in diameter) and an electric hand drill capable of a minimum speed of 2400 rpm. An area of skin in the eighth or ninth intercostal space of either side, at the appropriate position of the upper and middle third of the lung field, is shaved, disinfected, and anesthetized. The trephine is inserted as far as the pleura, the stylet is removed, the drill attached, and a cut is made with the trephine approximately 5 cm into the lung tissue. A core of lung tissue is aspirated by a large syringe containing 5 ml of sodium citrate and is immediately placed in fixative.

RADIOLOGY

Cattle can be x-rayed either standing or lying on their side with forelegs drawn forward. The total thorax of calves can be x-rayed, but only part of the chest can be done in adults; also part of the chest may be covered by the forelimb.

Angiocardiography can be performed to determine the vascular filling of the lungs. This procedure is accomplished by passing a 9 French angiographic catheter down the external jugular vein into the pulmonary artery, injecting diatrizoate meglumine* rapidly, and taking lateral radiographs at 0.5-second intervals starting at the time of injection.

Scintigraphy of the respiratory system, a nuclear technique used extensively in human medicine, can provide a measure of both total and regional ventilation and perfusion of each lung. Intravenous injection of technetium-99m-labeled albumin will distribute to the lung capillary bed in direct proportion to the regional blood flow, whereas inhaled 81m krypton gas will allow visualization of pulmonary airways.

OTHER LABORATORY PROCEDURES AND TESTS

A complete laboratory analysis is indicated when the animal with respiratory disease is representative of a herd problem or the economic value of the animal justifies in-depth investigation. Most total white blood cell counts will remain within the upper normal range, but immature white blood cell counts will increase with bacterial pneumonias, whereas sometimes a leukopenia or lymphopenia is present with an acute uncomplicated case of viral pneumonia. The blood chemistry values for blood fibrinogen usually are elevated and often are related to the severity of an inflammatory process of the respiratory tract. With the availability of venous and arterial blood gas analysis, a determination can be made of the pulmonary function status. Other more sophisticated lung function tests that are confined mostly to research but are occasionally used clinically are spirography for determination of respiratory volume, inspiratory and expiratory reserves, vital capacity, and residual air; continuous recording of carbon dioxide content of the breath; monitor-

*Renografin-60, E. R. Squibb & Sons, Inc., Princeton, NJ 08540.

ing of intrathoracic pressure; nitrogen wash-out test; and dynamic elasticity and compliance.

Following aspiration of the transtracheal wash or bronchopulmonary lavage, the specimen can be cultured on blood agar and MacConkey agar. Aspirates can also be submitted for a Gram's stain. When available, minimal inhibitory concentrations of the effective antibiotics can be determined to indicate the dose and frequency required to obtain an adequate tissue level. Smears for cytologic evaluation of the aspirate can be made in several ways, but specimens may need to be centrifuged and smears made from the resulting sediment. Air-dried smears can be stained using the common blood stains such as new methylene blue, Wright's stain, Wright's-Leishman stain, or Harleco's Diff-Quik.* Material obtained from the bronchial aspiration will include cellular elements that normally line the tracheobronchial tree; cells derived from inflammatory, hemorrhagic, congestive, neoplastic, or other pathologic processes; and background material composed of mucus, proteinaceous exudate, or degenerated cells. In many cases, the cause of the disease process can be recognized and identified, e.g., bacteria, fungi, parasitic larvae, viral inclusions, or neoplastic cells.

SEROLOGIC TESTS FOR VIRUSES AND BACTERIA

A serologic diagnosis can be made most accurately by paired serum samples taken at two- to four-week intervals and demonstrating at best a four-fold rise in titer. A less accurate diagnosis could be made by only a rise in titer.

Cattle

1. *IBR—Serum Neutralization.* Maternal antibody titers will last from four to six months. Following aerosol exposure to IBR, cattle will develop serum antibodies to the virus by 21 days and maximum levels of serum antibodies (titers of 1:16 to 1:64) by 28 days after exposure. Re-exposure will result in a two-fold increase in the titer. Infective titers will last for six months to one year. Serum titers resulting from intranasal vaccination commonly are less than 1:4, whereas intramuscular vaccination results in serum titers of 1:2 to 1:16.

2. *BVD—Serum Neutralization.* Immunologic tolerance can exist and can result in a very low serum antibody titer or no titer even though severe infection exists with the virus. Infective titers often range from 1:64 to greater than 1:256 and last for one year or longer. Vaccination serum titers for the commercial C24V and NADL vaccines range from 1:8 to 1:256 14 days following administration.

3. *Parainfluenza-3 Virus.* Circulating serum antibody titers after viral exposure most commonly range from 1:32 to 1:512, with maximal concentrations 14 to 20 days following exposure.

4. *Bovine Respiratory Syncytial Virus.* Infective titers commonly range from 1:10 to 1:640.

5. *DN599 (Herpes 3) Virus.* Infective titers range from 1:10 to greater than 1:640.

6. Pasteurella *Bacteria.* Serologic tests are available for these organisms at some laboratories, but interpretation is difficult.

7. Haemophilus somnus *Bacteria.* Infective titers of 1:256 and above indicate active infection. It should be kept in mind that vaccination of a susceptible animal will result in a titer of 1:064 to 1:128. If tested shortly after the booster, the titer in a few animals may rise briefly to 1:256.

Swine

1. *Pseudorabies, Swine Influenza, and* Haemophilus. These organisms can be diagnosed by serologic tests.

Sheep

1. *Parainfluenza-3 and Ovine Progressive Pneumonia.* These viruses are presently being diagnosed by serology. Future research may make serology more common for diagnosis of the respiratory syncytial and BVD viruses.

Supplemental Reading

Corstvet, R. E., Rummage, J. A., and Homer, J. T.: Recovery of pulmonary alveolar macrophages from nonanesthetized calves. Am. J. Vet. Res. 43:2253, 1982.

Dungworth, D. L., and Hoare, M. N.: Trephine lung biopsy in cattle and horses. Res. Vet. Sci. 11:244, 1970.

McGuirk, S. M.: Internal medicine diagnostics—thoracic cavity. Bovine Proc. 15:69, 1983.

McLaughlin, R. W., and Miske, F. R.: A technique for bronchial aspiration in the calf. Bovine Pract. 1:29, 1980.

Phillips, R. M.: Interpretation of serological results received from the diagnostic laboratory. Proc. Ann. Conf. Vet., Kansas State University, H-1, 1983.

Radostits, O. M.: The clinical examination of cattle. Part 1: The examination of the individual animal. Bovine Proc. 14:2, 1982.

Roudebush, P.: Lung sounds. J. Am. Vet. Assoc. 181:122, 1982.

Respiratory Therapeutics

C. A. HJERPE, D.V.M.

The general objectives of respiratory system therapy are as follows:
1. Control of bacterial infections.
2. Removal of causes of respiratory tract irritation.
3. Maintenance of normal intrapleural pressures.
4. Maintenance of airway patency.
5. Maintenance of tracheobronchial clearance.
6. Maintenance of adequate arterial oxygenation and carbon dioxide removal.

CONTROL OF BACTERIAL INFECTIONS

This subject is discussed in the section on bacterial diseases.

REMOVAL OF CAUSES OF RESPIRATORY TRACT IRRITATION

Animals affected with respiratory tract disease should not be exposed to irritants such as dust, smoke, or ammonia gas. If barns are used to house such animals, these structures must be adequately and uniformly ventilated so as to achieve a minimum of four air changes per hour and to avoid drafts and extreme temperatures and marked temperature fluctuations. Cattle affected with extrinsic allergic alveolitis (bovine farmer's lung) should

---

*Diff-Quik, American Scientific Products, Clay Street, Kansas City, MO 64116.

not be fed moldy hay, especially within a closed air space. Medicinal cough suppression is rarely, if ever, necessary in the food animal species. It is usually contraindicated, as tracheobronchial clearance is assisted by the cough reflex. Administration of corticosteroids for control of respiratory tract irritation and coughing may lead to respiratory secretion retention. Administration of analgesics may have a similarly deleterious effect.

MAINTENANCE OF NORMAL INTRAPLEURAL PRESSURE

When pleural effusion is diagnosed, thoracentesis and drainage are indicated, although rapid refilling is to be expected. Intrapleural instillation of antimicrobial drugs is unnecessary for treatment of infectious pleural disease, since all but polymyxin B cross the pleural membrane readily from the blood stream. Intrapleural administration of aminoglycoside antibiotics (dihydrostreptomycin, neomycin, kanamycin, gentamicin) is contraindicated because of the risk of respiratory arrest from neuromuscular blockade.

MAINTENANCE OF AIRWAY PATENCY

Glucocorticoids are used in the management of acute, severe necrotic laryngitis in cattle to help maintain airway patency while antimicrobial therapy is controlling the bacterial infection. Flumethasone is administered by intravenous or intramuscular injection in a dose of 1 mg/45 kg body weight. A single treatment with a glucocorticoid is usually sufficient.

Parasitic bronchitis in cattle is treated with levamisole phosphate, administered by subcutaneous injection, or levamisole hydrochloride, administered orally by drench, bolus, or gel or in feed or water in a dose of 8 mg/kg body weight. Fenbendazole is also effective as a drench in a dose of 5 mg/kg body weight. Ivermectin is effective at 200 mcg/kg, subcutaneously. Parasitic bronchitis in sheep and swine is treated by oral administration of levamisole hydrochloride or fenbendazole.

Tracheotomy may be indicated in cases of impending upper respiratory tract obstruction from necrotic laryngitis, pharyngeal abscessation, facial snakebite, nasal bone fractures, and so on. Laryngospasm and bronchospasm are not recognized as clinical entities in the food animal species.

MAINTENANCE OF TRACHEOBRONCHIAL CLEARANCE

A "clean," patent tracheobronchial tree is essential for normal gas exchange. Tracheobronchial exudates are cleared by the mucociliary apparatus, assisted by the cough reflex. Drying, thickening, and subsequent retention of tracheobronchial secretions may result from systemic dehydration, administration of nonhumidified oxygen, insertion of a tracheotomy tube, and prolonged treatment with anticholinergics. Clearance of thick exudates may be facilitated by inhalation therapy with steam humidification or ultrasonic nebulization with physiologic saline solution. The objective of these procedures is to loosen and liquify the exudates by increasing the volume and reducing the viscosity of tracheobronchial fluids. For nebulization to be effective, patients should be nebulized for 30 to 45 minutes on three to six occasions per day. Inhalation therapy by steam humidification or ultrasonic nebulization is usually palliative rather than curative and is generally impractical in food animals because of the problems of restraint and the close supervision required. Newborn animals can be treated in nebulization cages designed for dogs and cats. Steam humidification therapy involves inhalation of steam and is most effective in clearing nasal and laryngeal exudates, as little moisture actually reaches the tracheobronchial membrane. Bubble humidifiers are ineffective for therapeutic purposes. Ultrasonic nebulizers produce tiny droplets that reach the lower respiratory tract. Mucolytic agents and antibiotics can be administered, along with moisture, by nebulization but are no longer considered efficacious. Expectorants are now considered to be ineffective for improving tracheobrochial clearance. Maintenance of a normal state of systemic hydration is the most effective and practical way of assisting tracheobronchial clearance in food animal patients.

MAINTENANCE OF ADEQUATE ARTERIAL OXYGENATION AND CARBON DIOXIDE REMOVAL

Clinical signs that indicate possible need for oxygen (O_2) therapy include tachypnea, dyspnea, cyanosis, and tachycardia. However, an arterial partial pressure of O_2 value of less than 70 to 80 mm Hg is the definitive indicator of a possible need for O_2 therapy. O_2 therapy is indicated in anoxic anoxia from inadequate ventilation or severe lung disease. It is not likely to be beneficial in anemic anoxia, stagnant anoxia, or histotoxic anoxia. Oxygen therapy is usually impractical in food animals because of cost, problems of restraint, and the close supervision required. O_2 has been administered to valuable cattle by means of an O_2 therapy mask or nasal tube using flow rates of 12 liters/min and 4 to 8 liters/min/90 kg of body weight, respectively. The nasal tube should be inserted to a point one third of the way from the lateral canthus of the eye to the base of the ear. The newborn can be treated in nebulization or oxygen cages designed for dogs and cats.

Hypoxia from inadequate ventilation is usually the result of anesthetic overdose and depression of the medullary respiratory center. Intubation and mechanical ventilation with O_2 and/or intravenous administration of an analeptic such as doxapram is indicated.

In treating severe lung disease, ultrasonic nebulization therapy and O_2 therapy may be combined. Oxygen, together with artificial respiration, may be of value in helping to revive unconscious neonatal animals following dystocia.

MISCELLANEOUS OBJECTIVES IN RESPIRATORY SYSTEM MEDICATION

Epinephrine is specific for treatment of acute pulmonary edema from anaphylaxis in cattle. Epinephrine is administered in 1:1000 concentration by intravenous injection in a dose 5 ml/450 kg body weight.

Glucocorticoids appear to be of value in the treatment of atypical interstitial pneumonia. Flumethasone is administered once daily by subcutaneous or intramuscular injection in a dose of 5 mg/45 kg body weight until expiratory dyspnea is controlled, or for three days. If dyspnea is present on day four, flumethasone therapy is continued in a reduced daily dosage of 1 mg/45 kg body weight until dyspnea is controlled, or for four additional days. Virtually all animals that respond will do so within seven days.

Diuretics such as furosemide may be of value, together with glucocorticoids, in the management of early cases of acute bovine pulmonary emphysema (3-methyl indole toxicosis). Furosemide is administered twice daily, by intravenous or intramuscular injection or oral boluses, in a dose of 2.2 to 4.4 mg/kg body weight.

Supplemental Reading

Blood, D. C., Henderson, J. A., and Radostits, O. M.: Veterinary Medicine, 5th ed. Lea & Febiger, Philadelphia, 1979, 250–275.

McKiernan, B. C.: Principles of respiratory therapy. In Kirk, R. W. (ed.): Current Veterinary Therapy VIII: Small Animal Practice. W. B. Saunders Co., Philadelphia, 1983, 216–221.

DISEASES OF THE CARDIOVASCULAR AND HEMOLYMPHATIC SYSTEMS

DONALD R. CLARK, D.V.M., Ph.D.
Consulting Editor

Cardiovascular Pathophysiology

DONALD R. CLARK, D.V.M., Ph.D.

Each heartbeat with its associated bioelectric and mechanical events is termed a cardiac cycle. The cardiac cycle is divisible into phases of ventricular systole (contraction or emptying) and ventricular diastole (relaxation or filling). The interrelated events of venous, atrial, ventricular, and arterial pressure along with ventricular volume, heart sounds, and the electrocardiogram are depicted in Figure 1.

HEART SOUNDS DURING THE CARDIAC CYCLE

Vibrations produced during a cardiac cycle give rise to heart sounds. The first heart sound ("Lubb") is associated with atrioventricular valve (mitral and triscuspid) closure as systole begins. The second sound ("Dupp") is due to closure of the semilunar valves (aortic and pulmonic) as ventricular diastole begins. The third and fourth sounds, related to rapid ventricular filling and to atrial systole, respectively, are not ordinarily audible, but may be heard in circumstances such as A-V block or congestive heart failure.

In heart failure, exaggeration of the normally inaudible sounds produces a triplicate sound or cadence described as a gallop rhythm. A gallop rhythm is convincing evidence of congestive right or left heart failure and thus is a significant clinical finding.

CARDIAC MURMURS

Additional sounds generated in the heart and great vessels are murmurs and result from turbulent flow of blood. The turbulent or disturbed blood flow most frequently occurs as a result of change in the structure of the heart and vessels. Murmurs are systolic if they occur between heart sound 1 and 2, and diastolic if they occur between heart sound 2 and the following heart sound 1. Continuous murmurs may span the entire cardiac cycle.

Table 1 lists the various sounds and the usual causes of abnormal heart sounds.

NORMAL AND ABNORMAL CARDIAC OUTPUT

At rest, the heart pumps a basal volume of flow proportionate to the animal's body size. *Cardiac Index,* a general estimate of basal output, is approximately 3 to 3.5 L/m²/min. Greater rates are promoted by exercise, as neural and humoral influences increase heart rate or stroke volume or both. The combination of higher cardiac output and a greater extraction of oxygen allows oxygen delivery to tissues to increase during exercise by as much as 15-fold in healthy animals. Acute failure to deliver basal cardiac output produces circulatory shock; a more progressive and chronic inability to sustain adequate flow is the basis for congestive heart failure.

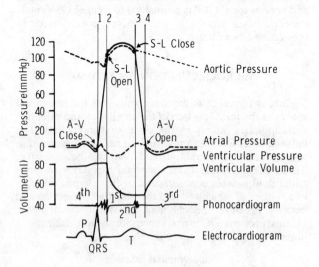

Figure 1. Events of the cardiac cycle. This figure depicts the systemic ventricular and atrial pressures as they interrelate with ventricular volume, heart sounds, and electrocardiogram. Ventricular ejection occurs between 2 and 3.

Table 1. *Heart Sounds and Likely Causes*

Heart Sound	Likely Causes
Splitting of second	Systemic or pulmonic hypertension
Accentuation of third or fourth ("gallop rhythm")	Congestive heart failure
Systolic murmur	Anemia, atrial septal defect, ventricular septal defect, aortic or pulmonic stenosis, mitral or tricuspid regurgitation
Diastolic murmur	Aortic or pulmonic insufficiency
Continuous	Patent ductus arteriosus

ARTERIAL AND VENOUS PULSES

The rhythmic intermittent discharge of blood into the arteries produces an abrupt rise in intra-arterial pressure, followed by a decline during the remainder of the cardiac cycle, as blood moves progressively forward through the capillaries. These events involve generation of the arterial pulse in which systolic and diastolic pressures represent the high and low pressure values during each cycle. Pulse pressure reflects the difference between systolic and diastolic values. Palpable pulse strength relates to pulse pressure. The pulse feels strong if the difference between systolic and diastolic values is great, as in conditions associated with a large stroke volume, and weak whenever the stroke volume is reduced.

Venous waves, most visible in the jugular groove, are a complex of 3 rapidly occurring fluctuations with each heartbeat. These are the A, C, and V waves, which represent atrial contraction (A), tricuspid valve retroversion during early ventricular systole (C), and venous distension during ventricular systole (V). Accentuation of venous pulses ("cannon waves" or "giant waves") takes place with ventricular premature beats, atrial fibrillation, and A-V block. The mean pressure in the large ventral veins, central venous pressure (CVP), reflects the interaction of cardiac pumping effectiveness, blood volume, and venous tone. CVP is normally 0 to 5 cm H_2O. Venous distention is a feature in constrictive pericarditis or in congestive heart failure.

MICROCIRCULATION AND EDEMA

Fluid is forced from capillary walls into the interstitial spaces in the initial portion of the capillaries and re-enters the capillaries largely in the distal or venous end. The balance of hydrostatic and osmotic pressures ensures that accumulation of interstitial fluids will not be excessive. Tissue edema results from abnormal elevations in interstitial fluid protein concentration or from hypoproteinemia, either of which reduces the effective plasma colloid osmotic pressure. Edema may also result from higher venous pressure, if either venous or lymph drainage is impaired, or if heart failure develops.

Supplemental Reading

Ettinger, S. J.: Textbook of Veterinary Internal Medicine. Philadelphia, W. B. Saunders Company, 1975.
Jubb, K. V. F., and Kennedy, P. C.: Pathology of Domestic Animals, 2nd ed. New York, Academic Press, 1970.

Diseases of the General Circulation

DONALD R. CLARK, D.V.M., Ph.D.

CIRCULATORY SHOCK

Circulatory shock is defined as severe insufficiency in capillary perfusion. Usual causes of circulatory shock are marked depletion of extracellular fluid volume (hypovolemic), loss of effective cardiac pumping action (cardiogenic), and excessive alteration in the caliber of vessels (vasculogenic). The effective circulatory blood volume may be diminished by actual loss of blood or plasma or by sequestration of blood in widely dilated vessels. Table 1 provides an etiologic classification of shock. Thus shock may result from such diverse causes as loss of blood (20 ml/kg or greater), acute emesis or diarrhea, myocardial depression, and vascular effects of circulating endotoxins from *Escherichia coli* and other organisms.

Clinical Signs

Certain signs of circulatory shock result from factors such as hypovolemia and endotoxin, while others result from physiologic responses, principally autonomic nervous system activity (Table 2).

Treatment

Early and effective correction of circulatory volume deficit is mandatory in shock therapy. Repletion of circulating fluid volume is most urgent in hypovolemic shock. The need for large volumes of fluids in shock involves the following considerations: (1) fluid losses may be hidden or inapparent, (2) capillary permeability may be increased, (3) loss of vascular tone may necessitate a greater than normal filling volume, (4) limited vascular overfilling (hypervolemia) ensures optimal stroke volume and cardiac output and, (5) crystalloid or electrolyte solutions given intravenously are distributed largely to the interstitial compartment and only to a limited extent, perhaps 25 per cent of total, are these fluids retained in vessels. Fluids may be given according to some predetermined dosage,

Table 1. *Shock*

Shock due to reduction in blood volume (Hypovolemic)
Loss of whole blood by external or internal hemorrhage.
Loss of plasma by exudation at body surface or into body cavities.
Loss of water and electrolytes by excessive sweating, diarrhea, diuresis, emesis, and transudation (e.g., acute intestinal obstruction).

Shock due to acute changes in cardiac pumping effectiveness (Cardiogenic)
Interference with effective cardiac filling. Cardiac tamponade, constrictive pericarditis, hydropericardium, positive pressure ventilation.
Restricted ventricular emptying. Acute cor pulmonale, increased vascular resistance, ruptured chordae tendineae, toxic myocardial depression, cardiac dysrhythmias.

Shock due to changes in venous capacitance or peripheral resistance (Vasculogenic)
Endotoxins and vasoactive agents of anaphylaxis.
Vasomotor paralysis from CNS trauma or paralysis.
Severe prolonged vasoconstriction from catecholamines.

Table 2. *Principal Signs of Circulatory Shock*

Rapid, weak pulse
Diminution of heart sounds
Mucous membranes pale or ashen, cold and dry
Prolonged capillary refill time ($\geq$ 3 sec)
Muscle weakness and depressed sensorium
Coldness of skin, particularly in extremities
Oliguria or anuria

or better, given in amounts and at rates shown to be appropriate by central venous pressure (CVP) monitoring. If plasma protein concentrations are not severely reduced, fluids may be safely given until CVP reaches 5 to 10 cm H_2O.

Blood, Plasma, and Plasma Expanders

Homologous blood may be of value if significant hemorrhage has occurred and if given before severe shock with capillary sludging and microthrombi formation (disseminated intravascular coagulation or DIC) has ensued. If blood transfusions are elected, they should be accompanied with infusion of balanced electrolytes. From 20 to 40 ml/kg of whole blood accompanied by 2 to 6 times this volume of balanced electrolytes is most effective.

Plasma is quite satisfactory for expansion of the blood volume. Plasma expanders such as dextrans are also effective, particularly low molecular weight dextran (LMD) solutions. LMD offers advantages of enhancing fluid shifts into vascular spaces and of preventing capillary sludging and DIC during severe shock states. Its chief disadvantage is high cost of treatment in large animals. An effective dosage is 10 ml/kg of 20 per cent solution along with electrolyte solutions.

Electrolyte Solutions

Treatment of shock should be based upon volume expansion in order to achieve optimal cardiac filling, cardiac output, capillary perfusion, and urine output. Ideally, this is achieved by monitoring the CVP as fluids are administered. In this way fluids can be given vigorously until CVP reaches 5 to 10 cm H_2O. It is unlikely that pulmonary edema or other complications will result if fluids are given under CVP guidance. Lactated Ringer's solution is preferred to normal saline whenever large quantities of fluids are required, except if hyperkalemia exists. The lactacidemia of shock does not preclude administration of lactated Ringer's solution. The solution may be buffered by addition of 0.75 gm $NaHCO_3$/L to raise the pH to 7.4.

If CVP is not monitored and fluid is given on an empirical dosage, 20 to 40 ml/kg is very conservative, and amounts equal to as much as 1 to 3 blood volumes (100 to 300 ml/kg) are often required. Dosage should be modified according to the severity of shock and response to treatment.

Cardiostimulatory and Vasoactive Drugs

Adrenergic drugs have limited usefulness in treatment of circulatory shock. Because they may be vasoconstrictive, arrhythmogenic, and likely to enhance tissue oxygen demands, catecholamines are generally contraindicated in shock. The only important exceptions to the total avoidance of catecholamines is their usefulness in shock of

anaphylaxis, and in other states of shock when they may appear critical for cardiac stimulation. Dopamine (Intropin*) and, even more particularly, dobutamine (Dobutrex†) have only modest vasoactive properties and can be used in an intravenous drip with greater safety than other catecholamines.

Steroids

Steroids in large or "pharmacologic" doses are indicated in shock but only after repletion of fluid volume. If given earlier, their vasodilatory action may produce a fall in arterial pressure and worsen venous pooling. An optimal dose of glucocorticoids is 4 to 6 mg/kg of dexamethasone or 25 to 30 mg/kg of prednisolone. Evidence exists that soluble steroid salts act more rapidly, but the cost differential makes their use questionable. Following volume repletion in cases of shock, however, these agents represent an effective means of promoting tissue perfusion by arterial vasodilation.

Other Measures

Broad-spectrum antibiotics should be utilized whenever shock is the result of sepsis or trauma. It is advisable, however, to consider the potential cardiodepressant effect of aminoglycoside antibiotics.

Heparin is sometimes employed at a dose of 250 units/kg to treat or to prevent DIC in shock. Cardiotonics other than catecholamines include glucagon (Glucagon†) at a dosage of 50 mcg/kg, repeated at 30 minute-intervals, and calcium gluconate at 10 to 20 mg/kg given slowly intravenously. Mannitol at 1 to 3 gm/kg may enhance urine flow in hypotensive shock and minimize cerebral edema in head trauma. Metabolic acidosis of shock may be minimized by administration of $NaHCO_3$. The amount required may be estimated from blood gas analysis results or from total CO_2 determination.

CONGESTIVE HEART FAILURE

Congestive heart failure results from the chronic inability of the heart to meet circulatory requirements and is characterized particularly by expansion of the extracellular fluid (ECF) volume and by edema. With the myocardium failing, the contractile vigor of the ventricles declines, resulting in diminishing of cardiac output and setting in motion of a series of compensatory mechanisms. The principal physiologic compensations are increases in heart rate and in ECF volume. Heart rate changes are autonomically controlled; expansion of the ECF volume is due principally to greater sodium and water reabsorption by the underperfused kidneys. Greater activity of the renin-angiotensin-aldosterone mechanism provides one important means for enhancement of salt retention by renal tubules.

Heart failure may be principally either left-sided or right-sided, depending upon which ventricle is most affected. In right-sided failure, the systemic veins and capillaries distend as a consequence of the right side of

*Available from American Critical Care, McGraw, IL 60085
†Available from Eli Lilly & Co., Indianapolis, IN 46206

the heart being unable to move the venous return forward. Higher systemic capillary turgor and pressure result in tissue edema with a likelihood of ascites, hydrothorax, and migration of fluids to dependent, ventral areas. Cattle with brisket disease are classic examples of right-sided heart failure. Left-sided heart failure is marked by high pulmonary capillary pressure and pulmonary edema. Common causes of left-sided heart failure are aortic or mitral valvular disease and myocardiopathy. Right-sided heart failure is more generally attributable to higher pulmonary vascular resistance (cor pulmonale), pericarditis, and myocardiopathy.

Treatment

The prognosis for successful recovery and the expense of treatment may discourage intense therapy except in selected cases. In general, therapeutic regimens should include restriction of exercise and salt; and the use of diuretics and digitalis glycosides. Aminophylline may be beneficial. Digitalis must be used with care and monitoring. Provisionally, the dose for digitalization of the ox could be estimated as follows:

1. Intramuscular digitoxin, 1.4 mg/100 lb.
2. Intravenous digoxin, 0.4 mg/100 lb.

The digitalization procedure sometimes employed is to administer one third of the calculated dose daily until proper responses are identified or until initial signs of toxicity are noted. Daily maintenance doses can be estimated at one-eighth to one-fifth of the digitalizing dose, given in 2 divided doses with careful and frequent examination for evidence of toxicity.

Excessively high venous and capillary pressures and the accompanying edema and cardiac distention can commonly be relieved by saluretic diuretics. The use of angiotensin-converting enzyme inhibitors such as epsilon-aminocaproic acid (Captopril*) may also prove to be an effective means of reducing hypervolemia.

ANAPHYLAXIS

Anaphylaxis is an acute, severe reaction to administration of an antigen to which an animal has been sensitized. Reactions involve the release of cellular histamine, kinins, and other vasoactive substances. The effects of these released substances, particularly histamine, is smooth muscle constriction, higher capillary permeability, and exocrine gland secretion. Results are urticaria, pruritus, hypotension, and bronchospasm. Respiratory distress and hypotensive shock may result.

Epinephrine is the drug of choice in treatment of anaphylaxis. Administration reverses the effects of histamine and limits the release of autocoids. Antihistamines act as competitive inhibitors of histamine at h_1 receptors but do not alter the effects of histamine already released and active. Corticosteroids potentiate the beneficial effects of epinephrine and exert other nonspecific anti-inflammatory actions. While recognizably beneficial, neither antihistamines nor glucocorticoids are the primary drugs to use in acute hypersensitivity reactions.

In general, a regimen for therapy of anaphylaxis is as follows:

1. Epinephrine (1:1000) SC or IM: 0.5 to 1.0 ml/100

---

*E. R. Squibb, Princeton, NJ 08540

lbs. Dilute to 1:10000 if used IV; may be repeated at 15-minute intervals.

2. Corticosteroids IV or IM: Equivalent to dexamethasone at 0.25 to 1 mg/kg. Larger doses are tolerated, and the dose given may be doubled in severe cases.

3. Diphenhydramine (Benadryl*) IM or IV: 0.5 to 1 mg/kg.

Adjunctive therapy may require intravenous electrolytes and bronchodilators such as aminophylline. Patients with severe and persistent collapse may benefit from therapy as decribed earlier for circulatory shock.

SPONTANEOUS ATHEROSCLEROSIS IN SWINE

The pig is susceptible to spontaneous atherosclerosis, a process that can be accelerated by feeding a high fat diet. The incidence of identifiable lesions has been reported to rise with age, ranging to 35 per cent in pigs more than 3 years of age. Although therapy for affected animals is not ordinarily feasible, brood animals to be maintained over a long period are known to be largely protected from atherosclerosis by high protein, low saturated fat diets.

---

*Available from Parke-Davis, Morris Plains, NJ 07050

Supplemental Reading

Skold, B. H., and Getty, R.: J. Am. Vet Med. Assoc. *139*:655, 1961.
Symposium on Drugs Affecting the Heart. J. Am. Vet. Med. Assoc. *171*:77–105, 1977.
Ettinger, E.: Textbook of Veterinary Internal Medicine, 2nd ed. Philadelphia, W. B. Saunders Company, 1983.

Conditions of the Pericardium, Myocardium, and Endocardium

CHRISTOPHER BUTTON, M.MED.VET. (MED.), Ph.D.

PERICARDIUM

Hydropericardium

Hydropericardium is an abnormal accumulation of serous fluid in the pericardial space. Hydropericardium is most common in malnourished or heavily parasitized animals, especially the young. Fluid accumulation in such animals is frequently secondary to lowered plasma oncotic pressure resulting from hypoproteinemia, especially hypoalbuminemia. Less frequently, hydropericardium may be secondary to local neoplasia, such as cardiac lymphomatosis of cattle, to congestive heart failure, or to toxic or inflammatory states, e.g., enterotoxemia of sheep, and edema disease and mulberry heart disease of pigs. In the latter diseases, the fluid often contains fibrin and tends to clot upon exposure to air.

A slowly developing hydropericardium does not influence circulatory dynamics appreciably. It is important to identify the primary etiologic agent or condition so that appropriate treatment or prophylaxis may follow.

Pericarditis

Pericarditis is an inflammation of the pericardium, generally accompanied by exudation into the pericardial space. Pericarditis (other than traumatic pericarditis) is

Table 1. *Infectious Diseases Associated with Pericarditis in Food-Producing Animals*

Cattle	Pigs	Sheep and Goats
Pasteurellosis and shipping fever complex	Pasteurellosis	Pasteurellosis
Streptococcal septicemia	Streptococcal septicemia	Streptococcal septicemia *Staphylococcus aureus*
Mycoplasmosis	*Mycoplasma* polyserositis (*M. hyorhinis*)	Mycoplasmosis
Chlamydiosis	Enzootic pneumonia (*M. hyopneumoniae*) Septicemic salmonellosis	Chlamydiosis
Tuberculosis	Glasser's disease (*Haemophilus parasuis*, *Haemophilus pleuropneumoniae*)	*Escherichia coli*
Contagious bovine pleuropneumonia	Hog cholera Encephalomyocarditis virus infection	

relatively rare in food-producing animals and is generally associated with signs or lesions in other organ systems. Diagnosis depends on thorough clinical and pathologic investigation, and appropriate therapy and prophylaxis can best be applied once the cause is known. A checklist of some infectious diseases resulting in pericarditis is given in Table 1. Traumatic pericarditis of cattle is discussed next.

Traumatic Pericarditis

Traumatic pericarditis (purulent pericarditis, hardware disease) is an acute, subacute, or chronic suppurative pericarditis of cattle, resulting from foreign body penetration of the reticulum, diaphragm, and pericardium. It causes a syndrome of toxemia and congestive heart failure.

Traumatic pericarditis is most common in older cows in poorly managed dairy operations and in feedlot cattle on chopped feeds. It is less common in range cattle. The incidence rises in the last trimester of pregnancy and shortly after parturition, presumably as a result of changes in intra-abdominal pressure. The foreign body, generally a nail or piece of wire, penetrates the reticulum, diaphragm, pericardium, and sometimes the myocardium. Organisms from the reticulum initiate a purulent pericarditis. The mass of exudate present and the adhesions formed between the pericardium and epicardium result in cardiac tamponade and congestive heart failure. Absorption of bacterial toxins and breakdown products from the process is responsible for fever, depression, and leukocytosis.

Clinical Signs and Lesions

Clinical signs in the acute stage, shortly after foreign body penetration (within 24 hr), are depression, fever, loss of appetite, a decline in milk production, rapid respiration, tachycardia of approximately 100 beats/min, reluctance to walk, a stiff gait with an arching of the back, elbow abduction, and signs of pain (e.g., grunting). Gastrointestinal disturbances, such as mild ruminal atony or bloat, constipation, or diarrhea, may be seen. A pericardial friction rub may be heard on auscultation. If the animal survives the acute phase, signs of pain become less evident, and appetite and milk production may improve. However, there is usually appreciable weight loss, jugular venous distention with an exaggerated pulsation, and brisket and sternal edema. Heart sounds become faint or even inaudible, and splashing or tinkling sounds are frequently audible. The area of percussable cardiac dullness is greater. Important laboratory findings are early neutropenia followed by leukocytosis with WBC counts of 15.0 to 30.0 × 10^9/L, reversal of the neutrophil to lymphocyte ratio, and a left shift.

Diagnosis

Diagnosis is based on history, clinical signs, and positive response to pain tests (grunting on deep palpation of the reticular area). A lateral radiograph of the cardiac and reticular areas with the subject in dorsal recumbency indicates the presence and position of metallic foreign bodies. The diagnosis is confirmed by the finding of a purulent exudate upon pericardiocentesis in the left fourth or fifth intercostal spaces. High altitude disease, congenital heart disease, thoracic or cardiac lymphomatosis, and valvular endocarditis are the most important differential diagnoses of advanced hardware disease. The prognosis is poor, especially when signs of congestive heart failure are present.

Treatment

Treatment is most successful when an early diagnosis is made, and the foreign body is removed by rumenotomy. A broad-spectrum antibiotic should be administered, and general supportive measures should be applied at this time. In chronic cases, digitalis glycosides and diuretics may also be administered; surgical removal of the foreign body and pericardiotomy may be attempted in such cases but are seldom successful, and slaughter is generally indicated.

Prevention

Prophylaxes include strict measures to prevent littering of the environment with nails or pieces of wire, the use of strong magnets to screen ground or chopped feeds, and the use of string instead of wire for baling. Magnets have been administered to cattle by mouth; they lodge in the reticulum, where they attract metallic foreign bodies and minimize the chances of reticular perforation.

MYOCARDIUM

Degenerative disease of the myocardium (myocardiopathy) is a fairly common histopathologic finding in food-producing animals, and inflammatory disease (myocarditis) and neoplastic disease are rare.

Myocardiopathy may be the result of intoxication (e.g., gossypol poisoning of pigs and monensin poisoning of ruminants) or of dietary deficiency (e.g., vitamin E and selenium deficiency in young animals); it may also be secondary to acute infectious disease (hog cholera, foot and mouth disease, blue tongue). Some myocardiopathies have no readily apparent cause (idiopathic). Focal suppurative myocarditis can result from bacteremia, septicemia, or septic emboli released from an infected focus (e.g., vegetative valvulitis).

Clinical Signs and Lesions

In addition to the signs of the primary condition, the signs of myocardiopathy or myocarditis may include fever, depression, weakness or exercise intolerance, congestive heart failure, cardiac arrhythmia, and sudden death. Four important conditions involving the myocardium of food animals are discussed next.

Nutritional Muscular Dystrophy. This is an acute or chronic syndrome of skeletal muscular and myocardial degeneration and necrosis in young food-producing animals. The syndrome is associated with a deficiency of selenium or vitamin E in the diet of pregnant and lactating females, in the milk their offspring receive, and in the diet of young animals. Only the cardiac syndrome of nutritional muscular dystrophy will be discussed here.

The cardiac manifestation of nutritional muscular dystrophy is one of acute cardiac failure with sudden death. Affected animals are frequently found dead, but, if seen, symptoms may include dyspnea, tachycardia, cardiac arrhythmia, a frothy, blood-tinged nasal discharge, weakness, dullness, collapse, and death. Symptoms may be precipitated by stress or exercise.

At necropsy, the subendocardium of mainly the calf's left ventricle or mainly the lamb's right ventricle show pale white areas of degeneration, necrosis, and mineralization. Histologically, the lesions are of hyaline degeneration and necrosis with calcification. The lungs are heavy and edematous (see pages 283–284).

Mulberry Heart Disease. This condition is an acute and usually fatal syndrome of cardiac failure in young (3 weeks to 4 months old), otherwise healthy pigs. A vitamin E and selenium deficiency is considered by some workers to be responsible for the condition.

Affected animals are commonly found dead, but if they are found alive, muscular tremor, weakness, dyspnea, cyanosis, and recumbency may be noted.

At necropsy, body cavities and the pericardium contain excessive fluid, fibrin threads, or clots. The liver is enlarged and mottled. There is edema of the lungs and hyperemia of the gastric mucosa. Multiple subepicardial, myocardial, and subendocardial ecchymotic hemorrhages account for the name of this disease. Histologically, there is widespread myocardial congestion, hemorrhage, and degeneration of muscle fibers. There is microangiopathy in the form of fibrinoid degeneration and necrosis of the tunica media of coronary arterioles.

The diet should have vitamin E added at 10,000 units/ton and selenium at 0.1 to 0.15 ppm. Individual animals may be given selenium injections at 0.06 mg/kg intramuscularly.

Encephalomyocarditis. This disease is a cardiovirus-induced syndrome of acute heart failure in young pigs 5 days to 20 weeks old. Morbidity varies between 2 and 50 per cent, and mortality approaches 100 per cent. The virus propagates as an enterovirus in rodents, which may act as reservoir hosts.

Affected pigs are usually found dead, but when observed, clinical signs are depression, anorexia, trembling, staggering, paralysis, vomiting, and dyspnea. Death is due to acute heart failure.

At autopsy, the skin of the underline is usually purple, and there are strands of fibrin on the pericardial, pleural, and peritoneal surfaces. The ventricular myocardium shows multiple, discrete, pale white areas, and necrotic streaks. Lesions are most common in the right ventricle, the interventricular septum, and the papillary muscles. Other macroscopic lesions are those of acute heart failure, e.g., lung and mesenteric edema and hepatic congestion.

Histologically, there is myocardial necrosis with or without mineralization accompanied by infiltration of lymphocytes, plasma cells, and macrophages. Individuals surviving myocardial necrosis develop myocardial scarring.

Diagnosis is based on the typical gross and microscopic findings and is confirmed by virus isolation. Recovered animals and infected herds can be identified serologically. Important differential diagnoses for the myocardial lesions include vitamin E and selenium deficiency and some viral strains of foot and mouth disease.

There is no treatment, but it is likely that vaccines will be developed. Prevention is based on general principles of hygiene and on effective rodent control.

Ionophore Intoxication. Monensin is a carboxylic ionophore antibiotic commonly included in ruminant rations at a concentration of 22 to 33 mg/kg as a growth promoter and coccidiostat. Field mixing errors have resulted in ingestion of excessive quantities of monensin with resultant toxicity to cattle and sheep: experimental ingestion of monensin has resulted in toxicity to pigs.

Clinical signs related to gastrointestinal disturbances and damage to skeletal muscle and the myocardium usually commence within 24 hr of consumption of rations containing excessive concentrations of monensin. Death may be sudden, or feed refusal may be accompanied by bloat, colic, diarrhea (sometimes bloody), and a stilted, stiff gait. Affected animals become weak, lethargic, and recumbent. Surviving animals show unthriftiness, gait abnormalities, and atrophy of skeletal muscles, especially over the hind quarters. There may be signs of congestive heart failure.

Macroscopic lesions may include diffuse hemorrhage of the intestinal tract. Skeletal muscle and the myocardium may show pale areas of necrosis. Other lesions are suggestive of congestive heart failure, e.g., pulmonary edema, fluid accumulation in body cavities, and an enlarged liver. Histologically, affected striated muscles show areas of hyaline degeneration and necrosis, a mixed cellular infiltrate, mineralization, and variable signs of organization.

Diagnosis is based on the history, symptoms, gross and microscopic pathology, and is confirmed by feed analysis. The primary differential diagnosis is nutritional deficiency of vitamin E or selenium. There is no specific treatment. Suspected feed should be withdrawn immediately.

Prevention

Prophylaxis should involve greater vigilance at feed mills and might involve test feeding of new batches of feed to a limited number of animals. Other ionophores—for example, salinomycin and lasalocid—produce a toxicologic syndrome similar to that of monensin.

ENDOCARDIUM

Endocarditis is an acute to chronic inflammatory condition of the endocardium. Mural endocarditis is rare, but vegetative valvular endocarditis is more common. Chronic bacteremia, secondary to such chronic septic conditions as metritis, mastitis, wounds, omphalophlebitis (navel ill), abscesses, cellulitis, or traumatic reticuloperitonitis, predisposes animals to endocarditis.

In cattle, the right atrioventricular (tricuspid) valve is most frequently involved, and *Corynebacterium pyogenes* is most often isolated, but staphylococci, streptococci,

Erysipelothrix insidiosa, coliforms, and the tuberculosis bacillus have also been isolated. In sheep, especially lambs, streptococci and *Escherichia coli* are most commonly incriminated. In pigs, the mitral valve is most frequently involved and *Erysipelothrix insidiosa* is the usual microbial agent, but *C. pyogenes,* streptococci, staphylococci, and salmonellae may also be involved.

Clinical Signs and Lesions

Endocarditis may be an incidental finding or it may produce fever and signs of cardiac embarrassment: tachycardia, venous distention, exercise intolerance, and subcutaneous edema. A primary septic focus may dominate the clinical signs. Loud, pounding heart sounds and a murmur of valvular insufficiency or stenosis may be auscultated. Fragments of the valvular vegetation may break loose, resulting in embolism and symptoms of central nervous, myocardial, skeletomuscular, renal, or pulmonary involvement. In addition, there is usually weight loss and, in cows, lowered milk production. Typical congestive heart failure may develop with time. Characteristic findings of laboratory tests in cattle are nonregenerative anemia, neutrophilic leukocytosis, and hyperglobulinemia.

Diagnosis

A diagnosis of endocarditis is based on history and clinical findings. A blood culture with positive results and persistent neutrophilic leukocytosis are additional important findings.

Treatment

The treatment of endocarditis involves attention to the primary focus and long-term (weeks to months) antibiotic therapy. The antibiotic should be chosen on the basis of culture results and sensitivity findings. If these are not available, high doses of penicillin are usually used. The prognosis is not favorable, although some animals have been cured with early diagnosis and prompt therapy. Chronic valvular fibrosis is present to some extent in many old animals. If severe, it may lead to insufficiency and a murmur. Congestive heart failure may supervene.

Supplementary Reading

Blood, D. C., Radostits, O. M., and Henderson, J. A.: Veterinary Medicine, 6th ed. London, Bailliére Tindall, 1983.
Jensen, R., and Mackey, D. R.: Diseases of Feedlot Cattle, 2nd ed. Philadelphia, Lea & Febiger, 1971.
Jensen, R.: Disease of Sheep. Philadelphia, Lea & Febiger, 1974.
Jones, T. C., and Hunt, R. D.: Veterinary Pathology, 5th ed. Philadelphia, Lea & Febiger, 1983.
Jubb, K. V. F., and Kennedy, P. C.: Pathology of Domestic Animals, 2nd ed. New York, Academic Press, 1970.
Leman, A. D., Glock, R. D., Mengeling, W. L., et al. (eds.): Diseases of Swine, 5th ed. Ames, Iowa, Iowa State University Press, 1981.

Evaluation of Anemia

ROBERT A. GREEN, D.V.M., Ph.D.

Anemia is a common complication of disease in food-producing animals. The condition is usually defined by a reduction in red blood cell count, hemoglobin concentration, or hematocrit value relative to normal for the species involved (values should also be adjusted for the animal's age, sex, and environment). The pathophysiologic significance of anemia is variable and depends on a balance between the severity of anemia and the extent that compensatory circulatory changes have augmented oxygen delivery to tissues. In addition to extreme variation in oxygen requirements associated with different levels of an animal's physical activity, the animal's need for oxygen is influenced by various environmental and physiologic factors. For example, hypothyroid animals have a lower metabolic rate leading to a reduction in oxygen demand that is manifested by mild anemia. In contrast, animals living at high altitudes with reduced oxygen tension develop mild polycythemia because of greater tissue oxygen demands. Various intrinsic erythrocyte metabolic changes can also influence oxygen delivery to tissues by altering the hemoglobin-oxygen dissociation curve (the relative affinity of hemoglobin for oxygen). Higher levels of erythrocyte 2,3-diphosphoglycerate (often present in anemia) decrease the affinity of hemoglobin for oxygen and thereby increase oxygen delivery to tissues.

Reduced oxygen delivery to the kidney in anemia causes elevated erythropoietin production. The marrow erythrocyte production rate can increase to about 6 to 8 times the basal rate in response to maximal erythropoietin stimulation. Various nutritional factors, particularly the availability of iron to developing erythroid precursors, also play important roles in determining the optimum rate of marrow erythropoiesis.

CLINICAL SIGNS

The clinical signs of anemia vary with the severity, the performance requirements placed on the animal, and the interaction with other debilitating problems caused by concurrent diseases. Compensatory physiologic changes for mild anemia may make detection difficult, as anemic animals tend to restrict their activity level. Often animals remain fairly bright and alert despite severe anemia, and only when the animal is exercised are clinical signs manifested. Despite lack of clinical signs, mild exercise or restraint procedures in animals with severe anemia may be sufficient to cause death. Therefore, caution is required when collecting blood for diagnostic tests and when administering supportive therapy to severely anemic animals. Usually some gradual weight loss, lethargy, and unthriftiness is manifested in animals with anemia characterized by gradual onset.

Marked hyperpnea or dyspnea is usually noted in animals having anemia of acute onset when the erythrocyte mass falls below 50 per cent of normal. Cows with anemia of acute onset may exhibit aggressive behavior or hyperexcitability when approached for examination. Pallor of the skin and mucous membranes becomes more evident as the anemia worsens. In cases characterized by marked erythrocyte destruction, icterus is apparent in mucous membranes as bilirubin levels approach 2 to 3 mg/100 ml. Hemoglobinuria is noted in animals with marked intravascular hemolytic anemia. In more chronic cases of hemolytic anemia, the ultimate severity is determined by the balance between the impact of the disease on erythrocyte survival and the ability of the marrow to increase erythroid production.

CLASSIFICATION OF ANEMIA

Since the causes of anemia are multiple, the most useful initial diagnostic procedure is to classify the patient's erythrocytic response.

In peripheral blood smears, greater erythrocyte production is usually indicated by a rise in the percentage of polychromatophilic erythrocytes (Wright's stain) or reticulocytes (New Methylene Blue* stain). The reticulocyte percentage should be adjusted for the animal's packed cell volume (PCV) according to the following equation:

$$\text{Adjusted Reticulocyte \%} = \text{Reticulocyte \%} \times \frac{\text{Patient's PCV}}{\text{Normal PCV}}$$

If the adjusted reticulocyte per cent is less than 0.5, a *nonresponding anemia* should be suspected, and if the adjusted reticulocyte per cent is greater than 2.0, a *responding anemia* should be suspected. Anemic animals with intermediate reticulocyte responses (0.5 to 2.0 per cent) are often in transitional states (marrow erythropoiesis has not had sufficient time to respond maximally) or have disease complications that limit their ability to respond. Determining the adjusted reticulocyte per cent serves as the primary basis for classifying anemia in all domestic animals except the horse. After anemia is classified, the etiologic possibilities are more restricted, and a logical basis for subsequent selection of diagnostic tests exists. Reviewing a blood smear for a potential cause of hemolytic anemia is futile in a patient with *nonresponding anemia*. In some instances, extensive diagnostic evaluation of anemia per se is unnecessary. For example, when anemia is secondary to another disease diagnostic and therapeutic efforts should mainly be directed towards resolving the primary disease, not the anemia. Extensive evaluation of anemia in patients with mild secondary anemia is expensive and usually unrewarding.

I. **Responding Anemia**—Adjusted Reticulocyte Percentage >2%.
  A. Plasma protein values are normal.
    (1.) Check for icterus, hemoglobinuria.
    (2.) Consider causes of hemolytic anemia.
    (3.) Review blood smear for abnormal erythrocyte morphology.
  B. Plasma protein values are decreased.
    (1.) Check for causes of acute hemorrhagic anemia.
    (2.) Evaluate hemostatic mechanism when cause of bleeding is not obvious.

II. **Nonresponding Anemia**—Adjusted Reticulocyte Percentage <0.5%.
  A. Normal marrow erythroid production is suppressed by pathophysiologic factors (usually characterized by marked erythroid hypoplasia of marrow).
    (1.) Check for renal disease.
    (2.) Check for other diseases causing sequestration of iron in reticuloendothelial cells (anemia of inflammatory disease).
    (3.) Check for myelophthisic disease (leukemia).
    (4.) Check for endocrine suppression of erythropoiesis.
    (5.) If marrow panhypoplasia exists, check for

suppression due to ingestion of myelotoxic drug or plant (bracken fern toxicosis).
  B. Defective erythroid maturation (ineffective erythropoiesis) is seen, usually characterized by marrow erythroid hyperplasia.
    (1.) Check for alteration in red blood cell indices.
    (2.) If microcytic hypochromic anemia is present, consider nutritional deficiency causing reduced hemoglobin synthesis (usually iron deficiency).
    (3.) If macrocytic normochromic anemia is present, consider factors interfering with normal mitotic division of erythroid precursors (folate, cobalt deficiencies).

LABORATORY FINDINGS

Laboratory test parameters play a major role in the classification of anemia (see previous outline). Initial detection of anemia is based on finding lowered levels of erythrocytic parameters, i.e., hematocrit value, red blood cell count, or hemoglobin level. Of these parameters, hematocrit value determination by the microhematocrit method is considered to be the simplest and the most accurate. The remaining methods are occasionally useful in determining red blood cell indices (see Ineffective Erythropoiesis, later in this article).

Diagnostic separation of *nonresponding anemia* from *responding anemia* is based on the reticulocyte percentage, a simple test performed using New Methylene Blue stain. As indicated previously, the reticulocyte per cent should be adjusted for the patient's hematocrit value. Some adjustment should also be made for prolongation in reticulocyte maturation time (which increases the reticulocyte per cent). This prolongation is caused by high erythropoietin levels in anemia, which induce premature release of reticulocytes from the marrow. Metarubricytosis should not be considered as an adequate "alternative" for reticulocyte enumeration for classifying anemia. Increased numbers of metarubricytes are often noted in blood smears from animals with either responding or nonresponding anemia. Indeed, higher numbers of metarubricytes are often noted in cases of *nonresponding anemia,* particularly those with greater extramedullary hematopoiesis. Metarubricytosis also accompanies marrow endothelial cell damage induced by certain toxemias, e.g., lead poisoning and endotoxemia.

When anemia appears to be nonresponding, bone marrow cytology is useful to establish the status of marrow erythropoiesis. Common sites for marrow aspiration in larger animals include sternum, ribs, and iliac crest. Employment of marrow cytology is not difficult, but some experience is necessary to obtain good samples and make "readable" smears. Although marrow cytology does not always help yield a final diagnosis, it limits diagnostic possibilities and provides a reasonable basis for selection of further diagnostic procedures.

If the anemia is responding, the plasma protein concentration should be determined with a refractometer. Simultaneously, the color of the plasma should be examined for possible icterus or hemolysis. If the responding anemia is associated with a reduced plasma protein level, evaluate the patient for possible causes of hemorrhagic anemia. Further laboratory tests may be necessary to help deter-

---

*Available from Sigma Chemical Co., St. Louis, Missouri 63178

mine if the animal has a hemostatic defect. Activated Coagulation Time* provides a simple, inexpensive screening test to detect abnormalities of the intrinsic coagulation cascade. Platelet numbers should also be estimated from the peripheral blood smear. If the patient has hemorrhagic anemia, a normal hemostatic mechanism, and no obvious external hemorrhagic lesions, occult gastrointestinal blood loss should be considered.

The presence of hemolytic anemia should be considered if the responding anemia is associated with normal plasma protein levels. The most useful laboratory aid in hemolytic anemia is careful review of a Wright's stained peripheral blood smear. The Diff-Quik† stain provides a practical stain for peripheral blood smears or bone marrow aspirates, which can be used in the small "office" laboratory. Abnormalities in erythrocyte shape, as well as any abnormal erythrocyte inclusions or parasites, should be identified. Although most causes of hemolytic anemia result in extravascular erythrocyte destruction, obvious hemoglobinemia and hemoglobinuria confirm intravascular hemolysis. Icterus results when increased erythrocyte destruction produces more bilirubin than the liver is able to excrete. In cattle, most cases of hyperbilirubinemia are due to hemolytic disease. Usually icterus is suspected by the finding of an increase in the icterus index. Mild elevations in bilirubin may be difficult to differentiate from the dietary carotenoids that impart a yellow color to serum. In such cases, quantitative serum bilirubin determination is required. Other serum chemistry tests or profiles are useful in the detection of underlying metabolic or organic diseases that induce anemia.

HEMOLYTIC ANEMIA

Acute hemolytic anemia is a prominent feature of various infectious, toxic, and immune-mediated diseases of food-producing animals. Clinical signs characteristic of hemolytic anemia are jaundice and hemoglobinuria. Depending on the acuteness of onset, other nonspecific signs of anemia may be present, e.g., pallor, lethargy, and dyspnea. Hemoglobinuria is a classic feature of hemolytic anemia characterized by a high rate of intravascular hemolysis. Diseases with marked intravascular hemolytic anemia are copper toxicosis, leptospirosis, babesiasis, and bacillary hemoglobinuria. Also, hemoglobinuria may accompany severe Heinz-body anemia caused by ingestion of certain toxic plants, e.g., kale, rape, or wild onions. Heinz bodies represent aggretates of denatured hemoglobin within the erythrocyte, which result from oxidation of hemoglobin by toxic metabolites originating from the ingested plants. The New Methylene Blue stain for identifying reticulocytes will also stain Heinz bodies in erythrocytes as dull blue inclusions that usually protrude slightly from the erythrocyte membrane. Hemoglobinemia is often accompanied by elevated levels of methemoglobin. Methemoglobin, an oxidized form of hemoglobin that cannot transport oxygen, imparts a brown color to the blood. Marked methemoglobinemia usually implies ingestion of a strong oxidizing substance, such as nitrate.

Hemoglobinuria must be differentiated from other conditions in which substances impart a red-brown color to urine. Hemoglobin is readily differentiated from myoglobin in urine through use of standard laboratory tests, e.g., solubility in saturated ammonium sulfate solution.

Hemolytic anemia characterized by marked extravascular hemolysis usually causes variable jaundice without hemoglobinuria. Examples of such types of anemia are anaplasmosis and eperythrozoonosis. Careful microscopic examination of erythrocyte morphology at high magnification is necessary to identify and differentiate abnormal inclusions or parasites from artifacts. In certain instances, the causes of anemia may not be apparent from the study of smears, and diagnosis may require serologic tests for confirmation.

Immune-mediated hemolytic anemia is generally seen in neonatal animals and results from ingestion of colostrum that contains antibodies against the neonatal animal's erythrocytes. In most cases, the dam was previously immunized with a whole blood origin vaccine that contained erythocyte antigens identical to those of the neonate. Such vaccines have typically been used in immunization programs against anaplasmosis and babesiasis. The affected neonatal calf usually develops acute intravascular hemolytic anemia, which often results in death during the first week of life. The severity of anemia depends on the antibody content of the colostrum and on the relative specificity of the antibody for the erythrocyte antigens of the neonate. Examination of blood smears from affected calves will often reveal marked erythrocyte agglutination.

HEMORRHAGIC ANEMIA

The cause of hemorrhagic anemia is clear when external blood loss occurs following traumatic injury. In other instances, blood loss may be insidious, but persistent, and ultimately result in severe anemia, e.g., bleeding due to gastrointestinal parasitism. Hemorrhagic anemia is characterized by reticulocytosis with variable hypoproteinemia. In occasional cases, persistent external blood loss may result in sufficient iron loss to cause iron deficiency anemia. The typical clinical signs of anemia are altered by the superimposed hypovolemic shock that accompanies acute hemorrhagic anemia. In addition, blood loss into body cavities or organs may cause further impairment of organ function and may compromise compensatory mechanisms, e.g., bleeding into the thoracic cavity would impair respiration. Bleeding into the central nervous system may cause paresis, ataxia, or even sudden death.

When the cause of bleeding is not obvious, the patient's hemostatic mechanism should be evaluated for potential abnormalities. Screening for disorders of platelet function is indicated when the patient has petechiation or notable bleeding from mucous membranes. The presence of thrombocytopenia can frequently be established by a careful microscopic count of the number of platelets per oil immersion field on a routine Wright's stained blood smear. Fewer than 7 platelets per oil immersion field indicate that the platelet count is below 100,000/µL. Bleeding due to thrombocytopenia is usually not important when the platelet count is above 50,000/µL, unless a qualitative defect in platelet function is also present. Screening for coagulopathy is indicated when the patient has subcutaneous or deep intramuscular hematomas. Activated Coagulation Time provides a useful screening test

---

*Available from Becton-Dickinson Co., Rutherford, NJ 07070 (Vacutainer #3206XF534. Test must be performed at 37°C.)

†Available from American Scientific Products, McGaw Park, IL 60085

to evaluate the severity of the coagulopathy, as well as the animal's response to therapy. Bleeding disorders associated with severe hepatic disease or with toxicity are due to generalized reduction in hepatic synthesis of coagulation factors, and poor response to vitamin K therapy is typical. In contrast, bleeding disorders due to ingestion of moldy sweet clover or anticoagulant rodenticides are caused by reduced synthesis of the vitamin K dependent coagulation factors, and good response to vitamin K therapy is expected. All drugs being administered for prophylaxis or treatment should be reviewed for potential interaction with the hemostatic mechanism. For a more complete discussion of bleeding abnormalities and their evaluation see Green, 1983.[3]

When the patient's hemostatic mechanism is normal, a search for occult blood is warranted. Often significant amounts of blood can be lost from the gastrointestinal tract without altering the normal color of feces. Heavy internal or external parasite loads can remove sufficient blood to cause rapidly developing, severe hemorrhagic anemia, particularly in animals that have not previously been exposed to the parasite. A few animals may have persistent blood loss related to gastrointestinal neoplasms or gastric ulcers. Blood originating from the upper gastrointestinal tract is digested and imparts a black tarry color to feces. Blood from the lower gastrointestinal tract is not digested and imparts a red color to feces. Therefore, fecal color is an important clinical aid in identifying the site of gastrointestinal bleeding.

ERYTHROID HYPOPLASIA

Anemia caused by erythroid hypoplasia has an insidious onset because of the long erythrocyte life span of food-producing animals. The condition is generally characterized by normal erythrocyte morphology with minimal reticulocytosis. As adequate time for physiologic compensation is given during the early stages of the disease, clinical signs of reduced exercise tolerance are only manifested under conditions that require greater cardiovascular performance. Some unthriftiness is usually apparent as the anemia worsens. If marrow erythroid hypoplasia is severe and persistent, the anemia will eventually cause obvious debilitation in the affected animal. Such cases of anemia may be associated with leukemia, renal disease, or suppression of marrow hematopoiesis associated with ingestion of myelotoxins, e.g., bracken fern toxicity.

Most chronic inflammatory diseases cause modest nonresponding anemia, often called the anemia of inflammatory disease. The mechanism of anemia is partially related to the elevated reticuloendothelial trapping of iron, and subsequently, inadequate iron release to support normal erythropoiesis. When the primary disease abates, anemia normally resolves during the convalescent stage, and specific treatment for the anemia of inflammatory disease is usually not required.

Bone marrow biopsy or aspiration is useful in evaluation of cases of hypoproliferative anemia. Establishing the relationship of erythropoiesis to the production of other hematopoietic cells is often helpful in differential diagnosis. Disease conditions accompanied by generalized marrow hypoplasia will have other major problems associated with bleeding or infections due to the lack of adequate platelet and white blood cell production, re-

spectively. Thorough evaluation of the animal's diet for potential myelotoxic drugs or plants is warranted when generalized marrow suppression is present. Selective erythroid hypoplasia is most often due to inadequate renal erythropoietin production, usually secondary to severe renal disease. In certain endocrinopathies, mild physiologic anemia may accompany lowering of the animal's basal metabolic rate, i.e., hypothryoidism.

INEFFECTIVE ERYTHROPOIESIS

When marrow erythropoiesis is elevated in the presence of persistent nonresponding anemia, conditions causing ineffective erythropoiesis should be considered. Deficiency of nutrients essential for normal erythropoiesis is the most common cause of this type of anemia. When deficiency of critical nutrients causes reduced hemoglobin synthesis in the developing erythrocyte, microcytic hypochromic anemia results. Evaluation of erythrocyte indices (mean corpuscular volume, mean corpuscular hemoglobin, and mean corpuscular hemoglobin concentration) is useful to help confirm the presence of hypochromic microcytes noted in peripheral blood smears. The usual cause of microcytic hypochromic anemia in animals is iron deficiency, resulting from either chronic blood loss in adult animals or inadequate dietary intake of iron in young growing animals (noted most frequently in baby pigs). Iron supplements will readily correct this type of anemia; however, a further search is needed in adult animals to establish the cause of bleeding, e.g., gastrointestinal parasitism and neoplasm.

Rare macrocytic normochromic anemia is encountered in diseases of animals. Nutrient deficiencies or diseases causing interference with normal mitotic division of erythroid precursors should be suspected in these instances. Evaluation of marrow erythroid precursors should reveal the presence of large erythroid cells called megaloblasts. Deficiencies in cobalt or folic acid can produce this type of anemia in animals, but its spontaneous occurrence is rare in food-producing animals.

TREATMENT

Once a diagnosis of anemia due to a specific cause is established, appropriate therapeutic and prophylactic recommendations may be obvious. This part of the article reviews the general approach to treatment of anemic patients. In food animals, treatment of anemia is usually influenced by economics. The decision to treat an animal is based on the salvage value of the animal as compared with the cost of treatment and the prognosis. In some cases, the primary medical consideration is only to prevent recurrence or further spread of the disease in the herd, and little attention is devoted to treatment of anemia in an individual animal.

Blood Transfusion

When a critical shortage of erythrocytes or total blood volume is present in a patient, transfusion of fresh whole blood provides the fastest correction of anemia. The necessity for transfusion is generally based not only on laboratory findings, but more importantly on the severity of clinical signs related to anemia. The hematocrit value may not reflect the severity of anemia, particularly during the first 12 hours following acute blood loss, because of inadequate fluid shifts from the extracellular compartment. Usually, transfusion of whole blood is utilized only in severe anemia of sudden onset, when cardiovascular compensation is inadequate. Appropriate measures to maintain adequate renal and cardiopulmonary functions are also indicated during treatment of the acutely anemic patient. If marked hemolysis is present, complications due to disseminated intravascular coagulation may be encountered.

Although blood transfusion is used less commonly in food animals than in companion animals, transfusion may be economically justified in treatment of acute anemia in valuable breeding animals. Cross-matching of whole blood from the recipient and donor is generally not performed if the recipient has not been transfused previously. Blood for transfusion may be collected in glass bottles, plastic bags, or large syringes containing an anticoagulant. Plastic containers are preferred over glass containers for blood collection because of reduced *in vitro* activation of hemostatic factors. Vacuum assistance may be required for collection of large volumes of blood from a donor's venous circulation. Acid-citrate-dextrose (ACD) solution is the anticoagulant most commonly used for blood that is to be transfused. The ratio of ACD to blood should be 14 ml ACD/100 ml of blood. When only small volumes are required, blood may be collected in a heparinized 50-ml plastic syringe (use 5 units of heparin/ml of blood) and transfused directly into the patient. Blood being administered intravenously should be given slowly to prevent circulatory overload and cardiac insufficiency, unless the animal has acute hypovolemia. Blood should be warmed to 37°C prior to administration. Sets with in-line filters are widely utilized to prevent infusion of clots in anticoagulated blood that might cause thrombotic complications.

Although uncommon, complications of transfusions are occasionally reported. Such complications include hemolytic reactions, microcirculatory blockades, cardiovascular overloads, and transmission of blood-borne diseases. Clinical signs of a transfusion reaction are fever, muscular tremors, salivation, dyspnea, and possibly hemoglobinuria. If a transfusion reaction is suspected, the transfusion should be stopped immediately, and administration of antihistamine and glucocorticoids may be beneficial.

Nutrition

In cases of chronic anemia with adequate circulatory compensation, treatment usually focuses on providing essential nutrients for normal marrow erythropoiesis. Occasional animals with anemia due to mineral deficiency may exhibit depraved appetite (pica). When malnutrition is suspected, the patient's diet should be evaluated not only for deficiency of essential vitamins and minerals but also for adequate caloric and protein intake. Young growing animals usually have limited iron stores and can rapidly develop iron deficiency when parasitism causes increased blood loss. A variety of iron dextran products are widely used in swine to prevent anemia in baby pigs. Short-term dietary supplementation with B vitamins, iron, copper, or cobalt may be beneficial in animals suffering from anemia related to chronic disease or malnutrition. Indiscriminate use of "shot-gun" multivitamin plus multimineral preparations, however, may produce toxic accumulation of trace minerals and should be used with caution in patients with cases of chronic nonresponding anemia. The clinician is best advised to administer only the deficient substance rather than administer multicomponent preparations in amounts that might induce toxicity.

Steroids

For chronic anemia that is caused by marrow stem cell damage and the subsequent failure of erythropoiesis, androgenic or anabolic steroids are generally considered to be the most useful nonspecific stimulant of erythropoiesis. Androgenic steroids appear to act primarily by elevating renal erythropoietin production. In most situations, erythropoietin levels are already high, and further erythropoietin elevation is usually of limited benefit to the patient. Compounds occasionally used to stimulate marrow hematopoiesis are stanozolol, oxymetholone, and testosterone enanthate. If the patient is also pancytopenic, the prognosis is generally poor. The primary effort should be to determine the cause of marrow damage and to initiate appropriate measures to prevent its further occurrence in the herd.

References

1. Riley, J. H., and Lassen, E. D.: Activated coagulation times of normal cows. Vet. Clin. Path. *8*:31–33, 1979.
2. Schalm, O. W., Jain, N. C., and Carroll, E. J.: Veterinary Hematology, 3rd ed. Philadelphia, Lea & Febiger, 1975.
3. Green, R. A.: Bleeding Disorders. *In* Ettinger, S. J. (ed.). Textbook of Veterinary Internal Medicine, 2nd ed. Philadelphia, W. B. Saunders Company, 2076–2098, 1983.

The Leukon

JOSEPH L. DORNER, D.V.M., Ph.D.

Interpretation of leukograms requires considerable knowledge about leukocyte populations, functions, kinetics, and pathophysiologic mechanisms responsible for leukocytosis and leukopenia. The leukogram includes a total white blood cell count (expressed as total white blood cells per μL of blood) and the relative number (percentage) of neutrophils, eosinophils, basophils, lymphocytes, and monocytes that make up the total.

Correct interpretation of the leukogram may reflect states of normalcy, physiologic leukocytosis, noninflammatory leukocytosis, inflammatory leukocytosis or leukopenia, convalescence, or leukemia. Except in cases of leukemia, the leukogram alone does not provide conclusive diagnostic information, but rather may support or refute a provisional diagnosis based on data obtained from a complete clinical history and physical examination.

LEUKOCYTE FUNCTIONS

Neutrophil. The primary function of the neutrophil is phagocytosis and enzymatic lysis of particulate matter and microorganisms, and it is an integral part of the host's defense mechanisms.

Neutrophils are bone marrow cells and exit the bone marrow storage pool by age, that is, mature, segmented neutrophils will leave first, followed by the band (stab) neutrophils, juvenile neutrophils, and so on. The finding of immature neutrophils in excess numbers implies, therefore, that the demand for neutrophils has exceeded the reserve capacity of the bone marrow. Once mature neutrophils exit the bone marrow, they enter the peripheral circulation where they are unevenly distributed between the circulating pool and the marginal pool. This phenomenon is brought about by the fact that neutrophils move slowly within blood vessels and have a tendency to form margins along blood vessel walls. These marginating neutrophils randomly enter the circulating pool, regardless of age, under the influence of physiologic or pathologic stimuli. They then enter the tissues at sites of injury or infection, where they act to neutralize infectious agents and to clear all debris in preparation for healing.

When a sample of blood is withdrawn from a normal animal, it will be the circulating pool from which cells are taken. However, numerous physiologic as well as pathologic conditions disturb the equilibrium that exists among the circulating, marginal, and bone marrow storage pool, and it is these disturbances that the clinician must recognize.

Eosinophil. All too frequently a rise of circulating eosinophils is wrongly interpreted as an indication of parasitism. While eosinophilia may result from some forms of parasitism, it occurs only after the host has become sensitized to the parasite. Sensitization leading to eosinophilia may result from any additional forms of antigenic stimulation.

The eosinophil is a phagocytic cell, albeit not as capable or versatile as the neutrophil, and functions principally in the ingestion of antigen-antibody complexes. Cellular constituents of the eosinophil neutralize the edema-producing and smooth muscle constricting properties of histamine and therefore modify the inflammatory reaction. Their appearance in excessive number in the blood indicates a possible antigen-antibody reaction as well as degranulation of mast cells.

Eosinophils are bone marrow cells, and their production parallels that of neutrophils. Once the cells enter the blood stream or tissues, they remain there.

Basophil. Basophils are bone marrow cells and perform their function in tissue. They are not mast cells but are comparable in that both the basophil and mast cell contain histamine and heparin, which are released through degranulation to initiate the inflammatory sequence. Basophils, like mast cells, are involved in delayed hypersensitivity reactions, and it is not unusual to observe mild basophilia in immune mediated disorders.

Lymphocyte. The lymphocyte functions in cell mediated immunity (T lymphocyte) and in humoral (antibody) immunity (B lymphocyte). Lymphocytes have variable life spans: short-lived lymphocytes have a life span of up to 3 days and are found primarily in the thymus and bone marrow. These short-lived cells are considered to be less active immunologically than long-lived lymphocytes, which have a life span ranging from several months to a year or more and are found in the blood, lymph nodes, and spleen. Long-lived lymphocytes are capable of mitotic activity and proliferate in response to antigenic stimulation.

Lymphocytes that have entered the blood may return to the lymphatic organs and re-enter the blood at a later time. The equilibrium between lymphocytes in the lymphatic organs and those in the blood may be altered by a variety of influences.

Monocyte. The monocyte is thought to be a bone marrow cell that has an important role in inflammation, since on entering the tissue it becomes an active phagocytic cell (macrophage). As such, monocytes remove dead or damaged cells, ingest particulate matter, and serve to process antigenic information. The monocyte also is a source of interferon and produces a granulopoietin referred to as colony stimulating factor.

LEUKOCYTIC AND LEUKOPENIC LEUKOGRAMS

These 2 terms imply the increase or decrease of total circulating white blood cells when compared with normal values. Total white blood cell counts, however, include all nucleated cells. Occasionally, nucleated erythrocytes will contribute to this total, and the count must be corrected according to the following formula:

Corrected WBC count =
observed WBC count $\times$ 100/(100 + number of nucleated erythrocytes)

The denominator of this formula is found by examining a stained blood smear and by recording the number of nucleated erythrocytes observed per 100 leukocytes. Differential white blood cell counts are recorded as relative values (percentage). Multiplying the relative value by the total white blood cell count results in an absolute count per μL.

In most instances, leukocytosis or leukopenia is directly related to changes in the circulating neutrophil population. Therefore, when the number of circulating neutrophils rises, there will be a concomitant leukocytosis. As neutrophils decline, leukopenia ensues.

Neutrophil to Lymphocyte Ratio. Food-producing animals are unique in that the leukograms of mature animals are characterized by lymphocyte leads, that is, lymphocyte populations are greater than the populations of other leukocytes. The normal neutrophil to lymphocyte (N:L) ratio for the cow, goat, and sheep is roughly 0.5:1, and for the pig it is 0.7:1. When N:L ratios are appreciably altered, the implication is that there has been a decrease or increase of either the neutrophil or the lymphocyte. This provides the clinician with a rapid method for assessing whether or not the leukogram is abnormal. When abnormalities are evident, absolute numbers are used to determine what cell type is responsible.

Physiologic Leukograms. When the absolute neutrophil count exceeds 4000/μL for the cow, 6000/μL for the sheep, 7000/μL for the goat, and 9000/μL for the pig, the animal has neutrophilia. This does not always imply inflammation, for there are numerous physiologic conditions that result in neutrophilia.

Physiologic neutrophilia is caused by the secretion of epinephrine, which causes cells to leave the marginal pool and to enter the circulating pool. The total number of neutrophils in the blood does not change nor does the half-life. This response is rapid and lasts roughly 20 minutes. The magnitude of neutrophilia (leukocytosis) is determined by the number of cells in the marginal pool. In food-producing animals, the marginal pool is approximately 1 to 1.5 times as great as the circulating pool. Therefore, if an animal is reluctant to be bled or is fractious, neutrophilia may have no clinical significance. There may be a slight accompanying rise in circulating lymphocytes, but all other leukocytes remain at essentially normal levels. The result is that the N:L ratio will approach or exceed unity (1:1), and absolute numbers will reveal greater numbers of neutrophils with no significant change in absolute numbers of lymphocytes, eosinophils, or monocytes.

Stress Leukogram. This is perhaps the most commonly encountered neutrophilic/leukocytosis in domestic animals and is referred to as noninflammatory leukocytosis. Corticosteroids, whether they are exogenous or endogenous, mobilize the marginal pool as in physiologic neutrophilia. In addition, circulating neutrophil half-lives and neutrophil exits from the bone marrow are increased. As a result, there may be a 1- to 4-fold increase in circulating segmented neutrophils.

Since the rate of release from the bone marrow storage pool is elevated, band neutrophils may be observed in the blood; however, the absolute band count should not exceed 300/µL. If the cause is due to a single episode or injection, neutrophil counts usually return to normal levels within 24 hr.

A rise in endogenous corticosteroids may result from trauma, pain, neoplasia, metabolic disorders, surgery, transportation, or any other stressful situation. Many diseases also elicit stress responses. Repeated leukograms as well as thorough physical examinations will aid in differentiating noninflammatory from inflammatory changes in leukocyte populations.

Corticosteroids affect not only segmented neutrophils but lymphocytes and eosinophils as well. Food-producing animals often have a 30 to 50 per cent reduction of circulating lymphocytes in 8 to 10 hr following a stressful situation, with a return to normal occurring between 24 and 30 hr after a single episode. This phenomenon, stress, is the single greatest cause for lymphopenia in all domestic animals. Eosinopenia, as a result of stressful experiences, is attributed to sequestration, to decreased production when stress is prolonged, or to corticosteroid therapy.

In summary, a stress leukogram is characterized by an N:L ratio equal to or exceeding unity, but, unlike the case with physiologic leukograms, lymphopenia, eosinopenia, and, occasionally, an absolute band neutrophil count of less than 300 cells/µL will be present.

Inflammatory Leukograms. Inflammatory processes and subsequent leukograms reflect cellular response to tissue injury. The more severe the inflammation, the greater the neutrophilic/leukocytosis. Localized inflammatory lesions, such as abscesses and metritis, result in greater neutrophilia than generalized inflammatory disease. Pyogenic bacteria produce more severe neutrophilia than other etiologic agents.

A leukogram generally reflects the ability of the host to respond to tissue demands for cells. As the inflammatory process develops, the marginal pool increases the size of the circulating pool, and neutrophils emigrate from the blood into the tissue. If the tissue demand exceeds the available supply of circulating neutrophils, leukograms will reveal leukopenia. This is frequently what is observed in acute bovine coliform mastitis. As a result of tissue changes and the activation and release of humoral factors, granulopoiesis and release rates from bone marrow are higher. If production exceeds the demand, leukograms will be characterized by more immature cells (left shift) with concurrent leukocytosis. This is defined as a regenerative shift or appropriate response. If the demand for neutrophils exceeds production capacity of the marrow, the leukogram will be characterized by the presence of immature cells without leukocytosis. This is defined as a degenerative shift or inappropriate response. If toxemia is generalized, the staining and morphologic characteristics of the circulating neutrophils will be altered. The cytoplasm of the cells will retain its basophilia but will become vacuolated and sustain a loss of granulation. Occasionally, "toxic" neutrophils may contain scattered red granules or, less frequently, blue-black granules as a result of precipitation of the basophilic ground substance. The finding of such changes may herald depression of granulopoiesis and progressive neutropenia.

Convalescence. As the inflammatory process abates, the left shift diminishes, and there is a tendency toward hypersegmentation of neutrophils (right shift). Monocytes may rise in proportion to the quantity of macromolecular matter that is to be removed from the tissues. Lymphocytes as well as eosinophils reappear in normal numbers. The reappearance of lymphocytes and eosinophils may result from diminution of the stress or from the development of an immunologic response to the disease entity, or both.

SPECIES DIFFERENCES

Cow, Sheep, and Goat. Leukograms of these species often exaggerate the inflammatory process because of their normal low N:L ratio, and because these species do not have a large bone marrow reserve of mature neutrophils. Early in the inflammatory process, normal white blood cell counts as well as leukopenia may be encountered. These leukograms reflect tissue demands as well as species-related relatively low numbers of neutrophils in the bone marrow storage pool. Leukograms may be characterized by a left shift within 24 hr, while the total white blood cell count may not have risen significantly. By definition, this is a degenerative shift or inappropriate response. The implication of such a finding does not hold true for these species unless repeated leukograms fail to indicate leukocytosis. In peracute inflammation, such as mastitis, leukograms are commonly characterized by an absolute reduction of neutrophils and the presence of immature neutrophils. The absolute immature count may not exceed 300 cells/µL as a result of the reduction in the total white blood cell count. A good history and a physical examination will assist in interpretation of this type of leukogram. Acute inflammatory leukograms of ruminants are typically in the 5 to 15,000 cells/µL range with rare counts exceeding 25,000.

Pig. Very little experimental work has been done in pigs, and knowledge of how this animal responds to inflammatory processes is limited. However, there appears to be no reason to assume that the response of such animals is unlike that of other domestic species. Since mature pigs, like the ruminants, are lymphocytic, it can be anticipated that in stressful and acute inflammatory processes, subnormal, normal, or only slightly elevated white blood cell counts may be encountered. Because pigs have a higher normal white blood cell count than ruminants and a greater number of circulating mature neutrophils, inflammatory leukograms may be characterized by total white blood cell counts of 30,000 to 40,000 cells per µL. In pyogenic infections, the white blood cell count may exceed 40,000.

LEUKOPENIA

Leukopenia, as in the case of leukocytosis, is related to neutrophil kinetics. That which causes neutropenia also causes leukopenia. Neutropenia results from excess utilization, decreased production, or increased sequestration of neutrophils.

Excess Utilization. Overwhelming bacterial inflammatory infections can cause an excessive tissue demand with resultant neutropenia and leukopenia. Diseases incriminated in such cases are coliform mastitis, peritonitis (hardware disease, intestinal rupture), pyometra, pneumonia, and any other suppurative process. Repeated leukograms are necessary to determine responsiveness, as persistence of neutropenia implies inability of the bone marrow to meet tissue demands and warrants a guarded to grave prognosis.

Decreased Production. This category of neutropenia and leukopenia is of a serious nature, as it implies bone marrow hypoplasia or aplasia. This type of response has been associated with bracken fern toxicity, hyperestrogenism, prolonged drug therapy, and neoplasia of the bone marrow (lymphosarcoma).

Certain viral diseases also can cause leukopenia as a result of decreased production and lymphocytic lysis. Swine suffering from hog cholera and rinderpest develop leukopenia. Sheep inoculated with blue tongue virus develop marked cases of leukopenia as a result of neutropenia and eosinopenia as well as lymphopenia. Cattle suffering from viral diarrhea develop leukopenia, as do ruminants exposed to Rift Valley fever. The mechanism responsible for these instances of leukopenia is questionable, since, in addition to decreased production, there exists the possibility that circulating leukocytes may be sequestered or utilized.

Sequestration. Anaphylactic or endotoxic shock causes a marked shift of cells from the circulating pool to the marginal pool, resulting in leukopenia. This effect is transitory and the normal response to inflammation occurs within hours.

Supplemental Reading

Coles, E. H.: Veterinary Clinical Pathology. 3rd ed. Philadelphia, W. B. Saunders Company, 1980.

Duncan, R. J., and Prasse, K. W.: Veterinary Laboratory Medicine—Clinical Pathology. Ames, Iowa State University Press, 1977.

Medway, W., Prier, J. E., and Wilkinson, J. S.: Veterinary Clinical Pathology. Baltimore, Williams & Wilkins Co., 1969.

Schalm, O. W., Jain, N. C., and Carroll, E. S.: Veterinary Hematology. 3rd ed. Philadelphia, Lea & Febiger, 1975.

Refer to the first volume of *Current Veterinary Therapy: Food Animal Practice* for the following: Smetzer, David L.: Cardiac Arrhythmias and Congenital Cardiac Defects, Section 12, Diseases of Cardiovascular and Hemolymphatic Systems.

DISEASES OF THE DIGESTIVE SYSTEM

DALE R. NELSON, D.V.M., M.S.
Consulting Editor

Pathophysiology of the Gastrointestinal System

ROBERT H. WHITLOCK, D.V.M., Ph.D.

Numerous physiologic processes take place in the gastrointestinal system, including glandular secretion, mucosal cell absorption, intestinal motility, and complex neuroendocrine activities. A disorder of any one facet could lead to serious disorder for the patient.

Visual inspection of the patient often provides the first clue as to the nature of the disease. If the cow has been "off feed" for several days, one would expect to find a gaunt or "tucked up" appearance. However, if the abdomen is full or distended despite the animal being anorectic for more than 48 hours, then obstructive disease, such as vagal indigestion, hydrops, ascites, and rumen overload, must be considered. A contracted abdomen or gaunt appearance would force consideration of other diseases, such as traumatic reticuloperitonitis, left abomasal displacement, ketosis, and salmonellosis, among others.

PREHENSION AND MASTICATION

Prehension and mastication are functions of the voluntary muscles of the lips, tongue, and jaw. Cranial nerve deficits to these muscles can interfere with their performance. The oral cavity, teeth, tongue, and pharynx should be carefully inspected for abnormalities. Local irritation, ulceration, or foreign body penetration can cause voluntary cessation of eating or drinking. It is important to differentiate between lack of desire to eat and inability to eat. The latter is often demonstrated by the animal showing interest in food and "picking" at it but retaining it in the mouth, as may occur with rabies, botulism, actinobacillosis, or moldy corn poisoning.[1]

DYSPHAGIA

Dysphagia can be caused by mechanical or functional pharyngeal disturbances and, clinically, is often characterized by apparent sialosis (drooling of saliva). Foreign body obstruction of the esophagus is a common cause of dysphagia, although choke may also be caused by tumors, enlarged mediastinal lymph nodes, or thoracic abscesses. Functional blockage of the swallowing reflex occurs with interference to the nervous supply of the muscles, as seen in rabies and botulism.

ABDOMINAL DISTENTION

Abdominal fullness or distention in a cow that is "off feed" is a relatively specific sign. The five "F's" must be considered: (1) fat, (2) fetus, (3) flatus, (4) feces, and (5) fluid. A rectal examination is important in differentiation. A fetus or distended uterus can easily be differentiated from ascites or a distended rumen. Visual inspection will differentiate fat, that is, the obese cow, from the flatus or gas accumulation seen in bloat. The majority of distended abdomens on an individual basis are due to fluid in the rumen. This can be confirmed by rumen ballottement that reveals a fluid or splashy consistency to the rumen in the upper left paralumbar fossa, which is normally doughy. If a fluid rumen is found with evidence of shock and tachycardia (pulse greater than 100/minute), then acute rumen overload (lactic acidosis) should be considered. Lactic acidosis can quickly be confirmed by measuring the rumen pH, which would be less than 5.0. If the pH is normal, other reasons for rumen distention, such as vagal indigestion or ingestion of a solute load, that is, salt or magnesium sulfate, must be sought. Diffuse peritonitis may also cause a distended abdomen and a fluid-filled rumen owing to ileus. A peritoneocentesis with a high WBC (greater than 10,000) and total protein (greater than 3.0 gm/dl) will confirm peritonitis. Additional evidence includes a high PCV (greater than 45 per cent) with a disparately lowered total protein (less than 7.0 gm/dl). The PCV is elevated due to the hemoconcentration, and the protein is lost into the peritoneal cavity.

A distended rumen in dairy cattle is usually secondary to one of several forms of vagal indigestion, including failure of eructation, failure of omasal transport, and abomasal impaction, or indigestion of advanced pregnancy. A plasma chloride will easily differentiate failure of omasal transport from abomasal impaction, which is consistently associated with hypochloremia (less than 80 mEq/L).

Table 1. *Acid-Base and Electrolyte Values in Cattle with Obstructive Gastrointestinal Disease*

Disease	No. Cases	Sodium*	Potassium*	Chloride*	Bicarbonate*
Left abomasal displacement	75	137 ± 0.6	3.5 ± 0.1	86 ± 4.0	27 ± 0.7
Right abomasal displacement	18	133 ± 1.0	2.9 ± 0.2	81 ± 3.0	34 ± 2.5
Abomasal impaction	12	136 ± 1.2	3.3 ± 0.2	86 ± 3.7	38 ± 3.0
Intussusception	5	134 ± 2.4	3.3 ± 0.4	86 ± 4.4	35 ± 4.4
Cecal volvulus	4	134 ± 2.1	3.1 ± 0.2	91 ± 3.0	32 ± 2.4
Normal values	—	134 ± 2.0	4.0 ± 0.5	103 ± 4.0	25 ± 5.0

*Values expressed as mEq/L.

ACID-BASE AND ELECTROLYTE CHANGES

Gastrointestinal obstructive diseases in cattle are usually associated with typical acid-base and electrolyte aberrations.[2] Obstructive diseases involving the area from the omasum to the colon include left abomasal displacement, right abomasal displacement, abomasal volvulus, abomasal impaction, pyloric stenosis, intussusception, cecal dislocation, cecal volvulus, and possibly small intestinal volvulus. The electrolyte and acid-base parameters of several diseases are presented in Table 1.

Hypokalemia with a normal sodium value is a common finding. The low potassium may be associated with decreased intake of roughage, which is high in potassium, along with continued renal potassium excretion. Renal potassium excretion continues despite the lack of intake and, in fact, may deplete the body of potassium. Another factor is the cellular shift of hydrogen and potassium. During alkalosis, potassium enters the cell and hydrogen moves out to neutralize the bicarbonate, resulting in the plasma hypokalemia. If this persists the cells become potassium-depleted because of decreased intake and continued renal loss.

Hypochloremia is the most significant change associated with obstructive diseases in cattle and occurs because of continued abomasal secretion despite the fact that the animals are ill and often anorectic. Abomasal juice, rich in chloride, is secreted into the lumen of the abomasum. The secretion is retained in the abomasum or is refluxed through the omasal canal back into the rumen, resulting in a large rumen chloride trap. Bicarbonate is generated by the kidney to provide anion balance. The abomasum secretes between 30 and 35 liters of a very low pH material in a 24-hour period. The bicarbonate increase results in a metabolic alkalosis typical of intestinal obstructions in cattle.

Clinically, abomasal reflux can be detected by ballottement of the rumen and rectal examination. The normal rumen occupies approximately the left half of the abdomen of a cow, whereas with abomasal reflux, the rumen continues to enlarge, taking on an almost L-shaped appearance in the ventral abdomen as the ventral sac enlarges toward the right side. Normally most anorectic cows are "tucked up," whereas the cow with obstructive disease is more rotund and has some fullness of the abdomen, especially when viewed from behind. This full appearance would not be expected from a cow that is "off feed" and anorectic. Quantitative estimation of the severity of clinical findings on a scale from 0 to 4+ aids in therapy.

A cow with obstructive gastrointestinal disease between the omasum and the cecum would be expected to have a hypokalemic, hypochloremic metabolic alkalosis, the severity of which varies with the chloride trap. The clinical signs of alkalosis are most often sunken eyes, lack of skin turgor, and change in rumen consistency. Ballottement of the rumen and the data in Table 2 provide guidelines as to the severity of the alkalosis associated with gastrointestinal stasis and, in fact, can offer a reasonable prediction of the bicarbonate value. Thus, with a 4+ dehydration and obstruction we would expect a base excess (BE) of approximately 25 mEq/L (see Table 2).[3]

Projectile diarrhea is often associated with a severe acidosis whether the diarrhea is due to salmonellosis, winter dysentery, bovine virus diarrhea, chemical or plant poisoning, or parasites. However, the diarrhea must be acute and profuse if acidosis is to be suspected. If the diarrhea is chronic and not profuse, the animal is likely to be metabolically compensated and, although severely dehydrated, may not be acidotic, since the loss of base is not acute.

Table 2. *Clinical Guide for Predicting the Acid-Base Status of a Bovine Patient**

Clinical Signs†	Hydration‡	Base Excess (mEq/L)	Estimated Bicarbonate (mEq/L)
Fluid distended rumen (very scant feces)	4+ dehydration	+20	50
Splashy rumen (scant feces)	3+ dehydration	+15	45
Moderate distention (scant feces)	2+ dehydration	+10	40
Doughy rumen (firm feces)	1+ dehydration	+5	35
NORMAL	NORMAL	0	25 ± 5
Slight diarrhea	1+ dehydration	−5	20
Mild diarrhea	2+ dehydration	−10	15
Moderate diarrhea (acute)	3+ dehydration	−15	10
Severe diarrhea (profuse, acute)	4+ dehydration	−20	5

*This guide is based on the slightest detectable change (1+) and the most severe change (4+).

†The correlating clinical sign for the prediction of alkalosis is abdominal distention; for acidosis it is the appearance of a gaunt, "tucked up" cow with diarrhea.

‡The hydration status is based on the combination of lack of skin turgor in the midneck area and the retraction of the eye in the socket.

HEMATOLOGIC ALTERATIONS

The determination of the microhematocrit and total plasma protein will often give much valuable information about the nature of an abdominal disorder. Most subacute to chronic inflammatory disorders are characterized by a low-normal PCV (25 to 32 per cent) and mild hyperproteinemia (total plasma protein greater than 7.5 gm/dl). The anemia is nonresponsive and is due to bone marrow depression by the chronic inflammatory process. Advanced or longstanding cases of chronic infection (hepatic abscesses, chronic reticulitis, or vagal indigestion) may have a total protein of 10.0 gm/dl or higher with a moderate anemia (PCV less than 25 per cent, normal 30 to 34 per cent).

A normal PCV with a low total protein (less than 6.0 gm/dl) has ominous prognostic value, suggesting a protein-losing enteropathy, body cavity sequestration of protein (diffuse peritonitis), or renal protein loss (amyloidosis). Usually a complete physical examination will provide adequate information for a tentative diagnosis. An elevated PCV and total plasma protein suggests acute massive dehydration, as may occur with acute grain overload, salt poisoning, or severe profuse diarrhea. Although a severe abnormality, the prognosis may be favorable if fluid therapy is adequate.

The leukogram reflects the status of neutrophil production by the bone marrow, tissue demand, and lymphocyte kinetics. A severe prolonged neutropenia may suggest inadequate marrow production, as may occur with bovine virus diarrhea or bracken fern poisoning. Chronic infections often provoke only mild hematologic alterations, that is, reversal of the neutrophil:lymphocyte ratio. A moderate leukocytosis (12,000 to 16,000 WBC) may be associated with an acute infectious process but rapidly returns to within normal range as the process becomes localized.

References

1. Michell, A. R.: Physiologic principles in the management of alimentary dysfunction. Vet. Rec. 80:375, 1967.
2. Whitlock, R. H., Tasker, J. B., and Tennant, B. C.: Hypochloremic, metabolic alkalosis and hypokalemia in cattle with upper gastrointestinal obstruction. Am. J. Digest. Dis. 20:595, 1975.
3. Whitlock, R. H.: Pathophysiology of lower gastrointestinal tract problems in the bovine. Proc. Ann. Mt., Am. Assoc. Bovine Pract. 9:43, 1976.

Emesis

ROBERT H. WHITLOCK, D.V.M., Ph.D.

Emesis, or vomiting, in ruminants is characterized by forceful ejection of forestomach contents through the mouth. Projectile vomiting is the most common form and is due to reverse peristalsis of the esophagus; it usually is not accompanied by the retching movements that characterize true vomiting. Emesis is associated with contractions of the musculature of the abdominal wall and neck with the head and neck extended. Vomiting may be of central or peripheral origin, depending on whether the stimulation arises from the vomiting center in the medulla or from irritation of afferent nerves that originate in various body organs and extend to the vomiting center.

PATHOPHYSIOLOGY

The initial phase of true vomiting consists of irregular, rapid, and deep respiration, followed by retching due to spasmodic contraction of all the muscles of respiration. The subsequent events consist of reflex mechanisms that prevent the vomitus from entering the respiratory tract and possibly causing inhalation pneumonia. Following deep inspiration, the glottis is closed and the nasopharynx sealed off by elevation of the soft palate. Expiration with contraction of the abdominal musculature forces ingesta into the esophagus and, with antiperistaltic contractions of the esophagus, propels it from the mouth.

Emesis with ingesta expelled from the mouth can be observed as a herd problem due to the consumption of spoiled corn silage,[1] green clover, moldy silage,[2] or high-acid silage found near the bottom of the silo. Toxic plants that cause vomiting include *Convallaria majalis* (lily of the valley), *Helenium hoopesii* (sneezeweed),[3] and *Veratrum viride* (skunk cabbage).[2] Other causes of emesis include an esophageal foreign body,[1, 4] overloading of the forestomach with ingesta (toxic indigestion, vagal indigestion, and so on), traumatic reticulitis,[2] diaphragmatic hernia, abomasal impaction, arsenic poisoning,[5] advanced stages of milk fever,[5] the use of a large-bore stomach tube,[5] papillomas in the esophageal groove,[5] obstruction of the omasal canal,[7] and megaesophagus.[6] Experimentally, alkaloidal extracts from *Veratrum* spp. have been used to induce eructation and vomiting in normal and bloated cows.[8] Thus, the natural ingestion of these plants would be expected to produce emesis.

Emesis has been observed in calves two to three months old affected with gastrointestinal catarrh and diarrhea.[2] The vomitus should be inspected for a foreign body, blood, or purulent exudate. Measurement of pH of the vomitus is of little diagnostic value. Emesis due to esophageal obstruction would be characterized by poorly masticated feed mixed with saliva, whereas vomitus from the rumen would resemble normal rumen contents. Serious complications of emesis in the ruminant are aspiration pneumonia and acute laryngeal obstruction.

THERAPY

Management of emesis caused by ingestion of toxic plants or feeds consists of diet alteration. Silage or forages that have been associated with vomiting may be tolerated if amounts are gradually increased over time. External palpation of the esophagus and passage of a stomach tube may confirm an esophageal foreign body. Foreign bodies lodged in the pharynx, larynx, or proximal esophagus may be removed by passing the hand into the mouth along the hard palate to the level of the esophageal opening. Foreign bodies can be removed from the proximal 6 to 8 cm of the esophagus manually. A probang or similar instrument can be used to remove foreign objects from the middle or distal esophagus. If traumatic gastritis or obstruction between the compartments of the forestomachs is suspected, a rumenotomy may determine the presence of any obstruction. Some cows with failure of omasal transport or abomasal impaction exhibit emesis as a major clinical sign along with abdominal distention and seem to respond to removal of the rumen contents. Sodium bicarbonate or magnesium hydroxide *per os* has been successful in relieving emesis in the individual cow in which no definitive cause can be ascertained.[1]

References

1. Fox, F. H.: Bovine Medicine and Surgery, 2nd ed. American Veterinary Publications, Inc., Santa Barbara, Cal., 1980, 662.
2. Udall, D. H.: *In* The Practice of Veterinary Medicine, 6th ed. George Banta Publishing Co., Menasha, Wis., 1954, 101–102.
3. Kingsbury, J. M.: *In* Poisonous Plants of the United States and Canada. Prentice-Hall, Inc., Englewood Cliffs, N. J., 1964, 409–412.
4. Stewart, S. L.: Vomiting in cows. Vet. Med. *34*:203, 1939.
5. Blood, D. C., Henderson, J. A., and Radostits, O. M.: *In* Veterinary Medicine, 6th ed. Williams & Wilkins Co., Baltimore, 1983, 137.
6. Kasari, T. R.: Dilation of the lower cervical esophagus in a cow. Can. Vet. J. *25*:177, 1984.
7. Hutyra, F., Marek, J., and Manninger, R.: *In* Special Pathology and Therapeutics of the Diseases of Domestic Animals, Vol. II, 5th ed. Alexander Eger, Inc., Chicago, 1949, 61–65.
8. Mullenox, C. H., Buck, W. B., Keller, R. F., and Binns, W.: Stimulating eructation and vomition in normal and bloated ruminants with alkaloid extracts of *Veratrum* spp. Am. J. Vet. Res. 27:211, 1966.

Tenesmus

ROBERT H. WHITLOCK, D.V.M., Ph.D.

Rectal tenesmus, or ineffectual straining to defecate, is a common sign of disease affecting the structures within the abdominal and/or pelvic cavity. The degree of tenesmus may be moderate to severe, constant or intermittent, productive or nonproductive, and of long or short duration, depending on the degree of inflammation, edema, and irritation present.

PATHOGENESIS

Common causes of tenesmus in the bovine include watery diarrhea, impending parturition, prolapsed vagina and/or rectum, urethral calculi, abdominal fat necrosis, obesity within the pelvic canal, estrogen toxicity, cystitis, vaginitis, and coccidiosis. Tansey ragwort in some geographic areas is commonly associated with tenesmus, and, although rare, rabies must always be a consideration in unexplained cases. Rectal irritation following manual examination of the rectum and pelvic area is a common iatrogenic cause of tenesmus. Cattle with diarrhea are very prone to develop tenesmus, so much so that some clinicians suggest that a rectal examination is contraindicated in a cow with watery diarrhea.[1] If a rectal examination must be done for diagnostic purposes, a smooth rubber glove rather than irritating plastic sleeves should be used following epidural anesthesia. Even with these precautions the animal may develop tenesmus.

An animal exhibiting tenesmus warrants a thorough physical examination. A visual and manual vaginal examination is indicated if the source of irritation is not apparent. If rectal and vaginal examinations fail to explain the tenesmus, further physical examination should be done. A neurologic assessment may reveal neurologic deficits suggestive of spinal cord compression due to vertebral body abscessation or rabies.[2] Unexplained tenesmus, along with bellowing, is often a feature of bovine rabies, but the signs of rabies are never consistent.

THERAPY

Clinical management of tenesmus involves regional or local anesthesia, therapeutic pneumoperitoneum, or tracheotomy. Epidural anesthesia (6 to 8 ml of 2 per cent procaine or lidocaine per 500 kg) has long been advocated for relief of tenesmus, but the short duration of anesthesia (one to two hours) dictates frequent administration of the anesthetic. Some veterinarians advocate the use of benzyl alcohol or ethyl alcohol (4 to 6 ml per 500 kg), which destroys nerve tissue, resulting in prolonged epidural anesthesia (two to six months). This technique has been employed in beef cattle but is not desirable for dairy cattle for sanitary reasons.[3] Internal pudendal nerve block, as used by Larson[4] for anesthesia of the bull penis and relaxation of the retractor penis muscle, will anesthetize the vulva and vestibular structures without affecting motor nerves.

Minor tenesmus from vaginal or rectal irritation can be relieved by local infusions of bland, protective antiseptics and local anesthetics in oil. These same local anesthetic gels (e.g., Xylocaine gel) may also be applied as a lubricant for rectal examination.

Therapeutic pneumoperitoneum has been described by Esperson[5, 6] and Svendsen.[7] The technique consists of insufflation of air into the peritoneal cavity; this is continued until the paralumbar fossa area is slightly distended or until the respiratory rate increases significantly. The therapeutic effect results from increased intra-abdominal pressure, which exerts pressure on the diaphragm and causes a secondary increased pressure within the thoracic cavity. The animal relaxes the abdominal musculature to reduce the pressure on the abdominal side of the diaphragm, and this facilitates respiration. Esperson reported satisfactory therapeutic effects in 108 of 157 cows. Tenesmus ceased immediately or gradually decreased in frequency and severity after 12 to 24 hours. One untoward effect of therapeutic pneumoperitoneum was subcutaneous emphysema. This is rarely a serious problem and will gradually be resorbed in two to four weeks. Tracheotomy with the insertion of a tracheal tube is considered the last resort in cases of uncontrolled tenesmus. This method is effective, as it prevents the animal from increasing the intra-abdominal pressure.

References

1. Argenzio, R. A., Whitlock, R. H., and Burroughs, C. F.: *In* Veterinary Gastroenterology. Lea & Febiger, Philadelphia, 1980, 524–525.
2. Blood, D. C., Henderson, J. A., and Radostits, O. M.: *In* Veterinary Medicine, 6th ed. Williams & Wilkins Co., Baltimore, 1983, 136.
3. Roberts, S. J.: *In* Veterinary Obstetrics and Genital Diseases, 2nd ed. Published by the author, Ithaca, N.Y., 1971, 195–196.
4. Larson, T. L.: The internal pudendal (pudic) nerve block for anesthesia of the penis and relaxation of the retractor penis muscle. J. Am. Vet. Med. Assoc. *123*:18, 1953.
5. Esperson, G.: Artificial pneumoperitoneum for treating tenesmus. Mod. Vet. Pract. *42*:42, 1961.
6. Esperson, G.: Artifizielles pneumatoperitonaeum gegen tenesmen beim rinde. Wien. Tierarztl. Mschr. *10*:825, 1962.
7. Svendsen, P.: Artificiel pneumatoperitonaeum. Nord. Vet. Med. *19*:163, 1967.

Constipation

ROBERT H. WHITLOCK, D.V.M., Ph.D.

Constipation is defined in *Dorland's Medical Dictionary* as "infrequent or difficult evacuation of feces." The criteria for the determination of constipation must be modified by the diet, use, and age of the animal. For example, heifers on a roughage diet often have very firm feces compared with lactating cows or beef cows on lush pasture. A more strict definition of constipation would be the abnormal retention of feces in the rectum, or unusually firm feces. Constipation is a symptom of an underlying disease. A distinct effort should be made to determine the underlying disease prior to therapy.

DIAGNOSIS

The common causes of constipation include starvation/malnutrition; severe debility; dehydration due to lack of water; partial intestinal obstruction, as may occur with fat necrosis; botulism; lymphosarcoma; intussusception; pelvic abscesses; acorn poisoning; paralytic ileus; fractured pelvis; lack of dietary bulk; and painful conditions of the anal sphincter. Each of these conditions can be better evaluated with a good history and complete physical examination, including rectal examination. Occasionally, a right flank laparotomy or fiberoptic endoscopy using a speculum may be needed to properly discern the nature of the lesion.

Constipation in the calf may rarely be caused by meconium retention; segmental atresia of the colon or atresia ani, both of which occur sporadically; umbilical hernia with an incarcerated intestine; and trichobezoar (hairballs) in the abomasum. Calves are more often plagued with diarrheal diseases and are only rarely affected with constipation.

Intestinal obstructions such as an intussusception, cecal volvulus, mesenteric volvulus, or an enterolith are rare causes of constipation in adult animals. In each case the predominant clinical sign would be abdominal pain manifested by kicking at the abdomen or getting up and down frequently. On a herd basis, constipation may be an important sign of lead poisoning, fluoride toxicosis, or chronic zinc poisoning.[1] Downer cows with spinal cord injury and musculoskeletal problems may have constipation as a secondary problem.

THERAPY

Simple constipation is best managed by providing adequate water with a mild laxative. Saline cathartics, including epsom salts ($MgSO_4$; 0.5 to 1 kg/500 kg orally) and magnesium oxide (0.5 to 1 kg/500 kg orally), will promote a mild catharsis. Some clinicians advocate 4 liters of mineral oil, or mineral oil with 0.5 liter of raw linseed oil. If the rumen is atonic, the mineral oil tends to float on top of the rumen liquor and may require a longer time to be effective. Cathartics are not to be administered if abdominal distention is present.

Cascara sagrada (10 to 20 ml of a 20 per cent solution for adult cattle, given subcutaneously or intramuscularly) is a safe, mildly irritant cathartic of the emodin group that will assist in treatment, but it should not be used as the only therapy.[2] If given rapidly intravenously it may cause transient collapse but rarely death; it rarely produces a profuse liquid stool. However, danthron (15 gm/500 kg orally), also an irritant cathartic, usually promotes an effective catharsis.

Emollient laxatives, such as dioctyl sodium sulfosuccinate (DSS) and olive oil or linseed oil, are not commonly used because of their expense and lack of clear superiority over traditional cathartics.

Parasympathomimetic cathartics are not indicated in cases of simple constipation but may be of value for paralytic ileus. Neostigmine methylsulfate (2 to 10 mg/500 kg subcutaneously or intramuscularly) may be of value in ileus. Carbachol (0.5 to 1 mg/500 kg subcutaneously) is a more potent parasympathomimetic "gut stimulant" but is more dangerous, occasionally even increasing the pain to the point of rupture of a distended viscus. Dexapanthenol, a precursor of coenzyme A, is a very mild, safe drug that is of questionable efficacy in the treatment of ileus. If used, the recommended dose range would be 2 to 5 mg/kg intramuscularly or intravenously.

Enemas are of questionable value in the treatment of constipation in that it is difficult to have the fluid flow sufficiently orad to be effective. Most cases of simple constipation respond to symptomatic treatment. The underlying cause of the problem must be corrected in complicated cases to bring permanent relief.

References

1. Blood, D. C., Henderson, J. A., and Radostits, O. M.: *In* Veterinary Medicine, 6th ed. Lea & Febiger, Philadelphia, 1983, 101.
2. Phillips, R. W., and Lewis, L. P.: *In* Jones, L. M., Booth, N. H., and McDonald, L. E. (eds.): Veterinary Pharmacology and Therapeutics, 4th ed. The Iowa State University Press, Ames, Ia., 1977, 725.

Lesions of the Oral Cavity and Surrounding Structures

WALLACE M. WASS, D.V.M., Ph.D.,
JAMES R. THOMPSON, D.V.M., M.S.,
EDWIN W. MOSS, D.V.M., M.S.,
JERRY P. KUNESH, D.V.M., Ph.D.,
PAUL G. ENESS, D.V.M.,
and LINDA S. THOMPSON, D.V.M.

Inflammation of the oral mucosa (stomatitis) is a primary characteristic of several diseases and a secondary feature of others. The term usually includes glossitis, palatitis, and gingivitis, but any of these conditions may occur separately.

Neoplastic changes are relatively rare in oral tissues. The resulting signs are similar to those seen with inflammation.

Oral lesions commonly cause signs of excessive salivation, altered chewing behavior, and decreased appetite.

In many cases there is close similarity between the signs of rabies and the highly contagious and destructive vesicular diseases such as foot-and-mouth disease and vesicular exanthema. Because of public health and disease control considerations, the possibility of these diseases must always be considered first whenever signs or characteristic oral lesions are observed.

ETIOLOGY

The most important causes of stomatitis are infectious. Vesicular stomatitis, vesicular exanthema, and foot-and-mouth disease are caused by viruses and are characterized by the formation of vesicles that rupture and become ulcerative lesions. Rinderpest, bovine viral diarrhea, and bovine malignant catarrh have primary erosions and ulcers in the oral mucosa.

Contagious ecthyma and ulcerative dermatosis are viral diseases of sheep and goats with lesions confined mostly to the lips. Viruses may cause proliferative lesions in the mouth. Blue tongue virus causes a catarrhal stomatitis in sheep and, rarely, in cattle.

Common bacteria causing primary lesions in the mouth and associated regions are *Actinomyces bovis*, *Actinobacillus lignieresii*, and *Fusobacterium (Spherophorus) necrophorum*. Secondary bacterial invasion commonly occurs in most other oral lesions.

Acute cellulitis frequently occurs in the intermandibular, sublingual, and retropharyngeal regions of cattle. The lesions spread rapidly and are often fatal. No single etiologic agent is involved, but *Fusobacterium (Spherophorus) necrophorum* organisms are sometimes isolated from the lesions. The usual route of invasion would appear to be extension of bacterial infection from lesions in the oral cavity.

Mycotic stomatitis caused by *Monilia* spp. appears to be a primary disease but probably results when the surface of the oral mucosa is altered owing to other causes or when the normal microflora is seriously disrupted.

Necrotic glossitis, a disease of unknown etiology, causes characteristic signs in feeder cattle. Necrotic lesions are confined to the tongue. The disease is thought to be transmissible and is probably viral in origin. All cases observed locally have been in animals that have had contact with swine.

Stomatitis of chemical origin occurs when irritating substances are accidentally ingested or are administered orally in too concentrated a form.

Physical causes of stomatitis are common and sometimes result in significant primary lesions or secondary complications. Injudicious use of balling guns, dose syringes, or stomach tubes is a common example. Ingestion of roughages containing sharp awns or spines can cause oral lesions. Sharp dental points also cause oral lesions but appear to be much less common in food animals than in equine species.

Ingestion of foods that are too hot can cause serious oral lesions, particularly in swine because of their voracious eating habits.

Foreign bodies lodged in the teeth or otherwise caught in the oral cavity will cause abrasive lesions on adjacent tissues and typical signs of stomatitis.

Developmental defects such as malocclusion of the teeth and cleft palate are occasionally observed in structures surrounding the oral cavity and are thought to be heritable traits in most instances.

CLINICAL SIGNS

Inflammatory lesions in the oral mucosa usually cause local pain in the early stages and have a depressing effect on the animal, resulting in a decrease in appetite. Abnormal chewing movements are seen, usually with some dripping of saliva from the mouth.

Animals with necrotic glossitis extend the head and neck and allow the tongue to protrude from the mouth while appearing to chew.

Depending on the extent of necrosis and the type of bacterial invasion, necrotic lesions impart an abnormal odor to the breath. Regional lymph nodes may be enlarged, and edematous swelling may be noted in soft tissues adjacent to the lesions.

Vesicles in the oral mucosa are usually thin-walled and rupture easily, leaving an ulcerated appearance. Erosions appear first as small, punched-out depressions that gradually become larger and may coalesce. Other clinical signs, such as fever and diarrhea, may be present, depending on the primary disease.

DIAGNOSIS

Any disease with stomatitis must be differentiated from the highly contagious and destructive vesicular diseases, principally foot-and-mouth disease. Laboratory confirmation is desirable, but a field diagnosis can be made with reasonable accuracy based on the number of animals and the species involved and by close examination of the oral and other lesions of the individual animals.

To protect against rabies exposure, proper precautions should be taken before inspecting the oral cavity. Protective rubber gloves should be worn and other salivary exposure avoided. Adequate restraint is necessary so that the animal is well controlled.

TREATMENT

Animals with oral lesions should be treated as infectious cases until that possibility has been ruled out. Isolation from unexposed animals should be maintained, and great care should be taken to disinfect contaminated gloves, boots, and instruments.

Specific treatment depends upon the findings in each examination. In most cases, nursing, elimination of stress, and provision of easily digestible and nutritious rations are indicated. Most lesions in the oral mucosa heal rapidly once the primary disease subsides or the inciting cause is removed.

Supplemental Reading

Blood, D. C., and Henderson, J. A.: Veterinary Medicine. Williams & Wilkins, Baltimore, 1974, 49–51.

Dorn, C. R., and Priester, W. A.: Epidemiologic analysis of oral and pharyngeal cancer in dogs, cats, horses and cattle. J. Am. Vet. Med. Assoc. *169*:11, 1976.

Examination of the Teeth and Diagnosis and Treatment of Dental Diseases

WALLACE M. WASS, D.V.M., Ph.D.,
JAMES R. THOMPSON, D.V.M., M.S.,
EDWIN W. MOSS, D.V.M., M.S.,
JERRY P. KUNESH, D.V.M., Ph.D.,
PAUL G. ENESS, D.V.M.,
and LINDA S. THOMPSON, D.V.M.

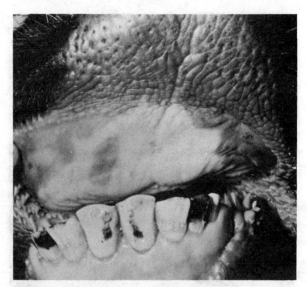

Figure 1. Extreme pitting and mottling of dental enamel in an adult Holstein-Friesian cow due to chronic fluorosis.

Treatment of individual dental problems in food animals is largely surgical and is not widely practiced at present. Exceptions are simple procedures such as removal of foreign bodies, clipping of needle teeth in newborn pigs, detusking of mature boars, and removal of benign growths. Fracture repair can be accomplished if the economic justification exists and if adequate facilities for after-care are available.

Inspection of the teeth should be done as part of any general physical examination since it often yields useful diagnostic information.

Extreme caution should be employed in examining the mouth of any animal of unknown history to protect against rabies exposure.

Protective rubber gloves should be worn, and other salivary exposure should be avoided. Restraint adequate to control the animal is necessary, and a mouth gag, dental wedge, or other speculum should be used to prevent damage to the examiner's hands and fingers or to instruments placed inside the mouth.

Evaluation of dental development is commonly employed to estimate the age of individual animals. This should be used only as an estimate of maximum stage of development. Dental development is likely to be delayed by inadequate or improper nutrition, disease, or adverse environmental conditions such as weather.

Deciduous teeth have little use in age determination. Calves are frequently born with fully erupted deciduous incisors, and most will have all of the deciduous incisors in place by two months of age.

Because of their ease of observation for emergence and development, the permanent incisors receive the most attention in cattle. However, information can be obtained from the molar and premolar teeth as well (Table 1).

Andrews[1] has shown the standard deviation to be approximately 10 per cent of the average age. Thus, for a given stage of development, such as 30 months (2.5 years), 67 per cent of the individuals examined will be 2.5 years ± 0.25 years and 95 per cent will be 2.5 years ± 0.5 years (between 2 and 3 years of age).

The eruption times of the incisor teeth of sheep and goats offer a more precise indicator of age than in the bovine. The central pair, or first permanent incisors, appear at 12 to 14 months of age; each succeeding year an additional pair of permanent incisors appears, replacing the smaller, shorter deciduous teeth. At four years of age the animal is said to have a full mouth. With advancing age the incisors spread apart and wear down. The degree to which this happens gives further indication of the age of the animal.

In all animals, mineral deficiency, particularly that of calcium, will cause delayed eruption and early, uneven wear. Excessive pitting and mottling of the enamel suggests prolonged intake of high levels of fluoride (Fig. 1).

A uniform reddish-brown discoloration of the deciduous teeth is observed with erythropoietic porphyria (Fig. 2), a hereditary disease of cattle and swine. It is characterized by photosensitization and anemia, and the teeth fluoresce red under ultraviolet light such as a Wood's lamp.

Table 1. *Estimating Age Using Dentition*

Tooth	Age at Eruption (mo)	Age at Maturity (mo)
1st molar	8	—
2nd molar	12	18
3rd molar	24	30
1st incisor	18	24–25
2nd incisor	24–25	30–32
3rd incisor	36	—
4th incisor	36–48	—

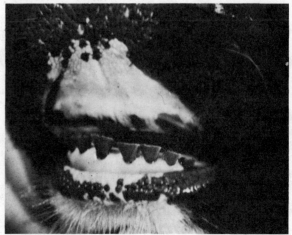

Figure 2. Reddish-brown discoloration of deciduous incisors in erythropoietic porphyria.

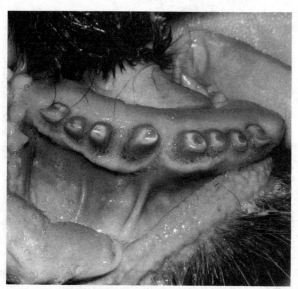

Figure 3. Extremely worn incisors in an aged Hereford cow.

Diseases of the Pharynx and Esophagus

WALLACE M. WASS, D.V.M., Ph.D.,
JAMES R. THOMPSON, D.V.M., M.S.,
EDWIN W. MOSS, D.V.M., M.S.,
JERRY P. KUNESH, D.V.M., Ph.D.,
PAUL G. ENESS, D.V.M.,
and LINDA S. THOMPSON, D.V.M.

Lesions in the pharynx and esophagus are important features of a number of systemic diseases and contribute significantly to the clinical signs. Primary lesions in the pharynx and esophagus are less common but present serious problems when they occur.

Infectious agents are the principal causes of lesions in the pharynx and esophagus, but physical trauma is also important. Chemical irritants, mycotoxins, and parasitic larvae also cause well-defined lesions. Neoplastic diseases and developmental defects are occasionally reported.

PATHOGENESIS

Since pharyngeal paralysis occurs with rabies, *primary consideration must be given to the possibility of rabies whenever signs of pharyngeal and/or esophageal paralysis or obstruction are observed.* Botulism may also cause pharyngeal paralysis.

The pharynx is frequently involved in acute and chronic bacterial infections and is a possible portal of entry for organisms that cause acute and often fatal cellulitis in the intermandibular and anterior cervical regions in cattle. Abscesses in the pharyngeal region sometimes interfere with the swallowing reflex. The pharynx shows signs of inflammation in upper respiratory infections.

Esophageal erosions are classic lesions observed in rinderpest, bovine viral diarrhea, and bovine malignant catarrh.

Careless use of balling guns, dose syringes, or stomach tubes commonly causes traumatic lesions in the pharynx and esophagus, often with serious consequences. Traumatic lesions also occur in the pharynx and esophagus owing to ingestion of large or sharp foreign bodies and some plants, particularly those with sharp awns or barbs.

If the larvae of *Hypoderma lineata* are killed while in the esophageal submucosa, severe tissue necrosis and serious illness may result. Some mycotoxins of the trichothecene group, including T-2 toxin produced by *Fusarium tricinctum* and stachybotryo toxin produced by *Stachybotrys atra*, are epithelionecrotic and can produce erosions and ulcers in the mouth, pharynx, and esophagus when ingested.

Attempted ingestion of certain foreign objects may cause obstruction in the pharynx, but such objects more commonly lodge in the esophagus. The most frequent sites are high in the cervical esophagus, at the thoracic inlet, over the base of the heart, and just anterior to the cardia of the stomach. Obstructions that are not promptly

Excessive wear or loss of the incisor teeth is a sign of advancing age in cattle and sheep (Fig. 3) and occurs more rapidly in animals that spend all or most of their life under range conditions. Sandy or semi-arid ranges are particularly likely to cause early dental wear. Periodontal disease causes premature loss of teeth in sheep in some regions.

Examination of the incisor teeth for loss and excessive wear is a common management practice in culling herds and flocks of cattle and sheep. However, valuable animals need not be eliminated from breeding programs because of advanced dental wear. If adequate nutrition can be supplied as dry concentrate or succulent forage, such animals can be successfully maintained as breeders for several years after the incisor teeth are worn down.

Capping of the incisor teeth with stainless steel prostheses has been used to prolong the useful life of range cattle but is not widely practiced at present.

In swine it is good practice to clip the needle teeth (canines) of baby pigs shortly after birth to avoid facial injuries caused by fighting between littermates during nursing and to protect the sow's teats from injury.

Mature boars should have their tusks clipped to prevent bite wounds. For best results, this is first done at one year of age and is then repeated every six months.

Reference

1. Andrews, A. H.: The use of dentition to determine age in British cattle. Bovine Pract. *10*:39, 1975.

Supplemental Reading

Cropsey, L. M.: Technical aspects of determining over-age in beef cattle. Bovine Pract. *9*:67, 1974.
Hartsock, T. G.: Effect of needle teeth on fighting behavior of newborn pigs. Can. J. Anim. Sci. *56*:4, 1976.
Suckling, G. W.: Periodontal disease in sheep. N. Z. V. J. *21*:1, 1973.
Turner, J. C.: Cemental annulations as an age criterion in North American sheep. J. Wildlife Man. *41*:2, 1977.

relieved cause necrosis or the later development of esophageal stricture.

Sheep and lambs may experience choke immediately following feeding on concentrate rations containing whole or coarsely ground cereal grains. These may appear dramatic but are usually self-correcting.

Lesions of lymphomatosis and peripharyngeal abscesses may cause dysphagia or obstruction in the pharyngeal or esophageal regions. Primary neoplasms in the pharynx and esophagus are rare.

CLINICAL SIGNS

Acute inflammation of the pharynx causes local pain, dysphagia, depression, and loss of appetite.

Obstruction or paralysis of either the pharynx or esophagus causes inability to swallow, regurgitation of ingested food and water through the nostrils, and ruminal tympany. Animals with acute cases of esophageal obstruction have signs of severe distress, anxiety, and obvious violent attempts at swallowing. Later they will be depressed and dehydrated and will drool saliva from the mouth. Signs of local pain subside and the animal makes repeated attempts to drink water and eat. Clinical signs will be modified if pharyngeal or esophageal obstructions are incomplete or temporary.

DIAGNOSIS

Diagnosis can be very difficult, particularly the differentiation of primary obstructive lesions from systemic diseases. Uncomplicated foreign body obstruction may be diagnosed from the clinical history alone or by inspection of the mouth and pharynx and exploration of the esophagus with a stomach tube.

Chronic lesions, such as enlarged lymph nodes, esophageal stricture, or developmental defects, are defined with greater difficulty. Radiographic examination or esophagoscopy may be useful, but accurate diagnosis may depend on necropsy.

TREATMENT

Lesions in the pharynx or esophagus associated with systemic diseases will resolve upon treatment of the primary condition.

Depending on location and type, foreign body obstructions can be relieved by various means including esophagotomy and esophagoscopy. Secondary complications, including necrosis, perforation, and stricture, develop if the lesions persist and the prognosis becomes more unfavorable.

Supplemental Reading

Blood, D. C., and Henderson, J. A.: Veterinary Medicine, Williams & Wilkins, Baltimore, 1974, 51–56.
Meagher, D. M., and Mayhew, I. G.: The surgical treatment of upper esophageal obstruction in the bovine. Can. Vet. J. 19:128, 1978.

Diseases of the Ruminant Forestomach

WALLACE M. WASS, D.V.M. Ph.D.,
JAMES R. THOMPSON, D.V.M., M.S.,
EDWIN W. MOSS, D.V.M., M.S.,
JERRY P. KUNESH, D.V.M., Ph.D.,
PAUL G. ENESS, D.V.M.,
and LINDA S. THOMPSON, D.V.M.

Simple indigestion is characterized by anorexia and atony of the forestomach. It is commonly seen in dairy animals and cattle in feedlots. Consumption of frosted feeds, too coarsely or too finely ground feeds, or too much concentrate contribute to this disorder. Other events might be sudden changes in feed such as switching from dry concentrate to lush pasture or from dry pasture to rich concentrate.

Simple indigestion is frequently seen in dairy cattle that have unlimited access to good quality silage. It may also occur in cattle that consume feed that has been permitted to spoil or sour in bunks or feeders. Prolonged or heavy oral dosing with sulfonamides or antibiotics inhibits the activity of rumen microflora, leading to indigestion in some cases. The abrupt withdrawal of these drugs may also cause indigestion.

The inappetence commonly observed in feedlot cattle when they are first introduced to rations containing ionophore antibiotics, such as monensin sodium, is appropriately described as simple indigestion. A similar syndrome of varying severity is observed when management errors lead to abrupt increases in ration levels of the additive or when it is unintentionally introduced suddenly, although at low levels, into cattle rations.

Pathogenesis

Relatively minor increases or decreases in rumen pH are likely to cause atony. Large intake of indigestible materials or the consumption of feeds containing large quantities of stale, sour, or putrefied materials will have a similar effect. Histamine, whether from intrinsic or extrinsic sources, will cause atony of the rumen. Often the exact sequence of events leading to rumen atony and inappetence is difficult to ascertain or explain. It does appear, though, that nearly any process that causes an abrupt alteration in rumen fermentation is likely to lead to the syndrome described as simple indigestion.

Clinical Signs

The first clinical sign will be diminished appetite. Reduction in feed intake may be as much as 50 per cent or more, with few other outward signs. In lactating dairy animals, milk production will decrease, closely paralleling the change in feed intake.

Some depression or dullness may also be observed. Decreased physical activity or alertness may appear if an entire herd or flock is involved but may be difficult to detect unless one is closely familiar with the behavior of that group.

Changes in body temperature are unlikely. Rumen

stasis or a reduction in the strength and frequency of contractions may be palpated or auscultated. Intestinal motility is likely to be decreased, but gaseous intestinal sounds may be increased, and diarrhea may be observed. Mild tympany will be seen in some cases.

Clinical Pathology

Changes in rumen pH suggest a diagnosis of simple indigestion in the absence of clinical evidence of other diseases. However, the absence of detectable pH changes does not necessarily rule out simple indigestion as a diagnosis. Other commonly employed laboratory tests are not likely to be helpful.

Diagnosis

Diagnosis of simple indigestion will usually be based on clinical examination and on ruling out other, more serious, diseases. Careful evaluation of the history is important, but the information necessary for diagnosis may not always be available. It is natural and logical to suspect a "feed problem" or feeding error when an entire herd or flock on a single ration is suddenly "off feed." In some instances, the error might be grossly apparent in the feed, but exact determination or confirmation is likely to depend on chemical analysis. The accidental introduction of ionophore antibiotics, such as monensin sodium, has been an occasional cause of herd inappetence in recent years in the United States.

When an individual animal is off feed, the cause may be more difficult to establish. In the lactating dairy cow the condition must be differentiated from the early stages of lactation ketosis. The simple laboratory or field test for urinary ketones will be very helpful.

Other diseases to consider are early hypocalcemia (milk fever), traumatic reticuloperitonitis, and displaced abomasum. Complete clinical examination and evaluation of the response to treatment will be necessary to eliminate each as diagnostic possibilities.

Treatment

A wide variety of treatments have been employed for simple indigestion. Rumenatoric drugs, widely used in the past, have fallen into some disfavor because of the lack of any rational scientific basis for their use.

Most animals will recover spontaneously from simple indigestion in three to four days. If the exact nature of the disturbance is known, symptomatic treatment can speed recovery. If the rumen is acidic, for example, oral doses of antacids such as magnesium hydroxide or magnesium carbonate, 0.5 to 1 lb (225 to 450 gm) per adult animal, would be indicated. If the rumen is alkaline, oral doses of acetic acid or vinegar (up to 1 quart/1000 lb, or 2 ml/kg) could be given. Mineral oil given orally in doses of one gallon (4 liters) or more will not directly affect the pH but might help passage of indigestible material and slow absorption of toxic materials.

If the rumen remains atonic for more than a day or so, rumen inoculum obtained from an abattoir or from a healthy animal can be administered orally. This would seem the most rational therapeutic approach for simple indigestion. It cannot be expected to succeed, however, if the agent or chemical responsible for inactivating the rumen initially is still active and present in effective quantities. Repeated administration is advisable, and results are not likely to be apparent in less than 36 to 48 hours.

Prevention

Prevention of simple indigestion is difficult because it depends on the vagaries of the entire management system as well as the special idiosyncrasies of the ruminant. Avoiding sudden changes in the ration and providing a balanced diet containing adequate coarse digestible roughage as well as other essential nutrients are vital. Regular consumption of approximately equal quantities of feed each day is desired.

Additives, particularly antibiotics, must be carefully metered so that approved doses are not exceeded and sudden changes in levels are avoided.

ACUTE RUMEN ENGORGEMENT (RUMEN IMPACTION, RUMEN OVERLOAD, RUMEN ACIDOSIS, GRAIN OVERLOAD, ENGORGEMENT TOXEMIA)

Definition

At least two distinct syndromes are recognized. Ingestion of excessive quantities of highly fermentable carbohydrate feed leads to lactic acidosis with acute dehydration and depression. It is by far the more common syndrome.

Ingestion of large quantities of highly fermentable proteinaceous material causes excess ammonium ion production, leading to alkalosis with excitement and hyperesthesia. (Consumption of soybeans and soybean derivatives is the most common cause in the midwestern region of the United States.) Either or both syndromes are commonly observed wherever intensive livestock management is practiced.

Mild lactic acidosis is extremely common in grain-fed cattle, and affected animals will frequently have other associated diseases as well, including liver abscesses, rumenitis or rumen parakeratosis, mycotic rumenitis, feedlot bloat, and laminitis.

Feeds or feed ingredients characteristically involved are brewers' grains, green corn, sweet corn, bakery bread, apples, sugar beets, and larger quantities than the animal is accustomed to of any of the feed grains. Finely ground grains are more likely to cause severe problems, although grinding is by no means a prerequisite.

Pathogenesis

The normal ruminant forestomach can be correctly visualized as a continuous culture fermentation receptacle. The normal microflora constitutes the culture: the ration being fed constitutes the medium or substrate on which the culture grows. The fermentation end-products are normally acetic, propionic, and butyric acid, short-chain volatile fatty acids that are absorbed from the rumen as the animal's primary energy source. Bacterial cell protein is also produced and is digested further down the tract as an amino acid source. Water-soluble vitamins are additional by-products.

When the ration is abruptly changed to larger than normal quantities of highly fermentable carbohydrate, normal fermentation patterns change. Gram-positive streptococcus and lactobacillus organisms become predominant and lactic acid (both D- and L-) becomes a principal fermentation end-product. Lactic acid production increases osmotic pressure within the rumen so that fluid is drawn into the rumen from the circulatory system and thus from other tissues as well (Fig. 1). The rumen

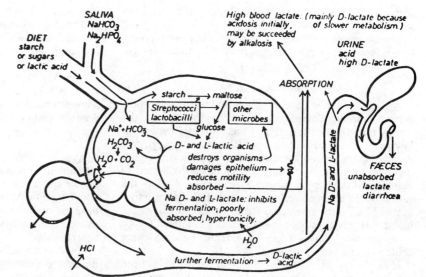

Figure 1. Schematic depiction of rumen lactic acidosis.

pH drops, resulting in rumen stasis, and a large percentage of the normal rumen microflora is destroyed. Most of the gram-negative microorganisms and protozoa disappear. Symptoms become severe when the pH reaches 4 to 5.

The D- and L-lactic acids are converted to sodium lactate. In the rumen they contribute to hypertonicity. Some becomes absorbed into the circulation (mainly D-lactate because of its slower metabolism) and contributes to a depression of the blood pH. There is some absorption of lactate from the omasum and abomasum and some as a result of continuing fermentation in the intestinal tract. An osmotic gradient is also established within the intestine, drawing fluid into the rumen and contributing to the profuse diarrhea.

Chemical damage to the surface epithelium of the rumen mucosa occurs and later results in adherence of debris and penetration by particulate matter from the rumen ingesta, such as hair and sharp pieces of plant material. Bacterial and mycotic organisms begin to invade the rumen wall, and absorption patterns are changed.

The urine volume will usually be greatly decreased owing to the dehydration, and secreted urine will be high in D-lactate and will be acidic.

The initial syndrome of acidosis is often followed by bacterial or mycotic rumenitis. Other possible sequelae are liver abscesses and peritonitis. Bloat may result from the decreased rumen motility and altered fermentation patterns. The development of acute, and later chronic, laminitis observed in some animals is thought to relate to the relative levels of histamine produced during the acute phases of the process.

Pregnant animals frequently abort some days or weeks after the acute phases of illness. Secondary rumenitis may cause an increased incidence of bloat, and this is thought to be a major cause of unexplained deaths in feedlots, commonly diagnosed as "sudden death syndrome."

The entire disease process is complex and variable, and a suggested additional component might be endotoxic shock from toxins released from the destruction of large numbers of gram-negative microorganisms from the rumen ingesta.[1, 2]

Clinical Signs

The rapidity of onset of clinical signs varies and depends on the nature and quantity of the feed consumed and the adaptation of the animal to that feed. Unadapted animals may die from quantities of feed that are readily consumed by animals conditioned to the feed. On the other hand, even animals on "full feed" will overeat and develop acute lactic acidosis under some circumstances.

Usually, clinical signs will become apparent in 12 to 36 hours following engorgement on grain or similar material. Incoordination and ataxia are first noticed, followed by profound weakness and depression. Anorexia will be apparent, and affected animals appear blind. Rumen stasis is complete, with abdominal pain evidenced by occasional grunting and grinding of the teeth. Abdominal fullness and fluid distention of the rumen are observed.

Significant dehydration will become apparent within 24 to 48 hours. Fetid diarrhea develops but may not be observed in animals that die early. Profuse diarrhea may be considered a sign of improvement if the animals are not seriously depressed.

In severe cases the animals may become recumbent in 24 to 48 hours owing to weakness and toxemia. The respiratory rate will most likely be increased because of acidosis. Body temperature may be subnormal by the time other signs are observed. The pulse is usually weak and thready in character.

Recumbent animals will lie quietly, often with the head tucked to the side, as in parturient paresis. Crusty mucus will be present on the muzzle because the animal fails to clean its nostrils.

When a herd problem is observed it is common to see several animals with profound depression and acute lactic acidosis. Animals with less severe cases will also be present and are likely to show only mild depression and diarrhea. Some animals may have acute laminitis with a characteristic lameness.

Acute deaths usually occur in 24 to 48 hours, but many animals have apparent recovery with later deterioration and death due to secondary complications. It is not unusual for losses to continue for three to four weeks in severely affected herds.

Some animals will partially recover but perform poorly in the feedlot owing to chronic rumenitis, liver damage, or laminitis.

Clinical Pathology and Necropsy

Affected animals have hemoconcentration and acidic rumen content. The pH of ingesta aspirated from the rumen may be 4 or lower, and the urine pH may be as low as 5. Blood pH changes within a narrow range and requires more precise conditions and sophisticated equipment for measurement. Samples should be collected in heparinized tubes containing a layer of mineral oil, or the tubes should be completely filled, sealed, and then refrigerated (4°C) until measured. Accurate assessment of the blood pH requires that bicarbonate or total CO_2 be measured also. Values below 7.2 generally indicate severe acidosis and a poor prognosis.

If soybeans or other high-protein feeds have been consumed, rumen pH may be alkaline owing to ammonia production. This will be reflected in the blood and urine pH as well.

Necropsy of acute cases demonstrates that the rumen is distended and filled with fluid content. The offending material is likely to be evident, but post-mortem measurements of pH levels are not likely to be valid owing to rapid changes in the dead animal.

Rumen engorgement of slightly longer duration will be characterized by rumenitis. However, post-mortem autolysis occurs rapidly in the rumen, so observations on the rumen mucosa must be interpreted carefully.

Diagnosis

Diagnosis will usually be based on history and clinical examination. The history alone is often sufficient, but often it may be misleading if the pattern of feed consumption is not known or not suspected. Laboratory evaluations, especially of the rumen ingesta, plasma, and urine pH, are particularly helpful.

The condition must be differentiated from polioencephalomalacia, urolithiasis, fulminating peritonitis, parturient hypocalcemia, and other diseases that cause profound depression.

Treatment

Animals with mild cases may recover without treatment, but in more severe forms the damage to the animal may be so extensive that even with intensive therapy only limited success will be achieved.

Emptying of the rumen by oral lavage or rumenotomy is indicated if circumstances permit.

The oral administration of antacids such as magnesium carbonate or magnesium hydroxide is indicated, but they should be mixed in 2 to 3 gallons (8 to 12 liters) of warm water and given by stomach tube to ensure dispersion throughout the rumen. Initial doses of up to 1 gm/kg body weight (454 gm for an adult bovine) should be followed by smaller doses repeated at 6- to 12-hour intervals. If the rumen has been evacuated, the initial dose should not exceed 0.5 lb (225 gm).

It is important that dehydration and acidosis be corrected as well. Balanced electrolyte and 5 per cent sodium bicarbonate solutions should be given intravenously. A 450-kg animal with 10 per cent dehydration may require as much as 50 liters of fluid over a 24-hour period. Sodium bicarbonate should be given at the rate of 0.5 mEq/kg body weight initially and repeated in 24 hours if necessary. Correction of blood pH to within the normal range is vital for survival even if the offending rumen ingesta is removed.

Administration of antihistamines is considered to be of value by some. Recent field experience indicates that oral administration of thiabendazole in normal anthelmintic doses helps in controlling secondary mycotic rumenitis.

Prevention

Avoiding sudden and drastic changes in the ration is paramount in preventing rumen acidosis. Bunk-fed cattle need regular quantities of ration at regular intervals, and adequate bunk space must be available so that all animals have an opportunity to feed normally. The ration must include adequate roughage (generally not less than 10 per cent) regularly.

Animals on self-feeder programs are particularly vulnerable to excessive consumption, especially early in the feeding program. Every precaution must be taken to ensure that roughage is available (mixed in the feed if possible) and that animals are brought onto full feed slowly. Feeders must be checked regularly and not permitted to run low or stand empty to avoid excessive intake by hungry animals after the feeders have been refilled.

RUMENITIS (RUMINAL PARAKERATOSIS)

Definition

The term *rumenitis* refers to a series of inflammatory changes that develop in the rumen mucosa and underlying tissues in cattle fed high-energy rations with inadequate roughage. Clinically, the syndrome includes the associated lesions of liver abscess and laminitis. The incidence may be as high as 100 per cent in cattle fed all-concentrate rations for prolonged periods or those that have not been carefully adapted to such rations. Rumenitis also occurs as a secondary stage of acute rumen engorgement with acidosis.

Pathogenesis

The association between liver abscess formation and ruminal lesions was first reported by Smith[3] and later by Jensen and colleagues.[4] A definite relationship between rumen adaptation to high-energy rations and the development of rumen lesions is now generally understood.

The exact pathogenesis of the rumen lesions has not been elucidated but it is commonly accepted that the end-products of rumen fermentation accumulate and change in relative quantity, causing an increase in hydrogen ion concentration and leading to inflammation of the rumen mucosa.

The sequence of events would appear to be (1) inflammation of the rumen mucosa, (2) adherence of debris to the mucosa, (3) ulceration and infection of deeper layers in the rumen wall, and (4) focal abscess formation in the rumen wall.

The appearance of abscesses in the liver follows sequentially. Chronic laminitis is a later sequela, but its relationship is uncertain and appears less well correlated with the preceding events. Other independent factors may be involved in the development of chronic laminitis. It is frequently observed in cattle fed high-energy rations for 60 to 90 days, but the incidence appears to be higher among females, and laminitis sometimes occurs in the absence of rumen and liver lesions. Likewise, there is nothing specific about the lesions in the rumen or the liver: either could arise from other causes.

Clinical Signs

Cattle do not necessarily become clinically ill during the early stages of rumenitis and liver abscess formation. Feed consumption is usually good and weight gains on all-concentrate rations for periods over 100 days are very acceptable. However, the addition of good-quality hay or silage for at least 10 to 20 per cent of the ration will often result in increased feed consumption and average daily gain.

Animals with advanced rumen and liver lesions may show reduced appetite and weight gains, usually late in the feeding period. Affected individuals show an apparent lack of fill, as evidenced by gauntness of the abdomen. Other clinical signs, possibly from developing peritonitis or septicemia, may be seen. There will be elongation and flatness of the hooves with a very apparent alteration in gait if there is a chronic laminitis.

An increase in the incidence of unrelated problems such as respiratory disease is likely in severely affected groups of cattle.

Necropsy

Lesions are usually observed only at slaughter and result in the condemnations of livers and rumens. The rumen mucosa will have edema and clumping of papillae in mild cases. More advanced cases demonstrate matting and necrosis of papillae with diffuse ulcerations. Hair and debris will adhere to the mucosa. Extensive thickening of the rumen wall with abscessation is also observed.

There is increased thickness of the cornified portion of the rumen epithelium and increased numbers of vacuoles on histologic examination. The lesion is characteristic of an acid burn.

Abscesses will be observed on cut sections of the liver and are apparent as light-colored spots on the uncut surface in severe cases.

Diagnosis

Chronic laminitis may be the first visible sign, but in many instances its appearance accompanies or precedes a noticeable reduction in feed consumption and rate of gain.

The condition can be suspected in any group of cattle being fed for maximal gains on high-energy or all-concentrate rations, but confirmation often depends on examination of rumens and livers at slaughter.

Treatment

Treatment and prevention depend upon the inclusion of adequate good-quality roughage in the ration. Stemmy hay is preferred as a roughage source and should equal at least 10 per cent of the dry matter in the ration. Chopped or finely ground hay is less effective in preventing rumenitis. Ensilage can be used, but greater quantities are necessary. Ground corn cobs are commonly used as roughage but should be supplemented with some hay.

Antibiotics fed at disease prevention levels reduce the incidence of liver abscesses but have no effect on the development of rumen lesions.

Individual animals that survive acute rumen engorgement develop secondary rumenitis, often with severe

mycotic involvement. Thiabendazole given daily (25 mg/kg B.W.) is helpful in reducing the severity.

TRAUMATIC RETICULOPERITONITIS

Definition

Small, sharp foreign objects are frequently swallowed by ruminants. These commonly lodge in the area of the reticulum, where they may penetrate the wall and cause an inflammatory reaction. The animal shows clinical signs when significant reticulitis develops or when penetration of the wall occurs with subsequent acute local peritonitis.

Swallowing of foreign objects is common in adult cattle, but its incidence has diminished with improved methods for handling feed, including the use of magnets on mechanical equipment and twine instead of wire for baling hay and straw. The condition occurs less commonly in sheep and goats because of their more discriminating eating habits.

Pathogenesis

Sharp objects lodge in the reticulum partly because of the honeycomb-like structure of the mucosal surface and partly because of its active contractions. Penetration by a foreign object exposes the tissues to infection and causes local peritonitis. The animal becomes clinically ill and develops anorexia and signs of acute abdominal pain. Lactating dairy cattle will have a sharp drop in milk production.

Sequelae to acute traumatic reticulitis include traumatic pericarditis, acute diffuse peritonitis, chronic localized peritonitis, chronic diffuse peritonitis, hepatitis, splenitis, pneumonia and pleuritis, and the vagus indigestion syndrome. In rare cases acute hemorrhage will cause sudden death.

Recurrences may be observed at any time but are more common during estrus, periods of increased physical activity, and late gestation.

Clinical Signs

The disease occurs in acute, subacute, and chronic forms, all with variations. The onset is sudden in the acute disease with complete anorexia and a precipitous drop in milk production. There will usually be a low grade fever (102.5° to 104°F [39.1° to 40°C]) and decreased rumen motility. Local pain in the region of the xiphoid cartilage is manifested by a characteristic grunt following reflex movements. The animal is reluctant to lie down or move. The thoracic spine is commonly elevated and the abdomen may appear to be "tucked up." Respiratory movements are mostly thoracic and characteristically shallow.

Affected animals will be constipated from reduced feed intake and dehydration, but animals that develop diffuse peritonitis may have diarrhea.

In subacute or chronic cases all of the typical signs will be less dramatic. Anorexia will be incomplete and the condition will resemble simple indigestion. Most animals have at least a short-term mild temperature elevation.

Clinical Pathology and Necropsy

During the acute phase and recurrences there is usually a measurable increase in circulating neutrophils with a shift toward immature types. Fibrinogen levels are also increased in some cases. Other changes, such as mild ketonuria, will be secondary to anorexia. Laboratory findings may be normal in cases of three to four days duration.

In acute diffuse peritonitis, the total circulating white blood cell count may be very low.

At necropsy the lesions will be characteristic of acute local peritonitis. However, most animals that die have developed diffuse peritonitis or involvement of the heart or lungs. An occasional animal will die from acute hemorrhage if the heart or a major blood vessel is punctured.

Diagnosis

Diagnosis is usually based on inappetence, temperature elevation, evidence of abdominal pain, and the absence of other diseases. Neutrophilia with a shift toward immaturity is helpful in diagnosis but is by no means pathognomonic.

Metal-detecting instruments have been used to detect metal in the reticulum. The procedure is useful but has serious limitations. The effective distance is limited, being approximately 10 cm (4 inches). Nonferrous materials are not detected, and the mere presence of metal is not diagnostic of the disease. The state of penetration is not indicated, and even iron filings will give a positive reading. A rumen magnet in the reticulum will also cause a positive reading on the metal detector.

Other conditions to consider in the differential diagnosis are lactation ketosis, abomasal displacement, rumen acidosis, and other acute inflammatory conditions, such as metritis, nephritis, and endocarditis.

Treatment

Treatment varies depending on the severity of the condition, the existing complications, economic considerations, and the available facilities.

Surgical removal of the offending foreign body by rumenotomy was very popular in the past. This is effective in cases in which the foreign body remains embedded in the wall of the reticulum or the problem is caused by nonferrous foreign material. Its disadvantage is the surgical stress imposed when the foreign object is no longer a problem but local peritonitis is the cause of the illness.

Most cases are now handled by more conservative methods. These include the administration of a rumen magnet to immobilize the foreign object and the use of antibacterial drugs to control infection. Restricting the physical activity of the animal and elevating the front quarters with a platform or other device are helpful in some cases.

Prevention

Installation of magnets at critical points in feed-handling equipment is helping to reduce the incidence of this disease. Oral administration of rumen magnets helps reduce the incidence of traumatic reticuloperitonitis. The magnets, administered with a balling gun, usually remain in the reticulum for prolonged periods, immobilizing ferrous foreign objects. An occasional animal will vomit a magnet, and magnets are sometimes expelled in the feces. The presence of a magnet in the reticulum can be determined with a compass. Magnets should not be administered to small calves, as they are not likely to be retained in the reticulum until the forestomach is well developed.

Cattle should not be exposed to areas of construction where nails and similar objects have been scattered.

PERITONITIS

Definition

Peritonitis in ruminants is a secondary complication of other diseases such as traumatic reticulitis, abomasal ulcers, liver abscesses, and rumenitis. It may also occur as an extension of metritis, rupture of the uterus or vagina during obstetric manipulations or delivery, or any perforating abdominal wound. It may be a secondary complication of acute bowel obstruction and abdominal surgery. Intraperitoneal injections of any kind commonly cause peritonitis. Fibrinous peritonitis is characteristic of sporadic bovine encephalomyelitis (transmissible serositis) and septicemia caused by *Haemophilus* spp. microorganisms.

Clinical Signs

The clinical signs in peritonitis will be modified or masked by those of the primary disease in many instances. Most types, however, will be characterized by abdominal pain and a slight to moderate temperature elevation in the early stages. In the later stages of diffuse peritonitis the temperature may be subnormal.

The abdominal musculature will be tense in early cases, and the animal will be reluctant to move. Intestinal sounds may be increased at first, but in diffuse peritonitis the abdomen becomes silent. Progressive weakness is apparent, with the animal becoming recumbent and possibly comatose. The pulse will be rapid and weak. Acute diffuse peritonitis is often a fulminating disease, with death occurring in 24 to 48 hours in the most severe cases. If the infection is mild or if effective treatment is instituted early, the course may be more prolonged or recovery may occur.

Clinical Pathology

Circulating neutrophils may increase with a shift toward immaturity early in the disease. If the condition advances rapidly the leukocyte count may decrease, possibly becoming subnormal.

Paracentesis of the abdominal cavity is useful in diagnosis but should be done with great care. Aseptic technique should be used and the site should be clipped and scrubbed as for surgery. A localized area should be anesthetized and the skin incised. Penetration of the abdominal wall should be made with a blunt needle or teat cannula to avoid puncture of internal organs. The rumen, reticulum, omasum, and abomasum are easily penetrated.

A properly performed paracentesis will yield only 1 to 2 ml of straw-colored fluid or possibly nothing at all in the normal animal. If peritonitis exists, a serosanguinous or purulent fluid will be withdrawn. Gastric or intestinal contents may be present, depending on the primary disease. The peritoneal fluid will contain urine if the bladder ruptures because of urolithiasis.

Necropsy

If peritonitis is localized or chronic the animal is not likely to be presented for necropsy unless it dies from the primary or other intercurrent disease. Multiple adhesions would be the characteristic lesions.

If the condition is acute and widespread, the serosal surfaces of the abdominal viscera will have hemorrhagic lesions. Fibrin and foul-smelling exudate will be present. Early adhesions will be easily broken down. Other lesions will vary with the primary disease.

Diagnosis

Diagnosis may be difficult. Advanced cases of diffuse peritonitis resemble other diseases characterized by extreme depression and weakness such as parturient hypocalcemia, toxic metritis, gangrenous mastitis, severe vagus indigestion, and advanced rumen acidosis. The history and clinical signs of temperature elevation and abdominal pain will be helpful, but abdominal paracentesis may be necessary to establish the diagnosis.

Peritonitis from perforations or lesions in the gastrointestinal or reproductive tract is usually characterized by the presence of a mixed bacterial flora. *Corynebacterium pyogenes* and *Fusobacterium (Spherophorus) necrophorum* are commonly isolated from such cases in cattle.

Treatment

In most instances treatment depends on the nature of the primary disease. Acute diffuse peritonitis will have a poor prognosis, and treatment is usually unrewarding.

Some success has been reported with intraperitoneal administration of antibacterial drugs. Solutions of antibiotics, sulfonamides, or nitrofurans can be mixed with saline or balanced electrolyte solution and administered into the peritoneal cavity by injection, using 2 to 3 liters of fluid to ensure good dispersion. Similar effects should be expected from intravenous administration, however, and antibacterial therapy will not be effective unless the primary lesion is walled off or otherwise closed.

RUMEN ATONY

Definition

Rumen atony refers to the state of reduced activity of rumen musculature that occurs as a characteristic feature of several disease syndromes. It does not occur as a primary disease and should be considered a clinical sign, not a diagnosis. Among the disorders commonly causing atony are acute feed engorgement, simple indigestion, parturient hypocalcemia, ketosis, vagus indigestion, hypomagnesemia, lymphosarcoma, abomasal ulcers, abomasal impaction, abomasal torsion (volvulus), traumatic reticuloperitonitis, and septicemic diseases. The rumen also becomes atonic in obstructions of the anterior intestinal tract or when the rumen itself becomes impacted with indigestible material.

RUMINAL TYMPANY (BLOAT)

Definition

Ruminal tympany, or bloat, refers to excessive accumulation of gas in the rumen. The gas may be in free form or may be mixed with ingesta in the form of froth. It occurs both on pasture and in feedlots and is a major cause of mortality in cattle wherever intensive farming is practiced. Additional losses include decreased milk production and reduced rate of gain. The reduced potential for using legume plants for pasture has a significant economic impact.

Pathogenesis

If the animal is able to eructate naturally, excessive production of gas in the rumen is of little consequence. Under some circumstances this mechanism becomes ineffective, particularly when the cardia of the stomach becomes obstructed by froth.

Frothing of rumen ingesta occurs when the viscosity of the fluid is elevated. Under some conditions several naturally occurring plant substances will have this effect. These include saponins, pectins, hemicelluloses, and certain proteins. The pH of the rumen contents is important in determining the stability of the foam. A pH of 6 is near optimum for maximum stability. Hypermotility of the rumen wall in the initial stages also contributes to the development of frothy bloat. Free gas bloat is commonly associated with rumen atony.

The bloat occurring in animals on pasture is most typical of frothy bloat. However, feedlot bloat may also be frothy.

Succulent plants, particularly young growing legumes in the pre-bloom stage, are leading contributors to pasture bloat. Alfalfa pasture is commonly involved. Harvested crops are less likely to cause bloat. The presence or absence of moisture on the plants does not appear to be a significant factor.

Animal factors can be important as well; particular strains of cattle have been shown to be more susceptible. This is probably related to the ability to or capacity for producing saliva. Adaptation of animals to a particular feed is an important factor. There may be short-term increased susceptibility due to changes in rumen microflora, but as animals become adjusted to a particular pasture or ration, the long-term effect is toward decreased susceptibility.

Secondary bloat may be caused by an obstruction of the esophagus or the cardia of the stomach. Anything that causes rumen atony will also cause tympany of the rumen. This is frequently observed in parturient hypocalcemia and may be part of the rumen acidosis–rumenitis syndrome. Bloat may be a terminal event in animals that die after several days or weeks of severe chronic rumenitis subsequent to rumen acidosis.

Isolated cases of chronic bloat are commonly seen in feedlot animals, often with no apparent cause. Numerous cases of chronic bloat are sometimes observed in animals that have recently suffered a respiratory disease epidemic. This will follow the acute infection by a few days to several weeks. This secondary bloat has been attributed to the necessary heavy use of oral and/or parenteral antibiotics to treat the respiratory disease. Rumen microflora may be altered, and this may lead to excessive gas production.

Greatly enlarged mediastinal and bronchial lymph nodes are often observed at necropsy. Mechanical compression and partial obstruction of the esophagus by these abnormal structures are possible explanations for the bloat. It is also possible that the enlarged lymph nodes interfere with vagal innervation of the rumen, causing rumen atony and subsequent tympany.

Clinical Signs

Severe ruminal tympany is readily apparent to the trained observer. In mild cases, however, it is necessary to differentiate between the rumen simply filled with ingesta and one distended with gas. In the latter case the skin over the left paralumbar fossa is very tight. The entire abdomen is distended but the upper left quadrant will be distorted so that it protrudes above the level of the bony prominences in the lumbar region.

Animals in the early stages of bloat will exhibit signs of colic. Increased rumen motility will also be noted. Animals with advanced cases will show dyspnea with open-mouth breathing, and rumen movements will be absent.

It is usually necessary to pass a stomach tube to differentiate free gas bloat from frothy bloat.

Necropsy

Post-mortem bloat in ruminants that die from other conditions causes some confusion in diagnosis if other findings are negative.

When bloat is the primary cause of death there will be congestion and hemorrhage in the anterior portions of the carcass and edema in the rear quarters, particularly in the scrotal and ventral perineal areas.

Also there will be congestion and possibly extravasated blood in the ventral sinuses of the spinal column and in the cranial cavity. The liver will be pale and the lungs will show signs of compression. The rumen will be distended, but usually the contents will be less frothy than before death.

Diagnosis

A preliminary diagnosis in the living animal is usually based on observation of the distended abdomen with extreme tightness of skin and distortion in the upper left rear quadrant. It may be necessary to pass a stomach tube to determine whether or not the bloat is frothy. Determination of the underlying cause will depend on complete clinical examination and careful evaluation of the history, particularly relative to recent consumption of feed or pasture plants.

Establishing a post-mortem diagnosis is frequently a problem. It is necessary to rule out clostridial infections, lightning strike, and other causes of sudden death. The diagnosis will depend, in part, on the absence of local or systemic lesions of such conditions.

Treatment

Free gas bloat can usually be treated by passing a stomach tube. If the bloat is frothy the stability of the foam must be reduced before the gas can be removed. Any bland oil, such as mineral oil, is useful for this purpose. Oil mixed with detergent will disperse faster in the rumen ingesta. Chemicals such as poloxalene and dioctyl sodium succinate are also effective in lowering the viscosity of the fluid ingesta, thereby reducing the stability of the foam.

Silicones have been used for treatment and prevention of bloat but are probably less reliable than oils. Orally administered turpentine is an old treatment that is reasonably effective but is highly irritating to the tissues and also imparts undesirable flavors to meat and milk.

It is important that the therapeutic agent be deposited in the region of the cardia or given in a sufficient quantity of fluid to ensure that it is well dispersed in the rumen. In this way a fluid line can be re-established and the obstruction relieved. Injection through the left flank into an atonic rumen is not likely to be adequate in severe cases.

In acute frothy bloat with the animal in severe distress, emergency rumenotomy may be necessary to save the animal's life.

Treatment of secondary bloat usually depends on removal of the primary cause. The bloat in parturient hypocalcemia will be rapidly relieved after the administration of intravenous calcium salts. Bloat in an animal that has become cast on its side or that is in dorsal recumbency will usually be relieved by shifting the animal to a more normal position.

Chronic bloat in feedlot animals can sometimes be treated by surgically establishing a small temporary rumen fistula, with or without the use of a prosthetic device. Rumen gas will escape through the fistula until it becomes closed by granulation tissue, usually in about four to six weeks. By then the primary condition will often have corrected itself and an uneventful recovery is made.

Prevention

Gradual adaptation to high-performance rations is of primary importance to avoid bloat. Animals going into lush legume pasture should be given an ample prefeeding of dry hay. Access to the new pasture should be limited to short intervals until the animals are well adjusted to the new feed. In some instances, mowing the forage and leaving it down for one or two days before pasturing is the best practical approach to prevent bloat. The same conditions apply to animals in feedlots. The change from starter feed to full feed should be made very gradually over a three- to four-week period. Self-fed cattle are particularly vulnerable, and it is wise practice to feed animals from bunks until they are well adjusted to the ration that will be supplied in the self-feeder.

Materials used for the treatment of bloat have been used for prevention. These include detergents, mineral oil, and poloxalene in various formulations. To be effective, however, these materials must be consumed by the animal the same day that the bloat-causing ration is fed.

In feedlot bloat, feeding more coarse roughage will often correct the problem. In other instances, it may prove practical to include an inexpensive detergent at the rate of 10 to 20 lb per ton of concentrate ration.

It has been suggested that preventive and therapeutic levels of antibiotics included in the ration may cause bloat. However, many feeders routinely use tetracycline at rates of up to 5 mg/lb (11 mg/kg) body weight for 7 to 14 days to prevent respiratory disease outbreaks with no increased occurrence of bloat. Some digestive upset may result, however, if the animals are not gradually introduced to the drug over a period of two to three days. Withdrawal of the antibiotics from the ration should also be made gradually to avoid digestive disturbances such as bloat.

References

1. Dougherty, R. W., Coburn, K. S., Cook, H. M., and Allison, M. J.: Preliminary study of appearance of endotoxin in circulatory system of sheep and cattle after induced grain engorgement. Am. J. Vet. Res. 36:6, 1975.
2. Mullenax, C. H., Keller, R. F., and Allison, M. J.: Physiologic

responses of ruminants to toxic factors extracted from rumen bacteria and rumen fluid. Am. J. Vet. Res. 27:119, 1966.
3. Smith, H.: Ulcerative lesions of bovine rumen and their possible relation to hepatic abscesses. Am. J. Vet. Res. 5:16, 1944.
4. Jensen, R., Deane, H. M., Cooper, L. J., Miller, V. A., and Graham, W. R.: The rumenitis-liver abscess complex in beef cattle. Am. J. Vet. Res. 15:55, 1954.

Supplemental Reading

Blood, D. C., and Henderson, J. A.: Veterinary Medicine. Williams & Wilkins, Baltimore, 1974, 84–113.
Clark, R. T. J., and Reid, C. S. W.: Foamy bloat of cattle; A review. J. Dairy Sci. 57:7, 1974.
Dougherty, R. W., Riley, J. L., and Cook, H. M.: Changes in motility and pH in the digestive tract of experimentally overfed sheep. Am. J. Vet. Res. 36:6, 1975.
Dunlop, R. H., and Hammon, P. B.: D-lactic acidosis of ruminants. Ann. N.Y. Acad. Sci. 119:1109, 1965.
Fell, B. F., Kay, M., Whitelaw, F. G., and Boyne, R.: Observations on the development of ruminal lesions in calves fed on barley. Res. Vet. Sci. 9:1968.
Harvey, R. W., Wise, M. B., Blumer, T. N., and Barrick, E. R.: Influence of added roughage and chlorotetracycline to all concentrate rations for fattening steers. J. Anim. Sci. 27:5, 1968.
Hofirek, B., Jagos, P., and Dvora, R.: Metabolic profile test of rumen fluid and its application in the diagnosis of rumen dysfunctions. Bovine Pract. (Abstr.) 11:90, 1976.
Jensen, R.: Diseases of Sheep. Lea & Febiger, Philadelphia, 1974, 209–262.
Jensen, R., et al.: Fatal abomasal ulcers in yearling feedlot cattle. J. Am. Vet. Med. Assoc. 169:5, 1976.
Kay, M., Fell, B. F., and Boyne, R.: The relationship between the acidity of the rumen contents and rumenitis in calves fed on barley. Res. Vet. Sci. 10:181, 1969.
Reid, C. S. W.: Causes and control of bloat. N. Z. J. Agric. 133:1, 1976.
Rowland, A. C., Wieser, M. F., and Preston, T. R.: The rumen pathology of intensively managed beef cattle. Anim. Prod. 11:499, 1969.

Gastric Ulcer Syndrome in Swine

WALLACE M. WASS, D.V.M., Ph.D.,
JAMES R. THOMPSON, D.V.M., M.S.,
EDWIN W. MOSS, D.V.M., M.S.,
JERRY P. KUNESH, D.V.M., Ph.D.,
PAUL G. ENESS, D.V.M.,
and LINDA S. THOMPSON, D.V.M.

The gastric ulcer syndrome has been recognized as a major disease problem in intensive swine-raising operations. A combination of environmental, nutritional, and other factors that cause stress are thought to be involved. Swine of all ages are affected, but the highest incidence appears to be in rapidly growing young animals. Factors that possibly increase the incidence of the disease are confinement housing, overcrowding, and the feeding of rations that have been too finely ground. Gastric ulcers are frequently found at necropsy as a secondary complication of other common swine diseases.

CLINICAL SIGNS

Most cases are subclinical or asymptomatic, as indicated by the high incidence reported in surveys taken at slaughter. In other instances animals in apparently good condition are unexpectedly found dead from massive hemor-rhage into the stomach. If observed before death, such animals progress rapidly into shock and become recumbent with fast, shallow breathing. The skin is cold to the touch and the entire body trembles. The animal may vomit blood or may pass bloody or tarry feces if death is delayed.

Animals with less acute cases show signs of severe anemia and will become unthrifty. If perforation of the gastric wall occurs peritonitis will develop and will be accompanied by fever, anorexia, severe depression, and possible recumbency. Death within 24 to 48 hours is likely, but some animals will recover.

Animals with chronic gastric ulcers remain unthrifty with poor appetites and poor growth rates.

NECROPSY

Gastric ulcers in swine are commonly multiple and are found most frequently in the esophageal portion of the stomach. The lesions begin as areas of proliferation and degeneration. Desquamation takes place, leaving an area of superficial erosion that may continue to develop into the deeper layers, forming an ulcer.

At necropsy the stomach is often distended with partially clotted blood, and the intestines contain dark, discolored ingesta. The amount and character of the hemorrhagic gastric and intestinal contents depend on the severity of the hemorrhage and the interval between bleeding and death.

Focal or diffuse peritonitis will be found if an ulcer has perforated.

DIAGNOSIS

Ante-mortem diagnosis can be very difficult. Many cases are asymptomatic or the signs are nonspecific. Hematemesis is considered a pathognomonic sign. Gastric ulcers should be suspected if intermittent passage of dark fecal material or undigested blood is observed and if other signs such as anemia and unthrifty performance are present.

Usually the diagnosis will be made at necropsy.

TREATMENT AND PREVENTION

Effective treatment of individual cases is usually hampered by the lack of early diagnosis. If possible the specific inciting causes must be identified and corrected. The ration should contain an adequate amount of vitamin K to support blood coagulation and should not be ground too finely.

In problem herds pelleted rations should be avoided, and at least 30 per cent coarsely ground oats should be included in the feed mixture.

Any factor that causes stress for the animal may serve as a precipitating influence.

Transportation of sows in late gestation should be avoided, and overcrowding of animals should be corrected. Adequate ventilation and other factors important to animal comfort must be considered.

In confinement operations, it may be helpful if foundation breeding stock can be obtained from other successful confinement herds.

Cimetidine has been used successfully to treat gastric ulcers in swine. A dose of 300 mg/animal given twice daily has proved to be highly effective if there is early diagnosis.

Supplemental Reading

Griffing, W. J.: A study of etiology and pathology of gastric ulcers in swine. Diss. Abstr. 24:1581, 1963.
Kowalczyk, T., Hoekstra, W. G., Puestrow, K. L., Smith, I. D., and Grummer, R. H.: Stomach ulcers in swine. J. Am. Vet. Med. Assoc. 137:339, 1960.
Kowalczyk, T., Olson, W. G., Zamora, C. S., and Schmidt, J. R.: Gastric ulcers in swine under modern intensified husbandry. VM/SAC 66:12, 1971.
O'Brien, J. J.: Gastric ulcers. In Leman, A. D., et al. (eds.): Diseases of Swine, 5th ed. Iowa State University Press, Ames, 1981, 632–646.

Diseases of the Abomasum and the Intestinal Tract

GLEN F. HOFFSIS, D.V.M., M.S.
and SHEILA M. McGUIRK, D.V.M., Ph.D.

Definition of Condition

In left displaced abomasum (LDA) the abomasum, which normally lies to the right of the ventral midline, assumes an abnormal position on the left side of the abdomen between the rumen and the body wall (Fig. 1). The diagnosis has been made with increasing frequency since the condition was first recognized in 1950.[1]

Accurate figures on the incidence of LDA in the cattle population are not available. The disease is limited almost exclusively to dairy cattle, with the highest occurrence in cows of the middle-aged group (four to six years of age) in early lactation. Approximately 80 per cent of all cases are diagnosed in the first month of lactation. The condition is rarely diagnosed in dairy bulls, young heifers, and beef cows. The incidence is also low in pregnant cows.

The incidence of the disease in individual herds may vary from less than 1 to 75 per cent of the cows being affected during their lifetime. Although genetic factors have been investigated,[2] recent evidence indicated no significant difference between the pedigrees of affected and unaffected cows.[3] The incidence is highest in cows during the stabled period, i.e., the winter months.[4]

The precise etiology of LDA is unknown, although it appears that primary factors that result in atony and gas distention of the abomasum can lead to displacement. The dietary factor associated with a high incidence of LDA is a low-roughage, high-concentrate diet.[4-7] Feeding high-concentrate diets increases production of volatile fatty acids (VFA) in the rumen. Unabsorbed VFAs pass into the abomasum and act directly on the smooth muscle to decrease motility.[8] As motility decreases, gas formation is increased by the liberation of CO_2 from the reaction between rumen bicarbonate and abomasal hydrochloric acid. Other gases, such as methane and nitrogen, are also found.

Concurrent disease may have a potentiating effect in further decreasing abomasal motility. Post-partum diseases such as hypocalcemia, metritis, mastitis, traumatic reticulitis, abomasal ulcers, fat cow syndrome, and simple indigestion have been associated with LDA in over 25 per cent of the cows.[4, 9] Likewise, cows treated for these postpartum diseases will often develop an LDA during the course of the disease.

Mechanical factors may also be involved in the etiology of the LDA. During pregnancy, the gravid uterus may elevate the rumen and other viscera from the abdominal floor, allowing the abomasum to move slightly to the left of the midline. Following parturition, with increased grain feeding, atony and gas formation may develop and the displacement becomes complete. The shape of the cow's abdomen is suggested as another mechanical factor. The incidence in dairy cows may be higher than that in beef cows because of their tendency to be larger and deeper bodied. Free-stall housing has also been incriminated because some cows have difficulty getting to their feet when the stalls are short. When the abomasum is already dilated, struggling to rise may cause a malposition of the abomasum. Regardless of the factors, once gas is trapped within the abomasum, it will move within the abdominal cavity. Displacement of the abomasum occurs only when the abomasum is dilated with gas.

Clinical Signs

Early signs are usually subtle. Usually some anorexia is present; most cows refuse grain but continue to eat some hay. If the condition is uncorrected, progressive weight loss will continue for several weeks and the cow is culled from the herd for poor body condition. Rarely, cows with LDA may be asymptomatic.[10] Clinical signs may be intermittent if the abomasum alternately displaces and replaces repeatedly.

Milk production gradually declines and may eventually cease. Because of the digestive malfunction and the inability to consume or digest adequate nutrients to support milk production, most cows will be ketotic at some time during the course of the disease. Ketones form from the resultant energy deficit. The ketosis associated with LDA is a classic example of secondary ketosis.

Feces may vary from more firm than normal (a sign typical of ketosis) to diarrhea. Cows with diarrhea have a much poorer prognosis than those with normal or dry feces.[11] Many cows with LDA have normal feces.

The vital signs are usually normal. An abnormal temperature, pulse, and respiratory rate are usually in response to concurrent diseases such as metritis. Dehydration usually occurs only late in the course of the condition or subsequent to other disease problems. Atrial fibrillation occurs frequently in a wide variety of gastrointestinal diseases including LDA. The heart should always be carefully auscultated for the characteristic arrhythmia.

Auscultation of the left abdominal wall for several minutes may reveal spontaneous tinkling and gurgling sounds. Simultaneous auscultation and percussion of the paralumbar area will yield a high-pitched, tympanic resonance ("ping") similar to that produced by a pebble dropped in a well. The area of the resonant ping may be as small as 10 to 12 cm (4 to 5 inches) or as large as 45 cm (18 inches) in diameter. The location of the ping will vary depending on the ingesta within the rumen, the position of the abomasum, and the amount of gas trapped within the abomasum. The ping may extend forward to the ninth or tenth rib or as far ventrally as a line between the stifle and the shoulder joint. Therefore the clinician should always auscultate and percuss the entire left side

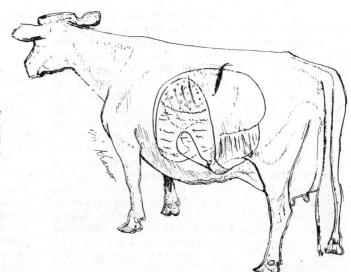

Figure 1. Left displaced abomasum. The presence of gas is indicated with circles to represent bubbles. The location of the gas cap is usually beneath the last rib and extends from the anterior aspect of the paralumbar fossa forward for a distance of 10 to 20 in.

of the abdomen. Rumen contractions, if present, are difficult to hear in the area occupied by the abomasum.

Occasionally an LDA will slightly distend the left paralumbar fossa just caudal to the last rib. Palpation of this area will reveal a balloon-like structure that springs back when the clinician removes his hand. In contrast, rumen gas usually causes a uniform bulge over the entire paralumbar fossa. A left displaced abomasum can rarely be palpated by rectal examination.

Many of the clinical signs seen in cows with LDA may be attributed to ketosis and other concurrent diseases as well as the LDA. Clinical signs vary because of the variety of other problems that can occur with LDA. In general, any dairy cow with ketosis, especially if it is persistent or nonresponsive to therapy, should be carefully and repeatedly examined for LDA.

Clinical Pathology

Most cows with LDA have a metabolic alkalosis. However, some have a normal acid-base balance, and, occasionally, metabolic acidosis may occur. The proposed mechanisms for the acid-base imbalance are discussed hereafter (see Abomasal Torsion).

Serum electrolyte alterations are usually small. Whitlock reported values of 137 ± 0.6 mEq/L for sodium, 3.5 ± 0.1 mEq/L for potassium, 86 ± 4.0 mEq/L for chloride, and $27 \pm$ mEq/L for bicarbonate in 75 cows with left abomasal displacement.[12] Serum calcium is usually slightly decreased. Serum phosphorus and magnesium levels may be normal or slightly increased. Electrolyte changes are discussed in more detail hereafter (see Abomasal Torsion).

Serum glucose levels may be decreased, increased, or normal. If serum glucose is elevated, glycosuria may be found. Ketonuria is often present and reflects ketonemia with elevation of serum nonesterified fatty acids. Approximately 50 per cent of the cows with metabolic alkalosis have paradoxical aciduria,[13, 14] the mechanism of which is discussed hereafter (see Abomasal Torsion).

Diagnosis

Auscultation of the characteristic ping produced spontaneously or by simultaneous auscultation and percussion of the left paralumbar fossa is very suggestive of LDA.[15] Occasionally, it is difficult to distinguish the ping associated with rumen gas or pneumoperitoneum from that of the LDA when the location is similar. In general, the rumen ping occurs over the entire left side and the pitch is lower. Rectal examination may determine that the gas is within the rumen. The ping of a pneumoperitoneum can be produced on both sides of the abdomen and along the transverse processes. The abdomen usually is not distended with this condition, and it rarely occurs except following abdominal surgery.

A Liptak test may distinguish between a rumen and abomasal ping. A needle (18-gauge $\times$ 5 cm) is inserted through an aseptically prepared site just beneath the lower extent of the ping. A few drops of fluid can be obtained and tested with pH paper. A pH less than 5 indicates that the abomasum has been entered, and a pH greater than 5 indicates that the rumen has been entered.

Another way to differentiate pings is to pass a stomach tube into the rumen. An assistant can blow into the stomach tube while the clinician auscultates and percusses the left side of the abdomen. If the characteristics of the sound produced by air forced through the rumen fluid are similar to the sounds obtained earlier by simultaneous auscultation and percussion, then the ping is most likely from the rumen. If there are two distinctly different pitches to the sounds, the abomasum is most likely responsible for one of the sounds.

Treatment

The goal in treatment of left displaced abomasum is to return the abomasum to its normal position so that normal digestive function can resume. The sooner this is accomplished, the quicker the cow will return to normal milk production and regain normal energy balance. Treatment should be accomplished as quickly, permanently, and inexpensively as possible.

Numerous conservative treatments have been tried. These increase gastrointestinal motility, which hopefully increases the tone of the abomasum, causing gas to be expelled and the abomasum to return to the normal position. Calcium solutions, neostigmine, and saline cathartics have been used. These drugs have given mixed results, and even when the abomasum does return to its normal position there is a high incidence of recurrence.

Mechanical replacement of the abomasum with or without concurrent drug treatment is another conservative approach. This has been done by forcing the cow to walk up a steep incline or taking a rough truck ride. Cows arriving at hospitals for LDA treatment often have very little gas in the abomasum, causing the ping to vanish. However, invariably the ping will return by the following day. The abomasum can be replaced more consistently by rolling the cow.[16] The cow is placed in lateral recumbency by reefing and then is moved to dorsal recumbency and rolled in a to-and-fro motion. Massaging the abdomen while rolling helps move the abomasum to the ventral midline. Finally, the cow is rolled to left lateral recumbency and allowed to get up from that position. Rolling is nearly always successful in replacing the abomasum except when adhesions are present that fix it in the LDA position. However, the recurrence rate from rolling the cow is high (approximately 75 per cent).

All surgical methods for the correction of the LDA involve fixation of the omentum or the abomasum to the body wall. The simplest procedure is the ventral closed-suturing technique, which is performed with the cow in dorsal recumbency. When the characteristic ping can be auscultated in the right paramedian area, the abomasum is blindly sutured to the abdominal wall with a long needle.[17] Recently a bar suture rather than a conventional suture has been recommended.[18]

The ventral paramedian abomasopexy is done with the cow in dorsal recumbency. After routine surgical preparation, a 20-cm (8-inch) paramedian incision is made. The wall of the abomasum, which should be visible immediately under the incision, is incorporated in the closure of the abdominal wall.[19, 20]

The left flank abomasopexy is performed via a left paralumbar laparotomy. A nonabsorbable suture, placed in the greater curvature of the abomasum, is carried along the peritoneum to the right paramedian area and inserted through the abdominal wall. The sutures are then grasped from the outside by an assistant and tied.[21]

The right flank omentopexy is performed from a right paralumbar laparotomy.[22, 23] After deflation and replacement of the abomasum, the omentum near the pylorus is incorporated into the incision line to hold the abomasum in normal position.

Minimal treatment should be required following surgical correction. Most cows begin eating within hours after correction. Cows that are dehydrated respond more rapidly with fluid therapy. Fluids can be easily administered orally. A commercially available formula high in chloride or a balanced electrolyte solution can be used. A satisfactory fluid can be made by dissolving 150 grams of sodium chloride and 30 grams of potassium chloride in 10 liters of water. Approximately 40 liters can be administered orally by stomach tube to most cows. Some cows will voluntarily drink the electrolyte solution, and in such cases it should be offered *ad libitum*. Oral fluids have an additional benefit in filling the rumen, thereby creating a barrier against redisplacement of the abomasum.

Special attempts to correct acid-base deficiencies are unnecessary in the uncomplicated LDA. Once the abomasum is surgically replaced, electrolyte and acid-base abnormalities will correct within 12 hours with no treatment other than good feeding practices. Ringer's or an equivalent balanced electrolyte solution is preferred for intravenous treatment in the severely dehydrated cow.

Prevention

Because the precise etiologic factors are unknown, prevention is equally imprecise. Nutritional counseling is currently the most effective approach.[24]

Dry cows should be separated from lactating cows so they can be fed according to their specific requirements. Dry cows should be maintained primarily on roughages to rehabilitate the digestive tract and reduce the level of volatile fatty acids. Roughages should provide 70 per cent or more of the total dry matter intake. Then, no more than 30 per cent of the total ration on a dry matter basis would be concentrates.[5, 24] Corn silage alone is not satisfactory for dry cows since it contains approximately 50 per cent concentrate on a dry matter basis. Corn silage provided *ad libitum* also leads to excessively fat cows (fat cow syndrome) that have a high incidence of LDA. Corn silage should not exceed 15 kg/cow/day during the dry period. Corn silage should be coarse-cut rather than fine-cut to provide maximum coarseness in the diet. Good quality grass hay, alone or with other feeds such as corn silage, is excellent for dry cows.[24]

A major nutritional change often occurs when cows are switched from dry cow to lactating cow rations. Ration changes should be made gradually to allow the rumen flora to adapt. Dry cows should become accustomed to grain feeding just prior to parturition. Feeding 5 kg of concentrates per head per day for about two weeks prior to parturition would help make a smooth transition. Once cows are milking, concentrates should be gradually increased to desired levels over several days. Concentrates are increased by about 1 kg per day until the cow is consuming the desired level.[24]

The prevention of post-partum diseases such as parturient hypocalcemia, retained placenta, and coliform mastitis will indirectly reduce the incidence of displaced abomasums. These and other diseases that decrease abomasal motility are responsible for the high incidence in many herds. Health programs that promote the general health of the herd often indirectly reduce the incidence of displaced abomasums.

Reducing mechanical obstacles may also aid in preventing displaced abomasums in some herds. Short free stalls may force cows to struggle when rising, causing a mechanical force that could be the final factor in causing a displaced abomasum. Steep and/or slippery entry and exit ramps for milking parlors may also have a similar effect. Any obvious obstacles should be corrected.

RIGHT DISPLACED ABOMASUM AND ABOMASAL TORSION (VOLVULUS)

Definition

The etiology and pathogenesis of right displaced abomasum (RDA) and right torsion of the abomasum (RTA) are similar to those described for LDA. The two conditions differ only in mechanical aspects. The abomasum moves within the abdominal cavity once it is atonic and dilated with gas. Usually it moves to the left side of the rumen to become a LDA. The clinical signs of LDA are relatively mild and very predictable. If the abomasum travels to the right side of the abdominal cavity, the signs

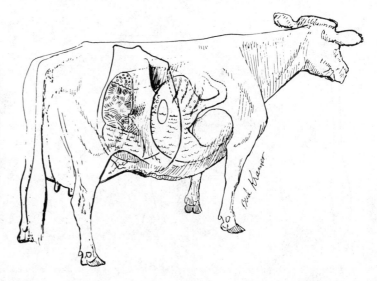

Figure 2. Right displaced abomasum. The abomasum may be rotated approximately 90° out of position as indicated. The presence of solid ingesta within the organ is represented as cross hatches. Fluid is represented as waves and gas is represented as bubbles. The area of resonant "ping" is identical to the size and location of the gas cap.

The circular line around the cow (see Figs. 2 to 9) indicates the shape of the abdomen in a cross sectional view at the level of the paralumbar fossa. Areas of enlargement are indicated. The cross section line represents the portion of various organs palpable rectally.

are very unpredictable and vary from mild to severe, depending on the amount of twist incurred by the abomasum.

RDAs and RTAs occur most frequently in dairy cows after parturition, as do LDAs.[25] However, RDAs are found much more frequently than LDAs in bulls, young animals, beef cows, and feedlot cattle. Occasionally the abomasum will initially displace to the left (LDA) and later move to the right, becoming an RDA or RTA.[26]

In North America, LDA occurs far more frequently than RDA and RTA. Gabel and Heath reported 147 cases of LDA compared with 18 cases of RTA during the same period.[25]

Clinical Signs

In RDA, sometimes called abomasal dilatation, the abomasum floats and rotates dorsally 90 to 180 degrees from its normal position. This is not sufficient to occlude the vasculature or put undue pressure on nerves and organ attachments. Two slightly different types of rotation may result in RDA as illustrated in Figures 2 and 3. The

clinical signs associated with RDA are identical to those of LDA.

With torsion of the abomasum (RTA), sometimes called volvulus, the signs are more pronounced and increase in severity as the degree of twist increases. These signs are attributed to pain, hypovolemia, and shock resulting from stretching of the organs and attachments, vascular impairment, and acid-base alterations.

The abomasum undergoes a variety of twists on the right side of the abdomen, but all are varying degrees of the same general motion. The range of motion varies from the slight twist in RDA[27] (see Figs. 2 and 3) to the most serious found in omasal-abomasal torsion (OAT)[28] (see Fig. 5). In RTA (Fig. 4), the twist involves a 180-degree rotation counterclockwise as viewed from above. If only the abomasum is involved, the twist is located in the abdomasal wall just caudal to the omasum and the duodenum will course posterior to the omasum. In omasal-abomasal torsion (OAT), the rotational motion is exactly the same as that described with RTA except that the omasum is also included in the organs, which are

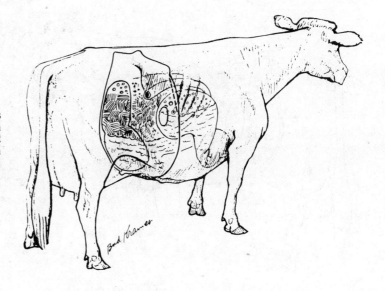

Figure 3. Right displaced abomasum. Rotation is approximately 180° counterclockwise as viewed from the rear. This entity and that represented in Figure 2 are different forms of right displaced abomasum, which are difficult to differentiate from each other clinically. Both are sometimes termed abomasal dilatation.

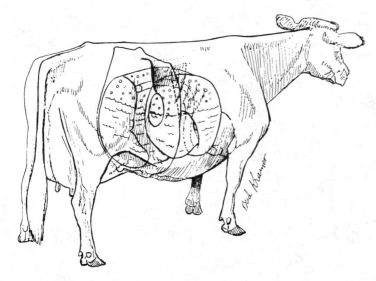

Figure 4. Abomasal torsion (volvulus). The abomasum is twisted 180° in a counterclockwise direction as viewed from the rear in addition to 180° in a counterclockwise direction as viewed from above. The abomasal contents are fluid, and, secondarily, rumen contents may become more fluid.

twisted. In this instance, the duodenum courses anterior to the omasum and the twist is in the reticulum (Fig. 5).

In RTA and OAT the abomasum occupies a position lateral to the liver. The liver is compressed by the distended abomasum and may show pressure changes.

At the onset of torsion, the cow usually has signs of discomfort and abdominal pain (see Abdominal Pain). Because the abomasum is partially or completely blocked at both ends, fluid and gas accumulate within a few hours, causing abomasal distention. The distention is most noticeable at the anterior ventral aspect of the right paralumbar fossa just behind the last rib.

If the abomasal vessels are sufficiently compromised, shock ensues, producing signs of rapid dehydration, cool extremities, and depression. The heart rate is usually elevated to about 100 beats per minute or more. The cow does not eat or drink, and milk production ceases.

The bowel movements may be normal for a short time after the torsion occurs but gradually reduce in volume and develop a dark brown to black color. The consistency of the feces is pasty, but diarrhea may be present in some cases. The black color is from extravasation of blood from the abomasal wall, which is digested in the intestines. Fecal volume and consistency depend on the amount of abomasal contents that can escape through the pylorus.

A large resonant ping will be located by simultaneous auscultation and percussion over the upper right rib cage.[29] The area begins behind the last rib and extends forward for 45 to 60 cm (18 to 24 inches). The area of resonance will become larger as the degree of torsion increases (see Figs. 4 and 5). In pregnant cows, the resonant area may be further anterior and audible over a smaller area. As the abomasum is pushed further forward, the diaphragm diverts it medially.

The abomasum can usually be palpated rectally with RTA or OAT and sometimes with RDA (see Figs. 3, 4, and 5). With careful palpation, the posterior aspect of the dilated abomasum will be felt at arm's length at the anterior aspect of the right paralumbar fossa. If the abomasum is palpable, torsion should be suspected.

Clinical Pathology

The acid-base imbalance is more pronounced with RTA or OAT than with LDA or RDA. The majority of these

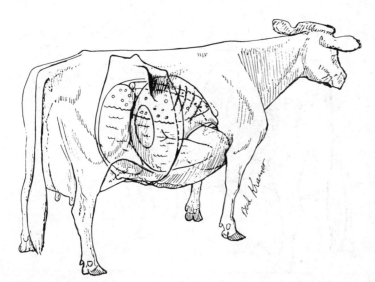

Figure 5. Omasal and abomasal torsion (OAT). The abomasum is twisted 180° as viewed from the rear as well as 180° as viewed from above and is identical to that illustrated in Figure 4. The only difference is that the twist includes the omasum and the point of rotation is located at the reticulo-omasal junction rather than at the omasal-abomasal junction as in Figure 4. The duodenum crosses the reticulum in this condition.

cows will have a severe metabolic alkalosis. The blood gas values in an extreme case in a steer were: pH, 7.528; pCO_2, 49.5 torr; pO_2, 33.2 torr; HCO_3, 40.5 mEq/L; base excess, +17.5. The metabolic alkalosis is generated by the sequestration of abomasal hydrochloric acid (HCl) secretions in the abomasum and forestomachs.[30] Normally, it is formed by the following reaction: $NaCl + H_2CO_3 \rightarrow NaHCO_3$ (plasma) + HCl (abomasum). The HCl must then move out of the abomasum to be absorbed in the intestine to buffer the $NaHCO_3$ in the plasma generated by this reaction. If the HCl is not moved to the intestines for absorption, the $NaHCO_3$ is not buffered and a metabolic alkalosis ensues. Reflux of abomasal contents into the forestomachs may also aid in the genesis of the metabolic alkalosis.[31]

Some cows with RTA or OAT may have a metabolic acidosis. In general, acidosis is seen after a longer duration and is due to dehydration and the subsequent lactic acid production by anaerobic metabolism in the peripheral tissues. Increased acid metabolite formation and absorption of endotoxins from the intestinal tract may contribute to the acidosis. Cows with RTA or OAT that have acidosis have a poor prognosis.

Electrolyte alterations are also more pronounced in RTA and OAT than in simple abomasal displacements. In the case previously illustrated, serum electrolyte concentrations were: sodium, 135 mEq/L; potassium, 2.8 mEq/L; chloride, 59 mEq/L; calcium, 8.3 mEq/L; phosphorus, 10.0 mEq/L; and magnesium, 2.5 mEq/L. The glucose concentration was 274 mg/dl.

Serum sodium concentration is usually within normal limits and, if abnormal, usually reflects the hydration of the animal. Potassium concentrations are usually low from decreased dietary intake and an intracellular shift where K^+ is exchanged with hydrogen in response to alkalosis. There may also be some urinary loss of potassium in spite of low serum levels. Serum chloride concentrations are often markedly low because of HCl sequestration in the abomasum and forestomachs. The calcium concentration is usually slightly decreased secondary to metabolic alkalosis. Serum calcium levels may be decreased from decreased dietary intake or decreased absorption due to functional pyloric obstruction. Increased serum phospho-

rus concentration occurs frequently, but the precise mechanism is not known. Dehydration with decreased renal perfusion probably plays a role. When the serum phosphorus concentration exceeds the calcium concentration, the prognosis is poor. Serum magnesium concentration may be normal or increased and probably reflects the hydration of the animal.

Glucose levels may be decreased, normal, or elevated in cows with RTA and OAT. The majority appear hyperglycemic from a massive glucocorticoid release secondary to the severe abdominal crisis. In most cases, the renal tubular threshold for glucose is exceeded and there is glycosuria. In hypoglycemia, anorexia has usually been prolonged and ketosis has occurred.

Ketonemia and ketonuria are frequently found (see LDA). Paradoxical aciduria occurs frequently as the result of the hypokalemia or hypochloremia.[13, 14] With dehydration, avid sodium retention might also contribute to the formation of acid urine. Recently, it has been thought that the excretion of undetermined anions, most likely acid metabolites, might be responsible for the paradoxical aciduria.[13, 14] There is no association between ketonuria and aciduria.

Diagnosis

Diseases that cause resonant pings in the right paralumbar fossa must be differentiated from RTA and OAT.[29] Gas in the colon or duodenum will sometimes produce a ping. The resonant area is usually small (less than 15 cm in diameter) and located high in the paralumbar fossa. These pings are incidental findings and are not responsible for clinical signs. A torsion of the cecum will produce a ping in the right paralumbar fossa. Cecal resonance is usually located in the dorsal and posterior aspect of the fossa (Fig. 6) as compared with the anterior ventral aspect of the fossa with RTA and OAT. Intestinal obstructions may also cause pings in various locations on the right side of the abdomen (Fig. 7).

Diseases that cause acute abdominal pain and intestinal obstruction must also be differentiated. These are discussed in more detail hereafter (see Abdominal Pain). Diagnosis of RTA or OAT is based on the clinical signs of dehydration and shock, the presence of a large ping on

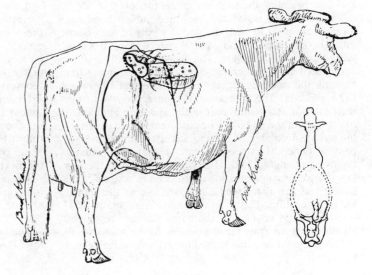

Figure 6. Cecal torsion. The blind end (apex) of the cecum may extend forward as in this view or be found in other positions. Sometimes the cecum is doubled on itself. The tympanic area has a size and location corresponding to the gas within the cecum. The cecum extends into the pelvic inlet and is easily palpated rectally.

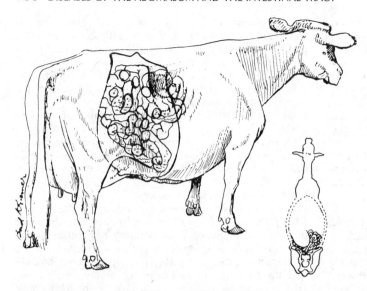

Figure 7. Intestinal obstruction. The small intestine is distended with gas and fluid proximal to the site of obstruction. The abdomen is distended on both sides and small tympanic areas may be audible on the right side in various locations. Rectal examination reveals distended loops of intestine in a wide area extending into the pelvis.

the right side of the abdomen, compatible rectal palpation findings, and a scant tarry stool. Hypochloremia and metabolic alkalosis support the diagnosis. In some instances, it may help to aspirate fluid from the abomasum via the right flank. A small gauge needle is inserted just below the area of the resonant ping. If the pH of the fluid is less than 4, the organ is most likely the abomasum. If the abomasum is very tightly distended, insertion of a needle may cause leakage of fluid or damage to the wall.

Treatment

Immediate surgery is indicated once RTA or OAT is diagnosed. Unlike LDA and RDA, torsions do not correct spontaneously and cannot be corrected by drug therapy, rolling, or the closed-suture technique. Time makes a great difference in the response of a cow to surgical correction. Delaying surgery increases the chances for irreversible damage to the wall of the abomasum or vagus nerves.

A laparotomy is done in the right paralumbar fossa in a standing animal[25] or the ventral paramedian site in a recumbent animal.[32] The paralumbar fossa approach offers the surgeon the best chance of maintaining his orientation and understanding the anatomy of the torsion.

The abomasum is deflated, and then the left hand and forearm are used to push the dorsal aspect of the abomasum in an anterior and ventral direction as if being tucked under the reticulum. The omasum is gently cradled and pulled in a posterior and lateral direction. After crossing the midline, the abomasum is essentially in an LDA position. The abomasum is then approached from the posterior and ventral part of the abdomen and pulled to the right of the midline. The omentum is used to retract the pylorus into view at the incision site and an omentopexy is done. Most torsions can be corrected without removing abomasal fluid. If fluid is not removed there is less chance of contamination, correction is accomplished faster, and the abomasal HCl is available to the animal for re-absorption. This is an advantage since the sequestered HCl that resulted in the hypochloremic metabolic alkalosis is once again made available to the animal.

Fluids should be administered intravenously during and following surgery, particularly if dehydration is apparent. The goal in fluid therapy is to replace the plasma and extracellular fluid deficit, provide chloride ion, and correct the metabolic alkalosis. Twenty or more liters of fluid will be necessary to correct the fluid deficit in very dehydrated adult cows.[12] The first 8 liters may be given as rapidly as possible in a severely dehydrated cow, whereas the remainder is given at the rate of about 5 liters per hour until normal hydration is restored. A balanced electrolyte solution high in chloride should be chosen. Ringer's solution or isotonic sodium chloride solution is preferred. Sodium bicarbonate and sodium lactate should not be used. Acidifiers, such as ammonium chloride, are not necessary if abomasal contents are not removed. Following surgical correction, the acid-base and electrolyte status of most cows will return to normal within about 12 hours if abomasal contents are not removed and a balanced electrolyte solution is administered during and after surgery. In fact, some animals will have a mild acidosis 12 to 24 hours after surgery due to the absorption of sequestered HCl. Antibiotics should be administered and glucose given intravenously to combat ketosis in dairy cows.

The prognosis depends on the severity of the torsion and the time lag between the onset of the twist and the correction. The volume of fluid within the abomasum and the serum chloride level can be indicators of the prognosis.[33] The volume of fluid within the abomasum will increase in direct proportion to the severity and duration of the twist. In general, if surgery is performed early a recovery rate of about 75 per cent can be expected for RTA and about 35 to 50 per cent for OAT. Diarrhea should be observed about 12 hours following surgery as the abomasal fluid enters the intestinal tract. Feces usually return to normal in one or two days in successful cases. Some cows will have a decreasing volume of feces over the next week followed by abdominal distention. These signs are identical to those described hereafter (see Vagus Indigestion [Functional Pyloric Stenosis).

Prevention

The prevention of abomasal torsion is identical to that for LDA.

VAGUS INDIGESTION

Definition

Vagus indigestion is a digestive disorder that occurs most often in adult cattle and only rarely in cattle under two years of age. The history is characterized by bouts of indigestion and anorexia. In lactating cows, milk production does not reach the expected potential. The primary signs of weight loss, dehydration, abdominal distention, and decreasing volume of bowel movements gradually become worse over several weeks or months.

The cause of vagus indigestion is thought to be interference with vagus nerve function. The specific form of vagus indigestion depends on the part of the vagus nerve that is malfunctioning. Clinical vagus indigestion syndromes were produced experimentally by Hoflund by sectioning various areas of the vagus nerves.[34] The specific causes of vagus nerve malfunction are not entirely identified. Most cases seem to result from adhesions formed in response to traumatic reticuloperitonitis (TRP). The vagus nerve courses through the diaphragm in the area of the reticulum, where adhesion, infection, and inflammation due to TRP or a perforated abomasal ulcer are most intense. The vagus nerve is easily damaged in this region. Other causes are actinobacillosis of the reticulum or rumen, inflammation of the mediastinal lymph nodes with diseases such as malignant lymphoma or tuberculosis, diaphragmatic hernia, and pleuritis. Cattle that survive surgery for abomasal torsion (RTA or OAT) but do not recover satisfactorily often have signs of vagus indigestion.[35]

Because of vagus nerve malfunction, transport of ingesta through the ruminant forestomachs or abomasum fails. Fecal output gradually decreases and the abdomen distends. The common features of the vagus indigestion syndromes are decreased fecal output, abdominal distention, dehydration, and weight loss.

Clinical Signs

The clinically recognized forms of vagus indigestion can be categorized as follows:

1. *Ruminal distention with hypomotility or atony of the rumen (Type I).*

There is an increase in rumen contents, which are more fluid than normal with a small gas cap at the top. It resembles simple bloat except that the distention is caused by fluid rather than gas. No rumen sounds are audible, and the heart rate is normal or increased. There is a functional blockage between the omasum and the abomasum, which has been referred to as a failure of omasal transport.

2. *Ruminal distention with hypermotility (Type II).*

This is identical to Type I except that the rumen has increased motility. The rumen wall can be seen to contract in waves, which are visible through the abdominal wall. Rumen contractions are not audible, so observation of the waves of contraction is important. The contractions are incoordinated primary or secondary rumen contractions, which often occur at the rate of four to six per minute (normal two per minute). Bradycardia may be present in some cases with the heart rate as low as 40 beats per minute.

3. *Functional pyloric stenosis (Type III).*

In this syndrome the abomasum fails to empty properly into the duodenum, causing accumulation of fluid or semisolid ingesta within the abomasum. Secondarily, the rumen distends with fluid because of the failure of ingesta to pass through the abomasum. The fluid that accumulates in the forestomachs results from reflux of abomasal secretions into the rumen and/or failure of transport of ingested fluids and saliva through the abomasum. This category of vagus indigestion is sometimes further divided into a partial pyloric stenosis.[34] This type of vagus indigestion often develops after surgery for abomasal torsion (volvulus).

In Types I and II the distended rumen will cause a symmetrically rounded left abdominal wall. If the rumen extends into the right side of the abdomen, the right abdominal wall will have a normal contour or may be slightly rounded.

The abdomen assumes a characteristic shape with Type III (functional pyloric stenosis). The right side of the abdomen is pear-shaped as viewed from the rear because the lower right quadrant of the abdomen is pushed outward by the distended abomasum, whereas the paralumbar fossa remains normally contoured. The left side of the abdomen would appear symmetrically rounded like an apple because of rumen distention. The characteristic shape of an apple on the left side and a pear on the right side of the abdomen has been termed as "papple"[31] (Fig. 8).

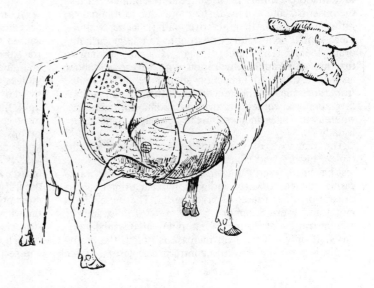

Figure 8. Vagus indigestion with functional pyloric stenosis. The abomasum is distended with contents that are fluid. The rumen and reticulum are secondarily filled with fluid. The left side of the abdomen is distended in a symmetric and round manner, while the right side is distended only in the lower right quadrant.

The clinical signs are similar in all three syndromes. The feces are decreased in volume and have a pasty consistency. There is dehydration, decreased milk production, and a gradual and progressive weight loss. In the later stages the animal usually refuses feed. The temperature, pulse, and respirations are normal. Ingested water is not adequately absorbed from the rumen.

On rectal examination the rumen is greatly distended and has a fluid consistency in all three syndromes. The posterior ventral blind sac of the rumen is so distended that it extends to the right side of the abdomen. The rumen has an "L" shape as viewed from the rear. Although the abomasum is usually not palpable, rumen distention and the "L" shape can be determined on rectal palpation. The fluid consistency of the distended rumen and abomasum can be appreciated by ballottement of the abdomen.

Clinical Pathology

Dehydration often increases packed cell volume and total serum protein. Advanced cases may have prerenal uremia in response to dehydration and poor renal perfusion. In functional pyloric stenosis, hypochloremic metabolic alkalosis will be found. Serum chloride is often decreased to 40 to 50 mEq/L. An elevation in rumen chloride concentration (above 30 mEq/L) indicates abomasal reflux into the rumen.[36] If the rumen chloride is normal, there are two possible explanations: either the abomasum is not pooling fluids, or the abomasum has a functional obstruction but is retaining rather than refluxing secretion into the rumen. In Types I and II the serum and rumen chloride levels are usually normal. Many affected cows will also be hypokalemic.

Diagnosis

The differential diagnosis should include the diseases that cause abdominal distention. Any disease that causes intestinal obstruction will eventually result in distention and must be differentiated by physical examination and laboratory findings. Accumulation of fluid within the abdominal cavity from ascites, peritonitis, or ruptured urinary bladder should be considered. These can be diagnosed by abdominal paracentesis. The clinician must also consider hydrops allantois or amnion as a cause for the distention. These can be differentiated by rectal examination. Primary bloat can be differentiated because the onset is acute and the distention is due to ruminal gas rather than fluid. In grain overload (D-lactic acidosis) there should be a history of exposure to a large carbohydrate source. The onset of signs is acute, leading to toxemia and rapid dehydration with severe metabolic acidosis. Abomasal impaction should be differentiated from functional pyloric stenosis. Ballottement will indicate firm abomasal contents in primary abomasum impaction, whereas in vagus indigestion the abomasal contents are usually fluid.

The diagnosis of vagus indigestion is based on the typical history and clinical signs. An atropine response test has been described as an aid in differentiating bradycardia related to vagus indigestion from primary heart disease or other causes of bradycardia. The pulse rate is monitored every 5 minutes for 30 minutes following the administration of 30 mg of atropine sulfate subcutaneously. If only a 5 per cent increase is noted, the bradycardia is probably due to an intracardiac lesion. If the heart rate increases by approximately 7 per cent, the bradycardia may have some vagal influence but does not indicate a major vagal lesion. If the heart rate increases by more than 16 per cent, a diagnosis of vagus indigestion is indicated.[31] The test is of limited value.

Treatment

Since most cattle are in poor physical condition when vagus indigestion is diagnosed, supportive therapy is important. A balanced electrolyte solution such as Ringer's solution should be administered intravenously to restore any chloride deficit and correct the dehydration. As much as 40 liters over one or two days may be necessary. More specific fluid therapy and chloride replacement can be accomplished if blood-gas and electrolyte data are available. In vagus indigestion, fluid and electrolyte therapy must be given intravenously, since fluids administered orally will not be absorbed from the rumen but will add to the rumen distention.

Once the animal is rehydrated, the clinician will be better able to assess the underlying causes of the disease. An exploratory laparotomy and rumenotomy are usually indicated in valuable individuals. The abdomen can be explored for adhesions or abscesses in the area of the reticulum, tumors, or other possible causes. The rumen can be evacuated and the reticulum, esophageal groove, and omasal orifice explored for foreign material and masses. Occasionally, abscesses can be drained and adhesions removed for specific correction of the condition. In the vast majority the underlying cause cannot be corrected. If there is ruminal tympany, a rumen fistula can be created to allow continued escape of gas from the rumen on a semipermanent basis. It also provides easy access to the rumen for administration of cathartics or fluids.

Prognosis in vagus indigestion is guarded to poor regardless of the clinical syndrome. A few animals respond favorably to rehydration and/or exploratory rumenotomy; however, extensive treatment is usually given only to valuable cattle. Less valuable cattle should be slaughtered before any drugs are given and dehydration increases.

ABOMASAL IMPACTION

Definition

Abomasal impaction may be defined as the abnormal accumulation of solid ingesta in the abomasum. It is caused by a failure of the abomasal musculature to contract properly ("abomasal pump"), the ingestion of foreign material, or dietary inadequacies such as coarse indigestible feeds. The history usually indicates a gradual onset of disease, and the disease frequently goes unnoticed until the terminal stages. Abomasal impaction is seen most commonly in commercial beef cattle fed marginal rations, but it also occurs in dairy calves. Specific forms of abomasal impaction could be categorized as follows:

1. Primary abomasal impaction results from ingestion of excessive amounts of coarse, indigestible roughages. It occurs in beef cows in many parts of the country from attempts to reduce feed costs for maintenance through the winter months. Cows fed late-cut hay, straw, and corn stover during the winter months are particularly vulnerable. These indigestible feeds accumulate in the abomasum and secondarily fill the reticulum and rumen. Because of

the indigestibility, a negative energy balance develops. Since adequate nutrients are not absorbed, cows retain a good appetite and consume the offending feed until the physical capacity of the rumen limits further intake. Affected cows are usually unthrifty and in a state of starvation.

Individually fed dairy calves may be similarly affected. Calves receiving inadequate nutrition from poor-quality milk replacers will sometimes eat bedding or other rough forages, causing impaction of the abomasum.

2. Foreign material may become entrapped in the abomasum, causing primary impaction. Cows frequently eat the placenta following parturition, which may occasionally become lodged in the abomasum, blocking the pyloric opening and leading to impaction. Large quantities of baling twine may be ingested, become entrapped in the abomasum, form a concretion, and lead to impaction. Unthrifty or louse-infected young cattle may ingest large quantities of hair by licking. The hair may become a trichobezoar in the abomasum, causing impaction.

3. Failure of the abomasal "pump" due to a lack of motility should be considered a secondary abomasal impaction. In vagus indigestion the abomasum is sometimes filled with semisolid material resembling an impaction. A similar situation complicates surgical correction of abomasal torsion when the abomasal musculature or nervous innervation is damaged sufficiently to prevent emptying. Often the abomasal contents are fluid.

Clinical Signs

Abomasal impaction usually occurs in the winter in beef cows. Long hair tends to mask the poor body condition. Also, the abdomen becomes distended because of the ingesta, giving the cow a round, fat appearance. Cows that are casually observed by owners are often thought to be fat and healthy, when upon closer examination they are found to be very thin. The disease may be advanced, and death may occur before owners realize that problems exist.

The major clinical signs are the characteristic shape of the distended abdomen (Fig. 9), poor body condition, and dehydration. The fecal output is reduced in volume and is hard and dry in most cases. Temperature, pulse, and respirations are normal.

Clinical Pathology

Hypochloremic metabolic alkalosis may occur but is not as predictable in abomasal impaction as in vagus indigestion. The catabolic state tends to produce metabolic acidosis, which modifies the overall acid-base status in the animal. Dehydration increases the packed cell volume and total protein, but these changes may be overriden by anemia and hypoproteinemia resulting from starvation. As a result, total protein and the packed cell volume may be in the normal range.

Diagnosis

Abomasal impaction produces a characteristic "papple"-shaped distention of the abdomen and should be differentiated from vagus indigestion, which may have a similar distention. Ballottement determines the fluid contents of the abomasum and rumen with vagus indigestion as compared with the firm contents in abomasal impaction. The history of a gradual onset of clinical signs and feeding poor-quality roughages will help confirm the diagnosis. A rumen distended with firm ingesta and the "L" shape may be found on rectal examination. The abomasum is usually beyond reach.

Malignant lymphoma may cause enlargement of the abomasal wall and accumulation of ingesta in the lumen. It can be differentiated in some cases by the presence of peripheral lymphadenopathy, circulation of neoplastic lymphocytes, and the serologic tests for bovine leukemia virus.

Treatment

Treatment of individual cattle is effective only in the early stages. In the earliest stages, saline cathartics, such as 0.5 kg of magnesium hydroxide or magnesium sulfate, effectively evacuate the abomasum. Fecal softeners, such as mineral oil and dioctyl sodium sulfosuccinate (DSS), may also be effective in softening the mass of ingesta. The rumen may be physically evacuated by rumenotomy in advanced cases, and the abomasum may be medicated by passing a stomach tube through the reticulo-omasal orifice and administering mineral oil or DSS directly into the abomasum. An indwelling nasogastric tube may be placed via rumenotomy for medication of the abomasum.[37] Physical removal of the abomasal contents by abomasotomy may also be done.[38]

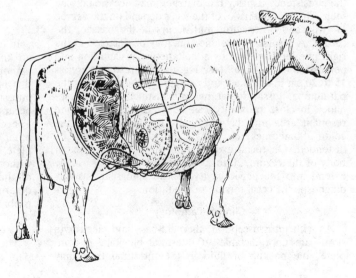

Figure 9. Abomasal impaction. The abomasum is engorged with firm feedstuffs and the rumen and reticulum are secondarily filled with similar material. The shape of the abdomen is identical to that illustrated in Figure 6.

As supportive treatment, intravenous and/or oral fluids re-establish hydration and provide nutritional support from glucose and amino acids. Animals with advanced cases suffering from starvation as well as abomasal impaction consistently respond poorly to therapy. To be successful, therapy should begin early.

Prevention

The welfare of the remainder of the herd should receive major emphasis when abomasal impaction is diagnosed. Foreign material, such as twine, should be removed from the environment when it is a cause. Nutrition should be improved by limiting coarse roughages and increasing the amount of high-quality hay or silage and, possibly, feeding concentrates. For calves, removing the bedding and improving the quality of milk replacer and starter rations are recommended.

CECAL TORSION

Definition

Torsion of the cecum occurs sporadically and is most frequently seen in dairy cattle in the immediate postpartum period. The cause is thought to be related to high concentrations of volatile fatty acids present in the lumen of the cecum.[39] Volatile fatty acids are passed in the ingesta from the rumen into the cecum or result from fermentation of undigested starch in the cecum. These acids cause atony of the cecum, leading to gas accumulation. The dilated cecum usually produces no clinical signs but predisposes to torsion. The cecum may twist at its base and involve the ileum as well as the colon.[40] The intestine and associated vasculature are obstructed. The apex of the cecum may extend caudally or cranially, depending on the nature of the twist. The exact degree and direction of the twist that occurs in cecal torsion have never been adequately described.

Clinical Signs

A dilated cecum without torsion is usually asymptomatic. At the onset of the twist signs of acute abdominal pain are consistently present[41] (see Abdominal Pain). Initially the feces may be normal but will decrease in volume and frequently develop a dark black color. Usually the consistency is pasty but diarrhea may occasionally be seen. The characteristics of the feces depend on the degree of twist and obstruction that occurs at the base of the cecum. A resonant tympanic area may be detected in the right paralumbar fossa by simultaneous auscultation and percussion of the area[41] (see Fig. 6). The resonant area is 15 to 20 cm in diameter and centered in the middle of the paralumbar fossa. Sometimes two distinct areas of resonance in close proximity can be detected. The second resonant area may be caused by gas distention in the colon. Sometimes the right paralumbar fossa will be distended. On rectal examination the gas-filled apex or body of the cecum, 20 to 25 cm in diameter, will usually extend into the pelvic cavity. These finings are usually diagnostic for cecal torsion or dilatation.

Clinical Pathology

As with intussusception, the acid-base and electrolyte status are unpredictable. If intestinal blockage is complete, the backup of fluid in the intestinal tract may ultimately prevent emptying of the abomasum. In these cases hypochloremic hypokalemic metabolic alkalosis will be present. With incomplete blockages or in the early stages of complete blockage when the abomasum can still empty into the intestinal tract, normal blood-gas parameters may exist. In such cases, serum chloride levels will be normal or only slightly decreased. Dehydration usually increases packed cell volume and total protein.

Diagnosis

The differential diagnosis of cecal torsion includes other diseases that cause a ping in the right paralumbar fossa. In right displaced abomasum or torsion of the abomasum, the ping is located in the most anterior aspect of the paralumbar fossa and extends further anteriorly than with cecal torsion. Gas within the colon may produce a ping in the same general vicinity; however, the animal is usually not as sick and the tympanitic area is usually smaller and does not extend as far posteriorly as with cecal torsion. Other causes of intestinal obstruction can be differentiated by rectal examination. In most cases, the rectal examination findings with cecal torsion are characteristic and diagnostic.

Treatment

Conservative treatments for cecal torsion are unrewarding, and immediate surgery is indicated. The best approach is from a right paralumbar laparotomy in a standing animal.[42] The cecum will be encountered just beneath the incision and frequently the apex can be exteriorized. The cecal contents should be completely removed. Not only does this aid detorsion, but it also removes the volatile fatty acids that predisposed to torsion and that could cause atony and dilatation of the cecum following surgery. In some animals, the cecum is degenerated and necrotic. Typhlectomy has proved successful.[42]

Supportive therapy includes antibiotics and fluids. If blood-gas data are available, the composition of the fluids can be specifically designed to combat the acid-base and electrolyte abnormalities. Otherwise, the use of balanced electrolyte solutions such as Ringer's solution is indicated. The volume to be administered depends on the degree of dehydration and shock in the animal.

INTUSSUSCEPTION

Definition

Intussusception occurs sporadically in cattle. There is no known breed, sex, or age group susceptibility. The pathophysiology in cattle is similar in most respects to that in other species. A major difference in cattle is that intussusception usually occurs in the jejunum and seldom occurs in the large intestine or ileocecal valve region.[42] The clinical course is more prolonged in cattle than in other species such as horses. Cattle have survived complete obstruction from intussusception as long as 12 days without showing extreme signs appropriate for the severity of the condition. The precise etiology has never been determined, and the history does not usually indicate the probable cause.

Clinical Signs

The animal will usually exhibit signs of acute abdominal pain and colic when intussusception first occurs. These signs gradually subside in 12 to 24 hours, and from then until death progressive depression and inactivity are observed. The animal does not eat or drink and becomes progressively more dehydrated.

The feces are normal in consistency, color, and volume at the onset of obstruction. After about 12 hours a small amount of blood and mucus, originating at the site of obstruction, gradually traverses the intestinal tract and appears in the feces. Fecal volume gradually decreases for several days after obstruction but may not cease for three or four days. Since intussusception is usually in the anterior intestinal tract, fecal output does not cease immediately. Feces are often fluid in the first 24 hours but gradually become firmer and by three or four days post obstruction will be dry or pasty. The feces are usually dark brown or black owing to the extravasation of blood at the site of intussusception.

Initially, the abdomen has a normal contour. Within about 12 hours, gas accumulation in the small intestine anterior to the area of obstruction (jejunum and duodenum) causes a progressive distention of the abdomen. The animal will have a symmetrically rounded shape on both the left and right sides of the abdomen. Auscultation and percussion of the right side of the abdomen may reveal small tympanic areas in various locations depending upon where the gas-distended intestines contact the abdominal wall. Resonant areas are usually absent on the left side of the abdomen because of the rumen.

Multiple loops of gas-distended small intestine located forward from the pelvic inlet are found on rectal palpation. The intussusception itself is rarely palpable.

Clinical Pathology

There is hemoconcentration with an increase in the packed cell volume and total protein. The total leukocyte count may be increased in advanced cases with necrosis at the intussusception. The leukocyte count and total protein may be increased in peritoneal fluid obtained by abdominal paracentesis, indicating a severe inflammatory process.

The acid-base status is not predictable. If the intussusception is in the anterior small intestine, there is a progressive backup of fluid into the abomasum, causing a functional pyloric obstruction that leads to hypochloremic hypokalemic metabolic alkalosis (see Abomasal Torsion). If the intussusception is situated posteriorly in the intestinal tract, abomasal fluid can escape into the small intestine for a long time and be absorbed. In these cases, normal acid-base status may be found. As with all obstructive diseases, the animal will eventually become acidotic in the terminal stages.

Diagnosis

The acute abdominal pain and abdominal distention associated with intussusception must be differentiated from abdominal pain caused by other diseases. Torsion of the root of the mesentery and strangulated hernias are particularly similar and difficult to differentiate. Hernias can be differentiated by palpation, but in many instances torsion of the root of the mesentery cannot be diagnosed until surgery.

Treatment

The treatment for intussusception is immediate surgery. An approach from the right paralumbar fossa in the standing animal allows for excellent exploration of the abdomen. The disadvantage of standing surgery is that the animal may attempt to lie down because of the intense pain that results from intestinal manipulation.

In the recumbent animal the right paralumbar fossa or the ventral midline approach may be used. It is more difficult to explore the abdomen in recumbent cattle with abdominal distention; however, the exposure of the intussusception may be better. There is better control of the animal in the recumbent position while the intussusception is exteriorized. In either case, the intussusception must be reduced and/or resected and an intestinal anastomosis performed.

Supportive therapy is essential during and following surgery. Intensive fluid therapy is usually required to combat dehydration and shock.

TORSION OF THE ROOT OF THE MESENTERY

Definition

This occurs sporadically and is usually seen in dairy cows; however, no specific age, sex, or breed predisposition has been found. The entire small intestine twists approximately 360 degrees around the mesenteric root. The cause is unknown, although it has occurred following rolling of cows to correct uterine torsion or LDA. It has also occurred after paramedian abomasopexy to correct LDA.[42]

Clinical Signs

Acute abdominal pain and decreasing fecal output are seen. A progressive and symmetric distention of the abdomen will occur. Tympanic areas can sometimes be auscultated on the right side of the abdomen. On rectal examination multiple gas-distended loops of small intestine will fill the abdominal cavity and extend into the pelvic cavity. The site of the twist in the mesentery is usually beyond reach.

Treatment

Immediate surgery is indicated.[42] The abdomen should be explored from the right paralumbar fossa in the standing animal. Most cases cannot be definitively diagnosed without surgery. With careful palpation, the twist in the mesentery can be located in the dorsal abdomen in the area of the left kidney. The direction of the twist can be determined by palpation, and most cases can be corrected by manipulation within the abdomen. Portions of the intestine may have to be decompressed, and a portion of the intestine may be exteriorized to facilitate correction of the twist. The prognosis is good where early diagnosis and surgery can be accomplished. Supportive therapy should include antibiotics and intravenous fluids.

STRANGULATED INGUINAL HERNIA

Definition

Strangulated inguinal hernia usually occurs in mature bulls. A loop of intestine may accidentally drop into the internal inguinal ring. A congenital enlargement of the internal ring probably predisposes to this accident. The left inguinal ring is almost always affected. Obstruction will not occur if the inguinal canal is large and the intestine can freely move within the ring and scrotum. In fact, some bulls may live for years with a large inguinal hernia without signs of intestinal malfunction. However, if the ring is small, the intestine will become entrapped and ingesta will not pass. External enlargement of the scrotum may not be apparent if the ring is small and a small amount of intestine drops into the inguinal canal. Because the inguinal hernia is not always apparent externally, it is important to consider this when examining bulls with intestinal obstruction.

Clinical Signs

The signs of acute abdominal pain, tympany, abdominal distention, and decreased fecal output seen in strangulated inguinal hernia are similar to those seen in torsion of the root of the mesentery and intussusception. Sometimes an enlargement may be visible at the neck of the scrotum.

Diagnosis

The diagnosis can be made in all cases by rectal palpation of the internal inguinal ring. In every case of intestinal obstruction in a bull, the inguinal rings should be thoroughly examined for a hernia.

Treatment

Immediate surgery is required using either a left paralumbar laparotomy on the standing bull or a ventral approach over the inguinal canal at the neck of the scrotum.

Prevention

The owner should be advised that inguinal hernias may be hereditary. He can than decide whether to continue using the bull for breeding.

ATRESIA COLI

Definition

Atresia coli is a congenital abnormality in calves in which the colon ends blindly in the region of the spiral colon. The distal portion of the colon is usually atretic or hypoplastic. The anus is usually normal, and the rectum is often normal for a distance of several inches.

Some believe that this is an inherited defect, although it has never been substantiated. A very high incidence of atresia coli has been found in unrelated calves in particular communities. It has also occurred in only one of a set of identical twins.[43] Early pregnancy diagnosis by rectal palpation has also been suspected as a cause. A similar condition has been produced in dogs by ligating intestinal vessels in the embryo. Because of these facts, there is considerable doubt that this is an inherited defect.[43]

Clinical Signs

The history and clinical signs present a characteristic pattern. The calf is born normal, active, and healthy and nurses normally. Approximately 12 to 24 hours after consuming colostrum the calf shows acute abdominal pain. The abdomen gradually distends symmetrically over the next two to three days. The acute abdominal pain subsides in about 24 hours and is replaced by depression and lethargy. A careful history will reveal that no bowel movements have ever been observed, and there will be no evidence of feces on the tail or rear parts of the calf.

Diagnosis

Acute indigestion from overfeeding of colostrum, acute peritonitis due to umbilical infection, intussusception, and *E. coli* septicemia from colostrum deprivation should be included in the differential diagnosis in a newborn calf. The diagnosis can be based on a history of no bowel movements, the onset of acute abdominal pain at 12 to 24 hours of age, and progressive abdominal distention.

Treatment

Calves can be saved by performing a colostomy or by anastomosis of the blind end of the colon to the rectum.[42]

Prevention

In advising clients, veterinarians should be cautious in discouraging the use of the sire and dam of the calf for breeding. It is probable that atresia coli is not inherited, and restricting the use of the sire and dam as breeders is not warranted in light of currently available information.

ABDOMINAL PAIN

Definition

Abdominal pain originates from stretch receptors in the serosal surfaces of all intestinal, urinary, and reproductive organs and the peritoneum. They are also located in the mesenteric attachments of these organs. Anything that stretches these organs, such as distention or torsion, will induce pain. Sometimes, manipulation of organs and mesenteries during surgery causes pain. Direct trauma to the surface of the organ, as in traumatic reticuloperitonitis or ulceration of mucosal surfaces, produces pain. The manifestations of abdominal pain are similar in all cattle regardless of the specific cause. It is important to recognize these signs and to differentiate the probable causes. Signs of abdominal pain are often the primary reasons clients seek veterinary service for their affected animals.

Clinical Signs

Cattle with abdominal pain have the overall appearance of discomfort. Frequently they may kick at their abdomen with their rear legs. Stretching, arching of the back, and frequent and alternate standing and lying down indicate discomfort. Cows may shift their weight from one hind leg to another in rapid fashion ("treading"). Cattle are sometimes reluctant to move and often have an anxious, wide-eyed expression. Affected cattle will usually isolate themselves from the remainder of the herd. They also refuse all feed and water, and milk production will be decreased or nearly absent in lactating cows. Some assume a crouching position as though they are attempting to lie down. The heart rate is usually increased to approximately 100 beats per minute. Respirations are increased but shallow in character, giving the impression that deep respiratory movements are painful.

Differential Diagnosis

Stretching of the abomasal wall causes pain in abomasal torsion. The diagnosis is based on a large area of resonant tympany (ping) audible on the right side of the abdomen.

The abomasum can also be palpated by rectal examination.

The abdominal pain in cecal torsion results from stretching of the wall of the cecum. A ping is auscultated in the right paralumbar fossa, and the cecum can be identified by rectal examination.

Intussusception induces pain from stretching of the intestine and mesentery as well as distention of the intestine proximal to the obstruction. Tympany may be present at several sites along the right side of the abdomen. Finding bilateral abdominal distention and gas-distended loops of intestine on rectal examination help differentiate this condition.

Torsion of the root of the mesentery results in abdominal pain because of stretching of the mesentery. Tympany, bilateral abdominal distention, and the rectal examination findings in torsion of the mesentery root are similar to those of intussusception. These two conditions are usually differentiated at surgery.

A strangulated inguinal or umbilical hernia causes pain from distention of the intestine with fluid proximal to the obstruction. In both conditions, gas-distended loops of intestine are found on rectal examination and the abdomen has bilateral distention. Inguinal herniation can be definitively diagnosed by rectal examination of the internal inguinal rings. Umbilical hernias can be diagnosed by external palpation of the umbilical area.

Penetration of the foreign body causes pain in traumatic reticuloperitonitis. Localization of pain in the anterior abdomen, the presence of a low-grade fever, a sudden decrease in milk production, mild neutrophilia, and a history of exposure to foreign bodies help differentiate this condition.

Urolithiasis with urethral or bladder distention induces pain due to distention of the serosal surfaces of these structures. A history of lack of urination, the presence of a distended bladder on rectal palpation, and an elevated BUN help to diagnose urolithiasis.

Blockage of the ureter with exudate results in pain in pyelonephritis. An abnormal urinalysis coupled with an enlarged ureter found on rectal palpation help with its differentiation.

Abomasal ulcers may induce pain from direct trauma to the abomasal wall or regional peritonitis from perforation. Ulcers usually bleed into the intestinal tract, resulting in dark, tarry stools (melena).

Abnormalities of the uterus frequently induce abdominal pain. Uterine torsion is the most notable uterine abnormality that consistently results in pain. This can be definitively diagnosed by rectal and/or vaginal examination. Diffuse peritonitis may also cause pain primarily owing to movement or disturbances of abdominal adhesions.

Differentiation of the various causes of abdominal pain is primarily accomplished by physical examination coupled with a skillfully obtained history. In some cases, clinical laboratory findings or exploratory surgery is necessary for a definitive diagnosis.

References

1. Begg, H.: Diseases of the stomach of the adult ruminant. Vet. Rec. 62:797, 1950.
2. Stober, M., Wegner, W., and Lunebrink, J.: Research on the familial occurrence of left-sided displacement of the abomasum in cattle. Bovine Pract. 10:59, 1975.
3. Martin, S. W., Kirby, K. L., and Curtis, R. A.: A study of the role of genetic factors in the etiology of left abomasal displacement. Can. J. Comp. Med. 42:511, 1978.
4. Robertson, J. M.: Left displacement of the bovine abomasum: Epizootiologic factors. Am. J. Vet. Res. 29:421, 1968.
5. Coppock, C. E., Noller, C. H., Wolfe, S. A., et al.: Effect of forage-concentrate ratio in complete feeds fed ad libitum on feed intake prepartum and the occurrence of abomasal displacement in dairy cows. J. Dairy Sci. 55:783, 1972.
6. Coppock, C. E.: Displaced abomasum in dairy cattle: Etiological factors. J. Dairy Sci. 57:926, 1974.
7. Svendsen, P.: Etiology and pathogenesis of abomasal displacement in cattle. Nord. Vet. Med. 21:Suppl. 1, 1, 1969.
8. Ash, R. W.: Inhibition of reticulo-rumen contractions by acid. Proc. Physiological Soc., July 10 and 21, 1956, 75–76.
9. Wallace, C. E.: Left abomasal displacement—A retrospective study of 315 cases. Bovine Pract. 10:50, 1975.
10. Ingling, A. L., Albert, T. F. and Schueler, R. L.: Left displacement of the abomasum in a clinically normal cow. J. Am. Vet. Med. Assoc. 166:601, 1975.
11. Wallace, C. E.: Prognostic significance of diarrhea in cows with left displacement of the abomasum. Bovine Pract. 11:62, 1976.
12. Whitlock, R. H.: Pathophysiology of lower gastrointestinal tract problems in the bovine. Proc. 9th Ann. Conv. Am. Assoc. Bovine Pract. 1976, 43–48.
13. Gingerich, D. A.: Paradoxical aciduria in bovine metabolic alkalosis. J. Am. Vet. Med. Assoc. 166:227, 1975.
14. Gingerich, D. A., and Murdick, P. W.: Experimentally induced intestinal obstruction in sheep: Paradoxical aciduria in metabolic alkalosis. Am. J. Vet. Res. 36:663, 1975.
15. Robertson, J. M.: Diagnosis of left displacement of the bovine abomasum. J. Am. Vet. Med. Assoc., 146:820, 1965.
16. Cote, J. F.: Displaced abomasum—A method of correction. Can. Vet. J. 1:58, 1960.
17. Hull, B. L.: Closed suturing technique for correction of left abomasal displacement. Iowa State Univ. Vet. 3:142, 1972.
18. Grymer, J., and Sterner, K. E.: Percutaneous fixation of left displaced abomasum, using a bar suture. J. Am. Vet. Med. Assoc. 180:1458, 1982.
19. Lowe, S. E., Loomis, W. K., and Kramer, L. L.: Abomasopexy for repair of left displacement in dairy cattle. J. Am. Vet. Med. Assoc. 147:389, 1965.
20. Robertson, J. M., and Boucher, W. B.: Treatment of left displacement of the bovine abomasum. J. Am. Vet. Med. Assoc. 149:1423, 1966.
21. Ames, S, II: Repositioning displaced abomasum in the cow. J. Am. Vet. Med. Assoc. 153:1470, 1968.
22. Hoffsis, G. F.: Right paralumbar omentopexy for the correction of left displaced abomasum. Proc. 4th Ann. Conv. Am. Assoc. Bovine Pract., 1971, 1979.
23. Gabel, A. A., and Heath, R. B.: Correction and right-sided omentopexy in the treatment of left-sided displacement of the abomasum in dairy cattle. J. Am. Vet. Med. Assoc. 155:632, 1969.
24. Staubus, S.: Management suggestions for preventing left displaced abomasums. Ohio State Univeristy, Dept. of Dairy Science, personal communication.
25. Gabel, A. A., and Heath, R. B.: Treatment of right-sided torsion of the abomasum in cattle. J. Am. Vet. Med. Assoc. 155:642, 1969.
26. Poulsen, J. S. D.: Clinical chemical examination of a case of left-sided abomasal displacement changing to right-sided abomasal displacement. Nord. Vet. Med. 26:91, 1974.
27. Pearson, H.: The treatment of surgical disorders of the bovine abdomen. Vet. Rec. 92:245, 1973.
28. Habel, R. E., and Smith, D. F.: Volvulus of the bovine abomasum and omasum. J. Am. Vet. Med. Assoc. 179:447, 1981.
29. Smith, D. F., et al.: The identification of structure and conditions responsible for right side tympanitic resonance (ping) in adult cattle. Cornell Vet. 72:180, 1982.
30. Hammond, P. B., Dzuik, H. E. Usenik, E. A., and Stevens, C. E.: Experimental intestinal obstruction in calves. J. Comp. Patho. Therap. 74:210, 1964.
31. Whitlock, R. H.: Bovine stomach diseases. In Anderson, N. V. (ed.): Veterinary Gastroenterology. Lea & Febiger, Philadelphia, 1980, 396–432.
32. Boucher, W. B., and Abt, D.: Right-sided dilatation of the bovine abomasum with torsion. J. Am. Vet. Med. Assoc. 153:76, 1968.
33. Smith, D. A.: Right-side torsion of the abomasum in dairy cows: Classification of severity and evaluation of outcome. J. Am. Vet. Med. Assoc. 173:108, 1978.
34. Neal, P. A., and Edwards, G. B.: Vagus indigestion in cattle. Vet. Rec. 82:296, 1968.

35. Rebhun, W. C.: Vagus indigestion in cattle. J. Am. Vet. Med. Assoc. *176*:506, 1980.
36. Ferrante, P., and Whitlock, R.: Chronic (vagus) indigestion in cattle: Comp. Cont. Ed. Prac. Vet. *3*:S231, 1981.
37. Baker, J. A.: Abomasal impactions and related obstructions of the forestomachs in cattle. J. Am. Vet. Med. Assoc. *175*:1250, 1979.
38. Merritt, A. B., and Boucher, W. B.: Surgical treatment of the abomasal impaction in the cow. J. Am. Vet. Med. Assoc. *150*:1115, 1968.
39. Svendsen, P., and Kristensen, B.: Cecal dilation in cattle. Nord. Vet. Med. *22*:578, 1970.
40. Jones, W. E., Johnson, L., and Moore, C. C.: Torsion of the bovine cecum. J. Am. Vet. Med. Assoc. *140*:167, 1957.
41. Whitlock, R. H.: Cecal volvulus in dairy cattle. Proc. Int. Cong. Dis. Cattle. 1976, 69–74.
42. Robertson, J. T.: Differential diagnosis and surgical management of intestinal obstruction in cattle. Vet. Clin. North Am. *1*:377, 1979.
43. Hoffsis, G. F., and Bruner, R. R.: Atresia coli in a twin calf. J. Am. Vet. Med. Assoc. *171*:433, 1977.

Enteritis and Diarrhea

ROBERT H. WHITLOCK, D.V.M., Ph.D.

Diarrhea, as defined by Hippocrates, is the abnormal frequency and liquidity of fecal discharges. This definition applies today regardless of species, but the characterization of normal feces depends on diet, age, and season of the year. For example, beef cattle on lush green spring pasture have very loose manure, whereas dairy heifers fed only dry hay during the stabling season have firm feces; both are normal.

PATHOPHYSIOLOGY

The pathophysiologic mechanisms that produce diarrhea include osmotic material in the gastrointestinal tract; secretory diarrhea; inhibited absorption; changes in mucosal permeability; and deranged motility.[1]

Osmotic diarrheas may be caused by three different mechanisms: (1) poorly absorbed solutes, such as magnesium sulfate or magnesium hydroxide, which are commonly administered saline laxatives; (2) maldigestion from pancreatic insufficiency (rare in cattle); and (3) intrinsic defects within the mucosa that may increase osmotic load within the lumen, therefore predisposing to diarrhea (rare in cattle). Calves, for example, lack the mucosal enzyme sucrase and when fed table sugar (sucrose) an enhanced osmotic load (unabsorbed solute) would be induced in the bowel with resultant diarrhea due to mucosal enzymatic defects.[2]

One cause of secretory diarrhea is increased passive secretion of electrolytes from the intestinal mucosa into the lumen of the bowel. Nutrients, electrolytes, and water are constantly being absorbed from the intestinal lumen through the tips of the villi and into the blood stream; simultaneously, water and electrolytes from the blood stream are secreted through the base of the villi into the lumen, establishing a bidirectional flux across the intestinal mucosa. Several inflammatory diseases (including salmonellosis,[3] bovine virus diarrhea, paratuberculosis [Johne's disease], and invasive *Escherichia coli*[4, 5]) and noninflammatory diseases (including heart failure, lymphosarcoma,[6] caudal vena caval obstruction, and systemic amyloidosis[7]) may increase intestinal secretion into the

bowel lumen, increasing the net flux into the lumen and thus causing diarrhea. Each of these noninflammatory diseases may be associated with increased hydrostatic pressure either by interference with venous return or by a decreased plasma oncotic (not osmotic) pressure (amyloidosis).

Mucosal permeability may be altered by a change in the surface area as occurs with sprue, coronavirus,[8, 9] malabsorption syndrome, and Johne's disease, and with lymphosarcoma when neoplastic cells infiltrate the mucosa.[6] Factors that increase effective tissue pressure, such as inflammation, lymphatic obstruction, and decreased plasma colloid oncotic pressure, change the permeability of the mucosa and lead to diarrhea.

ABNORMAL MOTILITY

Borborygmi, sounds resulting from the admixture of gas and fluid in the lumen of the bowel during auscultation of the abdomen, are not synonymous with effective peristalsis. Occasionally prominent borborygmal sounds may be heard in animals with the passage of normal feces, whereas some animals with diarrhea may have an absence of borborygmi. Many diarrheas attributed to disordered motility are more commonly associated with an increased intraluminal volume due to some of the factors listed previously. These increased intestinal fluid volumes result in a garden hose effect when the faucet is turned on, i.e., an increased flow or diarrhea. Increased intestinal propulsive activity has rarely been shown to cause diarrhea in animals.

THERAPY

The cornerstone of therapy in acute diarrhea is fluid and electrolyte replacement. Oral glucose and electrolyte solutions have been used successfully as aids in the correction of dehydration in human diarrheal diseases of diverse causes.[10] Most oral electrolyte solutions formulated to treat diarrhea contain approximately 100 mM/L glucose and 40 to 100 mM/L sodium. All currently available commercial oral electrolyte formulations* are marketed as nutritional aids, and their exact compositions are not widely advertised. Most formulations are based on the concept of glucose- and glycine-facilitated water absorption in the small intestine. Needless to say, cattle with severe dehydration are best treated with intravenous fluids. In most situations these fluids should be rich in bicarbonate, as the animals usually have a severe metabolic acidosis.[11, 12]

Nonspecific antidiarrheal therapy includes compounds (opiate derivatives) that alter intestinal motility, that is, increase segmental contractions so as to retard the flow of ingesta. Absorbants (kaolin and pectin) may absorb toxins, and bismuth subsalicylate (Pepto-BismolR†) has been shown to decrease intestinal hypersecretion.[13] *Lactobacillus acidophilus* cultures have been utilized to alter

---

*Glycolyte Powder, Summit Hill Laboratories, Avalon, NJ 08202; Re-Sorb, Beecham Laboratories, Bristol, TN 37620; Ion-Aid, Diamond Laboratories, Des Moines, IA 50317; Hydaid, Syntex, Des Moines, IA 50304; Life-guard, Norden Laboratories, Lincoln, NE 68501; Electroplus-A, Pitman-Moore, Washington's Crossing, NJ 08560.
†Available from Morton-Norwich Products, Norwich, NY 13815.

the gut flora but are of unproven efficacy.[14] Recent research has shown that *Lactobacillus acidophilus* is of no value in the treatment or prevention of induced diarrheal diseases.[15]

Broad-spectrum antibiotics have been used as primary therapeutic aids for infectious diarrheal diseases for years, but documentation to justify their usage is lacking, as most therapeutic trials in cattle have been uncontrolled.[16] Additionally, many question their use because (1) enteric pathogens (*E. coli* and *Salmonella*) are often resistant to most approved antibiotics and (2) their use does not always improve the survival rate.[17] Neonatal calf diarrheas are usually a complex of diseases due to the interaction of viruses, bacteria, and immune deficiency.[18, 19] Antibiotics are not of value for viral diarrheas but have been efficacious for enterotoxic colibacillosis in lambs.[20] This suggests that if oral antibiotics are beneficial, results should be obvious within the first 36 hours, and the indiscriminate and prolonged administration of antimicrobics should be avoided.

The major indication for parenteral antibiotic therapy in diarrheal disease is the suspicion of bacterial septicemia. Then a broad-spectrum antibiotic, such as gentamicin, or a nitrofuran may be indicated if the organism is susceptible. The indiscriminate use of antibiotics has brought about resistant strains and rendered even the most potent antibiotic of little value in some situations.

References

1. Fordtran, J. S.: Speculations on the pathogenesis of diarrhea. Fed. Proc. 26:1405, 1967.
2. Huber, J. T., Jacobson, N. L., McGilliard, A. D., and Allen, R. S.: Utilization of carbohydrates introduced directly into the omaso-abomasal area of the stomach of cattle of various ages. J. Dairy Sci. 44:321, 1961.
3. Giannela, R. A., Formal, S. B., Dammin, G. J., and Collins, H.: Pathogenesis of salmonellosis: Studies of fluid secretion, mucosal invasion and morphologic reaction in the rabbit ileum. J. Clin. Invest. 52:441, 1973.
4. Dupont, H. L., et al.: Pathogenesis of *Escherichia coli* diarrhea. N. Engl. J. Med. 284:1, 1971.
5. Grady, G. F., and Keusch, G. T.: Pathogenesis of bacterial diarrheas. N. Engl. J. Med. 285:831, 891, 1971.
6. Wiseman, A., Petrie, L., and Murray, M.: Diarrhea in the horse as a result of alimentary lymphosarcoma. Vet. Rec. 90:210, 1972.
7. Murray, M., Rushton, A., and Selman, I.: Bovine renal amyloidosis: a clinicopathological study. Vet. Rec. 90:210, 1972.
8. Mebus, C. A.: Pathogenesis of coronaviral infection in calves. J. Am. Vet. Med. Assoc. 173:631, 1978.
9. Mebus, C. A., Newman, L. E., and Stair, E. L. Jr.: Scanning electron, light and immunofluorescent microscopy of intestine of gnotobiotic calf infected with calf diarrhea coronavirus. Am. J. Vet. Res. 36:1719, 1975.
10. Bywater, R. J.: Evaluation of an oral glucose-glycine-electrolyte formulation and amoxicillin for treatment of diarrhea in calves. Am. J. Vet. Res. 38:1983, 1977.
11. Whipp, S. C.: Physiology of diarrhea—small intestines. J. Am. Vet. Med. Assoc. 173:662, 1978.
12. Whitlock, R. H.: Pathophysiology of lower gastrointestinal tract problems in the bovine. Proc. Am. Assoc. Bovine Pract. 1976, 43–48.
13. Ericsson, C. D., Evans, D. G., Dupont, H. L., Evans, D. J. Jr., and Pickering, L. K.: Bismuth subsalicylate inhibits activity of crude toxins of *Escherichia coli* and *Vibrio cholerae*. J. Infect. Dis. 136:693, 1977.
14. Dupont, H. L.: Interventions in diarrheas of infants and young children. J. Am. Vet. Med. Assoc. 173:649, 1978.
15. Mitchell, B.: Unpublished observations, 1979.
16. Tennant, B. C., Ward, D. E., Braun, R. K., Hunt, E. L., and Baldwin, B. H.: Clinical management and control of neonatal enteric infections of calves. J. Am. Vet. Med. Assoc. 173:654, 1978.
17. Radostits, O. M., Rhodes, C. S., Mitchell, M. E., Spotswood, T. P., and Wenkoff, M. S.: A clinical evaluation of antimicrobial agents and temporary starvation in the treatment of acute undifferentiated neonatal diarrhea in newborn calves. Can. Vet. J. 16:219, 1975.
18. Acres, S. D., Saunders, J. R., and Radostits, O. M.: Acute undifferential neonatal diarrhea of beef calves: the prevalence of enterotoxigenic E. coli, reo-like (rota) virus and other enteropathogens in cow-calf herds. Can. Vet. J. 18:113, 1977.
19. Moon, H. W., McClurkin, A. W., Isaacson, R. E., Pohlenz, J., Skartvedt, S. M., Gillette, K. G., and Baetz, A. L.: Pathogenic relationships of rotavirus, *Escherichia coli* and other agents in mixed infections in calves. J. Am. Vet. Med. Assoc. 173:577, 1978.
20. Smith, H. W., and Halls, S.: Observations by the ligated intestinal segment and oral inoculation methods on *Escherichia coli* infection in pigs, calves, lambs, and rabbits. J. Path. Bact. 93:499, 1967.

Supplemental Reading

Argenzio, R. A.: Physiology of diarrhea—large intestine. J. Am. Vet. Med. Assoc. 173:667, 1978.
Chen, L. C., Rohde, J. E., and Sharp, G. W. G.: Properties of adenyl cyclase from human jejunal mucosa during naturally acquired cholera and convalescence. J. Clin. Invest. 51:731, 1972.
Field, M.: Intestinal secretion: effect of cyclic AMP and its role in cholera. N. Engl. J. Med. 284:1137, 1971.
Gorbach, S. L.: Acute diarrhea—a "toxin" disease? N. Engl. J. Med. 283:44, 1970.
Moon, H. W.: Mechanisms in the pathogenesis of diarrhea: A review. J. Am. Vet. Med. Assoc. 172:443, 1978.

Colitis and Proctitis

ROBERT H. WHITLOCK, D.V.M., Ph.D.

Bovine colitis can be caused by salmonellosis, coccidiosis, winter dysentery, Johne's disease, and toxemias such as uremia, septic mastitis, and septic metritis among others.

Salmonellosis can be an individual or herd problem but commonly involves calves two to ten weeks of age. The clinical features include fever of 39 to 41°C, dullness, depression, profuse diarrhea with excessive mucus, and hematochezia. Definitive diagnosis is made by isolating the agent.

Coccidiosis typically involves young animals one month to two years of age. The feces contain more fresh blood than is seen in salmonellosis. Fever is usually absent in coccidiosis. For specific therapy of salmonellosis and coccidiosis please refer to other sections in the text.

Several other diseases that may result in colitis and proctitis include mycotoxicosis, Johne's disease, systemic amyloidosis with deposition of amyloid in the colon, eosinophilic enterocolitis, trichuriasis, and viral diseases, especially bovine virus diarrhea. A definitive diagnosis can best be made by a complete workup including virus isolation, bacterial culture, fecal cytology, and rectal biopsy, which is a safe procedure.[1]

PROCTITIS

Iatrogenic proctitis and tenesmus commonly occur in cattle with diarrhea following a rectal examination using plastic sleeves. The proctitis can be minimized with epidural anesthesia, the use of rubber surgeon's gloves over the plastic, and adequate lubrication. Both xylazine and Pro-Banthine bromide (30 mg/500 kg intravenously) assist in rectal relaxation, thus minimizing tenesmus.

A ruptured rectum may be due to sadism, careless rectal examination, or parturition.[2] Peritonitis is the sequela if perforation is complete; however, peripelvic abscesses may result from extraperitoneal rectal tears, whereas incomplete tears may leave only a cicatrix.

RECTAL STRICTURES

Rectal constriction is a form of proctitis and may occur as a result of (1) scarring due to a tear or traumatic injury to the mucosa; (2) stricture due to a nonexpanding circumferential lesion such as lymphosarcoma, peripelvic abscess, or fat necrosis; and (3) inherited defects associated with a rectal and vaginal stricture.[3] Jersey cows are particularly prone to this defect, which mechanically interferes with artificial insemination yet does not impair fertility. Dystocia is common, as are small, firm udders.

Rectal stricture of swine is an acquired annular fibrous rectal constriction (2.0 to 5.0 cm anterior to the anus) resulting in chronic obstipation.[4] Progressive emaciation and marked abdominal distention with intermittent foul, fetid feces characterize the disease.[5] Experimentally, both surgical manipulation of the arterial blood supply to the rectum and *Salmonella typhimurium* produce a prolonged enterocolitis and ulcerative proctitis with healed lesions, yielding an annular cicatricial ulcer of the rectum.[6] Rectal strictures often occur following an outbreak of enteric salmonellosis, and several swine in a group may be affected. No effective treatment is known.

RECTAL PROLAPSE

Rectal prolapse usually results from earlier bouts of tenesmus and has a higher incidence in the Hereford breed. The diagnosis is obvious, but successful treatment is often frustrating. The replacement of the prolapse is best accomplished following epidural anesthesia. Following replacement of the prolapsed tissue, a purse-string suture is usually necessary to prevent recurrence. In recurrent cases a submucosal resection may be needed to replace the prolapse or to prevent recurrence.

References

1. Morson, B. C.: Rectal biopsy in inflammatory bowel disease. N. Engl. J. Med. *287*:1337, 1972.
2. Van Kruiningen, H. J., Fox, F. H., and Weber, W. T.: Rupture of the rectum. Cornell Vet. *61*:557, 1961.
3. Leipold, H. W., and Saperstein, G.: Rectal and vaginal constriction in Jersey cattle. J. Am. Vet. Med. Assoc. *166*:231, 1975.
4. Lillie, L. E., Olander, H. J., and Gallina, A. M.: Rectal stricture of swine. J. Am. Med. Assoc. *163*:358, 1973.
5. Wilcock, B. P., and Olander, H. J.: The pathogenesis of porcine rectal stricture syndrome. I. The naturally occurring disease and its association with salmonellosis. Vet. Pathol. *14*:36, 1977.
6. Wilcock, B. P., and Olander, H. J.: The pathogenesis of porcine rectal stricture syndrome. II. Experimental salmonellosis and ischemic proctitis. Vet. Pathol. *14*:437, 1977.

Abomasal Ulcers

ROBERT H. WHITLOCK, D.V.M., Ph.D.

Abomasal ulcers can be classified as either perforating ulcers that cause peritonitis or nonperforating ulcers that may bleed and cause anemia. Abomasal ulcers may be classified into four categories labeled Types I through IV.

Although each type may vary dramatically according to the clinical signs, the pathogenesis of all types is probably very similar except for lymphosarcoma associated with ulcers.

PATHOPHYSIOLOGY

Increased gastric acid secretion may occur as a result of stress, which stimulates the adrenal gland and results in increased epinephrine release. Then more acid secretion by the stomach and/or stress will stimulate the hypothalamic-adrenal cortex axis to increase cortisol production. Cattle are as susceptible to stress factors as most other species. These stress factors may include high population density of cows, recent parturition, concurrent disease, high milk production, or severe weather changes. Any one of these or other factors or several stresses in concert may be sufficient to promote increased gastric acid or to decrease abomasal mucosal cell resistance, thus promoting an ulcer.

The major factors identified as requisites for ulcer formation in experimental animals are increased acid production and increased mucosal permeability to hydrogen (H^+) ions (induced by such agents as bile acids, aspirin, and VFA and by altered mucosal blood flow). Similar factors are probably operative in cattle. Neoplastic lymphoid cells infiltrate the abomasal wall and are likely to promote ulceration by interfering with the blood supply to the mucosa. The gastric mucosa of most species has two types of histamine receptors, Types I and II. Antihistamines block Type I receptors, which, when stimulated, produce vasodilatation, hypotension, and contraction of the smooth muscle of the gut and bronchi. Type II receptors, which are at least partially responsible for acid secretion, can be blocked with such drugs as cimetidine, ranitidine, and metiamide. These agents decrease acid production, thus preventing ulcerogenesis and facilitating ulcer healing.

Since the modern dairy or beef cow is being pushed for production, be it for milk or meat, some stress is always present. The abomasal mucosa is protected from normal levels of acid secretion by its mucus cover and the integrity of the mucosal cells; thus a delicate balance exists between the presence of acid and ulcer development. If one of the factors is absent or excessive, an ulcer may occur. In fact, nearly 100 per cent of calves at slaughter in one study had evidence of previous abomasal ulcers, most of which were clinically silent.

CLINICAL SIGNS

Type I Ulcer—Erosions and Ulcers

These ulcers usually occur secondary to other major disease processes such as septic mastitis or metritis. This ulcer type is most common in the early post-partum period and is recognized clinically by the presence of dark (occult blood positive) feces. Other causes of this type of ulcer include orally ingested nitrate, and other caustic agents and arsenic poisoning. As the animal recovers from the primary disease process, the ulcers and bleeding cease. Thus, the clinical symptomatology accompanying this type of ulcer is due to the primary disease rather than the ulcer.

Type II Ulcer—Bleeding Ulcers and Anemia

Affected cattle often have a history of dark, black stool and/or anemia as the major clinical sign. Occasionally these cows may have intercurrent disease, but the primary clinical sign may be related to the blood loss or dark stool. Benign bleeding ulcers are most common in two- to five-year-old cattle and occur uncommonly in cows over six years of age and rarely in nonlactating cows. The onset of clinical signs is rapid and response to therapy is prompt (two to five days if they survive).

Bleeding ulcers in older cows (more than five years) have a much greater likelihood of being associated with lymphosarcoma. Cows with lymphosarcoma-associated ulcers have a slower clinical onset (days or weeks) and often have weight loss. These ulcers occur throughout the lactational period, whereas 80 per cent of benign bleeding ulcers occur during the first month post partum.

A BLV titer would be of significant diagnostic value in these cases. The absence of a titer in a three-year-old cow would tend to rule out lymphosarcoma and indicate a better prognosis. Although a positive BLV titer is not diagnostic for lymphosarcoma, in combination with the clinical signs it should be of assistance. Most lymphosarcoma-associated ulcers occur in cattle over five years of age, whereas most benign bleeding ulcers occur in cows less than five years of age.

Type III Ulcer—Acute Circumscribed Peritonitis

Most ulcers that bleed do not perforate and most ulcers that perforate rarely bleed; thus the clinical signs associated with perforating acute ulcers are associated with peritonitis. Clinical signs of perforation with acute circumscribed peritonitis most closely resemble those seen with traumatic reticulitis. Localization of pain is the primary differentiating feature between acute peritonitis associated with abomasal perforation and reticulitis. The pain is present on the right side of the xiphoid with abomasal perforation, in contrast to a typical case of reticulitis where the pain is localized on the left side of the xiphoid. Similarly, these cows are reluctant to walk, have an abrupt decrease in milk production, tend to be "tucked up" (gaunt), and have decreased rumen motility. A peritoneocentesis is valuable in making a more definitive diagnosis of localized peritonitis.

Type IV Ulcer—Abomasal Ulcer Resulting in Perforation with Diffuse Peritonitis

Perhaps the most uncommon form of abomasal ulceration results in a fulminant peritonitis due to the perforated ulcer. Death often occurs 24 to 48 hours after the onset of clinical signs. The fulminant peritonitis is due to the extent of the ulcer with spillage of abomasal contents into the peritoneal cavity. The clinical signs are largely those of septic shock: severe tachycardia, hyperpnea, and precipitous drop in milk production.

THERAPY

The therapy of abomasal ulcers should be directed toward decreasing acid secretion if possible. Those cows with Type I ulcers usually respond as the primary disease is treated, i.e., the mastitis or metritis. Cows with bleeding abomasal ulcers should receive blood transfusions if they become significantly anemic, usually with a PCV of less than 15 and a heart rate greater than 100. Occasionally the blood loss may be so great that the PCV will not decrease although there is a tremendous loss of intravascular fluid. In these cases the heart rate and the pale mucous membranes may be the most important guides to therapy. It is not necessary to crossmatch the blood, but it is important to give large volumes of blood; usually several liters (6 to 10) will be required. The lifespan of transfused blood cells in cattle is relatively short and transfusions are only beneficial in emergency situations.

A decrease in acid secretion may be accomplished to some degree with the use of cimetidine or ranitidine. Cimetidine has been evaluated in cows and requires relatively large doses (8 to 16 mg/kg three times daily) to decrease acid secretion. This is a relatively large and expensive dose and may only be of minimal value. Ranitidine, used in human medicine, has not been evaluated in cattle. Another drug, carafate, a sulfated polysaccharide, has been effective orally in humans for gastric ulcers but has not been evaluated in cattle. It is expensive, yet relatively safe, and should be considered in a valuable animal.

Therapy for acute circumscribed peritonitis should be directed toward the use of antibiotics to minimize the infection and restricted exercise to prevent an extension of the peritonitis. Treatment would be similar to that given to cows for reticulitis with the exception of the use of a magnet.

Cows with perforated abomasal ulcers and diffuse peritonitis have a poor prognosis because of peritonitis, and death usually occurs. Even in cases where gastric resection has been attempted, lesions are so extensive that death is the result.

Supplemental Reading

Jensen, R., Pierson, R. E., Braddy, P. M., et al.: Fatal perforating ulcers in yearling feedlot cattle. J. Am. Vet. Med. Assoc. *169*:524–526, 1976.
Lahtinen, J., Aukee, S., Miettinen, P., et al.: Sucralfate and cimetidine for gastric ulcer. Scand. J. Gastro. *18*(Suppl. 83):49–51, 1983.
Palmer, J. E., and Whitlock, R. H.: Bleeding abomasal ulcers in dairy cattle. J. Am. Vet. Med. Assoc. *183*:448–451, 1983.
Palmer, J. E., and Whitlock, R. H.: Perforated abomasal ulcers in adult dairy cows. J. Am. Vet. Med. Assoc. *184*:171–174, 1984.
Whitlock, R. H., and Becht, J. L.: Probantheline bromide and cimetidine in the control of abomasal acid secretion. Proc. Am. Assoc. Bovine Pract. *15*:140, 1983.

Liver Disease (Hepatitis)

ROBERT H. WHITLOCK, D.V.M., Ph.D.

The clinical manifestations of liver disease in ruminants vary from obvious icterus to hepatoencephalopathy, epistaxis, chronic ketosis, emaciation, abdominal pain, and chronic diarrhea. Icterus in cattle is a relatively rare sign of liver disease, even in terminal liver failure. If icterus does occur it is more likely to be due to intravascular hemolysis, i.e., hemolytic anemia rather than liver disease.

LIVER ABSCESSES

The most common syndrome of liver abscess is, classically, the presence of clinically silent, occult lesions that are responsible for liver condemnation at slaughter but do not result in clinical disease. Most liver abscesses are associated with previous bouts of rumenitis caused by lactic acidosis and, as a result, are much more common in beef cattle than in dairy cattle. The anatomic location of the abscess in the liver determines the array of clinical signs. Several specific recognizable syndromes then develop, depending on the anatomic location of the abscess.

The second most common syndrome is one of gradual weight loss and a poor appetite without any localized signs. These abscesses can be located any place throughout the liver but cause problems because of their size or the organisms present. Some cows will give evidence of anterior abdominal pain by a failure to "scootch" when squeezed over the withers, but they do not show pain in the xiphoid region. This diagnostic feature helps differentiate traumatic reticulitis from liver abscess but is not specific for liver abscesses. Any inflammatory process in the thorax or high abdomen may cause pain. On occasion the Bromsulphalein (BSP T1/2) may be abnormal (greater than five minutes), suggesting a chronic parenchymatous lesion, but this is not specific for a liver abscess. The total protein, and specifically the gamma globulin, will be elevated as a reflection of chronic antigenic stimulation, i.e., an abscess.

The third, but less common, syndrome is acute anaphylactic shock and death due to release of purulent material from the liver abscess into the caudal vena cava. Once the abscess ruptures, the cow usually dies very suddenly. Collapse and death in minutes are usual, but some cows may show acute respiratory distress resembling atypical pneumonia and live for several days. This syndrome may resemble a heart attack, in that one minute the cow is normal and several minutes later it is dead. Few cows survive this syndrome despite intensive therapy.

The fourth most common syndrome of liver abscess is thrombosis of the caudal vena cava. This may also result in weight loss and emaciation, but one obvious difference is the development of mild ascites and chronic diarrhea. Both of these signs are associated with chronic passive congestion of the liver and decreased lymphatic flow from the abdominal viscera.[1] The clinical signs of emaciation and chronic diarrhea resemble those seen with paratuberculosis (Johne's disease). The almost pathognomonic clinical sign of this syndrome is the prominent distention of the mammary veins with obvious enlargement of collateral subcutaneous vessels in the ventral abdomen and lateral thoracic wall. The distention of the mammary veins without distention of the jugular veins helps differentiate thrombosis of the caudal vena cava from right heart failure (the other major diagnostic rule-out).

The fifth most common syndrome is epistaxis, which occurs as a result of a liver abscess that erodes into the caudal vena cava, producing a septic embolus that lodges in the lung, thus setting up an active infection in or around a pulmonary artery. Over a period of time, the lung abscess breaks into the bronchial tree, releasing blood and causing epistaxis.[2] An individual cow in a dairy herd with epistaxis should be suspected of having a lung abscess secondary to a liver abscess if it can be determined that the blood is not from the upper airways, for example, the sinuses owing to a nasal granuloma. Blood originating from the lung need not be frothy; in fact, many times it will drain from the nostrils as free blood. Most affected cows have intermittent periods of epistaxis, gradually lose

weight, and have decreased milk production. At some point following poor response to any treatment the cow is sent to salvage.

Therapy

The therapy of liver abscess (if attempted) should include the long-term use of antibiotics such as penicillin (10,000 I.U./kg). Penicillin should be effective, since more than 90 per cent of the abscesses contain *Fusobacterium Sphaerophorus necrophorum* and approximately 30 per cent of the abscesses contain *Corynebacterium pyogenes,* both of which are sensitive to penicillin.[3] Recently some veterinary clinicians have been using rifampin, a drug previously reserved for tuberculosis. Because of rifampin's ability to penetrate abscesses and its low toxicity, low cost, and unique mechanism of bacteriocidal activity (inhibits DNA-directed RNA polymerase), it is being used cautiously on animals with chronic abscesses, such as suspected liver abscesses. Its use should be in conjunction with another antibiotic.[4]

Experimentally, a toxoid from *Fusobacterium necrophorus,* when given prophylactically, reduced the incidence of liver abscesses more than 50 per cent.[5] Feed containing tylosin or chlortetracycline also has decreased the incidence of liver abscesses and has improved feed efficiency.[6] The overall prognosis for life or recovery from a clinical case of hepatic abscess is very low (less than 20 per cent); therefore, unless the animal is valuable, salvage is recommended.

FATTY LIVER SYNDROME (FAT COW SYNDROME)

Obese or overconditioned cows are predisposed to fatty liver syndrome, or fat cow syndrome, following a period of negative energy balance. Fatty liver can occur on a herd basis when dry cows are fed above energy requirements or in the individual cow having a long dry period or becoming overconditioned for other reasons. During a period of overconditioning, lipid (fat) is deposited in the hepatocyte and other body tissues, thus contributing to a mild physiologic fatty liver. During the dry period most overconditioned cows are clinically normal; however, following parturition with the initiation of lactation, new energy demands are placed on the liver.[7] Thus, as long as the cow consumes enough nutrients to meet her metabolic requirements, health may prevail. Should the cow go "off feed" for any reason, for example, mastitis, metritis, or left displaced abomasum, additional mobilized lipid is transported from the body stores to the hepatocyte, which then may compromise hepatocyte function. If the energy demands are not corrected or reversed, the cow may die of hepatic failure due to progressive fatty degeneration of the liver. Concurrent with increased hepatic lipid deposition is an increased intracellular neutral lipid deposition of skeletal muscle, which may explain some of the downer cows that have fatty livers.[8]

Clinical Signs

Physical examination usually reveals a cow in good to excellent condition but with partial anorexia, mild ketosis, and a depressed milk yield. The vital signs are often normal. As the disease progresses the cow may exhibit an "odd stare," hold its head high, have intermittent trembling, and eventually become recumbent. Cows with fatty liver are more susceptible to other diseases, such as left abomasal displacement, retained placenta, septic metritis, septic mastitis, and salmonellosis.

Laboratory examinations often indicate a low WBC count (less than 4,000/ccm), a mild hypoglycemia (less than 40 mg/dl), increased liver enzymes (SGOT, SDH, and OCT), and a prolonged BSP T1/2 (greater than seven minutes).[9] Mild ketolactia and ketonuria are to be expected. An elevated blood ammonia may be present in terminal cases. More definitive diagnostic methods include liver biopsy to measure hepatic lipid or triglyceride content chemically or histologically.[10] A simple estimate of hepatic lipid content can be based on the submersion of needle biposy specimens in water or copper sulfate solutions.[11] Cows with liver lipid concentrations above 34 per cent (biopsy specimen floated in 1.000 specific gravity solution with water) would be expected to have clinical manifestations of hepatic insufficiency.

Therapy

Treatment must be directed toward providing a positive energy balance, by either giving more energy to the cow or reducing her energy requirements. Corticosteroids (10 to 20 mg dexamethasone IM per 500 kg daily for three to five days) may promote a mild hyperglycemia and decrease milk production, which will reduce energy demands. However, these must be used judiciously since secondary or complicating diseases may be present concurrently.

Supplemental energy sources such as 200 gm glucose intravenously twice daily or an intravenous drip of 5 per cent dextrose in saline may be warranted. Oral propylene glycol (180 to 240 ml *per os* twice daily) is beneficial in that it promotes rumen protozoal activity and provides three carbon moieties that are glucogenic. Top dressing the feed with sodium proprionate may be counterproductive, as cows find it unpalatable. In advanced cases with complete anorexia, forcefeeding a gruel of electrolytes and alfalfa meal with propylene glycol may be advantageous. If the rumen analysis shows a few protozoa, then transfaunation of 10 to 20 liters of rumen liquor from a donor cow may prove very beneficial.

Lipotropic agents such as choline and methionine may be efficacious. If given, 40 to 60 gm methionine and/or 25 gm choline chloride orally BID has been indicated for the treatment of persistent ketosis in cattle with fatty liver syndrome.[12] Insulin (200 I.U. IM) of the protamine zinc preparation will help minimize further lipolysis. Cessation of milking or once daily milking will also reduce the energy demands.

The correction and treatment of complicating problems such as metritis, mastitis, or a displaced abomasum must be carried out if a response to the symptomatic therapy is expected.

Prevention

Fortunately this disease can easily be prevented by limiting caloric intake during the dry period. The body weight should not exceed 110 per cent of the cow's lactational weight during the dry period. Any cows that appear overweight should be fed less and not allowed *ad libitum* feed.

References

1. Rubarth, S.: Hepatic and subphrenic abscesses in cattle with rupture into vena cava caudalis. Acta Vet. Scand. *1*:363, 1960.
2. Selman, I. E., Wiseman, A., Petrie, L., Pirie, H., and Breeze, R. G.: A respiratory syndrome in cattle resulting from thrombosis of the posterior vena cava. Vet. Rec. *94*:459, 1974.
3. Thornsberry, C., Hill, B. C., and McDougal, L. K.: Rifampin: spectrum of antibacterial activity. Rev. Infect. Dis. *5*:(Suppl. 3)S412–417, 1983.
4. Scanlon, C. M., and Hathcock, T. L.: Bovine rumenitis-liver abscess complex: A bacteriological review. Cronell Vet. *73*:288, 1983.
5. Garcia, M. M., Dorward, W. J., Alexander, D. C., Magwood, S. E., and McKay, K. A.: Results of a preliminary trial with *Sphaerophorus necrophorus* toxoids to control liver abscesses in feedlot cattle. Can. J. Comp. Med. *38*:222, 1974.
6. Brown, H., Bing, R. F., Grueter, H. P., McAskill, J. W., Cooley, C. O., and Rathmacher, R. P.: Tylosin and chlortetracycline for the prevention of liver abscesses, improved weight gains and feed efficiency in feedlot cattle. J. Anim. Sci. *40*:207, 1975.
7. Morrow, D. A.: Fat cow syndrome. J. Dairy Sci. *59*:1625, 1975.
8. Roberts, C. J., Turfrey, B. A., and Bland, A. P.: Lipid deposition in different fiber types of skeletal muscle of periparturient dairy cows. Vet. Pathol. *20*:23, 1983.
9. Morrow, D. A., Hillman, D., Dade, A. W., and Kitchen, H.: Clinical investigation of a dairy herd with the fat cow syndrome. J. Am. Vet. Med. Assoc. *174*:161, 1979.
10. Reid, I. M., and Roberts, C. J.: Subclinical fatty liver in dairy cows. Irish Vet. J. *37*:104, 1983.
11. Herdt, T. H., Goeders, L., Liesman, J. S., amd Emery, R. S.: Test for estimation of bovine hepatic lipid content. J. Am. Vet. Med. Assoc. *182*:953, 1983.
12. Stober, M., and Dirksen, G.: Lipomobilization syndrome (fatty degeneration syndrome) in the dairy cow. Bovine Pract. *18*:152, 1983.

Pancreatitis

ROBERT H. WHITLOCK, D.V.M., Ph.D.

Pancreatic disease is rare in cattle and seldom produces clinical signs unless accompanied by insulin deficiency. Diabetes mellitus has been reported in cattle and is characterized by hyperglycemia, glucosuria, polydipsia, polyuria, and weight loss.[1-4] However, acute pancreatitis has not been reported in cattle; therefore, pancreatic islet destruction with subsequent insulin deficiency, as occurs in the dog and man, is not a common cause of bovine diabetes mellitus.

There is no one single cause of bovine diabetes mellitus; pathologic changes include absence of beta cells in pancreatic islets, neoplastic involvement of the pancreas, vacuolar degeneration of islets with lymphocytic infiltration, and chronic pancreatitis. Diabetes mellitus occurs as a complication of natural and experimental foot-and-mouth disease in which pancreatic islets undergo necrosis and disappear.[5, 6]

Treatment with protamine zinc insulin (0.25 to 0.5 I.U./kg subcutaneously twice daily) may be successful in some cases. However, blood glucose levels are difficult to control without dietary and exercise modifications, and often there is no improvement in clinical signs. Prognosis is generally not favorable.

PANCREOLITHIASIS

Pancreolithiasis (formation of concretions in the pancreatic excretory ducts) occurs sporadically in cattle; however, it is usually an incidental finding at slaughter and is rarely associated with clinical signs. In a survey conducted in Danish slaughter facilities,[7] the incidence was reported to be 19 per cent in animals less than four years old and 82 per cent in animals over four years old. Greater frequency was reported in red Danish cattle than in Holstein or Jersey breeds.

The major chemical constituents of pancreoliths are calcium carbonate and calcium phosphate, with traces of magnesium carbonate, fats, and protein.[7, 8] The cause of pancreolithiasis is not definitively known. The stones arise from precipitation of salts in pancreatic juice around nuclei, such as desquamated cells. The size, shape, and texture vary, but they are laminated, which suggests variable accretion. Pancreatic duct mucosa is chronically inflamed, and fibrosis of the lamina propria and submucosa results.[9] Salts in the pancreatic juice precipitate around nuclei, such as desquamated cells, obstructing the duct. Secretion is retained with atrophy of acinar tissue; however, the islets are preserved.

PANCREATIC PARASITES

Eurytrema pancreaticum, a trematode of ruminants, accepts the pancreatic ducts as its primary habitat, and its infestation can lead to chronic interstitial pancreatitis by extension of an inflammatory process from the ducts to the interstitium. It prefers the left lobe, and acinar tissue may be destroyed. This species is common in parts of Asia, Madagascar, and South America. Occasionally, other trematodes (*Dicrocoelium dendriticum* and *Metorchis conjunctus*) invade the pancreatic ducts and provoke interstitial inflammation when they are present in large numbers in the biliary system.[9]

PANCREATIC TUMORS

Pancreatic carcinomas and islet cell tumors occur in cattle.[10–13] Bovine islet cell tumors are reported to have an unusual tendency to invade the posterior vena cava.[9, 14] If the tumor is functional, weakness and convulsions from hypoglycemia may result.

PANCREATIC HYPOPLASIA

Hypoplasia of the pancreas occurs rarely in calves. Microscopically, islets and ducts are normal, but acinar tissue cells are undifferentiated and few in number. Clinically, steatorrhea and diarrhea may be observed.

References

1. Kaneko, J. J., and Rhode, E. A.: Diabetes mellitus in a cow. J. Am. Vet. Med. Assoc. *144*:367, 1964.
2. Phillips, R. W., Knox, K. L., Pierson, R. E., and Tasker, J. B.: Bovine diabetes mellitus. Cornell Vet. *61*:114, 1971.
3. Mostaghni, K., and Ivoghli, B.: Diabetes mellitus in the bovine. Cornell Vet. *67*:24, 1977.
4. Christensen, N. O., and Schambye, P.: Om diabetes mellitus hos kvaey. Nord. Vet. Med. 2:863, 1950.
5. Barboni, E., and Manocchio, I.: Pancreatic changes in cattle with diabetes mellitus after foot and mouth disease. Arch. Vet. Ital. *13*:477, 1962.
6. Barboni, E., Monocchio, I., and Asdrubali, G.: Observations on diabetes mellitus associated with experimental foot and mouth disease in cattle. Arch. Vet. Ital. *17*:339, 362, 1966.
7. Velling, K.: Bovine Pancreolithiasis in Denmark. Acta Vet. Scand. *16*:327, 1975.
8. Fitch, C. P., Boyd, W. L., and Billings, W. A.: Pancreatic lithiasis of cattle. Cornell Vet. *9*:68, 1919.
9. Jubb, K. V. F., and Kennedy, P. C.: The pancreas. In Pathology of Domestic Animals, Vol. 2. Academic Press, New York, 1970, 263–273.
10. Tokarnin, C. H.: Islet cell tumor of the bovine pancreas. J. Am. Vet. Med. Assoc. *138*:541, 1961.
11. Rowlatt, U.: Spontaneous epithelial tumors of the pancreas of mammals. Br. J. Cancer *21*:82, 1967.
12. Manocchio, I., Mughetti, L., and Ciorba, A.: Electron microscope study of adenocarcinoma of the beta cells of the pancreatic islets in cattle. Nuova Veterinaria *50*:106, 1974.
13. Priester, W. A.: Data from eleven United States and Canadian colleges of veterinary medicine on pancratic carcinoma in domestic animals. Cancer Res. *34*:1372, 1974.
14. Pelligrini, N., and Braca, G.: Functional beta cell insulomas in cattle. Postmortem findings and aspects relevant to meat inspection. Annali della Facolta di Medicina Veterinaria di Pisa *23*:225, 1971.

Supplemental Reading

Baker, J. S., Jackson, H. D., and Sommers, E. L.: Diabetes mellitus in a four-year-old pregnant holstein. Comp. Cont. Ed. *5*(6):S328, 1983.
Brody, R. S., and Prier, J. E.: Clinico-pathologic conference. J. Am. Vet. Med. Assoc. *139*:925, 1961.
Little, P. B.: Clinico-pathologic conference. J. Am. Vet. Med. Assoc. *143*:874, 1963.

Nematode Infections—Cattle, Sheep, Goats, Swine

R. P. HERD, M.V.Sc., Ph.D.

CATTLE

Young cattle are highly susceptible to worms and commonly have high worm burdens and high fecal egg counts and suffer severe production losses or mortality. Parasitism may be especially important in dairy calves because of the common practice of rearing successive groups of calves on the same area of contaminated pasture. Young cattle develop some immunity to worms after the first year at pasture, and this becomes stronger during their second grazing season. Most adult cattle have a high degree of immunity, which is reflected by low worm burdens, low fecal egg counts, and a low prevalence of clinical disease. Thus routine treatment and control programs are generally not needed for adult cattle. Even in a cow/calf operation, routine treatment is generally unnecessary because pasture contamination by calves is sufficiently diluted to make the occurrence of dangerous infection unlikely. In feedlots it appears that conditions are unsuitable for development of worm eggs to infective larvae, so treatment is required only at preconditioning or on arrival to eliminate infections previously obtained at pasture.

Parasite control programs should be aimed primarily at young cattle at pasture as indicated in the following:

Class of cattle	Routine control program
Adult dairy cattle	Seldom required
Dairy replacement heifers	Essential
Cow/calf operation	Seldom required
Beef replacement heifers	Essential
Feedlot	Precondition

The control programs presented here for the United States are based on the small amount of epidemiologic data available and will require modification as more data are collected for more regions in the future. In Britain and Australia much more epidemiologic data are available, and highly effective control programs have been formulated for many areas by utilizing those data. The reader is referred to the Supplemental Reading section for several publications detailing the British and Australian work.

Major Parasites

Although gastrointestinal parasitism in cattle may involve several species, the abomasal nematode *Ostertagia ostertagi* is the most pathogenic and economically important in the temperate regions of the world, including most areas of the United States. It is consequently important to understand the life cycle, epidemiology, and pathogenesis of this parasite and to plan control strategies with *Ostertagia* as a major target. Control strategies effective against *Ostertagia* will also be effective against most other trichostrongylid worms. Although *O. ostertagi* has been incriminated in most outbreaks of ostertagiasis, *O. leptospicularis* and *O. bisonis* may also cause disease.

Life Cycle

Ostertagia species have a direct life cycle. Eggs passed in the feces hatch first-stage larvae (L_1), which develop and molt to become second-stage larvae (L_2), which in turn develop and molt to the third-stage infective larvae (L_3). This development may occur within a week under optimal conditions, and L_3 may then migrate from the dung pat to herbage if there is adequate moisture. Following ingestion of infective L_3 by cattle, the parasitic cycle involves development through L_3–L_4–L_5 stages within the gastric glands. This usually takes 18 to 21 days, by which time the young adult emerges from the glands into the lumen of the abomasum. Under certain conditions to be discussed later, the parasite undergoes hypobiosis (arrested development, inhibited development) and does not develop to the adult stage for several months.

Epidemiology

Seasonal Development of Infective Larvae

In Britain, Western Europe, and northern United States, contamination of pastures with worm eggs starts early in the grazing season, but it is not until summer that conditions are ideal for rapid development of eggs to L_3. Hence there is an explosive increase of potentially dangerous L_3 in summer resulting from eggs passed over a period of several months. New populations of L_3 accumulate in the fecal pats through July, August, and September in northern temperate regions and become available to grazing cattle provided there is sufficient rainfall to assist the migration of L_3 from feces to herbage. This pattern may be modified in a dry summer when L_3 become trapped within the fecal mass and do not escape to herbage until autumn rains occur, resulting in a big increase in pasture infectivity in the fall when L_3 are likely to become conditioned for arrest. Most trichostrongylid worms survive the adverse winter conditions in a state of arrested or inhibited development within the host and resume development in spring when seasonal conditons are more favorable. In general, cattle are exposed to light infection in the first half of the grazing season and heavy infection in the second half.

Marked seasonal patterns of pasture infectivity and hypobiosis also occur in the southern hemisphere and southern United States. In many regions the hot dry summers or the alternating wet and dry weather in summer is adverse to larval survival. Even with irrigation systems, the alternating wet and dry conditions each day are lethal to larvae. In most regions with a mild winter there is a progressive increase in pasture contamination and infectivity from autumn through spring because of the combination of high worm egg output and favorable environmental conditions. In summer, there is likely to be a high mortality of pasture larvae and little transmission of infection. Most trichostrongylids survive the adverse summer in southern environments in a state of arrested development in the host and resume development in early autumn when conditions are again favorable.

Dairy cattle in confinement or beef cattle in feedlots are not exposed to significant numbers of infective larvae, although Type II ostertagiasis can occur if cattle were harboring massive numbers of arrested larvae when moved from pasture to confinement or feedlot. Although eggs may be passed in the feces of animals removed from pasture, it seems that conditions in confinement are inimical for development of eggs to infective larvae. It is possible that the high concentration of urine has an inhibitory effect in these situations. Infection with coccidia or *Strongyloides* sp. is a bigger problem in confinement housing and feedlots.

Longevity of Infective Larvae

Although contamination of pastures with worm eggs may be continuous throughout the year, development to infective L_3, migration of L_3 from dung pats, and the subsequent survival of L_3 on herbage differ markedly throughout the year in response to prevailing weather conditions. The fecal pat with its high moisture content acts as an important reservoir of infection and provides a safe haven for L_3 during dry periods. The migration of L_3 from dung pats to herbage is intermittent and dependent on sufficient moisture to provide a continuous film of water. Once a dung pat has dried out, rainfall of 50 to 100 mm over two or more days is needed to induce migration. When rainfall is intermittent, migration tends to occur in waves. Movement of L_3 usually extends 10 to 20 cm from the perimeter of the dung pat, but occasionally L_3 are recovered up to 1 meter away. Larvae may be spread over a wider area by temporary localized flooding after heavy rainfaill or by hooves, farm equipment, and so on. Preferred locations for L_3 are close to the ground on the undersides of legume leaves and in leaf axils of grasses that spread laterally.

In northern temperate regions, numbers of L_3 on pasture tend to be highest in summer and autumn following development from eggs passed in spring and summer. The L_3 survive until the following spring when rising temperatures trigger enhanced activity and death following exhaustion of food reserve. Infective L_3 of many trichostrongylid species survive well under winter snow and are then available to infect cattle turned out to pasture in early spring. The decrease in numbers in L_3 as they die in the spring is accentuated by the diluting effect of accelerated herbage growth. In southern temperate regions numbers of L_3 on pasture escalate in autumn, winter, and spring if there is adequate warmth and precipitation but die off rapidly under dry conditions in summer.

Hypobiosis (Arrested Development, Inhibited Development)

Hypobiosis is a temporary cessation of development of a parasite at a precise point in its early life; in the case of *O. ostertagi*, this occurs at the early L_4 stage. It has been reported in a large range of nematode parasites (at least 30 species). It has important practical implications because it enables the parasite to survive in a dormant state during adverse periods, when it would otherwise be eliminated by host immunity or when its progeny would be destroyed by adverse seasonal conditions. Many arrested larvae later resume normal development when the internal or external environment has become more favorable. They then seed pastures with eggs, often at a time when pasture infectivity may be quite low. A massive synchronous maturation of arrested larvae will cause clinical disease, such as Type II ostertagiasis. This has been hard to control in the past because most available anthelmintics have been ineffective against hypobiotic larvae.

The patterns of worm transmission tend to be reversed in the northern and southern temperate zones. Major accumulations of pasture L_3 occur in summer in the north, whereas major mortality of L_3 occurs at that time in the south. Major accumulations of pasture L_3 occur in spring in the south, whereas major mortalilty occurs at that time in the north. Type I ostertagiasis mainly occurs in the first half of the year in the south and in the second half of the year in the north. Pre-Type II ostertagiasis, the phase of arrested development, occurs in winter in the north and in summer in the south. Type II ostertagiasis, the clinical syndrome associated with the maturation of arrested larvae, occurs mainly in early spring in the north and early autumn in the south.

Host Immunity

Calves are most susceptible to worms during their first season at pasture but generally acquire a strong immunity during their second grazing season. Cattle exposed to *Ostertagia* infections normally have a strong immunity by the end of their second grazing season. Hence the disease is mainly a problem of dairy replacement heifers at pasture or beef calves grazing in contaminated pasture during the post-weaning period. Adult cattle are little affected because of their acquired immunity. Nevertheless problems can develop in cattle that have received minimal exposure to parasites as calves or in cattle suffering immunosuppression from a variety of causes, such as malnutrition, concurrent disease, or chemotherapy. Cattle raised indoors or on dry lots will have little exposure to nematodes and may not develop strong immunity. In general dairy calves develop immunity faster than beef calves because of their greater exposure to parasites. Consequently clinical parasitism is even less common in adult dairy cattle than in adult beef cattle

Pathogenesis

The major lesions, biochemical changes, and clinical signs associated with ostertagiasis usually occur immediately after emergence of young adults from the gastric glands. Initially cellular changes are confined to the parasitized glands, but when young adults begin to emerge the hyperplasia and loss of cellular differentiation become

more generalized, giving the abomasal wall a Moroccan leather appearance. Destruction of parietal HCl-producing cells often elevates the abomasal fluid pH from 2 to 7. This results in a failure to denature proteins, failure to activate pepsinogen to pepsin, and loss of bacteriostatic effect, leading to the onset of diarrhea.

The hyperplastic and undifferentiated mucosa also becomes more permeable to macromolecules, leading to elevated plasma pepsinogen levels ($>$3000 I.U. tyrosine) as nonactivated pepsinogen diffuses into the circulation. Plasma proteins also leak in the opposite direction from the circulation to the abomasal lumen. Necrosis and sloughing of surface epithelial cells may follow emergence of large numbers of worms, and congestion or edema of the abomasal folds may be encountered. The clinical consequences of all these changes are loss of appetite, impaired digestion, and diarrhea.

Clinical Disease

There are two main clinical forms of ostertagiasis: Type I and Type II.

Type I. This clinical entity results from the rapid acquisition of large numbers of L_3 that complete their development to the adult stage in three to four weeks. It occurs mainly in young cattle up to 18 months of age during their first season at pasture. It is most common from July to October in northern temperate regions and from January to April in southern temperature zones. Clinical signs coincide with the emergence of young adults from the gastric glands three weeks or more after cattle are exposed to heavily infected pastures. The main signs are anorexia, weight loss, diarrhea, and mortality. It is common for a large percentage of the group to be affected, in contrast to Type II disease in which only a small percentage show signs.

Pre-Type II. In this form, clinical signs are absent or mild in character, and the vast majority of *Ostertagia* worms (often $>$80 per cent) are arrested in their development at the early L_4 stage, slightly over 1.0 mm long. Pre-Type II ostertagiasis occurs in winter following acquisition of arrested-prone L_3 in late autumn in northern regions. In southern regions, pre-type II ostertagiasis occurs in late spring and summer after acquisition of arrested-prone L_3 in spring. It appears that hypobiosis of *Ostertagia* is largely a seasonal phenomenon triggered by falling temperatures in northern regions and other unknown stimuli in southern regions. Host immunity is thought to play a relatively minor role in this instance.

Type II. This clinical phase results from the emergence and maturation of large numbers of arrested larvae in the early spring in northern regions and early fall in southern regions. Clinical cases have been observed in grazing cattle, housed cattle, and feedlot cattle, most commonly two to four years of age. Diarrhea may be intermittent, coinciding with the emergence of successive waves of developing larvae. Anorexia, weight loss, hypoalbuminemia, moderate anemia, and submandibular edema (bottle jaw) may also occur. Clinical signs are usually seen in only a small percentage ($<$10 per cent) of animals coincident with massive emergence of larvae or loss of immunity. Type II ostertagiasis can be differentiated from Type I by the different seasonal occurrence, grazing history, older age of animals, small number affected, more protracted course, poorer prognosis, and insusceptibility to most anthelmintics. Although beef and dairy cattle both exhibit Type II ostertagiasis, a higher proportion of hypobiosis has been reported in beef cattle production systems. On many dairy farms the year-round pasture contamination by calves ensures continual transmission of worms, and there is probably less selection pressure for the parasite to undergo hypobiosis to ensure survival.

Diagnosis

A detailed history is helpful in arriving at a correct diagnosis, as there is a lack of specificity in clinical signs and a poor correlation between fecal egg counts and worm burdens. Knowledge of seasonal conditions, grazing history, likely levels of pasture infectivity, nutritional and reproductive status, managerial practices, anthelmintic treatments, and the expected degree of immunity to worms is helpful in making a decision. For example, Type I disease is most likely to be a herd problem in calves during their first grazing season, whereas Type II disease affects only a small percentage of animals at the time when there is emergence and maturation of hypobiotic worms, i.e., early spring (northern regions) and early fall (southern regions).

Clinical signs of anorexia, weight loss, diarrhea, rough coat, and submandibular edema are suggestive but not specific for ostertagiasis. Fecal egg counts may remain low in some animals in clinical outbreaks of disease and give no indication of the number of immature worms, inhibited worms, or adult worms in which egg laying has been suppressed by anthelmintic treatment or host immunity. Furthermore, it is difficult to differentiate eggs of *Ostertagia* from those of most other trichostrongylid species *(Haemonchus, Cooperia, Trichostrongylus)* or hookworms *(Bunostomum)*. Plasma pepsinogen concentrations are sometimes better correlated with *Ostertagia* burdens than fecal egg counts, but the test is not done by many laboratories and it also has interpretation problems.

The most positive way to make a diagnosis is by necropsy examination and total worm counts. The distinctive abomasal lesions can be observed and aliquots of abomasal contents and abomasal wall digests counted for worms. Adult *Ostertagia* are fine hair-like worms of only 1 cm length and are easily missed on macroscopic examination, even when many thousands are present. A moribund animal or one that is profusely scouring sometimes expels many of its worms in the feces, so that the worm count is artificially low at necropsy. Whereas moderate worm burdens are pathogenic in young cattle, heavy worm burdens may be required to cause clinical disease in adult cattle.

Control Strategies

Adult Dairy Cattle

Although most dairy cows pass worm eggs in their feces, worm burdens and egg counts are generally low because of their acquired immunity following exposure to nematodes when grazing pasture earlier in life. Clinical disease is uncommon, and the majority of trials have failed to support the claim that treatment results in significant increases in milk yield. There is no convincing evidence to justify mass treatment of dairy cows as an economic procedure. It is also illogical to expect that treatment at calving would have a prolonged effect on milk production over 305 days. With cows at pasture, the response would be very transient because worms removed by treatment would be quickly replaced from the environment. With cows in confinement, it is unlikely that they are exposed to appreciable infection.

Although mass treatment of dairy cows is not justified, there are some specific situations in which prophylactic treatment may be warranted. It may be beneficial to treat cows at the time of winter housing if they are transferred from autumn pastures carrying large numbers of arrested-prone larvae to a relatively worm-free environment indoors. This situation could arise if the pasture had been grazed by calves earlier in the year. Treatment with an anthelmintic effective against arrested larvae (e.g., ivermectin) would prevent Type II ostertagiasis in the following spring in northern regions. Prophylactic treatments might also be of advantage in cows that had lost immunity to worms under conditions of malnutrition, debilitating disease, or chemotherapy.

Dairy Replacement Heifers

OUTBREAKS

Treatment should be given promptly to reduce mortality and production losses. It is desirable to treat all heifers in the affected group, since productivity of animals not showing clinical signs is likely to be reduced. Whenever possible, young stock should be moved following treatment to less contaminated pastures or housed to avoid rapid re-infection. In outbreaks of Type I ostertagiasis, a reduction in worm burden of only 60 per cent will alleviate diarrhea within 48 hours of a single treatment.

The response to treatment of Type II ostertagiasis may not be immediate or satisfactory, especially if using thiabendazole or levamisole, although some benefit may be derived from repeated treatment at short intervals to kill sequential populations of adult worms that develop from arrested larvae. Ivermectin and the newer benzidimidazole drugs are more effective against arrested larvae and should be used in cases of Type II ostertagiasis.

PROPHYLAXIS

Using the epidemiologic data summarized previously, several control strategies have been developed for northern and southern temperate regions of the world. These strategies generally allow young cattle to be exposed to sufficient infection to induce a strong immunity but not sufficient to cause a significant loss in production. These strategies are mainly aimed at dairy heifers in their first year at pasture but are sometimes required during the second year at pasture.

Northern Temperate Zones

PROPHYLACTIC TREATMENTS IN THE SPRING. This consists of two prophylactic treatments administered three and six weeks after spring turnout. The rationale of this approach is that treatment kills new infections from overwintered L_3 before newly developed adult worms start shedding large numbers of eggs and contaminating pastures. By the time of the second treatment, most remaining overwintered L_3 on pasture will have died off because of rising temperatures. Although two treatments suffice in calves turned out in early May, an extra treatment might be needed in calves turned out in April, e.g., three treatments administered at three, six, and nine weeks after turnout. The period between treatments can be extended to 5 weeks with ivermectin because of its persistent anthelmintic activity.

This regimen minimizes worm eggs deposited in the early part of the grazing season and prevents heavy infection in calves in the second half of the grazing season. It is particularly useful on small intensive dairy farms with limited grazing areas. Although this regimen has resulted in significant weight gains so that heifers reach breeding size three months earlier than untreated heifers, pasture infectivity sometimes rises at the end of the grazing season, suggesting the need for an extra treatment at the time of winter housing with a drug effective against arrested larvae.

CONTROLLED-RELEASE DEVICE (CRD) AT SPRING TURNOUT. This is a labor-saving modification of the first strategy wherein a CRD is administered just before spring turnout, eliminating the need to yard cattle after turnout. The morantel CRD, marketed in Europe, was the first of these devices. It is an intraruminal bolus designed for continuous delilvery of a low dose of drug for at least 60 days. Although the cost is about double that of prophylactic treatments in the spring, it has the advantage of greater convenience to the farmer. There is a potential risk of strong selection for drug resistance with these devices, but the risk can be reduced by ensuring a high drug release rate, a sharp cutoff, and a low frequency of use as opposed to sequential treatments throughout the grazing season.

Future developments with CRDs are likely to include big technologic advances with controlled-release boluses, ear tags, and implants. It has been suggested that capsules alternating drug release for 7 days (giving newly ingested L_3 time to get out of the rumen) and no release for 10 to 20 days (less than the prepatent period) may be just as effective for field use as those devices that release the same rate continuously. Alternatively, a pulse-release bolus loaded with biodegradable polymer capsules containing a standard dose of anthelmintic could be formulated to release a therapeutic dose of anthelmintic at predetermined times, optimal for epidemiologic control, e.g., three and six weeks.

TREAT AND MOVE IN JULY. This is a simple control system developed by Michel in Britain, based on the knowledge that an explosive increase in Ostertagia L_3 occurs on pasture in mid-summer. The L_3 are derived mainly from eggs deposited from April through July. Thus, if susceptible calves that have grazed from early spring are moved to safe pasture in July, ostertagiasis can be avoided. Treatment with an effective anthelmintic at the time of the move serves two purposes: it removes a potentially harmful worm burden from the cattle, and it protects a safe pasture from new contamination. The move is more important than the treatment; a move without treatment gives almost as good results, but treatment without a move may end in disaster. The move to a safe pasture ensures several months of low worm burdens instead of a few days as the result of treatment alone.

This approach may not be so popular with farmers as it requires forward planning to provide a safe pasture of low infectivity at the appropriate time. A pasture used for hay, silage, or crops in the spring would generally be safe. Pastures grazed by sheep or other species are generally safe because of the small amount of cross-infection between host species. Pastures grazed by immune adult cattle should also have low infectivity.

ALTERNATE GRAZING SYSTEMS. Farms having both cattle and sheep can exploit alternate grazing of pastures for effective control of nematode infections in both host species. Best results have been obtained by a 6- or 12-month alternation. The combined effects of treatment to reduce egg counts at the time of changeover, the decrease in larval populations with time, and harvesting of L_3 by the opposite species ensure that levels of infection are reduced. Alternate grazing induces the same parasitologic advantages as leaving pastures unstocked, but it avoids the agronomic and economic disadvantages of the latter approach.

Alternate grazing of susceptible dairy calves with older immune cows may also be beneficial for herbage utilization and parasite control. In this system, the susceptible calves are grazed ahead of the immune adults to remove only the leafy upper herbage. The incoming adults then graze the lower more fibrous echelons of the herbage, which contain the majority of infective larvae. Feces passed by the immune adults contains fewer Ostertagia eggs, and this results in a dilution in pasture contamination and subsequent numbers of L_3 compared with paddocks permanently or rotationally grazed by calves. The ratio of calves to adults should not exceed three to one, and there must be sufficient fenced paddocks to prevent overgrazing by the young stock.

REPEATED ANTHELMINTIC TREATMENTS. The repeated use of anthelmintics has been exploited to suppress pasture contamination but is not always effective and has disadvantages of high cost, frequent handling of cattle, and selection for drug resistance. It may also delay the development of acquired immunity to worms. An intensive treatment schedule with monthly treatments does not prevent Ostertagia egg output nor guarantee significant live weight gains. Cattle given continuous daily access to molasses blocks containing phenothiazine have even developed clinical ostertagiasis.

Southern Temperate Regions

A consideration of the epidemiology in southern United States indicates a danger of Type I ostertagiasis in late winter and early spring (January to April) and Type II ostertagiasis in late summer and early autumn (August to September). The winter outbreaks of Type I ostertagiasis may be exacerbated by inadequate nutrition or liver fluke disease. It is therefore essential to start controlling pasture contamination in early autumn when a large egg-laying adult worm population develops from worms arrested through the summer. Treatment commencing in autumn would eliminate potentially dangerous worms prior to the period of nutritional stress, reduce the chances of outbreaks of Type I ostertagiasis, and ultimately lead to smaller numbers of arrested-prone L_3 on pasture in the spring, thus preventing Type II ostertagiasis in late summer or early fall.

Specific control strategies have not been worked out in detail in the southern United States, but many of the strategies adopted in northern temperate regions could be used if tailored to the epidemiologic characteristics of the region. For example, a small number of strategic anthelmintic treatments in autumn or a single application of a controlled-release device in early autumn should be of benefit in preventing a serious buildup of pasture infectivity through winter and spring and reduce the occurrence of both Type I and Type II ostertagiasis. Likewise, an alternate grazing system or a treat-and-move strategy prior to the major accumulation of L_3 on pasture could be used to an advantage.

Beef Cattle

Parasitic gastroenteritis is mainly a problem in weaned beef calves. Signs and effects of worm infection are rarely evident among suckling calves, and regular anthelmintic treatment of this class usually fails to demonstrate increased weight gains. These calves usually have a low intake of infective L_3 as a consequence of favorable stocking rates of cows and calves and the low level of contamination of pastures. Most adult beef cattle develop a strong immunity to nematode infection and do not require routine treatment for worms. Routine treatments are generally not required in cow/calf operations, as pasture contamination by nonimmune calves is sufficiently diluted to make the occurrence of dangerous infection unlikely. It has been claimed that treatment of cows before calving will result in heavier calves at weaning time, and properly controlled studies are needed to determine if this is true.

In northern temperate regions where spring-born calves run with their immune dams, the spring mortality of overwintered L_3 will have occurred before the suckling calves ingest significant quantities of grass. Furthermore, the low numbers of *Ostertagia* eggs passed in the feces of the immune cows would rarely be sufficient to produce dangerous numbers of L_3 on pasture later in the year. Worm problems would mainly arise when calves born early in spring ingested pasture before the spring mortality of L_3 occurred. This could lead to a big summer rise in L_3 and the need for anthelmintic treatments.

Autumn-born calves weaned in spring in northern regions would be at a considerably higher risk, since these calves would ingest larger numbers of L_3 in the spring, and eggs passed in their feces would contribute to the summer rise in pasture infectivity. A control strategy would be vital at the time of spring weaning. This could be achieved by alternate grazing, a treat-and-move strategy, prophylactic treatments administered at three-week intervals, ivermectin administered at five-week intervals, or administration of a controlled-release device. It is clear that decisions taken at weaning can have a profound effect on future herd health.

In southern temperate regions, spring-born calves are weaned in the fall. This is a time when it is vital to reduce the pasture contamination to prevent a winter and spring accumulation of L_3 on pasture. Control strategies at this time, when the weaned calves have only moderate worm burdens, might prevent the occurrence of ill thrift, weight loss, and diarrhea in winter or spring. Autumn-born calves weaned in spring are likely to be exposed to heavy infection and benefit from anthelmintic treatment. In parts of Australia, treatment of weaned calves in summer has been effective in reducing worm burdens at a time when re-infection from pasture is at a minimum. A second treatment three months later removes worms surviving the first treatment as well as the small number acquired since weaning. This results in a delayed onset of the autumn rise in egg counts and a lower availability of L_3 on pasture through winter and spring, thus avoiding clinical or subclinical disease.

Transmission of infection within feedlots appears to be negligible. The major concern is the worm burden carried by cattle on arrival if they have not been treated with effective anthelmintics in a preconditioning program. In the absence of re-infection within the feedlot, most infections will decline rapidly, even without anthelmintic treatment. If, however, cattle enter the feedlot carrying large numbers of arrested larvae there is a potential for an outbreak of Type II ostertagiasis. This can be avoided if calves are treated with a drug effective against arrested larvae before or soon after they enter the feedlot. Although untreated animals may eventually regain weight comparable to treated animals, there is still an economic advantage to be gained from treatment because of improved feed efficiency and reduced feed costs.

Anthelmintics

There are eight anthelmintics approved for general use in cattle in the United States: coumaphos, fenbendazole, haloxon, ivermectin, levamisole, morantel, phenothiazine, and thiabendazole.

Thiabendazole and levamisole have long been the most widely used cattle anthelmintics. They both have reasonably broad spectrums of activity and safety. Levamisole has the additional advantage of efficacy against lungworms and eyeworms and is available in an injectable formulation. Excitability and salivation are occasionally seen after treatment with levamisole. Thiabendazole and levamisole both have the disadvantage of being ineffective against arrested larvae of cattle when given at recommended doses. Most benzimidazole drugs are ovicidal for nematode eggs but are only likely to affect eggs in the gastrointestinal tract at the time of treatment, and this may be of trivial epidemiologic significance.

In recent years there have been reports of poor responses to both thiabendazole and levamisole. The commonly used dosage of 44 mg/kg of thiabendazole does not give high efficacy against all worms, and it is possible that some worms have now developed resistance to both thiabendazole and levamisole. In some studies, the efficacy of levamisole and thiabendazole has ranged as low as 23 to 56 per cent instead of the 80 to 90 per cent claimed by manufacturers.

The organic phosphate drugs coumaphos and haloxon do not have as broad a spectrum as the previously mentioned drugs, but coumaphos is effective against most trichostrongylid worms, including *Ostertagia,* and can be given to lactating dairy cows without having to withdraw milk from sale. Although mass treatment of dairy cows is not recommended, treatment of individual cows during lactation is sometimes needed.

A newly approved drug, morantel tartrate, has a broad spectrum of activity against gastrointestinal worms and high safety but, like most approved drugs, lacks activity against arrested larvae. A morantel tartrate sustained-release bolus that releases anthelmintic for at least 60 days has recently been marketed in Europe. It has obvious labor-saving advantages if used prophylactically and should be a useful device if it does not select unduly for the development of drug resistance.

Phenothiazine, the oldest of the anthelmintics, has been superseded by the modern broad spectrum drugs that have greater efficacy and safety. Phenothiazine has poor efficacy against *Ostertagia,* the most important cattle parasite. Cattle given continuous access to molasses blocks containing phenothiazine have developed clinical ostertagiasis. Treatments in feed are unreliable for parasitized animals because of the depression of appetite. Furthermore, the low and variable intake from blocks and licks is likely to lead to the development of drug resistance. Phenothiazine is also toxic to anemic or debilitated cattle.

Only the newer (less soluble) benzimidazole drugs and ivermectin have good activity against arrested larvae, although the activity of albendazole and fenbendazole tends to be erratic. A substantial percentage of animals treated with fenbendazole or albendazole have been found to harbor large numbers of arrested larvae after treatment. This may be linked to a faster passage of the drug through the alimentary tract of some animals. It is a serious deficiency from an epidemiologic point of view, since the wormy cattle remaining after treatment represent an important source of pasture contamination and infection for the subsequent grazing season. Some of the newer benzimidazole drugs (e.g., albendazole and parbendazole) are teratogenic and should not be used in early pregnancy. The insoluble benzimidazole drugs have long withdrawal times because of their slow excretion rate.

Ivermectin has been extensively tested throughout the world although it is not yet approved in all countries. It has high efficacy against nematodes and arthropods but not cestodes and trematodes. It is effective against both adult and immature nematodes with high efficacy against arrested *Ostertagia* larvae. It is effective against sucking lice, ticks, and mites when given by subcutaneous injection. It is safe in pregnant animals but should not be used in lactating dairy cows because of a prolonged withdrawal time. Ivermectin appears to be an ideal drug for treating southern cattle during summer hypobiosis or northern cattle at housing in late autumn, when hypobiotic larvae and ectoparasites are likely to be present.

SHEEP

Sheep in temperate nonarid regions frequently suffer severe clinical disease and production losses from worm infection. Generally, ewes and lambs are most susceptible to helminth infection, whereas dry ewes and wethers are more resistant. Consequently, ewes and lambs (pre- and post-weaning) should be given the highest priority in parasite control programs and safe grazing strategies. High concentrations of sheep at pasture and high fecal egg counts often lead to dangerous levels of pasture infectivity. The periparturient rise (PPR) in fecal egg counts is particularly important in lambing ewes, reaching much higher levels than in cattle. Sheep are less able than cattle to withstand the pathogenic effects of many thousands of worms, and serious outbreaks of helminthosis are common in sheep. A disastrous situation may occur if parasitized sheep are kept on a low plane of nutrition.

Parasite control is most satisfactorily achieved by reducing the exposure of sheep to infection by the integration of strategic anthelmintic treatments and judicious pasture management. This is dependent on a knowledge of the epidemiology for each region. This is lacking in many areas of the United States, and there is an urgent need for more research of this type. The accumulation of such data in Britain and Australia has led to the formulation of effective control programs, and the reader is referred to the Supplemental Reading section for further information.

Major Parasites

The trichostrongylid worms constitute the most important group of sheep worms in the temperate regions of the world. Three genera, *Haemonchus*, *Ostertagia* and *Trichostrongylus*, are the most abundant and most harmful in the northern and southern hemispheres. They are responsible for severe production loss, clinical disease, and mortality. *Haemonchus contortus*, a voracious bloodsucker, is the most damaging species in warm and wet regions, becoming less important in the colder zones where *Ostertagia* and *Trichostrongylus* spp. predominate. Nevertheless *Haemonchus contortus* is a major problem for sheep in the nonarid regions of both northern and southern United States. In England, *Nematodirus battus* is an additional problem in lambs in the first few months of life.

Life Cycle and Turnover

The trichostrongylid worms of sheep have a simple and direct life cycle. Eggs passed in feces hatch and develop through free-living L_1–L_2–L_3 stages within a week under optimal conditions. *Nematodirus* is an exception in that free-living development takes place entirely within the egg shell and hatching may be delayed until the following year. The trichostrongylid L_3 is the infective stage, and parasitic development from L_3 to egg-laying adult normally takes two to four weeks. Under certain conditions, development of *Haemonchus*, *Ostertagia*, and *Nematodirus* spp. in the gastrointestinal tract may be arrested at the early L_4 stage for several months and then resume development later when conditions are more favorable. As with the cattle nematodes, arrest is largely associated with larvae ingested from pasture in particular seasons of the year and has important implications for epidemiology and control.

It appears that *Ostertagia* and *Haemonchus* spp. have a short adult lifespan of only about one month and a rapid population turnover. Because of this short lifespan the number of worms present in the animal depends on the current intake of infective larvae from pasture. If the intake of L_3 is decreased, as when sheep are moved indoors or to drylot, their worm burdens will rapidly drop. However, anthelmintic treatment of animals that continue to be exposed to new infection at pasture will be of little value. It merely removes an adult population soon to be lost, and the lost worms are quickly replaced by new infection. Anthelmintic treatment gives better protection against long-lived species such as *Trichostrongylus*. Thus, a single anthelmintic treatment may remove a large adult population of *Trichostrongylus* spp. that has accumulated over a long period, and it would be only partly replaced when treated animals were returned to contaminated pasture.

Epidemiology

Seasonal Development of Infective Larvae

The sheep nematodes, like those of cattle, exhibit marked seasonal patterns of infectivity with only one or two disease-producing generations of worms per yer. In Britain, western Europe, and northern United States, most eggs passed in spring and early summer complete their development to infective L_3 in mid summer, resulting in an explosive increase of pasture infectivity at that time. In a dry summer, this may be delayed until autumn rains occur. Pasture infectivity then persists at high levels until the following spring, when L_3 start to die because of rising temperatures. Although L_3 on pasture successfully persist through the winter, any contamination of pasture after September rarely results in significant new infections. In the southern hemisphere and southern United States, major accumulations of L_3 on pasture occur from autumn through spring but decline rapidly in summer.

The Periparturient Rise (PPR)

The PPR appears to be of considerable importance in sheep and swine but is absent or moderate in horses and cattle. It has serious practical implications for sheep nematode control. It occurs any time from two weeks before lambing until eight weeks after lambing, irrespective of the season of lambing. At this time there is a general reduction in the immune response to worms, so that resistance to incoming larvae, controls on worm fecundity, and the capacity to expel worms are all diminished. It is suspected that lactogenic hormones are indirectly involved in bringing about these changes. The epidemiologic significance of the PPR is that it ensures heavy pasture contamination with worm eggs at the time of birth of the new host generation and transmission of worms from one host generation to the next. Although conditions may not be immediately suitable for the development of eggs to L_3, there may be a dangerous accumulation of L_3 later when lambs are relying less on milk and more on pasture. The PPR is often a major contributor to the sudden rise in second-generation (disease-producing) worms in the summer in northern regions.

Hypobiosis (Arrested Development)

Hypobiosis has important practical implications because it enables the parasite to survive in a dormant state in the host during adverse periods when there is a hostile immunologic environment or when its progeny would not survive in the outside environment. In contrast to the turnover of normally developing worms, arrested larvae tend to accumulate and may reach very large numbers, apparently unaffected by host immune responses. If a sudden resumption of development to adult worms occurs, it may produce a dramatic increase in pasture contamination and large worm burdens in the host at a time when pasture infectivity may be quite low. Hypobiotic larvae are also of practical importance because they are unaffected by some anthelmintics.

Studies in Ohio showed that hypobiosis occurred to a marked degree in early winter with almost the entire worm burden of *H. contortus* (98 to 100 per cent), *O. circumcincta* (89 to 98 per cent), and *N. filicollis* (77 to 90 per cent) affected. At this time the adult worm population was limited almost exclusively to *Trichostrongylus* spp. It appears that *Trichostrongylus* spp. have a long adult lifespan, which aids transmission from year to year, whereas *O. circumcincta* and *H. contortus* have short lifespans and a greater reliance on survival from year to year in the hypobiotic state. Hypobiosis is especially important to *H. contortus*, whose free-living stages survive poorly on pasture during winter. There is little information available on the occurrence of hypobiosis in sheep in southern states.

Host Immunity

Immune competence against gastrointestinal helminth infection is slow to develop in sheep and may not be fully expressed until about nine months of age. Thus, young sheep on infected pastures generally acquire heavy infections and exacerbate the situation by shedding large numbers of eggs in the feces. Although sheep eventually develop a strong resistance to *Nematodirus* spp. and moderate resistance to *Trichostrongylus* spp., resistance to *Haemonchus* and *Ostertagia* spp. is more labile, and outbreaks can occur in sheep of all ages. Immunologic unresponsiveness has been observed in the neonate, the periparturient ewe, and the nutritionally deprived. A genetic approach based on selection for responsiveness in young animals may offer the best approach to improve immunolgic responsiveness of young animals to parasite antigens.

Pathogenesis

Infection with *Haemonchus contortus* results in anemia and hypoproteinemia owing to the voracious blood sucking activities of adults and fourth stage larvae (L_4). Sudden death may occur as a result of severe blood loss. In addition, the migration of larvae into the pits of the gastric glands and the attachment of adult worms to the mucosa cause abomasitis. There is a significant rise in abomasal pH and plasma pepsinogen levels soon after infection but not to the same levels as those seen in ostertagiasis. The activities of the parasite are believed to interfere with the digestibility and absorption of protein, calcium and phosphorus. In chronic cases, death may result from exhaustion of protein and iron stores.

The other trichostrongylid worms have a variety of effects. The pathogenesis of ostertagiasis Types I and II is similar to that described for cattle. *T. axei* causes abomasitis, whereas *Trichostrongylus* and *Nematodirus* spp. in the small intestine cause villous atrophy and plasma leakage into the intestine. Anorexia is an important feature and exacerbates the hypoproteinemia resulting from the protein-losing enteropathy. Deficiencies in digestion and absorption may be partly due to the loss of enzymes normally found on the microvilli, which results when villous atrophy occurs. Most sheep acquire multiple infections, and there is evidence of a synergistic effect between *O. circumcincta* and *T. colubriformis*, so that the combined effects are more pathogenic than one would expect from the sum of the effects of the two parasites given alone.

Clinical Disease

Sheep infected with *H. contortus* may die suddenly without showing clinical signs, especially if driven. The main signs are marked anemia with pale skin and mucous membranes, anorexia, submandibular edema, and weakness. When driven, affected sheep may lag behind, breathe faster, stagger, and often go down and then rise and walk a little further after rest. In most cases there is no diarrhea; feces are drier and harder than normal and greatly reduced in quantity. In chronic cases there is extreme weight loss and the fleece may be lost. Sheep infected with other trichostrongylid worms show anorexia, ill thrift, weight loss, diarrhea, dehydration, staggering, weakness, recumbency, and death. In some cases there is a black scour. Lamb and yearling flocks are most seriously affected, and once mortality starts, a few animals may die each day.

Diagnosis

Gastrointestinal parasites are the most likely cause of ill thrift and diarrhea in sheep and should always be considered, especially in sheep suffering malnutrition. Diarrhea without ill thrift or loss of condition is not often due to worms. A detailed history including age, sex, reproductive status, likely immune status, seasonal conditions, nutritional status, managerial practices, and anthelmintic treatments is helpful in arriving at an accurate diagnosis.

There is a poor relationship between fecal egg counts and worm burden, and it is dangerous to make a diagnosis on the basis of a fecal egg count alone. A total worm count at necropsy should be done wherever possible. The trichostrongylid worms are fine, hair-like worms that can be easily missed by a cursory inspection, even when many thousands are present. In addition to examining aliquots of abomasal and intestinal contents under the microscope, it is desirable to examine digests of the abomasal wall for larval stages. The interpretation of the total worm count must take into consideration the fact that different species are pathogenic at different levels. Thus 1,000 *H. contortus* may be just as pathogenic as 10,000 *O. circumcincta*.

Control Strategies

Many control programs are guided by guesswork, convenience, or desperation after mortality occurs, and they ignore re-infection, the PPR, hypobiosis, and selection for drug resistance. Many control programs give sheep a few days without worms before the process of re-infection returns their worm burdens to pretreatment levels. At that stage, over 95 per cent of the total worm population is likely to be in the environment so that treatment removes less than 5 per cent of all worms and sheep are subject to immediate re-infection. These haphazard treatments may stop some deaths, but they do not stop production losses. To reduce worm burdens on a more permanent basis, it is necessary either to give repeated anthelmintic treatments at short intervals (e.g., every two weeks) or to reduce the rate of infection by some form of integrated control combining the prophylactic use of anthelmintics with appropriate grazing management. The latter approach is preferable because it involves less drug cost, less labor cost, and less selection pressure for the evolution of drug resistance.

The modern epidemiologic strategies are summarized hereafter.

Prelambing Treatments

This is a key strategy for lambing ewes to prevent the potentially damaging PPR and clinical and/or subclinical disease in both ewes and lambs. When given to ewes in winter in Northern regions, it is essential to use an anthelmintic (e.g., levamisole, ivermectin) that is effective against hypobiotic larvae, thus preventing maturation to adults and participation in the PPR. This treatment can be given at the time of winter housing or at any convenient period before the ewes go out to spring pasture. The object is to prevent them from contaminating spring pasture with worm eggs. Late-lambing ewes will require a second treatment just before or at lambing if they have already grazed spring pasture contaminated with overwintered larvae. In the case of both early- and late-lambing ewes, good results will be obtained only if ewes are kept indoors, in drylots, or are moved to safe pastures following treatment to avoid immediate re-infection. There is ample evidence in the literature that these strategies do not work if ewes are maintained on contaminated pastures. The "safe pasture" concept is discussed next.

Turnout of Lambs to Safe Pasture With No Treatment

Lambs raised indoors in a relatively parasite-free environment can be turned out to a safe pasture without the need for any anthelmintic treatment. A safe pasture is not necessarily "clean" or free of infective larvae but is one where infectivity is sufficiently low enough that the worm burdens of susceptible stock moved to it increase slowly. Regrowth after mechanical harvesting of hay, silage, or small grain crops can generally be considered safe. The use of electric fencing may facilitate maximum exploitation of safe pastures on many farms. Pastures previously grazed by cattle or other species are generally safe because of the small amount of crossinfection between species. Nevertheless, calves less than six months of age are susceptible to *H. contortus*. Rotational grazing is usually not effective for parasite control because of the prolonged survival of infective larvae on contaminated pastures.

Prophylactic Treatment in Spring in Northern Regions

The advantage of prophylactic treatment in the spring is that it prevents the occurrence of the summer buildup of pasture infectivity and resulting clinical and subclinical disease. When market lambs or ewe lamb replacements are turned out to spring pasture they are immediately exposed to L_3 that have survived over winter on pasture. Suckling lambs acquire infection from progeny of hypobiotic worms carried by ewes in winter as well as from overwintered L_3. By mid summer, they may be exposed to a massive buildup of second-generation worms and clinical helminthosis.

Recent Ohio studies showed that four treatments at three-week intervals, starting three weeks after spring turnout, were just as effective as eight treatments at three-week intervals for the entire grazing season. It was obvious that the early season treatments were highly beneficial, whereas the late season treatments were a waste of time and money. Studies in Ohio also demonstrated the value of prophylactic treatments in the spring for horses and dairy replacement heifers. In all three host-parasite systems, this strategy prevents the escalation of second-generation (disease-producing) worms.

Treat-and-Move Strategies

The rationale of this strategy is to extend the effectiveness of a single treatment by moving animals to a safe pasture to limit re-infection. Thus, if sheep are treated by July 1 and moved to a safe pasture in northern regions, they are unlikely to be exposed to the summer explosion in pasture infectivity. If they are treated and left on the same pasture, they will be exposed to heavy re-infection and derive little benefit from treatment. Thus, the move to a safe pasture is the key factor in this strategy. If a flock is moved to a safe pasture after treatment, it will enjoy several months of low worm burdens rather than only two or three worm-free days as the result of treatment alone. Infected sheep should not graze a safe pasture; they must be treated before being allowed to graze. The treatment serves two purposes: it removes a potentially harmful worm burden from the sheep, and it protects a safe pasture from new contamination.

In the Ohio studies, this strategy initially worked well, but a marked rise in pasture infectivity was observed in early October. It appeared that there had been a buildup of *H. contortus* larvae aided by the high fecundity of this parasite and late season rains favorable for development and survival of the free-living stages. It was concluded that a single treat-and-move strategy would provide safe pasture for a sufficiently long period for lambs to be marketed early, but a double treat-and-move system would be needed for lambs at pasture for longer periods of time. The latter would involve two anthelmintic treatments administered about six to eight weeks apart and the use of two pastures ungrazed by sheep that year. There is a need to study the selection pressure for drug resistance with this system because it can be argued that the safe pasture may eventually become populated with the progeny of resistant survivors.

Anthelmintics

There are only three anthelmintics approved for use in sheep in the United States (levamisole, thiabendazole, and phenothiazine) and one anthelmintic for goats (thiabendazole). It is likely that once ivermectin is approved, it will become an important anhelmintic in sheep. The cattle formulation causes a stinging reaction when injected in sheep.

Levamisole is the most widely used of the approved drugs because of its broad spectrum of activity and high efficacy against worms resistant to benzimidazole drugs and phenothiazine. Levamisole also has the advantage of being 97 to 100 per cent effective against arrested larvae of sheep at a dosage of 8 mg/kg. The efficacy against arrested larvae in sheep but not in cattle may reflect a better contact between parasite and drug because of reduced mucosal penetration by sheep larvae. A slower metabolism of anhelmintics in sheep than in cattle would also enhance efficacy toward hypobiotic worms. Levamisole is effective against *Dictyocaulus filaria* lungworms in addition to the major gastrointestinal nematodes, but it is not ovicidal. A small number of sheep may become excitable for a few minutes after treatment, and injectable levamisole may cause a transient inflammation at the site of injection. Field resistance of *O. circumcincta* and *T. colubriformis* to levamisole has been reported in Australia, but it has not been documented in the United States.

Thiabendazole was initially introduced as an effective, safe, and broad-spectrum anthelmintic in 1961. Its widespread use since that time has led to a serious worm resistance problem in many parts of the world including the United States. Because of cross resistance between pro-benzimidazole and benzimidazole drugs, all members of this family are now of limited usefulness for sheep. Phenothiazine is mainly effective against adult abomasal worms but lacks good activity against immature worms. Sheep nematodes have also developed resistance to this drug. Spilt drug, saliva, or urine containing the drug or its metabolites stains wool a red-brown color, which cannot be removed by scouring. The urine is reddish-brown for four or five days after treatment. Low-level daily administration has been used in an attempt to suppress and sterilize worm egg output to keep pasture contamination at a low level. Unfortunately, animals often fail to ingest the requisite amount, the continuous low-level administration of the drug has led to drug resistance, and growth of pasture grass may be inhibited by the excreted drug.

Drug Resistance

After the introduction of phenothiazine in the late 1930's, chemicals became the mainstay for nematode control in sheep, but haphazard use limited their effectiveness and often selected strongly for the development of drug resistance. Strains of *Haemonchus contortus* resistant to phenothiazine were reported in the United States in 1954 and 1957, and strains resistant to thiabendazole were reported in 1964, only three years after the introduction of that drug. Since then, there have been reports throughout the world of resistance by the major sheep pathogens (*Haemonchus, Ostertagia, Trichostrongylus* spp.) to the main classes of anthelmintics (benzimidazoles, organic phosphates, levamisole/morantel). Cross resistance between all benzimidazole and pro-benzimidazole drugs (thiabendazole, parbendazole, cambendazole, mebendazole, oxibendazole, fenbendazole, oxfendazole, albendazole, thiophanate, febantel) has also been reported.

Drug resistance represents a major problem for the sheep industry in the 1980's. A field strain of *H. contortus* in Australia now shows multiple resistance to all major groups of anthelmintics in use (benzimidazole, organic phosphate, levamisole/morantel). In the past it has usually been possible to switch to another drug with a different mode of action to kill resistant worms. However, the pharmaceutical companies cannot be expected to continue to discover or profitably develop new anthelmintics with different modes of action to temporarily salvage the situation. In any case, new drugs may offer only temporary solutions, since none have been shown to be immune to the development of resistance or to reverse already existing resistance. There is a need for veterinarians to become aware of the problem and to warn farmers against overuse of drugs or control strategies that are likely to select strongly for drug resistance. It is advisable to alternate anthelmintics in a slow rotation, using drugs from different chemical groupings rotated between and not within worm generations. In most situations this means an annual rotation of drugs.

GOATS

The major nematode pathogens of sheep are also the major pathogens of goats, and recommendations for parasite control in goats are frequently based on data obtained in sheep. This approach is not always the most effective, because it ignores differences in management, behavior, and epidemiology and illustrates the need for more studies on the dynamics of the goat/parasite relationship. Goats in the United States are usually kept on a small scale, except for a few large dairies. Many goats are kept in confinement and may spend only a short time at pasture each year. Browsing goats have little exposure to infective L_3 but can develop serious infections if given access to pasture at periods of peak L_3 accumulation. Angora goats appear to be especially susceptible to gastrointestinal nematodes under intensive grazing conditions.

It is not surprising that coccidiosis is a major problem with goats in confinement and that helminthosis due to

Haemonchus, Ostertagia, Trichostrongylus, and *Nematodirus* spp. is a bigger problem in goats at pasture. Signs of helminthosis include weight loss, ill thrift, anorexia, rough coat, anemia, diarrhea, coughing, and death. In the present state of limited knowledge, it appears rational to use some of the same nematode control strategies as discussed for sheep. These include prekidding treatments, turnout of kids to safe pastures, prophylactic treatments in spring in northern regions, and treat-and-move strategies. If an outbreak occurs and it is not possible to treat and move goats to safe pasture, it may be necessary to initiate intensive treatment at frequent intervals to counter the effects of continuous re-infection. With young kids in pens, coccidiosis and *Strongyloides* infections are likely to be bigger problems than trichostrongylid worms.

Thiabendazole is the only anthelmintic currently approved for use in goats in the United States. However almost all horse, cattle, and sheep anthelmintics have been used in goats. There has been a decline in the use of thiabendazole in recent years because of the occurrence of drug resistance, and the subsequent pro-benzimidazole and benzimidazole drugs have all suffered the consequences of the emergence of cross resistance. This problem has effectively ended the long period of dominance of the benzimidazole drugs and new non-benzimidazole drugs are now eagerly sought. Levamisole has a broad spectrum of activity against the trichostrongylid worms and can be given by subcutaneous injection. There appears to be little foundation for the view that levamisole causes abortion in pregnant does, as it failed to induce abortion in two recent studies after repeated treatments. Depression, hyperesthesia, and salivation may follow treatment, and the stinging reaction may agitate some goats. The cattle formulation of ivermectin also causes a stinging reaction when injected in goats.

SWINE

Nematode parasites remain a serious limiting factor to successful swine production, although the prevalence and intensity of infection vary with the region, type of housing, and management system. An increasing trend for total confinement of pigs has been associated with a decline in the incidence of the stomach worms (*Hyostrongylus, Ascarops, Physocephalus*) as well as the thorny-headed worm (*Macracanthorhynchus hirudinaceus*) and lungworm (*Metastrongylus* spp.). However, the prevalence of some parasites in confined swine is as high as that in pastured swine. There is an additional danger from waste disposal systems developed to recycle treated waste as feed supplement or fertilizer if not properly processed. In some regions, an increased incidence of *Strongyloides* has been associated with a change to permanent farrowing houses and liberal use of bedding.

Three intestinal species, *Ascaris suum, Oesophagostomum* spp., and *Trichuris suis,* remain as serious pathogens in swine both in confinement and at pasture, and newborn pigs in some areas suffer high mortality from *Strongyloides ransomi* transmitted via the colostrum. Liver condemnations due to *Ascaris suum* and *Stephanurus dentatus* have increased in some regions, and the stigma of trichinosis still persists over the swine industry in the United States.

Life Cycle and Epidemiology

Pigs become infected with ascarids (*Ascaris suum*) by ingestion of infective eggs. After hatching, L_3 penetrate the gut wall and commence the typical ascarid hepatic-tracheal migration. They reach the liver via the portal vein within 24 hours of infection, then pass via the bloodstream to the heart and lungs. Larvae reach the lungs about a week after infection, break out of the capillaries into the alveoli, molt to L_4, and migrate up the bronchioles, bronchi, and trachea. They are coughed up and swallowed, molt to L_5 in the small intestine, develop to maturity, and pass eggs in the feces six to eight weeks post-infection. Female *Ascaris suum* produce enormous numbers of eggs, up to half a million eggs/worm/day. The eggs may be infective after 30 days and are very resistant to external conditions, remaining viable for up to five years if protected from dessication.

Pigs become infected with the nodular worm (*Oesophagostomum* spp.) by ingestion of an infective larva (L_3). These invade the intestinal wall and are found in the mucosa and submucosa of the large intestine as early as 20 hours after infection. The third molt occurs in the gut wall, L_4 return to the gut lumen, molt to L_5, develop to maturity, and pass strongyle-type eggs in the feces seven to eight weeks post-infection. There is little host reaction to primary infection, but nodule formation may be marked in subsequent infections of sensitized animals. Sows commonly exhibit a periparturient rise (PPR) in fecal egg counts, reaching a peak six to seven weeks post-farrowing. Newborn pigs may be exposed to serious infection, as eggs can develop to infective L_3 within a week under optimal conditions.

The whipworm (*Trichuris suis*) life cycle is unusual in that eggs carry an infective L_1 (not L_3) when ingested by swine and all larval molts occur within the host. Larvae spend two to three weeks migrating within the cecal and colonic mucosa before reaching the surface epithelium and maturing to egg-laying adults six to seven weeks after infection. The long filamentous anterior end of the adult worm remains imbedded in the mucosa, forming subepithelial tunnels. The characteristic barrel-shaped, double operculated eggs become infective three weeks after being passed and can survive for up to six years in protected environments.

The threadworm (*Strongyloides ransomi*) can alternate between a free-living and a parasitic existence. Pigs may be infected prenatally, via colostrum, by ingestion of L_3 or by skin penetration of L_3. Transcolostral infection appears to be of considerable importance, with the greatest number of L_3 passed on the first day of lactation. Counts up to 50 L_3/ml of colostrum have been recorded. Sows apparently harbor arrested L_3 in their fat depots until farrowing time when they migrate to the milk cisterns of the mammae. Suffcient larvae may be stored in the fat deposits of the sow to infect four consecutive litters. The prepatent period is only four days following prenatal or transcolostral infection and seven to ten days following other routes of infection. Embryonated eggs or L_1 are passed in the feces, and the parasite persists indefinitely in muddy areas.

Pathogenesis

Penetration of the intestinal mucosa by nematode larvae (*Ascaris, Oesophagostomum, Trichuris, Strongyloides*) or tunnelling by adults (*Trichuris*) provides a portal of entry for bacteria, spirochetes, and viruses. Further migration within the gut wall may cause extensive destruction of tissue (*Trichuris, Strongyloides*) or a host nodular reaction, caseation, and calcification (*Oesophagostomum*) leading to interference with digestion and motility. Local peritonitis and adhesions sometimes result in intussusception or necrosis. Emergence of whipworm (*Trichuris*) larvae may produce dysentery three weeks after infection, well before eggs are passed in the feces, and be misdiagnosed as swine dysentery or proliferative enteritis. These cases do not respond to antibiotic therapy. Outbreaks of necrotic enteritis may be activated in pigs carrying *Salmonella* infections.

Migration of larvae through the liver (*Ascaris*) may result in interstitial hepatitis or "milk spots" and cause large-scale condemnation of livers at abattoirs. Larvae of gastrointestinal nematodes migrating through the lungs (*Ascaris, Strongyloides*) cause alveolar injury with edema and consolidation. Pigs become more susceptible to other diseases such as enzootic pneumonia and swine influenza. Severe gastric ulcers with fatal bleeding have been associated with both experimental and natural infection of *A. suum*, although the underlying mechanisms are not clear. Anemia sometimes occurs in pigs heavily infected with *Trichuris* as a result of blood-sucking and tissue destruction. Hypoproteinemia may be associated with any parasite where there is marked anorexia and/or a protein-losing enteropathy. Death of young pigs sometimes results from invasion of the myocardium by skin-penetrating *Strongyloides*.

Clinical Disease

Ascariasis may be manifest in young pigs by ill thrift, stunted growth, pot belly, and diarrhea. Adult worms may be vomited. Occasional cases of obstructive jaundice or intestinal obstruction and rupture occur. Larvae migrating though the lungs may cause "thumps" and elicit a soft cough. Nodular worms may cause weight loss and diarrhea in pigs of all ages but rarely death. The diarrhea is often khaki in color and contains undigested food. There may be a blood-stained mucoid diarrhea if massive numbers of larvae penetrate the gut wall. The bloody diarrhea of whipworm infection, starting three weeks after infection, may be confused with swine dysentery or proliferative enteritis. Affected pigs may also show anorexia, weight loss, straining, rectal prolapse, and a high mortality rate. Newborn pigs with a heavy threadworm infection may show stunted growth, pot belly, bloody diarrhea, and a high mortality rate.

Diagnosis

The history, clinical signs, and response to treatment are likely to be of value in making a correct diagnosis. The age of the affected pigs and their likely exposure to infective eggs or larvae are important considerations. Ascariasis is a disease of young pigs, and older animals rarely show clinical signs although they may be infected and an important source of contamination. Strongyloidiasis is mainly confined to baby pigs and may result from prenatal or transcolostral infection as well as from L_3 in the environment. The major nematodes discussed (*Ascaris, Oesophagostomum, Trichuris*) have a prepatent period of six to eight weeks, and it is possible for clinical signs to develop before the characteristic thick-shelled eggs (*Ascaris*), strongyle-type eggs (*Oesophagostomum*) or double-operculated eggs (*Trichuris*) are passed in feces. By contrast, the smaller embryonated eggs of *Strongyloides* may be passed as early as four days post-infection.

As with other host species, there is a poor correlation between fecal egg counts and worm burden. A small number of *Ascaris* females may produce millions of eggs, whereas *Trichuris* females are not prolific egg layers and a low or modest egg count may be associated with severe disease. The most positive way to make a diagnosis is by necropsy examination so that the intensity of the worm infection and the degree of tissue destruction can be accurately assessed.

Control Strategies

The North Carolina Swine Parasite Control Program or its modifications can be used effectively in many regions. In this program sows and gilts are given a broad-spectrum anthelmintic five to ten days before breeding and again five to ten days before farrowing to remove parasites from their digestive system, which serves as a source of the PPR and infection in the farrowing house. Boars are treated twice a year. Young pigs are treated at five to six weeks of age and treatment is repeated 30 days later. Anthelmintics to consider include levamisole or dichlorvos as a single treatment, fenbendazole for three days, and pyrantel tartrate or hygromycin B as continuous additives to the feed for a specified time during the period of greatest risk. Swine should be kept on well-drained open lots, or temporary pastures or on clean concrete or slats. Treatment is normally not needed for pigs in a clean operation on raised decks, but treatment of breeders once yearly offers a safeguard against accidental infection.

A major control problem is the great survival capacity of ascarid and whipworm eggs. Sometimes the only solution is to move range pigs to fresh ground and cultivate the old ground for three years before re-introducing swine. In housing, thorough cleansing with hot detergents or high-pressure water can be used to prepare surfaces for disinfection with agents such as hot lye (95 per cent sodium hydroxide). The disinfectant should be applied to walls and left for two to three days and then hosed away before pigs are returned. It is advisable to scrub sows thoroughly with hot detergent and water to remove eggs before moving them into a farrowing pen that has been cleaned and disinfected. Sows should also be treated a few days before they enter the farrowing pen so that feces containing viable eggs and expelled worms will not be introduced. Likewise, if young pigs are to be returned to pasture after treatment, it is preferable to confine them on concrete for one to two days and to destroy all feces and expelled worms before they are returned to pasture.

Feeder pigs can be given fenbendazole, dichlorvos, or levamisole, or continuous feed medication with pyrantel tartrate or hygromycin B. Where pigs are run on dirt and subject to continuous re-infection, it is more effective to provide a continuous feed additive. Baby pigs should be treated with thiabendazole or other appropriate anthelmintics at five and ten days of age if threadworm (*Strongyloides*) is a problem. It is imperative to keep breeding stock on dry, well-drained surfaces, because *Strongyloides* is capable of reproducing in a free-living cycle and will persist indefinitely in muddy areas. If swine kidney worm

(*Stephanurus dentatus*) is a problem, both adult and larval stages can be killed by fenbendazole and adults by levamisole. The "gilt only" farrowing system may also be considered, but it has the disadvantage of producing smaller litters.

Anthelmintics

Modern swine anthelmintics have high efficiency, high safety, and easy administration. The choice of anthelmintic should be based on the predominant parasite species present and the desired route of administration. Levamisole is effective against ascarids, nodular worms, threadworms, lungworms, and adult kidney worms but has low efficacy against whipworms. It can be injected subcutaneously or given in feed or water. Dichlorvos pellets are effective against ascarids, nodular worms, and whipworms. Feed premixes containing pyrantel tartrate or hygromycin B are effective against ascarids and nodular worms and hygromycin B also affects whipworms. Pyrantel tartrate has a prophylactic effect in killing ascarid L_3 in the gut and preventing their migration through the liver and lungs. Thiabendazole paste has high efficiency against threadworms only, whereas piperazine is effective against ascarids only. Ivermectin is not yet approved for swine in the United States. It is effective against a number of nematode species and are unique in that a single injection at low dose rate has high efficacy against arthropods.

Supplemental Reading

Armour, J., and Ogbourne, C. P.: Bovine Ostertagiasis: A Review and Annotated Bibliography. Miscellaneous Publication No. 7 of the Commonwealth Institute of Parasitology, Commonwealth Agricultural Bureaux, Farnham Royal, Bucks, England, 1982, 1–93.
Blood, D. C., Henderson, J. A., and Radostits, O. M.: Veterinary Medicine, 5th ed. Lea & Febiger, Philadelphia, 1979, 750–799.
Commonwealth Scientific and Industrial Research Organization, Australia: The Epidemiology and Control of Gastrointestinal Parasites of Sheep in Australia. Donald, A. D., Southcott, W. H., and Dineen, J. K. (eds.). CSIRO Publications, Victoria, Australia, 1978, 1–153.
Commonwealth Scientific and Industrial Research Organization, Australia: The Epidemiology and Control of Gastrointestinal Parasites of Cattle in Australia. Anderson, N., and Waller, P. J. (eds.). CSIRO Publications, Victoria, Australia, 1983, 1–90.
Herd, R. P.: A practical approach to parasite control in dairy cows and heifers. Comp. Cont. Ed. Pract. Vet. 5:S73–80, 1983.
Herd, R. P.: A practical approach to parasite control in sheep in the northern United States. Comp. Cont. Ed. Pract. Vet., 6:567–574, 1984.
Ministry of Agriculture, Fisheries and Food: Grazing Plans for the Control of Stomach and Intestinal Worms in Sheep and Cattle. Booklet 2154, Publications, Middlesex, England, 1980, 1–17.
Williams, J. C.: Ecology and control of gastrointestinal nematodes of beef cattle. Vet. Clin. North Am. 5:183–205, 1983.

Trematode Infections—Cattle, Sheep, Goats

R. P. HERD, M.V.Sc., Ph.D.

Fasciola hepatica is the most important trematode of livestock throughout the world. It is an increasing problem as new dams, irrigation projects, and improved water facilities provide new habitats for the lymnaeid snail intermediate hosts. Acute fluke disease causes high mortality in sheep, whereas chronic fluke disease causes substantial production losses in both cattle and sheep.

Several studies suggest that effective control can result in increased mature cow body weights, conception rates, milk production, and calf weaning weights. Feedlot studies have demonstrated increased weight gains and feed conversion rates, with reduced liver rejection rates at abattoirs.

In the United States, *F. hepatica* occurs primarily in the Gulf Coast states and western states, whereas *F. gigantica* occurs in Hawaii. *Fascioloides magna* is an additional problem in the Gulf Coast states, Great Lakes region, and northwestern states where cattle, sheep, or goats share pastures with deer, elk, and moose natural hosts. *Dicrocoelium dendriticum,* the small black lanceolate fluke, is restricted to foci in New York State. The paramphistomes, or stomach flukes, appear to be of minor economic significance in the United States, although heavy infections can cause severe enteritis and mortality in cattle and occasionally in sheep and goats. *Paramphistomum microbothrioides* is the most common species in the United States, although it appears that it has sometimes been erroneously described as *Cotylophoron cotylophorum* in the past.

LIFE CYCLE

Trematodes have an indirect life cycle, and most species of veterinary importance have a snail intermediate host. *F. hepatica, F. gigantica, F. magna,* and *P. microbothrioides* all have aquatic snail intermediate hosts. *D. dendriticum* has a land snail as its first intermediate host and a brown ant as its second intermediate host. One fluke egg passed by the cattle, sheep, or goat final host can give rise to thousands of infective cercariae or metacercariae. This is in marked contrast to the situation with nematodes, in which one egg produces only one infective larva. Eggs of *Fasciola, Fascioloides,* and *Paramphistomum* spp. hatch miracidia, which develop through sporocyst, redia, and cercaria stages after miracidia actively penetrate the appropriate snail intermediate host. Cercariae later emerge from the snail and encyst as metacercariae on herbage to be eaten by the final host. Eggs of *Dicrocoelium* are ingested by land snails, which later expel slime balls containing up to 400 cercariae. Whole colonies of brown ants may become infected from eating slime balls. The final host is infected by ingesting ants attached to herbage.

Although prenatal infection with *F. hepatica* has been reported in a small percentage of calves, most livestock are infected by ingestion of metacercariae from pasture. These excyst in the small intestine, and young flukes migrate through the gut wall and peritoneal cavity to reach the liver in six to seven days. They migrate in the hepatic parenchyma for four to six weeks, then enter the bile ducts and mature to egg-laying adults 10 to 12 weeks after infection. The life cycle of *F. gigantica* is similar to that of *F. hepatica. F. magna* completes the full life cycle only in deer, elk, or moose natural hosts. Adults are enclosed in thin-walled cysts, and eggs escape via fistulae to the bile ducts. In cattle, young flukes become completely encapsulated by a host reaction in the liver and there is no channel for release of eggs to the exterior. In sheep and goats, the young flukes tunnel extensively, causing severe damage to the parenchyma. Immature paramphistomes develop in the duodenal mucosa but migrate through the abomasum to the rumen and reticulum as they mature. *Dicrocoelium* migrates up the bile ducts from the duodenum and matures in the bile ducts and gall bladder without invading the liver parenchyma.

EPIDEMIOLOGY

The initiation of effective trematode control programs and the proper timing of treatment are dependent on an understanding of the epidemiology of the disease. Livestock most likely to be affected with *F. hepatica* are those grazing in low lying swampy areas, flood irrigation areas, or anywhere that surface water or small, slowly moving streams favor the propagation of lymnaeid snails. *F. hepatica* can survive for many years in sheep and shed up to 50,000 eggs per day, but cattle develop resistance and expel most flukes within a year. Cattle appear to have a natural immunity to liver fluke as well as an ability to develop acquired immunity, whereas sheep and goats seem to be lacking in both. Pastures become infective with metacercariae two months after being grazed by infected livestock, and metacercariae may survive on pastures for up to one year but die quickly under hot dry conditions. Housed animals will be protected against the disease unless they are fed hay with sufficient moisture to enable metacercariae to survive. Metacercariae are killed by ensiling the cut material.

Warm and wet conditions in the spring and early summer are highly favorable for massive proliferation of snails, hatching of fluke eggs, and development of cercariae within snails. If a wet season that allows rapid reproduction is followed by a dry season, livestock will be exposed to large numbers of metacercariae pastures after surface water recedes, resulting in heavy infection rates in the fall. The extent of production losses will also be influenced by the level of nutrition and concurrent nematode infections. In the Gulf Coast states, peak fluke burdens, adult *Ostertagia* burdens, and nutritional stress may all coincide in the winter. Whereas warm and wet conditions favor snail and fluke proliferation, cold conditions (below 10°C) inhibit their reproduction, and dry conditions kill large numbers of snails and metacercariae. In Britain, considerable success has been achieved in predicting high- or low-risk years for fascioliasis from meterologic data.

PATHOGENESIS

Acute fluke disease due to *F. hepatica* is caused by the sudden invasion of the liver by masses of young flukes. Severe destruction of parenchyma results in acute hepatic insufficiency as well as massive hemorrhage into the peritoneal cavity. Chronic fluke disease develops slowly and is caused by the activities of adult flukes in the bile ducts. In addition to cholangitis, biliary obstruction, and fibrosis, they cause anemia by their blood-sucking activities. Hypoproteinemia may also result from seepage of plasma proteins from the damaged bile duct epithelium. The pathogenesis of *F. gigantica* is similar to that of *F. hepatica*. Migration of immature flukes through hepatic tissue and production of anaerobic necrotic tracts may also trigger germination of latent spores of *Clostridium novyi* to cause Black disease. This occurs much more commonly in sheep than in cattle. Bacillary hemoglobi-

nuria due to exotoxins of *Clostridium hemolyticum* may also be triggered by migrating liver flukes.

F. magna infection in cattle is usually clinically inapparent because of massive encapsulation of flukes, but their unrestricted tunnelling in sheep and goats can be rapidly fatal. It is reported that a single fluke can cause death. In the wildlife natural hosts, there is only minor liver damage as the adults are enclosed in thin-walled cysts. *D. dendriticum* is relatively nonpathogenic because of its small size, smooth cuticle, and failure to invade the liver parenchyma. It may, however, cause cirrhosis of bile ducts and condemnation of livers. Clinical paramphistomiasis is caused by massive numbers of immature flukes in the duodenal mucosa, whereas adult flukes in the rumen and reticulum cause little harm in most circumstances.

CLINICAL DISEASE

Acute liver fluke disease due to *F. hepatica* is seen in sheep and goats but rarely in cattle because of both natural and acquired immunity. It is caused by massive hemorrhage and tissue destruction following ingestion of large numbers of metacercariae. Acute fluke outbreaks are likely to occur in seasons of very high rainfall. Death is usually sudden or occurs within 48 hours of the onset of symptoms. Clinical signs include anorexia, dullness, weakness, pale membranes, dyspnea, ascites, abdominal pain, and alternating standing up and lying down. It may be possible to palpate an enlarged liver. The feces are dry and are not diarrheic. Outbreaks may last only two to three weeks but involve high mortality, especially if the fluke migration triggers further deaths from Black disease. A subacute syndrome may also occur, with affected animals surviving for two weeks after the onset of clinical signs.

The chronic disease is a wasting condition caused by the blood-sucking activities of adult *F. hepatica* in the bile ducts. Sheep progressively lose weight over months and develop pale membranes, submandibular edema (bottle-jaw), ascites, or jaundice. Shedding of the wool may also occur. Cattle usually suffer the chronic disease only and experience weight loss, anemia, and a reduction of up to 10 per cent in milk yield. In Britain, most fluke infections are acquired by cows in the autumn and early winter, and the effects on lactation become apparent in mid winter. The poor body condition also contributes to lowered reproductive performance and a higher percentage of barren cows. A subacute disease sometimes occurs in dairy calves exposed to large numbers of metacercariae. Infection with *F. gigantica* causes clinical signs similar to those caused by *F. hepatica*. *F. magna* infection may cause a syndrome similar to chronic *F. hepatica* disease in cattle and acute *F. hepatica* disease in sheep. Paramphistomes may induce a severe enteritis with weight loss and diarrhea and may be clinically indistinguishable from ostertagiasis or Johne's disease. *D. dendriticum* infection is usually asymptomatic.

DIAGNOSIS

Clinical diagnosis of liver fluke disease is often complicated by the concurrent presence of gastrointestinal nematodes, which produce some of the same clinical signs.

A common experience in the Gulf Coast is that giving one or more treatments for nematodes has little effect. When a flukicide is given a dramatic clinical improvement occurs. A history of access to snail habitats, seasonal conditions favorable for snail reproduction, and an unexpected drop in milk yield are all important indicators in endemic areas. In outbreaks of acute *F. hepatica* disease in sheep and goats there will be no fluke eggs in the feces, and in cases of *F. magna* infection patency is unlikely to be reached in domestic animals. In subacute disease due to *F. hepatica,* a few flukes may reach adult stage and pass small numbers of eggs in the feces. In chronic *F. hepatica* infection in cattle, sheep, and goats variable numbers of eggs ranging from high to low occur in the feces. The immature paramphistomes that cause clinical signs do not betray their presence by eggs.

It is desirable to use a sedimentation technique for the detection of fluke eggs, as they do not float well in most flotation solutions. *F. hepatica* eggs are large (up to 150 μm), operculated, thin-walled, and yellow-brown. Eggs of *F. gigantica, F. magna,* and *P. microbothrioides* all resemble *F. hepatica* eggs but are a little larger, and those of *P. microbothrioides* have a transparent gray-green appearance. Immature stomach flukes are sometimes passed in the feces. They are 3 to 4 mm in size and can be detected by sedimentation and decanting techniques. The eggs of *D. dendriticum* are quite distinctive, being small (up to 45 μm), dark brown, and operculated, and contain a miracidium when passed in the feces.

In acute *F. hepatica* outbreaks, the main necropsy findings are an enlarged hemorrhagic liver covered with fibrinous strands, a large amount of blood-stained peritoneal fluid, and over 1000 immature flukes in the liver parenchyma. In the subacute disease, the liver is also enlarged and hemorrhagic, but some of the flukes will have reached the adult stage. The chronic disease is characterized by an emaciated carcass, a small, shrunken fibrotic liver, and 200 or more adult flukes in the bile ducts. In cattle infected with *F. magna,* flukes are found within a thick capsule and there is little general involvement of the liver, whereas in sheep or goats tunnels are seen in the parenchyma. In paramphistomiasis, immature flukes may cause thickening and hemorrhage of the duodenal wall but are sometimes overlooked because of their small size.

CONTROL STRATEGIES

Control is best achieved by strategic use of flukicides to remove flukes before productivity is affected and to prevent egg shedding before large numbers of susceptible snails are present. In some situations, the use of molluscicides, grazing management strategies, and fencing or drainage of snail habitats may be successfully integrated with strategic treatments. The timing, frequency, and choice of flukicides are best determined after consideration of the epidemiology of fluke disease in each area. The most appropriate timing may not always coincide with the times when livestock owners normally handle their stock for other purposes. However, the returns from improved weight gains, feed conversion, conception rates, milk production, or calf weaning weights may justify a change in management procedure to allow more effective fluke control. There may also be a need to offset winter

nutritional stress, since poorly nourished animals are more susceptible to the effects of liver fluke disease.

Studies in Louisiana suggest that an annual fall treatment with a flukicide is adequate for the sustained reduction of fluke burdens in low-risk years, but at least two treatments are needed in moderate and high-risk years. These studies were based on the use of albendazole (10 mg/kg), the only flukicide approved for use in the United States at that time. Although albendazole has a broad spectrum of activity against gastrointestinal nematodes, lungworms, tapeworms, and adult liver flukes, it has little or no efficiency against immature flukes. It is consequently most effective in the fall when flukes are adult, but is considerably less effective in the spring or early summer when a mixed, immature/mature population is present. The fall treatment is especially important in removing adult fluke burdens prior to the winter nutritional stress period as well as reducing environmental contamination with fluke eggs prior to the massive late winter-spring-early summer buildup of the snail population.

A second treatment in winter should be of benefit in removing residual flukes left after the fall treatment and in preventing heavy infection levels in the snail population. In some southern regions, substantial populations of adult *Ostertagia* and *F. hepatica* may coincide with a period of nutritional stress in the winter. Hence a winter treatment with albendazole would eliminate both trematode and nematode burdens and prevent the spring infection of snails as well as the accumulation of arrested-prone *Ostertagia* L_3 on spring pasture. Clorsulon has recently taken the place of albendazole as the only approved flukicide in the United States. It is effective against adult *F. hepatica* but not against immature flukes less than 8 weeks of age. Nematodes and cestodes are not affected by clorsulon. Effective management systems including grazing systems that avoid high-risk areas during periods of high transmission potential and the fencing off or drainage of snail habitats if practical.

The use of molluscicides has achieved only partial success, largely because of the high cost and the extreme rapidity of snail reproduction. Nevertheless, molluscicides may be of value when applied to relatively small snail habitats and integrated with strategic flukicide treatments. Toxicity to nontarget species and phytotoxicity are important constraints to molluscicide use. Molluscicides are best applied before the snail breeding season. Copper sulphate has been widely used in the past but has sometimes resulted in copper poisoning of livestock or killing of fish after drainage into nearby streams. Copper pentachlorphenate is more effective as it is not inactivated by organic matter like copper sulphate. Other potential molluscicides include niclosamide, nicotinanalide analogues, and N-tritylmorpholene. Biologic approaches to snail control have also been attempted, including the release of sciomyzid marsh flies, but the results have been disappointing.

FLUKICIDES

Clorsulon (7 mg/kg) is the only flukicide approved for cattle in the United States. It is 90 to 100 per cent effective against adult *F. hepatica* in the bile ducts but is not effective against immature flukes less than 8 weeks old. It is marketed as an oral drench for use in cattle of all ages and at any stage of pregnancy. There is a wide safety margin and a withdrawal period of three weeks. It is also effective against *F. gigantica* but not against *F. magna.* Albendazole (10 mg/kg) provides partial protection against *F. magna,* whereas an increased dosage (15 to 20 mg/kg) is effective against *D. dendriticum.* Drugs recommended for paramphistome therapy (brotianide, niclosamide, resorantel) are approved for food animals in the United States.

At the time of writing, a new benzimidazole drug, trichlorbendazole, shows great promise as a flukicide with potent activity against both mature and immature *F. hepatica* in ruminants. At a dosage of 12 mg/kg it is 90 to 100 per cent effective against flukes from one week of age to adulthood, except for a slight decrease in efficiency against four- to 6-week-old flukes entrapped in fibrous tissue in cattle livers. Trichlorbendazole has no effect against nematodes, cestodes, or paramphistomes, but its unique activity against all stages of liver fluke infection makes it a potent weapon for the control of *F. hepatica.*

Supplemental Reading

Blood, D. C., Henderson, J. A., and Radostits, O. M.: Veterinary Medicine, 5th ed. Lea & Febiger, Philadelphia, 1979, 750–799.
Malone, J. B., Loyacano, M. S., Armstrong, D. A., and Archibald, L. F.: Bovine fascioliasis: Economic impact and control in Gulf Coast cattle based on seasonal transmission. Bovine Pract. *17*:126–133, 1982.

Cestode Infections—Cattle, Sheep, Goats, Swine

R. P. HERD, M.V.Sc., Ph.D.

Gastrointestinal cestodes of food animals are of minor importance, but cystic larval stages of human and canid taeniids that occur in food animal intermediate hosts are of both economic and public health significance.

In the United States, *Moniezia* spp. of cattle, sheep, and goats are widely distributed owing to the ready availability of the oribatid pasture mite intermediate hosts. Livestock become infected by accidental ingestion of the mites, which are especially numerous on permanent pasture. The "fringed tapeworm" (*Thysanosoma actinioides*) is limited to western states because the appropriate intermediate host (psocid louse) is not so widely disseminated.

A discussion of cysticercosis and hydatidosis is outside the scope of a discussion of digestive system diseases, but it should be noted that *Taenia saginata* has become more common in the United States over the last decade as a result of the influx of migrant workers from enzootic areas, as a consequence of the use of raw sewage for the fertilization of pasture, and because of sewage contamination of irrigation water. There is a similar risk of the introduction of *T. solium* with migrant workers from Mexico and other enzootic areas. Cystic hydatid disease persists as a problem in sheep raising areas in Utah, California, Arizona, and New Mexico. Cysticercosis of sheep due to larval *T. ovis* and *T. hydatigena* causes carcass and organ rejection at abattoirs and adversely affects export markets.

LIFE CYCLE AND EPIDEMIOLOGY

Most cestodes of veterinary importance have an indirect life cycle with one intermediate host. There are no free-living larval stages. In the case of *Moniezia* and *Thysanosoma* spp., eggs disseminated from gravid proglottids passed in cattle, sheep, or goat feces are consumed by an arthropod intermediate host. The oncosphere or hexacanth embryo is released and burrows into the body cavity of the arthropod, where it develops to a cysticercoid (a small cyst with a single depressed scolex) within 100 to 200 days depending on the temperature. Each cysticercoid develops into a single tapeworm if the infected intermediate host is eaten by the appropriate final host.

Food animals become infected with the larval cysts by ingesting tapeworm eggs excreted by man or canids. After ingestion of the egg, the protective embryophore is digested in the gut and the released oncosphere activated by the bile salts. It penetrates the gut wall and is carried to the predilection site, where it grows into a cysticercus (a fluid-filled cyst with a single invaginated scolex), a coenurus (a fluid-filled cyst with numerous invaginated scoleces), or a hydatid (a fluid-filled cyst with numerous brood capsules and protoscoleces), depending on the species.

Moniezia tapeworms are relatively short-lived. They start shedding eggs about six weeks after infection, then disappear from the host after about three months. The eggs have a poor survival capacity and are infective for mites for only about three months after being passed. Development of cysticercoids in mites takes several months depending on the temperature, and it appears that cysticercoids can overwinter in mites. The prevalence of *Moniezia* infection in livestock shows a seasonal fluctuation coinciding with the active period of the vectors. At present it is not clear how much the transmission of tapeworm eggs is affected by wind, water, temperature, vectors, and fomites. Coprophagous flies probably play an important role in egg dissemination. Unlike *Moniezia,* *Thysanosoma* is a long-lived worm surviving for several years.

PATHOGENESIS

The intestinal tapeworms of cattle, sheep, and goats are not serious pathogens, although *Moniezia* infection is sometimes associated with poor growth and diarrhea. Adult tapeworms compete with the host for nutrients, interfere with gut motility, and excrete toxic substances. *M. expansa* has been associated with enterotoxemia outbreaks in lambs, and it has been suggested that it causes sluggish bowel movements and conditions suitable for the production of *Clostridium perfringens* exotoxins. Massive invasion of hepatic tissue by *T. hydatigena* oncospheres may create anaerobic conditions suitable for the propagation of *Clostridium novyi* and death from Black disease. There is evidence that tapeworm-infected sheep may be more subject to fly-strike. Young animals are most susceptible to tapeworm infection, and it is possible that older animals develop an acquired immunity. *T. actinioides* infection is not of clinical importance, but its presence in the bile ducts can result in the condemnation of livers.

CLINICAL DISEASE

There is some controversy over the importance of tapeworm infection of food animals, with a tendency for farmers to over emphasize their importance and be more concerned about tapeworms than the more pathogenic nematodes and trematodes. At the same time it is probably a mistake to totally ignore tapeworms and regard them as completely nonpathogenic. Most infections do not cause clinical disease, but heavy infections are sometimes associated with poor growth, diarrhea or clostridial infections. Clinical signs are usually not seen in cysticercosis or hydatidosis of food animals unless large cysts disrupt vital organs.

DIAGNOSIS

Diagnosis is usually made by finding proglottids or the characteristic thick-walled eggs in feces. *Moniezia* eggs contain a distinctive hexacanth embryo in a piriform apparatus. The much smaller *Thysanosoma* eggs have no piriform apparatus. *Moniezia* is a large cestode (200 cm), and it is common to recover masses of them at routine necropsy of lambs during the spring. In spite of their spectacular volume, tapeworms are much less pathogenic than the tiny hair-like trichostrongylid nematodes. The smaller *Thysanosoma* tapeworms (20 cm) are usually found in the duodenum or bile ducts at necropsy.

TREATMENT

As control of the arthropod vectors is impractical, periodic treatment with cestocides is the main method of control. In the past lead arsenate (0.5 gm for lambs, 1 gm for adult sheep, 0.5 to 1.5 gm for calves) was the main drug employed. It has now been superseded by more efficient and safer pro-benzimidazole or benzimidazole drugs, including albendazole, cambendazole, febantel, fenbendazole, mebendazole, and oxfendazole. Preliminary studies suggest that albendazole and fenbendazole at dosages of 10 mg/kg have excellent activity against gastrointestinal cestodes. There are no highly effective chemotherapeutic agents for the control of larval cestodes in ruminants, but several drugs (e.g., praziquantel, membendazole) have shown promising results under experimental conditions. At present, the best approach is to use drugs such as niclosamide and praziquantel to eliminate adult cestodes in the human and canid definitive hosts, with the object of reducing the environmental contamination with cestode eggs.

Drugs Affecting the Digestive System

LLOYD E. DAVIS, D.V.M., Ph.D.

Digestive disturbances are among the problems most commonly encountered in food animal practice. Precise diagnoses are often difficult, and, hence, an understanding of the underlying pathophysiologic features of a particular case frequently is lacking. This has led, in the past, to the marketing and use of various nostrums that had questionable efficacy in correcting the underlying medical problems. Drugs in modern use act to increase or decrease motility and/or secretion or to exert effects locally within the ingesta contained within the lumen.

DRUGS AFFECTING MOTILITY

Drugs modify motility and tone of the gastrointestinal tract by direct action on autonomic receptors in smooth muscle or reflexly by causing distention of the bowel. These drugs and their dosage are listed in Table 1.

The cholinergic drugs increase gastric emptying and propulsive activity of the intestines and colon while, at the same time, inhibiting the smooth muscle of sphincters. Pilocarpine and arecoline act primarily at muscarinic sites and exert marked pharmacologic effects on the heart, glands, eyes, bronchioles, and urinary tract stimulate motility of the gut. The effects of these drugs are readily antagonized by atropine. Carbachol has much less effect on the heart and bronchioles but stimulates nicotinic sites. This enhances its effects on the bowel, but fasciculation of skeletal muscle and stimulation of epinephrine release from the adrenal medulla may occur. The release of epinephrine may inhibit motility of the reticulorumen and intestine. These effects are dose-related, and the effects of carbachol are poorly antagonized by atropine.

Bethanechol is another synthetic choline ester that is more specific in its actions. It stimulates the smooth muscle of the gastrointestinal tract and the urinary bladder with minimal effects on the cardiovascular system or bronchioles. It has no nicotinic effects and is readily antagonized by atropine.

The anticholinesterases act at both muscarinic and nicotinic sites. All cholinergic receptors in visceral organs, ganglia, and skeletal muscle are stimulated. In addition to its ability to inhibit acetylcholinesterase, neostigmine also directly stimulates the cholinergic receptor. Because of their nicotinic actions, the effects of these drugs are only partially antagonized by atropine.

Cholinergic and anticholinesterase drugs should not be administered in the presence of mechanical obstruction of the gut, peritonitis, or doubtful viability of the intestinal wall. Whenever these drugs are employed, the therapist must have injectable atropine available to counteract excessive stimulation of the gut or untoward side effects.

The cathartics increase motility of the bowel by directly stimulating the smooth muscle, by activating receptors in the mucosa, which reflexly releases acetylcholine, or by modifying secretion and absorption of electrolytes and water. The drugs that are employed in food animals are listed in Table 1.

The irritant cathartics increase motility of the intestinal tract by directly stimulating smooth muscle in the wall of the bowel and by increasing secretion. The most commonly used drugs of this group are the anthraquinone derivatives. The pharmacologically inactive glycosides in aloin and senna are transported to the colon, where emodin, which stimulates motility, is released. This accounts for the delay of about 12 hours between ingestion and stimulation of defecation. Danthron is a synthetic, nonglycosidic anthraquinone that may be administered parenterally. The action of drugs in this group most nearly

Table 1. *Dosage of Drugs That Modify Gastrointestinal Motility*

Category and Drug	Cattle	Sheep and Goats	Swine	Comments
Cholinergics				
Pilocarpine	65–300 mg, SC	10–30 mg, SC	10–30 mg, SC	Stimulate motility
Arecoline	4–8 mg, SC	2–4 mg, SC	—	throughout GI tract
Carbachol	4 mg, SC	0.1–0.2 mg, SC	1–4 mg, SC	
Bethanechol	50 µg/kg, SC	50 µg/kg, SC	50 µg/kg, SC	
Anticholinesterases				
Physostigmine	30–50 mg, SC	5–20 mg, SC	5–20 mg, SC	
Neostigmine	1 mg/CWT	0.01–0.02 mg/kg	0.03 mg/kg	
Cathartics				
Senna	120–150 gm	30–60 gm	30–60 gm	Stimulate colon only
Aloin	10–20 gm	2–4 gm	1–2.5 gm	
Danthron	20–45 gm	2.5–5 gm	5–20 gm	
Castor oil	—	—	20–150 ml	Stimulate small
Magnesium sulfate	250–1000 gm	25–125 gm	25–125 gm	intestine motility
Sodium sulfate	500–750 gm	60 gm	30–60 gm	
Magnesium oxide	500 gm	5–10 gm	5–10 gm	
Magnesium hydroxide susp.	1–4 L	20–150 ml	10–50 ml	
Liquid petrolatum	250–500 ml	100–200 ml	100–200 ml	Lubricant
Docusate	5–15 gm	2–5 gm	2–10 gm	Surfactant
Anticholinergics				
Atropine	0.08 mg/kg	0.08 mg/kg	0.04 mg/kg	Inhibit motility
Methscopolamine	5 mg/CWT	5 mg/CWT	5 mg/CWT	
Opioids				
Morphine	—	—	0.25 mg/kg	Decrease propulsive
Paregoric	15–30 ml (calves)	—	—	movement but
Diphenoxylate	0.5 mg/kg	0.5 mg/kg	0.5 mg/kg	increase segmental resistance

mimics the physiologic act of defecation. The compounds are absorbed to some extent and are excreted into the urine and milk. They will color alkaline urine red and acidic urine a dark yellow.

Castor oil is a nonirritating triglyceride of ricinoleic acid. Following ingestion, castor oil is hydrolyzed in the small intestine to release ricinoleic acid, which increases secretion of electrolytes and water. The increased intraluminal volume stimulates motility of the small intestine, causing the elimination of liquid feces.

The irritant cathartics should not be administered to patients with possible obstruction, enteritis, or colitis. They should not be given to animals in late pregnancy, as they may initiate parturition. Their use in lactating animals should be attended with care as active fractions are secreted into milk, which may cause purgation in the nursing offspring.

The saline cathartics reflexly stimulate motility by distending the bowel. The magnesium and sulfate ions are poorly absorbed from the gut, thereby exerting an osmotic effect that causes movement of water from plasma into the lumen of the intestine. The increased volume stretches the mucosa and stimulates mechanoreceptors, reflexly increasing peristaltic activity.

Sodium sulfate is the most effective of the saline cathartics on a molar basis. It is inexpensive, safe, and best administered by stomach tube in a 6 per cent solution. Magnesium salts are effective and relatively inexpensive. Magnesium sulfate is generally employed in adults, whereas magnesium oxide or magnesium hydroxide may be used in calves, lambs, and piglets.

Drugs employed to lubricate the fecal mass in obstipation or impactions include liquid petrolatum ("mineral oil") and the surfactants. These substances are pharmacologically inert in usual doses, but docusate may stimu-late motor activity of the intestine when administered at high dosage. They are administered orally or may be incorporated in enemata to soften fecal masses in the colon. The principal untoward effects of liquid petrolatum are interference with absorption of fat-soluble vitamins, inhibition of healing of wounds in the anorectal area, interference with normal defecatory reflexes, and foreign body reactions at the gut wall, liver, and mesenteric lymph nodes following absorption. Liquid petrolatum and surfactants should not be used simultaneously, as emulsification of the oil might facilitate its absorption from the gut.

Appropriate uses of cathartics include (1) cleansing the bowel prior to elective surgery, (2) as an aid to eliminate parasites following administration of a vermifuge, (3) in poisoning to hasten elimination of unabsorbed toxin, (4) to facilitate reduction of impactions, and (5) to facilitate defecation in patients with prolapses or hernias where straining would be undesirable (lubricants or surfactants should be used).

Cathartics must not be given to patients showing signs of abdominal pain.

Several drugs have been advocated for use as rumenatorics. Increases in frequency and amplitude of ruminal contractions have been observed following administration of physostigmine, carbachol, and arecoline. Marked inhibition of ruminal motility follows administration of epinephrine, histamine, and atropine and high doses of carbachol or arecoline. The higher doses of carbachol and arecoline stimulate the release of epinephrine from the adrenal medulla, which, in turn, inhibits the ruminal musculature. Veratrine is an alkaloid derived from *Veratrum album* that stimulates reticuloruminal activity at low doses and vomiting at higher doses. The status of the drug in the treatment of ruminal atony has not been established, but subcutaneous doses of 40 mg in cattle and 20 mg in sheep have been suggested.

Frequently ruminal stasis is secondary to other conditions such as ketosis, acid-base disturbances, or infectious diseases. It is generally more rewarding to correct the underlying disturbances than to try to stimulate ruminal motility with drugs.

Drugs may be administered to decrease peristaltic activity or spasm within the gastrointestinal tract. The anticholinergic drugs occupy the cholinergic receptor at muscarinic sites and prevent the action of acetylcholine on smooth muscle and glands. Atropine blocks the effects of parasympathetic stimulation on smooth muscle, glands, and heart. At high doses it readily crosses into the brain, where it produces excitement. Methscopolamine is a more polar compound that does not cross the blood-brain barrier and that blocks ganglia in the gut as well as exerts antimuscarinic effects. Inhibition of excessive motility or spasm of the gut is frequently incomplete, as other mediators or autacoids such as serotonin, histamine, and prostaglandins may be involved in the abnormal activity of the gut.

The opioids paregoric (camphorated tincture of opium), morphine, and diphenoxylate decrease propulsive activity, delay gastric emptying, and increase the tone of the intestine and sphincters. The decrease in peristalsis occurs because of the spasmogenic effect of the opioids, which prevents the sequential contraction and relaxation characteristic of peristaltic movements. Tone of the colon is increased to the point of spasm, allowing time for desiccation of feces. Effective suppression of motility of the gut can be attained at doses that exert few systemic effects. It is questionable whether opioids should be administered for the treatment of diarrhea. The fundamental problem in most cases of diarrhea is hypomotility and excessive secretion of fluid and electrolytes into the lumen of the bowel.

DRUGS AFFECTING SECRETION

The glands associated with the digestive system are regulated by the autonomic nervous system and various hormones. Cholinergic drugs increase secretion of most glands and anticholinergic drugs decrease their secretion (Table 2).

Acid secretion by the abomasum of ruminants and the stomach of swine is controlled by the vagus nerves and gastrin secreted by the argentaffin cells. The anticholinergic drugs block gastric secretion mediated by vagal mechanisms but have no effect on gastrin- or histamine-induced secretion. The histamine H_2-receptor antagonist cimetidine decreases secretion induced by either histamine or gastrin. Its dosage and clinical use in food-producing animals remain to be established.

Of greater significance as a practical matter is the increased secretion by intestinal glands produced by enterotoxin-producing pathogens. The enterotoxins elaborated by *Vibrio* and *E. coli* increase secretion by altering cyclic nucleotide and calcium concentrations within intestinal glands. The excess secretion over absorption of water and electrolytes results in diarrhea. These mechanisms have been the target for drug therapy of severe infectious diarrheas. High doses of nicotinic acid affects cyclic nucleotide levels and have been shown to reduce scours in piglets. The search for new drugs that specifically antag-

Table 2. Drugs That Modify Glandular Secretion in the Gastrointestinal Tract

Organ	Drug	Action
Salivary	Pilocarpine Physostigmine Arecoline	Increase secretion
	Atropine	Decrease secretion
Gastric	Histamine Pentagastrin Betazole	Increase acid secretion
	Atropine	Partially decrease acid secretion
	Cimetidine	Decrease acid secretion
	ACTH Glucocorticoids Aspirin Phenylbutazone	Decrease secretion of mucus
Biliary	Bile salts Ouabain Theophylline Phenobarbital Magnesium sulfate	Increase bile formation
Pancreatic exocrine	Atropine Glucagon	Decrease secretion
	Bethanecol	Increase secretion
Intestinal	Bethanechol Pilocarpine Castor oil Prostaglandins	Increase secretion
	Atropine Chlorpromazine Aspirin Flunixin meglumine Lidamidine	Decrease secretion

onize the secretory effects of enterotoxins is being actively pursued. However, there are several new approaches to therapy that have been shown to be effective in diminishing secretion and mortality associated with infectious diarrhea.

Chlorpromazine (1 mg/kg, IM) decreases secretion and duration of diarrhea caused by *E. coli*. The mode of action is inhibition of the calcium-dependent regulator that stimulates secretion by the intestinal cells. Another effect of enterotoxins is to stimulate the production of prostaglandins, which, in turn, raise the intracellular concentration of cAMP, thereby causing secretion. Drugs such as aspirin and flunixin meglumine inhibit the production of prostaglandins and reduce mortality from coliform-induced diarrhea. For this purpose, aspirin was added to the feed or drinking water of piglets to provide a daily dose of 0.5 to 1.0 gm during the period of 9 to 20 days post partum.

Lidamidine is a newer drug with antiperistaltic and antisecretory activity that is effective against both prostaglandin- and enterotoxin-induced diarrheas. Experimentally, at a dose of a 8 mg/kg, this drug completely protected animals against the cathartic effects of castor oil.

These newer approaches to the inhibition of secretion, together with appropriate fluid, electrolyte, and antibacterial therapy, should enable us to markedly reduce neonatal losses associated with infectious diarrhea.

DRUGS ACTING WITHIN THE LUMEN OF THE GASTROINTESTINAL TRACT

Many drugs that have been administered orally to ruminants and swine for local effects have been shown to have little therapeutic value. These include compounds such as nux vomica, gentian, cassia, tartar emetic, capsicum, and so on. Mixtures containing such substances should be regarded as obsolete unless they are offered with placebo intent.

Surfactants, such as polyoxalene, are useful to reduce foaming of gastrointestinal contents as seen in frothy bloat of ruminant animals. They are best administered into the rumen via a stomach tube.

Adsorbents have been advocated for the treatment of gastroenteritis and diarrhea. They coat the surface of the inflamed mucosa and were thought to adsorb irritants and enterotoxins on their surface. Recently, it was found that adsorbents such as kaolin, attapulgite, and bentonite do not bind enterotoxin. The ion exchange resin, cholestyramine, avidly binds *E. coli* enterotoxin, but its efficacy is greatly reduced in the presence of milk. Bismuth subsalicylate, which possesses unique properties, is used in the treatment of enteritis. The bismuth is insoluble and exerts a demulcent effect by coating inflamed surfaces, and the salicylate exerts a local anti-inflammatory effect in the bowel.

Antacids such as calcium carbonate, magnesium hydroxide, aluminum trisilicate, sodium bicarbonate, and aluminum hydroxide have been employed in the treatment of gastric and ruminal hyperacidity. Care should be taken when using these drugs in the treatment of ruminal acidosis, as alkalization of the ruminal contents will enhance the absorption of histamine, ammonia, and other basic substances.

Antibiotics acting within the bowel are discussed elsewhere in the book.

SUMMARY

Although many drugs have been advocated for the treatment of various disorders of the digestive system, numerous agents have proved to be ineffective for their intended use. It is possible to modify motility and secretion, alter surface tension, and change pH with drugs. Many of the drugs employed exert widespread pharmacologic effects in the body that must be understood for their safe use in management of disorders of the gastrointestinal tract.

Supplemental Reading

Davis, L. E., and Baggot, J. D.: Gastrointestinal pharmacology. *In* Anderson, N. V. (ed.): Veterinary Gastroenterology. Lea & Febiger, Philadelphia, 1980, 277–310.

Jenkins, W. L.: Drugs acting on the digestive system. *In* Booth, N. H., and McDonald, L. E. (eds.): Veterinary Pharmacology and Therapeutics, 5th ed. Iowa State University Press, Ames, 1982, 593–606.

Jenkins, W. L.: Ruminant pharmacology. *In* Booth, N. H., and McDonald, L. E. (eds.): Veterinary Pharmacology and Therapeutics, 5th ed. Iowa State University Press, Ames, 1982, 607–619.

Yeoman, G. H.: Recent advances in the chemotherapy of neonatal diarrhea in farm animals. *In* Recent Advances in Neonatal Diarrhea in Farm Animals. Beecham Laboratories, Bristol, Tenn., 1980, 43–52.

Gastric Dilatation and Torsion in Swine

WALLACE M. WASS, D.V.M., Ph.D.,
JAMES R. THOMPSON, D.V.M., M.S.,
EDWIN W. MOSS, D.V.M., M.S.,
JERRY P. KUNESH, D.V.M., Ph.D.,
PAUL G. ENESS, D.V.M.,
and LINDA S. THOMPSON, D.V.M.

Gastric dilatation and torsion in swine can occur in slaughter hogs or breeding stock.[1] For the stomach to dilate and cause a serious problem, two major conditions must be met: (1) there must be a source for the distending gas, fluid, or food, and (2) an obstruction must prevent the relief of the distention by eructation, emesis, absorption, or passage of the gastric contents into the small intestine.[2, 3] As the stomach distends with gas or fluid, various anatomic and metabolic changes may occur, thereby causing a functional obstruction. The stomach wall may become atonic owing to antiperistaltic waves from the pyloric region (as a result of increasing intragastric pressure).[2] Hypovolemic shock can also be initiated by an obstructed portal vein causing a decreased venous return to the heart.[2]

The cause of this problem in swine is currently uncertain. The following factors have been incriminated: (1) irregular feeding, (2) feeding of gruel or whey rations, (3) low ambient temperature (causing an increase in sow uneasiness), (4) rapid ingestion of feed and air, and (5) excess excitement of animals during feeding time.[1, 4, 5] Death occurs rapidly with few premonitory signs. Postmortem examination reveals a greatly distended stomach (most often with watery contents), and the liver and spleen possibly being congested or hemorrhagic if involved in the torsion.

Owing to the rapid death, treatment is usually not attempted.

References

1. Leman, A. D., et. al. (eds.): Diseases of Swine, 5th ed. Iowa State University Press, Ames, 1981.
2. Anderson, N. V. (ed.): Veterinary Gastroenterology. Lea & Febiger, Philadelphia, 1980.
3. Wingfield, W. E., Betts, C. W., and Rawlings, C. A.: Pathophysiology associated with gastric dilatation—volvulus in the dog. J. Am. Anim. Hosp. Assoc. 12:136, 1976.
4. Blackburn, P. W., McCrea, C. T., Randall, C. J., and Thomas, G. W.: Torsion of the stomach in sows. Vet. Rec. 94:578, 1974.
5. Cedervall, A.: Gastric torsion in swine. Acta Vet. Scand. 12:142, 1971.

Terminal Ileitis (Porcine Proliferative Enteritis, Hemorrhagic Bowel Syndrome)

WALLACE M. WASS, D.V.M., Ph.D.,
JAMES R. THOMPSON, D.V.M., M.S.,
EDWIN W. MOSS, D.V.M., M.S.,
JERRY P. KUNESH, D.V.M., Ph.D.,
PAUL G. ENESS, D.V.M.,
and LINDA S. THOMPSON, D.V.M.

The syndrome called terminal ileitis of swine in the United States is probably the same as intestinal adenomatosis, necrotic enteritis, microproliferative enteritis, regional ileitis, proliferative hemorrhagic enteropathy, hemorrhagic bowel syndrome, and porcine proliferative enteritis in other parts of the world. *Campylobacter sputorum* subsp. *mucosalis* has been demonstrated within proliferated mucosal epithelial cells in all of these conditions, suggesting that all are manifestations of the same syndrome. The disease mainly affects young weaned pigs and pigs at market weight but can be seen anytime after weaning.

The clinical signs include pallor, anorexia, normal to subnormal temperature, and the passage of blood-tinged or tarry black feces 24 to 48 hours before death. Some individuals will be found dead without clinical signs of illness. Pigs surviving the initial stages have poor appetites, grow poorly or steadily lose weight, have periods of intermittent diarrhea, and may or may not pass mucus, fibrin, or blood in feces. Affected pigs become emaciated over several weeks and usually die.

Campylobacter sputorum subsp. *mucosalis* is found in many swine herds that show no clinical disease. This leads some researchers to believe that nutritional influences play some role in the precipitation of clinical signs. Attempts have been made to implicate specific feed ingredients. Further evidence is necessary, however, to substantiate specific nutritional effects on the occurrence of the syndrome.

Clinically ill pigs are treated orally with therapeutic levels of neomycin. Any of the aminoglycocide antibacterial drugs appears to be effective. Herd treatment is by medication of the feed or water with therapeutic levels of any of the tetracyclines. Many antimicrobial drugs are effective in controlling this condition. These choices are most commonly employed because of availability and F.D.A. approval for use in food producing animals in the United States.

Refer to the first volume of Current Veterinary Therapy: Food Animal Practice for the following: Whitlock, R. H.: Malabsorption Syndrome. Section 13, Diseases of the Digestive System.

Supplemental Reading

Lomax, L. G., and Glock, R. D.: Naturally occurring porcine proliferative enteritis: Pathologic and bacteriologic findings. Am. J. Vet. Res. *43:1608, 1982.*

DISEASES OF THE REPRODUCTIVE AND URINARY SYSTEMS

ROBERT S. HUDSON, D.V.M., M.S.
Consulting Editor

Mastitis

JOHN K. WINKLER, D.V.M.

Mastitis broadly defined is an inflammation of the mammary gland that alters its structure or function. The intensity and significance of the alterations are related to the cause (trauma or infection) and to the characteristics of the species, breed, or individual affected.

The effect of inflammatory changes in the mammary gland is the reduction of the quality and quantity of milk secretion. The economic significance of this is much greater in dairy cows and goats than in nondairy species. Mastitis caused by infection in any species of food-producing animals is of economic significance whenever it results in septicemia. Human exposure to pathogens causing intramammary infection in food-producing animals is also a significant public health concern.

ECONOMICS

Losses to the dairy cattle industry from mastitis are calculated to include lowered sale value, discarded milk, drug therapy, veterinary services, and labor. The dollar value of these factors may vary according to market prices. Currently, the loss estimated for the 11 million dairy cows in the United States exceeds a total of 2 billion dollars per year.

Although detailed loss estimates to the dairy goat industry from mastitis are not available, it can be assumed that losses would be proportionally similar to those for the dairy cow industry.

The economic significance of mastitis for beef cattle is based upon reduced milk production and rates of growth of calves, weak calves, debilitated or dead cows, and cull rate. Mastitis is not considered as being economically significant to the beef industry due to low incidence.

Significant losses to the swine industry result from mastitis. Inflammatory changes in the mammary gland cause agalactia, which may result in newborn deaths or uneconomical growth. Infected mammary glands and deaths of sows due to septicemia from mastitis pathogens

occur, but the incidence is low under current management conditions.

Losses for the sheep industry are similar to those for the beef cattle industry. Mortality due to acute intramammary infection is higher for ewes, and the problem of orphan lambs is more severe.

There is extensive public effort and expense to assure the safety and quality of meat and milk. Standards for the production, processing, and marketing of milk are prescribed and enforced by federal, state, and local regulations. Milk production is continuously monitored to meet standards for odor, taste, gross contaminants, bacteria, and somatic cells. At the present time, raw milk with 100,000 bacteria/ml or 1,500,000 somatic cells/ml is not acceptable for processing class I milk in the United States. Direct sale of raw milk is permitted in some states but is regulated by very stringent standards for quality and safety.

CAUSES OF MASTITIS

Predisposing Factors

Anatomy and Conformation

The location of the mammary glands of sheep, goats, and cattle in the inguinal area provides some protection from direct trauma, but recumbency exposes them to contamination and trauma. The glands of all 3 species are supported and held against the abdomen by median and lateral ligaments. Inherent anatomic differences in the strength of this support or the shape and size of the gland determine the vulnerability to trauma. Large pendulous glands with weak support are predisposed to trauma of parenchyma and teats. Tendency towards this type of conformation becomes exaggerated with age and more pronounced with each subsequent lactation.

Since the teat opening is the primary route of access for infection, teat structure and conformation may be factors in predisposition to mastitis. The structure of the teat end of bovine mammary glands is a natural defense mechanism. The streak canal or ductus papillaris leading to the opening is approximately 9 mm long, lined with stratified squamous epithelium. Fissures and ridges along

765

its long axis and desquamated keratinized epithelium in the lumen form a mechanical barrier to the entrance of bacteria. Furstenberg's rosette, at the junction of the streak canal and teat cistern, is formed by the convergence of longitudinal ridges of the cistern. Smooth muscle cells surrounding the area of the streak canal are credited with contracting to close and seal the opening.

Although the gross and cellular structures of the bovine teat have been studied in much more detail than those of other species, the teats of sheep and goats are similar. The duct system for cattle, sheep, and goats terminates in a single opening in the teat. The parenchyma of the goat gland is generally less dense than that of sheep, and the teats are more conically shaped and longer, but the basic structure for the 3 species is similar. There are 2 or more openings in each mammary gland of sows, and each opening is the termination of a duct system. This is a major difference in anatomic structure related to occurrence, control, and therapy for intramammary infection for swine as compared with ruminants.

Conformation characteristics that predispose animals to mastitis include the following:

1. Weak supporting ligaments causing mammary glands to be pendulous and vulnerable to contamination and injury.

2. Excessively large or long teats unadaptable to machine milking and also subject to injury.

3. Thin-walled or ballooned teats with a short, weak streak canal that reduces the effectiveness of protection from infection.

4. Very small, short teats that may require excessive time for removal of milk by machine, hand, or nursing.

Environment

Climate

Climatic conditions affecting the habitat of animals may predispose them to mastitis. Cattle, during extremely hot and cold weather, congregate in protected areas that become contaminated. Sunburn or frostbite also predispose animals to mastitis. Wet environmental conditions provide means for transfer of contaminants from the external surface of the animal, making sanitary harvesting of milk extremely hazardous as well as causing direct transfer of pathogens to the mammary gland. Wet or dry climatic conditions resulting in foot disease predispose animals to mastitis by excessive recumbency due to lameness. Responsibility for the selection, design, and maintenance of the environment for food-producing animals belongs to the managers. This responsibility includes both sanitation and safety of pastures, traffic lanes, housing, holding areas, and milking facilities for all stages in the productive life of the animal.

Examples of predisposing factors to mastitis are (1) contaminated areas that factilitate intramammary infection during the perinatal period, such as overused, manure-laden stalls or buildings as well as small lots or pastures with hazardous obstacles or poorly drained areas, (2) traffic lanes that require movement over obstacles, such as ditches, streams, roads, ledges, or surfaces that help produce foot disease, (3) slippery or too small holding areas for cows, (4) hazardous entrances and exits to milking parlors, (5) milking barns or parlors with slippery footing as well as unsanitary and maladjusted milking equipment, and (6) inadequate space per animal in holding areas, pastures, or feeding areas.

BREED. Although natural or designed environmental conditions may predispose animals to mastitis, there are individual breed and species differences in habits and adaptibility that may influence their susceptibility to environmental predisposing factors. For example, there are notable individual differences in the adaptibility of dairy cows to free stall housing or concrete footing. No matter what the condition of the environment, some individual dairy cows are almost persistently clean, while others are notoriously filthy. All other factors being equal, temperament of individual animals may determine the adaptibility to types of environment. Beef cattle breeds seem to be more careful and are more economical in the use of pastures and feeding areas than some dairy breeds that seem to make contaminated "lounging areas" out of forage.

Social dominance may become a predisposing factor when single animals are added to a group, or when breeds, species, or groups are mixed. Injuries or stress during the establishment of dominance are not uncommon.

Equipment

Design and function of milking equipment may indirectly or directly cause mastitis. Although modern facilities and equipment are designed to minimize the possibility of injury to the mammary gland during harvesting of milk, there are current intensive investigations to improve equipment. These studies and results are reported in the proceedings of the National Mastitis Council as well as in current dairy related literature.

Fundamental to equipment design and function is sufficient vacuum for milk removal and transport. Although malfunction is a potential predisposing factor, faulty milking techniques or procedures and poor sanitation may cause traumatic injury or cause equipment to become a fomite.

Techniques of milking as predisposing causes of mastitis include any action producing traumatic injury, such as (1) rough handling during preparation for letdown by overly rigorous massage, (2) excessive water pressure to "clean" the udder, (3) excessive machine or hand stripping, (4) removal of teat cups under vacuum, (5) application of teat cups and vacuum to teats prior to letdown, (6) incomplete removal of milk, and (7) delayed removal of teat cups.

Trauma and Infection

Trauma

Inflammatory changes without infection are due to trauma causing bruises or lacerations by environmental obstacles, contusions or bruises by high pressure water used to clean udders (especially of heifers), and abrasions or lacerations by unstable animals in a hazardous environment or by claws entangled with teats when rising. Sunburn, freezing, insect bites, snake bites, and chemical burns are infrequent but have resulted in mastitis.

Infection

Infection may follow a traumatic insult that causes a breakdown of protective mechanisms. Mastitis frequently occurs as a sequel to teat and udder lesions found in vesicular stomatitis, cowpox, or herpes mammilitis. Infection also occurs through the teat opening when there is no apparent compromise of natural defenses. Milk is a suitable growth medium for many pathogens.

CLINICAL SIGNS

The signs of intramammary infection range from no gross changes (subclinical) to severe septicemia and toxemia. The relative severity of mastitis produced by intramammary infection depends upon the types of pathogens, their virulence, and susceptibility and resistance of the animal. Classification of the signs as an aid to diagnosis may be in 4 categories: (1) *subclinical,* which is detected by tests for alteration of milk constituents or by presence of pathogens, (2) *chronic,* which is evident by intermittent gross alteration of milk without acute inflammatory signs, (3) *acute,* which includes the cardinal signs of inflammation of the gland plus systemic signs of anorexia and fever, and (4) *peracute,* which includes acute signs and signs of severe toxemia. It must be understood that any attempt to classify signs according to severity is somewhat arbitrary and useful only as a tool to diagnosis and prognosis.

DIAGNOSIS

Physical examination of the animal with inspection and palpation of the mammary gland and its secretions plus herd and individual history may yield a fairly accurate tentative diagnosis. Analysis of the secretion for constituents and pathogens is necessary for a definitive diagnosis.

History should contain a determination of the potential predisposing causes and the nature and incidence of previous episodes. Physical examination should involve examination of the animal for systemic signs as well as palpation of the gland for evidence of chronic signs (fibrosis) and more acute inflammatory changes. Examination of the milk secretion is needed for gross inspection of alterations such as the following:

1. Serous or watery consistency
2. Color
3. Viscosity
4. Tissue or mucoid debris
5. Odor
6. Sediment

Analysis of milk for alteration of constituents consists of determination of somatic cell content and identification of microorganisms. Tests for somatic cell content are used in the absence of gross (subclinical) alterations, whereas collection and culture of milk samples are necessary for identification of the causative organism. Tests for somatic cell content are the California Mastitis Test, Wisconsin Mastitis Test, Modified Whiteside Test, and Catalase Test as well as the Direct Microscopic Somatic Cell Count. There are many reference sources for the description of these and other procedures that are used to evaluate milk constituents.[5] These procedures would apply to any species.

DIFFERENTIAL DIAGNOSIS

Overzealous and unnecessary therapy may be administered if infectious mastitis is not differentiated from other common conditions of the mammary gland.

1. Bloody milk may result from trauma, causing undifferentiated whole blood to enter the duct system. It is seen most often as pink-tinged milk (not serum) early in lactation, especially in heifers, as a result of some capillary seepage into the alveolus. The condition is usually temporary and requires no therapy.

2. Hematoma of the mammary gland could be mistaken for acute swelling from infection or physiologic edema. The cause is trauma and may result in an extensive, blood filled cavity. Milk from the gland in the affected area is usually normal or slightly blood tinged. Infection is not necessarily present. Diagnosis is made by palpation of the fluctuant consistency as opposed to edema and by centesis to determine the contents. Management of hematoma is conservative to avoid further trauma and to allow time for reabsorption. Particular care must be taken to avoid infection, especially during diagnostic centesis.

3. Physiologic edema must be differentiated from inflammatory edema resulting from infection. Physiologic edema is symmetrical over the entire mammary gland area and may extend to adjacent areas of the abdomen and perineum. It is found during late gestation and early postpartum. Although milk secretion is inhibited and enlargement of the gland may predispose the cow to mastitis, there is no heat, pain, or alteration of secretion. Grossly, the swelling could be confused with mastitis, lymphatic obstruction, or hematoma. Absence of signs of acute inflammation and uniformity of characteristic swelling should be sufficient for differential diagnosis.

4. Obstruction of a duct system or teat opening by milk stones or proliferating epithelieum (spiders) will cause swelling of the area involved owing to milk retention and may be confused with inflammation.

5. Signs of intoxication due to peracute intramammary infection must be differentiated from signs of other severe systemic diseases, such as hypocalcemia, metritis, and ketosis. Examination of the mammary gland during routine physical examination should accomplish this.

THERAPY

Objectives for mastitis therapy are to (1) preserve the life of the animal, (2) restore function to the mammary gland, and (3) improve milk quality and efficiency of production. Specific therapeutic measures are directed at (1) removal of cause, (2) detoxification and support for systemically affected animals, (3) reduction and elimination of infectious agents, and (4) promotion of healing of damaged tissue. The recommendations that follow are modified according to the severity and extent of the disease process as well as expediency and cost effectiveness.

Peracute Mastitis

Peracute mastitis is characterized by rapid onset of a fulminating infection, painful swelling of the gland, alteration of secretion to serum-like consistency, severe systemic changes including anorexia, fever, depression, raised pulse and respiration rates, diminished pupillary reflexes, dark toxic mucous membranes, cold extremities, dehydration, and ataxia. All species may be affected, but this level of severity is more common for dairy cattle. Occurrence is more frequent during early postpartum and peak production or stress periods. *Diagnosis* is based upon clinical signs and identification of the organism cultured from secretion of the affected gland. The *causative organism* for cattle is most frequently a coliform (*Escherichia coli, Klebsiella pneumoniae, Aerobacter en-*

terobactum), or a hemolytic staphyloccus. All species are susceptible to intramammary coliform or staphyloccal infection, but other bacteria, such as *Clostridium perfringens* type C, *Pasteurella haemolytica,* and streptocci, are potential pathogens.

Therapy for peracute mastitis is primarily systemic.

Detoxification Therapy

1. Corticosteroids stabilize cell membranes, stimulate gluconeogenesis, and reduce inflammation. A single initial dose is recommended—not repeated unless necessary to relieve signs of endotoxic shock.
2. Parenteral fluids restore hydration, dilute toxins, and counter acidosis.
3. Exogenous oxytocin and frequent manual stripping remove toxic material from affected glands.
4. Antihistamines counter histamine accumulation.
5. Diuretics aid in elimination of toxins.

Antibacterial Therapy

1. Administer parenteral antibiotics or sulfonamides.
   a. Specific selection is based upon organism sensitivity.
   b. Broad-spectrum antibiotics if organism is unknown.
   c. Selection can be based upon previous therapeutic experience with the herd.
   d. Selection may be based upon clinical signs and environmental circumstances for presumptive diagnosis.
   e. Selection also may be based upon Gram's stain of secretion sample to differentiate coliforms from staphylococci.
2. Provide intramammary infusion.
   a. Select an agent identical to or compatible with the parenteral antibacterial agent.
   b. Intramammary infusion effectiveness is limited by the mechanical compression of the duct system produced by severe inflammatory swelling.
   c. Intramammary infusion is not practical for swine.

Anti-inflammatory Therapy

This reduces swelling and pain and enhances removal of toxic secretions as well as promotes diffusion of intramammary infusions.

1. Alternate hot and cold water or ice pack applications or hypertonic soaking may be of value but increases the risk of spreading infection to adjacent quarters.
2. Corticosteroid parenteral therapy may be contraindicated owing to suppression of defense mechanisms.
3. Anti-inflammatory drugs listed in Table 1 have had limited trials for all species.

Supportive Therapy

1. Clean, dry, weather protected environment.
2. Fresh drinking water and palatable hay available.
3. Limited grain and protein mix offered.
4. Force feeding of nutrients.
5. Rumen stimulants orally or parenterally.
6. Vitamin B complex administration parenterally.

Prognosis

Prognosis for peracute mastitis in all species is guarded to poor for recovery and very unfavorable for economic efficiency if the animal recovers.

Complications

1. Gangrene and sloughing of the affected tissue.
2. Abortion, retained placenta, and metritis.
3. Displaced abomasum in dairy cattle.
4. Pulmonary edema due to excessive rehydration therapy.

Acute and Chronic Mastitis

1. Therapy is moderated for intramammary infection producing systemic signs that lack the severe *toxic* signs described for peracute mastitis. Detoxifiction is unnecessary but timely, and persistent systemic antibacterial therapy is necessary to a degree dependent on the organism causing the infection.
2. Therapy for intramammary infection without systemic signs for cattle, goats, and sheep is effective by a combination of intramammary infusion of antibacterial medication and persistent removal of secretion by frequent hand stripping. Antibacterial agents should be selected according to the *in vitro* sensitivity of the organism. Removal of inflammatory debris may be aided by the use of oxytocin. Therapy for mastitis of sows is limited to systemic antibacterial and anti-inflammatory therapy.

Subclinical Mastitis

This level of mastitis is primarily of concern to owners of dairy cattle and goats. It is estimated that for every episode of clinical mastitis in cows there are 40 episodes of subclinical mastitis. These subclinical infections are detected by the presence of pathogens and by the increase of somatic cells in the milk. Subclinical infections are considered to be either a newly acquired infection or a nonclinical stage of an incompletely eliminated clinical infection. Therapy to eliminate or to control subclinical infections must be on a herd basis.

DAIRY HERD MASTITIS: PREVENTION AND CONTROL

Although therapy as a means of restoring function is necessary, the principle that "a problem in curative medicine has not been solved until the health maintenance program haš been adjusted to eliminate or reduce the probability of the problem's recurrence" is clearly applicable to mastitis.

Prevention

Elimination of all predisposing and direct causes as discussed earlier in this article would be ideal but not realistic. Control over all the variables of the environment and all the potential pathogens complicates any such effort beyond reason. The effort must concentrate on those factors and organisms most commonly causing the disease and the greatest economic loss. *Streptococcus agalactia* and *Staphylococcus aureus* are considered to cause 90 per cent of all intramammary infections in cattle. Prevention of infection by these organisms is the primary objective of control programs.

General Prevention Measures

I. Milking Procedure
   A. Pre-milking udder preparation.
      1. No washing unless teats are grossly contami-

Table 1. *Therapeutic Agents for Mastitis**

Name	Supplier	Species	Dosage	Route	Sensitive Organism
Detoxification					
Glucocorticoids					
Dexamethasone (Azium)	Schering Corp.	Bovine	0.1 mg/lb 0.2 mg/lb	IV IM	
Prednisolone (Solu-Delta-Cortef)	Upjohn Co.	Bovine	1–2 mg/lb	IV	
Fluid Therapy					
Plasma-lyte 148 (Ringer's) add NaCO₃ (approx. 0.5 oz/gal)	Travenol	All	To effect	IV	
PM Acidosis Formula A	Pitman-Moore Inc.	All	To effect	IV	
Antihistamines					
Tripelennamine (Recovr)	E.R. Squibb & Sons Inc.	Bovine	0.5 mg/lb	IM	
Anti-inflammatory Drugs					
Flunixin meglumine (Banamine)	Schering Corp.	—	0.5 mg/lb	IV or IM	
Phenylbutazone		—	0.1 mg/lb	IV only	
Diuretics					
Furosemide (Lasix)	National Laboratories Corp.	Bovine	0.5 mg/lb 2 gm daily	IM/IV Oral	
Trichlormethiazide and Dexamethasone (Naquasone)	Schering Corp.	Bovine	1–2 boluses 1st day, ½–1 bolus next 2 days	Oral	
Chlorothiazide (Diuril)	Merck Sharp & Dohme	Bovine	1–2 daily 2 gm, for 3–4 days	Oral	
Antimicrobial (Septicemia)					
Procaine penicillin G		All	10–25,000 units/kg, BID	IM	Gram-positive and some gram-negative
Ampicillin	Beecham Laboratories	All	5–10 mg/kg, BID	IM IV, SQ	Gram-positive and some gram-negative
Cloxacillin	Bristol Laboratories	All	10 mg/kg	IM	Gram-positive and some gram-negative, and penicillinase resistant
Oxacillin	Bristol Laboratories	All	10 mg/kg	IM, IV	Gram-positive, some gram-negative, and penicillinase resistant *Staphylococcus*
Gentamicin	Schering Corp.	All	1–3 mg/kg	IM tid	Gram-positive, some gram-negative, and penicillinase-resistant *Staphylococcus*
Oxytetracycline	Pfizer Inc.	All	2.5–10 mg/kg	IV or IM daily	Broad-spectrum antimicrobial
Erythromycin	Diamond Laboratories Inc.	All	2–5 mg/kg	IM every 24 hr	Gram-positive
Tylosin	Elanco Products Co.	All	5–10 mg/kg	IM or IV every 12 hr	Gram-positive
Lincomycin	Upjohn Co.	All (except horses)	2.5–5 mg/kg	IM every 24 hr	Gram-positive
Sulfonamides		All	Variable 1st dose, continue ½ dose/day	IV	Broad-spectrum antimicrobial
Antimicrobial (Intrammmary)					
Lactating Formula					
Penicillin G		Bovine	Mfr. formula	IM	
Cephalosporin (Cefa-lac)	Bristol Laboratories	Bovine	Mfr. formula	IM	
Cloxacillin (Dariclox)	Beecham Laboratories	Bovine	Mfr. formula	IM	
Tetracyclines (Liquamast)	Pfizer Inc.	Bovine	Mfr. formula	IM	
Novobiocin and Pencillin (SF 17900-Forte)	Upjohn Co.	Bovine	Mfr. formula	IM	
Hetacillin (Hetacin-K)	Bristol Laboratories	Bovine	Mfr. formula	IM	
Erythromycin (Erythromast)	Diamond Laboratories Inc.	Bovine	Mfr. formula	IM	
Dry Cow Formula (after last milking)					
Cephalosporin (Cefa-Dry)	Bristol Laboratories	Bovine	Mfr. formula	IM	
Cloxacillin (Dry-clox)	Bristol Laboratories	Bovine	Mfr. formula	IM	
Cloxacillin (Orbenin D.C.)	Beecham Laboratories	Bovine	Mfr. formula	IM	
Penicillin and Dihydrostreptomycin (Quartermaster)	Upjohn Co.	Bovine	Mfr. formula	IM	
Albacillin (Dry Guard)	Upjohn Co.	Bovine	Mfr. formula	IM	

*All of the therapeutic agents listed are *not* necessarily approved for unresricted use in food animals in the USA. The manufacturer's label must be consulted for current restrictions, contraindications, and potential side effects.

nated. Letdown established by herd familiarity with routine and hand stripping foremilk. Recent surveys indicate no increase in new infection.

2. Udder sprays in holding pens with sufficient time to "drip dry" prior to entering milking parlor. Proceed as in *1, 3,* or *4.*
3. Wash with fine spray with minimal water to clean teats. Use single service towels to dry. Wash only that which can be *completely dried.* Strip foremilk.
4. Reverse order in *3* by stripping foremilk and then washing. Advocates of this sequence cite manual manipulation of teats prior to stripping as causing redistribution of contaminants in foremilk.
5. Wash udder and teats using fine spray. Massage and clean with bare hands or with single service towels, dry completely, and strip foremilk.

B. Apply machine without allowing air intake during application.
C. Attend machine during milking to ensure immediate correction of slippage or "squawking."
D. Except in extreme instances of slow milking individual quarters, allow all 4 teat cups to remain until udder is milked out in preference to chancing the intake of air during individual cup removal. *Cut off vacuum to machine prior to removal.*
E. Immediately after removal of machine, dip teats in an effective solution (Table 2).
F. Rinse teat cups between cows to remove residual milk from previous cow using an approved sanitizing solution by one of the following:
   1. Commercial "back flush" system.
   2. Flush with teat cups inverted and vacuum off using udder sanitizing solution. Shake to remove excess water.
   3. Manually back flush through disconnected claw or milk tube and invert to remove sanitizing solution as an alternative to 2.
G. The use of a strip cup or plate to observe and evaluate foremilk is considered to be more time consuming than cost effective in large herds.

However, it provides a much safer and more accurate method. Spattering of milk can be minimized by holding the strip plate almost parallel to the direction of milk stream.

II. Post-milking Procedure
   A. Feed after milking to encourage cows to stand during the interval required for teat to close.
   B. Teats may be protected by use of teat sealant instead of regular teat dip solution when environment is conducive to exposure by coliforms (see Table 2).
   C. *Feeding area should be designed to discourage cows from using it as a sheltered loafing area.*

III. Dry Cow Infusion Therapy
   A. Select antibiotics for routine use based upon sensitivity of the predominant organisms infecting the herd.
   B. Infuse each quarter of all cows after the last milking prior to drying with a suitable commercial dry cow preparation.

IV. Postpartum Udder Management
   A. Provide uncontaminated, dry, and well drained parturition environment.
   B. Completely milk out cows as soon as possible after calving.

V. Milking Machine Function
   A. Provide for periodic inspection and testing of milking equipment by qualified personnel.
   B. Monitor the function of equipment in accordance with manufacturer's recommendations.

VI. Prevention of Iatrogenic Mastitis
   A. Remove all contamination from the teat end and disinfect with alcohol prior to infusion of dry or lactation product.
   B. Ensure that the equipment used and the preparations infused are free of all pathogens. Most yeasts, *Nocardia,* and *Mycoplasma* infections are spread by infusion with nonsterile cannulas or syringes using medication drawn from multiple dose vials. Commercially prepared individual infusion products should be used.

VII. Immunity for Prevention
   A. Select replacements on the basis of family history of *apparent* resistance to mastitis.
   B. Vaccination with bacterins or toxoids has not proved to prevent new infections. However, the recent work of Pankey and associates[6] indicates a rise in spontaneous cure rate for *Staphylococcus aureus* infections for cows vaccinated with a commerical staphyloccal bacterin (Lysigin*) over unvaccinated controls.

Control

I. Diagnosis and Analysis of the Problem
   A. Survey of entire operation for potential *predisposing* and *direct* causes.
   B. Evaluation of herd records and data to determine
      1. Incidence and occurrence of clinical cases
      2. Herd bacterial and somatic cell levels
      3. Identity of organisms previously involved
      4. Past and present control methods.
   C. Evaluation of milking facilities and equipment by application of standards and methods described in Section 14 of Volume 1 of this title.

Table 2. *Teat Dip Sanitizers and Sealant*

Compound	Strength* (%)	Efficacy Against S. agalactia and S. aureus
Iodophor	.25–1	+
Quaternary ammonia	.05–1	+
Chlorhexidine	.2–1	+
Sodium hypochlorite	4	+
DDBSA (Dodecylbenzene sulfonic acid)	2	+ (and some coliforms)
Lauricidin (1 per cent in acrylic latex;† Teat Shield‡ with Germicide)		+ (coliforms)

*Teat dip effectiveness is reduced if concentration of emollients incorporated in the compound exceeds 12%. Teat dips are classified and regulated as over-the-counter drugs by FDA and must be labeled as such to include adequate directions for use, storage, and expiration date.

†Disinfectant if latex has acrylic base.

‡A teat sealant and sanitizer effective against *S. agalactia, S. aureus,* and coliforms. Other compounds are sanitizers only.

*Available from Bioceutic Laboratories, St. Joseph, MO 64502

D. Evaluation of milking procedures and techniques previously described in this article.

E. Evaluation of the present infection status of the herd by the following:
   1. Bulk tank sampling for somatic cell count and organism identity.
   2. Individual cow status by California Mastitis Test (CMT) and composite quarter sampling if necessary.

F. Analysis of the relationship of the present herd status to production potential.

II. Recommendations Based upon Economic Feasibility
   A. Routine preventive measures described apply to control of all common organisms.
   B. Specific therapy for all clinical cases as they occur. See Table 1 for assistance with selection. Consider salvage or culling of cows infected with organisms resistant or unresponsive to therapy.
   C. Additional recommendations for herd infection as follows:
      1. *Streptococcus agalactia.* Since this organism does not exist in the environment, it can be controlled by eliminating infection from cows. Routine preventive measures as described will eliminate infection over a period of time. However, it is usually more economical to either identify and treat all infected cows simultaneously or "blanket" treat all the cows of the herd ("blitz") simultaneously.
      2. *Staphylococcus aureus.* This organism exists in the environment and invades tissue, making it a persistent potential infection resistant to therapy in a chronic case. Infected cows can be held to subclinical status and transmission minimized by routine preventive measures. Reduction of herd infection by dry cow therapy is more practical than treatment of subclinical infection during lactation. The cost of lost production due to *Staphylococcus aureus* infection may make it feasible to identify all infected cows and to form a separate infected herd to avoid transmission to uninfected cows. Cows in the infected herd that are cleared of infection can rejoin the clean herd, and those remaining infected can be culled when feasible.
      3. *Streptococcus uberis* and *dysgalactiae* exist outside the mammary gland and are persistently potential invaders. *S. uberis* is more resistant to therapy than *S. dysgalactiae.* Herd problems are best controlled by routine prevention and by dry cow therapy.
      4. Herd problems caused by coliforms are usually acute and require rigid environmental and milking management control measures. Control under confinement conditions and use of free stall housing must provide continuous maintenance of dry bedding, especially if wood shavings or sawdust are used.
      5. *Mycoplasma* infection necessitates immediate survey of the herd to identify, isolate, and cull infected cows. There is no effective therapy. Commercial back flush systems are reported as being beneficial to prevent transmission.
      6. Animals with *Nocardia* infections may be cured with therapy but once identified should be culled unless response is immediate and complete.
      7. Yeast infections are usually self-limiting when the cause is removed.

References

1. Schalm, O. W., Cavoll, E. J., and Jain, N. C.: Bovine Mastitis. Philadelphia, Lea & Febiger, 1971.
2. National Mastitis Council Proceedings, 1980–1983. Arlington, Virginia, National Mastitis Council, Inc.
3. Dairy Research Report. Homer, Louisiana, Hill Farm Experimental Station, 1983.
4. Heidrich, H. J., and Renk, W.: Diseases of the Mammary Gland of Domestic Animals. Philadelphia, W. B. Saunders Company, 1967.
5. National Mastitis Council Inc. Microbiologic Procedures for Use in the Diagnosis of Bovine Mastitis, 2nd ed. Ames, Iowa, Carter Press Inc., 1981.
6. Pankey, J. W., Boddie, W. T., and Watts, J. H.: Dairy Research Report, 1983, Homer, Louisiana.

Refer to the first volume of *Current Veterinary Therapy: Food Animal Practice* for the following:
Thompson, P. D., and Dahl, J. C.: Mastitis Control (Milking Machine).
Section 14, Diseases of the Reproductive and Urinary Systems.

Lactation Failure
Dysgalactia, Agalactia, Hypogalactia

THOMAS A. POWE, D.V.M., M.S.

Lactation failure is important in all food animals but is most common and is most important in swine because of the susceptibility of the young piglet to hypoglycemia. The principal symptom in most species is dysgalactia in varying degrees. In swine, however, agalactia syndrome (mastitis, metritis, agalactia or MMA) of sows is seen. Most dysgalactia problems are secondary to conditions that depress the secretion of milk, while some problems involve physical impairment of milk flow. The varied causes that are implicated make specific treatment and prevention difficult and usually treatment of symptoms must be used.

AGALACTIA SYNDROME OF SOWS (MMA)

A common disease of gilts and sows at 1 to 3 days postpartum, frequently characterized by the various clinical signs of mastitis, metritis and agalactia, is referred to as MMA. The condition is most often characterized by hypogalactia that lasts for 24 to 96 hr rather than by mastitis, metritis, or agalactia. The causes can generally be classified as infectious agents, more specifically as the toxin produced by the gram-negative agents; managerial deficiencies, including housing and feeding, endocrine imbalance, and possibly heredity for milking ability may also be involved. No specific treatment has been found, but most treatments involve the use of oxytocin, broad-spectrum antibiotics, and corticosteroids. The variation in possible causes generally renders prevention other than good management practices ineffective.

Clinical Signs

The sow or gilt that develops the agalactia syndrome will typically have normal milk production for 12 to 24 hr postpartum. This is followed by partial to complete agalactia. Some difficulty may arise in detecting agalactia postparturiently because many sows will not let down milk except during a 10 to 20 second period of time during the nursing cycle (oxytocin will override the letdown failure if milk is actually present in the glands). Close observation reveals hungry piglets and a restless sow that has a reduced mothering instinct or a complete loss of the nursing instinct. Sows seldom die unless the condition is complicated by severe toxemia.

Affected sows and gilts become anorectic, lethargic, constipated, and the body temperature is elevated (39.5 to 41°C). The elevated temperature can be misleading in that many postparturient sows will have slightly elevated temperatures; however, sows with temperatures of 40 to 41°C are more likely to have mastitis and to develop severe toxemia. Respiration and heart rates will be elevated, and some animals will show extreme discomfort and open-mouth breathing.

The entire mammary gland complex, including the periglandular tissue, may be involved. In the case of coliform mastitis, one or more glands may be indurated, and in white-skinned sows discoloration is quite obvious. The swollen, discolored tissue pits and blanches with pressure. Pain, lameness, and unsteadiness may be evident. The milk from the mastitic glands is thick and yellowish. Flakes are sometimes seen.

Lochia, a viscid nonodorous clear mucus that contains variable amounts of white pus, is common and usually does not correlate with agalactia. The evidence of lochia is frequently observed for 3 to 4 days postpartum and often leads to a misdiagnoses of metritis. Metritis produces a brownish foul-smelling discharge that occurs several times a day for several days and is accompanied by severe toxemia in the sow.

Agalactia without associated mammary gland swelling, discoloration, and infection is commonly secondary to other systemic diseases or food toxins.

ETIOLOGY

The precise etiology of lactation failure is undetermined. Over 30 different causes have been reported. An array of bacterial agents has been isolated from milk and mammary tissue with *Escherichia coli* and *Klebsiella* being the most commonly isolated agents. Beta-hemolytic streptococci and staphylococci are often isolated but do not produce agalactia as severe as that produced by coliforms. Some cases appear to be contagious, but experimental reproduction of the disease from cultured bacteria is often unsuccessful. Endotoxins from many of the gram-negative bacteria, when injected into the mammary gland, reproduce the agalactia syndrome. Speculation is that endotoxins from the mammary gland, uterus, and static gut can produce agalactia. Although mastitis is not the sole cause of dysgalactia in the sow, it appears to play a major role in the disease complex.

Hormones throughout the gestation and lactation periods influence the development of mammary tissue and the maintenance of lactation. Probably the most significant finding is that levels of prolactin, a hormone involved in proliferation and differentiation of mammary gland secretory cells, are usually low in serum and pituitary tissue of sows with agalactia. Thyroid hormone concentration has been found to be low in sows with agalactia. Adrenal gland weights are higher than normal in agalactic sows, as are serum cortisol levels. Estrogen is responsible for the inactivation of progesterone and cortisol through its effect on the production of the binding protein, alpha-1-globulin. Epinephrine blocks the effect of oxytocin at the myoepithelial level and the neurohormonal reflex arc at higher centers. Milk engorgement affects the feedback system that adjusts milk production response to demand.

Stress has been incriminated as a possible cause of lactation failure. Its association may be due to emotional changes or environmental changes (temperature, humidity, odors, ventilation, and exercise). Stress has a greater influence on first litter gilts than on sows. The effect of stress is believed to be the blockage of the action of oxytocin at the myoepithelial level by high cortisol levels.

Management procedures that produce stress as well as sudden changes in the ration may lead to dysgalactia. Problems have been observed following the feeding of alfalfa meal, changing to finely ground feed, omitting bulk in the ration, overfeeding during gestation (especially the last week), vitamin E or selenium deficiency, and feeding of excessive protein and imbalanced rations.

Toxic factors incriminated are ergotoxins, aflatoxins, and zearalenone (F2) from moldy feeds. Zearalenone produced by the fungus *Fusarium roseum* has estrogenic activity. Certain lines of swine are less stress prone than others, according to some research, and might be more resistant to lactation failure.

DIAGNOSIS

The major problem with clinical diagnosis of lactation failure is the differentiation of the acute infectious swelling and agalactia of mastitis from the noninfectious swelling or "caking" of the mammary glands, which also results in agalactia. Agalactia due to failure of milk letdown is most common in first litter gilts and is characterized by the inability of the gilt to feed the pigs. These gilts respond very well to oxytocin.

Some sows and gilts will exhibit parturient psychosis and will fail to allow the piglets to nurse and may even kill those that come around the head area. Tranquilizers or sedatives work very well in most sows and gilts. Some sows with parturient psychosis respond to the removal of the piglets' needle teeth.

NECROPSY FINDINGS

The lesions in lactation failure will vary from normal lactating glands to grossly pathologic lactating glands. Affected glands are firm or hard with gelatinous edema of the subcutaneous tissue. The skin may be red to blue. Generally, milk will not flow from cut surfaces of a mastitic gland but will flow freely from the normal gland. Each gland is composed of an anterior and a posterior segment served by separate teat canals, and it is not uncommon for one segment to be involved while the other remains uninvolved. Infected glands may have focal or diffuse lesions that vary from mild catarrhal inflammation to severe purulent and necrotizing mastitis.

Examination of uterine tissue generally is nonrevealing, as the uterus is normally postparturient and involuting, with normal mucus and some flakes of white pus. Bacteria may be isolated, but histologically there is no evidence of infection.

Enlarged adrenal glands may be seen, but consistent evidence of other tissue changes is absent.

TREATMENT

In general, treatment is aimed at the relief of symptoms. Many drugs, not all approved for swine, are used but none are better than oxytocin in relieving the failure of milk letdown. Each case is different, and many require more than oxytocin to re-establish normal milk flow. Even with temporary interruption (12 to 24 hr) of milk flow, the piglets need supplements. Hungry piglets learn to drink from a flat pan very quickly and can survive on whole cow's milk for a few feedings. For long-term feeding, a homemade mixture composed of 1 qt whole milk, 1 oz white syrup, and 1 oz corn oil is satisfactory if a commercial preparation is not available.

Drugs and treatments and the rationales for their use are listed as follows:

1. Oxytocin: 30 to 40 units per sow at 3- to 4-hr intervals for milk letdown.
2. Broad-spectrum antibiotics: Aimed at coliform bacteria.
3. Corticosteroids: Anti-inflammatory. (Synthetic corticosteroids are bound less by globulin than are natural corticosteroids.)
4. B vitamins: Appetite stimulants. (Beer and fresh yeast breads also seem to stimulate the appetite in less severely affected sows.)
5. Tranquilizers: To calm restless gilts or sows.
6. Forced exercise: The animal will frequently urinate, defecate, and then drink and eat afterwards.
7. Fresh feeds: Especially useful when moldy feeds are suspected.
8. Nonsteroidal anti-inflammatory drugs: Relieve pain and reduce inflammatory reactions.
9. Dipyrone: Reduces fever.
10. Antihistamines: Combat histamine release in cases of necrotizing mastitis.
11. Diuretics: Reduce edema.*

PREVENTION

Until a more precise etiology can be found, a prevention program that works with a high degree of success will be hard to implement. At present, the primary causes of agalactia seem to be stress and coliform mastitis or gram-negative bacterial endotoxin. Prevention must be directed toward controlling these factors.

Recommendations to help control stress and toxin-induced agalactia are as follows:

1. Provide proper sanitation, nutrition, environmental conditions, and protection from other diseases.
2. Select brood animals from lines known to be free of agalactia.

---

*Treatments 8 to 11 not approved for swine.

3. Exercise animals daily during preparturient periods.
4. Feed bulky diets or oral laxatives during the last 2 weeks of gestation and during early lactation.
5. Avoid sudden changes in feeding and housing. (Allow 2 to 3 days for adjustment to crates before farrowing.)
6. Select stress resistant replacements.
7. The use of autogenous bactrins is helpful in some herds.
8. Cull agalactic sows. (This is debatable and depends on the cause of agalactia.)

LACTATION FAILURE IN CATTLE, SHEEP, AND GOATS

The causes of lactation failure or dysgalactia in ruminants are usually associated with other diseases, especially those that produce toxemia, elevated temperature, metabolic disorders (ketosis, pregnancy toxemia, abomasal displacement, rumen acidosis, and mineral imbalance), mastitis, lameness, and those that produce anemia and congenital abnormalities.

In sheep and goats, a condition termed contagious agalactia is caused by *Mycoplasma mycoides*. It produces severe udder edema and high mortality in goats, and it may respond to treatment with tylosin or erythromycin if given early.

Other agents producing mastitis and dysgalactia in sheep and goats are *Pasteurella haemolytica* and *Chlamydia* spp. Tetracycline is generally useful against these agents.

Fungal-induced lactation failure, agalactia, or dysgalactia has been seen in cattle, sheep, and goats grazing pastures contaminated with ergot. Fescue pastures have been strongly suspected of producing lactation failure, but this has not been proved. When agalactia or dysgalactia is caused by ergot or is suspected to be caused by fescue, the only known treatment and prevention is the removal of the involved animal from the suspected contaminated pasture.

Retained Placenta

DAVID McCLARY, D.V.M., M.S.

Goats, sheep, swine, and cattle all may suffer from retained fetal membranes. The condition is most common and of the greatest economic importance in the cow. The bovine placenta is considered retained if not shed by 8 to 12 hr postpartum. Following normal parturition, the reported incidence of retained placenta is between 3 and 12 per cent (average 7 per cent) in dairy cattle. Beef cattle are less commonly affected. The retention rate is higher following dystocia, cesarean section, fetotomy, twinning, overdistention of the uterus, uterine inertia, premature parturition, and abortion.

Certain infectious diseases including brucellosis, campylobacteriosis, listeriosis, leptospirosis, and IBR may cause abortion or premature parturition, resulting in a greater incidence of retained placenta. Other direct causes are nutritional deficiencies in carotene, vitamin A, iodine, selenium, and vitamin E as well as imbalances in calcium and phosphorus. Nonspecific causes related to management problems such as contaminated calving areas, stress, and malnutrition in late gestation have all been implicated. Retained placenta should always be considered a sign of an underlying disease problem.

ETIOLOGY

Placental retention in ruminants is due to 1 of 3 basic defects: (1) detachment failures of the cotyledon and the caruncular unit, (2) expulsion failure due to uterine atony, and (3) expulsion failure due to mechanical blockage or entrapment. Failure of detachment of the cotyledons is the most common and important.

Changes in the placentome that contribute to eventual detachment begin in the last month of pregnancy. In the last few days of gestation, there is a significant reduction in the number of epithelial cells lining the caruncular crypts. Without this reduction detachment is less likely, raising the chance of membrane retention. Calving prior to the predetermined date by more than 4 days results in a higher incidence of retained placenta. This fact explains the greater rate of retained placentas in corticosteroid-induced parturition.

Other causes for detachment failure are injury, inflammation, or edema of the placentome. Nonspecific agents producing placentitis and cotyledonitis are pyogenic bacteria, such as *Corynebacterium pyogenes,* coliforms, staphylococci, streptococci, and molds. These organisms may originate from another diseased organ or body part. Pathologic changes vary from slight inflammation to severe necrosis. Noninflammatory edema of the chorionic villi as observed after cesarean section or uterine torsion may inhibit normal separation.

Atony often follows hypocalcemia or prolonged dystocia with exhaustion of the uterine musculature. Normal intensity of uterine contractions diminishes, resulting in a failure to expel the placenta. Normal detachment of the cotyledon from the caruncle usually occurs with simple uterine atony.

Occasionally, the placenta may be mechanically trapped in a rapidly involuting uterine horn, in the cervix, or on a fleshy horizontal band of tissue in the anterior of the vagina. Large placentomes often contribute to this type of retention. Simple manipulation and slight traction should easily correct this mechanical retention.

CLINICAL SIGNS

The clinical signs of retained placenta vary from uterine involvement alone to septic metritis. In the cow, the clinical syndrome is limited to the reproductive tract in most cases. The obvious clinical sign is the presence of fetal membranes protruding from the vulva. In some cases, the entire placenta is held in the uterus so there is no exposed portion. The condition may go unnoticed until the animal shows an abnormal uterine discharge or an odor characteristic of placental degeneration. Other possible signs are vulvar swelling, udder edema, and straining.

Septic metritis sometimes develops in the cow with a retained placenta. The affected animal may demonstrate the signs of septicemia and toxemia, including an elevated temperature, diarrhea, dehydration, anorexia, and general malaise. Any cow with a retained placenta should be closely monitored for changes in appetite, milk production, and general well-being, so septicemia can be identified immediately.

EXAMINATION

Since retained placenta may be a sign of an underlying disease, a complete history and physical examination should be made. If the animal's appetite, milk production, vital signs, and general well-being are normal, treatment can usually be delayed until 3 or 4 days postpartum. This delay allows for the normal uterine defenses to become better established and for autolysis of the placenta to proceed. Rectal examination of the reproductive tract should be made to determine if uterine tone is present and if early involution has begun. The normal uterus postpartum should be firm with prominent linear striations along the uterine body, indicating uterine contractions around the placenta. If the uterus is thin-walled, atonic, and the placentomes are readily palpable, there is a greater chance of delayed involution and uterine disease. Cows having a history of retained placenta should be closely examined for uterine disease 25 to 35 days postpartum.

TREATMENT

Treatment and management of animals with retained placenta often involves education of the client. In many cases, the client's main concern is elimination of the retained fetal membranes by whatever means necessary. With any treatment method, the prime consideration should be the well-being and the subsequent fertility of the affected animal. Prescribed treatments for retained fetal membranes have included combinations of forced manual extraction, intrauterine infusions, systemic therapy with antibiotics and hormones, and no treatment at all.

Manual Extraction

Although widely practiced and advocated at one time, manual removal of fetal membranes should be discouraged. Several studies have shown that the incidence of local and systemic metritis, uterine abscesses, and perimetritis is greater in cows subjected to forced manual extraction. This practice slows the normal involution rate and reduces the subsequent fertility of the animal.

Manual removal is indicated only if during a vaginal examination the placenta is loosely attached and easily removed by slight traction. If the placental retention is due to uterine atony or mechanical blockage, or if a majority of the attachments have released the placenta, it may be easily teased through the open cervix.

Intrauterine Therapy

Numerous antibiotics, antiseptics, and sulfonamides have been used for intrauterine therapy. These drugs are administered as boluses and as fluid douches. The product used should be relatively nonirritating and at least partially absorbed into all portions of the reproductive tract. Uterine boluses should dissolve rapidly in uterine fluids. Studies have shown that dairy cows with retained placentas treated with tetracycline boluses every other day plus one treatment after the placenta was expelled had a service per conception rate and an open interval similar to normal herd mates.

Some precautions should be taken with intrauterine treatment of retained placenta cases. Since some bacterial action is needed for autolysis and degeneration of the placenta, care should be taken not to overtreat with antiseptic and antibiotic preparations. Daily local therapy may actually prolong the time of retention. The uterus during early postpartum may be quite friable in the animal with retained placenta. Extreme care should be taken not to puncture the uterus during manipulation or while attempting to pass a pipette for an intrauterine infusion. Most antibiotics infused into the uterus are absorbed into the general circulation and redistributed to all parts of the body, including the mammary glands. The milk from infused dairy cattle should be discarded 2 to 4 days following treatment because of antibiotic residues.

Systemic Therapy

Systemic therapy is intended to either increase uterine contractions, thereby speeding expulsion time, or decrease the severity of infection. If the retention is due to uterine atony, ecbolic drugs may stimulate contractions. Hypocalcemia often contributes to uterine atony. Calcium borogluconate in conjunction with 40 to 60 units of oxytocin may be used every 2 hr to improve uterine contractions. Oxytocin is of limited value 48 hr postpartum when uterine sensitivity is reduced. A longer oxytocic effect can be derived with 1 to 5 mg of ergonovine. Estrogens have been shown to increase the blood supply to the uterus and to increase myometrial activity, but their use is controversial and of questionable value in the treatment of uterine disease. Excessive doses of estrogen may adversely affect normal cyclic activity in the cow.

In recent years, prostaglandins have been used as ecbolic drugs. Although more studies of efficacy need to be made, prostaglandins apparently have some ecbolic effect in the postpartum cow prior to development of the corpus luteum.

Researchers have found concentrations of oxytetracycline in all portions of the bovine reproductive tract following twice daily intravenous treatment of 11 mg/kg. While systemic treatment for retained placenta and genital tract infections reduces the chance of contamination of the uterus as compared with local therapy, it also requires daily treatment to maintain effective antibiotic levels. Once or twice daily treatment may not be a practical alternative. Long-acting oxytetracycline products may be of value in treatment of the beef cow with retained placenta.

No Treatment

If examination reveals the animal to be systemically normal and the uterus to be well contracted, treatment may not be indicated. Even if separation of the cotyledon and caruncle does not take place, the normal degeneration of the caruncle begins early in the postpartum period. In many cases, the placenta may be shed with the necrotic distal portion of the caruncle still attached. This process is usually completed by 10 to 14 days postpartum. If the animal is not treated, it should be closely monitored for signs of metritis and should be examined and possibly treated after passage of the placenta.

RETAINED PLACENTA IN OTHER FOOD-PRODUCING ANIMALS

Retained placenta in the ewe and doe is quite similar to the condition in the cow. Manual removal should always be discouraged. Ten to 20 units of oxytocin is of value in the first 2 days postpartum. Intrauterine boluses or pessaries on alternate days may reduce the chances of metritis. If signs of metritis develop, the animal should be given broad-spectrum antibiotics.

Retained placenta in the sow is relatively uncommon following normal delivery, but when it occurs the membranes are often retained in the apical portion of the uterine horn and thus not exposed. These sows often develop septic metritis. If retained placenta is suspected, the sow should be given repeated doses of oxytocin (20 to 30 units every 2 to 3 hr) and broad-spectrum antibiotics.

Supplemental Reading

Arthur, G. H., Noakes, D. E., and Pearson, H.: Veterinary Reproduction and Obstetrics, 5th ed. London, Bailliere Tindall, 1982.
Bretzlaff, K. N., Ott, R. S., and Korotz, G. D.: Distribution of oxytetracycline in the genital tract of cows. Am. J. Vet. Res. 43:12, 1982.
Morrow, D. A.: Current Therapy in Theriogenology, 1st ed. Philadelphia, W. B. Saunders Company, 1980.

Metritis

DAVID McCLARY, D.V.M., M.S.

Metritis is a problem in all food-producing animals, but it is of greatest importance in the cow. The condition is often secondary to complications of parturition, such as dystocia and retained placenta. The development and severity of metritis are related to the organism involved, and the animal's resistance to infection. Causative organisms are streptococci, staphylococci, and coliforms, with *Corynebacterium pyogenes, Fusobacterium necrophorum,* and *Bacteroides* spp. the most important.

Normal postpartum uterine discharges should not be confused with those of metritis. Immediately after parturition, the discharge or lochia should be clear to slightly red. Between days 8 and 14, normal uterine discharge should be mucoid with little or no odor. As the caruncles necrose, they impart a mahogany color to the discharge. By day 18, little or no fluid should be present in the uterus. The cow often eliminates infections during the postpartum period with no treatment if uterine tone and involution are near normal.

ACUTE METRITIS

Acute septic metritis usually is restricted to the first 5 to 10 days postpartum. Acute metritis is characterized by septicemia, elevated temperature (40 to 42°C), diarrhea, depression, anorexia, reduced milk production, elevated pulse and respiratory rates, and possible dehydration. Endotoxic shock may occur. In advanced cases, the animal may have a subnormal temperature and may be unable to stand. The uterine discharge is thin, watery, and reddish in color with an extremely foul odor. Rectal examination reveals a thin-walled, atonic, and fluid filled uterus. Excessive uterine manipulation should be avoided to prevent greater absorption of toxins and bacteria.

Prompt systemic treatment with broad-spectrum antibiotics or sulfonamides is indicated. Recent study indicates that oxytetracycline (11 mg/kg) reaches all tissues of the reproductive tract in therapeutic levels, but tetracylines are of limited value against *C. pyogenes, F. necrophorum,* and *Bacteroides* spp. Procaine penicillin G at 22,000 to 33,000 units/lb gives sufficient uterine concentration for effectiveness against these 3 organisms, however. Antibiotic therapy should be continued for at least 3 to 5 days. If dehydration or toxemia is present, fluids may be given parenterally.

If accomplished with minimal uterine manipulation, partial drainage of the sanguinopurulent uterine fluid may be helpful. An equine stomach tube passed transcervically via the vagina is useful in siphoning large volumes of fluid from the uterus. Extreme care must be taken not to puncture a friable, thin-walled uterus. Intrauterine infusions of antibiotics (oxytetracycline, 2 to 4 gm) may be indicated while the animal is being given systemic antibiotics.

Oxytocin (40 to 60 units) may induce uterine contractions, aiding evacuation during the first 48 hr postpartum. Estrogens increase uterine blood supply and tone, but they may also increase the absorption of organisms and toxins.

SUBACUTE METRITIS

Subacute metritis usually appears later in the postpartum period (days 8 to 14). It is characterized by a uterine infection with or without mild septicemia. Signs may consist of a slightly elevated temperature, mild anorexia, and a lowered milk production. One of the more prominent signs may be a swollen vulva and a thick red, yellow, or white malodorous discharge matted around the perivulvar hair or on the tail. The color and consistency of the discharge will vary depending on the infective organism. The appearance of discharge may be misleading, since the vaginal discharge may seem normal while the uterus contains a large volume of metritic fluid. On rectal examination, uterine tone varies from flaccid to turgid. Involution is usually retarded.

If treatment is indicated, broad-spectrum antibiotics may be given systemically or topically (intrauterine boluses or solutions). Tetracyclines are indicated for coliform, *Fusobacterium,* and *Bacteroides* infections, while penicillin may be used if a *C. pyogenes* infection is suspected. If an organism is resistant to treatment, it should be cultured and an antibiotic sensitivity test conducted.

Large volumes (250 to 500 ml) of broad-spectrum antibiotics every 2 to 3 days have been beneficial in treating subacute metritis. The volume of solution should never exceed the capacity of the uterus. In my opinion, 2 to 4 gm of tetracycline powder (Polyotic Powder*) in 200 to 400 ml hot water (65 to 70°C) gives good results in the treatment of subacute metritis at 10 to 14 days postpartum. The heat possibly causes an ecbolic effect by stimulating uterine prostaglandin production and release.

Oxytocin will have little or no effect on the uterus after 48 hr postpartum. Estrogens improve uterine tone but

should be used cautiously owing to their possible adverse effect on normal cyclic activity in the cow. Ergonovine (1 to 5 mg) may increase uterine tone and has minimal side effects.

Prostaglandins are beneficial in the treatment of pyometra when a functional corpus luteum is present. They may also be useful in stimulating ecbolic uterine activity prior to corpus luteum development. The degree and importance of this action is questionable and require more study.

CHRONIC METRITIS

Chronic metritis is seen later in the postpartum period following luteal development. It is usually a sequela to acute or subacute metritis. The most common organism isolated in chronic metritis is *C. pyogenes,* even though some other organism may have caused the original infection. Chronic metritis is usually a local infection. Slight vulvar swelling and a purulent discharge may be present if the cervix is open. Milk production may be slightly reduced.

On rectal examination the uterus is usually enlarged, with a thickened wall, and contains a few to several ml of fluid. Returning the animal to estrus, when uterine resistance to infection is greatest, is an effective means of therapy. First ovulation and corpus luteum development normally take place between days 14 and 20. If a corpus luteum is present, prostaglandin (25 to 40 mg Lutalyse*) is of therapeutic value in evacuating the uterus.

Treatment with intrauterine infusions may frequently be useful in the treatment of chronic metritis. Since the cervix is at least partially closed, infusions should be administered by pipette directed through the cervix by rectal palpation. Since the most common pathogen involved in chronic bovine metritis is *C. pyogenes,* penicillin (1 to 2 million units in 20 to 100 ml diluent) is the drug of choice. The uterus should not be overfilled.

Whenever the uterus is infused with antibiotics, residues must be considered. Milk should be discarded for 2 to 8 milkings, depending on the medication used.

Possible complications of metritis are perimetritis, uterine abscesses, tetanus, adhesions, and endometritis. Perimetritis and endometritis are discussed further.

PERIMETRITIS

Perimetritis is characterized by thickening and crepitance of the uterus. Adhesions of the uterus to surrounding structures are common. The condition frequently is secondary to an obstetric injury or is an extension of acute metritis through an atonic, compromised uterine wall. A guarded to poor prognosis in regard to subsequent fertility should be given. Systemic therapy as for peritonitis is indicated.

ENDOMETRITIS

Endometritis is the inflammation of the endometrium with minimal involvement of other portions of the reproductive tract. Endometritis is a possible cause for infertil-

---

*Available from American Cyanamid Co., Wayne, NJ 07470

*Available from The Upjohn Co., Kalamazoo, MI 49001

ity in the cow. There is usually no palpable change in the uterus, but observation of the estrous discharge may reveal some cloudiness or flakes of pus. Intrauterine infusions of an antibiotic or antiseptic solution 12 to 24 hr post-breeding have been used in treatment, but their value is questionable. Caustic or irritating solutions and excessive volumes (more than 40 to 60 ml) should be avoided. Although not documented, inducing short cycles with prostaglandin therapy may be of value.

METRITIS IN OTHER FOOD-PRODUCING ANIMALS

Metritis is not a common condition in swine. It is usually secondary to uterine inertia and retained placenta and may develop into a fatal septic metritis. Recovered animals often develop endometritis. C. pyogenes is the most common organism isolated. Systemic treatment with broad-spectrum antibiotics and 20 to 30 units oxytocin is indicated in clinical cases.

Metritis is a common occurrence in sheep and goats. It often results in a severe septic and often fatal condition characterized by tenesmus and deposition of a bloody, semisolid discharge. The animal should be treated at first indication of a problem with systemic antibiotics or sulfonamides, such as penicillin (40,000 units/kg, twice daily) or sulfamethazine (120 mg/kg once daily). Since tetanus is a common sequela, tetanus antitoxin should be administered.

Supplemental Reading

Arthur, G. H., Noakes, D. E., and Pearson, H.: Veterinary Reproduction and Obstetrics, 5th ed. London, Bailliere Tindall, 1982.

Ball, L., Olson, J. D., and Mortimer, R. G.: Bacteriology of the postpartum uterus. Proceedings of the Annual Meeting—Society for Theriogenology, 1984.

Callahan, C. J.: Bovine Medicine and Surgery, 2nd ed. In H. E. Amstutz, (ed.). Santa Barbara, American Veterinary Publications, Inc., 1980.

Pyometra in Cattle

JOHN McCORMACK, D.V.M.

Pyometra is characterized clinically by the accumulation of purulent material in the uterus, the retention of a corpus luteum, and anestrus.[1] Affected cows do not appear ill but often become economic liabilities, since long-term persistence of the disease leads to severe endometritis, which delays uterine involution. The end result is prolonged infertility or even sterility, possibly due to the destruction of uterine glands.[2] Animals with the disease do not recover spontaneously.

ETIOLOGY

Although pyometra usually occurs in the first 3 months postpartum following dystocia, retained fetal membranes, metritis, or perhaps other stresses in early lactation, it occasionally occurs post-breeding.[3] Infection introduced by insemination of pregnant cows thought to be in estrus often leads to embryonic death or abortion and subsequent pyometra. The indiscriminate infusion of cows in

the luteal phase of the estrous cycle likewise can cause pyometra.[3]

Culturing of the uterine contents or discharge reveals a variety of organisms. Hemolytic staphylocci, coliforms, Pseudomonas aeruginosa, Pasteurella sp. and Corynebacterium pyogenes are common. C. pyogenes is the organism most often implicated as the bacterial cause of pyometra.[2] Trichomonas foetus has also been incriminated as an etiologic agent in herds using natural breeding.

CLINICAL SIGNS AND DIAGNOSIS

A purulent discharge is often observed on the rear parts of the cow or on the ground or floor when the cow lies down. Rectal palpation of the reproductive tract reveals fluid-filled and thick-walled uterine horns, often of equal size, and a corpus luteum on 1 ovary. The corpus luteum may be difficult to detect upon palpation. It is thought that the corpus luteum is retained owing to the inhibition of prostaglandin $PGF_{2\alpha}$ from the diseased endometrium.[3]

To the inexperienced clinician, the pyometric uterus is sometimes confused with a pregnancy of 60 to 150 days. However, no membrane slips or placentomes are palpated in pyometric uteri. Sometimes the cervix will be closed, but it is usually narrowly dilated, discharging varying amounts of whitish-yellow or reddish-brown to gray pus.

TREATMENT

Treatment should be directed towards the re-establishment of the estrous cycle. Destruction of the corpus luteum can be accomplished in several ways.

Manual enucleation of the corpus luteum through the rectal wall is an effective but unacceptable method. Not only are the risk of excessive hemorrhage and subsequent ovarian adhesion considerable, but the corpus luteum is often not easily palpable.

Infusing with antibiotics and draining the uterus results in low clinical recovery rates and poor conception rates.

Various estrogens have been used as luteolytic agents. Estradiol cypionate injected at a dose of 5 to 10 mg generally produces contraction of the uterus within 24 to 72 hr, but the results are inconsistent and ovaritis, ovarian adhesions, relaxed pelvic ligaments, and cystic ovaries have been reported following its use.

The intramuscular administration of prostaglandins appears, at present, to be the method of choice for safely treating pyometra.

In one study, 26 cows with pyometra were injected with Dinoprost in doses ranging from 5 to 25 mg.[3] Complete evacuation of the uterine contents occurred in 22 cows (85 per cent) at estrus, which was observed 3 to 4 days after injection. The uteri began evacuating within 24 hr after the injections. A dose of 25 mg intramuscularly appeared to give the best results. Of the 22 cows that responded to the injections, 65 per cent became pregnant, requiring 2.2 services per pregnancy. Cows should not be inseminated during the induced estrus but at the next estrus.

Cloprostenol has also been successfully used.[4] When 93 pyometric cows were injected with 0.5 mg of cloprostenol, 90 (96.8 per cent) exhibited complete uterine evacuation within 3 to 9 days. In another trial in which 7 to 12 mg of estradiol cypionate was injected into 73 cows, 43 (58.9

per cent) responded with uterine evacuation.[5] By comparison, 72 of 79 cows (86.1 per cent) that received cloprostenol reacted to the drug. When 50 ml of nitrofurazone was infused into uteri of affected cows following evacuation, no benefit was observed in preventing relapses, and there was a decline in conception rates.

References

1. Roberts, S. J.: Veterinary Obstetrics and Genital Diseases. 2nd ed. Ann Arbor, Michigan, Edward Bros. Inc., 1971.
2. Hartigan, P. J., Griffin J. F. T., and Nunn, W. R.: Some observations on *Corynebacterium pyogenes* infection of the bovine uterus. Theriogenology. *1*:153–167, 1974.
3. Gustafsson, B., Backstrom, G., and Edqvist, L.: Treatment of bovine pyometra with prostaglandin $F_{2\alpha}$: An evaluation of a field study. Theriogenology. 6:45–50, 1976.
4. Gunzler, Ö., and Schmalfeldt, B.: Tierarztliche Umschau. Zur behandlung der pyometra des rindes mit dem prostaglandinanalog estrumate. *34*:477–481, 1979.
5. Fazeli, M., Ball, L., and Olson, J. D.: Comparisons of treatment of pyometra with estradiol cypionate or cloprostenol following infusion or noninfusion with nitrofurazone. Theriogenology. *14*:339–347, 1980.

Bovine Vaginitis

P. MICKELL DAVIS, D.V.M.

INFECTIOUS PUSTULAR VULVOVAGINITIS (IPV)

The causative agent of IPV is a virus indistinguishable from the IBR virus. The lesions of the vagina include a pronounced erythema punctuated with pustules that measure approximately 2 mm in diameter.

Clinical Signs

The affected cows often exhibit restlessness, standing with their tails slightly elevated. The vulva may become swollen, sensitive, and obvious pain or discomfort may be noted during the cow's frequent attempts to urinate. Advanced cases often have a yellowish, mucoid vaginal exudate, which may be observed on the ventral commissure of the vulva. Progression of the disease in some cows leads to coalescence of the pustules to form plaques. Hemorrhagic foci may also be present in these individuals. Resolution of the plaques results in erosions of the vaginal wall. IPV will advance to metritis in some individuals.

The duration of the clinical disease is generally 3 weeks. Primary healing is accomplished by the second week. A possible sequela to more advanced cases is endometritis, resulting in temporary infertility.

Once infected, a cow may be an intermittent shedder of the virus for an undetermined period. Reinfection may occur at any time. Transmission of the disease by coitus has been demonstrated. An infected bull can harbor the IPV virus for approximately 26 days. The disease is manifested in the bull as mild to severe balanoposthitis.

Treatment

Treatment of infected individuals is indicated to prevent secondary bacterial infection. Control of IPV within a herd involves cessation of natural mating, institution of artificial insemination if possible, and vaccination for IBR. Vaccination provides only short-term immunity due to the localized nature of the disease.

BOVINE GRANULAR VENEREAL DISEASE

Granular Vulvovaginitis (GVD)

The causative agents of GVD are *Mycoplasma bovigenitalium, Ureaplasma* spp., *Corynebacterium pyogenes,* and *Escherichia coli.*

The only consistent lesions are raised granular areas (1 to 2 mm) of hyperplastic lymphoid cells located primarily on the vestibular mucous membrane. Granular areas in severely infected individuals will coalesce causing a congested mucosa that will bleed with slight friction. Affected cows will exhibit uneasiness and frequent attempts to void urine.

GVD has an incubation period of 1 to 3 weeks after exposure. The granular lesions will decline in number but not in size as the cow recovers. Little is known about degree or duration of immunity.

Coitus is the primary method of transmission; however, improper artificial insemination technique in the presence of infection and contaminated bedding have been incriminated.

Treatment

There is no specific treatment for GVD. Cessation of natural mating and use of artificial insemination with good sanitary technique will aid in the control of the disease. Outbreaks are self-limiting and resolve with time.

CATARRHAL BOVINE VAGINITIS (CBV)

The causative agent of CBV is an enterovirus. Lesions of the disease include hyperemia of the vaginal mucosa and cervix, with edema of the cervix. Secondary bacterial infection is not uncommon.

Clinical Signs

An early clinical sign is a slight mucoid discharge from the vulva. Soiling of the tail and perineum is found with progression of the disease. A clear, yellowish, viscous exudate will be present on the vaginal floor. Secondary bacterial infection causes this exudate to become mucopurulent.

The incubation period for CBV is 2 to 3 days. The course of the disease is highly varied, ranging from 1 week to more than 1 month. Acquisition of immunity is questionable. If any immunity develops, it is of short duration. Delayed conception is a sequela to the disease.

Transmission is primarily by coitus. Bedding contaminated by vaginal discharges has also been incriminated.

Treatment

Treatment may be considered for secondary bacterial infection. Control measures are management oriented, including cessation of natural mating and frequent changes of bedding in the presence of infection.

OTHER CAUSES

Nonspecific vaginitis may appear in any of the food animal species. Etiology of nonspecific vaginitis is varied; fecal contamination and pneumovagina secondary to poor vulvar conformation, trauma secondary to dystocia, and vaginitis concurrent with metritis are examples. With the exception of conformation, these types of vaginitis are usually of short clinical duration and have no long-lasting detrimental effects.

Confinement swine operations have experienced cases of vaginitis associated with fecal contamination and un-associated with poor vulvar conformation. Contamination takes place when feces become trapped between the sow and the farrowing crate. Sows whose tails have been docked are more prone to infection because they are unable to remove the fecal material adhering to the vulva.

Haemophilus somnus isolations from the vagina and other areas of the reproductive tract of cows are recognized. More research is needed before the clinical disease is associated with the organism. The available reports associate some degree of decreased fertility as well as abortion in cows harboring *H. somnus.* "Nodular vaginitis" has been associated with *H. somnus,* but in general, published reports of clinical lesions and microscopic evidence are not available.

Supplemental Reading

Amstutz, H. E.: Bovine Medicine and Surgery, 2nd ed., vol. 1. Santa Barbara, American Veterinary Publications, Inc., 1980.

Doig, P. A., Ruhnke, H. L., Waelchli-Suter, R., et al.: The Role of *Ureaplasma* Infection in Bovine Reproductive Disease. The Compendium on Continuing Education, III. S324–S330, 1981.

Miller, R. B., Lein, D. H., and McEntee, K. E., et al.: *Haemophilus somnus* infection of the reproductive tract of cattle: a review. J. Am. Vet. Med. Assoc. *182*:1390–1392, 1981.

Roberts, S. J.: Veterinary Obstetrics and Genital Diseases, 2nd ed. Ann Arbor, Michigan, Edward Bros. Inc., 1971.

Bovine Ovarian Cysts

R. G. ELMORE, D.V.M., M.S.

Cystic conditions of the ovary are still an important infertility problem in dairy cattle. From 12 to 14 per cent of all problematic breeding cows have cystic ovaries. It has been estimated that between 10 and 40 per cent of all dairy cows develop cystic ovaries during their lifetimes and that 35 to 45 per cent of all dairy cows with ovarian cysts are affected with the condition repeatedly during their lifetimes.

CLINICAL SIGNS

Although nymphomania used to be the predominant sign of ovarian cysts in dairy cattle, anestrus is the most common sign today. Currently, most investigators report that 75 to 90 per cent of cows with ovarian cysts are anestrous. This change is probably due to the greater frequency of palpation of cows during the early postpartum period as a part of routine reproductive herd health programs. Without routine postpartum examinations, nymphomania would be more likely to attract the attention of dairy owners than anestrus. Because the incidence of ovarian cysts is relatively high during the early postpartum period, and because the only practical way to make a definitive diagnosis of ovarian cysts is rectal palpation, veterinarians should encourage their clients to establish a routine reproductive herd health program.

DIAGNOSIS

Diagnosis of ovarian cysts is based upon the finding of smooth, fluctuating, rounded structures on one or both ovaries measuring 2.5 cm or larger in diameter. These findings should be related to other genital tract findings and history. It is possible to confuse follicles of large diameter, soft corpora hemorrhagicae, and soft corpora lutea of pregnancy with ovarian cysts if one is not very careful and thorough in palpation. If the structure in question is a follicle, other signs of impending estrus (e.g., regressing corpus luteum, turgid uterus, mucus from the vulva, rough tail head, and so forth) should be evident. If the structure is a corpus hemorrhagicum, uterine edema will probably still be evident and metestrual bleeding may be seen. Corpora lutea of pregnancy can be extremely soft. A thorough palpation of the uterus to detect 1 of the 4 positive signs of pregnancy should aid in diagnosis. If the structure is in fact a cyst, the uterus will probably be flaccid, and there will not likely be a regressing corpus luteum. Although unusual, a cow may have an ovarian cyst and a corpus luteum at the same time. Ovarian cysts may be present in pregnant cows. The incidence in pregnant cows is higher during the first 90 days of gestation.

Types of Cysts

Veterinary pathologists generally recognize 3 types of ovarian cysts.

Follicular Cysts. These are anovulatory cysts, single or multiple on 1 or both ovaries, thin-walled, and clinical signs may be either nymphomania or anestrus.

Luteal Cysts. Luteal cysts are anovulatory cysts, commonly single structures on 1 ovary, thick-walled, and the clinical sign is almost always anestrus. Both follicular and luteal cysts are pathologic structures. It is normally very difficult to differentiate the 2 conditions clinically. It has been found that what often feels like a single, thick-walled structure on rectal palpation are actually multiple cystic structures located very close together. The walls of the adjacent structures make "the cyst" feel thick walled. It is not important to differentiate follicular cysts from luteal cysts clinically because both are treated the same way.

Cystic Corpora Lutea. These cysts are ovulatory, single structures with the characteristics of normal corpora lutea. They may be slightly larger with some fluctuation and contain vacuoles of varying size. In packing house specimens, approximately 30 per cent of the corpora lutea have vacuoles of 7 to 10 mm in diameter. Functionally, the estrous cycle is not affected. Cystic corpora lutea are entirely normal structures.

It was discovered during the 1940's that products high in luteinizing hormone (LH) activity have curative effects when administered to cows with ovarian cysts. Research has since raised some questions regarding the etiology of ovarian cysts. Whether there is a deficiency in production of LH by the anterior pituitary or a deficiency in the release mechanism of LH from the anterior pituitary is still not known. It has been postulated that in some cows, the ovaries are unable to respond to LH. This would explain why a small percentage of cows do not respond to LH therapy. Ovarian cysts are generally believed to be the result of a failure of production or release of adequate amounts of LH, or both.

ETIOLOGY

There is evidence demonstrating that a hereditary influence is involved in ovarian cysts in dairy cattle. In Sweden, the incidence of ovarian cysts declined from 11 per cent in 1954, to 5 per cent in 1964, and to 3 per cent in 1974 after adoption of a policy whereby bulls used at artificial insemination were culled if their daughters had a greater than average incidence of ovarian cysts. The 2 abnormalities of ovulation, cystic ovaries and twinning, are closely related and both are probably hereditary.

Many factors have been observed to be positively correlated with the incidence of ovarian cysts in dairy cattle. However, the cause and effect relationship of these factors has not been elucidated. Ovarian cysts are more common in closely confined, stabled animals during the winter. The condition is most frequent after the second to fifth parturition. Ovarian cysts appear more often in high producing cows. Many researchers state that greater feeding, especially rations high in protein stimulate lactation and the development of cystic ovaries.

TREATMENT

Currently, there are 3 approaches to treatment of ovarian cysts in dairy cattle: (1) spontaneous recovery, (2) manual rupture of cysts, and (3) administration of therapeutic drugs. Prior to 50 days postpartum, approximately 50 per cent of ovarian cysts will regress spontaneously. After 50 days postpartum, approximately 20 per cent of the ovarian cysts will spontaneously resolve. Several studies have demonstrated that waiting for self-recovery by the animal is not economically sound, since it usually lengthens the interval from calving to first breeding and conception.

Probably the earliest form of therapy for ovarian cysts was manual rupture via rectal palpation. Unfortunately, this is still done by some veterinarians. Controlled studies indicate that recovery after the manual rupture of ovarian cysts is approximately the same as spontaneous recovery rates. A false confidence in this practice has developed because self-recovery takes place coincidently in sufficient numbers to be misleading. Manual rupture of ovarian cysts can cause injury to the tissues of the ovary and its surrounding structures. This promotes adhesions of the ovary to its bursa and thus can be a source of infertility. In some cases, it can even produce sterility. Manual rupture of ovarian cysts should not be done.

Therapeutic Agents

Currently there are 3 forms of acceptable therapeutic products marketed in the United States for treatment of ovarian cysts in cattle. These are anterior pituitary extracts, human chorionic gonadotropin (HCG), and gonadotropin releasing hormone (GnRH). Anterior pituitary extracts and HCG have high levels of luteinizing hormone activity and provide the animal with an exogenous source of luteinizing hormone. GnRH causes the treated animal to release its own endogenous luteinizing hormone from the anterior pituitary gland. Several studies have demonstrated that exogenous sources of LH (anterior pituitary extracts and HCG) and the endogenous source of LH (GnRH) are equally effective in treating cows with ovarian cysts. There are several advantages, however, to using GnRH. Because of its small molecular size, GnRH is not likely to stimulate an immune response, as sometimes is produced by exogenous forms of luteinizing hormone. HCG and anterior pituitary extracts contain fairly large protein molecules upon which antibodies can be built. With these substances, it has been shown that anaphylaxis or refractoriness, or both, to repeated treatment may occur. More than one treatment with GnRH should not result in anaphylaxis nor should it likely result in refractoriness. HCG administered during mid-diestrus at the dosages used to treat cattle with ovarian cysts prolongs luteal function, whereas GnRH does not. Therefore if the ovarian cystic condition is misdiagnosed and normal cows in diestrum are treated with HCG, the estrous cycles will be prolonged. Similar use of GnRH will not alter the normal cycle. GnRH or HCG given to a pregnant cow should not produce any harmful effects.

After treatment with GnRH, HCG, or anterior pituitary extracts, (1) estrus will start normally, (2) palpable clinical changes in the cystic structures or the ovary will occur, or (3) no discernable changes in the cystic structures will be observed. Two weeks following treatment, the cow should be re-examined. If the cow is going to respond to treatment, changes in the ovaries should be detectable by then. If no changes are detectable at that time, the cow should be re-treated. The general response by the ovary is that the cystic structures become much firmer and usually smaller. Cows that respond to treatment frequently have a fertile estrus an average of 23 days post-treatment. Most researchers report that approximately 80 per cent of cows with ovarian cysts respond to initial treatment. Cows not responding to 2 or 3 treatments of GnRH should be given an exogenous source of LH (HCG or anterior pituitary extract).

Some clinicians have advocated the use of prostaglandins for resolution of ovarian cysts. Since most cows with ovarian cysts have very low levels of systemically circulating progesterone, it would seem likely that most cows with ovarian cysts would not respond to prostaglandin injections. The exception would be the cow with a luteal cyst. A most logical approach to incorporating prostaglandins into the treatment regime for ovarian cysts is to use it in combination with GnRH, HCG, or anterior pituitary extracts. For example, if LH products cause luteinization of the cystic structure by days 10 to 14 following treatment, prostaglandins could be used to cause regression of the luteal tissue. Following prostaglandin treatment, the cow should be in estrus within 2 to 5 days. This shortens the interval from initial treatment to first estrus from approximately 23 days to approximately 12 to 15 days. Prostaglandins will cause abortions in cows early in gestation. A cow thought to have a cystic ovary, but bred recently enough that a pregnancy examination cannot be accurately accomplished, should not be treated with prostaglandins. GnRH or LH agents should not endanger a pregnancy.

PREVENTION

Although cystic ovarian disease is one of the oldest recorded diseases, it still remains a major problem in modern United States dairies. Because of the complexities and the variations among animals, the efficient management of this malady is dependent upon complete reproductive records and a routine veterinary reproductive herd health program. Cows with cystic ovaries are highly responsive to treatment whenever it is administered early in the postpartum period.

Synchronization of Estrus

ROBERT L. CARSON, D.V.M., M.S.

Synchronization of estrus has the potential to be a tremendous management tool for the livestock industry. However, some attempts to synchronize livestock have had very disappointing results. Failure to respond, estrus at times other than expected, lack of true synchronization, and conception rates lower than expected are frequent. Many disappointments with synchronization are related to management factors and not to chemical agents. Such errors as poor heat detection, low quality semen, improper insemination timing and technique, inadequate sire power, poor herd health, improper nutrition, inadequate handling facilities, and failure of managers to understand normal reproductive expectancy can only lead to disastrous results when synchronization is attempted.

CATTLE

The products commerically available for cattle are prostaglandin $F_{2\alpha}$ ($PGF_{2\alpha}$) or its analogues and a combination of estradiol valerate-norgestomet injection and norgestomet implant. When cycling cows are injected with $PGF_{2\alpha}$ between days 5 and 17 of the estrous cycle the corpus luteum (CL) is destroyed, and the cow comes into a normal fertile heat in 2 to 5 days. This predictable response has allowed for several different synchronization schemes to be developed.

One of the first methods utilizes 2 injections of $PGF_{2\alpha}$ 10 to 11 days apart, with the cows being inseminated 80 hr after the last injection or following observed estrus. A similar method is to inject all the cattle and observe them for heat for 5 days. Those in heat should be bred. Those not bred 11 days after the first injection should be given another injection and bred 80 hr after the second injection or following observed heat. A method that conserves the amount of $PGF_{2\alpha}$ used is to palpate the cows and to inject only those with a mature CL. Another method that is sometimes utilized is observation of a group of cows for 5 days, breeding of those in heat, injecting of the remaining ones, and breeding in 80 hr or following observed estrus.

A major problem of synchronization with prostaglandins is failed or reduced response. One of the major causes is that animals are not cycling. In heifers this may be because they have not reached puberty, and they are

not at the proper age or weight, or both. Cows may not be cycling because they are recently postpartum, in high lactation, or fed low energy diets. Bovine females will not respond to prostaglandin if injected at the wrong time of the cycle. For lysis of the CL, the injection must be between days 5 and 17 of the estrous cycle. Mid-to-late diestrous animals respond better than do early diestrous animals. When injections are given on days 5, 7, and 10 of the estrous cycle, more animals come into heat when injected on days 7 and 10 than those injected on day 5. A slight improvement is seen on day 10 over day 7.

Very disappointing results have been obtained when synchronization with $PGF_{2\alpha}$ is followed by timed insemination. These disappointments are the result of variation in response to the drug, in that some of the animals may have been in heat prior to the planned insemination, some will be in heat afterwards, and some may not be in heat at all. Age, lactational status, and diestrous stage will influence when estrus occurs after injection. Heifers and dry cows tend to come into induced heat earlier than do lactating cows. Lactating cows show the most variability as to time of estrus. The stage of diestrus also has an influence on time of estrus. Animals injected early in diestrus (days 7, 8, 9) tend to come into heat earlier with less variation in time interval from treatment to estrus than those injected later in diestrus (day 10 or later). Early diestrual injection produces heat in 48 to 60 hr in heifers and dry cows and in 60 to 72 hr in lactating cows. Following late diestrual injection, heat is observed in 72 to 96 hr in heifers and dry cows and 96 hr or more in lactating cows. Low conception rates due to variability in time of estrus can be eliminated if animals are bred in accordance with estrus observation rather than timed insemination.

To use the injection-implant combinations to synchronize cattle, the animals are simultaneously given an intramuscular injection and implanted subcutaneously on the back of the ear. Nine days later the implant is removed and the animals come into heat in 24 to 36 hr. Basically, the estradiol valerate-norgestomet injection and norgestomet implant works by holding the cattle in an artificial diestrus until a designated time. The estradiol valerate component stops the formation of or causes the regression of the corpus luteum, while the norgestomet injection gives a rapid rise of this hormone inhibiting follicular development. The implant maintains this property until removed. Once the implant is removed rapid follicular development occurs, and all the animals come into heat at approximately the same time. Timed insemination can be utilized 48 to 54 hr after implant removal, or animals can be bred 12 hr after first observed estrus. The manufacturer suggests that this system will synchronize cattle in any stage of the cycle and will stimulate estrus in some animals that were not previously cycling.

Loss of the implant and infection at the implantation site are minor problems with this system and are not of any great significance. To be successful, when this system is applied to heifers they should be capable of cycling. Heifers that are not mature enough either because of age or weight will not respond or will show heat and not ovulate. A less than desirable response is seen in cows that are too recently postpartum or are in a poor nutritional state. Even though the injection-implant system may be capable of initiating cycling, animals should be on the verge of cycling or at least capable of cycling for satisfactory results.

There are data suggesting equal conception rates whether timed insemination or estrus observation breeding is used. It is my opinion that due to individual animal variability heat observation breeding might give better results.

First service conception rates are lower than control conception rates for both cows and heifers using the injection-implant system. The manufacturer suggests that this is compensated for by initiating cycling and by grouping subsequent heats, which results in a higher pregnancy percentage at the end of the breeding season.

SWINE

Estrus in swine can be grouped by various management procedures, such as boar exposure, transporting, mixing, regrouping, or somehow changing the routine of gilts and by simultaneously weaning pigs from a group of sows. These procedures often result in a less than desirable response over a wide and variable period of time, however. At present, there are not any drugs approved for estrus synchronization in swine available in the United States. There are some that have been used experimentally that show promise.

Feeding 15 to 20 mg of a synthetic progesterone for 18 days will result in estrus within a 3 to 5 day period after cessation of treatment with conception rates of 60 to 70 per cent. Another method involves breeding sows or gilts: when at 15 to 55 days of gestation they are given 15 mg $PGF_{2\alpha}$, followed in 12 hr by 10 mg $PGF_{2\alpha}$. They will abort and return to heat in 4 to 5 days without any detrimental effects on rebreeding or consequent farrowing rates. When normal cycling females are used in either treatment regime the response is usually good. However, estrus is being grouped not tightly synchronized, and close observation for animals in heat over several days is needed. Conception rates are acceptable but may be lower than desired. The synthetic progesterone treatment may stimulate estrus in some anestrous animals; however, the response percentage and conception rates are lower than in cycling animals. Estrus may be induced in anestrous animals by injecting 500 to 1500 units of pregnant mare serum gonadotropin followed in 72 to 96 hr with 250 to 1000 units of human chorionic gonadotropin. Estrus often will occur in 3 to 5 days. Response to this treatment is quite variable, and conception rates are somewhat lowered. Animals with functional ovaries will not respond, and this treatment may propagate poor reproductive performers.

SHEEP AND GOATS

The estrous cycle of sheep and goats can be controlled using progesterone and $PGF_{2\alpha}$ or its analogues, although these agents are not specifically approved for use in these species. Progesterone can be used throughout the year with limited success outside the natural breeding season. Sheep and goats, like all species, must have a functional corpus luteum for prostaglandins to work, therefore, use of these agents is limited to the true breeding season.

The most promising route of progesterone administration in sheep and goats is by vaginal pessary. In sheep, vaginal pessaries impregnated with 30 mg flurogestone acetate are left in place for 12 to 14 days, followed by an injection of 375 to 750 units PMSG (pregnant mare serum gonadotropin) at the time of pessary removal. In goats, pessaries containing 45 mg flurogestone acetate are left in place for 21 days, and 400 units PMSG are given at removal.

In cycling ewes and does, prostaglandin $F_{2\alpha}$ is luteolytic

Table 1. *Common Drug Dosages*

Drug	Supplier	Cattle	Sheep and Goats	Swine
Lutalyse* Dinoprost tromethamine	Upjohn Co. Kalamazoo, Michigan 49001	25 mg/head, IM	8 mg/head, IM	At 15–55 day of pregnancy, 15 mg/head followed in 12 hr with 10 mg/head, IM
Estrumate* Cloprostenol sodium	Haver-Lockhart BayVet Division Cutter Lab Shawnee, Kansas 66203	500 mcg/head, IM	125 mcg/head, IM	—
Synchro-Mate-B Estradiol valerate-norgestomet	CEVA Laboratories Overland Park, Kansas 66204	Estradiol, 5 mg and nogestomet 3 mg IM simultaneously. Nogestomet, 6 mg SQ ear implant. Remove in 9 days.	—	—
Regumate† Allyl trenbolone	Roussel-Uclef Paris, France	—	—	15 mg/head/day for 18 days in feed
Flurogestone acetate‡	Searle Laboratories Chicago, Illinois 60680	—	Vaginal pessary: sheep, 30 mg in place 12–14 days followed with 375–750 units PMSG at removal. Goats, 45 mg in place 21 days followed with 400 units PMSG at removal.	—

*Approved for use in cattle only.
†Swine only. Not approved for use in the United States at this time.
‡Approved for use in sheep and goats only.

and can be used to synchronize estrus. Prostaglandin is effective on day 4 of the estrous cycle in goats and on day 5 in sheep; therefore, 2 doses 11 days apart will synchronize estrus in both species. Estrus will begin approximately 2 days after the last injection of this regime.

The time of estrus and the response percentage are variable in both species with progesterone. Using prostaglandins in cycling animals in the natural breeding season, estrus is fairly predictable, and estrous response is good.

Conception rates in ewes are depressed using both progesterone and prostaglandin in that both transport and survival of spermatozoa in the reproductive tract of the ewe are reduced following the use of either of these agents. Conception rates in does range from 55 to 70 per cent using progesterone, while prostaglandins yield conception rates equal to natural estrus.

Regardless of the species involved or the treatment regime used, for satisfactory results a combination of normal, healthy animals capable of normal reproductive performance and good management is essential (Table 1).

Supplemental Reading

Momont, H., Seguin, B.: Temporal factors affecting the response to prostaglandin $F_{2\alpha}$ products in dairy cattle. Proceedings, Society for Theriogenology, 166–167, 1982.

Ott, R. S., Memon, M. A.: Sheep and Goat Manual. Society for Theriogenology. X: 19–23, 1980.

Webel, S. K., Scheid, J. P., Bouffault, J. C.: Estrus control in pigs. International Pig Veterinary Society, 49, 1980.

Wiltbank, J. N., Mores, S.: Breeding at a pre-determined time following Syncro-Mate-B treatment. National Association of Animal Breeders Beef AI Conference, Denver, 47–51, 1977.

Problems Associated with Artificial Insemination in Cattle

MARSHALL R. PUTNAM, D.V.M., M.S.

Problems with artificial insemination (AI) usually fall into one or more of the following categories: estrus detection, time of insemination, semen quality, semen placement or AI technique, and hygiene. Herd fertility, estrus synchronization, anestrus (especially in beef cattle), nutrition, and early embryonic death affect AI results but are not considered AI problems and are not discussed in this article. In reality, when dealing with a potential fertility problem in an AI program, each one should be investigated.

DETECTION OF ESTRUS

Failure to observe estrus is one of the major factors reducing reproductive efficiency in AI programs. In a dairy herd with a functional record system, evidence of estrus detection failure can come from several areas. DHIA (Dairy Herd Improvement Association) summary sheets show the number of cows more than 60 days postpartum at first breeding. Optimum estrus detection should yield 80 to 90 per cent of the cows being bred by 60 days postpartum. Herds that consistently show less than 80 to 90 per cent of the available cows in the breeding herd being bred are missing estrus. One can take the

problem cows and calculate interestrous intervals. Interestrous intervals falling into multiples of the 18 to 23 day-estrous cycle (36 to 46, 54 to 69 days between breedings) indicate missed heats. Practitioners can estimate the average number of cows that should be in heat each day by dividing the number of cycling cows in the breeding herd by the length of an estrous cycle. One hundred unexposed cows in the breeding herd divided by a 20-day estrous cycle equals an average of 5 cows in heat every day. A high percentage of the cows presented for anestrus should in fact be truly anestrus (with cysts, pyometra, and so forth) and should not be normal, open cycling cows. About 85 to 90 per cent of the cows presented for pregnancy should be pregnant and not normal, open cycling cows.

In beef cows, one must be careful to distinguish between estrus detection failure and anestrus. Records are usually not as available. To investigate the problem, divide the number of cows available for breeding by 20 days in an estrous cycle to determine the average number of cows expected to be in heat on a given day. Then take the last 5 days of breeding or heat dates and determine if that total approximates 5 days of expected heats. One must allow for some variation in how many cows cycle on each day. If the 2 numbers are not close, one must decide if estrus detection is the problem, or if the cows are anestrous. The question in beef cattle of estrus detection failure or anestrus can be answered in 2 ways, (1) palpation of ovaries for a functional corpus luteum and (2) estrus detection aids. When palpating ovaries, remember that a corpus luteum can be difficult to find on day 19 through day 5 of the next cycle. Thus, approximately 25 per cent of cycling cows may not have a palpable corpus luteum.

Heat Detection Aids

Heat detection aids are briefly listed and described. If visual observation fails, then these indicators may help. Veterinarians should try to tailor the use of aids to each situation.

Records. A record system that allows the manager to identify cows approaching 3 weeks post-breeding, cows greater than 40 days postpartum, and cows previously diagnosed as open is helpful. This gives the worker a list of cows to specifically check for heat.

Heat Detection Patches. Properly applied and observed these can aid in visual estrus detection. Breeding errors with these are high, since false-positive results, false-negative results, and missing patches are common.

Androgenized Cows with Chinball Marker. Expense of maintaining the cow and marker are deterrents. Again, accurate consistent visual observation is needed to find newly marked cows.

Teaser Bulls and Chinball Markers. In addition to maintenance expense, bulls have the added aspects of aggressive behavior and surgical costs.

Chalk on the Tailhead. Chalk on the tailhead is gaining popularity, but there may be a lot of mistimed breedings since the chalk is easily rubbed off for the wrong reason.

Estrus Synchronization Drugs. Provided a corpus luteum is present, prostaglandins allow the manager to concentrate on certain cows for a short period.

There are errors associated with different accepted estrus signs and estrus detection aids. Table 1 shows the per cent error associated with the different signs of estrus and heat

Table 1. *Errors in Heat Detection**

Sign	Per Cent Error (N = 4387 Cows)
Standing to be ridden	2.6
Riding other cows	2.9
Rough tailhead	3.6
Unusually active	4.5
Bawling	4.7
Mucus on vulva	6.1
Blood on vulva	7.1
No milk letdown	9.0
Fully activated mount indicator	12.4
Partially activated mount indicator	18.3

*From Reimers, T. J., Newmarz, S. K., Cowan, R. G., et al.: J. Anim. Sci. *53*:361, 1981.

mount indicators, and it shows the greater accuracy of good visual observation over heat detection indicators. Visual observation when combined with heat mount indicators gives very good results. Veterinarians may recommend that a bull be used in the herd while problems are being corrected.

INSEMINATION TIMING

Good conception rates are closely tied to correct insemination timing and are dependent on accurate estrus detection and a knowledge of estrus in the cow. Problems include insemination when the cow is not in estrus, early insemination, or late insemination. Using milk progesterone levels, European workers report that 14 to 26 per cent of dairy cows are inseminated when cows are not in heat. These cows had been incorrectly reported to be in estrus. This failure in estrus detection is mistakenly observing cows in estrus rather than missing cows in estrus and can be solved by training observers.

Variability in the length of estrus (6 to 20 hr), time of ovulation (8 to 18 hr post-estrus), and sperm capacitation time (4 to 8 hr) leads to the recommendation that insemination be 8 to 12 hr post-estrus detection. This was the basis for the original "AM-PM" rule. If one finds a cow in heat in the AM (early morning) then breed the cow in the PM (late afternoon) and vice versa. Breeder services now currently recommend once a day breeding if estrus detection is based on an early morning and late afternoon schedule. Research has shown that fertility is best when insemination is from the middle to the end of standing estrus. Fertility does not vary significantly when insemination is at the time of estrus detection or 12 to 24 hr after estrus detection. Estrus detection, at best, seldom provides an accurate determination of when estrus actually began. Most cows have been in estrus 5 to 6 hr when first detected. This is compounded by the fact that the majority of cows exhibit estrus at night, especially *Bos indicus*, when environmental temperatures are very high during the day. Most clinicians accept that more cows are bred too late rather than too early and that strict adherence to the AM-PM rule is unwarranted.

If the veterinarian suspects an insemination timing problem, a good, thorough investigation of estrus detection techniques and timing of insemination in relation to estrus detection are needed. Experienced veterinarians can check cows for breeding by palpable signs of estrus (e.g., turgid coiled uterus, absence of a corpus luteum,

and follicle development). Close examination of records may show that inseminations are not 18 to 23 days apart. Several inseminations in a given cycle may indicate improper timing, probably due to poor estrus detection.

Since milk progesterone levels mimic circulating progesterone levels, milk progesterone samples can be used to identify estrus. A sample taken at insemination can confirm estrus.

SEMEN QUALITY

In AI, semen quality is influenced by bulls and the level of expertise in collecting, evaluating, and freezing the semen for storage. Semen quality is also influenced by the expertise of those handling and thawing frozen semen after it leaves the distributor.

Provided that the semen was collected and processed by an established breeder's service, quality should be acceptable at that point. Custom frozen semen may provide more of a problem, especially when the owner wants frozen semen regardless of quality control. As a whole, semen is processed and frozen under good quality control conditions, because the company's reputation is vital to success. Problems with semen quality may begin during delivery. The owner should always check the liquid nitrogen level in the tank upon delivery to ensure that it was sufficient to hold the semen at the correct temperature. There should be enough liquid nitrogen in the tank to keep the temperature at $-130°C$ or lower. If the liquid nitrogen level is low, the temperature in the tank should be determined, and if it has risen above $-80°C$ significant damage has occurred to the semen. When the tank is empty of liquid nitrogen, the shipment should not be accepted.

Damage to Semen

The greatest potential for damage to semen quality is during semen handling on the farm. Inseminators should remember these following considerations:

1. There is an extreme temperature variation even within the neck of the tank, from $-196°C$ at the lower inlet to $+2°C$ at the upper opening.
2. Temperature of the frozen semen changes rapidly, and damage is additive on repeated exposures. The additive effect varies greatly, depending on the level of liquid nitrogen in the tank. If the level is low, as much as 10 minutes is needed after several exposures to lower semen temperature to $-196°C$.
3. When semen is exposed to air, as little as 15 seconds is needed to raise semen temperature to the critical zone. The veterinarian investigating a fertility problem should examine the handling and transferring procedures to see if they meet the following minimum requirements:
   a. Raise the canister to look for the desired semen no higher than 1 inch from the top opening in the tank neck. Ideally, the canister should be raised no higher than the frostline in the neck.
   b. If the correct semen rack cannot be located in 15 to 30 seconds, the canister should be lowered into the tank for 15 to 30 seconds before resuming.
   c. When removing a semen package, raise the rack only high enough to remove the package and not expose the lower packages to high temperatures.

d. Transfer of the semen packages should be done in 5 to 10 seconds. If it takes longer, too many obstructions or too much distance between vessels exist.

Thawing of semen packages should always be strictly based on the individual semen processing organization's recommendation. Each is a little different due to variations in processing and extenders.

One should be careful to observe both the minimum and maximum limits on thawing temperature and time. Variation of either affects fertility significantly.

Other thawing procedures commonly used have been investigated. "Pocket thaw," "cow thaw," and "gun thaw" have all been shown to significantly reduce fertility. Once the semen is thawed, it should be used as quickly as possible, taking precautions to avoid rapid changes in temperature, sunlight, and water. In winter, the AI gun should be warmed to body temperature before inserting the semen package. All water should be dried from semen packages since the drastic osmotic difference rapidly kills sperm cells. Semen should be transferred within 15 minutes after thawing. If there is a lag period between thaw and transfer, every effort should be made to protect the semen.

If damage to stored semen is suspected, do not try to evaluate the semen under field conditions. Evaluation of frozen semen requires special handling, knowledge, and equipment most practitioners do not have. An individual experienced in evaluating frozen semen should be enlisted. Most AI organizations will provide the service if requested.

SEMEN PLACEMENT ERROR

Next to estrus detection, semen placement error (by the technician) is most likely to affect fertility. Correct semen placement is very difficult to confirm in the field. Studies using dye deposition followed by slaughter have shown that up to 70 per cent of cows are inseminated incorrectly. The dye was placed in the vagina, posterior cervix, uterine horn, or bladder. The target for semen deposition is the anterior cervical os, a difficult site to find. Inexperienced inseminators often do not pass the pipette far enough, or they pass it too far into the uterine horns. Since the body of the uterus is only 1 to 2 cm in length, pipette passage 1 to 2 cm into the uterus results in most of the semen entering only one horn, effectively reducing conception. Semen deposition is often made too rapidly, and semen takes the avenue of least resistance. If one horn is not as open as the other, it does not receive enough semen. The plunger should be depressed over a 5-second period, allowing the semen to flow slowly and evenly, divided between horns.

Confirmation of semen placement is difficult at best. It is impossible to check pipette placement. The pipette position changes too easily. Postmortem tracts or examining culled cows inseminated with dye can be used to check semen placement at slaughter.

Professional technicians are more successful at insemination than owners or managers. Inseminators should periodically attend AI courses to improve or correct techniques.

HYGIENE

Hygiene during AI is another important consideration. The veterinarian should observe the inseminator's technique for possible contamination of the AI instrument. Equipment should be kept clean while handling and transferring. Generally, nothing should touch the AI instrument prior to entering the vagina. This can be accomplished by cleaning the cow and spreading the vulvar lips, allowing uncontaminated passage into the vagina. Double sheathing of AI instruments is an attempt to reduce contamination of the instrument up to the cervix but increases in conceptions using this technique are not significant, except when a known disease exists in the vagina.

Supplemental Reading

Bartlett, D.E.: What's new in A.I. of the bovine. Proc. of Soc. Therio. *128*:142, 1978.

Hock, P., Claus, R., Karg, H.: Milk progesterone determination as applied to the confirmation of estrus, the detection of cycling and as an aid to veterinarians and biotechnical measures in cows. Brit. Vet. J. *135*:541, 1979.

Robbins, R.K., Sullivan, J.J., Pace, M.M., et al.: Timing the insemination of beef cattle. Soc. Therio. *10*:247, 1978.

Sullivan, J.J.: Semen handling—a factor which affects fertility. Proc. of Soc. Therio. 81–98, 1982.

Management of the Repeat Breeder Female

DWIGHT F. WOLFE, D.V.M., M.S.

A female that fails to conceive after 3 or more regularly spaced services in the absence of detectable abnormalities is classified as a repeat breeder. The repeat breeder problem is best documented in dairy cattle. Various clinicians have reported the incidence of repeat breeders in large dairy cattle populations representing many herds, and it ranges from 5.0 to 15.1 per cent with an apparent average of 10.5 per cent. The problem is less frequent in beef cattle. Swine are also affected, although small litter size is more frequent. One study of swine indicated that of 550 sows culled for reproductive failure, 104 were culled because of return to estrus following breeding. The number of matings was not reported. The percentage of affected ewes and does appears to be less than that of affected dairy cattle.

A discussion of repeat breeders or conception failures must address normal reproductive expectancy. With normal healthy cycling cows a 63 per cent conception rate is expected on first service. Thus, in a herd of 100 cows, 37 cows (37 per cent) will be expected to return to estrus due to conception failure. On second breeding, 23 of these cows (63 per cent) will be expected to conceive, leaving 14 cows (37 per cent) that fail to conceive. On the third estrus, 9 cows (63 per cent) are expected to conceive, leaving 5 cows (37 per cent) as repeat breeders. Therefore, 5 per cent of a normal healthy cycling cattle population can be expected to be repeat breeders based on the previous classification of failure of conception after 3 services.

ECONOMICS

Repeat breeding is economically important to livestock producers. Each affected female suffers an extension of interparturition for at least 3 estrous cycles or approximately 2 months. In Holstein cattle in the United States, this extension of the calving interval causes an 8.8 per cent reduction in the annual income above feed cost and an average loss of 0.15 calves and 144 kg of milk per cow. Failure of conception may be less expensive than abortion or the production of inferior offspring.

CONCEPTION FAILURE

Conception failure is the result of either fertilization failure or early embryonic death. In cattle, early embryonic death must occur before day 16 in order to maintain regular estrous cycle lengths, and numerous studies indicate that the majority of embryonic losses are before day 15. In sows and ewes, embryonic death must be by day 12 to maintain regular cycle length. Fertilization failure and early embryonic death may result for a variety of reasons. Congenital or acquired anatomic abnormalities may preclude union of sperm and ovum. Age, season, several management factors, and semen quality alter fertilization rates.

FERTILIZATION FAILURE

Studies utilizing planned slaughter after breeding indicate that in first-service heifers, the fertilization rate approached 100 per cent as compared with 60 per cent in repeat breeder heifers. In normal cows, the fertilization rate was 83 to 85 per cent compared with only 60 per cent in repeat breeders. These studies have been substantiated utilizing embryo collection.

Congenital Defects in Fertilization Failure

Segmental aplasia of Müller's ducts is one of the more common abnormalities causing fertilization failure. The ovaries develop normally, and affected animals have normal estrous cycles. The developmental defects may involve the vagina, cervix, uterus, or oviducts. Imperforate hymen, imperforate cervix, aplasia of all or part of one or both uterine horns or oviducts, and double external or internal cervical ora are manifestations of this condition. Other forms of the abnormality are didelphia wherein each uterine horn connects by a separate cervical canal, and uterus unicornis wherein only one uterine horn has a lumen.

Diagnosis and Treatment

Many of these conditions can be confirmed with physical examination. Accumulation of normal cyclic secretions may occur anterior to an obstruction producing sac-like dilation of a portion of this tubular tract. Careful rectal palpation will distinguish this condition from pregnancy. Varying degrees of vaginal constriction, imperforate hymen, and anomalies of the external cervical os are detectable by speculum or digital vaginal examination. In slaughterhouse studies, the incidence of congenital anomalies is reported to be less than 1.0 per cent. Due to the suspected heritable nature of these anomalies, surgical repair is inadvisable.

ACQUIRED ABNORMALITIES

Acquired lesions of the genital tract are usually due to infections or parturient trauma. Adhesions between the ovary and fimbria may be mild or severe. The fimbria or bursa may be attached to the ovary at the site of a regressed corpus luteum or ovarian hematoma. In studies using culled specimens, the right ovary is more frequently involved, but the condition may be bilateral. Mild lesions may not affect fertility, but severe adhesions may prevent the ovum from entering the oviduct.

The prevalence of the condition increases with age and is uncommon in heifers. The adhesions are uncommon in sheep. Mycoplasmas have been isolated from a high proportion of ovarobursal lesions, and it has been suggested that there is a relationship between semen-borne mycoplasma and ovarobursal diseases.

Diagnosis and Treatment

Diagnosis of ovarian adhesions is difficult. Careful rectal palpation of the ovaries may detect a small percentage of the lesions that cause infertility. Exploratory laparotomy or laparoscopy may be indicated in valuable females. Therapy is considered unrewarding in the bilaterally affected cow. If the condition is unilateral, rectal palpation with breeding only when the ovulation is on the unaffected ovary may be helpful. An alternative is surgical removal of the affected ovary, so that all subsequent ovulations are of the normal ovary. If this option is chosen, the other ovary should be carefully examined during laparotomy to assure that there is no pathologic condition that is undetectable by rectal palpation.

OCCLUSION OR INFLAMMATION OF THE OVIDUCT

Occlusion or inflammation of the oviduct may be a cause of fertilization failure. Salpingitis, hydrosalpinx, pyosalpinx, or pachysalpinx may be a sequela to puerperal metritis. These conditions are not consistently palpable rectally. Two tests have been advocated as diagnostic aids for oviductal patency.

Diagnosis

One test involves the infusion of 20 ml of a 0.1 per cent sterile solution of phenolsulfonphthalein (PSP) into the uterine lumen of a cow during the mid-luteal phase of the cycle. PSP is not absorbed across the intact endometrium, and if the oviducts are patent the dye is passed through the oviducts to the peritoneal cavity. It is readily absorbed into the systemic circulation there and is excreted by the kidneys into the urine where a red or pink color is produced under alkaline conditions. The bladder should be catheterized and a pre-treatment urine sample collected. Urine should be collected 30 to 60 minutes after treatment, and 10 ml of urine added to 0.2 ml of 10 per cent trisodium orthophosphate buffer to alkalinize the urine. The urine becomes red or pink if PSP is present. False-positive results are seen if there is endometrial damage, and the test does not distinguish between unilateral and bilateral patency. False-negative results may occur in cows treated during the follicular phase of the cycle.

The second test utilizes sterilized starch granules to assess oviduct patency. With aseptic technique, an 18-ga

× 15-cm needle is inserted through the sacrosciatic ligament while the ovary is grasped rectally and stabilized. Ten ml of sterile water is injected with 1 gm of gamma-irradiated starch powder onto the surface of the ovary. Two to 4 days later, a small quantity of mucus is aspirated from the fornix of the vagina with a syringe attached to a sterile infusion pipette. A drop of mucus is placed on a clean dry slide to which is added a few drops of 2 per cent Lugol's solution. If present, starch granules stain blue-black and are readily identifiable under the 10× objective. This test should be performed during the mid-luteal phase of the cycle, as false-negative results may occur during the follicular phase.

The 2 tests may be helpful in assisting diagnosis of oviductal patency. Neither test, however, makes an assessment of oviduct function. Embryo transfer techniques may be utilized to assess patency and function of the oviducts with a considerable degree of accuracy. Methods exist for collecting embryos from single uterine horns of all food animal species. Collection of fertilized ova in the uterine horn is definitive for oviductal patency and function. False-negative results may be seen, if the veterinarian is not familiar with the techniques. If nonfertilized ova are collected, oviduct patency is assured, but other causes of fertilization failure should be considered.

IMPROPER TIMING OF INSEMINATION

Improper timing of insemination is one of the major causes of fertilization failure. This situation rarely occurs in females mated by natural service but in most instances is a management induced problem associated with artificial insemination. As determined by studies of serum or milk progesterone levels, in some herds up to 20 per cent of the inseminated cows are in the luteal phase of the cycle. If this problem is anticipated, client education, palpation of cows by a veterinarian, serum or milk progesterone samples collected at the time of insemination, and the use of estrus detection aids such as heat detection patches and surgically altered teaser males should be considered. Additionally, poor semen placement or semen handling during artificial insemination may be a cause of fertilization failure.

OVULATORY DISORDERS

Ovulation in the cow takes place 18 to 36 hr after the ovulatory luteinizing hormone (LH) peak and 10 to 12 hr after the end of behavioral estrus. Ovulation is 12 to 36 hr after the onset of standing estrus in the doe, 24 hr after the onset of estrus in the ewe, and 24 to 42 hr after the onset of estrus in the sow. Two disorders of ovulation may cause fertilization failure. These conditions probably are found in all species but are best documented in the cow. It is generally believed that ovulatory defects are due to endocrine disturbances. The quantity and timing of LH release from the anterior pituitary gland must be correct for normal ovulation.

With endocrine disturbances, inadequate or inappropriate LH release may lead to anovulation in the presence of behavioral estrus. Inseminating or mating at this estrus will cause failure of fertilization. The incidence of this condition is considered low. The follicle regresses and becomes atretic or cystic. Cattle with cystic degeneration of the ovaries either experience short estrus or anestrus and will not be considered.

Delayed ovulation may also take place in the presence of behavioral estrus. The incidence of this condition is reported to be 18 per cent in one study, but conflicting reports indicate that the percentage may be less than 2 per cent in repeat breeder cattle. The ovulation delay was less than 48 hr in 85 per cent of the cases reported. Insemination of delayed ovulating cows at the end of standing estrus results in unacceptably low conception rates due to the short fertile lifespan of sperm within the female tract. Diagnosis is based upon sequential rectal palpation of the same follicle on the same ovary at more than 24 hr after standing estrus. Treatment of this condition may be by repeated insemination every 12 to 24 hr until palpable ovulation occurs. Alternatively, the administration of gonadotropin-releasing hormone (GnRH), 0.15 mg, intramuscularly, or human chorionic gonadotropin (HCG), 3000 to 4500 units, intravenously, 6 hr before or at the time of insemination in the next ensuing estrus, may hasten ovulation.

INFECTIOUS INFERTILITY

Vaginitis, cervicitis, or endometritis may be lethal to sperm or impede sperm transport causing fertilization failure. The use of prostaglandin $F_{2\alpha}$ ($PGF_{2\alpha}$) causes loss of sperm motility and viability in the cervix of treated ewes. Low fertility following $PGF_{2\alpha}$ treatment in ewes apparently is caused by low sperm numbers in the oviducts around the time of ovulation. Vaginitis and cervicitis may be caused by numerous pathogenic organisms. Bovine herpesvirus and bovine venereal epididymitis and vaginitis virus (epivaginitis) are well documented as the causes of pustular vulvovaginitis in cattle. Mycoplasma, ureaplasma, and *Haemophilus* organisms may also be pathogenic in this portion of the female tract.

Diagnosis and Treatment

Diagnosis of these conditions is by rectal palpation, vaginal examination by speculum, and culture of infected tissues. The role of such conditions in infertility is uncertain, as they are frequently encountered in pregnant animals. Therapy consists of sexual rest to allow spontaneous recovery or topical administration of nonirritating antibiotics based on sensitivity patterns. It has been suggested that use of a double sheathing technique for artificial insemination of infected cattle may be beneficial.

An exception to this is epivaginitis virus, reported only in Africa. The virus, apparently related to bovine herpesvirus, is spread strictly by venereal transmission. Epivaginitis virus initially infects the vagina and vestibule, but later hydrosalpinx and perisalpingitis develop with up to 25 per cent of affected cattle becoming sterile owing to bilateral oviductal lesions. There is no therapy.

SEMEN AND FERTILITY

Bulls of high and low fertilities have been identified through artifical insemination records. The reason for the variation in conception rates among bulls with good semen quality is unknown. Fertilization failures or early embryonic deaths of defective zygotes may result from matings using bulls of low fertility. This condition presumably occurs in species other than cattle.

Careless handling of frozen semen can drastically lower fertilization rates. Proper care of the liquid nitrogen tank and proper handling of the semen from the tank to the female must be observed for optimum results. Fertility associated with faulty artificial insemination techniques is discussed elsewhere.

PHYSIOLOGIC CAUSES OF EARLY EMBRYONIC DEATH

Aging of the ovum may occur in delayed ovulating females or in females that are inseminated too late after ovulation. Generally, the aged ovum is still fertilizable, but a defective zygote develops that undergoes early embryonic death. Polyspermy (2 or more sperm entering 1 ovum), polyandry (fertilization by more than 1 sperm), and polygyny (1 sperm fertilizing a diploid ovum) all increase with aging of the gametes. The resultant polyploidy, more than the 2N number of chromosomes, is usually lethal. Lethal chromosomal aberrations are observed in all species. These lethal conditions are reported in up to 10 per cent of the ova of swine. Diagnosis is difficult and depends upon cytogenetic studies of the embryo or, occasionally, of the parents of the embryo. There is no treatment.

Genetic factors have been associated with the incidence of early embryonic death. Inbreeding has been shown to increase early embryonic deaths when the embryos are inbred. Daughters of dams conceiving at first service reportedly suffer a higher rate of embryonic death than daughters of dams not conceiving at first service. One researcher suggests that the genetic factors involved in embryonic mortality are not necessarily inherited by the parents but rather that most of the factors arise spontaneously in each parent generation and occur randomly in the gametes.

Hormone Influence

Improper balance of estrogen and progesterone during the early post-ovulatory period can affect ovum transport time in the oviduct. Excessive estrogen slows oviductal transport so that the ovum doesn't reach the uterus at the proper time. Excessive progesterone speeds ova transport through the oviduct. Either of these conditions may allow ova to leave the oviduct at a time when the uterine environment is not synchronous with the physiologic needs of the ovum so that early embryonic death occurs.

Progesterone deficiency has been suggested as a cause of conception failure in many species. The primary source of progesterone during early pregnancy is the corpus luteum. Milk or blood progesterone studies indicate that 2 to 50 per cent of cows that ovulate and fail to conceive have low progesterone levels. Some individuals with low progesterone levels do conceive, however. Diagnosis of this condition is difficult. Palpation of the corpus luteum for size and consistency is unreliable due to the wide variation in corpus luteum size. Multiple, frequent blood or milk samples must be assayed to accurately assess progesterone levels for an individual female.

Numerous empirical treatments have been used for progesterone deficiency. Injections of HCG or GnRH have been recommended to stimulate LH in the cow. Various regimens of exogenous progesterone have been administered to females of several species for pregnancy maintenance. One of the popular treatments is 500 mg repositol progesterone at 10 days after breeding and every 10 days thereafter. Administration of progesterone before the third day after breeding impairs fertility by decreasing oviductal transit time for the embryo. Definitive research is needed to ascertain the optimum dosage of exogenous progesterone necessary to maintain pregnancy in each species. Progesterone usage for estrus synchronization in sheep and goats is also associated with poor conception rates and resumption of estrus.

Environment

A decline in conception rates of cattle is well documented in the warm months of the year. Excessive solar radiation the day of insemination and high environmental temperature the day following insemination have a negative effect on conception rate. A rise of 0.5°C in the animal's body temperature means uterine temperature on those days also rises and causes a decline in conception rate. Ewes subjected to high ambient temperatures also suffer greater embryonic deaths. The high uterine temperature may cause fertilization failure by sperm or ova damage or early embryonic death may occur. Provision of shade and free access to feed and water is suggested to improve hot weather fertility. Shearing of sheep has been beneficial in periods of prolonged heat during the breeding season. Water mists and forced ventilation may be helpful in reducing thermal stress in swine, but some studies using large numbers of animals have failed to demonstrate reduction of summer infertility through the use of current cooling methods.

Nutrition

The effects of nutritional deficiencies and excesses on fertility are well documented. Little is known, however, of the pathogenesis. Energy restriction is probably the most common nutritional malady, and in heifers on inadequate energy diets a reduction of plasma progesterone levels and a reduction of normal fertilized ova have been documented. There is uncertainty as to whether the low energy intake alters sperm transport, fertilization, or growth and development of the early embryo. Low energy intake may also alter the endocrine function of the hypothalamus, anterior pituitary gland, or ovaries.

One clinician suggests there is a 1 per cent increase in conception rates at first service for every 1 per cent increase in live weight. This is applicable to females that are below normal body weight before the breeding season. Conception rates are depressed in females that are overweight at breeding. There is some evidence that feeding excessive amounts of protein is deleterious to conception. Selected nutrients of reproductive importance will be discussed next.

Nutritional Deficiencies

Several mineral deficiencies may be associated with failure of conception. Inadequate dietary copper, manganese, phosphorus, cobalt, and iodine have been associated with fertilization failure and early embryonic death in cattle and sheep. Vitamin A and beta-carotene deficiencies may be significant causes of infertility. Diets may have adequate vitamin A yet be low in beta-carotene. In cattle, delayed ovulation, silent estrus, and anovulation with follicular cyst formation have been associated with these deficiencies. Moreover, bovine luteal tissue has the highest beta-carotene content of any tissue. Defective corpus luteum formation and ovarian steroidogenesis may be associated with beta-carotene deficiency thereby causing ovulatory abnormalities or early embryonic deaths due to inadequate progesterone production.

Diagnosis of the nutrient deficiencies requires thorough ration analysis and possibly serum profiles for affected females. Vitamin A content of liver biopsy samples is most indicative of vitamin A stores in the body. Therapy consists of balancing the ration and supplying the appropriate nutrients in a form with high bioavailability. It appears that reproductive efficiency of dairy cows may be improved with the addition of 300 mg of beta-carotene/head/day, although the efficacy of this treatment is questioned by some researchers.

Age

It is generally agreed that fertility declines with the age of the female. In cattle, heifers have higher fertilization rates than mature cows but also experience higher incidences of early embryonic deaths. The number of repeat breeders is lowest in first-calf heifers and increases with age. It is reported that 13.3 per cent of cows more than 9 years of age are repeat breeders.

METRITIS AND ENDOMETRITIS

Postparturient metritis or endometritis has been incriminated as a cause of conception failure in cattle. This idea has been challenged because intrauterine therapy frequently fails to improve fertility in suspected females. Additionally, many pathogenic or nonspecific organisms have been isolated from the uterus of normal and pregnant females. Many females, especially cattle, suffer metritis in the early postpartum period. Most of these cases heal spontaneously by the second or third postpartum estrus. Metritis and endometritis cause fertilization failure due to sperm death in the hostile environment. Should fertilization occur, early embryonic death ensues because the uterine environment is detrimental to the embryo.

Diagnosis

Diagnosis of metritis is made by rectal palpation of an enlarged or fluid-filled uterus, or both. In sows, ewes, and does, ultrasonography may be useful. Endometritis is more difficult to diagnose because by 30 days postpartum only gross abnormalities are detectable by rectal palpation. Estrual mucus may have a cloudy appearance or contain flecks of purulent material. Examination of the vagina and cervix by speculum may reveal evidence of urovagina, pneumovagina, or other conditions that may incite endometritis. Material of the uterine lumen should be cultured to confirm the presence of pathogenic organisms.

With the cow adequately restrained, scrub and disinfect the vulva and perineal area. By rectal palpation, grasp and stabilize the cervix. As an assistant parts the vulvar lips, introduce a guarded culture swab through the cervix and into the body of the uterus. Advance the sterile swab out of its protective sheath, gently manipulate the tip within the uterus, and retract the swab back into the sheath. Retract the swab from the cervix, and with the vulvar lips parted withdraw the guarded swab. In heifers, sows, ewes, and does, position the guarded swab against the external os of the cervix and advance the swab into the uterus. Refrigerate or pack the sample on ice for immediate transport to a microbiologic laboratory.

Treatment

Therapy for metritis and endometritis may involve intrauterine or systemic therapy. Favorable results may be achieved by repeatedly shortening the estrous cycle with prostaglandins. This technique utilizes the natural immunologic response of the uterus during the estrogen dominated portion of the cycle. If intrauterine therapy is chosen, antibiotic selection should be based on culture and sensitivity. Mild antiseptics, such as 3 to 5 per cent povidone-iodine in sterile saline or chlorhexidine suspension, are often effective. Infusion of 2 to 5 ml of Lugol's solution in 30 ml of sterile saline is a popular treatment for chronic endometritis. This solution is mildly irritating to the uterus but is antiseptic. Numerous substances have been used for intrauterine infusion for treatment of endometritis. Provided the substances are not exceptionally irritating or damaging to the uterus, improved fertility often occurs because of, or in spite of, the treatment.

The degree of damage caused by endometritis cannot be determined by culture. Uterine biopsy, however, may be beneficial in assessing endometrial damage. By rectal palpation, grasp and manipulate the cervix while passing the biopsy instrument through the cervix and into the body of the uterus. Open the tip of the forceps and by rectal manipulation press the uterine wall into the jaws of the forceps. Close the jaws of the forceps, excising a small piece of endometrium. Withdraw the forceps and immediately place the specimen into Bouin's solution, which produces fewer shrinkage artifacts than formalin, and send to a laboratory with a staff experienced in interpreting endometrial biopsy specimens. A minimum of 3 samples should be collected, 1 sample from 3 to 6 cm anterior to the bifurcation on the medial surface of each uterine horn, and a sample from the uterine body taken as near the cervix as possible. The samples collected 5 to 10 days after estrus are best, as samples collected during estrus are difficult to evaluate for endometritis. Abnormal samples may contain cystic endometrial glands or lymph nodules. The degree of endometrial damage is determined by the extent of periglandular fibrosis.

The value of endometrial biopsy is in the diagnosis and prognosis of problem breeder females. The samples are collected during the luteal phase of the cycle when the cervix may be difficult to pass. There is no therapy for endometrial fibrosis or atrophy.

CAMPYLOBACTERIOSIS

A few particular diseases must be mentioned in a discussion of endometritis and early embryonic death. *Campylobacter fetus* subsp. *venerealis* is a significant venereal disease of cattle. Campylobacteriosis, formerly called vibriosis, is primarily a disease of the female, although bulls may be carriers and generally manifests as a herd infertility problem. The organism survives freezing, and individual cows can become infected by artificial insemination with semen from infected bulls.

At 10 to 14 days after infection, mild endometritis develops, and in 25 per cent of the cattle the infection enters the oviduct. Loss of fertility is due to early embryonic death, and salpingitis may cause fertilization failure at subsequent estrous cycles.

Diagnosis

Most infected females return to estrus 19 to 22 days following infection, but occasionally the interval will range 30 to 35 days. There are no palpable abnormalities in infected females, and the estrual mucus may or may not be cloudy. Definitive diagnosis is by isolation of the organism from an actively infected female. With the animal adequately restrained, grasp and immobilize the cervix by rectal palpation. Clean and disinfect the vulva and perineal area and introduce a guarded sterile infusion pipette, with a sterile 10-ml syringe attached, into the vagina, as an assistant spreads the vulvar lips. Place the tip of the infusion pipette into the external cervical os and by applying suction with the syringe, aspirate cervicovaginal mucus into the pipette. Cervical mucus, especially during diestrus, is quite viscous and may be difficult to aspirate into the pipette. Infusion of 2 to 5 ml of sterile saline into the cervix followed by aspiration may facilitate collection of the mucus sample, but undiluted mucus is preferred. Approximately 1 to 2 ml of mucus is adequate. Retract the pipette into the speculum, and withdraw both from the vagina avoiding vulvar contamination. Immediately inoculate the sample into a transport vial containing Clark's medium with an increased CO_2 concentration. If Clark's medium is unavailable, place the mucus in a sterile tube that can be sealed to avoid oxygen contamination. Refrigerate the sample and deliver to a laboratory as quickly as possible.

Treatment

Most infected females spontaneously recover from the disease after 3 to 6 estrous cycles, if they are not reinfected. Therapeutic administration of commercially killed bacterins may be useful. A single subcutaneous injection of streptomycin, 22 mg/kg, has been beneficial in bulls.

TRICHOMONIASIS

Trichomonas foetus, a protozoan, causes a venereal disease of cattle. Following infection, the protozoan produces vaginitis or endometritis or both in the female. Infected females remain infertile for 2 to 6 months probably due to early embryonic death caused by endometritis.

Diagnosis

Occasionally, postcoital pyometra from trichomoniasis may be palpable in infected females. These animals are usually acyclic and are not discussed here. Definitive diagnosis of trichomoniasis is dependent upon isolation of the organism. Examination of bull smegma is the preferred technique, but cervicovaginal mucus may be acceptable. Collect the mucus as previously described for campylobacteriosis and culture in Diamond's medium. The trichomonads may be identified by direct microscopic examination of the mucus at $100\times$ magnification by an irregular jerky movement associated with continuous rolling. At $400\times$ magnification, the presence of 3 anterior flagellae and an undulating membrane help confirm the diagnosis.

Treatment

Treatment of infected cows is usually not necessary because in most cases spontaneous recovery occurs after several estrous cycles. Dimetridazole, 50 mg/kg orally, for 5 days is effective for treating infected bulls. Metronidazole, 10 mg/kg up to 75 mg/kg intravenously, given once daily for 2 days is also effective. Neither of these drugs is approved for use in cattle in the United States.

SUMMARY

The repeat breeder female problem is complex. Frequently several abnormal conditions are involved, and the veterinarian is challenged to diagnose the condition. Extensive diagnostic tests are available that should be utilized on selected valuable individual females or on herds with repeat breeder problems. Successful therapy is satisfying. Reliable prognoses on individual females accompanied by judicious culling should be economically rewarding to the producer.

Supplemental Reading

Ayalon, N.: A review of embryonic mortality in cattle. J. Reprod. Fert. *54*:483–493, 1978.
Robert, S. J.: Veterinary Obstetrics and Genital Diseases. Ann Arbor, Edwards Bros., Inc., 1971.
Zemjanis, R.: "Repeat breeding" or conception failure in cattle. *In* David A. Morrow (ed.): Current Therapy in Theriogenology. Philadelphia, W. B. Saunders Company, 1980.

The Use of Embryo Transfer for Prevention of Disease Transmission

DWIGHT F. WOLFE, D.V.M., M.S.

Embryo transfer (ET) is a rapidly developing technology for animal breeding. It is anticipated that 180,000 calves will be produced by ET in the United States alone during 1985. The number of foals, pigs, kids, and lambs produced by ET is less but appears to be steadily expanding. The principal reason for the popularity of ET is the potential of increasing the reproductive capability of superior females. Selected females can be mated with superior sires, and multiple offspring can be carried by surrogate mothers. In some cases, females with acquired infertility due to aging, injury, or disease that precludes delivery of viable offspring may remain productive through the use of ET.

An added advantage of ET appears to be in its use for disease control in livestock. Considerable research has been directed towards the effects of various pathogens on pre-implantation embryos and the feasibility of transferring embryos from infected donor females to noninfected surrogate females. This concept is valuable for preserving genetic material of infected females and has been utilized to introduce genetic material into closed herds. Considerable economic return may be achieved by exporting embryos from infected herds or infected females, if in fact disease transmission can be precluded by ET.

INFECTION OF EMBRYOS

Contaminated equipment and media may serve as mechanical vectors for disease transmission by ET. Therefore, preventing disease transmission by ET depends on the organism in question not being transmitted via the gametes and not infecting the embryo during collection and transfer to recipient females.

Passage of pathogenic organisms from parents to embryos may occur by 2 means.

1. Embryos may become infected at fertilization when an organism is present inside or attached to the spermatozoon or ovum.

2. Organisms present in the oviduct, uterus, or seminal fluid may propagate in the embryonic environment and infect the embryo either through the zona pellucida or through the embryonic cells after the zona pellucida is lost.

It appears that transmission of bacterial disease by ET is of little concern because embryos may be exposed to efficacious antibiotics in flush or culture media thereby eliminating bacterial contamination. Viruses appear to be more difficult to eliminate. The addition of specific antisera to culture media containing infected embryos is plausible as a method of inactivating viruses adhering to the zona pellucida. Viruses may also be removed by partial enzymatic digestion of the zona pellucida. Repeated embryo washes can reduce bacteria or virus suspended in the flush media to noninfectious levels by serial dilution.

Brucella abortus

Brucella abortus is one bacterium that deserves special consideration. At present, no antibiotics are available that are consistently effective against this organism. The organism does not appear to penetrate or adhere to the intact zona pellucida of day 6 to 10 bovine embryos. Brucellae have been shown to adhere to zona pellucida–free embryos or to those with cracks in the zona pellucida. Brucellae may be shed in the uterine discharges of infected cows after parturition or abortion. It has been reported that in 1 group of heifers, the organism could not be cultured from the uterine flushings after the second post-abortion estrus, although 1 cow had been shown to remain positive by culture for 101 weeks post-abortion. A minimum of 6 serial washes of the embryos has proved reliable for removing the organism from embryos exposed *in vitro* to *B. abortus*.

It seems that *Brucella* infected cows may be used as embryo donors if they are at least 90 days postpartum at the time of embryo recovery. The embryos should be washed a minimum of 6 times, and the uterine flush and embryo transfer media should be examined by culture. Embryos should then be transferred to seronegative recipients that will be maintained in quarantine through gestation, and brucellosis status should be examined at parturition and up to 30 days postpartum.

VIRUSES INFECTING GAMETES

Bluetongue virus, an orbivirus of cattle and sheep, has been shown to infect semen in virus infected bulls. Virus-like particles have been observed by electron microscopy between the acrosome and nucleus or, in some instances, in the entire acrosome of spermatozoa. Epizootic hemorrhagic disease of deer, Colorado tick fever, and African horse sickness are also caused by orbiviruses, although there are no reports of their presence in the gametes of infected animals.

Oncornaviruses have been demonstrated in oocytes and early embryos of mice, guinea pigs, and primates. Mouse lymphocytic choriomeningitis virus, an arenavirus, has also been demonstrated in mouse oocytes and embryos. There is also evidence for the presence of mouse mammary tumor virus in oocytes and spermatozoa. Simian virus 40 (SV40) has been shown to absorb onto but not enter into rabbit spermatozoa.

VIRUSES PENETRATING THE ZONA PELLUCIDA

The zona pellucida is an effective barrier to many types of viruses. Some viruses have been shown to be capable of penetrating the zona pellucida. Bovine viral diarrhea virus (BVD) appears to penetrate the zona when infused into the uterus of superovulated cows, although *in vitro* studies indicate the virus does not penetrate the zona pellucida. There is *in vitro* evidence that coxsackievirus B3, human adenovirus type 5, and mouse meningoencephalitis virus penetrate the zona pellucida of mouse embryos, and feline leukemia viruses penetrate hamster embryos.

VIRUSES ADHERING TO THE ZONA PELLUCIDA

Disease can be transmitted by viruses attached to the zona pellucida without viral penetration into the embryonal cells. These viruses may infect the recipient or the embryo after hatching. Porcine parvovirus has been shown to adhere to the zona pellucida and to infect the recipients and kill or retard a majority of the embryos. Infectious bovine rhinotracheitis, a herpesvirus, also has been demonstrated to adhere to the zona. Porcine pseudorabies virus, another herpesvirus, apparently does not share this property. The viruses of African swine fever, swine vesicular disease, and foot and mouth disease also appear to adhere to swine embryos.

Embryos may be refractory to viruses that readily infect more differentiated cells. Zona pellucida–free bovine morulae appear to be refractory to bovine parvovirus *in vitro*. Two-cell zona pellucida–free mouse embryos are refractory to polyoma virus, but the morula is readily infected. Zona pellucida–free 2-cell and 8-cell stages and morula stage mouse embryos are refractory to cytomegalovirus infection, but later stages are susceptible.

EMBRYO TRANSFER FROM SEROPOSITIVE DONORS

Failure of virus absorption or penetration with *in vitro* exposure should not be accepted as evidence that the disease may be controlled by ET. Under *in vivo* conditions, viral penetration or absorption to the zona pellucida may occur. Each viral disease must be investigated by *in vivo* studies before decisions regarding the safety or efficacy of ET for prevention of disease transmission are made. Results of embryo transfers from seropositive donors to seronegative recipients are available for several viral diseases.

Transfer of embryos from cattle and sheep seropositive for bluetongue virus has been accomplished without inducing viral titers in seronegative recipients. Recipients of embryos from superovulated bovine leukemia virus infected donors remained seronegative as did the calves produced by the procedure. Embryos collected from sows seropositive for pseudorabies virus failed to produce seroconversion when transferred to seronegative recipients. The pigs farrowed from the procedure were seronegative.

Current health certification of embryos involves serological testing of donor females and sires for specific diseases. There appears to be little likelihood of predicting which viruses are amenable to control of transmission by embryo transfer. Methodical research is necessary for each pathogen utilizing serologic and cultural monitoring of donors, recipients, and progeny before deciding which disease may be controlled by ET.

Supplemental Reading

Eaglesome, M. D., Hare, W. C. D., and Singh, E.: Embryo Transfer: a discussion on its potential for infectious disease control based on a review of studies on infection of gametes and early embryos by various agents. Can. Vet. J. 21:106–112, 1980.

McVicar, J. W.: Embryo transfer and the possibilities of disease transmission. Proc. Livestock Cons. Inst. 150–156, 1983.

Stringfellow, D. A., Scanlan, C. M., Brown, R. R., et al.: Culture of bovine embryos after in vitro exposure to Brucella abortus. Theriogenology 21:1005–1012, 1984.

Waters, H. A.: Health certification for livestock embryo transfer. Theriogenology 15:57–66, 1981.

Abortion—An Approach to Diagnosis

DAN E. GOODWIN, D.V.M., Ph.D.

The purpose of this article is to describe abortion problems and to outline procedures that may lead to abortion diagnosis in food-producing animals. The diagnostic contributions of the animal owner, the practicing veterinarian, and the laboratory staff are discussed. Specific abortion-inducing diseases are presented in other articles of this volume.

Abortion (the act of giving untimely birth to offspring, O.E.D.) in animals causes anxiety in animal owners. Abortions represent genetic and economic losses and frequently cause a serious disposal problem, especially if the abortion resulted from disease that is transmissible to other animals and humans. Disposal is sometimes expedited by dogs, coyotes, buzzards, and other creatures who can spread parts of fetuses and placentas over wide areas.

Job, of the Old Testament, recognized the value of sound breeding bulls and nonaborting cows when he noted that his neighbors had escaped from the misery that beset him. "Their bull gendereth, and faileth not; their cow calveth and casteth not her calf." Job 21:10.

Although figures are not available to reveal losses due to abortion in the United States, the USDA (United States Department of Agriculture) collects and publishes information showing livestock production estimates (Table 1). This table should permit veterinarians in various states to estimate losses due to reproductive failure, a portion of which is a result of abortion. Comparison can be made among states as well as with the United States average shown at the bottom of the table. In Oklahoma, e.g., the table suggests that 11 per cent of cows eligible to calve in 1982 failed to produce a live calf, thus the reproduction failure rate was 11 per cent, a portion of which was due to abortion. The table also shows that Oklahoma equalled the United States average of 11 per cent. There is obvious room for improvement throughout the United States.

The livestock owner who has never had an abortion problem has not been in business very long or owns only a few animals. Occasional abortions are to be expected and can sometimes be beneficial, e.g., whenever the loss is caused by faulty genes that will not be perpetuated. Depending on economic and genetic considerations, single abortions may not be worthy of diagnostic investigation. Abortion losses of 2 to 3 per cent can be tolerated without undue concern in well managed livestock operations. A practical solution to low level abortion problems is to segregate and dispose of the aborting animals by slaughter; the loss of potentially valuable breeding animals is usually offset by the removal of defective genes and destructive pathogens.

Whenever losses continue or abortion storms occur there is no question about the need for a thorough investigation of the problems by the owner and the practicing veterinarian and, if indicated, the diagnostic laboratory staff. Although diagnoses are sometimes hard to establish, a thoughtful and accurate history, thorough clinical examination, and persistent laboratory investigation of numerous materials will usually yield facts that can be assembled to arrive at a diagnosis. The obstacles that sometimes stand in the way of successful investigations of abortions have been outlined by Kirkbride[1] as follows:

1. Abortion is frequently the result of an event that occurred weeks or months earlier and the cause, if it was ever present in the conceptus, is often undetectable by the time of abortion.

2. The fetus is often retained in utero for hours or days after death, resulting in autolysis that hides lesions.

3. Fetal membranes, which are commonly affected first and most consistently, are frequently unavailable for examination.

4. Toxic and genetic factors that may cause fetal death or abortion are not always discernible in the specimens available for examination.

5. Many causes of bovine abortion are unknown, or there are no routine diagnostic procedures for identifying them.

HISTORY

The value of a thorough history cannot be overstated. Veterinarians don't have to write books about the abortion problem, but they should gather essential information in a systematic way so that the livestock owner, the veterinarian and, if necessary, the diagnostic laboratory staff will have a map to follow as they consider diagnostic approaches. Questions should be asked objectively. Avoid asking leading questions that might influence the animal owner to give misleading answers. After recording information about owner's name and address, animal species, breed, and number of animals at risk, written answers need to be obtained for the questions listed in the abortion questionnaire (Fig. 1).

The history may yield answers that will give a strong

indication of the cause of abortion. If such is the case, then the veterinarian should direct the investigation at confirming this. It may require the collection of selected specimens for submission to a diagnostic laboratory. When accompanied by the written history and a request for specific tests, the specimens may generate the facts that will permit a diagnosis to be rendered.

CLINICAL SIGNS

If the history does not yield strong indications about the cause of abortion, the veterinarian should plan a broader investigation that would include an inspection of the animal's environment, clinical examination of aborting animals, and perhaps clinical examination of male and female herd mates. At the conclusion of the broader investigation, veterinarians may have obtained additional facts that will direct attention toward specific causes of abortion. At the least, they should have sufficient information at this point to suggest that the cause will fit into one of the following categories:

Venereal Infections
Nonvenereal Ascending Infection
Septicemia
Anemia
Nutritional Problem
Trauma
Genetic Defect
Toxic Problem
Endocrine Abnormality
Other

Depending on the category, the veterinarian may render a clinical diagnosis that will stand without the need for any additional investigation. Trichomoniasis, anaplasmosis, modified live-virus vaccine administration, trauma, and carbon monoxide poisoning are examples of abortion causes that can frequently be recognized without diagnostic laboratory assistance. Diagnostic laboratory tests should not be used as a crutch when the veterinarian is not lame. Laboratory investigations should never be used as a substitute for a poor history or for a poor clinical investigation.

MATERIALS FOR LABORATORY EXAMINATION

If it appears that laboratory assistance is needed and can be medically and economically justified, then specimens should be obtained for laboratory investigation. Laboratory staffs that are presented with good materials and good histories generally try harder. Rotten tissues and sorry histories frequently yield rotten and sorry results. The best specimens are freshly aborted fetuses and placentas. Dam serum samples delivered to the laboratory without delay along with a thorough written history or with a person who can provide the laboratory with a thorough history are also helpful. Because the average success rate for abortion diagnosis is around 25 per cent, it stands to reason that the laboratory staff is more likely to identify causative agents if it is able to examine several fetuses. Accordingly, if they are available, 3 to 4 fetuses and placentas and appropriate serum samples should be submitted. The failure of a laboratory staff to isolate

pathogens from several fetuses is probably significant—it suggests that the diagnostic search should lead to other considerations, e.g., genetic, endocrine, or toxic.

If it is impractical to submit whole fetuses, then the veterinarian should conduct necropsy examinations, collect clean or sterile fresh and fixed specimens, record the necropsy observations, and send the history, necropsy report, and specimens to the laboratory without delay. Gloves should always be worn during necropsy examinations to protect against infections from *Brucella, Salmonella,* and other pathogens. The veterinarian must assume the responsibility for protecting assistants who help with necropsy examination and specimen collection and shipment. The concern for protecting others must also extend to unwary postal and express service employees and laboratory employees who ultimately receive the package of abortion materials. Leaking packages travelling through public transport systems may sometimes constitute a serious public health hazard; they always constitute a powerful negative advertisement for the veterinary profession.

Any organ or tissue that appears to be abnormal should be collected along with generous portions of placenta, lung, thymus, heart, liver, adrenal gland, spleen, tied-off stomach and its contents, brain, bone marrow, eyelid, eyeball, and fetal blood or thoracic fluid (aqueous humor from the eyeball is useful for diphenylamine testing for nitrate; eyelids are useful for histopathologic demonstration of fungal spores; fetal blood and thoracic fluid may be of value for serologic testing). Fresh specimens of placenta and gastrointestinal tract should never be placed in the same containers with other tissues.

A serum sample collected from the dam should be submitted with the knowledge that single samples may have limited value. Another sample collected 2 to 3 weeks later will extend the usefulness of serology tests. When this is impractical or impossible, the veterinarian might consider submitting samples from several animals that have aborted recently along with samples from several animals that appear to be normal. A comparison of titers for various abortion diseases may allow inferences to be drawn that will point towards a specific disease as the abortion cause. The value of negative serologic results should not be overlooked for it is sometimes important to know that specific diseases are probably not present. The value of serologic investigations in individual herds can sometimes be enhanced by comparing test results from current serum samples with results obtained from reference serum samples that may have been collected several months or even years earlier. Some diagnostic laboratories routinely hold aliquots of serum samples for 1 to 2 years. Veterinarians should inquire if they are available. They may also want to advise livestock owners to consider having blood collected from selected valuable animals while they are healthy, so that serum can be held in the owner's freezers as reference standards for investigation of subsequent diseases that may develop. Serum samples should be collected in sterile tubes not containing residues that may be toxic for cell cultures used in some serologic tests. Brucellosis tubes and some commercial tubes are not satisfactory.

If the veterinarian thinks that it is indicated, he or she may wish to submit a blood sample in EDTA from the dam or fetus for hematologic studies. Other samples that may be of value include vaginal and uterine swabs and

Table 1. United States Livestock Production by State—1982*

State	All Cows That Have Calved Jan. 1, 1982-83 (1000 Head)		1982 Calf Crop		Breeding Ewes 1 yr. and Older Jan. 1, 1982 (1000 Head)	Lamb Crop/100 Ewes 1 yr. and Older Jan. 1, 1982 (Number)	Dec., 1981—May, 1982			June—Nov., 1982		
	1982	1983	1000 Head	Per Cent†	1000 Head	Number	Sows Farrowing (1000 Head)	Pigs/Litter (Number)	Pig Crop (1000 Head)	Sows Farrowing (1000 Head)	Pigs/Litter (Number)	Pig Crop (1000 Head)
ALA	1010	990	900	90		37	56	7.0	392	53	7.4	392
ALAS	4.1	4.0	3.0	74	1.9	77	.38	7.6	2.90	.35	7.7	2.70
ARIZ	355	360	285	80	235		18	7.7	139	18	8.0	144
ARK	1100	994	880	84			52	7.6	395	73	7.5	548
CALIF	2100	1970	1700	84	854	88	15	6.7	100	16	7.2	115
COLO	1020	1000	850	84	394	112	41	7.2	295	29	7.8	226
CONN	56	57	54	96	4.3	105	.90	7.5	6.8	.60	7.5	4.5
DEL	15	15	13	87			5.0	6.8	34	3.1	7.0	22
FLA	1410	1410	1150	81			30	7.5	225	38	7.3	277
GA	1032	953	840	85			145	7.08	1027	149	7.10	1058
HAW	93	95	71	76		123	5.2	6.7	35	5.3	6.8	36
IDAHO	730	760	735	99	389	107	9.0	7.9	71	10	7.3	73
ILL	1042	952	830	83	124	109	635	6.96	4419	660	7.18	4736
IND	670	650	585	89	96	120	410	7.30	2993	425	7.55	3210
IOWA	2124	1960	1900	93	283	98	1430	7.38	10557	1470	7.33	10771
KANS	1950	1627	1525	85	117	93	177	7.67	1357	174	7.51	1306
KY	1290	1330	1200	92	20	100	85	7.5	638	100	7.2	720
LA	860	750	590	73	6.7	120	11	6.7	74	14	6.8	95
MAINE	75	73	62	84	10	100	.90	5.4	4.9	1.5	6.0	9.0
MD	214	196	170	83	14	100	28	7.8	218	25	7.4	185
MASS	57	57	48	84	5.6	96	3.7	7.5	28	4.5	7.6	34
MICH	610	615	550	90	83		85	7.5	638	86	7.3	628
MINN	1490	1371	1300	91	199	123	440	7.43	3270	475	7.55	3588

	1	2	3	4	5	6	7	8	9	10	11	12
MISS	1050	970	840	83	87	123	30	7.5	225	31	7.6	236
MO	2450	2475	2340	95	455	103	360	7.16	2578	410	7.35	3015
MONT	1633	1549	1570	99	105	119	20	7.6	152	14	7.4	104
NEBR	2270	2150	1930	87	95	97	370	7.43	2748	380	7.55	2870
NEV	375	341	290	81	5.4	130	1.3	7.0	9.1	1.3	7.7	10
NH	36	36	32	89	6.8	115	.60	7.7	4.6	.60	7.6	4.6
NJ	55	52	43	80	468	80	3.0	5.3	16	2.5	6.3	16
N MEX	620	650	580	91	49	110	4.0	7.5	30	3.7	7.6	28
NY	1050	1055	960	91	5.4	104	10	7.7	77	10	7.7	77
NC	570	530	460	84	165	115	210	7.68	1612	222	7.70	1709
N DAK	1070	1130	1070	97	207	111	28	7.1	199	23	7.4	170
OHIO	770	765	715	93	70	100	191	7.54	1441	192	7.82	1502
OKLA	2450	2250	2100	89	350	103	18	7.2	130	17	7.5	128
OREG	827	770	720	90	95	84	11	8.0	88	11	7.5	83
PA	977	950	840	87			48	7.9	379	70	8.1	567
RI	4.4	4.4	4.0	91			.60	7.4	4.4	.40	7.5	3.0
SC	357	330	275	80			45	6.5	292	48	7.0	336
S DAK	1755	1795	1780	100	565	113	157	7.4	1162	156	7.5	1170
TENN	1225	1360	1180	91	7.5	100	100	7.3	730	95	7.0	665
TEX	6250	6600	5650	88	1605	75	60	6.6	396	61	6.9	421
UTAH	450	460	385	85	505	88	3.0	6.7	23	3.0	7.0	21
VT	202	204	190	94	7.0	147	1.6	8.3	13	1.4	7.5	11
VA	840	801	730	89	127	126	65	7.4	481	55	7.1	391
WASH	650	670	570	86	55	120	4.9	7.4	36	5.2	8.1	42
W VA	315	296	250	82	85	118	5.2	7.0	36	3.8	7.5	29
WIS	2087	2050	2000	97	81	130	160	7.7	1232	160	7.8	1248
WYO	685	704	675	97	750	88	2.7	7.7	21	3.0	6.8	20
US	50331	49146	44420	89	8787.6	97	5593	7.34	41035	5810	7.41	43057

*Sources: Crop Reporting Board, Statistical Reporting Service, USDA, Washington, D.C.

  Cattle—Released Jan. 28, 1983.

  Sheep and Goats—Released Jan. 26, 1983.

  Hogs and Pigs—Released Dec. 22, 1982.

†Percentage estimates for calf crop are based on the assumption that the 1982 calf crop was produced by the average of the Jan. 1, 1982 and by the Jan. 1, 1983, inventory of all cows that calved.

1. Are breeding records available to show length of estrous cycles and the numbers of services required for conception? (If practical, photocopies of the records should be obtained.)
2. How many abortions have occurred?
3. Is this a new problem or a continuing problem?
4. When did the abortions commence?
5. At what stages of gestation have abortions occurred?
6. Does the problem occur chiefly in young animals in their first pregnancy or in animals of all ages?
7. Do aborting animals appear to be sick before or after aborting?
8. Is dystocia a problem?
9. Are fetuses dead (fresh or autolyzed) or alive at time of abortion?
10. Are aborted fetuses of normal size for their gestational age?
11. Do they show developmental abnormalities?
12. Do they show signs of skin disease?
13. Are full term newborn animals weak?
14. Have mummies been aborted?
15. How long does it take for placentas to be expelled?
16. Do placentas show any abnormalities?
17. Have new breeding animals (male or female) been introduced in the last year?
18. Have aborting animals been hauled, worked, or otherwise stressed recently?
19. Were aborting animals treated with steroid drugs recently?
20. Is artificial insemination or embryo transfer practiced?
21. If so, what is the source of semen or embryos? (Sire health programs and semen as embryo processing techniques may need to be ascertained.)
22. Are clean-up sires used as a follow-up to artificial insemination? (Their breeding history and soundness may need to be ascertained.)
23. What type of vaccines and bacterins are used? At what ages and frequency are they used? Who manufactured them? (Dose level, expiration date, and methods of administration may need to be determined if history indicates abortions have resulted from vaccine breaks, vaccine infections, or vaccine misuse.)
24. What is the type and source of pasture, hay, protein supplement, grain, mineral supplement, and water?
25. What fertilizer applications were made to pastures or fields in the past year?
26. What heating or cooling methods are used in animal housing? (Carbon monoxide levels may need to be determined.)
27. What have previous abortion investigations disclosed?
28. What do you believe has caused the current abortion problem?

Figure 1. Questions aimed at obtaining answers from the livestock owner that will assist the veterinarian and, if necessary, the diagnostic laboratory staff in the investigation of abortions.

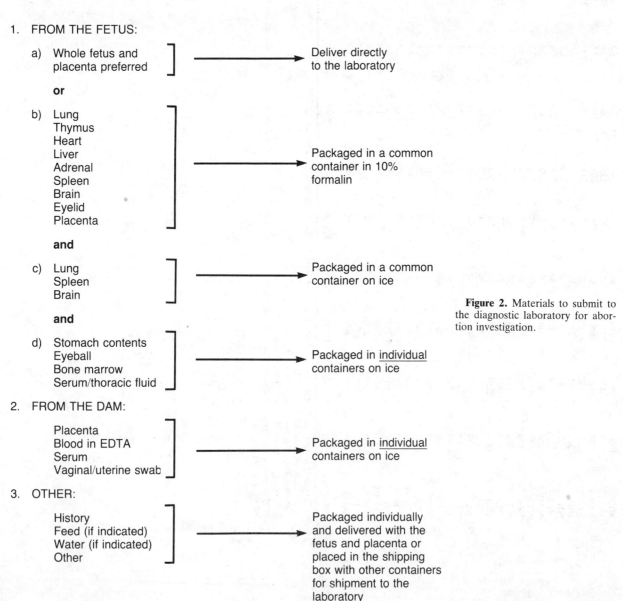

Figure 2. Materials to submit to the diagnostic laboratory for abortion investigation.

feedstuffs, water, or other materials from the animal's environment that might be related to the abortion problem. A summary of diagnostic materials that may be needed for the investigation is presented in Figure 2.

CONCLUSIONS

It is apparent that abortion investigations can require remarkable amounts of time, tedious work, and careful thought on the part of the animal owner, the veterinarian, and the diagnostic laboratory personnel. The animal owner that expects a blood sample collected from a recently aborted animal to yield information that will explain the abortion is usually going to be disappointed. The animal owner that is willing to spend the time and money for a thorough investigation is usually going to be rewarded with a presumptive or positive diagnosis that will permit effective treatment and preventive measures to be applied. Because of the limitations discussed previously, laboratory diagnostic success rates will probably never rise out of the minority range; however, the facts elucidated by the laboratory investigation combined with the facts contributed by the owner's history and the veterinarian's clinical examination will usually allow the veterinarian to render a useful diagnosis in the majority of the cases that are investigated.

Reference

1. Kirkbride, C. A.: The Compendium on Continuing Education, vol. 4, no. 8, August, 1982.

Elective Termination of Pregnancy

MAARTEN DROST, D.V.M.

COW

Early termination of pregnancy may be desirable in feedlot heifers, in very small heifers, and in cows and heifers bred accidentally. Therapeutic abortion is also indicated in cows carrying a mummy or a macerated fetus and, occasionally, in cows afflicted with hydrallantois, hydramnios, or a debilitating disease during the latter part of gestation. Induction of abortion should always be preceded by a rectal examination to confirm the presence and the stage of pregnancy. There are 3 basic ways to disrupt gestation in the cow, (1) destruction of the conceptus, (2) regression of the corpus luteum (CL) during the first 7 months, and (3) activation of mechanisms normally involved in the initiation of labor at term. The treatment employed largely depends on the stage of gestation.

After accidental breeding, particularly if the time for rebreeding is of essence, pregnancy may be terminated as soon as the CL becomes sensitive to the luteolytic action of prostaglandins on day 5 or 6 of gestation. Alternately, 30 per cent or more of the animals will fail to conceive and may return to estrus. If a cow does not show estrus following breeding, she may be treated immediately or after a later examination for pregnancy.

The developing embryo may be destroyed by the infusion of irritating substances (50 ml of a 2-per cent Lugol's solution, 500 mg tetracycline in 50 ml of saline, 50 ml of nitrofurazone, 50 ml of 70-per cent ethyl alcohol solution) into the uterus after day 4 of gestation. In addition to their direct effect on the early embryo, such irritating agents may also cause luteolysis, thus terminating gestation. Infusion after day 11 will lengthen the estrous cycle. From 30 to 65 days' gestation, the amniotic vesicle can be made to rupture by manual pressure per rectum. The membranes will be expelled 2 to 4 weeks later, and the animal will resume estrus approximately 1 month after disruption of the vesicle. From 65 to 90 days, and occasionally up to 120 days, the fetus may be decapitated per rectum. Regression of the CL may be effected by the intramuscular injection of 25 to 30 mg prostaglandin $F_{2\alpha}$ or 500 to 600 μg of a prostaglandin $F_{2\alpha}$ analogue. When treated between 5 and 150 days of gestation, the animal will generally abort within 5 days. The treatment is also effective for the expulsion of a mummified fetus. It is common to find the dry mummy lodged in the cervix 3 days after treatment with prostaglandins. Occasionally, a mummy, particularly the uncommon larger ones the size of a 7-month fetus, will not be expelled, and a hysterotomy must be resorted to.

Enucleation of the CL, though an efficient method of terminating pregnancy during the first 6 months, cannot be recommended because of the danger of excessive hemorrhage and the formation of ovarian adhesions.

Estrogens have also been used to cause regression of the CL. From 4 to 8 mg of estradiol or 40 to 80 mg of diethylstilbestrol are given intramuscularly. If administered within the first 4 days after the unwanted breeding, estrogens will usually prevent further gestation by interfering with the descent of the embryo into the uterus and by changing the synchrony between the developing embryo and the endometrium. Return to fertile estrus may be slower after estrogen treatment than after prostaglandin treatment.

During the fourth to seventh month of pregnancy, larger (20 mg) and repeated doses of estradiol are required, or intramuscular doses of 100 to 175 mg repositol diethylstilbestrol are required. Dystocia, retained placenta, and metritis are common sequelae to estrogen-induced abortion after 7 months' gestation.

Therapeutic abortion of cows carrying macerated fetuses or of cows afflicted with hydrops of the fetal membranes is an economically questionable procedure because of the poor prognosis for subsequent fertility and, in the case of hydrallantois, survival of the dam. The expulsion of the macerated fetal bones is generally ineffective because of their dry nature and their multiple sharp edges and protrusions.

Beyond 150 days of normal gestation, 25 mg dexamethasone may be combined with 25 mg prostaglandin $F_{2\alpha}$ to increase the efficacy of inducing abortion to approximately 95 per cent.

Premature parturition and labor may be induced with a single intramuscular injection of 20 mg dexamethasone or 5 mg flumethasone from the eighth month of gestation on. Earlier treatment can be effective if larger and repeated doses are used. Delivery generally occurs 48 to 72 hr after injection. Retained placenta is a common sequela. The closer to term the glucocorticoid treatment is used, the more rapid the response and the lower the incidence of retained placenta. Treatment of the retained placenta should be limited to removal of the exposed portion of the membranes by cutting it off at the vulva and, optionally, the systemic administration of broad-spectrum antibiotics.

Alternately, prostaglandin $F_{2\alpha}$ or its synthetic analogues may be used to initiate labor and parturition in cattle. Delivery is approximately 72 hr after intramuscular administration of 25 to 30 mg prostaglandin $F_{2\alpha}$ or 500 to 600 µg prostaglandin analogues. No adverse effects have been reported other than retention of the placenta.

Elective induction of parturition offers the advantage of scheduling the time of calving for a time when supervision is available. The calves born after induction are generally smaller in size, which reduces the percentage requiring cesarean section. Viability of the calf is directly proportional to its degree of maturity. Total milk production for the subsequent lactation and subsequent fertility of the cow are not adversely affected. The use of large doses of corticosteroids may be contraindicated in animals with infections, e.g., mastitis.

DOE

Early interruption of pregnancy (abortion) may be indicated in purebred does when they are bred to the wrong buck, particularly if the current breeding season is to be salvaged. Pregnancy in the doe is CL-dependent throughout its entire duration. Luteolysis can be induced with injection of 5 to 10 mg prostaglandin $F_{2\alpha}$ or 50 to 100 µg of a synthetic analogue. Abortion takes place within 4 to 5 days after injection. Estradiol is also luteolytic in the doe but is not recommended because of delayed return to estrus.

Parturition may safely be induced after 146 days of gestation with good viability of kids and without retention of fetal membranes. Kidding takes place 31.5 ± 1.5 hr after the intramuscular injection of 5 to 10 mg prostaglandin $F_{2\alpha}$, which permits rather precise scheduling, avoiding even middle of the night trips to the barn.

Glucocorticoids can be also used to precipitate labor and delivery in the pregnant doe. The efficacy of corticosteroid treatment rises as pregnancy becomes more advanced. Induction should not be attempted earlier than 1 week prior to term if the newborn is to survive. Intramuscular injection of 15 mg dexamethasone is generally followed by delivery within 72 hr.

EWE

The need for the induction of abortion in ewes is limited to the valuable purebred show animal that is bred to the wrong ram. The CL is essential for the maintenance of pregnancy during the first 2 months only. Regression of the CL can be effected by the intramuscular injection of 10 to 15 mg prostaglandin $F_{2\alpha}$, which leads to abortion within 72 hr.

During the last 9 days of gestation, parturition can be initiated in the pregnant ewe by the intramuscular administration of 15 mg dexamethasone. Delivery takes place 48 to 60 hr after injection. Retention of the fetal membranes, as is common in the cow, does not occur.

Corticosteroid induction of ewes suffering from ketosis of pregnancy is unsuccessful. This metabolic disorder apparently renders the pregnant ewe refractory to the action of glucocorticoids.

Table 1. Common Drug Doses

Drug	Supplier	Species	Dose
Azium (Dexamethazone)	Schering Corp. Kenilworth, NJ 07033	Bovine	20 mg IM
		Ovine	15 mg IM
		Caprine	15 mg IM
Flucort (Flumethasone)	Syntex Laboratories, Inc. Palo Alto, CA 94304	Bovine	5 mg IM
		Ovine	4 mg IM
		Caprine	4 mg IM
Lutalyse (Prostaglandin $F_{2\alpha}$)	The Upjohn Co. Kalamazoo, MI 49001	Bovine	25 mg IM
		Ovine	15 mg IM
		Caprine	8 mg IM
Estrumate (Cloprostenol)	BayVet Division of Cutter Laboratories Inc. Shawnee Mission, KS 66201	Bovine	500 µg IM
Bovilene (Fenprostalene)	Diamond Laboratories Inc. Des Moines, IA 50304	Bovine	1 mg SC

SOW

The relatively short gestation period of the sow reduces the need for therapeutic abortion in this species. Interruption of pregnancy may be indicated in a very valuable sow when she is inseminated or bred to the wrong boar. Active CL are required throughout gestation in the pig. CL are susceptible to the luteolytic action of prostaglandins after day 11. Intramuscular administration of 5 to 10 mg prostaglandin $F_{2\alpha}$ results in abortion in 24 to 48 hr and estrus 4 to 5 days later. Normal fertility appears at the second estrus after treatment. Estrogen should not be used in the sow, since it is luteotropic and prolongs the functional lifespan of the CL.

Timed parturition allows the scheduling of supervision during farrowing and may be labor saving by avoiding night and weekend parturitions. Furthermore, a reduction in the incidence of the MMA (metritis, mastitis, agalactia) syndrome has been found in sows in which parturition was induced. If farrowing takes places earlier than 3 days before term, the baby pigs will be small and weak and the survival rate will be poor.

Prostaglandins, especially prostaglandin $F_{2\alpha}$ and its analogues, may be used to initiate the physiologic process of parturition prematurely. From 10 to 25 mg prostaglandin $F_{2\alpha}$ are given intramuscularly from 2 to 6 days before expected parturition. Farrowing is within 24 to 36 hr after injection. Glucocorticoids such as dexamethasone must be administered in 100 mg doses for several consecutive days to advance the onset of parturition. The repeated injection and the potential danger of such pharmacologic doses of a potent corticosteroid in the presence of subclinical infection render this treatment undesirable if not contraindicated.

The duration of farrowing may be controlled with the use of parasympathomimetic agents such as dichlorvos, an organophosphate, or carbocholine hydrochloride. Treatment with these drugs reduces the mean "between-pig" interval and the incidence of stillborn pigs. Oxytocin stimulates contractions during parturition, but its action is not sustained. Oxytocin will not induce parturition in swine. (See Table 1 for Common Drug Doses.)

Supplemental Reading

Hormonal Control of Parturition: A symposium. Biol. Reprod. 16:1–94, 1977.
Morrow, D. A. (ed.): Current Therapy in Theriogenology, 2nd ed. Philadelphia, W. B. Saunders Company, 1985.

Diseases of the Internal Genitalia of Males

ROBERT S. HUDSON, D.V.M., M.S.

Infectious seminal vesiculitis is the most commonly diagnosed disease of the accessory genitalia in bulls. The disease merits concern because, in addition to its separate effect on reproduction, it is frequently the most obvious manifestation of a serious and complex disease syndrome, including elusive infections in other pelvic genitalia and concomitant or sequential epididymitis, orchitis, and periorchitis. The incidence of seminal vesiculitis varies from a sporadic 2 to 5 per cent in adult beef and dairy bulls to 5 to 50 per cent in groups of young bulls, suggesting contagion. Fewer middle-aged bulls incur vesiculitis than those less than 2 years old or more than 9 years old. Seminal vesiculitis is rare in boars, rams, and bucks.

In bulls, the relative ease of examination of the seminal vesicles (vesicular glands) and the more obvious response to insult may account for vesiculitis being reported more often than infections of other accessory genitalia. Although ampullitis, prostatitis, and bulbourethral adenitis appear frequently with vesiculitis at necropsy, ampullitis is less readily diagnosed clinically; prostatitis almost never. Greater size and firmness of the ampullae may escape detection, and the dense capsule of the bull prostate precludes enlargement. The bulbourethral glands are not palpable.

ETIOLOGY AND PATHOGENESIS

Essentially all the microorganisms mentioned in association with orchitis have been associated with seminal vesiculitis, stressing the complexity of infectious genital disease. The agent often eludes identification. In some cases, especially in outbreaks among young bulls, IBR or enteroviruses appear to initiate the insult and predispose the animal to opportunistic bacterial infections. *Chlamydia psittaci* has been reported to cause seminal vesiculitis in the buck. The predilection of brucellae for genital tissue includes the seminal vesicles of all the food animal species. The presence of *Brucella suis* in the seminal vesicles of boars without microscopic lesions causes concern in seminal transmission.

The pathogenesis is not clear. The outbreaks in groups of young bulls may be related to normal homosexual activity with oral and nasal entry of organisms and hematogenous spread. Likewise, extragenital foci of infection, especially in the lungs, appear to be a source of bloodborne infection. Ascending infection in the rare cases of generalized urinary tract disease must be considered. Seminal vesiculitis appears to follow orchitis and epididymitis, but it is difficult to determine which comes first. In practice, the veterinarian may not be able to determine the origin or route of infection.

Studies point to increased susceptibility of the seminal vesicles associated with discrete unpalpable congenital abnormalities, but bulls with satisfactory service records and no evidence of vesiculitis may have palpable unilateral hypoplastic or aplastic seminal vesicles or ampullae.

DIAGNOSIS

Overt clinical signs rarely arise. Acute vesiculitis may cause signs of peritonitis, tenesmus, and obscure rear limb lameness. The condition usually is discovered on routine rectal palpation or after purulent exudate is found in the semen. Affected vesicles are initially swollen, possibly painful, and often devoid of the normal lobulation. Advanced disease may cause abscessation and fibrosis. Caution is required in that there is normal variation in the size of the vesicles within and among bulls. Also, some diseased organs elude even careful palpation. Old bulls typically have firmer vesicles than young bulls.

Culture of fluid massaged from the vesicles and collected through a hygienically inserted sterile urethral catheter is preferable to culture of semen, which always contains contaminants. Even so, the vesicular fluid may be adulterated with the products of other organs.

PATHOGENESIS

Acute vesiculitis may regress spontaneously or may progress to a chronic state of bacterial infection. Abscessation and fibrosis may form adhesions extending to other organs or form tracts extending to the inguinal rings. Cases of long duration usually involve other foci of genital infection.

The effect of solitary seminal vesiculitis on reproduction is difficult to assess. Greater viscosity of vesicular fluid may reduce gross motility of sperm. Reports of more sperm abnormalities probably reflect concurrent disease in the testicles or epididymides. Survival of frozen-thawed semen is reduced.

Concern for transmission of disease through coitus or artificial insemination is logical, but the extent of risk is unknown. Many bulls with vesiculitis have been used without detectable suppression of herd fertility. In short, bulls with vesiculitis are classified as unsound but may not be infertile. The threat of infection to other genitalia, especially to the testicles and epididymides, outweighs the threat of vesiculitis alone.

TREATMENT AND CONTROL

Spontaneous recovery in many young bulls does not permit a good evaluation of treatment. Many bulls with well established bacterial infections resist antibiotic therapy. Confirmed and suspected chlamydial infections seem to respond to daily intravenous oxytetracycline, 5 mg/lb for 10 days. Regression of swelling is often dramatic. Surgical removal of the vesicles through the ischiorectal fossa is often disappointing. Easily replaceable bulls of marginal quality should be culled.

It may be that the recommendation to cull all bulls with the disease based on possible predisposition by congenital abnormalities merits consideration. The idea, however, is unlikely to gain popularity among producers working in free enterprise systems.

Management practices that help control infectious diseases of other bodily systems are thought to help reduce the prevalence of seminal vesiculitis.

Supplemental Reading

Arthur, G. H., Noakes, D. E., and Pearson, H.: Veterinary Reproduction and Obstetrics. London, Bailliere Tindall, 1982.

McCaulay, A. D.: Seminal Vesiculitis in Bulls. *In* Morrow, D. A. (ed.): Current Therapy in Theriogenology. Philadelphia, W. B. Saunders Company, 1980.

Diseases of the Testicle and Epididymis

ROBERT S. HUDSON, D.V.M., M.S.

Developmental abnormalities of the testicles include hypoplasia when one or both testicles are small (<30 cm scrotal circumference in postpubertal bulls) and more obscure defects when a variable portion of one testicle is involved. The condition is probably heritable in the food animal species and must be differentiated if possible from atrophy, usually by history or by long-term observation. Moderate hypoplasia involves subfertility but does not equate with sterility. Thus the condition may be insidious in its effect on breeding performance and male offspring. There is no treatment.

Among fertile males and breeds of the various species, there is wide variation in testicular size correlated with scrotal circumference, sperm output, age, and body weight. Scrotal circumference measurement affords practical evaluation of testicular size and has been standardized for bulls by the Society for Theriogenology.

Blind or aberrant efferent ductules cause sperm stasis and extravasation, thence sperm granulomas. In time, even after a period of service, granulomas in the epididymal head produce occlusion of the epididymal duct, retrograde pressure on the seminiferous epithelium, and testicular degeneration. The condition appears to be heritable in polled goats. If the head of the epididymis is enlarged and firm, it is usually because of sperm granulomas.

Aplasia of any portion of the epididymis blocks sperm transit, but blockage in the body or tail does not affect testicular function. Thus the testicle may appear normal. Bilateral granulomatous occlusion or epididymal aplasia constitute irreversible sterility.

TESTICULAR DEGENERATION

Varied insults, such as hormonal imbalance, hydrocele, infection, and ambient or local thermal interference with the testicular thermoregulatory system, cause the most commonly diagnosed disease of testicles, testicular degeneration. Cryptorchid and ectopic testicles are degenerate. Males experiencing insulation of the scrotum, e.g., scrotal dermatitis, periorchitis, or prolonged recumbency from lameness, rapidly sustain testicular degeneration. The condition may appear after a short febrile episode or during prolonged hot and humid weather. Scrotal frostbite affects many males. Boars may acquire testicular degeneration from prolonged exposure to cold floors or, infrequently, from torsion of a testicle.

At least a portion of the progressive degeneration that attends aging is likely due to multiple insults over time.

A larger proportion of old bulls with testicular degeneration has distal fibrosis of the testicle, indicating vascular lesions.

If not reversed, degeneration may progress to spermiostasis, inspissation of sperm, granulomas, fibrosis, and calcification.

Diagnosis

Degeneration often appears as a loss of the normal turgidity and elasticity, as the testicle is palpated superficially and gently. A tonometer has been devised to provide more objective evaluation but is not widely used. If deeper (firmer) palpation reveals fibrosis, degeneration is advanced, and the prognosis is worsened. Many of the previously listed local causes are self evident, but the causes of degeneration often escape detection.

Serial semen evaluations through the course of unchecked degeneration show a nonspecific progression from a minor increase in sperm abnormalities to oligospermia, to an increase in major head and midpiece abnormalities, and to the appearance of primitive germinal cells. In degeneration without obvious cause and with a vague history, evaluation of but a few ejaculates often fails to assist in differentiating the condition from moderate hypoplasia.

Radiography provides a valuable aid to palpation findings of fibrotic areas or masses, indicating especially the degree and pattern (isolated or diffuse) of calcification. Diagnostic radiography is not deleterious to spermatogenesis.

Treatment

There is no specific treatment. Hormones should be avoided, and known causes should be removed. Young sires with moderate degeneration often recover 60 to 90 days after removal of the insult.

ORCHITIS AND PERIORCHITIS

Trauma and occasional neoplasia aside, the common cause of inflammation of the testicle and surrounding tunica vaginalis is a myriad of infectious agents, including *Brucella abortus, Corynebacterium pyogenes, Escherichia coli, Pseudomonas, Proteus mirabilis, Actinobacillus seminis, Actinomyces bovis, Nocardia farcinca, Haemophilus,* and *Salmonella.* Bovine herpesvirus and cytopathogenic enterovirus cause orchitis in bulls. Chlamydial and mycoplasmal agents have been reported.

Infections are usually hematogenous but may invade punctures and lacerations. Either way the condition is usually unilateral. Acute inflammation of the testicle or tunica causes swelling and pain and frequently a stilted gait. Severe enlargement usually is due to fluid and fibrin in the cavity of the tunic. Suppurative organisms may cause abscesses. Chronic inflammation results in degeneration and its sequelae. Unilateral inflammation may reduce or destroy spermatogenesis in the contralateral testicle.

Diagnosis

If the testicle can be palpated, orchitis may be evident. A firm distended tunic cavity that prevents palpation of the testicle is evidence of periorchitis. An aid to diagnosis is radiography, as described for testicular degeneration.

Thermography and thermovision, which detect variations from the normal concentric color bands transformed from infrared surface emission, are particularly useful in detecting mild inflammation. Also ultrasound units, such as those used commonly for aid with rectal diagnosis of pregnancy in mares, provide an excellent means of non-invasive examination of scrotal contents.

Identifying microbial causes by culture of semen is hampered by contamination during collection but may be helpful. Testicular biopsy for culturing is usually regarded as a last resort.

Treatment

Gentle cold water sprays for 30 minutes twice daily help reduce the damaging inflammatory heat. While systemic antibiotics may traverse the normally impervious blood-testis barrier, reduced tissue perfusion makes penetration unlikely and probably ineffective.

Early in the course of unilateral inflammation of a testicle concern should be directed towards the unaffected testicle. While summary removal of a mildly inflamed testicle and adnexa might be overtreatment, careful aseptic hemicastration is indicated when the prognosis for the affected side is poor. Minimal additional inflammatory insult is caused by the surgery. A healthy or completely restorable remaining testicle can be expected to compensate for 60 to 80 per cent of the original sperm output of two testicles.

EPIDIDYMITIS

The tail of the epididymis is vulnerable to infection, especially in rams but also in bulls and bucks. It is less common in boars. Unilateral caudal epididymitis without testicular involvement is common in bulls. The opportunistic microorganisms of orchitis may be involved. Concomitant infections of the pelvic genitalia are common.

In adult rams, a specific severe epididymitis due to *Brucella ovis* causes significant loss of flock reproductive efficiency. The organism may exist in the epididymis without palpable enlargement, or there may be extreme swelling and fibrosis even with draining sinus tracts through the scrotum. The testicles may be involved. Transmission is by genital, oral, and respiratory routes and is enhanced by the animal's sampling of urine of other rams. The condition is often bilateral and causes sterility.

A separate epididymitis affecting ram lambs is attributed to a group of *lamb epididymitis organisms* mostly Brucellaceae but not including *B. ovis*. The epididymis appears to acquire particular vulnerability in the peripubertal hormonal environment. Both ascending and oral infections from sodomy and filthy environments are suspected. Infertility is the result.

Diagnosis

Palpation of swollen, painful, indurated epididymal tails is the best method of diagnosis. In endemic flocks, palpation several times a year helps identify new cases. Acute inflammation in bulls causes resistance to even gentle palpation.

B. ovis epididymitis of rams usually produces numerous leukocytes in the ejaculate and is relatively easily cultured from semen. Large numbers of leukocytes accompany detached sperm heads and low motility. Leukocytes in semen are not uniformly characteristic of lamb epididymitis.

Control

There is no good widely documented treatment for infectious epididymitis. Many bulls appear to recover spontaneously; unilateral castration is considered in severe cases.

Ram epididymitis requires palpation of epididymides, separation of clinically affected rams, and culling. Vaccination is of marginal value—it may reduce palpable lesions but usually not the inflammation and leukocyte content of semen. Lamb epididymitis appears to be controlled at times by feeding of tetracycline. There is no vaccine.

Supplemental Reading

Bulgin, M. S., Anderson, B. C., Kirk, J. H.: Ram epididymitis. Proc. Soc. Therio. 173–179, 1981.
McEntee, K.: Pathology of the testis and epididymis of the bull and stallion. Proc. Soc. Therio. 80–91, 103–109, 1979.
Memon, M. A.: Male infertility. Symposium on sheep and goat medicine. Vet. Clin. North Am., 5:619–634, 1983.

Diseases of the Penis and Prepuce

ROBERT S. HUDSON, D.V.M., M.S.

The large number and wide variety of significant lesions of the penis and prepuce of food animals dictate careful examination by the veterinarian. This may be done by close observation of the animal during coitus, during service with an artificial vagina, or during stimulation with an electroejaculator. Alternatively, the penis may be extended manually. This is easily done in the standing restrained ram or buck; bulls may require that an assistant place a hand in the rectum to help relax the retractor penis muscles. Once the technique of manual extension is mastered, there is little or no need for tranquilizers with their attendant risk of post-examination penile injury. Some boars, but not all, resist manual manipulation and require sedation or anesthesia.

BULL

Balanoposthitis primarily affects young bulls and may be due to specific IBR infection or nonspecific abrasions sustained during excessive service. The associated pain may cause bulls to refuse to serve. Healing is usually spontaneous, and service may be resumed in 2 weeks. The IBR infection is venereal, may shed virus in the semen, and may be prevented by vaccination.

Viral papillomas (warts) are found frequently on the penis but not on the prepuce of young bulls in groups. Abrasions admit the virus, and the wart grows rapidly and may surround the tip of the penis. Surgical removal is simple, the primary concern being preservation of the urethra. Ligating and suturing, if needed, are preferable to thermocautery, which may cause deep and serious necrosis. Vaccine, even if available, is of marginal value at best.

Young bulls commonly display matted rings of hair surrounding the free portion of the penis. The hair comes from the hair of other bulls, which have been mounted. The ring should be removed prior to service to avoid deep annular laceration of the penis.

Persistent frenulum, a congenital band-like attachment of the prepuce to the tip of the penis along the median raphe, is usually found in virgin bulls. The frenulum, not to be confused with a persistent prepubertal preputial adhesion, may cause ventral deviation of the erect penis. The impotence thus induced in *Bos taurus* breeds may not affect *Bos indicus* breeds that have excessive prepuce. Strong evidence for heritability dictates culling affected bulls from purebred herds. Otherwise, the frenulum is easily ligated at each end and excised.

Deep lacerations of the dorsum of the penis may interrupt the sensory nerve supply, which is very important for efficient intromission and ejaculation. Scars from lacerations should alert the examiner to possible impotence. Sensation may be tested by stimulation of the glans and dorsum with an electric prod while holding the retractor penis muscles. A positive response is a surprisingly mild contraction of the muscles. A better test is actual mating.

Lacerations of the glans and corpus cavernosum may result in fistulae that bleed only during erection, the blood being toxic to sperm. Immediate suturing after injury is indicated. Careful longitudinal wedge resection of the fistula, separate closure of the tunica albuginea and skin, and 3 weeks of sexual rest are usually successful. Fistulae of the glans are especially resistant to closure and require longitudinal resection, curettage of the cavity of the fistula, and deep suturing.

Lacerations or fistulae of the urethra, if more than 5 cm from the terminus, may reduce effective deposition of the ejaculate. Healing of sutured defects is categorically difficult because of the naturally vigorous wave-like movement of urination. A drastic but effective solution is concomitant ischial urethrotomy with indwelling catheter. After healing of the distal urethra, the ischial urethra is allowed to heal spontaneously.

Spiral and ventral deviations of the penis, observed during mating attempts, prevent intromission. Deviations usually appear in 3- to 4-year-old bulls, after a period of satisfactory service. Both types occur as defects of the penile apical ligament and may be repaired by surgically implanting a 2-cm × 12- to 15-cm strip of fascia lata from the patient to a plane between the tunica albuginea and apical ligament through a dorsal, penile midline incision.

Rupture of the corpus cavernosum penis (hematoma) is a common and serious accident during service. In some cases, it is caused by innately vigorous sexual behavior and is characterized by circumscribed symmetric swelling surrounding the penis just cranial to the neck of the scrotum. The prepuce is dark purple from extravasated blood and usually everted. The injury will heal spontaneously in many cases; ultrasound therapy is reported to improve results. I believe that surgical closure of the rent in the tunica albuginea provides less risk of recurrence and of some serious sequelae.

Surgery performed 1 to 2 days after injury allows easier repair. Under general anesthesia or deep sedation in right lateral recumbency with aseptic conditions, an incision of the cranioventral skin is made over the lateral aspect of the bulge of the hematoma. Subcutaneous tissue incision exposes the blood clot, which is removed. The affected portion of the penis is exposed and pulled through the incision in the skin. Multiple layers of peripenile elastic tissue are incised longitudinally and laterally to the penis to expose the dull ivory-colored tunica albuginea. The usually transverse rent will be found predictably at the dorsal aspect of the distal bend of the sigmoid flexure. Distraction of the torn edges may be 2 cm. The edges are débrided and sutured with a boot lace pattern using no. 1 polyglycolic acid suture. The multiple elastic layers are closed with a single simple continuous suture of 000 gut. Loose clots in the cavity are rinsed free with sterile saline at 37°C. The wall of the hematoma is sutured with 0 gut without closing space, then the skin incision is closed. Maximal healing requires 60 days sexual rest.

Because of the violence of the injury and frequent sequelae, the prognosis for rupture of the tunica albuginea is guarded, whether conservatively or surgically managed. Sequelae are peripenile adhesion, hematogenous abscess, disruption of the sensory nerve supply, and vascular shunts at the rupture site, causing erection failure. These shunts may be repaired by the technique for fresh rupture.

Failure of erection may arise from congenital and uncorrectable multiple shunts in the free portion of the penis. Both types of shunts may be confirmed by serial contrast radiography of the corpus cavernosum. Obstructive cavernositis, intracorporeal thrombosis, and dystrophic calcification are conditions that also cause erection failure. All are difficult to diagnose during life and are irreparable.

Preputial injuries, usually sustained in service, appear most frequently in *Bos indicus* breeds and their crosses, particularly in those individuals with excessively pendulous sheaths, long prepuces, and wide preputial orifices. Mild injuries may require little more than 2 weeks of rest but may become major wounds if the animals are left in service thus extending time loss as much as 2 months or more. The typical progression of the condition is traumatic edema, preputial prolapse, increased edema, attempted coitus, and laceration (splitting), usually on the ventrum of the prepuce.

Care of prolapse with or without laceration involves cleansing, applying of a lanolin-based protectant ointment, and bandaging with stockinette and adhesive elastic tape. Latex rubber tubing inserted into the preputial lumen and incorporated into the bandage provides urine drainage. The bandage protects the injury, reduces edema, and should be changed every 3 days or as needed. When reduction of edema allows reversion of the prepuce, bandaging without stockinette continues until the prepuce remains in place spontaneously.

If the prepuce is too long for containment or if a granulating deep laceration prevents the return to normal function, circumcision is indicated. One technique involves (1) full extension of the penis and prepuce, which may require cutting across stenotic areas of prepuce, (2) applying a latex rubber tourniquet at the preputial orifice, (3) resecting sufficient prepuce between proximal and distal annular incisions to reduce excessive length, (4) removing fibrotic tissue but still allowing full penile extension, (5) ligating all severed vessels, (6) removing the tourniquet and completing hemostasis, and (7) suturing superficial elastic tissue and skin with simple, interrupted stitches using 0 gut. A bandage similar to that described for simple prolapse is applied. The bandage should be removed in 3 days, the stitches in 10 days. Bulls usually can return to service in 60 days.

Retropreputial abscesses result from deep preputial laceration and immediate, complete retraction of the prepuce. The condition is common in *Bos taurus* breeds. Without prolapse, the injury may not be discovered until function is severely compromised by formation of peripenile adhesions. Abscesses should be drained through the original laceration in the prepuce. The prognosis is poor, but spontaneous recoveries occur in 60 to 90 days in a small proportion of affected bulls. Surgical excision of peripenile adhesions has been unrewarding.

Bulls regularly serving the artificial vagina occasionally sustain an avulsion of the prepuce from its attachment to the free portion of the penis. The prepuce is severely distracted and, contrary to the usual contraindication for suturing fresh but contaminated preputial wounds in range bulls, these avulsions should be repaired immediately.

BOAR

Penile congenital defects include persistent frenulum, which may be managed surgically as in the bull. Erection failure may be due to heritable micropenis and cavernosal venus shunts that are irreparable.

Failure of penile extension may also be due to infrequent or habitual "balling" in which the penis is inserted in the preputial diverticulum. Young boars may be corrected by forcing dismounting when the action is noted. Repeated mounting often results in correct extension. If the practice persists, culling should be considered in that there is some evidence of heritability. Surgical extirpation of the diverticulum is discouraged.

Lacerations of the distal portion of the penis are common in boars and usually result from biting females or other boars during breeding activity. Lacerations are also caused, especially in young boars, by raking the penis across the bristly hair of the rump of females or other boars during mounting attempts. Most lacerations heal with 2 weeks of sexual rest and no treatment. Severe wounds may require daily application of topical antibiotic ointments, or, rarely, surgical closure. Preputial injuries are rare in boars.

RAM AND BUCK

Penile and preputial injuries are quite rare in rams and bucks and usually can be managed similarly to those in bulls. Occasionally, the urethral process may be grossly traumatized or blocked with urinary calculi. Amputation of the process is simple and appears to have no suppressant effect on fertility.

Posthitis (pizzle rot) is a chronic necrotizing disease of the preputial orifice. Considered to be caused by the interaction of *Corynebacterium renale* infection and the high (4 per cent) urinary urea content of a high protein diet and reduced water intake, the condition is a serious cause of impotence. Early in the course of the disease, the orifice is ulcerated and exudes thick purulent debris. The condition may progress to fill the entire preputial cavity with exudate and necrotic tissue and occlude the prepuce. Early stages may respond to thorough cleansing and regular application of penicillin ointment. Systemic treatment is ineffective.

Supplemental Reading

Hudson, R. S.: Diagnosis of disturbances of mating ability in bulls. Auburn Vet. *37*:81–84, 1981.
Walker, D. F., and Vaughan, J. T.: Bovine and Equine Urogenital Surgery. Philadelphia, Lea and Febiger, 1979.

Dairy Herd Reproductive Efficiency

EDWARD T. HENRY, D.V.M.

What is dairy herd reproductive efficiency? Most clinicians involved in analyzing modern dairy herd reproductive performance probably would agree that a calving interval (CI) of less than 13 months for 90 per cent or more of the herd is a reasonable and obtainable goal. At the same time, it is hoped that the annual herd culling rate for infertility would be less than 6 per cent (Table 1). Now the next question is, what constitutes infertility? This can only be answered properly in light of the definition of reproductive efficiency. For those dairy operations utilizing artificial insemination (AI), infertility can be defined as a failure to conceive by a reasonable number of services or a failure to conceive within a reasonable period of time after calving or both. A reasonable number of services would be 3 to 4, and a reasonable period of time would be 130 to 140 days postpartum (see Table 1). Note that the word "reasonable" is not synonymous with "optimal." In order to meet the criteria of reproductive efficiency as stated in Table 1, one will have to go beyond reasonable and approach optimal.

HERD FERTILITY

Before pursuing a discussion of the 2 major factors (heat detection efficiency and conception rate) that affect reproductive efficiency, let's look at some useful parameters that indicate whether herd fertility is slipping into the area of inefficiency. Table 2 is a list of parameters available to dairy owners (and veterinary practitioners) through several sources, such as Dairy Herd Improvement Association (DHIA) records and reports, farm computer services, or their own calculations. The first 3 or 4

Table 1. *Definition of Dairy Herd Reproductive Efficiency*

What is Dairy Herd Reproductive Efficiency?	What is Infertility?*
Calving interval < 13 months for 90 per cent or more of the herd.	Failure to conceive by a reasonable number of services (e.g., 3 to 4 AI services).
Annual herd culling rate for *infertility* < 6%.	OR
	Failure to conceive within a reasonable period of time (e.g., 130 to 140 days postpartum).

*Whichever comes first.

Table 2. *Parameters Used to Evaluate the Magnitude of a Reproductive Efficiency Problem. Both Heat Detection Efficiency and Conception Rates Will Affect the Values for these Parameters*

Parameter	Value
Calving Interval (CI)	(12.4–12.7 mo.)*
Days Open or Calving to Conception Interval	(95–105 days)
Days in Milk (for herd)	(160–175 days)
Herd Reproductive Status (HRS) Index	(> 65)
% of Herd Diagnosed Pregnant per Month	(8–9%)
% of Cows Open More than 150 Days	(< 10%)
% Annual Culling for Infertility	(< 6%)

*Value in parentheses is the desired goal for that parameter.

parameters probably are more common than are the last 3 parameters. But what's important to recognize about all of these parameters is they indicate that an overall reproductive problem exists when the actual observed values exceed the ones in parentheses. They do *not* indicate which of the 2 major factors (heat detection rate and breeding or conception rate) is contributing to the problem. Abnormal values for these factors only serve to point out that there is a problem with reproductive efficiency. When approaching herd fertility problems, these indicators are a good starting point by which to note the magnitude of the overall problem.

Of the characteristics in Table 2, Days Open or Calving to Conception Interval, Days in Milk (DIM, for herd), Calving Interval (CI) and Herd Reproductive Status (HRS) Index are the more common and traditional ones used to assess reproductive performance. CI is good, but it is a historical parameter; computation of the CI requires 2 calvings. The reproductive factors that influence the second calving occurred 10 to 14 months ago or longer. To forecast a projected CI, just add a gestation (280 days) to the current Days Open figure. Remember, in order to achieve a CI of 13 months or less, the average Days Open will have to be 115 days or less. The CI and average Days Open only regard those cows that did in fact conceive. (What about those cows that fail to conceive—how do we account for them? More on those animals later.)

HRS Index is a good measure of the influence open cows are having on meeting the goals of reproductive efficiency. This index figure accounts for all cows that go beyond a specified period of time (e.g., 100 days or 120 days postpartum) and have not conceived. As long as this number stays relatively high (>65), then probably there are only a few cows that are outside of the reproductive goals with respect to Days Open. On the other hand, if this figure drops to the 40's or 30's or lower, there is a problem. It's an implication that there are either more problem cows, or there are individual cows with longer Days Open.

Since many dairies now are calving on a year-round basis, calculating the Percentage of Herd Diagnosed Pregnant per Month becomes useful. In order to maintain an equal number of lactating cows, the rate of freshening (calving) should equal the rate of drying off (also culling—a small percentage). This means there should be equal numbers of new pregnancies each month, i.e., one twelfth (8 to 9 per cent) of the herd should become pregnant each month. Usually, there isn't a problem with this percentage exceeding 10 per cent monthly, but when a reproductive problem arises this may be reduced by 50 to 60 per cent to 4 to 5 per cent.

No doubt another good starting parameter would be Days Open, but again this parameter only considers cows that conceive, so in order to get an initial handle on a herd fertility problem, all the parameters in Table 2 should be considered.

MAJOR FACTORS—HEAT DETECTION RATE AND CONCEPTION RATE

Now let's dissect reproductive efficiency into its basic components or factors and also look at those parameters used to measure or indicate problem areas related to those factors. (This discussion is based on the premise that AI is the major means of conception rather than natural service with bulls and that calving is essentially year-round.) Simply stated, there are 2 major factors that affect reproductive efficiency. First would be the efficiency or rate at which heat (estrus) is detected. The second major factor is breeding or conception efficiency.

Heat Detection Rate

Voluminous amounts of research have been conducted on the various factors contributing to the efficiency with which cows are detected in heat. When all is sifted, one of the key factors is the human being. Under the conditions of AI, a human assumes the responsibility of the bull (the expert detector), and due to some major biologic differences between humans and bulls, we of the human species are inadequately equipped to be a good substitute. This alone will lead to a decrease in efficiency.

Various researchers have shown that the postpartum interval to first ovulation (usually unaccompanied by detectable estrus) averages about 3 weeks, whereas the first detected estrus averages about 5 weeks postpartum.[1-3] King and coworkers, using a video recorder on a 24 hr observation basis during the first 90 days postpartum, were able to detect 100 per cent of the heats at a third ovulation whereas casual visual observation only detected 60 per cent of the heats at the same ovulation (Table 3).[2] Therefore to hear a complaint by a dairy owner that the cows are not cycling should most likely be interpreted as someone on the dairy just isn't doing a very adequate job of detecting heats. This can be confirmed biologically by rectal palpation for the presence of corpora lutea and milk or serum progesterone sampling of some of the cows in question.

Heat detection efficiency (rate) is defined as the percentage of eligible cows that are actually seen or detected in heat. A detection rate of 70 to 80 per cent should be very achievable and adequate for a dairy farmer to meet the goals of reproductive efficiency. It would appear that

Table 3. *Heat Detection Observation Rates by Continuous Monitoring and by Casual Observation**

Continuous Video Recorder— 24 hr/day		Casual Visual Observation	
Ovulation	% Heats Detected	Ovulation	% Heats Detected
1st	50	1st	20
2nd	94	2nd	44
3rd	100	3rd	60

*King, G. J., Hurnick, J. F., and Robertson, H. A.: J. Anim. Sci. 42:688–692, 1976.

Table 4. *Parameters Used to Evaluate Heat Detection Efficiency*

Days in Milk (DIM) at First Breeding	(60–65 days)*
24-Day Heat Detection Rate	(80–85%)
% Cows Pregnant at Pregnancy Examination	(80–85%)
% Cows Detected in Heat by 60 Days Postpartum	(> 80%)
% Cows Artificially Inseminated by 90 Days Postpartum	(> 90%)

*Value in parentheses is the desired goal for that parameter.

the time of day and the quality of the time spent in heat detection are of critical importance. Early morning and late evening (when combined) are the 2 periods in a 24-hr day that yield a high percentage of detected heats.[4]

The parameters listed in Table 4 are used to evaluate heat detection efficiency. They have no bearing on conception (breeding) figures. These strictly measure the efficiency or rate at which cows were detected in estrus. If a cow isn't seen in heat, she will not receive an AI service and therefore will not affect conception rate figures. Inefficiency in heat detection will lead to an increased calving to conception interval and ultimately an increased CI.

The 24-Day Heat Detection Rate is an excellent method to use. This is one that the dairy owner can implement immediately to prove just how efficiently (or inefficiently in some cases) heats are being detected. In order for cows to be included in this list, they must meet several criteria. First, they should be 30 days or longer postpartum. Second, they should be free of any pathologic conditions, such as cystic ovaries, pyometra, ovarian adhesions, and so forth. And third, they shouldn't have received a breeding (pregnancy is a good reason for anestrus). The time interval will be over the next 24 days. What is wanted is a group of cows most likely to display estrus within the next 24 days. Some of these cows in fact will be serviced during that interval, which will exclude them from the next 24-day list. At the end of the 24-day period, the number of cows seen in standing heat is divided by the total number eligible to cycle. If there were 50 cows on the list (meeting the 3 criteria stated earlier), and only 15 were detected, the heat detection rate would be 30 per cent—not too good. If a dairy owner is willing to face the facts about heat detection, this is an excellent way, and it only takes 24 days at most to get some good feedback.

The Per cent Cows Pregnant at Pregnancy Examination is also a very good parameter for evaluating heat detection and can be rapidly calculated at the time of a veterinarian's routine reproduction visit. I have had a few challenges that this finding isn't really evaluating heat detection but rather conception efficiency. It's true that if 25 cows are presented to the veterinarian for pregnancy diagnosis (in this example the last recorded breeding date being 45 days ago) and only 5 are pregnant, then there is likely to also be a conception problem. But what about those 20 open cows that were serviced 45 days ago or longer? They had a chance to have 2 heats (assuming that early embryonic death is in the range of 10 to 12 per cent—early embryonic death in all 20 of the open cows would be begging the question). Those 20 cows would have been in estrus 21 days postbreeding and had there been adequate heat detection, would have been serviced (AI) and would not have been included on a list for pregnancy diagnosis because they would be too early to be eligible for diag-

nosis. Therefore, the Per cent Cows Pregnant at Pregnancy Examination is a good parameter by which to measure heat detection efficiency.

Conception Rate

There are 4 subfactors that directly affect breeding or conception rates, (1) heat detection accuracy, (2) technician competency, (3) bull fertility, and (4) herd (female) fertility.

Heat Detection Accuracy. This is defined as the percentage of cows in a true physiologic heat. Under conditions of natural service, the bull and cow will usually come to an understanding as to where she is in her estrous cycle and her sexual receptivity, but under conditions of AI she doesn't have any say in the matter. A cow incorrectly declared in heat will receive an AI service and quite obviously the chance of conception is zero when this error occurs. (It's difficult enough when she is truly in heat.)

On dairies where management is pushing labor very hard to catch more cows in heat, this may become a significant problem. Rather than running the risk of missing a cow in heat, dairy personnel may declare a cow in heat that is showing less than positive signs of estrus. In this case, the heat detection efficiency may climb into the 90 per cent range, and yet the accuracy drop into the 70 per cent range. This is followed by an increase in services per conception and a decrease in first service (or more) conception rate.

Technician Competency or Ability. This factor is probably the most significant major contributor affecting conception efficiency. Work by Darlington[5] and Senger and colleagues[6] demonstrated that conception rates varied by as much as 22 per cent among AI technicians, and ranked number 1 (out of the 6 factors) as the factor most affecting conception performance (Table 5). The AI technician's major responsibilities are related to the proper handling of the semen from time of removal from the semen tank to correct placement (location) in the cow. Temperature fluctuations, rough handling of the straw, ampule and loaded gun or pipette, and improper placement in the reproductive tract will all dramatically lower the conception rates.

Bull Fertility. Such a characteristic has been shown to have a significant impact on conception rates.[5-7] One shouldn't be lulled into thinking that each straw or ampule of semen from different bulls has the same fertility. Research by Davidson and Farver in California demonstrated quite dramatically that the first service conception rate can vary as much as 36 per cent among AI bulls (range 34 to 70 per cent).[7] The combining of a bull with low fertility and a marginal AI technician's ability can

Table 5. *Factors Affecting Conception Performance**

Factor	Value
1. Inseminators	22%
2. Bulls	15%
3. Cystic Ovaries Reduce Conception; and	8%
Increase Interval to First Breeding	20 days
4. Retained Placenta Reduces Conception	12%
5. Age of Cow	—
6. Severe Uterine Infection Reduces Conception	8%

*Darlington, R. L.: Proc. Ann. Mtg. Soc. Therio., 1981.

Table 6. *Parameters Used to Evaluate Conception Rates*

Parameter	Value
First Service Conception Rate	(50–55%)*
Services per Conception	(1.5–1.8)
% Cows Pregnant by 3 or Less Inseminations	(85–88%)
% Cows Returning for 4th or More Insemination	(< 15%)

*Value in parentheses is the desired goal for that parameter.

have a profound impact on conception rates. With less than accurate heat detection, the effect is even more acute.

Herd (Female) Fertility. This parameter is the one in which the veterinarian plays the most direct role and probably has the most influence. The emphasis is to have as many cows as possible cycling and free of reproductive disease when they enter the breeding period. The major emphasis here is for the dairy owner to have an established ongoing reproductive program with a veterinarian to ensure that all cows are examined early, 21 to 35 days postpartum, to detect and to treat correctable reproductive problems, and also to identify that small percentage of cows that may have irreparable pathologic conditions of the genital tract. Not only is it important for cows to be free of reproductive diseases (ovarian cysts, endometritis, pyometras, and so forth), but the resumption of cyclic activity in the first 30 days postpartum has been shown to have a significantly positive effect on fertility.[3]

The parameters listed in Table 6 are used to measure and to evaluate conception rates. They will only indicate that there is a problem related to conceptions—they will not indicate which of the 4 is contributing to breeding inefficiency or failures. Also note that conditions influencing heat detection rates will not affect conception rates (and vice versa). For example, a situation could exist where heat detection efficiency is extremely poor—only 10 per cent of the heats are detected, and yet services per conception are 1.3 or 1.4. Not many cows are being detected, but the few that are detected are truly in estrus and being inseminated properly.

Even though I discourage using only 1 or 2 parameters to assess a reproductive problem, the use of Days Open and Services per Conception can be another initial starting point. For example, if Services per Conception are relatively low at 2.2 or less and Days Open are greater than 120, then one should be suspicious of inadequate heat detection. Should Services per Conception be 2.5 or greater, then further investigation is needed to determine which subfactor or combination of subfactors affecting conception rates is contributing to the conception problem.

Table 7 summarizes the major factors and subfactors affecting reproductive efficiency and lists the parameters used. The characteristics shown are not intended to be the only ones to be considered when evaluating reproductive performance. Should one choose to add to this list, it's important that critical evaluation be given as to which of the 3 groupings the new parameter would be added. Choosing 1 category (heat detection efficiency, conception rates, or magnitude evaluation (middle) category) will eliminate confusion and allow for better organization as to the problem.

MONITORING OF INFERTILITY

Many of the parameters (CI, Days Open, First Service Conception Rate, Services per Conception, and Per cent Cows Pregnant by 3 or less Inseminations) help evaluate

Table 8. *Parameters Used to Evaluate Cows That Fail to Meet the Reproductive Goals*

Parameter	Value
% Cows Open Greater than 150 days	(< 10%)*
% Cows Returning for 4th or More AI Service	(< 15%)
% Annual Culling for Infertility	(< 6%)
HRS Index	(> 65)

*Value in parentheses is the desired goal for that parameter.

Table 7. *Factors Affecting Dairy Herd Reproductive Efficiency*

Heat Detection Efficiency	Conception Rates

Frequency of Observation
  Dawn, Noon, and Evening, 86%
Time Spent in Observation
  20–30 min/corral
Use of aids or devices in heat detection, i.e.,
  chalking tailhead, Kmar patches,
  androgenized cows, penis-deviated bulls
	Heat Detection Accuracy
	  Timing of Insemination
	Technician Competency
	  Insemination Technique (Location)
	  Semen Handling Procedures
	Bull Fertility
	Herd Fertility—Veterinary Program
	  Resolution of cystic ovaries, endometritis,
	  and pyometra

Parameters Used to Evaluate Heat Detection Efficiency*	Parameters Affected by Either Heat Detection Efficiency or Conception Rates or Both	Parameters Used to Evaluate Conception Rates

Days in Milk at 1st Breeding
  (60–65 days)
24-Day Heat Detection Rate
  (80–85%)
% Cows Pregnant at Pregnancy Examination
  (80–85%)
% Cows Detected in Heat by 60 days
  (> 80%)
% Cows Inseminated by 90 days
  (>90%)
	Calving Interval
	  (12.4–12.7 mo)
	Days Open (95–105 days)
	
	% of Herd Diagnosed Pregnant per Month
	  (8–9%)
	Days in Milk
	  (160–175 days)
	HRS Index (> 65)
	% Cows Open Greater than 150 days
	  (<10%)
	% Annual Culling for Infertility (<6%)
		1st Service Conception Rate
		  (50–55%)
		Services per Conception
		  (1.5–1.8)
		% Cows Pregnant by 3 or Less Inseminations
		  (85–88%)
		% Cows Returning for 4th or More
		  Inseminations
		  (< 15%)

*Value in parentheses is the desired goal for that parameter.

the performance of cows that conceive and eventually calve. Table 8 lists 4 parameters used to evaluate the reproductive failures in a herd. A cow may eventually conceive, but because she falls outside of the limits established to maintain a 13 month or less CI she must be considered a reproductive failure.

One must accept the fact that there is always going to be a small percentage of cows that will be infertile, but as long as that percentage remains small, it will be tolerable. When the actual observed figures exceed the ones stated in Table 8, then concern and investigation as to the causes are needed.

INFLUENCE OF HEAT DETECTION RATE ON REPRODUCTIVE PERFORMANCE

In the previous discussion, it's been shown that maintaining a high level of heat detection and conception efficiency are absolutely necessary for optimum reproductive performance. Even though both factors are extremely important, does one factor such as Heat Detection Rate have more of an influence on reproductive efficiency than conception (breeding) efficiency? The answer is yes. Research by Barr demonstrated quite conclusively that Heat Detection Rate had a greater influence on Days Open (and ultimately on CI) than did conception rates.[8] In his study, there was a 92 per cent correlation between days lost due to heat detection failure (missed heat cycles) and days open. There was only a 38 per cent correlation between days lost due to conception failure and days open. Even though both factors are very important in maintaining optimal reproductive efficiency, heat detection plays a greater role in influencing days open than does services per conception (conception rate).

A formula (Table 9) was devised for computing days lost due to missed heats:[8]

Missed Heats (In Days) = Days Open − Voluntary Waiting Period (to start breeding cows) − ½ Heat Cycle (the average time to the next heat beyond the voluntary waiting period) − [(Services/Conception − 1) × 21]

This last part of the formula computes the days lost due to conception failure beyond the first service. Voluntary Waiting Period (VWP), ½ Heat Cycle (11 days), and days lost due to conception failure are all days for which a cow is open and can be accounted (see Table 10 for calculations). In the example in Table 10, 86 days can be accounted for, yet the days open are 149—there are 63 days which cannot be accounted for. Those 63 days represent days lost due to missed heat periods. Dividing

Table 9. *A Formula for Determining Missed Heats**

Missed Heats (in days) = Days Open
− Voluntary Waiting Period
− ½ Heat Cycle (11 days is the average time to the next heat beyond the voluntary waiting period)
− [(Services/Conception − 1) × 21]

(This accounts for days lost owing to conception failure by determining the services required beyond one, then multiplied by 21, the days normally required for a cycle.)

*Barr, H. L.: J. Dairy Sci. *58*:246–247, 1975.

Table 10. *Sample Calculation Using Missed Heats Formula**

Equation
Missed Heats = Days Open − Voluntary Waiting Period (VWP) − ½ Heat Cycle − [(Services/Conception − 1) × 21].

Example

Days Open	= 149 days
VWP	= 50 days
½ Heat Cycle	= 11 days (constant)
Services per Conception	= 2.2

Calculations
Missed Heats = 149 − 50 − 11 − [(2.2 − 1) × 21]
= 149 − 50 − 11 − 25
= 149 − 86
= 63 days
63 days ÷ 21 (length of heat cycle) = 3.0 missed heat cycles

Heat Cycles Accounted For
2.2 Heat Cycles from Services per Conception (observed)
3.0 Heat Cycles from Missed Heats (failed to observe)
—————
5.2 Total Heat Cycles

$$\text{\% Heats Missed} = \frac{3.0}{5.2} = 58\% \text{ of Heat Cycles Missed}$$

$$\text{\% Heats Detected} = \frac{2.2}{5.2} = 42\% \text{ of Heat Cycles Detected}$$

*In this example days lost owing to conception failure = 25 days; days lost owing to missed heats = 63 days.

63 by 21 days (average length of a heat cycle in the cow) converts days lost into cycles missed, which is 3 heats. Since services per conception are 2.2, it can be assumed that those 2.2 services per conception also represent 2.2 heats that were detected. Knowing now that there were 3.0 heats missed and 2.2 heats detected, gives a total number of heats possible of 5.2. Between day 50 (the beginning of the breeding period) and day 149 (the average days open) there were a potential total of 5.2 heats of which only 2.2 were detected. When stated in a percentage (2.2 ÷ 5.2 × 100), only 42 per cent of the heats were detected.

When comparing the days lost due to conception failure (25 days) and the days lost due to missed heats (63 days) in this example, there are more than twice as many days lost owing to heat detection failure than are lost owing to conception failure.

There are several limitations to the described formula that need to be clarified. First, the formula assumes that *all* cows will be cycling on or very shortly after the Voluntary Waiting Period. This isn't so, as there are a variety of conditions causing a small percentage (about 10 per cent) of cows to be truly anestrus. Secondly, the formula doesn't account for early embryonic deaths, which may have a small affect in appearing to contribute to an increase in days lost owing to missed heats. Thirdly, the formula assumes that the services per conception translate directly into accurate detection of heat. If heat detection accuracy were less than expected resulting in higher services per conception, then conception failure (days lost) would appear to contribute more than expected to days open. Even though these factors are not accounted for in the formula, the general trend shown by the calculated results is very meaningful. It can be used to illustrate where days are lost (from both conception failure and missed heats), the contribution of each to days open, and the relative efficiency of heat detection.

SUMMARY

Dairy practitioners of today need to be more than highly skilled technicians who have cows hanging off the end of their arms for 3 to 4 hr each morning. The actual reproductive examination, be it pregnancy, routine post-partum, or problem cow, is a data gathering technique. It's important for veterinarians to also understand and use the reproductive performance data that are available to them through a variety of sources.

The veterinarian needs to spend extra time in consultation with and giving advice to dairy owners concerning the level and progress of the herd's reproductive efficiency. While it is generally agreed that intensified dairy herd management has concurrently intensified reproductive problems, I fully realize the problems are usually subtle, often multifactorial, and sometimes politically difficult to deal with.

I also feel strongly that the practicing veterinarian is in a pivotal position for evaluating and advising the dairy owner as well as having a very positive influence on achieving efficient reproductive performance.

As important as hormones, drugs, and other medications are in assisting the veterinarian in a reproductive program, it is hoped that all those involved realize it is the human, and not necessarily the cow, who is often the major contributor to less than optimal reproductive efficiency.

References

1. Thatcher, W. W., and Wilcox, C. J.: Postpartum estrus as an indicator of reproductive status in the dairy cow. J. Dairy Sci. 56:608, 1973.
2. King, G. J., Hurnik, J. F., and Robertson, H. A.: Ovarian function and estrus in dairy cows during early lactation. J. Anim. Sci. 42:688, 1976.
3. Stevenson, J. S., and Call, E. P.: Influence of early estrus, ovulation and insemination on fertility in postpartum Holstein cows. Theriogenology 19:367, 1983.
4. Beerwinkle, L. G.: Heat Detection Programs and Techniques. Proc. National Assoc. Anim. Breeders. Eighth Conference on Artificial Insemination of Beef Cattle, 1974.
5. Darlington, R. L.: Research Summary of Factors Affecting Conception to First Service in Dairy Cows. Part III: Clinical Factors—Cystic Ovaries, Retained Placenta, Uterine Infections and Milk Fever. Proc. Ann. Meet. Soc. Theriogenology, 1981.
6. Senger, P. L., Hillers, J. K., Mitchell, J. R., et al.: Research Summary of Factors Affecting Conception to First Service in Dairy Cows. Part I: Bulls, Inseminators and Semen Quality. Proc. Ann. Meet. Soc. Theriogenology, 1981.
7. Davidson, J. N., and Farver, T. B.: Conception rates of Holstein bulls for artificial insemination on a California dairy. J. Dairy Sci. 63:621, 1980.
8. Barr, H. L.: Influence of estrus detection on days open in dairy herds. J. Dairy Sci. 58:246, 1975.

Breeding Season Evaluation of Beef Herds

MARK F. SPIRE, D.V.M., M.S.

A good beef cow and calf health program, while having many facets, should focus on the reproductive efficiency of the herd and have as its objective the improvement of the overall reproductive performance. The program should evaluate factors influencing the per cent calf crop, birth dates of the calves, and calf growth rates, i.e., factors that potentially influence the total pounds of calf weaned per cow. Failure of cows to display estrus and conceive early during the breeding season continues to be the major source of the reduction in pounds of calves weaned. Therefore, a major emphasis should be placed on a productive breeding season that results not only in a high pregnancy rate but also produces a tightly bred set of cows, which calve over a short period of time. The evaluation of the breeding season can be incorporated into a health program as a management technique. A breeding season evaluation should be flexible enough to evaluate the overall herd reproductive profile as well as the individual cow reproductive profile, bull performance, replacement heifer development, and herd nutrition.

Breeding season evaluations could become a forum for the exchange of management information between clients and veterinarians. The veterinarian should assume a role of responsible participation in the beef herd operation. Components of the evaluation can be outlined by the veterinarian into a workable format for an individual herd. A basic set of guidelines for the breeding season evaluation includes (1) herd reproductive information, (2) analysis of the reproductive information, (3) professional interpretation of the information, and (4) a decision or management position developed between the client and the veterinarian. This type of approach affords a systematic breakdown.

HERD INFORMATION

Herd information can be obtained from a herd survey provided by the veterinarian, records of actual calving dates provided by the owner, or records obtained from pregnancy examinations in which projected calving dates are made by the veterinarian. The recording of herd information generally must be encouraged by veterinarians, and their input into the establishment of a brief, concise record system must be made. The resulting record system can be used to analyze the progress or lack of progress in various phases of the overall breeding program and also can be used as a permanent data baseline.

The herd survey is primarily for new herds from which little previous reproductive information is available. Basic inputs (Fig. 1) should detail proportional breeding female ages, breed percentages, breeding season, basic feeding programs, and possible calf crop losses. This type survey becomes a starting point in determining reproductive problems and also serves as a primary data base.

Actual calving dates offer a look at factual information since they are obtained from calvings. This information shows the number of noncalving cows, the breeding pattern of the herd, the relative breeding dates of different age groups of cows and can be used to project calf growth. A disadvantage of the use of actual calving dates is a low probability of diagnosis of an infectious agent that causes early embryonic death or fetal loss. Other disadvantages are loss of identity of pasture breeding groups and loss of identity of bull placements. Waiting to evaluate the program until the end of calving season using this system delays the opportunity to correct nutritional problems prior to the next breeding season.

Projected calving dates from pregnancy examinations obtained 60 to 90 days after the breeding season have the potential to offer a systematic herd evaluation. By dating

1. From your spring calving herd, when was your first calf born this year?

   _____Approximately what percentage of your spring calves were born within 3 weeks of this calf? _____

   When was your last spring calf born this year? _____

2. Do you individually identify calves at birth? _____

3. How do you decide which cows will be culled from your herd? _____

4. How many heifers _____, cows _____, and total females _____were exposed to a bull last year?

5. How many calves did you wean last year? _____

6. Did you notice any bull problems last year? Yes _____No _____If yes, what kind of problem? _____

   _____

   Was breeding delayed from normal? Yes _____No _____

7. What vaccinations did you use last year on your:

   Cows _____

   Replacement heifers _____

   Calves _____

8. Did you pregnancy check last year? _____If so, how many heifers _____, cows _____, total herd _____were pregnant?

9. Do you provide extra feed in winter for:

   Open heifers? _____

   Young cows? _____

   Old cows? _____

10. Do you purchase replacement females?

    None _____Open heifers _____Bred heifers _____Open cows _____Bred cows _____

Figure 1. A partial example of a herd reproductive survey used for new clients.

the length of gestation at palpation, an estimate can be obtained on cyclic activity and conception during the previous breeding season. Estimated breeding values for the entire herd as well as individual evaluation of late breeding or open cows can be obtained. Detection of problems is made easier since such factors as breeding age variation, individual pasture differences, individual bull or bull battery performance, and losses due to disease can be observed prior to calving. Projected calving dates also allow time for nutritional management decisions to be made before the next breeding season, thus enhancing management potential. The primary disadvantages are individual palpator variances, actual calving date variances, and palpations preceding late gestational fetal losses. Basic information recorded at pregnancy examination on an individual cow should include date of palpation, cow's identification number, age, breed, condition, and estimated days pregnant. Additional data are breeding pasture and bull or bull battery identification. This information can be obtained and recorded at "chute side" the day a particular group of breeding females is processed.

ANALYSIS

The figures obtained by using a projected calving date system can be analyzed through 2 criteria. The first is by total breeding percentage, i.e., group pregnancy rates.

This is the traditional primary criterion used in evaluating the success of the breeding season. The total breeding percentage reflects the reproductive performance of the overall herd. Further grouping of information can be made to analyze breeding efficiency by cow age groups, by condition scores, and by pasture or bull batteries. The second criterion is the period breeding percentage, which is based upon pregnancy rates by 21-day intervals throughout the breeding season. This helps analyze the availability of cows for breeding based on defined intervals. The primary emphasis should be placed on factors that influence the first 21-day breeding interval, primarily the percentage of cows cycling at the start of the breeding season. Cow age, postpartum interval, and cow condition affect this percentage.

A workable format that can be presented to the client includes bar graphs (Fig. 2) depicting the percentage of pregnancy rates on the vertical axis and the breeding season interval on the horizontal axis. The sum total of the per cent of pregnant cows on the horizontal axis yields the total breeding percentage. This graphic depiction of the breeding season allows both pictorial and written data to be easily presented to the producer.

The actual percentages obtained from each year's herd should be compared with the goals previously established by the owner and the veterinarian. Commonly used figures are a 95 per cent pregnancy rate in a 63-day breeding period with 70 per cent of the pregnancies within the first 21 days for mature cows, and 81 per cent pregnancy rates after a 42-day breeding period for replacement heifers.

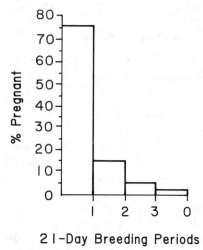

Figure 2. Bar graph of a breeding season evaluation analysis depicting the percentage of pregnancy rates in relation to the 21-day breeding periods.

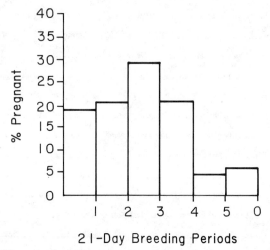

Figure 3. The effects of inadequate group nutrition resulting in a prolonged breeding season and low pregnancy rates per breeding interval.

These figures generally can only be reached by developing an intense reproductive program, which emphasizes rigid culling criteria, early postpartum estrual activity, development of an excellent replacement heifer program, and timely nutritional management. Failure to reach these goals results in losses of marketable product evidenced by declining weaning weights per cow exposed to breeding.

INTERPRETATION

Any downward shift in total pregnancy rates or any shift towards late-period breeding percentages from the established goals indicates reproductive management problems within the herd. When changes in these parameters are noted, the interpretation should be based upon research, diagnoses, and experience. Management recommendations are founded on the information gathered and implemented to prevent the recurrence of problems in subsequent breeding seasons.

In established herd programs, a reduction in overall total breeding percentages from previous years can reflect reduced bull fertility, inadequate group nutrition (Fig. 3), disease conditions caused by *Campylobacter* or *Hemophilus somnus,* or combinations of any of these factors. In a herd not on a routine program, a low total breeding percentage often accompanies an extended breeding season (Fig. 4). Management decisions, such as starting routine bull evaluation, nutritional consultation, and the initiation or modification of vaccination programs, can be made based on facts. This is a rational and knowledgeable approach to herd consultation.

A rise in the percentage of open cows or early pregnant cows at pregnancy examination offers the practitioner an opportunity to evaluate reproductive tracts and general condition of the cows, and to collect diagnostic samples for evaluation of common reproductive diseases. The difficulty of diagnosing the causes of early gestational losses increases as the time from breeding increases. This fact emphasizes the need to evaluate open cows thoroughly when the total breeding percentage fails to reach the established goal for the herd.

The grouping of cows to breed early and thus to calve early in the subsequent season influences the total pounds of beef produced by raising the average number of days from birth to weaning. Decline in the number of pregnancies during the first 21 days of the breeding season is generally influenced by the percentage of cows exhibiting estrus at the start of the breeding season as well as bull fertility. There are several factors, such as age, milk production, and precalving body condition, that influence early postpartum estrual activity, and their influence can be evaluated in the interpretive phase of the program.

Cow condition at calving (a reflection of group nutrition) has a significant influence on return to estrual activity. Cows in poor body condition have a delayed return to estrus compared with cows in good body condition. Studies of cow condition at pregnancy examination have shown a significant reduction in days pregnant as body condition scores decrease (Table 1). Low pre-calving energy levels have been shown to lengthen the time interval from calving to onset of post-calving estrual activity. Management recommendations can be made to

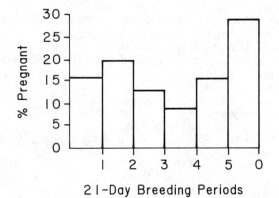

Figure 4. Results of a study of 50 yearling heifers not on a routine reproductive program that were developed on an inadequate nutritional program. Note the extended breeding season and high percentage of open cows. (From Proceedings of Annual Meeting, Society for Theriogenology, 1983.)

Table 1. *Influence of Body Condition on Rebreeding in 2 Kansas Cow Herds Under Routine Reproductive Programs**

Condition Score at Palpation	Total Number of Heads	Mean Gestation Length at Palpation (days, P < 0.05)
5	119	128
4	333	114
3	38	105

*From Proceedings of the Annual Meeting, Society for Theriogenology, 1983.

place cows in less than adequate condition at the time of pregnancy examination into a separate group and then improve nutrient levels to allow a gain in condition prior to calving. In addition, the energy levels should be elevated 50 to 100 days prior to calving thus reducing the effects of low prepartum energy on postpartum estrual activity.

Late calving and heavy lactating cows with a short postpartum period tend not to show estrual activity at the start of the subsequent breeding season and have lower conception rates if estrual activity does occur. In herds with longer than a 60-day breeding season, pregnancy rates are lower the first 21 days of the breeding season owing to an inadequate number of postpartum cycling cows. Correction should be aimed towards culling late calving cows and adding replacements that are bred to calve early. This will place emphasis on the selection of early calving females that will, in turn, lengthen the interval from calving to projected breeding and lessen the influence of suckling suppression on the return to postcalving estrual activity.

The effect of the age of the dam on subsequent rebreeding performance is frequently observed in intensified management programs. First-calf cows, 2 years of age, are particularly influenced, as evidenced by delayed onset of postcalving estrual activity and a lengthened postpartum interval. Mean gestational times at pregnancy evaluation are frequently shorter in this group of cows (Table 2). Additionally, the effects of dystocia in young cows have a negative influence on the percentage of cows cycling at the start of the breeding season and on subsequent pregnancy rates. Allowing this age group of cows a longer postpartum period by starting the breeding season 1 to 3 weeks ahead of the herd's breeding season will tend to allow 2-year-old heifers to fall into a comparable breeding pattern with the adult herd after their second breeding season. Additionally, the management of 2- to 3-year-old cows as a separate group from the adult herd will lessen grazing competition and allow young cows to

Table 2. *Influence of Age on Rebreeding in a Kansas Cow Herd Under a Routine Reproductive Program**

Age of Cow (years)	Total Number of Heads	Mean Gestation Length at Palpation (days)
1	62	135 (P < 0.01)
2	65	122 (P < 0.01)
3	12	134 (P < 0.1)
4–8	75	131 (P < 0.1)
9+	40	137 (p < 0.01)

*From Proceedings of the Annual Meeting, Society for Theriogenology, 1983.

reach their full reproductive potential prior to 4 to 5 years of age, as is frequently observed when all age groups are maintained in 1 breeding group.

DECISION OR MANAGEMENT POSITIONS

The first 3 components of a breeding season evaluation, e.g., herd information, analysis, and interpretation, give an overall performance evaluation of the herd in question. Careful interpretation of such data can allow the veterinarian to define areas of reproductive inefficiency in the herd. Management procedures to reduce the economic pressures of these inefficiencies can then be implemented. In most instances, advice from the veterinarian can be strengthened through the use of its direct and indirect influence on herd economics. Changes in management programs, such as nutrition, replacement development, bull evaluation, disease control, and culling of low productive cows can be implemented based on current economic losses by projecting the costs of modifying the current program and the resultant expected return on investment.

These herd management changes can be conveyed to the producer either verbally or in writing. Written documentation can be accumulated from year to year and will aid in the evaluation of the overall performance of the reproductive management program.

Developing a reproductive-based health program takes time. The degree of success of a program depends upon the experience of veterinarians, their willingness to continue learning animal husbandry techniques, their communication skills, and their commitment to marketing expertise. The greater economic pressures experienced by producers necessitate efficient reproductive management to achieve optimal performance in their herds. Through the use of management tools such as a breeding season evaluation, a veterinarian can offer additional services to clients that will allow an expansion into a herd management consultation role.

Supplemental Reading

Bellows, R. A., and Short, R. E.: Effects of precalving feed level on birth weight, calving difficulty, and subsequent fertility. J. Anim. Sci. *46*:1522–1528, 1978.

Burfening, P. J.: Effect of nutrition on future reproduction. Proc. Soc. Therio. Spokane, 63–77, 1981.

Wiltbank, J. N., and Spitzer, J. C.: Recent research on controlled reproduction in beef cattle. World Anim. Rev. *27*:30–35, 1978.

Breeding Management Problems in Sheep and Goats

RANDALL S. OTT, D.V.M., M.S.

Effective management of reproduction in sheep and goats is essential to the profitability of livestock enterprises utilizing these species. To help achieve the goal of effective reproduction management, a knowledge of basic reproductive characteristics is needed along with a general knowledge of those areas in which the veterinary practitioner can provide assistance to breeders and producers.

SHEEP

A program to maximize reproductive efficiency in sheep would encompass proper breed selection, ram breeding soundness evaluation, proper mating system, adequate nutrition program, an effective disease prevention program, and pregnancy testing.

Breeds vary in prolificacy. Selection of a productive breed that is adaptable to a particular environmental and management situation is an important consideration. Crossbred dams have been shown to have production advantages over purebreds; therefore, programs for maximum lamb production will most likely utilize a crossbred system.

As a service for clients, the fitness of individual rams and bucks may be assessed for breeding purposes. Highly fertile rams can increase lamb crops by causing conception in more ewes and by fertilizing more ova per ewe. Breeding soundness examinations can be valuable to help diagnose breeding problems in the flock. Finding that the males are satisfactory breeders may "rule out" this parameter and cause one to look for infections, infertility in the ewes, nutritional deficiencies, and so forth. Many times breeding soundness examinations may confirm a suspected case of male infertility and may allow the owner to receive compensation or a replacement animal from the seller if the ram is under warranty. One of the most important traits of the breeding ram is scrotal circumference, which is positively related to sperm production. Guidelines for breeding soundness examinations of rams are available from the Society for Theriogenology.

Most ewes are bred by natural service although selective or hand mating and artificial insemination are used in certain situations. A suggested mating system for maximum ewe fertility is the use of 3 rams in each breeding unit. It has been shown that significantly more ewes are detected in estrus when 3 rams are together rather than alone. Breeding pastures should be large enough so that dominant rams do not prevent subordinate rams from mating. A limit of 50 ewes/ram is recommended. Rams are frequently harnessed with tupping crayons so that ewes that have been served by the ram can be identified. The crayon color can be changed every 14 to 15 days. Introduction of the ram to the breeding flock at the beginning of the breeding season can result in partial synchrony of ovulation in the ewes several days later. Sheep tend to ovulate without showing overt signs of estrus, whereas goats have been reported to exhibit signs of estrus without ovulation at the beginning of the breeding season.

An average of 2 to 6 matings per estrus is reported, and when more than 1 ram is present, multiple sire matings occur. Males with good libido may mate 20 to 30 times a day. The duration of estrus in the ewe ranges from 10 to 40 hr with an average of about 24 hr. The length of the estrous cycle in sheep is 16 to 17 days. Ewes in estrus actively seek the ram. The need to learn how to find and successfully compete for the ram is thought to account for the poor performance of maiden ewes in pasture mating.

A common practice in sheep breeding is to flush the ewes just before and during the breeding season. Flushing ewes is thought to stimulate more ovulations during the early and late breeding season but is probably of little benefit during the middle of the season. Failure to meet energy requirements during gestation may result in pregnancy toxemia (ketosis) in late gestation in ewes or does carrying more than 1 offspring.

Early born ewe lambs can cycle and conceive in their first breeding season. Bringing ewe lambs into production as early as possible can decrease maintenance costs before the start of production and increase lifetime production. In order to accomplish early breeding, lambs must be large enough (65 per cent of mature weight is suggested) and in good condition. Age at puberty varies greatly among breeds. Female offspring from rams selected for large scrotal circumference reach puberty at a significantly younger age than female offspring from rams with small testes.

Care should be taken that animals added to the flock come from herds in which owners practice disease control. A program of reproductive disease prevention would include strict sanitation, early diagnosis of disease, and proper vaccination programs.

Determination of pregnancy in ewe lambs enables the nonpregnant ones to be culled and marketed while they can still command slaughter lamb prices. Use of transrectal Doppler and "real time" ultrasonography have been reported to be accurate methods of pregnancy testing in sheep. Although other methods are available, such as serum progesterone determinations, radiography, and vaginal biopsies, they are not considered practical or economical for general use at this time.

DAIRY GOATS

An important cause of infertility in dairy goats is the intersex condition or hermaphrodism. Female hermaphrodites may have a normal size vulva but an enlarged clitoris and a short or atretic vagina. A penile clitoris or even an ovotestis may occur in does that otherwise appear phenotypically female. Both hermaphrodism and congenital hypoplasia of the reproductive tract are found in naturally hornless (polled) goats and are more likely to occur when both parents are polled.

Selective or hand mating is the usual practice in dairy goat herds. It is not desirable to allow odorous bucks to run free with milking does. The duration of estrus in does is 32 to 40 hr. Does are usually mated with the buck at the onset of estrus and at 12-hr intervals until estrus subsides. In artificial insemination, the doe is inseminated when she first accepts mounting by a teaser buck and, again, 12 hr later.

Proper detection of estrus is the most important aspect of goat breeding when either hand mating or artificial insemination is practiced. Does actively seek the presence of the buck when in estrus. Bucks are sometimes descented at the time of dehorning by burning and destroying the odor glands located posteriorly and medially to the horn buds. This is probably a bad practice as does, when given a choice, will usually prefer a scented buck to a deodorized one. The mere presence of a buck may initiate and even synchronize the cyclic activity of does early in the breeding season.

Detection of estrus in does is best accomplished with the use of a buck. An intact buck may be penned in an area where does in heat can be spotted congregating near the pen. Bucks with breeding aprons, vasectomized bucks, testosterone injections of does, wethers, hermaphrodites, or bucks that have undergone penis deviations or preputial closures (teasers) may be used to aid estrus detection.

Signs of estrus in does are tail wagging, bleating, and urinating near the buck. There is some swelling of the vulva and mucous discharge. The reaction of the buck to the doe being teased is an indication of estrus in the does. Some does show few signs of estrus other than limited tail wagging and standing for mounting by the buck, and these signs are only present after teasing. Does will occasionally stand for mounting by other does; however, the level of homosexual activity in goats is low in reproductively normal females.

Length of the estrous cycle in dairy goats is usually 20 days. Abnormally short (5 to 8 days) estrous cycles may occur in does early in the breeding season. Cystic ovaries are thought to occur in dairy goats, although the inability to palpate the ovaries by rectal examination makes diagnosis difficult. Treatments that have been suggested are gonadotropin injections at one fourth of the bovine dose.

Retained fetal membranes and metritis may also occur. Intravenous broad-spectrum antibiotic therapy can be used for does with acute infection and elevated temperature. False pregnancy may occur in the doe with a large volume of clear fluid being passed at "parturition."

CONTROL OF REPRODUCTION IN SHEEP AND GOATS

A fundamental consideration in both species is the seasonal restraint of breeding. Sheep and goats are considered "short day breeders" as they initiate reproductive activity in response to decreasing length of daylight. Both are classified as seasonally polyestrous and usually stop estrus as the result of either pregnancy or the end of the breeding season.

Control of the time of breeding allows control of the time of lambing and kidding and control of milk production in does. Progestagens have been the most widely used agents for ovulation control. Fluorogestrone acetate has been administered by the intravaginal route using an impregnated polyurethane sponge. The vaginal pessaries are left in place for 14 days in sheep and for 21 days in goats and are followed by an injection of PMSG (pregnant mare's serum gonadotrophin) at the time of removal. Some success in accelerated lambing has been achieved using hormone therapy.

Prostaglandin $F_{2\alpha}$ or one of its analogues will induce luteolysis in the cycling ewe or doe during the breeding season. Estrous synchronization is of interest in goats as a tool that might facilitate artificial insemination. A 2-injection scheme of prostaglandin $F_{2\alpha}$ administered 11 days apart has been used for estrous synchronization of cycling does in research trials giving excellent fertility. A dose of 2.5 mg has been shown to be adequate for estrus induction in the doe. In sheep, dosages ranging from 6 to 15 mg have been used for estrus induction. However, fertility at the induced estrus has been reported to be reduced by some workers.

Control of the time of parturition in sheep and goats enables closer supervision of lambing and kidding during planned periods when labor could be used more efficiently. In one study, dexamethasone (16 mg) administered to ewes on day 143 of gestation resulted in lambs on days 144 to 146 with the largest litters being delivered

earliest. The use of exogenous prostaglandin has been demonstrated to be the drug of choice to induce parturition in the goat. In a recent study, does receiving either 2.5 mg or 5.0 mg prostaglandin $F_{2\alpha}$ on day 144 gave birth to kids within 28 to 57 hr. Retained fetal membranes have not been reported to be associated with induced parturition in ewes or in does.

A number of factors including light, temperature, and the presence of the male influence the seasonality of the estrous cycle. However, effects of the photoperiod are felt to be the most important. Control of the photoperiod with artificial lighting has received much attention in research with sheep but not much application in either sheep or goats. In the United States, the breeding season for sheep and goats generally extends from August to February, and both breed differences and geographic area account for wide variations. Some goat dairies have practiced exposing breeding animals to total darkness for 17 hr daily after the beginning of June to induce early onset of cycling. There is interest in developing breeds and strains in both species that under proper management might reproduce without seasonal restrictions, allowing accelerated lambing in sheep and year-round milk production in goats.

Supplemental Reading

Guss, S. B.: Management and Diseases of Dairy Goats. Scottsdale, Arizona, Dairy Goat Journal Publishing Corporation, 1977.
Ott, R. S.: Dairy Goat Reproduction. The Compendium on Continuing Education. Pract. Vet. 4:S164–S172, 1982.
Ott, R. S., and Memon, M. A.: Sheep and Goat Manual. Nebraska, Society for Theriogenology, 1980.

Use of some treatment regimens described in this article lack official regulatory approval. Refer to label instructions for proper usage.

Breeding Management Problems in Swine

THOMAS A. POWE, D.V.M., M.S.

Since the 1960s, the swine industry has emphasized greater production from larger numbers of swine, in smaller areas, at the shortest possible time, and on the most economical ration. This push for greater productivity has eliminated the pig's ability to alter its environment and maintain its natural physiologic and social functions. In order to meet the demands of the industry on the veterinarian, something more than mere culture testing and serologic testing must be done. Many of the swine's health problems are noninfectious and are related to breeding animal selection, environment, production goals, and how management operates the unit.

Solving breeding problems, of infectious or noninfectious origin, requires a sound approach to identifying the problems and differentiating the potential causes. Many check lists have been suggested, but each individual's needs will differ. However, the basic information is similar and includes the following:

1. Number, age, grouping, feeding, and housing of animals directly involved and of all animals in other phases of the life cycle in the unit.

Table 1. *Reproductive Problems Related to Management Procedures*

Problem	Cause	Normal	Abnormal	Treatment	Prevention	Remarks
Anestrus						
Gilts	Age	5½–6½ mo	7+ mo	Move and mix Put in presence of boar	Select breeding animals from early maturing animals	Fast growing, low backfat animals tend to be slower maturing
	Genetics		Up to 10% of all swine will have anatomic or hormonal defects		Close culling	
	Season	July, August, September	Other months with extreme cold periods or low energy diet	None	Schedule breeding of gilts for other season	Providing shade and cooling has not eliminated the problem
	Nutrition					
	Protein	14–15%	11–12%	Correct diet	Same as treatment	Flushing is of value with poor or borderline diets; of little value with good diets.
	Carbohydrate	3–4 lb	2 lb or less			
	Housing			Well ventilated (continuous air movement); < 75° F; humidity < 70%; adequate space with sight or sound exposure to boar	Same as treatment	Postweaning overcrowding delays puberty
Sows	Early weaning	21–35 days	< 21 days		High energy diets during lactation	Sows must have positive energy balance before estrus will occur; lactating sow may cycle on good diet
	Season				Schedule breeding	Extreme cold and heat may affect sows but not to the extent of gilts
Cystic ovaries	Continued recycling, conception fails to occur after several breedings					Treatment is of limited value; recommend culling
Repeat breeders	Infertile boar	10–20%	(See Remarks)		Reserve boar power	Examine boars when large numbers or all females recycle
	Heat detection and timing of breeding	Ovulation occurs 30 ± 9 hr after onset of estrus				For best results breeding should occur 30 ± 9 hr of onset of estrus
	Hormonal and anatomic deficits	10%			Culling	
	Zearalanone				Remove from diet	First sign may be seen in newborn; enlarged vulva and nipples at birth

Table continued on opposite page

Table 1. *Reproductive Problems Related to Management Procedures* Continued

Problem	Cause	Normal	Abnormal	Treatment	Prevention	Remarks
Resorption, abortion, mummies	Usually infection			See specific disease		
Stillbirth	Infection	3–6%	7–9%	See specific disease		
	Nutrition					
	Energy	3–4 lb during gestation	Full feed		Management of feed intake during gestation; feeding individually	Overfat female; prolonged labor; fat in the diet of sows and gilts increases viability of pigs
	Low calcium	16 gm/day		Injectable calcium at farrowing: slowly 1 ml/4 lb IV	Dietary intake	Aids in uterine contraction; may reduce need for cesarean section
	Prolonged labor	Total labor 3–3.5 hr; average 13–18 min between pigs	Total labor in excess of 4 hr; average 45–55 min between pigs	Assist farrowing	Use of Pg F$_{2\alpha}$ (10 mg); oxytoxin, 40 units after 4th or 5th piglet	85–90% farrowing within 36 hr of Pg F$_{2\alpha}$. Should not be used before day 111; 80–85% of stillbirths occur in last $\frac{1}{3}$ of litter
Small Litters						
Gilts		Lower than sows			Breed on third cycle; flushing ration, especially on marginal diets	No benefit beyond third cycle in increasing number of ova
Sows	Boar power	On pasture or pen mating 5 breedings/week			Mature boars	Although the problem may have resolved, clinical sign is increased litter scatter
	Overfeeding		Continuous flushing beyond 5th day after breeding or full feed during gestation			
	Genetics			Some breeds produce larger litters, e.g., Yorkshire and Landrace, 10–14 pigs; Duroc and Chesterwhite, 8–11 pigs		
Estrous Synchronization	(See article on Estrous Synchronization)					
Sows						
Gilts					Wean all sows at same time	Best results occur in animals on increased nutrition and weaned after 21 days; moving and mixing of gilts, placing in area of boars

2. Relationship of time of all events in the production cycle to the time of occurrence of problems.

3. Changes made in management, treatment, and the results associated with attempts to solve the problem.

Use the check list to center on the problems. Common problems are anestrus, repeat breeders with normal and abnormal cycle lengths, resorption, abortion, mummies, stillbirths, small litters, and estrous synchronization. Table 1 is an aid to determining cause, treatment, and prevention of many reproductive problems related to management procedures.

Supplemental Reading

Blood, D. C., Radostits, O. M., and Henderson, J. A.: Veterinary Medicine, 6th ed. Bailliere Tindall, 1983.
Hurtgen, J. P.: Large Animal Practice: Diagnosis and Treatment of Swine Diseases. Vet. Clin. North Am. 277–299, 1982.
Leman, A. D., Glock, R. P., Mengeling, W. L., et al.: Diseases of Swine, 5th ed. Iowa, Iowa State University Press, 1981.

Diseases of the Urinary System

THOMAS A. POWE, D.V.M., M.S.

Diseases of the urinary system are manifested by the abnormal constituents of the urine (proteinuria, hematuria, hemoglobinuria, pyuria, glycosuria, ketonuria, and creatinuria) and may cause abnormalities of volume (polyuria, oliguria, and anuria). Rupture of the renal pelvis (rare), bladder, and urethra, pain and dysuria, and defects of the neural control of the bladder are also possible.

The primary functions of the urinary system are the elimination of the end products of tissue metabolism and the maintenance of fluid and electrolyte balance in the body. Many clinical signs are associated with urinary diseases; however, the end result of most severe urinary diseases is uremia, produced by prerenal, primary renal, or postrenal diseases.

The prerenal diseases—cardiac failure, shock, and dehydration—produce renal ischemia and ultimately uremia. The primary renal diseases—glomerulonephritis, interstitial nephritis, pyelonephritis, embolic nephritis, and amyloidosis—are caused by immune reactions, toxemia, or infections. Postrenal diseases are associated with infections or obstructions or both that occur distal to the collecting ducts. The diseases diagnosed most often in food animals are urolithiasis in the male and cystitis and pyelonephritis in the female.

The sporadic appearance of renal disease in food-producing animals is not completely understood but is in part due to the early age at which most food animals are slaughtered, the failure to observe early clinical signs (especially in large groups of animals), the enormous compensatory ability of the kidney, and the diet, environment, and genetics of the herbivore.

DIAGNOSIS

Diagnosis is based on history, clinical examination, microscopic examination and culture of the urine, serum chemistry, and renal biopsy (valuable in regard to prognosis). The history generally reveals changes in volume of urine voided, frequency of urination, and presence of abnormal constituents in the urine. Clinical examination detects the presence of blood, pus, or other abnormal discharge. Rectal palpation aids in finding abnormal kidneys and thickened or distended bladder. Blood cells, casts, and bacteria can be observed on microscopic examination. Blood chemistry alterations usually indicate advanced disease and include hypochloremia, hypocalcemia, hypokalemia, hyponatremia, hypophosphatemia, hypermagnesemia, and elevated blood urea nitrogen levels. In chronic renal disease a nonregenerative anemia exists, and dairy cattle may have a history of repeated hypocalcemia.

TREATMENT

The principles of treating diseases of the urinary system are limited to supportive therapy, such as parenteral fluids containing sodium, glucose, and possibly calcium; relief of pain and obstruction, and the administration of appropriate antibiotics. Once the destruction of the nephrons has passed the critical stage (approximately 90 per cent destruction), little can be done other than to give temporary relief, as emergency slaughter is not recommended after uremia has developed. Diuretics may be useful in prerenal disease but are contraindicated in primary renal and postrenal diseases.

PRERENAL DISEASE—RENAL ISCHEMIA

In the early stages of prerenal disease, circulation to the kidney is reduced, the kidney remains normal, and the renal function is reduced. If the underlying cause is relieved, the kidney remains normal and normal function returns. When prerenal diseases are uncorrected, renal ischemia develops and treatment is frequently unsuccessful.

PRIMARY RENAL DISEASES

Glomerulonephritis

A primary renal disease of food-producing animals is glomerulonephritis, which is rarely diagnosed in food animals but may be more common than reported, especially in swine and sheep. It may be associated with the "thin sow" syndrome in swine and with pregnancy toxemia in sheep.

Nephrosis

Nephrosis in most cases is related to toxemia, is acute, and produces severe damage to nephrons, proteinuria, high specific gravity of the urine, and high blood urea nitrogen levels. Treatment is aimed at correcting the primary disease and providing support.

Interstitial Nephritis

Interstitial nephritis, caused by *Leptospira* spp. and chronic poisoning, is a debilitating disease that seldom causes death unless a large portion of nephrons is destroyed. It is difficult to diagnose.

Embolic Nephritis

Embolic nephritis is suppurative and may occur after septicemia. No clinical signs appear unless embolisms are very extensive. Such cases usually result in uremia and death. Sporadic instances of embolic nephritis show no observable renal dysfunction, but signs of toxemia are present and an enlarged kidney may be palpated. Microscopic examination of urine reveals pus and blood. Culture of the urine is indicated when proteinuria exists. Treatment with antibiotics for 10 to 14 days may be useful in early cases.

PYELONEPHRITIS

Most cases of pyelonephritis result from ascending bacterial infections from the lower urinary tract, notably *Corynebacterium renale* in cattle, sheep, and goats and *C. suis* in swine. In addition, pyelonephritis may result from the spread of embolic nephritis and *Escherichia coli*, staphylococci, and other bacteria may be involved. Pyelonephritis is present most commonly in the female and is usually associated with either breeding injuries or parturition. The lesion encompasses the renal pelvis and parenchyma. The ureters and bladder are also commonly involved.

Diagnosis

The course of urinary disease is usually chronic and the clinical signs may not be present for several weeks. Even though there are some species differences, most animals with pyelonephritis will have weight loss, hematuria, and pyruria that may or may not be detected early.

In swine, the first clinical signs are purulent vaginal discharge and hematuria along with weight loss and decreased appetite. As the condition becomes more severe, polydipsia, polyuria, pyuria, hematuria, inappetence, and rapid weight loss occur. The most reliable evidence of pyelonephritis is the frequent passage of blood in the urine. The presence of blood, pus, and bacteria in the urine on microscopic examination and culture provides confirmation.

Pyelonephritis in cattle, sheep, and goats usually has an insidious onset but may be acute, especially in sheep and goats. The first clinical signs may go unnoticed but usually include fluctuation of rectal temperatures from 40 to 41°C (104 to 106°F), hematuria, abdominal pain, and gradual weight loss. As the disease progresses dysuria may be manifested by signs, such as treading of the hand limbs, arching of the back, and dribbling of the urine. There may be periods of remission, but if undiagnosed and untreated the terminal signs of uremia will appear.

Confirmation of pyelonephritis depends on the results of the urinalysis, blood urea nitrogen levels, culture, and differential diagnosis (lymphosarcoma, cystitis, pericarditis), and the presence of other renal diseases. In cattle, a rectal examination is very useful in palpating the kidney, ureters, and the bladder. The kidney will be enlarged and alobular, the ureters will be enlarged, and the bladder will be thickened from cystitis. Blood urea nitrogen levels will be elevated only if there is less than 25 per cent normal renal function. Unilateral pyelonephritis may result in a renal abscess with variable clinical signs.

Treatment

Successful treatment is dependent on early diagnosis. Once the ascending infection progresses beyond a case of cystitis and involves the ureter and kidney, treatment is relatively unsuccessful and results in temporary remission. With early diagnosis appropriate antibiotics for 10 to 14 days may be effective 30 to 40 per cent of the time. Unless animals are extremely valuable, the best course of action is salvage by slaughter, which must be done before severe weight loss or uremia.

CYSTITIS

Cystitis is an inflammatory condition of the bladder that is sporadic in occurrence and is most common in females. Predisposing factors are obstruction to the urinary outflow, bladder paresis, and trauma. Cystitis is characterized by frequent and sometimes painful urination, blood, inflammatory cells, and bacteria in the urine. It is a predisposing case of ascending pyelonephritis and is impossible to differentiate from early pyelonephritis. Differentiation of cystitis and pyelonephritis is not important from the standpoint of treatment as treatment is the same, but it is important to differentiate the 2 for the purpose of prognosis. Early acute cystitis frequently is resolved with 10 to 14 days of antibiotic treatment. Chronic cystitis and pyelonephritis have guarded prognoses.

UROLITHIASIS
(Calculosis, Urinary Calculi, Waterbelly)

Urolithiasis of ruminants is a metabolic disease characterized by the formation of calculi composed of an organic matrix with crystals of mineral salts deposited in and on the matrix. The calculi may form equally in both the male and female, but the clinical sign, urinary obstruction, is seen almost entirely in the young castrated male. The formation of the calculi is complex and is caused by the interaction of diet, hormones, physical and chemical actions, and environment. Diagnosis of obstructive urolithiasis is based on the characteristic clinical signs and physical examination; however, many cases of urinary obstruction are not diagnosed until after the bladder or urethra has ruptured. Treatment consists of relieving obstruction, re-establishing urine flow, reducing toxemia, and preventing recurrence of calculi by dietary management.

Calculus formation begins with viruses, bacteria, epithelial cells, casts, or other urinary tract debris serving as a colloidal matrix upon which minerals deposit slowly. The important calculi are silica in the form of amorphous silicon dioxide, phosphate, or oxalate and carbonate salts in the form of calcium, ammonium, or magnesium. The type of calculus formed depends on the diet, and the frequency of calculus formation appears related to the diet, environment, and management of food and water intake. Animals in arid areas develop more calculi than animals in humid areas. Calculi are formed more frequently in animals with alkaline urine, borderline hypovitaminosis A, and hypervitaminosis D, and when water of high salinity is consumed.

The type of calculi varies both in shape and chemical composition with the diet. The 2 major types of calculi are silicates, usually single and irregularly shaped, in animals consuming large quantities of poor quality hay or grass stubbles (low in vitamin A), and the struvites (ammonium or magnesium phosphates), usually numerous and smooth, in feedlot animals (rapid tissue turnover, fast body growth, low vitamin A). All phosphate salt levels rise on high grain diets when there is a Ca:P ratio of less than 1:3. Oxalate calculi occur in animals on clover-rich pastures, or in animals consuming excessive oxalate-containing plants. Magnesium phosphate is most common in diets high in sorghum products or cottonseed meal.

All types of calculi tend to increase when there is a rise in the concentration of urinary constituents and when conditions are favorable for greater precipitation of urinary solutes. In urine, solubility is affected by the concentration of calculus-forming substances, the salt content of urine, pH of urine, the concentration of inhibitors of crystallization of urine, obstruction of urine flow, infections, and potentiators of crystallization. Crystal-forming substances may remain in solution in urine at concentrations that would exceed their solubility in water; thus most calculi are formed over a long period of time and when several contributing factors are present.

Some factors that aid in calculus formation include higher urinary calcium levels, sporadic eating (allows pH changes in urine), higher silica or phosphate in diet, excessive fluid loss or water deprivation, urinary stasis, lower urinary citrate levels, alteration in urinary colloidal particles or effectiveness, and greater matrix formation.

The formation of calculi is equally as common in the female, male, and the castrated male; however, urinary obstructions are almost exclusively in the castrated male or in the very young male. The reason for obstruction in the castrated male is attributed to the reduced diameter of the urethra of castrated males compared with intact males.

Anatomic features that contribute to urinary obstruction are the sigmoid flexure of the penis in bulls, rams, and bucks; the processus urethrae (vermiform appendage) in rams and bucks, and the swellings that may occur in the accessory sex glands when animals are on diets high in estrogens. Some clovers, *Fusarium* fungi, and, in the past, diethylstilbestrol accounted for much of the increased estrogen.

Clinically affected animals exhibit anorexia, ringing of the tail, stamping of the rear feet, and evidence of abdominal pain. The preputial hair is dry and often covered with crystals. The urethra may be dilated, and pulsation of the urethra may be observed over the ischial arch. In cattle, the distended bladder may be palpated per rectum. If the obstruction is not relieved, rupture of the bladder or the urethra will occur in about 48 hr. Immediate relief follows rupture of the bladder or urethra; however, the animal will become uremic in 2 to 3 days after rupture, and coma and death ensues in untreated animals. Urinary obstruction must be differentiated from ascites, bloat, acute indigestion, and pneumonia, especially after the bladder ruptures. Rupture of the urethra in the early stages must be differentiated from preputial abscess and penile hematoma. In the later stages of urethral rupture, the surrounding subcutaneous tissue necroses and sloughs.

Diagnosis is based on the clinical signs, physical examination, and elevated blood urea nitrogen levels. These levels may range from normal to near 175 mg/100 ml.

Treatment principles are basic: relieve obstruction, reestablish urine flow, and prevent or reduce uremia. The prognosis is dependent on the condition of the animal at the time of diagnosis, location of the calculi, type of calculi, and the intended use of the animal.

Steers may be slaughtered immediately if they are not uremic, or if their bladder urethra has not ruptured.

Sometimes temporary relief can be accomplished by a gentle back flush, or surgical removal may be required. Surgery involves a urethrotomy proximal to the calculi (90 to 95 per cent occur at the level of the distal sigmoid). In the case of silica calculi, the penis may be exposed at the level of the sigmoid and the calculi cracked with Bachus towel forceps forceps. In the bull, when continued usefulness is desired, an ischial urethrotomy is performed; a catheter is passed into the bladder with the aid of curved forceps, and the distal end of the catheter is passed distally and secured. The passing of the catheter into the bladder eliminates the need for laparotomy and suturing of the bladder, which will heal spontaneously if urine flow is returned.

In sheep and goats, the incidence of urethral obstruction at the level of the sigmoid is not as high as in cattle; however, there are numerous obstructions of the vermiform appendage that can be resolved by removing the obstructed end of the vermiform appendage. Calculi at the level of the sigmoid are relieved similarly to those in cattle. Because of the economic value of bucks and rams little attempt has been made to return those with high obstruction to breeding, and the attempts to do so have been of limited success.

The calculi that have formed are not likely to be dissolved, but appropriate steps may be taken to prevent enlargement or formation of additional calculi. The Ca:P ratio should be at least 1.2:1, adequate vitamin A should be provided, water intake should be increased, sodium chloride feed levels may be up to 4 per cent (creep feeding of nursing range calves up to 12 per cent near weaning). Ammonium chloride may be used to acidify the urine (steers 45 gm/head/day, lambs 10 gm/head/day; this has no effect on the formation of siliceous urinary calculi), and feedstuffs may be changed to reduce oxylates, silicates, phosphates, and estrogens.

Supplemental Reading

Blood, D. C., Radostits, O. M., Henderson, J. A.: Veterinary Medicine, 6th ed. London, Bailliere Tindall, 348–367, 1983.

Divers, T. J.: Diagnosis and therapy of renal disease in dairy cattle. Proc. Bov. Pract. *15*:74–78, 1983.

Jenson, R., Mackey, D. R.: Diseases of Feedlot Cattle, 2nd ed. Philadelphia, Lea and Febiger, 309–314, 1971.

Jenson, R., Swift, B. I.: Diseases of Sheep, 2nd ed. Philadelphia, Lea and Febiger, 167–169, 1982.

Jones, J. E. T.: *In* Leman, A. D., Glock, R. D., Mengeling, W. L., et al. (eds.). Urinary System in Diseases of Swine, 5th ed. Iowa, Iowa State University Press, 145–154, 1981.

Walker, D. F.: Bovine Urogenital Surgery in the Practice of Large Animal Surgery. *In* P. B. Jennings (ed.). Practice of Large Animal Surgery. Philadelphia, W. B. Saunders Company, 145–154, 1981.

DISEASES OF THE EYE

CECIL P. MOORE, D.V.M.
Consulting Editor

Ocular Diagnostic Techniques in Food Animals

R. DAVID WHITLEY, D.V.M., M.S.
and CECIL P. MOORE, D.V.M.

The eyes should be examined when primary or obvious ocular disease exists, during the routine physical examination, and when systemic disease is present, since the eye can serve as an index of the general health of the animal. Frequently, the ocular examination including ophthalmoscopy can be used as a convenient, inexpensive, and noninvasive means of assisting in the differentiation of systemic diseases in food animals.

The eye is unique in comparison to other body organs since the ocular media is normally transparent, and most of its structures can be directly visualized. An orderly sequence of evaluation is essential for a thorough and detailed assessment. The eye lends itself to examination from the superficial anterior structures to the deep posterior structures. A protocol is frequently incorporated into an ophthalmic examination form (Fig. 1).

It is hoped that this article will stimulate veterinary clinicians to more carefully scrutinize the eye of food animal patients and report findings. With practice in using the procedures and with continued careful observations, the value of the ophthalmic examination in assessing food animal patients with primary or secondary ocular diseases will be enhanced.

OPHTHALMIC HISTORY

Both general and detailed ophthalmic histories are critical to the examination. Sufficient time should be allotted to take a complete history. In instances when a primary ocular problem is the chief complaint, an ophthalmic history form may be completed by the owner or herder (Fig. 2). As part of the history, the herder should be questioned concerning the animal's visual status. Frequently, owners and other personnel can provide useful observations regarding an animal's vision; however, it should be noted that blind animals in a familiar herd environment often appear sighted, but when segregated from the herd or placed in an unfamiliar area exhibit obvious blindness behavior.

Signalment and genetic history are particularly important since certain disorders are known to be inherited or to occur more frequently in some breeds or lines. Any illness of the dam during gestation should be noted because congenital ocular anomalies may be secondary to gestational toxicity, infection, and vitamin deficiencies.

Intended uses of the animals may be a primary concern when animals receive ophthalmic examinations as part of prepurchase or breeding soundness evaluations.

GENERAL INSPECTION OF THE EYE

The orbit, ocular adnexa, and globe should be thoroughly inspected as part of the general physical examination. If possible, the animal should be observed moving about in its natural environment since unilateral or bilateral visual deficits are often more readily observed prior to restraint.

During the initial inspection and before restraint, the gross appearance of the head, face, and eyes should be assessed. Carriage of the head, position of the eyelids, amount and nature of discharges from the eyes, and the presence or absence of periorbital swelling should be noted. Frequently, position of the eyes within the orbit and direction of the gaze can be determined as well as relative size of the eyes. Ocular position within the orbit should be noted, i.e., whether the eyes are abnormally placed in the posterior aspect of the orbit (enophthalmos) or are protruding anteriorly (exophthalmos). Abnormal deviations of the eyes may also be evaluated (strabismus); these include esotropia (medial deviation), exotropia (lateral deviation), hypertropia (upward deviation), and hypotropia (downward deviation). With paralysis of the fourth (trochlear) cranial nerve, e.g., in cattle with polioencephalomalacia, there is frequently a resultant extorsion rotation of the globe dorsolaterally on the anterior posterior axis.

The size of the globe may be abnormal as a result of congenital defects or inflammatory processes. Eyes that are smaller than normal may be microphthalmic, nanophthalmic, or phthisical. Eyes that are larger than normal (macrophthalmia or megaloglobus) most commonly result from greater intraocular pressure secondary to inflammatory disease or injury. During initial observations, the animal's temperament may be assessed, and the methods of restraint should be determined. Restraint should be adequate to permit a close-up and detailed ophthalmic examination.

NEUROPHTHALMOLOGIC ASSESSMENT

Following general inspection and prior to a detailed examination, a neurophthalmic assessment should be performed. Although this may be performed quickly, it provides a reasonably thorough evaluation of a number of the cranial nerves. The palpebral reflex, elicited by touching or tapping the medial canthal area with the finger, should induce blinking and retraction of the globe.

Date: _____

History: _____

_____

_____

_____

_____

Diagnosis: _____ Prognosis: ☐ Favorable ☐ Guarded ☐ Poor

Reflexes and Neurologic Responses

Pupillary ☐ direct ☐ consensual
Blink ☐ palpebral ☐ corneal
☐ Oculocephalic
☐ Menace response
☐ Visual placing
☐ Vision testing

RIGHT EYE

Diagnostic Procedures

☐ Penlight examination
☐ Culture
☐ Schirmer's tear test
☐ Fluorescein
☐ N-L Fluorescein
☐ Rose bengal
☐ Topical anesthetic
☐ N-L Flush
☐ N-L Catheterization
☐ Cytology

Eyelids and Globe

☐ Tonometry—Schiotz
☐ Tonometry—Applanation
☐ Gonioscopy
☐ Tonography

External Eye and Cornea

☐ Mydriatic
☐ Biomicroscopy
☐ Direct ophthalmoscopy
☐ Indirect ophthalmoscopy

Lens

☐ Aqueous paracentesis
☐ Vitreous paracentesis
☐ Electroretinography
☐ Visual-evoked potential
☐ Dacryocystorhinography
☐ Orbital angiography
☐ Fluorescein angiography
☐ Ultrasonography

Fundus

☐ Other _____

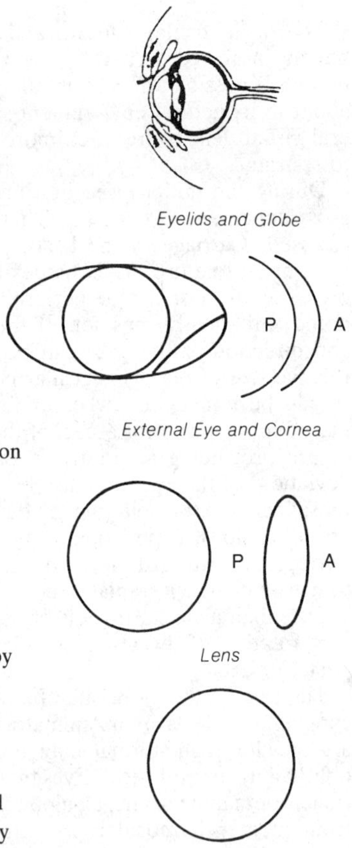

Examination Findings

Orbit
☐ Symmetry
☐ Palpable borders
☐ Retropulsion of globe

LEFT EYE

Eyelids
☐ Upper
☐ Lower
☐ Medial and lateral canthi
☐ Third eyelid

Tear Formation
☐ Meibomian glands
☐ Lacrimal lake
☐ Mucous thread

Eyelids and Globe

Tear Drainage
☐ Upper puncta
☐ Lower puncta
☐ Nasal orifice

External Eye and Cornea

Conjunctiva
☐ Palpebral
☐ Bulbar
☐ Nictitans

Cornea

Anterior Chamber
Iridocorneal Angle
Iris

Lens

Lens

Vitreous
Fundus
☐ Blood vessels
☐ Optic disk
☐ Tapetum
☐ Nontapetum

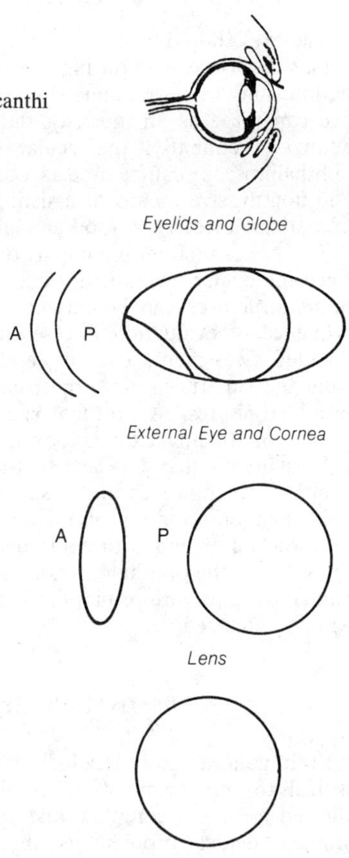

Fundus

Remarks/Recommendations: _____

_____

_____

Signature: _____

Figure 1. A form that incorporates a systematic approach to an ophthalmic examination.

Date: _____

_____
Signature of Person Completing This Form

1. What led you to believe your animal has an eye problem?
   ☐ Loss of vision
   ☐ Eye discharge
   ☐ Peculiar color of eye(s)
   ☐ Veterinarian noted problem
   ☐ Other, explain _____

2. How long has this problem been present? _____

3. Which eye(s) is(are) affected?   RIGHT   LEFT   BOTH

4. Has the character of the eye(s) changed since you first noticed it? .... NO   YES   UNKNOWN
   If YES, how? _____

5. Have you treated the eye(s)? .... NO   YES
   If YES, how, and with what? _____

6. How well do you believe your animal sees?
   ☐ Excellent   ☐ Poor in regard to moving objects
   ☐ Poor on all occasions   ☐ Poor in regard to stationary objects
   ☐ Poor especially in dim light or dark   ☐ Poor when turning to the right
   ☐ Poor especially in bright light   ☐ Poor when turning to the left
   ☐ Poor in regard to near objects   ☐ Poor when jumping or climbing down
   ☐ Poor in regard to far objects   ☐ Poor when jumping or climbing up

7. Do you think your animal sees well in familiar surroundings? .... YES   NO   UNKNOWN
   Strange surroundings? .... YES   NO   UNKNOWN

8. Has your animal had any other eye problems? .... NO   YES   UNKNOWN
   If YES, what type? _____

9. Has your animal experienced seizures, loss of balance, weakness, incoordination or personality change?   NO   YES   UNKNOWN

10. Is your animal receiving medication? .... NO   YES
    If YES, what? _____

11. Do you have other animals? .... NO   YES
    If YES, do they have eye problems? .... NO   YES
    If YES, what type? _____

12. Do you know your animal's dam or sire? .... NO   YES
    If YES, do either of them have eye problems? .... NO   YES   UNKNOWN

13. Is your animal consuming water and food normally? .... YES   NO   UNKNOWN

14. Is your animal urinating more frequently than normal? .... NO   YES   UNKNOWN

15. Has your animal had previous or present illness? .... NO   YES   UNKNOWN
    If YES, what type? _____

16. Has your animal been exposed to house or farm chemicals (cleaners, agricultural, industrial or automotive
    chemicals) or building supplies? .... NO   YES   UNKNOWN

CLIENT OPHTHALMIC HISTORY

Figure 2. An example of an ophthalmic history form that may be completed by the owner or herder.

The afferent arc of this reflex is via the fifth (trigeminal) cranial nerve. The efferent pathway is via the seventh cranial nerve for closure of the lids and the sixth cranial nerve for retraction of the globe. The corneal reflex is induced in a similar manner by touching the cornea with the finger or a piece of cotton. Neural pathways are the same as for the palpebral reflex. False-positive responses may occur when corneal sensation is abnormal, but the animal responds owing to visualization of the object near the eye. The menace response (opticofacial response) is tested by moving the hand in a vertical path in front of the eye. Movement of the hand in the vertical path minimizes the creation of air currents, which occur when the hand is advanced toward the eye or face, creating a false-positive response. An error in interpretation may also result if the examiner inadvertently touches the facial hair or vibrissae. The oculocephalic (doll's head) reflex should be elicited by moving the head from side to side. The normal response is for the eyes to move in a rhythmic fashion towards the direction of head movement. Abnormalities of the oculocephalic reflex are often associated with otitis interna and brain stem disorders. The pupillary light reflex (PLR) is tested as part of the detailed focal light examination. The PLR should be evaluated in a semi-darkened or darkened area using a consistent, bright focal light source. The examiner should use a well-charged penlight or, preferably, a 3.5-volt halogen light source, such as a Finoff transilluminator attached to a rechargeable handle. A normal PLR does not indicate vision, and, conversely, vision does not indicate normal PLR.

DETAILED INSPECTION OF THE EYE

Frequently, after only a preliminary inspection of the eye, the examiner must select additional diagnostic procedures. Certain of the ophthalmic diagnostic aids may interfere with other subsequent diagnostic aids. The addition of any topical solution to the eye, such as mydriatic, topical anesthetic, vital stain, or eye wash (collyrium) may interfere with corneoconjunctival cultures or the Schirmer's tear test. Many of the preservatives added to ophthalmic preparations are bacteriostatic or bacteriocidal and will prevent recovery of organisms from the eye. Also, mydriatics can interfere with the PLR and should not be instilled until after the PLR has been adequately evaluated and recorded. Topical anesthetic may invalidate the corneal reflex and will decrease reflex tearing.

Following restraint and the neurophthalmologic examination, a detailed inspection of the eye is performed and involves the following structures: orbit, eyelids, nictitating membrane, lacrimal system, conjunctiva, cornea, sclera, anterior chamber, iris, lens, vitreous, retina, choroid, and optic nerve. This portion of the examination is performed best in a semi-darkened area with a focal light source.

Examination of the orbit includes inspection and palpation. Visual comparison is made for symmetry, swelling, and ocular position (strabismus or nystagmus). The orbit is inspected in detail for abnormal swelling, retrobulbar masses, globe size, and ocular motility. The skin and bony rim should be palpated for masses, irregularities, and fractures. The globe should be retropulsed using digital pressure through the eyelids to evaluate the retrobulbar area for space occupying masses or abnormal decreases in orbital contents (fat and muscle). Retropulsion also allows inspection of the anterior surface of the nictitating membrane.

The eyelids are carefully looked at for position and movement across the cornea. Abnormalities of position or movement are entropion, ectropion, ptosis, lagophthalmos, blepharospasm, and inability to close the eyelids (poor or absent blink reflex, i.e., facial nerve paralysis). The skin of the eyelids should be examined for edema and inflammation (blepharitis). Other abnormalities include lacerations, discoloration, discharge, and alopecia. The eyelid margin and palpebral conjunctiva should be examined for abnormal eyelashes or hair; trichiasis, distichiasis, districhiasis, and ectopic cilia. Lacrimal drainage can be assessed by examining the lower eyelids for increased moisture associated with nasolacrimal duct obstruction or ocular irritation and increased lacrimation. Normally just above the lower eyelid and towards the medial canthus a lacrimal "lake" of fluid is noted, and a small thread of mucus may be present at the lacrimal caruncle.

The nictitating membrane (NM) should be inspected for conjunctivitis, protrusion, abnormal masses, foreign bodies, eversion of the cartilage, and hypertrophy of the gland. Manual retropulsion of the globe will cause protrusion of the NM and facilitate examination. Following topical anesthesia, nonlocking nontoothed forceps may be used to grasp and extend the NM for more detailed inspection of both the anterior and posterior surfaces.

The focal light examination of the anterior segment involves assessment of the eyelids, NM, palpebral and bulbar conjunctiva, cornea, anterior chamber, iris, pupillary margin, lens, and anterior vitreous. Examination of the lens and anterior vitreous requires that the pupil be chemically dilated. We prefer 1-per cent tropicamide* with adequate dilation, requiring a 15 to 30 min period following instillation. Topical atropine is not recommended for examination purposes to its relatively slow onset (1 hr) and long duration of effect. The focal light examination is best performed in a semi-darkened or darkened area in which light reflections and noisy distractions can be avoided. Several light sources are available for this examination, such as disposable pocket penlights, flashlights, direct ophthalmoscopes, otoscopes, transilluminators, and oculus side lights. Magnifying loupes also aid in the ocular examination; $1.5\times$ to $3.5\times$ are most useful.† The veterinary ophthalmologist frequently utilizes a handheld slit-lamp biomicroscope for this part of the ocular examination in food animals.

Use of the penlight is best in a darkened area, directing the light source into the eye at a 45-degree angle to the axis of the view of the observer. Penlight examination involves several diagnostic principles and techniques. A focusing slit-beam penlight or Finoff transilluminator is best. The slit-beam aperture on many direct ophthalmoscope heads may also be employed. Other illuminating techniques use diffuse light, direct focal illumination, retro-illumination, indirect illumination, sclerotic scatter, and zones of specular reflection. These methods are available to help localize lesions or opacities within the ocular media.

*Mydriacyl, 0.5% and 1.0%, Tropicamide, Alcon Laboratories, Inc., Fort Worth, Texas 76134 and Mydramide, 0.5% and 1.0%, Bio Products, Inc., Amityville, New York 11701.
†Optivisor, Donegan Optical Co., Inc., Lenexa, Kansas 66219

Due to the adjustable light intensity and variable magnification, the slit-lamp biomicroscope can be used to examine the transparent ocular media of the eye (preocular tear film, cornea, aqueous humor, lens, and vitreous) in optical section. Diffuse illumination utilizes a wide slit-beam or spot of light. This method is used initially to survey the patient's eye and to orient the observer. Direct focal illumination employs a narrow beam to examine the eyelid margin, tear film, NM, conjunctiva, cornea, anterior chamber, iris, and lens. Retro-illumination (direct and indirect) involves directing the light beam on an opaque surface that reflects light back through clear ocular media. Light reflected off the iris facilitates examination of the anterior chamber (aqueous) and the cornea. An increase in cells or protein or both in the aqueous, when viewed with a focal light source, gives the appearance of a light beam passing through smoke. This is known clinically as "aqueous flare" and results from the Tyndall phenomenon. Light reflected from the ocular fundus assists in detection of vitreal and lens opacities. Zones of specular reflection are observed when light is reflected from the smooth surfaces of the cornea and lens, which act as mirrors. Zones of discontinuity originate from the internal reflection within the lens and result in the appearance of successive reflecting zones of the various lenticular nuclei. This technique is useful to localize opacities and to determine approximate time or duration of the insult to the lens.

Focal illumination (direct and indirect) with a narrow beam helps to examine the eye in detail after a preliminary survey of the eye with diffuse light. Slit-beam light, magnification, and stereopsis offer virtually "visual palpation" of the ocular structures.

The conjunctiva should be examined for abnormal vascularity, hemorrhage, lacerations, foreign bodies, growths, and edema (chemosis). The conjunctiva, a true mucous membrane, can be used to assess the animal for the presence of anemia and icterus. Deep to the conjunctiva, the sclera should be scrutinized for change in color (i.e., dark appearance of hemorrhage or melanoma), abnormal masses, tears, and lacerations.

The cornea is normally transparent, avascular, moist, and unpigmented with a smooth even contour. It should be carefully examined with a focal light source for loss of transparency (edema or infiltrates), ulcerations, vascularization, pigmentation, dryness, masses, foreign bodies, lacerations, and changes of contour. If fluorescein application is considered at this point, the examiner is reminded that its use could interfere with other diagnostic tests; therefore, if a culture or Schirmer's tear test is indicated, it should be done prior to the instillation of fluorescein.

The anterior chamber should be examined for depth and abnormal material, which may include blood (hyphema), pus (hypopyon), fibrin, cells and protein (aqueous flare), or foreign bodies. Tissue abnormalities that may be detected are iris adhesions (synechiae or persistent pupillary membranes), iris cysts, neoplasia, lens, or granulation tissue. In some food animals, the filtration angle or iridocorneal angle can be directly visualized.

The iris is examined for congenital defects, color, topography, and position. Direct and consensual pupillary responses are evaluated. The pupils are examined for movement, constriction and dilation, size, position, symmetry, and shape. Hippus refers to the abnormal constriction and dilation of the pupil. Difference in size between the 2 pupils of greater than 1 mm is termed anisocoria. Contamination of the eye with Jimson weed may cause mydriasis. Abnormal location of the pupil within the iris is called corectopia, and abnormal shape is dyscoria. The iris is normally bowed forward slightly, owing to its support posteriorly by the lens. If this support from the lens is lost, as in lens subluxation or luxation, the iris will appear flat, the anterior chamber will appear deepened, and the iris may have "fluttering" type movements when the head moves. Abnormal movement or tremor of the iris is referred to as iridodonesis. When iritis is present, the iris may appear congested and swollen with loss of detail and may become darker in color.

The lens is normally a transparent avascular structure within the eye. It should be examined to determine presence, position, size, and the existence of opacities. Cataracts are opacities of the lens or its capsule. With aging in animals, the lens becomes more translucent or sclerotic as the lens fibers are compacted toward the center of the lens. This age change in the lens is called lenticular sclerosis and does not cause blindness in animals or prevent visualization of the ocular fundus by ophthalmoscopy. In general, if a fundus reflex is present or if the retina is clearly visible in a blind animal, the blindness is not due to lens changes.

Following the penlight examination, the posterior segment of the eye (the posterior vitreous and fundus) is inspected with a focal light source and a +20 diopter lens or with a direct ophthalmoscope. A provisory inspection can be performed in most food animals without chemical dilation of the pupil. However, to carefully scrutinize the lens, vitreous, retina, and optic nerve, pharmacologically induced mydriasis is recommended. One-per cent tropicamide is the drug of choice: 1 to 2 drops instilled topically in the eye will induce mydriasis in 15 to 30 min.

At referral centers, the veterinary ophthalmologist will commonly utilize a binocular, indirect ophthalmoscope, and +14, +20, and +28 condensing lenses to view the ocular fundus. In selected cases, fundus photography may be used for soundness and insurance examinations and for progression of undiagnosed or suspicious lesions.

The vitreous humor or vitreous body is the largest structure within the eye. It should be examined for congenital anomalies, such as colobomas, persistent hyaloid vessels, hemorrhages, hyaloid remnants, and detached retinas. Hyaloid remnants are frequently present in adult food animals and are considered normal. The hyaloid vessels may contain blood in calves and lambs up to 8 weeks of age. Acquired changes in the vitreous result in inflammatory cells, vitreous floaters, exudates, and opacities. Opacities that are suspended in the vitreous are referred to as asteroid hyalosis and are composed of a calcium lipid complex. Liquefaction of the vitreous is termed syneresis, and opacities in the liquified state are termed synchysis scintillans. These opacities, composed mainly of cholesterol, often rise and fall in the vitreous as the head moves. Examination of the anterior vitreous is best accomplished through a dilated pupil with a focal light source and magnification. The posterior vitreous is considered in the examination of the ocular fundus and is observed with ophthalmoscopy.

The retinas of the common food animals are vascularized throughout and therefore are classified as holangiotic. The ocular fundus should be examined for detachment of the retina, chorioretinal hypoplasia or dysplasia, vascular attenuation, vascular congestion, scars, hemorrhage, colobomas, alteration in tapetal coloration, nontapetal coloration, vascular pattern, changes in pigmentation, color and size of vessels, and foci of inflammation. Appearance of the optic nerve head (optic disc) should be noted and examined for shape, size, and color, and for the presence of pits, colobomas, or abnormal masses. Swelling of the optic disc without blindness is referred to as papilledema. Swelling can also occur with optic neuritis, which is characterized by blindness.

EVALUATION FOR BLINDNESS

Unilateral blindness is often not detected by the owner or herder. It may be confirmed by covering 1 eye at a time and by testing the animal's response in an obstacle course or maze. Ideally, this should be performed in both a well lighted area and a semi-darkened area. A pink-eye patch or shield or gauze taped over the eye works well as a blindfold. White gauze, cloth, or cotton dropped several feet in front of the animal within the visual field can also be used to assess vision by observing if the animal follows the movement. The items used for this test must not cause air currents or sound. The menace response is a crude test of vision, and, as previously pointed out, avoidance of air currents is mandatory.

Acute onset of blindness in food animals is usually associated with cautious movement, collisions with stationary objects, and altered behavior. Congenital blindness, long-standing blindness, or blindness of gradual onset can be much less obvious as many affected animals adjust well to their handicap and rely on other senses to ambulate in their environment. Only when they are removed from familiar surroundings does the blindness become obvious. Blind animals may be presented for skin lacerations and trauma due to entanglement in fences and other hazards.

Suggested Reading

Gelatt, K. N.: Textbook of Veterinary Ophthalmology. Philadelphia, Lea and Febiger, 206–261, 606–648, 741–763, 1981.

Rubin, L. F.: Atlas of Veterinary Ophthalmoscopy. Philadelphia, Lea and Febiger, 327–366, 1974.

Severin, G. A.: Veterinary Ophthalmology Notes, 2nd ed. Fort Collins, Colorado State University Publication Service, 1–24, 1976.

Slatter, D. H.: Fundamentals of Veterinary Ophthalmology. Philadelphia, W. B. Saunders Company, 111–170, 1981.

Basic Ophthalmic Therapeutics

STEPHEN BISTNER, D.V.M.

The use of ophthalmic drugs in food animals is somewhat limited, and the discussion of these drugs will be limited to those having clinical significance.

PRINCIPLES OF OPHTHALMIC DRUG ABSORPTION AND ADMINISTRATION

Before learning the routes of administration of ophthalmic pharmaceuticals, one should understand several basic principles pertaining to the absorption of topical ophthalmic drugs. The rate of delivery of an ophthalmic drug to the desired site is dependent on the following factors:

1. The vehicle in which the drug is suspended and the nature of the drug itself, including toxicity, pH, and stability. The cornea is covered by a precorneal tear film and in itself has variable permeability, the corneal epithelium being more permeable to fat soluble compounds, and the stroma being more permeable to water soluble compounds. If the corneal epithelium is damaged, a much higher level of drug absorption may be achieved in the corneal stroma. Ophthalmic drugs should possess biphasic solubility to maximize corneal penetration.

2. The degree of vascularization and inflammation in the eye can affect the level of drug present. A highly inflamed eye will carry away drugs more rapidly.

3. Drainage of ophthalmic agents through the nasolacrimal system can also influence the rate of disappearance of agents.

There are numerous ways by which ophthalmic agents can be delivered to the eye.

1. Topical solutions are easily instilled into the eye but do not remain in the eye for long periods of time. Therefore, if solutions are used, greater frequency of dosage is recommended. Solutions may be suspended in vehicles such as polyvinyl alcohol or methylcellulose to lengthen their contact time.

2. Ointments have advantages over solutions in that a longer ocular contact time is maintained, and they are carried away through the nasolacrimal system less rapidly.

3. Subconjunctival injections are a very effective way to achieve high levels of medication in the anterior ocular segment. The injections can be delivered via a tuberculin syringe with a 25- or 26-gauge needle, using topical anesthesia.

The route by which a subconjunctival injection enters the eye has not been clearly defined. Diffusion across the sclera and underlying tissues is one mechanism, as is leakage of the drug from the subconjunctival depot through the needle puncture site into the conjunctival sac. Recent experiments using topically applied prednisolone acetate drops indicate that the frequent application of drops achieved a higher level of prednisolone in the aqueous than did subconjunctival injection.

Newer developments in drug delivery systems have produced methods for slow release of medication by sustained release devices (Ocusert).* Although these devices are currently being developed and used in people, all tests performed would indicate that they will have equally good potential for sustained drug delivery in animals.

DRUGS AFFECTING THE AUTONOMIC NERVOUS SYSTEM

Adrenergic Drugs

Adrenergic agents are used for their mydriatic effects, which may also include cycloplegia. Mydriasis (dilation of the pupil) may be produced by sympathomimetic or parasympatholytic mechanisms.

Clinically, mydriatics are used to dilate the pupil to permit fundus and lens examination. Tropicamide, 0.5 to 1.0 per cent, is used for this purpose. The normal ungulate pupil will dilate in 20 to 30 min and remain dilated for 2

---

*Available from Ocusert Alza Pharmaceuticals, Palo Alto, California 94303

Table 1. *Onset and Duration of a Single Administration of Topical Anesthetic*

Anesthetic	Onset	Duration (min)
0.4% Benoxinate	15 sec	20
1.0% Butacaine	2–3 min	30–60
1.4% Cocaine	2 min	10
0.5% Dyclonine	2–4 min	30–50
1.4% Lidocaine	4–5 min	30
0.5% Proparacaine	15 sec	15
0.5% Tetracaine	2–3 min	20–30

to 3 hr. To achieve maximal dilation, 1 drop is instilled in the eye and then a second drop is instilled 10 min later. The longer acting mydriatic and cycloplegic agents are used most routinely in the therapy of anterior uveitis. Atropine sulfate, 1 to 4 per cent, produces mydriasis and cycloplegia. Cycloplegia causes relaxation of the ciliary body, prevents ciliary spasms, and reduces pain of uveitis. The major role of atropine in the ungulate is the treatment of anterior uveitis secondary to severe deep interstitial keratitis in bovine infectious keratoconjunctivitis.

TOPICAL ANESTHETIC AGENTS

There are numerous topical ophthalmic anesthetic agents available. The choice of which agent is best suited to a particular condition is left to the individual's discretion. I prefer proparacaine hydrochloride (Ophthaine drops*), 0.5 per cent. It should be refrigerated to prevent breakdown and discoloration. Topical anesthetics are used primarily for diagnostic and minor surgical procedures. Prolonged use of topical anesthetics may retard corneal healing and produce systemic toxicity. Onset and duration of some topical anesthetics are found in Table 1.

Local anesthetic block is frequently employed in the treatment of corneal disease or in performing enucleations in the bovine species. Akinesia of the lids can be achieved by use of an auriculopalpebral nerve block or a ring block. In enucleation procedures, a retrobulbar anesthetic block is necessary.

In the Peterson retrobulbar block in cattle, the optic, oculomotor, trochlear, abducens, and ophthalmic nerves and the maxillary divisions of the trigeminal nerve are blocked. An 8 to 10 cm, 18-gauge, slightly curved needle is inserted into the caudal angle between the supraorbital process and the zygomatic arch to the coronoid process of the mandible. The needle is manipulated off the rostral border of the coronoid process and is advanced to the pterygopalatine fossa and the orbitorotundum foramen. The syringe is aspirated to make sure the maxillary artery has not been entered, and 15 to 20 ml of local anesthetic are injected. Additionally, the auriculopalpebral nerve, located 5 to 7 cm caudal to the supraorbital process, is blocked where it crosses the zygomatic arch.

ANTIBIOTICS AND SULFONAMIDES

The major clinical ocular problem involving cattle is infectious bovine keratoconjunctivitis, an external disease condition produced by *Moraxella bovis*. Although the organism is susceptible to numerous antibiotics and chemotherapeutic agents, there are major problems in treat-

ing this clinical condition, and several points deserve emphasis:

1. The superficial keratitis associated with *M. bovis* infection results in edema of the epithelial cells and desquamation and necrosis of the epithelium. If the eye can be effectively treated at this time for 3 to 7 days with appropriate antibiotics, good results should take place with rapid growth of the epithelia of the cornea.
2. The major problem in treatment of this disease is that initial treatment is seldom carried out long enough, or it is instituted too late in the course of the disease when secondary changes have taken place that can result in severe structural damage to the cornea.
   a. Stromal inflammatory cellular infiltrates
   b. Intrastromal edema
   c. Necrotic sloughing of corneal stroma
   d. Neovascularization of the cornea
   e. Endothelial cell damage
   f. Secondary anterior uveitis
   g. Corneal perforation

Weber and colleagues have studied the antibiotic sensitivity of *M. bovis*. All strains of *M. bovis* are found to be resistant to cloxacillin. Sixty-eight per cent of hemolytic isolates are resistant to streptomycin. The mean minimal inhibitory concentration for triple sulfonamides and Tylosin are 7.13 and 6.69 mg/ml, respectively. Sulfonamide levels can be achieved in the blood of cattle by a single intravenous dose of sulfadimidine 100 mg/kg. Maximal achievable blood level of Tylosin is only 1 mg/ml, following intramuscular administration of 12 to 15 mg/kg.

In a recent study, long-acting tetracycline (OTC) given IM to calves at 20 mg/kg in 2 doses, 72 hrs apart, resulted in the elimination of the carrier state of *M. bovis* from calves that had been previously infected. Calves were treated with a single OTC IM injection, and culture results were negative by 24 hr after the first treatment. Based on pharmacokinetic studies, the concentration of OTC in the tears remained very low for a short period, whereas the concentration in the tissues (5.0 µg/ml) remained elevated. It appears to be the tissue concentrations that have eliminated the organism.

Subconjunctival injections can be given following akinesia of the lid with an auriculopalpebral nerve block and the administration of the topical anesthetic of choice. The bulbar conjunctiva at the 12 o'clock position approximately 5 to 7 mm from the limbus is the most efficient location for injection. A tuberculin syringe or 2.5 ml syringe can be used, and a 22-gauge to 25-gauge needle is recommended. No more than 1.0 ml of medication should be instilled in an individual. Antibiotics and dosages for conjunctival administration are found in Table 2.

With severe corneal stromal damage and structural disorganization with stromal inflammatory infiltrates, more extensive treatment may be required to bring the inflammation under control.

Reducing the degree of stromal inflammation as well as secondary uveal inflammation can be accomplished by the subconjunctival administration of corticosteroids. Using the higher concentrations of steroids, such as methylprednisolone acetate suspension (Depo-Medrol*), 40 mg/ml, triamcinolone acetonide suspension (Kenalog Injection†), 40 mg/ml, and betamethasone (acetate and disodium

---

*Available from E. R. Squibb Corp., Princeton, New Jersey 08540

*Available from Upjohn Co., Kalamazoo, Michigan 49001
†Available from E. R. Squibb Corp., Princeton, New Jersey 08540

Table 2. *Antibiotics and Doses for Subconjunctival Administration*

Antibiotic	Dose
Neomycin	100–500 mg
Bacitracin	10,000 units
plus polymyxin B	5–10 mg
Erythromycin	100 mg
Novobiocin	15 mg
plus polymyxin B	5–10 mg
Penicillin G	500,000 units
plus streptomycin	50 mg
Soframycin	250–500 mg
Other Agents	
Amphotericin B	15–125 µg
Carbomycin	2.5 mg
Chloramphenicol sodium succinate	50–100 mg
Kanamycin	10–20 mg
Oleandomycin	1.25 mg
Spiramycin	10–20 mg
Tetracycline	2.5 mg

phosphate combination*), 6 mg/ml, effective levels of anti-inflammatory agents can be administered subconjunctivally.

Cortisone injections may be repeated every 72 hr, if necessary, when antibiotics are given.

Very severe cases of deep interstitial keratitis are complicated by secondary uveitis. The use of a cycloplegic agent, such as 1- to 4-per cent atropine, can be beneficial in reducing pain and avoiding synechia formation. Again, frequency of application is important, and atropine ointment should be applied 3 times a day. If topical treatment is not feasible, subconjunctival injections of 0.5 ml of 1- to 4-per cent atropine sulfate are helpful. The higher concentrations (3 to 4 per cent) are advantageous in severe cases of uveitis, if they are available. When topical antibiotic preparations can be used in the bovine, ointments are preferred because of their prolonged contact time. Drugs of choice for topical application are chloramphenicol and sulfisoxazole ophthalmic ointments.

Other forms of medication have been evaluated in bovine infectious keratoconjunctivitis. Recent studies in humans and animals have shown that the use of membrane-controlled diffusion systems to release drugs can be very effective for ocular use. Recent work in cattle has demonstrated that ring devices slightly larger than the globe but smaller than the conjunctival fornix (135 to 140 mm in circumference or 42.9 to 44.5 mm in diameter) can be used to deliver a bio-available antibiotic, and the ring will be retained for up to a period of 19 days. Although not yet perfected, this form of treatment can provide a mechanism for continual administration of drugs.

Infectious ovine keratoconjunctivitis is a serious problem in sheep flocks. The cause may not be confined to a single infectious agent but rather numerous infectious agents, including *Chlamydia psittaci, Colesiota conjunctivae,* mycoplasma species, and a wide variety of bacteria, which have been isolated from conjunctival scrapings. Exfoliative cytology can be helpful in detecting the early stages of the disease when intracytoplasmic chlamydial inclusions of initial and elementary bodies may be present. Chlortetracyclines and sulfonamides are effective in treating *Chlamydia psittaci* agents. Nouws and Konig have reported that oxytetracycline administered as a single

*Available from E. R. Squibb Corp., Princeton, New Jersey 08540

intramuscular dose to sheep at 20 mg/kg achieves lacrimal fluid concentrations of 1.53 ± 0.70 µgm/ml, and that drug levels could be detected 25 to 30 hr post-injection. Both penicillin and dihydrostreptomycin have been shown to penetrate poorly into the lacrimal fluid of sheep.

CORTICOSTEROIDS

Corticosteroids produce generalized suppression of ocular inflammatory disorders and help to maintain ocular structure and physiology.

Action of Anti-inflammatory Agents

The beneficial effects of corticosteroids in the treatment of ocular disease can be summarized as follows:

1. They reduce cellular and fibrinous exudation and decrease tissue exudation.
2. They diminish the formation of scar tissue.
3. They limit neovascularization.
4. They reduce capillary permeability.

The major area of clinical use for corticosteroids is in controlling the inflammation associated with chronic superficial keratitis and the inflammation associated with uveitis.

Selection of Corticosteroids

The choice of corticosteroids may seem confusing to the practitioner, and several important points must be kept in mind

1. The ocular bio-availability of the drug (penetration of the steroid into the desired tissue).
2. The anti-inflammatory activity desired.
3. The duration of effect.

Following topical administration of corticosteroids to the eye, the highest levels are found in the cornea and conjunctiva. The penetration of topically applied steroids is determined by differential solubility characteristics and tissue factors. The derivative used in the corticosteroid preparation is significant because it increases corneal penetration and achieves the necessary levels in the aqueous humor. Changing the steroid derivative from the alcohol to the acetate greatly enhances the penetrating ability of the steroid. As an example, 1.0-per cent prednisolone acetate (Prednefrin Forte Drops*) provides higher concentrations of corticosteroids in the aqueous and corneal stroma than 0.1-per cent dexamethasone alcohol, 0.1-per cent dexamethasone phosphate, and 1.0-per cent prednisolone phosphate. However, if the corneal epithelium is severely damaged, other forms of steroids,

*Available from Allergan Pharmaceuticals, Irvine, California 92713

Table 3. *Steroids and Their Relative Anti-inflammatory Activities*

Steroid	Relative Anti-inflammatory Activity
Hydrocortisone	1
Prednisolone	4
Methylprednisolone	5
Betamethasone	25
Dexamethasone	25
Fluorometholone	40

Table 4. *Topical Glucocorticoid Ophthalmic Preparations*

Generic Name	Trade Name	Strengths Available (%)
Cortisone acetate ointment	Cortone Acetate	1.5
Hydrocortisone acetate suspension	Hydrocortone Acetate	2.5
Hydrocortisone acetate solution	Optef Drops	0.2
Hydrocortisone acetate ointment	Hydrocortone Acetate	1.5
Hydrocortisone ointment	Cortril	0.5 and 2.5
Hydrocortisone phosphate solution (as the disodium salt)	Corphos	0.5
Prednisolone phosphate solution (as the disodium salt)	Hydeltrasol, Optival	0.5
Prednisolone phosphate ointment	Hydeltrasol	0.25
Prednisolone alcohol solution	Prednefrin S	0.2
Prednisolone acetate suspension	Prednefrin Forte	1.0
Prednisolone acetate suspension	Prednefrin	0.12
Prednisolone sodium phosphate	Inflamase	0.125
Prednisolone sodium phosphate	Inflamase Forte	1.0
Dexamethasone phosphate solution (as the disodium salt)	Decadron	0.1
Dexamethasone phosphate ointment	Decadron	0.05
Dexamethasone suspension	Maxidex	0.1
Fludrocortisone hemisuccinate solution	Florinef Hemisuccinate	0.1
Betamethasone	Celestone	0.1
Triamcinolone acetonide	Kenalog	0.1
Fluorometholone	FML	0.1
Medrysone (hydroxymesterone)	HMS	1.0

especially prednisolone phosphate, may penetrate just as well.

Knowing the anti-inflammatory activity of various steroid compounds can also be helpful in selecting agents for treating ocular disease (Table 3).

Corticosteroids have their most dramatic effect in those diseases affecting the cornea, uveal tract, and external structures of the eye. They are ineffective in degenerative diseases of the corneal, retina, and uveal tracts.

The route of steroid administration is quite important. If the lesion is superficial—involving the lids, conjunctiva, or cornea—topical steroid drugs or ointments are usually effective. When the lesion is posterior to the iris, e.g., chorioretinitis and optic neuritis, systemic steroid therapy may be utilized to effect.

Topical Therapy with Steroids

In general, I prefer to use the ointments in treating animals because of the longer contact time and decreased frequency of administration. In treating superficial keratitis, the topical use of 0.1-per cent dexamethasone ointment or prednisolone ointment is effective.

Injection of Corticosteroids

Local injection of corticosteroids refers to subconjunctival injections, which provide a rapid way of delivering high concentrations. The repository forms of injections, such as methylprednisolone acetate, may provide a source of steroids that lasts for up to 2 weeks. Topical and injectable glucocorticoids are found in Tables 4 and 5.

Table 5. *Injectable Glucocorticoid Ophthalmic Preparations*

Generic Name	Trade Name	Strengths Available (%)
Cortisone acetate suspension	Cortone Acetate	25 mg and 50 mg/ml
Dexamethasone phosphate (as the disodium salt)	Decadron Phosphate	4 mg/ml
	Hexadrol Phosphate	4 mg/ml
Hydrocortisone injection (as the sodium succinate)	Solu-Cortef	100 mg, 250 mg, 500 mg, and 1000 mg vials
Hydrocortisone injection	Cortef (sterile solution)	5 mg/ml
	Infusion Hydrocortisone	5 mg/ml
Hydrocortisone suspension	Cortef (intramuscular)	50 mg/ml
Hydrocortisone acetate	Cortef Acetate	50 mg/ml
	Hydrocortone Acetate	25 mg/ml
	Cortril Acetate	25 mg/ml
Hydrocortisone butylacetate suspension	Hydrocortone-TBA	25 mg/ml
Methylprednisolone acetate suspension	Depo-Medrol	20 mg, 40 mg, and 80 mg/ml
Methylprednisolone sodium succinate	Solu-Medrol	40 mg, 125 mg, 500 mg, and 1000 mg vials
Prednisolone acetate suspension	Meticortelone (soluble)	25 mg/ml
	Nisolone (aqueous)	25 mg/ml
	Sterane (intramuscular and intra-articular)	25 mg/ml
Prednisolone butylacetate suspension	Hydeltra-TBA	20 mg/ml
Prednisolone phosphate	Hydeltrasol	20 mg/ml
Triamcinolone diacetate suspension	Aristocort (parenteral)	25 mg/ml
Triamcinolone acetonide suspension	Kenalog (parenteral)	10 mg/ml 40 mg/ml
Betamethasone (acetate and disodium phosphate combination)	Celestone Soluspan	6 mg/ml

Table 6. *Basic Ophthalmic Pharmaceuticals and Diagnostic Aids for Stocking a Veterinary Pharmacy*

Product	Supplier
Adrenergics	
0.5 and 1% Mydriacil (tropicamide drops)	Alcon Laboratories, Inc., Fort Worth, Texas
1–4% Atropine drops (ointment)	—
10% Neo-Synephrine Hydrochloride drops	Winthrop Laboratories, New York
Antibiotics	
Neomycin, polymyxin B, bacitracin-ointment of choice	—
Garamycin ophthalmic ointment (gentamicin sulfate)	Schering Corporation, Kenilworth, New Jersey
Chloromycetin ophthalmic ointment	Parke Davis and Company, Detroit, Michigan
Antibiotic-Steroid Combination	
Maxitrol ophthalmic ointment	Alcon Laboratories, Inc., Fort Worth, Texas
Topical Anesthetic	
Ophthaine (proparacaine HCl drops, 0.5%)	E. R. Squibb Company, Princeton, New Jersey
Ophthalmic Irrigating Solution	
Dacriose solution (4 oz)	Smith, Miller & Patch Division, Cedar Knolls, New Jersey and Cooper Laboratories, San German, Puerto Rico
Steroids	
Maxidex ophthalmic ointment	Alcon Laboratories, Inc., Fort Worth, Texas
Prednefrin Forte ophthalmic drops	Allergan Pharmaceuticals, Irvine, California

Contraindications for Corticosteroids

Purulent bacterial infections and ulcerations should not be treated with corticosteroids for a prolonged period of time because of the danger of superinfection with other bacterial or fungal agents. When severe corneal disease threatens to cause extensive visual loss, corticosteroids can be combined with effective antimicrobial therapy to prevent permanent visual alteration associated with scar tissue.

PRACTICAL DIAGNOSTIC AIDS

Fluorescein and rose bengal are 2 of the more commonly used dyes that aid in the diagnosis of external ocular disorders. Fluorescein is used primarily in the form of impregnated paper strips. Damage to the epithelium allows the underlying corneal stroma to stain with fluorescein dye. Fluorescein can also be used to test nasolacrimal patency by observing the passage of dye through the nasolacrimal system and its exit at the external nares. The use of cobalt-blue filtered light can be quite helpful in assessing the passage of dye. Some of the basic ophthalmic pharmaceuticals and diagnostic aids are found in Table 6.

References

1. Bistner, S.: Ocular Therapeutics. In Kirk, R. (ed.) Current Veterinary Therapy 8. Philadelphia, W. B. Saunders Company, 1983.
2. Hughes, D. E., and Pugh, G. W.: Infectious bovine keratoconjunctivitis: a ring device designed for prolonged retention in the bovine eye. Am. J. Vet. Res. 36:1043–1045, 1975.
3. Weber, J. J., Fales, W. H., and Selby, L. A.: Antimicrobial susceptibility of *Moraxella bovis* is determined by agar disc diffusion and broth microdilution. Antimicro. Agents and Chemo. 21:554–557, 1982.
4. Brightman, A., Theodorakis, M., Otto, J., et al.: Development of a Biodegradable Insert for the Treatment of Infectious Bovine Keratoconjunctivitis. Proceedings of the Fourteenth Annual Meeting of American College Veterinary Ophthalmologists, Chicago, Illinois, 1983.
5. Slatter, D. H., Costa, N. D., and Edwards, M. E.: Ocular inserts for the application of drugs to bovine eyes—*in vitro* and *in vivo* studies on the release of gentamicin from collagen inserts. Aust. Vet. J. 59:114–121, 1983.
6. Nouws, J. F. M., and Konig, C. D. W.: Penetration of some antibiotics into the lacrimal fluid of sheep. Vet. Quart. 5:114–121, 1983.
7. George, L. W.: Clinical infectious bovine keratoconjunctivitis. Comp. Cont. Ed. 6:712–722, 1984.

Congenital Ocular Defects in the Bovine

H. W. LEIPOLD, D.V.M., Ph.D.

Congenital defects are defined as abnormalities of structure present at birth that may affect a single structure such as the eye, or may affect multiple organs. Frequency of congenital ocular defects varies among species and breeds. Studies defining the incidence and importance of congenital ocular defects in the bovine are limited. The number of cases of anophthalmia-microphthalmia has been estimated for all breeds of cattle in the United States to range from as low as 1 in 50,000 births to as high as 1 in 7500 births. At highest risk are the Jersey and Holstein breeds. Of 1275 congenital defects in cattle, one series listed 238 ocular defects (18.6%). The most commonly diagnosed defects were heterochromia irides, anophthalmia-microphthalmia, and retinal dysplasia.

During embryogenesis of the eye a spectrum of developmental errors may occur, which may range from a focal blemish to an extensive defect that may involve single or multiple ocular structures. In addition, ocular defects may be part of syndromes with associated systemic defects, e.g., anophthalmia-microphthalmia with lumbosacral vertebral defects or high ventricular septal defects.

EMBRYOGENESIS

The anlage of the eye is seen first in the lateral wall of the developing diencephalon. Neuroectoderm produces the retinal layers, whereas surface ectoderm produces the optical components (cornea and lens). Mesoderm contributes the uveal stroma and blood vessels. Initially an optic vesicle is formed. Formation of the optic cup results from enfolding of the optic vesicle. The inner layer of the optic cup differentiates into the unpigmented ciliary epithelium and the sensory retina. Thus, the retina is considered an extension of the central nervous system and is connected to it via the developing optic nerve to the lateral geniculate body. The outer part of the optic cup differentiates into retinal pigment epithelium, ciliary pigment epithelium, and the pupillary sphincter and dilator muscles. The surface ectoderm that is in contact with the optic vesicles is the lens placode, which is induced to form a lens vesicle. Mesodermal tissue differentiates into nutritive and supportive ocular structures of the anterior and posterior uvea.

ETIOLOGY

Congenital ocular defects are rare in cattle but may assume major significance. They may be inherited or may result from environmental factors. Congenital eye disease is of particular concern to the veterinary practitioner involved in the management of breeding herds and artificial breeding service units because, if ocular defects are of genetic origin, expensive and extensive adjustment of breeding programs may be required. Although inherited defects usually have simple Mendelian patterns, such as an autosomal recessive gene or a dominant gene, polygenic modes of inheritance appear to be more important when considering the heritability of congenital ocular defects. Polygenic inheritance may be due to minor but additive effects of many genes. The phenotypic expression is influenced by small, usually undefined changes in the environment, spontaneous chromosomal mutations, teratogens, or other unidentified causes. A high incidence of defects in a single breed, bilateral expression of the defect, common ancestry, or independence from seasonal factors may suggest genetic transmission.

Studies have linked maternal hypovitaminosis A to blindness in calves due to optic foramen malformation. Experimental inoculation of BVD into susceptible heifers at 150 days of gestation caused acute ocular lesions in fetuses 17 to 21 days after inoculation. After 4 weeks, acute lesions resolve and in neonatal calves, focal or diffuse retinal atrophy is present. Cerebellar hypoplasia or degeneration may be seen in calves infected prenatally with BVD concurrent with cataracts, microphthalmia, and optic neuritis. Thus, calves may be born with ataxia and visual impairment. The signs may vary from mild to severe. Congenital defects may involve brain, skin, or bone structures, and intrauterine growth retardation, stillbirths, mummification, and abortions may also be encountered.

STRABISMUS AND NYSTAGMUS

Strabismus is defined as deviation of the eyeball from its axis and may include one or both eyes. In Jersey cattle, it has been shown to be due to homozygosity of a simple autosomal recessive gene. Convergent strabismus in Jersey cattle is not expressed at birth but is evident between 6 to 12 months of life. The condition has also been reported to have a high frequency in Shorthorn cattle, but genetic evidence is inconclusive. Abnormal ocular position may be caused by excessive tension of certain extraocular muscles and laxity of their opponents. However, primary lesions may be present in brain stem nuclei or in cranial nerves that innervate these muscles.

Undulatory nystagmus in the Finnish Ayrshire is likely due to autosomal recessive inheritance. Nystagmus is characterized by a high frequency, small amplitude tremor, which is usually symmetrical. Vision appears not to be impaired. In 1 study, 3 out of 5 bulls also had slight extensor rigidity of the posterior limbs. Histologic examination of vestibular nuclei and adjacent brain areas revealed no deviation from normal.

EYELID DEFECTS

Palpebral atresia, a lack of development of the palpebral fissure, is rare in cattle, as are other congenital defects of the eyelids, conjunctiva, and cornea. Distichiasis, defined as a second row of eyelashes usually directed against the cornea, may cause considerable ocular irritation. Entropion (inward rolling of the eyelids) has been postulated to be due to homozygosity of a simple autosomal recessive gene, whereas little is known regarding the genetics of ectropion (outward rolling of the eyelids). Transient conformational variations may predispose an individual animal to eyelid abnormalities. In entropion, both the upper and lower eyelids, including the canthral area, may be inverted. Surgical correction of the defect may be indicated and is usually successful; however, breeding of affected animals should be discouraged.

DERMOIDS

Ocular dermoids in cattle are solid, skin-like masses of tissue that may be found on eyelids, conjunctiva, nictitating membrane, and cornea. A number of breeds of cattle have been reported to be afflicted with dermoids. Usually the dermoids appear as a single mass adhering to the anterior surface of the globe astride the ventro-lateral limbus. They may range in their effect from a small blemish with no functional defect to a severe ocular irritation. Visual impairment may occur with large dermoid masses. Careful surgical excision can be accomplished, but breeding affected animals should be discouraged.

Ocular dermoids in Hereford cattle may be genetically transmitted, since features of autosomal recessive and polygenic inheritance have been observed. In Herefords, dermoids typically occur bilaterally as multiple, interconnected ocular masses. Clinically, histologically, and ultrastructurally these growths mimic normal haired skin. Sites most commonly involved are the ventro-lateral limbus, third eyelid, medial canthus, eyelids, and conjunctiva. Central corneal dermoids have also been observed in Hereford cattle.

MISCELLANEOUS EXTERNAL OCULAR DEFECTS

Hereditary corneal edema of German Black Pied and Friesian cattle in Great Britain is characterized by mild corneal edema at birth. The edema slowly worsens with age, causing visual impairment and blindness in advanced cases. The defect is transmitted as a simple autosomal recessive trait.

Supernumerary openings of the nasolacrimal drainage system have been reported in Holstein and Brown Swiss cattle. These patent supernumerary openings are located 2 to 3 cm distal to the medial canthus. The cause is not known. The effect of these openings may be a predisposition to infections and epiphora.

COLOR DILUTION DEFECTS

Albinism may be classified as complete, partial, or incomplete. Complete albinos have pure white to pink irides and no tapetum lucidum. Complete albinism is a simple autosomal recessive trait. Albino calves have pale skin and lack pigment. The pupils usually appear slit-like, and a red fundus reflex is present. Such calves often appear to be blind in bright light due to photophobia. Histologically, the complete absence of pigmentation of skin and eyes is characteristic of the albino.

Ocular defects of incomplete albino Hereford cattle include heterochromia irides, tapetum fibrosum hypoplasia, and typical coloboma of the nontapetal fundus. This incomplete albinism is transmitted as an autosomal dominant trait.

In partial albinism, the iris is blue and white centrally and brown peripherally, and the coat color is usually characteristic of the breed but may appear lighter. Partial albinism encountered in the Chediak-Higashi syndrome reported in Hereford cattle is recessively inherited. It includes, besides albinotic features, abnormally large, membrane-bound organelles in various cell types and greater susceptibility to infection.

Heterochromia irides has been described in various breeds of cattle, such as Holstein, Simmental, and Limousin. The iris is light blue in the center and whitish green in the outer zone. Photophobia and nystagmus usually are present. The fundi of affected eyes are generally light yellow in the tapetal area, and the nontapetal fundus appears gray. It is a hereditary defect, although the mode of transmission has not been described. The coat color is typical of the breed but may be dilute or more white than normal.

A new albinotic color deficiency recently identified in Angus cattle is inherited as a simple autosomal recessive trait. The Angus cattle involved have heterochromia irides and characteristic brown hair coats instead of typical black coats. The muzzles, hooves, and scrotum in males are also brown. The skin surface may be brownish to gray. This is particularly obvious in areas of glabrous skin, such as around eyelids, ear openings, muzzle, and anal and reproductive openings. The iris has an outer, faintly brown ring and an inner, light blue ring circling the pupil. The pupils always appear constricted in daylight. From a distance, the eyes appear white. The ocular fundus is albinotic.

LENS DEFECTS

Congenital defects of the lens in cattle are rare. Cataracts induced by prenatal BVD have been discussed. Absence of the lens, aphakia, may be found in anophthalmia-microphthalmia syndrome. Microphakia, or congenitally small lens, may also be part of this syndrome or may be associated with multiple eye defects in Jersey cattle. This syndrome in Jersey cattle is transmitted as a simple autosomal recessive trait and may include irideremia, lens luxation, and cataract.

Congenital cataracts have been reported in Jersey, Hereford, and Holstein cattle as due to homozygosity of a simple autosomal gene. These cataracts mature in animals by 4 to 11 months of age, thereby causing blindness in affected calves. Cataract surgery may be successfully performed in cattle.

Nuclear cataracts in 2 dairy herds have been observed with bilateral symmetry of opacity. Cataracts were confined to the nucleus of the lens, while the cortex was clear. Two distinct types were observed. The first type of cataract was characterized by a dense, opaque, white nuclear region visible on external eye examination without magnification. Although the second type distorted the light rays, upon close inspection the media was not totally opaque but had the appearance of the base of a clear glass bottle. Etiologic studies suggested environmental factors.

Glaucoma, cataracts, and lens luxations have been described in New Zealand Friesian cattle as autosomal dominant defects. Cataracts are relatively rare in cattle and when observed the main differential consideration should include intrauterine viral infection or genetic transmission.

FUNDUS DEFECTS

Defects of the ocular fundus have been observed in cattle. Retinal dysplasia has been discussed as an obligatory factor in Shorthorn and Hereford calves afflicted with internal hydrocephalus. Retinal dysplasia has also been reported to be caused by prenatal BVD infections.

Anomalies of the ocular fundus may occur in calves following maternal hypovitaminosis A. Optic nerve atrophy characterized funduscopically by avascularity, pallor, and loss of the myelin border is believed to be caused by a malformation of the optic foramen. Abnormal formation of the bony channel (optic canal) through the sphenoid bone apparently results from osteogenesis, which is not accompanied by normal osteolysis and osteoclastic resorption.

Typical colobomas are part of dominant incomplete albinism of Hereford cattle and may also be observed in Charolais calves. In Charolais, colobomas are bilateral but not necessarily symmetrical. There is usually no impairment of vision. The condition is inherited as an autosomal dominant trait.

OCULAR DEFECTS ASSOCIATED WITH SYSTEMIC ABNORMALITIES

Several descriptions of ocular defects in cattle include defects of other body organs, especially the central nervous system (CNS). Corneal opacity has been observed in Norwegian Red Poll calves affected with posterior paralysis, an inherited defect. Morphologic studies of a hydrocephalic syndrome in newborn Hereford calves revealed multiple defects in the CNS and associated mesodermal and ocular defects. Internal hydrocephalus was found in combination with enlargement of the cranium, narrowing of the Sylvian aqueduct due to a malformed mesencephalon, hypoplasia or dysplasia of the cerebellum, myelin deficiency of the cerebellum, spinal cord, and cerebrum, and atrophy of the optic nerve. Eye defects such as microphthalmia, retinal detachment, cataract, and liquefaction of the vitreous body were consistently present.

Congenital hydrocephalus in Shorthorn calves was accompanied by a stenotic aqueduct, cerebellar hypoplasia, myopathy and multiple ocular anomalies, retinal detachment and dysplasia, cataract, microphthalmia, and persistent pupillary membranes. Internal hydrocephalus combined with ocular and muscular defects is inherited as a single autosomal recessive trait.

In a series of 26 calves affected with microphthalmia-anophthalmia syndrome, 10 calves had other systemic defects, such as high ventricular septal defect of the heart and defects of the vertebral column.

In conclusion, a wide variety of congenital defects have been reported in cattle. Many, but not all, of these anomalies are genetic in origin. More studies are needed to carefully record types and frequencies of these ocular defects.

Supplemental Reading

Barkyoumb, S. D., and Leipold, H. W.: Nature and cause of bilateral ocular dermoids in Hereford cattle. Vet. Path. 21:316–324, 1984.

Leipold, H. W., and Huston, K.: Congenital syndrome with anophthalmia-microphthalmia and associated defects in cattle. Path. Vet. 5:407–418, 1968.

Ojo, S., Huston, K., Leipold, H. W., and Gelatt, K. N.: Ocular anomalies of incomplete albino Hereford cattle. Bov. Pract. 17:115–121, 1982.

Strasia, C. A., Johnson, J. L., Cole, D., and Leipold, H. W.: Partial albinism (heterochromia irides) in black Angus cattle. Bov. Pract., 128:147–149, 1983.

Infectious Bovine Keratoconjunctivitis

R. B. MILLER, D.V.M., M.S., Ph.D.
and W. H. FALES, M.S., Ph.D.

Infectious bovine keratoconjunctivitis (IBK) is a contagious infectious ocular disease of cattle caused by *Moraxella bovis*. The disease, also known as pinkeye, is characterized, clinically, by varying degrees of photophobia, lacrimation, conjunctivitis, and keratitis.

DISTRIBUTION AND INCIDENCE

IBK occurs worldwide and is enzootic in herds throughout the United States. Although IBK may occur during any season of the year, most epizootics of the disease are during the summer. The highest number of new cases coincides with the period of maximal solar radiation. This takes place in the north central United States from mid-June until mid-August; in the southern states this period of intense solar radiation is longer.

The herd incidence of IBK throughout the United States is not known. However, a survey of Missouri cattle owners in 1978 indicated that 45.35 per cent of the herds in that state had a clinical disease resembling IBK. Cattle more than 1 year of age are more resistant to both infection with *M. bovis* and development of clinical signs of IBK than cattle less than 1 year of age. In affected herds, up to 100 per cent of the calves and up to 85 per cent of the adults may have 1 or both eyes infected with *M. bovis*. The incidence of IBK with keratitis (corneal lesions) in herds will vary, with up to 100 per cent of the calves and 72 per cent of the cows affected. Bilateral lesions may be seen in 70 per cent of the calves and 50 per cent of the adults with IBK. Beef cattle have a higher incidence of IBK than do dairy cattle. A small but significant difference in susceptibility to IBK exists among breeds. Hereford and white-faced cattle are at the highest risk, while Angus, Charolais cross, and Indian breeds are less susceptible. Apparently, greater proportions of eye margin pigmentation reduce the incidence and severity of IBK. However, it is not known if this resistance is due to the amount of pigmentation or other genetic factors.

TRANSMISSION AND ETIOLOGY

Inapparent carrier cattle or cattle with IBK lesions may be sources of *M. bovis* that initiate epizootics of IBK. The *M. bovis* carriers may be herd residents, herd additions, or noncontact cattle from neighboring herds. The *M. bovis* organisms are present in ocular, nasal, and vaginal secretions. Transmission is by direct contact, nasal aerosols, insect vectors, and fomites. *M. bovis* has been isolated from the eyes of newborn calves. Apparently, the dam's reproductive tract was the source of infection.

The only recognized etiologic agent of IBK is *M. bovis*. Whether ultraviolet (UV) radiation from the sun or lamps enhances the development of IBK is not known for certain, but UV radiation does cause ultrastructural damage to the corneal epithelium. Certain strains of *M. bovis* will induce IBK without UV radiation. In addition to age, breed, and sunlight, other predisposing factors may include dust, vitamin A deficiency, mechanical irritants, i.e., tall grass and plant seeds, plant pollens, and the face fly (*Musca autumnalis*), the house fly (*M. domestica*), and the stable fly (*Stomxys calcitrans*), as mechanical vectors. *Moraxella bovis* grows as smooth or rough colonies and as hemolytic or nonhemolytic colonies on blood agar. The smooth hemolytic form is considered to be pathogenic, while the rough nonhemolytic form is not considered to be pathogenic. Rough colonies of *M. bovis* are isolated frequently during winter while smooth colonies are isolated frequently during summer. Isolates of *M. bovis* will change forms both *in vitro* and *in vivo*. All factors responsible for causing this change in colony form are not known, but UV radiation is thought to cause *M. bovis* to change from the nonhemolytic to the hemolytic form. Some workers classify the colony of pathogenic *M. bovis* as smooth while others classify this same colony as rough.

CLINICAL SIGNS

The eye is the only organ in the bovine in which lesions are known to be produced by *M. bovis* infection. The clinical signs of IBK are variable in severity and duration. They include lacrimation, photophobia, blepharospasm, spasm of the iris (miosis), conjunctivitis, blepharitis, and keratitis. Initial serous lacrimation (epiphora) may become slightly mucopurulent and copious. Photophobia may be expressed initially by the animal turning the affected eye away from light, by involuntary blinking, or by keeping the eye closed. Conjunctivitis may appear within 24 hr after lacrimation is evident. Slight edema and reddening of the mucous membranes of the eyes are signs of conjunctivitis. Keratitis usually develops during the height of photophobia and conjunctivitis, and may be observed as early as 2 to 4 days from the onset of the disease as evidenced by cloudiness, a white spot, or a vesicle in the center of the cornea. The condition may persist for 1 to 14 days and heal or become ulcerated. The ulcers may cover the entire cornea. The healing stage of corneal ulcers is shown by vascularization at the margins of ulcers. This vascularization may be perilimbal and circumscribe the cornea, or it may be limited to that area of the limbus immediately adjacent to the ulcer. As vessels reach the center of the cornea or ulcer, the corneal opacity often begins to clear peripherally. The final phase of healing is a recession of vascularization with resultant scarring, which is usually more dense in the central cornea.

DIFFERENTIAL DIAGNOSIS

IBK can usually be diagnosed by clinical signs alone. Within a herd, the number of cattle affected will vary and so will the clinical signs of the disease. There may be unilateral or bilateral eye involvement, and the severity of lesions in the affected eyes may also vary. Many other ocular infections of cattle are characterized by conjunctivitis and not by keratitis. Malignant catarrhal fever, a highly fatal disease, causes corneal opacity, and infectious bovine rhinotracheitis (IBR) virus occasionally causes lesions on the cornea near the corneal-scleral junction. Concurrent infections of *M. bovis* and IBR virus, *Neisseria*, *Listeria*, *Mycoplasma*, adenovirus, or *Thelazia* may cause an atypical or more severe form of the disease.

Eye swabs for the isolation and identification of *M. bovis* should be collected from both the upper and lower conjunctival sacs before treatment is attempted and before vascularization of the cornea. The swabs should be streaked onto plates at the time of collection. A semiselective media of brain-heart infusion agar with 5 per cent bovine or ovine red blood cells and 2.5 μg/ml of cloxacillin will decrease overgrowth by other organisms and increase the number of *M. bovis* isolations. If eye swabs are transported to a laboratory before plating, they should be placed in Stuarts* or Amies* transport media with 2.5 μgm/ml of cloxacillin and kept on ice during transit.

TREATMENT

Cases of IBK are frustrating for the practitioner to treat because owners usually do not appreciate or recognize the significance of the initial clinical signs. Veterinary assistance is usually sought after the cornea is ulcerated or vascularized. A factor that contributes to this lack of appreciation of clinical signs is the tendency for many infected eyes to resolve without corneal ulceration. The treatment of IBK is directed towards the elimination of *M. bovis* from the infected eyes to prevent development of lesions, or towards a shortening of the recovery time and a lessening of permanent damage to the eye. The cost effectiveness of treating IBK has not been documented but should be considered. Economic losses from the disease are due to (1) decreased growth rate, (2) reduced milk production, (3) treatment costs, (4) increased labor, (5) disfigurement of eyes in purebred cattle, (6) decline in dollar value of feeder calves, and (7) deaths. Reported average reductions in either weaning weights or in 205-day adjusted weaning weights of IBK affected calves varied from 3.6 kg to 18.2 kg. The variation in

*Regional Media Laboratories, Inc. (REMEL), 12076 Santa Fe Dr., P.O. Box 14428, Lenexa, Kansas 66215

effect of IBK was due to severity of disease and whether the disease was unilateral or bilateral. Growth suppression may be much greater in animals with severe disease and in baby calves with bilateral IBK. Most mortalities (4/1000 cases) from IBK occur in these baby calves.

Many of the commonly available antimicrobial drugs are effective against *M. bovis*. Antimicrobics suitable for topical instillation into the conjunctival sac include bacitracin, gentamicin, kanamycin, neomycin, nitrofurazone, polymyxin B, tetracycline, and 5 per cent sulfas. *M. bovis* is usually resistant to streptomycin and cloxacillin. Topical applications onto the eye should be at least 3 times a day for several days. Both eyes should be treated, taking care not to touch the eyes with the applicator, thus avoiding mechanical transmission of *M. bovis*. Topical treatment of early infections will prevent the development of keratitis. Intensive topical treatment of advanced cases will shorten the course of the disease. Affected cattle should be protected from exposure to sunlight, dust, and flies. Eye patches may be used to protect the affected eyes, but the eyes should be examined every few days for clinical response.

Ulcerated and vascularized eyes may also be treated with 1.0 per cent atropine ointment twice daily as supportive therapy for 2 or 3 days to reduce pain from ciliary spasms. The usual therapy for corneal vascularization is the subconjunctival injection of a mixture of antibiotic and corticosteroid, i.e., 1.0 to 2.0 ml of procaine G penicillin and 1.0 mg of dexamethasone. Other efficacious antibiotics for subconjunctival injection are gentamicin and ampicillin. With the animal restrained in a headgate, the nose is raised with a bull lead towards the affected side. The righting reflex will expose the sclera and the injection is made under the bulbar conjunctiva using a 23-gauge needle and a 3-ml syringe. A bleb several millimeters in diameter will be produced. The conjunctiva will act as a semipermeable membrane, which allows a slow release of the mixture onto the eye surface. Subconjunctival injections may be repeated daily for 3 days. Some practitioners prefer to inject 1 to 3 ml of the mixture into the palpebral conjunctiva using a 22-gauge needle. A mixture of 10 mg (0.5 ml) of methylprednisolone and 0.5 ml of procaine G penicillin has been used intrapalpebrally in an attempt to increase the duration of steroid activity. It is possible that intrapalpebral injection may result primarily in systemic absorption rather than in local activity because of the richly vascularized eyelids. Therefore the bulbar conjunctiva appears to be the preferred location for subconjunctival injections.

Deep corneal ulcers that appear likely to rupture (i.e., descemetoceles) should be treated by the use of a membrana nictitans flap after subconjunctival injection of an antibiotic. The skin around the lateral canthus is scrubbed with soap and water. A 2.0-per cent lidocaine solution is injected subcutaneously into each eyelid at the lateral canthus and into the base of the membrana nictitans. A needle holder, a cutting edge needle, a no. 3 chromic catgut, and a rat-tooth thumb forceps are needed for the procedure. The needle is inserted through the upper eyelid (1 cm dorsal to and 1 cm caudal to the lateral canthus) into the dorsolateral conjunctival fornix. The needle is then passed through the membrane nictitans from the backside to the frontside 1 cm from and parallel to the free margin. The suture is next passed into the ventral conjunctival fornix and out through the skin 1 cm ventral to and 1 cm caudal to the lateral canthus of the eye. The suture is tied so that the third eyelid completely covers the globe. An alternate approach is to place the suture 1 cm from the margin of the upper lid (entering the skin 2 cm from the lateral canthus) and after securing the third eyelid, exiting the skin near the same point as the point of entry. With each method, suture removal is in 10 days if it has not broken by that time. Nonabsorbable suture may be used, but this also needs to be removed in 10 days to prevent tearing of the membrana nictitans.

If systemic therapy is desired, sulfamethazine (100 mg/kg) either intravenously or orally for 1 to 3 days or 2 intramuscular injections (19.8 mg/kg) of oxytetracycline (200 mg/ml) given 3 days apart will eliminate most strains of *M. bovis* from the bovine eye. Other commonly used antimicrobics do not appear to be effective for the treatment of IBK by oral or parenteral routes.

PREVENTION

Prevention of IBK in a herd requires that efforts be directed toward (1) eliminating *M. bovis* carriers, (2) reducing the number of insect vectors, and (3) increasing the resistance of susceptible cattle by vaccination.

Systemic treatments that are beneficial in reducing the number of carriers in a herd include sulfamethazine and oxytetracycline, as described under treatment of IBK. A one time topical ocular application of 1.5-per cent silver nitrate solution has also reportedly been efficacious. To effectively eliminate carriers, all adult cattle in the herd should be treated during the nonvector season prior to calving. Prophylactically treating the eyes of newborn calves with topical antibiotics or 1.5-per cent silver nitrate will also reduce the incidence of IBK in young calves.

Of the insect vectors mechanically transmitting *M. bovis,* the face fly is the most important and the most difficult to control. Ocular secretions of cattle are an ideal diet for the female face fly, which must feed daily for 10 days. Face flies usually feed over a 1 mile radius, but they frequently fly up to 5 miles to feed. They feed only in open pasture and not in barns. *M. bovis* will remain viable in the digestive tract of face flies for 2 days. Dust bags will be approximately 60 per cent effective in controlling face flies if they are placed 18 in above the ground in a path or alley that the cattle must use daily. Insecticide tags placed in both ears of all cattle in a herd are probably as good as properly used dust bags and may be more convenient. To be useful, any method of face fly control must be initiated throughout an area early in the season (i.e., April) before a build-up of flies occurs.

Autogenous and commercial unlicensed intrastate bacterins or mixtures of the 2 have been used to vaccinate cattle against IBK. Bacterins have given variable results in the field. In controlled studies, the protection provided by homologous (autogenous) strain bacterins was not complete. At best, they reduced the total number of severe lesions and lessened the total number of days that eyes had lesions when vaccinated animals were compared with nonvaccinated herd mates. Bacterins should be administered subcutaneously in the neck with 2 doses given 21 days apart. For best results, *M. bovis* bacterins should be given 6 weeks prior to the time that IBK is usually seen in an area because at least 42 days are needed after the initial vaccination for cattle to develop antibodies.

A new type of *M. bovis* bacterin with pili as its major antigen was licensed by the USDA in 1983. Pili are involved in the attachment of bacteria to epithelial cells. An effective pili bacterin would stimulate production of host antibodies towards pili and inhibit bacterial attachment and colonization which, in theory, would prevent disease. The efficacy of this *M. bovis* pili bacterin has not been determined by widespread usage in the field. This bacterin would also require at least 42 days to stimulate host antibody formation.

Supplemental Reading

Anderson, J. F., Gelatt, K. N., and Farnsworth, R. J.: A modified membrana nictitans flap technique for the treatment of ulcerative keratitis in cattle. J. Am. Vet. Med. Assoc. *168*:706–708, 1976.

Baptisa, P. J. H. P.: Infectious bovine keratoconjunctivitis: a review. Br. Vet. J. *135*:225–242, 1979.

Pugh, G. W., Jr., and Hughes, D. E.: Bovine keratoconjunctivitis: carrier state of *Moraxella bovis* and the development of preventive measures against disease. J. Am. Vet. Med. Assoc. *167*:310–312, 1975.

Webber, J. J., and Selby, L. A.: Risk factors related to the prevalence of infectious bovine keratoconjunctivitis. J. Am. Vet. Med. Assoc. *179*:823–826, 1981.

Bovine Ocular Squamous Cell Tumors

ROBERT A. KAINER, D.V.M., M.S.

The term "cancer eye" has been used to designate any epithelial neoplasm of the bovine eye or its adnexa, whereas the term "epithelioma of the eye" has been used to imply squamous cell carcinoma. A more descriptive term, bovine ocular squamous cell tumors, includes both benign and malignant neoplasms.

CLINICAL SIGNS

Benign squamous cell tumors on the ocular bulb are either small, white, elevated hyperplastic plaques or large papillomas with verrucous or frond-like surfaces. In these dyskeratotic growths, the white color and firmness reflects the keratinization of the superficial layer of cells. The tumors are most frequent at the lateral or medial limbus, spreading from these sites over the cornea. Frequently, the benign growths are extremely keratinized. Ocular squamous cell carcinomas are more irregular and nodular with a pink hue, indicating greater vascularity of the increased stroma.

Benign keratocanthomas occur more often on the lower eyelid. They are hyperkeratotic growths coated with lacrimal secretions and debris. Palpebral papillomas are typically verrucous with fine surface projections. Except for those on the third eyelid, squamous cell carcinomas of the ocular adnexa tend to be invasive, particularly those in the region of the lacrimal caruncle. Adnexal squamous cell carcinomas tend to be more vascular and scirrhous.

Rapidly growing ocular carcinomas become ulcerated, necrotic, friable, and hemorrhage readily. Squamous cell carcinomas invading the orbit become massive and penetrate bone. In advanced cases, the parotid lymph node on the affected side, ordinarily nonpalpable, becomes palpable and even visible. Metastatic foci may be present in the enlarged lymph node. Clinical signs due to metastatic lesions in vital organs are rarely observed. Squamous cell carcinomas on the globe are less likely to metastasize owing to the barriers imposed by the cornea and sclera. Intraocular invasion usually results in containment of the tumor. Invasive carcinomas from the palpebrae and lacrimal caruncle metastasize more readily.

Not all benign ocular squamous cell tumors progress to carcinoma. About 30 per cent of observed tumors regress completely without any known intervention. Rarely, early squamous cell carcinomas may regress spontaneously. Squamous cell carcinoma can arise *ab initio* (without a grossly notable benign precursor lesion).

DIAGNOSIS

The gross appearance of ocular squamous cell tumors is usually pathognomic; however, it is often difficult to differentiate a benign tumor from a carcinoma *in situ*. In general, squamous cell carcinomas are larger, but size may not always be a reliable indicator of malignancy, as the large size of some hyperkeratinized benign tumors may be misleading. A smooth surfaced mass is not characteristic of a neoplasm of epithelial origin. Fine hairs projecting from a mass would suggest a dermoid cyst. Follicular hyperplasia of the third eyelid could be confused with a tumor. Granulomas must also be included in the differential diagnosis.

Confirmation of a diagnosis based on gross observations requires histopathologic or exfoliative cytologic examination. A biopsy specimen may be excised and fixed in 10 per cent buffered formalin solution; or a cytologic smear may be obtained with a spatula, spread on a slide, and fixed with polyethylene glycol spray or immersed in 95 per cent ethanol. On stained smears, anucleated, keratinized squamous cells from the surface layer and deeper cells with enlarged nuclei containing coarsely clumped chromatin indicate a benign squamous cell tumor. Cells with bizarre shapes and varying sizes with large hyperchromatic nuclei containing large clumps of chromatin and prominent nucleoli are pathognomonic for squamous cell carcinoma. The cytologic results are generally in agreement with the histologic results, 85 to 90 per cent of the time.

In advanced cases of invasive squamous cell carcinoma, necropsy may reveal metastatic lesions in the ipsilateral parotid and lateral retropharyngeal lymph nodes and in vital organs, most notably the lungs, where nodular, pinkish-white lesions occur within the parenchyma. Of all animals with ocular squamous cell carcinomas at slaughter, approximately 5 per cent will have metastatic lesions.

CONTRIBUTING FACTORS

Genetic and environmental factors contribute to the development of bovine ocular squamous cell tumors. Predisposition to the disease is highly heritable in Hereford cattle. Exposure to ultraviolet (UV) light is also a cause, and the amount of exposure is greater with increased altitude and decreased latitude. Reflection of light from snow and certain soil types, and irritation by wind, dust, and flies have been suspected of adding to the incidence of bovine ocular squamous cell tumors. A positive correlation between a high plane of nutrition and the incidence of ocular squamous cell tumors has been demonstrated in Hereford cows. Viruses have been associated with the disease but have not proved to be etiologic agents. Infectious bovine keratoconjunctivitis has not been shown to predispose cattle to these tumors.

INCIDENCE

Bovine ocular squamous cell tumors occur principally in older purebred or crossbred Hereford cattle. The tendency to develop this neoplastic disease is heritable. The tumors are seen also in Simmental cattle, occasionally in Holstein Friesians, and rarely in other breeds. They have not been reported in black Aberdeen Angus cattle. Peak incidence is between 7 and 8 years of age. Ocular tumors are infrequent in cattle less than 3 years of age, although squamous cell carcinoma has been observed in cattle 2 years of age.

Most of the squamous cell tumors originate at the lateral limbus (66 per cent) followed in incidence by the medial limbus, lower eyelid, third eyelid, and the lacrimal caruncle-medial canthal area. Nonpigmented regions are more predisposed to actinic changes caused by UV light and hence the growth of squamous cell tumors. Most of the tumors in Holstein Friesian cattle are on nonpigmented third eyelids.

In Hereford cow herds in semi-arid regions with abundant sunlight, especially at higher altitudes, the incidence of ocular squamous cell tumors may be from 20 per cent to more than 40 per cent. Three per cent to 10 per cent of these tumors are squamous cell carcinomas. Since cows with large ocular tumors are culled more often than treated, nearly 80 per cent of the ocular tumors of cows at slaughter are squamous cell carcinomas.

TREATMENT

Radiation Therapy. Implantations of radioactive isotopes emitting gamma radiation (cobalt-60, gold-198, cesium-137) are effective in treating ocular cell carcinomas. This method is expensive, however, and requires the services of a qualified veterinary radiologist. Beta radiation from a strontium-90 probe has been used with some success on surfaces of debulked circumscribed ocular tumors, although depth of penetration is limited.

Immunotherapy. Intratumoral injections of a modified tuberculosis vaccine (an oil-and-water emulsion of cell walls of the bacillus of Calmette-Guérin) and intramuscular injections of a phenol-saline extract of allogeneic ocular squamous cell carcinomas cause some regression of malignant tumors. Complete regression is found in about one fourth of the squamous cell carcinomas treated experimentally with mycobacterial cell wall emulsion, and about one third of the carcinomas regress completely following treatment with phenol-saline tumor extract. More recently, an adjuvant mycobacterial cell wall skeleton biologic (Ribigen*) has become available. Initial trials indicate that 2 doses at timed intervals using intratumoral injections of this biologic are effective in causing regression of smaller bovine ocular squamous cell tumors.

---

*Available from Ribi Immunochem Research, Inc., Hamilton, Montana 59840

Surgery. Surgical removal of benign and malignant bovine ocular squamous cell tumors is only moderately successful in managing the disease. Excision of small tumors from the eye can be accomplished under topical anesthesia with 0.5 per cent proparacaine following mechanical immobilization with a slotted ocular retractor or following regional anesthesia of the eyelids and orbit. Tumors can be removed from the eyelids, third eyelid, and lacrimal caruncle under local infiltrative anesthesia with 2 per cent lidocaine. Recurrence of tumor growth is common after these 2 procedures.

Anesthesia for exenteration of the eye and ocular adnexa may be achieved with a Peterson retro-orbital injection or a "four-point" injection of the orbit. Radical resection of the tissues of the eye, adnexa, adjacent orbital tissues, parotid and lateral retropharyngeal lymph nodes, and parotid and maxillary salivary glands requires prolonged general anesthesia. Generally, more extensive surgical methods are not cost effective for general practice.

When the orbit is invaded by an ocular squamous cell carcinoma or the parotid lymph node is enlarged, immediate shipment of the animal to slaughter is recommended.

Cryosurgery. A cryosurgical treatment protocol has been developed that is highly successful in causing regression of small (< 2 cm) bovine ocular squamous cell tumors. A double freeze cycle employing liquid nitrogen spray is recommended over a single freeze method. A double freeze cycle (rapid freeze to −25°C, unaided thaw to 5°C, and rapid refreeze to −25°C and thaw) results in a high percentage of complete regression of these tumors.

Lubricant may be applied to the skin, and styrofoam strips and plastic spoons coated with ophthalmic ointment may be used to cover the eye to protect the normal tissues from liquid nitrogen droplets. Thermocouple needles may be inserted into the base of palpebral tumors to monitor temperature, but they cannot be used with bulbar tumors.

Although the initial cost of cryosurgical instruments* is relatively high, the cost of liquid nitrogen is low. Protective materials add very little to the cost of treatment.

Hyperthermia. Hyperthermia induced in tumors by radio frequency current (RFC) is an effective, easily performed, and economically feasible procedure for the treatment of early benign and malignant ocular squamous cell tumors. Hyperthermia induced by localized current field (LCF), RFC in benign and malignant small tumors (< 25 mm in diameter) results in complete regression in a high percentage of the cases. Tumors thicker than 4 to 5 mm are debulked prior to hyperthermic treatment. The majority of the palpebral tumors are treated with the piercing probe of the LCF device or by a combination of the surface and piercing probes.

I have utilized 3 commercial LCF devices† and a prototype supplied by the inventor, J. D. Doss of the Los Alamos Scientific Laboratory. The instruments are calibrated to induce a temperature of approximately 50°C in tissues caused by RFC (2 MHz) passing between the electrodes. An audible pulse is emitted at 1-sec intervals when operating temperature is reached. Temperature is controlled by a thermister in one of the electrodes feeding back to the RFC generator. Owing to concentrated currents at the electrodes, the temperature usually peaks above 50°C before stabilizing. A low power mode is used for small tumors, and a high mode is used for large, well vascularized tumors. The RFC penetrates only about 4 mm.

Before hyperthermic treatment, the animal is restrained in a squeeze chute, and the head is secured with a halter. For local anesthesia of the globe and third eyelid, a small amount (0.3 ml) of 0.5 per cent proparacaine HCl solution (Ophthetic* and Alcaine†) is instilled into the conjunctival sac every 30 sec for 2 to 3 min. A slotted ocular retractor is slipped over the eye usually on the side opposite the lesion, and the eye is positioned and immobilized for treatment. Occasionally, a subconjunctival injection of 2 per cent lidocaine may be used at this time to supplement the topical anesthesia. The electrodes of the surface probe are pressed firmly to the lesion for 30 sec/application. At the moment of application, careful use of nose tongs may be needed for added restraint. If the surface of the lesion is too dry, a few drops of physiologic saline solution on the surface will assure conduction of the current. Multiple, overlapping applications of the electrodes will ensure coverage of larger areas.

Since the RFC penetrates effectively no more than 4 mm, thicker tumors must be debulked prior to application of the surface electrodes. The surgery may be performed under topical proparacaine anesthesia with the eye positioned and immobilized by the slotted ocular retractor. Tumors on the third eyelid may be treated following topical anesthetic instillation. The third eyelid is extended by gentle traction with forceps, and a finger may be inserted behind the lid for support. Local injections of 2 per cent lidocaine provide anesthesia for the hyperthermic treatment of tumors on the palpebrae and more extensive tumors in the area of the lacrimal caruncle. The electrodes of the piercing probe may be used to treat more deeply placed tumors in these locations. After treatment, ocular tissues are flushed with a 5 per cent solution of povidone-iodine (a 50 per cent solution of Betadine‡).

Healing is usually uneventful. The treated tumor and adjacent epithelium slough. Epithelial growth at the corneal sites occurs within a week. Following initial leukoma at the treatment site, corneal scarring is minimal or absent.

Prevention of further exposure of the carcinoma sites to UV light may be accomplished by the application of temporary eye shields, such as those used in the management of infectious bovine keratoconjunctivitis. This procedure is not necessary following routine treatment of small, mostly benign tumors.

Surgery vs. Hyperthermia. In a recent study comparing surgical removal with hyperthermia as the only treatment of similar ocular squamous cell tumors, the overall effectiveness of surgical removal was 46 per cent; hyperthermia effectiveness was approximately 92 per cent.

MANAGEMENT PROTOCOL

The following management protocol is recommended for controlling losses due to ocular squamous cell tumors in beef cow herds of predominantly Hereford or Simmental breeds:

*Available from Frigitronics, Inc., Shelton, Connecticut and Brymill Corporation, Vernon, Connecticut

†Available from Thermoprobe, Hach Company, Loveland, Colorado, Megatherm I, Western Instrument Company, Denver, Colorado, and Hypotherm, RDM International, Phoenix, Arizona

*Available from Allergan Pharmaceuticals, Inc., Irvine, California 92713
†Available from Alcon Laboratories, Inc., Ft. Worth, Texas 76101
‡Available from Purdue Frederick Co., Norwalk, Connecticut 06856

1. Two to 3 times each year, when the cattle are gathered for routine procedures, observe the eyes of susceptible animals (more than 2 years of age) for the presence of tumors and segregate the affected animals.
2. Treatment
   a. Treat all small, circumscribed ocular tumors with RFC induced hyperthermia.
   b. For large but noninvasive carcinomas of the globe or palpebrae, orbital exenteration may be indicated, depending on the productivity of the cow and market prices. Such an animal can be culled at a later date.
   c. Cows with invasive or metastatic squamous cell carcinoma, or both, should be considered for immediate shipment to slaughter.
3. Long-term genetic control of ocular squamous cell tumors may be achieved through careful record keeping and prudent culling of lines with greater predisposition to the disease.

This protocol will substantially reduce losses due to bovine ocular squamous cell tumors.

Supplemental Reading

Farris, H. E.: Cryosurgical treatment of bovine ocular squamous cell carcinoma. Vet. Clin. North Am. *104*:861–867, 1980.

Hoffman, D., Spradbrow, P. B., and Wilson, B. E.: An evaluation of exfoliative cytology in the diagnosis of bovine ocular squamous cell carcinoma. J. Comp. Path. *88*:497–504, 1978.

Kainer, R. A., Stringer, J. M., and Leuker, D. C.: Hyperthermia for treatment of ocular squamous cell tumors in cattle. J. Am. Vet. Med. Assoc. *167*:356–360, 1980.

Ocular Manifestations of Systemic Disease in the Bovine

WILLIAM C. REBHUN, D.V.M.

Ophthalmic lesions can provide clues to various systemic diseases in the bovine, as in other species. Since the eye is easily observed and examined, it is an important part of the physical examination of the patient. Ocular lesions that coexist with systemic diseases are discussed in this article.

THE ORBIT AND GLOBE

Exophthalmos

Although many breeds of cattle have hereditary bilateral, nonprogressive exophthalmos, a bovine patient that develops acquired *progressive* exophthalmos usually has an associated systemic illness. The bovine orbit can be affected by a variety of inflammatory and neoplastic disorders that result in progressive exophthalmos. Orbital cellulitis, actinobacillosis, actinomycosis, chronic frontal sinusitis, chronic maxillary sinusitis, lymphosarcoma, and other neoplasms of the bovine oral or nasal cavity can produce exophthalmos.

Clinical Signs

Progressive unilateral exophthalmos is the hallmark of the above listed diseases. Exophthalmos is bilateral in many cases of lymphosarcoma. If exophthalmos is acute and associated with fever and anorexia, orbital cellulitis should be suspected. When exophthalmos has been gradual over several weeks, sinusitis, granulomatous infection, or neoplasm is more probable. The one exception to this time related difference would be lymphosarcoma, in which exophthalmos can progress quickly over a few days to total proptosis of the globe. Although a retrobulbar tumor may have been present for some time, it may result in only a subtle case of exophthalmos. Thus, when exophthalmos reaches a point where the cornea suffers damage, rapid deterioration occurs, as proptosis results in exposure keratitis and severe chemosis within 1 to 3 days. Therefore, if the owner reports observing a cow with severe exophthalmos for only a few days, lymphosarcoma should still be included in the differential diagnosis.

Other signs of orbital or systemic disease are often found during a thorough physical examination. Frontal or maxillary sinus distention or dullness to percussion may suggest sinusitis or sinus neoplasm. Soft tissue masses in the oral or nasal cavity may indicate granulomatous or neoplastic conditions. Lymphadenopathy, melena, masses associated with the reproductive tract or kidneys (found on rectal examination), or cardiac abnormalities might support a diagnosis of lymphosarcoma. Lymphosarcoma tends to occur in cattle 3 to 8 years of age. Older cattle with neoplasms in the oral or nasal cavity and exophthalmos are frequently afflicted with carcinomas.

Ophthalmic lesions of these orbital diseases are usually limited to exophthalmos unless exposure keratitis exists. Once exposure keratitis develops, regardless of the primary disease, ophthalmic lesions may develop rapidly and include chemosis, eyelid swelling, lacrimation, photophobia, blepharospasm, corneal dessication, corneal edema and vascularization, and possible rupture of the globe.

Diagnosis

Diagnosis is usually possible based on physical examination findings. If following examination, the clinician is uncertain of the diagnosis, ancillary procedures, such as skull radiographs and aspirates from the retrobulbar space, may be indicated. In cases of obvious sinus distention, as in chronic frontal sinusitis secondary to dehorning infections, trephination of the sinus is necessary for diagnostic cytologic and culture techniques. Biopsy of oral or nasal cavity masses is indicated to differentiate granulomatous lesions (actinomycosis, actinobacillosis) from neoplastic lesions.

Treatment

For chronic sinusitis, trephination and flushing of the affected sinus coupled with systemic antibiotics are indicated. In most cases of chronic frontal sinusitis, pyogranulomatous tissue rather than frank pus fills the sinus, complicating surgical drainage. Bony expansion and infection frequently extend towards the interior of the skull with erosion into the calvarium, and an associated, often fatal, meningitis results.

For actinobacillosis, 20-per cent sodium iodide should be administered intravenously at the rate of 30 g/450 kg. This can be repeated once or twice weekly until iodism occurs. For actinomycosis, sodium iodide at the above rate is given, and 5 gm of streptomycin is administered intramuscularly 3 times daily for at least 1 week.

For orbital cellulitis, systemic antibiotics, warm compresses on the orbit, and topical antibiotics and lubricants to protect the cornea are indicated. Drainage should also be provided if possible, and this will depend upon whether the cellulitis originated from the eyelids (puncture wounds), from the oral cavity, or elsewhere.

For lymphosarcoma and other neoplastic diseases, no treatment is practical unless enucleation must be performed for the patient's comfort (i.e., a cow in late gestation that is to be kept alive until calving).

Suturing the eyelids together (temporary tarsorrhaphy) may provide short-term relief from exposure. Regardless of the cause of exophthalmos, if severe exposure damage to the eye has occurred, enucleation may be necessary.

Strabismus and Nystagmus

Aside from congenital esotropia or exotropia that tends to be bilateral and nonprogressive, acquired strabismus in cattle usually signals neurologic disease. Unilateral medial strabismus may be observed occasionally in cattle affected with listeriosis. This is caused by inflammatory injury to the abducens nucleus and results in loss of innervation to the lateral rectus muscle, thereby allowing medial strabismus. Bilateral, dorsomedial strabismus is common in calves affected with polioencephalomalacia and is thought to be due to a particular sensitivity of the trochlear nerve nuclei to this encephalopathy. Therapy is based on the specific neurologic disease and is discussed in this volume under that particular disease.

Similarly, acquired nystagmus is usually indicative of neurologic disease, and a complete neurologic examination should be performed. Congenital pendular nystagmus that is present bilaterally in some cattle should not be confused with acquired nystagmus.

THE EYELIDS

Lesions of the eyelids that may reflect systemic disorders are urticaria and denervation associated with neurologic disease.

Urticaria may cause bilateral eyelid and conjunctival edema. The affected animal may have other signs of acute allergic disease, such as hives, swelling of the mucocutaneous junctions, and dyspnea. Urticaria in cattle is commonly caused by new feeds, toxic plants, drugs such as oxytetracycline, penicillin, and sulfas, and milk allergy. Treatment consists of systemic antihistamine, epinephrine, and corticosteroid in the nonpregnant animal.

In cattle, facial nerve palsy may be due to trauma or may reflect ipsilateral inflammatory disease, such as listeriosis or otitis media interna (in calves). Treatment is directed towards the primary neurologic disorder.

The prominence of the third eyelid in cases of tetanus is due to tetany of the retractor oculi muscles, which pull the globe caudally and therefore deeper into the orbit, allowing a passive prolapse of the nictitans.

THE CONJUNCTIVA

Conjunctivitis

Inflammation of the conjunctiva has been associated with several organisms that cause systemic diseases. These are *Mycoplasma* sp., *Ureaplasma* sp., bluetongue virus, and IBR virus. It is important to differentiate these organisms in a herd endemic.

Clinical Signs

In the early stages of inflammation, the conjunctiva is injected, edematous, and a serous discharge is present. Affected cattle may have unilateral or bilateral signs, and morbidity within the herd varies from 10 to 80 per cent. With mycoplasmic or ureaplasmic conjunctivitis, the discharge remains serous, and the condition is mild to moderate. Mild upper respiratory signs may accompany conjunctivitis.

With IBR virus, the signs quickly advance, and multifocal white plaques may appear on the palpebral and bulbar conjunctiva. As conjunctival inflammation increases, the ocular discharge becomes mucopurulent. In addition, systemic signs of fever, depression, decreased appetite, and reduced milk production appear. Respiratory lesions typical of IBR virus may or may not be present. After 7 to 10 days, the conjunctivitis culminates in a very edematous, inflamed conjunctival surface, and the white plaques begin to coalesce and disappear. At this time, peripheral corneal edema and vascularization may appear in some cases.

In bluetongue infection, serous conjunctivitis may advance to keratoconjunctivitis with serous or mucopurulent discharge.

Diagnosis

In cases of *Mycoplasma* or *Ureaplasma* induced conjunctivitis, samples should be submitted to diagnostic laboratories that have the capability of culturing these organisms. IBR conjunctivitis can usually be diagnosed clinically due to the pathognomonic lesions and can be confirmed by results of fluorescent antibody testing of conjunctival scrapings. Scrapings are best obtained from animals with acute cases with the typical white plaque lesions, since such eyes are heavily infected with virus. Viral isolation can also be performed at this time but seldom is necessary and may be quite costly.

In bluetongue, mucosal lesions on the muzzle and in the oral cavity should alert the clinician to a possible mucosal disease. Laminitis, fever, and edematous swelling of the lips may be present. Serologic testing is necessary for confirmation of the diagnosis.

Treatment

Treatment may not be practical in herd endemics if large numbers of cattle are affected. If culture results confirm *Mycoplasma* or *Ureaplasma*, tetracycline or tylosin ophthalmic products could be applied topically as frequently as practical. If respiratory signs are present as well, the same antibiotics would be indicated parenterally. In most instances, the disease runs its course through the herd and results in no permanent ocular damage. Recurrences are possible, and new animals introduced into an affected herd often acquire the infection.

Treatment is not necessary for the conjunctival form of IBR virus. Certainly, if feasible, cattle would benefit from cleansing the eyes of ocular discharges and from the application of broad-spectrum antibiotic ophthalmic ointment to affected eyes. However, these measures are seldom practical. Specific antiviral ophthalmic products have not been used because of expense, concern about milk and meat residues, and the fact that most cases resolve within 14 to 21 days without any permanent ocular damage. If the respiratory form of IBR virus coexists with the conjunctival form, infected cattle may need treatment with broad-spectrum antibiotics to prevent secondary bacterial pneumonia. The important aspect of IBR viral conjunctivitis is that the herd is at risk to other IBR virus conditions, including abortion, respiratory problems, infectious pustular vulvovaginitis, and neonatal viremia. Therefore, the herd and any nearby unexposed groups of animals should be vaccinated on a routine yearly basis. If uninfected animals exist on a farm with infected animals, they should immediately be vaccinated with an intranasal modified-live IBR vaccine to establish protection within 72 hr.

Treatment for bluetongue is primarily supportive.

Conjunctival Color Change

Pallor or Anemia

Pale mucous membranes in young cattle or calves frequently result from anemia due to ectoparasites or endoparasites. These parasites should be identified and eliminated appropriately. Hemolytic causes of anemia, such as water intoxication and leptospirosis, should be considered in older calves that also have hemoglobinuria.

In adult cattle, anemia is associated with many diseases or conditions, such as caudal vena caval syndrome with hemoptysis due to rupture of a lung abscess, splenic rupture secondary to lymphosarcoma of the spleen, bleeding abomasal ulcers, rectal enucleation of a corpus luteum, anaplasmosis, babesiosis, and bacillary hemoglobinuria.

Treatment of anemia consists of supportive whole blood transfusions and any specific measures as related to the cause. Whole blood should be administered when anemia is judged to be severe: a heart rate of 120/min or greater, a respiratory rate of 60/min or greater, and extreme pallor of the membranes. The standard transfusion volume for a calf is 1 to 2 L and for a cow is 4 to 6 L. Each liter container should have 25 to 35 ml of 20-per cent sodium citrate as an anticoagulant before blood collection from a suitable donor starts. Specific therapy directed at the primary cause of the anemia should be instituted as soon as the patient is stable.

Jaundice

Except in anaplasmosis of cattle, jaundice is an uncommon finding. When apparent, the differential diagnosis should consider toxic plant hepatopathy, diffuse liver abscessation, severe hemolytic disease, severe babesiosis, and, rarely, *Dicrocoelium dendriticum* proliferation within the biliary system.

Treatment must be supportive and determined by the specific cause of the illness.

Hemorrhage

Conjunctival hemorrhage in a newborn calf is usually associated with trauma due to dystocia. Acquired conjunctival petechial hemorrhages in neonatal calves are often associated with septicemia. In older calves and adult cattle, petechial and ecchymotic hemorrhages are most common in thrombocytopenia as seen in bracken-fern intoxication, BVD, septic mastitis, septic metritis, and *Pasteurella* septicemia. Disseminated intravascular coagulation may also occur as a complication of bovine septicemia. Warfarin toxicity rarely causes hemorrhage in cattle.

Specific therapy will depend upon the exact cause. Platelet-rich whole blood transfusions would be indicated as supportive therapy.

THE CORNEA

The bovine cornea seldom develops lesions in response to systemic conditions. One exception is corneal edema that develops in phenothiazine toxicity in cattle. This edema occurs because of photochemical damage to the corneal endothelium that is bathed by the phenothiazine-laden aqueous humor, and it may occur in one or both eyes. Treatment consists of removal of the source of phenothiazine.

Corneal opacity has been described in conjunction with BVD infection but has not been observed in my experience. It has been suggested that bilateral corneal edema is pathognomonic for malignant catarrhal fever; however, the basic ophthalmic lesion in that disease is ophthalmitis, which is discussed later.

Corneal opacities secondary to severe conjunctivitis have been observed in bluetongue. This disease is not often observed in the northeastern United States.

UVEITIS

Inflammation of the uveal tract involves the iris, ciliary body, and choroid. In cattle, uveitis primarily involves the anterior uveal tract, but the posterior segment can be involved as well. Most uveitis in cattle is of endogenous origin and, therefore, is suggestive of systemic diseases that affect many parts of the body in addition to the eyes.

Etiology

In neonatal calves (1 to 14 days of age), the most common cause of unilateral or bilateral uveitis is septicemia or endotoxemia. The source of septicemia or endotoxemia is usually a navel infection or enteritis caused by gram-negative organisms. Calves that have had inadequate colostral transfer of immunoglobulins are very prone to this condition. *Pasteurella* sp. and *Streptococcus* sp. have been identified as the cause in some instances.

In adult cattle, unilateral or bilateral uveitis is occasionally observed in patients with septic mastitis, septic metritis, endocarditis, traumatic reticuloperitonitis, tuberculosis, and peritonitis. Malignant catarrhal fever causes severe bilateral uveitis and ophthalmitis with prominent corneal opacity.

Clinical Signs

Uveitis is characterized by conjunctival and ciliary injection, miosis, a dull, discolored iris, fibrin, white cells and occasionally red cells in the anterior chamber, and signs of ocular pain, such as blepharospasm, lacrimation, and photophobia. Peripheral corneal edema and vascularization may be present, but the cornea is free of ulceration. Therefore, in brief, a painful red eye or an eye with anterior chamber opacities would typically be present.

In neonatal calves with uveitis, fever, depression, and dehydration are common. These same calves may also show signs of meningitis, joint ill, or embolic pneumonia due to septicemia. Adult cattle with uveitis generally have a primary site of infection, such as the endocardium, which can be identified during a thorough physical examination. In cattle with malignant catarrhal fever, obvious mucosal lesions, depression, extremely high fever, and lymphadenopathy are present along with bilateral uveitis.

Diagnosis

In most instances, uveitis is simply one sign of a systemic disease process; therefore, a primary diagnosis is required to define the cause. In cattle, uveitis can be confused with other ocular lesions that result in corneal opacity or lenticular opacity. Corneal ulcers from trauma and infectious bovine keratoconjunctivitis can readily be ruled out by negative results of a fluorescein dye test. In uveitis cases with severe hypopyon, a cataract can be eliminated as the cause by transilluminating the anterior chamber to establish that the opacity is anterior to the anterior lens capsule and, therefore, not a cataract.

Treatment

Treatment should be directed towards the primary problem. Neonatal septicemic calves should receive appropriate broad-spectrum systemic antibiotics and fluid therapy. If inadequate transfer of colostral immunoglobulins is confirmed by evaluation of serum proteins, a plasma or whole blood transfusion may be necessary as well. Topically applied broad-spectrum antibiotics and 1-per cent atropine ophthalmic ointment twice or four times daily are indicated for treatment of the uveitis. I prefer to use gentamicin topically. The combination of ampicillin and gentamicin is indicated for systemic therapy when meat residues of antibiotics are not a concern.

Adult cattle should be treated for the primary infectious disease with appropriate systemic and local agents. Uveitis in these cattle should be treated with topical and subconjunctival antibiotics as well as atropine to relieve ciliary spasm and to prevent synechiae formation.

The acute or peracute form of malignant catarrhal fever is highly fatal and therapy is seldom practical. In the occasional mild or chronic form of the disease, I have used topical antibiotic-corticosteroid ophthalmic drugs and 1-per cent atropine ophthalmic ointment several times daily with some success.

The prognosis for eyes affected with uveitis secondary to septicemia is good if the primary cause of the septicemia can be corrected, and if the patient is observed within 24 hours of the onset of disease. If the primary disease cannot be controlled, or if the uveitis has existed for 48 hours or more prior to therapy, the prognosis is guarded owing to continued inflammation and sequelae to uveitis within the eyes.

THE LENS

In utero infection with BVD during days 76 to 150 of gestation has resulted in congenital cataracts in calves. These calves may also have cerebellar hypoplasia. Although infrequently observed, such lesions could provide a key to the diagnosis of a herd problem for which BVD infection is a consideration in a newborn calf. Precolostral serum would demonstrate BVD antibodies if BVD was the cause.

THE FUNDUS

Although fundus lesions are uncommon in cattle, examination of the fundus can provide clues to certain systemic diseases. Ophthalmoscopic examination should definitely be performed if a patient shows evidence of poor vision or dilated pupils that respond poorly to direct light stimulation. Although lesions are uncommon, they certainly cannot be identified unless funduscopic examination is performed.

Etiology

In cases of severe chorioretinopathies or optic neuropathies, general signs are reduced vision or obvious blindness and dilated, nonresponsive pupils, or pupils that are poorly responsive to direct light. If the anterior segment is clear, ophthalmoscopic examination should be performed. In acute inflammatory chorioretinitis, transudates, hemorrhages, or perivascular exudates may be apparent. In the tapetal zone, these inflammatory lesions usually appear as dull, grey, focal areas that are raised. In the nontapetal zone, the lesions are raised, greyish-white, and focal. In TEM [thromboembolic meningoencephalitis], hemorrhage and severe inflammation may be present due to septic thromboemboli in the retinal or choroidal vessels. In chronic cases, the tapetal areas take on a hyper-reflective appearance, often with a central zone of hyperpigmentation. The nontapetal lesions are observed as depigmented focal areas with central hyperpigmentation. In malignant catarrhal fever, anterior segment lesions usually preclude the ophthalmoscopic examination of the fundus.

Bilateral severe papilledema, retinal edema, and peripapillary hemorrhages are present when blindness is due to vitamin A deficiency or prolonged anterior cervical compressive lesions. Intoxication due to *Dryopteris filix-mas* (male fern) can cause optic neuritis, papillitis, peripapillary exudates, hemorrhage, and edema. This condition is seen mainly in animals in England.

Diagnosis

Lesions observed with ophthalmoscopy coupled with historical data and systemic signs should allow a diagnosis. Vitamin A deficiency is extremely rare today, since most feedstuffs contain adequate levels. Septicemia that results in fundus lesions is frequently accompanied by systemic signs of fever, depression, and possibly shock. TEM occurs primarily in feedlot animals in which neurologic deficits and fevers are often associated findings. Prolonged anterior cervical compression by a restraining device (chute) or accidental trauma might explain peripapillary retinopathy and optic neuropathy (papilledema) in a solitary blind animal.

Treatment

Therapy for the primary problem and therapy for the ocular symptoms are required. Septicemia should be treated with appropriate systemic antibiotics and supportive care. TEM is poorly responsive to treatment unless provided in the very early stages. Subconjunctival, topical, and systemic antibiotics would be indicated in bacterial septicemia. Papilledema due to anterior cervical compression should be treated with corticosteroids and diuretics in acute cases. If a case is chronic, the prognosis is guarded.

CORTICAL BLINDNESS

Bilateral blindness with intact pupillary light reflexes is consistent with cortical blindness. This clinical finding is observed most commonly in polioencephalomalacia, lead poisoning, and occasionally in severely ketotic hypoglycemic cattle.

Clinical Signs

In calves with polioencephalomalacia, depression, opisthotonus, seizures, and dorsomedial strabismus may accompany blindness. In adult cattle, profound depression and blindness are often the only signs. Ophthalmoscopic lesions are not present. In lead poisoning, seizures, grinding of the teeth, and salivation are often seen along with cortical blindness. In severe ketosis and hypoglycemia, a multitude of neurologic signs may exist as expected in cases of nervous ketosis merely depression, decreased milk production, and refusal of high energy feed may exist.

Diagnosis

Physical examination findings and laboratory data may be necessary to distinguish these diseases in adult cattle. In calves, polioencephalomalacia is the most common problem and, in acute cases, the cerebrospinal fluid (CSF) is usually normal or has slightly elevated protein values. Basophilic stippling may be observed in the erythrocytes in cattle affected with lead poisoning, and mild to moderate elevations in renal biochemical values may be present. The CSF is usually normal or has slightly elevated protein levels in lead poisoning and in polioencephalomalacia of adult cattle. However, if the disease is chronic, pleocytosis of the CSF may be evident owing to cerebral cortical necrosis. In severe ketosis, characteristic physical signs and severe ketonuria are generally sufficient evidence for a diagnosis to be made.

Treatment

For polioencephalomalacia, thiamine should be administered at 500 to 1000 mg intravenously for calves and 3000 to 4000 mg intravenously for cows. This treatment is then continued on one half the dose intramuscularly once daily for 5 to 7 days. The prognosis is fair to good in acute cases and poor in chronic cases because of cerebral cortical necrosis. Blindness is often the first sign to appear and the last sign to resolve. Therefore, it can take several days for vision to return, and the animal should not be deemed hopelessly blind for at least 1 week following resolution of the neurologic signs.

In lead poisoning, EDTA preparations should be administered at recommended dosages, and the source of lead eliminated. After several days of therapy, EDTA should be discontinued to allow lead in bone to be released into the blood stream and to be available for chelation when therapy is reinstituted. A rumenotomy may be indicated if acute intoxication has occurred because of consumption of a massive amount of lead. Supportive therapy and sedatives may be necessary to control seizure activity. The prognosis generally is poor in chronic cases.

In severe ketosis, intravenous glucose solutions and systemic corticosteroids are indicated. The prognosis for resolution of ketosis is excellent but in rare cases of blindness, the prognosis for return of vision is poor. The pathophysiology of the visual loss is unknown.

Supplemental Reading

Barnett, K. C., Palmer, A. C., Abrams, J. T., et al.: Ocular changes associated with hypovitaminosis A in cattle. Br. Vet. J., 126:561–573, 1970.
Bistner, S. I., Rubin, L. F., and Saunder, L. Z.: The ocular lesions of bovine diarrhea-mucosal disease. Path. Vet., 7:275–286, 1970.
Bistner, S. I., Shaw, D., and Sartori, R.: Ocular manifestation of low level phenothiazine administration in cattle. Transactions of the Eleventh Annual Scientific Program of the College of Veterinary Ophthalmologists. 84–94, 1980.
Dukes, T. W.: The ocular lesions in thromboembolic meningoencephalitis (ITEME) of cattle. Can. Vet. J., 12:180–182, 1971.
Hughes, J. P., Olander, H. J., and Wanda, M.: Keratoconjunctivitis associated with infectious bovine rhinotracheitis. J. Am. Vet. Med. Assoc., 145:32–39, 1964.
McConnon, J. M., White, M. E., Smith, M. C., et al.: Pendular nystagmus in dairy cattle. J. Am. Vet. Med. Assoc., 182:812–813, 1983.
Rebhun, W. C., Smith, J. S., Post, J. E., et al.: An outbreak of the conjunctival form of infectious bovine rhinotracheitis. Cornell Vet., 68:307, 1978.
Rebhun, W. C.: Diseases of the bovine orbit and globe. J. Am. Vet. Med. Assoc., 175:171–175, 1979.
Rebhun, W. C.: Viral diseases of the bovine eye. Bovine Pract. 14:139–142, 1979.
Rebhun, W. C.: Orbital lymphosarcoma in cattle. J. Am. Vet. Med. Assoc., 180:149–152, 1982.
Rosen, E. S., Edgar, J. T., and Smith, J. L. S.: Male fern retrobulbar neuropathy in cattle. Trans. Ophthalmol. Soc. U.K., 89:285–299, 1969.
Rosenbusch, R. F., and Knudtson, W. U.: Bovine mycoplasmal conjunctivitis. Cornell Vet., 70:307, 1980.
Smith, J. S., and Mayhew, I. G.: Horner's syndrome in large animals. Cornell Vet., 67:529–542, 1977.
Timoney, P. J., and O'Conner, P. J.: An outbreak of the conjunctival form of infectious bovine rhinotracheitis virus infection. Vet. Rec., 89:370, 1971.
Weaver, L. D.: Malignant catarrhal fever in two California dairy herds. Bovine Pract. 14:121–127, 1979.
Whitten, L. K., and Filmer, D. B.: A photosensitized keratitis in young cattle following use of phenothiazine as an anthelmintic. Aust. Vet. J., 23:336–340, 1974.

Ocular Diseases of Sheep and Goats

CECIL P. MOORE, D.V.M.
and R. DAVID WHITLEY, D.V.M., M.S.*

EYELIDS

Entropion

Inversion of the eyelids in lambs may cause frictional rubbing of the cornea and conjunctiva, resulting in lacrimation, photophobia, blepharospasm, corneal opacity, and blindness. In some flocks, congenital entropion may affect three fourths of the lambs from 2 days to 3 weeks of age. Treatment consists of everting the eyelids and applying topical antibiotic ophthalmic ointment to control secondary bacterial infections. Eversion of the eyelid may be accomplished with mattress skin sutures or Michel metal wound clips† placed in the skin to turn back the eyelid margin. When large numbers of lambs are treated, absorbable sutures or metal clips will remain in place a few weeks to be spontaneously expelled. Alternate methods of treatment are injecting minor irritants under the eyelid skin (i.e., repositol penicillin), pinching or crushing the periocular skin, or removing an elliptical strip of skin from the entropic area and suturing the skin margins. In severe cases of entropion, topical ophthalmic antibiotic ointment is beneficial to corneal healing when applied 3 times daily. Topical 1-per cent atropine sulfate ophthalmic ointment applied 2 to 3 times daily will benefit those eyes with severe corneal ulcers and concurrent uveitis.

---

*We wish to thank Dr. Julia Wilson of Gainesville, Florida, for critical review of this article.

†Available from Propper Mfg. Co., Inc., Long Island, New York 11101

Periocular Dermatoses

Infections, parasites, sunlight-induced irritation, neoplasia, and trauma are the major causes of periocular dermatoses in sheep and goats. A number of viral diseases may cause periocular dermatitis in small domestic ruminants. Contagious ecthyma (sore mouth or ORF) is a pox virus that may infect both sheep and goats. Ulcerative dermatostis and sheep pox may affect the eyelids of sheep. Ulcerative lesions of the eyelids may be a common feature of these viral diseases. Transmission is by direct contact. Owners and veterinarians must be cognizant of the public health significance of contagious ecthyma. Treatment of ocular lesions is empirical and involves the use of topical antibiotic ophthalmic ointment 3 times daily to prevent secondary bacterial infections and corneal involvement.

Blepharitis and conjunctivitis have been observed with bluetongue, an arbovirus infection. Retinopathy (discussed later) is a more severe ocular manifestation of bluetongue virus.

Viral papillomas (warts) are generally uncommon in sheep and goats but sometimes involve the eyelids. The papillomatous lesions are usually self-limiting but occasionally may enlarge to become problematic, requiring removal. Surgical excision or cryosurgical excision may serve as immune potentiators in animals with extensive involvement.

Bacterial and fungal organisms may cause periocular dermatologic lesions in small ruminants. *Clostridium novyi* causes "big head" secondary to butting and head trauma in rams. Streptothricosis, caused by *Dermatophilus congolensis,* may occur during rainy seasons and produces chronic exudative dermatitis. Penicillin is the antibiotic of choice to treat these infections. Pyogranulomatous cutaneous nodules associated with draining tracts may occur secondary to cutaneous punctures. "Gritty" sulfur granules from such lesions are characteristic of actinobacillosis. Streptomycin and systemic iodides are the preferred drugs for actinobacillosis treatment.

Trichophyton verrucosum, the most common dermatophyte isolated from sheep and goats, may cause crusty alopecic areas of the periocular skin, particularly in young animals. Although lesions are frequently self-limiting, topical antifungals may still be applied. Owners should be reminded of possible zoonoses.

Ectoparasites may incite self-trauma, resulting in blepharodermatitis in sheep and goats. Sarcoptic and demodectic mange mites may cause facial lesions. Intense pruritus with crusty, ulcerated areas of facial skin may be an early sign of sarcoptic mange. Lime sulfur may be applied locally; however, generalized cases require dipping in insecticide solutions. In North America sarcoptic mange is quite rare, and in the United States it is a disease that must be reported to the appropriate agency. Usually nonpruritic, demodicosis may manifest as nodular or pustular eyelid dermatitis. In young goats, nodules may have to be surgically drained. Keds, lice, and ticks are common ectoparasites of sheep and goats that may cause self-trauma and anemia in the host. Ocular involvement is minimal and usually limited to blepharitis secondary to self-trauma.

Sorehead is a parasitic disease of domestic and wild ruminants caused by the filarid parasite *Elaeophora schneideri.* Adult sheep are most frequently affected and may have alopecic, ulcerated, and encrusted lesions of the face. Additional discussion of elaeophorosis is found under Keratoconjunctivitis and Uveitis.

Sunlight-induced periocular skin disease may appear as a direct solar irritation (sunburn) or as a result of photosensitization. Erythema, edema, pruritis, necrosis, and sloughing of nonpigmented skin characterizes both primary and secondary forms of photosensitization. *Thamnosma texana* (Dutchman's breeches) may cause severe photosensitization in sheep of the southwestern United States. Ocular squamous cell carcinoma (OSCC) may occur on nonpigmented facial skin and is presumed to be stimulated by long-term solar (UV) irritation. Treatment of OSCC consists of local excision, cryosurgery, hyperthermia, radiation therapy, or enucleation, depending on the location and extent of the tumor.

Eyelid injuries and lacerations are most common when wire or exposed nails puncture or hook the eyelid. These lacerations can usually be surgically repaired to allow satisfactory eyelid function. It is extremely important not to amputate any lacerated tissues but rather to perform minimal débridement or scarification of the margins before surgical repair. The reader is referred to ophthalmic surgical texts for principles of eyelid surgical repair.

CONJUNCTIVA AND CORNEA

Conjunctival Color Variation

Pallor, icterus, cyanosis, and hyperemia are variations from the normal pink coloration of the conjunctival mucosa. Pale and jaundiced conjunctiva may occur simultaneously and are characteristic of a number of infectious and toxic diseases, e.g., *Clostridium perfringens* type A, leptospirosis, anaplasmosis, babesiosis, eperythrozoonosis, trypanosomiasis, theileriasis, liver flukes, copper poisoning, and plant poisoning (*Brassica* sp.). Anemia in the absence of icterus suggests acute or chronic blood loss or inadequate bone marrow activity. Dark purple coloration of the mucosa is seen in cyanotic states, e.g., pneumonia, congestive heart failure, respiratory obstruction, or shock. A murky brown discoloration of the conjunctiva may result from nitrite intoxication due to methemoglobinemia. A bright cherry red conjunctiva is typical of cyanide poisoning. Conjunctival injection and hyperemia may indicate inflammatory disease of the external eye or systemic toxemia.

Infectious Keratoconjunctivitis

Numerous infectious agents have been incriminated as causes of infectious keratoconjunctivitis of sheep and goats. Rickettsia, chlamydia, mycoplasma, and aerobic bacteria have been isolated from sheep with diseased eyes, while mycoplasma and aerobic bacteria are the predominate isolates from goats with external eye disease. Viral and fungal keratoconjunctivitis of small ruminants are quite rare.

Ovine chlamydial conjunctivitis is caused by *Chlamydia psittaci* and manifests as chemosis, hyperemia, and ocular pain (blepharospasm and epiphora). Lymphoid follicle formation and corneal opacification may also be observed. In a given flock the incidence may reach 90 per cent with nursing and feedlot lambs having the highest morbidity. Chlamydial conjunctivitis is highly contagious and spreads rapidly by direct contact, insect transfer, and contact with ocular discharge and contaminated fomites. Arthritis may also be a major component of this disease, which is prevalent throughout the United Kingdom and North America. In most sheep with chlamydial infections, the clinical course of the disease is 6 to 10 days. Severely affected animals may be blinded by extensive corneal opacity but usually regain vision.

Diagnosis of ovine chlamydial conjunctivitis is based on clinical observations and laboratory findings. Intracellular gram-negative inclusions in conjunctival epithelial cells are pathognomonic of chlamydial keratoconjunctivitis. Immunofluorescence of conjunctival scrapings is also pathognomonic. Complement fixation antibodies are often detectable in serum of affected animals in 7 to 10 days. Expressing lymphoid follicles provide material for inoculation into yolk sacs of chick embryos.

Colesiota conjunctivae (also named *Rickettsia conjunctivae*), *Mycoplasma* spp., and *Neisseria* spp. are other important causes of ovine keratoconjunctivitis. Additional aerobic bacteria, including *Staphylococcus* spp., *Streptococcus* spp., *Escherichia coli*, *Pseudomonas* spp., *Corynebacterium* spp., and *Listeria monocytogenes,* have been isolated from clinical cases of infectious keratoconjunctivitis in sheep and goats. The precise role of specific organisms may be difficult to assess, since the external eye is continually exposed to environmental irritants (noxious gases, dust, pollens, chemicals, and flies) and an array of microorganisms.

A common feature of these infections is that clinical signs may range from mild conjunctivitis to corneal ulceration with diffuse corneal opacity. Generally, conjunctival hyperemia and chemosis are the predominant clinical findings. However, in some instances purulent keratitis (which may begin as punctate lesions) with extensive corneal ulceration and perilimbal corneal vascularization may be observed. Usually in 2 to 3 weeks, the corneal neovascularization clears with minimal scar formation and with nearly complete recovery of vision. Fortunately, only a small percentage of infected animals develop severe keratitis with keratomalacia, descemetocele formation, or staphyloma formation.

Mycoplasmal septicemia in sheep and goats may be caused by *Mycoplasma conjunctivae* and may result in keratitis and uveitis in addition to systemic manifestations. Other species have been incriminated in goats with septicemia and ocular disease: *M. conjunctivae, M. arginini, Acholeplasma oculi,* and *M. mycoides* subsp. *mycoides.*

Diagnosis of infectious keratoconjunctivitis of sheep and goats is based on clinical signs and laboratory findings. Cytologic assessment of stained conjunctival scrapings and isolation of specific organisms are the most useful diagnostic tests. Results of scrapings stained with Wright, Giemsa, and Gram's stains are most informative. In addition to identifying bacterial organisms, cytologic examination may reveal large intracytoplasmic basophilic inclusions (chlamydial bodies), small rod-shaped intracytoplasmic inclusions (rickettsia), coccobacillary organisms attached to the epithelial cell membranes (mycoplasma), or fungal elements. Isolation of *Chlamydia, Rickettsia,* or *Mycoplasma* requires media and techniques available through specially equipped diagnostic laboratories.

It is fortunate that even in complicated cases ocular lesions may heal spontaneously with full resolution within 3 weeks. Antimicrobial therapy will markedly shorten the course of infectious keratoconjunctivitis. Ideally, any choice of antimicrobials for treating infectious keratoconjunctivitis caused by bacteria is based on *in vitro* susceptibility testing. *Chlamydia, Rickettsia,* and *Mycoplasma* are generally susceptible to tetracycline. Erythromycin and chloramphenicol have also been recommended but appear to be less efficacious in field studies.

For topical therapy to be effective, antibiotics must be applied 3 times each day. Although topical therapy may be quite beneficial, it is often impractical. Injectable oxytetracycline (5 to 10 mg/kg) has been a satisfactory treatment for infectious keratoconjunctivitis of sheep and goats. Injectable and topical therapy may be combined. In outbreaks where a number of animals must be treated, administration of antibiotic medication by injection is preferable. In cases with severe corneal involvement, protecting the eye with a temporary tarsorrhaphy or nictitans flap may also be beneficial.

Since environmental irritants make the symptoms more severe, and since the spread of infection is by direct contact or contact with contaminated fomites, the following practices may be recommended: clip pastures with long-stemmed grasses or weeds, implement fly control, provide ample shade, dispose of contaminated bedding, and maintain clean feed and water troughs. The owners or husbandry workers should isolate infected or recently exposed animals and avoid overcrowding, transporting, or exhibiting infected or exposed animals. Easy access to sources of food and water is also important, as severely affected animals may be temporarily blinded.

Parasitic Keratoconjunctivitis

Thelazia spp., *Oestrus ovis,* and *Elaeophora* sp. may cause external eye disease in sheep and goats. *Musca* spp. are the intermediate hosts for *Thelazia* spp., which may cause mild conjunctivitis and keratitis in sheep and goats. Usually thelaziasis is subclinical. *O. ovis* may cause conjunctivitis in sheep if larvae aberrantly invade ocular mucous membranes. Domestic sheep may develop corneal opacities from *Elaeophora* sp.

Treatment for *Thelazia* spp. consists of oral levamisole 5 mg/kg or topical echothiophate iodide. Worms may be manually removed with fine forceps after local anesthetic application. Ivermectin at a dose of 50 μg/kg has been reported to be effective in treating *O. ovis.* The efficacy of ivermectin in treating *Elaeophora* sp. is unknown. Oral piperazine (50 mg/kg) has been reported to produce satisfactory results.

Miscellaneous Causes of Keratoconjunctivitis

Phenothiazine may induce photosensitization in sheep and goats. Lacrimation begins 12 to 36 hr after treatment followed by severe corneal edema, blepharospasm, and photophobia. Treatment of photosensitization keratitis involves preventing additional exposure to sunlight by confining affected animals to shaded areas and eliminating the source of the photosensitizing substance. If properly managed, animals with corneal edema will recover in 4 to 7 days.

Locoweed poisoning has been observed as a cause of keratoconjunctivitis sicca in sheep. It is speculated that drying of the eyes may be due to chronic degenerative neurotoxicoses, resulting in failure of neurogenic stimulation of tear secretion and inadequate blink response. Behavioral and sensory abnormalities, muscular incoordination, weight loss, abortion, and fetal abnormalities are also found with locoism in sheep.

Blunt and penetrating trauma to the eye may result in corneal opacities and ulcerations. Following ocular trauma, corneal ulceration may be identified by instillation of fluorescein dye to the eye. Topical or subconjunctival antibiotics and atropine are indicated when a corneal ulcer is present. Blunt injury may result in corneal edema (without ulceration), blepharoedema, conjunctival hemorrhage, or hyphema. Confinement in a dark area will allow many cases of blunt ocular trauma to resolve spontaneously. Patients with cases of traumatic corneal edema with hyphema (in the absence of corneal ulceration) may benefit from topical instillation of antibiotic corticosteroid ointment and atropine. For surgical repair of corneal lacerations and ruptured globes, the reader is referred to appropriate texts for descriptions of principles of intraocular surgery.

UVEITIS

A number of systemic infectious diseases of sheep and goats may result in uveal involvement. Lambs and kids may become septicemic with *E. coli*, *Staphylococcus* sp., *Streptococcus* sp., *Salmonella* sp., or *Corynebacterium* sp. infections. Hematogenous spread of these organisms to the eye results in fibrin and inflammatory cell accumulation in the anterior chamber accompanied by miosis and iris edema. Lesions are usually bilateral and opacification may be sufficient to result in blindness. The septicemic form of *Listeria monocytogenes* may produce hypopyon or endophthalmitis in sheep in addition to associated abnormal neurologic signs. *Mycoplasma* spp. may cause septicemia in sheep and goats with iridocyclitis and keratoconjunctivitis being the predominant ocular signs. Secondary glaucoma may result from severe anterior uveitis induced by *M. agalactiae,* and chorioretinal lesions have also been reported.

Treatment of anterior uveitis secondary to systemic infectious disease in sheep and goats involves the use of appropriate systemic antibiotics and the application of topical antibiotic corticosteroid combinations and atropine sulfate. Systemic nonsteroidal anti-inflammatory preparations may also be used in these cases.

Parasitic causes of uveitis in sheep and goats appear to be less common than bacterial causes. Toxoplasmosis has produced inflammatory changes of the iris, ciliary body, choroid, and retina of sheep. Trypanosomiasis of sheep may cause signs of severe uveitis, including corneal opacities, hypopyon, chorioretinitis, and optic neuritis. The inflammation with resultant blindness is due to invasion of the eye by the parasite. *Elaeophora schneideri* is an intra-arterial parasite of deer, elk, and domestic sheep of North America. Ocular lesions may be unilateral or bilateral and include iridocyclitis and chorioretinitis as well as diffuse keratitis, cataracts, and vitreous clouding. Affected domestic sheep may be less prone to blindness than wild ruminants. Treatment for anterior uveitis discussed previously also applies to treatment for parasitic uveitis.

RETINOPATHIES AND OPTIC NEUROPATHIES

Inflammatory diseases causing lesions of the posterior segment of the eye include those bacterial and parasitic diseases discussed under uveitis, i.e., mycoplasmosis, listeriosis, elaephorosis, trypanosomiasis, and toxoplasmosis. Acute nonspecific inflammatory lesions are manifest funduscopically as hemorrhage, edema (hazy or grey areas) or exudates, and inflammatory infiltrates (beige or white areas). Chronic changes include zones of hyperreflection or hyperpigmentation. Retinal detachment or fibrosis and optic nerve atrophy may be sequelae to posterior segment inflammatory diseases, which result in permanent vision loss.

Bluetongue and scrapie are viral organisms that may cause retinal disease. Vaccination of pregnant ewes with attenuated bluetongue virus vaccine during the first half of pregnancy results in a necrotizing retinopathy and central nervous system malformation. Necrosis and inflammatory cell infiltrates with retinal rosette formation (dysplasia) occur in prenatal lambs infected at 50 to 58 days of gestation. Other developmental defects that follow live virus vaccination of ewes at 4 to 8 weeks of gestation are hydrocephalus, cerebellar hypoplasia, and supernumerary sulci and gyri.

Retinopathy appears following natural infection with scrapie virus in sheep and goats, accompanying the generalized neurologic disease. Oval, blister-like lesions have been observed scattered throughout the tapetal fundus. These distinct raised areas may vary from one fourth to three fourths the size of the optic disc. Similar lesions have also been associated with branches of retinal vessels. These are apparently accumulations of lipid between the pigment epithelium and the photoreceptors. Rod and cone outer segment degeneration is found at these foci.

Of the toxic neuroretinopathies of small domestic ruminants, "bright blindness" of sheep is the most notable. This toxic retinopathy is caused by ingestion of bracken (*Pteris aguilina*). In bright blindness there is no external ocular disease or opacity of the refractive media. Pronounced tapetal hyperreflectivity in ewes 3 to 4 years old is the predominant clinical feature. Pupils are nonresponsive to light. The fundus appears mirror-like with fine lines and spots of grey. Initially, the optic disc may appear normal but slowly becomes pale and appears greyish-pink. In severe cases, choroidal blood vessels may be observed. Lowered platelet and leukocyte counts have been reported. Thiaminase is believed to be the toxic principle of bracken.

Stypandra imbricata or "blind grass" is a plant that grows in western Australia, which, if ingested, may cause damage to photoreceptor cells, optic nerves, and optic tracts of sheep.

Antiparasitic drugs may cause retinal or optic nerve neurotoxicity and resultant loss of vision in sheep. Hexachlorophene, used to treat liver flukes, may cause edema of the optic disc 24 hr after intoxication. Pupillary light responses are lost at 72 hr and are not regained owing to degeneration and gliosis of the retina and optic nerve. Rafoxanide may be neurotoxic, causing progressive optic nerve edema and vacuolation that can produce blindness.

Other causes of photoreceptor cell degeneration are vitamin A deficiency and a presumed inherited retinal degeneration. As with larger ruminants, sheep and goats may experience night blindness as a early sign of vitamin A deficiency. Spontaneous retinopathy believed to be a rod and cone dysplasia has been reported in a young goat.

CORTICAL BLINDNESS

Hesitation or inability to pass through a gate, reluctance to move, separation from the flock, or carriage of the head close to the ground is behavior suggestive of blindness. This may be confirmed by directing the animal through a maze or noting response (or lack of response) to menacing hand gestures. Visual deficits in the presence of normal ocular findings, including normal pupillary light responses, are indicative of deficits of the higher visual pathways. Encephalopathies that may involve vision loss as an important component include metabolic, inflammatory, toxic, and traumatic neurologic diseases.

CONGENITAL OCULAR DISEASE

The precise cause of many congenital ocular lesions in lambs and kids is not known; however, a number of these lesions do have known causes. These are categorized as infectious, toxic, nutritional or heritable. Hydranencephaly and retinal dysplasia in lambs have resulted from the administration of modified live virus bluetongue vaccine to the ewe during the second trimester of pregnancy (see Retinopathies). Hydranencephaly is an encephalopathy characterized by reduction of the cerebral hemispheres to membranous sacs filled with cerebral spinal fluid. Affected lambs are ataxic and blind and referred to as "dummies."

Severe cephalic malformation in newborn lambs is caused by *Veratrum californicum*. This plant, also known as "skunk cabbage," contains 3 alkaloids that are poisonous to the developing fetus. If a pregnant ewe ingests the plant on day 14 of gestation, facial hypoplasia with the eyes developing very close together or fused (cyclopia) takes place in the lamb. Poisoning later in gestation may cause embryonic death. During the early part of the breeding season, ewes should be restricted from grazing areas where this plant is known to grow.

Anophthalmos and microophthalmia with multiple ocular cysts have been reported with selenium and apholate toxicity in sheep. From 70 days gestation to parturition, severe iodine deficiency in ewes causes reduction of fetal brain weight. Abnormal cell densities of the visual cortex of lambs have also been noted.

Entropion is perhaps the most common and most significant congenital abnormality of sheep. A high incidence of entropion in lambs in specific flocks has been associated with the use of certain rams and suggests a genetic cause. The clinical disease and management of entropion in lambs were discussed at the opening of this article.

A number of other ocular anomalies are occasionally seen in neonates and do not have a clearly defined cause. These are dermoids, microphthalmia, heterochromia, colobomata, and persistent pupillary membranes. The extent of vision loss ranges from none to total blindness, depending on the severity of the defect. Although dermoids may be surgically excised, the other anomalies mentioned are not treatable.

Supplemental Reading

Koning, C. D. W.: Keratoconjunctivitis Infectiosa Ovis (KIO), "pink eye" or "zere oogjies" (A Survey). Vet. Quart. 5:127–130, 1983.
Moore, C. P., and Whitley, R. D.: Ophthalmic diseases of small domestic ruminants. Vet. Clin. North Am. 6:641–665, 1984.
Rasmussen, R. E.: Repair of entropion in lambs. Mod. Vet. Pract. 61:943–944, 1980.
Wyman, M.: Eye diseases of sheep and goats. Vet. Clin. North Am. 5:657–675, 1983.

Porcine Ophthalmology

W. A. VESTRE, D.V.M., M.S.

Ophthalmic disease in the pig has received little attention and is often overlooked both as an entity in itself and as a part of systemic disease, presumably due to difficulty of adequately examining the often uncooperative patients, lack of facilities to examine them in their usual surroundings, and economic considerations. As with other species, the pig is subject to infectious, congenital, and degenerative ocular diseases.

ANATOMY AND PHYSIOLOGY

The porcine orbit is open and continuous with the temporal fossa with considerable variation among breeds. The orbital axes are separated by roughly 90 degrees and the visual axes by 60 to 70 degrees, leading to an asymmetric location of extraocular muscles. The pig has prominent eyes with a forward position that allows a wide field of vision: 260 to 280 degrees with a small binocular field above the prominent snout. Binocular vision is estimated at 30 to 50 degrees. The orbit of the pig is conical in shape with the extraocular muscles firmly anchored in a deep sphenoid fossa in front of the optic foramen. The muscle origins in this fossa have a limited tendinous connection with each other but no true annulus zinnii.

The pig is one of the few animals to possess both a Harder's gland and a nictitans gland. The Harder's gland is large, lobulated, and situated infralaterally within the orbit. It rests close to the periorbital membrane within its own connective tissue capsule but outside the extraocular muscle cone. The gland is enclosed in a venous sheath or reservoir through which its ducts pass from its dorsal aspect to empty onto the bulbar surface of the nictitating membrane and the conjunctival sac. The nictitans gland is large and active, being more prominent on the palpebral side of the cartilage. The gland is tubuloalveolar with primarily a mucous secretion.

The pig's sclera is highly pigmented, with the deepest pigmentation at the limbus. The conjunctiva is also pigmented at its limbal attachment, contributing to the pigment ring bordering the cornea.

The pupil of the pig's eye is almost circular, being only slightly oval horizontally with an irregular margin. When dilated, it assumes a circular shape. There is no corpora nigra, but considerable pigment is found on the anterior surface of the iris. The highly pigmented ciliary body has an easily distinguishable pars plana and pars plicata. The main structure of the ciliary body is not well developed having an absence of circular muscle fibers. The drainage channels are part of a scleral venous plexus with no single Schlemm's canal.

The retina of the pig is well endowed with cones, an extensive vascular tree, and an area sufficiently free of blood vessels to suggest an area centralis at the posterior pole. The fundus has a uniform light red-brown appearance and lacks a tapetum. The blood vessels pass through the optic papilla either centrally or near its border. There are usually major retinal arteries and veins and a capillary network in multiple layers. There is no true macula, fovea, or tapetum. The retinal arteries derive from the main ciliary artery that divides rapidly and crosses over the papilla to enter the retina as the superior and inferior nasal and temporal arteries. The papillary margin is not discrete, and medullated nerve fibers commonly extend from the margin.

The pig eyelid is thick and heavy due to abundant subcutaneous fat cells. This produces a deep palpebral fold on the skin of the upper eyelid a few millimeters from and following the contour of the eyelid margin. The cilia of the upper eyelid are long, numerous, coarse, and extend along the whole eyelid margin. The lower lid is free of both cilia and palpebral folds. The eyelids have only a sheet of connective tissue as the equivalent of a tarsal plate. The main glands of the eyelid are not meibomian glands, as in most animals, but modified sweat glands among muscle bundles of the very extensive orbicular oculi muscle.

Lacrimal fluids drain through a single superior puncta in most animals, with an inferior puncta present only occasionally.

CONGENITAL ANOMALIES

The overall incidence of ocular congenital defects in swine is not well documented, although the pig is subject to the same malformations as other animals. There are a few reports of ocular defects, but an estimate of the relative percentage awaits study. Ocular defects such as dermoid and congenital glaucoma, common to most species, have been reported. Other frequently reported ocular defects are cyclopia, anophthalmia, and microphthalmia. The incidence of additional anomalies appears to be quite low. Optic nerve coloboma and choroid and optic nerve hypoplasia have been documented in miniature swine.

Optic atrophy and associated abnormalities, including staphyloma, hydrophthalmos, retinal and choroidal atrophy, retinal calcification, and microphthalmia have been documented in a male boar and his offspring. This syndrome appeared to be hereditary, but the mode of inheritance was not proved.

Hereditary microphthalmos has been known in Yorkshire pigs. The defect varied from extreme microphthalmos, with ocular tissue found only on dissection, to almost normal appearing globes. No true anophthalmos was found. The inheritance in this line was thought to be due to a dominant gene with low penetrance. A litter with both microphthalmos and macrophthalmos from a Yorkshire breeding pair has also been reported. All eyes had multiple intraocular defects suggestive of arrested development. No nutritional or infectious causes could be demonstrated. Varying degrees of microphthalmos and multiple intraocular defects have been documented in piglets with a suspected hereditable etiology.

Vitamin A deficiency has been documented as a cause of blindness in newborn pigs by several investigators. The deficiency may produce anophthalmos or varying degrees of microphthalmos. The ocular defects were present even when the deficiency was mild enough to produce viable piglets that were able to be reared. In the least severely affected animals, the eye was of normal size and shape although the iris and sclera were abnormally formed. As the deficiency was ameliorated, the clinical changes detected tended to be confined to the eye. Deficiency during the first month of pregnancy caused the ocular defects.

Cerebrospinal lipodystrophy in Yorkshire pigs has been reported and may serve as an appropriate model for the disease in humans. The affected neurons have round osmiophilic cytoplasmic inclusions that show as concentrically laminated membranous bodies on histologic and electron microscopic evaluations. Clinically, these deposits may show as focal white spots scattered throughout the retina.

Heterochromia irides in swine has an estimated incidence of 5 to 7 per cent. This appears unrelated to color of coats in some breeds but closely related to white coats in Yorkshires. In miniature pigs, heterochromia irides has been documented in both colored and white-coated animals with an incidence of 1.1 and 26.9 per cent, respectively. The overall incidence was 15.8 per cent. When affected animals are mated, the incidence in offspring increased as it would if both parents were light colored. Heterochromia irides in miniature swine appear to be inherited as a simple autosomal recessive trait, but its expression appears to be influenced by other factors, e.g., coat color, as the incidence rises to 38.3 per cent in totally white pigs.

TOXICITIES

Phenothiazine

Phenothiazine has been used as an anthelmintic in various species with the potential toxic effects appearing to vary widely among species. Ocular changes reported with phenothiazine overdose are blindness and corneal opacity either unilaterally or bilaterally, first noticed 48 hours after the overdose. Eyelid edema has also been reported. The mechanism appears to be a photosensitization reaction leading to iritis, uveitis, and corneal edema. Marked corneal edema may allow fibrovascular infiltrates (keratitis) to develop. Pigs should not be exposed to direct sunlight for 3 days after treatment with phenothiazine. Lesions are reversible if detected early.

Arsanilic Acid

Widely used as a food additive for growth promotion and for control of swine dysentery, arsanilic acid has been well documented as a cause of blindness when given in excess or for a prolonged time, or during periods of restricted water intake.

Symptoms are blindness, weakness, torticollis, and incoordination. These signs may appear within 1 week of administration of a high dose. Ocular lesions consist of pupil dilation with a clinically normal appearing globe. Blindness develops in 25 to 30 days in animals given 1000 ppm arsanilic acid. The blindness appears to be permanent. No pupillary light response is present. Ophthalmoscopically, optic nerve atrophy is apparent as pallor of the disc and loss of the normally vacuolated appearance of the central disc. The margins are well defined. Arteriolar constriction of vessels crossing the optic disc is also present. The electroretinogram remains normal in affected animals, but the visually evoked response is absent. Lesions of arsanilic acid blindness are characterized by parenchymatous neuropathy with demyelinization and axonal destruction of the optic nerves and tracts. Microscopically demonstrable lesions are present 3 or more days after the onset of clinical blindness and will continue to develop even after the arsanilic acid has been withdrawn.

CATARACTS

Cataracts have been reported in both control and treated swine exposed to neutron, gamma, and x-ray irradiation. These took the form of irregularly shaped plaques in the posterior subcapsular lens. The changes were not significant enough to cause visual disturbance in the animals.

Punctate opacities, vacuoles, and prominent suture lines in the lenses have been seen following prolonged starvation in swine. Riboflavin deficiency can cause cataracts.

Bilateral cortical cataracts in mature sows (over 2½ years of age) have been found with Hygromycin B as the suspected cause. The severity of the cataracts varied from early posterior polar opacities to dense, mature cortical cataracts. Visually, pupillary responses were normal as were the retinas. No systemic abnormalities were associated with the lenticular changes. Histologically, ocular changes were confined to the lens, which had posterior migration and proliferation of lens epithelium, cortical water clefts, and Morgagnian globule formation. Approximately 30 per cent of all brood sows more than 2½ years of age were affected in the treated herds.

INFECTIOUS DISEASES

Pseudorabies (Aujeszky's Disease)

An ocular sign in some animals acutely affected with pseudorabies is loss of vision. The degree of visual loss may be total or partial with some affected pigs able to distinguish between light and dark but unable to navigate around obstacles and other animals to compete for food. Other clinical signs, such as fever, depression, disorientation, head pressing, nystagmus, and eventually convulsions are present with the visual loss. Permanent blindness is a sequela in the small number of pigs that recover. Histologic findings are of nonsuppurative meningoencephalitis. The ganglion cell layer of affected eyes has decreased cell numbers. Remaining cells had degenerative changes characterized by indistinct cell outlines and fading and brownish granularity of the cyctoplasm. Within the optic nerve, perivascular cuffing with mononuclear and neutrophilic cells occurred. In recovered animals, examined 4 months after the acute phase, there was a marked reduction of cell numbers of the ganglion cell layer of the retina and a reduction of the density of the inner plexiform and nerve fiber layers.

All acutely ill pigs had derangement of the central nervous system and a significant degree of blindness. If blindness persisted for 6 to 7 days, the loss of sight was permanent. The presence of ocular lesions of systemic pseudorabies appears to be extremely variable.

In a review of experimentally induced pseudorabies (and in some natural outbreaks), the pathologic findings included ocular involvement, but the clinical signs did not include visual loss. Principal central nervous system changes were diffuse nonsuppurative meningoencephalomyelitis and ganglioneuritis with perivascular cuffing, diffuse and focal gliosis, and neuronal and glial necrosis. Meningitis extended along the optic nerve to the sclera. Intraocular changes consisted of lymphoreticular proliferation in the adventitia of retinal veins and gliosis associated with neuronal degeneration in the ganglion cell layer.

Pseudorabies-induced keratoconjunctivitis has also been studied as a potential animal model for human herpes simplex keratitis. Viral inoculation onto traumatized corneas produced keratoconjunctivitis characterized by corneal ulcers and persistent opacities. The disease was usually nonfatal with a predictable self-limiting course. The punctuate corneal ulcers may spread rapidly, progressing to disciform or geographic forms, accompanied by follicular conjunctivitis, chemosis, blepharospasm, corneal anesthesia, purulent exudate, transient blindness, edema of the iris, miosis, and fever. Corneal vascularization is well developed 12 days post-inoculation and coincides with regression of the ulcer. Histologically, there was necrosis and erosion of epithelium through post-inoculation day (PID) 11 and regeneration of a thin epithelial layer by PID 14. Epithelial degeneration was accompanied by corneal edema, deep stromal vascularization, and heavy inflammatory infiltration of the cornea and bulbar conjunctiva. Transient iritis characterized by edema, perivascular mononuclear cuffs, and stromal infiltration of mononuclear cells developed. There was also a moderate inflammatory reaction in the areas of the optic nerve characterized by mononuclear perivascular foci in the meninges. The inflammation intensified through PID 9 to 11, then subsided beginning at PID 14. A few corneal ulcers progressed to perforations with anterior synechia and hypopyon.

The keratoconjunctivitis induced by pseudorabies virus appears to be self-limiting, as encephalitis rarely occurs with this form of the disease. The virus does not spread to the noninfected eye. Conjunctivitis and central corneal ulceration have also been reported in pigs infected with pseudorabies virus intranasally.

Experimentally, optic nerve inflammation did not appear extensive enough to cause the blindness noted clinically. The visual loss was attributed to chemosis and corneal edema.

Pseudorabies virus persists in the diseased eye through PID 7 and is gone by PID 10 in all animals treated with topical antiviral agents. Swine antibody titers peak at about PID 18. Virus persists in the tear film throughout PID with decreased isolates until PID 18. The disappearance of virus from the eye and the appearance of antibodies correlates well with the clinical course of the disease.

HOG CHOLERA

Histologic studies of both field and experimental cases of hog cholera indicated that one might expect to detect perivascular cuffing ophthalmoscopically. Early in the course of the disease, the eyes show a copious conjunctival discharge and inflammation, which occur 4 to 7 days after exposure to the virus. This is readily observed in white pigs and may progress to the point where the eyelids adhere together owing to the exudate. The ocular discharge may begin as excess tearing and is often the first indication of hog cholera in white pigs. Pigs may appear blind. Inflammatory changes in the retina and uvea develop if the animals survive 7 days or longer. Congestion, edema, and occasionally hemorrhage of the iris and ciliary body are accompanied by mononuclear cell infiltration. Choroidal infiltration is focal and mild. There is acute retinitis with secondary neural damage. Retinal gliosis is observed in proximity to perivascular cuffing with random distribution. Optic neuritis is present with diffuse glial proliferation but without papilledema or destruction of the myelin.

The virus has been shown to invade both the retina and uveal tract, but significant changes do not occur before the sixth day of infection and are most significant after the ninth day of infection.

African Swine Fever

Blindness with keratitis and phthisis bulbi in some cases has been reported in pigs affected with Africa swine fever. The clinical course and histopathologic changes of ocular involvement have not been well documented, but findings include conjunctival hemorrhages early in the febrile stage of the disease. Later, serous to mucopurulent conjunctival and nasal discharges may be present.

Listeriosis

In adult swine, listeriosis occurs in association with other diseases and is rarely reported as a primary disease. In neonatal pigs, however, the disease is reported as a primary infection. It is believed that swine are normally quite resistant to the disease.

The liver and lungs appear to be the first organs affected in neonatal pigs, but evidence of ocular involvement was noted as early as 36 hr after oral inoculation. The lesion is a necrotizing vasculitis with occasional thrombosis. Multiple focal inflammatory areas are either primary thromboses or extensions of inflammation from other septic thrombi. The development of phlebitis in the choroid is thought to be related to direct invasion of the vessels by the organism. Foci of inflammation may be noted using ophthalmoscopy.

Toxoplasmosis

Toxoplasmosis can be found in both acute and chronic forms with chorioretinitis reported in all species in which intraocular infection has been seen. Although not documented, it is speculated that active chorioretinitis and perivascular cuffing, well described in other animals, should be visible ophthalmoscopically in the pig and might serve to aid diagnosis. Histologically, nonsuppurative iridocyclitis is the most frequently observed lesion. The mildest lesions consist of monocytes around small venules. Large aggregates of inflammatory cells are found with necrotic cells and small foci of coagulative necrosis. Retinal lesions are frequent and are always accompanied by cyclitis or iridocyclitis. Histiocytes and monocytes infiltrate inner retinal layers and adhere to the inner limiting membrane of the retina and adjacent vitreous. The nerve fiber and ganglion cell layers are edematous with focal areas of coagulation necrosis. Severe lesions show focal disorganization and loss of retinal pigment epithelium (RPE) with some areas of detached RPE, and macrophages, neutrophils, and lymphocytes in the subretinal space. Several foci of chorioretinitis are usually present, characterized by loss of retinal architecture, detachment, folds, edema, necrosis, and subretinal exudate. Chorioretinal fusion and atrophy are also observed. The focal inflammatory lesions extend centripetally from small necrotic venules or capillaries to involve all retinal layers.

Coagulation necrosis and retinal gliosis are often present. Choroidal lesions similar to the iris and ciliary body foci occasionally will be found without adjacent retinal involvement. These will lead to depigmentation of focal areas, which should be visible on ophthalmoscopic examination. Other lesions are focal aggregates of histiocytes and monocytes in muscle and fat and focal gliosis of optic nerves.

Glässer's Disease

Intraocular signs associated with this acute systemic polyserositis of pigs have been documented. The meningoencephalitis with fibrinous exudation can have uveal involvement with similar exudation.

Erysipelas

Uveal and retinal involvement with erysipelas in the acute systemic stage is expected but unfortunately rarely looked for. Signs expected would be focal chorioretinitis and iritis.

Conjunctivitis

Chlamydial conjunctivitis of pigs, similar to that reported in sheep, has been described. The organism has been recovered and can be grown in yolk-sac culture. Elementary and initial bodies can be seen in conjunctival scrapings.

The pig is assumed to be susceptible to various bacterial conjunctival infections, as are other species, but studies on the normal conjunctival flora and that of affected eyes in pigs remain to be done.

Edema Disease and Mulberry Heart Disease

Eyelid edema is a common feature of edema disease and endotoxemia produced by *Escherichia coli* in pigs. Other ocular lesions are chemosis and conjunctival inflammation. Exophthalmos has also been documented. All of these are seen in mulberry heart disease.

Cysticercosis

Ocular cysticercosis in swine commonly involves the conjunctiva and extraocular muscles. Intraretinal, subretinal, and subchoroidal cases of cysticercoses have also been documented.

Teschen Disease

Retinitis characterized by foci of gliosis has been documented in encephalomyelitis. Clinically, nystagmus and blindness are the ocular components of the disease associated with other abnormal central nervous system signs.

Swine Pox

Ocular involvement of swine pox includes conjunctivitis, blepharitis, and keratitis.

Swine Adenovirus

Keratoconjunctivitis associated with pharyngitis and pneumonia caused by adenovirus has been reported.

Supplemental Reading

Blogg, J. R.: The Eye in Veterinary Practice: Extraocular Disease. Philadelphia, W. B. Saunders Company, 1980.
Saunders, L. Z., and Rubin, L. F.: Ophthalmic Pathology of Animals. Basil, S. Harger, 1975.
Williams, L. W., and Gelatt, K. N.: Food Animal Ophthalmology. *In* K. N. Gelatt (ed.). Veterinary Ophthalmology. Philadelphia, Lea & Febiger, 1981.
Williams, L. W., and Gelatt, K. N.: Ocular Manifestations of Systemic Disease, part 3. Food Animals. In K. N. Gelatt, (ed.). Veterinary Ophthalmology. Philadelphia, Lea & Febiger, 1981.

NEUROLOGIC DISEASES OF FOOD ANIMALS

W. C. REBHUN, D.V.M.
Consulting Editor

Neurologic Examination of Cattle

THOMAS J. DIVERS, D.V.M.

The initial objective of the neurologic examination of cattle is to determine if the nervous system is indeed abnormal, or if the clinical signs are caused by an abnormality of another system. It is not always easy to differentiate clinical signs of musculoskeletal dysfunction from those of neurologic dysfunction. If the animal's nervous system is abnormal, every effort should be made to determine the neuroanatomic location of the dysfunction. Clinical signs of neurologic diseases are best divided into those of the cerebrum, cerebellum, brain stem, spinal cord segments C1–C5, C6–T2, T3–L3, and L4–S2, coccygeal nerves, and peripheral nerves. Each anatomic area has specific clinical signs that suggest dysfunction of that particular area. Of course, many nervous diseases in cattle affect more than one area simultaneously. Every effort should be made to determine the symmetry of the neurologic signs.

CLINICAL SIGNS

Cerebrum

Behavioral changes and central blindness are characteristic clinical signs of cerebral dysfunction. The behavioral changes vary from coma and stupor to convulsions and belligerence. Cattle with cerebral disease most often are dull and depressed, circle with compulsive walking (usually towards the side with the lesion), or are pressing their heads against stationary objects. Although the cattle may be blind, the pupillary response to light is normal. If only one cerebral hemisphere is involved, blindness would be contralateral. Ataxia is absent or minimal with cerebral disease alone, although many cattle with acute cerebral disease and blindness may appear weak and walk with a short, shuffling gait. If the cerebral disease causes secondary compression of the brain stem, then ataxia would be expected.

848

Brain Stem

Ataxia, paresis, and cranial nerve deficits are usually present with brain stem dysfunction. Depression is variable and may be severe. If the brain stem disease is unilateral and in the more rostral area (midbrain), then ataxia and paresis may occur in the contralateral limbs. Signs of ipsilateral cranial nerve III deficits are common with lesions in this region. If the disease is in the medulla or pons, the ataxia and paresis frequently are ipsilateral, and irregular respiratory patterns may be observed.

Cerebellum

The cerebellum modulates movement of the head, limbs, and body. Clinical signs of cerebellar dysfunction are motor ataxia without paresis, head tremors, truncal ataxia, and base wide stance. Vision should be present, but the menace response may be absent or delayed. Because of the close proximity and communication between the cerebellum and the vestibular system, some signs characteristic of central vestibular disease may also be observed, such as head tilt, strabismus, and changing nystagmus. Opisthotonus with forelimb extension is common with lesions in the rostral cerebellum.

Spinal Cord

C1–C5

Spinal cord disease in this region commonly causes tetraparesis and ataxia of all 4 limbs or recumbency. With mild to moderate disease, paresis may not be easily noted. Ataxia may be slightly more obvious in the rear limbs than in the forelimbs. The animal may be recumbent but should be able to lift its head and neck even when there are severe lesions in the lower cervical area. With severe lesions of the upper cervical area (e.g., atlanto-occipital disease), however, the animal may be recumbent and unable to lift its head or neck. Cattle with cord diseases in the C1–C5 region have normal or exaggerated limb reflexes, unless secondary muscle damage from recumbency has occurred. If the cervical disease is a result of a fracture or abscess, obvious signs of cervical pain, such as head extension, stiff neck, and reluctance to eat from the ground, may be observed. If disease is more pronounced on one side of the cord, paresis and ataxia are more advanced on the ipsilateral side.

C6–T2

Spinal cord disease in this region will also cause ataxia and paresis in all 4 limbs or recumbency. The clinical signs should be worse in the forelimbs than in the hind limbs. If the duration of the disease is greater than 7 days, atrophy of shoulder or forelimb muscles may be noted. Some spinal reflexes of the forelimbs will be depressed, while those of the hind limbs will be normal or exaggerated, unless secondary muscle damage has developed.

T3–L4

Neurologic disease in this region will cause ataxia and paresis only in the rear limbs. If the lesion is severe and if the animal is recumbent, it should be able to get onto its sternum and move its front limbs. The spinal reflexes of the hind limbs are usually normal or exaggerated, unless secondary muscle damage has occurred because of recumbency. If the disease is a result of a fracture or of an abscess in this region, careful palpation may reveal an area of deformity or signs of pain, or both. In cattle, the panniculus reflex may, on rare occasions, be helpful in localizing the site of the lesion within this region. Radiographs, including myelograms, can be performed even in adult cattle if warranted to aid in diagnosing spinal fractures or compressive cord lesions, or both.

L4–S2

Disease of the spinal cord segments in this area (which are usually contained within the fourth, fifth, and sixth lumbar vertebrae in adult cattle) cause ataxia, paresis, and hyporeflexia of the rear limbs and anus. Abnormal micturition may be present and is most often characterized as a "lower motor neuron bladder" with frequent dribbling of urine while the animal is walking and easy expression of urine during a rectal examination.

Coccygeal Nerves

Diseases of the last sacral nerves and the coccygeal nerves cause paralysis of the tail, perineal analgesia, hyporeflexia of the anus, and abnormal micturition. Cattle that have been pulled by the tail may develop secondary paresis and hyporeflexia.

Peripheral Nerves

Diseases of the peripheral nerves cause lower motor neuron disease (paresis) of the muscles or tendons, or both, which they supply. Usually, peripheral nerve disease in cattle is a result of traumatic injury and is unilateral. The peripheral nerves most commonly damaged in cattle are the sciatic, obturator, femoral, radial, and cranial nerves VII and VIII. Damage to the peripheral portion of cranial nerves VII and VIII is usually caused by trauma or middle ear infections. Occasionally, a disease may affect the motor function of a peripheral nerve without any visible microscopic lesions or clinical signs that suggest lower neuron disease (e.g., spastic paresis syndrome in calves). Neuromuscular disease, such as botulism, may cause diffuse lower motor neuron signs in cattle. Electromyography may be used to substantiate the presence of neuromuscular disease in cattle.

HISTORY AND CLINICAL SIGNS

An accurate and complete history along with consideration of the signalment is an important antecedent to the neurologic examination. A visual and historical investigation of the environment may provide important clues for the diagnosis of neurologic diseases, such as pseudorabies, malignant catarrhal fever, and lead poisoning. Information on both past and present feeding problems aids diagnoses, such as grass tetany, listeriosis, botulism, grass staggers, and fractured spine resulting from metabolic bone disease. Careful questioning of the herd manager about prior illness in the affected animal or the herd may be helpful (e.g., cattle suspected of having vertebral body abscessation commonly have a history of pneumonia or other chronic suppurative processes.) Prior knowlege of the incidence of listeriosis or lymphosarcoma in the herd may be germane to making a diagnosis.

The therapy an animal is receiving could also be responsible for neurologic dysfunction (e.g, nitrofurazone toxicity in calves).

The age of the animal is an essential consideration when trying to diagnose congenital anomalies of the nervous system, polioencephalomalacia, and lymphosarcoma. On occasion, knowlege of the incidence of a particular disorder in a breed is crucial (e.g., cerebellar abiotrophy in Holsteins or hereditary neuroaxial edema in polled Herefords). A careful documentation of the onset and course of the neurologic disorder is often helpful in distinguishing between traumatic lesions and progressive inflammatory or neoplastic diseases involving the nervous sytem.

NEUROLOGIC EXAMINATION

A complete physical examination, including rectal examination, should be performed at the time of the neurologic examination. The nervous dysfunction may be determined to be secondary to a disease of another system. A complete examination is also essential in order to provide an assessment of the mental status, gait (including proprioception and strength), cranial nerve function, and spinal reflexes. The examination may need to be curtailed, depending upon environmental circumstances or the size and disposition of the animal. Rabies must always be considered in cattle with neurologic dysfunction, especially those with paresis, ataxia or behavioral changes, or both, and necessary precautions should be taken during the examination.

Examination of Mental Attitude

Deranged behavior and a change in mental status associated with a disease of the nervous system suggest cerebral or brain stem dysfunction, or both. The change in attitude may range from depression and stupor to belligerence and mania. The entire range of signs can be present within the same disease (e.g., lead poisoning). Abnormal behavior is easily recognized in those cattle with chronic or severe disease. Observing the affected animal within the herd during feeding and after other stimulation (sound and so forth) is helpful in determining abnormal behavior. The owner's impression is of the utmost assistance in many instances of mild behavior changes.

Evaluation of Gait

The gait should be scrutinized in the ambulatory patient to determine the presence of ataxia, proprioceptive deficit, and weakness. The number of limbs involved and the severity of the deficit in each limb should be determined. Ataxia is an incoordianted movement of the limbs and may result from sensory (proprioception) or motor deficits. Although abnormal motion may occur with musculoskeletal disease, the movement is not incoordinated. Clinical signs of ataxia include delayed protraction of the limbs, dragging of the toes, spasticity (usually exhibited by a stabbing gait), hypermetria, circumduction, crossing over of the limbs, stepping on the opposite foot, pivoting on the inner hind foot when turning, and falling. Affected cattle should be observed in motion on a surface with good footing. They should be led or chased in a straight line and circled in both directions. For more subtle disorders, the ataxia may become more pronounced and thus more easily recognized if the animal is backed up or made to go down an incline. Absence of normal proprioception (sensory awareness of the position of the limbs) can usually be determined while the animal is moving. Abnormal positioning of the limbs when the animal is standing may also suggest a proprioception deficit.

Incoordination complicated by weakness would suggest brain stem, spinal cord, or peripheral nerve disease. This is particularly important in differentiating peripheral vestibular disease (ataxia without paresis) from central vestibular disease (ataxia with paresis). Ataxia without weakness is also seen with cerebellar disease and certain diseases that affect release mechanisms of the spinal cord (tetanus and spastic paresis). Although most diseases of the spinal cord cause both ataxia and paresis, paresis may be difficult to appreciate in cattle with mild to moderate cases. Paretic cattle generally walk with a short, shuffling, incoordinated gait and, on occasion, appear to be slightly crouched in the rear limbs while walking and standing. They may have difficulty rising and may be easily pushed or pulled from side to side. Some severely affected cattle may collapse when pressure is applied to the loin region. Each ataxic and paretic limb should be palpated carefully for evidence of muscle atrophy.

Evaluation of Cranial Nerves

Cranial Nerve II. Optic nerve function is best tested by performing both the menace reflex and the pupillary response to light. A menacing gesture with the side of the hand should cause a rapid closure of the eyelids in normal cattle. This reflex requires a functioning retina, optic nerve, contralateral geniculate nucleus, contralateral occipital cortex, and ipsilateral facial nucleus and nerve. If the menace response is absent but a direct pupillary response is present, dysfunction within the opposite cerebral cortex or lateral geniculate nucleus, or both, is suggested. Normal newborn calves and cattle with cerebellar disease may be slow to respond to a menacing gesture, however.

Fundoscopic examination should be performed on all cattle with nervous disorders. Obvious papillary edema is seldom seen except in animals with vitamin A deficiency. Retinal hemorrhages are frequently observed in cattle with thromboembolic meningoencephalitis.

Cranial Nerve III. The oculomotor nerve provides parasympathetic innervation to the iris (pupillary constric-tion) and motor innervation to the dorsal rectus, ventral rectus, medial rectus, and ventral oblique muscles of the globe. The oculomotor nerve is best evaluated by the pupillary response to a strong light; this is very difficult to evaluate outdoors and is best done indoors with a strong flashlight. Newborn calves, very excited cattle, or cattle with milk fever may be slow to constrict their pupil despite having normal oculomotor nerve function. Although rarely appreciated clinically, strabismus may occur with oculomotor nerve deficits.

A slight upper lid ptosis also may be noted with cranial nerve III dysfunction, probably due to loss of innervation to the levator palpebrae muscle. The oculomotor nerve may be damaged with progressing cerebral disease (most often edema) and compression of the midbrain. The development of nonresponsive dilated pupils in animals being treated for cerebral disease is an unfavorable sign. If the oculomotor nerve deficit is asymmetrical, anisocoria may be present.

Cranial Nerve IV. The trochlear nerve has efferent fibers to the dorsal oblique muscles of the eye, and damage to the nerve can cause dorsomedial strabismus. This is best determined by evaluating the position of the eye while the head is moved in different directions. It is a fairly common finding in calves with polioencephalomalacia.

Cranial Nerve V. The trigeminal nerve supplies sensory fibers to the face and motor fibers to the muscles of mastication. The sensory component is best evaluated by touching the inside of the nose and ear on both sides of the face. The animal with normal cortical function will jerk the head away and back up. The motor function evaluation is more subjective but can be determined by observation of the animal eating, by palpating the masseter muscles for evidence of atrophy, by encountering resistance when opening the jaw, and by shaking the animal's head with the jaw open to determine jaw tone. Sialosis is commonly observed with trigeminal nerve deficits. Bovine listeriosis frequently damages this nerve. Although the IBR virus often infects and damages the nerve, loss of function is seldom appreciated clinically.

Cranial Nerve VI. The abducens nerve innervates the retractor bulbi and lateral rectus muscles. Medial strabismus and inability to retract the eye are indicative of abnormal function.

Cranial Nerve VII. The facial nerve provides motor input to the muscles of facial expression, lacrimal glands, and salivary glands. Abnormal function should be suspected when the lower lip, ear or eyelid, or both, on the same side of the face, droop. Damage to the facial nerve often results in exposure keratitis.

Cranial Nerve VIII (Vestibulocochlear Nerve). The vestibular portion of the eighth cranial nerve provides input to the vestibular nuclei and, along with the cerebellum, helps control balance, orientation of the head, body, and eyes. Abnormal function should be suspected in an animal with a head tilt, circling, and ataxia. The head will tilt towards the side on which the lesion is located. Because of greater extensor tone contralateral to the side of the lesion, circling is toward the side containing the lesion. Resting strabismus and nystagmus may also be observed, but found consistently only in the early periods of vestibular disease in cattle. Abnormal nystagmus and strabismus may occur if the head is moved rapidly. Central vestibular disease is characterized by head tilt (usually toward the side with the lesion), variable nystagmus, ataxia and paresis, and the likelihood of multiple cranial nerve deficits. The quick phase of the nystagmus is away from the side with the lesion in peripheral vestibular disease and is variable in central vestibular disease.

Cranial Nerve IX and X. The glossopharyngeal and vagus nerves supply motor innervation to the pharynx and larynx; damage to either nerve results in pharyngeal and laryngeal paresis. Difficulty in swallowing food and saliva with reflux through the nose, coughing, and a change in voice are characteristic clinical signs.

Cranial Nerve XII. The hypoglossal nerve provides motor input to the tongue. The function of the hypoglossal nerve is best determined by pulling the tongue to each side of the mouth.

Some cranial nerves (e.g., facial and vestibular) easily suffer peripheral damage. When cranial nerves are damaged peripherally, there is usually only one nerve affected except for the concurrent damage to nerves VII and VIII, which often occurs with diseases of the middle ear region. There should be no paresis or proprioception deficit of the limbs, and ataxia is present only if the vestibular nerve is affected. This is in contrast to central (brain stem) damage of the cranial nerve nuclei where ataxia and paresis occur, and multiple cranial nerves are more likely to be affected.

Evaluation of Spinal Reflexes

The panniculus reflex may be evaluated in standing or recumbent cattle. The skin along the topline is pricked gently with a needle to evaluate this reflex. Sensory input enters the cord at the site of the skin prick, ascends to cervical thoracic intertumescence and there synapses with lower motor neuron cell bodies, causing stimulation of the cutaneous trunci muscle. A skin prick on either side of the backbone between T2 and L4 should cause a reflex movement of the cutaneous trunci muscle on the same side. Many normal cattle do not exhibit an obvious response.

The anal reflex can also be evaluated in standing or recumbent cattle. The anus or perineal region should be pinched, causing a mild to moderate contraction of the anus and tightening of the tail against the body. The function of sacral nerves 1, 2, and 3 and the coccygeal nerves are tested by this reflex. This reflex may be absent in cattle with abnormal neurologic signs caused by lymphosarcoma.

Most spinal reflexes can be assessed accurately only in calves or in recently recumbent cows. Adult cattle that have been recumbent for any period often develop ischemic myopathy and, therefore, secondary hyporeflexia. However, this is variable, so the reflexes should be evaluated in all recumbent cattle. The size of the animal, the period of recumbency, and so forth should be considered when interpreting reflexes. A pair of pliers and an instrument used as a plexometer are the only equipment necessary for evaluation of the commonly tested spinal reflexes.

Both upper limbs should be tested while the animal is in lateral recumbency; the animal should then be rolled over, and the opposite limbs should be tested. Squeezing a dewclaw with the pliers will test the withdrawal reflex of the forelimbs. A sudden withdrawal of the limb and movement of the shoulder is normal and suggests integrity of lower motor neurons in the C5–T2 region. While holding the limb gently in a relaxed and slightly flexed position, the tendonous attachment of the triceps muscle above the olecranon may be tapped lightly with the plexometer for the triceps reflex. An extension of the limb during the triceps reflex suggests normal function of the radial nerve. In many normal cattle, the triceps reflex is not easily elicited.

Rear limb withdrawal may be tested in the same manner, but since the response is usually more exaggerated, the clinician should stay at a safe distance. The sudden withdrawal of the rear limb suggests function of the sciatic nerve (L6–S2). The femoral nerve (L4–L6) may be tested by tapping the middle ligament of the patella gently with the plexometer. The normal response in an extension of the stifle. This reflex is more dependable than the reflex of the triceps but less so than either withdrawal reflex. Exaggerated reflexes, indicative of a lesion rostral to the nucleus of the tested reflex arch (upper motor neuron), are not easily determined in cattle. Resistance to the flexion of each limb should be judged. Weak or absent resistance in the front or rear limbs is compatible with lower motor neuron dysfunction of the brachial plexus or pelvic plexus, respectively.

Collection of Spinal Fluid

Spinal fluid collection should be attempted in cattle with neurologic disorders whenever the diagnosis is obscure or an etiologic agent is being sought. Cerebrospinal fluid can easily be obtained from the cisterna magnum or lumbosacral space of recumbent or well-restrained cattle. Mechanical restraint will suffice in most cattle, but small amounts of intravenous xylazine (0.05 mg/lb or 0.11 mg/kg) may be required in some. The skin over the poll should be clipped and surgically scrubbed. The head is flexed, and an area on the midline and just rostral to an imaginary line between the cranial edges of the wings of the atlas is anesthetized. A puncture is made with a 14-gauge needle through the skin at this site. A 3½-inch (8-cm), 18-gauge spinal needle* is then introduced through the skin perforation and slowly advanced; particular care should be taken to remain on the dorsal midline. The needle will pass through the nuchal ligament before contacting the dura and entering the subarachnoid space. A change in resistance usually can be felt both when the needle tip completes penetration of the nuchal ligament and when it enters the subarachnoid space. If any change in resistance is encountered, the stylet should be removed and examined for free-flowing spinal fluid. By using nose tongs, the head usually can be kept in a ventral flexed position during this procedure. Attention should be paid to the animal's respiration and, should it become obstructed, mechanical flexion should be decreased.

A lumbosacral tap is preferred in ambulatory patients with spinal cord dysfunction or in patients that cannot be safely or sufficiently restrained for a cisternal tap. The ambulatory animal may be restrained in a chute or stanchion for the procedure. The lumbosacral tap can be performed in recumbent cattle by positioning them squarely in sternal position or in lateral recumbency. Usually, a small depression can be palpated at the lumbosacral space in calves and dairy cows. The area should be clipped and prepared, and a skin puncture made

---

*Available from Becton Dickinson and Company, Rochelle Park, NJ 07662

initially with a 14-gauge needle. A 3½-inch, 18-gauge spinal needle is adequate for calves and most dairy cows; a longer needle may be needed for bulls and large cows. The needle should be advanced slowly, and great care should be taken to remain at the midline. Usually, the needle can be felt penetrating the interarticular ligament. When the dura is punctured, there may be a slight but suddent movement of tail or hind limbs. In the standing or sternal animal, slight aspiration with a syringe may be necessary to collect the sample.

SUMMARY

A good history and a complete physical and neurologic examination should enable the clinician to localize the disease. The collection and interpretation of the results of spinal fluid examination may help characterize the disease process in some cases. With a knowledge of differential diagnosis of central nervous system disease in cattle, the veterinarian may make a rapid but reliable decision concerning prognosis and therapy.

Infectious Causes of Meningitis and Encephalitis in Cattle

THOMAS J. DIVERS, D.V.M.

Infections of the central nervous system (CNS) in cattle may be caused by bacteria, viruses, or fungi. These infections are often limited to the covering of the brain (meningitis) but may involve the parenchyma of the brain (encephalitis). In most instances, the clinical signs are more reflective of the location and duration of the disease within the CNS than the cause of the disease. Regardless of the etiologic agent, infections of the CNS are serious, and the prognosis is usually guarded. If the animal is to be treated successfully, therapy should be prompt and exact. Seldom can a confirmation of the disease agent be established before therapy is begun. Therefore, knowledge of the most common etiologic agents, their antimicrobial sensitivities, and the pharmokinetics of selected drugs used for treating CNS infections is essential.

BACTERIAL MENINGITIS

The most common infectious disease of the CNS of young calves is bacterial meningitis. Bacterial meningitis in young calves most often results from bacteremia and may, therefore, be only one part of a multisystem disease. Meningitis may occur in combination with arthritis, omphalitis, panophthalmitis, enteritis, pneumonia, and nephritis in calves. The disease is most prevalent in calves that do not receive adequate colostrum. The most frequent etiologic agents are *Escherichia coli*, *Pasteurella* spp., *Corynebacterium pyogenes*, *Staphylococcus aureus*, *Proteus* spp., *Streptococcus* spp., and *Salmonella* spp. The most common age for onset of clinical signs is less than 14 days. *Listeria monocytogenes* and *Haemophilus somnus* are frequent causes of CNS infection in yearlings and in adult cattle. Bacterial meningitis may also occur sporad-

ically in adult cattle and is usually secondary to sinusitis, skull injury, or septicemia.

Clinical Signs

Clinical signs are directly related to the location of the infection within the CNS as well as to the duration and severity of the infection. They are also reflective of caudal brain stem and cerebellar dysfunction common in young calves. These signs include depression, tetraparesis, and ataxia with head tremors, abnormal nystagmus, and terminal opisthotonus. Abnormal respiratory patterns may be apparent. Marked stupor or blindness may be present in cases of encephalitis. Calves with more chronic cases of meningitis may only exhibit continual recumbency, apathy, and anorexia. Hyperalgesia, muscular rigidity, and marked incoordination are frequent findings of spinal meningitis and nerve root involvement. The temperature of affected animals is usually elevated early in the disease but may be normal or even subnormal by the time of examination.

Diagnosis

The diagnosis is based on clinical signs and on higher levels of neutrophils and protein in the cerebrospinal fluid (CSF). The normal values for white blood cells and protein in the CSF of cattle are <5 cells/mm^3 and <40 mg/100 ml, respectively. Fibrin may be observed within the CSF of some calves with meningitis. Culture of the fluid should be attempted as should culture of any other infected areas (joints, umbilicus, and so forth). The meningeal vessels are congested, and the meninges are thickened in calves dying of acute meningitis. Infarcted areas of the brain may be observed in some calves that had survived for several days. The primary differential diagnosis in young calves with bacterial meningitis would include metabolic diseases (e.g., hypoglycemia), toxic encephalopathies (e.g., lead), viral encephalitis, and congenital anomalies involving the CNS.

Treatment

The recommended treatment of bacterial meningitis is prompt and intensive antimicrobial therapy and supportive care. Bacterial infections of the CNS are usually life threatening and resistant to conventional therapy. Therefore, antimicrobial drugs that are not approved for use in food-producing animals and higher doses of drugs that are approved may be listed. Initial antimicrobial therapy in valuable calves should include intravenous penicillin, 40,000 units/kg, 4 times daily and either intravenous gentamicin, 2 to 4 mg/kg, 4 times daily or, preferably, intravenous amikacin, 6 mg/kg, 4 times daily. The CSF concentration of gentamicin and penicillin in the normal neonatal calf, when given at this dosage, is high enough to be effective *in vitro* against most of the common pathogens. Antibacterial concentration should be much higher in calves with meningitis than in normal calves. Amikacin (80 mg) may also be given intrathecally (lumbosacral) every 12 hr when higher CSF concentrations of an aminoglycoside are needed. Intravenous chloramphenicol (20 to 40 mg/kg) 4 times daily or intravenous sulfadiazine trimethoprim (20 mg/kg) 4 times daily is another choice. Both drugs cross into the CSF well and have broad-spectrum activity. Sulfadiazine trimethoprim may also be combined with ampicillin or an aminoglycoside. Chloramphenicol is not metabolized well in the neonatal calf, and oral solutions or parenterally administered ones may reach toxic levels with daily doses of 80 mg/kg or more. Chloramphenicol is not to be used in food-producing animals in the United States. Steroids should only be used if progression of clinical signs is rapid. Since many calves with meningitis are hypogammaglobulinemic, the administration of 1 to 2 L of bovine plasma may be indicated. Maintenance of fluid balance, caloric intake, and adequate ventilation are important. Calves with meningitis may be unable to suckle, and fluid and caloric intake is best maintained by intravenous administration, if feasible. When the calf is fed by stomach tube, accumulation of excess milk in the rumen may occur. Abdominal distention should be monitored and, if it occurs, force feeding should be discontinued.

All other infected areas of the body (umbilicus, joints, and so forth) should be treated appropriately.

Prevention

All precautions must be taken to ensure that calves are born in a clean environment and receive adequate colostrum. The calves should be raised in clean, well ventilated, individual pens and should receive whole milk or good quality milk replacer. The umbilical area should be inspected, and the calf should be scrutinized daily for signs of illness.

LISTERIOSIS

Listeriosis is a zoonotic disease primarily affecting ruminants (in order of prevalence: cattle, sheep, and goats). In cattle, the disease is most frequent during the winter and spring and often involves a history of feeding improperly fermented silage. The etiologic agent is *Listeria monocytogenes,* an aerobic, beta hemolytic, gram-positive rod. The natural reservoir is soil or animal feces, or both, but it may be passed in milk. The organism may get into feed sources from the soil or manure. Improperly fermented silage or silage with urea that never attains a pH of <5.5 during the ensilage period appears to offer an ideal substrate for the organism's growth. Bunker silos may allow more improperly fermented silage and more soil contamination than other types of silos. The organisms survive repeated freezing and thawing for years in silos, soil, and feces. It has been proposed that infected cattle ingest the organism, which then enters a buccal wound and infects a cranial nerve (most often the trigeminal nerve). The organism may then migrate up the cranial nerve to the brain stem, where multiple microabscesses occur. It is also postulated that a decline in cell mediated defense mechanisms allows the establishment of infections. There are 5 serotypes of *L. monocytogenes;* type 4B is the cause of encephalitic listeriosis.

Clinical Signs

The encephalitic form of *Listeria* is usually seen in adult cattle. Circling and localizing unilateral brain stem signs are frequent. Facial nerve paralysis is common, and affected cattle have an ear droop, lip droop, saliva loss, and failure to blink on one side of the face. Ipsilateral exposure keratitis is a common finding. Unilateral trigeminal nerve paralysis frequently occurs and is best demonstrated by lack of sensation on the affected side of the face and nose. If bilateral trigeminal nerve involvement occurs, there may be an obvious jaw droop. The vestibular nucleus is often involved, resulting in varying degrees of head tilt, circling, strabismus, and resting nystagmus. The hypoglossal, vagal, or glossopharyngeal nerves may also be involved, resulting in a protruding tongue or dysphagia, or both with persistent loss of saliva. Vomiting may occur as an early sign in some cattle.

Some cows affected with listeriosis do not have obvious localizing brain stem signs and circling but instead have behavior changes and unusual stances (pressing forward in their stanchions or against other objects). Cows with listeriosis are depressed, ataxic, and paretic, but their weakness is not always easily appreciated. The temperature is usually normal by the time clinical signs become obvious. Although the disease is usually sporadic, occasional herd outbreaks take place, wherein several cows in a herd may be affected over a period of several weeks.

Diagnosis

A tentative diagnosis is made based on history and clinical findings. The collection of CSF is very helpful in establishing a diagnosis since most cows with listeriosis have mild to marked pleocytosis, which is predominantly of mononuclear cells. The CSF protein level is usually elevated. Isolation of the organism is difficult and therefore not usually attempted. Histopathologic examination of the brain confirms microabscesses within the white matter of the brain stem, cerebellum, and rarely the cerebrum. Serologic test results are of little benefit in helping to confirm the disease. Differential diagnosis in adult cattle with similar signs should include thromboembolic meningoencephalitis, rabies, pseudorabies, brain abscess, sinusitis with associated leptomeningitis, and nervous ketosis. In young calves being sucked on the ears by other calves or in cattle with a foreign body in the ear, inner ear infections may occur, and cattle may have clinical signs similar to listeriosis. Usually, these cattle are not paretic and only have involvement of nerves VII and VIII. An otoscopic examination is usually diagnostic in these exogenous middle ear infections. Similarly, endogenous inner ear infections in calves and feeder calves with concurrent pneumonia can be confused with listeriosis.

Treatment

Administration of high levels of penicillin is the preferred therapy for encephalitis listeriosis. (The levels are higher than those approved by the FDA.) The absence of any marked lesions to the dura suggests the "blood-brain barrier" may still be functional. Penicillin does not readily cross the blood-brain barrier, which necessitates high serum concentrations. This is best established by the administration of intravenous penicillin, 40,000 to 80,000 units/kg, 4 times daily for the initial 3 to 5 days. Therapy can then be continued with intramuscular penicillin, 20,000 units/kg, twice daily, for another 14 to 21 days. If treatment is inadequate or discontinued too early, a chronic case of encephalitis may result. Intramuscular penicillin (40,000 units/kg) 2 times daily alone may be effective if administered early. Tetracycline has also been used effectively in treating *Listeria* encephalitis of cattle. Because of the difficulty in drinking and swallowing as well as the loss of saliva, cattle may become dehydrated and acidotic. Oral fluids and bicarbonates may be administered by stomach tube as needed. The prognosis is fair to good if cattle are treated prior to becoming recumbent; if untreated, most cattle die within 14 days.

INFECTIOUS THROMBOEMBOLIC MENINGOENCEPHALITIS (TEME)

TEME is caused by *Haemophilus somnus,* a gram-negative pleomorphic organism. *H. somnus* may cause an acute septicemic disease of cattle, affecting predominantly the lungs, joints, or CNS. The highest incidence of the disease appears during the winter and is greatest in yearling feedlot cattle. There also seems to be a marked increased incidence in certain areas of North America, particularly Canada. Some areas in North America have not reported any TEME cases, although the organism has been cultured frequently from normal animals. Thromboembolic meningoencephalitis is apparently rare in dairy animals in the eastern United States. In certain animals, *H. somnus* may invade the respiratory tract, evade phagocytosis, and produce bacteremia. Organism adherence to endothelial cells produces the characteristic vasculitis, which leads to infarction and abscessation. Postmortem findings are multifocal hemorrhage and fibrinopurulent necrosis throughout the brain and spinal cord as a result of vasculitis. Interstitial pneumonia with thrombosis of vessels, neutrophil invasion, fibrinous pleuritis, pericarditis, and arthritis may be found.

Clinical Signs

A large number of cattle with TEME die without observable clinical signs. TEME may contribute to sudden death observed in feedlot cattle during the winter. Cattle with clinical signs of TEME are most frequently depressed, sleepy, or convulsing because of cerebral dysfunction. Affected cattle are ataxic and weak and may have localizing signs of brain stem disease. Fever and retinal hemorrhages are common. Clinical signs of respiratory disease may be or may have been present in cattle with TEME or in their herdmates.

Diagnosis

A history of previous respiratory disease in the herd as well as related information about geography, age, and seasonal predisposition is helpful in making a tentative diagnosis. The finding of retinal hemorrhages in cattle with CNS disease and a compatible history are also highly suggestive. The CSF characteristically has neutrophilic pleocytosis with an abnormally high protein concentration. Surviving animals or herdmates have an increase in *Haemophilus* spp. complement-fixing antibodies. The organism may be cultured from the CSF, lungs, or urine.

Although many animals die before therapy can be initiated, antibiotic therapy may be successful in some cases. Intravenous tetracycline (10 mg/kg) twice daily or intravenous penicillin (40,000 units/kg) 4 times daily, or intramuscular penicillin (20,000 units/kg) twice daily is recommended. Intravenous or subcutaneous chloramphenicol (20 mg/kg) 4 times daily has been a successful treatment but is not approved for use in food-producing animals in the United States. Aspirin (0.4 grains/kg, orally, every other day) may be helpful in reducing thrombosis. Antibiotic therapy in some animals may only interrupt the progression of clinical signs, and some affected animals may survive but remain blind or ataxic or both. The use of bacterins has proved useful in decreasing the incidence of the disease in both field trials and control studies. The vaccine must be administered twice, 2 to 4 weeks apart, in order to provide clinical protection.

PITUITARY GLAND ABSCESS

Pituitary gland (hypophysis) abscesses occur sporadically in cattle and are most common in those 1 to 3 years of age. Abscesses may develop in this area by one of several mechanisms. The most likely is that of bacterial embolization, arising from abscessation elsewhere in the body (e.g., chronic enzootic pneumonia or hardware disease), causing meningoencephalitis that localized within or around the hypophysis. The etiologic agent is usually *Corynebacterium pyogenes* or *Pasteurella* spp. In bulls, the use of nose rings has occasionally been incriminated as a source of bacterial embolization.

Clinical Signs

The clinical signs are generally a result of the pressure on and inflammation of the hypophysis, midbrain, and surrounding cranial nerves. Affected cattle are most often dull, depressed, weak, and ataxic. Some may circle continuously and hold their heads in extension. A "stargazing" attitude with the head held in extension and the muzzle pointed dorsally is common. The oculomotor nerve may be involved with resulting anisocoria. Although cattle have a restrictive dura, the abscess may extend to the optic chiasm and result in blindness. The trigeminal nerve may also be involved, causing decreased sensation to the face and loss of normal movement of muscles of mastication. The abscess has also been reported to compress the mesencephalic aqueduct, resulting in internal hydrocephalus and causing bradycardia, which is thought to result from interference with the hypothalamus' role in autonomic function.

Diagnosis

The disease should be considered in any adult cow with bradycardia, signs of cerebral disease, aniscoria, and blindness. Plasma fibrinogen concentration is usually elevated, as are CSF protein levels and white blood cell counts. Because of chronicity, pleocytosis may consist predominantly of either neutrophils or mononuclear leukocytes. Other areas of abscessation within the body are occasionally found at necropsy. Abscesses within the cerebrum and not associated with the pituitary gland may cause similar clinical signs, especially unilateral blindness, circling, and depression. These cerebral abscesses are most often caused by *Corynebacterium pyogenes.*

Treatment

Successful therapy of pituitary and cerebral abscesses is unlikely once clinical signs are observed. Treatment with high levels of penicillin may be attempted.

MALIGNANT CATARRHAL FEVER

Malignant catarrhal fever (MCF) is believed to occur in 4 clinical forms in cattle: peracute, head and eye, intestinal, and mild. Neurologic signs may predominate in the commonly fatal head and eye form. In the United States, MCF primarily is a sporadic disease in cattle that have been in contact with lambing ewes or wildlife ruminants. Affected cattle have a severe necrotizing vasculitis with pronounced mononuclear infiltration of various tissues and organs along with lymphoid necrosis. The etiologic agent is thought to be bovine herpesvirus 3.

Clinical Signs

Most cattle with the head and eye form of MCF have an acute onset of high fever (40 to 42°C), depression, disorientation, mucopurulent nasal and ocular discharges, conjunctivitis, oral mucosal hyperemia and erosions, lymphadenopathy, and corneal opacity. Diarrhea or constipation and generalized skin lesions are seen sporadically. Usually, the CNS signs consist of severe depression, ataxia, and tremors. Most cattle with the head and eye form of MCF die within 1 to 7 days.

Diagnosis

Definitive diagnostic tests, such as virus isolation, are not readily available. However, a tentative diagnosis can be made based upon clinical signs, postmortem findings, and a history of previous exposure to sheep. Bluetongue virus and BVD virus can cause vascular lesions in cattle but can be differentiated from MCF by their milder vascular lesions, serologic test results, and virus isolation. The sporadic incidence of MCF resembles sporadic bovine encephalomyelitis (BUSS disease). BUSS, caused by a chlamydia agent, frequently occurs in animals younger (less than 6 months of age) than those with MCF and has a lower mortality. There are also no ocular or mucosal lesions with BUSS.

BOVINE HERPESVIRUS 1 ENCEPHALITIS

Encephalitis caused by bovine herpesvirus 1 (infectious bovine rhinotracheitis, IBR) appears sporadically in calves. The virus is thought to be a neurotropic strain of the IBR virus. It is most common in calves 4 to 7 months of age but may also be found in neonatal calves.

Clinical Signs

Calves with IBR encephalitis are usually depressed, blind, and anorectic. Convulsions and fever may be present at the onset of clinical signs. Many of the affected calves become comatose and die within 1 to 3 days after onset of clinical signs. Signs suggestive of severe respiratory disease or other organ system involvement are seldom present.

Diagnosis

A tentative diagnosis of any viral encephalitis in calves can be based upon the characteristic clinical findings of encephalitis and the presence of mononuclear pleocytosis in the spinal fluid. A definitive diagnosis of IBR encephalitis can be confirmed by the microscopic findings of nonpurulent meningoencephalitis, by the results of fluorescent antibody studies of the brain, by the presence of inclusion bodies, and by the isolation of bovine herpesvirus 1. The signs of encephalitis associated with heavy coccidial infections may be similar to the signs of IBR encephalitis, e.g., similar history, similar chemical signs, young calves affected, and a herd problem.

PSEUDORABIES (AUJESZKY'S DISEASE)

Pseudorabies, caused by a herpesvirus *(Herpesvirus suis),* primarily affects pigs and rarely cattle. Affected cattle have usually been in contact with pigs. There is no known contagion among cattle.

Often there is intense local pruritus in affected cattle, causing violent licking, chewing, and rubbing of the body. Itching may be present anywhere on the body, but it is most common about the head, flanks, and feet, and is generally unilateral. During this stage, cattle appear excited, with convulsions and constant bellowing. The great majority of cattle with pseudorabies die or are in the terminal stages within a day after onset of clinical signs. The temperature is usually elevated. Young calves with pseudorabies are more likely to have clinical signs of encephalitis and erosions of the oral cavity without pruritus.

Diagnosis

Pseudorabies should be considered in any cattle exhibiting neurologic signs that have been in contact with swine. If the affected animal is intensively pruritic, a tentative diagnosis of pseudorabies is reached easily. Microscopic examination of nerve trunk and spinal cord tissues in the areas of intense pruritus commonly reveals neuritis and myelitis. Cattle may die before the virus reaches the brain. A definitive diagnosis may be reached using virus isolation from edematous fluid of the local lesion or from nervous tissue. Intranuclear inclusion bodies are not consistently found in cattle with pseudorabies.

Supplemental Reading

Blood, D. C., Radostits, O., and Henderson, J. A.: Neonatal Infection. *In* Veterinary Medicine, 6th ed. London, Bailliere, Tindall, 95–107, 1983.
Burrows, G. E.: Disposition of selected antibiotics in experimental *Pasteurella* pneumonia of calves. Am. Vet. Med. Assoc. Conference, New York, 1983.
Carrillo, B. J., Popischil, A., and Dahme, E.: Pathology of a bovine viral necrotizing encephalitis in Argentina. Zbl. Vet. Med. *30*:161–168, 1983.
Cradle, R. A., Mesfin, G. M., and Mock, R. E.: Horizontal transmission of pseudorabies virus in cattle. Am. J. Vet. Res. *43*:326–328, 1982.
deLahunta, A.: Veterinary Neuroanatomy and Clinical Neurology, 2nd ed. Philadelphia, W. B. Saunders Company, 401–406, 1983.
Espersen, G.: A hypophysis—abscess syndrome in cattle. I. Clinical investigation. Nord. Vet. Med. 27:266, 1975.
Espersen, G., and Moller, T.: A hypophysis—abscess syndrome in cattle. III. Pathogenesis. Nord. Vet. Med. 27:627, 1975.
Mebus, C. A., Kafunda, M., and Ferris, D. H.: Malignant catarrhal fever. Bovine Pract *14*:130–132, 1979.
Petrov, M., and Anglov, A. K.: Symptoms and pathology of *Corynebacterium* infections in cattle. Nanke. *19*:30–40, 1982.
Stephens, L. R., Little, P. B., Wilkie, B. N., and Barnum, D. A.: Infectious thrombolic meningoencephalitis in cattle: a review. J. Am. Vet. Med. Assoc. *178*:378–384, 1981.
Wiseman, A., Allan, E., Selman, E. I., et al.: Encephalitis and infectious bovine rhinotracheitus. Vet. Rec. 151–152, 1981.

Toxic Encephalopathies in Cattle

JOHN A. SMITH, D.V.M., M.S.

AMMONIA (UREA) TOXICOSIS

Excessive consumption of urea or other nonprotein nitrogen (NPN) sources by unadapted ruminants may lead to ammonia toxicosis. Urea is the most common and most toxic of the NPN sources. Others are biuret, gelatinized starch-urea (Starea), urea phosphate, diammonium phosphate, ammonium polyphosphate solution, ammoniated rice hulls, ammoniated cottonseed meal, ammonium sulfate, and monoammonium phosphate. The amount that can be safely fed depends on a number of factors. A general rule of thumb is that NPN should not comprise more than one third of the total nitrogen in the ration. Toxicity is most likely to occur when there are errors in the mixing of NPN into rations, when NPN is offered to unadapted animals, when NPN is used in energy deficient rations (such as high roughage rations), or when animals are allowed free access to palatable liquid supplements. Ruminants quickly adapt to the feeding of NPN but also quickly lose this adaptation (in as little as 2 to 3 days). By gradual introduction of urea into the feed, ruminants can tolerate as much as 1 gm/kg/day. However, at such high levels, even a short period of anorexia may result in toxicosis when feeding is resumed due to loss of adaptation. High rumen pH, high body temperature, restricted water intake, and liver disease will all lessen the amount of NPN needed to produce toxicosis.

Ammonia toxicosis may also occur if animals are exposed to fertilizers with ammonium salts as the nitrogen source. Gross errors in the use of ammonium chloride to prevent urolithiasis in feedlot animals could also contribute to ammonia toxicosis.

Clinical Signs

Ammonia toxicosis is always acute. The onset is rapid, from 10 min to 4 hr after ingestion. Initial signs are colic manifested by grinding of the teeth, groaning, treading, kicking at the abdomen, and restlessness. Salivation, polyuria, muscle tremors, jugular pulsation, forced rapid respiration, and bloat are often evident. Terminally, signs of central nervous system (CNS) involvement become prominent and include weakness, staggering, and incoordination, which progress to violent struggling, bellowing, and tetanic spasms just prior to death.

Diagnosis

Diagnosis of ammonia toxicosis is based on a history of consumption of NPN followed shortly by the typical clinical signs. If possible, the NPN content of the feed should be determined, intake estimated, and calculations made to determine if a presumably toxic dose has been ingested. Confirmation of the diagnosis can be made by determination of ammonia levels in blood, serum, rumen fluid, or urine. Samples should be frozen immediately and kept frozen until analyzed, or preserved with saturated mercury chloride to stop autolysis and resulting ammonia production. Toxic levels are 80 mg/100 ml of rumen fluid or 2 mg/100 ml of blood or serum. Differential diagnoses for the typical combination of gastrointestinal and nervous signs might be toxic indigestion (grain overload), lead toxicosis, organomercury toxicosis, salt toxicosis–water deprivation, and organophosphate toxicosis.

Treatment

The source of toxicity should be removed. Further absorption may be inhibited by administration of large volumes of very cold water orally by stomach tube (4 to 8 L/100 kg). Oral acetic acid (5 to 6 per cent) or vinegar may be added to the water (1 to 2 L/100 kg). Supportive therapy is relief of bloat and administration of intravenous fluids to counteract shock, dehydration, and acidosis. Normal saline with added sodium bicarbonate would be a rational choice. There is no specific antidote.

LEAD

Lead is one of the most common causes of poisoning in cattle. Oral consumption is the major route of exposure. The sources of lead are many and varied. Although most modern paints are lead-free, cattle may have access to old, flaking paint on barns, fences, equipment, and so forth, which may contain up to 50 per cent lead, or to discarded buckets of lead-based paints. Other sources are machinery grease (up to 50 per cent lead), used motor oil (30 per cent of the tetraethyl lead in gasoline is deposited in the motor oil), discarded lead storage batteries, plumbing lead, window caulking material, linoleum, lead-lined tanks, roofing felt, cable coverings, and veterinary "white lotion" (lead acetate). Lead arsenate pesticides commonly poison cattle, but the gastrointestinal effects of the arsenic predominate. Motor vehicle pollution of forage is very unlikely to result in overt signs of poisoning but can contribute to the background level of body lead. Pastures near lead mines, smelters, or lead reclaiming operations may become significantly contaminated. Lead shot in the body becomes encapsulated and is unlikely to cause poisoning.

Lead is ubiquitous, and almost all animals will have a background level; the toxic dose is therefore the amount that will add to the background level, producing a toxic level in a given individual. A single dose of 50 to 400 mg/kg may kill a calf, as calves are more susceptible; 600 to 800 mg/kg will kill an adult. A daily intake of 6 to 7 mg/kg of lead appears to be the minimum dosage that will eventually cause death in cattle.

Clinical Signs

Regardless of whether the ingestion of lead has been chronic or acute, the onset of signs in cattle is relatively acute. Signs may appear from a few days to several weeks after ingestion of a single toxic dose. The most outstanding manifestations of lead toxicosis in cattle are the nervous signs. A smaller though still considerable percentage of cases will exhibit gastrointestinal signs, which may precede the nervous signs. Animals with cortical blindness (absence of menace response but intact pupillary responses) are common in lead ingestion cases; such animals are presented for examination because of wandering aimlessly and walking into objects. Other nervous signs are circling, pressing against objects, ataxia, rhythmic twitching of the ears and bobbing of the head, violent blinking of the eyelids, and muscle tremors. Periods of excitement, with bellowing, staggering, muscular spasms, tetany, and convulsions may occur periodically, and usually signal impending death within several hours. In some cases, only the convulsive phase may be seen, followed by rapid death, or animals may simply be found dead. Anorexia, constipation followed by diarrhea, colic, grinding of the teeth, rumen atony, salivation, and a tucked abdomen are gastrointestinal signs. The body temperature may be normal or markedly elevated. The course may range from several hours to 10 days.

Clinical Pathology and Necropsy Lesions

Liver enzyme and serum urea nitrogen levels may be elevated because of liver and kidney damage. The cerebrospinal fluid (CSF) pressure, protein level, and white blood cell count may also be mildly elevated. Anemia and

...g of erythrocytes seen in some species ... in cattle. Necropsy lesions are usually ...wing to the sudden nature of death.

Diagnosis

...gns and the demonstration of a probable ...ead ingestion are important in establishing a ...iagnosis. The diagnosis may be confirmed by ... blood, liver, renal cortex, feces, and stomach ... for lead. Blood should be collected in oxalate ...gulant; tissues may be fresh or in formalin. Urine ... too variable for use in helping to establish a ...osis. Background lead levels will vary with the ...lity but are generally in the range of 0.1 ppm for ...ood, 1 to 2 ppm for liver, kidney, and rumen contents, and 12 ppm for feces. Significant levels are 0.30 ppm in whole blood, 10 ppm (wet weight basis) in liver and kidney, and 35 ppm in feces. Kidney is probably preferable to liver, as confirmed cases of lead poisoning have been seen in which liver lead was less than 10 ppm. Fecal lead levels respond more quickly to decreases in intake of lead; therefore, a high level in blood or tissues with a low level in feces indicates exposure 1 to 3 weeks prior to sampling. Differential diagnoses for those cases with gastrointestinal and nervous signs would be similar to those for urea toxicosis. Differential diagnoses for cases with predominantly nervous signs are polioencephalomalacia, thromboembolic meningoencephalitis, listeriosis, nervous coccidiosis, vitamin A deficiency, rabies, tetanus, pseudorabies, nervous ketosis, hepatic encephalopathy, hypomagnesemia, organochloride toxicosis, strychnine toxicosis, toxic plant ingestion, brain abscesses, hemorrhage, and edema.

Treatment*

The toxic source must be removed from the animal's environment. Further absorption may be reduced by the repeated use of purgatives, such as sodium or magnesium sulfate at 0.5 to 3.0 gm/kg orally in water. Rumenotomy may be extremely beneficial, especially if lead ingestion has occurred recently. The specific treatment is calcium disodium edetate (CaEDTA.†) The recommended dose ranges from 75 mg/kg daily to 110 mg/kg twice daily, as a 1 to 2 per cent wt/vol solution in 5 per cent dextrose subcutaneously, intraperitoneally, or preferably by slow intravenous injection. In my experience, the higher dose rate is preferable. Further division of this total daily dose (i.e., 220 mg/kg/day in 3 or 4 doses) may be more beneficial but is often impractical. This treatment is given for 2 days, withheld for 2 days, and repeated for 2 more days. Several treatment series may be necessary. CaEDTA is a chelating agent that exchanges calcium for lead in blood, tissues, and bones. CaEDTA may also chelate other micronutrients, particularly zinc, and parakeratosis may result with prolonged therapy. Oral zinc supplementation (1 mg/kg/day) and provision of trace mineralized salt may therefore be indicated. Other supportive therapy may be necessary. Poisoned animals are usually anorectic, and force feeding is indicated. A gruel made by soaking alfalfa pellets can be given orally with a large tube and a bilge pump. Convulsions can be con-

*Most treatments are not approved.
†Available from Haver-Lockhart, Shawnee, KS 66201

trolled with intravenous pentobarbital up to 30 mg/kg to effect or chloral hydrate (50 to 70 mg/kg, as a 5 to 7 per cent intravenous solution), repeated as necessary. Dexamethasone (0.1 mg/kg intravenously) may be indicated for cerebral edema, usually as a once only dose. Daily thiamine (1 mg/kg intravenously or intramuscularly) and ascorbic acid (200 mg orally) have also been recommended.

MERCURY

Mercury toxicosis is no longer common in cattle. Most cases of poisoning in the past involved the accidental feeding of waste seed grains that had been treated with organomercurial fungicides. Inorganic and aryl (aromatic) mercury compounds, such as those used for medicinal purposes (calomel, Mercurochrome, thiomersal, phenylmercuric nitrate, and others) cause gastrointestinal and renal signs. Only the alkyl organic mercurials (methylmercury and ethylmercury compounds) cause neurologic disease. (See the section on Physical and Chemical Disorders for a further discussion of mercury toxicosis.)

WATER DEPRIVATION–SALT TOXICOSIS

Water deprivation–salt toxicosis is not as common in cattle as in swine but can occur under conditions in which the intake of sodium ions is high in relation to the intake of water. Such conditions may occur when cattle are fed a grain mix or protein supplement that contains excessive salt either as an error in mixing or as a means of limiting intake. There also have been instances of milk replacers that contained excessive salt. The amount of salt required to produce toxicosis depends on the amount of water available. Water restriction may occur in freezing weather, if the water source is too far from the feeding areas, if the water is distasteful due to pollution, medication, and so forth, or if automatic watering devices fail. Another possibility is the water may have a high salinity, as may occur in coastal areas or oil fields. Drinking water should contain less than 0.5 per cent total salts. The acute toxic dose of sodium chloride in the cow is 2.2 gm/kg. The pathogenesis of water deprivation–salt toxicosis is not firmly established. (See the section on Physical and Chemical Disorders for a further discussion of salt toxicosis.)

ORGANOCHLORINES

Organochlorine insecticides (chlorinated hydrocarbons) are relatively nontoxic to cattle if used properly. However, they are very persistent in both the body and the environment. Most cases of poisoning in cattle therefore result from either human error or cumulative poisoning. These compounds are supplied as sprays or powders for animal housing; as sprays, powders, or dips for use on animals; and as crop sprays. Simple physical contact with treated crops is unlikely to cause toxicosis, but spray drift onto animals or ingestion of treated plants may result in toxicosis. The relative toxicity varies widely among the numerous compounds. DDT, methoxychlor, Perthane, TDE, and Dilan are relatively less toxic, while chlordane, heptachlor, aldrin, dieldrin, lindane, and toxaphene are relatively more toxic. For specific data consult the supplemental readings at the end of this article.

Toxicity may be acute or chronic. The relative danger of chronic toxicity depends on the rate of removal from the fat, which also varies (see Clarke, Harvey, and Humphries). Fat animals are more resistant to acute toxicosis than thin ones, owing to their ability to sequester more of a toxic dose in the fat. Fasting may precipitate clinical signs in an animal with organochlorines stored in the fat. Calves are more susceptible than adults, and dairy calves appear more susceptible than other calves. The form in which the compound is taken also influences toxicity. Organochlorines are insoluble in water and soluble in fat. They are poorly absorbed from the gastrointestinal tract and are most rapidly absorbed from oily solutions. They can penetrate skin when applied as oily solutions or emulsions. Dieldrin is absorbed from the skin in the powder form. Once absorbed, organochlorines are stored to varying degrees in the body fat, with the exception of methoxychlor. They do not tend to accumulate in any other organ, including the brain. The route and rate of excretion varies with the compound. Some (DDT in particular) may be excreted in the milk.

The exact mechanism of toxicosis is not clear and probably varies with the compound. Generally, the toxins are diffuse central nervous system stimulants or depressants. Organochlorines may act by releasing hydrochloric acid, by interfering with enzyme processes, or, as in the case of DDT, by affecting nerve cell membrane potentials. Their site of action may be central or peripheral, or both. Most organochlorines, and particularly aldrin and dieldrin, have effects similar to those of organophosphates in that they also appear to stimulate the parasympathetic nervous system, probably by inhibition of cholinesterase.

Clinical Signs

The signs of acute and chronic toxicosis are similar. The onset of signs of acute toxicosis may be from a few minutes to a few days after exposure but averages 4 to 5 hr; delays of up to 2 weeks after a single dose have been reported. Chronic toxicosis signs take longer to appear. Progressive signs may be seen in chronic toxicosis in which full development of signs may take 2 to 5 days or more. Given the variety of compounds, there is no single, typical set of clinical signs, but a general pattern may appear as follows: changes in the animal's attitude, such as apprehension, hypersensitivity, or belligerence may be the first obvious abnormality. These changes are not usual in chronic toxicosis. Neuromuscular signs then appear, often in this order: (1) twitching of the eyelids, facial muscles, and cervical muscles, (2) clonic spasms of the cervical muscles, (3) clonic spasms of the forequarters, and, finally, (4) clonic spasms of the hindquarters. These spasms may be almost continuous, or may be repeated at regular or irregular intervals, and may be accompanied by salivating and chewing. Other neurologic signs are frenzy, incoordination, stumbling, aimless wandering, circling, jumping over imaginary objects, and abnormal posturing, such as resting on the sternum with the hind legs standing or keeping the head between the forelegs. These signs may progress to clonic-tonic convulsions, which may persist until death or may be regularly or irregularly interrupted by periods of depression, paddling, nystagmus, grinding of the teeth, and groaning. Convulsions sometimes begin explosively, with the animal either charging into an object and falling into a convulsion or rearing its head and backing and twisting in a circle before falling into a convulsion. With some organochlorines such as toxaphene, convulsions may be induced by external stimuli. Some animals will become comatose several hours prior to death. Although the foregoing signs of diffuse stimulation are typical, signs of depression, drowsiness, anorexia, and reluctance to move may predominate in some animals, leading to emaciation and dehydration. Some cases may also alternate between stimulation and depression. Patients with mild cases of poisoning might not exhibit tremors and convulsions but might walk with extended pasterns (on tiptoes) with short, choppy steps. Later they may appear to have laminitis, walking very gingerly on all 4 feet. The reflexes become slow, and the animals lose weight rapidly.

Necropsy Lesions

Findings at necropsy are generally nonspecific and can usually be related to agonal death. These are random hemorrhages, pulmonary congestion, hemorrhage and edema, and congestion and edema of the brain and spinal cord. Chronic exposure may cause fatty degeneration of the liver and kidneys.

Diagnosis

A tentative diagnosis of organochlorine toxicosis may be made on the basis of a history of probable exposure, an occurrence of neuromuscular signs, and a lack of definitive lesions at necropsy. The diagnosis may be confirmed by demonstration of excessive levels of organochlorines in the tissues, particularly the liver, kidney, stomach contents, hair, and brain. The mere presence of an insecticide in these tissues, and especially in the fat, does not confirm the diagnosis, since animals exposed to recommended levels may accumulate detectable amounts. Differential diagnoses would be similar to those of ammonia and lead toxicoses.

Treatment and Prevention

The source should be eliminated. If the exposure was oral, a saline cathartic such as sodium or magnesium sulfate (0.5 to 3.0 gm/kg orally) should be administered. Activated charcoal may be used as an adsorbent. A vegetable-origin charcoal (Norit,* Nuchar C,† or Darco G-60‡) should be given at 2 to 9 gm/kg, orally as a slurry of 1 gm charcoal/3 to 5 ml water. The charcoal should be given first, followed by the cathartic in 30 min. Mineral oil should be avoided. If the dermal route is involved, the animals should be washed with soap and water. Neuromuscular signs may be controlled by sedation or light anesthesia with chloral hydrate (50 to 70 mg/kg intravenously to effect) or pentobarbital (30 mg/kg intravenously to effect) repeated as needed. Phenobarbital (5 gm/head/day orally for 3 to 4 weeks, off 3 to 4 weeks, repeated for 3 to 4 weeks) stimulates the liver microsomal enzymes and may also increase the rate of detoxification. Calcium borogluconate (1 ml/kg of a 23 per cent solution subcu-

---

*Available from American Norit, Jacksonville, FL 32208
†Available from West Virginia Pulp and Paper, Richard, WV 23225
‡Available from Atlas Chemical, Wilmington, DE 19899
Note: Most treatments are not approved.

(anteriorly or slow intravenous injection) has also been recommended. If long-term barbiturate or chloral hydrate therapy is necessary, frequent intravenous infusions of saline or lactated Ringer's solution and 5 to 10 per cent dextrose may be indicated for maintenance and for avoidance of liver damage. Feeding of activated charcoal (0.9 kg/head/day) may adsorb some of the insecticide in the gut and help break the cycle, speeding elimination.

ORGANOPHOSPHATES AND CARBAMATES

The organophosphates are organic derivatives of phosphoric and diphosphoric acids, and the carbamates are organic derivatives of carbamic acid. These compounds are supplied as dusts and sprays for plants, granules for soil treatment, topical preparations for animals (dusts, sprays, dips, and pour-ons), and oral forms for animals (anthelmintics and systemic insecticides in liquid, granular, tablet, and paste forms). Exposure may occur by the oral, dermal, or respiratory routes. Cattle may consume treated plants or seed grains mixed with soil insecticides. Feed or water containers may be contaminated by prior use as insecticide containers. Crop sprays may drift onto animals or into feed, water, or feeding equipment. Improper use of external or oral organophosphates, such as simultaneous use of the 2 forms, may also result in toxicosis.

Organophosphates and carbamates vary widely in their toxicity to cattle and, in general, are more toxic than the organochlorines. The least toxic organophosphates have an order of toxicity similar to that of DDT. Cattle are less susceptible than cats but more susceptible than dogs, pigs, and horses. Zebu type breeds appear to be more susceptible, and young animals are more severely affected than adults. Sex differences are also noted, some compounds being more toxic in males and others in females. One of the most notable examples is the extreme sensitivity of mature bulls to chlorpyrifos (Dursban), with older and larger bulls being most sensitive. Some organophosphates may potentiate the toxicity of others, possibly by inhibiting the liver enzymes responsible for detoxification. Drug interactions with organophosphates are also common, most notably succinylcholine and phenothiazine-derivative tranquilizers. For specific toxicity data, consult the Supplemental Reading.

Organophosphates are readily absorbed by all routes. The solvent may affect the rate of dermal absorption. Organophosphates and carbamates inhibit the action of acetylcholinesterase and pseudocholinesterase. Acetylcholinesterase is an enzyme present at cholinergic nerve endings, myoneural junctions, and in erythrocytes. Pseudocholinesterase is present in the brain and plasma. These enzymes hydrolyze the neurotransmitter acetylcholine, thereby preventing extended action from a single nerve impulse. Organophosphates cause irreversible inactivation of cholinesterases by phosphorylation. Carbamic acid causes a reversible inactivation by carboxylation of cholinesterases. The result is a build-up of acetylcholine with overstimulation of the parasympathetic nervous system. Muscarinic, nicotinic, and central nervous system effects are clinically evident. Recovery is achieved by hydrolysis of the phosphorylated or carboxylated cholinesterase or by synthesis of new cholinesterase.

Clinical Signs

The clinical signs of organophosphate and carbamate toxicosis are similar. The onset of signs may vary from minutes to hours, and may be as long as 7 to 10 days. The muscarinic (parasympathetic) signs tend to occur first. These include salivation, lacrimation, coughing, nasal discharge, miosis, dyspnea, colic, diarrhea, and polyuria. The nicotinic signs are muscle fasciculation and a sawhorse stance, followed by weakness and paralysis. Central effects in cattle consist mainly of severe depression, but some may exhibit hyperactivity. These animals rarely convulse with organophosphate toxicosis. Death is usually due to the muscarinic effects of bronchoconstriction, respiratory hypersecretion, and slowed, erratic heartbeat, all causing hypoxia.

The systemic organophosphates such as coumaphos and nonsystemic pour-on organophosphates often cause a preponderance of gastrointestinal signs in adult cattle. The signs generally reflect gastrointestinal stasis and include ruminal atony, bloat, anorexia, diarrhea, and dehydration. Many commercial products contain organophosphates or carbamates in combination with organochlorines and may therefore produce a combination of signs. Coumaphos alone will produce signs similar to organophosphate toxicosis plus organochlorine toxicosis. Signs of delayed neurotoxicity may occur days to weeks after exposure to triorthocresyl phosphate, mipafox, leptophos, haloxon, and chlorpyrifos. The sign consists of posterior paresis with knuckling and ataxia, which may proceed to total paralysis of the rear limbs. The lesion is a "dying back" of the axons of long nerves, especially the sciatic nerve.

Necropsy Lesions

Necropsy findings are usually minimal and nonspecific. The effects of muscarinic stimulation may be evident, such as saliva and excessive fluid in the respiratory and gastrointestinal tracts.

Diagnosis

A history of possible exposure and characteristic parasympathomimetic signs suggests the diagnosis of organophosphate toxicosis or carbamate toxicosis. Analysis of tissues is usually unrewarding owing to rapid metabolism. Feed, stomach contents, or the suspected poison will generally yield better results. The most useful test for confirmation of the diagnosis is a blood or tissue cholinesterase activity assay. Depletion of cholinesterase activity in the blood does not cause clinical signs nor does it always correlate with the severity of signs; however, since the changes in the blood usually reflect those in the nervous tissue, and since blood is more easily obtained, the test is useful for diagnostic assistance. If brain tissue is available, it is superior to blood for accurate results. Most laboratories use the modified Michel method on whole blood, which measures the hydrolysis of acetylcholine.

Differential diagnoses for the typical combination of gastrointestinal and nervous disorders would be similar to those listed for urea toxicosis. Differential diagnoses for the delayed neurotoxicity syndrome should include peripheral nerve trauma (sciatic nerve) and spinal cord lesions, such as vertebral abscess, tumor, fracture, or aberrant *Hypoderma* larval migration.

phorylating the acetylcholinesterase as well as reacting
with the organophosphate. It should be given at 25 to 50
mg/kg, as a 20 per cent solution during a 6-min intravenous
injection or as a maximum of 100 mg/kg by intravenous
drip. This can be repeated as needed, usually twice a day.
Pralidoxime is not useful for carbamate toxicosis. Other
supportive therapy may include fluid administration and
multiple vitamins.

NITROFURANS

Nitrofurans are synthetic broad-spectrum antimicrobial
compounds that may be bacteriostatic or bacteriocidal,
depending on concentration. Their exact mechanism of
action is unknown, but they appear to inhibit several
oxidative enzymes. Nitrofurans are not approved for use
in cattle in the United States but are nevertheless occasionally used in the treatment of calves with diarrhea.
The most commonly used preparation is Nitrofurazone.
Toxicosis has been reported for oral doses as low as 3
mg/kg, which resulted in paralysis of the hind limbs in the
animal. Chronic toxicosis results at doses of 10 to 15 mg/
kg for 3 to 5 weeks, and acute toxicosis may result at 30
mg/kg, usually within 24 hr. The pathogenesis is unknown.

Clinical Signs

Chronic toxicosis is characterized by anorexia, hyperexcitability, and intermittent convulsions. The sign of
acute toxicosis is weakness that progresses to total paralysis and death within 5 days to 2 weeks. Acute tremors,
circling, and convulsions may also develop.

Clinical Pathology and Necropsy Lesions

Laboratory findings include pancytopenia, high plasma
pyruvate levels, and serum chemical changes suggestive
of hepatic or renal dysfunction. Necropsy findings are
nonspecific.

Diagnosis

The diagnosis must be based on a history of systemic
(usually oral) treatment with nitrofuran, followed by signs
of paralysis and central nervous system involvement.
Plasma nitrofuran levels have not been helpful for establishing the diagnosis. Differential diagnoses would consist
of enterotoxemia, enteric-toxemic colibacillosis, lead or
mercury ingestion, water deprivation, organophosphate

---

*Treatment not approved.

with oral nitrofurans.

RODENTICIDES

Rodenticide toxicosis in cattle is uncommon, probably
because of the usual packaging and use of these compounds in small quantities. Inadvertent incorporation of
large quantitites in a feed mix is a possible source of
toxicosis in cattle. Malicious poisoning is also an unfor-
tunate possibility. Strychnine, thallium, and zinc phosphide are 3 commonly used rodenticides that may produce
prominent neurologic signs in cattle. Of these, strychnine
produces the most profound nervous signs, while thallium
and zinc phosphide are general systemic toxicants. (These
compounds are discussed in the section on Physical and
Chemical Disorders.)

ANTITREMATODAL DRUGS

Two antitrematodal drugs, carbon tetrachloride and
hexachlorophene, may produce prominent neurologic
signs when misused. With the advent of safer antitrematodal drugs, cases of toxicosis caused by such drugs should
decline.

Carbon Tetrachloride

Carbon tetrachloride (CCl_4) is a volatile, colorless liquid
with an odor similar to that of chloroform. CCl_4 is given
orally or parenterally for elimination of flukes; the parenteral dose in cattle is 1 ml/9 kg. There appears to be a
wide variation in the toxic dose. As little as 5 ml has
caused fatal poisoning in 400 kg cattle. Low temperature
conditions, high fat or high protein diets, toxic plants
(clover, kale, crushed beet tops, lucerne, marigolds, he-
liotrope, stinkwort, and oxalate accumulators), chemicals
(phenobarbital, organochlorines), overconditioning, and
aspiration during drenching will all increase the toxicity
of CCl_4. CCl_4 is slowly absorbed from the gut. Being fat
solvent, it apparently alters the selective permeability of
membranes, allowing the escape from cells of essential
substances, such as coenzymes.

Clinical Signs

Poisoning is commonly acute. Signs may occur immediately, or they may be delayed for 2 to 3 days. Anorexia,

---

*Treatment not approved.

depression, drowsiness, staggering, incoordination, bloody feces, constipation followed by diarrhea, cardiovascular collapse, fibrillation, and death within 24 hr are observed.

Necropsy Lesions

Necropsy findings are gastroenteritis, fatty degeneration of the liver, and renal congestion. If death was sudden, liver and kidney lesions may be absent.

Diagnosis

Diagnosis is based on the history of exposure followed by signs of central nervous system and gastrointestinal disturbances. Differential diagnoses would be similar to those listed for ammonia toxicosis.

Treatment

Oral activated charcoal followed by a saline purgative should be administered as described for organochlorines. Intravenous calcium borogluconate (1 ml/kg of a 23 per cent solution intravenously or subcutaneously) and 5 to 10 per cent dextrose by continuous intravenous drip will help counteract hypocalcemia and hepatic and renal damage. B vitamins, especially nicotinic acid, are also indicated.

Hexachlorophene

Hexachlorophene is a phenol used as a disinfectant and soil and plant fungicide as well as an antitrematodal drug. Cattle may be overdosed with the drug, may consume treated plants or contaminated water, or may absorb hexachlorophene from udder disinfectants. Calves have been poisoned by the use of milk buckets that had earlier contained hexachlorophene. The acute oral LD_{50} in ruminants is 30 to 60 mg/kg. Hexachlorophene is rapidly absorbed from the skin and gut. It uncouples oxidative phosphorylation, inhibits a number of respiratory enzymes, and damages cell membranes.

Clinical Signs

Fever, depression or hyperexcitability, incoordination, muscle tremors, stiffness, tetanic spasms, convulsions, sudden respiratory failure, and death are characteristic signs.

Necropsy Lesions

Gross lesions are not remarkable. The most important lesions are microscopic status spongiosus and edema of the cerebral white matter.

Diagnosis

A history of exposure is essential for diagnosis. Feces, stomach contents, blood, or tissues may be submitted for analysis; any level of hexachlorophene is considered suspicious. Differential diagnoses with similar clinical signs and microscopic lesions are ammonia and lead toxicoses, viral encephalopathy and hepatic encephalopathy from aflatoxins or pyrrolizidine alkaloids.

Treatment

For oral poisonings, oral activated charcoal and saline cathartics should be administered as described previously for organochlorines. The animal with dermal exposure should be washed with soap and water. Cold water sprays and whirlpool can be used to control the fever. Antipyretics are not indicated. Pentobarbital (30 mg/kg intravenously to effect) should be used to attempt control of convulsions but is not always successful.* Volume diuresis with intravenous fluids (saline, lactated Ringer's solution) may help speed elimination. Intravenous urea as a 30 per cent solution in 10 per cent dextrose, given in a slow drip, has been used experimentally with success in cats at a total dose of 2 gm urea/kg. This treatment has not been tested in cattle.

NICOTINE

Nicotine sulfate has been used as an anthelmintic and as a horticultural spray. Cattle may be poisoned by ingesting a spilled solution, treated foliage, or food or water from contaminated containers. It is also readily absorbed through the skin. Approximately 1 gm of nicotine sulfate will poison young (12- to 18-month-old) cattle. Nicotine causes an initial stimulation followed by a depolarizing-type blockade of all nicotinic cholinergic receptors (i.e., acetylcholine receptors of motor end-plates, autonomic ganglia, and the central nervous system).

Clinical Signs

The signs consist of an initial parasympathetic stimulation, similar to organophosphate toxicosis, followed by depression and paralytic signs. They may appear within minutes of exposure and consist initially of excitement, rapid respiration, salivation, irritation of the mouth and pharynx, and diarrhea. Depression, incoordination, tachycardia, shallow and slow respiration, coma, flaccid paralysis, and death from respiratory paralysis follow. Death from a lethal dose usually is during or shortly after a severe clonic-tonic seizure. Cattle may succumb to latent effects hours after recovery from the paralytic effects. Recovery from sublethal doses usually is within 3 hr.

Necropsy Lesions

Findings at postmortem examination are unremarkable. Cyanosis, subcutaneous vessel engorgement, failure of the blood to clot, congestion of the gastrointestinal mucosa, and a distinct, pungent nicotine odor in the rumen (similar to an old smoking pipe) may be encountered.

Diagnosis

Diagnosis is made by a history of exposure, clinical signs, and nicotine odor. Organophosphate and carbamate toxicoses and certain plant toxicoses (yellow jessamine and spotted hemlock) produce similar signs.

Treatment

Treatment is usually unsuccessful. Oral tannic acid (5 to 25 gm in 2 to 4 L of water for an adult cow) or potassium permanganate (1:5000 solution as a gastric lavage) may aid in removal of unabsorbed nicotine sulfate.* Artificial respiration may keep the animal alive until the effects of the drug subside, but this is rarely practical in cattle.

---

*Treatment not approved.

Activated charcoal	Norit	No	1 gm/3–5 ml H_2O	Jacksonville, Florida 32208
	Nuchar C	No	Same as Norit	West Virginia Pulp and Paper Richard, West Virginia 23225
	Darco G–60	No	Same as Norit	Atlas Chemical Wilmington, Delaware 19899
Ammonium chloride	—	Yes	130 mg/kg po, sid	Various
Ascorbic acid	Vitamin C	Yes	200 mg po	Various
Atropine sulfate	—	Yes	For organophosphate toxicosis: 0.5 mg/kg, 1/4 IV, 3/4 SC or IM	Fort Dodge Laboratories 800 Fifth Street NW Fort Dodge, Iowa 50501 (and others)
Calcium borogluconate	Various	Yes	1 ml/kg of 23% solution IV or SC	Various
Calcium disodium edetate [CaEDTA]	Havidote	No	75–220 mg/kg SC or IV in 2 or more divided doses daily, 2 days on, 2 days off, 2 days on	Haver-Lockhart Laboratories Box 390 Shawnee, Kansas 66201
Chloral hydrate	Chloropent Injection	No	40–100 ml/100 kg to effect	Fort Dodge Laboratories 800 Fifth Street NW Fort Dodge, Iowa 50501
Dexamethasone	Azium	Yes	0.1 mg/kg IV	Schering Corp. Animal Health Division Kenilworth, NJ 07033
Dimercaprol	BAL in oil	No	3 mg/kg IM qid	Hynson, Westcott & Dunning Becton Dickenson Charles & Chase Streets Baltimore, Maryland 21201
Glyceryl guaiacolate	Guaifenesin	No	110 mg/kg IV	Summit Hill Laboratories Avalon, New Jersey 08202
Magnesium sulfate	Epsom salts	No	Cathartic 0.5–3.0 gm/kg po	Various
Mineral oil	—	No	8 ml/kg po	Various
Pentobarbital	—	No	Up to 30 mg/kg IV to effect	Fort Dodge Laboratories 800 Fifth Street NW Fort Dodge, Iowa 50501
Potassium permanganate	—	No	1:5000 solution for lavage	Various
Potassium Prussian Blue	—	No	100 mg/kg/day po	Various
Pralidoxime chloride	Protopam chloride	No	25–50 mg/kg IV as a 20% solution given over 6 min	Ayerst Labs American Home Products Co 685 Third Avenue, New York 10017
Selenium-tocopherol	BO–SE	Yes	5.0–7.0 ml/100 kg SC or IM	Burns-Biotec Laboratories Omaha, Nebraska 68103
Sodium sulfate	Glauber's Salts	No	Cathartic 0.5–3.0 gm/kg po	Various
Sodium thiosulfate	Scarlet Drench	Yes	30–40 mg/kg of sodium thiosulfate po	Haver-Lockhart Laboratories Box 390 Shawnee, Kansas 66201
Tannic acid	—	No	5–25 gm in 2–4 L H_2O po (cow)	Various
Thiamine	Vitamin B1	Yes	1 mg/kg IM or IV	Various
Zinc	—	No	1 mg/kg po, sid	Various

prominent, hyperesthesia, muscle spasms that tend to proceed from the rump to the head, stiff legs, ataxia, incoordination, and later, continuous tonic seizures with opisthotonus, paddling, and unconsciousness. Cattle may fall forward on their nose during typical uncontrolled activity. Animals may recover if the coma is not too deep but may succumb to liver failure several days later.

Necropsy Lesions

Postmortem findings are hepatic, renal, and pulmonary congestion; pulmonary edema and hemorrhage, gastrointestinal and cardiac hemorrhage, liver and brain cell degeneration, and a formaldehyde-like odor in the stomach.

Diagnosis

History of exposure and clinical signs, especially ascending spasms, and a formaldehyde-like odor in the stomach suggest the diagnosis of metaldehyde toxicosis. The stomach contents can be analyzed for acetaldehyde for confirmation. Differential diagnoses may consist of ammonia, lead, organomercurial, organochlorine, strychnine, and zinc phosphide toxicoses.

Treatment

Mineral oil (8 ml/kg orally) apparently slows absorption and can be used in conjunction with a saline cathartic (sodium or magnesium sulfate at 0.5 to 3.0 gm/kg orally).* Fever should be controlled with cold water rinses and enemas. Excitement and convulsions should be treated with pentobarbital (30 mg/kg intravenously to effect) unless the animal is already depressed. Fluid therapy is indicated for volume diuresis and acidosis. A 1.6 molar sodium lactate solution at 22 ml/kg given over 12 hr has been recommended for the dog.

Supplemental Reading

Buck, W. B., Osweiler, G. D., and VanGelder, G. A.: Clinical and Diagnostic Veterinary Toxicology, 2nd ed. Dubuque, Iowa, Kendall/Hunt Publishing Co., 1976.
Clarke, M. L., Harvey, D. G., and Humphreys, D. J.: Veterinary Toxicology, 2nd ed. London, Bailliere Tindall, 1981.
Hatch, R. C.: Veterinary Toxicology, sect. 17. In Booth, N. H., and McDonald, L. E. (eds.). Veterinary Pharmacology and Therapeutics, 5th ed. Ames, Iowa, The Iowa State University Press, 976–1021, 1982.

*Treatment not approved.

Cerebellar Disease in Cattle

MAURICE E. WHITE, D.V.M.

The cerebellum coordinates and regulates movement. The cerebellar nuclei facilitate brain stem neurons but are themselves regulated by inhibitory signals from Purkinje's cells in the cerebellar cortex, which receive information from several neuronal systems. Since the cerebellum does not initiate movement, loss of voluntary movement is not a clinical sign of uncomplicated cerebellar disease; there is instead a general lack of coordination of muscle groups. Ataxia with preservation of strength, spasticity, and a dysmetric, usually hypermetric gait, and often a loss of balance are present. Newborn calves with congenital cerebellar disease may be unable to stand, and adults with progressive disease may reach the point where they cannot stand without assistance. A head tremor that worsens when the animal reaches for food or water (intention tremor) is frequently present. Because the ocular muscles are among those coordinated by cerebellar nuclei there is sometimes nystagmus. With severe disease, opisthotonus may occur. Affected animals often appear to be anxious, wide-eyed, and hyperexcitable. A unique finding in some animals with cerebellar disease is a reduction or absence of the menace (blink) response despite normal vision and facial muscle strength. Before careful examination, this may give the observer the impression that the animal is blind. Almost all cerebellar disease in cattle is bilateral, but in the occasional case with unilateral disease, signs are usually ipsilateral to the lesion. To summarize, the presence of ataxia, spasticity, and dysmetria in a strong, bright, and alert animal, often associated with tremor, nystagmus, and a decreased menace response in a sighted animal, should suggest cerebellar disease.

This article will discuss diseases that cause primary cerebellar signs, or diseases in which cerebellar signs are a prominent part. Diseases are divided into 3 categories: (1) disease in which signs are present at or near birth, (2) late onset disease, and (3) generalized neurologic disease with a major cerebellar component.

CONGENITAL CEREBELLAR DISEASE

Bovine Virus Diarrhea (BVD) Induced Cerebellar Degeneration with Hypoplasia

The most common cerebellar disease in North American cattle is probably congenital cerebellar degeneration due to infection with BVD between days 100 and 200 of gestation. Affected calves show signs of cerebellar disease from birth that are occasionally associated with ocular lesions, such as cataracts, retinal inflammations, and retinal hemorrhages. At necropsy, there are uniform reductions in cerebellar size and multiple histologic lesions, including cavitation of white matter, disorganization of cortical structure, dysmyelination, and other changes. Several affected calves are sometimes born over a short time span, reflecting exposure to BVD at similar times during the spread of the agent through the herd. The owner often does not recall any signs of BVD in adult cattle during the time when the fetuses were exposed. Diagnosis is usually made on the gross and histologic changes found in affected calves. Evidence of a titer of BVD in precolostral serum would help confirm the diagnosis but is difficult to obtain under routine management conditions. Although there is no treatment, mildly affected calves often learn to compensate for the disorder.

Sporadic Congenital Cerebellar Ataxia with Hypomyelinogenesis

Cerebellar disease associated with hypomyelinogenesis of the cerebellum, brain stem, and spinal cord, and degeneration of Purkinje's cells and other neurons has been reported in several breeds, including Jersey, Shorthorn, Hereford, Angus, Angus-Shorthorn, and Sofia Brown. Severe whole body tremor and dysmetric ataxia may be present at birth or may begin at 2 to 3 weeks of age. Most cases are suspected to be due to autosomal recessive transmission. Diagnosis is by histologic examination and by exclusion of BVD-induced disease.

Several calves sired by an Ayrshire bull in an artificial insemination unit in Great Britain were ataxic at birth. One of the 6 cases had cerebellar hypoplasia at necropsy. This is probably because of an autosomal recessive gene.

Absence of the Cerebellar Vermis

Sporadic cases involving the absence of the caudal portion or entire cerebellar vermis have been seen in cattle, sometimes associated with hydrocephalus. The cause is unknown.

Multiple Central Nervous System Malformation

Cerebellar degeneration is occasionally seen in association with other central nervous system malformations such as hydranencephaly, in which signs of cerebellar disease are part of a syndrome of multiple neurologic defects. Akabane virus and bluetongue virus can cause this syndrome, and idiopathic outbreaks have also been reported. Diagnosis is by evidence of viral infection, and confirmation may require necropsy.

Neurofilamentous Degeneration of Horned Hereford Calves

A syndrome in horned Hereford calves was recently described that was characterized by the birth of 6 calves, in a 180-cow herd, that were unable to rise at birth and had fine tremors, most prominent in the hind limbs and neck. Stimulation of these calves led to worsening of signs, and progressive muscle weakness developed after stimulation and movement. Weakness is not seen in uncomplicated cerebellar disease and, although the initial signs resemble those of cerebellar disease, this finding should aid in diagnosis in the field. At necropsy, there was histologic evidence of neurofilamentous neuronal degeneration of multiple cell groups in the central nervous system and ganglion cells within the peripheral and autonomic nervous system. A recessive mode of inheritance is suspected.

Arnold-Chiari Malformation

The Arnold-Chiari malformation consists of herniation of caudal cerebellar tissue through the foramen magnum with displacement and elongation of the caudal brain stem. This malformation is usually associated with other severe neurologic malformations, such as hydrocephalus and spina bifida, but can occur alone. While this may be found on necropsy, it has not been directly associated with clinical signs of cerebellar disease in cattle.

since 1979. There is no treatment.

Hereditary Congenital Ataxia in Holstein Calves

A syndrome of progressive cerebellar disease was reported in 6 female and 2 male Holstein calves from 2 related herds. Calves with the syndrome were traced to a single ancestor, and the problem ceased when bulls related to the suspected carrier were removed from the herd. Signs developed at 5 to 6 weeks of age and progressed until the calves were destroyed. At necropsy, there was degeneration of Purkinje's cells and mild neuronal degeneration in other areas of the brain, but the syndrome differed from the abiotrophy described earlier because there was a reduction in the size of the brain associated with distortion of the cranial cavity and small convolutions of the cerebellum. No further reports of this condition have appeared in the veterinary literature.

Solanum Poisoning

Some plants of the Solanaceae family, including *Solanum dimidiatum* in the United States, *S. fastigiatum* and *S. bonariensis* in South America, and *S. kwabense* in Africa cause a syndrome of cerebellar degeneration when they are ingested in large quantities by cattle. Such animals show signs of severe cerebellar disese, which are precipitated by excitement. Animals may appear normal when left to quietly graze, but signs develop rapidly when they are disturbed, and the sudden development of ataxia, opisthotonus, tremor, and nystagmus can cause the animal to fall into what appears to be a seizure. At necropsy, there is vacuolization, degeneration and loss of Purkinje's cells, with axonal spheroids in the cerebellar granular layer and white matter in some cases. The disease has been reproduced with prolonged feeding of toxic plants. Morbidity and mortality can be high, with cattle dying because of loss of body condition or accidents secondary to severe ataxia and falling. Recovery seems to be rare, even when animals are removed from pasture containing these plants, but some compensation occurs.

Familial Convulsions and Ataxia

Familial convulsions and ataxia syndrome is a disorder of purebred and crossbred Angus cattle, which may be inherited as a dominant trait. Newborn and young calves develop intermittent seizures, with calves surviving the seizures developing signs of cerebellar disease, such as ataxia and dysmetria, over a 2- to 3-month period. If the animals survive until 15 months of age seizures decrease, and most animals are normal at 2 years of age. There is histologic evidence of degeneration of the cell bodies and axons of Purkinje's cells. Diagnosis is made by history and histologic results. No treatment has been described. A similar disease has been reported in a Charolais calf.

Cerebellar Neoplasia

Neoplasms of the cerebellum are rare in cattle but have been reported. The most frequently described cerebellar tumor is the medulloblastoma, which has been found in calves between 1 and 9 months of age and has been reported in a pair of twins. With signs of progressive asymmetric cerebellar disease developing at such a young age, it is probable that development of the tumor starts in utero. Confirmation is made at necropsy.

Parasitic Infections

Coenurosis

Invasion of the cerebellum by the intermediate stage of *Taenia multiceps* may produce signs of progressive cerebellar disease.

Hypoderma bovis

Injury due to larvae of parasites such as *Hypoderma bovis* causing unilateral cerebellar disease has been described but is rare.

Cerebellar Trauma

Cerebellar trauma without accompanying signs of involvement of other parts of the brain is rare in cattle. The onset of signs in trauma is sudden, and there may be external signs of injury or blood in the cerebrospinal fluid. Animals may learn to compensate following cerebellar injury.

Cerebellar Abscess

Abscess of the cerebellum without generalized meningoencephalitis is rare in cattle. Signs of progressive cerebellar disease would resemble those of cerebellar neoplasia. Confirmation is made at necropsy.

GENERALIZED NEUROLOGIC DISEASE WITH A PROMINENT CEREBELLAR COMPONENT

Polioencephalomalacia

Thiamine-responsive polioencephalomalacia is one of the most common ruminant neurologic disorders. The lesions in this disease are widespread, and the cerebellum is affected along with the cerebral tissue. Signs of cerebellar involvement, such as ataxia, dysmetria, and tremor, may be present along with signs of cerebral involvement, which predominate. Response to thiamine treatment is pathognomonic.

Paspalum Staggers

Grasses of the genus *Paspalum,* including *P. dilatatum* (dallis grass), *P. notatum* (Argentine bahia grass), and *P. distichum* (water couch) may be parasitized by the ergot *Claviceps paspali.* Cattle eating infected grasses can develop cerebellar disease, including tremor, ataxia, and dysmetria. In the early stages of poisoning, signs may be mild but become worse when the animal is excited, with the animal falling into what appears to be a seizure, followed by recovery when the animal is left alone.

Diagnosis rests on finding signs in cattle grazing grasses infected with the ergot, and treatment consists of removing them from the infected pasture.

Canary Grass and Ryegrass Staggers

Phalaris species of grasses, such as Toowoomba canary grass (*P. tuberosa*) and pissing *P. minor* and *P. arundinacea* of ryegrass (*Lolium perenne*), can cause a syndrome of tremor and ataxia. *Phalaris* poisoning is found in Australia, New Zealand, and South Africa, while *Lolium perenne* poisoning is found primarily in New Zealand but is also found in Australia and Great Britain. Diagnosis is based on dietary history, and treatment consists of removing animals from pastures with poisonous plants.

Storage Disease

GM$_1$ gangliosidosis in Friesians, mannosidosis in Angus and Murray Grey, and glycogenosis in Brahman are storage diseases in cattle in which intraneuronal lesions develop because of enzyme deficiencies. Signs such as ataxia and tremor may be seen early in these conditions, but all progress to include more diffuse signs of central nervous system involvement, such as seizures or blindness. Diagnosis is made by enzymatic studies, and confirmation is at necropsy.

Bilateral Peripheral Vestibular Disease

Middle and inner ear infections cause some of the most common neurologic disorders seen by practitioners. In one study, 1 in every 5 weaned calves in a feedlot had evidence of otitis media. Damage to the peripheral vestibular receptors in the ear leads to signs of ataxia with preservation of strength. Facial weakness due to facial nerve impairment and head tilt are also present in most cases. When both ears are affected, the clinical signs resemble those of cerebellar disease. Animals develop wide head excursions that look like a tremor, but there is no spasticity and no dysmetria. The inability to blink, which develops owing to facial weakness, can be mistaken for the loss of menace response occurring with cerebellar disease. *Pasteurella multocida* and *Corynebacterium pyogenes* are commonly isolated from patients with otitis media, and treatment with antibiotics is usually effective.

Supplemental Reading

Barlow, R. M.: Morphogenesis of cerebellar lesions in bovine familial convulsions and ataxia. Vet. Pathol. *18*:151–162, 1981.

Blood, D. C., Radostits, O. M., and Henderson, J. A.: Veterinary Medicine, 6th ed. London, Bailliere Tindall, 1983.

Cho, D. Y. and Leipold, H. W.: Arnold-Chiari malformation and associated anomalies in calves. Acta Neuropath. (Berl.) *39*:129–133, 1977.

Cho, D. Y. and Leipold, H. W.: Congenital defects of the bovine central nervous system. Vet. Bull. *47*:489–504, 1977.

Cyswski, S. J.: *Paspalum* staggers and tremorgen intoxication in animals J. Am. Vet. Med. Assoc. *163*:1291–1292, 1973.

deLahunta, A.: Veterinary Neuroanatomy and Clinical Neurology, 2nd ed. Philadelphia, W. B. Saunders Company, 1983.

Donnelly, W. J. C. and Sheahan, B. J.: GM$_1$ gangliosidosis of Friesian calves. Irish Vet. J. *35*:45–55, 1981.

Jensen, R., Maki, L. R., Laverman, L. H., et al.: Cause and pathogenesis of middle ear infection in young feedlot cattle. J. Am. Vet. Med. Assoc. *182*:967–972, 1983.

Johnson, K. R., Fourt, D. L., and Ross, R. H.: Hereditary congenital ataxia in Holstein-Friesian calves. J. Dairy Sci. *41*:1371–1375, 1958.

Leipold, H. W., Smith, J. E., Jolly, R. D., et al.: Mannosidosis of Angus calves. J. Am. Vet. Med. Assoc. *175*:457–459, 1979.

caused by bovine viral diarrhea virus. J. Am. Vet. Med. Assoc. *183*:544–547, 1983.

Metabolic Diseases that Cause Neurologic Syndromes

RAYMOND W. SWEENEY, V.M.D.

Many metabolic diseases of cattle cause neurologic syndromes. These are hypomagnesemia, hypoglycemia, nervous ketosis, vitamin A deficiency, hypocalcemia, hepatoencephalopathy, and renal failure. Polioencephalomalacia and salt toxicity are discussed elsewhere in this volume.

HYPOMAGNESEMIA

Hypomagnesemic tetany (lactation tetany, grass tetany, milk tetany) can affect all ruminants but is most common in lactating cattle. Occasionally, 2- to 4-month-old calves on a milk only diet will develop this syndrome. Hypomagnesemia is often associated with hypocalcemia.

The pathogenesis of hypomagnesemia is generally thought to be due to insufficient dietary intake of magnesium, such as in animals grazing lush grass pastures or cereal grain pastures, or in 2- to 4-month-old milk-fed calves. Lush grass pastures, especially those that have been heavily fertilized, have been shown to have lower magnesium contents than mature pastures. Heavy fertilization with nitrogen- and potassium-containing substances is thought to reduce the availability of soil magnesium to plants. High potassium levels in the diet may reduce the absorption of magnesium from the gastrointestinal tract. In addition to dietary effects, other factors involving stress, such as transit and cold exposure, may precipitate the disease.

The decreased plasma levels of magnesium are thought to enhance neuromuscular conduction, increasing the excitability of the muscle cells, accounting for uncontrolled muscle contractions and tetany. Early signs of the disease are muscle twitching and hyperesthesia, excitability, belligerence, and frequent urination and defecation. A staggering gait develops, progressing to recumbency, opisthotonus, and convulsions. Death will occur if the disease is left untreated

magnesium-containing solutions, often with calcium added. Among the recommended treatments are 25 per cent calcium borogluconate + 5 per cent $MgCl_2$ at 1 ml/kg* and 20 per cent $MgSO_4$ at 0.5 ml/kg. Care should be taken when administering these solutions that heart and respiratory rates remain regular. Excessive magnesium levels can cause medullary depression with respiratory arrest as well as cardiac irregularities. The therapeutic effect of the parenteral magnesium treatment is temporary, and dietary supplementation should be started.

Dietary supplementation can be achieved by adding 60 gm to 120 gm of MgO/head/day to the concentrate. In grazing operations the provision of hardened molasses-magnesium lick or a trace mineral salt containing magnesium will accomplish this.

HYPOGLYCEMIA

Hypoglycemia is most common in neonates less than 4 weeks old and is usually the result of inadequate carbohydrate feeding. This can be caused by lack of appetite secondary to another disease, reduced availability of milk (underfeeding or less production by the dam), or feeding with a poor quality or improperly prepared milk replacer. Low environmental temperatures compound the problem in 2 ways. Neonates exposed to cold ambient temperatures have higher energy requirements for thermoregulation and rapidly become hypothermic when deprived of milk. In addition, the digestibility of certain feedstuffs in cold-exposed animals may be reduced, exacerbating hypoglycemia. Finally, concurrent diseases may also increase metabolic energy requirements. A typical case history might involve diarrhea in a cold-exposed neonate. Frequently, the young animal has been treated with commercial oral electrolyte solutions and deprived of milk for several days. These solutions do not provide adequate energy and, after 2 to 3 days, the neonate becomes malnourished, debilitated, perhaps hypothermic, and hypoglycemic.

Clinical signs are severe depression, coma and, on rare occasions, seizures. Bradycardia, if present, is helpful in differentiating primary hypoglycemia from the coma of shock or septicemia (which is usually present with tachycardia). Treatment consists of immediate administration of 0.5 to 1 ml/kg of 50 per cent dextrose solution.

---

*Available from Bio-Ceutic Laboratories, St. Joseph, MO 64502 as Forcal or from Med Tech, Inc., Elwood, KS 66024 as Cal-Phos no. 2, among others.

However, several hours after a single intravenous glucose bolus severe hypoglycemia may again occur owing to the "rebound effect" caused by high insulin release. This may be prevented by following the initial bolus with slow intravenous administration of glucose (5 per cent dextrose in water, 1 to 2 ml/kg/hr) and oral carbohydrate (milk). Adjunct therapy should consist of gradual warming of hypothermic calves and of gradual reintroduction of milk to the diet (even if diarrhea persists). Healthy neonates may require 1½ to 1½ per cent of body weight per day of milk in cold weather.

NERVOUS KETOSIS

Ketosis (acetonemia) may result from the negative energy balance that is present when a cow's intake does not meet production requirements ("underfeeding ketosis") or when a relative imbalance of lipogenic to glucogenic nutrients in the diet ("spontaneous ketosis") is present. Underfeeding ketosis may result when the cow is not offered sufficient quantities of acceptable feed, or when her appetite is reduced secondary to a concurrent disease (e.g., displaced abomasum). It has also been shown that peak levels of milk production precede peak feed intake levels in post-parturient cows. While peak milk production occurs by 4 to 6 weeks postpartum, peak feed intake may not occur until 6 to 8 weeks postpartum. This leads to a relative energy deficiency in high-producing dairy cattle. Regardless of the cause, body fat is mobilized as an energy source, and hepatic ketogenesis develops.

Clinical signs are reduced appetite and milk production and, if present, localizing signs referable to the primary disease process. Neurologic signs range from depression and apathy to delirium, propulsive activity, hyperesthesia, blindness, and staggering. Cows frequently chew on inanimate objects or on themselves, resulting in self-mutilation. Ketonuria or ketolactia, or both, are frequently present and may be confirmed by a positive nitroprusside reaction (Acetest*). The pathophysiology of the neurologic signs in nervous ketosis is not known but is thought to be in part related to hypoglycemia. The nervous form of ketosis seems to have a higher incidence during the summer.

Nervous signs may be temporarily relieved by intravenous administration of chloral hydrate, 20 to 40 mg/kg. Treatment of ketosis is aimed at providing glucose or glucose precursors to the cow in the form of intravenous glucose (50 per cent solution 1 ml/kg) or oral glycerine or propylene glycol (0.25 to 0.50 mg/kg, twice daily). The majority of cows with nervous signs due to ketosis will respond to chloral hydrate and intravenous glucose therapy. Oral propylene glycol should be continued for several days to prevent recurrence of neurologic deficits. In addition, if the cow is inappetent, force feeding of alfalfa meal gruel or donor cow rumen contents, or both, may become necessary. Corticosteroids (dexamethasone, 0.02 mg/kg intramuscularly or intravenously once daily) are recommended for several days, as they will increase gluconeogenesis and improve the availability of glucose. Corticosteroids are contraindicated if bacterial infection is present. Finally, regular insulin (0.2 to 0.3 units/kg

---

*Available from Ames Company, Division of Miles Laboratories, Inc., Elkhart, IN 46514

subcutaneously once daily) may aid in reducing ketogenesis by preventing peripheral lipolysis and may be given in conjunction with glucose.

VITAMIN A DEFICIENCY

Hypovitaminosis A, caused by a dietary deficiency of that fat soluble vitamin, can cause neurologic signs in cattle. Animals on poor quality pasture or housed animals fed insufficient quantities of poor quality forage without vitamin A supplementation are susceptible. It is most frequent in beef calves 6 to 8 months old after feeding on dry pastures.

Most green plants contain large quantities of beta carotene, which is cleaved in the intestinal mucosa and liver to form vitamin A (retinal). Retinal is a component of the visual pigment (rhodopsin) necessary for dim light vision, and one of the early signs of vitamin A deficiency is night blindness.

Vitamin A is also essential for normal bone growth and for maintenance of normal epithelial tissues. In adult animals, neurologic signs are due to increased cerebrospinal fluid (CSF) pressure, which results from the decreased permeability to CSF of the epithelial cells of the arachnoid villi. In growing animals, hypovitaminosis A also causes abnormal skull bone growth, dural fibrosis with secondary overcrowding of the cranial cavity, and greater CSF pressure. Compression of the cerebellum, brain stem, spinal cord, optic nerves, and peripheral nerve roots can occur.

The changes described cause the characteristic clinical signs of blindness and papilledema. Syncope and convulsions are occasionally seen. Weakness, ataxia, and paresis may result from spinal cord and peripheral nerve compression but are uncommon.

Diagnosis may be confirmed by the determination of plasma vitamin A levels (abnormal is less than 10 μgm/100 ml). Elevated CSF pressure is also pathognomonic. Normal CSF pressure is less than 100 mm of water, and vitamin A deficient calves may have CSF pressures greater than 200 mm H_2O. Postmortem confirmation is based on the determination of vitamin A levels in frozen hepatic tissue and histologic examination of the formalin-fixed parotid salivary gland.

Clinically affected animals should be treated parenterally with an aqueous vitamin A preparation (400 units/kg). It is recommended that vitamin A be added to the diet of normal animals at a rate of 40 units/kg.

MISCELLANEOUS METABOLIC CAUSES OF NERVOUS DISEASES IN CATTLE

Hepatoencephalopathy must be considered in cattle showing bizarre behavior, central blindness, head pressing behavior, or severe mental depression. It may be observed occasionally in cows with fatty liver syndrome. It is more common secondary to acute hepatic necrosis (e.g., chemical intoxication) or chronic liver disease (e.g., pyrrolizidine alkaloid ingestion). Diagnosis is based on clinical signs in combination with laboratory evidence of liver disease. Prolonged sulfobromophthalein (BSP) excretion half life (>5 min) is common. Elevated serum levels of liver enzymes may be present in acute hepatic necrosis

and sluggish pupillary responses. Signs usually resolve after treatment with solutions containing calcium (23 per cent intravenous calcium borogluconate, 1 ml/kg).

Acute renal failure and azotemia may appear as a result of a toxic insult (mercury, arsenic, aminoglycoside antibiotic) or as a result of renal ischemia following hypovolemic shock. Severe cerebral depression or coma are the chief neurologic signs. These signs may be due to changes in plasma concentrations of phosphorus, magnesium, and calcium as well as the accumulation of urea and other metabolic by-products normally cleared by the kidneys.

Supplemental Reading

Baird, G. D.: Primary ketosis in high-producing dairy cows: clinical and subclinical disorders, treatment, prevention outlook. J. Dairy Sci. 65:1–10, 1982.
McMurray, C. H., Rice, D. A., O'Neill, D. G., Chestnut, M., and McGaughey, J.: Hardened calcined magnesite-molasses block for preventing hypomagnesemia in beef cows. Vet. Rec. 109:471–472, 1981.
Whitaker, D. A., and Kelly, J. M.: Incidence of clinical and subclinical hypomagnesemia in dairy cows. Vet. Rec. 110:450–451, 1982.
Williams, P. E. V., and Innes, G. M.: Effects of cold exposure on the digestion of milk replacer by young calves. Res. Vet. Sci., 32:383–386, 1982.

Polioencephalomalacia in Ruminants

STEPHEN G. DILL, D.V.M.

Polioencephalomalacia (PEM), also commonly referred to as cerebrocortical necrosis, is characterized by cerebral edema and necrosis of the gray matter of the brain. PEM occurs in young cattle, sheep, goats, antelope, and deer that are between 2 months and 2 years of age. The disease has a worldwide distribution, and it can appear sporadically or as a herd problem. PEM is due to a reduced availability of biochemically active thiamine (vitamin B_1) to the cells of the body. Thiamine is necessary to the biosynthesis of certain enzymes, especially various ones involved in carbohydrate metabolism. Neurons are dependent upon carbohydrate metabolism as an energy source. Significant inhibition of carbohydrate metabolism can result in neuronal dysfunction and death.

The decreased availability of thiamine can take place in a number of ways. Thiamine is normally produced by rumen microflora and, therefore, is not usually required in the diet of ruminants with normal rumen function. PEM has been reproduced by feeding 1-week-old lambs prevent coccidia infections in ruminants. It is a structural analogue of thiamine and has been used experimentally to reproduce signs of PEM in sheep. Experimental reproduction was successful with the oral administration of amprolium at dosages of 880 mg/kg for 4 to 6 weeks and at 1 gm/kg for 3 to 5 weeks. This dosage is 17 to 20 times the recommended dosage of 50 mg/kg for 21 days. Amprolium-induced PEM lambs also had cessation of erythrocyte production in the bone marrow. Anemia following recovery from PEM has not been reported in field cases. Herd outbreaks of PEM in the field and experimental reproduction of PEM have occurred in cattle fed a predominantly molasses and urea diet. It has been commonly observed that there is a greater incidence of PEM in ruminants on a high concentrate, low fiber diet. Significantly increased fecal thiaminase levels have been measured in sheep on a similar diet. Diets high in sulfate or low in cobalt may also cause the incidence of PEM.

CLINICAL SIGNS

Anorexia and depression are the first clinical signs displayed. These rapidly progress to ataxia, blindness, and, frequently, to dorsomedial strabismus (medial aspect of the pupil rotates dorsally). Such signs may be followed by an inability to rise, coma, and death. Nystagmus, muscle tremors, head pressing behavior, and opisthotonus are common. Blindness is typical of diffuse cortical disease in that vision is lost, but pupillary light responses are normal. The period of time from onset of signs to death may vary from 2 to several days. A presumptive diagnosis should be made on the basis of history and physical examination findings to facilitate early institution of therapy.

CLINICAL PATHOLOGY

In acute cases, the cerebrospinal fluid (CSF) usually contains normal (<40 mg/100 ml) to mildly elevated protein levels and normal (<5 WBC/mm^3) numbers of cells. In chronic cases, mild to moderate elevations in protein concentration and white blood cell count may occur owing to cerebrocortical necrosis. Thiamine diphosphate is necessary for the formation of the enzyme transketolase. Blood transketolase activity declines before the onset of clinical signs and remains low until after treatment. Fecal thiaminase levels are frequently elevated in affected ruminants. Blood pyruvate and lactate levels may be elevated, but these changes are less reliable than the decrease in transketolase activity or the increase in focal thiaminase activity.

NECROPSY

When present, gross postmortem changes are swelling and edema of the cerebrum with thickened and occasionally flattened gyri. Congestion of cerebral meningeal vessels may be present. The gray matter of the cerebral cortex, especially the occipital lobes, may have focal or laminar areas of necrosis. Microscopic changes also are found primarily in the gray matter and consist of neuronal necrosis, gliosis, neurophagia, and pericellular edema. The thalamus, cerebellum, and brain stem may at times be affected histologically.

DIFFERENTIAL DIAGNOSIS

The differential diagnosis of ruminants with the signs previously described include heavy metal toxicity (especially lead), a space occupying mass, such as an abscess or neoplasm, hepatic encephalopathy, nervous ketosis, *Clostridium perfringens* type D enterotoxemia, parasite migration, or inflammatory disease. The signs of lead toxicity may be indistinguishable from those of PEM unless dorsomedial strabismus is detected, which would be more indicative of PEM. A history of lead exposure and blood or urine samples tested for lead concentration may be necessary to differentiate these 2 diseases. The signs of ruminants with hepatic encephalopathy are very similar to those of ruminants with PEM. Ruminants with hepatic encephalopathy may be maniacal or depressed. Icterus may be present. Gamma glutamyl transpeptidase, succinate dehydrogenase, serum glutamic oxaloacetic transaminase, alkaline phosphatase, and bilirubin values should be elevated. Nervous ketosis can cause excitable behavior or depression and appears early in lactation or late in pregnancy. Blood glucose levels are usually reduced in cattle with nervous ketosis. Ketones are present in the plasma and urine. *C. perfringens* type D (overeating disease) can result in focal cerebral necrosis. Occurrence is more common in ruminants on a high concentrate diet or in those receiving a high volume milk diet. Signs may include pyrexia and diarrhea.

Parasitic migration occurs more commonly in the spinal cord but also appears in the brain. *Parelaphostrongylus tenuis* migration is found in goats and sheep, and *Hypoderma bovis* is found in cattle. Parasitic migration is more likely to cause focal asymmetrical signs than diffuse symmetrical signs. CSF in these cases may have eosinophils. Bacterial meningitis is associated with pyrexia, hyperesthesia, normal vision, and a dramatic rise in protein level and neutrophils in the CSF. Cattle are affected with thromboembolic meningoencephalitis secondary to *Haemophilus somnus* septicemia, which can be differentiated from PEM in a fashion similar to meningitis. Listeriosis causes unilateral brain stem signs with no visual deficit. Acute viral encephalitides include rabies in all species, malignant catarrhal fever (MCF) in cattle, and arthritis encephalitis in goats. Animals with rabies can be depressed or excitable; they generally are visual. Cattle with MCF are febrile and have other lesions of MCF, such as keratitis, uveitis, dermatitis, lymphadenopathy, mucosal lesions, salivation, and diarrhea. The encephalitic form of caprine arthritis encephalitis affects young kids, is usually asymmetrical, and causes no visual deficit; it often has a more chronic course than PEM. CAE in goats with viral encephalitis typically will have a mild to moderate rise in white blood cell counts and protein values, with mononuclear cells being the predominant cell type.

TREATMENT AND PREVENTION

Thiamine hydrochloride should be administered intravenously as early in the course of the disease as possible at a dose of 10 mg/kg initially, repeated intramuscularly twice daily for 2 to 3 days. An improvement in clinical signs should be noted in 1 to 3 days. If no improvement has occurred after 3 to 4 days, it may be advisable to recommend slaughter. Complete resolution of signs may be observed in 1 to several days, or cerebral damage may be irreversible, resulting in some degree of blindness, depression, or ataxia. Blindness may be the last sign to resolve, and it may require 1 to 7 days.

Because cerebral edema appears grossly and histologically, anti-inflammatory and anti-edema drugs may also be helpful. Therapeutic agents given for this purpose are mannitol* (1 to 3 gm/kg intravenously), dexamethasone (1 to 2 mg/kg intravenously), prednisolone (1 to 4 mg/kg intravenously), furosemide (0.5 to 1.0 mg/kg), or dimethyl sulfoxide (DMSO†) (90 per cent medical grade: 1 gm/kg diluted to a concentration of 20 to 40 per cent with 5 per cent dextrose and given slowly intraveneously). Mannitol and furosemide adminstration will cause dehydration. DMSO therapy may cause muscle fasciculations or slight hemolysis. If anti-inflammatory drugs are used, they should be administered only once or twice. Affected animals should be placed in a well-bedded stall. If the animal is anorectic or dehydrated, fluids, electrolytes, and nutrients should be administered by stomach tube or intravenously. Antibiotics should given to animals that are down or dysphagic to prevent aspiration pneumonia.

If a specific cause can be identified, it should be eliminated. Ruminants on a high concentrate diet need to have the diet altered slowly to include more roughage and less carbohydrate. If many animals are affected, dietary supplementation of thiamine at a rate of 3 to 5 mg/kg of feed should decrease the incidence of disease. Dietary cobalt and sulfate levels should be evaluated and changed accordingly if abnormal.

If the signs of PEM are recognized early in the course of the disease, therapy can be instituted promptly, improving the prognosis significantly.

Supplemental Reading

Blood, D. C., Radostits, O. M., and Henderson, J. A.: Veterinary Medicine, 6th ed. London, Bailliere Tindall. 1267–1275, 1983.
Spicer, E. M., and Horton, B. J.: Biochemistry of natural and amprolium-induced polioencephalomalacia in sheep. Aust. Vet. J. 57:230–235, 1981.

---

*Available from Abbott Industries, North Chicago, IL 60664
†Available from Diamond Laboratories, Inc., Des Moines, IA 50304

encountered in Europe and Asia well before the United States was established. Today it exists almost worldwide with some notable exceptions, such as Great Britain, New Zealand, Australia, and other areas (such as islands) which have been able to remain free by quarantine of potential vectors such as dogs.

In confirmed cases that have occurred in farm animals in the United States during the past 15 years, the numbers have not been relatively large, ranging from 200 to 600 per year. Moreover, there is usually a geographic distribution or focus of infection that generally exists in an area for 3 to 5 years before being eliminated. Currently, the eastern United States "rabies areas" include portions of Virginia, Maryland, and southern Pennsylvania as well as a 2 county area in northern New York. Generally speaking, rabies will persist in an area until a substantial reduction in numbers of the responsible vectors of transmission has been accomplished either by self-elimination (disease) or by reduction in population by means of qualified wildlife management programs and personnel. (See the article Rabies (Lyssavirus), in the section Viruses, Chlamydiae, Mycoplasma.)

ETIOLOGY

The causative virus is a rhabdovirus and, because of its concentration in the salivary glands of an infected vector, transmission readily occurs by means of inoculation of the virus in the saliva when a victim is bitten by a rabid carrier. In the past, this included principally the domestic dog and cat populations but presently, because successful attempts at reducing or eliminating rabies from these animals have been accomplished by vaccination programs, the most common source is wildlife, particularly the fox, raccoon, and skunk. Additionally, both vampire bats and insectivorous bats have proved to be the principal sources of the spread of the disease in some areas. The incubation period is extremely variable. In an epidemic, it seems to range from 1 to 3 weeks; however, in isolated cases, much longer periods have been reported.

IMPORTANCE

Compared to almost all other recognized diseases in food animals, the number of cases of rabies is virtually insignificant. However, it is agreed that the real importance lies in the fact that once clinical signs develop, death becomes a certainty. This is essentially as true in

will not demonstrate multiple typical signs. This makes the disease one of the most difficult to teach about and continually challenges the expertise of the most experienced clinician. Therefore, when one describes a "typical" case, it must be approached in the hypothetical sense with a warning that all of the signs might be demonstrated, but a case with none of the signs or different signs does not eliminate the possibility of rabies as the correct diagnosis. Some of the signs that are noted with a relative degree of frequency could be exemplifed in a case study of a cow as follows:

Day 1. The patient preferred isolation; she had to be driven to the milking parlor from the far end of the freestall barn, barn lot, or pasture. She showed a slight drop in milk production (20 per cent). The appetite appeared normal. Upon complete physical examination, everything seemed to be normal. (If rabies is in the area, the experienced clinician would insist, at this point, that the animal be walked and would observe the rear fetlocks in particular.) A very slight, uniformly bilateral knuckling of the fetlocks was noted.

Day 2. The patient has consumed about half of her feed, and her production has dropped about 50 per cent. Knuckling of the rear fetlocks is more pronounced, and the cow's tail is overactive, actually snapping from side to side. As the day progresses, the ability to snap the tail diminishes and, by evening, the tail head remains active, but the rest of the tail loses motor tone and can be shaken like a dish rag, similar to the state following epidural anesthesia.

Day 3. The patient appears overly alert, and posterior paresis has progressed to the point of producing an unsteady or staggering gait. Anorexia is complete, and milk production has virtually ceased. Tenesmus (as seen in normal parturition or in some cases of coccidiosis) has begun. Also, the animal bellows intermittently, particularly when no one is close by; it is a peculiarly low pitched and hoarse sound, probably because of the developing pharyngeal paralysis.

Day 4. The patient is unable to rise from sternal recumbency; she is depressed and does not attempt to drink or eat. Tenesmus has intensified, and the early signs of rectal prolapse have appeared. Bellowing is less frequent but is more hoarse—almost "bubbly." The tail and rear extremities are devoid of all sensation and motor function. The cow died "during the night" on Day 4½ from the appearance of the first sign.

In addition to these signs, or in cases in which few or none of them ever appear, a variety of other signs may appear. For example, the cow may be found down and unable to rise as the first sign. She will remain alert and will eat and drink until she dies in 3 to 5 days. The cow may demonstrate an apparently prolonged estrus, extending until paresis or death on the fourth or fifth day. She may suddenly demonstrate a nervous disorder, sometimes approaching mania, and she attacks anything that moves, including herdmates, humans, pets, and, if outside, may give chase to any birds that fly overhead. If the affected animal is a bull or steer, prolapse of the penis and sheath will appear on about day 2 or 3.

These signs are by no means a complete list of all the ones that are possible in the "atypical" case. In our area (New York State), death occurs from 1 to 9 days from the onset of signs, with an average being 4½ days.

Pigs generally demonstrate a more standard set of signs, including head and ear shaking and twitching, front limb trembling, frequent chewing movement, and excessive frothy salivation. A hoarse, high pitched squeal is usually heard when the pig is forced to move. In my experience, however, extremely different manifestations may sometimes be present. A 700 kg sow was presented to the Ohio clinic by an owner with the only complaint being that of the sow's inability to stand. The animal remained in lateral recumbency with no other signs. Death was on day 32. The results of the autopsy were negative except for positive identification of Negri bodies.

In sheep and goats, anorexia and depression are usually the first signs. Excessive salivation and pharyngeal paralysis soon follow. As one worker has stated "in many instances little may be observed beyond vague signs of digestive disturbances followed by paralysis."

DIAGNOSIS

Because the virus has an affinity for nervous tissue, brain tissue (especially brain stem) examination by the fluorescent antibody technique (FAT) is the standard laboratory test today. Its accuracy is superior to both mouse inoculation and Negri body demonstration tests that it has replaced.

It becomes clear, after consideration of the variety of unrelated signs that each case may or may not demonstrate, that a positive diagnosis may not be made easily. It is true that in the presence of an epidemic, when a number of cases have received confirmation of rabies by laboratory testing in an area or on a farm, subsequent cases with similar appearances can be diagnosed with a high degree of accuracy. However, when rabies has not been diagnosed in an area for a number of years, the first case, particularly if almost completely atypical, becomes a challenge. For example, I first knowingly became exposed to rabies 24 years after beginning to practice, although a 5- to 6-year long epidemic had appeared in the state 15 to 20 years previously, during which time I had not become exposed. The animal was a mature Holstein cow; the owner's complaint was that she was unable to stand in her tie stall. She was moved to the platform behind a row of cows, where she died on the fourth day. The only signs she demonstrated from onset to death were posterior paresis from day 1 and anorexia from day 2. Because the clinician failed to obtain a complete history prior to the patient's death, rabies had not even been suspected. Only because of the lack of gross lesions at autopsy was rabies positively identified by means of ancillary laboratory tests, including FAT. Upon further questioning of the owner, it was revealed that this cow had been a purchased addition 90 days earlier. She had originated from a province in which rabies was endemic at the time.

Conditions that may have some of the same signs as rabies are numerous. Any evidence of encephalitis, meningoencephalitis, or meningitis can have specific infectious agents as causes or can have toxic or metabolic causes. Examples would be thromboembolic meningoencephalitis, listeriosis, nervous ketosis, and organophosphate poisoning. Because of the frequency of excessive salivation and the inability to swallow in cases of rabies, choke is often suspected in the initial part of the examination. This similarly has resulted in direct exposure of many veterinarians, herd owners, and farm workers to rabies. The bottom line seems to be "always suspect rabies until another diagnosis can be proved."

TREATMENT

There is no treatment for rabies in any animal once the clinical signs have developed. For many years, fresh bite wounds inflicted on farm animals by subsequently proven rabid animals have been cleansed and cauterized by agents ranging from tincture of green soap or tincture of Zepharin to caustic potash and fuming nitric acid, but the efficacy of these methods is impossible to prove. If the bite victim ultimately developed rabies, the logical conclusion was that the cleansing and cauterizing methods had been ineffective. If the victim remained healthy for at least 6 months, one could never conclude positively that rabies would have developed regardless of attempts at prevention.

PREVENTION

The most successful preventive method against the spread of rabies has been the required vaccination of dogs in several states as well as the recommended or required vaccination of house cats and barn cats in endemic areas. Cooperative wildlife reduction programs are effective when a specific species is identified and its numbers reduced in an area of outbreak. It invariably takes a longer period of time to effect control when the vectors are wildlife than when the vectors are pets.

Fortunately, spread from one domestic herbivore to another does not seem to occur. When a clinical case is diagnosed, isolation is preferred, but in epidemics, this sometimes is impractical. Affected dairy cattle in stanchions or tie stalls standing next to healthy animals have not been shown to spread the disease. Strong recommendations should be made to the owner to guard against human exposure to saliva from feed, water, mangers, halters, or utensils that have become contaminated. Before the FAT became accepted as the diagnostic method of choice, it was recommended that the victim be allowed to die so that Negri bodies would have developed, and a positive identification could be made. This procedure had an economic significance as well; if a positive laboratory confirmation was not made, the owner would receive no indemnity. With the advent of the FAT, however, the rabid patient is euthanized as soon as the clinical diagnosis of rabies is made, since the test is as accurate in cases with early signs as it is in cases with late signs.

Vaccination of food animals against rabies is not widely practiced for 2 reasons. The first is that the chance of rabies developing in a large number of domestic animals, even in an endemic area, is rather small. Secondly, the

Spinal Cord Problems in Cattle

KAREN H. BAUM, D.V.M.

An essential part of diagnosing spinal cord problems in cattle involves locating the lesion. Involvement of C1-C5 causes conditions ranging from tetraparesis to tetraplegia and ataxia in all 4 limbs, although the pelvic limbs may be more severely affected. Tone and reflexes are normal or exaggerated in all limbs. Hypalgesia may be detectable caudal to the lesion.

Ataxia and tetraparesis or tetraplegia are also seen with a lesion at the cervical intumescence (C6-T2), but thoracic limb reflexes and tone are depressed to absent. There may be muscle atrophy in the thoracic limb. The pelvic limbs will be spastic with normal or exaggerated reflexes and tone. Hypalgesia or analgesia caudal to the lesion may be detectable. Thoracolumbar (T3-L3) involvement causes pelvic limb ataxia and paresis or paraplegia with normal tail and anal tone and reflexes. The pelvic limb reflexes and tone may be normal or exaggerated. Hypalgesia or analgesia caudal to the lesion may be detectable, and urinary incontinence may be observed. The thoracic limbs are normal, as with any lesion caudal to T2.

Decreased or absent tail, anal, and pelvic limb tone and reflexes indicate a lumbosacral intumescence lesion (L4 through caudal segments). There may be atrophy of pelvic limb muscles, hypalgesia or analgesia, urinary incontinence, and obstipation. The pelvic limbs will be ataxic, paretic, or paralyzed.

TRAUMA

Trauma may cause vertebral fractures or subluxations with resultant spinal cord contusion and acute onset of signs. Cows in estrus may be ridden, causing caudal, sacral, or lumbar injury. Rectal palpation should confirm estrus as well as possible areas of pain or luxation. The pelvic limbs often display bilateral knuckling and, frequently, reduced anal and tail tone are detectable. The tail head appears lower because of crushing. Cerebrospinal fluid (CSF) analytical results are generally normal.

Therapy should be aimed at keeping the animal quiet, and anti-inflammatory agents should be administered as indicated. Prognosis depends upon the severity of the neurologic injury. Full recovery may take weeks to months.

damage to the spinal cord may occur from an acute(?) fracture.

In acute trauma of open cows, 20 to 40 mg of dexamethasone* may be given. Intramuscular flunixin meglumine† (500 mg once or twice daily) in an adult cow, for 2 to 3 days, is also indicated as an anti-inflammatory agent and analgesic. Aspirin‡ or phenylbutazone§ are inexpensive analgesics that are practical for long-term use. Aspirin may be given at 240 to 480 grains orally, twice daily, for an adult cow, while 1 to 2 gm twice daily of phenylbutazone may be administered orally. One adverse effect of nonsteroidal anti-inflammatory agents is abomasal ulcers; therefore, treatment should be discontinued if melena or abomasal pain becomes evident. Treatment of nervous ketosis, hypocalcemia, or any concurrent disease is a must, as animals with these conditions are prone to further injury when excited.

INFLAMMATION

Vertebral body abscesses are present in calves as well as adults. They have been reported in animals from 2 weeks to 5 years of age. The signs are dependent upon the location of the lesion. Most animals have an acute or subacute onset of posterior ataxia, progressing to posterior paralysis or tetraparalysis.

The most common organisms isolated in such cases are *Corynebacterium pyogenes* and *Fusobacterium necrophorum*. Other organisms isolated include *Streptococcus* sp., *Staphylococcus* sp., *Pseudomonas* sp., and *Escherichia coli*. Some animals have concurrent infections, such as omphalitis, hepatic abscesses, and traumatic reticulitis.

Diagnosis of a vertebral abscess is based upon a history of acute onset of paresis or paralysis without evidence of trauma, a previous illness that may have resolved, and laboratory findings indicating hyperglobulinemia and elevated serum alkaline phosphatase levels. The animal is usually alert, appetent, and afebrile. Radiographs may be pathognomonic, especially in young animals. A CSF analysis is usually unremarkable as is the complete blood count. Differential diagnoses include trauma, fractured vertebrae, and other compressive spinal cord lesions.

---

*Available as Azium from Schering Corp., Kenilworth, NJ 07033
†Available as Banamine from Schering Corp., Kenilworth, NJ 07033
‡Available as aspirin boluses (240 gr) from Professional Veterinary Laboratories, Minneapolis, MN 55437
§Available as Butazolidin tablets (1 gm) from Jen-Sal Laboratories, Division of Burroughs Wellcome Co., Kansas City, MO 64141

Treatment is generally unrewarding, as a few animals respond to high doses of penicillin (20,000 to 40,000 units/kg twice daily) or oxytetracycline (10 to 20 mg/kg twice daily) for 10 to 21 days. Concurrent use of nonsteroidal anti-inflammatory drugs, such as phenylbutazone and aspirin, may result in temporary improvement. A low dose of aspirin (240 grains orally twice daily in an adult cow) is warranted for analgesia. Poor response to treatment is thought to be due to poor penetration of antibiotics, irreversible spinal cord damage, leptomeningitis, or secondary fractures of the abscessed vertebra.

Epidural abscesses cause progressive posterior paresis or tetraparesis. The onset is commonly insidious, unlike trauma or vertebral body abscesses. Adult animals are usually affected, although age alone cannot rule out the possibility of an epidural abscess in a calf. The exact neurologic deficits depend upon the lesion's location. Appetite, attitude, feces, and temperature tend to be normal.

Clinicopathologic analysis may demonstrate hyperglobulinemia, a normal complete blood count, and protein elevation in the CSF. Bacteria associated with epidural abscesses include *Corynebacterium pyogenes*, *Staphylococcus* sp., and *Streptococcus* sp. Although the prognosis is guarded once neurologic deficits are obvious, high levels of penicillin or oxytetracycline (as with vertebral abscesses) may be given for a minimum of 7 to 10 days. As with any spinal cord condition, good footing and adequate bedding are essential. Osteomyelitis may be a secondary complication, leading to less chance of recovery.

Improper epidural injections, deep tail lacerations, and tail amputation may lead to ascending myelitis. When left untreated, animals develop progressive posterior paresis followed by paralysis, tetraparesis, and tetraparalysis. The animal may be febrile with an "inflammatory" leukogram (neutrophilia with immature neutrophils or neutropenia with immature neutrophils if demand is overwhelming). A complete history and clinical examination will usually identify the cause.

A CSF sample obtained by a tap may demonstrate numerous nucleated cells, especially neutrophils in an acute case, as well as an elevation of the protein concentration. The prognosis is dependent upon duration and severity of signs. High levels of penicillin, sulfonamides or oxytetracycline, or all three, may result in improvement. Sulfonamides given at a loading dose of 1.5 grains/lb followed by 1 grain/lb once a day may be administered intravenously or orally. They are compatible with penicillin or tetracycline.

Posterior paralysis and paresis may be seen in middle-aged breeding bulls with vertebral osteophytosis or ankylosing spondylosis. The bull is usually alert, appetent, and afebrile with a normal or "stress" leukogram (neutrophilia without "left-shift" and lymphopenia) and normal CSF. Therapy is supportive, and prognosis is grave.

Rabies, malignant catarrhal fever (MCF), and possibly *Hypoderma* migration may cause inflammatory spinal cord lesions. Geographic location, other clinical signs, and recent treatments (as with organophosphates) must be considered. Since MCF causes vasculitis, the CSF may demonstrate numerous red blood cells as well as elevations of white blood cells and protein levels. The CSF analysis in rabies is variable but may be normal.

NEOPLASMS

Although lymphosarcoma is the most common neoplasm to cause extradural spinal cord compression, schwannomas and neurofibromas have also been reported. Adults are most often affected, although occasionally calves have neoplastic spinal cord compressions. Intramedullary neoplasms are rare.

The animal is usually appetent, afebrile, and alert with a history of an insidious onset of progressive ataxia, posterior paresis, or tetraparesis. There may be tail paresis, perineal hypalgesia, or "dog-sitting" posture. Physical examination is critical when lymphosarcoma is suspected. External or internal lymph nodes may be enlarged; the heart may have an irregular rate, rhythm or intensity; the uterus may have palpable neoplastic masses; and melena may be present owing to infiltration of the abomasum, leading to bleeding ulcers. Lymphosarcoma masses in the orbit may lead to unilateral or bilateral exophthalmos. Sometimes, neurologic signs due to lymphosarcoma may be present without any other detectable lesion.

The complete blood count may demonstrate lymphocytosis that would be suggestive, but not pathognomonic, of lymphosarcoma. A positive bovine leukosis virus agar gel immuno diffusion (AGID) test would lend further support to a diagnosis of lymphosarcoma. A negative BLV-AGID would be more valuable in helping to rule out a diagnosis of lymphosarcoma, as cattle with tumors are infrequently AGID negative. CSF analysis may be normal or may demonstrate elevation of protein concentration. Serum globulin levels are usually normal in cattle with neoplastic spinal cord compression.

Steroid therapy of cattle affected with neoplasms may result in temporary improvement. An exceptional animal may improve enough to allow embryo transfer, but this would be rare. Dexamethasone may be given to an open cow in diminishing doses, in combination with penicillin or ampicillin. A dose of 20 to 40 mg of dexamethazone could be given the first day, followed by half the dose the next 2 days. Treatment every other day with one fourth to one eighth the initial dose could continue for 3 to 4 more treatments. A relapse of abnormal neurologic signs should be expected within 1 to 4 weeks after cessation of steroid therapy. Duration of signs from onset to an inability to rise may range from 1 day to several weeks.

DEGENERATIVE AND MISCELLANEOUS PROBLEMS

Diffuse or focal spinal cord signs have been reported with organophosphate toxicity, ammoniated mercury toxicity, thrombotic meningoencephalitis, and consumption of cycad palm (*Cycas media*). Progressive ataxia may be present in young Charolais cattle (8 to 24 months of age) and appears as ataxia and hindlimb weakness. Congenital malformation and hypomyelogenesis occasionally cause abnormal spinal cord signs in the neonate.

Myopathies, neuromuscular disorders (botulism, tick paralysis, tetanus), and musculoskeletal conditions may be confused with spinal cord diseases. These must be eliminated from the differential diagnoses before deter-

laneous disorders. Agri-Practice. 4.10, 1983.

Hartley, W. J., and Webb, R. F.: A suspected new storage disease in cattle. Vet. Path. 19:616–622, 1982.

Hooper, P. T., Best, S. M., and Campbell, A.: Axonal dystrophy in the spinal cords of cattle consuming the cycad palm, Cycas media. Aust. Vet. J. 50:146–149, 1974.

Irving, F., and Butler, D. G.: Ammoniated mercury toxicity in cattle. Can. Vet. J. 16:260–264, 1975.

Khan, M. A.: Significance of "spinal-stage" Hypoderma larvae in systemic insecticide toxicity. Res. Vet. Sci. 10:355–360, 1969.

Leipold, H. W., Strafuss, A. C., and Blauch, B.: Congenital defect of the atlanto-occipital joint in a Holstein-Friesian calf. Cornell Vet. 62:646–653, 1972.

Mozier, J. O.: Advances in cattle ectoparasite control with a discussion of some problems related to treatment with systemic insecticides. J. Am. Vet. Med. Assoc. 154:1206–1213, 1969.

Nicholson, S. S.: Bovine posterior paralysis due to organophosphate poisoning. J. Am. Vet. Med. Assoc. 165:280–281, 1974.

Palmer, A. C., Blakemore, W. E., Barlow, R. M., et al.: Progressive ataxia of Charolais cattle associated with a myelin disorder. Vet. Rec. 91:592–594, 1972.

Rebhun, W. C., deLahunta, A., Baum, K. H., et al.: Compressive neoplasms affecting the bovine spinal cord. Comp. Con. Ed., 6:S396–400, 1984.

Rolfe, D. L.: Aortic thromboembolism in a calf. Can. Vet. J. 18:321–324, 1977.

Weisbrode, S. E., Monke, D. R., Dodaro, S. T., and Hull, B. L.: Osteochondrosis, degenerative joint disease, and vertebral osteophytosis in middle-aged bulls. J. Am. Vet. Med. Assoc. 181:700–705, 1982.

White, M. E., Pennock, P. W., and Seiler, R. J.: Atlanto-axial subluxation in five young cattle. Can. Vet. J. 19:79–82, 1978.

Diseases of the Peripheral Nerves

WILLIAM C. REBHUN, D.V.M.

The clinically important peripheral nerves of the thoracic and pelvic limbs that are responsible for normal locomotion and weight bearing in ruminants are subject to injury from trauma, inflammation, and compartmental syndromes that cause combined neurologic-muscular disease. Each major nerve will be discussed individually, although combinations of neurologic injury are always possible. It is important to recognize that myopathies may mimic peripheral nerve disease and that spinal roots or spinal nerve injuries may be confused with peripheral neuropathies. Therefore, it is recommended that readers also peruse the article on spinal cord diseases to appreciate the similarities as well as the differences in these neurologic disorders.

of the forelimbs. Therefore, the clinical signs of radial nerve dysfunction reflect inability to extend the lower forelimb and digits. The affected limb cannot support weight and may be difficult to advance. In some cases, the toe drags, and the skin on the dorsum of the digit may be traumatized. In other cases, the limb is carried off the ground. In most acute cases, the elbow may be slightly "dropped" or located more ventrally than in the opposite normal limb. However, the elbow in affected limbs usually does not drop to the severe degree observed in cases of brachial plexus damage. There may be analgesia at the dorsal digit.

Treatment

Treatment for radial nerve injury should include anti-inflammatory agents and analgesics. Except in pregnant cows, dexamethasone* should be administered in moderate doses, such as 20 to 40 mg intravenously or intramuscularly for animals 400 to 800 kg. For calves, 10 mg of dexamethasone is sufficient. Analgesics such as aspirin† (240 to 480 grains for adults, twice daily orally), phenylbutazone‡ (1 to 2 gm for adults orally twice daily) or flunixin meglumine§ (250 to 500 mg intramuscularly or intravenously twice daily per adult), should also be used. Steroid and analgesic therapy is tapered or discontinued after 2 to 3 days in most cases, and many cases require only 1 treatment.

Where facilities and labor allow, hydrotherapy with a hose and running water twice daily is very helpful as supportive treatment. If treatment is instituted quickly after the injury, the prognosis is good in most cases. When treatment is delayed several days or longer after the injury, it may be ineffective, and the course may be prolonged. Mild cases may require no treatment, but it is usually better to treat intensively in all cases to avoid any possibility of residual nerve damage. Radial nerve damage secondary to humeral fractures has a much poorer prognosis and should be considered separately.

Many radial nerve injuries can be avoided by improved padding for tilt tables and by proper foreleg padding when cattle are kept in lateral recumbency for surgery.

---

*Available as Azium from Schering Corp., Kenilworth, NJ 07033

†Available as aspirin boluses (240 gr) from Professional Veterinary Laboratories, Minneapolis, MN 55437

‡Available as Butazolidin tablets (1 gm) from Jen-Sal Laboratories, Division of Burroughs Wellcome Co., Kansas City, MO 64141

§Available as Banamine, Schering Corp., Kenilworth, NJ 07033

SCIATIC NERVE INJURY

Etiology

Damage to the sciatic nerve is usually due to iatrogenic injuries by intramuscular injections in the hind leg. Multiple injections or injections of irritating material into the gluteal muscles of calves and dairy cows are the most common cause in my experience. Similar injection injuries may occur to the sciatic nerve or its major divisions (tibial and peroneal nerves) in neonatal calves due to improper injections into the biceps femoris muscle.

Clinical Signs

With complete sciatic nerve paralysis, the limb supports weight, but the hip and hock are slightly dropped in the affected limb. The digit may not advance normally (drag), and knuckling of the fetlock is present. The animal may stand on the dorsum of the digit and fetlock. Analgesia of the limb is present distal to the stifle except on the medial surface.

Complete sciatic nerve paralysis is more common with fractures of the ilium and femur. Iatrogenic sciatic nerve damage due to improper injection techniques usually results in an incomplete paralysis in adult cattle. These cattle are usually able to bear weight on the digit but have marked knuckling of the fetlock and a dropped hock. In neonatal calves, however, injection injuries generally cause a rather complete paralysis, with dragging of the digit on its dorsal surface as the limb advances and weight bearing on the dorsum of the fetlock.

Swelling over the gluteal region or "tell-tale" injection sites should be looked for, since most of these injections have been administered by lay persons who may be reluctant to provide the veterinarian with a complete history.

Treatment

Treatment is symptomatic with anti-inflammatory agents and hydrotherapy when possible. If the animal was being treated for an infectious problem corticosteroids may not be indicated, but nonsteroidal anti-inflammatory drugs could be considered in appropriate dosages (see Radial Nerve Injury). Further injections into the affected limb should be avoided. A support bandage or a "gutter pipe" splint should be applied to the limb from the toe up to the distal hock in an effort to prevent knuckling or further trauma to the dorsum of the fetlock. These injuries may be transient or may respond quickly in cases of minor sciatic damage. Direct damage, multiple injection injuries to the nerve, or neglected injuries, however, may result in prolonged or permanent nerve damage. In certain severe cases, the nerve may take weeks or months to fully recover.

PERONEAL NERVE INJURIES

Etiology

The classic cause of peroneal nerve injury to the cow is pressure due to prolonged recumbency as a result of milk fever or some other "down" condition. This pressure may represent direct neurogenic injury or may be due to a compartmental syndrome, as recent evidence suggests.

The recumbent cow does exert pressure on the lateral surface of the crus and proximal lateral tibial area of the down limb. This is demonstrated by the typical abrasions and decubital sores that develop just distal to the stifle on the lateral surface of the limb in downer cows.

Improper intramuscular injections into the distal biceps femoris muscle, especially in calves, can also damage the peroneal nerve. There is a fine line between sciatic and peroneal nerve damage in cattle since this differentiation requires careful neurologic examination.

Clinical Signs

The affected limb is knuckled at the fetlock and may bear weight on the dorsum of the fetlock. The hock does not drop as in sciatic nerve paralysis but, rather, appears overextended or less flexed than the opposite hock. Analgesia is usually present in the dorsum of the digit.

Treatment

Because this condition is often associated with recumbency, principles of nursing care are the most important means of treatment and prevention. Recumbent cows should have good footing and be well bedded to cushion the peroneal nerves and prevent compartmental syndrome. Cows that are recumbent should be rolled to their opposite side at hourly intervals to prevent pressure damage to the down limb. Physical therapy with massage, warm compresses, and local applications of DMSO to the lateral crus and stifle area are all helpful to cattle with peroneal paralysis.

In addition, anti-inflammatory agents are indicated in acute cases or in cases where peroneal paralysis is likely to follow prolonged recumbency. Dexamethasone (10 to 30 mg parenterally) is helpful in acute cases, when its use is not contraindicated by concurrent infectious diseases or pregnancy. Nonsteroidal anti-inflammatory agents, such as aspirin of flunixin meglumine, are also helpful in standard dosages. Caution is advised with the use of phenylbutazone or flunixin meglumine, since repeated use or high dosages of these drugs may result in abomasal ulcerations. Good bedding is the single best prevention for this condition in cattle.

FEMORAL NERVE PARALYSIS

Etiology

In calves, femoral nerve paralysis has been reported following dystocia, wherein excess traction stretches or damages the femoral nerves. Femoral nerve paralysis has been suspected in "creeper" cows that struggle to rise while having their hind limbs extended caudally. These cows struggle to place their hind limbs under their bodies and create exertional myopathies in the quadriceps femoris muscles. The myopathy and the associated hemorrhage and edema may affect the femoral nerve directly or as part of a neuromuscular compartmental syndrome.

Clinical Signs

Total femoral nerve paralysis is characterized by an inability to support weight. Since the extensors and stay apparatus are affected, the stifle and all joints distal to the stifle tend to flex. With incomplete paralysis or with

bedding, and intermittent lifting is indicated in calves to encourage them to bear weight. In adult cows, good bedding and footing are imperative. In addition, if myopathy is suspected, massage, hydrotherapy, topical DMSO* applications, and assistance in rising should be provided. This assistance, once the cow can support weight, may be accomplished by manual support on the tail while the cow rises or by the judicious use of mechanical support devices. Cows that continue to struggle to rise have poorer prognoses than cows that lie quietly and await assistance. The course of the malady may be days to weeks, and a slow, gradual improvement in the ability to support weight is the desired result. In cattle with myopathy, vitamin E and selenium preparations† should be administered parenterally at recommended dosages to ensure adequate levels of these compounds.

OBTURATOR NERVE PARALYSIS

Etiology

Obturator nerve paralysis is usually caused by dystocia, wherein a large fetus or excess traction exerts direct pressure on the nerve as it courses down the medial surface or the shaft of the ilium. This is most common in heifers with the first calf where either the small size of the heifer's pelvis or the large size of the calf results in dystocia. Fractures of the shaft of the ilium may also create obturator nerve damage. A similar syndrome can occur in cattle that "split" by slipping on ice or slippery concrete and tear their adductor musculature in the hind limbs.

Clinical Signs

The affected limb is slightly abducted in the standing animal and will abduct or slip laterally when the cow stands or walks on a slippery surface. In first-calf heifers, bilateral signs may be observed, and the animal may be unable to rise without assistance. In these instances, both legs are abducted when standing and move noticeably laterally when the patient attempts to walk. These animals will continually slip when walking on a slippery surface and, therefore, are prone to tearing or stretching of their abductor musculature in the hind limbs.

---

*Available as Domoso (90% medical grade) from Diamond Laboratories Inc., Des Moines, IA 50304

†Available as Bo-Se, Mu-Se from Burns-Biotec Laboratories Inc., Omaha, NE 68103

Corticosteroid therapy should be administered once daily for 2 to 3 days and then discontinued. If diagnosed early, the prognosis is good. If diagnosis is delayed or if adductor muscle damage has occurred from repeated attempts to rise, the prognosis is poor.

Supplemental Reading

Cox, V.S.: Understanding the downer cow syndrome. Compend. Cont. Educ. Pract. Vet 3:5472–5478, 1981.

deLahunta, A.: Veterinary Neuroanatomy and Clinical Neurology, 2nd ed. Philadelphia, W.B. Saunders Company, 1983.

Tryphonas, L., Hamilton, G.F., and Rodes, C.S.: Perinatal femoral nerve degeneration and neurogenic atrophy of quadriceps femoris muscle in calves. J. Am. Vet. Med. Assoc. 164:801–806, 1974.

Inflammatory Neurologic Diseases of Small Ruminants

MARY C. SMITH, D.V.M.

The practitioner often considers the diagnoses of neurologic diseases of sheep and goats to be among the most frustrating of problems. When a weak, disoriented, or convulsing animal is first examined, it is often difficult to differentiate between metabolic or toxic conditions and primary neurologic diseases. Pregnancy toxemia, hypoglycemia, enterotoxemia, acidosis, hypocalcemia, and transport tetany are among the disease processes that have apparent neurologic components. Polioencephalomalacia (described elsewhere) is so common in sheep and goats that the experienced veterinarian hardly dares not to give an animal showing vague or perplexing signs 100 to 300 mg thiamine. An alert animal with posterior paresis is no easier to evaluate. While the trained neurologist is arguing about which segment of the spinal cord is involved, the average practitioner, although very serious about performing a complete neurologic examination, is still struggling to differentiate the weakness of starvation or white muscle disease, or the pain and dysfunction of polyarthritis from true spinal cord disease.

There is no easy way out of this quagmire. Veterinarians cannot afford to treat patients with one drug at a time until there is a response. If the best guess happens to be wrong, a patient may die because of irreversible damage to nervous tissue. This is especially true of polioencephalomalacia and listeriosis. If a "shotgun" approach to therapy is adopted and the patient recovers, the veterinarian has gained experience with neurologic disease in

general and not with any specific condition. If the animal
dies, a complete necropsy, including histologic examination of brain and spinal cord, must be performed to arrive
at even a tentative cause of death. Unfortunately, the
laboratory is often far away, the sheep decompose quickly,
and the metabolic or nutritional problems that mimic
neurologic diseases often leave no lesions.

The great number of neurologic diseases to which the
sheep or goat are susceptible have been reviewed in a
recent symposium on sheep and goat medicine (see Supplemental Reading, Neurologic disease in sheep and
goats). This article will be limited to consideration of
common conditions that, because of their inflammatory
nature, can be at least diagnosed if not cured.

HISTORY AND PHYSICAL EXAMINATION

The diagnosis of neurologic diseases of small ruminants
is often based on history and signalment, as much as it is
on physical examination. The age, diet, and stage of
production are extremely important facts to obtain. After
a complete physical examination and neurologic evaluation, the task of arriving at a tentative diagnosis often
consists of comparing the history and signs of the patient
with textbook descriptions of various diseases.

One must not overlook the possibility of using cerebrospinal fluid (CSF) analysis to narrow the list of differential
diagnoses. A lumbosacral tap is of minimal danger to the
patient. No sedation is required for the animal with
marked posterior paresis. Struggling animals may be
briefly quieted with 4 to 8 mg intravenous xylazine hydro-
chloride/100 kg. *This drug is unapproved for small ruminants, and larger doses may be fatal to animals with central
neurologic diseases.* The animal may be restrained with
the pelvic limbs hanging over the edge of a table or a
bale of hay, or with the animal in lateral recumbency with
the spinal column flexed. The lumbosacral area is clipped
and prepared with alternating povidone-iodine and alcohol swabs. A 20-gauge, 1½-inch or 18-gauge, 3½-inch
spinal needle is inserted into the depression just caudal
to the level of the tubera coxarum. It is advanced through
the supraspinous ligament towards the center of the
lumbosacral space. Alternatively, CSF may be removed
from the atlanto-occipital site if the head is flexed ventrally. The animal may be standing or may be in lateral
recumbency for this procedure. The needle enters the
skin exactly on the midline at the level of the cranial
border of the wings of the atlas and is directed slightly
forward while being slowly advanced. At least 1.5 ml of
fluid should be collected and placed in an EDTA blood
collection tube for determination of protein concentration,
total white blood cell (WBC) count, and WBC differential
determination. If the sample is hemorrhagic, another tap
should be performed 2 days later. In most instances of
inflammatory CNS disease, the protein level or WBC
count, or both, will be elevated. Minimal or no changes
from normal values (protein <40 mg/100 ml and 0 to 4
WBC/mm³) are expected with toxic, metabolic, or non-
neurologic diseases.

POST-DEHORNING ENCEPHALOMALACIA

Post-dehorning encephalomalacia is a problem of the
young goat kid. There is a history of recent disbudding

by heat or caustic product, or cauterization. Sometimes the
previously normal animal acts dull and has to be taught
to drink again. In other cases, the animal is found dead
within a few days after disbudding, and the owner suspects
enterotoxemia. Because of the thinness of the calvarium
and the absence of a cranial sinus at the appropriate age
for disbudding (approximately 1 week), the cerebrum is
easily damaged by excessive heat or cold. Treatment
consists of steroids to reduce swelling of the cerebrum
and antibiotics to protect against bacterial penetration of
the brain through damaged tissue. Tube feeding is performed several times a day until the ability to suckle
returns. Meningitis, cerebral abscess, and tetanus are
possible sequelae. Tetanus antitoxin (250 units subcutaneously) is indicated prophylactically if the kid did not
receive colostrum from a doe given a tetanus toxoid
booster during late pregnancy.

MENINGITIS

There are 2 different ways in which meningitis may
occur independently of disbudding. The first involves the
neonatal lamb or kid with septicemia, perhaps originating
from omphalophlebitis. Septic arthritis or anterior uveitis
may also be present. Fever, nystagmus, convulsions or
depression, and pain on manipulation of the neck may
occur.

The second situation involves acute onset of meningitis
without an obvious pre-existing focus of infection. The
animals are either growing or mature, frequently die in
less than 24 hr from the onset of signs, and may be part
of a herd or flock problem. The veterinary literature is
scanty, but the most commonly isolated organism appears
to be a *Streptococcus.* It has been postulated that one or
more members of the herd are asymptomatic carriers. In
one herd of goats that I have seen, the outbreak ceased
after all the goats were injected with benzathine penicillin
to which the isolated *Streptococcus* sp. was sensitive.

Aggressive antibiotic therapy should be instituted at
once. Penicillin and tetracycline are possible choices.
Anticonvulsants should be used if indicated. Cooling with
iced water is advised if the body temperature is above
42°C. When facilities permit, CSF should be obtained to
help document the presence of purulent meningitis and
to attempt a culture of the causative organism. Because
animals in convulsions due to polioencephalomalacia may
develop an elevated temperature, thiamine must be part
of the therapy for suspected meningitis.

LISTERIOSIS

Listeria monocytogenes is the most common bacterial
cause of brain stem inflammation in small ruminants.
Listeriosis has traditionally been associated with silage
feeding because the organism has the capability of multiplying in spoiled (high pH) silage at low temperature. In
areas where silage feeding is not practiced, listeriosis still
occurs, and thus other sources of the organism such as
hay, wet pasture, and even carrier animals are possibilities.

If the *Listeria* organism is instilled into the conjunctival
sac or inoculated into the oral mucous membrane, it
travels along cranial nerves such as the trigeminal nerve

they are not observed when ill. Determination of cause of death rests upon brain culture results and histologic demonstration of microabscesses and glial nodules. Perivascular cuffing and meningeal infiltration with mononuclear cells and a few neutrophils and eosinophils also occur.

Although young lambs and kids can be experimentally infected, most animals with listeriosis are more than 6 months of age. Stress or nutritional inadequacies may lower an animal's resistance to *L. monocytogenes;* thus listeriosis is sometimes a sequela to the dehorning of an adult goat. Most workers believe that the disease is more common during the winter. As winter is also the time for advanced pregnancy, differentiation from pregnancy toxemia is important. Facial nerve paralysis does not occur with pregnancy toxemia, but ketonuria can be expected once the animal is not consuming feed causing listeriosis. Glucosuria is common in any animal with central neurologic disease, especially if convulsing, and thus is not pathognomonic for enterotoxemia.

Examination of CSF will help document the inflammatory nature of a suspected case of listeriosis, but findings cannot be used to rule out caprine arthritis encephalitis (CAE) virus infection or cerebrospinal nematodiasis. Typically, there is an elevation in both white blood cell count and protein level, with the increase in white blood cell numbers being relatively greater (white blood cell to protein ratio greater than 1). However, completely normal CSF is sometimes obtained from an animal with listeriosis.

The prognosis is guarded at best if signs have advanced to the point where walking or swallowing is not possible. Treatment with antibiotics must be aggressive. Initial intravenous sodium penicillin can be followed by 40,000 units/kg. procaine penicillin G subcutaneously twice daily. Antibiotics should be continued for at least 7 to 10 days. If no improvement is seen in 2 weeks, the down or dysphagic animal should be euthanized. Corticosteroids should be avoided, as they predispose the animal to relapse. In a small herd or flock of valuable animals, prophylactic penicillin for 3 days may help other animals that may be incubating the disease.

The affected animal's stall should be well bedded. Some animals benefit from a canvas sling. If facial nerve paralysis prevents closure of the eyelids, ophthalmic ointments and protective bandages or suturing of the lids will limit exposure keratitis. Exposure keratitis often obscures primary uveitis. Force feeding with a mash or a gruel of cooked cereal, alfalfa pellets, and so forth, using a spoon, turkey baster, or stomach tube is necessary if the animal cannot eat unassisted. Sodium bicarbonate (1 to 2 tablespoons/day) is added if loss of saliva has led to acidosis.

febrile. Most (but not all) animals with clinical signs of CAE have positive agar gel immuno diffusion test results to the virus. As the prevalence of titer to the virus in goats in the United States is approximately 80 per cent, the blood test is of no aid in establishing a diagnosis. CSF changes are similar to those of listeriosis except that there is typically a smaller increase in white blood cells. The white blood cell to protein ratio is generally less than 1.0.

Gross lesions consist of single to multifocal areas of discoloration. Histologically, primary demyelination and perivascular mononuclear cell infiltration are present. A trained pathologist is required to distinguish CAE from listeriosis. Prior to 1974, all such cases were called listeriosis.

There is no effective treatment for CAE but because the confirmation of a diagnosis is uncertain during life, treatment for other possible neurologic diseases is indicated. In addition, if dysphagia is the predominant sign in a kid or lamb, vitamin E and selenium should be administered because of the possibility of white muscle disease.

CEREBROSPINAL NEMATODIASIS

In the United States, the nematode generally incriminated in diseases of the CNS of sheep or goats is *Parelaphostrongylus tenuis.* The natural host of the adult worm is the white-tailed deer; numerous snails and slugs on pasture grazed by deer carry the infective larval stage. The larvae of *P. tenuis* migrate to the spinal cord of small ruminants after ingestion of the snails or slugs. A brief sojourn in the dorsal gray columns is normal and apparently asymptomatic in the deer, but inflammation and malacia may attend aberrant migration through the spinal cord or brain of sheep and goats.

The clinical signs of *P. tenuis* migration vary with the number of larvae and the portion of the CNS invaded. If the parasite is migrating through the medulla, signs mimic those of listeriosis or CAE. Most affected animals are more than 6 months of age. Exposure to infected pasture several months earlier is a prerequisite, although the presence of the deer may have escaped notice. Examination of CSF is quite helpful, as approximately 70 per cent of samples from goats clinically affected with *P. tenuis* contain eosinophils. The other 30 per cent of CSF samples are indistinguishable from CSF samples obtained from either listeriosis or CAE cases.

Treatment of cerebrospinal nematodiasis is empirical; controlled clinical trials have not been performed. Various anthelmintics have been used, and some animals have appeared to respond to thiabendazole, fenbendazole (15 mg/kg/day for 3 days), levamisole (8 mg/kg, subcutaneous administration achieves higher plasma levels than does oral administration), and diethylcarbamazine. Dexamethasone for the first few days is advised to limit the inflammation associated with destruction of the parasite.

SPINAL CORD DISEASE

If clinical signs suggest involvement of the spinal cord and if CSF examination supports a diagnosis of inflammatory disease, then CAE and *P. tenuis* migration are the most common causes. The young kid with paraparesis or hemiparesis (often initially mistaken for lameness) that progresses to tetraparesis is apt to be afflicted with CAE. Radiographs will help to rule out a vertebral body abscess. Spinal cord abscesses are most common in animals with previous cases of omphalophlebitis. These abscesses may be located in a vertebra above the heart or above the kidneys. Lambs with ascending paralysis beginning at the perineum may have a post-docking infection of the cauda equina.

The older lamb or kid, or the adult with spinal cord disease, may be infected with CAE or *P. tenuis*. As with brain stem disease, the presence of eosinophils in the CSF is highly suggestive of parasitic migration. Another clinical sign that has been associated with *P. tenuis* is the self-excoriation by the animal of a narrow, vertically-oriented strip of skin, presumably due to irritation to a dorsal nerve root by the parasite. Some animals that have been treated for cerebrospinal nematodiasis stabilize or improve but retain a gait deficit for the rest of their lives. The goat with CAE of the spinal cord is not expected to recover. With either disease, cerebral signs may occur later in the course of the disease, and histologic examination will confirm the presence of the disease.

Supplemental Reading

Asahi, O., Hosoda, T., and Akiyama, Y.: Studies on the mechanism of infection of the brain with *Listeria monocytogenes*. Am. J. Vet. Res. *18*:147–157, 1957.

Brewer, B. D.: Neurologic disease in sheep and goats. Vet. Clin. North Am.: Large An. Pract. 5:677–700, 1983.

Cork, L. C.: Differential diagnosis of viral leukoencephalomyelitis of goats. J. Am. Vet. Med. Assoc. *169*:1303–1306, 1976.

Mayhew, I. G., de Lahunta, A., Georgi, J. R., et al.: Naturally occurring cerebrospinal parelaphostrongylosis. Cornell Vet. *66*:56–72, 1976.

Norman, S., and Smith, M. C.: Caprine arthritis-encephalitis: review of the neurologic form in 30 cases. J. Am. Vet. Med. Assoc. *182*:1342–1345, 1983.

Smith, M. C.: Diagnostic value of caprine cerebrospinal fluid analysis (Abstract). Proc. Third Intl. Conf. Goat Produc. and Dis. 294, 1982.

Neurologic Disease in Swine

BARBARA STRAW, D.V.M., Ph.D.

Neurologic disease in pigs may result from infections, toxicities, nutritional imbalances, traumas, or genetic causes. Because of the short life span of pigs kept for production, neoplastic and degenerative diseases are rare. In swine, disorders of the nervous system appear as changes in behavior, states of consciousness, and loco-motion, or as involuntary motor activity. Economically, neurologic disease can be important on an individual animal basis when it occurs in a sow or boar, but particularly when it affects a large proportion of the herd.

PHYSICAL EXAMINATION

Because of the uncooperative nature of the pig, most of the physical examination is done by observation. First animals should be observed from outside the pen to watch for changes in posture, gait, mental state, reflex activity, and sensory perception, and occurrence of involuntary movement. Typical behavior exhibited by normal swine when a newcomer enters the barn is to move to the far end of the pen and then to turn to face the newcomer. If the stranger seems nonthreatening, the pigs will become curious and will approach to investigate. Sudden movements may send then scampering to the other end of the pen again only to repeat the process of cautious approach and investigation. The pen should be entered, and all pigs should be made to get up and move about. When assessing locomotor ability, the type of flooring must be taken into consideration. Even normal pigs take occasional missteps on slotted floors or on floors with especially uneven surfaces; however, pigs with locomotor disturbances are unable to compensate for these types of floors and, when forced to move, disturbances are obvious. Typical normal values for rectal temperatures of pigs at different ages are as follows: baby pigs, 39.5° C; nursery pigs, 39.3° C; and adult pigs, 38.3 to 38.8° C. Activity and environmental temperature will cause the body temperature of pigs to vary widely; therefore, temperature readings should be taken on both affected and apparently normal animals. Examining several pigs in the herd may reveal the true extent of disease as well as provide baseline data for normal temperatures of pigs on a given day and at a given location.

When individual pigs are affected, they are given an examination similar to that used in other animals. In order to define the course of a disease in the case of a herd problem, pigs that are newly affected should be examined as well as those showing typical signs and those in the stage of recovery. Dead pigs and newly affected pigs are chosen for necropsy examination. Pigs should be killed by electrocution or injection. Avoid the common practice of knocking a pig on the head, since artifacts from such trauma complicate examination of the brain and spinal cord. Gross postmortem examination of the central nervous system in swine includes removal of the dorsal portion of the skull and observation of the meninges for congestion or accumulation of pus. The brain is examined for gross malformations. Samples for bacterial cultures and impression smears should be taken from the choroid plexus of the fourth ventricle. The hypothalamus and olfactory bulbs are recommended specimens for virus isolation. The brain stem is collected for histologic examination in pigs suspected of cerebral angiopathy and malacia secondary to *Escherichia coli* enterotoxemia. Spinal cord sections are taken at the cervical thoracic and lumbar levels for histologic examination in cases of toxicities, nutritional deficiencies, baby pig myelin dysgenesis, and visceral larva migrans. Samples should be fresh (bacterial isolation), frozen (virus isolation), or fixed (histologic examination), depending on the test.

Table 1. *Differential Diagnosis of Neurologic Disease in Unweaned Pigs**

Conditions	Proportion of Litters Affected	Proportion of Affected Piglets within a Litter	Mortality	Age at Onset	Signs in Sow	Signs	Necropsy Findings
Hypoglycemia	Sporadic	May be 1 or 2 if large litter with more pigs than teats; or whole litter if sow not milking	High: 90 to 100% of affected pigs	Usually 2 to 3 days but any age	May be off feed, not milking, in sternal recumbency	Ataxia, sternal or lateral recumbency, convulsions, paddling of the forelegs, gasping and chomping of the jaws, bradycardia, subnormal temperature	No food in stomach; absence of body fat; mahogany-brown muscles
Pseudorabies	High: up to 100%	High: up to 100% in pigs from nonimmune sows; 20 to 40% in pigs from immune sows	High: up to 100%	Initial outbreak affects all ages of unweaned pigs	Abortion, vomiting, sneezing, coughing, constipation, neurologic signs	Dyspnea, fever, hypersalivation, vomiting, diarrhea, ataxia, nystagmus, convulsions, coma; younger pigs more severely affected	Few visible gross lesions; congestion of nasal mucosa and pharynx, pulmonary edema, necrotonsillitis, small white necrotic foci in liver and spleen
Congenital tremors	High	80% or more	Low: 0 to 25%	Birth	None	Severe tremors at birth gradually diminish within 3 wks; tremors disappear when pigs are asleep; tremors most severe in pigs infected at the beginning of the outbreak	No gross lesions
Streptococcal meningitis	Low: down to 50%	Up to 2/3 of litter	High in affected pigs	2 to 6 wks	None	Elevated temperature, hindquarter weakness, stiff gait, stretching movements, tremors, incoordination, paddling, paralysis, opisthotonus, convulsions, blindness, deafness, lameness	Congestion of brain and meninges, suppurative meningitis, excess turbid cerebrospinal fluid, suppurative polyarthritis

NEUROLOGIC DISEASE IN SWINE   001

Disease				Age at onset		Clinical signs	Lesions	Diagnosis
Iron toxicity	As many as were given iron injections	Entire litter	High	Age at iron administration	None	Apathy, drowsiness, dyspnea, coma	Edema around the injection site; pallor of muscles, swollen kidneys, epicardial hemorrhage, hydrothorax, liver necrosis	History of iron injection; recognition
Organophosphate toxicity	Can be high, depending on how many were treated	High: up to 100%	High	At birth when sow treated prior to farrowing	Usually none	Salivation, vomiting, stiff, sawhorse stance, diarrhea, colic, lacrimation, sweating, dyspnea, muscle tremors	Pulmonary edema	History
Vitamin A deficiency of sow	High	High	High	At birth	None	Incoordination, head tilt, hind leg paralysis, paddling, eye lesions	Yellow-gray liver, kidney abnormalities; fluid accumula- or in body cavities	History of liver ration topography; formation of anomaly
Congenital malformation	Sporadic	Low	High	At birth	None	Variable; hydrocephalus,‡ cyclops, brain hernia,‡ eyeless,‡ catlin mark,‡ hind leg paralysis,‡ string halt,‡ cerebellar hypoplasia (2 degrees to prenatal swine fever infection), spina bifida	Anomaly of nervous and other systems	Physical examination and necropsy; includes gestation that can be

*Not in the United States: enterovirus, Teschen and Talfan diseases, hemagglutinating encephalomyelitis, Japanese B encephalitis, hog cholera and African swine fever.
†Fluorescent antibody.
‡Trait is heritable.

	weaning		and staggering gait; ataxia, tremors, paddling, paralysis, palpebral edema		in SC and stomach	hemolytic *E. coli* from small intestine and colon
Salt poisoning (water deprivation)	Any age	Affected by pens	Blindness, muscle weakness and fasciculations, dullness, anorexia, vomiting, diarrhea, seizures = head tremor, opisthotonus, back up, fall over, paddle and chomp. Hemoconcentration, eosinopenia: [Na] > 160 mEq/L	High	Gastritis, gastric ulcers, enteritis, constipation	Pathognomonic eosinophilic cuffing of vessels, especially in cerebrum
Brain stem malacia	Nursery pig or occasionally finisher	Sporadic	Dullness, mild incoordination, unthriftiness, failure to grow	Low	None	Histologic evidence of brain stem malacia
Meningitis due to Streptococcus (Salmonella)	Usually in nursery pigs; occasionally in finishers	A few pigs affected over a few weeks; occasionally large outbreaks	Elevated temperature, hindquarter weakness, stiff gait, stretching movements, tremors, incoordination, paddling, paralysis, opisthotonus, convulsions blindness, deafness, lameness	High	Congestion of brain and meninges; suppurative meningitis, excess turbid cerebrospinal fluid, suppurative polyarthritis	Isolation of α and β hemolytic streptococcus from lesion of suppurative meningitis in Lancefield group D, I and II; (isolation of *Salmonella cholerasesuis*)
Middle-ear infection	Any	Sporadic	Abnormal head carriage, tendency to circle	Low	Inflammation, suppuration or both in middle ear	Clinical signs and necropsy findings
Haemophilus para-suis *meningoencephalitis*	Usually nursery pigs 5 to 8 wks old	10 to 50% of pigs in a group, especially if recently commingled	Fever, muscle tremors, incoordination of hind legs, recumbency, paddling	Moderate, 20 to 50%	Fibrous meningitis with pleuritis, pericarditis, peritonitis and arthritis	Isolation of organism
Organic arsenical toxicity	Any age; in finishing pigs treated for swine dysentery or in sows treated for eperythrozoonosis	Several to many pigs affected	Ataxia, posterior paresis, goose-stepping, blindness, paralysis	Low	None	Sciatic nerve demyelination; kidney and liver arsenic levels > 2 ppm
Brain or spinal cord injury (trauma, skull or vertebrae fracture, abscess, parasite migration; Stephanurus dentatus, fibrocartilagenous emboli	Any	Sporadic	Local neurologic deficit tendency	Low	Localized damage to brain or spinal cord	Necropsy findings
Tetanus	Any, but most common in recently castrated pig	Sporadic	Stiff gait, erect ears and tail, protrusion of nictating membrane, progresses to lateral recumbency, opisthotonus, rigid muscle, stiff legged spasms	High	No gross lesions	At site of infection see gram-positive bacilli with terminal spores

882

Table continued on opposite page

Condition	Ages Affected	Distribution of Affected Pigs	Clinical Signs	Mentality	[illegible]	Diagnosis
Rabies	Usually in pigs older than 2 mo	Sporadic	?? ??????? ?? and twitching of nose, prostration, chewing, salivation, generalized clonic muscle spasms	High, ????	??? ????? ??????	Fresh brain for animal inoculation, histopathology, Negri bodies, FA* test
Listeriosis	Any; signs more severe in younger pigs	Sporadic	Fever, trembling, incoordination, dragging hind legs while showing stiff gait with foreleg, hyperexcitability	High in young pigs to 100%, older pigs may recover	Meningitis, focal hepatic necrosis	Isolation of organism from brain, spinal cord, liver, or spleen
Toxicities			See Table 3			
Non-Metal Imbalances			See Table 4			

*Fluorescent antibody

Table 3. Toxicities Resulting in Neurologic Disease

General Clinical Signs	Toxic Agent	Other Signs	Neurologic Signs	Source
Largely gastrointestinal	Inorganic arsenic	Vomiting, diarrhea	Convulsions	Herbicides Insecticides Cotton Defoliants
	Lead (rare)	Vomiting, diarrhea, salivation, anorexia	Muscle tremors, ataxia, clonic seizures, blindness	Motor Oil Paint Grease Batteries
Frequently characterized by violent activity	Chlorinated hydrocarbons		Hyperexcitability, hyperesthesia, muscle tremors, tono-clonic seizures	Insecticides
	Strychnine		Tetanic seizures	Rodenticide
	Sodium fluoroacetate		Convulsions, running fits	Rodenticide
	Water intoxication	Anorexia, diarrhea	Depression, blindness, muscle tremors, hyperesthesia, ataxia, convulsions, coma	Unrestricted access to water after deprivation
Cholinesterase inhibition	Dichlorvos Organophosphates Carbamate	Lacrimation, miosis, cyanosis, reddening of skin, salivation, diarrhea, vomiting	Muscle rigidity, tremors, paralysis, depression	Wormer Insecticides
Generalized central nervous system signs	Nitrofurans		Hyperirritability, tremors, weakness, convulsions	Antibacterial used to treat swine enteric diseases
	Ammonium salts		Depression, tono-clonic seizures	Cattle feed
	Mercury	Vomiting, diarrhea	Ataxia, blindness, paralysis, coma	Grain treated with mercury as a fungicide, paint, batteries
	Pentachlorophenol	Vomiting	Depression, muscle weakness, posterior paralysis	Wood preservative
	Phenoxy herbicides	Anorexia	Depression, muscle weakness, ataxia	Herbicides
Pigs with access to pasture	Pigweed		Muscle weakness, tremors, ataxia, posterior paralysis, coma	Pasture
	Cocklebur	Vomiting	Depression, muscle weakness, ataxia, muscle tremors	Pasture
	Nightshade	Anorexia, vomiting, constipation	Depression, ataxia, muscle tremors, convulsions, coma	Pasture
	Nitrate, nitrite	Salivation, polyuria, miosis	Muscle weakness, ataxia, convulsions	Lamb's quarters, Canada thistle, jimsonweed, sweet clover
Deafness	Hygromycin		Deafness	Wormer
	Streptomycin		Deafness	Antibiotic

pigs can reach them, and supplied so that there are no more than 10 pigs per waterer. The owner should be asked whether there is any medication in the water and, if so, at what level. Feed should be examined for proper nutritional balance. If it is mixed on the farm, determine the content of all the components and the method of mixing. Feed problems generally involve all of the pigs given the feed and thus can be ruled out tentatively if another group of pigs is eating the same feed and is not affected. Mixing procedures should also be checked to see if feed additives (particularly arsenic, nitrofurans, and hygromycin) are being provided at the proper levels. The owner should also be questioned as to recent processing of pigs, such as iron injection, castration, weaning, and any medication used and the response to it. When an infectious disease is suspected, it is important to know if there have been any recent additions to the herd, if animals have been taken to a show and returned to the herd, or if skunks or wild animals have had access to the pigs or have been in proximity.

DIAGNOSIS

A tentative diagnosis of neurologic disease is based on history, clinical signs, distribution of affected pigs, and gross postmortem findings (Tables 1 to 4). Confirmation is usually by results of laboratory examination of submitted specimens.

	stiff gait, lordosis, hyperexcitability, muscle spasms, night blindness, paralysis.
	Pregnant sows: see Table 1
Niacin or riboflavin deficiency	May result in demyelinization of nerves, but lameness, skin lesions, cataracts and poor growth prominent signs
Pantothenic acid deficiency	Goose-stepping, incoordination, diarrhea, coughing, hair loss, and poor growth
Vitamin B$_6$ deficiency	Poor growth, diarrhea, anemia, hyperexcitability, ataxia, epileptiform convulsions

TREATMENT

When neurologic disease appears sporadically in individual pigs, it is treated by daily injections of 20,000 units/kg of benzylpenicillin for 3 days. On a herd basis, treatment for neurologic disease is straightforward when the cause is known. Pending diagnosis, palliative measures are instituted. Providing warm, dry, comfortable quarters with easy access to palatable feed and water will help minimize secondary complications. When only a few pigs in a pen are sick, they should be moved to a separate pen to avoid competition and possible cannibalism by their healthier penmates. If signs of suppuration, such as purulent meningitis or polyserositis, were seen on necropsy, surviving pigs may be placed on broad-spectrum antibiotics. Severely diseased pigs should be treated parenterally, while the rest of the pigs should be given antibiotics in the feed or water.

DISEASES OF THE
MUSCULOSKELETAL SYSTEM

BRUCE L. HULL, D.V.M., M.S.
Consulting Editor

Introduction to the Musculoskeletal System

BRUCE L. HULL, D.V.M., M.S.

Examination of the musculoskeletal system should begin with observation of the animal in motion. If this is not possible, the animal should be observed while it is quietly standing. At rest, the animal will shift its weight away from affected limbs. Lowering the head with extension of the neck forward will shift weight away from the rear legs, while elevating the head with flexion of the neck will shift weight away from the front legs. In rear leg lameness, the weight is shifted forward giving the shoulders a prominent appearance. Front leg lameness causes the animal to support most of the weight on the rear legs, giving a sickle-hocked appearance.

If a single digit is involved, the animal will stand base wide or base narrow to protect the affected claw. The classic example is bilateral medial claw sole abscess, which leads to a cross-legged stance.

When in doubt, one should always start the examination for lameness with the cow's foot because 90 per cent are lame in the foot. Of these foot lameness cases, approximately 90 per cent are located in the rear feet.[1] Rear foot lameness problems are often seen in the lateral toes.

Reference

1. Pinsent, P. J. N.: The management and husbandry aspects of foot lameness and dairy cattle. Bovine Pract. *16*:61–64, 1981.

Stifle Injuries and Patellar Luxations

DALE R. NELSON, D.V.M., M.S.
and S. K. KNELLER, D.V.M., M.S.

A thorough physical examination will help provide a diagnosis of many stifle problems. The problem should first be localized to the stifle joint, and then the specific disorder can be determined. Radiographic examination and laboratory evaluation may provide valuable information, particularly for prognosis. It should be recognized that although clinical signs may be acute, they may actually be delayed indications of chronic disease, which will affect prognosis and treatment.

With stifle lameness, the animal avoids flexing the stifle, and the hock and the stifle are held in a "fixed" position when walking. Weight is borne on the tip of the toe when walking or standing. The heel will not be in contact with the ground, and the fetlock may be slightly flexed. Both front and rear legs are placed ("camped") under the body. Periarticular swelling and increased synovial fluid are evident, particularly in acute injuries. Heat in the joint may indicate infection. Abnormal movement in the joint is found by palpating the stifle while the animal walks. Muscle atrophy will result from any lameness or lack of use of the leg. The quadriceps femoris and gluteal muscle groups are particularly affected by stifle lameness.

Lameness in the foot closely resembles stifle lameness, so hoof testers and a knife should be used to examine the foot thoroughly. Crepitation in the hip may appear to originate in the stifle, so the hip joint should be palpated externally and internally from within the rectum while the leg is manipulated.

It is normally difficult to physically displace the patella in adult cattle. Palpating the patella while the animal walks allows comparison of abnormal patellar movement with abnormal gait. Dorsal luxation or upward fixation may cause a "catch" at the end of stifle extension and at the beginning of flexion, producing a "jerky" gait or rarely, the leg may be locked in extension. A crouching stance with inward rotation of the stifle is characteristic of lateral luxation of the patella. Atrophy of the quadriceps femoris muscle can cause secondary patellar luxation.

Manipulation of the lower leg while palpating the collateral ligaments causes them to tense and to be more easily located. The lateral collateral ligament can be found by deep palpation but may be difficult to locate in heavily muscled animals. The medial collateral ligament is found by following the proximal edge of the tibia back from the medial patellar ligament. Widening or "gaping" of the joint indicates a stretched or torn collateral ligament.

The medial meniscus is palpated between the medial patellar ligament and the medial collateral ligament at the proximal edge of the tibia. Abnormal movements of the meniscus from torn attachments are detected by palpating the medial joint space while manipulating the lower leg. Locating the lateral meniscus by palpation is difficult.

tibia is pulled backward for a drawer sign. Sometimes severe distention of the joint capsule prevents drawer movement until synovial fluid is drained to relieve pressure. The cranial drawer test used in dogs may be used in sheep and goats.

Rotary movement in the stifle joint is increased with cranial cruciate ligament rupture. Crepitation may be felt, and "knocking" or "cracking" sounds may be heard when the leg is manipulated or when the animal is walking. The tibial crest is more prominent, and periarticular swelling is present.

Pathognomonic radiographs of the stifle joint in mature cattle can be difficult to obtain. The thickness of the joint and associated muscles requires more exposure than for distal extremities, and the relationship of the adjacent abdomen and udder produce problems in cassette positioning in standing animals. In a standing animal, lateral-medial and caudo-cranial views are most useful. Because of positioning difficulties and proximity of bony structures to the cranial surface rather than to the posterior surface of the stifle, the cranio-caudal view is of limited value. Animals that are reluctant to bear weight on the affected limb are difficult to evaluate radiographically because the malposition of the femur and tibia may not be demonstrated on the lateral view and because the increased muscle thickness may obstruct the caudo-cranial view in the nonextended stifle. Precise lateral alignment is necessary on a lateral view to evaluate the position of the femoral condyles relative to the tibial spine for confirmation of cranial cruciate ligament rupture. Administration of tranquilizers and lateral recumbency may be required, and in such cases, medial-lateral views are more beneficial. Loss of the meniscus may reduce the width of the joint space in the posterior-anterior view; however, variations of position must be minimized for accurate evaluation. Early degenerative joint disease may not be visible radiographically.

Examination of synovial fluid may be beneficial. Color, turbidity, viscosity, cell counts, and cell types are minimal tests. A Gram's stain of a centrifuged sample may reveal bacteria. Often trauma causes hemorrhage into the stifle joint, and the fluid will be red or brown but will have normal viscosity. The normal number of polymorphonuclear cells is $<1000/mm^3$.

Arthrocentesis is usually done at 2 sites because the lateral femorotibial compartment does not always communicate with the femoropatellar space. To enter the lateral femorotibial space, a needle is inserted behind the lateral patellar ligament and directed backward. The other compartments can be reached by inserting the needle between the medial and middle patellar ligaments distal patella can be a significant problem in cattle and buffalo, particularly draft animals. Trauma, poor nutrition, and heavy work in immature animals are suggested causes. Immature bulls and rams with a "post-legged" conformation may develop problems if used excessively for breeding. Hereditary predisposition has also been proposed as a cause.

Adults are usually afflicted, and one or both legs are involved. An intermittent or continuous "jerky" gait in the affected legs is similar to stringhalt in horses. A "catch" at the end of extension and at the beginning of flexion may be felt on the patella when walking. Occasionally, the leg locks in extension similar to ponies and horses. The tips of the toes may be rounded from dragging the foot forward. Medial patellar desmotomy, preferably on the standing animal, will correct the problem. The ligament is transected near its insertion on the tibial crest.

Lateral Luxation

Lateral luxation is infrequent in cattle, sheep, and goats. Usually congenital, one or both legs can be affected although unilateral luxations may not be obvious for several weeks after birth. Severe cases have persistent lameness, while less severe cases show intermittent lameness. Bilateral luxations cause a crouching stance with inward rotation of the stifles, and animals may have difficulty standing without help. Sometimes the patella can be repositioned easily, otherwise the leg must be extended to return the patella to the trochlear groove. Primary patellar luxation must be differentiated from that of atrophy of the quadriceps femoris muscle caused by lack of use or femoral nerve injury.

Surgical repair has involved reducing the laxity of the medial femoropatellar ligament by gathering excess tissue with sutures. Results have varied because of the lateral tension on the patella from the biceps femoris tendon. A procedure successfully used in foals and calves overcomes this problem by transecting the insertions of the biceps femoris muscle and the origin of the lateral patellar ligament and releasing them from the patella.

Femoral Nerve Injury

The femoral nerve innervates the quadriceps femoris muscle, the extensor of the stifle. Injury to the nerve can cause atrophy of the muscle that will affect the action of the patella (the sesamoid bone within the tendon of insertion).

Calves are more commonly affected than adults. Trauma or overextension of the hip because a hind leg is caught can damage the nerve. Traction during dystocia with "hip-lock" can overextend the femurs.

Clinical signs indicate stifle malfunction. The legs may not support weight. The stifle and hock are flexed while walking. The stride is shortened because of difficulty in bringing the leg forward. Lateral patellar luxation may result. The quadriceps femoris muscle may atrophy in a week after injury, and this becomes severe in several weeks so that the muscle is a fibrous bundle. A "hollowed out" appearance replaces the muscle mass.

Little can be done for the injury caused by distocia. Trauma on or near the nerve should be treated before muscle atrophy results.

STIFLE

Degenerative Joint Disease

Degenerative joint disease or osteoarthrosis is common in older animals, particularly bulls. Trauma or the aging process causes degenerative changes in the articular cartilages, such as fibrillation, pitting, ulceration, and erosion. Damage to the menisci and ligaments often is associated with the degenerative processes. Osteophytosis of the bone and calcium deposition in the joint capsules and ligaments may be found. Cattle are particularly prone to excessive mineralization in soft tissues in and around injured joints. The stifle is especially vulnerable because of the desire for straight hindlegs in many breeds of livestock. Straightness in the stifle predisposes this joint to persistent trauma from normal movement as well as to acute trauma. Clinical signs indicate acute lameness but, morphologically and radiographically, the joint may have severe chronic changes. All species are affected, but most information is related to cattle.

Pathogenesis of degenerative joint disease has been studied in bulls. Initially, fibrillation and rupture of the lateral meniscus may result from trauma, and incongruity of the joint follows. Degenerative changes begin in the articular cartilage. Subsequent damage to the medial meniscus produces further joint instability. Cartilage degeneration becomes more severe, osteophytes develop on the bone at articular margins, and minerals are deposited in the joint capsule and ligaments. The cranial cruciate ligament may rupture. Clinical signs may be mild until the cranial cruciate ligament ruptures, and signs may be acute and severe.

Phenylbutazone and aspirin may help alleviate lameness, but the disease is progressive.

Cranial Cruciate Ligament Rupture

Rupture of the cranial cruciate ligament can occur as a result of an acute traumatic injury or, as previously described, as a sequelae to degenerative joint disease. With an acute injury, the menisci and collateral ligaments may also be damaged.

Lameness is moderate to severe, and signs indicating stifle lameness are seen. Periarticular swelling may be present from associated muscle or tendon injury. Joint fluid is increased in quantity; and the color may be yellow, red, or brown, but viscosity is normal. The tibial crest is more prominent. Sliding of the femoral condyles over the tibial articular surfaces may be heard or felt while the animal is walking. The drawer test produces positive results.

Radiographs of the stifle will confirm the rupture of the cranial cruciate ligament. The animal must bear weight on the leg to displace the joint alignment. In some cases, the animal may have to be placed in lateral recumbency with anterior stress placed on the proximal tibia because the animal will not bear weight on the limb. For radiographic examination, the femoral condyles should be identified behind the tibial spine. The femoral condyles must be completely superimposed on the lateral view, or it will be misleading. A posterior-anterior view may show changes in joint width or intra-articular mineralization, indicating damage to the menisci or collateral ligaments. This finding can be dependable, but minimal differences should not be overinterpreted.

Corrective surgical procedures have been developed. A modified Paatsama procedure using skin to replace the ligament has been used in cattle. Imbrication has been used in cattle and sheep. Results have been reasonable from surgery if no secondary pathologic changes are present. Lightweight animals have higher rates of successful surgeries than heavyweight animals.

OSTEOCHONDROSIS

A disease of rapidly growing individuals, osteochondrosis is a disturbance of cell differentiation and maturation in joint cartilage and metaphyseal growth plates, resulting in a thickened cartilage layer in the joint. Localized necroses of deeper layers of cartilage occur, and secondary changes occur in the surrounding bone. Fissures and ulcerations of cartilage develop. A cartilagenous flap at the edge of the fissure may subsequently mineralize (osteochondritis dessicans). Detachment of the flap causes a loose body in the joint (joint mouse). Lesions may involve multiple sites and are usually bilateral.

Hereditary factors, particularly rapid growth rates, are important in the development of osteochondrosis. Nutrition, especially as it influences rapid growth, has a significant role.

Osteochrondrosis has been recognized in swine (as leg weakness) and cattle. The stifle may be one of several joints involved. Lesions have been in both femoral condyles in cattle, while the medial femoral condyle appears more frequently involved in swine. Lesions may or may not be associated with lameness; they may heal or progress to secondary degenerative joint disease.

MEDIAL COLLATERAL LIGAMENT INJURY

Injury to the collateral ligament is usually associated with trauma. Often the ligament is stretched rather than torn, and lameness is temporary. If the medial meniscus becomes detached from the collateral ligament and the joint capsule, excessive movement causes permanent damage to the meniscus. Dairy heifers are more frequently affected.

Clinical signs suggest stifle injury. The affected leg is held away from the body to relieve pressure on the medial side of the joint. When the leg is abducted, there is a widening or "gaping" of the medial side of the joint. Palpation of the medial collateral ligament will usually find it intact but lengthened. The medial meniscus, palpated between the medial patellar and medial collateral ligaments, has excessive movement, sliding in and out

or sex predisposition exists.

Clinical signs suggestive of stifle injury are present. The leg may be abducted when standing, and more weight is placed on the medial toe when walking. Lateral to medial movement of the lower leg is increased as compared with medial to lateral movement of the lower leg when manipulated. Widening or "gaping" of the joint may be felt by deep palpation on the lateral side, which may be difficult. Posterior-anterior radiographs with the limb adducted may indicate a widening of the joint space on the lateral side.

Imbrication of the fascia over the lateral collateral ligament has improved the condition.

RUPTURE OF PERONEUS TERTIUS MUSCLE

The peroneus tertius and long and medial digital extensor muscles originate in a common tendon in the extensor fossa of the femur. The extensor muscles insert on the digits, while the peroneus tertius muscle inserts on the tarsus and metatarsus.

The tendon of origin ruptures more frequently than the muscle bellies. This allows overextension of the hock. Affected cattle show some evidence of stifle lameness. The stifle is "fixed" during movement, and the foot is pulled forward with difficulty. Weight is borne on the leg. A localized swelling may develop on the lateral side of the stifle. If the leg is pulled to the rear, the hock can be overextended so that the tibia, metatarsus, and phalanges form a straight line at a 90-degree angle to the femur. The gastrocnemius tendon will be slack.

Improvement often occurs with rest. The swelling over the tendon may become firm and persist, causing slight lameness.

EPIPHYSEAL SEPARATION

Separation of the distal femoral and the proximal tibial epiphyses may result from trauma. Separation of the proximal tibial epiphysis is characterized by a Salter-Harris Type II fracture. Animals less than 18 to 20 months of age are affected.

Crepitation may be produced by manipulation. Pain may not be as evident as with a midshaft fracture. A medial deviation of the stifle is observed with a proximal tibial epiphyseal separation. Radiographs will provide a basis for differential diagnosis.

Satisfactory repair presents problems, since epiphyseal fragments are small and very near the joint. Intramedul-

Jensen, R., Park, R. D., Lauerman, L. H., Braddy, P. M., et al.: Osteochondrosis in feedlot cattle. Vet. Pathol. 18:529–535, 1981.
Leitch, M., and Kotlikoff, M.: Surgical repair of congenital lateral luxation of the patella in the foal and calf. Vet. Surg. 9:1–4, 1980.
Nelson, D. R., and Koch, D. B.: Surgical stabilization of the stifle in cranial cruciate ligament injury in cattle. Vet. Rec. 111:259–262, 1982.
Reiland, S.: Pathology of so-called leg weakness in the pig. Acta Radiol. Suppl. 358:23–44, 1978.
Reiland, S., Stromberg, B., Olsson, S. E., et al.: Osteochondrosis in growing bulls. Acta Radiol. Suppl. 358:179–196, 1978.
Tryphonas, L., Hamilton, G. F., and Rhodes, C. S.: Perinatal femoral nerve degeneration and neurogenic atrophy of quadriceps femoris muscle in calves. J. Am. Vet. Med. Assoc. 164:801–806, 1974.
Weaver, A. D.: Disease of the bovine stifle joint. Bovine Pract. 7:41–45, 1972.
Weisbrode, S. E., Monke, D. R., Dodaro, S. T., and Hull, B. L.: Osteochondrosis, degenerative joint disease and vertebral osteophytosis in middle-aged bulls. J. Am. Vet. Med. Assoc. 181:700–705, 1982.

Septic Arthritis

N. KENT AMES, D.V.M., M.S.

Septic arthritis can be defined as inflammation of a joint with the presence of pathogenic microorganisms or their toxins. It is classified as to the source of the infectious organism. Primary septic arthritis results from direct penetration of a contaminated foreign object into the joint. Secondary septic arthritis is the spread of pathogenic microorganisms into a joint from a localized infection adjacent to the joint. Tertiary septic arthritis is the systemic or hematogenous spread of infection from some other part of the body into the joint.

Although primary septic arthritis does occur in food animals, it is relatively rare and is generally caused by an accidental injury from a sharp object, such as a nail, wire, or pitchfork. The organisms associated with primary septic arthritis would include the common environmental contaminants. Secondary septic arthritis is found more frequently than primary septic arthritis. It would develop as an extension of infections of periarticular tissues. Skin, bone, ligament, and tendon infections could spread to the adjacent joints to cause secondary septic arthritis. This is common in proximal and distal interphalangeal joint infections in cattle. The organisms that are involved are *Corynebacterium, Fusobacterium, Streptococcus* and *Staphylococcus* species, and coliforms. Tertiary septic arthritis usually will affect many animals and multiple joints. Polyarthritis and navel ill are common names for tertiary septic arthritis. It is often seen in young animals when the joint appears to be less resistant to microbial invasion. The organisms associated with tertiary septic

...dulds are many and varied. Viruses, such as caprine arthritis encephalitis (CAE) virus, as well as certain *Mycoplasma* and *Chlamydia*, have been isolated.

DIAGNOSIS

The signs associated with an inflammation of septic arthritis are varied but are similar. There is a localized area of inflammation around the affected joint. There is pain, as evidenced by the associated lameness and by the reluctance to move. The joint capsule is generally distended, with the range of motion of the joint diminished. The animal will show varied manifestations of systemic disease, including fever, depression, and anorexia.

Any patient with a joint suspected of having septic arthritis should undergo radiography for evidence of degenerative joint disease including lytic areas and roughening of the bone or bone proliferation. These findings will be helpful prognostic aids as well as enabling the practitioner to remain informed about the progress of the animal.

Arthrocentesis is a valuable aid in the diagnoses of septic arthritis. Care must be taken in performing arthrocentesis to avoid contamination of the sample or introduction of infection into the joint.

Joint fluid evaluation should include amount, color, viscosity, spontaneous coagulation, mucin precipitation, protein, nucleated cells, and per cent neutrophils (Table 1). Other tests to indicate the presence of microorganisms in joint fluid are culturing, glucose levels as compared with serum glucose levels, and direct microscopic examination.

Culturing of joint fluid or of synovial membrane may be difficult and unrewarding. Many of the septic joints produce no bacterial growth when cultured, and lack of bacterial growth does not eliminate infection as a cause. Negative culture results may indicate a chronic infection or prior treatment for the disease. Synovial fluid has some antibacterial properties that may inhibit bacterial growth. Also, many organisms found in joint fluid require special culturing techniques (i.e., *Mycoplasma* and *Chlamydia*).

PROGNOSIS AND TREATMENT

The prognosis for any animal with an infected joint should be guarded. Although some cases respond nicely to minimal therapy, many require long-term therapy and have less than total return to function. Treating septic arthritis involves (1) providing antimicrobial agents to control the infection and (2) returning the integrity of the joint to normal as far as is practically possible and soon done.

The choice and route of administration of the antimicrobial solution should be made with the help of culture and sensitivity testing results. Since this is often impractical or impossible, the veterinarian must rely on sound medical principles and experience.

Animals with a single infected joint may respond to intra-articular injections of broad-spectrum, nonirritating antibiotics repeated at 2 day intervals for 4 treatments. An equal amount of fluid should be removed from the joint before injecting the antibiotic to avoid excessive pain from joint capsule distention. This treatment may be used with or without concurrent systemic antimicrobial solutions; however, systemic treatment usually helps to improve the prognosis.

More severe infections may require joint lavage. Large amounts of warm saline can be used to flush out debris. This lavage may be repeated every 3 to 4 days followed by antimicrobial agents into the joint. Extremely severe joint infections will require arthrotomy to remove devitalized tissue that cannot be flushed through a needle.

Livestock with polyarthritis are generally given systemic treatment to control the cause of the infection as well as to control the joint problem. The duration of therapy is generally long, and the prognosis is poor.

Support of the affected joint with bandages, splints, and casts may be necessary to rest the area, control the pain, and allow the animal to function. Systemic analgesics should be used both to control pain but, more importantly, to encourage early return to normal function.

Supplemental Reading

Brown, S. G.: Infectious arthritis and wounds of joints. Vet. Clin. North Am. *8*:501–510, 1978.

Firth, E. C.: Current concepts of infectious polyarthritis in foals. Equine Vet. J. *1*:5–9, 1983.

Rosenberger, G.: Clinical Examination of Cattle. Berlin and Hamburg, Verlag Paul Parley, 377–381, 1979.

Shiel, M. J., Coloe, P. J., Worotniuk, B., and Burgess, G. W.: Polyarthritis in a calf associated with a group 7 *Mycoplasma* infection. Aust. Vet. J. *59*:192–193, 1982.

Van Pelt, R. W., and Langham, R. F.: Nonspecific polyarthritis secondary to primary systemic infection in calves. J. Am. Vet. Med. Assoc. *149*:505–511, 1966.

Van Pelt, R. W., and Langham, R. F.: Synovial fluid changes produced by infectious arthritis in cattle. Am. J. Vet. Res. *29*:507–516, 1968.

Van Pelt, R. W.: Traumatic arthritis in cattle. Am. J. Vet. Res. *29*:1883–1889, 1968.

Woodard, J. C., Gaskin, J. M., Poulos, P. W., et al.: Caprine arthritis-encephalitis: clinicopathologic study. Am. J. Vet. Res. *43*:2085–2096, 1982.

Tendon Injuries

N. KENT AMES, D.V.M., M.S.

Tendon injuries in food animal species may be acquired or congenital. Acquired tendon injuries are usually the result of trauma or rupture. The flexor tendons are often lacerated or severed in the mid-metacarpal or metatarsal region, as a result of trauma or of the animal kicking a sharp object. The most notable tendon ruptures in cattle involve the gastrocnemius and peroneus tertius tendons. Contracted tendons in the newborn calf are the most common congenital conditions involving the tendons seen by the practitioner.

Table 1. *Evaluation of Normal and Abnormal Synovial Fluid*

Parameter	Normal	Abnormal
Amount	Small	Increased
Color	Colorless to slightly yellow; clear	Yellow to brownish: cloudy
Viscosity	Strings of 4 cm	Decreased
Spontaneous coagulation	No clots at 48 hr	Clots within few minutes
Mucin precipitation	Elastic clump in clear fluid	Flocculent in cloudy fluid
Protein	<2 gm/100 ml	>2 gm/100 ml
Nucleated cells	<300/mm³	Increased
Per cent neutrophils	<10 per cent	Up to 90 per cent

appropriate antimicrobial drugs. Bandages, casts, and splints afford adequate immobilization. Adhesion, weakness, and stretching of the healed tendon still present major problems.

CONTRACTED TENDONS

The majority of contracted tendons in calves are noted within the first 1 to 2 weeks after birth. They vary in severity from a slight "bucking" of the knee to complete flexion of the fetlock with inability to straighten the limb. They occur more commonly in the forelegs, but all legs may be involved. Contracted tendons may appear with other congenital or heritable abnormalities, such as cleft palate and arthrogryposis. Therefore, a calf with contracted tendons should have a thorough physical examination to eliminate the possibility of other more serious problems.

Most cases of contracted tendons are mild and correct themselves as the calf exercises and as the tendons stretch. Calves that show little or no improvement after a few days of exercise or calves that cannot place the foot flat on the ground require therapy.

Splinting the leg is generally adequate treatment. The splint should run from just above the level of the ground to the elbow in the forelegs and to the hock in the rear legs. A polyvinyl chloride pipe split sagitally or other firm material makes excellent splints. The splints should be well padded and tight enough to place some tension on the tendons. The toes should be left unbandaged to support the weight of the calf and to further stretch the tendons. Splints may be left in place for 1 to 3 days then changed to check for complications, such as skin necrosis and swelling. The prognosis of contracted tendons is generally favorable unless the condition requires tenotomy. In severe cases, tenotomies may need to be performed to initially extend the legs. Tenotomies must be performed under aseptic conditions, and poorer prognoses should be given in these severe cases.

Older animals may acquire contracted tendons, as a result of disuse of limbs. This disuse is often secondary to fractures, tendon injuries or nutritional deficiencies. The treatment is generally the same as for younger animals, except the inciting cause must also be corrected.

RUPTURED TENDONS

Spontaneous rupture of tendons rarely occurs in food animals owing to the enormous tensile strength of the tendons and the general lack of stress to the tendons.

be dropped. Palpation frequently reveals swelling in the area of the rupture. Although this injury may be a true tendon rupture, it is usually viewed as a muscle-tendon separation.

The prognosis for rupture of the gastrocnemius is poor, and salvage must be considered as an alternative. Treatment is most successful in cases of partial rupture and consists of confinement to a well-bedded stall. The recovery period is prolonged, and one should plan on resting the animal at least 3 months in a stall.

Rupture of the peroneus tertius is also identified by physical examination. The classic rupture of the peroneus tertius will allow flexion of the stifle, while extending the hock. This permits wrinkling of the Achilles tendon. Although the prognosis is guarded, the tendon will often heal with rest by the animal in a stall, if the animal is able to advance the leg and support weight.

LACERATED TENDONS

Suturing of flexor tendons in large animals is difficult, as the suture material tends to pull out of the tendon without external support. If suturing is attempted, a tendon suture pattern, such as the Bunnell or the Locking Loop, should be used. Because the wounds are traumatic and grossly contaminated, they require extensive débridement using sterile technique to remove all contaminated and devitalized tissue. Copious amounts of warm sterile saline should be used to flush debris out of the wound. After proper débridement, a large gap may occur between the tendons' ends that cannot be closed with suture. It is then necessary to allow the wound to heal by filling the gap with scar tissue. If the flexor tendons are cut, the leg should be placed in flexion to decrease the size of the gap and to allow the healing, which may require up to 3 months. Casts, splints, and shoes have all been used to place the leg in flexion. The major complications from these devices are broken casts, pressure necroses of the skin with increased lameness, and inability to monitor and treat the open wounds. The flexed joint must continue to be supported after the casts or splints are removed to allow the muscle to regain its strength after this prolonged disuse.

A method theorized to strengthen the healing tendon is the use of a substance within the wound to act as a scaffold for fibroblasts to align themselves and extrude collagen in a linear fashion. The resulting scar would emulate normal tendon. Extruded carbon fiber used for repair of tendons has met this objective. Carbon fiber has been successful in food animals, although much more investigation is needed to substantiate claims.

Supplemental Reading

Ames, N. K., and Coy, C. H.: Repair of Bovine Tendon Lacerations with Carbon Fiber Implants. Proceedings XIII World Congress on Diseases of Cattle. The Netherlands 1763-1765 1982.

McCullagh, K. G., Goodship, A. E., and Silver, I. A.: Tendon injuries and their treatment in the horse. Vet. Rec. 105:54-57, 1979.

Valdez, H., Clark, R. G., and Hanselka, D. V.: Repair of digital flexor tendon lacerations in the horse, using carbon fiber implants. J. Am. Vet. Med. Assoc. 177:427-435, 1980.

Valdez, H., Coy, C. H., and Swanson, T.: Flexible carbon fiber for repair of gastrocnemius and superficial digital flexor tendons in a heifer and gastrocnemius tendon in a foal. J. Am. Vet. Med. Assoc. 181:154-157, 1982.

Williams, I. F., Heaton, A., and McCullagh, K. C.: Cell morphology and collagen types in equine tendon scar. Res. Vet. Sci. 28:302-310, 1980.

Fractures

N. KENT AMES, D.V.M., M.S.

Fractures of food animal species are common problems facing practicing veterinarians. Although practitioners may have a thorough knowledge of the skeletal anatomy and principles of fracture treatment, the size and weight of the patient, plus the extreme muscle pull with distraction of the fracture, often make treatment unrewarding and futile. The location and character of the fracture and the economic value of the animal must be critically evaluated before treatment is attempted.

FIRST AID TO THE PATIENT WITH FRACTURE

When a case involving a fracture is encountered, a thorough physical examination should be completed to determine serious complications. Appropriate therapy should then be initiated. All open fractures should be cleansed and débrided within the first few hours to prevent contaminated wounds from becoming infected. Débridement is accomplished with mild soap and water, followed by removal of all devitalized tissue, using copious amounts of warm sterile saline to flush out debris and contaminates. These procedures should be performed in a sterile manner, using surgical gloves, sterile instruments, and sterile materials. Care should be taken to avoid opening tissue planes or creating pockets of dead space. Radiographs in 2 planes are essential to determine the location and the character of the fracture and are mandatory in determining the method of fixation.

After initial evaluation, it may be decided to refer the patient for definitive treatment. Do not attempt to transport the patient with a fracture without adequate immobilization of the fracture site; further soft tissue damage, opening of a previously closed fracture, and discomfort to the patient are major concerns. Splints made from polyvinyl chloride pipe split lengthwise are very effective as temporary immobilization devices. The splint should be well padded and should immobilize the joint above and below the fracture. A modified Robert Jones bandage or Thomas splint may also be used for temporary immobilization.

PRINCIPLES OF FRACTURE REPAIR

The principles of fracture repair in food animals are similar to those in other species. The fracture must have anatomic reduction and rigid fixation, and the patient must continue to have normal body functions for a sufficient period of time to allow healing. Reduction of the fracture should be accomplished without delay to prevent distraction and overriding. General anesthesia with traction and countertraction is often necessary to reduce fractures in large animals.

Internal fixation may be required for adequate stabilization of some fractures. Bone plates, screws, intramedullary pins, and wires are advantageous in comminuted, oblique, and spiral fractures as well as in fractures involving joints. These aids may also be used when external fixation is impossible or impractical. Strict aseptic technique must always be practiced during internal fixation. The major disadvantages of internal fixation are exposure of the fracture and difficulty of the surgical procedure, and the cost of the implants and equipment. The use of bone plates and screws in very young calves is often unrewarding owing to the soft nature of the bones and thin cortices, which allow screws to loosen and come out. Intramedullary pins are effective when used in simple midshaft fractures. They are available in sizes up to ½-inch diameter. A stack-pinning technique may be more effective than the use of a large single pin that will allow rotational instability.

Kirschner devices and cross-pinning methods have met with some success. The major problems associated with these techniques are infections that travel down the pins into the bone and subsequently loosen the devices.

A large animal fracture patient must be able to stand comfortably immediately after fracture repair for a successful outcome. Analgesics may be indicated to control the pain. Although food animals generally do not tolerate mechanical assistance with hip lifts or slings, the animal should be assisted to its feet early during the convalescence period. Animals that remain recumbent for more than 2 days postoperatively have a grave prognosis for recovery.

LOWER LIMB FRACTURES

The majority of fractures in food animals are those of the lower limbs. Fractures of the metacarpal and metatarsal bones generally can be adequately immobilized with external fixation alone. The prognosis for healing of these fractures is favorable when proper reduction and adequate stability are provided. If the fracture is compound, the prognosis should be guarded.

When placing a cast on the leg, the animal must be adequately restrained. General anesthesia is the method of choice; however, tranquilizers and sedatives plus physical restraint may be adequate. Holes may be drilled into the hoof and a wire passed through them to allow traction to be placed on the fracture, facilitating reduction. The leg should be clean and dry before a cast is applied. Stockingette can be applied over the leg; however, judicious use of cast padding is necessary to minimize decubital ulcers.

Although plaster rolls are easy to apply, the products that are currently available will not cure fast enough for use in large animals. The newer resin casts have the advantage of being strong, lightweight, and waterproof but are more difficult to apply and are slightly more expensive. At least 4 layers of cast material are necessary to form a rigid cast with more layers needed at the top,

adult animals may last from 6 to 8 weeks without complications. However, casts on rapidly growing animals may need to be changed every 2 to 3 weeks for calves and every 1 to 2 weeks for lambs and goats.

The healing of a fracture depends upon the type, the reduction, the stabilization, and the age of the patient. Most fractures are adequately healed in 8 to 10 weeks. Before removal of the cast, radiographic evaluation is necessary for accurate determination of healing.

TIBIA, RADIUS, AND ULNA FRACTURES

Fractures of the tibia, radius, or ulna are too high to be adequately immobilized with a cast. The tibia as well as the radius and ulna are also well suited for internal fixations. A modified Thomas splint has the advantages of availability, ease of application, and low cost. They may be heavy and cumbersome to the patient, however. Splints must be well padded to avoid pressure that causes necrosis in the axillary or inguinal regions.

HUMERUS AND FEMUR FRACTURES

Fractures of the humerus and femur present special problems. Adequate stability is generally not accomplished by external fixation. Internal fixation with intramedullary pins and plates is useful in younger, lightweight animals but provides inadequate stability in larger, heavy-weight animals. It is difficult to apply pins to the femur unless the fracture is simple and midshaft due to the shape of the bovine femur.

The humerus may be the most problematical long bone to immobilize in the bovine. The radial nerve plus the brachialis muscle make the approach difficult. Fortunately, humeral fractures are relatively rare and owing to the musculature surrounding the area, the animal may heal spontaneously with rest in a stall and conservative treatment. When one decides upon the conservative approach for humeral fractures, the carpus should be supported to prevent secondary contracture.

OTHER FRACTURES

Fractures of the digits are often diagnosed and treated successfully. First and second phalanges fractures are rare but can be treated with casts on the lower leg and foot. Third phalanx fractures are alleviated by elevating the affected digit off the ground with a wooden block or shoe

Mandibular fractures heal satisfactorily with the use of internal fixation. Intramedullary pins can be used successfully with mandibular fractures. Plates and screws also are effective in mandibular fractures. Fractures of the symphysis can be wired together easily and effectively. The major complications are associated with osteomyelitis and dysmasesis during convalescence.

Fractures of the carpal and tarsal bones create a number of complications. Arthritis is a common sequela, as are infection and sequestration. External fixation may reduce the amount of lameness during fracture healing; however, the prognosis remains guarded.

COMPLICATIONS OF FRACTURE TREATMENT

Inadequate stabilization and osteomyelitis are major complications in fracture of food animals and can result in nonunion, malunion, and delayed union. The inability to stand and walk are common secondary complications that result from the size and weight of the animal plus the type of fixation employed. Arthritis, nerve and vascular injuries, and pressure necrosis are less common but severe complications of food animal fractures.

Supplemental Reading

Adams, O. R.: Lameness in Horses, 2nd ed. Philadelphia, Lea & Febiger, 1972.

Adams, S. B., and Fessler, J. F.: Treatment of radial-ulnar and tibial fractures in cattle, using a modified Thomas splint-cast combination. J. Am. Vet. Med. Assoc., 183:430–433, 1983.

Ames, N. K.: Comparison of methods for femoral fracture repair in young calves. J. Am. Vet. Med. Assoc. 179:456–459, 1980.

Catcott, E. J., and Smithcors, J. F. (eds.): Equine Medicine and Surgery. 2nd ed. Wheaton, Illinois, American Veterinary Publications, Inc., 1972.

Gibbons, W. J., Catcott, E. J., and Smithcors, J. F. (eds.): Bovine Medicine and Surgery. Wheaton, Illinois, American Veterinary Publications, Inc., 1970.

Greenough, P. R., MacCallum, F. J., and Weaver, A. D.: Lameness in Cattle. Philadelphia, J. B. Lippincott Company, 1972.

Smith, H. A., Jones, T. C., and Hunt, R. D.: Veterinary Pathology, 4th ed. Philadelphia, Lea & Febiger, 1972.

Osteomyelitis

N. KENT AMES, D.V.M., M.S.

Osteitis is defined as inflammation of the cortex and medullary cavity of bone, while osteomyelitis is defined as septic inflammation of bone.

Osteomyelitis in food animals may be chronic, or it

may be acute, with severe pain, swelling, and systemic signs, including fever, depression, and anorexia.

Therapy consists of systemic antibiotics with support bandages, splints, or casts. Surgical drainage and curettage with removal of dead and infected bone may also be necessary.

ETIOLOGY

The causative organisms of osteomyelitis are varied and can originate from many sources, including contaminated open fractures, wounds, extension of existing infections, and the blood. If a segment of bone is separated from its blood supply and becomes septic, a sequestrum is formed that serves as a nidus for continued infection. Coliform organisms, *Staphylococcus* spp., *Streptococcus* spp., and *Corynebacterium* spp. are often isolated in cases of osteomyelitis that began as contamination of open fractures or wounds. *Actinomyces* spp. cause maxillary and mandibular osteomyelitis (lumpy jaw) after gaining entry through small lacerations in the mouth of cattle. Other wound infections that may lead to osteomyelitis are sinusitis as a result of dehorning and ascending infections as a result of tail docking and tail biting.

Osteomyelitis may also be spread by the hematogenous route or by extension of existing infection. Septic arthritis may lead to infection of the epiphysis (E type osteomyelitis) or of the physis (P type osteomyelitis). Respiratory, enteric, or navel infections may spread *Pasteurella* spp., *Salmonella* spp., plus other organisms to bone or to joints through the blood.

CLINICAL SIGNS

The clinical signs of osteomyelitis vary with the location of the infection, the causative organism, and the duration of the infection.

Chronic draining tracts that are slow to heal despite vigorous local and systemic treatment are often indicative of osteomyelitis. Radiographs of infected bone often show areas of lysis, while sequestra and dead bone appear radiopaque. Animals with such cases may exhibit signs of local swelling and pain with few systemic signs. Young growing animals that develop osteomyelitis often show severe lameness with fever, depression, and reluctance to stand and walk. Osteomyelitis within a fracture may produce systemic signs and may lead to delayed healing or nonunion.

Cattle with actinomycosis may exhibit little systemic involvement, and the maxilla or mandible progressively increases in size and sometimes drains. Animals with sinus infections as sequelae to dehorning develop anorexia and depression, which are attributed to infection and pressure within the sinus. Complications of tail docking and tail biting (i.e., extension of infection to the vertebral column) may progress to paresis, paralysis, and death.

TREATMENT

Treatment of osteomyelitis is often difficult, and an extended period of time may be required for complete resolution. Principles of osteomyelitis treatment include the following.

1. Control of existing infection with appropriate levels of systemic antibiotics effective against the causative organism.

2. Surgical removal of devitalized infected bone or bone fragments.

3. Support of the area with splints, casts, or bandages when the patient is physically unstable.

4. Supportive care of the animal, including analgesics to control pain.

Culture techniques and susceptibility to antibiotic results should be used to identify the infective agent and antibiotic of choice, respectively. Care must be exercised in observing withdrawal times for milk and slaughter standards, when administering antibiotics to food-producing animals. It may be necessary to continue antibiotic therapy for extended periods (i.e., 2 to 5 weeks) to control existing bone infections.

Surgical removal of a sequestrum, foreign body, or devitalized bone is essential in the management of osteomyelitis. Curettage is employed to remove nonviable bone and necrotic tissue.

An animal with sinusitis as a sequela to dehorning is best managed by trephination of the affected sinus, thus establishing drainage and a mechanism for lavage of the sinus with antimicrobial solutions.

Successful treatment of cattle that have actinomycoses has been achieved using antibiotics or 200 to 300 ml of 20 per cent sodium iodide solution intravenously, repeated in 3 to 4 days. Care must be taken to avoid this regimen in pregnant cows due to reported abortions. Local and systemic antibiotics have also been effective if used early in the course of the disease. Radiation therapy may be useful in some cases but requires special techniques and is expensive.

Ascending infections of the spinal cord and vertebrae as sequelae to tail docking and tail biting are not responsive to treatment unless therapy is instituted early.

PREVENTION

Prevention is the best mode of treatment for osteomyelitis. Early vigorous treatment of all open fractures and of all wounds with bones exposed is necessary to prevent osteomyelitis. Any wound that potentially involves bone should be completely debrided, and the animal should be placed on appropriate antibiotics. Puncture wounds should be flushed with antibacterial solutions after thorough débridement without recontaminating the area.

Supplemental Reading

Gibbons, W. J., Catcott, E. J., and Smithcors, J. F. (eds.): Bovine Medicine and Surgery. Wheaton, Illinois, American Veterinary Publications, Inc., 1970.

Greenough, P. R., MacCallum, F. J., and Weaver, A. D.: Lameness in Cattle. Philadelphia, J. B. Lippincott Co., 1972.

Hirsh, D. C., and Smith, T. M.: Osteomyelitis in the dog: microorganisms isolated and susceptibility to antimicrobial agents. J. Small Anim. Pract. 19:679–687, 1978.

Rose, R. J.: Surgical treatment of osteomyelitis in the metacarpal and metatarsal bones of the horse. Vet. Rec. 102:498–500, 1978.

Silverman, S., and Ackerman, N.: Postoperative osteomyelitis. Mod. Vet. Pract. 59:843–848, 1978.

that there are a number of specific disease entities that are known collectively as foot rot. An understanding of their etiologies and pathogeneses will help the veterinarian to diagnose and to provide some method of relief for clients.

The foot rot complex can be divided into 4 clinical entities.

1. Interdigital phlegmon
2. Contagious interdigital dermatitis
3. Digital dermatitis
4. Interdigital dermatitis

INTERDIGITAL PHLEGMON

Synonyms for this condition include acute foot rot, chronic foot rot, and infectious pododermatitis. Interdigital phlegmon is an acute or subacute necrotic infection of the interdigital skin that extends into the underlying soft tissues with resulting swelling and lameness. It is caused by a synergistic infection of 2 anaerobic gram-negative bacteria, *F. necrophorum* and *Bacteroides melaninogenicus.*

Interdigital phlegmon is seen in both dairy and beef cattle and affects all age groups. The occurrence is usually sporadic with only 1 or 2 animals in a herd affected at a time, although epizootics involving up to 90 per cent of the animals in a pen have been reported in feedlot operations.

The etiologic agents, *F. necrophorum* and *B. melaninogenicus,* are part of the normal flora of the digestive tract. They are noninvasive to the normal skin, so predisposing factors interfering with the integrity of the skin must be present before disease develops. These include (1) wet, muddy lots that cause softening and maceration of the skin; (2) trauma to interdigital skin from dried or frozen mud, stones, and stubble in the area where cattle must walk; (3) trauma from foreign bodies caught in the interdigital space; (4) nutritional deficiencies, especially of vitamin A and trace minerals; (5) the existence of the other entities of the foot rot complex (especially in dairy cattle); and (6) possible (but not proved) systemic infections, such as septicemic *Haemophilus somnus* or viral diseases that may predispose an animal to epizootic foot rot by causing local vascular damage.

Clinically, interdigital phlegmon is characterized by lameness in affected feet that may vary from slight to very severe. There is usually mild to severe swelling of tissues above the coronet. There is early superficial necrosis of the interdigital skin that progresses to severe necrosis with open fissures into the subcutaneous tissue. The exudate

methoxine (55 mg/kg intravenously). Often one treatment is enough in animals with acute cases, but animals should be re-examined after 24 hr to evaluate responses. In epizootic outreaks, beef cattle may be treated with sulfathiazole in water (454 gm/379 L for 3 days) or sulfamethazine in water (454 gm/758 L for 3 days), or chlortetracycline in feed (2.2 mg/kg of body weight for 7 days, then 1.1 mg/kg body weight for 7 days).

Local treatment is usually not required but, if required, it should be applied when individual animals have been restrained for examination. The lesion should be cleaned with a mild disinfectant solution, and any loose necrotic tissue should be removed. Antibacterial powders or solutions such as Koppertox* should be applied. A bandage may be placed around the foot, or the toes may be wired to keep the claws together.

The best means available for prevention of interdigital phlegmon is to identify and alleviate any potential predisposing conditions. This includes examining the ration for nutritional deficiencies, especially deficiencies of vitamins and trace minerals. Ethylenediamine dihydroiodine (EDDI) at a level of 50 to 60 mg/head/day fed continuously has been widely used as a prophylactic agent, although its efficacy has not been proved. EDDI is not approved for use in dairy cattle rations because of potential iodine toxicity to children drinking the milk.

CONTAGIOUS INTERDIGITAL DERMATITIS

This condition is also known as chronic foot rot. Contagious interdigital dermatitis is defined as a contagious, long-term and chronic infection of the interdigital skin, with secondary changes in the bulbs of adjacent claws. The primary transmissible etiologic agent is *Bacteroides nodosus,* although *F. necrophorum* and spirochetes are present in the lesions and contribute to their formation.

Clinically, contagious interdigital dermatitis is a slowly progressing, long-term herd infection in dairy cattle. The disease tends to be quiescent during dry summer pasture periods, but symptomatic disease appears during high environmental moisture periods or during continuous housing on moist litter in the winter and spring. Usually, the majority of the cattle in a herd will be infected, but only a few will show overt clinical signs at any one time. The early lesion is characterized as a mild, moist interdigital dermatitis without lameness. As the disease progresses, the lesions become necrotic, and there is often an abundance of foul odor-producing exudate, although

---

*Available from Fort Dodge Laboratories, Fort Dodge, Iowa 50501

interdigital fissures do not form. The infections will often extend posteriorly and laterally into bulbs of the heel, causing under-running of the horn, horn erosion, cleft formation in the bulbs, and deep black necrotic pockets in the bulbs. Interdigital hyperplasia is a common secondary manifestation of this disease.

Diagnosis is based on a typical herd history of a long-term infection of the feet, with most clinically apparent cases during periods of wet weather and confinement. Examination of the feet of the more severely affected animals would show interdigital dermatitis with typical deep necrotic black pockets and clefts on the bulbs of the heels. The diagnosis in a herd is aided by the finding of bacteria typical of *B. nodosus* in Gram's stain smears. Exudate should be obtained from active cases of interdigital dermatitis and used to make a smear on the slide. The Gram's stain slide should be examined under oil immersion magnification for the presence of very large uniformly staining barbell-shaped or club-shaped gram-negative bacteria and for the presence of spirochetes. The spirochetes are usually quite numerous and easy to find, but *B. nodosus* is usually present in very small numbers, so several fields may have to be examined before they are found. Culture procedures are difficult and thus are not used as diagnostic aids in this condition.

Therapeutic and preventive procedures for herds with contagious interdigital dermatitis are often frustrating to the owner and to the veterinarian. The condition is chronic and probably cannot be eliminated from the herd. Treatment of individual animals is usually limited to the more severely affected ones with the horn at the bulbs of the feet involved or with deeper secondary infections. These animals should be moved to clean, dry quarters. Radical foot trimming is mandated to clean and drain the necrotic processes and to bring the foot back to its normal confirmation. Antimicrobials recommended for local and systemic treatment of interdigital phlegmon can be used for the more severely affected animals. Footbaths (3 to 5 per cent formalin or 2 to 5 per cent copper sulfate) can be used for the herd, but the bath must be cleaned on a regular basis. There are reports from Europe that zinc sulfate aids in controlling this condition. Initially, $ZnSO_4 \cdot 7H_2O$ should be given to the affected herd at 7.5 mg/kg/day to a maximum of 3 gm/animal for 3 to 4 weeks. A maintenance level of 1 gm/animal/day or 111 ppm zinc in dry matter of feed is then provided. Changes in management conditions aimed at keeping the feet dry should be instituted.

DIGITAL AND INTERDIGITAL DERMATITIS

The last 2 conditions, digital dermatitis and interdigital dermatitis, do not have a defined bacterial origin. They are acute, subacute, or chronic inflammatory conditions of the digital or interdigital skin. These are usually herd conditions with a common predisposing cause that compromises the digital skin or initiates the inflammatory process in a number of animals, allowing invasion by a variety of fecal bacteria, including *F. necrophorum*, *Bacteroides* sp., and *Corynebacterium pyogenes*. Initial lameness may be slight, but invasions of the deeper tissues by the bacteria can result in severe lameness because of the pathologic conditions involved. Common secondary manifestations of this condition are interdigital phlegmon,

interdigital and digital hyperplasia, including wart-like growths, interdigital dermatitis, and abscesses in adjacent soft tissues. The most important step in treatment of the herd is to identify and to eliminate the predisposing causes. Consideration should be given to the predisposing causes listed for interdigital phlegmon and contagious interdigital dermatitis. Also there is some evidence that ingested toxins present in the feed or that toxins produced in digestive upset may predispose animals to these conditions. Where appropriate, foot baths and zinc sulfate therapy may be of value. Individual therapy is aimed at eliminating the deeper septic processes and consists of the systemic and local antibacterial therapy previously listed and appropriate surgical procedures where indicated for septic arthritis and interdigital hyperplasia. If diffuse septic laminitis or deep abscesses are present, prolonged antibiotic therapy is necessary, although the prognosis must be considered poor.

Supplemental Reading

Berg, J. N., and Loan, R. W.: Fusobacterium necrophorum and Bacteroides melaninogenicus as etiologic agents of foot rot in cattle. Am. J. Vet. Res. 36:1115–1122, 1975.

Greenough, P. R., MacCallum, F. J., and Weaver, A. D.: Lameness in Cattle, 2nd ed. Philadelphia, J. B. Lippincott Co., 151–169, 1981.

Jensen, R., and Mackey, D. R.: Diseases of Feedlot Cattle. Philadelphia, Lea & Febiger, 325–330, 1971.

Toussaint-Raven, E., and Cornetisse, J. L.: The specific contagious inflammation of the interdigital skin in cattle. Vet. Med. Res., 2:223–247, 1971.

Contagious Foot Rot of Sheep

JOHN N. BERG, D.V.M., Ph.D.

Contagious foot rot (contagious digital epidermatitis) of sheep is an acute or chronic contagious infection of the epidermal tissues of the foot. It is characterized by an initial case of interdigital dermatitis with extension into the adjacent epidermal tissues underlying the hard horn, causing hoof separation and overgrowth. Usually more than one foot is involved. Merino sheep are more susceptible than other breeds, although all breeds will contract the infection. All ages are susceptible, but older sheep tend to have the most severe disease.

ETIOLOGY AND PATHOGENESIS

Foot rot of sheep is considered to be a synergistic infection of 2 gram-negative anaerobic bacteria, *Bacteroides nodosus* and *Fusobacterium necrophorum*. Motile fusiforms, spirochetes, and *Corynebacterium pyogenes* are also commonly found in the lesions and may contribute to the pathogenesis. *B. nodosus*, one of the primary pathogens, is an obligate parasite of the epidermis of the digits. The only source of *B. nodosus* to noninfected sheep is the feet of infected sheep, which is why this is called a contagious disease. The bacterium can survive for short periods of time on wet, cool pastures. Predisposing factors, such as prolonged contact with moisture causing a soft macerated skin surface, are considered essential for initiation of the infection.

The disease starts as an infection of the interdigital skin

CLINICAL SIGNS

Contagious foot rot is seen as a flock condition, with as many as 50 to 75 per cent of the sheep showing signs of active infection. The disease is chronic and progressive with more severe lesions usually in the older animals. Severe cases are more common during periods of wet weather and confinement. Newly affected animals develop lameness in one or more feet. As the disease progresses, the lameness may become very severe with the animal "carrying" a foot, walking on its knees, or refusing to get up. Severely affected animals lose weight, and milk production declines owing to an inability to graze.

Examination of the interdigital skin of infected feet will show small areas of moist necrotic inflammatory processes in mild cases. As the disease progresses, separation of the horny tissue along the distal axial and abaxial walls and bulbs will become evident. Deep pockets of black necrotic tissue with a characteristic fetid odor will underlie the horny tissues and occur in the bulbs. The hoof will be overgrown and have a distorted shape.

DIAGNOSIS

Diagnosis is usually based on flock history and clinical signs. A key factor in diagnosis includes a history of a high percentage of involved animals typically affected in 2 to 4 feet. Confirmation using laboratory test results is usually not necessary, but confirmation can be based on the presence of B. nodosus in Gram's stain smears of the exudate from acute cases. The bacterium appears as very large club-shaped or barbell-shaped gram-negative rods. They are usually few in number, although large numbers of spirochetes are frequently observed in the stained sections. Cultural procedures for B. nodosus involve very specialized techniques and are not generally available for diagnostic purposes.

THERAPY AND CONTROL

Control efforts in infected flocks are dependent on a diligent examination and therapy program. The sheep in the flock should be examined individually. Each infected foot must be radically trimmed to expose all visible infected tissues and to return the distorted hoof to an approximation of its normal shape. Chloramphenicol (10 per cent in 70 per cent ethanol), zinc sulfate (10 per cent

or iodine.

The disease can be eliminated from some flocks by sorting the animals into infected and noninfected groups after culling of all severely infected animals. Infected animals are treated and re-examined at 2-week intervals until 2 successive examinations produce negative results. The sheep must not be placed in infected pens or on infected pastures.

Zinc sulfate added as a feed supplement has been reported by European investigators to be effective for therapy of infected flocks. Therapy consisted of 0.5 gm $ZnSO_4 \cdot 7 H_2O$ (100 mg Zn)/head/day for 8 weeks.

Vaccination with oil adjuvant and alum precipitated B. nodosus bacterins has been reported by investigators in Australia, New Zealand, and Europe which helped control the disease in infected flocks when combined with good management practices. Unfortunately, these vaccines have not worked in trials conducted in the United States. Pili vaccines for B. nodosus and bacterins for F. necrophorum are being developed and tested and may be available in the future. There is, at present, no vaccine commercially available in the United States.

Supplemental Reading

Cross, R. F.: Response of sheep to various topical, oral and parenteral treatments for foot rot. J. Am. Vet. Med. Assoc. 173:1569–1570, 1978.
Demertzis, P. N., Spais, A. G., and Papasteriadis, A. A.: Zinc therapy in the control of foot rot in sheep. Vet. Med. Rev. 1:101–106, 1978.
Jensen, R., and Brinton, L. S.: Diseases of Sheep, 2nd ed. Philadelphia, Lea and Febiger, 265–267, 1982.
Schmitz, J. A.: Ovine foot rot: a review. Proc. U.S. Anim. Health Assoc. 78:385–392, 1974.
Thomas, J. H.: The bacteriology and histopathy of foot rot in sheep. Aust. J. Agri. Res. 13:725–732, 1962.

Aseptic Laminitis of Cattle

JOHN N. BERG, D.V.M., Ph.D.

Laminitis (diffuse aseptic pododermatitis, founder) is an acute, subacute, or chronic aseptic inflammation with consequent degenerative changes that affect the sensitive and horny laminae of the foot. Laminitis may occur as a primary condition but more often occurs as a secondary condition to rumen acidosis, metritis, mastitis, and acetonemia. Laminitis is worldwide, although the incidence is usually sporadic. The disease is most common in the younger animals of intensive animal husbandry systems. In dairy cattle, the condition is common in the immediate postparturient period.

ETIOLOGY AND PATHOGENESIS

The specific causes and pathogenic mechanisms of laminitis in cattle have not been delineated, but vascular changes are probably primary to the disease. The local features associated with acute laminitis are hyperemia, hemorrhage, thrombosis, and edema. Vascular damage results in stagnant hypoxia in the laminar tissues. As the disease becomes chronic, degenerative changes appear in the vessel walls, and fibrous tissue forms throughout the corium and dermal laminae. This causes severe hypoxia that interferes with the production and nutrition of the keratogenic tissues, with subsequent degeneration or even necrosis in the sensitive laminae. The whole process leads to a loss of cohesion between the sensitive and horny laminae, with resulting deformities in the hoof. Cattle that have undergone an incidence of laminitis are more prone to other disease conditions of the foot, such as sole ulcers, white line separations, and foot rot.

The factors inciting these changes are unknown. It has been postulated that toxins or allergens are absorbed from primary sites with disease, such as the digestive tract with rumen acidosis or the uterus with metritis. These toxins may directly affect the vasculature of the foot or may indirectly cause the local release of substances such as histamine.

CLINICAL SIGNS

The initial signs of acute and subacute laminitis are associated with foot pain. The animal may have a very slight stiffness or may have severe enough pain that it is reluctant to stand. Affected cattle move stiffly, with arched back, hind limbs well under the body, and forelimbs in front of the body. They are reluctant to walk on hard surfaces. There is often increased heat in affected feet, greater pulsation in the digital arteries, and marked venous distention of the hind legs. The onset of acute laminitis is often accompanied by sweating, shivering, muscular tremors, and higher respiratory rate. Systemic temperature is usually normal unless predisposing conditions cause an elevated temperature.

Gross changes in the hoof are not seen in acute laminitis but are evident as the disease becomes chronic. The hoof tends to appear elongated, flattened, and widened. The lamellar border is usually exposed at the toe. When the sole is pared, the horn along the lamellar border is usually soft with a waxy yellow discoloration and reddish brown patches from previous hemorrhages. Sagittal sections of infected digits reveal varying degrees of deviation of the third phalanx from its normal confirmation of the hoof.

DIAGNOSIS

Diagnosis is based on observation of the typical clinical symptoms associated with pain in 2 to 4 feet. Differential diagnosis includes such conditions as traumatic pleuritis and pericarditis, in which the cattle have a similar stiff gait with arched back. The feet should be examined for the presence of infectious conditions such as the various types of foot rot. Diffuse septic laminitis clinical signs mimic many of the aseptic laminitis clinical signs. In septic laminitis, there are usually signs of a predisposing infec-

tious condition in the foot, such as necrotic interdigital dermatitis, and there are often signs of necrotic separation of the hoof wall from the underlying tissues, especially at the coronary junction.

Cattle with laminitis should always be examined for toxic and infectious predisposing conditions, such as rumen acidosis and other digestive disturbances, acetonemia, mastitis, metritis, and retained fetal membranes.

TREATMENT

The first step in therapy of acute and subacute laminitis in cattle is to eliminate the source of the toxin by administering appropriate treatment for the underlying causes, such as digestive upset and metritis. Regardless of the underlying cause, concentrates should temporarily be reduced in quantity or removed from the diet. If the digestive tract appears to be the source of the toxin, a laxative such as magnesium hydroxide (1 to 2 lb in 2 to 3 gal warm water) should be given orally. In the acute stage, laminitis is treated by administration of antihistamines, such as diphenhydramine (55 to 110 mg/100 kg intravenously or intramuscularly) or pyrilamine maleate (55 to 110 mg/100 kg intravenously or intramuscularly), and corticosteroids, such as dexamethasone (5 to 20 mg intravenously or intramuscularly) or prednisolone (100 to 200 mg intravenously or intramuscularly). Antiprostaglandin drugs, including aspirin (100 mg/kg twice a day) and intravenous flunixin meglumine (110 mg/100 kg), have been used to relieve pain. These drugs must be administered within the first 24 hr after the onset of symptoms to be effective. Antihistamine administration should be repeated 2 to 3 times per day. Therapy should continue for 2 to 3 days; there will be a noticeable response during this time if the drug is effective.

Two other practices that have been recommended for treatment of acute laminitis are autogenous blood therapy (draw 50 ml of jugular blood and inject it into the pectoral muscles) and jugular phlebotomy (3 to 5 L of blood are drawn from the jugular vein and discarded). The rationale of these procedures is not known. The latter procedure (phlebotomy) is widely used in Europe and is reported to be as successful as antihistamines and corticosteroids in per cent recovery obtained.

Chronic laminitis with outgrowth of horny tissue should be treated by hoof trimming. The claw should be trimmed so that it approximates its original shape and confirmation. Hoof trimming should be repeated on a 6 month basis in those animals retained for breeding purposes.

If the disease becomes a herd problem, special attention should be given to management practices that might help prevent the disease. Diet is especially important. The herd owner should be advised to avoid sudden changes in diet, to use a high concentrate (roughage ratio of 50:50 or 40:60), and to avoid overfeeding of concentrate, silage, and haylage. Plenty of exercise should be provided. These practices are especially important in the 3 to 4 weeks before and after parturition.

Supplemental Reading

Edwards, G. B.: Acute and subacute laminitis in cattle. Vet. Ann. 22:99–106, 1982.

Greenough, P. R., MacCallum, F. J., and Weaver, A. D.: Lameness in Cattle, 2nd ed. Philadelphia, J. B. Lippincott Co., 219–227, 1981.

Fescue foot, a noninfectious disease sometimes observed in cattle that graze tall fescue, is characterized by lameness, reddening of the area of the coronary band, swelling of the lower rear limbs, and in severe cases gangrene of the extremities with sloughing of the affected part. It occurs where Kentucky-31 or fescue varieties derived from it are grown and grazed.

Some fescue fields have a history of fescue foot outbreaks, but in general outbreaks are nonrecurring. Though fescue foot has never been a problem on many established fescue pastures, a low level of toxin may still be present. In such cases, animals may not ingest enough of the toxin to develop visible symptoms, or some herds or individuals within a herd may be less susceptible than others.

Fall regrowth and total yearly accumulated fescue have usually caused the problem. A correlation seems to exist between the length of time of stockpiling and the frequency of outbreaks. Noticeable lameness appears with the onset of cold weather and snow or ice cover and has occasionally been reported during warm weather. Cattle on a low-quality ration or "in thin flesh" prior to being turned onto fescue pasture are more often affected. A single animal or the whole herd may be involved. The etiologic agent has not been identified. A fungus may be involved, but this has not been proved.

CLINICAL SIGNS

Noticeable symptoms usually appear 5 to 15 days after turning cattle into a new pasture: several weeks' exposure on a pasture of low toxicity may be required. Cases have occurred, however, on fields pastured continuously. Forelimb involvement, which is found very infrequently in our experience, is restricted to cattle less than 1 year old.

In older cattle, early signs are a slight arching of the back, roughened hair coat, and soreness in one or both rear limbs. Many times the left hind leg is the first affected. Younger stock, such as yearlings, may show a pronounced tendency to shift from one rear foot to the other. Symptoms are more noticeable early in the morning before animals have moved about. Knuckling of the pastern is also observed in the early stages of mild cases or in the recovery phase of those more severely affected. All animals may show slight to severe loosening of the stool, resembling that of animals on lush spring pasture.

Reddening of the coronary band and the area between the dewclaws and hooves is accompanied by mild swelling as the severity increases, and lameness may become more pronounced. The distal end of the tail may undergo similar between the hock and dewclaws, leaving only the long bone intact. Emaciation is common in moderately to severely affected animals. Although they will eat, feed intake appears reduced, and there is a tendency to nibble or roll the food around.

In the more southern states of the United States, where winter is less severe, one sees less serious foot involvement and more general effects, such as a rough, dull hair coat, higher respiration and heart rates, and elevated body temperature.

DIAGNOSIS

Fescue foot resembles several other conditions in which lameness or gangrene, or both, of the extremities are prominent: chronic ergotism, infectious pododermatitis, chronic selenium poisoning, frozen feet, and traumatic injury, such as stone bruising.

Lame cattle that show no gross lesion will generally recover, often slowly, when removed from toxic fescue. Animals receiving a massive dose of the toxin prior to their removal from toxic fescue will become progressively worse. Those showing signs of permanent injury, such as continuous swelling in the dewclaw region, development of a deep lesion in the affected area, or loosening or sloughing of an affected part, should be salvaged through normal marketing channels.

PREVENTION

Although there is no specific treatment for fescue foot, many problems can be avoided or losses minimized by proper management.

Cattle should be observed daily for signs of lameness or stiffness during the first month on pasture and in cold weather, especially when rain, snow, and ice are prevalent. Affected individuals should be moved to another field or should be placed on different feed. In severe weather, removal to a barn or protected area will minimize additional stress, secondary frostbite, and additional discomfort. Removal to an area that is reasonably clean also reduces the chances of secondary infection in any skin lesions.

In experimental grazing trials over a period of several years, 400-lb calves receiving 1 to 2 lb of ground shelled corn/head/day have shown much milder symptoms than those receiving no supplements. Animals requiring additional protein should be fed a protein supplement and should have access to a mineral mix. Energy, however, appears to be the most important factor mitigating fescue foot.

Mixed pasture of fescue and legumes seem to create some than pure stands. Rotational grazing using fescue and another grass would be helpful but may not be practical for winter grazing. Removal of all vegetable growth once a year by pasturing, cutting and baling, or clipping appears to reduce problems. Fescue stockpiled after July 1 seems to cause fewer problems than that accumulated for the season. Grass accumulated over several years is even more likely to produce greater toxicity. Grazing of fall regrowth or yearly accumulated growth before severe weather in January and February also reduces the chance for fescue foot.

Heavy nitrogen fertilization may increase the toxin. Therefore, no more than 200 lb of nitrogen/acre should be applied/year, in a split application. Toxicity also rises when severe summer droughts are followed by limited fall rains. Fall regrowth can be just as toxic in the presence of the excessive nitrogen of soil nitrification in limited moisture that prevents full growth of the fescue plant as that of excessive nitrogen application.

Feeding hay to cattle grazing fescue, even fescue hay, will tend to dilute the effect of toxic pasture by reducing the consumption of grass containing the toxin. Field-cured fescue hay processed in the early dough to boot stage, when quality is maximal, is considered safe for feeding to cattle. Although a number of cases have been reported in which hay has been implicated in an outbreak, generally this has been hay cut in October or later. Our experience and the experience of others indicate that toxic fescue cut for hay remains toxic.

Supplemental Reading

Garner, G. B., and Cornell, C. N.: Fescue Foot in Cattle. In Wyllie, T. D., and Morehouse, L. G. (eds.): Mycotoxic Fungi, Mycotoxins, Mycotoxicoses: An Encyclopedic Handbook. New York, Marcel Dekker, vol. 2, 45–62, 1978.

Garner, G. B., Tookey, H. L., and Jacobson, D. R.: Proceedings of Fescue Toxicity Conference, Lexington, Kentucky, 1973. Columbia, Missouri, Extension Publication, University of Missouri, 1–139, 1973.

Interdigital Fibromas

GLEN F. HOFFSIS, D.V.M., M.S.

Interdigital fibromas, also called corns, interdigital overgrowths, interdigital cysts, and interdigital skin hyperplasias, occur in all breeds of cattle in all parts of the world. They are common and frequently produce signs of lameness.

Interdigital papillomas should be differentiated from fibromas because papillomas may have an infectious etiology. Papillomas usually have a rough surface with numerous wart-like projections, and they sometimes develop in epizootics.

ETIOLOGY

Interdigital fibromas consist of a growth and protrusion of connective tissue covered by skin epithelium between the digits. They originate from the skin in the interdigital space and proliferate in response to trauma, excessive motion or moisture, and abnormal foot and hoof conformation, such as splay toes and protrusions of the interdigital fat pad. There may be a hereditary predisposition in some animals.

Interdigital fibromas usually begin as smooth proliferations of skin arising originating from tissues located near the coronary band. Hyperplasia is in response to one of the aforementioned etiologic factors over a period of months. Regression can sometimes take place if the inciting factor is removed. When the fibroma has grown to the extent that it protrudes approximately one half the length of the hoof wall, spontaneous regression is rare.

Dairy cows tend to have a higher prevalence of interdigital fibromas in the rear feet, probably owing to the rear feet contacting more moisture from manure and urine than the front feet. Bulls, particularly beef bulls, appear to have a higher prevalence of interdigital fibromas in their front feet, probably because of the higher weight and greater stress placed on this area, and because heavy bulls tend to walk with more movement on their front feet than do cows. Beef cattle, particularly those that have been fed to excessive body condition, may be predisposed to fibromas by an excessive interdigital fat pad. One or all 4 feet may be affected. Usually both front feet or both rear feet are involved.

CLINICAL SIGNS

Lameness is caused when the interdigital fibroma has protruded approximately half way down the hoof wall. Once it reaches this size, the 2 claws will put lateral pressure on the fibroma as the animal walks. Periodically, the fibroma will contact the floor or protrusions from the floor, which induce pain. Once these 2 events occur, another source of irritation is introduced, which will cause further irritation and therefore further proliferation. Eventually, the fibroma will reach a size where it contacts the ground continuously. At this point, painful ulcerations may develop on the surface, and organisms may be introduced to the deeper tissues. An infectious process located beneath the surface of a fibroma may become localized with abscess formation, or it may invade through the connective tissues of the interdigital space. Such infections may also cause infectious arthritis of the coffin or other joints. An infectious process will contribute to the production of pain and lameness.

TREATMENT

The course of therapy will be determined by making a judgment on whether the fibroma will regress spontaneously if the inciting cause and irritation is removed, or if an infectious process is eliminated. Fibromas may sometimes regress if they are not excessively large. Cows with such fibromas should be placed in a clean environment. The foot should be thoroughly washed and bandaged after application of an antibacterial ointment. Systemic antibiotics may be indicated if the fibroma is infected.

If the fibroma is sufficiently large or if conservative treatment has failed, surgical excision is indicated. The

excised. Following complete excision, the interdigital space should be packed with an antibacterial ointment and bandaged heavily. The bandage should be applied carefully, since it accomplished hemostasis as well as protection to the surgical site. Following surgery, the animal should be kept in a dry area for approximately 2 weeks. At that time, the bandage should be removed. A bed of granulation will have filled the defect and the risk of infection is minimal even without further bandaging. The rate of recurrence following surgical excision is very low, probably on the order of 1 per cent. Another means of therapy is removal by cautery.

PREVENTION

Prevention can be accomplished only by assuring that cattle are kept in a clean environment free of irritants. Trimming overgrown hooves promptly may be helpful in prevention. It should also be kept in mind that there may be a hereditary predisposition for interdigital fibromas within some breeds and some blood lines.

Supplemental Reading

Chivers, W. H.: An investigation of bovine interdigital overgrowth. Vet. Med. Dec.:579–580, 1957.

Greenough, P. R., MacCallum, F. J., and Weaver, A. D.: Lameness in Cattle, 2nd ed. Philadelphia, J. B. Lippincott Co., 162–168, 1981.

Rebhun, W. C., and Pearson, E. G.: Clinical management of bovine foot problems. J. Am. Vet. Med. Assoc. 181:572–577, 1982.

Salsbury, D. L., and Lyons, L. J.: A simplified procedure for removing interdigital cysts of cattle. Vet. Med./Small Anim. Clin. Dec.:609–612, 1969.

Shideler, R. K.: Surgical excision of bovine interdigital fibroma. Vet. Med./Small Anim. Clin. July:609–612, 1969.

Studer, Erich: Surgical treatment of corns in cattle. Vet. Med./Small Anim. Clin. Oct.: 1295–1298, 1974.

Coxofemoral Luxation

BIMBO WELKER, D.V.M.

Coxofemoral luxation or hip joint dislocation is the condition in which the femoral head has become displaced from its position within the pelvic acetabulum. It is a fairly common musculoskeletal disorder reported in almost all older cattle, with 2 to 5 years being the most frequent age. Though no true predisposition by sex or breed is reported, most clinical reports and clinical experiences involve adult dairy cows. The dislocation is usually unilateral, with bilateral dislocation being much less common.

Congenital malformation or underdevelopment of the acetabulum or supporting structures is reported and may be a predisposing factor in some cases, particularly the young. The inherent instability of the hip joint makes it vulnerable to injury. Any sudden, forceful insult to the coxofemoral joint is capable of resulting in luxation. The sudden force applied during mounting or the sudden splaying of the leg laterally or medially during a fall can result in dislocation. More commonly, however, coxofemoral luxation is associated with metabolic dysfunctions that result in weakness and ataxia. The laxity of the ligamentous structures at parturition coupled with the weakness and ataxia induced by metabolic diseases, (i.e., milk fever, toxic metritis and mastitis, or obturator nerve problems) make the cow much more susceptible to injury.

Displacement of the femoral head is most commonly in a craniodorsal direction. Caudoventral luxation of the head of the femur into the obturator foramen is the next most common direction of displacement. Cranioventral and caudodorsal displacements appear with much less frequency.

CLINICAL SIGNS

Regardless of the direction of displacement, a "supporting and swinging leg" lameness is exhibited if the cow is ambulatory. Craniodorsal displacement will result in shortening of the affected limb with outward rotation of the toe. This is the classic abnormality described; but descriptions are not adequate of the variations produced by dislocations in the other positions. Coxofemoral luxation cannot be excluded as a diagnosis based on the absence of these specific deviations of the limb.

The limb will be used in a crutch-like fashion. Cows usually show difficulty in lying down or standing up and may become unable to rise if the affected limb is positioned under the animal. Some swelling may be visible in the coxofemoral joint area, and crepitation may be detected on movement. If the cow remains ambulatory, a false joint may form at the new location of the femoral head, but the lameness persists and the cow becomes unthrifty.

Because luxation produces severe pain initially, many cows are reluctant to use the leg and become downer cows. Cows that become recumbent may be bright and alert or depressed, depending on the severity of pain and the presence of or absence of concurrent metabolic diseases. In late pregnancy, cows are often unable to rise because of the additional weight of the calf. All downer cows should be examined for coxofemoral luxation.

DIAGNOSIS

Diagnosis of coxofemoral luxation in the ambulatory animals is tentatively based on the clinical signs described: abnormal appearance of the hip joint area, swelling, displacement of the greater trochanter, and crepitation heard or felt externally or palpated rectally during movement. The presence of a supporting and swinging leg lameness of sudden onset and a shortened leg with a turned out toe, characteristic of a craniodorsal displacement, should suggest coxofemoral luxation. Other diagnoses that show similar clinical signs and symptoms must be considered. Coxofemoral subluxation produces swelling, crepitance, and lameness that may be indistinguishable from complete luxation. Fractures of the capital physeal, fractures of the neck of the femur, other proximal fractures of the femur, and fractures of the pelvis may all produce lameness that must be considered in the differential diagnosis. Other coxofemoral joint lesions that should be considered include septic arthritis, degenerative arthropathy, and osteochondrosis. Stifle injuries should also be considered as a source of lameness because they may produce crepitation in the coxofemoral area.

Rectal palpation is the most helpful diagnostic tool in the field to differentiate these problems. In many cases the displaced head of the femur can be palpated in its abnormal position outside the acetabular fossa. The area above or below the wing of the ileum and within the obturator foramen should be palpated. Complete rectal examination of the pelvis should also be performed to look for the existence of pelvic fractures. A diagnosis of coxofemoral luxation cannot be ruled out based on the failure to find the femoral head in an aberrant location. Radiologic evaluation is the primary means of differentiation between fractures and luxations when *feasible* and economical.

Diagnosis of luxation in the recumbent animal is based on rectal examination findings, abnormal or bizarre posture of the rear limbs, and radiographic evidence. Manual manipulation of the limb while palpating rectally or during deep external palpation over the greater trochanter area will simulate the motion of walking and may aid in differentiating the disease processes. Another helpful diagnostic manipulation is to abduct the limb as laterally as possible. In cows with luxations or fractures, the limb can often be manipulated to a 90-degree angle with the body. Occasionally, the cow will be observed in sternal recumbency with the limb splayed perpendicularly to the lateral body wall. This abnormal position, while not pathognomonic for coxofemoral luxation, is certainly evidence of severe abnormality of the musculoskeletal system.

TREATMENT AND PREVENTION

Attempts to manipulate and reduce a luxation is justifiable in all cases within the first 24 hr of luxation. Beyond this time, the degree of muscle contraction makes replacement exceedingly difficult. The direction of displacement also plays a key role in the ultimate success of replacement. Craniodorsal displacements are most amenable to external traction and replacement and have the best prognosis, at least for initial correction.

Replacement is facilitated by some type of muscle relaxation, such as general anesthesia, deep sedation, or lumbar epidural anesthesia. The c̶___ with the affected limb uppermo̶___ should be fixed so they are not___ limb. A rope passed around t̶___ region and secured behind th___ will work well. Traction can t̶___ limb. Craniodorsal displacem___ by placing a fulcrum (wood___ on the medial side of the___ and by putting downward___ leg is under traction. Th___ femur and move it in a caud___ ments in other directions are more difficult ___ and to attain proper directions of pull. The operator should be persistent, however, and continue to change manipulative techniques, as the alternatives to replacement by this method are less rewarding. For instance, surgical correction of coxofemoral luxation is generally not successful in the bovine by techniques currently being used.

Reluxation is a common problem in all cases. Factors that contribute to reluxation are damaged muscle masses, ruptured ligamentous supporting structures and joint capsules, fractures of the rim of the acetabulum, and debris within the acetabular fossa. Effective measures to prevent redisplacement are not available. Confinement of the animal to permit time for periarticular tissue to reorganize may be helpful.

Because of the poor prognosis, if reduction is not successful, if repeated reluxation occurs, or if the animal becomes a downer, slaughter or culling should be considered. Unfortunately, the majority of cases will fit into this category.

The overall prognosis for coxofemoral luxation is extremely poor, and therefore attempts at prevention are the best treatment. Prevention primarily involves providing optimal footing at all times, especially in those animals weakened by disease. Additional support can be given to sick animals by hobbling the rear legs to prevent splaying and by possible isolation to prevent trauma by other cows.

Supplemental Reading

Adams, O. R.: Preliminary report on repair of coxofemoral luxations and coxofemoral subluxations in cattle. J. Am. Vet. Med. Assoc. 130:515–519, 1957.

Fretz, P. B., Dingwall, J., and Horney, F. D.: Excisions arthroplasty in calves. Mod. Vet. Pract. 54:67–69, 1973.

Greenough, P. R., MacCallum, F. J., and Weaver, A. D.: Lameness in Cattle, 2nd ed. Philadelphia, J. B. Lippincott Co., 269, 1981.

Malmo, J.: Coxo-femoral dislocations in dairy cattle. Contr. Ther. Gen. Pract., 68:1971.

Rees, H. G.: Coxo-femoral dislocation in dairy cattle. Vet. Rec. 76:362, 1964.

Horizontal Wall Cracks

BRUCE L. HULL, D.V.M., M.S.

Horizontal wall cracks have also been called "thimble toe." The loss of continuity of the hoof wall is parallel to the coronary band and extends around the circumference of the toe. The heel area is usually not involved. The lesion usually affects all 8 toes of an animal.

ETIOLOGY

Horizontal wall cracks usually follow a severe systemic infection that has been accompanied by an acute febrile response. This febrile episode causes imperfect horn growth at the coronary band that later splits or separates. This imperfect hoof does not usually split until it nears the wear surface (2 to 3 cm from the coronary band). Nutritional deficiencies and metabolic diseases are also considered to be a cause by some investigators. When the split occurs, the distal shell of the hoof is attached only by the sensitive laminae. As the animal walks, this shell moves back and forth causing severe pain. In addition to this pulling on the sensitive laminae, dirt and manure may work into the cracks and cause septic laminitis.

CLINICAL SIGNS

Before the split occurs, clinical signs are minimal. A small horizontal groove may be noted on the hoof, but the animal shows no pain. Once the split occurs, the animal becomes very sore and is often reluctant to move because walking causes the shell of the hoof to move and pull against the sensitive laminae. This stage may be accompanied by weight loss and sudden drop in milk production.

TREATMENT

The treatment of choice is a foot trim. The trim should be accompanied by removal of any undermined wall to prevent dirt and debris from accumulating. In doing this, care should be taken to avoid injury to the sensitive laminae. Also the toe should be "dubbed" as short as possible. This helps prevent the shell of the toe from rocking back and forth on the sensitive laminae as the cow walks.

Although this treatment will alleviate pain, it usually takes 4 to 6 weeks for the new hoof wall to reach the wear surface and for the outer shell to fall off. Occasionally, another foot trim, as described, will be needed during this time.

Supplemental Reading

Amstutz, H. E.: Hoof wall fissures. Mod. Vet. Pract. 59:906–908, 1978.
Greenough, P. R., MacCallum, F. J., and Weaver, A. D.: Lameness in Cattle. 2nd ed. Philadelphia, J. B. Lippincott Co., 1981.

Vertical Wall Cracks

BRUCE L. HULL, D.V.M., M.S.

Vertical wall cracks, also called quarter cracks, are usually seen on the cranial aspect of the claws of the front feet. These cracks are a loss in the continuity of the hoof wall. The cracks start at the coronary band and extend for a variable distance towards the wear surface.

ETIOLOGY

Vertical wall cracks are most common in the front foot of beef bulls. Dry weather and hoof brittleness are definitely involved in the pathogenesis. Laminitis has been suggested as a cause but is certainly not a consistent finding. Occasionally, damage to the coronary band due to external trauma may initiate a wall crack. Since overly dry or brittle hooves are the prime cause of vertical wall cracks, a higher incidence of the condition can be expected in late summer or early fall.

CLINICAL SIGNS

Vertical wall cracks range in severity from partial thickness cracks that are incidental findings, to deep cracks that become infected and lead to septic laminitis. The range in lesion severity is accompanied by a wide range in clinical signs, from a normally moving animal to an abnormally moving or lame animal. In any animal having vertical wall cracks and evidence of lameness, hoof testers should be used to ascertain if the lameness is indeed caused by the cracks.

TREATMENT

If an animal with vertical wall cracks is not lame, one should not be too vigorous in treatment. Excessive grooving out of the cracks will expose the sensitive laminae and lead to lameness. A good foot trim with special emphasis on shortening the toes is indicated to help relieve abnormal stress on the hoof wall. Also, the hoof wall should be sealed (grease, tar, Koppertox,* or varnish) to help it retain moisture and become more pliable. Resealing is indicated periodically until the crack grows out.

In addition to these procedures, any lame animal should have the crack cleaned out and widened with a hoof groover. Often this treatment will reveal an abscess (septic laminitis). Abscesses are most prevalent distally and in some cases may extend into a sole abscess. If the abscess can be pared out nicely and leave a dry defect in the hoof wall, this defect can be filled with hoof acrylic.† However, if the defect has draining tracts it should be kept open.

When fissures extend from the coronary band to the wear surface, a wooden block should be applied to the normal digit with hoof acrylic.† This block prevents excessive pull on the hoof wall, as the crack starts to heal.

Supplemental Reading

Amstutz, H. E.: Hoof wall fissures. Mod. Vet. Pract.: 59:906–908, 1978.
Greenough, P. R., MacCallum, F. J., and Weaver, A. D.: Lameness in Cattle. 2nd ed. Philadelphia, J. B. Lippincott Co., 1981.

---

*Available from Fort Dodge Laboratories, Fort Dodge, Iowa 50501
†Available as Technovit from Jorensen Laboratories, Loveland, Colorado 80537

Sole Abscesses

BRUCE L. HULL, D.V.M., M.S.

A sole abscess is located between the sensitive laminae and the horny sole of the foot. The purulent exudate in these abscesses varies in color from pinkish-yellow to gray-brown and is usually under considerable pressure. Depending upon duration, a variable amount of the sole is undermined.

ETIOLOGY

Abscesses result from damage to the integrity of the sole. This damage may be caused by foreign bodies, puncture wounds, laminitis, and white line separation, and cracks are due to overgrown claws. As these breaks in the integrity of the sole are contaminated, they lead to bacterial growth beneath the sole.

CLINICAL SIGNS

The prime sign of a sole abscess is severe pain. This pain is often severe enough to cause the animal to be "three-legged lame." Due to this lameness and its sudden onset, sole abscesses have often been confused with fractures. With sole abscesses, the animal is reluctant to bear weight on the affected toe. This will lead to a base-wide or base-narrow stance to relieve pressure on the involved toe. Because sole abscesses are most frequent in the lateral toe of the rear foot, the base-wide stance and gait of the animal can easily be confused with that of stifle injury.

A simple sole abscess is usually not associated with any swelling or inflammation above the coronary band. However, later in the course of the disease a sole abscess may break out and drain at the coronary band. Any time a draining lesion is found at the coronary band, one should evaluate the PII-PIII joint.

Hoof testers may be employed to evaluate pain over a given digit or over a given area of a digit. Radiographic evaluation is not indicated and is often unrewarding in the diagnosis of sole abscesses.

Although the signs and symptoms as described may make one suspicious of a sole abscess, the diagnosis is dependent on a foot trim. The foot trim should include the following out of any black lines or puncture wounds, which may be encountered. Although these may appear small and insignificant, they often lead to large sole abscesses.

TREATMENT

While following out the aforementioned black lines or puncture wounds, dry lines will often become moist shortly before the abscess is opened. Opening the abscess will drain the pus, which is often under considerable pressure and may be accompanied by gas. Often there is a thin layer of new sole deep in the abscess. Because this new sole is thin and soft, care must be taken in removing the undermined sole so that the sensitive laminae is not exposed. All undermined sole should be removed. If undermined sole is left, inadequate drainage may occur due to occlusion by a pack of manure or mud, and the abscess may reform. The undermined sole is usually removed with a hoof groover.

Although all undermined sole should be removed, the wall of the claw should be left intact to serve as a weight bearing surface. This wall should be trimmed so that it extends only about 1 cm below the reforming sole. A long wall promotes the accumulation of manure and mud over the pared out abscess. After paring off the undermined sole, the foot may be wrapped with an antiseptic ointment. If the wrap becomes soaked with manure and urine, wrapping is undesirable. Consequently, it is probably preferable to leave the abscess area open and treat it with a drying agent. It is usually best to clean this abscess area every day or two and apply a drying agent such as Koppertox* for 7 to 10 days.

Following this treatment, there is usually dramatic relief from the lameness within 12 to 24 hr. The animal is usually back to normal and needs no further treatment after 7 to 10 days.

Supplemental Reading

Greenough, P. R., MacCallum, F. J., and Weaver, A. D.: Lameness in Cattle, 2nd ed. Philadelphia, J. B. Lippincott Co., 1981.
White, M. E., Glickman, L. T., and Embree, I. C.: A randomized trial for evaluation of bandaging sole abscesses in cattle. J. Am. Vet. Med. Assoc. 178:375–377, 1981.

*Available from Fort Dodge Laboratories, Fort Dodge, Iowa 50501

Rusterholz Ulcer

Pododermatitis Circumscripta

BRUCE L. HULL, D.V.M., M.S.

A Rusterholz ulcer is a lesion at the junction of the sole and bulb that starts as a bruise, develops into a devitalized area, and later produces granulation tissue and even osteoarthritis. This lesion is usually located near the axial border of the involved toe and overlies the attachment of the flexor tendons. The ulcerated area is characterized by the presence of a mass of granulation tissue protruding through the sole. This granulation tissue is the result of the piston-like effect of PIII, forcing the sensitive laminae out through the defect in the sole. Rusterholz ulcers are most common in the lateral rear toes of mature animals.

ETIOLOGY

Although Rusterholz ulcers may occur in pastured animals, they are more frequent in animals confined on concrete. Wet concrete appears to be associated with a higher incidence of Rusterholz ulcer cases. Chronic bruising is definitely associated with their pathogenesis. Some workers have incriminated nutritional problems, especially calcium and phosphorus imbalance, genetics, and conformation as possible causes. The role of these various etiologic factors is not completely understood at the present time.

CLINICAL SIGNS

The lameness associated with Rusterholz ulcer is usually severe and sudden in onset. As this condition often involves the lateral toe of the rear foot, the animal usually walks and stands base wide to relieve pressure on the lateral digit. Stanchioned animals will often stand back, so only the toe bears weight on the curb of the manure gutter.

Hoof testers will elicit pain when applied over the bulb to sole junction of the affected digit. As with sole abscesses, the final diagnosis must be made in conjunction with a foot trim. The foot trim may reveal granulation tissue, a crack in the sole, or merely a discolored area of the sole. As with a sole abscess, the crack or discolored area must be pared out to reveal the lesion. Although a true sole abscess is possible in this area (axial sole and bulb junction), a Rusterholz ulcer characterized by granulation tissue is usually found.

Untreated Rusterholz ulcers often lead to weakness and necrosis of the flexor tendon near its attachment to PIII. This weakening eventually (3 to 4 weeks) causes a rupture of the tendon attachment. When the tendon ruptures, the toe of the hoof suddenly tips upward owing to the absence of the flexion of PIII.

TREATMENT

Treatment of a Rusterholz ulcer is time consuming and frustrating. After paring out all of the undermined sole, one must gently probe the underlying granulation tissue for fistulous tracts. These tracts, if found, must be explored for any evidence of deep abscesses or osteomyelitis. The presence of deep tracts, especially in suspected cases of osteomyelitis, is a reason for radiographic evaluation of the foot. If PII-PIII joint involvement is found, digit amputation is the most economical treatment, although drainage and ankylosis can be considered in valuable animals.

The granulation tissue that protrudes through the sole must be debrided to the level of the sole and cauterized to prevent excessive hemorrhage. The sole around the ulcer must be "feathered" as to be thinner and pliable near the ulcer and thicker and less pliable away from the ulcer.

Although bandaging the foot, or drying it as is done with a sole abscess, may lead to a successful outcome, this is very tedious and time consuming. It is certainly preferable to apply a wooden block to the normal digit with hoof acrylic.* Alternatively, a plaster block and cast may be applied to the normal digit. In either case, this relieves pressure on the affected digit. Relief of pressure allows the animal a more pain-free recovery period but, more importantly, prevents the "piston effect" of PIII, which would lead to new granulation tissue. A block or cast also alleviates stretch on the flexor tendon, which may be weak.

Antiseptic dressings or drying agents such as Koppertox† should be used in conjunction with a wooden or plaster block. Even with the help of a block, a Rusterholz ulcer will take 3 to 6 weeks to heal.

---

*Available as Technovit from Jorgensen Laboratories, Loveland, Colorado 80537

†Available from Fort Dodge Laboratories, Fort Dodge, Iowa 50501

Supplemental Reading

Greenough, P. R., MacCallum, F. J., and Weaver, A. D.: Lameness in Cattle, 2nd ed. Philadelphia, J. B. Lippincott Co., 1981.

Rebhun, W. C., and Pearson, E. G.: Clinical management of bovine foot problems. J. Am. Vet. Med. Assoc. 181:572–577, 1982.

Verrucose Dermatitis

BRUCE L. HULL, D.V.M., M.S.

Verrucose dermatitis is a proliferative lesion that appears "wart-like" and usually originates above the bulbs of the heel. Rarely, this lesion can be seen on the dorsal surface of the foot above the interdigital area. Verrucose dermatitis is a distinct clinical entity and should not be confused with stable foot rot that actually originates in the interdigital area and is often an erosive lesion.

ETIOLOGY

Although *Fusobacterium necrophorum* can be cultured from verrucose dermatitis, it is a mixed bacterial and fungal problem that is precipitated by filth and moisture. It is often associated with long toes and shallow heels, which cause the bulbs of the heels to be constantly exposed to water and manure.

CLINICAL SIGNS

Verrucose dermatitis is almost exclusively found on the rear feet. The wart-like growths characteristic of this lesion are often matted together by an exudation of dried serum. Although the lesion may extend as high as the dewclaws, it rarely causes lameness.

TREATMENT

A foot trim should always be performed as part of the treatment for verrucose dermatitis. This trim should be aimed at shortening the toes while preserving as much of the heel as possible. One should also consider either cleaning the environment or removing the affected animal from the environment until the lesion heals.

The wart-like lesions and affected skin should be radically excised and heat cautery used to control hemorrhage. A dry antiseptic dressing should then be applied until healing is complete.

Spondylitis

BRUCE L. HULL, D.V.M., M.S.

Spondylitis means inflammation of the vertebrae. When applied to the disorder in cattle, the term spondylitis is generally synonymous with ankylosing spondylitis, as ankylosis and its sequelae are the causes of the clinical syndrome.

ETIOLOGY

Spondylitis is seen mostly in mature bulls housed in confinement situations. The lesion has been observed in older cows, but is most common in older bulls. Degeneration of the intervertebral disc, allowing excessive intervertebral motion, is probably the initiating cause. This excessive motion in turn stimulates new bone formation around the vertebral bodies. New bone formation is most extensive ventrally but also occurs laterally. The exostosis typically affects the last 2 or 3 thoracic and first 2 or 3 lumbar vertebrae. However, the entire lumbar spine back to and including the lumbosacral joint may be involved.

CLINICAL SIGNS

Although bridging exostosis may be palpated rectally along the ventral surface of the vertebral bodies, it is not what causes the clinical signs. In fact, palpation of exostosis on ventral vertebral bodies could almost be considered a normal finding in an older bull. In one study, 21 of 25 middle-aged dairy bulls showed evidence of vertebral osteophytosis.[1] In some animals, exostosis becomes extensive enough to actually bridge the vertebral bodies and to form a splint along these bodies.

Fracture of this splint of exostosis leads to the clinical signs. Some reports indicate that the splint fractures after a clumsy mount or after a slip. In some cases, the splint may fracture with no apparent predisposing trauma. The clinical signs generally appear suddenly and vary in severity, depending on the extent of the injury. Mild signs include difficulty in rising, reluctance to mount, and a stiff gait. The stiffness of the gait may be quite severe, to the point that the animal drags its rear feet. In its most severe form, spondylitis causes complete posterior paralysis and even absence of spinal reflexes.

Rectal palpation of the exostosis is a helpful diagnostic sign; however, not all cases of spondylitis extend into the posterior lumbar region.

TREATMENT

Treatment, especially in more severely affected animals, is probably hopeless, and destruction of the animal should be considered. Mildly affected animals may respond to stall rest and analgesics; however, the symptoms are very likely to recur, often more severely.

Reference

1. Weisbrode, S. E., Monke, D. R., Dodaro, S. T., et al.: Osteochondrosis, degenerative joint disease and vertebral osteophytosis in middle-aged bulls. J. Am. Vet. Med. Assoc. *181*:700–705, 1982.

DERMATOLOGIC DISEASES

PETER C. MULLOWNEY, M.V.B., M.R.C.V.S.

The Pathophysiology of Dermatologic Diseases of Food-Producing Animals

PETER C. MULLOWNEY, M.V.B., M.R.C.V.S.

Although skin diseases of food-producing animals have received relatively little attention in veterinary education, they can be economically significant.

Heavy louse infestation in cattle causes skin irritation and scratching, which leads to restlessness, damage to hides, and loss of weight gain or milk production. Cattle heavily infested with sucking lice may develop fatal anemia. Losses due to lice infestation in the U.S amount to more than $30 to $50 million annually. Lesions of demodectic mange, although often insignificant to the animal, cause pinpoint holes in the hide and markedly decrease its value.

In commercial cattle feedlots, psoroptic mange was found to cause a reduction in daily feed consumption of 21.5 per cent and a decrease in weight gain of 0.15 kg/head/day. More heavily infested cattle lost 70 kg in the course of the infestation and required 100 additional days feeding at an increased cost of $45 to restore weight losses. When treated with toxaphene, cattle must be withheld from slaughter for 28 days, thus adding to feed costs. Accidents with pesticides may result in losses owing to organophosphate toxicity. Infested cattle are more prone to respiratory problems and often sustained injuries during dipping. Hides damaged by infested mite wounds bring lower prices. The constant pruritus causes animals to rub against fence posts and housing, damaging these structures.

Damage to hides and the resulting carcass trimming at slaughter caused by warble fly larvae were responsible for a loss of $192 million in 1960. Screwworm infestations were responsible for a further $100 million loss.[1]

Sarcoptic mange in swine is of worldwide importance because of its ability to arrest growth rate and reduce feed efficiency. Severely affected animals are often anemic, which can result in lower conception rates and reproductive problems in gilts and sows.

Other skin diseases may have an effect on production and feed efficiency. Greasy pig disease can cause death in young pigs and can markedly reduce weight gain in pigs up to eight weeks of age. Swine vesicular disease and foot-and-mouth disease can lead to slaughtering of the whole herd to control the spread of the disease. Contagious ecthyma (or orf) markedly interferes with rate of weight gain in lambs and kids.

ANATOMY OF THE INTEGUMENT

The skin serves as an anatomic and physiologic barrier between the animal and its environment. It provides protection from physical, chemical, and microbiologic injury, and its sensory components enable the animal to perceive heat, cold, pain, touch, and pressure. It is important in heat regulation and in the deeper layers acts as an important fat storage depot, which provides the animal with insulation. It is also involved in the synthesis of vitamin D by the ultraviolet light conversion of 7-dehydrocholecalciferol to cholecalciferol within the sebaceous glands. In food animals, skin is also an important by-product that is used in the manufacture of leather. The hair covering the skin plays an important role in decreasing exposure of the skin to noxious agents and in insulation and is a most valuable by-product in the sheep and Angora goat.

The skin is composed of two major layers—the outer layer (or epidermis) and the inner layer (or dermis). The epidermis is made up of five layers: the horny layer (or stratum corneum); the clear layer (or stratum lucidum), found only in nonhairy areas; the granular layer (or stratum granulosum); the prickle layer (or stratum spinosum); and the basal layer (or stratum basale).[2]

Epidermal appendages consist of sebaceous glands, apocrine sweat glands, merocrine sweat glands, hair, hooves, and horns. Beneath the epidermis is the dermis (or corium), and beneath this is the hypodermis (or subcutis), where the adipose stores can accumulate. The stratum corneum consists of anuclear, completely keratinized cells that are in the process of being exfoliated. This layer may be up to 30 cells thick. Lipid is formed on and between the squamae of the outer two-thirds of the stratum corneum. The absence of sudanophilic staining in the lower corneum, the living epidermis, and the sweat gland; the presence of a continuous column of lipid from the sebaceous gland duct to the interfollicular stratum corneum; and the fact that surface lipid composition closely resembles that of sebum indicate that the sebaceous gland is the major source of this material. Lipid is also present on the surface of hairs both within the hair follicle and on the hair shaft above the epidermis. This may provide a nutrient media for lipophilic microorganisms.[3]

The protective properties of the outer layers of the

epidermis are probably due to the inertness and cohesiveness of the cornified cells, the hydrophobic and antimicrobial properties of the skin surface lipid, and the activity of soluble proteins including immunoglobulins derived from sweat. The intact skin is highly resistant to infection by microorganisms, but the superficial stratum corneum is readily damaged. Wetting and increased humidity are known to result in swelling and disruption of the stratum corneum and loosening of the attachments between its cell layers. Disruption and removal of the outer layers of the corneum has also been shown to result from treatment with organic solvents.[3]

The basal layer (stratum basale) is a single row of columnar to cuboidal cells resting on the basement membrane and separating the epidermis from the dermis. Most of the cells are keratinocytes, but a few are melanocytes. Melanocytes are responsible for pigmenting the skin by forming melanin. In areas of white skin there is not a decreased number of melanocytes; the melanocytes produce less melanin. Animals with nonpigmented skin are more susceptible to squamous cell carcinoma and photosensitization because melanin protects the skin from ultraviolet radiation. In albino animals, the melanocytes fail to form melanin because of a congenital absence of tyrosinase. The kernatinocytes are continually reproducing and pushing upward to replenish the epidermal cells above and are ultimately shed as dead horny cells. They produce the dead fibrous protein, keratin, which is the main constituent of the outermost horny layer of the skin.[2]

There are two types of keratin: soft keratin, which forms the epidermal horny layer, and hard keratin, which forms the outer layer of hairs, hooves, and horns. In the process of keratinization, the keratohyaline granules form an intercellular cement substance high in lipoprotein but low in sulfur that cements the tonofibrils of adjacent keratinocytes of the epidermal horny layer together. This substance is called the glycocalyx. Keratin containing high amounts of glycocalyx is soft keratin. It also contains phospholipids and cholesterol. Hard keratin of the hair and claws is relatively free of glycocalyx.[4]

The major function of the dermis is to support and nourish the epidermis and its appendages. It consists of collagen bundles, ground substance, and dermal cells.

Cutaneous asthenia, dermatosparaxis (or Ehlers-Danlos syndrome), has been reported in the bovine and is related to a defect in enzyme production rather than to production of abnormal collagen. This results in fragmented, shortened collagen bundles that lack uniformity of size and orientation. This causes hyperelasticity of skin and articular ligaments, cutaneous fragility, and delayed healing of skin wounds.[5]

The dermal cells are mainly fibroblasts, mast cells, and histiocytes. Fibroblasts are responsible for formation of the ground substance and collagen. Mast cells are degranulated in response to tissue injury and histamine, heparin, and proteases released. Histamine is associated with allergic states and anaphylaxis and causes vasodilation and wheals as a result of increased extravasation of fluids from the capillaries into the extracellular fluid space. Heparin acts as an anticoagulant to prevent formation of thrombi. This enhances removal of extravasated blood by lymphocytes or by phagocytosis by connective tissue macrophages. Histiocytes are derived from blood monocytes and are also called wandering macrophages. They are responsible for phagocytosis of bacteria and particulate matter.[2]

The hypodermis functions to store fat, acts as heat insulation, and supports the overlying dermis and epidermis to give body contour.[6]

Sebaceous glands are simple alveolar holocrine glands that appear as evaginations of the hair follicle. Sebum production is increased by small doses of androgens and decreased by large doses of estrogens. Underproduction of sebum (asteatosis) leads to a dull coat, whereas overproduction of sebum (seborrhea) produces hairs covered with fatty flakes similar to bran. An excess of sebum production is seen in exudative epidermitis of pigs.

The sweat glands are simple tubular structures. There are two general types—merocrine and apocrine. The merocrine tubular glands are the primary sweat glands of man but are found only on the carpus of pigs and in the nasolabial area of pigs and ruminants. The apocrine tubular gland is the predominant sweat gland in domestic animals. In ruminants, rather than being coiled, it is straight and dilated and appears duct shaped. Sweat glands serve as a cooling mechanism for the body as well as an excretory organ. The secretory product is mostly water, which is slightly alkaline. In domestic animals except for the horse, the secretion is scant and rarely perceptible. The activity of the sweat glands is controlled by the sympathetic nervous system and is usually a reflection of body temperature but may also be affected by excitement and pain. Localized areas of abnormal sweating may arise from peripheral nerve lesions or obstruction of sweat glands.

Hair covers almost the entire body in food animals and is a flexible, keratinized structure produced by the hair follicle. The distal (or free) part of the hair above the surface of the skin is the hair shaft. The part within the hair follicle is the hair root, which has a hollow terminal knob. The hair bulb is attached to a dermal papilla, which ensures the close association of the vascular bed with the rapidly growing epidermis in this region. The hair shaft is composed of three layers: an outer cuticle, a cortex of densely packed keratinized cells, and a medulla of loose cuboidal or flattened cells. The pattern of the surface of the cuticular cells, together with the cellular arrangement of the medulla, is characteristic for each species. The hair (or fleece) of sheep is referred to as fibers. There are three types of fiber: (1) wool fibers, tightly crimped fibers of small diameter lacking a medulla; (2) kemp fibers, which are coarse and have a characteristic medulla; and (3) coarse hairy fibers of intermediate size relative to wool and kemp fibers. The various breeds of sheep produce wools with different ratios of these fibers, and these wools are utilized for different purposes. This also makes some breeds more susceptible to skin conditions such as fleece rot.[4] The character of the wool fiber may vary with changes in the internal environment. In copper deficiency, the crimp of the fine wool fibers is lost and the wool becomes straight and steely.

The epidermal cells at the apex of the dermal papilla give rise to cortical cells and cuticular cells. The cells at the depths of the epidermal pegs give rise to the inner root sheath, whereas more laterally located cells give rise to the outer root sheath. The growth of a hair is achieved by apposition of new cells from the depths of the follicle. The hair pigment is derived from the epidermal melanocytes, located over the dermal papillae. A paleness of pigmented skin and hair may be noted with copper deficiency and molybdenum poisoning, following burns and freeze branding, and during recovery from zinc deficiency.

The normal growth and shedding of hairs occurs in cycles that are influenced by the photoperiod. A complete hair cycle consists of three stages—anagen, catagen, and telogen. Anagen is the period within the cycle during which hair growth is accomplished. Catagen is the transitory stage that occurs before the resting, or telogen, phase. The hair coat reflects the state of health and disease of the animal. Many disease conditions are characterized by a lusterless or dull hair coat; the cuticular cells are not flattened against the cortex, and thus light is not reflected normally.

Part of the hair coat is shed every spring, and regrowth commences in the fall. A delay in changing the coat is a sign of a disorder in hair growth that may be associated with chronic conditions affecting the respiratory or digestive systems or chronic nutritional deficiency.

SKIN LESIONS

The description of lesions and the depth at which they occur may aid the clinician and pathologist in determining the diagnosis. The presence or absence of pruritus is most important in the differential diagnosis.

The identification and differentiation of lesions are important in the diagnosis. Lesions should be recognized as either primary or secondary. A primary lesion is one that develops spontaneously, whereas a secondary lesion evolves from a primary lesion or is caused by trauma or medication. Lesions should be described according to distribution, arrangement, configuration, depth, consistency, quality, and color. Primary lesions consist of macules, papules, pustules, nodules, tumors, vesicles and wheals.

A macule is defined as a circumscribed flat spot up to 1 cm in size characterized by change in color of the skin. Patches and echymoses are similar to macules but are larger than 1 cm in diameter. A petechia is a pinpoint-sized macule, and purpura is a type of macule caused by bleeding into the skin.

A papule is a small solid elevation of the skin up to 1 cm in diameter that can be palpated as a solid mass. A plaque is larger and is formed by the coalescence of several papules.

A nodule is a small circumscribed solid elevation larger than 1 cm in diameter that usually extends into the deeper layers of the skin.

A tumor is a neoplastic enlargement that may involve any structure of the skin or subcutaneous tissue. A cyst is an epithelium-lined cavity containing fluid or a solid material.

Pustules are small circumscribed elevations of the skin filled with pus, whereas abscesses are defined as demarcated fluctuant lesions resulting from a dermal or subcutaneous accumulation of pus.

Vesicles are sharply circumscribed elevations, smaller than 1 cm in diameter, of skin filled with clear free fluid that are rarely seen since they are fragile and transient. Vesicles larger than 1 cm in diameter are called bullae.

Secondary lesions are scales, crusts, scabs, ulcers, excoriation, lichenification, hyperpigmentation, comedo, hyperkeratosis, and fissures.[2]

Abnormal colorations of the skin, including jaundice, pallor, erythema, and the bluish color of gangrene, should also be noted.

Alopecia is defined as absence of hair from skin areas where it normally is present. Congenital alopecia has been reported in all food-producing animals. Alopecia can be due to either lesions in the follicle, which result in failure of the follicular epithelium to produce a hair fiber, or damage to the fiber itself, resulting from trauma or infectious processes such as ringworm.

Follicular alopecia may be temporary, as when due to severe systemic disease or nutritional deficiency. It can be permanent if scarring occurs following trauma or burns or following radiation or dermatitis. An irreversible alopecia known as *symmetrical alopecia* occurs in Holstein cattle. It is genetically determined but is not expressed until the animal is an adult.[5] The skin biopsy can be utilized to determine whether alopecia is permanent or temporary.

Hypertrichosis, which is an abnormal length of hair fiber, occurs congenitally and may also be acquired with hypophyseal tumors, undernutrition, or chronic debility. Hypotrichosis, or the presence of less than a normal amount of hair, has been reported in all domestic species as a congenital finding.[5]

PATHOLOGIC CHANGES IN THE SKIN

Skin biopsy and other diagnostic aids are extremely important in the diagnosis of dermatologic diseases of food animals but are not utilized as often as they should be.[7]

Skin biopsy for histologic, immunofluorescent, electron microscopic, parasitologic, virologic, and bacteriologic examination may not confirm a specific diagnosis but is frequently very useful in the elimination of other differential diagnoses. Poor sampling, in both the site selection and mechanical technique, limits the ability of the pathologist to interpret the section. The biopsy material should include abnormal, marginal, and normal skin. However, if the punch biopsy is used, normal skin should not be included to eliminate the possibility that incorrect orientation or trimming may omit the lesion from the face of the block sectioned. It is important to give full details of history, previous treatments, possible diagnosis, and differential diagnoses when the biopsy sample is submitted to a diagnostic laboratory. It is only when the clinician and pathologist develop good communication and an understanding for each other's difficulties that each can make a maximum contribution to the final diagnosis.[7]

Other diagnostic aids that should be considered are as follows:

1. Skin scraping for demonstration of external parasites and dermatophytes.

2. Bacterial and fungal culture. Numerous diseases of bacterial and fungal etiology can be diagnosed if care is taken to utilize media and culture conditions that allow the organisms to grow and that avoid overgrowth with nonpathogens.

3. Viral isolation from vesicles of vesicular skin disease.

4. Demonstration of rising antibody titer to viral antigens.

5. Allergy testing is not as significant in large animals as in small animals owing to the very large number of possible allergens to which large animals are exposed. Patch testing may, however, be useful in the confirmation of contact allergy.[8]

6. Cytologic examination by aspiration or impression smear is useful in the diagnosis of several conditions.

7. Autoimmune skin diseases probably occur in food animals as they do in the horse and small animals, but reagents are not readily available for testing for these conditions.

8. The use of the Wood's lamp is of limited usefulness in the diagnosis of ringworm in food animals, as *Trichophyton* sp. and several pathogenic *Microsporum* sp. do not fluoresce.

HAIR ANALYSIS

Analysis of hair for confirmation of trace element deficiencies or molybdenosis is carried out by some laboratories. Several laboratories conduct hair analyses and make dietary recommendations based on these analyses. Utilization of hair or a biopsy material for this purpose is controversial. A large portion of clean hair must be submitted. Normal values for the bovine are 6.6–10.4 mg copper/kg, 90–140 mg zinc/kg, 8–20 mg manganese/kg, over 5 mg iron/kg, over 0.05 mg cobalt/kg, and less than 0.3 mg molybdenum/kg.[9]

The mineral content of hair is affected by season, breed, hair color within and between breeds, sire, age, and body location. Seasonal effects may be due to stage of hair growth and changes caused by perspiration, surface contamination, and diet. Hair from young animals may be lower in zinc, manganese, and iron but is higher in sodium, calcium, copper, and potassium than is hair from older animals. Pigmented hair is higher in calcium, magnesium, potassium, and sodium than white hair, but trace mineral concentrations are similar in hair of different colors. The effect of body location or mineral content may be due to differences in surface contamination, hair growth cycles and hair texture. Concentrations of calcium, phosphorus, and copper in hair are not affected by dietary intake of these minerals. Zinc and selenium concentrations in hair may reflect dietary intake. Hair analysis has also been used to assess exposure to arsenic, lead, and cadmium.[10]

References

1. Mullowney, P. C.: Dermatologic diseases of cattle. Part I. Parasitic diseases. Comp. Cont. Ed. Pract. Vet. *3*:S334–S344, 1981.
2. Muller, G. H., Kirk, R. W., and Scott, D. W.: Small Animal Dermatology, 3rd ed. W. B. Saunders Co., Philadelphia, 1983.
3. Lloyd, D. H., Dick, W. D. B., and Jenkinson, D. M.: Structure of the epidermis in Ayrshire bullocks. Res. Vet. Sci. *26*:172–179, 1979.
4. Calhoun, M. L., and Stinson, A. W.: Integument. *In* Dellman, H. D., and Brown, E. M. (eds.): Textbook of Veterinary Histology, 2nd ed. Lea & Febiger, Philadelphia, 1981, 378–411.
5. Mullowney, P. C.: Dermatologic diseases of cattle. Part III. Environmental, congenital, neoplastic and allergic diseases. Comp. Cont. Ed. Pract. Vet. *4*:S138–S150, 1982.
6. Banks, W. J.: Applied Veterinary Histology. Williams & Wilkins. Baltimore, 1981, 341–372.
7. McGavin, M. D., and Fadok, V. A.: Factors limiting the usefulness of histopathological examination of skin biopsies. Vet. Clin. North Am. *6*:203–213, 1984.
8. Byars, D. T.: Allergic skin disease in the horse. Vet. Clin. North Am. *6*:87–90, 1984.
9. Rosenberger, G.: Clinical Examination of Cattle, 2nd ed. Verlag Paul Pavey, Berlin, 1977.
10. Combs, D. K., Goodrich, R. D., and Meiske, J. C.: Mineral concentrations in hair as indicators of mineral status: A review. J. Anim. Sci. *54*:391–398, 1982.

Ticks Commonly Infesting Livestock

PETE D. TEEL, Ph.D., R. P. E.

Ticks utilize livestock as a blood source and are present in such species diversity and numbers that they diminish animal health and production in many areas of the U.S. Tick feeding results in severe irritation and accompanying blood loss. Infested animals reduce their feed intake and may experience weight loss. Lesions produced by feeding ticks predispose animals to secondary infection and myiasis. The importance of ticks is further punctuated by their transmission of rickettsiae, spirochaetes, haemoprotozoae, and viruses to livestock.

Both hard ticks (Ixodidae) and soft ticks (Argasidae) attack livestock, and knowledge of their biologies is fundamental to control strategies. General information on the distribution, hosts, and predilection feeding sites on host animals is summarized in Table 1. Most hard ticks and some soft ticks, such as *Otobius megnini,* feed for long periods (days to weeks) on their hosts as immature or adult ticks, enabling on-animal applications of ectoparasiticides for effective control. There are many other tick species (not listed in Table 1) that attack wild animals and birds that may be found parasitizing livestock, however not normally in such numbers or for sufficient time to justify on-animal use of acaricides. The pajaroello tick, *Ornithodoros coriaceus,* for example, attack deer and cattle in animal bedding grounds and is believed to be the vector of epizootic bovine abortion in California. With the exception of larvae that feed for seven days, this multihost tick feeds only for short periods (15 to 30 minutes), limiting the effectiveness of any conventional on-animal acaricide treatment.

Several acaricides have been approved for use on livestock by the Environmental Protection Agency. Properly applied, these acaricides can provide a safe means of reducing a tick infestation on the host and offer a degree of protection against re-infestation. The active compounds and delivery systems now available provide some flexibility in application intervals and methods depending on the tick species. Most tick species feed indiscriminately on livestock (see Table 1), attaching to the axillae, tail head, udder/scrotum, and dewlap, making it necessary to treat the entire body via a spray or dip. Tables 1 and 2 can be used as indexes for selecting appropriate treatments for the subject livestock and tick species.* Certain species are predisposed to feeding on the ears of livestock animals: *Amblyomma maculatum, Otobius megnini,* and *Dermacentor (Anocentor) nitens.* Cattle ear tags or tapes and

---

*Mention of a tradename does not constitute endorsement or warranty by the author or Texas A&M University.

Table 1. *Partial List of Ticks That Parasitize Livestock in the U.S.*

Tick Species	Generalized Life Cycle	Principal Hosts	Feeding Areas on Domestic Hosts	Distribution
Lone star tick (*Amblyomma americanum*)	3-host	Cattle, horses, dogs, and man as well as a wide variety of birds and wild mammals	Indiscriminant (all areas of the body subject to attack)	Southern and southeastern U.S.
Cayenne tick (*Amblyomma cajennense*)	3-host	Cattle, horses, sheep, goats, and dogs as well as wild birds and mammals	Indiscriminant	Southern Texas
Gulf Coast tick (*Amblyomma maculatum*)	3-host	Adults: cattle, sheep, deer, and coyotes Immatures: ground-dwelling birds and small mammals	Outer portion of cattle ears	Gulf States north through Oklahoma to southeastern Kansas
Cattle tick (*Boophilus annulatus*)*	1-host	Cattle, horses, sheep, goats, dogs, and deer	Indiscriminant	Southern Texas and Mexico
Tropical cattle tick (*Boophilus microplus*)*	1-host	Cattle, horses, sheep, goats, dogs, and deer	Indiscriminant	Southern Texas and Mexico
Winter tick (*Dermacentor albipictus* [In synonymy with *D. nigrolineatus*])	1-host	Horses, mules, cattle, elk, deer, and moose	Indiscriminant	Southern, southwestern, and northwestern regions of U.S.
Rocky Mt. wood tick (*Dermacentor andersoni*)	3-host	Adults: cattle, horses, dogs, man, elk, deer, and other wild mammals Immatures: small mammals	Indiscriminant	Rocky Mts. from northern New Mexico to Canada, eastern slopes of the Cascade and Sierra Nevada Mts.
Pacific Coast tick (*Dermacentor occidentalis*)	3-host	Adults: cattle, horses, sheep, dogs, man, and deer Immatures: many species of small mammals	Indiscriminant	Oregon and California, western slopes of the Cascade and Sierra Nevada Mts.
Tropical horse tick (*Dermacentor (Anocentor) nitens*)	1-host	Equines	Outer ear	Coastal regions of states from southern Texas to Florida and Georgia
American dog tick (*Dermacentor variabilis*)	3-host	Adults: prefer canines; will feed on man, cattle, and horses Immatures: small rodents	Indiscriminant	Texas to Montana and east to the Atlantic; also Pacific seaboard from Washington to California
Blacklegged tick (*Ixodes scapularis*)	3-host	Adults: cattle, horses, sheep, swine, man, and deer Immatures: small mammals and birds	Indiscriminant	Eastern, central, and southern U.S.
Spinose ear tick (*Otobius megnini*)	Modified 1-host	Immatures: cattle, horses, sheep, cats, dogs, rabbits, elk, and mountain sheep	Inner portion of outer ear	Western and southwestern U.S.

*Ticks suspected of being *Boophilus annulatus* or *B. microplus* should be reported to state animal health agencies and/or USDA, APHIS, Veterinary Services officials. State and federal regulations require quarantine and eradication procedures for these species.

Table 2. *Partial List of Acaricides Approved for Tick Control*

Acaricide	Strength of Final Preparation			
	Spray	*Dip*	*Ear Device*	*Other*
Coumaphos (Co-Ral, Bay Vet, Haver-Lockhart)	0.125%*, ‡, §	0.125*, §		30% spray foam and 50% dust for ear application*, ‡
Crotoxyphos (Ciodrin, SDS Biotech)	1.0%* 0.25%†, §			
Dioxathion (Delnav, NoRAM, Cooper)	0.15%*, ‡	0.15%*, ‡		
Dioxathion and Diclorvos (Lintox-D, Stauffer Chem. Corp.)	0.11%*, ‡			
Fenvalerate[1] (Ectrin, Diamond Shamrock, SDS Biotech)	0.05%*		0.8% ear tag*	
Flucythrinate (Guardian, American Cyanamid Co.)			7.5% ear tag*	
Lindane				3.5% aerosol for ear application*, ‡
Permethrin[1] (Atroban, Cooper, Wellcome Animal Health, Inc.; Ectiban, ICI Americas, Inc.; Overtime, Bio Ceutic Labs., Inc.; Permectrin, Anchor Labs.)	0.0125%*, ‡		10.0% ear tag and ear tag tape*	

Notes: Symbols in the table denote the following species: beef cattle and nonlactating dairy cattle (*), lactating dairy cattle (†), horses (‡), and sheep and nonlactating goats (§). Read all labels closely for appropriate use of product and safety precautions.

aerosol formulations are available and offer labor-saving approaches to control these three species. It is necessary to treat both ears of the host with the selected treatment as opposed to single-ear application, which is recommended for fly control. The synthetic pyrethroids available in slow-release ear tag/tape devices are lipophilic and are distributed over the animal body through self-grooming. Their application can provide four to five months of ear tick control on cattle.

Safe use of acaricides is paramount to both the applicator as well as livestock. Before using any acaricide, read the label and follow directions for preparation, application, and clean up. In addition, note any specific requirements or precautions regarding use of the acaricide for the specific livestock species and breed. Manufacturers will note limitations on treating certain species. Some acaracides are not recommended for treatment of Brahman bulls and, in some cases, Brahman cattle. Limitations may also be given for lactating cattle and goats or nonlactating animals within a minimum number of days before freshening. Animal age limitations, application frequency, total number of applications, and withdrawal periods to slaughter should be noted. Check labels for precautions against concomitant administration of external and internal parasiticides where possible synergistic effects may produce toxicosis.

The list of acaricides in Table 2 is *not* comprehensive, and changes are periodically made by the EPA regarding current labels and availability of new and old products. In addition, other products or formulations may become available to specific states through special local need permits. Refer to product labels for current use and instructions.

Rapid livestock marketing and transportation enables ticks to be moved great distances, therefore it is not uncommon to find these parasites outside of their normal geographic distribution. Surveillance and identification of ticks infesting livestock are important for adoption of appropriate control measures as well as identification of foreign species that may be introduced into the U.S. Producers, veterinarians, extension personnel, and others can assist in a National Tick Surveillance Program by sending ticks to their State Animal Health Organization or to the National Veterinary Services Laboratory, USDA, APHIS, P. O. Box 844, Shipping and Receiving, Ames, Iowa, 50010, for identification. Ticks should be placed in 80 per cent ethanol and labeled as to collection date, location, host, and collector.

Muscoid Flies of Range Cattle

DARRELL E. BAY, Ph.D., R. P. E.

The horn fly, *Haematobia irritans,* and the face fly, *Musca autumnalis,* are the two most common muscoid flies of cattle on pasture and rangeland throughout much of the United States. The face fly, however, introduced into the New England area in 1952, has not yet extended its range into the southwestern U.S. Although both species are somewhat similar in appearance, the horn fly is approximately one-half the size of the face fly and may be further distinguished by its characteristic beak, or proboscis, carried anteriorly in saber-like fashion, whereas the larger face fly possesses a nonbiting, or sponging, mouthpart. Identification may also be facilitated by distinctive behavioral attributes of each species. Both sexes of the horn fly ordinarily remain on a host continuously, although feeding occurs only intermittently; individuals usually cluster on the sides and back of cattle, over which they swarm when disturbed. A characteristic resting position with the head pointed downward is frequently assumed except when congregation on the underside on an animal occurs during hot or rainy weather. Female face flies, on the other hand, gather about the head where they feed on secretions from the eyes and muzzle as well as on blood oozing from open wounds and the bites of other insects. Both of these species frequently may be confused with house flies, *Musca domestica,* and/or stable flies, *Stomoxys calcitrans;* however, populations of the latter two insects are usually associated with livestock in dry lot or feedlot operations rather than rangeland.

ECONOMIC IMPACT

Although both sexes of the horn fly are obligatory blood feeders, daily blood loss for an animal infested with a population of 500 flies is estimated to be only 7 ml/day. Economic losses attributable to this pest, therefore, are probably due primarily to annoyance and irritation, which may be subsequently manifested in decreased weight gain and/or milk production. Calves weaned from infested dams, for example, have been reported to weigh an average of 5.5 kg less than those from treated dams. The horn fly is also an intermediate host of *Stephanofilaria stilesi,* a filarid worm responsible for producing a circumscribed dermatitis along the midventral line of cattle.

Female face flies are incapable of taking a blood meal directly owing to the nature of their mouthparts; however, this species is also responsible for considerable host annoyance and irritation as a result of its characteristic feeding behavior around the eyes, lips, and nostrils. Face flies occur on animals only when they are outdoors; darkened buildings and other similar areas are avoided by the flies. Male face flies feed on pollen produced by flowering vegetation, which they frequent, and are not found in direct association with an animal host. Protective and evasive actions of cattle undoubtedly reduce milk flow and/or weight gains. More importantly, however, face flies are important mechanical vectors of the bacterium *Moraxella bovis,* which is responsible for bovine infectious keratoconjunctivitis (pinkeye), and the virus of infectious abortion. The species may also serve as an intermediate host of the eye worm, *Thelazia rhodesii.*

CONTROL

Successful control of horn flies and face flies involves the administration of EPA-approved insecticides by one or more of several recommended techniques. *Direct application* consists of applying an insecticide, usually of a residual nature, to an animal by a method such as spraying, dipping, or dusting. *Self-treatment devices,* such as dusting stations and oilers, provide control on a daily basis when situated and maintained properly. The use of *slow-release insecticides* impregnated into soft plastic devices such as ear tags is a fairly recent innovation that offers the potential for seasonal fly suppression. *Feed-through insecticides* or *oral larvicides* prevent the development of larval stages in the manure.

Direct Application. Since horn flies remain on cattle almost continuously, they may be controlled relatively easily by a program of regular host treatment (e.g., spraying, dipping) with approved WP or EC formulations of residual insecticides mixed with water (Table 1). Mist or low-pressure spray applications of 1 to 2 quarts of material per animal are usually sufficient for horn fly control. Care should be exercised, however, to ensure uniform coverage. In addition, certain pour-on applications of materials recommended for cattle grub and louse control are also effective against horn flies. Treatment should be initiated in the early spring when fly populations reach 50 to 100 per head and continued at intervals, based upon population resurgences, throughout the duration of the fly season.

The achievement of adequate face fly control, on the other hand, is difficult at best since this species spends a significant amount of time away from the host. Moreover, when present on cattle, face flies congregate on the face, a location difficult to treat. Direct spray applications, therefore, are generally regarded to be ineffective against this species.

Self-Treatment Devices. The use of self-applicatory devices (e.g., dust bags, oilers) offers a convenient method of horn fly control and also aids in the control of face flies when such devices permit contact with the face. Dust bags are usually purchased ready-to-use (see Table 1). Insecticide formulations for backrubbers and/or facerubbers (see Table 1) must be mixed with No. 2 diesel fuel or a

Table 1. *Suggested Insecticides for Muscoid Fly Control on Range Cattle**

Insecticides	Manufacturer	Strength of Finished Preparation		
		Spray	Dust	Oiler
Coumaphos (Co-Ral)	Haver-Lockhart	0.06%	1.0%	1.0%
Crotoxyphos (Ciodrin)	Shell Animal Health	1.0%	3.0%	1.0%
Dichlorvos (Vapona)	Shell Animal Health	1.0%		
Dioxathion (Delnav)	Cooper Corporation	0.15%		1.5%
Famphur (Warbex)	American Cyanamid		1.0%	
Malathion		0.5%	5.0%	2.0%
Methoxychlor (Marlate)	E.I. DuPont de Nemours & Co., Inc.	0.5%	10.0%	5.0%
Permethrin (Ectiban)	ICI Americas, Inc., Agricultural Chemicals Division	0.015%	0.25%	0.15%
Ronnel (Korlan)	Dow Chemical	0.5%		1.0%
Stirofos (Rabon)	Shell Animal Health	0.35%	3.0%	

*Read the label closely to determine appropriateness of a product. Some materials should not be used on lactating dairy cattle; others require specific preslaughter intervals.

Table 2. *Pyrethroid Insecticide Ear Tags for Muscoid Fly Control on Range Cattle*

Trade Name	Manufacturer	Attachment System
8% Fenvalerate (10 gm/tag)	Diamond Shamrock	Allflex
Ectrin Insecticide Ear Tag	Diamond Shamrock	Allflex
Purina Insecti-Shield Cattle Ear Tag	Diamond Shamrock	Allflex
Moorman's Ear Tag Plus	Diamond Shamrock/Zoecon	Temple
Starbar Insecticide Cattle Ear Tag	Diamond Shamrock	Allflex
Great Plains Chemical "Vet Shack" Insecticide Ear Tag		
10% Permethrin (9.5 gm/tag except Anchor Tag @ 11.5 gm)	Burroughs-Wellcome	Allflex
Cooper Atroban Insecticide Ear Tag	Burroughs-Wellcome	Allflex
Purina Insecti-Gard Insecticide Ear Tag	Burroughs-Wellcome	Allflex
Coop Insecticide Ear Tag	Y-Tex	Y-Tex
Gard-Star Insecticide Ear Tag	Fearing	Fearing
Fearing Insecticide Ear Tag	Anchor	Allflex
Anchor Permectrin Ear Tag		

special backrubber oil; motor oil should be avoided, as toxic products therein may produce irritation.

Since the degree of control is closely associated with the frequency of application, self-treatment devices must be situated so that cattle are forced to utilize them. Recommended locations are near, although not directly over, mineral or salting stations, over gates leading into watering areas, along alley ways, and in loafing areas. Regular maintenance is essential to ensure such devices are charged and in proper working order. Face fly control may be enhanced by lowering dust bags and oilers after animals have become accustomed to them as well as constructing oilers with suspended flaps at least 12 inches in length. Additionally, salt or mineral holders equipped with dust bags or oilers such that the face of the animal contacts the material during feeding may be constructed or purchased.

Insecticide-Impregnated Ear Tags. The use of slow-release insecticides impregnated into plastic ear tags or tapes is a fairly recent innovation in the control of horn flies and face flies. Presently available ear tags contain 13.7 per cent stirofos (Rabon), 10 per cent chlorpyrifos (Dursban*), or one of the newly approved synthetic pyrethroids, fenvalerate or permethrin, sold under various trade names (Table 2). In addition to providing season-long fly control, such tags are also effective against spinous ear ticks (*Otobius megnini*) and Gulf Coast ticks (*Amblyomma maculatum*). Although published reports exist of horn fly control in herds with only 10 to 20 per cent of the animals tagged, current recommendations are for one or two such tags per head. Face fly control is generally unsatisfactory with only one tag per head, but 50 to 70 per cent control has been obtained with a pyrethroid tag in each ear. Control failures have generally been the result of loss or breakage, particularly in heavy brush, although recent reports suggest the development of resistance that may seriously jeopardize future usefulness.

Oral Larvicides. Oral larvicides, or feed-through insecticides, operate by passing through the animal's digestive tract to kill fly larvae in the feces. Phenothiazine may be fed in salt or mineral supplements to control both horn flies and face flies; it also aids in the control of certain helminthes. Rabon oral larvicide is available as either a feed premix or a mineral mix in loose or block form and is also labeled for both horn fly and face fly control.

Methoprene (Altosid*), an insect growth regulator (IGR) labeled only for horn fly control, is available in loose mineral or mineral block form.

As with self-treatment devices, oral larvicides require a minimum of human labor. Performance in the laboratory has generally been excellent; however, fly control in the field is often less than satisfactory since not all animals in the herd consume the product at a uniform rate. Augmentation by more traditional control measures therefore may be required.

Supplemental Reading

Beadles, M. L., Ginrich, A. R., and Miller, J. A.: Slow-release devices for livestock insect control: cattle body surfaces contacted by five types of devices. J. Econ. Entomol. 70:72–75, 1977.
Bruce, W. G.: The history and biology of the horn fly, *Haematobia irritans* (Linneaus); with comments on control. N. C. Agric. Exp. Stn. Tech. Bull. No. 157, 1964, 32.
Harvey, T. L., and Brethour, J. R.: Effect of horn flies on weight gains of beef cattle. J. Econ. Entomol. 72:516–518, 1976.
Teskey, H. J.: A review of the life history and habits of *Musca autumnalis* DeGeer (Diptera:Muscidae). Can. Entomol. 92:360–367, 1960.

*Available from Zoecon Corp., Dallas, Texas 75234.

Fly Infestations

J. P. SMITH, D.V.M., M.S.

CULICOIDES

Culicoides ("punkies," "no-see-ums," "gnats," "moose flies," "biting midges") comprise at least 80 species recorded from all major land areas of the world. Morphologically they are among the smallest of the hematophagous flies (measuring 0.5–5.0 mm in length), which easily pass through screens that exclude mosquitoes. Preferred breeding sites are springs, streams, shorelines of lakes, and tidal marshlands. Female flies deposit their eggs in moist manure, wet hay, mud, and compost. Larvae remain viable for weeks or even months when completely submerged during flooding. Some species maintain uniform numbers throughout the warm months, whereas others exhibit two peak population periods, one in the spring and one in the fall. Adult flies are not strong fliers, and dispersal rarely exceeds 8 km (5 miles). Dispersal

*Available from Ft. Dodge Laboratories, Fort Dodge, Iowa 50501.

may be enhanced, however, by wind currents, and pupae of intertidal species may be translocated great distances by water currents.

Adults feed most actively during the evening, night, and early morning hours. Adult activity is reduced at temperatures below 13° C (55° F) and wind velocities above 5 miles per hour. Species attack both man and animals including birds, reptiles, and certain amphibians. Although some species have been collected only from mammals, others show a marked preference for birds. Host specificity is not a marked characteristic.

ECONOMIC IMPORTANCE

The bite is extremely painful, and dermatologic effects (rashes, wheals, and so on) often persist for longer periods than mosquito bites. In addition, the blood-sucking habits of *Culicoides* make them potential vectors of several livestock diseases. *Culicoides* are successful vectors for *Onchocerca* spp. in horses and cattle. The virus of blue tongue is transmitted by *Culicoides* spp. in many livestock regions of the world including the United States. *Culicoides* is a suspect vector of ephemeral fever in cattle, and outbreaks of fowl pox have been associated with large populations of *Culicoides*.

PREVENTION AND CONTROL

In some situations long-term control directed toward destruction of breeding sites has been successful. Mosquito abatement programs are usually successful against *Culicoides*.

STOMOXYS CALCITRANS

General Morphology and Biology

Stomoxys calcitrans ("stable fly," "biting house fly") is widely distributed throughout the livestock-producing areas of the world. Morphologically, stable flies are similar to and often mistaken for the common house fly, *Musca domestica;* the former may be readily identified by its saber-like mouthparts, or proboscis. Stable flies can be distinguished from horn flies, *Haematobia irritans,* by their larger size. The lower extremities and flanks of the host appear to be the preferred feeding sites.

Stable flies are day-biting flies and both sexes suck blood; however, they are in direct association with a host only during the process of feeding. In temperate regions fly abundance peaks during the warm months. The greatest fly density is found in close proximity to suitable breeding sites.

Economic Importance

Although there are no established values for effects that stable flies have on production, there is widespread agreement that they are the most important pest of dairy cattle and are economically important pests of beef cattle in total or partial confinement. Cattle response to this "parasitic worry" is reflected in decreased milk production and weight loss. In addition, the wounds inflicted by the feeding fly bleed freely, creating an attraction for other muscid flies and the screwworm fly.

Frequent changes of hosts during a single blood meal make the stable fly an excellent mechanical vector of anthrax and trypanosomiasis ("surra").

Prevention and Control

Practices to control stable flies, especially in dairy cattle, are controversial. The advantages (i.e., net returns) are not always significant when cows have access to a liberal supply of supplemental feed and a high-energy ration. Economic thresholds have been determined to be approximately 25 flies per animal per day. The most satisfactory control of stable fly populations results from using effective control practices incorporated in an integrated pest management (IPM) program.

Successful IPM programs make use of various combinations of the following control measures. The choice(s) may be dictated by current management practices.

Insecticides. Residual and area sprays are applied to resting areas to control adults and to breeding sites to control larval maturation. Insecticides are applied directly to the host. Residual sprays appear to be the most efficient chemical control method with respect to adult fly kill and the period of effectiveness on the premises where animals are in continuous confinement. Area sprays should be considered when animals have access to pasture and briefly visit pens and barns, as adult flies may be widely dispersed resting on vegetation in fields adjacent to confinement premises.

Feed Additives. Currently larvicidal feed additives have not been very successful primarily because strong fly populations may develop in areas other than in manure piles. Favorable stable fly control has been noted when mineral blocks containing 0.94 per cent methoprene were offered to cattle free choice. Experimental doses given to cattle at 20 µg/kg/day with an avermectin resulted in greater than 90 per cent kill of stable fly larvae in manure.

Insect Growth Regulators and Juvenile Hormone Mimics. An insect growth regulator, diflubenzuron 1.0 per cent, sprayed on adult resting sites may reduce egg hatch and larval development by 80 per cent. When applied as a water-soluble liquid, effective control may last up to six weeks, whereas wettable powder formulations have less residual properties. Juvenile hormone mimics are still in the experimental stage. They may be mixed in the ration or sprayed on the surface of breeding sites. Juvenile hormones prevent emergence of adults from the pupal case and in some situations have been shown to be as effective as residual insecticides.

Attractant-Toxicants. Attractant-toxicants using baits and insecticide-impregnanted panels have given satisfactory levels of fly control in buildings and adjoining lots where cattle are confined. Other adjunct control measures of fly suppression when incorporated in IPM systems consist of sterile fly release and pupal parasites.

TABANID FLIES

Two genera of the family Tabanidae, *Tabanus* ("horse flies," "greenheads," "breeze flies") and *Chrysops* ("deer flies"), are economically important vectors of disease and pest flies of livestock and man.

General Morphology and Biology

Tabanids are large-bodied flies, 5 to 25 mm in length, with prominent, brightly colored eyes that project laterally. Adult females are blood suckers (males feed on plant nectar) and feed during late afternoon and evening hours. Populations are greatest during the warm summer months, and peak populations occur in the vicinity of favorable breeding sites, which are located along the flood plains of water courses. The larval stages develop in water-logged soils for several months before pupation. In the world temperate zones, there is usually one generation per year.

Economic Importance

Tabanids have been incriminated in the mechanical transmission of such important livestock diseases as anaplasmosis, anthrax, vesicular stomatitis, bovine leukemia, and surra. As biologic vectors, they may transmit the filarid worm *Elaeophora schneideri* to sheep and wild cervids.

The feeding habits of these voracious blood-sucking flies contribute heavily to livestock production losses. Their bites are painful and irritating. Significant weight loss and reduced milk production follow perpetual and unprotected attacks. Recent feeding sites that ooze blood predispose cattle to infestations by the primary screwworm. Blood loss, which in some cases may exceed 100 ml daily, is often imposed upon concurrent depletion resulting from gastrointestinal helminthiasis.

Prevention and Control

Tabanids are among the most difficult livestock insects to control. Insecticide applications, such as area or animal sprays, have met with limited success. The high concentrations and total amount of chemical pesticides necessary for satisfactory area sprays are environmentally hazardous. Synergized pyrethrins applied daily by backrubbers and automatic mist sprayers near mineral boxes and water supplies reduce fly populations when the equipment is kept in working condition. Water emulsion sprays of the synthetic pyrethroid permethrin 0.1 per cent give satisfactory fly kill for up to 14 days after treatment. Similar dust applications of permethrin 0.25 per cent give satisfactory fly kill for up to ten days post treatment.*

SIMULIUM spp.

Simulium spp. ("black flies," "buffalo gnats," "turkey gnats") are responsible for deaths of domesticated animals throughout the world. Attacks by these insects are especially important where suitable waterways exist for the immature developmental stages.

General Morphology and Biology

"Black flies" may be up to 5 mm in length and are characterized by a well-developed scutum on the thorax, appearing as a prominent "hump," hence the common term "buffalo gnats." Not all species are black, as some tropical species are shades of yellow and orange. "Black flies" are day-biting flies that congregate in huge swarms in close proximity to breeding sites such as swift, shallow, well-aerated waterways. Tropical and subtropical species successfully develop along large rivers. In northeastern Texas, Arkansas, Louisiana, and Mississippi, larval stages are periodically observed in enormous numbers clinging to underwater vegetation and debris during the winter months. The adult flies emerge during late winter and early spring and abruptly subside with warm weather.

Economic Importance

When feeding, "black flies" are vicious and persistent biters. Enormous numbers attack cattle, interrupting grazing behavior as hosts seek relief in any available shelter. Milk yield in dairy cattle may be reduced by 50 per cent, and lowered milk production in beef cattle is reflected in decreasing calf weaning weights. In Canada, swarms of "black flies" carried by favorable winds have killed cattle 140 miles from breeding sites near large rivers. Weight losses in pastured cattle may reach 1 kg (2.2 lb) per day during peaks of fly activity. Losses reported from Bowie County, Texas, in 1979 were estimated at $750,000.

Cattle exposed to "black fly" attack may suffer an acute disease syndrome characterized by a vesicular dermatitis and edema of the dewlap, brisket, and ventral abdominal wall. Udder and teat lesions may be severe, and range cows are reluctant to allow their calves to nurse. In beef herds, fatalities from massive fly attacks have been attributed to inhalation pneumonia from inhaled flies, generalized toxemia, and anemia, especially in young stock. Tolerance to "black fly" feeding has been observed in native cattle that have been previously exposed to the flies. In addition, some species serve as vectors of onchocerciasis in cattle and man and a hemoprotozoon *(Leucocytozoon)* infecting turkeys, ducks, and geese.

Prevention and Control

Aerial sprays with Abate* have been used successfully to suppress "black fly" numbers in Texas and Arkansas. In Canada, methoxychlor at 0.3 ppm injected into streams and rivers as a larvicidal agent was effective in reducing two-thirds of the target species 100 miles downstream from the point of injection. Ethanolic solutions of the synthetic pyrethroid permethrin at 2, 4, and 6 mg per kg body weight have been reported to have repellent effects, preventing 70 per cent of the flies from taking a blood meal from cattle for up to eight days. The repellent action of aqueous mixtures, as emulsifiable concentrates, and dusts are reportedly less effective.

STEPHANOFILARIA STILESI

Stephanofilariasis occurs worldwide and is referred to as "cascado" in Indonesia, "hump sore" in India, and "filarial sore" in Malaya. In the United States and Canada *Stephanofilaria stilesi* is the etiologic agent for a verminous dermatitis, the greatest prevalence of which is found in range cattle of the Southwest.

Biology

The adult filarid worm inhabits small cysts near the base of hair follicles in the epidermis of cattle. The female discharges live larvae, microfilariae, that concentrate in close proximity to the adult worms. The horn fly, *Haematobia irritans,* is the biologic vector. Ingestion of microfilariae and their development to the infective stage

---

*Note: The synthetic pyrethroids, when applied to livestock to control horse flies, reduce the time spent on the host, thus diminishing the blood meal. Fly mortality occurs after host contact.

---

*Available from American Cyanamid Co., Princeton, New Jersey 08540.

takes place within the horn fly while it feeds along the ventral abdominal wall. Infective larvae are present in the salivary glands of the fly 18 to 21 days following a blood meal. During subsequent blood meals infective larvae leave the fly and gain access to the skin tissues of the final host. Adult worms persist in the skin for two to three years before spontaneous remission takes place.

PATHOGENESIS

Lesions, single or multiple, may occur along the ventral abdominal wall from the brisket to the pubic region. Small pea-sized papules, often in close proximity, coalesce to form a single, large, hairless lesion. Developing lesions are deep red in color, and dermal crevices exude copious amounts of blood-tinged serum. Mature lesions are characterized by alopecia and hyperkeratosis covered with thick crusts and deep fissures. Pruritus is mild, but excoriation of the lesion from self-mutilation has been observed. Teat lesions may predispose the affected quarter to mastitis.

Diagnosis

A reasonably accurate diagnosis may be made on the basis of anatomic location and characteristic gross lesions. A definite diagnosis may be confirmed by observing adult worms or microfilariae in skin scrapings or skin biopsy. Several areas from the lesion should be sampled by first removing superficial crusts and scabs and scraping deeply enough to cause bleeding. A differential diagnosis should include the nematode *Pelodera strongyloides* (syn. *Rhabditis strongyloides*). *P. strongyloides,* more commonly associated with confined cattle, produces lesions characterized by hair loss, and the exposed skin is reddened and exudes serum. Various developmental stages of the worm may be observed in skin scrapings. From biopsy material cross sections of the uterus of *P. strongyloides* will reveal eggs, whereas microfilariae are observed in cross sections of the uterus of *S. stilesi.* The two parasites may occur concurrently.

Treatment

Effective anthelmintic agents are not yet commercially available. Benefit/cost ratios do not justify treatment in range cattle.

Prevention and Control

Effective measures to reduce the transmission and prevalence of this parasite depend on the effectiveness of the horn fly control program. The general health and performance of cattle are not noticeably affected by the parasite. Minor losses may be related to hide damage and trim. Active lesions attract flies, including the screwworm fly, and severe myiasis may contribute to substantial losses to the producer.

Supplemental Reading

Bay, D. E., et al.: Evaluation of a synthetic pyrethroid for tabanid control on horses and cattle. Southw. Ento. *1*:190–203, 1976.
Fredeen, F. J. H.: Controlling blackfly outbreaks. Can. Agric. *20*:15–17, 1975.
Graham, O. H.: Eradication programs for the arthropod parasites of livestock. J. Med. Ento. *13*:629–658, 1977.
Hall, R. D.: Stable fly, *Stomoxys calcitrans* (L.), breeding in large round hay bales: Initial associations (Diptera: Muscidae). J. Kan. Ento. Soc. *55*:617–620, 1982.
Hansens, E. J.: Review: Tabanidae of the east coast as an economic problem. N. Y. Ento. Soc. *LXXXVII*:312–318, 1979.
Hawkins, J. A.: Mechanical transmission of anaplasmosis by tabanids (Diptera: Tabanidae). Am. J. Vet. Res. *43*:732–734, 1982.
Jorgensen, N. M.: The systemics, occurrence, and host preference of *Culicoides* (Diptera: Ceratopogonidae) in southeastern Washington. Melanderia *3*:1–47, 1969.
Miller, J. A.: Larvicidal activity of Merck MK-933, an avermectin, against the horn fly, stable fly, face fly and house fly. J. Eco. Ento. *74*:608–611, 1981.
Ohshima, K.: Evidence on horizontal transmission of bovine leukemia virus due to bloodsucking tabanid flies. Jpn. J. Vet. Sc. *43*:79–81, 1981.
Shemanchuk, J. A.: Repellant action of permethrin, cypermethrin, and resmethrin against black flies (Diptera: Simuliidae) attacking cattle. Pestic. Res. *12*:412–416, 1981.
Smith, K. G. V.: Insects and Other Arthropods of Medical Importance. The Trustees of the British Museum (Natural History), London, 1973.
Soulsby, E. J. L.: Helminths, Arthropods and Protozoa of Domesticated Animals. 7th ed. Lea & Febiger, Philadelphia, 1982.
Steelman, C. D.: Effects of external and internal arthropod parasites on domestic livestock. Ann. Rev. Ento. *21*:155–178, 1976.
Stott, J. L.: Bluetongue virus in pregnant elk and their calves. Am. J. Vet. Res. *43*:423–428, 1982.
Wright, J. E.: Diflubenzuron: ovicidal activity against adult stable flies exposed to treated surfaces or to treat animals. Southw. Ento. *3*: 1978.

Myiasis

DARRELL E. BAY, Ph.D., R.P.E.

Myiasis is a term applied to the infestation of animal tissues or organs by dipterous (fly) larvae. As with other types of parasitism, myiasis may be classified as obligatory, in which the larva is dependent upon a host to successfully complete its developmental cycle, and facultative, in which the larva, although usually free-living, becomes associated with a host, usually in diseased tissue of the latter. Various descriptive terms have been used to define the localization of myiasis; however, in the present context, we will limit ourselves primarily to traumatic myiasis or the infestation of wounds by members of the families Calliphoridae (blow flies) and Sarcophagidae (flesh flies).

SCREWWORMS

The larva of the screwworm *Cochliomyia hominivorax* is an obligatory parasite of the family Calliphoridae that feeds on the healthy tissues of warm-blooded animals, including man, in subtropical regions of North and South America. Adult females characteristically deposit batches of 200 to 400 eggs in slightly overlapping rows, resulting in a shingle-like appearance, near wounds or, less frequently, in moist areas such as natural body openings. The navels of newborn cattle and many other large mammals are highly susceptible to infestation, as are wounds resulting from horns, barbed wire, and such routine ranching practices as castration, dehorning, and branding. Bites of other ectoparasitic arthropods such as horn flies, horse flies, and ticks are also predisposing factors. It has been estimated that as many as 85 per cent of cases of screwworm infestations in cattle during a recent resurgence in southern Texas occurred in the ears as a result of previous infestations by Gulf Coast ticks, *Amblyomma maculatum.*

Embryonic incubation occurs fairly rapidly, and eggs usually hatch within 12 hours or less. Newly hatched larvae are gregarious and burrow into exposed muscle, forming pocket-like cavities in the host tissue. Larvae orient themselves with the tapered head down, abrading

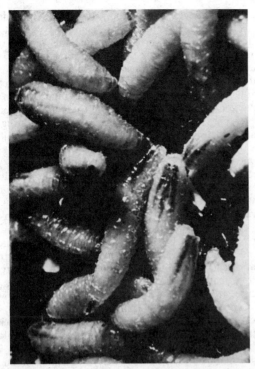

Figure 1. Screwworm larvae with characteristic pigmented tracheal trunks. (Courtesy of United States Department of Agriculture, Animal and Plant Health Inspection Service.)

and cutting the host tissues with their mouthparts, and probably secrete proteolytic enzymes, which aid in the digestive process. Once infested, wounds exude profuse quantities of an odorous discharge and increase in attractiveness to further ovipositional activity by adult screwworm flies as well as secondary invaders. Screwworm larvae, however, can be readily distinguished in such mixed infestations by their characteristic paired pigmented tracheal trunks at the blunt posterior end (Fig. 1). Infested animals cease grazing and attempt to hide in heavily shaded areas or similarly secluded sites. As the infestation increases in size and number of larvae, the host becomes gaunt and harried and may be recognized as "wormy" by its appearance and behavior. If untreated, death usually results although the exact mechanism is unknown. Intraperitoneal injections of larval metabolic products have been shown to produce severe anaphylaxis, and frequently death, in laboratory animals. Moreover, most screwworm infestations are accompanied by secondary bacterial infections (e.g., *Proteus, Streptococcus,* and *Staphylococcus*).

Treatment consists of applying insecticides, approved for such use by the Environmental Protection Agency, to infested wounds. Currently labeled compounds include 3 per cent spray foam 5 per cent dust formulations of coumaphos (Co-Ral*); 2.5 per cent aerosol or 5 per cent smear, dust, or pressurized spray formulations of ronnel (Korlan†); and a 3 per cent smear formulation of Lindane. Lindane, however, may not be applied to lactating dairy cattle. Appropriate ranch-management practices may also be utilized to minimize the threat of screwworm infesta-

tion. Surgical procedures such as branding, castration, and dehorning should be performed during the winter when adult flies are less active, and calving dates should be planned for early spring. Animals may also be sprayed with 0.25 or 0.5 per cent formulations of coumaphos or ronnel, respectively, as preventive measures.

A program to eradicate the screwworm by mass releasing laboratory-reared sterilized flies to mate with native flies was initiated in 1962 under the auspices of the Southwestern Screwworm Eradication Program. This program was so successful that eradication from the United States was officially declared by 1964. Periodic re-infestations from Mexico, estimated at approximately 0.1 per cent of rates previously reported, continued to be experienced however, and, for reasons not fully understood, much of Texas was re-infested by numbers probably equaling those of the most severe preprogram years during 1972. A joint eradication program between the United States and Mexico was subsequently established with facilities in Tuxtala Gutierrez, Chiapas, operative in 1976. It is to be hoped that this effort will finally end the threat of screwworm in the United States. However, constant vigilance by all people involved in animal production will be necessary to achieve this end.

OTHER WOUND INVADERS

Although much less injurious, other species of blow flies and some species of flesh flies may also occur in wounds of living animals. Larvae of these species most commonly infest necrotic lesions in the absence of the true screwworm, but both types may occur simultaneously. Treatment for both types is the same; however, identification of the true screwworm is very important as part of the eradication program now being conducted by the United States and Mexico. A differential diagnosis may be made by sending samples of suspected larvae preserved in 70 per cent ethanol to laboratories with personnel trained in screwworm identification.

WOOL MAGGOTS (FLEECE WORMS)

A highly specialized type of dermal myiasis often occurs in sheep and goats due to attack by several species of blow flies or flesh flies termed *wool maggots* or *fleece worms*. Typical infestations develop when wool or mohair becomes soiled with urine, fecal material, or bloody fluids, thus creating conditions conducive to oviposition. Effective treatment involves shearing of the affected areas followed by applications of insecticides such as a 0.5 per cent dust or 0.125 per cent spray or dip formulation of coumaphos (Co-Ral) or a 2.5 per cent aerosol or 0.5 per cent spray or dip formulation of ronnel (Korlan). "Tagging" or shearing of the rear legs and tail as well as routine spraying or dipping facilitates prevention.

Supplemental Reading

Bushland, R. C.: Screwworm research and eradication. Bull. Entomol. Soc. Am. *21*:23–26, 1975.
Cocke, J. Jr.: New advances against the screwworm. Tx. Agr. Ext. Serv. Publ. L-1089, 1981.
Harwood, R. F., and James, M. T.: Entomology in Human and Animal Health. Macmillan Publishing Co., Inc., N.Y., 1979.
Patrick, C. D.: Suggestions for controlling external parasites of livestock and poultry. Tx. Agr. Ext. Serv. Publ. B-1306, 1981.

---

*Available from Haver-Lockhart Laboratories, Shawnee, Kansas 66201.
†Available from Dow Chemical Company, Indianapolis, Indiana 46268.

Cattle Lice (Pediculosis)

DALLAS L. NELSON, D.V.M., Ph.D.

The parasitic lice of cattle are divided into two suborders. Anoplura are sucking lice that have pointed heads and mouth parts that are adapted for sucking tissue fluids and blood of the host. Mallophaga are biting lice that have mouth parts adapted for biting and chewing the skin.

Injury caused by biting lice is, for the most part, restricted to birds. However, biting lice cause irritation to the skin of all host species when present in large numbers. The cattle-biting louse *Bovicola bovis* can be distinguished by its reddish-brown color. If present in large numbers, the lice group around the tail and withers, which results in a loss of hair, dermal irritation, and scab formation (Fig. 1).[1]

The sucking lice are the most important, as their presence is more pathologic to the host animal because of the anemia they can cause. They may also be vectors of infectious diseases. The three most important species of sucking lice that infest cattle in North America are *Haematopinus eurysternus* (short-nosed cattle louse), *Linognathus vituli* (long-nosed or blue cattle louse), and *Solenopotes capillatus* (little blue cattle louse). The sucking lice congregate around the head, neck, and shoulders of cattle. With heavy infestations they spread over the entire body.

The life cycles of all species of cattle lice are very similar. The female louse attaches eggs to the base of hairs, and the eggs hatch in 8 to 15 days. The cycle from egg to egg requires 20 to 30 days. The infestation is spread by direct contact among animals or by bedding or objects that affected animals rub against to relieve their itching sensation. Crowding of animals gives an excellent opportunity for the spread of lice.

Both internal and external parasites are more of a problem in poorly nourished animals than in well-nourished animals. This appears to be especially true for lice.

The young animal usually harbors the heaviest infestations and is the most severely affected.

Lice are a greater problem during the winter, when nutrition may be poorer than in summer and crowding facilitates the spread of infestation. The thick hair coat of winter provides better protection for lice reproduction. During the warmer seasons when the animal sheds, the protection and numbers of the parasites are reduced. A severe louse problem is seldom enountered during the summer. This is especially true for range cattle that are exposed to rain and direct sunlight.

One or two per cent of the animals in any given herd carry a heavier infestation of lice than other members. These animals are designated as "carrier animals." They remain heavily infested the year round. Although the carriers have an unthrifty appearance, the infestation may not cause debilitation among these animals. Bulls are more often carriers than cows. In controlling lice, special consideration should be given to identification and treatment of carrier animals. It is seldom necessary to treat a herd of cattle during the summer when they are on pasture. It is advantageous to treat carrier animals when they are removed from pasture in the autumn. This procedure may slow the spread of lice during the winter when the whole herd is more susceptible to severe louse problems.

Lice manifest their pathogenicity by sucking blood and causing irritation to the skin. Blood loss that leads to anemia can result in loss of productivity.[2, 3] The resulting anemia comes at a time of year when cattle are subjected to the greatest stress. The parasitic anemia may potentiate or complicate other disease conditions. Phenomenal improvement in production is seen when heavily infested animals are treated. Improved efficiency following treatment would depend on the degree of infestation present at the time of treatment.

All of the currently available products for treating lice are organophosphorus compounds. The dipping vat and sprays are the most efficient treatment methods. During cold weather, dusts and pour-on preparations are useful.

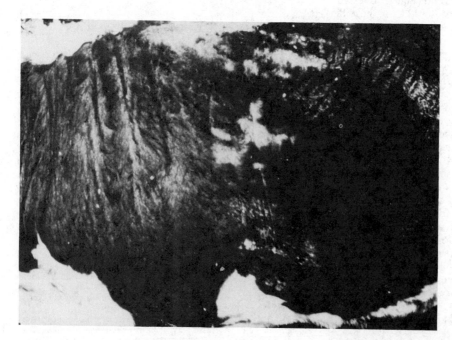

Figure 1. Heavy lice infestation results in irritation of the skin and hair loss due to rubbing.

When treating cattle for lice, two applications two weeks apart should be given. The second application controls lice that have hatched from eggs present when the first treatment was given.

References

1. Matthysse, J. G.: Cattle Lice, Their Biology and Control. Bulletin 832, Cornell University Agricultural Experiment Station, Ithaca, New York, 1946.
2. Collins, R. C., and Dewirst, L. W.: Some effects on the sucking louse, *Haematopinus eurysternus,* on cattle on unsupplemented range. J. Am. Vet. Med. Assoc. *146*:129–132, 1965.
3. Freer, R. E., and Gahan, R. J.: Controlling lice in beef herds—is it economic? Agri. Gazette 308–309, 1968.

Cattle Grubs (*Hypoderma Myiasis*)

DALLAS L. NELSON, D.V.M., Ph.D.

Adult heel flies are active over a variable period of time, starting in early spring and continuing to late summer or autumn. The adult female deposits eggs on the hairs of the legs and lower parts of the body. In two to six days the eggs hatch and the maggots burrow directly through the skin into the subcutaneous tissue. The larval penetration causes a variable amount of irritation to the skin. For approximately four to five months, the larvae migrate through the connective tissue of the body, apparently by the use of a potent proteolytic enzyme. In the case of *Hypoderma lineatum,* they migrate to the submucosal tissue of the posterior third of the esophagus. The migration of the larvae results in greenish edematous tracts. Small swellings in the connective tissue containing larvae and a greenish-yellow exudate are sometimes noted. Also, localized areas of edematous connective tissue are attributed to larval migration. The larvae of *H. bovis* migrate to the fat in the epidural space between the periosteum of the vertebrae and the dura mater. Anatomically the larvae are most often found between the eighth thoracic and first lumbar vertebrae. The larval tracts are found in the intermuscular connective tissue of this area and in the fascial planes through which the spinal nerves and their branches emerge from the spinal canal. At this stage of migration, the larvae are located in such an anatomic position that they pose their greatest potential problem to the host animal. Meningitis, periosteitis, and osteomyelitis in addition to connective tissue disorders have been attributed to the migration of *H. bovis* larvae.[1]

After a period of development that lasts from two to three months, the larvae continue their migration from the region of the esophagus or epidural space until they arrive in the subcutaneous tissue of the back. Here they are able to produce a breathing hole through the skin, presumably by the use of the same proteolytic enzyme. The larvae remain in this position for a period of around two months. A fibrous connective tissue capsule is formed around the larvae. The larvae penetrate through the breathing hole, fall to the ground, and immediately go into the pupal stage. They remain as pupae for one to three months before emerging as adult flies. The length of the pupal stage depends on weather conditions.[2]

TREATMENT

There are a number of effective products for the treatment of cattle for *Hypoderma* infections. All of the active ingredient compounds belong to the organophosphorus chemical family. They are systemic in that they are absorbed by the host animal and are carried by body fluids to the parasite.

In large feedlots, the use of dipping vats is a popular treatment method for grubs. In former times, the total body spray was popular. Pour-on formulations are widely used. The active compound is formulated so that treatment can be given by pouring the formulation down the middle of the animal's back. A comparatively recent development is the formulation of an insecticide at a higher concentration so that smaller volumes of the formulation can be used per animal treated.

Regardless of the method or the product used to treat cattle for grub control, the label on the product should be read each time before use. The prescribed interval between the time of treatment and slaughter should be adhered to strictly. The regulations regarding the treatment of dairy cattle are especially important.

The systemic insecticides used for grub control are capable of causing systemic intoxication if used in amounts greater than those stated in the manufacturer's directions. When cholinesterase is rapidly and severely depressed in the host animal, typical cholinergic symptoms can result.

After organophosphorus compounds became widely used to treat cattle for grub control, a syndrome was described that did not have typical cholinergic symptoms.[3] In this syndrome, symptoms appear a few hours after treatment, reaching their maximum severity around 24 to 48 hours post treatment. The symptoms are the result of dead and dying grubs. In some cases there is enough similarity between the host-parasite reaction and cholinergic symptoms to cause confusion in diagnosis. When cattle are treated at a time when larvae are located in an especially sensitive anatomic position, a variable number of animals will manifest symptoms indicative of a reaction to the larvae. In most cattle herds, the morbidity is low, with less than 10 per cent of animals developing a reaction.

Cattle treated when *Hypoderma lineatum* are in the esophageal tissue are vulnerable to a type of host-parasite reaction, the early symptoms of which are frothy salivation and the spitting out of partially masticated feed. These symptoms result from a swelling of the esophageal tissue, making it difficult or impossible to swallow. Partially masticated feed is often seen on the ground. In severe cases there is swelling of the esophagus into the jugular furrow. Gastric tympanites results from an inability to eructate. On necropsy the esophagus is extremely edematous. Within the edematous tissue are found streaks of hemorrhage. Grub larvae are closely associated with hemorrhage. If the condition is long standing, there will be evidence of emaciation and dehydration. In most herds the mortality is low and most cattle return to normal in 72 hours.

The treatment of gastric tympanites poses a problem. If the esophagus is extensively involved, the stomach tube should not be used, as additional trauma or puncture may result. In most cases, tympanites should be treated by the use of a cannula. Anti-inflammatory therapy, such as the use of adrenal corticosteroid preparations, is indicated, as are antibiotics, to prevent secondary infection. Animals should be placed on a ration that can be easily swallowed. Correctly differentiating between a host-parasite reaction and intoxication from the insecticide is important. When gastric tympanites results from a swollen esophagus, the use of atropine (with its resulting lowered rumen motility) only aggravates the condition.

When *Hypoderma bovis* larvae are in the region of, or are actually in, the spinal canal, treatment with a systemic insecticide may result in conditons that vary from weakness to paraplegia of the posterior limbs. On necropsy examination, a large amount of hemorrhage and inflammation is seen in the spinal canal in the area where the larvae are found. It is thought that chemical trauma (from the larval digestive enzymes) and compression (from hemorrhage) cause nerve impairment. This condition has occurred as long as three days after grub treatment.[4] Animals that have only motor impairment to the posterior limbs have a good prognosis. Some paraplegic animals will recover, but the prognosis is not good. Good husbandry practices and anti-inflammatory and antibiotic therapy are indicated. In mild cases, the animals are usually asymptomatic by two to three days post treatment.

It is obvious that cattle should not be treated when *Hypoderma* larvae are in a vital anatomic position. Considerable effort has been expended trying to develop safe and effective treatment dates for different geographic areas.

The question of correct timing of grub treatments is very complicated. In our modern beef industry, cattle are moved over wide areas of the country. Some cattle being fed in western feedlots have probably been trucked several hundred miles to the lot. Their actual place of origin may not be known. There are many recent reports of territory overlap of the two species of *Hypoderma*. This may have resulted from the movement of cattle and the establishment of grubs in new territories. The result of this has been the reporting of adult fly activity from early spring to late autumn.

Treatment should be given soon after fly activity ceases. The commercial feed lot operator may know little about the time of adult activity in the area where the cattle originated. Many operators treat cattle soon after they arrive at the lot and before they are placed on full feed. This reduces the potential for gastric tympanites associated with the host parasite reaction. Some operators are making a second treatment 90 to 120 days after the first for larvae resulting from late season adult fly activity.

References

1. Wolfe, L. S.: Observations on the histopathological changes caused by the larvae of *Hypoderma bovis* (L.) and *Hypoderma lineatum* (De Vill.) (Diptera:Oestridae) in tissues of cattle. Can. J. Anim. Sci. *39*:145–157, 1959.
2. Scharff, D. K.: Cattle grubs, their biologies, their distribution and experiments in their control. Technical bulletin 471, Montana State College Agricultural Experiment Station, Bozemen, Montana, 1950.
3. Scharff, D. K., Sharman, G. A. M., and Ludwig, P.: Illness and death in calves induced by treatments with systemic insecticides for the control of cattle grubs. J. Am. Vet. Med. Assoc. *141*:582–587, 1962.
4. Cox, D. D., Mozier, J. O., and Mullee, M. T.: Posterior paraylsis in a calf caused by cattle grubs (*Hypoderma bovis*) after treatment with a systemic insecticide for grub control. J. Am. Vet. Med. Assoc. *157*:1088–1092, 1970.

Bovine Mange

PETER C. MULLOWNEY, M.V.B., M.R.C.V.S.

Four genera of mange mites affect cattle: *Chorioptes, Demodex, Sarcoptes,* and *Psoroptes*. Other mites isolated from cattle include harvest mites, Psorergatic mites, and ear mites. Colloquial terms for diseases caused by mange mites are mange, scab, itch, and barn itch. Mites are minute acarids that live permanently on (or in) the skin of the host animal. Chorioptic, sarcoptic, and psoroptic mange mites are similar in appearance. The adults are eight-legged, oval, whitish parasites 0.5 mm in diameter. They can be differentiated on the basis of examination of the pretarsi (Figs. 1 through 6). Demodex mites are elongated, alligator-shaped parasites 0.2 to 0.4 mm long. Mange mites are generally host specific. As they feed, multiply, and die, they injure the host's skin. The resultant lesion may be due to mechanical damage, secretion of irritant substances by the mite, or an immunologic hypersensitivity to the foreign antigens of the mite. The skin wounds may also become infected secondarily with bacteria. The appearance and location of the lesions are usually characteristic for the particular species of mite, especially in the early stages. The extent of lesions depends on the number of mites, their reproductive activity, and the host's reaction. Affected animals may lose weight, be less productive, and have damaged hides.

Several types of mange are reportable diseases; whenever a diagnosis is made or suspected, the state veterinarian should be notified and will supervise treatment. Definitive diagnosis is made by taking a deep skin scraping at the periphery of the lesion.[1]

CHORIOPTIC MANGE

Chorioptic mange *(Chorioptes bovis)* is spread by direct contact or by grooming tools. Infestation of bedding is not a common method of transmission. It is most evident in the winter in stabled cattle, particularly dairy animals in the northeastern states. The lesions are generally confined to the perineum and back of the udder, extending in severe cases to the backs of the legs and over the rump. Itching may be present, but it is never as severe as it is in psoroptic or sarcoptic mange. Wounds caused by the mites are small, the skin under the thin scabs is only slightly swollen, and inflamed lesions are often not noticed until the disease is well advanced; as hair is rubbed off, the skin appears thick, wrinkled, and ridged. A rapidly spreading syndrome characterized by coronitis, intense irritation, and a marked fall in milk production has been described. In summer months, mites persist in the area above the hooves, particularly on the hindlegs, where they cause crusty scabs. These may also be present on the muzzle.

Diagnosis is based on skin scrapings and should be differentiated from infestation with *Psoroptes ovis*. Chorioptic mange is probably the most common form of

KEY TO PARASITIC MITES OF BOVINES

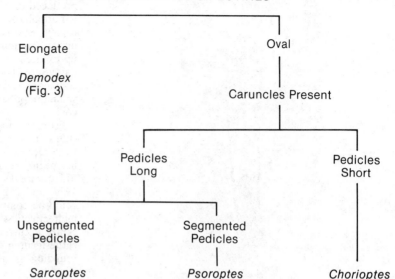

Figure 1. Pretarsi consists of suckers (caruncles) on a stalk (pedicle).

mange in cattle, and mites can be found in the absence of clinical signs. The life cycle takes three weeks to complete and is spent entirely on the host animal.[2]

Treatment consists of application of 0.25 per cent solution of crotoxyphos once or 0.03 to 0.06 per cent twice. Application of lime sulfur is also effective, but some sources suggest that it must be applied on six occasions, six to ten days apart, to all animals to eradicate the parasite in a herd.

DEMODECTIC MANGE

The average incidence of bovine demodiciosis in the United States was estimated as greater than 87 per cent from an examination of cattle hides.[3] *Demodex bovis* mites live in hair follicles and can usually be detected by deep skin scrapings or examination of the waxy material

that can be expressed from the pustular lesions. The adult mite is elongated and alligator-shaped (see Fig. 1).

Under both stable and pasture conditions, the extent and severity of *Demodex bovis* infestations increase with higher concentrations of animals. On some large farms over 30 per cent of cattle have been found to be clinically affected. Although the lesions are of little clinical significance, they can damage the hides and result in significant economic loss. The disease occurs in animals of any age, especially those with poor nutrition, but most cases occur in adult dairy animals, particularly in late winter and spring.[3]

The life cycle of *D. bovis* is usually spent entirely on the host animal; the mites may live for a few days off the host. Although transmission can occur via inanimate objects, it usually occurs by direct contact. The common method of spread is from infested dam to her offspring, but mites may not be transmitted from an infected dam

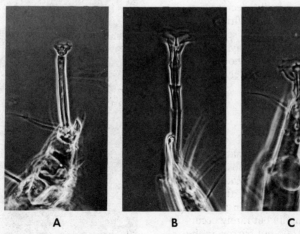

Figure 2A. *Sarcoptes* pretarsi. (Figures 2A to 6 from Georgi, J. R.: Parasitology for Veterinarians. W. B. Saunders: Philadelphia, 1984. With permission.)

Figure 2B. *Psoroptes* pretarsi.

Figure 2C. *Otodectes* pretarsi, very similar to *Chorioptes* pretarsi.

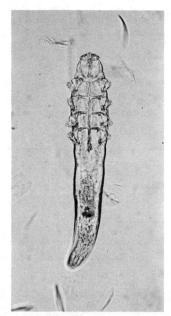

Figure 3. *Demodex canis.*

to all her offspring equally. Reducing the period of contact between dam and offspring is thought to lower the incidence of infection, but experiments have shown that calves can acquire demodectic mites after being exposed to their dams for as little as 12 hours.[4] The disease does not spread rapidly on individual animals or between adults. It may seem to disappear spontaneously in the summer, but lesions usually re-appear the following winter.

Invasion of hair follicles causes chronic inflammatory loss of hair fibers and secondary pustular infection with staphylococci giving a nodular appearance. Scabs or crust-like lesions are also observed. Nodules are commonly found on the brisket, axillae, neck adjacent to the shoulders, and the withers. In heavily infested cattle, nodules are found in other areas of the body such as the sides, back, hips, the side of the face, and intermandibular region. Nodules vary in size from a grain of sand to a pea or larger. Some cattle show considerable sensitivity to palpation of the smaller nodules.[5] These lesions cause pinpoint holes in the hide and markedly decrease its value. The lesions generally do not cause pruritus. On rare occasions, they may cause death due to secondary bacterial invasion. Repeated dipping or spraying with acaricides is usually carried out; however, although this will limit the spread of the condition, it is unlikely to cure existing lesions.

PSOROPTIC MANGE

Psoroptes ovis in cattle causes a severe dermatitis with heavy scab formulation. Heavily infested cattle lose weight or do not gain as much weight as uninfested cattle. The mite that infests cattle is believed to be of the same species as the mite that attacks sheep, and transfer from cattle to sheep can occur experimentally but rarely occurs under natural conditions.[6] The mites do not burrow in the skin but live at the base of hairs and cause irritation by piercing the skin and injecting toxic saliva, which produces severe inflammation. An exudate forms and scabs are produced on the skin surface. The life cycle of the mite is normally spent entirely on the host, but all stages are capable of survival away from the host for up to ten days; under optimum conditions, adult females may survive for up to three weeks. The complete life cycle takes 10 to 11 days. Spread occurs by contaminated fomites and by direct contact. The condition is more common in winter than in summer, possibly as a result of shedding of the winter coat.

Psoroptic mange is most common in the western central states. It was almost eradicated in the 1950's (no cases were reported in 1950, 1951, and 1952); however, there has been a resurgence of the disease recently. There were 313 outbreaks in 1978 (in 15 states), 238 outbreaks in 1979, and 252 in 1980. The reasons for the resurgence could be complacency about the eradication program or ineffectiveness of acaricides used; also changes have recently occurred in the intensity and complexity of the cattle-feeding industry in the Texas panhandle and surrounding areas. Systemically active organophosphates, which are not as effective as toxaphene against mange mites, are more popular owing to their shorter withdrawal period. Dips and acaricides have been added to the USDA-approved list of substances known not to eradicate mites on a single dipping. Some authors suggest that lime sulfur may need to be applied five times before all mites are eliminated.[7]

Currently in the United States, coumaphos, hot lime sulfur, phosmet, and toxaphene are permitted dips. The reported resistance of lice and mites to known dip-active ingredients suggests the need for new ectoparasiticides. *Psoroptes ovis* mites and sucking lice were eliminated from light to heavily infested calves within ten days with a single subcutaneous injection of 20 mg/kg of nifluridide, an amino-anilide precursor of perfluoroalkylbenzimadazole, with no evidence of toxic effects.[8] Ivermectin (22,23-dihydroavermectin B, [Merck MK-933]), injected intramuscularly at the rate of 200 mg/kg, completely eliminated psoroptic mites from cattle within two weeks after treat-

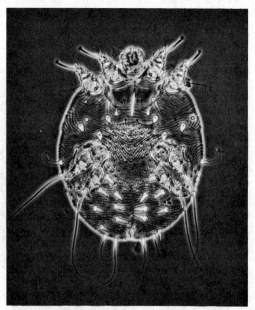

Figure 4. *Sarcoptes* (female).

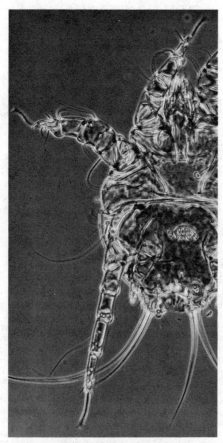

Figure 5. *Psoroptes* (male).

ment. However, mites surviving one, three, and five days after treatment were viable and infective when transferred to untreated cattle. Cattle treated with ivermectin should be isolated from other cattle for at least five days after treatment. At the time of writing, neither ivermectin nor nifluridide had been approved by the FDA for use in food-producing animals.[9]

In commercial cattle feedlots, psoroptic mange was found to cause a reduction in daily feed consumption of 21.5 per cent and an average decrease in weight of 0.15 kg/head/day. More heavily infested cattle lost 70 kg in the course of infestation and required 100 additional days feeding at an increased cost of $45 to restore weight losses. When treated with toxaphene, cattle must be withheld from slaughter for 30 days, thus adding to feed costs. Infested cattle are more prone to respiratory problems and often sustain injuries during dipping. Hides damaged by infected mite wounds bring lower prices.

The initial lesions may be found on only part of the body, most often on the shoulders and withers and around the tailhead. In severe cases, a large part of the skin is affected. Scabby areas become thick, wrinkled, and fissured. Secondary bacterial or fungal infections can occur. Animals lose weight or do not gain weight as well, and if the herd is not treated the condition spreads rapidly. Persistent licking, rubbing, and scratching occur as well as swishing of the tail and signs of nervousness. The presence of hair patches on barbed wire fences is an indication that cattle may be affected. Badly affected animals may become weak and die. The cause of death is

not completely understood but it may be due to (1) loss of body heat as a result of the considerable loss of hair that occurs in heavily infested animals; (2) development of a secondary infection wtih a pathogenic organism or an organism that under normal circumstances is nonpathogenic; (3) loss of fluid and electrolytes; or (4) secretion by the mites of a toxin that poisons the animal or affects a vital organ. Damage to vital organs such as the liver, kidney, and so on can be partially determined by serum biochemistry.[10]

The epidemiologic investigation of outbreaks of psoroptic mange, especially the tracing of infested cattle back to their herds of origin and the identifying of herds to which cattle have been sold, is very important in the eradication of the disease. One of the major factors interfering with the tracing of the disease is the delay between the time the herd becomes infested and the reporting of the disease; this averaged four to six months in 1978.[7] Precipitating antibodies have been demonstrated in sheep and cattle infested with *Psoroptes ovis* and may be of some benefit in epidemiologic investigations.[11]

If the disease could be eradicated, the costs of dipping cattle as well as the direct costs of the disease could be eliminated. Pesticide can cost up to $1.00 per head. Three men are required to dip 100 cattle per hour, and trucks must be cleaned and disinfected after transporting infested animals.

SARCOPTIC MANGE

Sarcoptic mange is caused by *Sarcoptes scabiei* var. *bovis*. However, the parasite is not completely host-specific, and this must be taken into account when attempting eradication. The disease is most common in poorly fed, poorly housed, and overcrowded animals. It occurs regularly in the northeastern states. The disease is most active in cold, wet weather and spreads slowly during the summer months.

The female mite burrows in the superficial layers of the

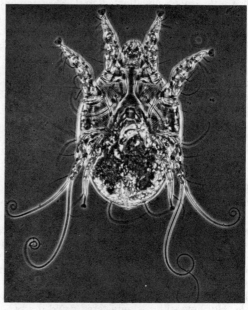

Figure 6. *Chorioptes* (female).

skin. The resulting irritation and hypersensitivity of the host to the parasite can cause severe pruritus. The mite's complete life cycle is spent on the host, although spread can occur via inanimate objects as well as by direct contact.

The intense pruritus causes loss of condition and production and a decrease in grazing time. Animals can injure themselves by constant scratching. Udder and teat injuries are common in closely confined animals. Estrus detection is difficult because of constant scratching. In advanced cases, animals scratch and bite themselves constantly, become emaciated, and may die if not treated properly. Skin over the neck and sacrum is most commonly affected, but lesions may develop anywhere on the body. Continual irritation of the skin leads to excessive keratinization, connective tissue proliferation, and edema. The thickened skin becomes wrinkled, fissured, denuded, and stiff. Secondary bacterial infections are common. The course is acute and the entire body surface may be involved within six weeks. Calculated losses from the disease range from $100 to $200/head, but production increases 5 to 10 per cent after treatment that costs approximately $2 per head.[12]

Because lesions are caused by a hypersensitivity reaction, the severity of the lesions is not always related to the number of mites present. Several deep skin scrapings should be examined directly and by the potassium hydroxide digestion flotation method before such a diagnosis is discounted.

HARVEST MITE INFESTATIONS (CHIGGER MITES)

The larvae of several species of harvest mites are parasitic on cattle. The natural hosts are usually small rodents, but nymphs and adults are free-living predators feeding mainly on arthropods in grain and hay. They usually infest domestic animals secondarily and then only transiently. The larvae are most active in the autumn at harvest time and may cause dermatitis in animals grazing at pasture or those confined being fed newly harvested grain. Cattle are usually affected on the face and lips and about the feet and lower limbs. Affected areas are itchy and scaly, but with rubbing, small fragile scabs and absence of hair may become apparent. The infestation is usually self-limiting, and treatment is usually not necessary but the legs can be washed in 0.25 per cent maldison. Area control of the mite may be obtained by the use of either chlorpyrifos granules at 1.1 kg/ha or as a 22.4 per cent spray of a chlorpyrifos at 1.6 kg/ha or a 12.8 per cent spray of propoxur at 1.0 kg/ha.[13]

PSORERGATIC MITES

The bovine psorergatic mite Psorergates bos has been identified in cattle in New Mexico, Texas, California, Kansas, Minnesota, and Wyoming. Infestation does not cause economic loss or lesions similar to mange but resembles those caused by lice. Alopecia and desquamation have been noted, but pruritus or deep dermal lesions do not occur. The mite has also been isolated from areas of normal skin.

The mite is extremely small and is difficult to detect on a slide. Hot lime sulfur administered twice at a two-week interval as a dip or spray is the acaricide of choice.[14]

CATTLE EAR MITES (Raillietia auris)

Ear mites cause ulceration of the external auditory canal and blockage with a plug of pus that may result in loss of hearing. Although no clinical signs of discomfort such as head shaking, rubbing and anorexia are detected, it would appear from the severity of the lesions that some discomfort would occur with swallowing and chewing that might affect an animal's ability to gain weight or produce milk.[15] The mite may give rise to secondary infections, which can result in debilitation and death of the animal. The loss of hearing may impair the detecting of predators that threaten the survival of free-ranging cattle. Once R. auris becomes established within a herd, they infest nearly all its members. Treatment for these mites is not mentioned in the literature but, presumably, acaracides effective against other mites would be suitable.[15]

References

1. Nelson, D. L.: Mites (mange). In Howard, J. L. (ed.): Current Veterinary Therapy: Food Animal Practice, 1st ed. W. B. Saunders Co., Philadelphia, 1981, 1143–1144.
2. Gaafar, S. M.: Parasitic dermatoses. In Amstutz, H. E. (ed.): Bovine Medicine and Surgery. American Veterinary Publications, Wheaton, Ill., 1980, 887–911.
3. Blood, D. C., Radostits, O. M., and Henderson, J. A. (eds.): Veterinary Medicine, 6th ed. Bailliere Tindall, London, 1983, 963–969.
4. Fisher, W. F., Miller, R. W., and Everett, A. L.: Natural transmission of Demodex bovis to dairy calves. Vet. Parasit. 7:233–241, 1980.
5. Smith, H. J.: Bovine demodicidosis. II. Clinical manifestations in Ontario. Can. J. Comp. Med. 25:201–204, 1951.
6. Graham, O. H., and Hourrigan, J. L.: Eradication programs for the arthropod parasites of livestock. J. Med. Entomol. 13:629–658, 1977.
7. Hourrigan, J. L.: Spread and detection of psoroptic scabies of cattle in the United States. J. Am. Vet. Med. Assoc. 175:1278–1280, 1979.
8. Boisvenue, R. J., and Clymer, B. C.: Systemic activity of Nifluridide against sucking lice and the common scabies mite on cattle. Vet. Parasit. 11:253–260, 1982.
9. Guillot, F. S., and Meleney, W. P.: The infectivity of surviving Psoroptes ovis on cattle treated with Ivermectin. Vet. Parasit. 10:73–78, 1982.
10. Fisher, W. F., and Crookshank, H. R.: Effects of Psoroptes ovis on certain biochemical constituents of cattle serum. Vet. Parasit. 11:241–251, 1982.
11. Fisher, W. F., and Wilson, G. I.: Precipitating antibodies in cattle infested with Psoroptes ovis. J. Med. Entomol. 14:146–151, 1977.
12. Nusbaum, S. R., et al.: Sarcoptes scabiei bovis—A potential danger. J. Am. Vet. Med. Assoc. 166:252–256, 1975.
13. Mount, G. A., et al.: Area control of chigger mites with granules and concentrated spray of Chlorpyrifos. J. Econ. Ent. 71:27–28, 1978.
14. Bergstrom, R. C., and Etherton, S. L.: Psorergatid mites from cattle in Wyoming. VMSAC 78:1761–1762, 1983.
15. Heffner, R. S., and Heffner, H. E.: Occurrence of the cattle ear might (Raillietia auris) in South Eastern Kansas. Cornell Vet. 73:193–199, 1983.

Dermatophytosis
ALLAN C. PIER, D.V.M., Ph.D.

DEFINITION

Dermatophytosis is a disease of the skin and its appendages (i.e., hair and nails) caused by infection by a specific group of pathogenic fungi, the dermatophytes. Synonyms for the disease in animals include ringworm, dermatomycosis, trichophytosis, microsporiosis, and girth itch. Dermatophytosis is the oldest and most frequently recognized of the fungal infections. Various forms of the disease involve animals and humans the world over.

Dermatophytes are keratinophilic fungi that invade or

reside in the skin, hair, and nails where keratinization has occurred. They rarely penetrate below keratinized levels of the skin because of lack of keratin and nutritional inhibition by serum proteins.

Dermatophytic pathogens are contained in the genera *Trichophyton*, *Microsporum*, and *Epidermophyton*. There are approximately 28 species of dermatophytes known. Many of them are obligate parasites of animals or humans; some live freely in the soil and occasionally invade keratinized tissues of animals or humans.

Dermatophyte species that have a proclivity to parasitize animals are called zoophilic dermatophytes; those that perferentially parasitize humans are called anthropophilic; those that live freely in the soil are called geophilic. However, these perferences in residence are not absolute, and zoophilic dermatophytes often infect humans, anthropophilic dermatophytes occasionally infect animals, and geophilic dermatophytes may occasionally infect either animals or humans. The dermatophytoses are among the few mycoses that are truly contagious, and animal-to-animal or animal-to-human contagion often occurs.

Of the 28 known dermatophytes, 8 are of real consequence in animals. These organisms have highly predictable animal hosts and origins of infection. Thus, identification of the infecting dermatophyte species permits determination of likely sources of infection that must be eliminated to effect control of the spread of new infection to other animals in the herd, flock, or animal colony. The dermatophytes of major importance to domestic animals are listed in Table 1.

CLINICAL SIGNS

Clinical signs of dermatophytosis in animals are confined to involvement of the skin of infected animals. Most of the dermatophytes listed in Table 1 invade the hair as well as the skin (e.g., *T. mentagrophytes* [granulare], *T. verrucosum*, *T. equinum*, *M. canis*, *M. equinum*, and *M. gypseum*); *M. canis* also has been known to invade the nails of cats and dogs. The remaining dermatophytes in Table 1 (e.g., *M. nanum* and *M. gallinae*) involve only the skin; invasion of the hair or feathers by these latter two agents is not observed.

Typically the lesions of dermatophytosis (ringworm) of the haired skin of animals begin to appear one to two weeks after an exposure of a susceptible animal to infected animal or to infectious materials in the environment (common sources are listed in Table 1). The lesions begin as thickening and scaling of the skin; soon an area of hair loss appears as the hairs are invaded and break off in the developing lesion. The lesion expands in size for about four to eight weeks and then begins to resolve as the animal develops an immune response to the invading dermatophyte. The lesion regresses in size and hair growth resumes after 8 to 16 weeks. Calves with *T. verrucosum* infections develop multiple lesions 2 to 6 cm in diameter, often around the head and neck; the lesions typically consist of an area of alopecia and a prominent whitish asbestos-like accumulation of scales. Lesions caused by *T. mentagrophytes* (dogs, horses), *T. equinum* (horses), and *M. canis* (dogs and cats) are usually multifocal and small (0.5 to 2 cm in diameter), and develop less encrustation than those seen with *T. verrucosum* infections in calves. Older, partially immune animals may have occult infections in the absence of obvious lesions (e.g., cats with *M. canis*). The lesions of *M. gypseum* on horses, dogs, and other animals are usually isolated (1 to several per animal), medium to large (up to 4 to 8 cm in diameter) foci of hair loss. Pigs infected with *M. nanum* develop large brown scaly areas of the skin reaching 8 to 12 cm in diameter without hair involvement. Seldom do animals infected with either *M. gypseum* or *M. nanum* develop a

Table 1. *Major Dermatophytes of Domestic Animals*

Dermatophyte	Affected Animals	Frequency Index	Common Source
Trichophyton			
T. mentagrophytes (granulare)	Rural dogs	1	Infected hair or scales from rodents (i.e., grain bins,
	Rural cats	2	etc.) or other infected animals
	Horses	2	
	Cattle	3	
	Sheep	3	
	Swine	4	
	Rural people	2	
	Lab animal colonies	1	
T. verrucosum	Cattle	1	Infected hair or scales (remain viable on wooded
	Rural people	2	stanchions, calf pens, etc., for several years)
T. equinum	Horses	1	Infected hair or scales on tack, brushes, etc.
	Horsemen	3	
Microsporum			
M. canis	Urban dogs	1	Infected hair and scales from dogs, cats on bedding,
	Urban cats	1	brushes, etc.
	Horses	3	
	Primates	3	
	Urban people	2	
M. gypseum (complex)	Horses	2	Soil (geophilic dermatophytes)
	Dogs	3	Occasionally infected hair or scales
	Cats	4	
M. nanum	Swine	1	Soil (geophilic dermatophyte)
			Occasionally infected skin scales
M. gallinae	Poultry	3	Infected skin scales

1 = Usual agent; 2 = frequent; 3 = occasional; 4 = rare.

myriad of small discrete lesions as is often seen with *M. canis*, *T. mentagrophytes*, or *T. equinum* infections. Poultry infected with *M. gallinae* develop scaly to scabby lesions on the comb and wattles; the feathers are not involved.

Clinical dermatophytic involvement is usually more prominent in young animals; presumably mature animals in the herd are less frequently involved clinically owing to actively acquired immunity. A degree of seasonality is seen with some infections (e.g., *T. verrucosum* and *M. canis* infections: winter and spring prevalence; *T. mentagrophytes* [granulare] and *M. gypseum* infections: summer and fall prevalence). Infection around the eyes or mouth may affect the animal's ability to forage and slow its rate of growth, and secondary bacterial invasion of active lesions may also occur; however, often the clinical course is uneventful but infected animals pose a threat of contagion to other animals and their human attendants.

DIAGNOSIS

All of the scaly, hairless lesions on animals are not necessarily ringworm. Specific criteria of diagnosis are needed here as with other infectious diseases. Dermatophytosis is diagnosed by microscopic examination of wet mounts of hair, skin scales, or nail parings taken from the periphery of active lesions. Mycelial activity is greater at the periphery of skin lesions, so hairs and skin scales selected with care from these areas yield the best results. A wet mount is made using 20 per cent KOH and equal parts of ink (e.g., permanent black Super Quink*). The preparation is covered with a coverslip, heated gently, and examined microscopically. Parasitic forms can be seen as septae hyphae approximately 2 to 3 μ wide and chains of arthrospores in skin scales and within the hairshaft. On the external surface of the hairshaft, just distal to the root, chains or sheaths of arthrospores may be seen; this condition is called ectothrix. If no diagnostic forms are seen, the KOH-ink preparation should be put in a Petri dish with a moist piece of paper towel or filter paper, covered, left at room temperature overnight, and re-examined microscopically the next day. Fungal elements will be distinct and blue-colored in such preparations.

Recognition of dermatophytes in a microscopic preparation indicates the existence of dermatophytosis but does not identify the causative agent. There is no difference in treatment for dermatophytes, but it is helpful to identify the infecting agent culturally to predict the source of infection (for other animals in the herd, flock, or colony) and the degree of contagion that might be anticipated for human attendants (e.g., *T. mentagrophytes* versus *M. gypseum*). Cultural isolation of dermatophytes is best accomplished by implanting selected hairs and scales on Sabouraud's dextrose agar to which inhibitors (e.g., cyclohexamide and chloramphenicol) have been added to control the growth of bacterial and fungal contaminants. A number of commercially available mediums in disposable containers are satisfactory (e.g., Mycobiotic agar, Difco or Mycosel agar†). Species identification is made after one to four weeks of growth at room temperature

---

*Available from Parker Pen Company, Janesville, Wisconsin 53545.
†Available from Baltimore Biologics, Cockeysville, Maryland 21030.

(37°C for *T. verrucosum* suspects). Identification is based on colony morphology and color, macroconidia (large multicelled spores) morphology, and occasionally nutritional requirements for specific vitamins. (The latter is a task reserved for a well-equipped mycology laboratory.) Some commercial mediums rely on color change (i.e., alkaline reaction) to signify the presence of a dermatophyte. However, these are subject to error through false positive reactions. Like those listed previously, media can be used to culture scales or hair and the color change can be considered only presumptively from suspect lesions. Positive diagnosis of the presence of dermatophyte infection is best made by microscopic examination of the KOH wet mount of hair and scales, and positive identification of the type of infecting dermatophyte is usually made from microscopic morphology of the mature culture and other indications discussed previously.

TREATMENT

Perhaps the most important concepts to remember when considering therapy of dermatophytic lesions of the haired skin of animals are these:

1. There are a multiplicity of remedies to choose from, in part owing to the fact that few are highly successful. This statement is particularly appropriate to topically applied preparations.

2. Regardless of what preparation is used, lesions of the haired skin can be expected to ameliorate after approximately 8 to 16 weeks, probably because of the development of actively acquired immunity. (Where immunologic competence is defective, or where infection involves nails or other slow-growing keratin, recovery may be delayed.) Thus, the apparent clinical progress may be influenced by the age of the lesion treated as well as the remedy selected.

3. The propensity for contagion often dictates use of topical agents to reduce the infectivity to other animals and humans of hair and scales from the lesion.

The most effective therapy for dermatophytosis is orally administered griseofulvin, an antifungal antibiotic with a high level of specific activity against dermatophytes. Griseofulvin is fungistatic rather than fungicidal, so treatment must be continued until the infected hairs and keratinized epithelium grow out and are sloughed or clipped off. Recommended dosage is 10 to 20 mg/kg of the ultrafine-particle preparation given daily for a period of one to two weeks. A reduced dosage rate of 1.25 to 2.5 gm/day for seven to ten days has been reported to be effective in horses. Two or more large doses (ca. 100 mg/kg) given a week apart have also been reported to be effective in limited trials. Side effects from griseofulvin therapy may include gastritis in some individuals. Currently, griseofulvin is not licensed for veterinary use in animals intended to be used for food. This fact and the expense of treatment relegate the use of griseofulvin to valuable show stock or breeding animals on an individual basis.

A new avenue of therapy in certain mycoses has been offered by the advent of a group of drugs known collectively as imidazoles. Thiabendazole, the anthelminthic, has been used in a 2 to 4 per cent ointment for topical treatment of dermatophytoses in animals. More recently ketoconazole has been used effectively on selectively deep and superficial mycoses in man.[1] Oral ketoconazole has been effective specifically in human dermatophytosis, including infections of both skin and nails, when given at doses of 200 to 600 mg/day.[2] Related drugs, sulconazole nitrate in a 1 per cent cream and miconazole nitrate in a 2 per cent cream, have been beneficial when applied to human dermatophytoses of the glabrous skin.[3] Oral ketoconazole* has been used effectively in dogs at a dosage 10 to 30 mg/kg/day for the treatment of deep mycoses. Specific data on the use of ketoconazole in cattle are not available. However, this compound and others of the imidazole group appear to offer much needed alternatives for fungal therapy including the dermatophytoses.

Topical preparations are numerous. Many may have some beneficial effects but, generally speaking, their main value is in reducing the infectivity of hairs and scales shed from active lesions. Thus, they can be used to hasten the actual "cure time" when used in conjunction with hair clipping toward the end of a period of oral griseofulvin therapy or to reduce the spread of infection to other sites on an individual or to other animals. Most of these preparations do not actually reach the dermatophytes located deeply in keratinized tissue.[6] Several are considered moderately effective for use on dermatophytoses in food-producing animals. These include:

1. *Technical captan* (N-trichloromethylmercapto-4-cyclohexene-1, 2-dicarboxamide). A 1:200 to 1:400 suspension of 45 per cent active powder applied preferably as a spray or as a rinse directly on the infected body surface. Re-treat in a week. (This is not a currently approved product for use on animals intended for food).

2. *Iodine.* Among the oldest and most commonly used preparations are tincture of iodine and Lugol's solution applied directly to lesions. More recently, organic iodine complexes (e.g., ethanol-iodine complexes) with less irritating properties have been used at concentrations of 25 to 50 ppm iodine.

3. *Other topical antidermatophytic agents.* Tolnaftate (1 to 2 per cent solution) and various fatty acid creams, including undecylenic acid preparations, aid in curtailing the spread of dermatophytosis of the glabrous skin when applied to individual lesions. However, their effectiveness on multiple lesions in haired skin is moderate at best.

From the above, it is obvious that treatment of dermatophytoses in food-producing animals is either very expensive or marginally effective. The major reason for treating affected animals is to reduce spread of infection to other individuals, to their environment (e.g., fence posts, wooden stanchions, and so on) or to their human attendants. The growth rate or other productivity of infected individuals will not usually be greatly affected unless the eyes or muzzle are involved or secondary bacterial infection intervenes.

In summary, selected individuals may be effectively treated orally with griseofulvin; groups of calves and so on can be rendered less infective and recovery enhanced by spraying with captan or topical application of one of many preparations. Barring re-infection, lesion remission should be apparent after 8 to 16 weeks.

*Nizoral, Janssen Pharmaceutical, New Brunswick, New Jersey 08903.

PREVENTION

Of primary importance in any treatment or control program is to remove the infectious source of the dermatophyte. Zoophilic dermatophyte spores may remain viable on sheltered stable supports, posts, and so on for several years, effecting exposure of subsequent groups of calves or other young stock. Prevention includes rodent-proofing animal quarters *(T. mentagrophytes),* disinfecting tack, brushes, blankets, and so on *(T. equinum, T. mentagrophytes, M. canis);* and disinfecting wooden stanchions, posts, and so on *(T. verrucosum).* Disinfection may be accomplished by spraying or dipping contaminated objects with technical captan, with agricultural Bordeaux mixture (commercially available at most nurseries), or with fungicidal solutions of high phenol coefficient (e.g., 2% Amphyl*).

The greatest hope for control of dermatophytosis in food-producing animals appears to rest in the use of active immunization. An effective vaccine for *T. verrucosum* has been developed in Russia. Two intramuscular injections of this modified viable low virulence preparation (TF 130) at a ten-day interval was shown to be 96 per cent effective in immunizing 1.4 million young calves.[5] The vaccine is not currently available in the United States.

References

1. Borelli, D., Bran, J. L., Fuentes, J., et al.: Ketoconazole, an oral antifungal: laboratory and clinical assessment of imidazole drugs. Post. Grad. Med. J. *55*:657–661, 1979.
2. Foy, W., Cox, R. W., Stiller, R. L., et al.: Oral ketoconazole for dermatophyte infections. J. Acad. Derm. *6*:455–562, 1982.
3. Gip, L. and Forsstrom, S.: A double-blind parallel study of sulconazole nitrate 1 per cent cream compared with miconazole nitrate 2 per cent cream in dermatophytoses. Mykosen *26*:231–241, 1982.
4. Dunbar, M., Pyle, R. L., Boring, J. G., and McCoy, P.: Treatment of canine blastomycosis with ketoconazole. J. Am. Vet. Med. Assoc. *182*:156–157, 1983.
5. Rotermund, H.: LTF 130: an effective vaccine against bovine trichophytosis. (In German.) Monatschr. Vet. Med. *35*:334–335, 1981.
6. Gentles, J. C.: Treatment and prophylaxis of Ringworm. Proc. VII Intl. Soc. Human and Animal Mycology. Int. Cong. Series *480*:3–8, 1979.

Supplemental Reading

Anderson, C. E.: Veterinary Pharmaceuticals and Biologicals 1978/1979. Harwal Publishing Co., Media, Pa., 1978.
Blood, D. C., Henderson, J. A., and Radostits, O. M.: Veterinary Medicine, 5th ed. Lea & Febiger, Philadelphia, 1979.
Jensen, R., and Mackey, D. R.: Diseases of Feedlot Cattle, 3rd ed. Lea & Febiger, Philadelphia, 1979.
Rippon, J. W. (ed.): Medical Mycology. W. B. Saunders Co., Philadelphia, 1974.

*Available from National Laboratories, Montvale, New Jersey 07645.

Differential Diagnosis of Virus Infections of the Ruminant Skin

E. PAUL J. GIBBS, B.V.Sc., Ph.D., F.R.C.V.S.

Skin disease may be the only feature associated with a virus infection or it may be part of a generalized disease. A clinical examination of the skin often provides valuable information to assist the clinician in the differential diag-

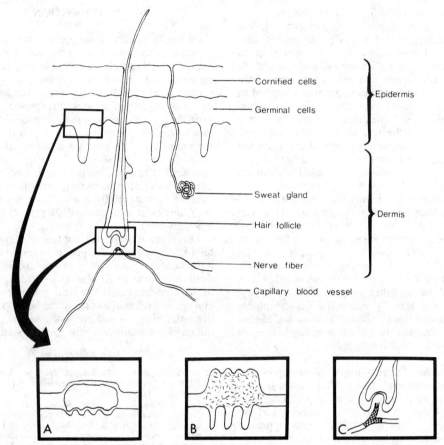

Figure 1. Pathogenesis of virus infections of the skin. The histologic structure of the skin is simple with only slight modification in specialized areas of the body. The skin and epidermoid mucous membranes of the upper alimentary tract and the external genitalia are stratified squamous epithelia and have similar structural and physiologic features.

The skin becomes infected by direct inoculation of virus through an abrasion or insect bite or through the viremia associated with a generalized infection. Normal skin is resistant to topical infection with virus.

Localized virus infections, such as those caused by the papilloma viruses and some of the poxviruses, result from direct introduction of the virus into the skin. With diseases such as foot and mouth disease and swine vesicular disease, the primary site of virus replication is often in the respiratory or alimentary tract, and the skin lesions result from the subsequent viremia. However, on occasion, even with these viruses, the primary site for virus replication may be the skin itself.

Although viruses may attack different parts of the skin *(A—C)* there is only limited variation in the primary response of the skin to a virus infection, but the appearance of the lesion may be modified by the environment, secondary bacterial or mycotic infection, and by self-inflicted trauma provoked by irritation.

A, Several viruses (e.g., those in the pox and herpes groups, foot and mouth disease virus, and swine vesicular disease virus) replicate in the germinal cells of the epidermis and produce vesicles or pustules. Virus is present in high titer in the vesicular-pustular fluid. Some of the viruses also involve the dermal connective tissue, e.g., sheep pox.

B, Papilloma viruses replicate in the germinal cells of the epidermis, causing hyperplasia of the epidermis over the dermal papillae.

C, Viruses such as bluetongue virus replicate in the endothelium of capillary blood vessels, causing hemorrhage or impairment of hair and wool growth.

nosis of several virus diseases, not only those traditionally associated with the skin, such as pox and herpes infections. Regrettably, the attention paid to the skin during a clinical examination of a diseased animal can often be said to be in inverse relation to the size of the skin: the skin is the largest organ of the body.

The majority of the virus diseases mentioned in this review have been described individually in a previous section of the book. For this reason, emphasis is placed on the differential diagnosis of virus diseases of the skin. To simplify the text and to facilitate cross reference, most of the information is presented in tables or as short notes.

PATHOGENESIS OF VIRUS INFECTIONS OF THE SKIN

A knowledge of the pathogenesis of virus infections of the skin is not essential for diagnosis but it is often helpful and is summarized in Figure 1.

CLINICAL DIAGNOSIS OF VIRUS INFECTIONS OF THE SKIN

Many of the virus diseases listed in Tables 1 and 2 do not normally occur in North America, Europe, or Australia. It is to be hoped that the veterinarians practicing in these areas will not encounter diseases such as rinderpest; however, to omit them from consideration in this review would be unwise. The freedom—or relative freedom—from major virus diseases that these areas enjoy depends, in part, upon the practicing veterinarian recognizing them should they occur and promptly informing the appropriate veterinary authorities.

The following general points should be remembered:

1. The appearance of virus lesions in the skin is often modified by the environment or by secondary bacterial and mycotic infections.

2. Vesicular diseases are sometimes difficult to differentiate on clinical signs alone even for experienced clinicians.

3. Skin infection may be a reflection of systemic infection; other organ systems should be examined.

4. The examination should extend, where applicable, to affected and superficially normal animals in the group and to other species in contact with the disease. The early clinical stages of several virus diseases are pathognomonic,

Table 1. *Virus Infections of the Skin of Cattle*

Disease	Virus Classification (Family and Genus)	Geographic Distribution of Virus	Clinical Signs	Epidemiology
Skin Disease Predominates				
Lumpy skin disease (LSD)	Pox (Capripox)	Africa south of a line from Sudan to Senegal.	Cutaneous nodules 1–4 cm diam over entire skin. Dysgalactia, lymphadenitis, and edema of limb(s) may occur. Convalescence protracted.	Disease seasonal and probably spread mechanically by biting insects. In recent years, LSD has spread extensively within Africa. Pseudo lumpy skin disease (see below) and LSD may coexist in an epidemic. LSD virus is antigenically related to sheep and goat pox virus.
Cowpox	Pox (Orthopox)	Europe	Pustular lesions usually restricted to teats or muzzle of calf suckling affected dam.	Uncommon disease. Epidemiology unknown but cattle may be atypical host for virus. Natural host may be a rodent. Cowpox causes a localized infection in humans.
Bovine vaccinia mammillitis	Pox (Orthopox)	Worldwide	Same as for cowpox.	Uncommon disease. Infection arises from attendants recently vaccinated against smallpox with subsequent transmission among cattle.
Pseudocowpox	Pox (Parapox)	Worldwide	Mild proliferative disease usually restricted to teats, or muzzle of calf suckling affected dam.	Very common disease. Cattle are susceptible to re-infection, and virus persists within milking herds. The virus causes a localized infection in humans—milker's nodule.
Pseudo lumpy skin disease (PLSD) and bovine herpes mammillitis	Herpes	Worldwide	Similar to lumpy skin disease but lesions have slightly depressed center and do not involve subcutis. No lymphadenitis. Convalescence is not protracted. With bovine herpes mammillitis, lesions restricted to teats and udder skin. Edema of teats, vesication, and ulceration lead to scabs forming over most of teat surface.	Disease seasonal and probably spread by biting insects. Epidemics occur. Morbidity can be high but mortality low. Mammillitis more commonly seen than PLSD in countries with high production dairy cows. As with other herpes infections, infected cattle may become carriers.
Warts/papillomatosis	Papova (Papilloma)	Worldwide	Proliferative, slowly growing lesions often present at sites where skin abrasion occurs. May be single or numerous.	Very common disease. Infection is spread by fomites and close contact with infected animals. Several types exist.
Skin Disease as Part of a Generalized Infection				
Foot-and-mouth disease	Picorna (Aphtho)	Worldwide except for N. America, most of Europe, and Australasia.	Vesicles occur in mouth and on lips, muzzle, teats, coronary band, and interdigital clefts of feet. Depression and loss of condition. Convalescence protracted.	Infection transmitted by aerosol and fomites. Seven antigenic types exist.
Vesicular stomatitis	Rhabdo (Vesiculo)	Americas	Same as for foot-and-mouth disease.	Epidemiology not fully known. Transmission may occur by arthropods as well as by direct contact. Two antigenic types exist.
Rinderpest	Paramyxo (Morbilli)	Africa, Middle East, and Indian subcontinent.	Epithelial necrosis in mouth and alimentary tract. Erosions can occur on muzzle, lips, and teats. Diarrhea and pneumonia may cause death. On occasion macules, which later lead to vesicopustules, cause erection and tufting of the hair.	Infection transmitted by direct contact and by aerosol over short distances.

Localized skin disease may result from direct extension of lesions from the mouth, nose, or genitalia with infectious bovine rhinotracheitis/infectious pustular vulvovaginitis (herpes), malignant catarrh (herpes), blue tongue and related diseases (orbi), mucosal disease/bovine virus diarrhea (pesti), and bovine papular stomatitis (parapox). Occasionally these diseases may produce generalized skin disease.

Self-inflicted injury to the skin may result from the pruritus associated with Aujeszky's disease (herpes) and other virus infections of the central nervous system.

Table 2. *Virus Infections of the Skin of Sheep and Goats*

Disease	Virus Classification (Family and Genus)	Geographic Distribution of Virus	Clinical Signs	Epidemiology
Skin Disease Predominates				
Sheep/goat pox	Pox (Capripox)	Eastern Mediterranean, Africa and Asia.	Pocks over entire skin surface, especially around head and genitalia. Internal organs also infected, and sequelae include pneumonia and death.	Transmission of infection probably by respiratory tract. Sheep and goat pox viruses currently considered indistinguishable; both related to lumpy skin disease virus.
Contagious pustular dermatitis (contagious ecthyma; orf)	Pox (Parapox)	Worldwide	Pustules and scabs, particularly around muzzle and lips. Lesions may be present on teats and in mouth of lambs.	Very common disease. Transmission through skin abrasions such as caused by dry and prickly pasture. The virus causes a localized infection in humans—orf.
Warts/papillomatosis	Papova (Papilloma)	Probably worldwide	Proliferative, slowly growing lesions often present at sites where skin abrasion occurs.	Uncommon disease. Virus considered different from cattle wart virus. Infection probably spread by fomites.
Skin Disease as Part of a Generalized Infection				
Foot-and-mouth disease	Picorna (Aphtho)	Worldwide except for N. America, most of Europe, and Australasia.	Vesicles occur in mouth and on lips, teats, coronary band, and interdigital clefts of feet. Clinical disease usually milder than in cattle or pigs.	Infection transmitted by aerosol and fomites. Seven antigenic types exist.
Rinderpest and peste des petits ruminants (PPR)	Paramyxo (Morbilli)	Africa, Middle East, and Indian subcontinent.	Epithelial necrosis in mouth and alimentary tract; erosions can occur on muzzle, lips, and teats. Diarrhea and pneumonia may cause death. Rinderpest and PPR are clinically indistinguishable.	Infection transmitted by direct contact and by aerosol over short distances. Rinderpest infection of sheep generally uncommon and occurs after contact with infected cattle. PPR restricted to sheep and goats; cattle do not develop disease.
Blue tongue	Reo (Orbi)	Africa, Asia, N. and S. America, and parts of Australasia.	Epithelial erosions on muzzle, lips, and teats. Edema of head. In acute stage generalized erythema of skin and coronary band leads to subsequent "wool break."	Virus transmitted by insect vector (*Culicoides*). Currently 22 antigenic types recognized.

Abnormal hair growth may be a sequela to an *in utero* infection with border disease virus (pesti), and self-inflicted injury to the skin may result from a viral infection of the central nervous system—for example, Aujeszky's disease (herpes) and scrapie.

but animals at this stage of the disease may not be causing concern to the client and are not presented for examination.

5. The extent and severity of the skin lesions are sometimes obscured by the coat. With some virus diseases the coat is itself an indicator of previous infection; in border disease in lambs, which is a pestivirus infection acquired *in utero,* the wool has a higher percentage of hair than is normal; in sheep previously infected with blue tongue virus, "wool break" may occur.

6. The epidemiology of several virus diseases of the skin is characteristic (Tables 1 and 2). A full history of the disease outbreak may assist the clinician in making a diagnosis—for example, diseases that are insect transmitted are often seasonal; some are diseases related to infection of animal attendants.

COLLECTION AND EXAMINATION OF SAMPLES FOR LABORATORY DIAGNOSIS OF VIRUS INFECTIONS OF THE SKIN

When collecting samples for virus diagnosis it must be remembered that the clinician's suspicion that the disease is caused by a virus may be incorrect; samples should be collected for alternative diagnoses.

Assuming that it is a virus disease, the following should be remembered:

1. The titer of virus is usually highest at affected sites and during the early stages of disease.

2. Viruses replicate only in living cells and their stability is adversely affected by exposure to light, desiccation, extremes of pH, and most common disinfectants.

3. Secondary bacterial or mycotic infection is a common sequela of virus disease; samples taken from the later stages of disease are less likely to contain virus.

To overcome the problems mentioned above, the sample should be protected by storage at 4°C in virus transport medium.

More than one virus infection of the skin can be present in a group of animals at the time of sampling; these may be unrelated to the disease under investigation or may be exacerbating the problem. To avoid an erroneous or incomplete diagnosis, different types of lesions and more than one animal should be sampled.

When collecting a skin scraping or obtaining a biopsy the areas should be washed with water or saline—not with alcohol, as this inactivates most viruses. Scraping of the skin and mucous membranes should be extended to the periphery and base of the lesion. It is helpful to wet the lesion and scalpel blade with virus transport medium before sampling, as this helps to prevent the tissues from falling from the blade.

LABORATORY DIAGNOSIS

Descriptions of the laboratory procedures for the diagnosis of virus infections of the skin as listed in Tables 1 and 2 are given in the section on individual virus diseases.

Electron microscopy is particularly useful for the rapid diagnosis of virus diseases of the skin, but attempted isolation of the causal virus in tissue culture is probably the most widely used and most sensitive technique available.

Nonviral Teat Lesions

R. L. SIEBER, D.V.M., M.S.

Teat lesions originate from a variety of sources: trauma, environmental conditions, exposure to irritating chemicals, viral infections, and improperly functioning milking equipment. Teat lesions can have a severe economic impact on a dairyman by interfering with the milking routine and by increasing the likelihood of intramammary infection and culling of animals.

ENVIRONMENTAL LESIONS

Chapping is the most common teat lesion seen in the northern United States and Canada. The condition appears as horizontal fissures in the skin near the base of the teat. A slight weeping of serum results in the formation of a light brown linear scab, unless the lesion becomes infected, resulting in a much darker scab. Teat chapping is frequently associated with cold and damp weather but can be exacerbated by chemicals and milking equipment. In most cases the skin appears dry and leather-like and may flake.

Teat chapping problems can frequently be resolved by using a good quality teat dip. Teat dips in use in the dairy should be critically examined for their skin conditioning ability and changed if necessary. Application of hydroscopic skin-softening agents such as glycerin or lanolin as salves or in teat dips will result in marked improvement within two weeks.

Freezing is one of the most severe environmental causes of teat lesions. The appearance of the lesion depends on the severity of the insult. Initially the teat will appear reddened or pale in color. In severe cases a thimble-shaped scab will encase the distal half of the teat. After several days, the scab will slough, leaving a raw and denuded teat that rapidly forms a second scab. The teat orifice may be occluded, making milking difficult. In less severe cases, the skin becomes leather-like and takes on an orange-red coloration. In these cases a scab does not form, and after several days the condition does not appear to bother the cow during milking. Sores on the teat end are frequently seen in herds where the cows are sent outside immediately after milking. The lesion appears in the area where a drop of liquid froze or evaporated.

Treatment of frozen teats is aimed at preventing intramammary infection during the healing process. The application of skin-softening agents is beneficial in milder cases. Prevention requires drying the teats after milking, providing windbreaks or protected areas for the cows to go to immediately after milking, preventing winds from blowing through sheds, and providing shed entrances that cannot be blocked by one belligerent animal. Consideration should be given to discontinuing teat dipping in severely cold weather if teats cannot be adequately dried.

Sunburn is an occasional environmental problem affecting the teats and udder. Sunburn appears as a severe reddening and drying of the teats and udder, usually affecting only the lateral teat surfaces on one side of the udder and the distal medial surfaces on the other teats. The condition is quite painful for several days, followed by peeling of the skin in approximately one week. In severe cases, blistering may occur.

Diagnosis of sunburn is made from the appearance of shade lines and the dry reddened skin. Treatment consists of applying moisturizing salves or ointments.

CHEMICAL LESIONS

The appearance of chemically induced lesions is dependent on the severity of the insult, not on the chemical involved. In most cases the offending chemical is applied as a teat dip or udder wash, but it may be added to the bedding. The problem is commonly seen as a drying and flaking of the teat skin or the appearance of scab-like lesions on the teat end. The teat orifice often becomes discolored from stains in teat dips or udder washes. The stained tissue appears similar to a scab when iodine-based products are used.

Chemically induced dryness of the teat skin is seen most often in winter. The problem is similar to chapping, with horizontal cracking of the teat skin in mild cases and vertical cracking in severe situations. It is frequently caused by teat dips with poor conditioning ability. Iodine teat dips appear to be the most frequent culprit, most likely owing to their widespread use. The problem has also been seen with the use of quaternary ammonium dips, chlorhexidine-based dips, dodecyl benzene sulfonic acid, and hypochlorite teat dips. The characteristic staining of the teat end is present on 40 to 50 per cent of the teats in affected herds. Changing to a teat dip with better skin-softening qualities will result in marked improvement in 10 to 14 days.

On dairies where lime is added to the bedding a similar condition will occasionally occur on the lateral surfaces of the teats and udder. The problem is often blamed on the use of incompletely slaked lime. This condition may also result from the interaction between teat dips and udder washes with lime and premise disinfectants such as paraformaldehyde.

The application of a concentrated udder wash or cleaning solution or a teat dip that has been frozen may result in a more severe lesion over the distal 1 to 2 cm of the teat. Approximately 80 to 90 per cent of the dipped teats will develop scabs over the teat end, with about 5 per cent exhibiting a unique mushroom-shaped appearance, with the stem of the mushroom extending up the teat canal. If the teat was chapped or scratched, scabs will form over the cracks in the skin.

MACHINE-INDUCED LESIONS

The milking equipment can affect the teat by causing abrasions in the areas of contact, by disrupting the normal blood and tissue fluid flow through the teat and udder parenchyma, and by placing pressure or stress forces unevenly on the teat, resulting in distortion or stretching of the teat tissue.

Machine-induced abrasions are usually confined to the

area where the mouthpiece of the inflation contacts the teat. The problem is rare with the type of equipment on the market today. Most machine-induced abrasions are a combination of problems, like sunburn or chapping, that have been complicated by the rubbing action of the inflation mouthpiece.

The effects of vacuum on the fluid dynamics of the teat result in some of the most significant machine-mediated lesions. During machine milking, blood and tissue fluids pool in the portion of the teat exposed to vacuum. Machine factors that result in inadequate reversal of this process will result in congestion, pain, and hemorrhage over the distal third of the teat. Overmilking has a similar effect. Chronic exposure to these conditions may result in a palpable thickening of the distal third of the teat.

A common condition seen in most herds is the development of a ring-shaped callous around the teat orifice ranging from 1 to 4 mm in thickness and up to 1 cm in diameter. The callous tissue may appear cracked and scab-like. The condition has been historically termed a prolapse or eversion of the teat meatus and was assumed to be due to machine milking. Recently it has been found on hand-milked cows and beef cows, indicating that other factors are involved in its formation. The condition is widespread, appearing to some degree on most cows. The condition is commonly found in herds where tests of the milking equipment reveal no mechanical faults, but it is more prevalent in herds that are overmilked. The condition varies from herd to herd, and high-producing cows are more frequently affected. It is more prevalent at the peak of lactation than during stages of low production. Comparison of the levels of intramammary infection for teats with this condition and those without it reveals no appreciable difference.

SUMMARY

Many teat lesion problems are seasonal in occurrence. The problem will frequently subside in the spring, only to recur in mid fall. In the midwestern United States most teat lesion problems occur from November to April.

When investigating a teat lesion complaint a large proportion of the herd should be examined, including heifers and dry cows. Environmental factors, husbandry practices, and secondary bacterial infection can markedly affect the appearance of the teats and make it difficult to find typical lesions.

In almost all cases treatment consists of removing the causative agent and using skin moisturizers. Improving the teat skin condition will markedly decrease secondary bacterial infection and subsequent intramammary infection.

Supplemental Reading

Baumann, L. E.: Milking Machine Influence on Blood Flow in the Bovine Teat. M.S. Thesis, University of Minnesota, 1982.

Francis, P. G.: Mastitis Control and Herd Management. Technical Bull. 4, Nat. Inst. for Res. in Dairying, Reading, England, 1981.

Sieber, R. L., and Farnsworth, R. J.: Prevalence of chronic teat-end lesions and their relationship to intramammary infection in 22 herds of dairy cattle. J. Am. Vet. Med. Assoc. 178:1263–1267, 1981.

Environmental Skin Conditions
Photosensitization with Gangrene

LEONARD BLACK, B.V.Sc., Ph.D., F.R.C.V.S.

Although most pathologic conditions of the skin, and indeed of all other systems, can be assigned to environmental causation, this article will be limited to the consideration of photosensitization and other conditions that produce superficial ischemia and gangrene. Photosensitivity is excessive sensitivity to light owing to the presence of photodynamic agents in the skin. These agents cause dermatitis when exposed to ultraviolet light.

CLINICAL SIGNS

Onset may be as early as one day after dosing phenothiazine to pigs or, where plant toxins are concerned, four to five days after changing pasture. In Southdown sheep suffering a hereditary biliary excretion defect the signs appear when the lambs first start grazing.

Afflicted animals seek shade or, if none is available, turn away from the sun. Sunlight produces swelling, cracks, serum ooze, necrosis, and sloughing of the lightly pigmented areas of the skin, which are only sparsely covered with hair or wool. In cattle lesions appear on the udder, back, and flanks, whereas in sheep the face and ears are usually affected. In sheep jaundice is generally prominent. Phenothiazine may provoke photophobia, blepharospasm, lacrimation, and keratitis. Wasting and lethargy are features of chronic hepatotoxic damage (crotolariasis).

PATHOGENESIS

The Extrinsic Form

The signs occur after intake of preformed photodynamic agents or their immediate precursors. Plants that may cause the condition include St. John's wort (*Hypericum perforatum*), buckwheat (*Polygonum fagopyrum*), wild carrot (*Cymopterus watsoni*), perennial rye grass (*Lolium perenne*), clover, alfalfa, lucerne (*Trifolium* spp.), rape (*Brassica* spp.), and others. Consumption of the aphids that often infest trefoil (*Medicago denticulata*) and phenothiazine sulfoxide, a product of the helminthic phenothiazine, have also been implicated.

The Intrinsic Form

Two varieties can be distinguished. *Congenital porphyria* has been reported in cattle in Argentina, England, Jamaica, South Africa, and the U.S. and in pigs in Denmark and New Zealand. It is a rare condition transmitted by a simple recessive autosomal gene in cattle and a dominant gene in pigs. A hereditary defect in metabolism causes aberrant breakdown products of hemoglobin to be formed. Type I porphyrin, an iron-heme catabolite, accumulates in the tissues of cattle and, in addition to photosensitization, causes pink discoloration of the teeth and bones. The urine is also pink on excretion but darkens on exposure to light. In pigs the teeth are tinged pink and may fluoresce in UV light. In this species, however, photosensitization is not a feature nor is the urine discolored in any but the most severe cases.

Skin conditions can also take a *hepatotoxic form*. Normal metabolites accumulate in the tissues in excessive quantities as a result of liver damage and/or deranged biliary function. Phylloerythrin, the photodynamic substance involved, is derived from chlorophyll and in health is metabolized in the liver and excreted in the bile. The plants possibly responsible for liver damage include *Tribulus terrestris, Lantana camara, Lippia rehmanni, Narthrecium ossifragum, Panicum miliaceum, Agave lecheguilla, Crotolaria retusa, Senechio jacobeus, Holoclyx graziovii, Kochia scoparia, Myoporum laetum, Tetradymia* spp., *Nolina texana,* and *Lupinus angustifolius.* Poisonous algae *(Microcystis aeruginosa, Microcystis flosaquae,* and *Anabaena flosaquae),* mineral poisons (copper, phosphorus), and certain helminthic and trypanocidal therapeutic agents (carbon tetrachloride and phenanthradinium) have also been implicated.

DIAGNOSIS

Typical distribution of lesions on the light-colored and unprotected areas of the skin is highly suggestive. In congenital porphyria pink discoloration of the bones, teeth, and urine is characteristic. Methods for quantitative determination of porphyrins have been published. When hepatotoxins are responsible jaundice and liver degeneration are usually evident.

Gangrene and sloughing due to other causes should be differentiated. These include:

1. *External pressure:* Decubial sores form on boney protruberances owing to pressure, for instance in parturient paresis when animals are obliged to lie on hard surfaces for prolonged periods.

2. *Internal pressure:* This is due to swelling, for instance around the hocks of stanchioned animals.

3. *Snake venom:* The venom of Viperidae (Russels viper, puff adder, European adder, rattlesnake, cottonmouth moccasin, and fer-de-lance) contains coagulant and necrotizing agents that produce sloughing at the site of the bites.

4. *Ergot poisoning: Claviceps purpurea,* a fungus that infests rye (and occasionally other cereals and grasses), causes constriction of the arterioles. Cattle are usually affected although other species are also susceptible. The condition manifests itself as sloughing of the extremities (ears and tail) and of those parts of skin where the circulation is constricted (Fig. 1). Lameness and recumbency may also be evident.

5. *Burns, scalds, and rope galls.*

6. *Frostbite:* The teats are especially vulnerable if cows are turned out in the cold after washing but not drying of the udder.

7. *Bacterial toxins: Staphylococcus aureus* (alpha toxin) produces gangrene of the udder. Clostridial infection

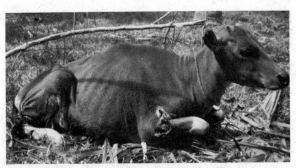

Figure 1. Ergot *(Claviceps purpurea)* poisoning. Note sloughing of the ears and of the joints, where circulation to the skin has been impeded. Recumbency is another feature. (Courtesy of Drs. I. Gde Sudana, D.V.M., D.T.V.M., Director, Balai Penyidikan Penyakit Hewan Wilayah VI, Bali and F.J.R.R. Menard, D.T.V.M., M.R.C.V.S.)

produces gangrenous and emphysematous lesions in the muscles that may smell of butyric acid (butter-like).

8. *Viral infections:* Bovine ulcerative mamillitis (herpes virus) is responsible for gangrenous lesions in the udders of cows and heifers.

9. *Type III hypersensitivity:* Antigen-antibody complexes, deposited in the arterioles, produce thrombosis, ischemia, and sloughing (see Hypersensitivity).

TREATMENT

Prevent exposure to sunlight. Prevent further ingestion of toxic plants or minerals. Remove green feed. Laxatives (liquid paraffin, 1 to 2 ml/kg body weight or magnesium sulphate, 0.5 to 1 gm/kg dissolved in water) should be given as a drench to prevent additional absorption of toxic substances from the gut.

Local lesions should be débrided. Streptokinase-streptodornase (Varidase*) injected beneath the scab hastens separation. Iodine tincture, 2 per cent, stimulates healing of dormant lesions. Demulcents (calamine lotion), insect repellents, and steroid-antibiotic cream (Panalog†) are helpful. An aerosol spray of crystal violet and chloramphenicol both shields the lesions from light and combats infection.

Hydrocortisone (100 to 600 mg in 1000 ml of 10 per cent dextrose saline) injected IV or SC for cattle as well as penicillin G by IM injection is recommended.

Supplemental Reading

Blood, D. C., and Henderson, J. A.: Diseases of the skin: Photosensitisation. *In* Veterinary Medicine, 4th ed. Bailliere, Tindall, London, 1974, 245–247.
Schwartz, S., Berg, M. H., Bossenmaier, I., and Dinsmore, H.: Determination of porphyrins in biological materials. Methods in Biochem. Anal. *8*:221, 1960.

---

*Available from Lederle Laboratories, Pearl River, New York 10965.
†Available from E. R. Squibb, Princeton, New Jersey 08540.

Bovine Hypersensitivity Skin Disease

THOMAS O. MANNING, D.V.M., M.S., A.C.V.D.
and VICKI JO SCHEIDT, D.V.M., A.C.V.D.

The bovine skin diseases associated with hypersensitivity reactions are few in number (Table 1), but their small number belies their veterinary medical importance. Hypersensitivity is a state of altered reactivity. The body reacts with an exaggerated response to a foreign agent. Hypersensitivity reactions are disadvantageous to the animal. The type of hypersensitivity (immediate or delayed) is of importance because it may affect the type of clinical signs, pathogenesis, diagnosis, and therapeutic management. Hypersensitivity reactions may also be mixed. The skin is only one organ involved in hypersensitivity reactions. These skin reactions are usually not life-threatening. However, the skin is important in that it may forewarn the animal's attendant or veterinarian of foreboding and disastrous hypersensitivity reactions involving other organ systems (respiratory, gastrointestinal, and so on).

CLINICAL SIGNS

Immediate Hypersensitivity

Clinically, hypersensitivity reactions may be divided into immediate and delayed reactions. Hypersensitivity reactions have also been classified by Campbell on the basis of their etiology:[1] (1) directly attributable to administration of the allergen (induced allergies), (2) human intervention playing some part in induction of disease, and (3) spontaneous (naturally occurring) allergies (atopies) (see Table 1). The causes of spontaneous allergy are obscure. Such reactions are frequently unpredictable and mild. They seem to appear for no obvious reason, last three to four hours, and resolve without a trace or clue as to the cause.

Immediate hypersensitivities are mediated by certain types of antibodies (IgE and IgG). These antigen-specific antibodies are a result of previous sensitization to an allergen and expedite the immediate release of pharmacologically active substances (histamine, serotonin, and so on). Classification of anaphylaxis using the traditional Gell and Coombs categories (atopy, Arthus-serum sickness, immune complex) has received little attention in bovine hypersensitivity.

Skin reactions associated with immediate hypersensitivity reactions usually begin within 30 minutes of exposure. The common presentation of urticaria (erect tufts of hair) has led many to the misconception that all erect tufts of hair or edematous papules-plaques are associated with allergic reactions. Follicular diseases (demodex, dermatophytosis, bacterial) and insect bites must be ruled out. Systemic hypersensitivity may progress from the milder stage of urticaria to confluent plaques of edema and angioedema. Cutaneous edema is most obvious about the face (eyes, muzzle, ears) and the perineal region (anus and vulva). Urticaria may be associated with pruritus and

The authors wish to acknowledge with thanks the consultation of Dr. Tom Divers and Dr. Maurice (Pete) White.

Table 1. Causes of Bovine Hypersensitivity Skin Disease

Induced Allergies	Human Intervention	Spontaneous
Vaccines	Milk allergy	Feedstuff
Leptospira pomona	*Hypoderma bovis*	Milk
bacterins (rabbit sera)	*Hypoderma lineatum*	Grain
Brucella abortus strain 19		Hay silage
Foot-and-mouth disease		Pasture
vaccine		Bedding (moldy)
Shipping fever vaccine		Plants
Antibiotics		Molds
Penicillin		Insects
(methylcellulose)		Cobwebs
Penicillin-streptomycin		
Neomycin		
Oxytetracycline		
Corticosteroids		
Chorionic gonadotropins		

pain. Cattle may sweat profusely and, in cases of severe allergic shock, become so cyanotic that the white hairless portions of the body (udder, vulva, and anus) develop a purple hue.

Diagnosis

Skin testing as a diagnostic tool for the immediate type of bovine hypersensitivity has been reported in the veterinary literature. Its practicality and efficacy are of question. A small volume (0.05 to 0.1 ml) of a dilute solution (1:10 to 1:1000) injected into the skin of an allergic animal will produce swelling, pain, and erythema. Which types of immediate hypersensitivities produce the strongest reaction to diagnostic intradermal skin testing has not been reported. When testing the skin, it is highly desirable to include normal cattle as controls. Skin tests should be performed with care to avoid severe anaphylactic reactions.

Delayed Hypersensitivity

Delayed hypersensitivities are mediated by lymphocytes. These leukocytes migrate to the site of allergen deposition, where they mediate a tissue reaction. Delayed reactions usually take one to three weeks to develop after initial exposure. Once the initial hypersensitivity reaction has developed, the delayed response requires two to three days to express itself upon re-exposure. The tuberculin test, based on delayed hypersensitivity, is very effective in cattle. This test demonstrates that cattle are capable of hypersensitivities of this type. Clinical allergies of the delayed type are uncommon. The differentiation between allergic contact dermatitis and irritant contact dermatitis presents a perplexing clinical problem.

Delayed skin hypersensitivity reactions usually present as papular dermatitis. Papules may coalesce to form plaques. Papules develop between the hindlegs and on the dewlap, neck, and back. They often spread to cover most of the body. The hair in the affected area becomes sparse, and lesions exude serum and crust over. This delayed reaction seems to be a generalized Arthus-like reaction caused by antigen-antibody deposition on blood vessel endothelium.

CONTROL

Avoidance of the particular suspected allergen is the ideal method of controlling the hypersensitive individual.

An in-depth history may indicate the responsible allergen. In most spontaneous hypersensitivity reactions, however, avoidance of the allergen may be difficult or impossible.

Because of the acute onset and unpredictable course of most allergic reactions, veterinarians tend to consider them as emergencies. The first impulse should be to remove the animal from the offending allergen and stabilize the patient. This may be accomplished by discontinuing the administration of a suspect drug or, in the case of milk allergy, milking the cow dry. When the reaction is spontaneous and the agent is not as obvious, it is advisable to remove the animal from its environment. A well-ventilated area with plenty of water and a simple diet is ideal.

Drugs

The choice of anti-allergic/anti-inflammatory drugs for the control of hypersensitivities may be perplexing for the veterinarian. This broad category of drugs (Table 2) has been described by Eyre and is divided into four groups.[2]

Functional or Physiologic Antagonists

The sympathomimetic amines act by physiologically counteracting the pathologic events induced by the vasoactive chemical mediators of inflammation. Adrenaline has been widely employed in the treatment of acute anaphylactic shock and acute pulmonary edema. Adrenaline also reverses the fall in blood pressure and cardiac insufficiency and additionally causes constriction and decreased permeability of the microvasculature. Indirect-acting sympathomimetics include methylxanthines (aminophylline, theophylline) and amphetamines. These agents possess properties similar to adrenaline. Aminophylline may be employed in circumstances similar to those in which adrenaline is used. Salbutamol, a specific beta-2 antagonist, may be used as a specific bronchodilator without the significant cardiovascular actions of adrenaline and aminophylline.

The anticholinergic agent atropine is an effective bronchodilator and antisecretory agent. Mediators of anaphylaxis stimulate pulmonary vagal reflexes, which contribute significantly to the pathogenesis of airway obstruction. Atropine antagonizes vagal tone.

Selective Pharmacologic Inhibitors

The H_1 antagonists of histamine (pyribenzamine, promethazine, pheniramine) are of little value in veterinary medicine, especially in ruminants. Antihistamines only interfere with histamine. They lack the ability to reverse (repair) the inflammatory process or inhibit the release of other mediators of inflammation. Although some Type I hypersensitivities involving the skin and nasolacrimal areas may respond to antihistamines, the response of antihistamines is slower but lasts longer than that of sympathomimetic drugs. Antihistamines are of no value in the treatment of anaphylactic shock in the bovine. The H_2 class histamine antagonist cimetidine principally blocks the stimulation activity of histamine on the myocardium and gastric secretion. However, because H_2 receptors effect bronchodilation and modulate mediator release of other anaphylactic agents, H_2 antagonists may actually potentiate Type-1 anaphylaxis. Cimetidine has been reported to cause abomasal ulceration in ruminants.

Anti-Inflammatory Drugs

Glucocorticosteroids of all types are similar in chemical structure and mode of action. The physiologic effects of these drugs are complex. The anti-inflammatory actions of these compounds suppress all aspects of early inflammation (vasodilation, edema, migration of leukocytes), late inflammation (collagen deposition, fibroblast formation), and scar formation. Inflammation is inhibited irrespective of the inciting cause. Glucocorticoids act by stabilizing lysosomal and cellular membranes. Therefore, they prevent the release of chemical mediators and proteolytic enzymes. Two important features of glucocorticoids include their ability to (1) potentiate the effects of endogenous adrenaline resulting in bronchodilation, and (2) inhibit prostaglandin production.

Nonsteroidal anti-inflammatory drugs (phenylbutazone, acetylsalicylic acid, indomethacin, ibuprofen) block the enzyme cyclooxygenase, thereby inhibiting the biosynthesis of prostaglandins and endoperoxidases, which are essential in the major pathways of inflammation. Although primarily used for musculoskeletal disorders, recent studies have shown their effectiveness in controlling

Table 2. *Drugs For the Control of Bovine Hypersensitivity Skin Disease*

Drug	Dosage	Precaution/Comment
Functional/Physiologic Antagonists		
Adrenaline (epinephrine) (1:1000 solution)	4–8 ml/cow	
Aminophylline	PO 3–5 gm QID	Little benefit
	IM 1 gm QID	IM—painful
Atropine	1 gm/cow SID followed by 0.5 gm/cow in 2–3 days	Atypical interstitial pneumonia and organophosphate toxicity
	100 mg/cow	Acute bronchial constriction
Selective Pharmacologic Inhibitors		
Tripelennamme	1.0 mg/kg	
A-H solution	25 ml/cow SC or *slow* IV BID	
Aspirin	PO 100 mg/kg BID or TID	
Phenylbutazone	PO 6 mg/kg every 48 hrs	
Wide-Spectrum Anti-Inflammatory Drugs		
Dexamethasone	IM or IV 5–20 mg	Caution: latent IBR or advanced pregnancy (abortion)

cardiorespiratory manifestations of hypersensitivity and helminth-induced interstitial pneumonia in cattle. Nonsteroidal anti-inflammatory drugs are both antipyretic and analgesic.

Miscellaneous Inhibitors of Inflammation

These include diethylcarbamazine citrate (DECC) and disodium cromoglycate (DSCG). DECC is used as an anthelmintic for bovine lung worms. Its efficacy in helminth-induced hypersensitivity pneumonia may be explained by its ability to control the release of prostaglandins, histamine, and SRS-A rather than its anthelmintic activity. DSCG interferes with the release of histamine and SRS-A. Although of limited use in bovine pulmonary hypersensitivity, DSCG may be useful in controlling clinical allergies in the horse.

References

1. Campbell, S. G.: Allergic reactions. *In* Amstutz, H. E. (ed.): Bovine Medicine and Surgery. American Vetenary Publications, Wheaton, Ill., 1980, 503–509.
2. Eyre, P.: Pharmacological aspects of hypersensitivity in domestic animals: a review. Vet. Res. Commun. 4:83–98, 1980.

Bovine Neoplastic Skin Diseases

ELAINE HUNT, D.V.M.

The primary cutaneous neoplasms in the bovine include papilloma, fibropapilloma, squamous cell carcinoma, fibroma, melanoma, and cutaneous lymphosarcoma. Squamous cell carcinoma is most commonly associated with the ocular structures and is discussed in the section concerned with ophthalmic disorders; the majority of the remaining tumors are benign. Anatomic sites of predisposition are listed in Table 1.

PAPILLOMA, FIBROPAPILLOMA (WARTS)

Warts—the contagious, hairless, self-limiting tumors of the skin—are caused by bovine papilloma virus (BPV). Four of the five identified strains of BPV share some antigenic similarity but lack immunologic cross-reactivity, thus explaining some of the commercial vaccine failures. BPV-5, -2, and -1 are the most common tumor types in the U.S. The infections are of greatest economic significance when young, valuable animals are barred from overseas sales, competitive shows, or placement in bull-test stations; severe infestations may contribute to ill thrift, especially if complicated by fly strike or louse infestation.

Clinical Signs

Affected cattle are often 18 months of age or less; spontaneous regression occurs in 1 to 12 months. Dose and method of exposure affect rapidity of lesion development; most appear within four months of exposure. The firm, gray, protruding masses usually have a horny surface, may be as small as 1 mm in size or several inches in diameter, may be singular or clustered, and may be broad-based or pedunculated. If over 20 per cent of the body is affected, the animal may show concurrent signs of ill thrift. Lesion localization is a characteristic of each virus strain and is outlined in Table 1.

Diagnosis

Generally this is by inspection and recognition; histopathologic examination is rarely necessary. If required, excised tumors can be fixed in 10 per cent formalin or Bouin's fixative. Serologic techniques are available but are rarely used for routine diagnosis.

Table 1. *Predisposed Anatomic Sites for Bovine Neoplastic Skin Diseases*

Neoplasia	Location	Comments
Warts, typical		
BPV-1	Glans penis of male; filamentous or frond-like on nose or teats	Transmitted at coitus
BPV-2	Head, neck, withers, face, dewlap of young animals	Usually regress; common form of warts
BPV-5	White, smooth elongated nodules or "rice grains"	
Ocular papilloma	Long, frond-like, branching growths attached to eyelid or corneoscleral junction or rounded protuberance	May regress spontaneously or give rise to carcinoma
Atypical warts		
BPV-3	Nonpedunculated, flat circular growths; delicate and frond-like on cut section	Herd outbreaks, large numbers affected, adults and young; do not regress
Bovine leukosis, skin form	1–3 years old; widespread nodules or plaques in skin	Frequent regression and recurrence
Vulvar squamous cell carcinoma	5 years or older; only on unpigmented skin of vulva; rough surface, roughly circumscribed, foul smelling, ulcerated; Ayrshires and Holsteins especially affected	Thought due to ultraviolet rays; no therapy if large; rare in U.S.
Melanoma	May be predilection toward Angus; cattle 18 months or younger; usually benign; no site of predilection; firm, dome-shaped, appear jet black on cut surface or can be diagnosed by histologic tests	Fairly uncommon in U.S.
Mastocytoma	Calves as well as mature animals; subcutaneous, generally nodular, multiple masses 1–10 cm	Often in conjunction with mast cell infiltrates of internal organs; rare
Cutaneous angiomatosis	Hemangioma-like lesion frequently on dorsum of the back; often multiple reddish gray to pink, soft, sessile or pedunculated, up to 2.5 cm; recurring hemorrhage can be profuse; 5 year olds or older	Seen in U.K. and France

Treatment

Vaccination in ongoing cases of the common head and neck form is reported to have no positive benefit and may even increase the size of the warts and prolong the clinical disease course if the vaccine is administered in the early stages of infection. Autogenous vaccination, wart maceration, and cryosurgical wart destruction have all been utilized in attempts to stimulate an immune response and hasten wart resolution; documentation of the real success of these techniques is lacking.

Prevention

Repeated exposure to one strain of BPV will usually result in resistance to further infection, although animals may then develop infection from another strain. Elimination of sharp or abrasive structures in the environment (splintered feed bunks, wooden fencing, or barbed wire); proper sanitation of tattooing and dehorning equipment; prevention of interchange of ropes, brushes, and halters; segregation of affected cattle; and repeated use of commercial or autogenous wart vaccines in *uninfected* cattle may decrease the incidence of clinical disease. Autogenous vaccines can be derived from excised warts that are ground up and formalin-treated or by mincing and freeze-thawing the tumor tissue two to three times, then mixing one part of minced tumor with nine parts of 0.85 saline solution and filtering through gauze. This vaccine can be stored at 4°C. Either vaccine is administered intradermally, 1 to 5 ml once weekly for three weeks, in calves two to three months of age or older.

GENERALIZED WARTS

Extensive, generalized tumor development (especially over the head, neck, shoulders, dewlap, and brisket) occurs in occasional animals. These may persist for months and show no evidence of tumor regression despite therapy. When more than 20 per cent of the body is affected, prognosis for recovery is poor; failure of cell-mediated immunity is suspected in such cases.

ATYPICAL WARTS

These are fragile, nonpedunculated, circular growths that do not protrude from the skin as prominently as regular warts and often have hair growing between the delicate fronds. These may coalesce to cover such large areas that excision is impossible. Cases occur in young and mature animals; the papillomas usually do not regress. Interdigital papillomas may also be caused by the same virus. On cross section, atypical warts will demonstrate fine, delicate fronds; histopathologically, there is an absence of dermal fibroplasia. There is no known means of treatment or prevention other than surgical excision.

BOVINE LEUKOSIS

The skin form of bovine leukosis is very *rare* and is considered to be a type of sporadic bovine leukosis (as opposed to enzootic bovine leukosis). As such, serum submitted for bovine leukosis virus antibody will be negative, so this diagnostic test cannot be utilized and histologic diagnosis is necessary. Affected cattle are reported to be one to three years old with widespread 1- to 5-cm nodules or plaques *in* the skin of the neck and back and on the dorsal and lateral surfaces of the head, perineum, and thighs. Hair loss frequently occurs owing to the cutaneous infiltration of neoplastic cells. Frequent regression and recurrence of dermal nodules occur eventually accompanied by lesions of the multicentric form.

Supplemental Reading

Bastianello, S. S.: A survey on neoplasia in domestic species over a 40-year period from 1935 to 1974 in the Republic of South Africa. I. Tumours occurring in cattle. Onderstepoort J. Vet. Res. *49*:195–204, 1982.
Garma-Aviña, A., Valli, V. E., and Lumsden, J. H.: Cutaneous melanomas in domestic animals. J. Cutan. Pathol. *8*:3–24, 1981.
Hunt, E.: Infectious bovine skin diseases. *In* Mullowney, P. G. (ed.). The Veterinary Clinics of North America: Symposium on Large Animal Dermatology. W. B. Saunders, Philadelphia, 1984.
Moulton, J. E. (ed.): Tumors in Domestic animals, 2nd ed. University of California Press, Berkeley, California, 1978.
Onuma, M., Honma, T., and Mikami, T.: Studies on the sporadic and enzootic forms of bovine leukosis. J. Comp. Path. *89*:159–167, 1979.
Priester, W. A., and Mantel, N.: Occurrence of tumors in domestic animals. Data from 12 United States and Canadian colleges of veterinary medicine. J. Nat. Cancer Inst. *47*:1333–1344, 1971.
Theilen, G. H., and Madewell, B. R. (eds.): Veterinary Cancer Medicine. Lea & Febiger, Philadelphia, 1979.

Parasitic Skin Diseases of Sheep

CHARLES W. LIVINGSTON, JR., D.V.M., Ph.D.

The problem of ovine ectoparasites has been increasing in recent years because many livestock producers have failed to apply insecticides regularly for the control of ectoparasites. The eradication of the screwworm removed the absolute necessity for spraying newly sheared sheep. Certain insecticides have been removed from the market as unsafe products, and some producers have been reluctant to use the remaining approved insecticides because of either fear of producing health problems in animals or man or a belief that the approved insecticides are not sufficiently effective to offset the costs of application. Whatever the reason, routine application after shearing has not been practiced regularly and treatment considered only when heavy parasitism was obvious, usually when the sheep were in heavy fleece and treatments were less effective.

CLINICAL SIGNS AND LESIONS

Other than flies, sheep may harbor four types of ectoparasites: mites, lice, ticks, and keds. The clinical signs observed result from the feeding of the ectoparasites on the skin. With the exception of the biting louse *(Bovicola ovis)*, all of the ectoparasites ingest blood, and, in addition to skin irritation and discomfort, large numbers of ectoparasites may produce anemia and general unthriftiness. Sheep will rub, bite the wool, scratch, stamp feet, or kick at legs and abdomen, causing the fleece to become thin, ragged, and dirty. It is possible that blood-borne diseases

Table 1. *Control of Lice, Ticks, and Keds on Sheep and Goats*

Drug	Withdrawal Period (Days)	Amount to Apply	Remarks
Crotoxyphos (Ciodrin, Shell Chemical Co.) 0.25% spray	0	2–4 qt/animal	Repeat as needed but not more often than once a week
Crotoxyphos and dichlorvos (Ciovap, SDS Biotech; Simax, Shell Chemical Co.)	1	1 gal/animal	Repeat in 10–14 days but not within 7 days
Dioxathion and Dichlorvos (Lintox-D, Stauffer Chemical) spray or dip (lice and keds)	0	Wet animals thoroughly	Do not use on dairy goats
Coumaphos (Co-Ral, Haver Lockhart) 0.06% spray or dip (lice and keds) 0.125% spray or dip (ticks and keds) 0.5% dust (keds)	15 15 15	Wet animals thoroughly Agitate dip fluid before using 1–2 oz rubbed into wool over entire body	Do not use on lactating dairy goats or dry animals within 15 days of freshening
Diazinon 0.03% spray (high pressure) 0.06% spray (low pressure)	14 14	1 gal/animal 1 qt/animal	Apply to sheep only Apply to sheep only
Dioxathion (Delnav, Cooper) 0.15% spray or dip	0	Spray or dip thoroughly	Do not use more than once every 14 days, do not use on dairy goats, do not dip animals less than 3 months old
Lindane (MoorMaFume, Moorman Manuf. Co.) 0.05% spray	30	Spray thoroughly	Do not use on emaciated or lactating animals; do not use on dairy goats
Lindane (Isotox, Rhone Poulene; MoorMaFume) 0.03% spray 0.03% dip	30 30	Spray thoroughly Dip thoroughly	Do not treat dairy goats Do not treat dairy goats
Malathion 0.5% spray or dip or 5.0% dust	0	Spray or dip thoroughly	Do not apply to lactating dairy goats
Methoxychlor (Marlate, E.I. DuPont de Nemours & Co.) 0.5% spray or dip (lice) or 5.0% dust (lice)	0	Work thoroughly into wool or hair	Do not apply to lactating dairy goats
Fenvalerate (Ectrin, SDS Biotech; Vet Shack Insecticide WDL) (Synthetic Pyrethroid) 10% water dispersible liquid and 0.025% spray		1 to 2 pints per animal	Angora goats for mohair production only (state label in many states)

such as tularemia and bluetongue can be transmitted by various ectoparasites.

Three species of lice, *Bovicola ovis* (biting louse), *Linognathus ovillus* (sucking louse), and *L. pedalis* (sucking foot louse), are found in sheep flocks. Lice can survive off the host for several days, but direct contact with infested sheep is the usual means of transmission. Eggs attached to individual wool fibers hatch within two weeks and develop to adults in three to four weeks. The high temperatures occurring in the wool during the summertime decrease the number of lice on the host. Peak numbers of lice are present during the wintertime when the wool is long. Shearing during the spring removes large numbers of lice with the fleece. The foot louse is usually found in circumscribed areas on the feet or limbs and migrates to the abdominal or scrotal areas only when large populations develop. High populations of foot lice can cause lameness in sheep.

The sheep ked or "tick" *(Melophagus ovinus)*, a bloodsucking ectoparasite approximately 7 mm in length, is reddish-brown in color and has a sack-like leathery body covered with short bristly hairs. The female ked does not lay eggs but gives birth to a single fully developed larva, which is cemented to the wool and which pupates within 12 hours. After a 23-day pupal period, the adult ked emerges from the pupal case. The male ked has a life span of approximately 80 days, whereas the female ked's life span is usually from 100 to 120 days, during which time approximately ten larvae are produced. The entire life cycle of the ked is spent on the host.

Sheep mange mites are of little economic importance in the United States. Psoroptic mange (sheep scab) apparently has been eradicated in the United States, and if one suspects or observes mites infesting sheep, the state veterinarian and USDA officials should be notified. Psoroptic ear mange mites occasionally are found on goats, and chorioptic mange mites may occur on the feet of sheep and goats. Although only mild lesions are usually produced, the proper authorities should be notified.

Losses resulting from tick infestation are increasing, particularly in those geographic areas in which changes in stocking rates promote the growth of underbrush on rangeland. Dense stands of underbrush promote the multiplication of the tick population. Several species of hard ticks may be found on sheep. *Dermacentor andersoni* (Rocky Mountain fever tick), *Amblyomma americanum* (lone star tick), *Amblyomma cajannese* (cayenne tick), and *Rhipicephalus sanguineus* (brown dog tick) appear to be the more common ticks identified. One soft tick, *Otobius megnini* (spinose ear tick), is found often in the ear canal of sheep. While biting to obtain a blood meal, ticks permanently damage the skin, producing "cockles" that decrease the value of the pelt in a manner similar to the damage produced by sheep keds. The salivary fluids from engorged female ticks produce a severe ascending paralysis in an occasional sheep. The removal of the ticks will result in a dramatic recovery. Ticks in the ear canal can result in temporary deafness, dullness, and loss of weight.

DIAGNOSIS

The diagnosis of ectoparasitism depends upon the observation and identification of the species involved. One should consider scrapie, photosensitization, myiasis (blowfly larva), and hornfly damage, particularly to the poll and ear areas, in making a differential diagnosis.

TREATMENT AND CONTROL

Sheep keds and lice can be easily controlled by shearing and spraying or dipping with an approved insecticide. Two treatments at 14- to 21-day intervals are advisable. Insecticides approved for sheep ked, lice, mite, or tick control in the United States include those listed in Table 1. One should read the product label and follow the instructions completely when using these insecticides.

Ticks are more difficult to control because they do not remain on the host for the entire life cycle. Spraying immediately after shearing and at selected intervals with an approved insecticide is recommended. The use of fire as a means of improving pastures for grazing purposes should decrease the tick population in the burned areas and should be considered where feasible.

Supplemental Reading

Patrick, C. D.: Suggestions for Controlling External Parasites of Livestock and Poultry. Texas Agricultural Extension Service Publication B 1306, College Station, Texas, 1981.
Price, M. A., Newton, W. H., and Harman, P. J.: External Parasites of Texas Sheep and Goats. Texas Agricultural Extension Service Publication MP 834, College Station, Texas, 1972.

Nonparasitic Skin Diseases of Sheep

CARL A. KIRKER-HEAD, M.A., Vet. M.B., M.R.C.V.S. and PETER C. MULLOWNEY, M.V.B., M.R.C.V.S.

Skin diseases of sheep have recently been reviewed.[1, 2] The most significant skin diseases are caused by ectoparasites, and these are covered in Article 15. Other skin diseases of sheep can be divided by etiologic agents into those of bacterial, viral, fungal, neoplastic, environmental, and congenital origin (Table 1). Skin diseases may result in significant economic loss if the correct treatment and preventive measures are not employed.

A thorough history and physical examination are essential when investigating a dermatologic problem. In addition, it may become necessary to employ other diagnostic aids such as skin scrapings, bacterial and fungal cultures, and skin biopsies before a correct diagnosis can be reached.

References

1. Lofstedt, J.: Dermatologic diseases of sheep. Vet. Clin. North Am. 5:427–448, 1983.
2. Fubini, S. L., and Campbell, S. G.: External lumps on sheep and goats. Vet. Clin. North Am. 5:457–476, 1983.

Supplemental Reading

Mullowney, P. C.: Skin diseases of sheep. Vet. Clin. North Am. 6:129–140, 1984.

Table 1. Nonparasitic Skin Diseases of Sheep

Condition	Etiology	Predisposing Factors	Lesions	Diagnosis	Treatment
Bacterial					
Actinobacillosis	*Actinobacillus lignieresii.*	Wounds and abrasions of the skin or mucosa as caused by fighting rams, plant awns, thorns.	Pyogranulomatous inflammatory reaction. Nodule development in soft tissue of head. Local lymph node involvement. Occasional hematogenous spread systemically.	Gram stain. Culture. Sulfur granules seen in pus.	Surgical excision or drainage. Sodium iodide 80 mg/kg in a 10% solution IV. Streptomycin 20 mg/kg intravenously.
Swelled head (big head)	*Clostridium novyi.* Occasionally *C. sordelli* or *C. edematiens.*	Skin wounds permitting entry of soil-borne organism. Seen especially in fighting, butting rams near to breeding season.	Nongaseous, nonhemorrhagic edema initially under eyes, spreading to head and neck. Subendocardial and subepicardial petechial hemorrhages at necropsy.	Clinical signs: tissue edema, anorexia, fever, pain, toxemia. Gram stain. Anaerobic culture.	Surgical incision to provide drainage. Antitoxin if available. Systemic tetracycline or penicillin. Isolation of infected sheep. Vaccination.
Caseous lymphadenitis	*Corynebacterium pseudotuberculosis* (ovis).	Introduction of infected animal into previously unexposed group. Contamination of skin wounds. Ingestion of contaminated feed material.	Chronic abscess formation at site of entry or in draining lymph nodes, especially in head and neck region. Deeper organs may abscess. Ruptured abscesses drain thick pus. Peripheral lymphadenitis may develop up to 6 months after first exposure.	Clinical signs: Gram stain. Culture. Serology: serum antitoxin, serum agglutination, rabbit skin test, mouse protection test, synergistic hemolysis inhibition, immunodiffusion, and ELISA test.	Open surgically to permit drainage. Flush with H$_2$O$_2$ or disinfectant. Pack emptied capsule with swabs. Alternatively carry out complete surgical excision. Control by isolation and eradication or autogenous vaccination.
Dermatophilosis (streptothricosis, lumpy wool)	*Dermatophilus congolensis*	Skin trauma, shearing injuries, intercurrent disease, malnutrition, contaminated sheep dip. Wet weather permitting release of motile zoospores from lesions. Long fleece maintains a damp, favorable environment for zoospore proliferation.	Inflammatory reaction due to zoospores penetrating dermis. Initial erythema on back and sides progressing to crusting and matting of fleece. Occasional transient pruritus. Secondary bacterial invaders common.	Impression smear with Gram, Wright, or Giemsa stain. Microscopic examination of macerated crusts in saline to identify zoospores. Culture on blood agar. Histopathologic evaluation of skin biopsy.	Early infection: spray with zinc sulfate, copper sulfate, or potassium aluminum sulfate. Established infection: oral and systemic iodides. Penicillin and streptomycin. Long-acting tetracyclines. Shear fleece when scab lifts.
Fleece rot	Nonspecific. *Pseudomonas aeruginosa* commonly isolated. Other bacterial agents can, however, predominate.	Prolonged wetting of long, dense, or heavily folded fleeces, especially in sheep with irregular fleece fiber size. Low fleece wax content favors wetting.	Superficial dermatitis over withers and back. Hyperkeratosis, acanthosis, edema, focal spongiosis, and polymorphonuclear leukocyte infiltration of dermis. *P. aeruginosa* initiates microabscess formation. Occasional fleece discoloration.	Clinical signs: culture may reveal *P. aeruginosa*.	Of little value. Select for suitable fleeces and hardly skin. Shear fleece prior to wet season. Use of *P. aeruginosa* vaccine may reduce severity of dermatitis.
Staphylococcal dermatitis	*Staphylococcus aureus*	Small skin penetrations, primarily of the head.	Suppurative dermatitis involving facial and periorbital skin.	Clinical signs: Gram stain. Culture. Histopathology.	Topical or systemic antibiotics. Topical antiseptics. Isolate infected animals.
Ulcerative posthitis	*Corynebacterium renale.*	High-protein diet, especially with high legume content favoring ammonia production. High-estrogen content diet favors preputial swelling.	Initially small, thick, adherent scabs on external surface of prepuce. Deeper tissues involved with chronic irritation. Preputial swelling. Blowfly strike. Adhesions.	Clinical signs: bacterial isolation.	Topical penicillin, bacitracin, cetrimide, or copper sulfate. Oral thiabendazole may be beneficial. Surgery may be required.
Viral					
Blue tongue	Orbivirus. Group: Diplornavirus.	Immune status of sheep (no crossimmunity between strains). Presence of dipterous midge, *Culicoides varipennis*, essential to transmission. U.K. and Merino breeds more susceptible than African breeds. Cattle may act as reservoir of infection.	Swelling of lips, muzzle, and ears. Hyperemia and eczema of woolless skin. Breaks in staple of the fleece. Coronitis. Laminitis. Later the hooves may slough, and deep fissures and cracks may develop on lips and muzzle.	Clinical signs: fever, collapse, salivation, lacrimation, oral erosion and ulceration, diarrhea, and pneumonia. Viral isolation from chick embryo cell culture or susceptible sheep.	Reduction of insect population. Vaccination with attenuated live virus vaccine. Passage of vaccine virus through vector may increase its pathogenicity for sheep. Use in early pregnancy can cause deformity. Follow recommendations.
Border disease	Togavirus. Antigenically similar to bovine viral diarrhea virus.	Immune status, stage of gestation, and size of infectious dose modify the severity and frequency of teratogenic effects. Some suggest cattle may act as reservoir of infection. Lateral and vertical transmission possible.	Hypertrophy of primary skin follicles. Presence of kempy fibers. Persistence of halo hairs and protrusion above the normal level of the fleece.	Clinical signs: low fertility and abortion in ewes; neonates exhibiting dysmorphogenesis, domed head, short limbs, thick trunk, tonic-clonic contractions. Histopathology. Viral isolation. Serology.	Slaughter lambs at birth or at market weight before weight loss occurs. Retain exposed ewes (who develop immunity) but separate from unexposed pregnant sheep. Separation of breeding ewes from cattle and use of BVD vaccine of questionable value.

Disease	Etiology	Epidemiology	Clinical Signs	Diagnosis	Treatment/Control
Contagious ecthyma (contagious pustular dermatitis, sore mouth, orf)	Poxvirus. Group: Parapoxvirus.	Abrasions of skin or mucous membrane, especially in animals previously unexposed or unvaccinated. Use of vaccine in CPD disease-free flocks. Housing of nonimmune sheep in a pox contaminated environment (virus can survive several years on old scabs).	Epithelial hyperplasia and granulomatous inflammation of the dermis. Papules progress to form vesicles and later pustules that ulcerate and crust over. Lips, mouth, eyelids and feet primarily affected. Occasional respiratory and alimentary involvement. Secondary bacterial infection and screwworm myiasis common. Mastitis, lameness, anorexia are common sequelae.	Clinical signs. Histopathology: epithelial proliferation, ballooning degeneration, eosinophilic intracytoplasmic inclusions. Electron microscopy. Fluorescent antibody testing of cell culture inoculates. Test inoculation of susceptible sheep.	Isolate affected sheep. Do not remove scabs. Control secondary bacterial infection with topical tetracycline or gentian violet. Use live virus vaccine only in affected flocks. Vaccinate lambs at 6–8 weeks. Solid immunity developed.
Scrapie	Prion. Infectious protein.	Introduction of carrier animal into a previously unexposed flock. Possible hereditary component. Epidemiology requires further investigation. Lateral and vertical transmission possible.	Rarely seen clinically in sheep less than 1 year old. Wool loss and excoriation due to nibbling or rubbing against fixed objects. No dermatitis. Affected sheep also exhibit an exaggerated and incoordinated gait.	Clinical signs. Histologic examination of medula oblongata, showing vacuolation of nerve cells.	Quarantine and slaughter of all sheep in affected flock. Identification and slaughter of all exposed sheep moved from flock and their progeny.
Ulcerative dermatitis (lip and leg ulceration, venereal balanoposthitis and vulvitis)	Unclassified virus. Similar but antigenetically distinct from CPD virus.	Skin abrasions of face, feet, prepuce, and vulva. Autumn breeding contributes to genital form. Winter snow and abrasive plants predispose to lip and leg forms.	Epithelial necrosis, ulceration, and scab formation. Genital lesions characterized by moist exudate covering a moist and swollen surface. Granulating ulcers seen on lips, face, and feet. Secondary bacterial infection common. Sequelae include arthritis, ankylosis, phymosis, paraphymosis, and urethral fistula development.	Clinical signs. Histologic examination. Inoculation of sheep vaccinated for CPD aids in differentiation of the two diseases.	Isolate affected sheep until all lesions are healed. Confine sheep with pedal lesions to minimize further trauma. Minimize secondary infection with broad-spectrum antibiotics.
Environmental Photosensitivity	May be *primary* owing to ingestion of preformed photodynamic agents or *secondary* owing to failure of hepatic excretion of phylloerythrin.	Exposure to sunlight. Grazing of pasture containing primary photodynamic agents (e.g., St. John's wort [*Hypericum perforatum*]), which produces the toxin hypericin) or ingestion of hepatotoxic plants or molds (e.g., ragwort [*Senecio jacobaea*]). Use of some phenothiazine anthelmintics. Heritable component related to congenital liver insufficiency seen in some Southdown and Corriedale sheep.	Primarily on areas unprotected by wool or hair. Initial photophobia followed by erythema of lips, eyelids, face, vulva, and coronets. Skin lesions intensely pruritic. Edema develops, causing dyspnea and inability to eat. Dry gangrene and skin sloughing may later become complicated by secondary bacterial infection.	Clinical signs. History of access to toxic plants. Administration of some phenothiazine anthelmintics.	Remove from offending pasture. Keep in shade. Topical application of demulcents, antibiotics, steroid-antibiotic combinations, and fly repellents. Systemic corticosteroids and antibiotics.
Facial eczema	*Pithomyces chartarum*. A fungus. Active principle is sporidesmin, which is hepatotoxic and leads to retention of phylloerythrin, a breakdown product of chlorophyll, in the circulation.	Warm and humid climate. Short pasture containing recently killed plant material. The fungus, which proliferates on the dead plant material, is particularly common on rye-grass pasture.	Edema of ears, eyelids, and submaxillary tissue follows on from early signs of lethargy, head shaking, sniffing, conjunctivitis, and keratitis. Dermatitis of coronets, vulva, and medial aspect of hindlimbs follows. Exudation, scabbing, and sloughing of skin occurs. Secondary bacterial infection and fly strike often seen. Sheep commonly die.	Clinical signs. Identification of fungus on dead foliage.	Supportive care. Antibiotics. Antihistamines. Zinc sulfate helps minimize effects of sporidesmin. Summer irrigation and hard grazing reduce the dead grass available for fungal growth. Fungicidal and fungistatic agents aid in prevention.
Fescue poisoning	*Fusarium* spp., a fungus. Active principle may be ergotamine, a strong vasoconstrictor.	Grazing of pasture containing tall fescue (*Festuca arundinacea*) that is harboring the *Fusarium* fungus. Commonly seen in winter owing to lack of availability of other pasture species.	Gangrene of the lower limbs. Hindlimbs usually affected earlier and more severely than forelimbs.	Isolation of *Fusarium* spp. fungus from the foliage.	Oral thiabendazole (5 gm/100 lb) just before grazing and every 7 days thereafter while on fescue pasture.
Frostbite	Exposure to very cold temperatures.	Freezing cold weather. High winds. Lack of shelter. Young lambs and anemic or dehydrated sheep especially susceptible.	Primarily seen on distal extremities, teats, and tips of ears. Local necrosis of affected skin and ischemic dry gangrene of that part.	History and clinical signs.	Symptomatic and supportive.

Table continued on following page

Table 1. Nonparasitic Skin Diseases of Sheep Continued

Condition	Etiology	Predisposing Factors	Lesions	Diagnosis	Treatment
Mycotic Disease *(italic)*					
Dermatophytosis (ringworm)	*Trichophyton verrucosum. T. gypseum. T. Mentagrophytes. Microsporum canis.*	Direct contact with infected or carrier animals and indirect contact through a contaminated environment.	Fungi invade stratum corneum and hair fibers, causing autolysis of hair shaft and consequent alopecia. Fungal hyphae and epithelial debris accumulate on skin surface to cause crust formation. Lesions disappear spontaneously in 4–5 weeks.	Clinical signs. Microscopic examination of skin scrapings to identify arthrospores. Culture of skin scrapings on Sabouraud's dextrose agar.	Iodine shampoos. Fungicidal ointments. Captan powder spray solution (30 gm of 45% Captan powder in 5 gal water). 2–4% thiabendazole topical ointment.
Neoplastic *(italic)*					
Squamous cell carcinoma	Exact etiology unknown.	Poor hair or wool cover. Exposure to high levels of ultraviolet light. Presence of photosensitizing agents in pasture. Trauma as caused by ear tagging or Mules operation. Increased incidence seen with increasing age of sheep. Merino sheep especially susceptible.	Primarily seen on ears, muzzle, lower lip, perineum, and vulva. Early tumors of the ear show as cutaneous horns. Advanced tumors are frequently ulcerated. Secondary bacterial infection and fly strike common. Mastitis seen in 12% of cases.	Clinical signs. Histopathology; acanthosis and pseudoepitheliomatous hyperplasia present in the hyperkeratotic lesions. Lymphocyte and plasma cell inflammatory infiltrate commonly seen.	Surgical amputation or excision where possible.
Papilloma (warts, fibropapillomatosis)	Papilloma virus. Family: Papovavirus.	Cutaneous abrasions facilitate entry of virus. Direct contact required for transmission.	Benign. Papillomas found primarily on hairy skin of limbs and face (1–4 cm in diameter and 0.5 cm in height). Surface consists of multiple horny spines. Secondary bacterial infection and trauma exacerbate lesions. Position of lesion may lead to lameness or deficiencies in prehension, breathing, and vision.	Clinical signs. Histopathology; central core of fibrous tissue covered by hyperplastic epidermis. Identification of virus by electron microscope.	Lesions regress spontaneously after several months. Surgical excision can be employed if necessary but may recur.
Nutritional *(italic)*					
Iodine deficiency	Iodine deficiency.	Inadequate uptake of iodine in food and water; more commonly seen in areas with sandy soil and heavy rainfall. Conditioned iodine deficiency follows excessive consumption of cruciferous plants, continuous low level ingestion of cyanogenetic glycosides, or ingestion of pasture with high calcium levels. Merinos have inherited tendency to develop goiter.	Congenital iodine deficiency in neonates characterized by alopecia, a thick scaly skin, enlarged thyroid gland, and generalized weakness. Older sheep show poor reproductive efficiency and a high incidence of abortion or neonatal death.	Determination of protein-bound iodine in serum. Normal levels are 2.4–4.0 μg/dl.	Prevent by administration of 250 mg potassium iodide orally to ewes 60 and 30 days before lambing.
Copper deficiency	Copper deficiency.	Sandy soils and peat soils recovered from swamps are commonly deficient in copper. Secondary copper deficiency follows reduced absorption or utilization due to presence of molybdenum or other interfering agents.	Fine wool becomes limp and glossy and loses its crimp. Black wool may undergo depigmentation to gray or white. Defects in hematopoiesis, osteogenesis, and myelination of CNS also occur. Lambs may develop enzootic ataxia.	Determination of blood copper level (deficiency if less than 0.7 mg/dl) or liver copper level (deficiency if less than 80 mg/dl). Analysis of pasture copper and molybdenum levels.	Weekly oral administration of 1.5 gm copper sulfate. Addition of copper to concentrate ration (5 mg/kg of feed). Make 0.5% copper sulfate mineral licks available.
Zinc deficiency	Zinc deficiency.	Sheep have poor zinc storage capacity, but zinc deficiency rarely seen except when produced experimentally. Excessive dietary calcium may predispose to the condition.	Skin wrinkling. Parakeratosis of face, feet, and scrotum. Open lesions around hooves and eyes. Reduced growth rate, salivation, swollen hocks, impaired testicular development, and spermatogenesis also seen.	Clinical signs. Histopathology. Determination of serum zinc levels (often unreliable) and dietary composition.	Provide mineral licks containing zinc. Alternatively add zinc to diet at 50 mg/kg of total dietary dry matter.

External Parasites of Swine

KEVIN J. DOBSON, B.V.Sc., M.A.C.V.Sc.

External parasites of swine of economic importance include mites, lice, fleas, and mosquitoes. All are harmful because they irritate the animal, interfering with growth and sometimes transmitting disease-producing microorganisms. Associated problems can include condemnation at the slaughterhouse and insecticidal residues associated with the treating of these parasites. Sarcoptic mange is by far the most important parasitic infestation.

SARCOPTIC MANGE

Definition

Sarcoptic mange resulting from infestation with the mite *Sarcoptes scabiei* var. *suis* clinically manifests itself as either a chronic skin condition affecting only a few pigs or, more commonly, an allergic pruritus causing rubbing in a great number of pigs.

The occurrence of sarcoptic mange is widespread. In most countries in which surveys have been carried out, mange has occurred in 50 to 90 per cent of all herds.

The etiologic agent *Sarcoptes scabiei* var. *suis* is a small, grayish-white, circular parasite about 0.5 mm in length and just visible to the naked eye when placed on a dark background. It has four pairs of short stumpy legs, some of which have long unjoined pedicles that terminate in sucker-like organs.

The life cycle in the pig has not been fully investigated. Adults develop below the surface of the skin through egg, larval, and nymphal stages. The cycle from egg to ovigerous female requires 10 to 15 days. Research studies suggest that mite activity is mainly confined to the inner surface of the ear, and in established infestations this material may contain very large numbers of mites. In contrast, it is often very difficult to find mites in other parts of the body.

The importance of sarcoptic mange is now undisputed. In badly affected herds individual pigs may become stunted and unthrifty. In better managed herds in which there are individual carrier animals with chronic ear mange, the syndrome of mite hypersensitivity occurs in a large proportion of pigs, resulting in the growth rate and efficiency of feed conversion being reduced by approximately 10 per cent. The cost of chemicals and labor for control can be considerable in these herds.

Clinical Signs

Pruritus is the only constant clinical sign. Although the newborn piglet of an infected dam may initially exhibit intermittent body scratching, true generalized pruritus does not occur until some weeks later.

The intensity and duration of pruritus vary considerably. When control measures are inadequate, itching and rubbing are common in pigs in most pens of growers up to the time of slaughter.

Pathogenesis and Lesions

Lesions appear initially as plaque-like encrustations about 5 mm in diameter, and these may coalesce to cover up to 70 per cent of the luminal surface of the ear. These tend to regress and disappear in 12 to 18 weeks.

Skin papules (red pimples) associated with hypersensitivity follow and can be seen on the rump, flank, and abdomen. They contain large numbers of eosinophils, mast cells, and lymphocytes but there is no evidence of mites.

Continual rubbing causes a proliferation of connective tissue and keratinization so that the skin appears thickened and wrinkled. Hair loss and skin abrasion may occur over the flanks of animals.

Lesions of chronic mange develop only in a few animals. In the ear they are seen as thick asbestos-like scabs loosely attached to the skin and very rich in mites. Chronic scabs may progressively cover the head, neck, and other parts of the body, although this is uncommon.

Epidemiology

Mange is perpetuated within a herd owing to the presence of animals with chronic ear lesions containing large numbers of mites. Usually these are breeding animals (including boars) on which treatment is not carried out or has been ineffective.

Spread from the affected breeder animal to the growing pig is by direct contact soon after the sow farrows. There is maximum opportunity for spread because pigs huddle together for warmth. Spread to a large part of the herd can occur because dry sows are often housed together. Spread and the hypersensitivity syndrome are also assisted by regrouping of weaned litters according to size.

The ability of the mite and eggs to survive away from the host is limited to a few days, although the mite can live longer experimentally at cooler temperatures. Other hosts have not been shown to sustain reproducing population of mites as a source to pigs.

Diagnosis

Herds other than those derived from specific pathogen-free (SPF) sources are likely to be infested with mange unless special measures have been taken to eradicate this parasite. Clinical signs of rubbing in grower pigs in association with small red papules on the body are the most consistent and reliable indications of sarcoptic mange.

Confirmation of sarcoptic mange can only be made by demonstrating the presence of the mite within the herd, which is best achieved by examining the inside of the ears of breeding animals with a flashlight until some are found with chronic ear scab. A sample scratched out with the finger or a blunt instrument should be collected. The presence of mites can be demonstrated on the farm by breaking up the material onto a sheet of black paper. After a few minutes the scab residue can be gently blown off, leaving mites adhering to the paper by suckers on their feet. Mites can be observed directly or with a magnifying glass.

The usual laboratory technique is to break down ear scab with 10 per cent potassium hydroxide and observe the debris under a low-power microscope.

Differential diagnosis from other skin conditions may be required, and the reader should consult other parts of the text.

Parakeratosis is associated with a low zinc–high calcium diet and presents with scaly skin lesions on the buttocks and legs of grower pigs. It is comparatively uncommon.

Exudative epidermitis, or greasy pig disease, caused by *Staphylococcus* infection affects one or more piglets of a litter prior to weaning, causing skin darkening and a greasy appearance.

Swine pox caused by the vaccinia virus occasionally is seen in epidemic form affecting suckers and weaners and is characterized by discrete vesicles and papules over the whole body.

Sunburn and photosensitization can affect white pigs exposed to the sun for the first time, and the lesions appear on those parts most exposed to the sun.

Ringworm, particularly that caused by *Microsporum nanum,* is characterized by large circular lesions in which the skin is slightly darker in color with a fine scale and should not be confused with sarcoptic mange.

Treatment and Control

Insecticidal treatments mainly in the form of sprays, dips, dusts, and pour-ons containing the active ingredients amitraz, ciodrin, coumaphos, diazinon, dioxathion, fenchlorphos, ivermectin, lindane, maldison, polysulphides, phosmet, ronnel, rotenone, toxaphene, and trichlorophon are available to treat external parasites. A list of known products is given in Table 1. The precise products available and their registered use are dependent on local legislation. The manufacturer is required to give instructions on dilutions, preslaughter withholding periods, and any special precautions.

The relative effectiveness of remedies from the author's experience suggests that all products are effective if mange is kept well under control but most are not fully effective once mange is out of control. Failure to control mange is due to a poor understanding of the epidemiology, lack of appreciation of economic loss, and general apathy. Effort is often concentrated on animals with hypersensitivity, and chronic carrier animals are ineffectively treated.

Lindane marketed as a wettable powder and applied as a 0.06 per cent high-pressure spray is very effective because of its residual toxicity. It has the disadvantage of not being recommended for young pigs and sows near farrowing. A withholding period of 30 days is required prior to slaughter.

Organophosphorus compounds are generally less effective, particularly in established mange, but have the advantage of a very short or nil withholding period.

Several newer products or new formulations of older products are reported to be quite effective. Amitraz used as a 0.05 per cent spray has been shown to be efficient. Phosmet, a pour-on product used as a 20 per cent oily solution at rate of 1 ml/10 kg B.W. is effective, and it is recommended that a small amount of the pour-on be placed in the inner aspect of each ear. The ivermectin products have been shown to be very effective when given orally or subcutaneously at 300 to 500 μg or 200 μg/kg B.W., respectively, for the control of sarcoptic mange and lice.

An effective mange control program is dependent on identifying the chronic carrier animals, culling these animals and treating all other animals. To meet this end individual breeding animals including boars should be restrained, examined, and treated at least twice at a weekly interval and thereafter as required. Grower pigs may require intermittent treatment at intervals of one to three months depending on the effectiveness of control in the breeding herd. Freedom from mange in the growing pig is possible provided all sows are clean and the growing pigs are segregated from other infested pigs.

Prevention

The most effective method of preventing losses due to mange is the development of SPF herds through hysterectomy. Breakdowns are rare in these herds.

Eradication of mange from infected herds is possible but requires diligence and dedication. The breeding stock are treated simultaneously at weekly intervals for three consecutive weeks with an efficient insecticide prior to farrowing, and the progeny of treated animals are raised in isolation from nontreated animals to break the mange cycle.

DEMODECTIC MANGE

Demodectic mange is a relatively unimportant condition of pigs occasionally identified at meat inspection but seldom seen as a clinical entity in the field. Its distribution is probably widespread although not well documented, with reports of identification from many countries.

The demodex mite *Demodex phylloides* is a spindle-shaped organism about 0.25 mm in length with four pairs of short stumpy legs. It is usually located in the hair follicle, where the female lays her eggs. The life cycle includes three nymphal instars prior to adulthood and takes about two weeks to complete.

The precise method of spread is not known but it is probably by direct contact, as mites do not survive very long away from the host.

Lesions in the pig are not obvious and may be seen as red pinpoint areas around the snout and eyelids. Occasional cases are seen as a scaly nodular condition of the mammary gland and flanks resembling old pox lesions and containing a thick, white, cheese-like material with many mites. This is usually identified at meat inspection.

Diagnosis is made by demonstrating demodectic mites from the lesion. Treatment has not been successful and is usually unnecessary. Severely affected animals should be culled from the herd.

LICE

Definition and Pathogenesis

The pig louse (*Haematopinus suis*) is the only species that affects pigs. It is about 6 mm long, has black markings, has piercing and sucking mouth parts and is grayish-brown in color.

The distribution of the pig louse is widespread but is now seen less often because many herds are treated routinely for the more resilient mange mite.

In the life cycle the adult female lays three to four eggs (nits) each day. Each egg is about 1 to 2 mm long and is attached by a clear cement to the hair. Eggs hatch in 12 to 20 days. The nymphs develop through three instars, all of which feed on blood. The third instar develops into an adult. The whole cycle requires 20 to 30 days.

The economic importance of lice is less well-defined than that of sarcoptic mange. Heavy infestations result in anemia in young pigs, and constant irritation from lice can interfere with growth rate and food conversion. Lice may act as the vector in the spread of swine pox and have

Table 1. *Guidelines for Insecticidal Treatments of External Parasites*

Active Chemical	Concentration and Form	Parasites Affected	Directions For Use	Slaughter Withholding Time
Amitraz	0.05% sol	Lice, mites	Spray pigs, pens, and surroundings; repeat in 7–10 days	Nil
Ciodrin	0.25%	Lice	Spray	Nil
Coumaphos	0.06% sol	Lice	Spray and repeat but not more than once every 10 days	Nil
(Co-Ral,	0.10% sol	Mites		7 days
Haver-Lockhart)	1% dust	Lice	Apply to hogs and dry bedding at 20 gm/m²	
Diazinon	0.05% emul	Lice, mites	Spray pigs 3 times at 10-day intervals	14 days (Aust.)
Dioxathion	0.15% sol	Lice	Spray or dip; do not treat sows within 2 weeks of farrowing or while nursing	Nil
(Delnav Cooper Corp.)				
Fenchlorphos	0.0014% sol	Lice, mites	Spray pigs thoroughly	14 days
Ivermectin	Oral dose	Lice	300–500 µg/kg B.W.	28 days
	SC inj.	Mites	200 µg/kg B.W.	
Lindane	0.06% emul	Lice, mites	Dip or spray	60 days (dip)
	1% dust	Fleas	Dust head, neck, and backs	30 days (spray)
Maldison	0.5% emul	Lice, mites	Spray animals	Nil
	2.5% emul	Fleas	Spray houses and premises	—
	6% dust	Lice, fleas	Dust animals thoroughly	Nil
Polysulphides	2% sol	Mites	Spray pigs	Nil
Phosmet	20% oily sol	Mites	Pour-on: 1 ml/10 kg B.W. along back, place some in inner ear	
Ronnel	0.25% emul	Lice	Spray thoroughly	Nil
(Korlan, Dow Chemical)	5% granules	Lice	Apply over bedding at 25 gm/m²	
Rotenone	1% powder	Fleas	Dust head, neck, and backs	Nil
Toxaphene	0.5% emul	Lice, mites	Spray thoroughly	28 days
Trichlorophon	0.125% emul	Lice, mites	Spray thoroughly	Nil
(Neguvon, Haver-Lockhart)				

been reported as causing damage to the hide if used for manufacturing purposes.

The pig louse is host-specific and cannot live for more than two to three days away from the host. Lice may be found on all parts of the body but are seen more frequently on the skin of the head, jowl, flanks, and the inside of the legs. They often shelter inside the ears, where they are sometimes seen in "nests."

The method of spread is by direct contact from one pig to another during the period of huddling, although clean pigs placed in a yard just vacated by lousy pigs could become infested.

A diagnosis of lousiness should always be considered when pigs scratch and rub. Confirmation is readily made by identification of adult lice on the pig and of nits attached to the lower parts of hairs. Examination inside the ears of a number of breeding animals will assist in finding lice if they are present and will enable differential diagnosis from sarcoptic mange.

Treatment and Control

Lice are destroyed by all treatments used for sarcoptic mites. In addition, granules containing insecticides in the bedding and some aerosols are used to treat lice.

Older treatments have been largely replaced by chemical insecticides. The range of treatment is given in Table 1.

Successful treatment of lice, as with mange, is dependent on attention to detail including special attention to ears, not forgetting the boars, multiple treatments, and segregation of infested introduced or adult animals from the young, recently weaned pigs.

Eradication of lice from a herd is a goal readily achievable by simple but sound management.

FLEAS

The two flea species most commonly associated with swine are *Pulex irritans,* the human flea, and *Echidnophago gallinacea,* the stickfast flea. Species occasionally encountered are *Ctenocephalides felis,* the cat flea, and *Tunga penetrans,* the jigger flea (Africa).

Fleas are widely distributed in nature and are not host-specific. They will generally choose any convenient mammal or bird for a blood meal. They seldom present a serious problem in a well-managed piggery.

The flea is a wingless insect about 2 to 4 mm in length with a thick brown chitinous exoskeleton. It has powerfully developed legs.

The life cycle of all fleas is similar and includes an egg-laying stage in which eggs are dropped and hatch in the bedding of the host; a larval stage dependent on moderate temperature and high humidity; and a pupal stage. The cycle can be completed in 18 days but may take in excess of one year under adverse environmental conditions.

Host dependency of the flea is only partial and is confined to the adult, which requires periodic blood meals. However it can survive many months without a host, although the stickfast flea spends most of its adult life on a host animal.

Problems with fleas are uncommon but reports have been recorded where pigs were seriously disturbed. In addition, they can transmit infectious diseases such as swine pox in pigs and bubonic plague in humans. An allergic dermatitis similar to mite hypersensitivity in pigs has also been recorded. The jigger flea has been reported as causing agalactia in sows and death of piglets in the Republic of Zaire owing to the ovigerous female (jiggers) obstructing the teat duct.

Unless fleas are abundant, the diagnosis of a flea infestation is difficult, as the adult flea (other than the stickfast) leaves the host animal. Larvae and eggs are not easily seen and fleabites are not readily differentiated from those of lice, mosquitoes, and mites. Differential diagnosis is assisted by eliminating other specific pig external parasites.

Treatment and control are dependent on locating and destroying the flea breeding area and include application of an insecticide, on the pigs and surroundings. Therefore litter, bedding, dirt, and manure should be removed from the pig sheds and burned and the housing thoroughly cleaned. Insecticidal sprays with 2 to 5 per cent malathion or dusts with 1 per cent rotenone, 1 per cent lindane, or 6 per cent malathion will destroy residual fleas (see Table 1).

MOSQUITOES

Aedes spp. of mosquitoes have been reported to have attacked swine in large numbers in Florida and South Australia. The latter case was associated with brackish pools of sea water left by high tides.

Lesions observed by the author were in the form of raised edematous weals on the legs and abdomen of several or all the pigs within a pen. Lesions disappeared spontaneously within one to two days.

Attacks from mosquitoes on any livestock are relatively infrequent, but in affected piggeries the pigs suffer discomfort and irritation. Affected pigs, if marketed, may have to be skinned at slaughter.

Control within an enclosed piggery is possible by routinely using an aerosol spray containing diazinon in the late evening. Mosquito screening and insect repellents are also useful adjuncts.

Prevention can be attempted by identifying the breeding ground of the mosquito and destroying the larvae by draining the water reservoirs or covering the surface with oil. A wide range of insecticides have been used successfully in breeding grounds.

Supplemental Reading

Dobson, K. J.: External parasites. *In* Leman, A. D., Glock, R. D., Mengeling, W. L., Penny, R. H. C., Scholl, E., and Straw, B. (eds.): Diseases of Swine, 5th ed. Iowa State University Press, Ames, 1981, 579–584.

Hewett, G. R., and Heard, T. W.: Phosmet for the systemic control of pig mange. Vet. Rec. *111*:558, 1982.
Johansson, L. E., Nilsson, O., and Olevall, O.: Amitraz (Tactic) for the control of pig mange. Nordsk Vet. Med. *32*:161, 1980.
Lee, R. P., Dooge, D. J. D., and Preston, J. M.: Efficiency of invermectin against *Sarcoptes scabiei* in pigs. Vet. Rec. *107*:503, 1980.
Stewart, T. B., Marti, O. G., and Hales, O. M.: Efficiency of ivermectin against five genera of swine nematodes and the hog louse *Haematopinus suis*. Am. J. Vet. Res. *42*:1425, 1981.

Nonparasitic Skin Diseases of Swine

PETER C. MULLOWNEY, M.V.B., M.R.C.V.S.
and RALPH F. HALL, D.V.M.

Diseases of the integumentary system are not the most important diseases of swine from an economic standpoint but can affect feed conversion efficiency and profitability in the herd. The most common skin diseases, sarcoptic mange and diseases caused by other ectoparasites, were responsible for a loss of $35 million in the national pig herd in 1980 and ranked seventh in importance as economic diseases behind pneumonia, internal parasitism, neonatal diarrhea, atrophic rhinitis, reproductive failure, swine dysentery, and arthritis.[1] The conditions have been covered in Article 17. Other skin diseases, some of which may be confused with infestation with external parasites, can be divided by etiology into bacterial, viral, fungal, congenital, neoplastic, environmental, allergic, and diseases of unknown origin (Table 1). These have recently been reviewed.[2, 3]

References

1. King, N. B.: Contributions and needs of animal health and disease records. Am. J. Vet. Res. *42*:1093–1108, 1981.
2. Penny, R. H. C., and Muirhead, M. R.: Skin diseases. *In* Leman, A. D., et al. (eds.): Diseases of Swine. Iowa State University Press, Ames, 1981.
3. Mullowney, P. C., and Hall, R. F.: Skin diseases of swine. Vet. Clin. North Am. *6*:107–129, 1984.

Table 1. Nonparasitic Skin Diseases of Swine

Condition	Etiology	Predisposing Factors and Age	Lesions	Diagnosis	Treatment and Prevention
Infectious Skin Diseases					
Actinobacillosis	*Actinobacillus equuli* or *Actinobacillus suis*.	Contact with horses in some cases of *A. equuli*. Young pigs.	Septicemia, multiple hemorrhages on ears and ventral abdomen, necrosis of tail and skin over joints, swollen joints, arthritis, cyanosis of extremities, subcutaneous abscesses, pericarditis, endocarditis, pleural effusion, pneumonia, petechiae in kidneys.	Clinical signs, lesions on necropsy, bacterial culture. Differentiate from other septicemias, *Strep.* and *Corynebacterium* abscesses.	Tetracycline, ampicillin, cephalosporins, chloramphenicol, trimethoprim/sulfamethazole, streptomycin.
Actinomycosis	*Actinomyces bovis*.	Bites and scratches of udder. Sows.	Extensive granulomas of skin especially over udder. Secondary mastitis. Wasting due to visceral infection. Most common in sows.	Clinical signs, bacterial culture. Differentiate from ulcerative granuloma caused by *Borrelia suilla*.	Oral potassium iodide, streptomycin.
Corynebacterial abscesses	*Corynebacterium pyogenes*.	Trauma, lacerations, bite wounds, faulty injection technique, castration, tail biting. Any age.	Abscesses.	Bacterial culture. Differentiate from streptococcal abscesses.	Surgical drainage, antibiotics generally ineffective. No vaccines.
Erysipelas	*Erysipelothrix rhusiopathiae*.	Contamination of environment by pig feces, surface water, turkey manure, flies. Subclinical aflatoxin toxicity, poor nutrition, changes in nutrition, stress, fatigue, temperature changes. Not common under 3 months and over 3 years.	Generalized septicemia, T 40–43°C. Diamond-shaped skin lesions, anorexia, firm, dry feces, abortion, conjunctivitis, vomition, arthritis, endocarditis.	Clinical signs, bacterial culture, serology in chronic cases.	Erysipelas antiserum. Procaine penicillin 50,000 units per kg. Tetracycline, tylosin, vaccination. Improve sanitation, remove chronically affected animals.
Exudative epidermitis	*Staphylococcus hyicus*.	Entry via umbilicus, abrasions on feet and legs, lacerations, vesicular virus lesions, bite wounds, biotin deficiency, agalactia. 5–35 days of age.	Marked erythema, greasy skin exudate, erosions of coronary band, brown skin scabs, white precipitate on papillary ducts and renal pelvis.	Clinical signs, bacterial culture, slide agglutination with absorbed antisera.	Systemic antibiotics. Cloxacillin in lanolin base locally, dip in Clorox or Nolvasan. Improve sanitation, supplement diet with soybean oil, vitamins A, B, D, and E. Clip needle teeth. Keep surgical instruments clean. Tetracycline in feed. Control external parasites. No vaccine commercially available.
Oral necrobacillosis	*Fusobacterium necrophorum*.	Fight wounds, spread by teeth-cutting instruments, poor hygiene. Suckling pigs 1–4 weeks of age.	Necrotic ulcers of cheeks, lips, gums, tongue, and legs; listlessness, necrotic odor to lesions.	Clinical signs.	Curette and swab lesions with hydrogen peroxide or antibiotic spray. Sulfadimidine, penicillin, or streptomycin systemically for 3 or 4 days. Remove milk teeth. Improve sanitation. Sterilize teeth-cutting instruments.
Cervical lymphadenitis, jowl abscesses, streptococcal abscesses	Beta hemolytic *Streptococcus* sp., Lancefield group E.	Carrier animals, contaminated feed or water, concurrent swinepox and lice infestation. 10–50 weeks of age.	Enlarged lymph nodes rupture and discharge pus. Anorexia, moderate depression, diarrhea, retarded growth.	Clinical signs, slaughter inspection, culture. Differentiate from *Corynebacterium* abscesses.	Surgical drainage. Chlortetracycline, sulfamethazine, or tylosin in feed. Modified live vaccine. Eliminate lice.
Ulcerative spirochaetosis	*Borrelia suilla*.	Poor hygiene. Most common in sows.	Ulcers on udder up to 30 cm in diameter. Secondary mastitis.	Clinical signs. Examine smears of lesion under dark-field illumination, smears from formalin-fixed tissue stained with silver stain. Bacterial culture. Differentiate from actinomycosis.	Oral potassium iodide, penicillin systemically. Dust lesions with sulfanilamide, arsenic trioxide, or tartar emetic. Intralesional injection of sodium arsenite. Tetracycline, tylosin, erythromycin, and spectinomycin orally may be beneficial.
Swinepox	Pox virus.	Lice infestation. Dry scabs in environment. More common in young animals.	Pustular lesions on back and sides, may spread to ventral abdomen. No lesions on mucosal surfaces.	Clinical signs, presence of lice, histology and serology.	Improve hygiene. Control lice.
Foot-and-mouth disease	Picorna virus (Rhino). Not present in U.S. since 1929.	Spread by direct contact, aerosol, animal products such as meat, milk, or hides. All ages.	Vesicles and erosions on oral mucosa, tongue, snout, lips, gums, pharynx, palate, coronary band, interdigital space, dewclaws, and teats. Lameness, anorexia.	NOTIFIABLE DISEASE. NOTIFY FEDERAL VETERINARIANS. Cannot distinguish clinically from vesicular stomatitis, vesicular exanthema, and swine vesicular disease. Identify virus.	Eradication policy. Prevent import of animals and animal products from enzootic countries. Avoid feeding garbage. Vaccination in enzootic countries.

Table continued on following page

Table 1. Nonparasitic Skin Diseases of Swine Continued

Condition	Etiology	Predisposing Factors and Age	Lesions	Diagnosis	Treatment and Prevention
Infectious Skin Diseases Continued					
Swine vesicular disease	Picorna virus (Entero). Not present in U.S.	Similar to foot-and-mouth disease.	Similar to foot-and-mouth disease. No ruminants affected.	NOTIFIABLE DISEASE. NOTIFY FEDERAL VETERINARIANS. Identify virus, serology, demonstration of virus antigen.	As for foot-and-mouth disease.
Vesicular exanthema	Picorna virus (Calici). Not reported since 1959.	As for foot-and-mouth disease.	As for foot-and-mouth disease.	As for foot-and-mouth disease.	As for foot-and-mouth disease.
Vesicular stomatitis	Rhabdo virus. Two antigenic strains: New Jersey and Indiana.	Spread by direct contact and arthropod vectors.	Similar to foot-and-mouth disease.	Isolation of virus, serum antibody titers.	Keep water and soft feed in front of animals at all times. Antibiotics for secondary infections.
Ringworm	Most cases *Microsporum nanum*, also *M. canis*, *M. gypseum*, *Trichophyton verrucosum*, *T. mentagrophytes*.	Persists in environment for up to 12 months. Carrier animals. All ages affected. *M. nanum* adults.	Circular lesions coalesce. On most parts of body but not ventral abdomen. Some lesions pruritic. Thin, dark, crusty scabs.	Clinical signs, examination of skin scraping, culture in Sabouraud's dextrose agar. If on ventral midline, probably pityriasis rosea.	Nystatin locally. Griseofulvin in feed. Spray with iodine, captan, or salicylic acid.
Noninfectious Skin Diseases					
Melanoma	Possibly hereditary.	More common in Durocs, young pigs.	Single or multiple black nodular cutaneous tumors.	Clinical signs, histologic examination.	Surgical removal if individual nodule.
Feed-ingredient deficiency	Several deficiencies reported causing dermatologic lesions.	Biotin, inositol, linoleic acid, protein, riboflavin, vits. A, C, E, K, selenium deficiencies. Growing pigs.	Various. A scurfy hair coat is often present. Long hair with protein deficiency. Subcutaneous hemorrhages with vit. K deficiency.	Clinical signs and ration analysis.	Correct deficiencies.
Zinc deficiency, parakeratosis	Zinc deficiency in ration.	Excess calcium, copper, and phytic acid. Deficiency in unsaturated fatty acids. Concurrent T.G.E. or intestinal clostridial infections. Growing pigs.	Small circumscribed erythematous areas on ventral abdomen, papules, keratinous crusts. Differentiate from sarcoptic mange, exudative epidermitis, pityriasis rosea.	Clinical signs, zinc ration <40 mg/ kg, serum zinc and alkaline phosphatase decreased. Response to supplementation.	Supplement ration with 200 gm zinc carbonate/ton. Correct calcium levels.
Skin necrosis	Trauma to knees and teats.	New concrete farrowing crates, alkaline disinfectants, estrogens in feed in teat necrosis. Congenital splayleg. 1–14 days.	Reddish-brown areas followed by necrosis on fetlock coronets, elbows, hocks, and teats.	Clinical signs.	Extra bedding alongside farrowing crate. Adhesive bandages or acrylic resin-reinforced plastic skin on anterior teats.
Photosensitization	Many plants, phenothiazine, tetracycline, sulfas, chlorothiazide.	Grazing pigs. Secondary photosensitization if liver disease. All ages.	White parts only affected. Erythema, edema, pain, serum exudate, lameness, dry, hard, cracked skin, pruritus.	Clinical signs, history. Differentiate ergotism, sunburn, erysipelas in nursing piglets.	Remove from pasture, house in dark area. Laxative orally, emollients to skin.
Sunburn	Unacclimatized to bright sunlight.	Severity depends on length of exposure. All ages.	Erythema, edema, and pain.	Clinical signs. Less severe than photosensitization. No exposure to photodynamic agents.	Protect from sun, provide shade.
Pityriasis rosea	Unknown, possibly hereditary.	1–14 weeks.	Small papule with brown scab surrounded by reddened zone, spreads centrifugally, lesions coalesce. No loss of hair. Most on ventral midline.	Clinical signs. Negative skin scraping. Differentiate from ringworm.	None effective. Spontaneous cure in 6–8 weeks.

Common Skin Diseases of Goats

VICKI JO SCHEIDT, D.V.M., A.C.V.D.
and THOMAS O. MANNING, D.V.M., M.S.,
A.C.V.D.

The recent emergence of the dairy goat as a popular companion and show animal has opened a new and exciting area in the field of food animal medicine. As a result, the practitioner is confronted with evaluation and treatment of numerous caprine diseases, many of these involving the skin. This article briefly reviews several of the more common skin diseases of the goat.

BACTERIAL SKIN DISEASES

Bacterial infections of the skin are common in the goat.[1, 6] Predisposing factors include stress of parturition, environmental sanitation, and trauma. Coagulase-positive staphylococci bacteria are isolated in the majority of cases, with Corynebacterium pseudotuberculosis and C. pyogenes occasionally present.[1, 2, 6]

Staphylococcal impetigo is a superficial pustular dermatitis clinically observed as vesicles or pea-sized pustules that rapidly rupture and form yellow-brown crusts. Hair follicles are not involved. The udder, base of the teats, and intramammary sulcus are the common areas affected; however, lesions may spread to the medial thighs, ventral abdomen, and undersurface of the tail. Systemic signs are uncommon except in those cases in which a staphylococcal mastitis has developed.

Treatment with topical antibiotic ointments or antiseptics (2 per cent boric acid, iodine, or chlorhexidine solutions) is effective in localized infections.[1, 2] For generalized infections, systemic antibiotics should be administered for one to two weeks based on culture and sensitivity testing. Penicillin is effective in the majority of cases. Although not approved for use in the goat, procaine penicillin G can be given intramuscularly at a dose of 22,000 to 88,000 U/kg. The infection may spread to other goats by the milker; therefore, affected animals should be milked last and good milking hygiene utilized. In recurrent, chronic cases, autogenous bacterins may help shorten the course and severity of the infection.[1, 3]

Bacteria commonly invade hair follicles and cause inflammation or folliculitis. Furunculosis develops when affected follicles rupture and the infection spreads to the surrounding dermis and subcutis. Clinically, affected animals present with deep pustules or firm nodules that are often painful.

These nodules eventually become fluctuant, rupture, and release a hemorrhagic, purulent exudate that dries as a crust or scab. The caudal aspects of the udder are commonly affected; however, lesions may spread to the medial thighs, face, ventral abdomen, flanks, and perineum. Demodectic mange should be considered when firm nodules are present on the face, neck, or shoulders of the goat.[1, 2] A sterile abscess may develop following injection of a vaccine or medication and must be considered in the differential diagnosis.

Diagnosis of bacterial folliculitis-furunculosis can be made from direct smears or culture of a lesion. As in cases of caprine impetigo, coagulase-positive staphylococci are the common pathogens isolated, with C. pseudotuberculosis, C. pyogenes, and Pseudomonas aeruginosa rarely present.[1-3]

Therapy includes administration of a systemic antibiotic in conjunction with an appropriate topical preparation as described for impetigo.[1-3] Systemic antibiotic therapy often is required for a minimum of three to four weeks. Autogenous bacterins may be helpful in chronic, recurrent cases. Strict sanitary measures during milking will prevent transmission by the milker to nonaffected animals.

Caseous Lymphadenitis

Corynebacterium pseudotuberculosis is the most common cause of caseous lymphadenitis and bacterial abscessation on the head and neck of the goat.[1-6] Mode of transmission of the organism is unknown but may be associated with ingestion of infectious material, secondary invasion of open wounds, or accidental inoculation with contaminated needles. Firm nodules involving lymph nodes may develop on the jaw, head, neck, chest, or ventral abdomen. Pain is noted when nodules become fluctuant and rupture. A thick, yellowish-green, paste-like material is released. This material is highly contagious; therefore, affected animals should be isolated. Systemic signs may be present in animals with multiple or internal abscesses resulting in emaciation, weakness, and death.[2-4]

Differential diagnosis of abscessation of the head and neck in the goat should include salivary cyst, impacted cud, goiter, and neoplasm. Diagnosis of caseous lymphadenitis can be made by direct smear or culture of the exudate. Gram-positive coccobacilli, forming bizarre configurations, are noted on a Gram's stain of a direct smear. C. pseudotuberculosis forms small (2 to 4 mm in diameter), whitish-yellow colonies on blood agar that are catalase-positive within 36 to 96 hours at 37°C. Serologic tests are not diagnostic.

Therapy includes surgical drainage or wide excision and frequent daily flushing with antiseptics such as hydrogen peroxide, iodine, or chlorhexidine solutions.[2, 4] Lesions should be treated daily until completely healed. Systemic antibacterial therapy based on culture and sensitivity testing is rarely indicated. Penicillin or oxytetracycline injections have been recommended with varied results.[2, 3] Isolation of affected animals and proper disposal of infectious material are mandatory owing to the contagious nature of the organism.

Prophylactic measures using commercial bacterins are controversial.[4] Successful control has been associated with good management programs that include isolation or culling of infected animals, immediate isolation of kids from affected dams, purchasing abscess-free herds, and thorough cleaning and disinfection of the premises.

Dermatophilosis

Dermatophilosis in the goat is a superficial, exudative dermatitis caused by the actinomycete Dermatophilus congolensis.[1, 2] This organism is easily identified on direct smears made from the undersurface of crusts or scabs stained with Giemsa or Gram stain or new methylene blue. Typically, D. congolensis has the appearance of rows or chains of gram-positive cocci in a "railroad track–like" pattern. The organism can be cultured on blood agar for definitive diagnosis.

D. congolensis is not found in the environment under

natural conditions and depends on the presence of carrier animals confined under moist conditions to produce disease. Normal skin is more resistant to infection and serves as a barrier against invasion by the organism. Therefore, the disease is most commonly seen during the rainy seasons and in association with traumatic abrasions (insect bites, open wounds) that alter or destroy the normal mechanical and physiologic barriers of the skin.[2, 7]

Dermatophilosis has been reported in both kids as young as five days old and adult goats.[1, 2] In kids, 2- to 4-mm scabs or crusts have been seen on the inner surface of the pinna, haired surface of the ear, underside of the tail, and bridge of the nose. Beneath the crusts and scabs are dry, scaly depressions. Lesions commonly seen on adults include focal, raised crusts involving the muzzle, dorsal midline, rump, scrotum, ears, and thighs.[1, 2, 5] Removal of the crusts reveals moist, erythematous erosions that may be painful. Secondary infections with staphylococci, streptococci, or corynebacteria may develop. Interdigital infection with *Fusiformis nodosus* or *F. necrophorum,* alone or in association with *Dermatophilus* sp., must be considered when lesions are limited to the feet.[1] Papilloma-like lesions confined to the muzzle and lips may be confused with contagious ecthyma or goat pox.[1, 2] Dermatophilus infection of the lower limbs in sheep is called proliferative dermatitis or "strawberry foot rot."

Because dermatophilosis is contagious, therapy includes removal and proper disposal of crusts. Daily application of topical disinfectants (iodine solutions, 2 per cent lime sulfur, or chlorhexidine) will facilitate crust removal and promote healing.[1, 2] Systemic antibiotics may be indicated in severe, chronic cases. Penicillin (22,000 to 88,000 U/kg, IM) given twice a day for five to seven days is effective.[2, 8] Elimination of predisposing factors is mandatory to prevent recurrence and ensure recovery of affected animals. Reducing skin trauma (adequate ectoparasite control) and keeping all animals dry and well-groomed will limit the spread of infection and reduce recurrence. Because dermatophilus can survive in crusts for up to 40 months at temperature ranges of 26 to 31°C, proper disposal of contaminated material is vital.[2, 7]

Dermatophytosis

Caprine dermatophytosis is reportedly an uncommon disease.[7] An increased incidence has been reported in young goats under one year of age and on certain goat farms.[2, 7] *Trichophyton verrucosum* is the most common dermatophyte isolated from affected goats; however, cases of *Microsporum canis* have been reported.[2, 7]

As in other species, skin lesions associated with dermatophytosis in the goat are variable and include circumscribed or patchy areas of alopecia, erythema, scaling, and yellowish-gray crusts.[2] Generalized infections may occur. The ears, face, and neck are most commonly affected; however, lesions may spread to the extremities or entire body.[2, 5, 7]

Diagnosis of dermatophytosis can be made by Wood's light examination, microscopic examination of affected hair and scale, and fungal culture. A positive fluorescence using a Wood's light is only seen in cases caused by *M. canis.*[7] Microscopic examination of affected hair is a better screening test in the goat since the majority of cases are caused by *T. verrucosum.* All suspected cases of caprine dermatophytosis require a fungal culture for accurate and definitive diagnosis.[7]

Therapy of dermatophytosis in all species is aimed at reducing environmental contamination and decreasing the severity and course of the infection. Owing to the self-limiting nature of this disease, topical therapy is necessary and often all that is required. A 2 to 5 per cent lime sulfur solution (Orthorix*), 3 per cent captan (Orthocide*), or iodine solution (Betadine†) can be applied as a spray or dip to the entire body surface.[2, 3, 5, 7] These solutions are highly effective antifungal agents. Daily application is recommended for the first seven days, followed by weekly application until clinical remission is achieved. Affected goats should be isolated from nonaffected animals. All exposed animals should be treated.

The environment should be disinfected to eliminate the potential for re-infection. Sodium hypochlorite (Clorox), iodine (Betadine), or Nolvasan‡ preparations can be used on bedding, indoor and outdoor pens, and other environmental materials.[2, 3, 5, 7]

VIRAL SKIN DISEASE

Contagious ecthyma (orf, soremouth, contagious pustular dermatitis) is a viral dermatitis of sheep and goats caused by a pox virus.[1] The disease is encountered throughout the world and most commonly occurs in late summer, fall, and winter.[9] In young kids, papules develop on the gums, lips, or nostrils and progress to vesicles, pustules, and scabs, which eventually fall off. Although adult goats are less severely affected, similar lesions may be seen on the muzzle, tongue, gingiva, perineum, scrotum, and teats.

The course of the disease is one to four weeks. Lifelong immunity is common following exposure.[1, 9] Transmission of the virus to man is common.[9] Lesions have been commonly reported on the hands of sheep handlers and milkers exposed to affected goats.

Secondary bacterial infections may be present and should be considered in cases that are predominantly pustular in form. Dermatophilosis and staphylococcal dermatitis must be considered in atypical or persistent cases.

Therapy is not indicated in uncomplicated cases.[1] Severely affected kids may fail to eat adequately and lose weight. Such cases may require supportive therapy. Live virus vaccines are not recommended in closed, noninfected herds, since scabs from both vaccinated and infected animals may fall to the ground and remain viable for a year or longer.[9] Vaccinated or infected animals should be isolated and affected does milked last. Because the virus is infectious to humans, owners should avoid excessive contact.

ECTOPARASITIC SKIN DISEASES

External parasitism is a common cause of skin disease in goats resulting in poor condition and performance.[1, 10]

---

*Available from Chevron Chemical Co., Ortho Division, San Francisco, California 94119.
†Available from Purdue Frederick, Norwalk, Connecticut 06856.
‡Available from Ft. Dodge Laboratories, Fort Dodge, Iowa 50501.

Louse Infestations

Pediculosis, an infestation of lice, is the most common ectoparasitic skin disease of dairy and Angora goats.[1, 10] Lice are divided into two suborders based on different morphologic characteristics associated with their mouthparts.[11] Anoplura, or sucking lice, have mouthparts adapted for sucking tissue fluids and blood from the host. Mallophaga, or biting lice, have mouthparts adapted for biting and chewing hair and skin. Lice are host-specific, spending an entire life cycle on one host.[1, 3, 11] Transmission often results from overcrowding and contaminated grooming instruments. An increased incidence is seen in the winter months.

Sucking lice *(Linognathus stenopsis, L. africans)* may produce anemia, especially in goats with concurrent endoparasitism, malnutrition, or paratuberculosis.[1, 3] The blue-colored adults and their eggs (nits attached to hair follicles) are easily visualized during close examination with a bright light.

In the goat, the biting louse *(Damalina [Bovicola] caprae)* is responsible for broken hair follicles and poor quality coats, which result from excessive scratching and rubbing.[3] Severe economic losses are encountered in heavily infested young Angora herds.

Signs of pediculosis include scratching, rubbing, restlessness, weight loss, and decreased milk production. Various degrees of hair loss, scaling, and dry crusts are present along the lateral and ventral aspects of the body and neck.

Treatment with an effective topical insecticide (powders, sprays, dips) is recommended; however, it is important to remember that few insecticides have been licensed for use in the goat. Rotenone or flea powders used on cats and dogs are convenient and safe for young kids.[1] Sprays or dips are effective in adult goats and include coumaphos (0.25 per cent in water), crotoxyphos (1 per cent in water), and crotoxyphos-dichlorvos as listed in Table 1.[1, 10] These chemicals are considered safe for lactating animals in most states; however, individual state regulations vary and should be checked prior to use.[1, 3, 10] Regardless of the method selected, treatment should be applied every seven to 10 days.[1, 3] Clipping the hair prior to treatment will increase the efficiency of the dip or spray. Treatment of the environment (bedding, barns) is not indicated, since lice must live on their host to survive. Successful control should include improvement of housing facilities to prevent overcrowding.

Psoroptic Mange

Psoroptes cuniculi is a common problem in dairy goats causing ear irritation and disease.[1, 3, 11, 12] Clinical signs of an ear mite infestation in the goat include behavioral changes, head shaking, ear scratching, and excessive wax accumulation. In adult goats, visualization of mites by gross or otoscopic examination requires tranquilization or anesthesia. Most cases are benign and confined to behavioral signs. In severe cases, hair loss, scale, and crusts on the pinnae may be present.

Treatment with rotenone (Canex*) is effective. A mixture of one part rotenone to three parts mineral oil is recommended.[1, 10] Drops should be applied to the ear canal every 3 days for 21 days. Other ear mite formula-

Table 1. Common Ectoparasites of the Goat, Symptoms, and Treatment

Parasite	Symptom	Treatment
Pediculosis *Linognathus* sp. *Damalina* [*Bovicola*] sp.	Restlessness, rubbing, scratching, weight loss	Malathion dust Apply q 7–10 days for 2 to 4 treatments
Ear mites *Psoroptes cuniculi*	Head shaking and ear scratching	Rotenone (Canex) 1 part to 3 parts mineral oil 5 drops in ear canal q 3 days for 21 days
Mange *Choroptes caprae*	Intense pruritus—tail base, back, and flank	Coumaphos (Coral, Haver-Lockhart) 4 T of 25% conc in 4 gal water, saturate until wet q 10 days for 2 to 4 treatments
Sarcoptes scabiei var. *caprae*	Intense pruritus—head, ears	Coral (as for choroptic mange) 2% Lime Sulfur (Orthorix) diluted 1 part to 4 parts water, applied to entire body, weekly for 4 treatments
Demodex caprae	Nonpruritic nodules on head, neck, shoulders	Amitraz (Mitoban) Mix 1 bottle (10.6 ml) in 2 gal water; paint individual nodules weekly or apply as a dip over entire body every 7 to 14 days for 6 to 10 treatments

tions used for ear mite infections in cats and dogs (Ridamite*, Cerumenex*, Tresaderm†) can be used.[11]

Sarcoptic Mange

In the goat, sarcoptic mange initially begins on sparsely haired areas (face, lips, nose, and ears) and progresses to the entire body.[1, 3, 10] The skin is erythematous, crusty, thickened, and wrinkled owing to the intense pruritus caused by the mites as they burrow into the epidermis. Lymphadenopathy, secondary bacterial infections, and emaciation may be present in chronic cases.

Transmission is by direct contact between animals. Human infections have been reported.[13] Diagnosis is based on clinical signs and demonstration of the mites or eggs in skin scrapings. Because of the difficulty associated with demonstrating mites in skin scrapings from affected goats, diagnosis is often confirmed by response to therapy.

Many insecticides are reportedly effective against *Sarcoptes scabei* var. *caprae*.[1, 10] A 2 to 5 per cent lime sulfur solution is a very effective, nontoxic drug and can be applied on lactating animals. Weekly lime sulfur dips are given for four to six treatments. Antiseborrheic shampoos (Sebbafon‡) can be used prior to application of the dips to remove excessive crusts and scabs. A lime sulfur concentrate (Orthorix§) is diluted 1:40, applied to the entire body, and allowed to dry. A 0.2 per cent trichlo-

---

*Available from Parlam Division, Ormont Drug, Englewood, New Jersey 07631.

†Available from MSD AGVET, Division of Merck & Co., Inc., Rahway, New Jersey 07065

‡Available from Winthrop Laboratories, New York, New York 10016.

§Available from Chevron Chemical Co., Ortho Division, San Francisco, California 94119.

---

*Available from Pitman-Moore, Inc., Washington Crossing, New Jersey 08560.

rofon solution has been reported as an effective treatment for sarcoptic mange.[1]

Chorioptic Mange

Chorioptes caprae produces an intensely pruritic dermatitis in goats involving the neck, base of the tail, and flank.[1, 3, 10] Lesions have also been reported around the base of the feet, face, scrotum, and udder.[1, 3, 10] As in sarcoptic mange, the skin is scaly, thickened, and wrinkled. Grayish crusts may develop in the later stages. Diagnosis is made by clinical signs and demonstration of the mite in skin scrapings. Unlike scabies mites, chorioptes mites do not burrow into the epidermis and are more easily identified in skin scrapings. Therapy includes insecticidal dips as in sarcoptic mange.

Demodectic Mange

In the goat, demodectic mange is manifested by firm cutaneous nodules, 0.2 to 2.5 cm in diameter, involving the face, neck, shoulders, and sides of the trunk.[1, 3, 10] Unlike sarcoptic and chorioptic mange, demodicosis is usually benign, nonpruritic, and often undetected. Lesions may range in number from one to several hundred. Economic losses result when hides are severely damaged.[1, 10] These nodules commonly rupture and release a grayish-white, caseous material. Microscopic examination of the exudate reveals numerous cigar-shaped *Demodex caprae*. This form of demodex is reported in the United States and France.[1] Nodules commonly occur at 10 to 15 months of age and continue to increase in size and number until 3 years of age. Decreased milk production, inappetance, and weight loss commonly develop. As the affected goat becomes older, these nodules become firmer and the general condition of the body improves. The mechanism of transmission is unknown. Contamination between animals by mangers has been reported.

In East Germany and Africa, caprine demodicosis is different clinically and involves up to 30 per cent of the goat population. Small papules and nodules in the skin have resulted in severely damaged hides and subsequent economic losses by the leather industry.

The recommended therapy for demodectic mange when few nodules are present includes clipping the hair over the affected area, lancing each nodule with a scalpel blade, and removing the caseous material inside the cavity. Each nodule is then flushed or swabbed with a tincture of iodine.[1] In severe cases, the affected goat can be treated with ronnel (Ectoral*, Korlan E†) dips as described in the dog.[12] Two treatments with a 0.5 per cent malathion solution, at six-day intervals, have been reported. Amitraz (Mitoban‡) has been reported effective when applied over the entire body as a dip or painted over localized nodules. One bottle of the amitraz concentrate (10.6 ml) is diluted in two gallons of water and applied every 7 to 14 days as in the dog.[8]

NEOPLASMS

The incidence of skin tumors in the goat is uncommon compared with other large animal species.[14]

---

*Available from Pitman-Moore, Inc., Washington Crossing, New Jersey 08560.

†Available from Dow Chemical, Indianapolis, Indiana 46268.

‡Available from Upjohn Co., Kalamazoo, Michigan 49001

Cutaneous papillomas (warts) in goats are atypical compared with papillomas in other species because they do not spontaneously regress.[1, 9] Two clinical forms have been reported in the literature, both affecting a herd of Saanen dairy goats. In the first report, a herd of 100 milking goats developed papillomas on the head, neck, shoulders, and front limbs above the carpus.[1] A viral etiology was suspected but not identified. In the second case, only the white-colored, adult Saanen goats were affected with no involvement of the black goats.[1] Warts were confined to the teats and udder. Remission was not observed during a five-month period.

The papillomas reported in these goat herds were elongated, cone-like structures, approximately 3 cm in length. Histologically, some of these lesions appeared as typical papillomas, whereas others failed to reveal viral inclusion bodies.[1] Isolation of virus from affected tissue has not been reported.[9]

Single or infected papillomas may be surgically excised. Recurrence is reportedly rare.[8] Both cryosurgery and electrocautery are effective and convenient methods of treatment. Reported results with the commercial bovine vaccine have been poor.[1, 9]

Other cutaneous neoplasms reported in the goat include fibroma, fibrosarcoma, squamous cell carcinoma, and melanoma.[1] Squamous cell carcinoma commonly involves sparsely haired areas of the body exposed to sunlight, which include the vulva, perineum, udder, ears, and base of the horns.[1] Matting of the hair, ulceration, and myiasis may be the first signs noted. Melanomas have been reported on the udder and coronet region of the foot. Melanomas have a tendency to metastasize.[14]

NUTRITIONAL SKIN DISEASES

Nutritional diseases in goats, as in other species, can cause nonspecific coat and skin changes such as scaling, brittle or broken hair follicles, and dry, lusterless pelage. Conditions such as chronic malnutrition, endoparasitism, or chronic infection can cause relative protein, vitamin, and mineral deficiencies and are responsible for unthriftiness.

Vitamin A deficiency in goats produces emaciation, seborrhea, and hair loss.[1] Goat herds being fed a selenium-deficient diet and varied amounts of vitamin E have developed hair loss and scaling around the eyes. Injections of vitamin E–selenium alleviated these signs within a four-week period.

Iodine deficiency in goats has been reported to cause goiter and stillbirths in pregnant does.[1] Prophylactic treatment with mineralized or iodized salt added to the diet is effective. Diffuse alopecia and weakness have been reported in newborn kids with goiter.[1]

Goats fed purified diets deficient in zinc developed testicular hypoplasia, decreased growth rate, and a dull, rough coat.[1] Skin changes included alopecia and thick crusts on the head, neck, scrotum, and distal extremities. Pruritus was not observed. Histologic examination of skin biopsies revealed extensive hyperkeratosis and parakeratosis compatible with zinc deficiency. In most cases, natural diets are sufficient in zinc providing intestinal absorption is normal. Therefore, goats fed a poor diet will commonly respond when started on an adequate natural or commercial ration. Diets containing large amounts of calcium and/or cereal products (associated with increased levels of phytates) bind with zinc in the intestinal tract and prevent absorption. Goats fed diets containing excessive amounts of calcium or cereal products may have poor zinc absorption and develop clinical signs. Changing the diet and providing supplementation with 100 ppm of daily dietary zinc is recommended.[1] Oral supplementation with zinc oxide, zinc sulfate, or zinc carbonate at 0.5 to 1.0 gm once daily is effective.[1, 12]

Diagnosis of zinc deficiency in goats is based on history (daily diet), clinical signs, histopathologic findings, and response to treatment.

ENVIRONMENTAL SKIN DISEASE

Severe environmental conditions can cause alterations in the skin and hair coat of goats primarily housed outdoors. Freezing temperatures may cause frostbite of the distal extremities and tips of the ears, especially in young kids.

Sunburn most commonly affects the teats and the lateral aspects of the udder of dairy goats, especially the Saanen breed.[1] Human sunscreen preparations and teat dips containing iodophors provide some protection from excessive sunlight. Sunscreens must be washed off prior to milking. Reducing exposure to sunlight during the peak periods of the day (noon) is recommended.

Photosensitization may occur when photodynamic agents, such as the pigments present in St. John's wort and buckwheat, are ingested and the animal is exposed to sunlight. Severe liver disease and accumulation of phylloerythrin in the skin produce a secondary photosensitization. Sparsely haired and lightly pigmented areas on the ears, muzzle, eyelids, lateral aspects of the udder, and vulva are most commonly affected in both forms.[1] Initially, erythema and edema develop and progress to skin necrosis, pruritus, and pain. Diagnosis is based on history, clinical signs, and serum liver enzyme levels. Treatment is directed at removal of the hepatotoxic or photodynamic plant. Supportive therapy may be indicated in cases associated with severe liver disease.

REFERENCES

1. Smith, M.: Caprine dermatological problems: A review. J. Am. Vet. Med. Assoc. 178:724–729, 1981.
2. Scott, D. W., Manning, T. O., and Smith, M. C.: Caprine dermatology I. Normal skin, bacterial, and fungal disorders. Comp. Cont. Ed.: Submitted for publication.
3. Guss, S. B.: Management and Diseases of Dairy Goats. Dairy Goat Journal Publication Corp., Scottsdale, Ariz., 1977.
4. Ayers, J. L.: Caseous lymphadenitis. In Howard, J. L. (ed.): Current Veterinary Therapy. Food Animal Practice, 1st ed. W. B. Saunders Co., Philadelphia, 1981, 660–662.
5. King, N. B.: Skin Diseases. Univ. Sydney Postgrad. Comm. Vet. Sci. Proc. 52:199–201, 1980.
6. Ayers, J. L.: Corynebacterium infections. In Howard, J. L. (ed.): Current Veterinary Therapy. Food Animal Practice, 1st ed. W. B. Saunders Co., Philadelphia, 1981, 658–660.
7. Jungerman, P. F., and Schwartzman, R. M.: Veterinary Medical Mycology. Lea & Febiger, Philadelphia, 1972.
8. Sweeney, C. L.: Personal communication.
9. Merck & Co., Inc.: Merck Veterinary Manual, 5th ed. Merck & Co., Inc., Rahway, N.J., 1979.
10. Watkins, A. B.: Dairy Goat Management, External and Internal Parasites. International Dairy Goat Research Center, Prairie View A & M University Technical Bulletin, 1982.
11. Soulsby, E. J. L.: Helminths, Arthropods and Protozoa of Domesticated Animals, 6th ed. Lea & Febiger, Philadelphia, 1968.
12. Smith, M.: Selected problems in goat medicine. 72nd Ann. Conf. Vet., Ithaca, N.Y., Dept. Clin. Studies, Cornell Univ., 1980.
13. Chakraverty, A. N., Gash, S., and Banerjie, A. K.: Case notes of scabies in a family transmitted from goats. Ind. Med. Gaz. 99:153–154, 1953.
14. Damodaran, S., and Parthasarathy, K. R.: Neoplasms of goats and sheep. Ind. Vet. J. 49:649–657, 1972.

MISCELLANEOUS SYNDROMES

JIMMY L. HOWARD, D.V.M., M.S.
Consulting Editor

Congenital Tremor
(Myoclonia Congenita)

MARTIN E. BERGELAND, D.V.M., Ph.D.

Congenital tremor is a disease of neontal pigs characterized by rapid, repeated contraction and relaxation of one or more skeletal muscle groups. The myoclonus usually abates and ceases within two to eight weeks but may persist several months and occasionally can be detected in adult swine. Other names for the disease include trembles, shaky pigs, dancing pigs, jumpy pigs, and shivers.

The condition was observed in 1854 in Germany and since has been reported in the United States, Europe, and Australia.[1] Although congenital tremor is not a major economic problem, it continues to occur sporadically and can result in significant piglet mortality in farrowings with a high incidence of the disease.

ETIOLOGY

The cause of the common sporadic form of congenital tremor has not been firmly established, but existing evidence favors prenatal viral infection. A small (20 nm) virus with cuboidal symmetry has been isolated from affected piglets, and the syndrome has been reproduced in the offspring of pregnant gilts experimentally inoculated with this virus.[2] At present, it seems likely that this virus is an important cause of the disease.

Since tremor is a clinical sign, it is reasonable that it may be caused by different etiologic factors. A condition in newborn male Landrace pigs characterized by coarse tremors, epileptiform convulsions, and a high-pitched squeal has been attributed to inheritance by a sex-linked, probably lethal, recessive gene.[3] Congenital tremor together with cerebellar hypoplasia, hypomyelinogenesis, and other fetal malformations has been associated with prenatal hog cholera virus infection.[4, 5] Myoclonus and cerebellar demyelination have been observed in newborn pigs from which pseudorabies virus was isolated.[6] In each of these instances, however, the mortality has been greater and the lesions different from those seen in the common form of congenital tremor.

There is convincing circumstantial evidence that congenital tremor is boar transmitted.[1] It usually does not recur in subsequent litters from identical matings, but it rarely occurs in subsequent litters from sows bred to different boars. Whether the disease is transmitted by virus-infected semen or by some other means remains to be elucidated.

CLINICAL SIGNS

Rhythmic clonic contractions of one or more skeletal muscle groups of the neck, legs, or trunk begin at or within a few hours of birth. Depending upon the location and number of affected muscles, the tremor may be generalized or may mainly affect the head or legs. All or part of a litter may be affected. The severity of the signs varies considerably among litters and littermates, ranging from a barely perceptible quiver to violent jerking movements. The tremor is heightened by muscular activity and subsides dramatically when the pigs are asleep or at recumbent rest.

When the cervical muscles are severely affected, violent head shaking can interfere with or prevent nursing. Piglets with severe tremors of the hind limbs tend to shift their weight forward, sometimes walking only on their front legs.

In some herds, there are numerous pigs with rather mild tremors that have spastic contractions of the pelvic limb muscles, causing them to sit with their hind limbs rigidly extended forward and slightly laterally, with the pectoral limbs placed vertically between the rear legs. It is not clear at this time whether this is a clinical variation of the same disease or if there is some difference in the cause and pathogenesis of this syndrome.

Mildly affected pigs may recover within hours, days, or several weeks. More severely affected pigs may have persistent signs for several months, and some adults may have a stiff-legged gait and may develop tremor when excited.

The mortality is variable but usually does not exceed 10 to 20 per cent under good management.

LESIONS AND PATHOGENESIS

There are no gross lesions specific for the disease. The only microscopic lesion that has been found with any consistency is spinal hypomyelinization.[7, 8] The degree of hypomyelinization is variable and is not closely correlated with the severity of clinical signs.[8] Casual examination by routine histologic methods often does not reveal any definite lesions. The spinal lesion is best detected by comparing special myelin-stained sections with sections of corresponding levels of spinal cords from normal pigs of the same age.

Some pigs with tonic spasms of the pelvic limbs have edematous thigh muscles, which, on histologic examination, have undergone varying degrees of coagulative necrosis. This appears to be a postnatal lesion and probably is an exertion myopathy.

The pathogenesis of the disease is obscure. Since the lesion is basically noninflammatory, the virus presumably interferes with spinal myelin formation by some unknown mechanism.

Death is due to starvation or from other diseases that commonly affect piglets that do not consume adequate colostrum and milk at normal nursing intervals.

PREVENTION, TREATMENT, AND CONTROL

If the assumption that congenital tremor is caused by boar-transmitted viral infection is correct, prevention should be based on elimination of carrier boars from the herd. Unfortunately, no method of detecting carrier boars has yet been developed.

There is no specific therapy for congenital tremor. Keeping the pigs warm is helpful, since cold accentuates the tremor. Assisting the pigs to nurse promptly after birth and frequently during the first few days may allow many of the affected pigs to survive. Providing a clean, comfortable environment to prevent or minimize skin abrasion and its complications also is helpful.

References

1. Gustafson, D. P.: Congenital tremors. In Leman, A. D. et al. (eds.): Diseases of Swine, 5th ed. Iowa State University Press, Ames, Iowa, 335–338, 1981.
2. Gustafson D. P., and Kanitz, C. L.: Experimental transmission of congenital tremors in swine. Proceedings 78th Meeting U.S.A.H.A., 338–345, 1974.
3. Harding, J. D. J., Done, J. T., Harbourne, J. F., and Gilbert, F. R.: Congenital tremor type III in pigs: a hereditary sex-linked cerebrospinal hypomyelinogenesis. Vet. Rec. 92:527–529, 1973.
4. Emerson, J. L., and Delez, A. L.: Cerebellar hypoplasia, hypomyelinogenesis, and congenital tremors of pigs, associated with prenatal hog cholera vaccination of sows. J. Am. Vet. Med. Assoc. 147:47–54, 1965.
5. Harding, J. D. J., Done, J. T., and Darbyshire, J. H.: Congenital tremors in piglets and their relation to swine fever. Vet. Rec. 79:388–390, 1966.
6. Mare, C. J., and Kluge, J. P.: Pseudorabies virus and myoclonia congenita in pigs. J. Am. Vet. Med. Assoc. 164:309–310, 1974.
7. Christensen, E., and Christensen, N. O.: Studies on "trembling in newborn pigs." Nord. Vet-med. 8:921–934, 1956.
8. Fletcher, T. F.: Ablation and histopathologic studies on myoclonia congenita in swine. Am. J. Vet. Res. 29:2255–2262, 1968.

Sudden Death Syndrome of Feeder Cattle

ROGER J. PANCIERA, D.V.M., M.S., Ph.D. and DON E. WILLIAMS, D.V.M., M.S.

By the term sudden death syndrome we refer to a syndrome that occurs in feedlot cattle fed diets high (80 per cent or greater) in grain. It is characterized by peracute death that is preceded by few or no signs of illness and, at necropsy, by congestion of the vasculature of the thoracic and cervical tissues, tracheal and peritracheal hemorrhage, and rapid autolysis.

The disease occurs year-round but is much more prevalent in warm months and is limited to cattle that have been on high concentrate diets for several weeks. It is more prevalent when management errors or adverse weather brings about irregular consumption of feed, leading to overeating. Major outbreaks have occurred immediately following the refilling of feeders after periods of enforced fasting; the disease is generally more prevalent when daytime feed consumption is diminished owing to extremely high ambient temperatures followed by overeating during the cooler night period. Observations indicate that the feeding of high proportions of grain that are processed to enhance fermentability in the rumen—for example, by rolling, grinding, and steam flaking—increases incidence of disease. Monthly death loss in large feedyards (10,000 to 60,000 capacity) may reach 0.15 per cent to 0.2 per cent in months of greatest incidence and as high as 1.5 to 2 per cent annually.

Clinical illness is rarely noticed. The common event is for animals to be observed feeding normally and to be found dead minutes or hours later. Necropsy findings are nonspecific and reflect rapid post-mortem autolysis. Cadavers have gaseous distention of the gastrointestinal tract if not examined within minutes after death. If necropsy is delayed an hour or more, there may be accumulations of gas in fascial planes and throughout the subcutis. Tissues posterior to the diaphragm tend to be blanched, and those cranial to the diaphragm are engorged with blood. The liver and kidney are severely autolyzed—that is, pale, friable, or mushy—and contain gas bubbles. There are petechial and ecchymotic hemorrhages in the tracheal mucosa and peritracheal connective tissue. The lungs are variably congested and edematous.

The cause of the disease is not known. Various clostridial organisms have been suspected. Although outbreaks of sudden death syndrome are reported to have been interrupted by vaccination with polyvalent clostridial toxoid (Turner, 1971), vaccination of tens of thousands of cattle with similar biologics in controlled field trials has not resulted in reduced incidence of disease. Furthermore, specimens from cases of sudden death syndrome, when obtained very shortly after death, do not yield clostridial organisms nor have assays for clostridial toxin in intestinal content been positive. Rumenal tympany has been considered but tympany is not present in ill animals or animals observed immediately after death.

Those who have studiously observed the disease believe onset is related to excessive intake of high concentrate feed. Whereas they do not believe the disease to be simple lactic acidosis, they do believe that subclinical rumenal acidosis is a triggering factor. Huber and Williams (1976) have observed rumen pH below 5 and the presence of demonstrable endotoxin in rumen content of affected cattle as compared with cattle dead of other causes. An existing hypothesis is that the syndrome is a fatal hypersensitivity (anaphylactoid) to unusually high levels of endotoxin liberated in the rumen by the rapid die-off of gram-negative flora caused by acute subclinical rumenal lactic acidosis.

The disease can be controlled by feeding rations with a higher ratio of roughage to concentrate, but that practice is not considered economical because of the decreased feed conversion and increased cost of weight gain when roughage content of rations is increased. Measures that ensure orderly and continuous rather than irregular consumption of high concentrate rations will minimize disease. Combining less rapidly digestible grain preparations with the, more disease-provocative, more rapidly digestible processed grains should be beneficial. A 75 per cent reduction of disease was obtained in one trial by adding calcium carbonate to the ration at the rate of 112 gm per animal per day. The use of the feed additive monensin appeared to dramatically reduce incidence of the disease when its use was initiated in feedlot cattle rations.

Supplemental Reading

Cecil Reedy Workshop on Sudden Death. *In* Proceedings, Academy of Veterinary Consultants, March 19, 1976.
Cecil Reedy Workshop on Sudden Death. *In* Proceedings, Academy of Veterinary Consultants, March 11, 1977.
Discussion of Sudden Death Syndrome. *In* Proceedings, Academy of Veterinary Consultants, March 14, 1975.
Nagaraja, T. G., et al.: Relationship of rumen gram-negative bacteria and free endotoxin to lactic acidosis in cattle. J. Anim. Sci. *47*:1329, 1978.
Turner, T. N.: The sudden-death syndrome in feedlot cattle. Vet. Med./SAC *88*:803, 1971.

Winter Dysentery

ROBERT B. HILLMAN, D.V.M., M.S.

Winter dysentery is an acute, highly contagious disease of adult stabled cattle characterized by an explosive, usually brief, attack of diarrhea and/or dysentery. The disease occurs most commonly during the winter months in the northern United States and Canada but has also been reported in many European countries, Australia, and Israel. Although this disease has been seen on rare occasions during the warmer seasons, it is most prevalent and most severe during the extended periods of close confinement.

The incidence within a herd is influenced by recent previous experience with winter dysentery and by the number of young adults (two- and three-year-olds) in the group, as a moderate, short-lasting immunity appears to develop following a natural attack. It is unusual for herds to encounter recurrent attacks at less than two- to three-year intervals. When affected, herds having experienced winter dysentery the previous year or two have a lower attack rate with only the new young adults seriously involved, whereas herds with a history free of the disease may have nearly 100 per cent involvement. Stresses such as abrupt changes in feeding and sudden weather changes have been suggested as inciting factors that increase the incidence and severity of the disease, but many severe outbreaks are seen with no history of stress. The condition commonly occurs as a localized enzootic, with the disease spreading rapidly from farm to farm in a small area.

The cause of winter dysentery remains unresolved. *Vibrio jejuni* has been proposed as the causative agent, but recent work contradicts this theory. Workers in Israel, France, and Canada have isolated viruses from winter dysentery outbreaks, but extensive work in the United States, while indicating a viral etiology, has failed to produce an etiologic agent. Comparative studies with the virus isolated in France indicate this virus is not involved in New York State outbreaks. These studies also elimi-

nated as the etiologic agent the viruses of infectious bovine rhinotracheitis, bovine virus diarrhea, parvoviruses, enteroviruses, and coccidia.

The mortality rate in winter dysentery is low (less than 1 per cent) unless complicated by additional disease problems such as shipping fever pneumonia, coccidiosis, and so on. In spite of this, economic losses can be severe owing to reduction of body condition and, particularly, milk production. Estimates of milk production loss for individual cows vary from 25 to 95 per cent, averaging over 50 per cent. The marked production loss persists for up to two weeks, and cattle rarely return to full predisease levels for the remainder of the lactation.

CLINICAL SIGNS

The characteristic sign of winter dysentery is the explosive onset of a projectile diarrhea. After an incubation period of three to seven days, 10 to 20 per cent of the herd suddenly exhibits a profuse diarrhea that is homogenous, watery, brown in color and has a distinctive fetid odor. The diarrhea spreads rapidly and within four to seven days all the susceptible animals in the herd are affected. In very large herds it may take two weeks or more for complete involvement. Many cattle pass some blood that appears on the second or third day of diarrhea as red flecks widely dispersed in the copious fluid feces. About 5 to 10 per cent of the affected animals develop more severe hemorrhaging that turns the diarrhea completely red. In most cases, the marked reduction in milk production and a mild loss of body condition are the only consistent additional clinical signs, as appetite, temperature, pulse rate, and respiratory rate remain normal. The diarrhea typically lasts only two to three days, but milk production, although tending to increase following recovery, rarely attains predisease levels during that lactaton. Another frequently mentioned sign that is not consistently observed is a mild cough that, although not seriously affecting the outcome of the disease, adds considerable risk to the clinician attempting to remain clean while diagnosing and treating affected animals. Severely affected cattle suffering extensive blood loss exhibit additional signs including depression, anorexia, dehydration, anemia, and weakness.

CLINICAL PATHOLOGY

Most cases of winter dysentery require no clinical pathologic examination, but monitoring electrolytes as a guide to fluid therapy may be useful treating severely affected valuable animals.

NECROPSY LESIONS

Uncomplicated cases of winter dysentery are rarely fatal. In experimental cases lesions are limited to a catarrhal inflammation of the gastrointestinal tract.

DIAGNOSIS

The season, explosive onset, local enzootic distribution, high morbidity within a herd, and short duration combine to make the diagnosis of winter dysentery uncomplicated. Other causes of diarrhea that must be eliminated include parasitosis, which usually has a more insidious onset, affects young cattle, and has numerous ova in the feces. Bovine virus diarrhea has a lower morbidity, often presents with characteristic oral lesions and a high fever, and is frequently fatal. Dietetic gastroenteritis has a history of a dramatic change in diet or the feeding of spoiled forage. Salmonellosis usually affects fewer animals at a time, has a longer duration, and is a much more severe disease.

TREATMENT

Many mild cases of winter dysentery require no treatment, and the course does not appear to be altered, since return to normal occurs in two to three days with or without therapy. Treatment in animals exhibiting moderate amounts of blood seems to hasten recovery and in severely affected animals may prevent a fatal outcome. Intestinal astringents and antiseptics are usually employed. Homemade concoctions such as 5 per cent copper sulfate solution (30 to 60 ml every 12 hours), pine oil and creolin mixed in equal parts (30 to 60 ml every 12 hours) and Gibbons cow scour powder (gum catechu, 45 parts; sodium bicarbonate, 45 parts; and zinc phenolsulfonate, 10 parts; 30 to 90 gm twice a day), although still effective, have largely been replaced by convenient, commercially available cow scour boluses. These boluses are readily available from most veterinary pharmaceutical suppliers and contain similar combinations of astringents and antiseptics. Intestinal sulfonamides are also used to treat winter dysentery.

Severely affected animals should be placed on intensive fluid therapy with replacement of electrolytes dictated by monitoring serum levels. Intravenous administration should be supplemented by oral electrolyte solutions to which alfalfa pellets or calf starter can be added to supply nourishment.

Although controlled studies have failed to reveal any benefit from various vaccines, mixed bovine bacterins have been used by many practitioners both as a preventative for winter dysentery and as a treatment in the face of an outbreak with reported beneficial results. Because mixed bacterins are no longer available, some practitioners now use *Pasteurella* bacterins in the same manner.

PREVENTION

Failure to isolate the etiologic agent and produce a specific vaccine precludes an effective immunization program. Prevention therefore relies on strict measures controlling traffic, particularly in endemic areas. Careful disinfection of footwear and equipment is essential for people such as feed salesman, artificial inseminators, and veterinarians who must travel from farm to farm.

Supplemental Reading

Campbell, S. G., and Cookingham, C. A.: The enigma of winter dysentery. Cornell Vet. *68*:432–441, 1978.

Fox, F. H.: Winter Dysentery. *In* Gibbons, W. J., Catcott, E. J., and Smithcers, J. F. (eds.): Bovine Medicine and Surgery and Herd Health Management. American Veterinary Publications, Inc., Wheaton, Ill., 1970. 438–440.

Kahrs, R. F., Scott, F. W., and Hillman, R. B.: Epidemiologic observations on bovine winter dysentery. Bov. Pract. *6*:36–39, 1973.

Porcine Stress Syndrome

DAVID G. TOPEL, Ph.D.

Stress adaptation is a physiologic response to noxious stimuli or stressors. The stress conditions encountered from the pig's environment or its husbandry systems and the pig's ability to adapt to these conditions determine its degree of stress susceptibility. A small number of pigs in specific genetic lines have abnormal stress resistance and when they are exposed to stress conditions they exhibit a series of signs that have been reported as the porcine stress syndrome (PSS).

CLINICAL SIGNS

When stress-susceptible pigs are exposed to a severe stress, the initial observable response is muscle and tail tremors. The muscle tremors are associated with a rapid breakdown of muscle adenosine triphosphate (ATP) and a high production of lactic acid. Further stress usually results in marked dyspnea, irregular breathing, alternating blanched and reddened areas of the skin, rapid increase in body temperature, and development of an extreme lactic acidosis.

The next stage in the syndrome results in a total collapse, marked muscle rigidity, and extreme hyperthermia. Death usually occurs during this stage of the syndrome. Once a pig enters the final stages of the syndrome, death occurs in 80 per cent or more of the pigs in 20 to 90 minutes if no treatment is administered. A similar syndrome is triggered by the anesthetic halothane and is referred to as malignant hyperthermia syndrome.

DIAGNOSIS

Energy Metabolism

The energy required for skeletal muscle to contract is supplied by the available adenosine triphosphate (ATP) and creatine phosphate. This phase of muscle metabolism is abnormal in stress-susceptible pigs. During extreme exertion of skeletal muscle, the major source of ATP is from the biochemical breakdown of glycogen. An end product of these reactions is lactic acid, and stress-susceptible pigs have extremely high levels of blood lactic acid (250 to 300 mg/100 ml, blood pH of 7.0 or lower) when they enter the final stages of the syndrome. The extreme lactic acidosis is a major cause of death from the stress syndrome. The large quantity of lactic acid in the postmortem muscle of pigs that have died from the stress syndrome or were sacrificed in the later stages of the syndrome results in a pale, soft, watery condition of specific skeletal muscles such as the *gluteus medius,* portions of the *biceps femoris* and *semitendinosus,* and the *longissimus.*

Calcium Metabolism

The rate of Ca^{2+} release from the binding sites of the sarcoplasmic reticulum and mitochondria is much greater in the skeletal muscle of stress-susceptible pigs when they are subjected to stressors such as severe exercise or certain anesthetic agents such as halothane. This response results in an excess of Ca^{2+} in the sarcoplasm of skeletal muscle, and this excess Ca^{2+} activates the glycolytic cycle and the extreme production of lactic acid. At the middle and final phases of the stress syndrome, the blood Ca^{2+} levels increase greatly. Under normal conditions, no differences in blood Ca^{2+} exist in stress-susceptible and normal pigs.

Liver Metabolism

The lactic acidosis associated with the porcine stress syndrome is the result of excess lactate produced in the muscle tissue and also a lower rate of lactate metabolism by the liver. When the stress-susceptible pigs develop the stress syndrome, changes occur in the liver metabolism that result in a lower conversion of lactate to glucose and a lower oxidation of lactate to CO_2.

Hormone Function

The adrenal gland hormones have been extensively studied in an attempt to elucidate the etiology of the stress syndrome. A number of other hormones, such as growth hormone and thyroxine, have also been studied. The hormones studied to date appear to have a small influence on triggering the syndrome but may play an important role in the recovery phases of affected pigs.

MUSCULARITY AND GENETIC MECHANISMS

Several research reports show a positive association between extremely heavy-muscled animals and the stress-susceptibility traits, whereas other reports show a poor relationship. This variation is related to genetic differences in breeds or lines. The porcine stress syndrome is the result of a recessive type inheritance, and the incidence is higher in very muscular pigs. Only a small percentage of the very muscular pigs have the genetic abnormality, however, and it is possible to remove the stress problem from very muscular pigs by good genetic selection. The stress syndrome is found in most swine breeds and also in other species, including humans. The incidence is higher in certain lines of Yorkshires, Hampshires, and Landrace and very high in the Pietrain. The incidence is very low in the Duroc breed.

DETECTION AND PREVENTION

An objective, rapid, and simple test to accurately predict which pigs are stress-susceptible or which appear normal and carry the recessive stress gene(s) is not available. Of the methods evaluated, plasma CPK levels after stress, the use of the anesthetic halothane to screen small pigs (18 to 27 kg), and blood typing methods have some usefulness. The halothane screening and the blood CPK tests will detect which pigs have the abnormal stress syndrome, but they cannot detect the pigs that are the heterozygotes (PSS carriers). The blood type test can detect the heterozygotes, but it is a more expensive and difficult test to determine. Because it is a genetically controlled syndrome, producers can select against the condition by knowing which lines within a breed carry the recessive genes and then preventing the use of these animals in the breeding program. If pigs have the stress syndrome, careful handling conditions should be practiced when pigs are moved to reduce potential stress. Also, tranquilizers can be administered in advance if stress-susceptible pigs are going to be subjected to stress conditions.

TREATMENT

Dantrolene is an effective drug for the treatment of porcine stress syndrome. If pigs have entered the middle or later stages of the syndrome, an intravenous injection of dantrolene sodium is required. A procedure was reported by Gronert and colleagues (1977) that can be used to convert a relatively insoluble dantrolene to a sterile, intravenous solution.

If the stress condition is observed in the early stages of the syndrome, the pig should be removed from the impending stress and allowed to rest. If the syndrome has not developed too far, the pig will recover without further treatment. Also, intravenous administration of a tranquilizer, fast-reacting hydrocortisone, and a bicarbonate is sometimes helpful.

Supplemental Reading

Christian, L. L.: Halothane test for PSS-field application. Am. Assoc. Swine Practitioners Proc. 6–11, 1974.

Gronert, G. A., Milde, J. H., and Theye, R. A.: Dantrolene in porcine malignant hyperthermia. Anesthesiology 44:488, 1976.

Gronert, G. A., Mansfield, B. S., and Theye, R. A.: Rapidly soluble dantrolene for intravenous use. In Antonia, J., and Britt, B. A. (eds.): 2nd Int. Sym. Malignant Hyperthermia. Grune and Stratton, New York, 535, 1977.

Nelson, T. E.: Excitation-contraction coupling: a common etiology pathway for malignant hyperthermia susceptible muscle. In Antonia, J., and Britt, B. A. (eds.): 2nd Int. Sym. Malignant Hyperthermia. Grune and Stratton, New York, 23, 1977.

Rasmusen, B. A., and Christian, L. L.: H blood type in pigs as predictor of stress-susceptibility. Science 191:947, 1976.

Topel, D. G., Bicknell, E. J., Preston, K. S., Christian, L. L., and Matsushima, C. Y.: Porcine stress syndrome. Mod. Vet. Prac. 49:40, 1968.

Refer to the first volume of *Current Veterinary Therapy: Food Animal Practice* for the following:

Panciera, R. J., and Williams, D. E.: Tracheal Edema (Honker) Syndrome of Feeder Cattle. Section 10, Miscellaneous Disease Syndromes.

Smith, A. R.: Hypoglycemia in Swine. Section 2, Neonatal Diseases and Disease Management.

Ward, J. K.: Weak Calf Syndrome. Section 2, Neonatal Diseases and Disease Management.

Ward, J. K.: White Muscle Disease (Stiff Lamb Disease). Section 2, Neonatal Diseases and Disease Management.

APPENDIX

A PARTIAL LIST OF NORMAL VALUES

WALTER E. HOFFMANN, D.V.M., Ph.D.

Normal values often depend on age, sex, breed, and the emotional status of the animal at the time of sampling. The values given here are from adult animals, unless otherwise indicated, and are derived from standard texts, the veterinary literature, and, in some cases, our own laboratory (University of Illinois College of Veterinary Medicine).

Table 1. Normal Blood Values for Adult Animals[1]

	Cattle		Sheep		Goats		Swine	
	Range	Average	Range	Average	Range	Average	Range	Average
Erythrocytes								
Erythrocytes ($10^6/\mu L$)	5–10	7.0	9–15	12.0	8–18	13	5–8	6.5
Hemoglobin (gm/100 ml)	8–15	11.0	9–15	11.5	8–12	10	10–16	13
PCV	24–46	35.0	27–45	35.0	22–38	28	32–50	42
MCV	40–60	52.0	28–40	34.0	16–25	19.5	50–68	60
MCH	11–17	14.0	8–12	10.0	5.2–8	6.5	17–21	19
MCHC	30–36	31.0	31–34	32.5	30–36	33	30–34	32
Reticulocytes (%)	0	0	0	0	0	0	0–1	0.4
ESR (1 hr)	0	0	0	0	0	0	Variable	
RBC diameter	4–8	5.8	3.2–6	4.5	2.5–3.9	3.2	4–8	6.0
Fibrinogen (gm/L)	3–7		1–5		1–4		1–5	
Leukocytes								
Leukocytes (μL)	4000–12,000	8000	4000–12,000	8000	4000–13,000	2000	11,000–22,000	16,000
Neutrophils (band)	0–120	20	rare	—	rare	—	—	—
Neutrophils (bands, %)	0–2	0.5	rare	—	—	—	0–4	1.0
Neutrophils (mature)	600–4000	2000	700–6000	2400	1200–7200	3250	—	—
Neutrophils (mature, %)	15–45	28	10–50	30	30–48	36	28–47	37
Lymphocytes	2500–7500	4500	2000–9000	5000	2000–9000	5000	—	—
Lymphocytes (%)	45–75	58	40–75	62	50–70	56	39–62	53
Monocytes	25–840	400	0–750	200	0–550	250	—	—
Monocytes (%)	2–7	4	0–6	2.5	0–4	2.5	2–10	5
Eosinophils	0–2400	700	0–1000	400	50–650	450	—	—
Eosinophils (%)	2–20	9	0–10	5	1–8	5	0.5–11	3.5
Basophils	0–200	50	0–300	50	0–120	50	—	—
Basophils (%)	0–2	0.5	0–3	0.5	0–1	0.5	0–2	0.5
Neutrophil/lymphocyte ratio	0.45/1		0.48/1		0.65/1		0.7/1	

Table 2. Normal Blood Values for Young Animals

	Calves (4–8 mo)[2]		Lambs (2–6 mo)[14]		Kids (3–12 mo)[6]		Piglets (3 mo)[4]	
	Range	Average	Range	Average	Range	Average	Range	Average
Erythrocytes								
Erythrocytes ($10^6/\mu L$)	6.3–11.5	8.26	—	10.6	—	17.77	—	6.6
Hemoglobin (gm/100 ml)	—	—	—	11.4	—	10.5	—	11.1
PCV	—	—	—	34.9	—	27.2	—	—
Leukocytes								
Leukocytes (μL)	4.9–19.5	9.1	—	7.69	—	13.53	—	18.3
Neutrophils (%)	10–53	26.55	—	26.8	—	32.5	—	25.2
Neutrophils (bands, %)	0–4	0.67	—	—	—	—	—	8.9
Lymphocytes (%)	39–77	61.79	—	64.4	—	67.5	—	54.8
Monocytes (%)	1–18	7.11	—	6.4	—	—	—	2.7
Eosinophils (%)	0–14	3.9	—	2.0	—	—	—	7.3
Basophils (%)	0	0	—	0	—	—	—	0.5

Table 3. *Serum Enzyme Levels**

Enzyme	Cattle	Sheep	Goats	Pigs	Reference
Alkaline Phosphatase					
IU/L	0–38	5–30	7–30	9–31	12
mU/ml (SMA 12/60)	28–277	—	—	119–175	18
King Armstrong	0.3–114	3–166	—	—	1
Arginase					
IU/L	0–4.7	0–70	1–30	0–4.5	12
Lactic Dehydrogenase					
IU/L	176–365	60–111	31–99	96–160	12
Sorbitol Dehydrogenase					
IU/L	4.3–15.3	5.8–27.9	14–23.6	1–5.8	12
Transaminase (SGOT)					
IU/L	20–34	79 ± 11	43–132	8./2–21.6	12
Sigma-Frankel Units	42–70	164 ± 23	90–275	17–45	12
Transaminase (SGPT)					
IU/L	4–11	11 ± 1	7–24	9–17	12
Sigma-Frankel Units	8–24	23 ± 2	15–50	19–35	12
Gamma Glutamyl Transpeptidase					
IU/L	11.2–24.3	—	—	—	8

*Values will vary depending upon the procedure.

Table 4. *Serum (S) or Plasma (P) Constituents**

Test Parameter	Cattle	Sheep	Goats	Pigs	References
Glucose (mg/100 ml)	35–55	35–60	45–60	65–95	11
BUN (mg/100 ml)	6–27	8–20	13–28	8–24	5
Creatinine (mg/100 ml)	1.0–2.07	1.2–1.93	0.9–1.82	1–2.7	5
Cholesterol (mg/100 ml)	80–120	52–76	80–130	36–54	3
Bilirubin					
Total (mg/100 ml)	0.1–0.47	0–0.39	0–0.1	0–0.6	3
Calcium (mg/100 ml)	10.2 ± 0.28	12.16 ± 0.28	10.7	10.1 ± 1.08	13, 9, 16, 15
Phosphorus (mg/100 ml)	5.5 ± 0.8	5.2 ± 0.11	—	7.87 ± 1.42	13, 9, 15
(calves)	8.9 ± 0.6				
Sodium (P) (mEq/L)	132–152	146.9 ± 4.9	142–155	135–150	12, 17, 7, 12
Potassium (P) (mEq/L)	3.9–5.8	4.85 ± 0.39	3.5–6.7	4.4–6.7	12, 17, 7, 12
Chloride (P) (mEq/L)	97–111	107.5 ± 4.0	99–110	94–106	12, 17, 7, 12
Magnesium (P) (mg/100 ml)	2.89 ± 0.25	2.5 ± 0.3	3.2 ± 0.35	3.2 ± 0.49	8

*Normal values may be dependent on the procedure used.

Table 5. *Normal Values for Serum Protein (gm/100 ml)*[3]

Protein	Cattle	Sheep	Goats	Pigs
Total protein	6.74–7.46	6.00–7.90	6.40–7.90	7.90–8.90
Albumin	3.03–3.55	2.70–3.90	2.70–3.90	1.80–3.30
Globulin	3.00–3.48	3.50–5.70	2.70–4.10	5.29–6.43
Alpha-1	0.75–0.83	0.30–0.60	0.50–0.70	0.32–0.44
Alpha-2				1.23–1.54
Beta-1	0.80–1.12	0.70–1.20	0.70–1.20	0.13–0.33
Beta-2		0.40–1.40	0.30–0.60	1.26–1.68
Gamma-1		0.70–2.20	0.90–3.00	2.24–2.46
Gamma-2	1.69–2.25	0.20–1.10		
Albumin:globulin ratio	0.84–0.94	0.42–0.76	0.63–1.26	0.37–0.51

Table 6. *Additional Normal Values*

	Cattle	Sheep	Reference
BSP Clearance (T½)	3.1 ± 0.6 min	2 ± 0.3 min	3
Activated Clotting Time	74–100 sec		10

References

1. Allcroft, W. M., and Folley, S. J.: Observations on the serum phosphatase of cattle and sheep. Biochem. J. *35*:254–266, 1941.
2. Benjamin, M. M.: Blood cytology of shipping fever in beef cattle. J. Am. Vet Med. Assoc. *123*:209–212, 1953.
3. Benjamin, M. M.: Outline of Veterinary Clinical Pathology, 3rd ed. Ames, Iowa State University Press, 1978.
4. Calhoun, M. L., and Smith, E. M.: Hematology and hematopoietic organs. *In* Dunne, H. W., and Leman, A. D. (eds.). Diseases of Swine, Ames, Iowa State University Press, 1975.
5. Coles, E. E.: Veterinary Clinical Pathology, 3rd ed. Philadelphia, W. B. Saunders Company, 1980.
6. DeShaw, J. R., Brown, S. O., and Szabuniewicz. M.: Hematology of the developing juvenile Spanish goat. Southwestern Vet. *22*:287, 1969.
7. English, P. B., Hardy, L. N., and Holmes, E. M.: Values for plasma electrolytes, osmolality and creatinine and ovarious P_{CO_2} in normal sheep. J. Am. Vet Res. *30*:1967, 1969.
8. Eueleth, D. F.: Comparison of the distribution of magnesium in blood cells and plasma of animals. J. Biol. Chem. *119*:289, 1937.
9. Hackett, P. L., Gaylor, D. W., and Bustad, L. K.: Blood constituents in Suffolk ewes and lambs. Am. J. Vet Res. *18*:338, 1957.
10. Hoffmann, W. E., and Dorner, J. L.: Unpublished data, Urbana, University of Illinois, 1978.
11. Kaneko, J. J.: Carbohydrate metabolism. *In* Kaneko, J. J., and Cornelius, C. E. (eds.). Clinical Biochemistry of Domestic Animals, 2nd ed. New York, Academic Press, 1970.
12. Kaneko, J. J.: Standard Values in Domestic Animals. Davis, University of California, 1974.
13. Mylrea, P. J., and Boyfield, R. F.: Concentrations of some components in the blood and serum of apparently healthy dairy cattle. I. Electrolytes and minerals. Aust. Vet. J. *44*:565, 1968.
14. Schalm, O. W., Jain, N. C., and Carroll, E. J.: Veterinary Hematology, 3rd ed. Philadelphia, Lea & Febiger, 1975.
15. Simesen, M. G.: *In* Cornelius, C. E., and Kaneko, J. J. (eds.). Clinical Biochemistry of Domestic Animals, 1st ed. New York, Academic Press, 1963.
16. Spector, W. S. (ed.): Handbook of Biological Data. Philadelphia, W. B. Saunders Company, 1956.
17. Tasker, J. B.: Fluid, electrolyte and acid-base abnormalities in cattle. J. Am. Vet Med. Assoc. *155*:1906, 1969.
18. Veterinary Reference Laboratory. Report Form. Fullerton, California, 1977.

AVAILABILITY OF SOME COMMON PRODUCTS

PRODUCT	COMPANY
Abate	American Cyanamid Co.
Acepromazine	Ayerst Laboratories, Inc.
Acetest Tablets	Ames Company
Acetobols	Parnell Laboratories
Albacillin	The Upjohn Company
Albamast	The Upjohn Company
Albendazole	SmithKline Animal Health Products
Albon	Roche Laboratories
Alcaine Ophthalmic Solution	Alcon Laboratories, Inc.
Altosid	Zoecon Industries Inc.
Ambilhar	Ciba Pharmaceutical Co.
Ames Media	Reginal Media Labs.
Amphyl	National Laboratories Corp.
Amprolium	Merck & Co., Inc.
Anaplaz	Fort Dodge Laboratories
Ancobon	Roche Laboratories
Anthrax Spore Vaccine	Colorado Serum Company
Antivenin (Crotalidae)	Wyeth Laboratories
Antrycide	Imperial Chemical Ltd. (ICI)
Antrypol	Imperial Chemical Ltd. (ICI)
Anvax	Jensen-Salsbery Laboratories
Aquamephyton	Merck & Co., Inc.
Aqua-Pen and Four-Pen	G. C. Hanford Mfg. Co.
Arbo III	Armour Baldwin Laboratories
AS 700	American Cyanamid Co.
Atgard	Shell Chemical Co.
Aureomycin	American Cyanamid Co.
Aureo S-700	American Cyanamid Co.
Azium	Schering Corporation
Atroban Ear Tags	Cooper Corporation
Bailey Ejaculators	Western Serum Co.
BAL	Hynson, Wescott & Dunning Inc.
Banminth	Pfizer Laboratories
Baymix	Bayvet Division of Cutter Laboratories
Berenil	Hoechst-Roussel Pharmaceuticals Inc.
Betadine	Purdue Frederick Co.
Betamethasone	E. R. Squibb & Sons Inc.
Betavet Soluspan Aqueous Suspension	Schering Corporation
Bicillin Fortified	Wyeth Laboratories
Biodry	The Upjohn Company
Biosol	The Upjohn Company
Biosol-M	The Upjohn Company
Bloat Guard	SmithKline Animal Health Products
Bo-Se	Burns-Biotec Laboratories Division
Bovaflavine	Farbwerke Hoechst, AG
Bovatec	Hoffmann-La Roche, Inc.
Bovi-clox	E. R. Squibb & Sons Inc.
Braunamid	B. Braun Melsungen, AG
Bright-Line	American Optical Corporation
Butterfly Tubing	Abbott Laboratories
C-76	Frigitronics Incorporated
Cable Wire Suture	United Surgical Supplies Co.
Cambendazole	Merck & Co., Inc.
Canex	Pitman Moore Inc.
Cap-chur Rifle	Palmer Chemical & Equipment Co., Inc.
Caricide	American Cyanamid Co.
Cefa-Dri	Bristol Laboratories
Cefa-Lak	Bristol Laboratories
Chloromycetin Ophthalmic	Parke-Davis
Chloropent	Fort Dodge Laboratories
Chorisol	Burns-Biotec Laboratories
Ciodrin	Shell Chemical Co.
Ciovan	Shell Chemical Co.
Ciovap	SDS Biotech Corporation
Coral	Cutter Laboratories
Co-Ral Pour-on	Haver-Lockhart Laboratories
Corid	Merck & Co., Inc.
Coumaphos	Bayvet Cutter Laboratories
Cryogun	Brymill Corporation
Cuprate	Burns-Biotec Laboratories
Dacriose Solution	Smith, Miller & Patch Division
Dairi-Clox	Beecham Laboratories
Dantrium	Norwich-Eaton Pharmaceuticals
Darco G-60	Atlas Chemical
Decadron	Merck & Co., Inc.
Deccox	Rhodia, Inc.
Delnav	Anchor Laboratories
Del-Tox	Burroughs Wellcome Co.
Dental Wedge	Jorgenson Laboratories
Depo-Medrol	The Upjohn Company
Dexamethasone	Sussex Drug Products Company
Diquel	Jensen-Salsbery Laboratories
Diuril	Merck & Co., Inc.
D-L Batyl Alcohol	Sigma Chemical Company
Dopram V	A. H. Robins Company
Dry Clox	Bristol Laboratories
Dursban	Fort Dodge Laboratories
ECP	The Upjohn Company
Ectiban	ICI Americas, Inc.
Ectrin	Diamond Shamrock
Electrosulf-3	Affiliated Laboratories
Eltradd	Haver-Lockhart Laboratories
Emblax Powder	Haver-Lockhart Laboratories
Emtryl	Salsbury Laboratories
Eqvalan	Merck & Co., Inc.
Erythro-200	Abbott Laboratories
Erythrocin Lactobionate	Abbott Laboratories
Estradiol	Sigma Chemical Company
Estrumate	ICI United States, Incorporated
Ethidium	Imperial Chemical Ltd. (ICI)
Etorphine	D-M Pharmaceuticals
Fenbendazole	Hoechst-Roussel Pharmaceuticals, Inc.
Fenthion	Bayvet Cutter Laboratories
Fenvalerate	SDS Biotech Corporation
Flagyl	G. D. Searle and Company
Flo-Cillin	Bristol Laboratories
Flucort	Diamond Laboratories, Inc.
Fingajet	Hoechst-Roussel Pharmaceuticals Inc.
Formula #1200	G. C. Hanford Mfg. Co.
Formula A-34	Masticure Products Co., Inc.
FSH-LH	Armour Baldwin
Fungicidin	Parlam
Fungizone	E. R. Squibb
Furacin Soluble Powder	Eaton Laboratories
Furacin Solution	Norwich-Eaton Pharmaceuticals
Gallimycin 36	Abbott Laboratories
Gecolate	Summit Hill Laboratories
Ganaseg	E. R. Squibb
Garamycin Ophthalmic	Schering Corp.
Gentocin	Schering Corporation

PRODUCT	COMPANY
Glauber's Salt	Fisher Scientific
Glucagon	Eli Lilly Company
Glyceryl Guaiacolate	Summitt Hill Laboratories
Gonadovet	Jensen-Salsbery Laboratories
Gonamone	Fort Dodge Laboratories
Guardian Ear Tags	American Cyanamid Co.
GX-118	Starbar
Halox	Burroughs Wellcome Company
Hava-Span	Haver-Lockhart Laboratories
Havidote	Haver-Lockhart Laboratories
Hetacin-K	Bristol Laboratories
Hetrazeen	Heterochemical Corporation
Hexasol 40	Whitney and Company
Hi-Amine	Pitman-Moore, Inc.
Huchar C	West Virginia Pulp & Paper Co.
Hygromix	Elanco Products
Hypnodil	Janssen Pharmaceuticals
Hypothermia (Radio-frequency Current) Equipment (Thermaprobe)	Hatch Co. or (Megatherm) Western Instrument Co.
Imidocarb	Burroughs Wellcome Company
Imizol	Burroughs Wellcome Company
Immobilon	Rickett and Colman Pharmaceutical Div.
Injacon	Hoffmann-La Roche, Inc.
Injacon 100 + B	Hoffmann-La Roche, Inc.
Innovar-Vet	Pitman-Moore, Inc.
Iron-Dextran	Med-Tech, Inc.
Isotox	Rhone Poulenc
Ivomec	Merck & Co., Inc.
Kantrim	Bristol Laboratories
Kenalog	E. R. Squibb
Keflin	Eli Lilly and Company
Ketaset	Bristol Laboratories
Ketostix	Ames Co.
Kopertox	Ayerst Laboratories
Korlan	Dow Chemical Company
Kymar	Burns-Biotec Laboratories
LA-200	Pfizer, Inc.
Labstix	Ames Co.
Lasix	National Laboratories
Levasol	Pitman-Moore, Inc.
Lindex	Tech America
Linspray	Norden Laboratories
Lintox	Zoecon Corporation
Lintox-D	Zoecon Corporation
Liquamast	Pfizer, Incorporated
Liquamycin	Pfizer, Incorporated
Lomadine	May & Baker Ltd.
Longicil	Fort Dodge Laboratories
Loridine	Elanco Products Company
Loxon	Burroughs Wellcome Co.
Lutalyse	The Upjohn Company
Marlate	E. I. DuPont de Nemours & Co., Inc.
Maxitrol Ophthalmic	Alcon Labs., Inc.
Maxidex Ophthalmic	Alcon Labs., Inc.
Mannitol	Abbott Laboratories
Menadione	Heterochemical Corporation
Methoxychlor and Malathion	Anchor Laboratories
Metrazol	Knoll Pharmaceutical
Mich Wound Clips	Propper Mfg.
Mikedimide	Parlam Corp.
Monoacetin	Fisher Scientific
Monoject	Sherwood Medical Industries
Morantel	Pfizer, Incorporated
Moor Ma Fume	Moorman Manufacturing Co.
Multistix	Ames Co., Division of Miles Laboratories

PRODUCT	COMPANY
Mycobiotic	Difco
Mycosel	Baltimore Biologics
Mycostatin	E. R. Squibb
Mydramide	BioProducts, Inc.
Mydriacyl	Alcon Laboratories
Naganol	Bayer
Nasalgen	Jensen-Salsbery Laboratories
Neguvon	Haver-Lockhart Laboratories or Bayvet
Nematel	Pfizer, Incorporated
Neo-Aristovet	American Cyanamid Co.
Neosynephrine HCl drops	Winthrop Laboratories
Neo-Terra	Pfizer, Incorporated
Nicotinamide	Fisher Scientific
Nizoral	Janssen Pharmaceutical
Nolvasan	Fort Dodge Laboratories
Norit	American Norit
Novidium	May and Baker Ltd.
Nuchar	West Virginia Pulp & Paper
Ocusert	Ocusert-Alzo Pharmaceuticals
Omnizole	Merck & Co., Inc.
One-Stroke-Environ	Vestal Laboratories
Ophthaine	E. R. Squibb
Ophthetic Ophthalmic Solution	Allergan Pharmaceuticals, Inc.
Optivisor	Donegan Optical
Orbenin-DC	Beecham Laboratories
Orthocide	Chevron Chemical Co.
Overtime	Bioceutic Laboratories
Oxfendazole	Suntex, Incorporated
Panacur-American	Hoechst-Roussel Pharmaceuticals, Inc.
Panalog	E. R. Squibb
Pentothal	Abbott Laboratories
Permectin II	Anchor Laboratories
Permethrin	ICI Americas, Inc.
Permount	Fisher Scientific
Plastic Insemination Pipette	NASCO
Polyflex	Bristol Laboratories
Polyotic Soluble Powder and Oblets	American Cyanamid Co.
Pour-on Insecticide	Tech America
Prednefrin Forte Ophthalmic Solution	Allergan Pharmaceuticals, Inc.
Pro-Fixx	Scientific Products
Prolate	Zoecon Corporation
Quartermaster	Hamilton Laboratories
Rabon	SDS Biotech Corporation
Ralgro	International Minerals and Chemical Corp.
Re-COVR	E. R. Squibb
Revivon	Rickett and Colman Pharmaceuticals
Ribigen	Ribi Immunochem Research Inc.
Ridamite	Ormont Drug and Chemical Co. Inc.
Ringer's Solutions	Abbott Laboratories
Ripercol	American Cyanamid Co.
Robaxin	A. H. Robins Company
Rompun	Haver-Lockhart Laboratories
Rumensin	Elanco Products Company
Safeguard	American Hoechst Corp.
Saffan	Schering Corporation
Samorin	May and Baker Ltd.
Sandril (Reserpine)	Eli Lilly and Company
Scarlet Drench Powder	Haver-Lockhart Laboratories
Sebbafon	Winthrop Laboratories
SEZ	American Cyanamid Co.
Simax	Zoecon Corporation
Solu-Delta-Cortef	The Upjohn Company

PRODUCT	COMPANY	PRODUCT	COMPANY
Somato-Staph Bacterin	Anchor Laboratories	Toxiban	Vet-A-Mix
Spanbolets II	Norden Laboratories	Tramisol	American Cyanamid Co.
Sparine	Wyeth Laboratories	Tranvet	Diamond Laboratories, Inc.
Special Formula 17900 Forte	The Upjohn Company	Traxel-2	Bayvet Division of Cutter Laboratories
Spottan	Haver-Lockhart Laboratories	Tresaderm	Merck & Co., Inc.
Starbar Insecticide Cattle Ear Tag	Diamond Shamrock Corp.	Tribressen	Burroughs Wellcome Co.
		Trypamidium	Specia
Stewart's Media	Reginal Media Laboratories, Inc. (Remel)	Tween 20	Fisher Scientific
		Tygon	Norton, Plastics and Synthetics Div.
Stresnil	Pitman-Moore, Inc.		
Sulfabrom	Merck & Co., Inc.	Tylan 200	Elanco Products Company
Sulfa-Lite	Bio-Ceutic	Tylosin	Elanco Products Company
Surital	Parke-Davis and Company	Valbazen	Norden Laboratories
Synchromate	G. D. Searle and Company	Valium	Hoffmann-La Roche Laboratories
Synovex-H	Syntex Agri. Business, Inc.		
Synovex-S	Syntex Agri. Business, Inc.	Valsyn GEL	Eaton Laboratories
Tactik	F & B Chemicals Pty. Lyd. or Schering Corp.	Vanodyne-FAM	Vanodyne International Ltd.
		Vapona	SDS Biotech Corp.
Taractan	Hoffmann-La Roche Laboratories	Vebonol	Ciba Geigy Ltd.
		Vetafil	Dr. S. Jackson
TBZ	Merck & Co., Inc.	Vetalog Parenteral	E. R. Squibb
Technovit	Jorgensen Laboratories	Vetame	E. R. Squibb
Telmin	Pitman-Moore, Inc.	Vetibenzamine	Ciba Geigy Ltd.
Terramycin Injectable	Pfizer, Incorporated	Vetidrex	Ciba Pharmaceutical
Thiabendazole Paste	Merck & Co., Inc.	Vetisulid	E. R. Squibb
Thorazine	Pitman-Moore, Inc.	Vetrophin	Abbott Laboratories
Tiguvon	Bayvet Division of Cutter Laboratories Inc.	Vitamin K_1	Merck & Co., Inc.
		Voren	Boehringer Ingelheim
TODAY	Bristol Laboratories	Warbex	American Cyanamid Co.
Tomanol	Intervet Pty. Ltd.	XLP-30	SDS Biotech Corporation
Tonophosphan	Hoechst U.K. Ltd.	Yomasan	Haver-Lockhart Laboratories

ADDRESSES OF SOME COMPANIES MANUFACTURING COMMON DRUGS

Abbott Laboratories
Professional Veterinary Products
North Chicago, Illinois 60064

Affiliated Laboratories
Myerstown, Pennsylvania 17067

Alcon Laboratories, Inc.
Forth Worth, Texas 76101

Allergan Pharmaceuticals
Irvine, California 92713

American Cyanamid Company
P.O. Box 400
Princeton, New Jersey 08540

American Hoechst Corporation
Agricultural Division
Route 202–206
North Somerville, N.J. 08876

American Optical Corporation
Buffalo, New York 15215

Ames Company
Div. of Miles Laboratories
Elkhart, Indiana 46514

Anchor Laboratories
St. Joseph, Missouri 64502

Atlas Chemical
See ICI United States, Inc.

Ayerst Laboratories
685 Third Avenue
New York, New York 10017

Baltimore Biologics
Cockeysville, Maryland 21030

Bayer
Bayerwerk, Federal Republic of Germany

Bayvet-Cutter Laboratories
P.O. Box 390
Shawnee Mission, Kansas 66201

Beecham Laboratories
501 Fifth Street
Bristol, Tennessee 37620

Bio-Ceutic Laboratories, Inc.*
P.O. Box 999
St. Joseph, Missouri 64502

Bio Products, Inc.
369 Bayview Avenue
Amityville, New York 11701

Boehringer Ingelheim,
Sydney, Australia

Bristol Laboratories
P.O. Box 657
Syracuse, New York 13201

Burns-Biotec
8530 K Street
Omaha, Nebraska 68127

Burroughs Wellcome Company
50 Park Drive
Research Triangle Park, North Carolina
 27708

Chevron Chemical Co.,
Ortho Division
San Francisco, California 94119

Ciba Pharmaceutical
Summit, New Jersey 07901

Ciba-Geigy Ltd.
Basel, Switzerland

Colorado Serum Company
4950 York Street
Denver, Colorado 80216

Cooper Corporation
Parsippany, New Jersey 07054

Cutter Laboratories
Shawnee, Kansas 77230

Diamond Laboratories, Inc.
2538 SE 43rd Street
Des Moines, Iowa 50303

Diamond Shamrock†
Animal Health Division
1100 Superior Ave.
Cleveland, Ohio 44114

D-M Pharmaceuticals
P.O. Box 1584
Rockville, Maryland 20850

Donegan Optical Co.
Kansas City, MO 64108

Dow Chemical Company
Indianapolis, Indiana 46268

E. I. DuPont de Nemours & Co., Inc.
Wilmington, Delaware 19698

Eaton Laboratories
17 Eaton Ave.
Norwich, New York 13815

Elanco Products Company
P.O. Box 1750
Indianapolis, Indiana 46206

F&B Chemicals Pty. Ltd.
102/160 Rowe St.
Eastwood NSW 2122
Australia

---

*Recently merged with Anchor Laboratories.

†Recently purchased by SDS Biotech.

Farbwerke Hoechst AG
Frankfurt, Germany

Fisher Scientific
Pittsburgh, Pennsylvania 15219

Fort Dodge Laboratories
800 Fifth Street NW
Fort Dodge, Iowa 50501

Frigitonics, Inc.
Shelton, Connecticut 06484

GLA Company
Agricultural Electronic Division
4743 Brooks Street
Montclair, California 91763

Glaxo Laboratories
Greenford Middlesex, England

Hamilton Laboratories
Spring Street Rd. #2
Hamilton, New York 13340

G. C. Hanford Mfg. Company
304 Oneida Street
Box 1055
Syracuse, New York 13201

Hatch Company
Loveland, Colorado 80537

Haver-Lockhart Laboratories
Box 390
Shawnee, Kansas 66201

Heterochemical Corporation
Valley Stream, New York 11580

Hoechst U.K. Ltd.
Middlesex, United Kingdom

Hoechst-Roussel Pharmaceuticals, Inc.
Somerville, New Jersey 08876

Hoffmann-La Roche, Inc.
Roche Chemical Division
Nutley, New Jersey 07110

Hynson, Wescott, and Dunning, Inc.
Charles and Chase Sts.
Baltimore, Maryland 21201

ICI United States, Inc.
3411 Silverside Road
P.O. Box 751
Wilmington, Delaware 19897

International Minerals and Chemical
 Corp. (IMC)
Terre Haute, Indiana 47808

Intervet Pty. Ltd
34 Hotham Parade
Artarmon N.S.W. 2064
Australia

Janssen Pharmaceutical
New Brunswick, New Jersey 08903

Jensen-Salsbery Laboratories
P.O. Box 167
Kansas City, Missouri 64141

Jorgenson Laboratories
2198 West 15th Street
Loveland, Colorado 80538

Eli Lilly and Company
307 E. McCarty Street
Indianapolis, Indiana 46225

Masticure Products Company, Inc.
P.O. Box 1188
Norwich, New York 13201

May and Baker Ltd.
Dageham, United Kingdom

B. Braun McIsungen AG
West Germany

Merck & Co., Inc.
MSD-AGVET Division
Rahway, New Jersey 07065

Moorman's Manufacturing Co.
Quincy, Illinois 62310

Nasco
Fort Atkinson, Wisconsin 53538

National Laboratories
Montvale, New Jersey 07645

Norden Laboratories
601 W. Cornhusker Highway
Lincoln, Nebraska 68521

Ocusert-Alzo Pharmaceuticals
Palo Alto, California 94303

Norton, Plastics and Synthetics Division
Akron, Ohio 44309

Norwich-Eaton Pharmaceuticals
Norwich, New York 13815

Palmer Chemical and Equipment Co.,
  Inc.
Douglasville, Georgia 30134

Parke, Davis and Company
Joseph Campau at the River
Detroit, Michigan 48232

Parlam Division
Ormont Drug and Chemical Co., Inc.
520 South Dean Street
Englewood, New Jersey 07631

Parnell Laboratories Pty. Ltd.
6 Norman Street
Peakhurst NSW 2210
Australia

Pitman-Moore, Inc.
Washington Crossing,
New Jersey 08560

Pfizer, Incorporated
235 East 42nd Street
New York, New York 10017

Propper Mfg. Co., Inc.
Long Island, New York 11101

Purdue Frederick
So. Washington St.
Norwalk, Connecticut 06856

Rhodia, Inc.
Ashland, Ohio 44805

Rhone Poulenc
Agrochemical Division
Monmouth Junction, New Jersey 08852

Rickett and Colman Pharmaceutical Division
Hull, England

A. H. Robins Company
1407 Cummings Drive
Richmond, Virginia 23770

Ribi Immunochem Research, Inc.
Hamilton, Montana 59840

Reginal Media Laboratories, Inc.
  (REMEL)
12076 Santa Fe Drive
P.O. Box 14428
Lonexa, Kansas 66215

Salsbury Laboratory
2000 Rockford Rd.
Charles City, Iowa 50616

Schering Corportion
Galloping Hill Rd.
Kenilworth, New Jersey 07033

Scientific Products
McGraw Park, Illinois 60085

SDS Biotech Corporation
1100 Superior Avenue
Cleveland, Ohio 49114

G.D. Searle and Company
P.O. Box 5110
Chicago, Illinois 60680

Shell Animal Health
P.O. Box 3871
Houston, Texas 77001

Shell Chemical Company
San Ramon, California 94503

Sherwood Medical Industries
St. Louis, Missouri 63103

Sigma Chemical Company
St. Louis, Missouri 63178

SmithKline Animal Health Products
West Chester, Pennsylvania 19380

Smith, Miller & Patch
Division, Cooper Laboratories
Cedar Knolls, New Jersey 07927

Specia
Rhone Merieux, 69002
Lyon, France

E. R. Squibb
P.O. Box 4000
Princeton, New Jersey 08540

Starbar
Dallas, Texas 75234

Summit Hill Laboratories
P.O. Box 1
Avalon, New Jersey 08202

Sussex Drug Products Company
Edison, New Jersey 08817

Syntex Laboratories, Inc.
Stanford Industrial Park
Palo Alto, California 04304

Tech America
P.O. Box 338
Elwood, Kansas 66024

The Upjohn Company
7000 Portage Road
Kalamazoo, Michigan 49001

United Surgical Supplies Company
Mamaroneck, New York 10543

Vanodyne International Ltd. Eccles
Manchester M30 OWT, England

Vestal Laboratories
St. Louis, Missouri 63166

Veta-A-Mix
Shenandoah, Iowa 51601

Western Serum Co.
Denver, Colorado 80201

Western Instrument Co.
Denver, Colorado 80201

Winthrop Laboratories
90 Park Avenue
New York, New York 10016

Wyeth Laboratories
P.O. Box 8299
Philadelphia, Pennsylvania 19101

Zoecon Corporation
12200 Denton Drive
Dallas, Texas 75234

TABLE OF COMMON DRUGS: APPROXIMATE DOSES

Name of Drug	Ruminants	Swine
Acepromazine	0.05 to 0.1 mg/kg IV, IM, or SC	0.1 to 0.2 mg/kg IV, IM, or SC
Acetazolamide	6 to 8 mg/kg orally in food or water	Same
Acetic acid (5% solution)	In 20% glucose give 1 to 4 L orally for urea toxicity	None
Acetylsalicylic acid (aspirin)	10 to 20 mg/kg	Same
Adrenal corticotropic Hormone (ACTH) (Adrenomone)	200 units daily IM	Same
Albacillin	Intramammary infusion	None
Albamast (L)	Intramammary infusion (Novobiocin, 150 mg)	None
Albendazole	Cattle: 7.5 mg/kg oral paste	None
Ammonium chloride	200 mg/kg orally for urolithiasis prevention	None
Amphetamine (5% solution)	0.5 to 4 mg/kg IV, SC, or IP	Same
Ampicillin	4 to 10 mg/kg IM or IV	Same
Amprolium	10 mg/kg orally	100 mg/kg/day in food or water
Antivenin (Crotalidae) polyvalent	10 to 200 ml IV	Same
Aquamephyton	10 to 50 mg IV, IM, or SC	10 to 30 mg IV, IM, or SC
Atropine sulfate	0.1 to 1.0 mg/kg IV, IM, or SC	Same
Bacitracin plus polymyxin B	B.: 10,000 units and P.: 5 to 10 mg subconjunctival injection	None
BAL	4 mg/kg q 4 h IM until recovery	Same
D-L Batyl alcohol	0.5 to 1.0 g/adult animal daily IV as bone marrow stimulant	None
Baymix crumbles	60 g/100 kg orally on feed for 6 consecutive days	None
Bemegride (Mikedimide)	10 to 20 mg/kg IV	Same
Betavet soluspan	1 to 5 ml intra-articular	Same
Bicillin	1 ml/35/kg SC only	None
Biosol	5 to 10 mg/kg orally; 2 to 4 boluses, intrauterine	Same ½ to 1 bolus, intrauterine
Biosol-M (liquid)	1 ml/18 kg/day orally	Same
Butacaine sulfate (1% solution)	Topically in eye; duration 30 to 60 min	Same
Butazolidin	5 to 10 mg/kg orally, IV	None
Calcium EDTA (20% solution)	Max. safe dosage is 75 mg/kg/day IV drip	None
Calcium gluconate (23% solution)	1 ml/kg IV, SC, Im	Same
Calcium hydroxide (Slaked lime)	0.5 mg/kg daily as a 15% supplement in feed	None
Calcium hypophosphite	30 mg in 100 ml in 10% glucose IV	None
Cambendazole	20 mg/kg orally	None
Carbomycin	2.5 mg as a subconjunctival injection	None
Caricide	50 to 100 mg/kg	Same
Carmilax	1 to 4 bolets orally; 100 to 454 g powder in 4 L water	None
Cefa-Lak (sodium cephapirin)	Infuse one syringe into each infected quarter, 200 mg	None
Cephaloridine (Loridine)	10 mg/kg q 12 h IM or SC	Same
Cephapirin benzathine (Cefa-Dri)	300 mg/tube for mastitis	None
Charcoal, activated	2 to 9 g/kg in a concentration of 1 g charcoal in 3 to 5 ml water orally	None
Chloral hydrate	50 to 70 mg/kg IV	4 to 6 ml of 5% solution/kg IV
Chloramphenicol	20 to 50 mg/kg q 8 h orally; 10 mg/kg q 12 h IM or IV; 50 to 100 mg as a subconjunctival injection	Same
Chloropent injection	0.4 to 1.0 ml/kg IV	None
Chlorothiazide (Diuril)	4 to 8 mg/kg once or twice daily given orally for adult cattle	None
Chlorpromazine (Thorazine)	0.22 to 1.0 mg/kg IV; 1.0 to 4.4 mg/kg IM	0.55 to 3.3 mg/kg IV; 2.0 to 4.0 mg/kg IM
Chloretetracycline	6 to 10 mg/kg IV or IM; 10 to 20 mg/kg orally	Same
Choline chloride	Adult cow: 50 g daily orally; 25 g in 10% solution SC	None
Chorionic gonadotropin solution	Bov.: 5000 units IV: Cap.: 3000 units IV	2000 to 3000 IU IV
Chorisol	2500 to 5000 USP units IV (cattle); 10,000 USP units IM	None
Cloprostenol	Adult cow: 0.5 mg IM	None
Cloxacillin (Dairi-Clox)	200 mg/tube for mastitis	None
Cloxacillin, benzathine (Dry-Clox; Bovi-Clox)	500 mg/tube for mastitis	None
Copper glycinate	60 mg for calves; 120 mg for mature cattle SC for Cu def.	None
Copper sulfate	0.4% solution; 2 to 4 l orally for phosphorous toxicity; 1 g/adult cow daily orally for the Cu def.	None
Co-Ral Pour-On	0.3 mg/kg—pour uniformly along back	None
Depo-Medrol	20 to 240 mg intrasynovial injection	Same
Dexamethasone	1 to 10 mg IV or IM	Same
Diazepam	0.5 to 1.5 mg/kg IV or IM	Same
Diethylstilbestrol	Abortifacient in cattle; 40 to 80 mg IM; 100 to 175 mg in late pregnancy	None
Digoxin	0.2 to 0.6 mg/kg IV	None
Dimercaprol (BAL)	10% solution in oil; 2.5 to 5.0 mg/kg IM every 4 hours for 2 days; T.I.D. on 3nd day; then B.I.D. for next 10 days or until recovery	None
Dipyrone (Novin)	5 ml/50 kg IM, IV, or SC	Same
Diquel	0.55 to 1.10 mg/kg IV or IM	1.25 to 4.4 mg/kg IV or IM
Doxapram (Dopram V)	5 to 10 mg/kg IV	Same

Name of Drug	Ruminants	Swine
Dry-Clox	Infuse contents of one syringe into each infected quarter (Benzathine cloxacillin, 500 mg)	None
Electrosulf-3	0.22 g/kg	Same
Eltradd IV-4000	Dissolve one packet in 4 liters of water—give 50 to 100 mg/kg/day IV or SC	Same
Emblax powder	Mix 454 g with 4 liters of water—administer intrarumenally	None
Epinephrine (1:1000 solution)	0.02 to 0.03 mg/kg SC, IM, or IV	Same
Ergonovine maleate	Cows: 1 to 3 mg; ewes and goats: 0.4 to 1.0 mg	Sows: 0.4 to 1.0 mg
Erythromycin (Erythro-100-200)	2 to 5 mg/kg IM, SC	Same
Erythromycin	300 mg/tube for mastitis	None
Erythromycin, novobiocin, plus polymyxin B	E.: 100 mg; N.: 15 mg; P.: 5 to 10 mg as a subconjunctival injection	None
Estradiol cyclopropionate	Adult cow: 4 to 8 mg IM abortifacient late pregnancy 20 mg IM. Repeat for 2 to 3 days	1 to 3 mg not for abortifacient
Fenthion (Triguvon) (Spottan)	30 ml/100 kg pour-on; 4 ml/150 kg one-spot	None
Fenbendazole	Cattle: 5 mg/kg oral suspension	None
Finajet (Trenbolone acetate)	Cattle: 125–250 mg; sheep: 30 mg IV or IM	None
Flo-Cillin	2 ml/70 kg	None
Flucort solution	1.25 to 5.0 mg daily IV or IM	Same
FSH-P	Cattle: 10 to 50 mg; sheep and goats: 5 to 25 mg	5 to 25 mg
Fungicidin	Apply liquid liberally morning and night	Same
Furacin dressing	Apply directly on the lesion	Same
Furacin soluble powder	Dust on lesion directly	Same
Furaltadone (Valsyn Gel (L,O))	500 mg/tube for mastitis	None
Furosemide (Lasix)	2.2 to 4.4 mg/kg q 12 h IV	Same
Gallimycin 36 Sol. (L,D)	Intramammary infusion (erythromycin, 300 mg)	None
Glucagon	25 to 50 μg/kg IV	None
Glucose (40% solution)	Cattle: 500 ml; sheep: 50 ml IV	50 ml IV
Glycerol monoacetate (Monoacetin)	0.1 to 0.5 mg/kg IM hourly for several hours for fluoroacetate poisoning	None
Glyceryl guaiacolate (Gecolate) (5% solution)	110 mg/kg IV	None
Gonadotropin, pituitary (Vetrophin)	3 to 5 mg IV	None
Gonadotropin releasing hormone (Gonadorelin)	100 μg IV	None
Gonadovet	Cows: 50 to 100 units; sheep and goats: 25 units	Sows: 50 units
Griseofulvin	20 mg/kg/day once daily orally for 6 weeks	Same
Halox drench	Add one packet to one liter of water; 1 ml/2.5 to 3.5 kg; do not use on goats	None
Hava-Span	1 bolus/50 to 100 kg	None
Hetacillin (Hetacin)	5 to 15 mg/kg IM or SC	Same
Hi-Amine	Cattle: 15 to 20 g/day for 2 to 3 weeks; sheep: 7.5 to 15 g/day for 2 to 3 weeks	None
Hydrochlorothiazide	0.25 to 5.0 mg/kg IV or IM	None
Hygromix	None	Mix in feed according to label
Hypnodil	None	Give to effect
Injacon	Cattle: 0.5 to 6 ml/head IM sheep and goats: 0.25 to 2 ml/head IM	0.25 to 3 ml/head IM
Injacon 100 + B complex	Cattle: 2.5 to 10 ml/head IM; sheep and goats: 1 to 5 ml/head IM	1 to 5 ml/head IM
Innovan-Vet	None	1 ml/12 to 25 kg IM
Insulin	Adult cow: 150 to 200 units every 36 hr SC	None
Iron-dextran injection	None	100 to 200 mg IM for 1 to 3 day old pigs
Isoflupredone acetate (Predef)	0.1 to 0.15 mg/kg	None
Jenotone	2 mg/kg q 12 h IM or SC	Same
Kanamycin (Kantrim)	6 mg/kg q 12 h IM; 10 to 20 mg subconjunctival	Same
Ketamine (Ketaset)	2.0 mg/kg IV	2.0 to 3.0 mg/kg IV
Kopertox	Apply to hoofs	Same
Kymar aqueous	Cattle: 25,000 USP units q 24 h IM; sheep: 5000 to 10,000 USP units	None
Levamisole (L-Tetramisole) (Levasole)	3.3 to 8.0 mg/kg SC; 5.5 to 11.0 mg/kg drench or bolus	8 mg/kg in feed or water
Liquamast	Injection into udder immediately after milking (Oxytetracycline HCl, 426 mg)	None
Luteinizing hormone (P.L.H.)	Sheep and goats: 2.5 mg IV; cows: 25 mg IV	5 mg IV
Magnesium gluconate	0.44 mg/kg of a 15% solution IV or SC	None
Magnesium lactate	2.2 ml/kg of a 3.3% solution IV or SC	None
Magnesium oxide	1 g/45 kg orally as a supplement to prevent grass tetany; 2 to 3 g/45 kg orally for acid antidote	None
Magnesium sulfate	0.44 ml/kg of a 20% solution IV or SC for grass tetany; 1 to 2 g/kg orally as cathartic	Same for cathartic
Mannitol (20% solution)	5 to 10 ml/kg IV	Same
Menadione (Vitamin K)	0.5 to 2.5 mg/kg q 12 h IM; 5 mg/kg orally	None
Methocarbamol (Robaxin)	110 mg/kg IV	None
Methoxyflurane	Induce 1%; maintain 0.5%	Same
Methylene blue	1 to 4% solution; 4.4 to 8.8 mg/kg IV drip for nitrate poisoning	None
Metrazol	10 mg/kg IV or 100 mg orally	Same
Milk of magnesia	3.0 to 30.0 ml/45 kg orally	Same
Mineral oil	Cattle: 1 to 4 liters orally; sheep and goats: 100 to 500 ml orally	50 to 100 ml orally
Molybdate (ammonium or sodium salt)	50 to 100 mg/head/day orally in copper toxicosis	None
Molybdenumized superphosphate	Apply 114 g per acre to molybdenum deficiency pastures	None
Neguvon Pour-On	30 ml/100 kg—apply along the back	None
Neo-Aristovet	Apply to lesion once or twice daily	Same
Neo-Terramycin	1 to 3 boluses/50 to 100 kg orally	Same

Table continued on following page

Name of Drug	Ruminants	Swine
Neomycin	7 to 12 mg/kg q 12 hr orally	Same
Nitrofurazone (0.2% ointment or solution)	Topically	Same
Neostigmine methylsulfate	Solution 1:2000 to 1:5000; 1.1 to 2.2 mg/50 kg SC or IV	Same
Nicotinamide	2 to 3 mg/kg every 4 h	None
Norgestamet (Synchromate B)	Cow: day one—6 mg ear implant plus daily injections of 5 to 6 mg IM 7 days	None
Novobiocin (Albamast [L]) (Biodry [D])	150 mg/tube for mastitis infusion; 400 mg/tube for mastitis infection	None
Oleandomycin	1.25 mg as a subconjunctival injection	None
Orbenin-DC (D)	Intramammary infusion (Benzathine Cloxacillin, 500 mg)	None
Oxfendazole	None	3 mg/kg orally
Oxytetracycline HCl	6 to 11 mg/kg IV or IM; 10 to 20 mg/kg q 6 h orally	Same
Oxytocin	20 to 100 USP units (1 to 5 ml) IM or IV	20 to 50 USP units IM or IV
D-Penicillamine (Cupramine)	Antidote for copper and mercury; dose for man: 15 to 50 mg/kg daily in divided doses orally	None
Penicillin		
Pen G, procaine	40,000 units/kg q 24 h IM;	Same
Pen G and Pen benzathine	40,000 units/kg once	Same
Penicillin G + streptomycin	P.: 500,000 units; S.: 50 mg as a subconjunctival injection	None
Pentobarbital	30 mg/kg IV to effect	Same
Pentylenetetrazol (Metrazol)	6 to 10 mg/kg IV mild stimulant; 10 to 20 mg/kg IV barbiturate antidote	Same
Phenylbutazone	4 to 8 mg/kg orally; 2 to 5 mg/kg IV	Same
Piperazine	100 to 200 mg/kg orally	Same
Pituitary gonadotropin	5 mg/adult cow IV	None
Poloxalone (Therabloat)	100 mg/kg orally	None
Posterior pituitary extract	Cow: 10 to 20 USP units IV, IM	5 to 20 USP units IV, IM
Potassium chloride	50 g daily orally; 1.0 Meq/kg/hr IV drip	None
Potassium permanganate	Solution 1:5000 to 1:10,000 for lavage	None
Pralidoxime chloride	20 mg/kg IV for organic phosphate poisoning	None
Prednisolone sodium succinate (Solu-Delta-Cortef)	0.2 to 1.0 mg/kg IV or IM	Same
Progesterone suspension	Cows: 150 to 200 mg IM	None
Promazine (Sparine)	0.44 to 1.0 mg/kg IV or IM	Same
Proparacine HCl (Ophthaine)	0.5% solution; topically in the eye	Same
Propiopromazine (Tranvet)	0.22 to 1.0 mg/kg IV or IM	Same
Propylene glycol (50% solution)	Cattle: 500 mL; sheep 50 mL orally	None
Prostaglandin F_2 alpha	Cow: 25 to 30 mg IM; ewe and doe: 8 to 10 mg IM—often second injection in 11 to 12 days	None
Protamine sulfate (Heparin antagonist)	100 mg/adult animal IV in a 1% solution for Bracken fern toxicosis	None
Saffan	None	2 to 3 mg/kg IV
Scarlet drench powder	200 to 400 ml as a drench	None
Selenium tocopherol (BO-SE)	5.0 to 7.0 ml/100 kg SC or IM	Same
Sodium acetate phosphate	Cattle: 60 gm in 300 ml water IV	None
Sodium bicarbonate (7.5% solution = 0.89 mEq/ml of bicarbonate	2 to 5 mEq/kg IV for 4 to 8 h period	Same
Sodium formaldehyde sulfoxylate	5% solution as lavage as mercury poisoning antidote	None
Sodium nitrate (1% solution)	16 mg/kg IV, follow with 30 to 40 mg/kg IV sodium thiosulfate for cyanide poisoning	None
Sodium sulfate (Glauber's salt)	1 to 3 g/kg orally	None
Sodium thiosulfate	As arsenic antidote: 10 to 20% solution; 30 to 40 mg/kg IV or orally	None
Soframycin	250 to 500 mg as a subconjunctival injection	None
Spectinomycin	None	10 mg/kg orally q 12 h
Spiramycin	10 to 20 mg as a subconjunctival injection	None
Sulfabromomethazine (Sulfabrom)	130 to 200 mg/kg orally	None
Sulfachlorpyridazine (Vetisulid)	65 to 95 mg/kg orally	45 to 75 mg/kg orally
Sulfadimethoxine (Albon)	55 mg/kg orally (initial dose); 27.5 mg/kg orally (daily)	Same
Sulfaethoxypyridazine (S.E.Z.)	200 to 400 mg/kg	Same
Sulfa-Lite	214 mg/kg initially followed by 107 mg/kg for the next 3 to 5 days	Same
Sulfamethazine	200 mg/kg orally (initial dose); 100 mg/kg orally (daily)	Same
Sulfisoxazole diolamine (Gantrisin)	Ophthalmic ointment	Same
Synovex-S	Steers: implants pellet in ear last 60 to 150 days of fattening period	None
Synovex-H	Heifers: implant pellet in ear last 60 to 150 days of fattening period	None
Taractan	None	0.3 to 1.0 mg/kg IV; 3.3 mg/kg IM
Tannic acid	5 to 25 g in 2.0 to 4.0 L of water orally	None
Tetracaine	0.5% solution; topically in eye; duration 20 to 30 min	Same
Tetracycline HCl (polyotic)	11 mg/kg orally	None
Thiabendazole	40 to 60 mg/kg	None
Thiabendazole paste	75 mg/kg	None
Thiamine	For polio: 0.25 to 0.5 g IM or IV for 3 to 5 days	None
Thiamylal sodium (Suritol)	3 to 5 mg/kg IV	Same
Triamcinolone (Vetalog)	0.02 to 0.04 mg/kg IM; 6.0 to 18.0 mg intra-articular	None
Tribrissen	30 mg/kg daily orally	Same
Tripelennamine HCl (Re-Covr)	1 mg/kg IV or IM	Same
Tropicamide (Mydriacil)	0.5 to 1.0 solution; topically in eye; one drop in eye followed in 10 min with another drop	Same
Tylosin (Tylan)	2 to 4 mg/kg IM	Same
Valium	None	5.5 to 8.5 mg/kg IM
Valsyn Gel (L,D)	Intramammary infusion (Furaltadone, 500 mg)	None

Name of Drug	Ruminants	Swine
Vebanol	200 to 300 mg IM	None
Vetame	Cattle: 0.1 to 0.2 mg/kg;	0.88 to 1.3 mg/kg
	Sheep: 1.0 mg/kg IM or IV	IM or IM
Vitamin E—Selenium	0.1 mg/kg SE and 1.36 IU/kg vitamin E IM	Same
Vitamin K (Aquamephyton)	1 mg/kg IV or IM	Same
Xylazine (Rompun)	Cattle: 0.05 to 0.33 mg/kg IM: sheep: 0.01 to 0.22 mg/kg IM	None
Zeranol (Ralgro)	Cattle: 36 mg SC (ear); lambs: 12 mg SC (ear)	None

CONVERSION TABLES

Table 1. *Household Measures**

Measure	Approximate Equivalents			
	Metric		*Apothecaries'*	
1 drop	1/20 ml	1	minim	
1 teaspoon	5 ml	1+	dram	
1 dessertspoon	8 ml	2	drams	
1 tablespoon	15 ml	½	ounce	
1 wineglass	60 ml	2	ounces	
1 glass	250 ml	8	ounces	

*From Kirk, R. W., and Bistner, S. I.: Handbook of Veterinary Procedures and Emergency Treatment. 3rd ed. Philadelphia, W. B. Saunders Co., 1981.

Table 2. *Conversion Factors**

1 milligram	=	1/65	grain	(1/60)†
1 gram	=	15.43	grains	(15)
1 kilogram	=	2.20	pounds	[avoirdupois]
		2.68	pounds	[Troy]
1 milliliter	=	16.23	minims	(15)
1 liter	=	1.06	quarts	(1+)
		33.80	fluidounces	(34)
1 grain	=	0.065	gm	(60 mg)
1 dram	=	3.9	gm	(4)
1 ounce	=	31.1	gm	(30+)
1 minim	=	0.062	ml	(0.06)
1 fluid dram	=	3.7	ml	(4)
1 fluid ounce	=	29.57	ml	(30)
1 pint	=	473.2	ml	(500−)
1 quart	=	946.4	ml	(1000−)

*From Kirk, R. W., and Bistner, S. I.: Handbook of Veterinary Procedures and Emergency Treatment. 3rd ed. Philadelphia, W. B. Saunders Co., 1981.

†Figures in parentheses are commonly employed approximate values.

Table 3. *Approximate Conversions— Pounds to Kilograms*

Pounds	Kilograms
11	5
22	10
33	15
44	20
55	25
66	30
88	40
110	50
132	60
154	70
176	80
198	90
220	100
242	110

Table 4. *Conversion from Fahrenheit to Centigrade Thermometric Readings**

Cent. Deg.	Fahr. Deg.	Cent. Deg.	Fahr. Deg.	Cent. Deg.	Fahr. Deg.	Cent. Deg.	Fahr. Deg.
−40	−40.0	−4	24.8	32	89.6	68	154.4
−39	−38.2	−3	26.6	33	91.4	69	156.2
−38	−36.4	−2	28.4	34	93.2	70	158.0
−37	−34.6	−1	30.2	35	95.0	71	159.8
−36	−32.8	0	32.0	36	96.8	72	161.6
−35	−31.0	+1	33.8	37	98.6	73	163.4
−34	−29.2	2	35.6	38	100.4	74	165.2
−33	−27.4	3	37.4	39	102.2	75	167.0
−32	−25.6	4	39.2	40	104.0	76	168.8
−31	−23.8	5	41.0	41	105.8	77	170.6
−30	−22.0	6	42.8	42	107.6	78	172.4
−29	−20.2	7	44.6	43	109.4	79	174.2
−28	−18.4	8	46.4	44	111.2	80	176.0
−27	−16.6	9	48.2	45	113.0	81	177.8
−26	−14.8	10	50.0	46	114.8	82	179.6
−25	−13.0	11	51.8	47	116.6	83	181.4
−24	−11.2	12	53.6	48	118.4	84	183.2
−23	−9.4	13	55.4	49	120.2	85	185.0
−22	−7.6	14	57.2	50	122.0	86	186.8
−21	−5.8	15	59.0	51	123.8	87	188.6
−20	−4.0	16	60.8	52	125.6	88	190.4
−19	−2.2	17	62.6	53	127.4	89	192.2
−18	−0.4	18	64.4	54	129.2	90	194.0
−17	+1.4	19	66.2	55	131.0	91	195.8
−16	3.2	20	68.0	56	132.8	92	197.6
−15	5.0	21	69.8	57	134.6	93	199.4
−14	6.8	22	71.6	58	136.4	94	201.2
−13	8.6	23	73.4	59	138.2	95	203.0
−12	10.4	24	75.2	60	140.0	96	204.8
−11	12.2	25	77.0	61	141.8	97	206.6
−10	14.0	26	78.8	62	143.6	98	208.4
−9	15.8	27	80.6	63	145.4	99	210.2
−8	17.6	28	82.4	64	147.2	100	212.0
−7	19.4	29	84.2	65	149.0	101	213.8
−6	21.2	30	86.0	66	150.8	102	215.6
−5	23.0	31	87.8	67	152.6	103	217.4
						104	219.2

*From Catalogue 65, Hospital and Surgical Equipment. V. Mueller, Chicago.

INDEX

Numbers in italics refer to illustrations. Numbers followed by (t) refer to tables.